Manual of Dietetic Practice

Manual of Dietetic Practice

Sixth Edition

Edited by Joan Gandy

In conjunction with

The British Dietetic Association

WILEY Blackwell

BDA The Association of UK Dietitians

Edition History
Blackwell Science Ltd (1e, 198; 2e, 1994; 3e, 2001); Blackwell Publishing Ltd (4e 2007); The British Dietetic Association. Published by John Wiley & Sons, (5e 2014)

Registered Offices
John Wiley & Sons, Inc., 111 River Street, Hoboken, NJ 07030, USA
John Wiley & Sons Ltd, The Atrium, Southern Gate, Chichester, West Sussex, PO19 8SQ, UK

Editorial Office
9600 Garsington Road, Oxford, OX4 2DQ, UK

For details of our global editorial offices, customer services, and more information about Wiley products, visit us at www.wiley.com.

Wiley also publishes its books in a variety of electronic formats and by print-on-demand. Some content that appears in standard print versions of this book may not be available in other formats.

Library of Congress Cataloging-in-Publication Data

Names: Gandy, Joan, editor. | British Dietetic Association, issuing body.
Title: Manual of dietetic practice / edited by Joan Gandy in conjunction with the British Dietetic Association.
Description: Sixth edition. | Hoboken, NJ : John Wiley & Sons, Inc. : The British Dietetic Association, 2019. | Includes bibliographical references and index. |
Identifiers: LCCN 2018039798 (print) | LCCN 2018041076 (ebook) | ISBN 9781119235903 (Adobe PDF) | ISBN 9781119235910 (ePub) | ISBN 9781119235927 (hardcover)
Subjects: | MESH: Diet Therapy | Dietetics | Nutritional Physiological Phenomena
Classification: LCC RM216 (ebook) | LCC RM216 (print) | NLM WB 400 | DDC 615.8/54–dc23
LC record available at https://lccn.loc.gov/2018039798

Cover design by Wiley

Set in 9.5/11.5pt ITC Garamond by SPi Global, Pondicherry, India
Printed and bound by CPI Group (UK) Ltd, Croydon, CR0 4YY

C9781119235927_220825

The manufacturer's authorized representative according to the EU General Product Safety Regulation is Wiley-VCH GmbH, Boschstr. 12, 69469 Weinheim, Germany, e-mail: Product_Safety@wiley.com.

This book is dedicated to Edith Elliot (BDA member number 001)
for her outstanding and continuing contribution to dietetics.

This edition is also dedicated to Briony Thomas (Editor of the first three editions and Co-editor of the fourth edition of the Manual of Dietetic Practice*) 1950–2019.*

Contents

APPENDICES

Contributors

Editor and Contributor

Joan Gandy *Dietetics Department, School of Life and Medical Sciences, University of Hertfordshire, Hatfield, Hertfordshire*
Address for correspondence: c/o The British Dietetic Association, 5th Floor, Charles House, 148/9 Great Charles Street Queensway, Birmingham B3 3HT, UK

Contributors

Sarah Adam *Metabolic Dietitian, Royal Hospital for Children, Queen Elizabeth Hospital, Glasgow*

Phil Addicott *Mental Health Dietitian, Cardiff and Vale University Health Board, Cardiff, Wales*

Lindsey Allan *Macmillan Oncology Dietitian, Royal Surrey County Hospital, Guildford*

Ursula Arens *Freelance Nutrition Writer, London*

Sarah Armer *Specialist Dietitian – Home Enteral Feeding, Community Nutrition and Dietetic Service, South West Yorkshire NHS Foundation Trust, Barnsley, South Yorkshire*

Lisa Baker *Catering Dietitian, Medirest (Compass Group), London*

Melanie Baker *Clinical Lead, Nutrition Support Team (Leicester Intestinal Failure Team), Department of Nutrition and Dietetics, University Hospitals of Leicester NHS Trust, Leicester*

Eleanor Baldwin *Specialist Dietitian – Adult Refsum's Disease, Nutrition and Dietetic Department, Chelsea and Westminster Hospital NHS Foundation Trust, London*

Rachael Barlow *Clinical Academic, Cardiff and Vale University Health Board and Cardiff University, Faculty Member for Enhanced Recovery after Surgery (ERAS) Society, UK*

Tahira Bashir *Freelance Specialist Dietitian, Unique Inspiration Ltd, Birmingham*

Julie Beckerson *Specialist Haemato-Oncology Dietitian, Hammersmith Hospital, Imperial College Healthcare NHS Trust, London*

Jason Beyers *Lead Paediatric Dietitian, Department of Nutrition & Dietetics, Bristol Royal Hospital for Children, Bristol*

Ruth Birt *Regulatory Affairs Consultant, Regulatory Solutions Ltd, Glasgow*

Jamie Blackshaw *Team Leader: Obesity and Healthy Weight, Public Health England, London*

Caroline Bovey *Advanced Public Health Dietitian, Department of Nutrition and Dietetics, Aneurin Bevan University Health Board, Caerleon, Cardiff*

Lauren Bowen *Head of Patient Catering, ISS Facility Services Healthcare, London*

Rachel Bracegirdle *Oncology Dietitian, Guy's and St Thomas' NHS Foundation Trust, London*

Emily Bridge *Clinical Lead Burn Dietitian, Nottingham University Hospitals NHS Trust, Nottingham*

Claire Bullock *Paediatric Dietitian, Department of Nutrition and Dietetics, Derriford Hospital, Plymouth, Devon*

Gaynor Bussell *Freelance Dietitian Specialising in Women's Health, Cardigan, Ceredigion, Wales*

Sarah J. Cameron *Specialist Dietitian in Neurorehabilitation, Wolfson Neurorehabilitation Centre, Queen Mary Hospital, Roehampton*

Helen Campbell *Dietitian, Nutrition and Dietetics Department, The Alfred Hospital, Melbourne, Victoria, Australia*

Rachel Carruthers *Metabolic Dietitian, Charles Dent Metabolic Unit, University College London Hospitals, London*

Elaine Cawadias *Dietitian, Ottawa, Ontario, Canada*

Abbie Cawood *Visiting Research Fellow, Faculty of Medicine, University of Southampton, Southampton*

Heidi Chan *Senior Medical Affairs Advisor for Inherited Metabolic Diseases, London*

Saira Chowdhury *Senior Specialist Upper GI Oncology Dietitian, Department of Nutrition and Dietetics, Guy's and St Thomas' NHS Foundation Trust, London*

Angela Cleaver *Senior Gastroenterology Dietitian, University Hospital Llandough, Cardiff*

Barbara Cochrane *Paediatric Metabolic Dietitian, Queen Elizabeth University Hospital, Glasgow*

Peter Collins *Senior Lecturer/Course Coordinator, Nutrition and Dietetics, School of Exercise and Nutrition Sciences, Faculty of Health, Queensland University of Technology, Brisbane, Australia*

Lisa Cooke *Head of Paediatric Dietetics, Nutrition and SALT, Bristol Royal Hospital for Children, Bristol*

June Copeman *Principal Lecturer, Nutrition and Dietetics, Leeds Beckett University, Leeds, West Yorkshire*

Kathy Cowbrough *Nutrition and Dietetic Consultant, Retford, Nottinghamshire*

Emma Craig *Clinical Lead Dietitian, Dietetics Department, The Royal Hospital for Neuro-disability, West Hill, London*

Julie Crocker *Lead Cystic Fibrosis Dietitian, Royal Hospital for Children, Glasgow*

Helen Croker *Senior Research Associate and Unit Manager of the Obesity Policy Research Unit, Faculty of Population Health Sciences, Great Ormond Street Institute of Child Health, Great Ormond Street Hospital NHS Foundation Trust, London*

Alison Culkin *Lead Intestinal Failure Dietitian, St Mark's Hospital, Harrow, London*

Janeane Dart *Senior Lecturer, Department of Nutrition and Dietetics and Food, Monash University, Melbourne, Australia*

Vicky Davies *Professional Lead for Nutrition and Dietetics, Therapy Services, The Walton Centre, Liverpool*

Adri De Sousa *Respiratory Specialist Dietitian, Dietetic Department, Royal Papworth Hospital NHS Trust, Cambridge*

Mhairi Donald *Macmillan Consultant Dietitian, Sussex Cancer Centre, Royal Sussex County Hospital, Brighton, Sussex*

Sarah Donald *Metabolic Dietitian, Cambridge University Hospitals NHS Foundation Trust, Addenbrookes Hospital, Cambridge*

Pauline Douglas *Senior Lecturer, Ulster University, Coleraine, Northern Ireland*

Jennie Dunwoody *Senior Dietitian, Dietetics Department, The Royal Hospital for Neuro-disability, West Hill, London*

Pamela Dyson *Research Dietitian, University of Oxford, Oxford Centre for Diabetes, Endocrinology & Metabolism (OCDEM), Churchill Hospital, Oxford*

Shelley Easter *Specialist Paediatric Dietitian, Bristol Royal Hospital for Children, Bristol*

Lucy Eldridge *Dietetic Team Leader, Department of Nutrition and Dietetics, The Royal Marsden NHS Foundation Trust, London*

Charlotte Ellerton *Specialist Metabolic Dietitian, National Hospital for Neurology & Neurosurgery, London*

Kiri Elliott *Policy Officer – Education and Professional Development, British Dietetic Association, Birmingham*

Clare Ewan *Paediatric Dietitian, Musgrove Park Hospital, Taunton*

Lydia Fletcher *Senior Dietitian, Dietetics Department, The Royal Hospital for Neuro-disability, West Hill, London*

Suzanne Ford *Specialist Metabolic Dietitian, North Bristol NHS Trust, Bristol*

Lynette Forsythe *Specialist Paediatric Dietitian – Intestinal Failure and Neonates, Royal Manchester Children's Hospital, Central Manchester Hospitals NHS Foundation Trust, Manchester*

Joan Gandy *Dietetics Department, School of Life and Medical Sciences, University of Hertfordshire, Hatfield, Hertfordshire*

Elaine Gardner *Freelance Dietitian, Module Organiser for Nutrition and Infection, The London School of Hygiene & Tropical Medicine, London*

Emma Gaskin *Specialist Senior Dietitian, Therapies; Nutrition and Dietetics, Medway NHS Foundation Trust, Medway Maritime Hospital, Gillingham*

Gillian Gatiss *Specialist Hepatology and Research Dietitian, Department of Nutrition and Dietetics, Cambridge University Hospitals NHS Foundation Trust, Cambridge*

Samantha K. Gill *Research Associate, King's College London, London*

Jenny Gillespie *Practitioner, Paediatric Overweight Service Tayside, Perth Royal Infirmary, Perth, Scotland*

Eva Glass *Macmillan Head and Neck Dietitian, ABMU Local Health Board, Swansea*

Jane Green *Specialist Community Dietitian, Doddington Hospital, Doddington, Cambridge & Peterborough NHS Foundation Trust, Cambridgeshire*

Karen Green *Senior Specialist Dietitian (Neurosciences), Department of Nutrition & Dietetics, The National Hospital for Neurology & Neurosurgery, London*

Poonam Gulia *Specialist Dietitian – Gastroenterology, GutCare Clinic at Dr Ashok's Ayurveda Medical Group, Birmingham*

Vanessa Halliday *Senior Lecturer, Public Health Section, School of Health and Related Research (ScHARR), University of Sheffield, Sheffield*

Catherine R. Hankey *Senior Lecturer in Human Nutrition, University of Glasgow, Glasgow Royal Infirmary, Glasgow*

Lynn Harbottle *Freelance Consultant in Nutrition, Dietetics and Well-being, Bournemouth, Dorset*

Kathryn Hart *Lecturer in Nutrition and Dietetics, Department of Nutritional Sciences, Faculty of Health and Medical Sciences, University of Surrey, Guildford, Surrey*

Michelle Harvie *Lead Research Dietitian, Prevent Breast Cancer Research Unit, University Hospital South Manchester, Manchester*

Jennette Higgs *Director, Food to Fit Ltd, International Nutrition and Dietetics Consultants, Towcester, Northamptonshire*

Julie Hinchliffe *Cardiovascular Rehabilitation Specialist Dietitian, Salford Royal NHS Foundation Trust, Salford*

Linda Hindle *Deputy Chief Allied Health Professions Officer, National Engagement Lead for Police, Fire and Ambulance Services, Public Health England, London*

Richard Hoffman *Senior Lecturer (Retired), School of Life and Medical Sciences, University of Hertfordshire, Hatfield, Hertfordshire*

Michelle Holdsworth *Professor of Public Health, School of Health and Related Research (ScHARR) – Public Health Section, University of Sheffield, Sheffield*

Sandra Hood *Diabetes Specialist Dietitian and Community Lead, Dorset County Hospital NHS Foundation Trust, Dorchester, Dorset*

Sarah Howe *Specialist Dietitian in Inherited Metabolic Disorders, Department of Nutrition and Dietetics, University Hospitals Birmingham NHS Foundation Trust, Birmingham*

Rosanna Hudson *Policy Officer – Education, British Dietetic Association, Birmingham*

Joana Jardim *Regional Healthcare Dietitian, ISS Facility Services Healthcare, Kettering*

Yvonne Jeanes *Principal Lecturer, Clinical Nutrition, Department of Life Sciences, University of Roehampton, London*

Judith John *Consultant Dietitian in Public Health, Public Health Wales, Cardiff, Wales*

Katie Johnson *Clinical Team Manager, Community Neurological Rehabilitation Service, St Mary's Hospital, Leeds Community Healthcare NHS Trust, Leeds*

Katie Keetarut *Highly Specialist Dietitian (Inflammatory Bowel Disease), University College London Hospital, London*

Sue Kellie *Deputy Chief Executive, British Dietetic Association, Birmingham*

Katie Kennedy *Company Dietitian, Dr Schär, Warrington*

Natasha Kershaw *Burns Dietitian, St Andrew's Burn Centre, Chelmsford*

Karen Klassen *Post-doctoral Research Fellow, Department of Nutrition, Dietetics and Food, Monash University, Melbourne, Australia*

Annemarie Knight *Programme Lead, Dietetics, King's College, London*

Edwige Landais *Researcher in Nutrition, Institut de Recherche pour le Développement (IRD), UMR 204 'Nutrition et Alimentation des Populations aux Suds', France*

Martin Lau *Services Development Manager and Dietitian, Arthritis Action, London*

Anne Laverty *Community Dietitian (Learning Disability) (retired), Northern Health and Social Care Trust, Northern Ireland*

Judy Lawrence *Research Officer, British Dietetic Association, Birmingham*

Sherly X. Li *Research Dietitian, MRC Epidemiology Unit, University of Cambridge, Cambridge*

Rebecca Lindstrom Sowman *Specialist Gastroenterology & Lower GI Surgery Dietitian, St Mary's Hospital, Imperial College Healthcare NHS Trust, London*

Miranda Lomer *Senior Consultant Dietitian in Gastroenterology, Guy's and St Thomas' NHS Foundation Trust, London*

Jacqueline Lowdon *Clinical Specialist Paediatric Dietitian, Leeds Children's Hospital, The Leeds Teaching Hospitals NHS Trust, Belmont Grove, Leeds*

Marjory Macleod *Dietitian FBDA (retired), Learning Disabilities Service, NHS Lothian, Edinburgh, Scotland*

Angela Madden *Lead for Nutrition and Dietetics, School of Life and Medical Sciences, University of Hertfordshire, Hatfield, Hertfordshire*

Bruno Mafrici *Lead Renal Dietitian/Team Leader, Dietetics, Nottingham University Hospitals NHS Trust, Nottingham*

Linda Main *Freelance Dietitian, Drummond Consultants Ltd & Dietitian at HEART UK – The Cholesterol Charity*

Kwunita Man *Lead Dietitian for Neurology, Nutrition and Dietetics Service, Hertfordshire Community NHS Trust, Hertfordshire*

Sara Mancell *Lead Children's Dietitian, Nutrition & Dietetics Department, King's College Hospital NHS Foundation Trust, London*

Tanita Manton *Senior Dietitian, The Royal Hospital for Neuro-disability, West Hill, London*

Luise V. Marino *Clinical Academic Paediatric Dietitian, Paediatric Intensive Care, HEE/NIHR ICA Clinical Lectureship, Department of Dietetics/SLT, University Hospital Southampton NHS Foundation Trust, Southampton*

Alison McGlone *Clinical Specialist Lead Dietitian, Royal Victoria Hospital, Belfast Health and Social Care Trust, Belfast*

Jennifer McIntosh *Allied Health Professional Lead/ Specialist Dietitian, Specialist Services and Learning Disability Care Group, Leeds and York Partnership NHS Foundation Trust, York, North Yorkshire*

Yvonne McKenzie *Specialist Dietitian in Gastrointestinal Nutrition and IBS, Clinical Lead in IBS for the Gastroenterology Specialist Group of the British Dietetic Association, Oxford*

Annette McLean *Dietetic Lead for Mental Health, and Deputy Head of Nutrition and Dietetics, Llandough Hospital, Cardiff and Vale University Health Board, Cardiff, Wales*

Helen McNair *Older-Adults Dietitian, Community Nutrition and Dietetic Service (Barnsley), South West Yorkshire Partnership NHS Foundation Trust, Barnsley, South Yorkshire*

Lauren McVeigh *Specialist Paediatric Dietitian, Bristol Royal Hospital for Children, University Hospitals Bristol NHS Foundation Trust, Bristol*

Christina Merryfield *Lead Dietitian, Bupa Cromwell Hospital, London*

Rosan Meyer *Honorary Senior Lecturer, Department of Paediatrics, Imperial College, London*

Emma Mills *Mansfield, Nottinghamshire*

Hayley Moroney *Specialist Dietitian, The National Hospital for Neurology and Neurosurgery, London*

Alison Morton *Consultant Dietitian (retired) (Adult Cystic Fibrosis), Formerly at Leeds Teaching Hospitals NHS Trust, Leeds*

Charlene Mulhern *Childhood Obesity Workforce Delivery Manager, Health Intelligence Division, Public Health England, London*

Camille Newby *Regional Specialist Paediatric Dietitian in Inherited Metabolic Disease, Bristol Royal Hospital for Children, University Hospitals Bristol NHS Foundation Trust, Bristol*

Heather Norris *Neonatal Dietitian, St Michael's Hospital, University Hospitals Bristol NHS Foundation Trust, Bristol*

Mary O'Kane *Consultant Dietitian (Adult Obesity), Leeds Teaching Hospitals NHS Trust, Leeds*

Siân O'Shea *Freelance Dietitian, Cardiff*

Fionna Page *Independent Nutrition Consultant and Registered Dietitian, First Page Nutrition Ltd, Wiltshire*

Katherine Paterson *Clinical Lead Specialist Cardiology and Obesity Dietitian, Department of Nutrition and Dietetics, Norfolk and Norwich University Hospitals NHS Foundation Trust, Norwich*

Dympna Pearson *Freelance Dietitian & Behaviour Change Trainer, Leicester, Leicestershire*

Sue Perry *Deputy Head of Dietetics, Hull and East Yorkshire Hospitals NHS Trust, Hull, East Yorkshire*

Mary Phillips *Advanced Specialist Dietitian (Hepato-pancreato-biliary Surgery), Royal Surrey County Hospital, Guildford*

Ursula Philpot *Level Lead and Senior Lecturer, Nutrition and Dietetics, School of Clinical and Applied Sciences, Leeds Beckett University, Leeds, West Yorkshire*

Gail Pinnock *Specialist Bariatric Surgery Dietitian, Stone Allerton, Somerset*

Vicki Pout *Deputy Acute Dietetic Manager, Clinical Nutrition and Dietetics, Queen Elizabeth The Queen Mother Hospital, Kent Community Health NHS Foundation Trust, Margate, Kent*

Charlotte Proctor *Advanced Specialist Critical Care Dietitian, Northwick Park Hospital and St Mark's Hospital, Harrow, Middlesex*

Najia Qureshi *Head of Education and Professional Development, British Dietetic Association, Birmingham*

Jean Redmond *Scientific Director, Real-World & Analytics Solutions, IQVIA, London*

Gail Rees *Associate Professor in Human Nutrition, School of Biomedical and Healthcare Sciences, Plymouth University, Plymouth*

Claudia Rueb *Specialist Dietitian, Upper GI Surgery & Cancer, St Mary's Hospital, Imperial College Healthcare NHS Trust, London*

Alan Rio *The Royal Marsden Hospital, Fulham Road, London*

Sarah Ripley *Country Manager (UK), Cambrooke Therapeutics, Manchester*

Louise Robertson *Specialist Dietitian in Inherited Metabolic Disorders, Department of Nutrition and Dietetics, University Hospitals Birmingham NHS Foundation Trust, Birmingham*

Martina Rooney *Doctoral Researcher, Nutrition Innovation Centre for Food and Health (NICHE), Ulster University, Coleraine, Northern Ireland*

Laura Rowe *Nutrition & Dietetics Professional Lead/Specialist Diabetes Dietitian, Airedale General Hospital, Steeton, West Yorkshire*

Lisa Ryan *Head of Department of Natural Sciences, School of Science and Computing, Galway-Mayo Institute of Technology, Galway, Ireland*

Gurpreet Sagoo *Specialist Paediatric Dietitian, Great Ormond Street Hospital, Great Ormond Street Hospital for Children NHS Foundation Trust, London*

Inez Schoenmakers *Senior Lecturer, Department of Medicine, Norwich Medical School, Faculty of Medicine and Health Sciences, University of East Anglia, Norwich, Norfolk*

Laura Sealy *Specialist Paediatric Dietitian (Oncology, Haematology and BMT), Nutrition & Dietetics Department, Bristol Royal Hospital for Children, Bristol*

Clare Shaw *Consultant Dietitian, Department of Nutrition and Dietetics, The Royal Marsden NHS Foundation Trust, London and Sutton*

Katherine Singleton *Paediatric and Metabolic Dietitian, Department of Nutrition and Dietetics, University Hospital of Wales, Cardiff*

Isabel Skypala *Consultant Allergy Dietitian, Clinical Lead for Food Allergy, Department of Allergy & Clinical Immunology, Royal Brompton & Harefield NHS Foundation Trust, South Kensington, London*

Lynsey Spillman *Specialist Hepatology and Research Dietitian, Department of Nutrition and Dietetics, Cambridge University Hospitals NHS Foundation Trust, Cambridge*

Laura Stewart *Weight Management and Diabetes Service Lead, Perth Royal Infirmary, NHS Tayside, Perth*

Rebecca Stratton *Visiting Research Fellow, Faculty of Medicine, University of Southampton, University Hospital Southampton NHS Foundation Trust, Southampton*

Louise Sutton *Head of Sport and Exercise Nutrition, Carnegie School of Sport, Leeds Beckett University, Leeds*

Bella Talwar *Clinical Lead Dietitian, Nutrition & Dietetics, Head and Neck Centre, University College London Hospitals NHS Foundation Trust, London*

Ella Terblanche *Advanced Dietitian for Critical Care, Imperial College Healthcare NHS Trust, London*

Laura Thomas *Gastroenterology Dietitian, Department of Nutrition and Dietetics, University Hospital Llandough, Penarth, Wales*

Karen Thomsett *Dietitian, Dent Community Health NHS Trust, Whitstable and Tankerton Community Hospital, Whitstable, Kent*

Sarah Trace *Specialist Paediatric Dietitian (Nephrology), Paediatric Dietetic Department, Bristol Royal Hospital for Children, University Hospitals Bristol NHS Foundation Trust, Bristol*

Helen Truby *Professor of Nutrition and Dietetics, Director of Dietetics, Department of Nutrition, Dietetics and Food, Monash University, Melbourne, Australia*

Anthony Twist *Specialist Dietitian, The Robert Jones and Agnes Hunt Orthopaedic Hospital NHS Foundation Trust, Oswestry, Shropshire*

Sarah Wallis *Senior Dietitian, Frimley Park Hospital, Frimley Health NHS Foundation Trust, Portsmouth Road, Frimley*

Mary Ward *Professor of Nutrition and Dietetics, Nutrition Innovation Centre for Food and Health (NICHE), School of Biomedical Sciences, Ulster University, Northern Ireland*

C. Elizabeth Weekes *Senior Consultant Dietitian, Department of Nutrition and Dietetics, Guy's & St Thomas' NHS Foundation Trust, London*

Ailsa Welch *Professor of Nutritional Epidemiology, Department of Population Health and Primary Care, Norwich Medical School, University of East Anglia, Norwich, Norfolk*

Kevin Whelan *Professor of Dietetics, Head of Department of Nutritional Sciences, King's College, London*

Rhys White *Principal Oncology Dietitian, Department of Nutrition and Dietetics, Guy's and St Thomas' NHS Foundation Trust, London*

Kirsten Whitehead *Lecturer in Dietetics University of Nottingham, School of Biosciences, Division of Nutritional Sciences, Sutton Bonington Campus, University of Nottingham, Loughborough, Leicestershire*

Harriet Williams *Area Head of Dietetics, Department of Nutrition and Dietetics, Betsi Cadwaladr University Health Board, Ysbyty Gwynedd, Bangor*

Kate Williams *Lead Dietitian, Adult Eating Disorders Service, South London and Maudsley NHS Foundation Trust, London*

Lisa Williams *All Wales Nutrition Training Facilitator, Cardiff and Vale University Health Board, Cardiff, Wales*

Nicola Williams *Team Lead Dietitian, Royal Manchester Children's Hospital, Central Manchester Foundation Trust, Manchester*

Samford Wong *Lead Dietitian for Spinal Injuries and Research, National Spinal Injuries Centre, Stoke Mandeville Hospital, Aylesbury*

Paula Wood *Principal Scientist, Research Dietitian, Personal and Human Performance Team, Defence Science and Technology Laboratory, Porton Down, Salisbury, Wiltshire*

Philippa Wright *Lead for Paediatric Rehabilitation and Therapies, The Royal Brompton & Harefield Foundation Trust, South Kensington, London*

The BDA Specialist Groups

- Critical Care
- Diabetes
- Food Allergy
- Food Services
- Freelance Dietitians
- Gastroenterology
- HIV Care
- Mental Health
- Neurosciences
- Obesity
- Older People
- Oncology
- Paediatric
- Parenteral & Enteral Nutrition
- Public Health
- Renal Nutrition
- Sports Nutrition

Sub-Groups

- Autism (sub-group of Paediatric)
- Haematology (sub-group of Oncology)
- Paediatric Oncology (sub-group of Paediatric)
- Prescribing Support Dietitians (sub-group of Older People)
- Trauma (sub group of Critical Care)

Other contributors

- Paul Appleby
- Kerrie Boyd
- Neasa Forde
- Heather Russell
- Alison Smith
- Jill Stewart
- Malgorzata Szychta
- Emma Tovey
- Tazmin Wisudha-Edwards
- Sue Wolfe

Foreword

Dietitians are highly trained professionals who work in a wide variety of settings. While most dietitians work in clinical areas and public health, they also have key roles in an increasing range of areas, including research, teaching, journalism and the media, sport, industry and public relations. Their education and training are based on a core curriculum which uses many resources, including the British Dietetic Association's (BDA) *Manual of Dietetic Practice* (MDP).

The MDP is the core text, and as such it essential that it be revised periodically. This, the sixth edition, has been completely revised by experienced practitioners from all related fields of practice. Some chapters have been completely rewritten, including 'Assessment of nutritional status', 'People in low-income groups' and 'Public health nutrition'. Embracing the need to work in an increasingly diverse environment, a new chapter, 'Working with minority ethnic groups', replaces 'Dietary patterns of black and minority ethnic groups'.

Dietitians from all areas of practice and all levels of experience, from students to professors, have contributed in varying degrees to this publication. In addition, many of the authors have also contributed the BDA's series of specialist texts, thereby ensuring that MDP dovetails into more advanced texts and practice. As such, the MDP is an essential text for all students and qualified dietitians, and other health professionals.

Richard Balfe

The Lord Balfe of Dulwich, Honorary President of the British Dietetic Association

Preface

This is the sixth edition of the *Manual of Dietetic Practice*, and it is part of a range of resources available to dietitians, dietetic students and others. The range includes an increasing number of specialist dietetic texts, and this edition of the manual is written, as far as possible, to complement these texts. Some specialisms are too small to warrant a separate text, and are therefore included in the *Manual of Dietetic Practice*, e.g. inherited metabolic disorders in adults. This edition of the manual is aimed mainly at non-specialist dietitians and dietetic students, and is intended for use as a standard textbook in dietetic departments. Since the publication of the fifth edition of the manual, a book of case studies in dietetics and nutrition has also been published.

Dietetics is a dynamic profession, which means that knowledge and practice change rapidly, and dietitians are working in more diverse areas. All the chapters have been updated and revised, and some have been completely rewritten. The shift towards prevention and primary care is reflected in the rewritten chapter *Public health nutrition*. As the demographics of the population change, dietitians need to be able to work with more diverse groups. This is reflected in the revised chapter *Working with minority ethnic groups*. It is important that dietitians are up to date with changes in social systems, and the chapter *People in low income groups* has therefore been rewritten to reflect this.

In keeping with the previous edition, dietitians from across the width of the profession, from students to professors, have contributed to this edition. The systemic approach of the manual has been maintained to be in line with the specialisms of the BDA specialist groups and other dietetics groups and networks.

The *Manual of Dietetic Practice* is constructed to be cohesive, and, as such, there is considerable cross-referencing between chapters. It is divided into two parts, encompassing seven sections with appendices, as follows:

Part 1 General topics
Section 1 – Dietetic practice
Section 2 – Nutritional status
Section 3 – Nutrition in specific groups
Section 4 – Specific areas of dietetic practice
Section 5 – Other topics related to practice

Part 2 Clinical dietetic practice
Section 6 – Nutrition support
Section 7 – Clinical dietetic practice

The area of paediatric dietetics is always challenging, as well as interesting, and Chapter 3.8 provides an appropriate level of knowledge for non-paediatric dietitians who work with children in general settings. It is hoped that dietitians will find this useful, and that it will provide student dietitians with an introduction to another exciting and satisfying area of practice.

There is a dedicated *Manual of Dietetic Practice* website (www.manualofdieteticpractice.com/default.asp) that has additional resources, including figures and tables that can be downloaded.

Although editing the manual has been a challenge, the level of support has been overwhelming and inspiring. I am indebted to the many people who have written or revised the book's chapters, the many reviewers and other contributors. Finally, I would like to thank Mirjana Misina, project manager, who has worked alongside me throughout and made the process so much easier than the last time!

Joan Gandy

About the companion website

This book is accompanied by a companion website:

www.manualofdieteticpractice.com

The website includes:

- Figures and tables in PowerPoint
- Web resources
- Appendices
- References from the book

PART 1
General topics

SECTION 1

Dietetic practice

1.1 Professional practice

Najia Qureshi, Judy Lawrence, Rosanna Hudson, Samantha K. Gill, Kiri Elliott, Sue Kellie and Joan Gandy

Key points

- UK dietitians must be graduates of an approved education programme and registered with the Health and Care Professions Council.
- The British Dietetic Association is a professional association that aims to inform, protect, represent and support its members.
- Dietitians are autonomous practitioners who work within an ethical framework of conduct.
- The nutrition and dietetic process is central to dietetic practice.
- Dietetics is an evidence-based profession with research and outcome evaluation at its core.
- Dietitians engage in continuing professional development throughout their careers to ensure that their practice is robust, effective and innovative.

Dietetics is a well-respected and established profession, albeit a relatively new one. The first UK dietitian, Ruth Pybus, a nursing sister, was appointed in 1924 at the Royal Infirmary in Edinburgh. She initially sought to demonstrate that a dietetic outpatient clinic could significantly reduce the number of admissions and therefore benefit the hospital. She was successful and, after a 6-month trial, her appointment as a dietitian was confirmed. The development of other dietetic departments quickly followed, especially in London, and the first non-nursing dietitians were appointed in 1928. From these early days, dietetics has been a science-based profession and, in the 1980s, became the first of the allied health professions (AHPs) to become a graduate profession.

The British Dietetic Association (BDA) was founded in 1936 as the professional association for registered dietitians in Great Britain and Northern Ireland. The BDA promotes the vital work of its members in order to raise the profile of the profession. It represents the best interests of dietitians collectively when working with national organisations, stakeholders and key partners, and aims to influence government policy. This in turn drives demand for evidence-based nutrition and dietetics.

Dietetics is both an art and a science that requires the application of safe and evidence-based practice, reflective practice and systematic clinical reasoning. A dietitian needs to combine these skills with knowledge and experience, together with intuition, insight and understanding of the individual (or specific) circumstance, in order to maintain and improve practice. Following several public enquiries at the end of the last century, it was recognised that there needed to be greater priority given to nonclinical aspects of care, such as skills in communicating with colleagues and service users, management, development of teamwork, shared learning across professional boundaries, auditing, reflective practice and leadership. Subsequent legislative changes were implemented with the establishment of the Health and Care Professions Council (HCPC).

Dietetics as a profession

A degree of responsibility and expectation are part of being a professional. A member of any profession, including dietetics, must, within their practice, agree to be governed by a code of ethics, uphold high standards of performance and competence, behave with integrity and morality, and be selfless in the promotion of the public good (Cruess *et al.*, 2004). Furthermore, these commitments form the basis of an understanding that results in professions, and their members, being accountable to service users and to society.

Professional regulation

To use the title of dietitian, and to practise as one, it is mandatory to have completed an approved programme of education and be registered with the HCPC. The HCPC

Manual of Dietetic Practice, Sixth Edition. Edited by Joan Gandy.

Companion website: www.manualofdieteticpractice.com

was set up in 2001 to protect the health and well-being of people using the services of the health professionals registered with them. It aims to:

- Maintain and publish a public register of properly qualified members of the professions.
- Approve and uphold high standards of education and training and continuing good practice.
- Investigate complaints and take appropriate action.
- Work in partnership with the public and other groups, including professional bodies.

To remain on the HCPC register, dietitians must continue to meet the standards that are set for the profession. The professional standards are:

- Good character of health professionals.
- Health.
- Proficiency (dietetics).
- Conduct performance and ethics.
- Continuing professional development (CPD).
- Education and training.

The HCPC uses these standards to determine if a registrant is fit to practise. If the HCPC finds that there are concerns about a dietitian's ability to practise safely and effectively, and therefore fitness to practise is impaired, it has the legal right to take action. This may mean that such registrants are not allowed to practise, or that they are limited in what they are allowed to do. The HCPC can legally take appropriate action to enforce this (HCPC, 2010).

The British Dietetic Association as a professional body

The distinction between a regulatory body (HCPC) and a professional body (BDA) is often misunderstood. It is important that dietitians be fully aware of the differences from the beginning of professional training. Much like the HCPC, the BDA is committed to protecting the public and service users. However, the two organisations achieve this in very different ways (Table 1.1.1). The HCPC has the ultimate authority to prevent dietitians from practising if, following investigation, they are deemed to be unsafe or untrustworthy. However, the BDA provides guidance, advice, learning and networking opportunities, and professional indemnity insurance cover, all with the aim of supporting the development of safe and effective practitioners. This ultimately helps protect the public and service users. The BDA also provides a trade union function and supports members throughout their working life on issues such as pay and conditions, equal opportunities, maternity rights, and health and safety.

Table 1.1.1 Remits of the Health and Care Professions Council (regulatory body) and the British Dietetic Association (professional body)

Health and Care Professions Council	British Dietetic Association
Protect the public and service users	Protect the public and service users
Set professional standards of practice	Membership support
Approve education programmes that train and educate graduates to meet these standards	Advance the science and practice of dietetics
Register graduates of these programmes	Promote education and training in the science and practice of dietetics
Ensure registrants meet professional standards	Regulate the relationships between dietitians and their employers through the trade union
Sanction registrants who do not meet these standards	Provide professional indemnity insurance

Autonomy

Autonomy can be defined as the right of self-governance. As independent practitioners who practice autonomously, dietitians are accountable for their decision-making, given that they have a moral and legal obligation for the provision of safe and competent service delivery (BDA, 2017). This means they are answerable for their actions and omissions, regardless of advice or directions from another health professional. Dietitians have a duty of care for their service users and clients, who are entitled to receive safe and competent care or service. The HCPC states that, as autonomous and accountable professionals, dietitians '*… need to make informed and reasonable decisions about their practice. This might include getting advice and support from education providers, employers, professional bodies, colleagues and other people to make sure that you protect the wellbeing of service users at all times*' (HCPC, 2016).

It is important that dietitians be aware of the boundaries of their autonomy, which will never be limitless but confined to their scope of practice. As with all health professionals, dietitians must never practise in isolation. Up-to-date knowledge skills and experience are the cornerstones of safe and effective practice, and as such dietitians should always have access to a support network of learning, development and peer review. In the National Health Service (NHS) setting, the system for learning and development is usually already established via internal processes, e.g. supervision, appraisal, local training programmes, library services and journal clubs. Outside of the NHS, these processes are not automatically in place, and it is essential that healthcare professionals actively establish a network of support and learning to match their scope of practice, e.g. freelance practice (see Chapter 4.1, Freelance dietetics).

Scope of practice

Identifying individual scope of practice is not easy as the boundaries will be different for each practitioner and

Table 1.1.2 Factors that define dietetic scope of practice

Factor	Example
Occupational role	Clinician, researcher, educator, writer, consultant
Sector	Private practice, industry, higher education, commercial
Environment	Acute, community, GP practice, industry, media
Client group	Children, elderly, people with learning difficulties, public, supermarket
Speciality	Diabetes, public health, obesity, product development
Approaches	Behavioural therapy, group education, anthropometry, cook-and-eat session
Types of cases for referral elsewhere	Other dietitians or other healthcare professionals, social services

will evolve over time (BDA, 2009). The description of a dietitian's scope of practice is often broad and may describe some or all of the factors shown in Table 1.1.2.

A much more specific scope of practice is described in relation to specific service users. When presented with a service user, the dietitian should undertake a personal risk assessment as part of the overall assessment, asking key questions before proceeding. These questions include:

- Is the service user safe?
- Am I safe?
- Can I justify the decision I have made during the assessment (e.g. has the research, evidence, standards and guidance been considered)?
- Can I identify the most appropriate approach for the service user group?
- Do I have the correct balance of skills, knowledge and experience to be competent in my chosen approach?
- Do I need to seek advice from a peer/team lead/professional body?

Extended scope of practice

The extended roles that a dietitian will undertake are those outside their core and specialist roles. They are usually (but not exclusively) roles traditionally carried out by other health professionals of at least specialist or advanced level, either as a core duty or role extension. Additional skills and knowledge are acquired through formal training. The extended role practitioner must advance dietetic practice and contribute to improving outcomes. Examples of extended roles include:

- Replacing gastrostomy tubes in the community.
- Inserting peripheral midlines for intravenous feeding.
- Supplementary prescribing of medicines.

Activities such taking blood pressure or a finger-prick test of blood to test for blood glucose are not included in the extended roles of a dietitian. Whatever role a dietitian commits to, extended or otherwise, they must constantly be aware of their individual scope of practice, and practice within this. Extended roles and pushing the boundaries of nutrition and dietetic practice are not new. It is actively encouraged by the BDA, and is part of what continues to make dietetics the relevant, dynamic and resourceful profession it is.

Ethics and conduct

Conduct is the manner in which a person behaves, especially in a particular place or situation, while ethics are moral principles that govern an individual's or a group's behaviour. However, it is essential to put these definitions into context for them to have any meaning. In professional practice, professional ethical conduct is of paramount importance. Outside of their professional role, dietitians have the right to behave how they choose, within the limits of the law, and this will be limited only by personal ethical boundaries. In professional practice, it is the professional codes of conduct that provide the framework for how, and the benchmark by which, ethical conduct will be measured. A major function of a code of conduct is to enable professionals to make informed choices when faced with an ethical dilemma. For the dietetic workforce, the key guidance is laid out in the HCPC's *Standards of conduct, performance and ethics* (2016) and *Guidance on conduct and ethics for students* (2009).

The BDA's *Code of Professional Conduct* (2017) builds on the generic standards of the HCPC with more dietetic-specific guidance. They apply to the whole dietetic workforce from unregulated students and support workers to qualified dietitians. This code is necessarily broad and cannot provide definitive answers to every situation that members may encounter over the course of their careers. They have been written in such a way as to provide members with the freedom to advance, develop and innovate practice in their chosen area of nutrition and dietetics, centred on the needs and expectations of their service users.

Purpose of dietetics

The primary purpose of the practice of dietetics is to optimise the nutritional health of the service users, be they an individual, group or community, or population. By optimising the nutritional health of the service users, the dietitian expects to positively influence health outcomes. In dietetics, it is common for the dietitian to seek to influence or change other aspects of care or treatment, e.g. medication or the psychological well-being of the service user. However, the primary purpose of the dietitian is to identify and take action to improve the nutritional status of the service user and to improve those symptoms that are amenable to dietetic intervention.

Any single consultation or professional activity is incredibly complex and involves a number of different and varied strands of knowledge – from biological and social sciences to food and medicine, alongside communication and clinical decision-making skills and attributes such as empathy and respect. These are applied within professional and legal frameworks and boundaries and within organisational and social norms and standards. Most of this thought process is invisible to other professionals (and often to the user) as it takes place rapidly in the dietitian's mind. The integration of all these components in a systematic way is what differentiates between dietitians and other professionals who provide some nutrition services. Service users, health professionals, healthcare organisations and governments demand high-quality healthcare. Quality in healthcare can be measured in domains such as patient experience, effectiveness and safety.

Process for nutrition and dietetic practice

The BDA's Process for Nutrition and Dietetic Practice (PNDP) (the Process) (2016) demonstrates how dietitians integrate professional knowledge and skills into evidence-based decision-making, and hence the Process could be described as the cornerstone of practice. The Process describes the fundamentals of the dietetic intervention and is a tool in facilitating the profession to provide a consistent quality of care. It is applicable to all areas of practice including clinical, public health and health promotion, and whether working with individuals, groups or communities.

The Process is shown in Figure 1.1.1, and it clearly shows the central role of the service user in dietetic practice. Service users bring their culture, beliefs and attitudes to the intervention, and these values guide shared decision-making. Within statutory regulated health services, this focus on the service user is described as patient-centred care. There are many and varied definitions for patient-centred care, but that of the Institute of Medicine (2001) '*Providing care that is respectful of, and responsive to, individual patient preferences, needs and values and ensuring that patient values guide all clinical decisions*' encompasses all the concepts.

While providing a concept for a systemic method for practice, the Process does not undermine the professional autonomy of the dietitian, who is required to make decisions at every step. The Process clearly identifies the steps within a dietetic intervention and the skills, resources and knowledge used by the dietitian, but does not replace the dietitian's decision-making. The BDA nutrition and dietetic process consists of five steps (Table 1.1.3):

- Assessment.
- Nutrition and dietetic diagnosis.
- Formulation and planning of the intervention.
- Implementation of the intervention.
- Monitoring and evaluation.

Dietetic diagnosis

As previously stated, dietitians are autonomous professionals, and therefore responsible for their actions. One of the ways in which a dietitian demonstrates this autonomy is the identification of a nutritional and dietetic diagnosis. The diagnosis step may be considered the most important step in the Process, but it is often the

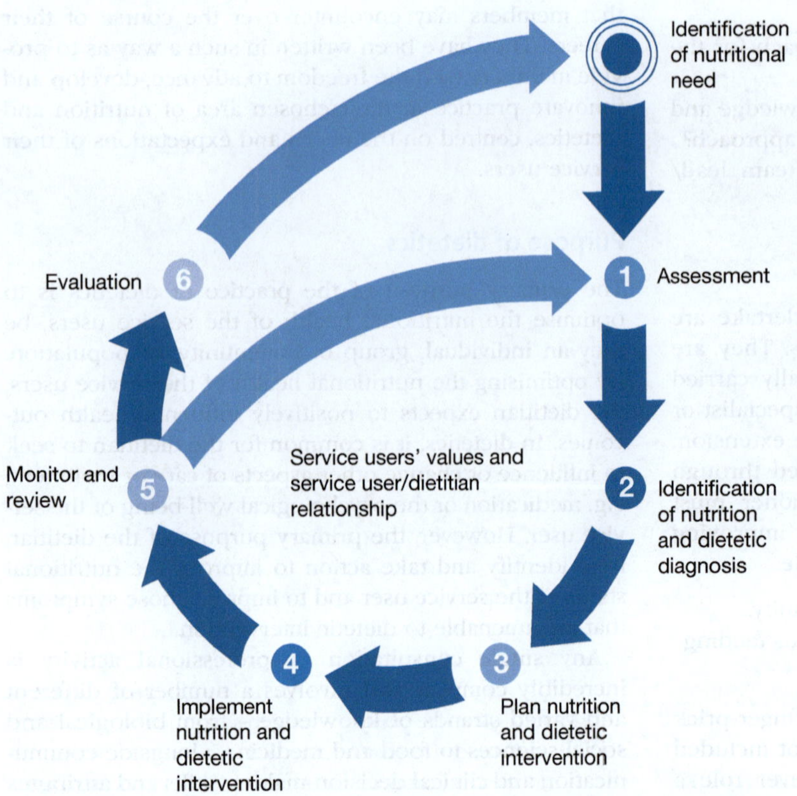

Figure 1.1.1 Nutrition and Dietetic Process (source: The British Dietetic Association 2016. Reproduced with permission from The British Dietetic Association)

Table 1.1.3 Definitions of the steps in the Model and Process for Nutrition and Dietetic Practice (BDA, 2016)

Step	Definition
Assessment	A systematic process of collecting and interpreting information to make decisions about the nature and cause of nutrition-related health issues in an individual, a group or a population Its purpose is to obtain adequate and relevant information to identify nutrition-related problems and to inform the development and monitoring of the intervention It is initiated by the identification of need, e.g. screening, referral by a health professional, self-referral, high-level public health data, epidemiological data or other similar process
Identification of nutritional and dietetic diagnosis	Identification of nutritional problems that impact on the physical, mental and/or social well-being where the dietitian is responsible for action **Individual** It requires therapeutic or educational action as determined by the dietitian and service user Based on scientific evaluation of physical and psychological signs, symptoms, dietary and medical history, procedures and test results, and the priorities of the service user **Groups** In a therapeutic group, there will be a diagnosis for the individuals in the group (as individuals). In a public health group, the diagnosis step will be the same as for the population **Populations** Within a public health needs assessment framework, the nutritional diagnosis is defined as assessing a nutritional health priority for action. It involves choosing (for action) the nutritional health conditions and determinant factors with the most significant size, impact and severity At all levels, it includes the identification and categorisation of the occurrence, risk or potential for the development of a nutritional problem that the dietitian will be responsible for treating independently or of leading the strategy to manage
Plan intervention	A set of activities and associated resources that are used to address the identified nutritional and dietetic diagnosis, designed with the intent of changing nutrition-related behaviours, risk factors, environmental factors or aspects of physical or psychological health or nutritional status of the individual, group or population. All interventions are planned with the communities, service users and carers who are the recipients of the intervention. This client-centred approach is a key element in developing a realistic plan that has a high probability of positively influencing the outcome. This will usually involve describing: • Overall measurable and specific outcomes • Intermediate goals that will achieve the outcomes, determined by the diagnosis statement and assessment information • Plan designed to meet the goals and outcomes – interventions, provision of food, provision of nutritional support, education package, counselling, coordination of care, social marketing campaigns, food availability, food shopping and cooking skills • Roles and responsibilities of individuals, professionals and organisations in delivering the plan
Implementation	The action phase of the nutrition and dietetic process. Dietitians may carry out the intervention, or delegate to or coordinate with another health or social care professional; patient, client or carer; voluntary organisation or member of the nutrition and dietetic team
Monitoring	The review and measurement of the client, group or population's nutritional status at planned intervals with regard to the nutritional diagnosis, intervention plan, goals and outcomes. It includes monitoring the implementation processes of the plan
Evaluation	The systematic comparison of current findings against previous status, intervention goals and outcomes or a reference standard, and usually takes place at the end of the process

step that is missed. In making a diagnosis, the dietitian uses critical reasoning skills to evaluate the assessment information and to make judgements as to the risks to the service user(s) of taking action, or not. The dietitian will prioritise the nutritional issues identified and make a judgement as to whether taking action on these issues will make a difference to the health and outcomes for the service user (individual, group or population).

In developing the diagnosis, the dietitian identifies the relevant aspects of the assessment, and clearly states the nutritional problems that he or she and the service user have prioritised, the nutritional issues the dietitian can influence and the impact the nutritional and dietetic intervention will have on the service user's health (physical, mental or social well-being). The benefits from making a nutritional and dietetic diagnosis include:

- Sharing with the others involved with the service user the nutritional issue(s) that the dietitian and service user have prioritised.
- Identifying the specific nutritional issue(s) that the dietitian can influence.
- Identifying the indicators in the assessment process that will form the basis of monitoring and evaluation.
- Demonstrating the thoroughness of the assessment process and clearly communicating this to other professionals.

The diagnostic statement should clearly record for all service providers the problem, its cause (aetiology) and why the dietitian considers that it is a problem (symptoms). This statement also forms the basis of the monitoring and evaluation step as dietitians will also have identified the most important indicators from their description of the symptoms.

Recording and information management

Another fundamental aspect of professionalism is the accurate recording of the nutrition and dietetic process. The HCPC (2013) standards of proficiency require dietitians to be able to maintain records appropriately. The information in records, including dietetic records, is used for many different purposes. Most importantly, it provides a permanent account of the dietetic process, especially the intervention, and a means of communication between all professionals and others involved, including the service user. Information contained within records is also used for several other purposes, including demonstrating the overall effectiveness of the dietetic service and, possibly, organisation, quality monitoring and service improvement, research and public health purposes. While the increasing use of electronic health records requires more systematic record keeping, there is evidence that using a systematic format in any record, paper or electronic, improves the quality of care and service user outcomes (Mann & Williams, 2003). It is therefore important that the information in professional records be recorded accurately, systematically and consistently.

Quality improvement

Quality (Donabedian, 1980) has many dimensions. In the health service, patients, the public and carers expect safe, effective and consistent high-quality care and treatment. For the individual dietitian, this is a requirement of registration with the HCPC. Quality improvement involves a series of activities undertaken to reduce the gap between current practice and desired practice.

As a result of the need to account for its management and clinical efficiency, effectiveness and value for money, the NHS developed the concept of clinical governance. Clinical governance is defined as '*the system through which NHS organisations are accountable for continuously improving the quality of their services and safeguarding high standards of care, by creating an environment in which clinical excellence will flourish*' (Scally & Donaldson, 1998, p. 61). The principles of clinical governance are embedded within the organisation and encompass:

- Clinical audit.
- Evidence-based practice.
- Information governance (including record keeping).
- Patient and public involvement.
- Patient safety.
- Revalidation and performance.
- Risk management and medicolegal issues.

The term clinical effectiveness was developed as a response to demands to provide evidence of effectiveness. Health professionals have developed measures to report on the quality of clinical services and assess the effectiveness of medical interventions. These include:

- Clinical or medical audit.
- Outcome measures.
- Evidence-based practice.
- Guidelines.

Clinical audit is carried out locally and nationally, and provides a method for systematically evaluating, reflecting upon and reviewing practices against evidence-based standards.

Dietetic outcome measurement

The provision of safe, effective and good-quality care, or intervention, is fundamental to dietetic practice and is a HCPC registration requirement. A dietitian needs to know that an intervention is evidence based and effective, i.e. that it achieves the predicted outcome and makes effective use of the available resources. To demonstrate this, dietitians need to be able to systematically and consistently identify and predict what the desired outcomes of their interventions will be, the timescale involved and to what extent this has been achieved from the viewpoint of both the dietitian and the recipient. Measuring outcomes and sharing this information demonstrate the value of a dietetic service to commissioners and to the wider health community. Systematic collection and analysis of outcome data can facilitate decision-making and enhance the quality of healthcare.

Measurement of outcomes can take place at the individual, service, multidisciplinary team, organisational or national level. Measuring healthcare outcomes is a developing field, and no single methodology is universally applicable to all situations or able to capture all dimensions of care. Outcome measurement should use SMAART principles (systematic, measurable, appropriate, acceptable, realistic and timely). There are several approaches to measurement, and an increasing number of validated tools are available. Measures may be patient reported – such as patient reported outcome measures (PROMs) (see Chapter 2.2, Assessment of nutritional status) or patient reported experience measures (PREMS). Putting the patient at the centre of care is a central feature of health policy across the UK, so measuring the patient experience has to be a key component of outcome measurement. Therapy outcome measures are those where the professional measures a change in a specified domain. The use and development of validated outcome measures in dietetics is an emerging methodology, and one that is underpinned by application of the Process to enable a consistent approach to the provision of dietetic care.

Digitalisation

Information technologies are revolutionising healthcare delivery. Traditionally, face-to-face or telephone consultations were the mainstay of dietetic contacts but now video consultations are becoming more common, providing flexibility and efficiency to meet the needs the service user. Across the profession, and indeed throughout the whole of healthcare, electronic care records with a range of interoperable functions are replacing paper records, thus enabling fast data collection and analysis. Standardised language and clinical coding are also important features of digital dietetic records, widening the scope for the secondary use of records.

Clinical terminology is a type of standard language that consists of structured lists of coded concepts and their descriptors. These concepts can be used in clinical practice to enable standardised recording of patient information. A clinical terminology can be embedded in electronic systems and makes possible clear and consistent communication of clinical information, improves record sharing and speed of entry of information. The coding enables the concepts and related information to be communicated efficiently and unambiguously between the different digital systems used by health and social care workers.

In the UK, Systematized Nomenclature of Medicine Clinical Terms (SNOMED CT) is the chosen clinical terminology to be used across all care settings and clinical domains. A list of concepts for the PNDP (have been developed in USA and are known as the nutrition care process terminology (NCPT)). Some NCPT terms have been adapted for use in patient records across the world. In the UK, work is ongoing to incorporate such concepts into SNOMED CT.

Remarkable breakthroughs in the medical world as a result of new technologies continue to transform the care available, e.g. digital imaging, surgical apparatus and meters to monitor a range of conditions. Dietetic practice evolves around these advances, with modified dietetic interventions alongside tailored patient pathways. Mobile devices including smartphones have also played a role in both the increase in the number of health applications (apps) and the rise in social media as a platform to share nutritional messages. Dietitians have a significant role to play in contributing to online discussions to help promote evidence-based facts and dispel myths. Dietitians must understand the latest guidance on information governance and how it applies to their own specialist areas of work. Information governance includes rules and processes to ensure that personal data is held securely and only used for legitimate purposes, and that service users are provided with consent options regarding who can access these data.

Evidence-based practice

Evidence-based practice is not a single activity but must be continuous throughout a dietitian's professional career. It is what distinguishes a dietitian from an alternative practitioner, and is an essential element in the nutrition and dietetic process. Evidence-based practice can be broken down into five key stages:

- Formulating the question.
- Finding the evidence.
- Critical appraisal.
- Using and acting on evidence.
- Evaluation and reflection.

The first three stages have been carried out in many cases by Practice-based Evidence in Nutrition (PEN) (www.pennutrition.com/bda). The PEN system aims to support dietitians to use evidence-based practice in their day-to-day roles. PEN applies the concept of knowledge translation by summarising the evidence base on a nutrition- or dietetic-related topic and providing the practical guidance for implementation into practice. Each topic in the PEN system is collated under a knowledge pathway, which is subdivided into sections such as background or practice questions. A number of training modules are available on PEN. The dietitian needs to use clinical judgement to apply the evidence to the individual situation and the clients' needs. It is important that dietitians be research-active in order to contribute to PEN and other sources of clinical guidelines. Dietitians are in a unique position to understand the areas of their work that are lacking in terms of an evidence base and to formulate the most relevant research questions. PEN is a worldwide resource, so UK dietitians can work with their international colleagues to formulate the questions most pertinent to clinicians. PEN evidence analysts use Grading of Recommendations, Assessment, Development and Evaluations (GRADE), a systematic way of making judgements and evaluating the evidence base, developed by the GRADE working group, to evaluate the evidence.

Clinical guidelines are recommendations on the appropriate treatment and care of patients with specific diseases and conditions. Guidelines can be generated at an international level, e.g. the World Health Organization; nationally by organisations such as National Institution for Health and Clinical Excellence (NICE) or Scottish Intercollegiate Guidelines Network (SIGN) in the UK, or by other clinical specialist organisations and professional bodies, e.g. BDA, Royal College of Physicians; and associated clinical working groups, e.g. Intercollegiate Stroke Working Group. Some, such as those developed by NICE, also consider cost-effectiveness. Guideline developers are increasingly using GRADE to assist in linking their evaluation of the evidence to the clinical recommendation. GRADE provides both an assessment of the quality of the evidence – high, moderate, low and very low – and the strength of the recommendations.

Routine activities that aid practitioners include keeping a portfolio and reading and evaluating new evidence. A portfolio is vital evidence of CPD and should be used to reflect and evaluate practice and the effect of any change. Simple electronic tools are available to provide information on new evidence. These include:

- *Application software (apps)* – including EBM toolkits from publishers (e.g. BMJ), books, journals, searchable databases (e.g. PubMed) and critical appraisal tools.
- *Electronic table of contents (eTOC) from appropriate journals* – current contents pages are sent to subscribers (this is usually a free service).

- *Alerts, updates and newsletters* – from professional bodies and organisations, e.g. TRIP (www.tripdatabase.com), which includes Bandolier and Cochrane, and the Centre for Reviews and Dissemination (CRD), York.

Most of these services are available as email alerts or really simple syndication (RSS) feeds; once set up, they are automatic.

Research, audit and service evaluation

The skills required to conduct research can also be applied to conduct audit and service evaluation. However, research is used to generate new evidence, while audit and service evaluation evaluate care. It is important to remember that a survey conducted in clinical care cannot be called an 'audit' unless the results are compared with a standard; standards are generated by research. An important distinction between research, audit and service evaluation is that research requires ethical approval from the appropriate research ethics committee (REC), while audit and service evaluation do not. Within the NHS, they all require review and approval by the appropriate department, i.e. research and development or clinical governance. Table 1.1.4 gives a brief summary of the key differences between the categories of studies. If the categorisation of the study is unclear, it is important to consult the appropriate department or committee before commencement.

Research *'means the attempt to derive generalisable new knowledge by addressing clearly defined questions with systematic and rigorous methods'* (Health Research Authority, 2016). It underpins evidence practice and is a vital component of a dietitian's professional role. The HCPC (2013) requires that dietitians must be able to *'recognise the need to monitor and evaluate the quality of practice and the value of contributing to the generation of accurate data for quality assurance, governance, clinical audit, research and improvement programmes'*. The essential nature of research and audit as part of professional practice is embedded within both the BDA's Code of Professional Conduct (2017) and the Curriculum Framework for the Pre-registration Education and Training for Pre-registration Dietitians (BDA, 2013a). The BDA (2013b) defines four stages of research involvement, and details the skills required at each stage. On qualification, all dietitians should have the necessary skills to understand, interpret and apply research. If dietitians maintain and build upon these basic skills, some will eventually lead research and supervise others (Whelan, 2007).

Research governance and ethics

Research governance encompasses regulations, standards and principles of good research practice, thereby ensuring that research is conducted to high ethical and scientific standards. It applies to everyone involved in the research process, including researchers at all levels, employers and support staff. In a clinical setting, this will include care providers. In 2015, the Health Research Authority took responsibility for replacing the research governance framework with a new UK policy framework for health and social care

Ethical approval from an appropriate committee is essential for any research involving humans, clinical data, human organs or tissues; it is a legal requirement in the NHS. Informed consent and confidentiality are central to ethical research. The review process will vary depending on the organisation. Within the NHS, the Health Research Authority offers a central and consistent service, including the integrated research application system (IRAS) (www.myresearchproject.org.uk). This is a single system of applying for permissions and approvals for health and social care and community research in the UK without unnecessary duplication. Each university will have its own system for ethical approval.

How to do research

This section gives a brief overview of research; more detailed information can be found in Ray *et al.* (2016). Further resources are listed at the end of the chapter.

Planning research

The first step is developing the research question, and the PICO principle can be used to generate a concise question. The aims and objectives of the research should relate directly to the research question; the methodology will be determined by the aims and objectives. When disseminating the results of the research, the discussion and conclusion of a paper or abstract should relate to the question and aims and objectives. The research question may arise from clinical practice or from the literature. A research question will lead to a hypothesis.

The research question plays a crucial role when reviewing the literature for the project. The literature review may stem from the aims and objectives, or serve to formulate the aims and objectives. The research aim is usually a broad statement outlining the goal, while objectives are more detailed statements of how the aim will be achieved. Each objective should be simple, straightforward and achievable. Well-thought-out objectives suggest a methodology and thus help determine the methodology. It is good practice to include potential participants when planning research; INVOLVE (http://www.invo.org.uk/) has more information about public involvement in health and social care research. The actual method is how the study will be carried out and includes details such as where the research will take place, who will be involved, how the participants will be recruited, the actual data collection and how the data will be analysed. It is quite acceptable to include both quantitative and qualitative methodologies in a study, but often such a study will be divided into two stages, with one stage informing the other. Table 1.1.5 gives an overview of research methodologies.

It is essential to write a research protocol when planning the project and include details of the study rationale, aims and objectives, methods with specific measureable outcomes, statistical analysis, dissemination plans and timeline. The protocol can be used when

Table 1.1.4 Differentiating clinical audit, service evaluation, research and usual practice/surveillance work [source: Health Research Authority. Reproduced with permission from the Health Research Authority, 2017 (www.hra.nhs.uk)]

Research	Service evaluation*	Clinical audit	Surveillance	Usual practice
The attempt to derive generalisable new knowledge, including studies that aim to generate hypotheses as well as studies that aim to test them.	Designed and conducted solely to define or judge current care.	Designed and conducted to produce information to inform delivery of best care.	Designed to manage outbreak and help the public by identifying and understanding risks.	Designed to investigate outbreak or incident to help in disease control and prevention.
Quantitative research – designed to test a hypothesis. Qualitative research – designed to identify/explore themes following established methodology.	Designed to answer: 'What standard does this service achieve?'	Designed to answer: 'Does this service reach a predetermined standard?'	Designed to answer: 'What is the cause of this outbreak?'	Designed to answer: 'What is the cause of this outbreak?' and treat.
Addresses clearly defined questions, aims and objectives.	Measures current service without reference to a standard.	Measures against a standard.	Systematic, statistical methods to allow timely public health action.	Systematic, statistical methods may be used.
Quantitative research – may involve evaluating or comparing interventions, particularly new ones. Qualitative research – usually involves studying how interventions and relationships are experienced.	Involves an intervention in use only. The choice of treatment is that of the clinician and patient according to guidance, professional standards and/or patient preference.	Involves an intervention in use only. The choice of treatment is that of the clinician and patient according to guidance, professional standards and/or patient preference.	May involve collecting personal data and samples.	Any choice of treatment is based on clinical best evidence or professional consensus.
Usually involves collecting data that are additional to those for routine care but may include data collected routinely. May involve treatments, samples or investigations additional to routine care.	Usually involves analysis of existing data but may include administration of interview or questionnaire.	Usually involves analysis of existing data but may include administration of simple interview or questionnaire.	May involve analysis of existing data or administration of interview or questionnaire to those exposed.	May involve administration of interview or questionnaire to those exposed.
Quantitative research – study design may involve allocating patients to intervention groups. Qualitative research – uses a clearly defined sampling framework underpinned by conceptual or theoretical justifications.	No allocation to intervention: the health professional and patient have chosen intervention before service evaluation.	No allocation to intervention: the health professional and patient have chosen intervention before audit.	Does not involve an intervention.	May involve allocation to control group to assess risk and identify source of incident but treatment unaffected.
May involve randomisation.	No randomisation.	No randomisation.	No randomisation.	May involve randomisation but not for treatment.
Normally requires REC review. Refer to http://www.hra.nhs.uk/resources/before-you-apply/is-nhs-rec-reviewrequired/ for more information.	Does not require REC review.	Does not require REC review.	Does not require REC review.	Does not require REC review.

*Service development and quality improvement may fall into this category.

Table 1.1.5 Research methodologies

Descriptive	Cross-sectional survey	
	Qualitative, e.g. grounded theory, discourse analysis, ethnography, narrative research and phenomenology	
Empirical	Experimental	Randomised parallel groups
		Randomised crossover
	Observational	Cohort
		Cross-sectional
		Case control

applying for governance and ethical approval, and funding and will form the basis of the eventual dissemination. When using questionnaires, or other instruments to measure variables, it is important to consider the population for which they are validated and how the results obtained from them will be analysed. If results require statistical analysis, it is sensible to consult a statistician at this stage so that any necessary modifications can be made to the planned data collection.

Conducting research

This stage of the research process is usually constrained by time and money. A Gantt chart detailing delivery dates and deadlines is a useful organisational tool. Difficulties in obtaining ethical approval or with recruitment of research staff and participants often delay projects, so sufficient time should be built in at the planning stage to avoid missing deadlines later. Communication is key to keeping the research process on track, e.g. if recruitment is slower than anticipated, it is helpful to let funders know before deadlines are missed; funding bodies often have a wealth of experience and can be a source of help and advice if necessary. Meticulous record-keeping will also help the research process to run smoothly. Data collection sheets that are easy to complete will be less likely to contain errors. Data collection methods should be piloted and necessary changes made. Research logs or diaries can act as a cross-check to reference dates and times during which certain activities took place. Keeping a research diary may be a requirement of an organisation.

Data analysis will probably involve transferring data into a software analysis program, and particular care should be taken at this stage to avoid introducing errors. If possible, double data entry should be used, where two people enter quantitative data on separate spreadsheets and compare them for differences. Qualitative data often need to be transcribed; this time-consuming task can be delegated to professional transcribers, although this step can be a valuable part of the process of becoming familiar with the data.

Dissemination

It is essential that dietitians disseminate all the evidence generated, including research, audit and service evaluation. There are vehicles for every type and size of study; small and negative studies are valuable as they add to the evidence base and may inform others of potential difficulties. Dissemination can occur internally, within the department or institution, or externally, at conferences and in peer-reviewed journals. Conferences are the best way to disseminate small studies and initial findings. The most important way to disseminate work is as a manuscript published in a peer-reviewed journal. Guidance on how to write a conference abstract or a manuscript for publication can be found at www.bda.uk.com/conference/research. Publication guidelines, e.g. consolidated standards of reporting trials (CONSORT), have been produced in order to improve the quality of research reporting and are available from the Equator Network (www.equator.org.uk).

Continuing professional development

Professional practice develops over time, and individual professionals must strive, and expect, to develop and improve their practice so that services and the outcomes for their service users improve. This process is known as continuing professional development (CPD). CPD is an active process by which every day and more formal experiences are critically reflected upon to identify learning points, which are then recorded in a useful format. The BDA (2013a) defines CPD as '... *a systematic on-going process which allows individuals to maintain, update and enhance their knowledge and expertise in order to ensure that they are able to carry out work safely and effectively*'.

As defined by the HCPC (2013), CPD is how '... *professionals maintain and develop throughout their career to ensure that they retain their capacity to practice safely, effectively and legally within their evolving scope of practice*'. All healthcare professionals are expected and required to work within their scope of practice, with the understanding that this usually changes over time – from broad practice across the profession to a deeper understanding and more expert practice in a narrower, more specialist field. CPD is obviously the route to this expert practice, and the range of CPD activities is extensive. It includes work-based learning, such as reflective practice, clinical audit or journal club; professional activities, including active membership of a specialist group, mentoring or teaching; or formal education, from short courses to higher degrees. The need for different blends of learning will vary with the practice and career aspirations of the individual and the demands of their current post or practice.

A dietitian has a responsibility to meet the HCPC Standards for CPD (2013). All HCPC registrants are required to undertake CPD and record their activities within a portfolio. In line with other registered professions, the HCPC carries out an audit of dietitians on a biyearly basis, selecting 2.5% of the profession for review. Those selected are required to complete the HCPC's profile-mapping CPD activity directly to the HCPC standards. Each audit covers CPD activity from the preceding 2 years. All dietitians on the HCPC register have an equal chance of selection, regardless of where they are based, within Britain or overseas, or their current work situation, e.g. part-time, full-time or on maternity leave.

Both the HCPC and the BDA identify CPD as the responsibility of the autonomous professional, i.e. the individual dietitian. Whilst many employers are supportive, it is the registered professional's personal responsibility to ensure that CPD activities and documentation are kept up to date. This may need to be met using personal time and resources. Those working outside the NHS, particular those working as freelance dietitians, will need to be proactive in sourcing opportunities for themselves. CPD helps to maintain current competence and to develop new competence, thereby ensuring that dietitians can continue to work in an evidence-based manner. If all dietitians embrace CPD, as they should, this will create departments where there is a strong learning culture with active involvement in student and staff supervision, mentoring and team and individual reflection.

Continuing professional development activities

An individual's CPD should reflect a wide range of learning activities and be relevant to the individual's current or developing scope of practice. CPD does not only refer to traditional training or courses. It can be applied to any activity outside of an individual's day-to-day practice, which develops the individual's practice and allows professionals to reflect upon their own learning. Further examples of CPD are shown in Table 1.1.6. Further guidance on CPD activities is available with both the BDA and the HCPC.

Reflective practice

Reflective practice has been defined as '... *the capacity to reflect on action so as to engage in a process of continuous learning*' (Schon, 1991), and it is essential for the development of professional practice in dietetics. The purpose of reflection is to enable a practitioner to apply a systematic approach to consideration of a particular experience, thereby developing practice through analysis and consideration of points of learning for the future. Thus, dietitians use reflective practice as a method through which to make sense of their practice and development needs. Initially, the situation or experience is analysed, with consideration given to the knowledge and skills used and the individual's reaction to the experience. Subsequently, learning from experience is explored in order to facilitate professional development for future practice. During the process, further learning needs are often identified. This reflection on practice is also one method by which a professional may identify new theories of practice and so integrate the technical science basis and the practice and art of dietetics.

Reflection is a skill that requires development and practice. It requires individuals to be open to their feelings and to what they can learn from the experience.

Recording continuing professional development

Dietitians have a responsibility to maintain an accurate, continuous and up-to-date record or portfolio of CPD activities (HCPC, 2013). There are a number of models that provide a structured process to aid the process of reflection and for building a portfolio (Gibbs, 1988; Rolfe *et al.*, 2001). The BDA provides tools to support the development of a portfolio and pro formas to record

Table 1.1.6 Examples of continuing professional development (CPD) activities

Work-based learning	Professional activity	Formal/educational	Self-directed learning
Learning by doing	Involvement in a professional body	Courses	Reading journals/articles
Case studies	Membership of a specialist interest group	Further education	Reviewing books or articles
Reflective practice	Lecturing or teaching	Research	Keeping a file of progress
Clinical audit	Mentoring	Attending conferences or seminars	
Discussions with colleagues	Being an examiner or tutor	Writing articles or papers	
Gaining and learning from experience	Organising journal clubs or other specialist groups	Distance-learning	
Work-shadowing	Membership of other professional bodies or groups	Planning or running a course	
Secondments	Presenting at conferences		
Job rotation	Supervising research		
Journal club	Being promoted		
In-service training			
Supervising staff or students			
Analysing significant events			
Project work or project management			

CPD, based on this particular framework that uses the following questions:

- What?
- So what?
- Now what?

This translates to a process by which an individual can identify an activity or incident (the *what* element), consider the impact of the activity on practice and whether, as an individual, he or she dealt with the situation appropriately (the *so what* element). Finally, the individual will consider the *now what* element, i.e. what can be learned from the incident to improve professional practice, going forward. This model enables the dietitian to describe the CPD activity, explain what is learnt and reflect on the benefits to the service user alongside the use of new skills, in addition to investigating any areas for development or improvement.

Critical analysis and evaluation refocuses the dietitian's thinking and helps generate new knowledge and ideas. As a result, individuals may modify their actions, behaviour, treatments and learning needs. As part of their professional commitment to CPD, dietitians must make time to record their reflections, a process which often helps clarify thoughts and provides written evidence to share with others at a later date. It is important to note that reflection is undertaken from a personal perspective. This is not a team exercise but about the individual practitioner and the development of their professional knowledge, skills and competence. A professional development toolkit of support can be found in the BDA's learning zone (www.bdacpd.co.uk).

Practice supervision

Dietitians should also seek practice supervision throughout their professional training and career. Supervision is the process of professional learning and support involving a range of activities. It enables individuals to develop knowledge and competence, assume responsibility for their own practice and enhance service user protection, quality and safety of care (BDA, 2014). The supervision process can directly influence CPD, providing a structured process of professional support that facilitates lifelong learning and personal development, and highlights training needs. Practice supervision is integral to delivering good-quality service, and should be included in working practices where work-based scenarios are explored, reflection upon practice takes place and evidence of CPD is gathered. This process of supervision will start with students in practice education and continue throughout the working life of dietitians. Examining performance, identifying strengths and weaknesses, and seeking to improve are key attributes of a professional.

Preceptorship

Ideally, professionals in the first year of practice, particularly within the NHS, should work within a structured development programme called preceptorship. The aim of preceptorship is to enhance the competence and confidence of newly registered practitioners as autonomous professionals (DH, 2010). During this time, the new practitioners, supported by preceptors, will develop their skills, behaviour and attitude to become more confident practitioners. Within the UK, access to preceptorship programmes varies at the local level. While some benefit from a structured programme incorporating a mix of theory and guided reflection, other graduates are less fortunate in their ability to access this level of support. Further guidance is available from a number of different sources, including the BDA.

Conclusion

Dietetics has a proud tradition of upholding safe, effective, evidence-based nutritional expertise, and this is fundamentally owing to the professionals who work within the discipline. The profession's commitment to constantly be innovative, while striving for the highest standards of technical and ethical competence, have seen it evolve into the internationally respected profession it is today.

Dedication

This chapter is dedicated to the memory of Rosanna Hudson (1972–2017).

Acknowledgement

The editor acknowledges the prior contribution of Ingrid Darnley and Julie Farmer.

Further reading

Greenhalgh T. (2010) *How to Read a Paper: The Basics of Evidence-Based Medicine*. Oxford: Wiley Blackwell.

Hickson M. (2008) *Research Handbook for Health Care Professionals*. Oxford: Wiley Blackwell.

Lawrence J, Douglas P, Gandy J (2016) *Dietetic & Nutrition Case Studies*. Oxford: Wiley

Internet resources

BDA How to prepare a conference abstract for BDA events, https://www.bda.uk.com/events/research_symposium/abstract_guidance_2016

Centre for Evidence-Based Medicine, www.cebm.net/

Centre for Reviews and Dissemination (CRD), York, www.york.ac.uk/inst/crd/

Enhancing the Quality of Health Research (EQUATOR), www.equator-network.org

Health and Care Professions Council, www.hcpc-uk.org

Healthcare Improvement Scotland, www.healthcareimprovementscotland.org/welcome_to_healthcare_improvem.aspx

Healthcare Quality Improvement Partnership (HQIP), www.hqip.org.uk

NHS Evidence, www.evidence.nhs.uk/

NICE Guidance and Scotland, www.healthcareimprovementscotland.org/programmes/nice_guidance_and_scotland.aspx

National Research Ethics Service, www.myresearchproject.org.uk

Practice-Based Evidence in Nutrition (PEN), www.pennutrition.com/bda

Scottish Intercollegiate Guidelines Network, www.sign.ac.uk

Trip Database – Clinical Search Engine, www.tripdatabase.com/

References

NB: BDA documents can be accessed by members via the member's page. Non-members should contact the BDA directly.

BDA. (2009) *Guidance Document on Extended Scope Practice*. Birmingham: BDA.

BDA. (2013a) *Curriculum Framework for the Pre-registration Education and Training for Preregistration Dietitians*. Birmingham: BDA.

BDA. (2013b) *Continuing Professional Development Position Statement*. Birmingham: BDA.

BDA. (2014) *Practice Supervision*. Birmingham: BDA.

BDA. (2016a) *Model for Dietetic Outcomes*. Birmingham: BDA.

BDA. (2016b) *Model and Process for Dietetic Outcomes*. Birmingham: BDA.

BDA. (2017) *Code of Conduct*. Birmingham: BDA.

Cruess SR, Johnston S, Cruess RL. (2004) 'Profession': a working definition for medical educators. *Teach. Learn. Med.* 16(1): 74–76.

DH. (2010) *Preceptorship framework for newly registered nurses, midwives and allied health professionals*. Available at https://hee.nhs.uk/sites/default/files/documents/DoH%20Preceptorship%20Framework%20for%20newly%20registered%20nurses%20midwives%20and%20allied%20health%20professionals%202010.PDF. Accessed 27 June 2017.

Donabedian A. (1980) *The Definition of Quality and Approaches to its Assessment*. Ann Arbor, MI: Health Administration Press.

Gibbs G. (1988) *Learning by Doing: A Guide to Teaching and Learning Methods*. Oxford: Further Educational Unit, Oxford Polytechnic.

HCPC. (2009) *Guidance on Conduct and Ethics for Students*. London: HCPC.

HCPC. (2010) *Information for Employers and Managers: The Fitness to Practice Process*. London: HCPC.

HCPC. (2013) *Standards of Proficiency – Dietitians*. London: HCPC.

HCPC. (2016) *Standards of Conduct, Performance and Ethics*. London: HCPC.

Health Research Authority. (2016) *Defining research*. Available at http://www.hra.nhs.uk/documents/2016/06/defining-research.pdf. Accessed 27 January 2017.

Health Research Authority. (2017) *Differentiating clinical audit, service evaluation, research and usual practice/surveillance work*. Available at http://www.hra.nhs.uk/documents/2016/06/defining-research.pdf. Accessed 21 July 2017.

Institute of Medicine. (2001) *Crossing the Quality Chasm: A New Health System for the 21st Century*. Washington, DC: National Academy Press.

Mann R, Williams J. (2003) Standards in medical record keeping. *Clin. Med.* 3: 329.

Ray S, Fitzpatrick S, Golubic R, et al. (2016) *Oxford Handbook of Clinical and Healthcare Research*. Oxford: OUP.

Rolfe G, Freshwater D, Jasper M. (2001) *Critical Reflection for Nursing and the Helping Professions – A User's Guide*. Basingstoke: Palgrave.

Scally G, Donaldson LJ. (1998) Clinical governance and the drive for quality improvement in the new NHS in England. *BMJ* 317: 61–65.

Schon D. (1991) *The Reflective Practitioner: How Professionals Think in Action*. Surrey: Ashgate Publishing Limited.

Whelan K. (2007) Knowledge and skills to encourage comprehensive research involvement among dietitians. *J. Hum. Nutr. Diet.* 20: 291–293.

SECTION 1

1.2 Dietary modification

Annemarie Knight

Key points

- Dietary modification is defined as the elimination, manipulation or introduction of dietary components to achieve dietary goals.
- Skilful assessment is required to identify the individual and psychosocial factors that may influence the success of dietary interventions.
- Dietary modification requires the use of a range of dietetic skills, including communication and health behaviour change skills.
- A total diet approach should be adopted, and dietary advice should be given in terms of food choice, not nutrients.

Dietary modification is a cornerstone of dietetic practice and employs a range of dietetic skills. When undertaking dietary modification, dietitians need in depth knowledge of food composition, food availability and factors that determine what people eat. It is well acknowledged that dietary interventions are more likely to be effective when they are based on a sound understanding of the factors influencing the food choice of individuals or communities, and not on the principles of changing health behaviour alone. An integrated approach to dietary counselling that considers all the relevant factors can improve compliance, satisfaction and clinical outcomes (Fine, 2006). The impact that these factors have on developing the most effective dietary intervention strategies will vary depending on the situation.

In the assessment step of the process for nutrition and dietetic practice, the dietitian uses skills in nutritional, dietary and clinical assessment in order to decide the goals of dietary intervention (BDA, 2016) (see Chapter 1.1, Professional practice). Key to deciding how best to achieve these goals is an assessment of the interaction between the individual, or community, and their social situation. This assessment can also aid the identification of potential barriers that may impact the effectiveness of the intervention. Service users can and should be actively involved in their own healthcare, and the dietitian's role is to advise and help facilitate negotiated patient-centred goals. When monitoring and evaluating the effectiveness of any dietary intervention, ongoing reassessment of the factors contributing to the achievement of dietary goals will be necessary.

Principles of dietary modification

Dietary modification can be defined as the elimination, manipulation or introduction of dietary components to achieve dietary goals. Dietary interventions are aimed at individuals, groups or communities and vary greatly in complexity. Modifications that are considered simple, e.g. increasing the fruit and vegetable intake of a community, may in fact be very difficult to achieve and require significant dietetic input. Similarly, those considered more complex, e.g. meeting an individual's nutritional requirements via the parenteral route, might be more straightforward to achieve.

Whether total or partial control of an individual's nutritional intake is required, challenges will almost certainly arise. A detailed knowledge of food and its composition is vital, together with an excellent understanding of the available tools and resources, to reach achievable results. Once the requirement for dietary modification is highlighted and the level of regulation has been determined, four keys factors should be considered to achieve the required result: knowledge, achievability, motivation and communication.

Knowledge

In order for dietary modification to be effective, both the dietitian and service user (and any other healthcare professionals, or supporting individuals) must be knowledgeable regarding the rationale for the changes proposed. It is part of the dietitian's role to ensure that all those involved understand why change is necessary and

Manual of Dietetic Practice, Sixth Edition. Edited by Joan Gandy.

Companion website: www.manualofdieteticpractice.com

how the proposed dietary modification will contribute to achieving treatment goals. From a service user's perspective, this can encourage compliance and also empower individuals to take some responsibility (NESTA & Health Foundation, 2016) for their own health and lifestyle. This process can be demonstrated through programmes such as Dose Adjustment for Normal Eating (DAFNE) and Diabetes Education and Self-Management for Ongoing and Newly Diagnosed (DESMOND), which focus primarily on the education and empowerment of the patient to allow for ongoing dietary modification that compliments individual lifestyles (see Chapter 7.12, Diabetes mellitus). Patient-centred counselling can promote collaboration between the patient and the dietitian, resulting in tailored interventions that can enhance adherence (Rosal *et al.*, 2001).

Achievability

It is the dietitian's responsibility to ensure that the goals set for diet modification are achievable, both from the clinical and service user's perspectives. The provision of practical, tailored advice and support are useful in this process. Excellent communication and, in some cases, counselling skills are required to assess the service user's lifestyle and level of understanding, to ensure that the goals set are appropriate (see Chapter 1.3, Changing health behaviour). Within a clinical or institutional setting, dietary modification is arguably more achievable due to the more controlled environment. Meals are generally provided and nutritionally regulated, so more specific guidance is easily accessible. There may however be barriers to ensuring an individualised approach to dietary modification in an institutional setting. With regard to artificial enteral and parenteral nutrition, a prescribed regimen is normally provided and amended as required, usually resulting in greater compliance.

Working alongside service users in outpatient or community settings can pose different challenges. Dietary interventions may be targeted at individuals or groups, and, in both cases, the optimum duration and frequency of contact needed to build effective relationships will need to be considered. More frequent or longer consultations may be necessary to ensure that the dietitian can provide adequate support.

Motivation

As evident in many areas of dietetic practice, the motivation levels of both the service user and the dietitian is key to success. The Transtheoretical Model (Stages of Change Model) (Prochaska & DiClemente, 1986) demonstrates this process, highlighting those stages where successful dietary modification may be optimised. Identifying that individual service users will differ in terms of their motivation to adopt potential dietary modifications is also key, and, in all cases, targeting and tailoring of advice will probably increase effectiveness (Thomas, 1994). It may be appropriate to first make smaller dietary changes, allowing additional time and support for the adoption of more substantial dietary changes. The dietitian can use skills such as rapport building, motivational interviewing, reflective listening and problem solving to assess and increase the motivation to change (Fine, 2006; Gable & Hermann, 2016).

Communication

Effective, clear communication underpins successful dietetic practice. The way in which dietary advice is communicated can have an important impact on its effectiveness. An individualised approach should be adopted to ensure that messages are tailored to the individual or group and that the most effective communication strategies are adopted. Recognising that dietary choices are mostly made on the basis of foods rather than nutrients and communicating actions using food terms enable the individual to take control of their dietary changes. When communicating dietary strategies to individuals, groups or communities, the dietitian may use written, verbal, audiovisual, electronic or interactive forms of communication, although a combination of these will often be used. Advances in technology have allowed for changes in how patients are supported to make dietary changes, and telehealth-delivered interventions can help improve diet quality (Kelly *et al.*, 2016). Knowledge of tools such as dietary exchange systems and resources can also facilitate the communication of dietary modifications. Skills in changing health behaviour and effective communication are central to successful dietary modification (see Chapter 1.3, Changing health behaviour).

Types of dietary modification

Modifying dietary intake can provide a methodical and practical solution to wider health issues, and encourage an individualised and problem-solving approach. This can range from the elimination of nutrients through to the reintroduction of dietary components, and can also include the manipulation of foods (Table 1.2.1).

Manipulation of dietary components

Dietary components can be manipulated in the following ways.

Texture

The texture or consistency of the diet may be modified, e.g. in the management of swallowing disorders.

Composition

It may be necessary to alter the chemical composition of the diet in the management of conditions such as food hypersensitivity. Modification may require the use of dietary products whose macronutrient composition

Table 1.2.1 Approaches to dietary intervention

	Dietary intervention	Example of dietary modification to achieve dietary goals
Elimination	Weight management	Eliminate energy-dense foods
	Food hypersensitivity	Eliminate foods containing allergens
		Eliminate foods causing intolerance
Manipulation	Weight management	Manipulation of portion size
	Oral nutritional support	Substitute foods to increase energy density
	Texture modification	As per the *The Nutrition and Hydration Digest: Improving Outcomes through Food and Beverage Services* (BDA, 2017)
	Artificial nutritional support	Manipulation of chemical composition of dietary components, e.g. elemental feed
	Restrict nutrients	Low-fat diet, electrolyte restriction in renal disease, metabolic disorders
Introduction or reintroduction	Healthy, balanced diet	Ensuring intake is balanced, including all food groups
	Elimination diet	Foods are eliminated and reintroduced slowly, assessing symptoms (e.g. FODMAP diet, suspected allergies)
	Weight management	Introduce substitutions for high-energy-density foods
	Oral nutritional support	Introduce substitutions for low-energy-density foods

has been manipulated, e.g. amino acid or medium-chain triglyceride–based formulae.

Quantity

When modifying the quantity of a dietary component, it is necessary to consider the frequency of consumption, portion size and any appropriate food substitutions that can be made in the diet to achieve dietary goals.

Elimination of dietary components

Where possible, dietary interventions should always take a total diet approach and focus on the overall pattern of foods eaten rather than on specific foods or nutrients (Freeland-Graves & Nitzke, 2013). In the majority of cases, the elimination of individual foods will not be necessary; instead, modifying the quantity of the food consumed alongside the frequency of consumption will be sufficient to achieve dietary goals. The elimination of dietary components will be necessary in some conditions, e.g. inborn errors of metabolism. Where dietary components are excluded, it is important to assess the role they play in the individual's diet and what substitute foods need to be recommended to ensure that nutritional requirements are met.

Introduction and reintroduction of dietary components

A starting point for dietary modification is often to base recommendations on an individual's current dietary intake, although achieving dietary goals will involve the introduction of new foods. The introduction of dietary components will range from simple to complex recommendations, all of which should meet individual requirements. Where foods have been eliminated from the diet, it will be necessary to plan their reintroduction, e.g. a food challenge with an identified allergen in the management of food hypersensitivity (see Chapter 7.11.2, Food hypersensitivity).

Process of dietary modification

Rationale

The first step in dietary modification is to ascertain the purpose of the modification based on a comprehensive assessment and the identification of the nutritional problem. The aim of dietary modification may be to:

- Achieve a nutrient profile that offers greater health benefits.
- Meet dietary needs in a safer way.
- Correct a dietary deficiency or surplus.
- Avoid the consumption of a particular dietary component.
- Achieve symptom relief.
- Achieve specific metabolic or clinical effects.

Key dietetic skills of clinical reasoning and evidence-based practice are employed to develop a dietary intervention plan. Dietary modification should provide benefit to the individual or group, but it should be noted that the interactions between foods and nutrients are complex, and altering one dietary component may affect another, e.g. increasing the energy density of a diet in oral nutritional support may increase the intake of saturated fat with the associated cardiovascular consequences. A total diet approach allows for an overall view of the likely consequences.

Factors that influence food choice

In deciding the most effective dietary intervention, any factors that will potentially influence adherence to the proposed modification should be identified.

Access to food

This will include factors such as purchasing patterns, budgetary constraints and cooking skills. To achieve dietary change, it will be necessary to identify whether the foods that have been recommended are available where the individual shops, if support is needed with shopping or if the individual has the required skills to prepare the foods in the modified diet, e.g. for a texture-modified diet, it is important to assess if the necessary equipment is available to modify foods to the correct consistency. At a community level, shopping and leisure facilities available in the local area may influence the effectiveness of interventions.

Taste and food preferences

Individual food preferences and the role food plays in an individual's life need to be considered when making dietary modifications.

Lifestyle influences

The lack of time and the burden of juggling work and home commitments can be significant constraints in adopting healthy eating practices or dietary advice. It is important that the burden of the proposed dietary modification in terms of time and effort be considered.

Cultural background

Developing effective dietary intervention strategies for individuals and groups from minority ethnic backgrounds requires an understanding of their relevant health behaviours (Thomas, 2002). The factors affecting food choice and health are complex, and dietitians should ensure their cultural competence. When developing dietary interventions for minority ethnic groups, it is necessary to take account of dietary patterns and acknowledge the variations in health beliefs, attitudes and practices within each cultural group (Bronner, 1994; Satia-Abouta *et al.*, 2002) (see Chapter 3.5, Working with minority ethnic groups).

Religious or ethical beliefs

In order to ensure that dietary modifications are compatible with an individual's or group's beliefs, it is necessary to establish them and the extent to which they are followed. There can be a wide variation in the interpretation of and adherence to the dietary restrictions associated with a particular faith.

Media

The media plays an important role in influencing food choice and shaping beliefs about nutrition and the role of the dietitian. It is important that dietitians keep abreast of media reporting on nutrition and diet in order to ensure that dietary education is effective and targeted, and that incorrect dietary beliefs are addressed.

Practical aspects of dietary modification

All dietary modifications should be individualised and based on a detailed assessment. Box 1.2.1 presents information on how dietary modification can be approached in order to achieve a range of dietary goals. In addition, a range of other modifications may be used in order to achieve dietary goals, including:

- *Meal patterns* – the timing or frequency of meals may be adjusted, e.g. the provision of small, frequent meals may promote dietary intake. It may also be necessary to also consider whether or not foods or fluids should be consumed together.

Box 1.2.1 Practical examples of dietary modification strategies

Macronutrient modification

- Aim of dietary modification is to decrease the percentage energy contribution of dietary fat:
  - Identify foods contributing to dietary fat intake
  - Limit frequency of consumption of high-fat foods
  - Limit portion size of high-fat foods
  - Recommend lower-fat alternative foods
  - Recommend lower-fat cooking methods
- Aim of dietary modification is to increase dietary intake of protein:
  - Increase frequency of consumption of high-protein foods, including between-meal snacks
  - Increase portion size of high-protein foods
  - Fortify commonly consumed foods with additional protein
  - Consider need for supplements to achieve dietary aim

Micronutrient modification

- Aim of dietary modification is to increase dietary intake of iron:
  - Increase frequency of consumption of high-iron foods
  - Increase portion size of high-iron foods
  - Consider foods that increase or decrease the bioavailability of dietary iron
  - Consider need for supplements to achieve dietary aim
- Aim of dietary modification is to decrease dietary intake of potassium:
  - Eliminate or limit frequency of consumption of high-potassium foods
  - Recommend cooking methods to reduce potassium content of foods

Single/multiple food exclusion

- Aim of dietary modification is to exclude cow's milk protein and egg:
  - Eliminate all food sources of cow's milk protein and egg, including where these are present as ingredients
  - Advise alternatives to foods eliminated in order to ensure nutritional adequacy
  - Consider need for supplements to ensure nutritional adequacy of diet

- *Meal environment and eating behaviour* – altering the environment in which food is consumed may be an effective modification strategy. Changing feeding behaviour may be an important part of achieving dietary targets, and may involve other healthcare professionals.

Dietary modification underpins many aspects of dietetic practice, and it is vital that dietitians understand the principles detailed in this chapter, so that they can then be applied in practice.

Acknowledgement

The book editor acknowledges the prior contribution of Katherine Law.

References

BDA. (2016) *Model and process for nutrition and dietetic practice*. Available at https://www.bda.uk.com/publications/professional/model_and_process_for_nutrition_and_dietetic_practice_. Accessed 21 December 2016.

BDA. (2017) *The nutrition and hydration digest: improving outcomes through food and beverage services*, 2nd edn. Available at https://www.bda.uk.com/publications/professional/NutritionHydrationDigest.pdf. Accessed 22 January 2018.

Bronner Y. (1994) Cultural sensitivity and nutrition counselling. *Top. Clin. Nutr.* 9: 13–19.

Fine J. (2006) An integrated approach to nutrition counselling. *Top. Clin. Nutr.* 21: 199–211.

Freeland-Graves JH, Nitzke S. (2013) Position of the academy of nutrition and dietetics: total diet approach to healthy eating. *J. Acad. Nutr. Diet.* 113(2): 307–317.

Gable J, Hermann T. (2016) *Counselling Skills for Dietitians*, 3rd edn. London: Wiley-Blackwell.

Kelly JT, Reidlinger DP, Hoffmann TC, *et al.* (2016) Telehealth methods to deliver dietary interventions in adults with chronic disease: a systematic review and meta-analysis. *Am. J. Clin. Nutr.* 104(6): 1693–1702.

NESTA and the Health Foundation. (2016) *Supporting self-management: A guide to enabling behaviour change for health and wellbeing using person- and community-centred approaches*. Available at https://www.health.org.uk/sites/health/files/RtVSupportingSelfManagement.pdf. Accessed 18 September 2018.

Prochaska J, DiClemente C. (1986) Towards a comprehensive model of change. In: Miller W, Heather N (eds) *Treating Addictive Behaviours: Processes of Change*. New York: Plenum.

Rosal MC, Ebbeling CB, Lofgren I, et al. (2001) Facilitating dietary change: the patient-centered counseling model. *J. Am. Diet. Assoc.* 101(3): 332–341.

Satia-Abouta J, Patterson RE, Neuhouser ML, *et al.* (2002) Dietary acculturation: applications to nutrition research and dietetics. *J. Am. Diet. Assoc.* 102(8): 1105–1118.

Thomas J. (1994) New approaches to achieving dietary change. *Curr. Opin. Lipidol.* 5: 36–41.

Thomas J. (2002) Nutrition intervention in minority ethnic groups. *Proc. Nutr. Soc.* 61: 559–567.

1.3 Changing health behaviour

Dympna Pearson and Helen Croker

Key points

- The art of dietetic practice is to integrate the science of food and medicine with psychosocial aspects of people's lives in the context of changing health-related behaviours.
- An integrated approach embraces the underlying theory, principles, skills and processes necessary to initiate and maintain change.
- A behavioural approach is directive and client centred. Consultations are structured and focused, with both practitioners' and patients' agendas taken into consideration through collaborative working.
- Increasing self-awareness is important for becoming an effective change agent.

> 'I do not understand my own actions. For I do not do what I want, but I do the very thing I hate'
> (Romans 7:15 Revised Standard Version).

Dietetics was originally based on the traditional medical model of expert-led advice-giving with the expectation that, once people are told what to do, they will follow this advice. However, it is well established that advice alone does not automatically change behaviour (e.g. Contento *et al.*, 1995). The challenge for dietitians is to develop an understanding of what influences health behaviour and acquire the necessary skills to facilitate change. Traditional medical care has moved towards a patient-centred model, which takes into account the psychosocial aspects of care, as well as the clinical picture (Stewart, 1995). The National Institute for Health and Care Excellence (NICE) recommends such an approach (NICE, 2014). Although not universal, patients attending dietetic consultations tend to prefer this approach (Hancock *et al.*, 2012).

However, changing behaviour is inherently difficult; behaviours are complex and result from the interplay of habit, unconscious responses to the environment, and conscious choices, influenced by complex social environments and cultures (Kelly & Barker, 2016). It is therefore important to consider the broader context; the environment in which people live has a major influence on their health. This chapter focuses on achieving change in individuals and maximising interventions by enhancing traditional practice to form an integrated approach.

An integrated approach to changing health behaviour

There is a range of approaches for facilitating change. Different approaches may work for different people at different times. An integrated approach:

- Aims to enable patients to take the next concrete, practical step to change eating or other lifestyle behaviours.
- Combines a directive and nondirective patient-centred approach by using a 'guiding' style (Rollnick *et al.*, 2010).
- Should be evidence-based (drawn from relevant theories of behaviour change or clinical approaches, using appropriate behaviour change techniques).
- Includes a range of tools and approaches adapted from the world of psychology to provide information, strengthen motivation and facilitate change.
- Integrates the most relevant approach for that individual at a given time, e.g. exploring motivational difficulties or working on modifying behaviour.
- Treats the whole person, taking into account the environment in which the individual lives, what matters to the individual and the factors likely to influence the individual's health behaviour.
- Recognises that the skills and mindset of practitioners will influence how effective they are as behaviour change agents; practitioners should engage in ongoing self-development and self-awareness as part of continuing professional development (CPD).

Manual of Dietetic Practice, Sixth Edition. Edited by Joan Gandy.

Companion website: www.manualofdieteticpractice.com

Differences between traditional advice giving and an integrated approach

Traditional medical approaches often consist of advice giving and guiding patients towards a preferred course of action. Advice giving has a role, but advise must be delivered in the context of a helping relationship with a solid foundation of engagement. Authoritarian advice is unlikely to be well received and may induce defensiveness (Miller & Rollnick, 2013). Practitioners need to be mindful of the patient's personal circumstances and viewpoint rather than just following the clinical agenda. If the patient has not asked for advice, ask permission before doing so, e.g. '*Would you like me to suggest some options … ?*'.

A consultation based on an integrated approach has the following characteristics:

- The patient and practitioner are working together equally.
- The patient is treated with courtesy and respect.
- There is a sharing of information and ideas.
- The language and approach is collaborative.
- The patient is actively involved – there is a two-way conversation.
- The practitioner is actively listening and interpreting what the patient says, checking for understanding.
- There is common agreement and a clear plan about the way forward.

Foundations underpinning behaviour change approaches

The foundations of an integrated approach to changing health-related behaviours are its theoretical underpinning, guiding principles, interpersonal skills and ongoing practitioner development. An overview of each is provided in the following text.

Theoretical underpinning

What is theory, and why use it?

Interventions are more likely to be effective if based on good understanding of the behaviour in question and the conditions in which it takes place. Health behaviours are particularly complex as they are usually several (e.g. achieving good diabetes control comprises numerous dietary, activity and monitoring behaviours) with differing social contexts. Interventions are correspondingly complex, which can be challenging. Theories of behaviour change seek to '*explain why, when and how a behaviour does or does not occur, and the important sources of influence to be targeted in order to alter the behaviour*' (Michie *et al.*, 2014b). These are conceptualised as health behaviour models. The actual strategies used are called behaviour change techniques, and these are informed by the theory underpinning the dietetic interaction. Many of these techniques cut across different approaches, e.g. behavioural goal setting. In addition to making change more likely, good use of theory to inform practice means that interventions have the potential to be described accurately and replicated. NICE guidelines specifically recommend that interventions be evidence-based and use proven behaviour change techniques (NICE, 2014). Interventions should ideally be developed in a structured way using theory; theory can also be used less formally to inform clinical practice.

Models

There are a number of health behaviour models that contribute to the understanding of human behaviour in relation to health. A model attempts to understand and describe factors affecting a behaviour, and, from this, specific approaches can be developed to influence it. The model that has probably had the most influence on dietetic practice is the Transtheoretical Model of Change (Prochaska & DiClemete, 1986). While somewhat out of favour now, as it was difficult to apply to complex behaviours (being originally designed for addictions), the spirit of the approach is still useful (i.e. that change is complex, comprises different stages each requiring differing approaches, usually involves relapse and is influenced by self-efficacy). A newer model, the COM-B model, conceptualises behaviour as part of an interacting system involving capability (C), opportunity (O) and motivation (M) (Michie *et al.*, 2011; Michie *et al.*, 2014a). In this model, one or more must be changed for behaviour (B) change to occur. It is useful as it is an overarching framework that is compatible with other models and approaches. Also, it is mentioned in the NICE (2014) review, and hence may increase in prominence over the coming years. For a comprehensive overview of behaviour change theories, see Michie *et al.* (2014b).

Although not a theoretical behaviour change model, Egan's three-stage helping model is a problem management framework that has had considerable impact on dietetic practice (Egan, 2013). It helps to form a structure for the dietetic consultation:

- Stage 1: Current scenario (described as the 'assessment' in clinical practice).
- Stage 2: Preferred scenario (exploring options and goal setting).
- Stage 3: The action stage (involves the patient implementing a plan of action).

Counselling and psychological approaches

A counselling approach uses active listening skills to work in a patient-centred way. Approaches from the world of motivational interviewing, behavioural therapy and cognitive behavioural therapy are the most commonly used psychological approaches in dietetic practice. Rather than being theories *per se*, these clinical approaches draw upon several behaviour change theories.

Motivational Interviewing (MI)

Motivational difficulties are often the greatest challenge for people struggling with change. The task of the healthcare professional (HCP) is to tap into the intrinsic motivation that exists within each individual and help build and strengthen that motivation to facilitate change. Patients often express a desire to change but get stuck in *'I want to, but I can't …'*. MI aims to help individuals explore and resolve the discrepancy between where they are and where they want to be in relation to their health behaviours, through the use of a collaborative conversation style of consulting for strengthening a person's own motivation and commitment to change (Miller & Rollnick, 2013). It is part of an integrated approach, rather than a standalone therapy, and consists of a range of therapeutic strategies underpinned by a person-centred approach. The use of high-level interpersonal skills in this context enables the client to build commitment and reach a decision to change if appropriate (Miller & Rollnick, 2013; Rollnick *et al.*, 1992).

Behavioural Therapy (BT)

BT helps patients identify unhelpful behavioural patterns and develop ways of modifying them. It is largely drawn from behavioural learning theories (see Michie *et al.*, 2014b). These relate to identifying and modifying the triggers and responses to a behaviour. This can be conceptualised as an A–B–C model; behaviours (B) have antecedents (A) and consequences (C), and changes to one or both of these can bring about change in behaviour. These behaviours may be eating or activity related and could be targeted for increase (e.g. vegetable eating, walking) or decrease (e.g. sugary drinks, sedentary time). The behaviour change techniques most commonly used by dietitians with these theories are self-monitoring (to identify triggers), stimulus control (to modify or avoid triggers), response substitution (to learn to respond differently to triggers), reinforcement (use of rewards) and goal setting (particularly the gradual shaping of behaviours). NICE (2014) recommends that such techniques be used to support change. There is a wide range of practical techniques commonly used in dietetic practice that help patients manage eating and activity behaviours (Pearson & Grace, 2012). The techniques used will depend on what is appropriate for the person and condition at that time. Some examples are listed in Box 1.3.1, and other techniques are described later in this chapter.

Box 1.3.1 Examples of behavioural strategies used in dietetic practice

- Do nothing else while eating; sit down at a table
- Do not eat when watching TV or reading
- Chew each mouthful thoroughly
- Put down the knife and fork between mouthfuls
- Use a smaller plate or bowl
- Put food away – out of sight
- Plan menus for the week ahead
- Always shop from a list
- Never shop on an empty stomach
- Do not sit for longer than half an hour
- Plan activity for the week ahead
- Eat little and often
- Do not overfill the plate

Cognitive Behavioural Therapy (CBT)

This includes behaviour modification techniques as well as cognitive restructuring, which aims to help patients identify and then change unhelpful thoughts, ideas and beliefs that might maintain unhelpful, undesirable behaviours. Rapoport (1998) has described the application of these approaches to dietetic practice. Gable and Herrmann (2016) describe specific situations when CBT approaches may be useful, e.g. when the patient uses all or nothing language (*'I can't'*, *'it always goes wrong'*, *'I never…'*). In these situations, it can be helpful to work with the patient to distinguish thoughts from feelings (as feelings cannot be challenged but thoughts have the potential to be challenged) and then generate new, more helpful ways of thinking. It is essential that appropriate clinical supervision be in place for practitioners using this approach.

Guiding principles

Health professionals ideally base their practice on underlying principles, ethics and beliefs. Good communication skills play a major role in the outcome of a consultation, and underlying these skills are principles that guide the practitioner and influence how they apply any skills they have acquired. These principles provide a foundation for any model, theory or skills, and include the following:

A person-centred approach

A person-centred approach forms the basis of the helping relationship. Carl Rogers (1951) described the core conditions that must be present to work in a person-centred way:

- *Empathy* involves caring in a truly genuine and accepting way and developing a sensitive and accurate understanding of how patients perceive their experience. It means sharing another person's experience as if it were our own, while being aware throughout that it is not. From the patients' perspective, they feel heard and understood.
- *Genuineness* (congruence) is important for forming a helping relationship built on trust. It means being who we truly are, being honest and matching what we say with how we say it, both verbally and nonverbally.
- *Acceptance* (unconditional positive regard) means having respect for others as human beings, regardless of who they are or what they have done. This means accepting the patient unconditionally and being nonjudgmental. We find it relatively easy to accept someone we like or who does what we want. It is more difficult to accept someone we dislike or who does not act as we would wish. Health professionals need to guard against forming judgments about patients who do not adhere to recommended treatments and should seek to understand their perspective, rather than labelling them as noncompliant.

These core conditions are not always easy to adhere to, and their importance highlights the need for continual reflection on practice. When consultations do not go well, a natural response is to blame the patient as being difficult. It may be more productive to first look to oneself and consider if any of the core conditions were absent.

In an effort to address the limitations of the biomedical model, Stewart *et al.* (2014) combined it with a patient-centred approach to create a patient-centred clinical method. This went beyond the conventional biomedical approach to include consideration of the patient as a person. The method comprises four interactive components:

1. Exploring health, disease and the illness experience.
2. Understanding the whole person.
3. Finding common ground.
4. Enhancing the patient–clinician relationship.

A patient-centred approach has been associated with improved health status, increased efficacy of care and reduced costs (Stewart *et al.*, 2000, 2011). It contains many of the elements outlined in the following text.

Respecting patient autonomy

This is key for facilitating change; it is an acceptance of the right of individuals to make choices about their own actions. Practitioners need to resist the urge to 'fix it' or to tell people what to do, in the belief that they know what is best. Experience and expertise need to be shared in a collaborative way in order to achieve the best outcomes for each individual. Patients need to be fully involved in any decisions about their own future.

Client responsibility

This principle acknowledges that people are responsible for their own actions. However, practitioners need to try to understand the difficulties that people experience with change while respecting patient autonomy.

Social influence

HCPs have a remit to influence health behaviour. This influence can be very powerful, even when time is limited. Practitioners may feel that a situation is hopeless when the patient has multiple problems, e.g. poor relationships, low income and poor health. Although everybody has the ability to change, this does not necessarily mean that everyone will, but they may be able to take some steps towards improving their health.

Collaboration

The principle of collaboration helps to accommodate both the patient's and the practitioner's agenda. It recognises that two people with expertise have met; one with expertise about themselves (the client) and one with expertise in the topic area, along with specific helping skills (the practitioner). A collaborative helping relationship is built on trust and mutual respect; both parties are equals in exploring the possibilities for change (Pearson, 2010).

Self-efficacy

In order to change, people need to believe that change is possible. The practitioner's task is to help people develop self-belief in their ability to make changes. This can be achieved by helping to build the patient's confidence and competence (Bandura, 1977).

Empowerment

Empowerment is a process through which people gain greater control over decisions and actions affecting their health. This principle has especially influenced the development of care offered in diabetes management (Funnell & Anderson, 2003). It recognises that patients are in control of and responsible for the daily self-management of diabetes, and that, to succeed, a self-management plan must fit patients' goals, priorities and lifestyle, as well as their diabetes.

Interpersonal skills

Effective patient care relies heavily on good communication skills which can be applied in any setting, e.g. during consultations and while discussing patient care with medical staff, relatives, administrators, etc. These skills are variably described as counselling, consultation, interviewing, active listening, reflective listening and communication or inter-personal skills. Many practitioners are naturally good listeners; others develop their listening skills through years of practice. These skills should be continually developed and refined. Using these skills throughout the consultation can facilitate health behaviour change. There is good evidence to support the use of communication skills in healthcare generally (e.g. Najavits & Weiss, 1994; Stewart, 1995), but less so in dietetics. Surveys of UK dietitians show that a majority view communication skills as very important, and, encouragingly, the proportion receiving training appears to have increased over time (Whitehead *et al.*, 2009; Rapoport & Nicholson Perry, 2000).

Attending behaviour

This conveys acceptance by actively listening, both verbally and nonverbally. Attending also involves being aware of our own verbal and nonverbal behaviour, which reflects our thoughts, feelings and attitudes.

Nonverbal communication

In addition to the words we speak, we give powerful messages through nonverbal communication. This has been shown to be extremely important and may account for as much as 85% of communication (Ivey *et al.*, 1997). The practitioner can learn a lot by taking note of patients' nonverbal cues.

Important aspects of nonverbal communication include:

- Body language needs to be appropriate for the context of the conversation. An open, relaxed posture, leaning slightly forward, is generally recommended, rather than an unnatural or stiff posture. It is also important to avoid distracting behaviours such as constant nodding, fiddling with pens, swinging feet or looking at a watch. Hand movements are a normal part of nonverbal communication, but they should not be invasive. Sit at an appropriate distance so as not to invade the other person's space, but not being too far away.

- Eye contact that is varied and without staring.
- Facial expressions that convey empathy and provide encouragement, e.g. an encouraging smile or nod. Facial expressions should match the mood of the conversation, e.g. not smiling when the person is describing something sad.
- The pace of an interview is important. Rushed consultations can leave the patient feeling confused or unsure about what has been discussed. It is important to allow time for patients (and practitioners) to think clearly and express their thoughts. The use of a brief silence or a pause can help achieve this.
- Tone of voice and general demeanour also influence the meaning of what is said. It is important for practitioners to take note of these factors as patients may be communicating something different from the actual words said. Practitioners need to be aware that their own tone of voice and body language can convey meaning in either a more or less helpful way (e.g. it can communicate disapproval or encouragement).

Practitioners need to be familiar with and take into account cultural differences, along with the age and gender of the person they are working with. Disabilities such as hearing, sight or cognitive impairment also impact on communication.

Minimal encouragers

These indicate to patients that they are being actively listened to and encourage them to talk. This includes nonverbal language such as nodding, an encouraging smile or minimal utterances, e.g. '*mm, mm*', '*ah-hah*', '*and*', 'so…', etc. Finding the right balance of how and when to use (and not to overuse) minimal encouragers is a skill requiring practice. Some words used in everyday conversations such as '*right*' and '*ok*' can convey the wrong meaning or become irritating if constantly repeated.

Verbal following

This consists of a word, a phrase or a sentence (sometimes phrased as a question) that repeats what the patient has just said (although not in a parrot-like fashion). For example:

> *Patient*: 'I'm really struggling to fit this diet in with the rest of the family.'
> *Dietitian*: 'Family?' or 'You are struggling to fit the diet in with the family.'
> *Patient*: 'Yes, they all like…'

It encourages the person to expand on what they have said, and needs to be used skilfully and not overused, but combined with other skills to convey accurate empathy.

Paraphrasing

Paraphrasing means rephrasing the factual content of what has been said, and is used to reflect back the essence of the conversation in pieces, e.g.:

> *Patient*: 'This diet is just too hard to follow when I'm eating out.'
> *Dietitian*: 'You are struggling to manage with eating when you are not at home…'

To be effective, it requires a level of accuracy, which helps provide clarity for both the patient and practitioner. A paraphrase should be used tentatively, so that the client can agree or correct any inaccuracies. A succinct, accurate paraphrase is very powerful in helping clients feel understood.

Reflecting feelings

A reflection of feeling conveys to patients that the practitioner is trying to understand what they are experiencing emotionally. People can show their feelings in different ways: verbally, nonverbally or a combination of these. Asking people how they feel is not always helpful as people can struggle to express their emotions, so avoid questions such as '*How do you feel?*' It is more useful to reflect tentatively, and at the right intensity, what the person appears to be experiencing, e.g.:

> *Patient*: 'And then he told me that I have got diabetes!'
> *Dietitian*: 'It sounds as if the news was upsetting for you…'

Many dietitians are wary of addressing feelings (for fear of 'opening a can of worms'), but to neglect how people are feeling in relation to their health is to miss a vital element of what is likely to influence their behaviour. However, dietitians need to recognise their limitations in this area and know when and how to refer on.

Questions

Questions are useful for eliciting important information. Closed questions are efficient for gathering specific information, e.g. '*Do you take milk in your tea?*', whereas open questions encourage patients to explain things from their perspective, e.g. '*Can you fill me in on what led up to your doctor suggesting you come to see me?*' Most consultations require a combination of open and closed questions. However, questions need to be used selectively to avoid what can feel like an interrogation. In general, try to ask open questions (unless specific information is required), avoid asking two questions in a row and, for every question, offer at least two responses (Miller & Rollnick, 2013).

Summarising

Summarising helps to pull things together at different points in the consultation, and is especially useful at the beginning and end of the session. Short summaries help to clarify the situation as the consultation proceeds, e.g.:

Dietitian: 'Can I check what we have covered so far? You went to see the doctor because you were feeling unwell, and the result of all the tests was that he told you that you have diabetes, which was unexpected, and the news has left you feeling upset and worried. Is that right? (Pause) Is there anything else?'

Longer summaries may be needed to clarify long and complicated stories. They provide a pause, time to think and help give direction on what to focus on next. Summaries are also useful to help dietitians remember what needs to be recorded in notes.

Potential pitfalls for practitioners

Dietitians and health professionals often feel an obligation to make patients change, but we cannot make people change. Despite the best of intentions, this can get in the way of facilitating change. In an integrated approach, the dietitian aims to enable the patient to choose and implement changes to their health-related behaviour. Anything which leaves the patient feeling disempowered or criticised may inhibit this. Examples of common pitfalls are:

- Trying to persuade or force patients to change, e.g. '*Your blood pressure is raised; you really must make some changes…*'. Using pressure to try and convince someone to change assumes that the practitioner knows best. If a person feels under pressure, they are less likely to make a free choice.
- Trying to solve the problem, e.g. '*I think you need to cut out chocolate and go walking instead*'. This is often portrayed as well-meaning advice or a solution offered from the practitioner's point of view. In practice, however, patients are their own experts and are best at finding a solution that will work for them. They may need some guidance, but the practitioner should facilitate rather than dictate.
- Underplaying the real health risks, e.g. '*The situation could be worse…*'. This may take the form of trying to appease patients. It arises from a desire to protect patients and is often due to fear of upsetting them or a fear of not knowing how to cope with a patient's distress if they become upset. How information about health risks is presented is of vital importance.
- Presenting information in a threatening manner, e.g. '*If you don't lower your cholesterol, you risk getting…*'. Fear can motivate some people, but others may become defensive.
- Hiding behind or dictating policy, e.g. '*If you don't lose more than a couple of pounds by your next appointment, you will be discharged*'. This strategy may be an attempt to control caseload by discharging anyone who is not succeeding, but in practice is likely to reinforce a person's sense of failure and may put him or her under unrealistic pressure. Policies need to incorporate negotiation and flexibility.
- Interrogating, e.g. '*Why didn't you follow your eating plan?*' The why question is difficult to answer and may induce defensiveness. Asking lots of questions, often in a desire to get to the heart of the problem so that it can be solved, or to try to get the patient to be truthful, is counterproductive. It does not encourage patients to talk openly as the agenda is practitioner-led and can close down the conversation.
- Blaming and/or judging, e.g. '*You must be eating more than you have said or you would have lost weight*'. This assumes that the patient is lying and that the practitioner knows better than the patient.

Ongoing practitioner development

In psychology and counselling, practitioners routinely receive supervision on developing their own responses and understanding as well as improving how they work with their patients. This is not generally the case with other health professionals. It is unrealistic to expect anyone to be totally empathic, unconditionally accepting and genuinely collaborative, while also being free from judgement, blame and criticism, and having the desire to want to rescue, protect or fix it for their patients. Although dietitians can aspire to these qualities, they are not necessarily given. Some elements can be acquired through skills training and can be further enhanced through self-development (Gable & Hermann, 2016). Ongoing self-evaluation, developing self-awareness and life management skills can help this process. A tool to assess communication skills in dietitians has recently been developed and validated, which could facilitate CPD (Whitehead *et al.*, 2014). Regular supervision is essential, and all health professionals should ideally be involved in ongoing self-development work as an essential foundation to their practice and as part of CPD.

The dietetic consultation in practice

The setting

A dietetic consultation has the explicit intention of discussing the person's diet in relation to the individual's health. It is clearly very different from an informal meeting, and therefore needs to operate within certain boundaries, but should not be so formal that it feels uncomfortable. The environment or setting in which people are seen clearly needs careful consideration. Is the waiting room arranged in a way that is welcoming, with suitable seating and reading material? Is the consultation room arranged in the best way? Has clutter been removed, and telephones or other interruptions diverted? The dietitian (as the patient's advocate) has a professional responsibility to seek optimal consultation settings.

The proposed framework for the consultation

The dietetic consultation comprises a series of elements. Suggested frameworks for initial and follow-up consultations are shown in Figures 1.3.1 and 1.3.2, but

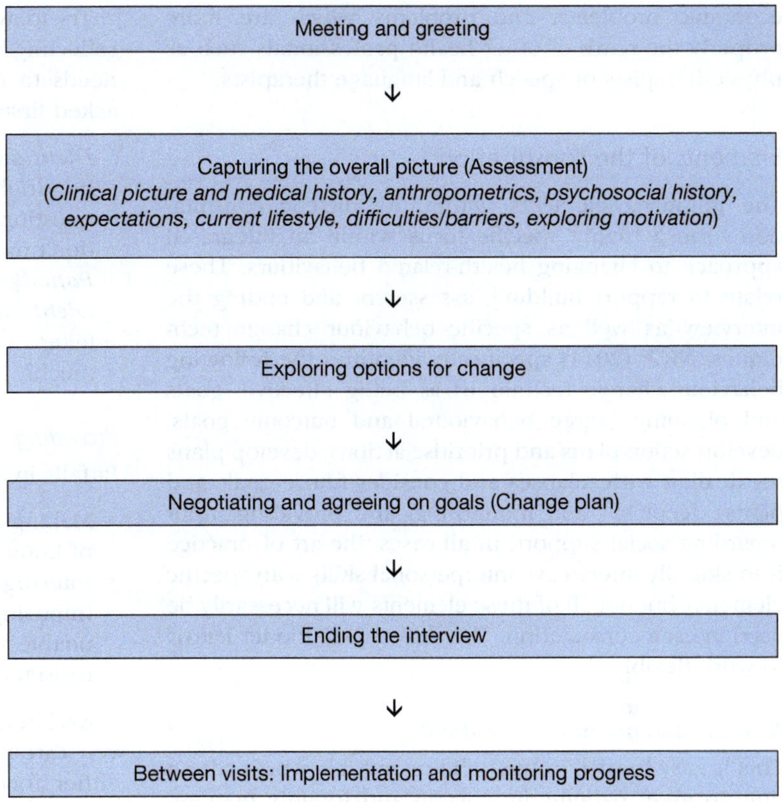

Figure 1.3.1 A suggested framework for an initial dietetic consultation

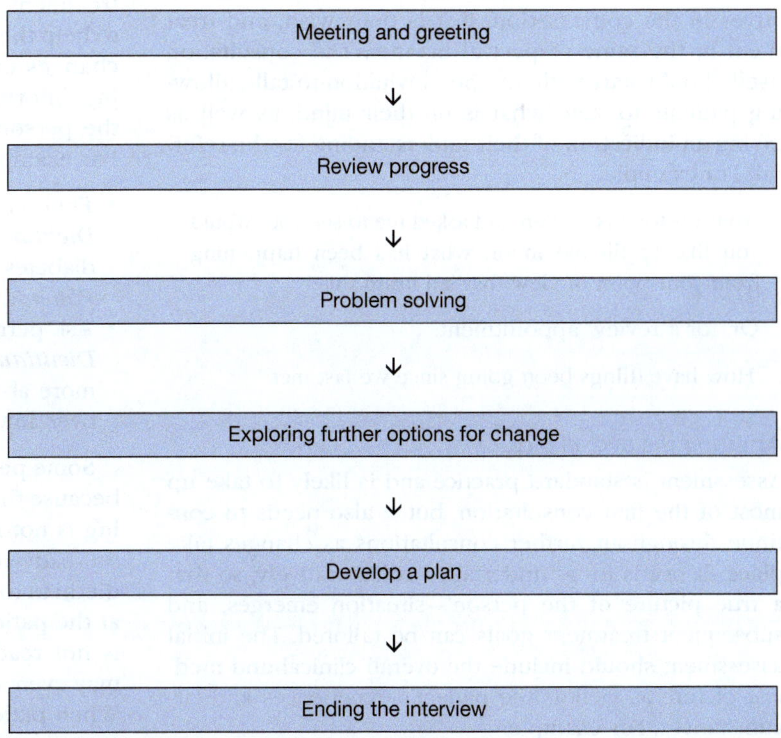

Figure 1.3.2 A suggested framework for a follow-up dietetic consultation

should be used flexibly, with different elements applied interchangeably within each interview, depending on the patient's needs. Not all elements are necessarily included in all interviews. For example, if someone is very ambivalent about making changes, the whole of the first session may involve exploring this. The following text explores how interpersonal skills link to the elements involved in the consultation, and how to manage difficulties. It is important to be aware of one's limitations and to refer on appropriately. Difficulties generally outside a dietitian's expertise include psychiatric or psychological problems, relationship problems, bereavement, stress, social and economic problems, and problems which are more properly the remit of other health professionals such as physiotherapists or speech and language therapists.

Elements of the consultation

The following elements within the dietetic consultation form a highly specific focus within an integrated approach to changing health-related behaviours. These relate to rapport building, assessment and ending the interview as well as specific behaviour change techniques. NICE (2014) specifically identifies the following behaviour change techniques as being effective: goals and planning (agree behavioural and outcome goals, develop action plans and prioritise actions, develop plans for dealing with relapses and consider future goals and plans), feedback and monitoring, and providing input regarding social support. In all cases, the art of practice is to skilfully interweave interpersonal skills with specific elements, but not all of these elements will necessarily be used in each consultation. The skilled practitioner learns to work flexibly.

Meeting and greeting the patient

This is easy to rush in busy clinics, but it is worth taking time to greet patients in a warm and friendly manner. Introductions are important, including checking how the patient wishes to be addressed and stating the amount of time available. It is important to involve patients' relatives in the conversation, if it is their wish, and treat them in the same respectful manner. The consultation itself should start with an open invitation to talk, allowing patients to state what is on their mind, as well as giving an indication of their understanding for the referral. For example:

> 'Your doctor has written and asked me to see you. Would you like to fill me in on what has been happening from your point of view that led up to this?'
>
> Or, for a review appointment:
>
> 'How have things been going since we last met?'

Assessing the overall picture

Assessment is standard practice and is likely to take up most of the first consultation, but it also needs to continue throughout further consultations as changes take place. It needs to be undertaken collaboratively, so that a true picture of the person's situation emerges, and subsequent treatment goals can be tailored. The initial assessment should include the overall clinical and medical picture as well as the patient's experiences and circumstances. For example:

> *Dietitian*: 'Can you tell me a bit about your current situation – family, job, that kind of thing – so that we can see how any dietary or lifestyle changes may fit in...?'
> *Patient*: 'Well, I work part-time...'
> *Dietitian*: (paraphrase/reflect this information)

Try to avoid asking several questions in a row without reflecting back responses. If a series of closed questions needs to be asked, it is less intrusive if permission is asked first, e.g.:

> *Dietitian*: (assessing calcium intake): 'Would it be alright with you if we go through a number of questions, so that we both get a clear picture and don't miss anything important?'
> *Patient*: 'That's fine'.
> *Dietitian*: 'Can you tell me how much milk you take? ... do you eat cheese? ... how often? ... how much? ... what about yogurt?'

Providing information

Pitfalls in a dietetic consultation include:

- Making assumptions about the patient's current levels of knowledge or understanding.
- Interrogating them.
- Imposing information that they do not want or are unable to assimilate at that time. This may increase resistance to change.

Exchange of information needs to be interwoven through every aspect of the consultation. It can either focus on providing information to patients or gathering information about their overall situation. The aim is to assess what patients know about their own condition – biochemistry results, approaches to treatment, etc. – and to offer information based on this to help them in their decision-making regarding making changes or managing their condition better. Exchanging information needs to be patient-centred, so that the person feels free to disclose relevant information. For example:

- Find out what they know (e.g. about their diabetes)
  Dietitian: 'Has your doctor/nurse explained what diabetes is?'
  Patient: 'Yes...' (Sounding unsure).
- Ask permission to give them further information
  Dietitian: 'Would it be helpful if we talked a bit more about that now?' or 'Would you like me to go over any of it again?'

Some people do not want or need information, either because they already know the facts or because the timing is not right. If someone is genuinely not interested or ready to know more, asking permission alerts the dietitian to this and enables the consultation to progress at the patient's pace. Information given when someone is not ready for it can seem like undue pressure and may even stop people from engaging or from returning. When patients agree to receive information, they listen more carefully.

- Provide the information in an objective, neutral manner. Information should relate to current scientific understanding and be given simply and objectively, e.g.:

> 'There is good evidence that losing weight can help lower blood pressure'.

- Try to avoid long, complicated explanations and the use of jargon or technical language. Find out what their interpretation is of the information you give them.
  'What do you think about that?' or 'Does that make sense?'

Motivation

Motivation is affected by many factors and can fluctuate. The amount of importance people attribute to a change, in terms of their overall life, will affect the likelihood of them implementing it, and this should be explored, e.g.:

Dietitian: 'Would you say that making changes to your diet in order to lose weight is a priority for you at the moment?'
Patient: 'Oh, yes, I mean if it will help with my blood pressure…' or 'I'm not sure it will make any difference…'.
Dietitian: (Reflecting the response and continuing to explore) 'You are keen to get your blood pressure down' or 'You can't see much point in making any changes to your diet…'

This is part of establishing a common agenda. It is the responsibility of practitioners to ensure that patients are offered accurate information. This helps to raise awareness in a nonthreatening manner about unhelpful behaviours and their implications. Increasing concern about a behaviour may increase its importance, making change more likely. This can be done by providing information in a helpful way (see the preceding text).

If the change is important for the individuals, the next step is to explore whether they feel confident in their ability to change and to offer support, e.g.:

Dietitian: 'Do you feel able to make some change to your eating at the moment?'
Patient: 'I know I should if it will help with my blood pressure, but I have tried lots of times…'
Dietitian: (Reflecting the response and continuing to explore) 'You have tried lots of times, and are feeling a bit disheartened by that experience?'
Patient: 'Yes'
Dietitian: 'Is there anything that we could we do together that would help?'

It is possible to use scaling questions to explore motivation (e.g.: 'On a scale of 0–10, where 0 is not important/not confident at all and 10 is extremely important/confident, where would you place yourself?') (Mason & Butler, 2010). This approach needs to be used with a high level of good interpersonal skills, and applied sensitively; it should not be used simply as a tick box approach. It can be a helpful way to broadly establish where change sits on the patient's agenda but should not be a rigid assessment tool. Responses should be met with reflective statements rather than judgments.

Eliciting information on current health-related behaviours

A picture of current eating and activity levels can be gained by asking the patient to describe a typical day, e.g.:

Dietitian: 'Can I ask you to describe a fairly typical day, in terms of how food (or activity) fits into that day, starting from when you get up in the morning to the last thing at night?'
Patient: 'Well, the mornings are always a rush…'.
Dietitian: (Follow the person's description with reflective responses and summarise to capture what has been said).

Taking a diet history is another way of gathering detailed information about current diet. It is traditionally the mainstay of dietetic practice, but has pitfalls:

- It involves lots of questions, so can feel interrogative and risks damaging the helping relationship. People who eat for emotional reasons are less likely to disclose this with intensive questioning. They may feel vulnerable, and being under the spotlight can expose this and increase defensiveness.
- All methods of assessing dietary intake, and especially dietary recall, have inaccuracies (see Chapter 2.3, Dietary assessment). People are likely to report what they think the professional wants to hear rather than what they actually do.

Initially, general information about how diet fits in with their overall life (typical day) can be gathered, and further necessary information can be uncovered when options for change are discussed. Self-monitoring (see the following text) is another tool that can be used to gather information about diet; this can be informative and illuminating. Once a supportive alliance is formed, patients are more likely to offer accurate information. By threading the process of exchanging information about dietary intake and activity into different aspects of the interview, patients are less likely to feel they are being judged.

Exploring options for change and help with decision-making

Once someone decides to make changes, it is helpful to explore the possible options. It is initially helpful to identify the change most favoured by the patient, and then assess how realistic this is for them. Focusing on this makes it more likely that the change will be implemented and maintained. However, it may be necessary to concentrate on the option that will have most impact on the immediate health concern (e.g. reducing saturated fat intake when cholesterol level is raised). Generally, the following approach can be helpful:

Dietitian: 'There are a range of possibilities which would help your overall health – changing the types of fat you eat, eating more fruit and vegetables, eating less sugar, etc. – where do you think you would like to start?'

Visual aids are useful, e.g. the Eatwell Guide (see Chapter 2.1, Dietary reference values and food-based dietary guidelines). The recommendations for each food group can be discussed and further information about a person's diet gathered at the same time, e.g.:

Dietitian: 'The recommendations are to eat five portions of fruit and vegetables per day. How does that compare with what you are doing at the moment?'

Negotiating goals and developing a change plan

Setting appropriate behavioural goals is the basis to achieving a successful outcome. These should be negotiated with patients so that they are actively involved in deciding what is realistic. Goals set by practitioners may not take account of other factors in people's lives. Unrealistic goals can set patients up for failure and undermine the confidence of both the patient and the practitioner. Patients should be encouraged to use a stepwise approach to achieve a particular goal.

Goals should ideally fulfil SMART criteria (i.e. be specific, measurable, achievable, relevant and time specific). For example:

- *Specific* – eating less fat might be achieved by spreading fat more thinly on bread.
- *Measurable* – eating five portions of fruit and vegetables each day.
- *Achievable and realistic* – reducing chocolate intake by only consuming one bar each day instead of two.
- *Relevant to the goal of treatment* – if the aim of treatment is to decrease fat intake, patients need to concentrate on eating foods that are low in fat.
- *Time specific* – setting a goal to be achieved within an agreed time frame.

For a goal to make a difference in the time set to achieve it, it needs to be as far reaching as possible. For example, if the main goal is to reduce fat intake, the main dietary source of fat intake needs to be identified and reduced to a level that will make a difference. If fried foods are eaten daily, an appropriate weekly goal may be to use fat-free methods of cooking. This would have a bigger effect than a goal of, say, not eating doughnuts if doughnuts are only consumed once a fortnight. Only two or three specific, realistic and achievable changes should be chosen. Successful negotiation of each of the smaller steps gives people a sense of achievement and helps maintain motivation.

Once a specific goal has been agreed on and the ways of implementing it explored, it is helpful to summarise this in a change plan (an example is shown in Figure 1.3.3). Any change plan should be a starting point which is regularly reviewed and updated in light of what works in practice. Once goals have been established and a change plan agreed on, other strategies can be implemented to support behaviour change, e.g. rewards and support.

Identifying and implementing rewards

Rewarding behaviour change is a way of reinforcing new behaviours and is commonly used in BT. It is important that rewards be contingent on carrying out specific behaviours (as set out in SMART goal setting) rather than abstract outcomes such as weight loss or eating more healthily. Such discussions must be carefully negotiated as patients may find it difficult to identify appropriate rewards or indeed consider that they are worthy of receiving them (often encountered in weight management). Suitable rewards include doing enjoyable leisure time activities and hobbies, being with favourite people, buying small things they want or doing whatever they find relaxing or fun (Holli & Calabrese, 1998). Rewards need to be truly pleasurable (and non-food based). Practitioners should avoid suggesting rewards that would appeal to them personally. People should also be encouraged to mentally congratulate themselves

Name: ____________________ **Date:** ____________

What do I want to achieve overall?

Why is it important to me?

Specific goal (*What* exactly am I going to do?)

Steps to achieve this (*How* am I going to do it?)

What needs to be in place?

What might get in the way?

I will ask for support to help me work towards my goal from:

What will help to reinforce new habit (reward or encouragement)?

How will I keep a record of progress?

When will I review progress?

When will I start?

Figure 1.3.3 Step-by-step guide to making changes

on every effort and achievement, however small, to help build feelings of self-esteem and self-efficacy. Other methods of reinforcing new habits may not necessarily be pleasurable, e.g. asking the family to remind you to go for a walk each evening, but can still be effective.

Building support

The importance of social support from a range of sources cannot be underestimated. In addition to dietitians and other health professionals, support from family members, friends and colleagues can be key. Responsibility for enlisting support from elsewhere lies with the patient, but they may need guidance. Relatives can be included in consultations, and leaflets produced for family members outlining how they can support the patient. The patient may need to clarify the type of support that would be most helpful, e.g.:

> 'I really appreciate your support. It would help me even more if you don't nag me but offer practical support and encourage me – such as helping me with the planning and preparation of meals'.

Other sources of support include self-help groups, books, telephone help lines, websites and social networking platforms. Dietitians can link patients up with these as appropriate.

Self-monitoring/Developing self-awareness

Self-monitoring or diary keeping supports behaviour change. The prime purposes are to increase self-awareness of current behaviours, highlight problem areas and reinforce successes. A willingness to observe behaviour often indicates a willingness to come to terms with it and change it if appropriate.

Self-monitoring can be used in many ways, e.g. to identify:

- Time and place of eating.
- What a person was doing prior to eating.
- With whom eating occurred.
- How the person felt and what they were thinking.
- Symptoms.
- The behavioural outcome.

However, it would not be realistic or appropriate to ask patients to record all these, all the time. Diary keeping should focus on the behaviour currently being targeted, e.g. timing of meals, nutritional content of the diet or portion sizes. It is a difficult skill that needs practice. To be effective, the individuals should know what is expected of them and the purpose of monitoring; they need to agree to do it and be able to use their preferred method, i.e. pre-printed sheets or their own notebook. It should not be used to check up on patients. In order to reinforce that self-monitoring is for the patient's benefit, it is helpful to ask what they have learnt from it. Diaries should be used collaboratively and not simply sent to patients without prior discussion and agreement. Any monitoring needs to be regularly reviewed by the patient, so that they can use it to adapt and update their change plan. Difficulties with self-monitoring may indicate that unresolved motivational issues exist which need to be addressed (see the section 'Managing common difficulties' in the following text).

Ending the interview

This is just as important as a good beginning. Sufficient time is needed to ensure that the main points of the consultation are summarised and that agreements are clear about goals set, monitoring, review and follow-up. The patient should be given the opportunity to ask questions to clarify anything unclear.

Managing common difficulties

Clients who want advice

Patients usually come to see a dietitian recognising that they have expertise in an area. They will often ask, '*what do you think I should do?*' It is important to give information when patients are seeking it (can be an indication of readiness to change), but at the same time drawing on the expertise that patients have about themselves. For example:

> *Dietitian*: 'You would like me to tell you exactly what to eat in order to …?'
> *Patient*: 'Yes, what I need is a diet sheet; that is what I have come for'.
> *Dietitian*: 'It sounds like an eating plan would really help, as well as being clear which foods are best to avoid and which ones to include. I can certainly give you that information, and we can work out what would be the best eating plan for you, together. That way, we can make sure that we include some of the foods you really like and make sure that the plan fits in around your life. How does that sound?'

Referred patients who do not want advice

Sometimes patients feel that they have been sent to the dietitian, rather than choosing to come. Engaging in such a consultation is likely to be met with resistance. It can help to explore their understanding of what led to the referral. It is more helpful to ask '*Can you tell me what led up to your doctor suggesting that you come to see me*' than '*Do you know why this appointment was made?*' It is useful to find out what their thoughts are about the referral – '*I wonder what your thoughts were when the doctor suggested coming to see me?*' – rather than '*How do you feel about coming here?*' Clarify that your role is to explore the situation with them and to consider possible options, but not to tell them what to do. Ask permission to progress on that basis and explain what service you can offer.

Clients who cannot come up with their own solutions

Patients should be given the opportunity to make their own suggestions but not all patients can come up with ideas. It is tempting to jump in with suggestions, but the dietitian's ideas might be inappropriate, and patients may feel under pressure to agree without thinking it through, later finding that they cannot do it in practice. In this situation, it can help to present possible solutions in the context of what has worked for others; options which may or may not work for them. This still leaves a space for them to either take up a particular option or decline it. Always ask permission before making suggestions, e.g. '*Would you like me to tell you about some of the things that have worked for other people?*'

Ambivalence about change and motivational difficulties

Ambivalence about change is normal – patients often feel torn between wanting better health and not wanting to change established habits. Sometimes people get stuck thinking, '*I want to, but I can't*'. The task of the practitioner is to listen out for and reflect back any talk about change, e.g. '*I want to …, I could …, I should …, I need to …*'. This is described as 'change talk' in motivational interviewing, which signals movement towards a commitment to change (Miller & Rollnick, 2013).

A decision not to make a change at the present time is a viable option, as it may be better not to start making changes before the patients are ready. If they have already tried and failed many times, a further half-hearted attempt and failure might reinforce their already low levels of self-esteem. Providing unwanted advice in this situation may be met with resistance. It is important to respect patient autonomy regardless of the decisions made.

Motivation for change can be triggered by helping a person become more aware of the discrepancy between where they are and where they would like to be. But this needs to happen in their own mind (facilitated by a skilled practitioner who highlights the discrepancy between their intentions and their actual behaviours), rather than having it exposed as a product of their inadequacy. For example, instead of '*You need to keep away from the biscuits, you know the effect it has – you need to work on your will power*', a reflective response can be more helpful '*So although you want to lose weight, you are finding it hard to keep away from the biscuits*'.

Importance and confidence

Importance and confidence are key constructs of motivation. Exploring the importance of change can help build motivation by encouraging patients to talk about their reasons for wanting to change. How confident people are about their capacity to make and sustain a change is also key (Miller & Rollnick, 2013). The dietitian can assist by:

- Exploring what worked in the past.
- Encouraging patients to talk about their past and present successes.
- Drawing attention to success in other areas of life.
- Helping to devise a change plan with small, achievable steps.
- Looking for opportunities to support patients' confidence in their ability to change.
- Conveying optimism, e.g. '*It sounds like that would work for you*'.
- Using affirmations, e.g. '*You have made good progress; you must be pleased*'.

Internal and external triggers that get in the way of planned change

A number of feelings, thoughts, beliefs, events and situations can influence the likeliness of behaviours happening (or not happening). As discussed in the preceding text, techniques from BT can help to change the environment to make it more conducive to desired behaviours and less conducive to undesired ones. Such techniques can be implemented at the planning stage (i.e. people may be able to anticipate problems likely to arise) or when particular problems arise. Planning ahead can help draw attention to problems that could be addressed in advance, and also makes revising the plan easier, as they know clearly what they are expecting of themselves. Any changes need to be worked out collaboratively with the patient, rather than presented as solutions from the practitioner's viewpoint, e.g. '*Why don't you…*', '*Do you think you could…*', '*How about…*'.

The following are examples of strategies for modifying external triggers (also called stimulus control techniques) to eating for weight management, but they can be adapted for other conditions:

- Planning meals and shopping in advance so that appropriate foods are available to eat regularly.
- Planning daily eating times in advance.
- Carrying suitable snacks.
- Asking a friend, partner or colleague to change at the same time, or to be encouraging.
- Avoiding tasting when cooking, as this may result in overeating.
- Limiting the opportunities for seeing tempting foods other than at mealtimes, e.g. put things away in cupboards; do not shop when hungry.
- Taking a route home which does not involve passing a tempting food shop/bakery.
- Always making sure there are suitable foods (e.g. fruit and vegetables) available at home to avoid being tempted to eat less suitable foods if hungry.
- Not buying, or only occasionally buying, tempting/calorie-dense foods such as chocolates, cakes and crisps.

Strategies for modifying internal triggers include:

- Asking in response to an urge to eat, '*Am I really hungry?*' Urges to eat (sometimes called cravings) need to be distinguished from hunger. The former are psychological triggers to eating and distinct from physical hunger. Real hunger needs to be responded to but a number of strategies can be learned to help overcome psychological urges. Some people find it helpful to use a hunger score ('*How hungry am I on a scale of 0–10 where 0 is not at all hungry and 10 is extremely hungry*') to check if they are truly hungry. Cravings are sometimes described as waves; they build until they are at their peak, but then break on the shore and fade away within 15–30 minutes (Brownell, 2004). A craving can be withstood by doing something incompatible with eating until it has faded away.

- Making a list of activities that are incompatible with eating (called response substitution, e.g. walking, reading, phoning a friend, cleaning the car, planning a holiday, running, having a relaxing massage or bath, painting or practicing a relaxation exercise). When faced with an urge, patients can choose something from this list.
- Modifying unhelpful thoughts. The way people think can have a huge impact on their subsequent actions. People can be helped to identify unhelpful thoughts and to replace these with more helpful, coping thoughts. As this process can be complex, further training, accompanied by appropriate supervision, is recommended. Referral to specialist practitioners may be necessary.

Steps involved in modifying unhelpful thoughts include:

1. Identifying unhelpful thoughts through diary keeping, e.g. 'What were you thinking at that time?'
2. Generating alternative ways of thinking, and testing out if these alternatives are more helpful in everyday life.

Sometimes mood changes can be due to other worries, e.g. relationship problems, being depressed about one's job or long-term effects of an illness. These may need to be addressed, and it may be necessary to refer the patient for more in-depth counselling/therapy.

Problem solving

Problems can arise at all stages of making change, and need to be addressed. It is important to address any difficulties related to change and to encourage patients to generate solutions to the perceived difficulties themselves. This helps to increase their sense of confidence and competence. There is no one right option; it is a question of experimenting to find what works best for each person. The following steps are key elements of problem solving and can be used at any stage in the intervention:

1. Identify and clearly define the problem.
2. Explore all possible options and weigh up the pros and cons of each.
3. Choose the preferred option/s.
4. Develop a plan.
5. Implement and monitor the plan.
6. Review the plan.

Setbacks

Lapsing from a planned change or a change one has made is normal, but patients frequently see it as a failure (Marlatt & Gordon, 1985). Prevention and management of lapses need to be anticipated and worked with throughout the whole consultation process. Many of the strategies already outlined can help. Lapses often lead to feelings of guilt, which increases susceptibility to other slips and the possibility of complete abandonment of changes and a return to previous patterns.

How a person thinks about a lapse is likely to determine the outcome. It can be helpful to explain the following:

- Lapses are a natural and accepted part of change. Eating an unplanned food is a slip and not a personal failure.
- High-risk situations (ones which present an increased and significant risk of returning to old behaviours) are either triggered by internal states (e.g. anxiety, boredom, anger, loneliness) or external events (e.g. social situations, passing a bakery, smell of food) – or a combination of both. Individuals can learn to cope by identifying their particular high-risk situations and learning how best to manage these.
- Change is an ongoing evolving process, a goal in itself. The process should be the focus rather than perceived failure or success at any given step. Every small change in behaviour along the way in the desired direction is a step forward and a sign of important progress.
- Lapses can be a learning experience.
- Even if patients abandon their change plan for now, all is not lost.

Dietitians can help people to identify what leads to lapses, so that plans can be made in advance to prevent them, rather than just relying on will power. A list of coping strategies can be established which could be accessed when necessary, akin to a first aid plan. The way a person copes after a setback can affect the likelihood of further lapses. The following six steps can be offered to help the person cope during a lapse:

- *Stop*: Go away from the situation to a safe place to think about what has happened.
- *Say*: It is not a catastrophe. One error does not mean the end of the world.
- *Learn*: What was happening before the lapse? Analyse the situation to see why it happened.
- *Plan*: What can be done in the same situation to avert another lapse? Use the preceding information to plan in advance to reduce the risk of it happening again. Decide what can be done immediately to stop the slip spiralling out of control. Put these strategies into practice at once.
- *Be positive*: Has anything really changed? Review personal goals and motivation for change.
- *Ask*: Is there anything that can be done to balance up the slip? For example, do some extra exercise. (It is not recommended that patients skip a subsequent meal as this can trigger overeating.)

Implications for practice

Integrating a behavioural approach to changing health-related behaviours involves using a wide range of skills. Behaviour change interventions have been described as combining art and science (Hunt & Pearson, 2001).

In other words, not only the message but also the way in which it is delivered is important. Dietitians need to ensure that they equip themselves with the necessary skills to integrate a behavioural approach into practice. This includes having appropriate training and clinical supervision and ensuring that this way of working becomes an integral part of CPD. This also has implications for future preregistration training and research.

References

Bandura A. (1977) *Social Learning Theory*. Englewood Cliffs, NJ: Prentice Hall.

Brownell KD. (2004) *The Learn Programme for Weight Management*, 10th edn. Dallas, Texas: American Health Publishing Company.

Contento J, Balch GI, Bronner YL, *et al.* (1995) The effectiveness of nutrition education and implications for nutrition education policy, programs, and research: a review of research. *J. Nutr. Educ.* 27(6): Nov/Dec Special Issue.

Egan G. (2013) *The Skilled Helper. A Problem Management and Opportunity-Development Approach to Helping*, 10th edn. USA: Brooks/Cole Publishing Company.

Funnell MM, Anderson RM. (2003) Patient empowerment: a look back, a look ahead. *Diabetes Educ.* 29: 454–458.

Gable J, Herrmann T. (2016) *Counselling Skills for Dietitians*, 3rd edn. London: Wiley-Blackwell.

Hancock REE, Bonner G, Hollingdale R, et al. (2012) 'If you listen to me properly, I feel good': a qualitative examination of patient experiences of dietetic consultations. *J. Hum. Nutr. Diet.* 25: 275–284.

Holli BB, Calabrese RJ. (1998) *Communication and Education Skills for Dietetics Professionals*. Philadelphia: Williams and Wilkins.

Hunt P, Pearson D. (2001) Motivating change. *Nurs. Stand.* 16: 45–52.

Ivey AE, Gluckstern N, Ivey MB. (1997) *Basic Attending Skills*, 3rd edn. North Amherst, MA: Microtraining Associates.

Kelly MP, Barker M. (2016) Why is changing health-related behaviour so difficult? *Public Health* 136: 109–116.

Marlatt GA, Gordon JR. (1985) *Relapse Prevention: Maintenance Strategies in Addictive Behaviour Change*. New York: Guilford Press.

Mason P, Butler CC. (2010) *Health Behaviour Change: A Guide for Practitioners*, 2nd edn. Edinburgh: Churchill Livingstone: Elsevier.

Michie S, van Stralen MM, West R. (2011) The behaviour change wheel: a new method for characterising and designing behaviour change interventions. *BMC Implement Sci.* 6: 42.

Michie S, Atkins L, *West R*. (2014a) The Behaviour Change Wheel: A Guide to Designing Interventions. Sutton, Surrey: Silverback Publishing.

Michie S, West R, Campbell R, et al. (2014b) *ABC of Behaviour Change Theories*. Silverback Publishing.

Miller WR, Rollnick S. (2013). *Motivational Interviewing. Helping People Change*. New York: Guilford Press.

Najavits LM, Weiss RD. (1994) Variations in therapist effectiveness in the treatment of patients with substance use disorders: an empirical review. *Addiction* 89: 679–688.

NICE. (2014) *Behaviour change: individual approaches (PH49)*. Available at https://www.nice.org.uk/guidance/ph49. Accessed 30 December 2016.

Pearson D. (2010) *Changing Behaviour in Advancing Dietetics and Clinical Nutrition*. Edinburgh: Churchill Livingstone, pp. 17–22.

Pearson D, Grace C. (2012) *Weight Management: A Practitioners Guide*. Oxford: Wiley Blackwell.

Prochaska JO, DiClemente CC. (1986) Towards a comprehensive model of change. In: Miller WR, Healther N (eds) *Treating Addictive Disorders: Processes of Change*. New York: Plenum, pp. 3–27.

Rapoport L. (1998) Integrating cognitive behavioural therapy into dietetic practice: a challenge for dietitians. *J. Hum. Nutr. Diet.* 11: 227–237.

Rapoport L, Nicholson Perry K. (2000) Do dietitians feel that they have had adequate training in behaviour change methods? *J. Hum. Nutr. Diet.* 13: 287–298.

Rogers CR. (1951) *Client-Centered Therapy*. Boston: Houghton Mifflin.

Rollnick S, Healther N, Bell A. (1992) Negotiating behaviour change in medical settings: the development of brief motivational interviewing. *J. Ment. Health.* 1: 25–37.

Rollnick S, Butler C, Kinnersley P, et al. (2010) Motivational interviewing. *BMJ* 340: 1900.

Stewart M. (1995) Effective physician–patient communication and health outcomes: a review. *CMAJ* 152: 1423–1433.

Stewart M, Brown JB, Donner A, *et al.* (2000) The impact of patient-centered care on outcomes. *J. Fam. Pract.* 49: 796–804.

Stewart M, Ryan BL, Bodea C. (2011) Is patient-centred care associated with lower diagnostic costs? *Health. Policy* 6(4): 27–31.

Stewart M, Brown JB, Weston WW, et al. (2014) *Patient-Centred Medicine. Transforming the Clinical Method*, 3rd edn. London: Radcliffe Publishing Ltd.

Whitehead K, Langley-Evans SC, Tischler V, *et al.* (2009) Communication skills for behaviour change in dietetic consultations. *J. Hum. Nutr. Diet.* 22: 493–500.

Whitehead KA, Langley-Evans SC, Tischler VA, *et al.* (2014) Assessing communication skills in dietetic consultations: the development of the reliable and valid DIET-COMMS tool. *J. Hum. Nutr. Diet.* 27(2): 321–332.

SECTION 2

Nutritional status

2.1 Dietary reference values and food-based dietary guidelines

Joan Gandy

SECTION 2

Key points

- Dietary reference values (DRVs) are estimates of the nutritional requirements of a particular population and assume that requirements are normally distributed.
- DRVs are devised for healthy populations and may not be applicable in some clinical situations.
- Dietitians should understand the guiding principles of establishing DRVs and their limitations.
- Food-based dietary guidelines (FBDGs) present recommendations in a user-friendly manner for the general public.

Dietary reference values (DRVs) are established within a population as a measure of nutritional adequacy. As such, they are aimed at preventing deficiencies rather than preventing nutrition-related diseases. They have many uses, including forming the basis of food labelling (see Chapter 4.5, Food law and labelling), food-based dietary guidelines (FBDGs), such as the Eatwell Guide, and dietary recommendations that are aimed at optimising health and preventing disease related to over- and undernutrition.

The first DRVs were devised in the late nineteenth century, and international values were established by the League of Nations (the forerunner of the United Nations) in 1936–1938 to prevent deficiencies in population groups (Beaton, 1991). Many countries have their own values, and international values have been published by the Food and Agriculture Organization of the United Nations (FAO), World Health Organization (WHO) and United Nations University (UNU). In Europe, the European Food Safety Agency (EFSA) has published scientific opinions on DRVs for water, carbohydrates, fats, fibre, energy, proteins and micronutrients (EFSA, 2017).

In a separate initiative, the European Commission funded the EURopean micronutrient RECommendations Aligned (EURRECA) project to harmonise micronutrient recommendations across Europe. This project included scientists from 17 countries and aimed to deliver an aligned set of standards that provided a robust scientific basis for establishing micronutrient requirements and for devising micronutrient recommendations. It focused on the needs of specific vulnerable groups, e.g. infants, children and adolescents, adults, pregnant and lactating women, the elderly, people with low income and immigrants. In addition, EURRECA evaluated the impact of socioeconomic status, ethnic origin, inter-individual variability and vulnerability due to genetics, environmental factors and epigenetic phenomena on dietary requirements. A full list of publications is available at http://ilsi.eu/eurreca.

In the UK, the Department of Health (DH) Committee on Medical Aspects of Food Policy (COMA) revised DRVs for all nutrients in 1991 (DH, 1991). Since then, the Scientific Advisory Committee on Nutrition (SACN) have revised the recommendations for energy (SACN, 2011), vitamin D (SACN, 2016) and carbohydrates (SACN, 2015). The committee have also reviewed the recommendations for iron, but, due to lack of convincing evidence, the DRVs were not changed (SACN, 2010). A methodological framework for the review of nutrient references intakes was published by the DH in 2015. Public Health England (PHE) (2017) have produced a summary of the UK government's dietary recommendations for energy and nutrients.

Development of dietary reference values (DRVs)

DRVs are developed by an expert group, e.g. WHO, by reviewing the evidence; DRVs are then derived by the expert group for the specific population of a country or a group of countries. The values are based on the assumption that individual requirements for a nutrient within a population or group are normally distributed, and that 95% of the population will have requirements within two standard deviations of the mean (DH, 1991). They assume that the individuals are healthy, and also

Manual of Dietetic Practice, Sixth Edition. Edited by Joan Gandy.

Companion website: www.manualofdieteticpractice.com

Table 2.1.1 Definitions of dietary reference values

Definitions used in the UK (DH, 1991)	
Recommended daily amount (RDA)	Average amount of the nutrient that should be provided per head in a group of people if the needs of practically all members of the group are to be met
Recommended intakes	Amounts sufficient, or more than sufficient, for the nutritional needs of practically all healthy persons in a population; intake emphasises that the recommendations relate to food actually eaten
Requirement	The amount of a nutrient that needs to be consumed in order to maintain normal nutritional status
Estimated average requirement (EAR)	The mean requirement of a nutrient for a population or group of people; on average, 50% will consume more than the EAR, and 50% will consume less than the EAR
Lower reference nutrient intake (LRNI)	The level at which approximately 2.5% of the population or group will have an adequate intake; it will not be enough for most people; individuals with this intake may be meeting their requirement, but it is highly probable that they are not
Reference nutrient intake (RNI)	At this level, intake will be adequate for 97.5% of the group or population; it is possible that the intake of individuals at this level will not meet their requirement, but it is highly improbable
Safe level	This is given when insufficient information is available to derive requirements; it is an average requirement plus 20%, and is believed to be adequate for most people's needs; the panel judged that there is no risk of deficiency at this level, and that there is no risk of undesirable effects above this level
Other values used for dietary reference values (DRVs)	
Protective nutrient intake (PNI)	Amount > RNI for some micronutrients that may be protective against a specified health or nutritional risk of public health relevance; PNI are expressed as daily value or an amount to be consumed with a meal
Upper tolerable nutrient intake level (upper limit, UL)	The maximum intake of some micronutrients that is unlikely to pose risk of adverse health effects in almost all (97.5%) apparently healthy individuals in a gender- and age-specific population
Recommended dietary allowance (RDA)	Average daily dietary intake that meets the requirements of nearly all (97–98%) healthy persons
Adequate intake (AI)	Established for a nutrient when available data are insufficient to estimate an intake that would maintain adequacy; the AI is based on observed intakes by a group of healthy persons
Estimated energy requirement (EER)	The average dietary energy intake that is predicted to maintain energy balance in a healthy adult of a defined age, gender, weight, height and level of physical activity consistent with good health
Dietary reference intake (DRI)	A term used in the USA and Canada to broaden the use of RDAs, particularly in food labelling and fortification
Daily value (DV)	These were developed by the US Food and Drug Administration to help consumers compare the nutrient contents among products within the context of a total daily diet

consider their gender, age, growth and physiological status, i.e. pregnancy and lactation. Guiding principles for the development of recommendations for micronutrients have been established by EURRECA (van't Veer *et al.*, 2012). Table 2.1.1 gives the definitions of the DRVs used in the UK and by other expert groups, such as WHO and the Institute of Medicine (USA).

Limitations

While DRVs are useful, they are open to misuse, and the inherent problems associated with developing recommendations for an entire population should be considered. It is assumed that nutrient requirements are normally distributed for a population; however, the data may be skewed, or sufficient data may not be available to establish normality. Robust data are required for the expert group to evaluate requirements; these data may be derived from tissue levels, balance studies, body pool size, amount required to prevent symptoms of deficiency, or a measure of function of the nutrient. However, these data are not always available. When there is insufficient data, the expert group will recommend a safe level or adequate intake (AI) rather than a recommended intake value. It is important to remember that DRVs are recommended for healthy populations, and that many factors may affect dietary requirements, as shown in Table 2.1.2.

In particular, it is important to consider bioavailability; while the majority of macronutrient intake is absorbed, the absorption of micronutrients is more variable. This is recognised to an extent in DRVs, e.g. DRVs for iron are calculated to reflect the fact that only 15% of dietary iron is absorbed. However, they cannot take into account other factors that affect bioavailability, such as the amount consumed, body stores, presence or absence of other nutrients or dietary constituents, form of the nutrient (e.g. haem or non-haem iron) and the food source from which it is derived (Hurrell & Egli, 2010). These factors may have considerable impact on the adequacy of dietary intake.

Reference values are devised to cover the requirements of the majority of a population, and therefore will overestimate the needs of a significant part of that population. It is important to remember that DRVs

Table 2.1.2 Factors affecting dietary requirements

Factor	Example
Metabolic requirements	Age, gender, body size
	Lifestyle (smoking, obesity, physical activity, etc.)
	Disease, e.g. fever, catabolism
	Trauma
	Growth
	Pregnancy and lactation
Bioavailability	Malabsorption or altered absorption, e.g. milk calcium is better absorbed than non-milk calcium
	Reduced utilisation
	Increased losses, e.g. diarrhoea, burns, renal disease
	Environment, e.g. heating of nutrients
	Drugs, e.g. diuretics
	Dietary concentration
	Dietary interactions
	Drug–nutrient interactions

reflect the needs of healthy people and may not be appropriate in many clinical circumstances. While they are a useful basis to calculate individual needs, they cannot be used alone, and other factors, including those shown in Table 2.1.1, must be considered. This is discussed further in Chapter 6.1 (Nutritional requirements in clinical practice).

Uses of dietary reference values

They should be used with caution in the dietary assessment of individuals as it must be remembered that DRVs are based on populations and groups, and the nutritional needs of individuals within that group or population, as well as the factors discussed earlier, will vary. Within a population, the nutritional requirements of individuals form a continuum, and where a particular individual lies on that continuum will be unknown. It is therefore impossible to determine whether an individual's needs are being met on the basis of a DRV. It is only possible to assess the degree of probability that an individual's needs will or will not have been met. If the estimated average requirement (EAR) for a nutrient is being consumed, there is an approximately 50% chance that needs will be met. If intake is at or above the reference nutrient intake (RNI), it is highly likely that needs are being met (and probably exceeded). If intake is below the lower RNI (LRNI), it is highly unlikely that sufficient is being consumed, unless that person is part of the 2.5% of the population with unusually low requirements.

The diet of groups or populations may be assessed by comparison with DRVs; however, it is important that the group or population be comparable to that for which the recommendations are derived. DRVs are also used for the development of diets for groups of people, e.g. prisoners, and the provision of supplies, e.g. school meals. Nutrient reference values are also used in food labelling (see Chapter 4.5, Food law and labelling), fortification and formulation.

UK dietary reference values for specific nutrients

DRVs have been set for many nutrients, but not all have an EAR, RNI and LRNI. It is clearly inappropriate to set an RNI (covering the needs of 97.5% of the population) for energy, because such an amount would far exceed the needs of most people and, if consumed, would lead to weight gain and associated health problems. The DRV for energy is therefore only set as an EAR. Similarly, the DRVs for the main energy-yielding nutrients (such as fat, carbohydrate and starch) are also expressed in terms of average needs. In addition, recommendations for free sugars are given in weights.

Energy

EARs for energy are based on regression analyses of the measured basal metabolic rate (BMR) against gender, age and weight. The analyses have been used to generate prediction equations. Numerous equations are available, and they should ideally be population specific. In 1991, DH used the equations of Schofield *et al.* (1985), but SACN in 2010 recommended the use of Henry's (2005) equations for this purpose. Energy prediction equations are discussed further in Chapter 6.1 (Nutritional requirements in clinical practice). Increments are also added for the last trimester of pregnancy and for lactation. As energy requirement is given as an average, 50% of a population will need more than the EAR, and 50% less.

In healthy populations, the total daily energy expenditure (TEE) is traditionally calculated by the factorial method, where BMR is multiplied by a physical activity level (PAL), e.g. a sedentary 40-year-old man, weighing 90 kg, with a PAL of 1.4, and BMR (as derived from prediction equations) of 7.97 MJ (1880 kcal), would have a

TEE of 11.16 MJ (2665 kcal). In their report on DRVs for energy, SACN (2011) do not recommend this approach, but recognise that no viable alternative is currently available. In 1991, the DH defined the following PALs:

1.4 – inactive men and women
1.6 – moderately active women
1.7 – moderately active men
1.8 – highly active women
1.9 – highly active men

The methodology for deriving the current UK dietary recommendations for energy is described in more detail by Millward (2012).

Protein

DRVs for protein (EAR and RNI) are based on estimates of the amount needed to maintain nitrogen balance, with an allowance for the fact that only about 70% of the protein consumed is incorporated into the body tissue. Incremental amounts are added to these figures for pregnancy and lactation. It is recommended that protein intakes not exceed twice the RNI. The DRVs for protein assume that energy requirements are met, as protein will be used preferentially for energy when the body is in negative energy balance. The DRVs also assume that the protein is of high biological value.

Fat and carbohydrate

These nutrients cannot be given EARs or RNIs as there is no absolute requirement for them (other than for small quantities of essential fatty acids), and they do not cause specific signs or symptoms of deficiency or toxicity. However, it is recognised that the proportion of fat and carbohydrate in the diet has important health implications; therefore, values are given as the percentage of total food energy they should provide. It is assumed that 5% of energy intake is from alcohol, and values are expressed as percentage of food-only energy. These figures are recommended averages for populations, and are not necessarily appropriate for all individuals (see Chapter 4.2, Public health nutrition).

In 2008, SACN (2008) endorsed the recommendations that total dietary fat should be <35% of food energy, with saturated fat not exceeding 11% of food energy. Trans fatty acids should be less than 1.2% of food energy intake. The recommendations for carbohydrate were reviewed in 2016, and SACN recommended that the recommendation for intake of starchy carbohydrate, wholegrain where possible, should be maintained at 50% dietary energy. Free sugars should, on average, not exceed 5% of daily dietary energy intake, i.e.:

- 19 g (5 sugar cubes or 3–5 teaspoons) for children aged 4–6 years.
- 24 g (6 sugar cubes or 4–6 teaspoons) for children aged 7–10 years.
- 30 g (7 sugar cubes or 5–7 teaspoons) for children aged 11 years and older, and for adults.

Dietary fibre

By definition, dietary fibre is not a nutrient, and therefore no specific requirement exists, although its importance in the diet is unequivocal. However, as there is debate regarding the terminology, analysis and physiological significance of what is a heterogeneous group of compounds, recommendations regarding fibre intake are difficult to formulate. In the DH (1991) report, the DRV for a specifically defined form of dietary fibre, non-starch polysaccharide (NSP), as analysed by the Englyst and Cummings method, was expressed as a recommended average intake for the adult population (18 g/day). For individuals, the recommended minimum (12 g/day) and maximum (24 g/day) intakes of NSP were also given. However, it should be noted that these recommended intake figures are not comparable with the dietary fibre declared on many food labels (see Chapter 4.5, Food law and labelling). These are now usually derived from the Association of Official Analytical Chemists (AOAC) method of analysis, which measures a range of components in addition to NSP, and results in figures that are about 30% higher than those obtained by the Englyst and Cummings method.

In the 2016 review, SACN recommended a new definition of fibre, as one which '*… encompasses all carbohydrates that are naturally integrated components of foods and that are neither digested nor absorbed in the small intestine and have a degree of polymerisation of three or more monomeric units, plus lignin*'. This replaces the term NSP. In addition, they recommended that the AOAC method should be used for the chemical determination of fibre. The revised recommendations for fibre intake are:

- 15 g for children aged 2–5 years.
- 20 g for children aged 5–11 years.
- 25 g for children 11–15 years.
- 30 g for those aged 16 years and older, and for adults.

Micronutrients

For most vitamins and minerals, DRVs are given as the EAR, RNI and LRNI. Insufficient information was available for establishing the distribution of requirement for pantothenic acid, biotin, vitamin E, vitamin K, manganese, molybdenum, chromium and fluoride, and guidance only on safe intakes is given. In 2003, in response to concerns regarding supplemental intakes of some micronutrients, the Food Standards Agency's Expert Group on Vitamins and Minerals (EGVM) has reviewed the available evidence on the safety of 31 vitamins and minerals, and has made recommendations on the safe upper levels of their consumption (EGVM, 2003). EFSA (2017) have recently published an overview of tolerable safe upper intake levels.

In 2003, SACN reviewed the evidence on the role of sodium in cardiovascular disease, and made recommendations on salt, as opposed to sodium, intake. The recommended intake of salt in adults should be <6 g/day (see Chapter 4.2, Public health nutrition). More recently, SACN (2015) reviewed the recommendations for vitamin D and health. The recommended daily vitamin intake for adults and children over 1 year of age is 10 μg/day. As a precaution, babies aged less than 1 year should have an intake of 8.5 μg/day. PHE (2016) have gone on to recommend that supplements be taken universally to achieve these intakes in autumn and winter when the skin's ability to absorb sunlight and endogenously produce vitamin D is reduced. Groups at high risk of deficiency, i.e. those with little or no exposure to the sun or who have dark skin, are advised to take supplements throughout the year.

Food based dietary guidelines

Food based dietary guidelines (FBDGs) are designed to give simple messages to help the general public eat healthily. They are based on DRVs, but are presented as foods, making them more understandable and applicable to the population than nutrient-based recommendations. They should be designed to be appropriate to each population group, i.e. country, age and/ culturally specific. The WHO (2003) has summarised FBDG as '*the expression of the principles of nutrition education mostly as foods intended for use by individual members of the general public, and if not expressed entirely as foods, written in language that avoids, as far as possible, the technical terms of nutritional science*'.

Development of food based dietary guidelines

In 1996, the FAO/WHO produced guidelines on the production of FBDG that are still valid. These were summarised by EFSA (2007) as a seven-step process:

1. Identification of diet–health relationships.
2. Identification of country-specific diet-related problems.
3. Identification of nutrients of public health importance.
4. Identification of foods relevant for FBDG.
5. Identification of food consumption patterns.
6. Testing and optimising FBDG.
7. Graphical representation of FBDG.

It cannot be stressed enough that, to be effective, FBDG must be specific to the population they are aimed at. Examples of country-specific FBDG can be found in a report from EUFIC (2009).

The Eatwell Guide – UK

The Eatwell Guide (Figure 2.1.1) is the UK's FBDG, and was produced in 2016; it was an update of the Eatwell plate, originally produced in 1996 by Hunt and colleagues. Detailed information on healthy eating, as well as on the development of the Eatwell Guide, can be found on this NHS website: https://www.nhs.uk/live-well/eat-well/the-eatwell-guide/. It is applicable to almost everyone above 2 years of age in the UK, including minority ethnic groups and vegetarians. It is based on five food groups:

- Potatoes, bread, rice, pasta and other starchy carbohydrates.
- Fruit and vegetables.
- Beans, pulses, fish, eggs, meat and other proteins.
- Dairy and alternatives.
- Oil and spreads.

The following information is taken from the guide:

- Choose wholegrain or higher-fibre versions with less added fat, salt and sugar.
- Eat at least five portions of a variety of fruit and vegetables every day.
- Eat more beans and pulses, two portions of sustainably sourced fish per week, one of which is oily. Eat less red and processed meat.
- Choose lower fat and lower sugar dairy and alternatives.
- Eat less foods that are high in fat, sugar and salt, i.e. cakes, sweets, chocolate, crisps, etc.
- Check the label on packaged foods; choose foods lower in fat, salt and sugars.
- Drink plenty of fluids, i.e. >6–8 glasses of fluids per day, including water, low-fat milk and sugar-free drinks and tea coffee. Limit fruit juice and/or smoothies to <150 mL/day.

Unlike the UK, some countries also incorporate physical activity into their FBDG, e.g. Switzerland.

Conclusions

DRVs are generally based on the best evidence available at the time of publication, and should therefore be constantly reviewed. There is a paucity of evidence for some nutrients, and the requirements for optimal health are continuously being researched; therefore, it is important to use DRVs as reference points rather than definite, set values. It is essential that dietitians understand the guiding principles used in the derivation of DRVs, as well as their limitations and applications. The DRVs in the UK and other countries are revised periodically, and further details can be found on the relevant websites. FBDGs translate DRVs into easily understandable messages about healthy eating that are based on foods rather than nutrients. These must be population specific to be effective; they require full evaluation and regular revision. The UK's Eatwell Guide forms the basis of many, if not most, dietetic interventions.

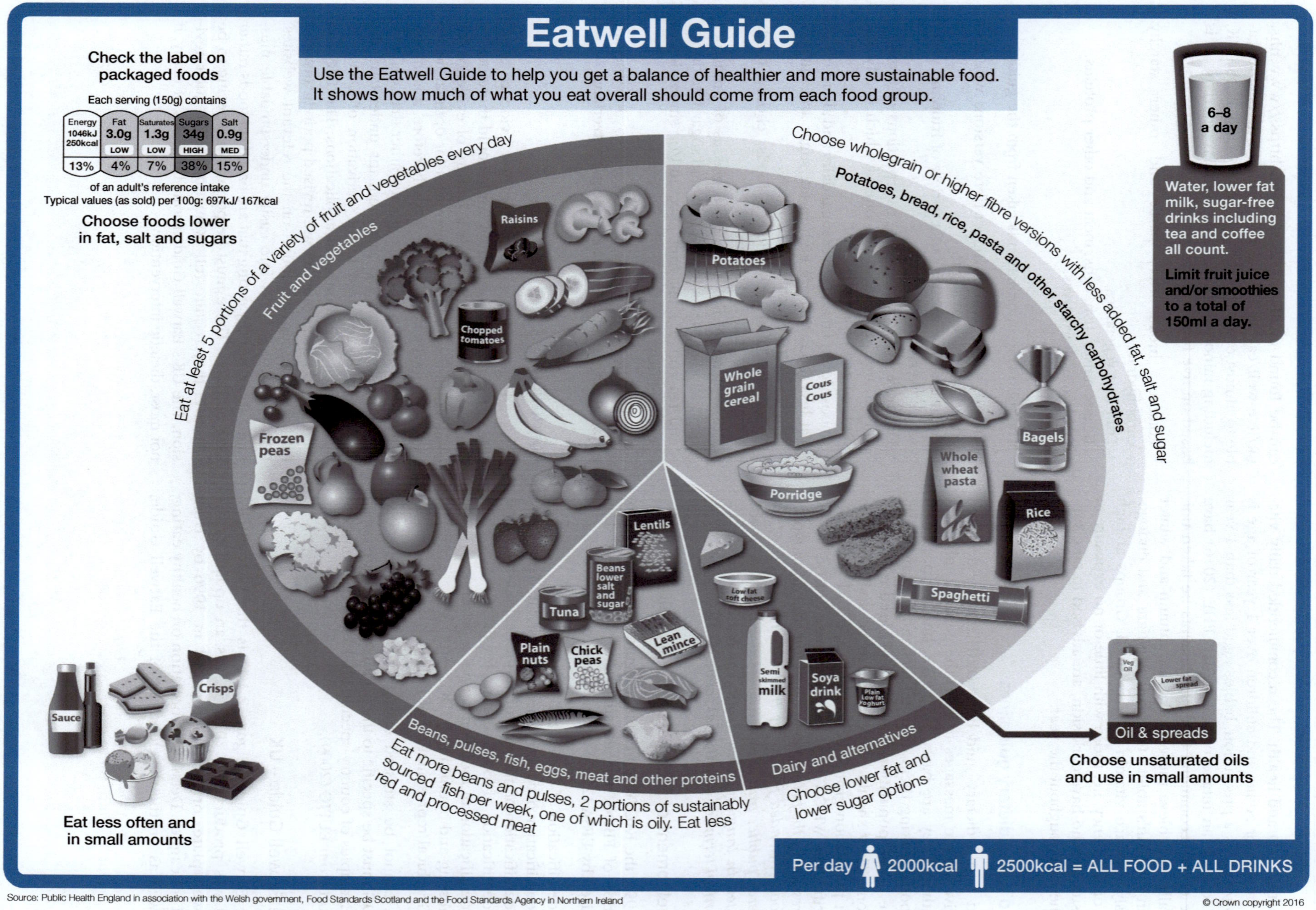

Figure 2.1.1 The Eatwell Guide (source: Public Health England in association with the Welsh government, Food Standards Scotland, and the Food Standards Agency in Northern Ireland. Reproduced with permission.)

Further reading

Food and Agriculture Organization of the United Nations (FAO). (1991) *Nutrient Requirements*. Available at www.fao.org/docrep/u5900t/u5900t00.htm.

Institute of Medicine (Food and Nutrition Board). (2000) *Dietary Reference Intakes: Applications in Dietary Assessment*. Available at www.nap.edu.

Institute of Medicine (Food and Nutrition Board). (2003) *Dietary Reference Intakes: Guiding Principles for Nutrition Labeling and Fortification*. Available at www.nap.edu.

Institute of Medicine (Food and Nutrition Board). (2003) *Dietary Reference Intakes: Applications in Dietary Planning*. Available at www.nap.edu.

Internet resources

UK

Public Health England: The Eatwell Guide, https://www.gov.uk/government/publications/the-eatwell-guide

Scientific Advisory Committee on Nutrition, https://www.gov.uk/government/groups/scientific-advisory-committee-on-nutrition

Europe

European Food Information Council, www.eufic.org/en

European Food Safety Authority, www.efsa.europa.eu

EURopean micronutrient REcommendations Aligned, www.eurreca.org

USA

Institute of Medicine (USA),

US Department of Agriculture: Dietary Reference Intakes, https://www.nal.usda.gov/fnic/dietary-reference-intakes

Australia and New Zealand

National Health and Medical Research Council, www.nhmrc.gov.au/guidelines/publications/n35-n36-n37

International

Food and Agriculture Organization of the United Nations (FAO), www.fao.org

World Health Organization, www.who.int

References

Beaton GH. (1991) *Derivation, Interpretation and Application in Evolutionary Perspective*. Rome: FAO. Available at www.fao.org/docrep/u5900t/u5900t00.htm. Accessed 15 January 2013.

DH. (1991) *Dietary Reference Values for Food Energy and Nutrients for the United Kingdom. Report of the Panel on Dietary Reference Values of the Committee on Medical Aspects of Food Policy. Report on Health and Social Subjects 41*. London: HMSO.

EFSA. (2007) *Development of Food-based Dietary Guidelines. EFSA Scientific Colloquium No 5 Summary Report*. Parma, Italy: EFSA.

EFSA. (2017) *Overview on Tolerable Upper Intake Levels as derived by the Scientific Committee on Food (SCF) and the EFSA Panel on Dietetic Products, Nutrition and Allergies (NDA)*. Available at www.efsa.europa.eu/sites/default/files/assets/UL_Summary_tables.pdf Accessed 22 September 2017.

EUFIC. (2009) *Food-based dietary guidelines in Europe*. Available at www.eufic.org/en/healthy-living/article/food-based-dietary-guidelines-in-europe. Accessed 22 September 2017.

Expert Group on Vitamins and Minerals (EGVM). (2003) *Safe Upper Levels for Vitamins and Minerals*. London: Food Standards Agency. Available at https://cot.food.gov.uk/sites/default/files/vitmin2003.pdf. Accessed 19 September.

Food and Agricultural Organization, World Health Organization (FAO/WHO). (1996) *Preparation and use of Food-Based Dietary Guidelines. Report of a joint FAO/WHO consultation*. Nicosia, Cyprus: WHO. Available at www.fao.org/docrep/X0243E/x0243e00.htm. Accessed 22 September 2017.

Henry CJ. (2005) Basal metabolic rate studies in humans: measurement and development of new equations. *Public Health Nutr.* 8: 1133–1152.

Hunt P, Rayner M. Gatenby S. (1995) A national food guide for the UK? Background and development. *J. Hum. Nutr. Diet.* 8: 315–322.

Hurrell R, Egli I. (2010) Iron bioavailability and dietary reference values. *Am. J. Clin. Nutr.* 91: 1461S–1467S.

Millward DJ. (2012) A new approach to establishing dietary energy reference values. *Curr. Opin. Clin. Nutr. Metab. Care*. 15: 413–417.

PHE. (2016) *A summary of the UK Government's dietary recommendations for energy and nutrients*. Available at https://assets.publishing.service.gov.uk/government/uploads/system/uploads/attachment_data/file/618167/government_dietary_recommendations.pdf Accessed 8 February 2019.

SACN. (2003) *Salt and Health*. Avaialble at https://assets.publishing.service.gov.uk/government/uploads/system/uploads/attachment_data/file/338782/SACN_Salt_and_Health_report.pdf Accessed 8 February 2019.

SACN. (2008) *The Nutritional Well-being of the British Population*. Available at https://webarchive.nationalarchives.gov.uk/20090108192101/http://www.sacn.gov.uk/pdfs/nutritional_health_of_the_population_final_oct_08.pdf Accessed 8 February 2019.

SACN. (2010) Iron and health. Available at https://assets.publishing.service.gov.uk/government/uploads/system/uploads/attachment_data/file/339309/SACN_Iron_and_Health_Report.pdf. Accessed 19 September 2018.

SACN. (2011) *Dietary Reference Values for Energy*. Available at https://assets.publishing.service.gov.uk/government/uploads/system/uploads/attachment_data/file/339317/SACN_Dietary_Reference_Values_for_Energy.pdf Accessed 8 February 2019.

SACN. (2015) Carbohydrates and health. Available at https://assets.publishing.service.gov.uk/government/uploads/system/uploads/attachment_data/file/445503/SACN_Carbohydrates_and_Health.pdf. Accessed 19 September 2018.

SACN. (2016) Vitamin D and health. Available at https://assets.publishing.service.gov.uk/government/uploads/system/uploads/attachment_data/file/537616/SACN_Vitamin_D_and_Health_report.pdf. Accessed 19 September 2018.

Schofield WN, Schofield C, James WPT. (1985) BMR – review and prediction. *Hum. Nutr. Clin. Nutr.* 39(Suppl. 1): 1–96.

van't Veer P, Hesekerb H, Grammatikakic E, *et al.* (2013) EURRECA/WHO Workshop Report: deriving micronutrient recommendations: updating best practices. *Ann. Nutr. Metab.* 62: 63–67.

World Health Organization European Region (WHO). (2003) *Food Based Dietary Guidelines in the WHO European Region*. Copenhagen: WHO, Europe.

2.2 Assessment of nutritional status

Angela Madden and Richard Hoffman

SECTION 2

Key points

- Assessment of nutritional status is fundamental to dietetic practice; it is a detailed, specific and in-depth evaluation undertaken by a trained and competent health professional.
- Nutrition assessment considers many different aspects which vary depending on the individual assessed, and single measures should not be evaluated in isolation.
- Tools for nutritional assessment can be simple (e.g. visual assessment) or more complex (e.g. anthropometry), but, to be effective, require correct techniques and critical evaluation of the findings that are relevant to the context in which they are used.
- Nutritional assessment is an ongoing process that is essential for monitoring nutritional status and for planning and evaluating dietetic interventions.

A multidisciplinary approach to nutritional assessment is important to ensure that timely and effective intervention can be planned. Nutritional status can be assessed in both populations and individuals. This chapter describes the process in individual adults, with specific focus on the process and interpretation of data, and Chapter 3.8.2, Growth, nutritional assessment and nutritional requirements provides details of assessment in children. The assessment process evaluates a number of aspects, e.g. physical and dietary assessments, and is used in a variety of settings, e.g. clinical, sport and research. A desirable nutritional status can be described as when the patients' dietary intake meets or exceeds their needs, keeping their body composition and function within the normal range for healthy individuals (Jeejeebhoy *et al.*, 1990).

The assessment of nutritional status is a comprehensive and detailed procedure that should be conducted by highly trained and experienced professionals with expertise in both gathering and interpreting relevant data. As such, it should be a fundamental part of dietetic practice. The BDA (2016) defines *assessment* as *'a systematic process of collecting and interpreting information in order to make decisions about the nature and cause of nutrition-related health issues that affect an individual, a group or a population'*. Assessment is the first step in the Process for Nutrition and Dietetic Practice (Chapter 1.1, Professional practice), but also contributes to the stages of monitoring, review and evaluation that follow.

It is important not to confuse nutritional assessment with nutritional screening. Nutritional screening is a simple procedure that uses tools designed and validated for use by all healthcare professionals (HCPs), specifically to identify individuals at risk of malnutrition (over- and undernutrition), e.g. 'MUST' (BAPEN, 2012) (Chapter 6.2, Malnutrition). Individuals identified as being at risk of malnutrition may then be referred to dietitians, according to local or national guidelines, who are trained and experienced in the full range of nutritional assessment techniques.

Nutritional assessment should be structured, standardised and focussed on the service user and, therefore, it usually follows the ABCDEF format:

- Anthropometry, body composition.
- Biochemical, haematological tests.
- Clinical, physical.
- Dietary.
- Environmental, behavioural and social.
- Functional.

Finally, patient-centred nutrition-related goals should be planned.

Table 2.2.1 gives examples of what may be assessed in each aspect. The tools used and information collected in the assessment will vary depending on the practice setting, i.e. individual, group, community or population. While defining these aspects provides a useful structure for undertaking nutritional assessment, it is important to realise that these do not stand independently, and that factors interrelate, so maintaining a holistic and whole-patient-centred view is important.

An individual's clinical status has the potential to affect nutritional status in many ways (Table 2.2.2). Acute or chronic illness, injury, surgery and other treatment can have considerable impact on nutritional status, both

Manual of Dietetic Practice, Sixth Edition. Edited by Joan Gandy.

Companion website: www.manualofdieteticpractice.com

Table 2.2.1 Aspects of nutritional assessment

Aspects	Example procedure
Anthropometry and body composition	Weight, height, body mass index, skinfold thickness, mid-upper arm and waist circumference Bioelectrical impedance analysis
Biochemical and haematological	C-reactive protein Iron status – haemoglobin, ferritin, etc. Hydration status and electrolytes
Clinical	Physical appearance, blood pressure, medication, indirect calorimetry
Dietary	24-hour recall Food frequency questionnaires
Environmental, behavioural and social	Shopping habits, housing, cooking facilities, education
Functional	Handgrip strength dynamometry Walking speed Timed sit-to-stand tests

Table 2.2.2 Examples of the effects of illness, injury and surgery on nutritional status

Increased nutrient requirements	Increased nutrient losses	Impaired nutrient ingestion, digestion and/or absorption
The metabolic response to trauma or surgery The metabolic costs of repairing tissue damage, e.g. wounds, pressure ulcers Sepsis or infection Certain conditions, e.g. cystic fibrosis, liver cirrhosis	Vomiting Diarrhoea Renal excretion Surgical drains Bleeding Wound or fistula exudates Dermal or other surface losses	Lack of appetite Lack of digestive enzymes, e.g. pancreatitis Loss of absorptive surfaces, e.g. resection of any part of the gastrointestinal (GI) tract, e.g. coeliac disease Effects of treatments on GI tract, e.g. radiotherapy Effects and symptoms of other conditions on food intake, e.g. dysphagia, breathlessness Difficulty self-feeding, chewing or maintaining food in the mouth

directly (due to the effects of the disease or injury itself) and indirectly (via possible effects on food intake). These effects may result in increased nutritional requirements, increased nutrient losses and/or impaired nutrient ingestion, digestion and/or absorption. Drug therapy may further affect nutrient intake, absorption, metabolism and excretion (Chapter 5.3, Medicines management). Each chapter in Section 7 details assessment of nutritional status in specific conditions.

Anthropometry and body composition

Anthropometry is one of the most frequently used assessment methods, with weight and height forming basic, but still useful, assessments. Accurate measurement of body composition is more complex, especially in the presence of illness or disease, and traditionally has been confined to the research setting. However, with developing technology and increasing availability of the necessary equipment, e.g. bioelectrical impedance, dietitians are increasingly including these techniques in clinical nutritional assessment as well as in research.

Anthropometry is the external measurement of the human body and reflects health and nutritional status; it can be used to predict risk of ill health and survival and assess the response to nutrition interventions (Madden & Smith, 2016). Anthropometric measurements are influenced by nutritional and other factors, including age, gender and ethnicity and are frequently compared with standards or used in prediction equations; wherever possible these standards or equations should be derived from the same or comparable population. The most commonly used anthropometric measures are height, weight, waist and limb circumferences and skinfold thickness. The accuracy of measurements depends on the expertise of the assessor and the quality of the equipment used. It is essential that all equipment is calibrated and serviced, e.g. weighing scales, or replaced as appropriate, e.g. tape measures; in some settings, calibration is a statutory requirement.

Training is essential to ensure that all measurements are made using the correct, standardised procedure so that accurate and reproducible results are obtained. Guidance on procedures and reference data used for comparison is described for each measurement below. Good practice requires that those undertaking anthropometric assessments should check the technical error of their measurements (Ulijaszek & Kerr, 1999) and

Table 2.2.3 Examples of documentation required for anthropometric assessment

Context	Explanation of relevance
Procedure	Confirmation that standardised procedure followed or not.
	Any deviation from standard procedure should be explained, e.g. patient unable to stand on scales unaided; left arm swollen so right arm measured.
Time of measurement	On waking vs late afternoon may impact on height.
	Before or after meals, haemodialysis or paracentesis will influence weight.
Patient	Clothing and footwear, e.g. wearing nightwear / light clothes / bare feet may influence height and weight; long tight sleeves may impact on arm anthropometry.
	Before or after voiding bladder / bowels.
Equipment used	Wall-mounted height measure vs portable stadiometer in clinic.
	Bariatric weighing scales vs bed scales.
	Precision skinfold callipers vs plastic version.
Assessor	Identify assessor to facilitate continuity of measurements and minimise inter-observer error.
Reference data	Where comparison is made to reference data or cut-off values, these should be referenced (author, year), noting relevance, e.g. age, gender or ethnic group.

where possible, that the same person should take repeat measurements. In addition to the measured values, the context of the measurements should also be documented (Table 2.2.3).

Body weight

Weighing scales, including bed scales and bariatric platforms, must be maintained and calibrated regularly. In the UK, class III scales are required in medical premises for medication, treatment and monitoring of patients, and the maximum permitted error should typically be <200 g for a 70 kg patient (DH, 2008; UK Statutory Instrument, 2000). The procedure for weighing a person should be standardised, e.g. using the protocol of the National Diet and Nutrition Survey (NDNS) (Public Health England (PHE), 2014).

Reference data are not used for body weights, and a single measurement is not particularly useful in assessing nutritional status, other than to determine an individual body mass index (BMI) category. Measurement of body weight at regular intervals is vital to identify changes in weight over time and to calculate percentage increase or decrease. Changes occurring over days are likely to reflect change in fluid balance, while changes in body weight over weeks or longer indicate changes in body composition but does not identify whether this is associated with fat stores, fat-free mass (FFM), fluid or a combination of these, but may indicate the need for more detailed assessment.

Factors that affect body weight include:

- *Fluid retention, oedema or ascites* – small fluctuations of <1.5% body weight occur in response to physiological changes in fluid balance. Pathological changes in fluid balance (e.g. associated with hypoalbuminaemia; renal, cardiac and hepatic dysfunction; and with some medication) may be much larger, and may therefore obscure weight change associated with loss or gain of fat or FFM (Madden & Smith, 2016). Excess fluid can be estimated (Table 2.2.4) and used to give a dry weight to facilitate BMI calculation. If used, this method should be documented, and the limited accuracy recognised.
- *Amputations* – body weight can be adjusted to include estimated weight of a missing limb (Table 2.2.4); this should be documented.
- *Plaster casts, splints and replacement joints* – can add significant weight, and adjustment for this should be made and documented (Table 2.2.4). Fibreglass casts weigh less than those made from plaster of Paris.

Table 2.2.4 Weight adjustments for fluid retention, amputations and plaster casts

Clinical description	Estimated change in body weight
Fluid retention (Madden & Smith, 2016; Mendenhall, 1992)	
Ascites:	
Minimal	+2.2 kg
Moderate	+6.0 kg
Tense	+14.0 kg
Oedema:	
Barely detectable	+2 kg
Severe	+10–25 kg
Amputation (BAPEN, 2012)	
Upper limb	–4.9 %
Forearm	–1.6 %
Hand	–0.6 %
Lower limb	–15.6 %
Lower leg	–4.5 %
Foot	–1.4 %
Cast (BAPEN, 2012)	
Upper limb	+<1 kg
Lower leg or back cast	+0.9–4.5 kg

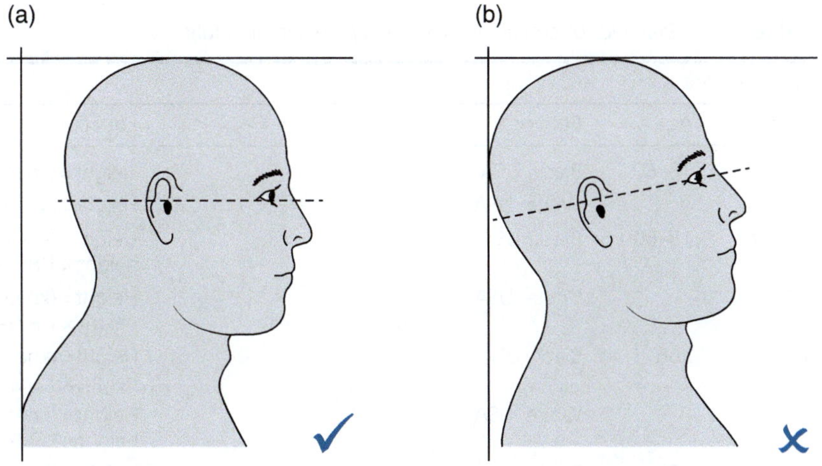

Figure 2.2.1 Position of head for measuring height using: (A) Frankfort plane, where lower eye socket is horizontally level with upper ear canal; and (B) typical but incorrect position (source: Madden *et al.*, 2012, figure 1, p. 122. Reproduced with permission from John Wiley & Sons, Ltd)

The weight of a replacement joint is not usually significantly different from that of the bone it is replacing. If there are concerns, advice should be sought from an orthopaedic specialist.

When weight cannot be measured

If it is not possible to weigh a patient due to his or her clinical condition or lack of accessible scales, body weight may be estimated. The limitations of this approach should be recognised:

- *Self-reported weights* – the accuracy of patient-reported weight varies, with a tendency to underestimate, with mean differences between reported and measured body weight of up to 6.5 kg (Connor Gorber *et al.*, 2007). The reported figure is unlikely to take into account any change in weight since admission or from when the illness began.
- *Estimates by others* – weight of hospitalised patients aged ≥16 years estimated by HCPs may be less accurate than self-reported weight, with error by HCPs exceeding 10% of weight in nearly half of estimates (Hendershot *et al.*, 2006). Estimates of weight provided by first-degree relatives may be within 3–5% of measured weight (Reed & Price, 1998).

Weight loss

Weight loss is an important indicator of the risk of malnutrition, and is expressed as percentage weight loss (Cederholm *et al.*, 2015):

$$\%\text{Weight change} = \left[\frac{\text{Usual or previous weight(kg)} - \text{Actual weight(kg)}}{\text{Usual or previous weight(kg)}}\right] \times 100$$

Unintentional weight loss of >10% habitual weight over any time period, or loss of >5% over 3 months, is considered diagnostic of malnutrition (Cederholm *et al.*, 2015). In clinical situations, weight loss may be more detrimental in lean individuals than in those who are obese, even when the same percentage weight loss has occurred. However, it is important to remember that rapid weight loss in obese individuals also makes them vulnerable to malnutrition-associated morbidity, i.e. sarcopenic obesity (Wannamethee & Atkins, 2015).

Height

Height is usually measured using a free-standing or portable stadiometer or wall-mounted measure, which should be checked regularly for accuracy (Madden & Smith, 2016). The procedure for measuring height should be standardised, e.g. using the protocol of the UK NDNS (PHE, 2014). Subjects should stand upright with their heels against the vertical measure and their head positioned in the Frankfort plane (i.e. upper ear canal and lower eye socket are horizontally level) (Figure 2.2.1). The measuring plate is lowered until it lightly touches the top of the head.

When height cannot be measured

If it is not possible to measure a patient, height may be estimated or derived using a prediction equation. The limitations of this approach should be recognised, and the alternative method documented.

- *Self-reported height* – accuracy of patient-reported height varies with a tendency to overestimate, with mean differences between reported and measured height of up to 7.5 cm (Connor Gorber *et al.*, 2007). Loss of height with age is associated with greater inaccuracy of self-reports, with mean overestimates of 2.3–5.0 cm in adults aged ≥65 years. The inaccuracy of self-reported height in most adults may not influence malnutrition screening outcome (Stratton *et al.*, 2003), except in women aged ≥70 years where BMI is underestimated (Reidlinger *et al.*, 2014).
- *Estimates by others* – the height of hospitalised patients aged ≥16 years estimated by HCPs may be less accurate than self-reported height, with only 41% of HCPs estimating within 2.5 cm of measured height (Hendershot *et al.*, 2006); estimates provided by relatives may be within 1% of measured height (Reed & Price, 1998).
- *Recumbent height* – may be accurate if the person is able to lie flat, but measurements are approximately

Table 2.2.5 Examples of equations for estimating height in adults

Knee height				
Gender	Age	Ethnicity	Equation	Author
Men	18–60	Black, USA	Height = (knee height × 1.79) + 73.42	Chumlea *et al.* (1994)
		White, USA	Height = (knee height × 1.88) + 71.85	
Women	18–60	Black, USA	Height = (knee height × 1.86) – (age × 0.06) + 68.10	
		White, USA	Height = (knee height × 1.87) – (age × 0.06) + 70.25	
Men	≥60	Black, USA	Height = (knee height × 1.85) – (age × 0.14) + 79.69	Chumlea *et al.* (1998)
		White, USA	Height = (knee height × 1.94) – (age × 0.14) + 78.31	
Women	≥60	Black, USA	Height = (knee height × 1.61) – (age × 0.17) + 89.58	
		White, USA	Height = (knee height × 1.85) – (age × 0.21) + 82.21	
Demi-span				
Gender	Age	Population	Equation	Author
Men	20–45+	European	Height = 57.8 + (1.40 × demi-span)	Bassey (1986)
Women		Nottingham, UK (*n* = 125)	Height = 60.1 + (1.35 × demi-span)	
Men	≥65	Living at home (Health Survey for England); 98% white; England, UK (*n* = 2469)	Height = 73.0 + (1.30 × demi-span) – (0.10 × age)	Hirani and Aresu (2012)
Women			Height = 85.7 + (1.12 × demi-span) – (0.15 × age)	

All lengths in centimetres; age in years.

2% greater than standing height (Gray *et al.*, 1985). For patients with contractures who need to be measured in a more complex lying position, a method proposed by Finch and Arumugam (2014) provides useful values.

- *Ulna length* – the most practical and quickest way to estimate height in adults who cannot stand is from the ulna length. The measurement of ulna length requires a non-stretch tape, and the standard procedure involves placing the left arm diagonally across the chest with the palm facing inwards and fingers pointing towards the shoulder. The measurement is taken between the central and most prominent parts of the styloid process and the centre (tip) of the bony prominence (olecranon) at the elbow (Figure A3.1 in Appendix A3). This is validated for use on the left side, but, as no systematic differences have been found, either side can be used. Height can then be estimated from the ulna length (Table A3.4 in Appendix A3). However, caution should be used in non-White populations, as predicting height from ulna length has been shown to overestimate height in Asian and Black adults (Madden *et al.*, 2012).
- *Knee height* – can be used in adults who cannot stand for height measurement, and requires the use of either an anthropometric calliper or non-stretch tape. The procedure requires the person to bend both their knee and ankle to 90° either while sitting with their foot flat on the floor or lying on their back. The measurement is taken parallel to the tibia from underneath the heel to the top of the thigh immediately above the condyles of the femur (i.e. above the patella) on the left side where possible (Chumlea & Guo, 1992; Hickson & Frost, 2003). Height can be estimated from knee height using population-based equations (Table 2.2.5).
- *Demi-span, half-span and arm-span* – can be measured in adults while standing, sitting or lying on their back, and requires a non-stretch tape. The person stretches out his or her arm perpendicular to the body, and demi-span is measured between the centre of the sternal notch and the finger-root between middle and ring fingers on the left side where possible (Bassey, 1986; Hickson & Frost, 2003). Half-span is measured with the arm in a similar position but from the sternal notch to the tip of the middle finger, and arm-span is measured between finger tips while both arms are extended (Kwok & Whitelaw, 1991). The arms should be horizontal and straight, with the palm facing forward (or up, if lying). For elderly and those with weaker arms, support may be needed to hold the position during measurement. Height can be estimated from demi-span and arm-span using equations from different populations (Madden & Smith, 2016) (Table 2.2.5).

Body mass index (BMI)

BMI is a weight-for-height indicator that is used to provide a quick evaluation of overweight or underweight, and is calculated as weight (kg)/height squared (m^2). It is a simple, widely used measure for use in nutritional assessment of individuals and populations, and forms part of many screening tools. BMI does not differentiate between components of body weight (i.e. fat mass), FFM or their location (i.e. central or peripheral adiposity), which are important determinants of health risk. As a result, BMI values tend to underestimate obesity in individuals with reduced levels of FFM (e.g. the elderly), and overestimate obesity in muscular individuals (e.g. athletes). Other anthropometric assessments provide better evaluation of health risk (see waist-to-height ratio in the following text).

The classification of BMI is based on the effect that body weight has on morbidity and mortality (see Table A3.5 in Appendix A3). Increasing BMI is associated with greater risk of developing type 2 diabetes, cardiovascular disease, osteoarthritis and some cancers (Chapter 7.13.1, General aspects and prevention of obesity). Conversely, low BMI values are indicative of malnutrition and associated clinical risk. Factors influencing the risk associated with BMI include:

- *Ethnicity* – the classification of BMI (see Table A3.5 in Appendix A3) is based on studies undertaken in mostly White adults. Equivalent metabolic and cardiovascular risk is observed at lower and variable BMI values in Asian adults (WHO, 2016). The additional cut-off points provided by the WHO allow for this variation. In the UK, BMI >23 kg/m^2 is used to identify risk of type 2 diabetes in adults of South Asian and Chinese descent (NICE, 2012) and in Asian Americans in the USA (American Diabetes Association, 2017).
- *Age* – BMI classification is derived from studies on adults mostly aged 18–65 years, so care should be taken when interpreting values for people outside this range. Systematic review of mortality in nursing-home residents aged ≥65 years indicates that being overweight and obese (but with BMI <40 kg/m^2) is associated with a reduced risk of death, and suggests that ≤21 kg/m^2 should be considered a threshold for identifying undernutrition in this population (Veronese *et al.*, 2015). This classification of BMI is not appropriate for children, where age-specific BMI centiles should be used (Chapter 3.8.2 Growth, nutritional assessment and nutritional requirements).
- *Body composition* – BMI should be interpreted with caution in people who have fluid retention (Table 2.2.4) or a high proportion of muscle mass, e.g. athletes, body builders and military personnel (Prentice & Jebb, 2001). It will also be affected by over- or underestimates of weight or height as discussed earlier.
- *Setting* – BMI can be used in both public health and clinical settings. However, it must be used as part of the overall assessment and not as a standalone result. Clinical judgement should override BMI category where necessary.

Other indices of adiposity or undernutrition based on weight

Several other indices of adiposity have been derived in an attempt to overcome the limitations associated with determining or interpreting BMI (Madden & Smith, 2016). Those based on weight include a body shape index (Krakauer & Krakauer, 2012), demiquet (Lehmann *et al.*, 1991), fat-mass index (Schutz *et al.*, 2002), mindex (Lehmann *et al.*, 1991) and Ponderal index (Cole *et al.*, 1997). Some indices require more complex calculation or the measurement of fat mass, and hence are less practical. As a result, most are not in common practice and have not been evaluated to the same extent as BMI. Fat-free mass index (FFMI) is calculated from FFM (kg) / height squared (m^2), and values <17 and <15 kg/m^2 are diagnostic of undernutrition in men and women, respectively (Schutz *et al.*, 2002; Cederholm *et al.*, 2015), and predict the survival rates of hospital patients (Rondel *et al.*, 2016).

Evaluation of central adiposity

The health risk associated with excessive body fat stores varies depending on the location of the fat, with central deposition (visceral adiposity) associated with worse outcomes than peripheral deposits (Kuk *et al.*, 2006). BMI and similar whole-body indices do not evaluate distribution, so measuring abdominal girth may add useful information.

Waist circumference

A non-stretch tape is required for measuring waist circumference, and a standardised procedure should be followed, e.g. the protocol of the UK NDNS (PHE, 2014). In summary, subjects should remove bulky outer and tight garments and stand upright with arms hanging loosely by the side. The tape is positioned midway between the iliac crest and costal margin, i.e. lower rib, ensuring that it is untwisted and horizontal. The subject is asked to look straight ahead and breathe out, and the measurement is made at the end of expiration. Measurement is not possible in pregnancy or in those unable to stand or with a colostomy. Increasing waist circumference is associated with greater risk of cardiometabolic morbidity and mortality (Ashwell *et al.*, 2012; Taylor *et al.*, 2010). NICE (2016) recommends the use of waist circumference in the assessment of obesity-related health risks, with measurements >102 and >88 cm identifying very high risk in men and women, respectively. Ethnicity-specific cut-offs for identifying low risk/high risk are also available (Table A3.6, Appendix A3). There are no age-specific cut-offs, but measurements typically increase with age (Ford *et al.*, 2003). Waist circumference is a useful tool for monitoring weight loss programmes and can predict changes in risk, even if weight has remained stable. However, when BMI >35 kg/m^2, measuring the waist circumference adds little predictive power.

Waist-to-height ratio

Meta-analyses indicate that waist-to-height ratio (WHtR) is a better predictor of diabetes, hypertension, dyslipidaemia, metabolic syndrome and cardiovascular disease than BMI (Ashwell & Gibson, 2016). Risk is identified at values ≥0.5, facilitating a simple public health message to ***keep waist circumference at less than half height*** (Ashwell & Gibson, 2014).

Waist–hip ratio

Waist-to-hip ratio (WHR) is a predictor of health risk that is comparable with BMI or waist circumference alone (Huxley *et al.*, 2010). WHR values ≥0.90 in men and ≥0.80 in women are associated with substantially greater risk of metabolic complications (WHO, 2008). It is used less frequently in individual assessment, mainly due to difficulties in locating the appropriate place to measure hip circumference.

Sagittal abdominal diameter

Sagittal abdominal diameter (SAD) is measured using a portable sliding beam abdominal calliper which is used to quantify the anterior–posterior thickness of the abdomen while subjects are lying supine (Gletsu-Miller *et al.*, 2013) or standing (Iribarren *et al.*, 2006). SAD values are predictive of cardiometabolic risk. SAD-to-height ratio in adults aged 20–64 years is a risk predictor comparable with WHtR and better than BMI (Kahn & Bullard, 2016).

Body adiposity index

Body adiposity index (BAI) is used to estimate percentage body fat without measuring weight, and is calculated as (Bergman *et al.*, 2011):

$$\text{BAI} = \frac{\textit{Hip}}{\textit{Height}\sqrt{\textit{Height}}} - 18$$

Its value in predicting health risk varies in different populations, but, overall, it is no better than BMI and more difficult to calculate (Dhaliwal *et al.*, 2014; Snijder *et al.*, 2012).

Mid-upper arm circumference

Mid-upper arm circumference (MUAC) is measured using a non-stretch tape and standardised procedure, e.g. NDNS protocol (PHE, 2014). The measurement is undertaken with the patients sitting or standing, with their arm bare and the top of the shoulder accessible. The forearm is placed across the body, bending the elbow at 90°. The midpoint between the acromium process on the top of the shoulder and the olecranon process of the elbow is identified and marked. The arm is then allowed to hang loosely by the side, and the circumference measured at the marked midpoint. MUAC has three roles (Madden & Smith, 2016):

- MUAC is required for the assessment of mid-arm muscle circumference (MAMC) (see the following text).
- It can be used to provide a crude estimate of BMI, although errors may vary between –6 and +4 kg/m^2.
- Its ability to independently predict clinical risk is variable, depending on the clinical population. Reference values for MUAC derived from a USA population (Bishop *et al.*, 1981) are given in Table A3.2 in Appendix A3. More recent data is available (McDowell *et al.*, 2008), but reflect secular changes in obesity prevalence and is not suitable for assessment of undernutrition. Data for the UK population are not currently available.

Skinfold thickness

Measurement of subcutaneous fat using skinfold callipers facilitates the estimation of total body fat and, by calculation, evaluation of muscle stores. As intra-abdominal fat cannot be assessed this way, the measurement is difficult in obesity where skinfolds are >40 mm. Therefore, skinfold anthropometry is most useful in assessing undernutrition. Precision callipers, e.g. Harpenden or Holtain, are needed for accuracy. The measurement procedure requires training and practice to allow the observer to identify the correct anatomical site and provide reliable values. These are described clearly with diagrams in books (Frisancho, 2008; Lohman *et al.*, 1988, Stewart & Sutton, 2012), and are available online for triceps and subscapular sites (Centers for Disease Control and Prevention (CDCP), 2005). To minimise the effect of error, three measurements should be made and an average used; for monitoring, the same person should take repeat measurements. A skilful practitioner should aim for intra-observer error of ≤5% (Perini *et al.*, 2005). The potential uses of skinfold measurement are:

- Triceps skinfold (TSF) is required for the assessment of MAMC.
- TSF can be used to evaluate body fat stores by comparison with reference data. Values derived from a USA population (Bishop *et al.*, 1981) are given in Table A3.1 in Appendix A3. Data for the UK population are not currently available.
- Percentage body fat can be estimated from skinfold measurements based on regression equations, e.g. Durnin and Womersley (1974). Alternative equations use seven sites (Jackson & Pollock, 1978; Jackson *et al.*, 1980). Determining body fat using anthropometry is less accurate than other methods described in the following text.

Mid-arm muscle circumference (MAMC)

MAMC can be used to evaluate muscle mass, an indicator of protein stores, and is also an outcome measure to evaluate nutrition interventions. It is calculated as:

$$\text{MAMC(cm)} = \text{MUAC(cm)} - \left[\text{TSF(mm)} \times 0.314\right]$$

It is an independent predictor of clinical outcome in many clinical populations, and low values are associated with adverse outcomes (Madden & Smith, 2016). As such, it is a more important anthropometric variable than MUAC

Table 2.2.6 Summary of methods for the determination of body composition (source: adapted from Gibney *et al.*, 2009. Reproduced with permission from Wiley-Blackwell Publishing for 6th edition)

Method	Accuracy	Cost	Radiation	Time	Convenience for subject
Anthropometry	+	+++++	None	++++	++++
BIA	++	+++	None	+++++	+++++
CT scanning	+++	++	High	+++	++
Densitometry	++++	+++	None	++	++
Dilution	+++	++	Variable	++++	+++
DXA	+++	++	Negligible	+++	+++
IVNAA	+++++	+	Very high	+	+
MRI scanning	+++	++	None	+++	++
TBK	+++	++	None	+++	++

+++++, excellent; ++++, very good; +++, good; ++, satisfactory; +, bad.
BIA, bioelectrical impedance analysis; CT, computer assisted tomography; DXA, dual energy x-ray absorptiometry; IVNAA, in vivo neutron activation analysis; MRI, magnetic resonance imaging; TBK, total body potassium.

and TSF used independently. Reference data for MAMC derived from a USA population (Bishop *et al.*, 1981) are given in Table A3.3 in Appendix A3 and were used in most studies examining the predictive value of MAMC. There is no consensus on which arm should be measured. In view of this, the arm used should be recorded, and repeat measurements undertaken on the same side. Comparisons with reference data derived using the opposite arm should be interpreted with caution (Madden & Smith, 2016).

Calf circumference

Although arm circumference is more commonly measured, more skeletal muscle is associated with the lower limbs, so measuring calf circumference may provide a useful alternative. The measurement is undertaken with the person seated or lying supine, and either leg can be used and values compared to reference values (Corish & Kennedy, 2003; McDowell *et al.*, 2008). A calf-circumference of <31 cm is considered indicative of risk of impaired function (Rolland *et al.*, 2003).

Body composition

Nutritional assessment requires dietitians to have a good understanding of body composition methodology because, in addition to validating bedside or field, new technologies are increasingly being used to assess body fat and FFM in clinical and public health settings. These include bioelectrical impedance analysis (BIA) and imaging techniques. While they provide valuable opportunities, their validation in non-healthy populations is currently limited (Smith & Madden, 2016). By contrast, accurate body composition assessment in research settings is best undertaken using a four-component model which reduces errors associated with variable fluid and bone mineral (Heymsfield *et al.*, 2015). A four-component module typically comprises fat, water, protein and mineral, and can be determined by measuring body density (e.g. air displacement plethysmography – BodPod, COSMED UK), body mineral (e.g. dual energy xray absorptiometry, DXA) and total body water (TBW) (e.g. deuterium dilution) (Fuller *et al.*, 1992). Each of these methods can be used individually to provide a two-component assessment of body fat and FFM, but with loss of accuracy in clinical populations (Morgan *et al.*, 2006; Woodrow *et al.*, 1996). When deciding which method to use to assess body composition, practical issues, convenience to participant and cost need to be weighed up against the accuracy required (Table 2.2.6).

Bioelectrical impedance analysis (BIA)

BIA is an easy, non-invasive bedside measure used to estimate TBW and body composition. It is based on the principle that fat does not contain water and that the water content of FFM is constant. Therefore, when a small electrical current passes through the body, it flows predominantly through tissues containing water and ions but not through fat. Measurements of resistance to the electrical current allow TBW to be estimated using regression equations, and, from this, FFM and fat mass can be calculated. In practice, assumptions made about the inverse relationship between resistance and TBW may be false (Smith & Madden, 2016). Newer single-frequency BIA monitors can undertake whole-body measurements in the vertical position and may also be able to undertake segmental measurements, i.e. upper or lower body. Cheaper models are also available, but the accuracy and reliability of their results have been questioned (Jaffrin, 2009). Multi-frequency BIA monitors can be used in both vertical and supine positions, and also facilitate segmental measurements and estimation of intra- and extracellular water – thus, in theory, providing more useful estimates in clinical populations with varied hydration status. In practice, their use and validity is limited (Smith & Madden, 2016).

Monitors usually compute raw data and provide body composition results immediately. However, practitioners should appreciate which regression equations are being used to calculate results to ensure that these are appropriate for the person undergoing assessment. Equations vary with age, gender and ethnicity, and most have been developed in healthy, non-obese, White populations. Use of demographically inappropriate equations can lead to inaccurate results. Equations may also include other variables, e.g. height, weight and exercise level, and inputting incorrect values for these will also adversely affect results. BIA monitors are unlikely to be suitable for use in nutritional assessment if they do not provide raw data (i.e. resistance) or state the equation used.

When a suitable BIA monitor and appropriate equations are available, a standardised procedure is required to optimise the accuracy of results. Typically, this should include overnight fasting (Tinsley *et al.*, 2016); avoiding exercise, alcohol and caffeine for 12 hours; and voiding urine prior to measurement. BIA is most useful in the collection of population data (rather than in individuals), providing that a consistent procedure is followed, an appropriate population-specific equation is used and those being measured are in good health and not under- or over-hydrated. The equipment required is portable and of relatively low cost, while repeatability and inter-observer variation are lower than in anthropometry. Recent developments in BIA include:

- *Bioelectrical spectral analysis* – used to determine extra- and intra-cellular water by modelling BIA data at ≥50 frequencies. In theory, this has potential application in clinical populations with abnormal hydration but has limited clinical value at present (Cloetens *et al.*, 2015, Tangvoraphonkchai & Davenport, 2017).
- *Phase angle* – can be determined during BIA measurement and is independent of regression equations, so it is theoretically more useful in patients with abnormal hydration status. In healthy individuals, phase angle is usually 5°–7°, and higher values are indicative of greater cellular health (Norman *et al.*, 2012). It has been shown to have prognostic value in clinical populations (Gonzalez *et al.*, 2016; Grundmann *et al.*, 2015). Current evidence does not yet facilitate its use in clinical practice.
- *Bioimpedance vector analysis (BIVA)* – can facilitate evaluation of tissue hydration. Reference values have been derived, and healthy individuals are usually positioned between the 75th and 95th centiles (Smith & Madden, 2016). This has been used to assess nutritional status in gastrointestinal disease and anorexia nervosa (Khalil *et al.*, 2014), but practical guidance for using this in clinical practice is limited at present.

Biochemical and haematological markers

Clinical chemistry provides objective results for nutritional assessment and in the monitoring of nutritional status and nutritional support. Biochemical and haematological measurements must be interpreted with care, since they may be influenced by homeostatic mechanisms, disease and age. However, clinical chemistry is essential to determine the status of specific nutrients, e.g. vitamin B_{12} or iron deficiency. Laboratory tests are not carried out on every individual but are patient-specific as guided by the clinical situation or research protocol. Table A5.4 in Appendix 5 gives reference ranges for some variables; however, these ranges vary depending on laboratory standards and protocols, and it is essential to refer to local reference ranges (Raghavan *et al.*, 2016).

Visceral protein status

Most (30–50%) body protein is found in skeletal muscle (also called somatic protein). Skeletal muscle wastes during disease, malnutrition and inactivity. Visceral protein is found in organs such as the liver, heart, pancreas and kidneys, and in blood (plasma proteins). Plasma proteins, such as albumin and prealbumin, are sometimes measured as an indicator of visceral protein status. Synthesis of these proteins is compromised in malnutrition. However, non-nutritional factors, such as injury, sepsis, liver disease and altered fluid state, can have a greater effect than nutritional influences.

Albumin

Albumin in plasma has a half-life of approximately 20 days; therefore, it is not sensitive to short-term changes in protein status. Albumin levels are affected by age, infection, zinc depletion (causing decrease) and dehydration (causing increase). Therefore, low levels correlate poorly with nutritional status (Anderson & Wochos, 1982; Friedman & Fadem, 2010). However, an albumin level of <35 g/L indicates an impaired ability to cope with major illness, surgical intervention or sepsis, and can be a useful part of a nutritional assessment (Scott *et al.*, 1998).

Prealbumin

Prealbumin has been used to monitor nutritional status and can be a sensitive index of early response to nutritional support due to its short half-life of <2 days (Shenkin, 2006). It is affected by changes in hydration status and acute changes in liver and renal function, but the fluctuations are smaller than for albumin. Levels may be depressed in inflammatory states independently of nutritional status. It is wise to consider prealbumin results with C-reactive protein (CRP) values to distinguish between reduction due to illness or malnutrition (Robinson *et al.*, 2003).

Other plasma proteins

Transferrin (half-life 8–10 days) and retinol binding protein (half-life 1–2 hours) have been suggested as alternatives to albumin because of their shorter half-lives and thus greater sensitivity to protein depletion. However, they are of little value in assessing nutritional status as they are extremely sensitive to changes in stress or disease and, in the case of transferrin, to iron status (Casati *et al.*, 1998).

Nitrogen balance

Measurement of nitrogen excretion over time will reflect nitrogen balance and changes in total body protein mass. It is a useful tool, in theory, to assess and monitor catabolism, and is used to assess protein requirements. However, accurate techniques are complex, and hence rarely undertaken outside research settings. Most nitrogen is excreted as urinary urea, and urea-nitrogen is measured using a 24-hour urine collection in clinical practice. Total nitrogen output can be estimated by taking into account faecal and skin nitrogen losses.

Micronutrients

Vitamins, minerals and trace elements are assessed, usually after fasting overnight, if deficiencies are suspected or to check the adequacy of intake during supplementation. Tests for micronutrients required for haematopoiesis (so-called haematinics, i.e. folate, vitamin B_{12}, iron, transferrin and ferritin) are widely available in clinical laboratories, but other micronutrients may require specialist facilities. Other vitamins that may be monitored for signs of specific or general nutritional deficiencies are A, C, D, E, B_1, B_2 and B_6. Minerals and trace elements bind to plasma proteins and, since some plasma proteins change in response to disease, i.e. during the acute phase response (APR), measuring the APR is important to distinguish between changes due to nutritional status and changes due to disease. APR is usually assessed by measuring CRP. Periodic measurements of blood levels are, however, useful as a way of monitoring long-term nutritional support, e.g. in home enteral feeding. Webster-Gandy *et al.* (2011) discuss the measurement of vitamin, mineral and trace element status further.

Calcium status can be monitored by measuring blood levels. Total plasma calcium is a measure of both the physiologically active ionised form and non-ionised calcium; the latter is mainly bound to albumin, and some is also complexed with citrate or phosphate. When plasma albumin is low, total calcium will also appear low. The biochemistry result for corrected calcium takes into account the reduction in circulating calcium secondary to low circulating protein levels, and is the better value to use. Plasma pH will influence calcium binding, and, in acidosis, less calcium is albumin-bound and more exists in the ionised form. Calcium balance is influenced by hormonal and biochemical factors, including parathyroid hormone, calcitonin and calcitriol (the active metabolite of vitamin D) (Chapter 7.9.1, Osteoporosis).

Hydration status and serum electrolytes

Iatrogenic, dietetic and clinical interventions can influence hydration status and serum electrolytes (Chapters 6.6, Fluids and electrolytes and 7.17.1, Critical care). Commonly used markers of hydration status include serum sodium, potassium and urea. However, results need to be interpreted alongside fluid balance charts and clinical examination for indications of over- or under-hydration. Urinary sodium levels can be measured to check salt depletion. This is useful in conditions with large fluid loss, e.g. Crohn's disease.

Dehydration

Dehydration concentrates the extracellular fluid, reflected in the blood results as hypernatraemia, uraemia and raised serum haemoglobin. If sodium and urea rise concurrently, dehydration should be suspected even in the presence of fluid overload, e.g. oedema. Fluid balance can be monitored by daily measurement of body weight. Dehydration with raised urea may occur without raised sodium levels if patients are losing both sodium and fluid, yet are having a low sodium intake, e.g. diarrhoea while being enterally fed.

Refeeding syndrome

Prior to feeding an at-risk patient, blood levels of potassium, calcium and phosphate should be checked. If these are low, magnesium should also be measured, and all acted upon according to local protocols. Once feeding has commenced, low blood levels of phosphate, potassium and magnesium indicate possible refeeding syndrome (Chapter 6.4, Enteral nutrition).

Dietary biomarkers

There is increasing interest in the development of laboratory dietary biomarkers that can be used to verify food records or as an alternative (O'Gorman & Brennan, 2017). At present, these are research tools and not yet used in practice.

Other variables

Other biochemical or haematology results may provide further clinical information relevant to nutritional assessment in specific clinical conditions:

- Renal function, e.g. creatinine, urea.
- Inflammation, e.g. CRP.
- Infection and immune, e.g. white blood cells, CD4 count.
- Liver function, e.g. bilirubin, gamma glutamyl transferase.
- Coeliac disease, e.g. anti-tissue transglutaminase antibodies.

Clinical assessment

Clinical assessment should comprise both reported information and physical examination.

Reported information

Information may be obtained directly from the person undergoing assessment, their family and/or carers, or documented in medical, nursing, allied health professional, pharmacy or social care records. Careful questioning may be needed to determine reliable information, especially in those who are sick, anxious or with poor memory. The information required will vary depending on the reason for the assessment, the individual and the context, but is likely to include past and current medical history and a history of weight change and physical activity.

Information on nutrient intake is described in more detail in the following text and in Chapter 2.3 (Dietary assessment). Information on clinical tests might be relevant, e.g. blood and urine tests, biopsy or scan results. Current medication, including prescribed and over-the-counter medicines, should be identified and considered for drug–nutrient interactions (Chapter 5.3, Medicines management). Information on ability to swallow may be relevant in older people and in those with neuromuscular disorders (Park *et al.*, 2015).

Physical examination

It is not possible to overestimate the importance of physical observations and of undertaking additional examination where necessary. Traditionally, dietitians rely on clinical assessments undertaken by other HCPs rather than directly examining their patient. There is increasing interest in dietitians developing examination skills that are relevant to assessing nutritional status (Mordarski, 2016). Adherence to high standards of professional practice relating to patient consent and dignity and infection control procedures is essential.

Examples of physical signs of nutritional problems are listed in Table 2.2.7 (Shaw & Lawson, 2008). Some overt vitamin deficiencies have visible signs, such as xerophthalmia (vitamin A) and Casal collar (niacin deficiency). However, it is important to understand that sub-clinical micronutrient deficiencies are more common than overt deficiencies; hence, absence of specific signs does not indicate an adequate status.

Physical examination should also consider:

- General physical appearance
  - Does the person look thin, of acceptable weight or overweight? Emaciation, pale complexion and hair loss suggest long-term undernutrition.
  - Loose clothing, rings and ill-fitting dentures indicate weight loss.
- Facial appearance, e.g. sunken eyes, dry mouth and fragile skin are indicative of dehydration. Hollowing around the temples indicates possible undernutrition.
- Mouth, including lips and tongue, may reveal problems affecting eating, e.g. poor dentition, dry mouth, sore or painful mouth, orofacial surgery or radiotherapy, or provide evidence of possible iron or vitamin B deficiency. Loss of taste and ability to chew or swallow food should be considered.
- Hands, e.g. badly damaged nails and surrounding tissue (Russell's sign), may be an indication of self-induced vomiting in bulimia nervosa.
- Oedema, usually in the lower limbs or sacral area, may reflect underlying disease, or heart failure secondary to prolonged protein or thiamine deficiency. The presence of oedema may mask loss of lean tissue.
- Breathlessness may be due to a clinical condition or be a symptom of anaemia and may raise concern about iron status. If severe, it may make eating difficult.

Table 2.2.7 Examples of physical signs of nutritional problems (source: Shaw & Lawson, 2008. Reproduced with permission from Wiley Publishers)

Assessment	Clinical sign	Possible nutrient(s)
Hair	Thin, sparse	Protein and energy, zinc, copper
	Colour change – flag sign	
	Easily plucked	
Skin	Dry, flaky	Essential fatty acids, B vitamins
	Rough 'sandpaper' texture	Vitamin A
	Petechiae, bruising	Vitamin C
Eyes	Pale conjunctiva	Iron
	Xerosis, keratomalacia	Vitamin A
Lips	Angular stomatitis	B vitamins
	Cheilosis	
Tongue	Colour changes	B vitamins
Teeth	Mottling of enamel	Fluorosis (excess fluoride)
Gums	Spongy, bleed easily	Vitamin C
Face	Thyroid enlargement	Iodine
Nails	Spoon shape, koilonychias	Iron, zinc, copper
Subcutaneous tissue	Oedema, over-hydration	Protein, sodium
	Depleted subcutaneous fat	Energy
Muscles	Wasting	Protein, energy, zinc
Bones	Craniotabes	Vitamin D
	Parietal and frontal bossing	
	Epiphyseal enlargement	
	Beading of ribs	

- Poor wound healing may indicate impaired immune function as a consequence of undernutrition and/or vitamin deficiencies, and/or lack of mobility.
- Adverse effects of illness or treatment, such as nausea, vomiting, diarrhoea.
- Repeated medical investigations, treatments and medications requiring fasting (nil-by-mouth) or dietary change may impact negatively on nutrient intake.

Dietary assessment

Dietary assessment is discussed in detail in Chapter 2.3, Dietary assessment. Establishing the extent to which nutritional needs are being met is central to the nutritional assessment. This requires the quantitative comparison of estimated nutrient intake with estimated individual nutrient requirements (Chapter 2.1, Dietary reference values and food-based dietary guidelines), and the identification of possible reasons for inadequacy or excess which can then be used to inform subsequent interventions. Factors that need to be considered include:

- Current food – quantity and variety of foods. Are all food groups represented?
- Fluid intake.
- Duration and extent of any changes in oral intake.
- Presence of factors potentially affecting food and fluid intake.
- Changes in appetite.
- Alterations in meal pattern or timings.
- Alteration of food preferences or food consistency.

The greater the extent and duration of any changes, the more marked the effect on nutritional status will be. It is important to link the aspects of dietary assessment described earlier with the practical and social aspects of food provision described in the following text. Nutritional requirements are available for healthy population groups (dietary reference values) or can be estimated for an individual, taking into account age, gender, level of physical activity and clinical condition (Chapters 2.1, Dietary reference values and food-based dietary guidelines and 6.1, Nutritional requirements in clinical practice). As estimating both nutrient intake and individual requirements is challenging, especially in people who are unwell, the conclusions from dietary assessment at a single time point may often need to be interpreted with caution. However, this should not lead to complacency over possible nutritional inadequacy, and follow-up dietary assessment, e.g. by monitoring food intake through food charts, should be considered.

Environmental, behavioural and social assessment

These factors can have a significant impact on the nutritional status of some individuals and may be identified from the information reported by them or their family and/or carers, or documented by other health or social care professionals. As some factors are potentially sensitive or associated with stigma, a delicate approach should be employed when exploring them directly. Factors that may affect food and fluid intake include:

- Psychological status
  - Depression or apathy, e.g. following bereavement, relationship breakdown or loss of employment.
  - Confusion and/or memory loss, e.g. in dementia.
  - Loss of autonomy due to chronic illness, bullying or social anxiety.
  - Severe or chronic pain.
  - Anxiety about health, prognosis or other related factors.
- Ability to buy, prepare and cook food
  - Sudden change in domestic arrangement, e.g. loss of partner who organised meals, or moving from a catered institution into the community.
  - Difficulty accessing shops due to distance, lack of transport or inability to pay fares or carry provisions.
  - Lack of secure food storage, e.g. shared accommodation, or limited freezer space for home-delivered meals.
  - Inadequate cooking facilities, e.g. bed-and-breakfast accommodation.
  - Impaired mobility may affect the ability to prepare and cook food.
  - Ill health, pain and weakness may contribute to loss of interest in eating.
  - Lack of previous experience in planning or cooking meals may impact on young adults leaving looked-after care and on those with learning disabilities.
- Social factors
  - Living conditions and recent changes, e.g. an elderly person moving into sheltered accommodation or an evicted family re-housed in a hostel.
  - Cultural and religious beliefs, especially if living away from communities with shared beliefs and unable to access specific foods, e.g. halal meat or kosher products.
  - Employment patterns including multiple low-paid jobs, working away from home and shift work.
  - Low income and recent changes in income, e.g. redundancy, recent immigration.
  - Impact of alcohol, illegal-substance abuse and the use of psychoactive substances.
  - Education, e.g. the inability to read (or read English) or severe dyslexia will impact the ability to read food labels, cooking instructions, nutrition labelling and to understand health messages.

In addition to informing nutritional assessment, gaining a good understanding of environmental, behavioural and social factors helps dietitians to plan their dietetic intervention by understanding the unique circumstances of the individual.

Functional assessment

There is increasing interest in assessing function during the assessment of nutritional status. This is based on the growing evidence that functional data are closely associated with clinical outcomes. The measurements can often be easily undertaken and provide numerical values that facilitate interpretation and monitoring. In addition, many patients engage enthusiastically with some functional assessments, and they may also have motivational value. Some functional measures, e.g. handgrip strength, can be easily evaluated in clinical or community practice, while others may be undertaken by other members of the multidisciplinary team.

Muscle strength

Handgrip strength

Impaired handgrip strength is associated with increased post-operative risk, hospitalisation (Norman *et al.*, 2011), cardiovascular and all-cause mortality (Leong *et al.*, 2015) and cognitive decline and mortality in adults aged >60 years (Rijk *et al.*, 2016). Handgrip dynamometry is the functional test that is most frequently used by dietitians in clinical practice. Dynamometers are portable, easy to use and relatively cheap, but their use requires the co-operation of the person being assessed, and they are not suitable for assessing those with hand injuries and pre-existing muscle or nerve damage. Frail or very elderly patients may find lighter, digital dynamometers easier to use.

Handgrip strength is measured with the person seated, shoulder abducted, elbow flexed at 90° and forearm in a neutral position. They are then asked to squeeze the handles of the dynamometer, as tightly as possible, three times on both sides. The pressure exerted is read off the scale, usually expressed in kilograms, and the maximum value is recorded to allow comparison with published data. Normative values expressed as population centiles have been derived using meta-analysis from UK studies of >60,000 participants aged 4 to >95 years (Table A3.7 in Appendix 3), Dodds *et al.*, 2014). Weak handgrip strength is defined as values lower than the age- and gender-specific population mean grip strength minus 2.5 standard deviations.

Knee strength

Knee extensor strength provides an assessment of lower limb muscle strength, and is also associated with disability and mortality (Izawa & Watanabe, 2016). It requires more complex and expensive equipment, which may only be available in a research setting, and takes longer to assess than measuring handgrip strength. Population values can be used to predict future mobility limitation (Manini *et al.*, 2007).

Measureable activities of daily living

Walking speed

Walking speed or gait speed is predictive of adverse clinical outcomes and mortality (Cheung *et al.*, 2016; Kim *et al.*, 2016). This is usually measured over 4 m, and a cut-point of <0.6 m/s is used to identify dysmobility (Cummings *et al.*, 2014). A stopwatch is required, and a measured distance can be marked out in a clinic or ward. In patients with chronic kidney disease, each reduction in walking speed of 0.1 m/s is associated with a 26% increase in risk of mortality (Roshanravan *et al.*, 2013). Changing gait potentially provides a method of evaluating nutrition interventions (Smith & Madden, 2016).

Sit-to-stand

Sit-to-stand tests evaluate either the number of times a person can rise, with his or her arms crossed, from sitting to standing and then repeating this within a timed period (usually 30 or 60 seconds), or measures the time taken for repeating the sit-to-stand process five times (Centers for Disease Control and Prevention (CDCP), 2016a; Jones *et al.*, 2013). A stopwatch and an armless, straight-backed chair placed against the wall, with its seat approximately 43–48 cm from the floor, are required. Occupational therapists and physiotherapists have expertise in carrying out the assessment, but dietitians could undertake this with the appropriate training. Five sit-to-stand repetitions taking ≥12 seconds are indicative of increased risk of falling in older people (Lusardi *et al.*, 2017). Age- and gender-specific norms for the 30-second sit-to-stand test are available for adults >60 years (CDCP, 2016a). Changes in the sit-to-stand score potentially provide another method of evaluating nutrition interventions.

Timed-up-and-go tests are similar to those discussed in the preceding text but combine rising from sitting on a chair with walking approximately 3 metres and then returning to the chair and sitting down (CDCP, 2016b). Taking ≥12 seconds to complete the procedure is indicative of increased risk of falling in older people (Lusardi *et al.*, 2017). Functional measures are sometimes combined to provide an overall assessment of a person's ability to undertake activities, e.g. Barthel Index (Mahoney & Barthel, 1965).

Self-reported measures

In addition to the assessments described in the preceding text, many questionnaires are available to assess patients' functional ability, some of which are self-reported, e.g. Duke activity status index (Hlatky *et al.*, 1989). Most are designed for use in a specific clinical context, and many are not validated (De Saint-Hubert *et al.*, 2010; O'Caoimh *et al.*, 2015; Yang *et al.*, 2014). In theory and following validation, questionnaires have the potential to be developed into instruments to evaluate outcomes following nutritional intervention, but, at present, more supporting evidence is needed.

Patient-reported outcome measures

Patient-reported outcome measures (PROMs) are questionnaires specifically designed to evaluate factors that patients perceive as important. To be effective, they need to be designed and evaluated in the specific population in which they are intended for use, and should be developed in partnership with patients. To date, few dietetic-specific PROMs have been developed, but there are condition-specific PROMs that might be useful in some patient groups, e.g. coeliac disease (Crocker *et al.*, 2016).

Table 2.2.8 Monitoring nutritional status in clinical settings

Assessment	Rationale	Method	Frequency
Weight	Assess change in body mass – intentional or unintentional Calculate percentage change Calculate BMI Determine whether nutritional goals are achieved	Scales Alternative measures, e.g. self-reported usual weight from patient, family, carer	At initial assessment, then as clinically indicated: Daily to assess change in fluid balance Twice a week initially, reducing to monthly
Weight history	To assess recent and long-term weight change Ascertain normal weight for an individual	Medical notes Dietetic records Recall by patient, family, carer	At initial assessment
Height	To calculate BMI	Stadiometer Self-reported height Tape measure Alternative measure, e.g. ulna length	Once only unless shrinkage has occurred, e.g. osteoporosis
Other anthropometric measurements	Assessing fat or muscle status Monitor nutrition support	MUAC TSF Waist circumference	At assessment and then weekly or monthly, depending on clinical status
Biochemistry and haematology	To assess hydration and protein status Monitor nutrition support	Medical notes Pathology systems	Daily initially, then twice weekly Longer intervals, e.g. monthly according to individual circumstances
Clinical, medical and drug factors	Assess risk to nutritional intake, metabolism and requirements	Relevant notes Pharmacy chart	Every 2–3 days acutely, then weekly Long-term, as required
Diet and nutritional intake	To establish usual intake To ensure oral and/or artificial intake are meeting requirements	Interview Food diary Food intake chart Fluid balance chart Discussion with patient, carer, family, ward staff	At assessment, then at considered intervals thereafter Dependent on patient's condition
Environmental, behavioural and social factors	Establish factors affecting nutritional intake	Dietetic record cards Consultation with patient, family, carer	Initial assessment and thereafter as required
Functional assessment	To assess muscle strength and ability to undertake activities of daily living and assess response to nutritional intervention	Handgrip strength dynamometry Walking speed Timed sit-to-stand tests	At assessment, and then weekly until discharge

BMI, body mass index; MUAC, mid-upper arm circumference; TSF, triceps skinfold thickness.

As the importance of behaviour change is increasingly recognised in long-term conditions, understanding the patient's perspective is vital, and PROMs provide a mechanism to systematically facilitate this.

Monitoring nutritional status

Following initial nutritional assessment in clinical settings, ongoing monitoring of nutritional status must be undertaken regularly to ensure any nutritional intervention is effective. The patient, dietitian or other HCP can monitor the nutritional status, depending on the clinical status and location of the patient. Suitable methods and suggested frequency of assessment are summarised in Table 2.2.8, but frequency should be adapted to individual circumstances and take account of local policies and standards. To facilitate comparison of serial assessments, systematic and accurate documentation is required which should comply with local standards. This may include specific details of how data have been collected, and explain any deviation from standard procedures. Identifying the assessor will allow data to be clarified and facilitate consistent observations.

Acknowledgement

The Editor acknowledges the prior contribution of Joan Gandy.

Further reading

Alberti KGMM, Zimmet P, Shaw J. (2007) International Diabetes Federation: a consensus on type 2 diabetes prevention. *Diabet. Med.* 24: 451–463.

Frisancho AR. (2008) *Anthropometric Standards: An Interactive Nutritional Reference of Body Size and Body Composition for Children and Adults*. Ann Arbor: The University of Michigan Press.

Gibson RS. (2005) *Principles of Nutritional Assessment*, 2nd edn. Oxford: Oxford University Press.

Heymsfield S, Lohman TG, Wang ZM, et al. (2005) *Human Body Composition*. Illinois: Champaign, Human Kinetics.

NICE. (2013) *BMI: Preventing ill health and premature death in black, Asian and other minority ethnic groups*. Available at https://www.nice.org.uk/guidance/ph46. Accessed 20 February 2017.

Provan D. (2010) *Oxford Handbook of Clinical and Laboratory Investigation*, 3rd edn. Oxford: Oxford University Press.

Internet resources

Lab Tests Online, http://labtestsonline.org.uk

Parenteral and Enteral Nutrition Group (PENG) of the British Dietetic Association, Outcomes toolkit, http://www.peng.org.uk/pdfs/publications/peng-dietetic-outcomes-toolkit.pdf

References

American Diabetes Association. (2017) Classification and diagnosis of diabetes. *Diabetes Care*. 40(S1): S11–S24.

Anderson CF, Wochos DN. (1982) The utility of serum albumin values in the nutritional assessment of patients. *Mayo Clin. Proc.* 57(3): 181–184.

Ashwell M, Gibson S. (2014) A proposal for a primary screening tool: 'Keep your waist circumference to less than half your height'. *BMC Med.* 12: 207. doi: 10.1186/s12916-014-0207-1.

Ashwell M, Gibson S. (2016) Waist-to-height ratio as an indicator of 'early health risk': simpler and more predictive than using a 'matrix' based on BMI and waist circumference. *BMJ Open.* 6: e010159. doi: 10.1136/bmjopen-2015-010159.

Ashwell M, Gunn P, Gibson S. (2012) Waist-to-height ratio is a better screening tool than waist circumference and BMI for adult cardiometabolic risk factors: systematic review and meta-analysis. *Obes. Rev.* 13: 275–286.

BAPEN. (2012) *The MUST report – nutritional screening of adults: a multidisciplinary responsibility. Executive summary [Online]*. Available at http://www.bapen.org.uk/screening-for-malnutrition/must/must-report/the-must-report-executive-summary. Accessed 22 December 2016.

BDA. (2016) *Model and process for nutrition and dietetic practice*. Available at https://www.bda.uk.com/publications/professional/model_and_process_for_nutrition_and_dietetic_practice_. Accessed 20 February 2017.

Bassey EJ. (1986) Demi-span as a measure of skeletal size. *Ann. Hum. Biol.* 13: 499–502.

Bergman RN, Stefanovski D, Buchanan TA, *et al.* (2011) A better index of body adiposity. *Obesity* 19: 1083–1089.

Bishop CW, Bowen PE, Ritchey SI. (1981) Norms for nutritional assessment of American adults by upper arm anthropometry. *Am. J. Clin. Nutr.* 34: 2530–2539.

Casati A, Muttini S, Leggieri C, *et al.* (1998) Rapid turnover proteins in critically ill ICU patients. Negative acute phase proteins or nutritional indicators? *Minerva Anesthesiol.* 64: 345–350.

Cederholm T, Bosaeus I, Barazzoni R, *et al.* (2015) Diagnostic criteria for malnutrition – an ESPEN consensus statement. *Clin. Nutr.* 34: 335–340.

Centers for Disease Control and Prevention (CDCP). (2005) *NHANES anthropometry and physical activity monitor procedures manual*. Available at https://www.cdc.gov/nchs/data/nhanes/nhanes_05_06/BM.pdf. Accessed 30 December 2016.

Centers for Disease Control and Prevention (CDCP). (2016a) *The 30-second chair stand test*. Available at https://www.cdc.gov/steadi/pdf/STEADI-Assessment-30Sec-508.pdf. Accessed 19 September 2018.

Centers for Disease Control and Prevention (CDCP). (2016b) *The timed up and go (TUG) test*. Available at https://www.cdc.gov/steadi/pdf/STEADI-Assessment-TUG-508.pdf. Accessed 19 September.

Cheung CL, Lam KS, Cheung BM. (2016) Evaluation of low lean mass and slow gait speed in predicting death in the National Health and Nutrition Examination Study 1999–2004. *J. Gerontol. A Biol. Sci. Med. Sci.* 71: 90–95.

Chumlea WC, Guo SS, Steinbaugh ML. (1994) Prediction of stature from knee height for black and white adults and children with application to mobility-impaired or handicapped persons. *J. Am. Diet. Assoc.* 94: 1388–1391.

Chumlea WC, Guo S. (1992) Equations for predicting stature in white and black elderly individuals. *J. Gerontol.* 47: M197–M203.

Chumlea WC, Guo SS, Wholihan K, *et al.* (1998) Stature prediction equations for elderly non-Hispanic White, non-Hispanic Black, and Mexican–American persons developed from NHANES III data. *J. Am. Diet. Assoc.* 98: 137–142.

Cloetens L, Johansson-Persson A, Helgegren H, *et al.* (2015) Assessment of body composition in subjects with metabolic syndrome comparing single-frequency bioelectrical impedance analysis and bioelectrical spectroscopy. *Metab. Syndr. Relat. Disord.* 13: 91–98.

Cole TJ, Henson GL, Tremble JM, *et al.* (1997) Birthweight for length: ponderal index, body mass index or Benn index? *Ann. Hum. Biol.* 24: 289–298.

Connor Gorber S, Tremblay M, Moher D, *et al.* (2007) A comparison of direct vs self-report measures for assessing height, weight and body mass index: a systematic review. *Obes. Rev.* 8: 307–326.

Corish CA, Kennedy NP. (2003) Anthropometric measurements from a cross-sectional survey of Irish free-living elderly subjects with smoothed centile curves. *Br. J. Nutr.* 89: 137–145.

Crocker H, Jenkins C, Churchman D, *et al.* (2016). The coeliac disease assessment questionnaire (Cdaq): development of a patient-reported outcome measure. *Value Health*. 19(7): A595.

Cummings SR, Studenski S, Ferrucci L. (2014) A diagnosis of dismobility – giving mobility clinical visibility: a Mobility Working Group recommendation. *J. Am. Med. Assoc.* 311: 2061–2062.

De Saint-Hubert M, Schoevaerdts D, Cornette P, *et al.* (2010) Predicting functional adverse outcomes in hospitalised older patients: a systematic review of screening tools. *J. Nutr. Health Aging* 14: 394–399.

DH. (2008) *Patient weigh scales*. Available at http://webarchive.nationalarchives.gov.uk/20130107105354/http://www.dh.gov.uk/prod_consum_dh/groups/dh_digitalassets/documents/digitalasset/dh_085721.pdf. Accessed 21 December 2016.

Dhaliwal SS, Welborn TA, Goh LG, *et al.* (2014) Obesity as assessed by body adiposity index and multivariable cardiovascular disease risk. *PLoS One*. 9: e94560. doi: 10.1371.

Dodds RM, Sydall HE, Cooper R, *et al.* (2014) Grip strength across the life course: Normative data from twelve British Studies. *PLoS One*. 9: e113637. doi: 10.1371.

Durnin JVGA, Womersley J. (1974) Body fat assessed from total body density and its estimation from skinfold thickness: measurements on 481 men and women aged from 16 to 72 years. *Br. J. Nutr.* 32: 77–97.

Finch H, Arumugam V. (2014) Assessing the accuracy and reliability of direct height measurement for use in adult neurological patients with contractures: a comparison with height from ulna length. *J. Hum. Nutr. Diet.* 27(S2): 48–56.

Ford ES, Mokdad AH, Giles WH. (2003) Trends in waist circumference among US adults. *Obes. Res.* 11: 1223–1231.

Friedman AN, Fadem SZ. (2010) Reassessment of albumin as a nutritional marker in kidney disease. *J. Am. Soc. Nephrol.* 21: 223–230.
Frisancho AR. (2008) *Anthropometric Standards: An Interactive Nutritional Reference of Body Size and Body Composition for Children and Adults*, 2nd edn. Ann Arbor: University of Michigan Press.
Fuller NJ, Jebb SA, Laskey MA, *et al.* (1992) Four-component model for the assessment of body composition in humans: comparison with alternative methods and evaluation of the density and hydration of fat-free mass. *Clin. Sci.* 82: 687–693.
Gibney MJ, Lanham-New SA, Cassidy A, *et al.* (2009) *Introduction to Human Nutrition*, 2nd edn. Oxford: Wiley Blackwell.
Gletsu-Miller N, Kahn HS, Gasevic D, *et al.* (2013) Sagittal abdominal diameter and visceral adiposity: correlates of beta-cell function and dysglycemia in severely obese women. *Obes. Surg.* 23: 874–881.
Gonzalez MC, Barbosa-Silva TG, Bielemann RM, *et al.* (2016) Phase angle and its determinants in healthy subjects: influence of body composition. *Am. J. Clin. Nutr.* 103: 712–716.
Gray DS, Crider DS, Kelley C, *et al.* (1985) Accuracy of recumbent height measurement. *J. Parenter. Enteral Nutr.* 9: 712–715.
Grundmann O, Yoon SL, Williams JJ. (2015) The value of bioelectrical impedance and phase angle on the evaluation of malnutrition and quality of life in cancer patients: a comprehensive review. *Eur. J. Clin. Nutr.* 69: 1290–1297.
Hendershot KM, Robinson L, Roland J, *et al.* (2006) Estimating height, weight and body mass index: Implications for research and patient safety. *J. Am. Coll. Surg.* 203: 887–893.
Heymsfield SB, Ebbeling CB, Zheng J, *et al.* (2015) Multi-component molecular-level body composition reference methods: evolving concepts and future directions. *Obes. Rev.* 16: 282–294.
Hickson M, Frost G. (2003) A comparison of three methods for estimating height in the acutely ill elderly population. *J. Hum. Nutr. Diet.* 16: 13–20.
Hirani V, Aresu M. (2012) Development of new demi-span equations from a nationally representative sample of older people to estimate adult height. *J. Am. Geriatr. Soc.* 60: 550–554.
Hlatky MA, Boineau RE, Higginbotham MB, *et al.* (1989) A brief self-administered questionnaire to determine functional capacity (the Duke Activity Status Index). *Am. J. Cardiol.* 64: 651–654.
Huxley R, Mendis S, Zheleznyakov E, *et al.* (2010) Body mass index, waist circumference and waist: hip ratio as predictors of cardiovascular risk – a review of the literature. *Eur. J. Clin. Nutr.* 64: 16–22.
Iribarren C, Darbinian JA, Lo JC, *et al.* (2006) Value of the sagittal abdominal diameter in coronary heart disease risk assessment: cohort study in a large, multiethnic population. *Am. J. Epidemiol.* 164: 1150–1159.
Izawa KP, Watanabe S. (2016) Relation of nutritional status to physiological outcomes after cardiac surgery in elderly patients with diabetes mellitus: a preliminary study. *Aging Clin. Exp. Res.* 28: 1267–1271.
Jackson AS, Pollock ML. (1978) Generalised equations for predicting body density in men. *Br. J. Nutr.* 40: 497–504.
Jackson AS, Pollock ML, Ward A. (1980) Generalised equations for predicting body density in women. *Med. Sci. Sports Exerc.* 12: 175–182.
Jaffrin MY. (2009) Body composition determination by bioimpedance: an update. *Curr. Opin. Clin. Nutr. Metab. Care* 12: 482–486.
Jeejeebhoy KN, Detsky AS, Baker JP. (1990) Assessment of nutritional status. *J. Parenter. Enteral Nutr.* 14: 193S–196S.
Jones SE, Kon SS, Canavan JL, *et al.* (2013) The five-repetition sit-to-stand test as a functional outcome measure in COPD. *Thorax* 68: 1015–1020.
Kahn HS, Bullard KM. (2016) Beyond body mass index: advantages of abdominal measurements for recognizing cardiometabolic disorders. *Am. J. Med.* 129: 74–81.
Khalil SF, Mohktar MS, Ibrahim F. (2014) The theory and fundamentals of bioimpedance analysis in clinical status monitoring and diagnosis of disease. *Sensors* 14: 10895–10928.
Kim HJ, Park I, Lee HJ, *et al.* (2016) The reliability and validity of gait speed with different walking pace and distances against general health, physical function and chronic disease in aged adults. *J. Exerc. Nutrition Biochem.* 20: 46–50.
Krakauer NY, Krakauer JC. (2012) A new body shape index predicts mortality hazard independently of body mass index. *PLoS One* 7: e39504.
Kuk JL, Katzmarzyk PT, Nichaman MZ, *et al.* (2006) Visceral fat is an independent predictor of all-cause mortality in men. *Obesity* 14: 336–341.
Kwok T, Whitelaw MN. (1991) The use of armspan in nutritional assessment of the elderly. *J. Am. Geriatr. Soc.* 39: 492–496.
Lehmann AB, Bassey EJ, Morgan K. *et al.* (1991) Normal values for weight, skeletal size and body mass indices in 890 men and women aged over 65 years. *Clin. Nutr.* 10: 18–22.
Leong DP, Teo KK, Rangarajan S, *et al.* (2015) Prognostic value of grip strength: findings from the prospective urban rural epidemiology (PURE) study. *Lancet* 386: 266–273.
Lohman T, Roche AF, Martorell R. (1988) *Anthropometric Standardization Reference manual.* Champaign, IL: Human Kinetics.
Lusardi MM, Frirtz S, Middleton A, *et al.* (2017) Determining risk of falls in community dwelling older adults: a systematic review and meta-analysis using post-test probability. *J. Geriatr. Phys. Ther.* 40: 1–36.
Madden AM, Smith S. (2016) Body composition and morphological assessment of nutritional status in adults: a review of anthropometric variables. *J. Hum. Nutr. Diet.* 29: 7–25.
Madden AM, Tsikoura T, Stott DJ. (2012) The estimation of body height from ulna length in healthy adults from different ethnic groups. *J. Hum. Nutr. Diet.* 25: 121–128.
Mahoney FI, Barthel DW. (1965) Functional evaluation: the Barthel Index. *Md. Med. J.* 14: 61–65.
Manini TM, Visser M, Won-Park S, *et al.* (2007) Knee extension strength cutpoints for maintaining mobility. *J. Am. Geriatr. Soc.* 55: 451–457.
McDowell MA, Fryar CD, Ogden CL, *et al.* (2008) *Anthropometric reference data for children and adults: United States, 2003–2006. National Health Statistics Reports 10.* Available at www.cdc.gov/nchs/data/nhsr/nhsr010.pdf. Accessed 26 February 2017.
Mendenhall CL. (1992) Protein–calorie malnutrition in alcoholic liver disease. In: Watson RR, Watzl B (eds) *Nutrition and Alcohol.* Boca Raton: CRC Press, pp. 363–384.
Mordarski B. (2016) Nutrition-focused physical exam hands-on training workshop. *J. Acad. Nutr. Diet.* 118: 868–869.
Morgan MY, Madden AM, Jennings G, *et al.* (2006) Two-component models are of limited value for the assessment of body composition in patients with cirrhosis. *Am. J. Clin. Nutr.* 84: 1151–1162.
NICE. (2012) *Type 2 diabetes: prevention in people at high risk.* Available at https://www.nice.org.uk/guidance/ph38. Accessed 28 December 2016.
NICE. (2016) Obesity in adults: prevention and lifestyle weight management programmes. Available at https://www.nice.org.uk/guidance/qs111. Accessed 29 December 2016.
Norman K, Stobäus N, Gonzalez MC, *et al.* (2011) Handgrip strength: outcome predictor and marker of nutritional status. *Clin. Nutr.* 30: 135–142.
Norman K, Stobäus N, Pirlich M, *et al.* (2012) Bioelectrical phase angle and impedance vector analysis: clinical relevance and applicability of impedance parameters. *Clin. Nutr.* 31: 854–861.
O'Caoimh R, Cornally N, Weathers E, *et al.* (2015) Risk prediction in the community: a systematic review of case-finding instruments that predict adverse healthcare outcomes in community-dwelling older adults. *Maturitas.* 82: 3–21.
O'Gorman A, Brennan L. (2017) The role of metabolomics in determination of new dietary biomarkers. *Proc. Nutr. Soc.* 16: 1–8.
Park YH, Bang HL, Han HR, *et al.* (2015) Dysphagia screening measures for use in nursing homes: a systematic review. *J. Korean Acad. Nurs.* 45: 1–13.

Perini TA, de Oliveira GL, Ornellas JD, *et al.* (2005) Technical error of measurement in anthropometry. *Rev. Bras. Med. Esporte* 11: 86–90.

PHE. (2014) *National Diet and Nutrition Survey: Appendices and Tables.* Available at https://www.gov.uk/government/statistics/national-diet-and-nutrition-survey-results-from-years-1-to-4-combined-of-the-rolling-programme-for-2008-and-2009-to-2011-and-2012. Accessed 21 December 2016 (see appendix L for measurement protocols).

Prentice AM, Jebb SA. (2001) Beyond body mass index. *Obes. Rev.* 2(3): 141–147.

Raghavan R, Ashour FS, Bailey R. (2016) A review of cutoffs for nutritional biomarkers. *Adv. Nutr.* 7: 112–120.

Reed DR, Price RA. (1998) Estimates of the heights and weights of family members: accuracy of informant reports. *Int. J. Obes. Relat. Disord.* 22: 827–835.

Reidlinger DP, Willis JM, Whelan K. (2014) Resting metabolic rate and anthropometry in older people: a comparison of measured and calculated values. *J. Hum. Nutr. Diet.* 28: 72–84.

Rijk JM, Roos PR, Deckx L, *et al.* (2016) Prognostic value of handgrip strength in people aged 60 years and older: a systematic review and meta-analysis. *Geriatr. Gerontol. Int.* 16: 5–10.

Robinson MK, Trujillo EB, Mogensen KM, *et al.* (2003) Improving nutritional screening of hospitalized patients: the role of prealbumin. *J. Parenter. Enteral Nutr.* 27: 389–395.

Rolland Y, Lauwers-Cances V, Cournot M, *et al.* (2003) Sarcopenia, calf circumference and physical function of elderly women: a cross sectional study. *J. Am. Geriat. Soc.* 51: 1120–1124.

Rondel AL, Languis JA, de van der Scheuren MM, *et al.* (2016) The new ESPEN diagnostic criteria for malnutrition predict overall survival in hospitalised patients. *Clin. Nutr.* 34: 335–340.

Roshanravan B, Robinson-Cohen C, Patel KV, *et al.* (2013) Association between physical performance and all-cause mortality in CKD. *J. Am. Soc. Nephrol.* 24: 822–830.

Schutz Y, Kyle UU, Pichard C. (2002) Fat-free mass index and fat mass index percentiles in Caucasians aged 18–98 y. *Int. J. Obes. Relat. Metab. Disord.* 26: 953–960.

Scott A, Skerratt S, Adam S. (1998) *Nutrition for the Critically Ill: A Practical Handbook.* London: Arnold.

Shaw V, Lawson M. (2008) Nutritional assessment, dietary requirements and feed supplementation. In: Shaw V, Lawson M (eds) *Clinical Paediatric Dietetics*, 3rd edn. Oxford: Blackwell Science.

Shenkin A. (2006) Serum prealbumin: is it a marker of nutritional status or of risk of malnutrition? *Clin. Chem.* 52: 2177–2178.

Smith S, Madden AM. (2016) Body composition and functional assessment of nutritional status in adults: a narrative review of imaging, impedance, strength and functional techniques. *J. Hum. Nutr. Diet.* 29: 714–732.

Snijder MB, Nicolaou M, van Valkengoed IG, *et al.* (2012) Newly proposed body adiposity index (BAI) by Bergman *et al.* is not strongly related to cardiovascular health risk. *Obesity* 20: 1138–1139.

Stewart AD, Sutton L. (2012) *Body Composition in Sport, Exercise and Health.* Abingdon, UK: Routledge.

Stratton RL, Dixon R, Longmore D, *et al.* (2003) Effect of recalled weight and height on malnutrition risk. *Clin. Nutr.* 22(S1): S9–S10.

Tangvoraphonkchai K, Davenport A. (2017) Changes in body composition following haemodialysis as assessed by bioimpedance spectroscopy. *Eur. J. Clin. Nutr.* 71: 169–172.

Taylor AE, Ebrahim S, Ben-Shlomo Y, *et al.* (2010) Comparison of the associations of body mass index and measures of central adiposity and fat mass with coronary heart disease, diabetes, and all-cause mortality: a study using data from 4 UK cohorts. *Am. J. Clin. Nutr.* 91: 547–556.

Tinsley GM, Morales FE, Forsse JS, *et al.* (2017) Impact of acute dietary manipulations on DXA and BIA body composition estimates. *Med. Sci. Sports. Exerc.* 49:823–832..

UK Statutory Instrument. (2000) *Weights and Measures. The Non-automatic Weighing Instruments Regulations.* London: HMSO. (S.I.No.3236) Available at http://www.legislation.gov.uk/uksi/2000/3236/contents/made. Accessed 21 December 2016.

Ulijaszek SJ, Kerr DA. (1999) Anthropometric measurement error and the assessment of nutritional status. *Br. J. Nutr.* 82: 165–177.

Veronese N, Cereda E, Solmi M, *et al.* (2015) Inverse relationship between body mass index and mortality in older nursing home residents: a meta-analysis of 19,538 elderly subjects. *Obes. Rev.* 16: 1001–1015.

Wannamethee SG, Atkins JL. (2015) Muscle loss and obesity: the health implications of sarcopenia and sarcopenic obesity. *Proc. Nutr. Soc.* 74: 405–412.

Webster-Gandy J, Madden A, Holdsworth M. (2011) *Oxford Handbook of Nutrition and Dietetics*, 2nd edn. Oxford: Oxford University Press.

WHO. (2008) *Waist circumference and waist–hip ratio.* Available at http://www.who.int/nutrition/publications/obesity/WHO_report_waistcircumference_and_waisthip_ratio/en/. Accessed 29 December 2016.

WHO. (2016) *BMI classification.* Available at http://apps.who.int/bmi/index.jsp?introPage=intro_3.html. 28 December 2016.

Woodrow G, Oldroyd B, Turner JH, *et al.* (1996) Four-component model of body composition in chronic renal failure comprising dual-energy X-ray absorptiometry and measurement of total body water by deuterium oxide dilution. *Clin. Sci.* 91: 763–769.

Yang M, Ding X, Dong B. (2014) The measurement of disability in the elderly: a systematic review of self-reported questionnaires. *J. Am. Med. Dir. Assoc.* 15: e1–9.

2.3 Dietary assessment

Ailsa Welch

Key points

- Methods for estimating dietary intake in individuals can be retrospective measures, e.g. 24-hour recalls (24 HR), diet histories or food frequency questionnaires (FFQs), or current measures, e.g. weighed or estimated food records.
- There have been recent developments in digital, online and computerised methods for measuring dietary intake.
- The differences between methods and the impact of measurement error need to be considered when planning to use dietary methods.
- It is essential to understand the advantages and limitations of dietary assessment methods both for use in clinical practice and when reading and interpreting the scientific literature.

Dietary assessment methods are used for a variety of purposes, from individual assessments in clinical situations, through to use in epidemiology. In epidemiology, they are used to estimate intakes of populations and establish associations between nutrition and disease. They are also used as a basis for developing dietary guidelines and health policy, for monitoring change in intervention studies and for monitoring the effectiveness of public health interventions. Dietary assessments have traditionally been used to estimate intakes of foods and nutrients, but more recent interest has arisen in estimating the intake of bioactive phytochemicals, e.g. flavonoids, additives and contaminants. Ideally, assessment methods should have a low burden on respondents and investigators, and should be rapid and cheap, but also result in accurate, precise data with minimal measurement error.

There are a number of dietary assessment methods available for measuring food consumption at the national, household and individual levels. This chapter focuses on assessment methods suitable for individual intakes. At the national level, food balance sheets can be used to assess dietary intakes. Household level methods include the food account method, inventory method, household record method and list recall methods, and further information on these methods can be found in Gibson (2005).

Table 2.3.1 describes the advantages and limitations of the main types of dietary assessment methods used for individuals. Although many methods are available for estimating dietary intake in individuals, they can mainly be divided into two types: retrospective measures of intake, such as 24 HR, diet history or FFQs; and current measures of intake, such as weighed or estimated food records. Qualitative information is available from all methods, but quantitative estimates for nutrient consumption are possible only if data for weighed or estimated portion weights are available.

Weighed records, estimated food records, 24 HR and dietary histories are the most intensive methods. The quantity of food consumed may be weighed directly or estimated using household measures such as cups and spoons, photographs, standard units or average portions (Food Standards Agency, 2001; Nelson *et al.*, 1997). Data for portion sizes should be derived from weighed intakes, government surveys and research groups in populations similar to the one to be studied. Food models/replicas (three-dimensional models representing foods) can also be used, particularly in clinical practice.

More recently, methods are being developed that utilise photographs of portion size recorded with mobile phones or digital cameras (Penn *et al.*, 2010). For all methods, the amount consumed can be measured or described, either including or excluding wastage material usually discarded during food preparation, e.g. outer leaves and peel from vegetables or bones from cuts of meat. Several newer methods for recording food intake are being developed that involve digital, online and computer technology, including methods that scan barcodes on packaged food.

Manual of Dietetic Practice, Sixth Edition. Edited by Joan Gandy.

Companion website: www.manualofdieteticpractice.com

Table 2.3.1 Characteristics of dietary assessment methods

Method	Advantages	Limitations
Retrospective methods		
24 HR (single or multiple days)	Not reliant on long-term memory; interview length 20–45 minutes	Single 24 HRs can be used for group assessments but not for estimating intake of individuals; people may not recall all items of food or drink
Diet history	Respondent literacy not required	Report of past intake is influenced by current diet; trained interviewers required
FFQ (if portion estimates included, termed semi-quantitative FFQ)	Useful for large sample sizes; relatively straightforward to complete	Needs to be developed for specific population groups to ensure important food items are covered and requires updating to accommodate changes to supply of foods; responses governed by cognitive, numeric, and literacy abilities of respondents, also by length and complexity of the food list Not easy to develop for clinical practice since specific computer programs need to be developed
Short frequency questionnaires	Targeted at specific food types, administration simpler and easier than long questionnaires	Need to be developed for specific population groups to ensure questions are relevant
Current methods		
Weighed food record (weighed inventory technique)	No requirement for memory retrieval, as it records current intake; food intake weighed, so estimates of quantity consumed not required	Literate, cooperative respondents required as burden is high; possible that respondents change usual eating patterns to simplify the record; high data entry costs
Food record with estimated weights	No requirement for memory retrieval as it records current intake	Literate, cooperative respondents required as burden is high; possible that respondents change usual eating patterns to simplify the record
Duplicate analysis	Greater accuracy	Very labour intensive; requires laboratory to do food composition analysis
Records using electronic equipment, e.g. mobile phones, digital cameras	Visual records of foods Avoids need for paper records Data can be sent to investigators electronically	Currently involves labour-intensive programs to convert to usable data, i.e. quantities and types of foods, although systems are in development to deal with this; limited use in older people who experience difficulties with using newer technology

Number of days of recording

The number of days of reporting required for adequate measurement of nutrients using 24 HRs, weighed or estimated records varies depending on the day-to-day variability of nutrient consumption (Lanigan *et al.*, 2004; Mennen *et al.*, 2002; Nelson *et al.*, 1989). The number of days is partly dependent on the variation in nutrient concentration in foodstuffs. In foods, the concentration of macronutrients such as protein and carbohydrate varies less than that of micronutrients such as vitamin C or iron. The number of days required to classify adult individuals into the correct third of the percentage distribution for usual intake for 80% of individuals has been calculated (Mennen *et al.*, 2002; Nelson *et al.*, 1989). Up to 7 days of recall are required for energy, protein, sugars and calcium. Nutrients with greater variability, including alcohol, vitamin C, riboflavin, and iron, require 4–14 days of records. Fewer days of data collection are required to capture habitual diet in children (Lanigan *et al.*, 2004). More recent estimates of the number of days to estimate energy intake (using the doubly labelled water technique) suggest that 3 days of records are optimal, of which 1 day should be a weekend day (Ma *et al.*, 2009).

Dietary assessment methods

24 hour recall

24 HR determines intake during the preceding 24 hours and can be recorded on paper or using interactive computerised software (Slimani *et al.*, 1999). Day-to-day variability in nutrient intake is large, and a single day will not categorise individuals correctly within a distribution of intake. Particular issues are the capture of episodic (infrequently eaten) foods such as fish and liver; therefore, single 24 HR are better used for group assessments than estimates for individuals. However, multiple 24 HR can be used to overcome this problem. Newer methods of online recording of 24 HR are under development for self-completion by participants in studies. Examples are the Automated Self-Administered 24-Hour (ASA24®) Dietary Assessment Tool for the USA and Australia; the Oxford WebQ, which has been used in the UK Biobank Study, a national survey of 500,000 people in the UK; and myfood24, which has recently been developed for use in the UK (Cade, 2017; Galante *et al.*, 2016; Subar *et al.*, 2012).

The 24 HR method is useful for assessment in clinical situations, but the difficulties in assessment and accurately reporting intake due to the variations in nutrient concentrations of foodstuffs need consideration. This will affect the number of days required to obtain adequate measures of nutrient intakes (see the previous section).

Diet history

The diet history consists either of an interview administered 24 HR or establishing usual eating pattern over a 1-week period, followed by a frequency questionnaire to provide additional information. The dietary history provides a representative pattern of usual intake and is interview administered only. Diet histories are traditionally used in clinical practice and may take up to 1.5 hours to complete.

Food frequency questionnaires

FFQs consist of a list of specific foods or food types associated with the frequency of consumption to record average consumption over the previous month or year. They are termed semi-quantitative if portions are included. FFQs are thought to provide estimates of habitual intake, and are widely used in nutritional epidemiology (Cade *et al.*, 2004; Welch *et al.*, 2005). They need to be specific to a population group to ensure coverage of important foods, and the population must be literate and numerate, as some mathematical ability is necessary to calculate relative frequencies (Smith, 1993). Factors influencing response to FFQs are the length and complexity of the food list and current diet (Smith, 1993). For clinical use, it is necessary to develop specific software and databases to obtain nutrients, and therefore record methods are likely to be preferable (Welch *et al.*, 2005). In general, the amounts of foods eaten calculated from FFQs are greater than with current measures of intake (Dehghan *et al.*, 2007; Welch *et al.*, 2005).

Short frequency questionnaires

Short frequency questionnaires have been developed to estimate intakes of specific foods or nutrients, and these can be useful in clinical practice to determine where eating habits require change; examples include the Dietary Instrument for Nutrition Education (DINE) and the 5 A DAY Community Evaluation Tool (FACET) questionnaires (Ashfield-Watt *et al.*, 2007; Roe *et al.*, 1994; Welch *et al.*, 2006).

Weighed food record inventory and estimated food record

For weighed food records, all food and drink consumed over a period is weighed and recorded on forms or in booklets, with details of food type and method of preparation, to obtain consumption over a period of days. Portable scales need to be supplied. Leftover food should be weighed and deducted. The recommended time period for records is 4–7 days or more, although the number of days depends on the nutrient of interest, study population and objectives of the study. As some populations have different eating habits at weekends, weekend days should be included proportionately. For estimated food records, all foods consumed over a period of days are recorded with details of food type, method of preparation and estimated portion sizes. If recorded over 7 days, this is often called a 7-day diary.

Both these methods have a high respondent burden and need cooperative, literate respondents. Respondents require training in the level of detail needed to describe foods. It is also possible that respondents may change usual eating patterns to simplify the process of the record and may also find this method tedious. It is also beneficial to include a review of weighed records during the period of recording either after the first day or at the end.

Duplicate sample technique

Duplicate samples of all foods consumed are made and the nutrient content analysed chemically. This method is used for metabolic studies and, although providing greater accuracy than other methods, its use is only feasible for certain purposes. Studies are conducted in hospital metabolic units or research centres; they are expensive, time consuming and require considerable technical support.

Choice of dietary method for research or clinical use

Dietary methodology for clinical practice requires rapid assessments of nutritional intake in order to prescribe dietary change or to improve nutritional status. Traditionally, 24 hours of usual intake or diet histories have been used for this purpose. FFQs and weighed or estimated food records are not generally used due to the more intensive burden on respondents and on the resources required for coding and processing the data. For research purposes, a number of methods maybe used from FFQs to multiple 24 HR.

When designing a research study, it is advisable to obtain expert advice to decide on the optimum method. Online advice is available through the Dietary Assessment Primer, which has been developed in the USA by the National Institutes of Health and National Cancer Institute. This website guides researchers and other users through the choices of dietary methodology for estimating food and nutrient intakes in groups of individuals (Dietary Assessment Primer, 2017).

Recall of remote diet – current intake biases recall of past diet

When designing studies or reading the literature, dietitians need to be aware that recall of diet in the remote past is heavily influenced by current dietary habit. Studies have found that the correlations between recalled past diet and current diet are higher than the correlations between actual past diet and recall of past diet (Willett, 2012). The onset of diseases such as cancer may affect appetite and dietary assessment, as recall of remote diet is strongly related to current diet. Therefore, studies where diet was measured prior to the onset of disease are less likely to suffer from bias than, for instance, case–control studies in which the diet of cases with disease is compared with controls.

Use of data and conversion of reported intake to nutrients and food types

Qualitative data

Dietary method data can be used qualitatively, e.g. during the process of reviewing nutritional intake for the purpose of dietary treatment, as in clinical practice. However, the majority of uses of dietary methods are targeted towards quantitative analyses.

Quantitative data

Food composition databases, data entry and nutrient calculation systems

The data collected by dietary methods are converted into food and nutrient consumption data by calculating the amount of food eaten and linking this to a database with values for the nutrient composition of foods. The governments of many countries provide the databases of nutrient composition of foods. The UK National Nutrient Database consists of *McCance and Widdowson's The Composition of Foods* (2014) and its supplements. It is essential to read the information distributed with the printed or electronic versions of databases to determine the uses and limitations of the data (see Chapter 2.4, Food composition tables and databases).

Nutrient databases vary in the coverage and comprehensiveness of the foods and nutrients, and in the conversion factors used for certain nutrients. Care should be taken when comparing values from different sets of food tables because the definition and expression of nutrients may not always be the same. Different conversion factors may have been used to prepare the values, e.g. to calculate protein from nitrogen or to convert the major nutrients to energy. The same nutrient may be quoted in different ways, e.g. carbohydrate may be expressed as monosaccharide equivalents, actual weights or by difference. In the UK food tables, carbohydrate is expressed as monosaccharide equivalents, but, for food labelling purposes, carbohydrate should be provided as actual weight.

The nutrient values provided in food tables are generally averages of representative samples of foods or selected values from literature surveys. However, like any other biological material, the composition of food can vary considerably, and so the values in food tables are only representative of the true biological range of values and should not be considered as having the accuracy of atomic weights. Values in nutrient composition databases are expressed as either per 100 g of food or per common household measure. The most up-to-date information on the UK, European, US and international nutrient databases can be found on the follow websites: Public Health England (https://www.gov.uk/government/publications/composition-of-foods-integrated-dataset-cofid), European Food Information Resource Network (EuroFIR) (http://www.eurofir.org), US Department of Agriculture (http://ndb.nal.usda.gov) and the INFOODS Food and Agriculture Organization of the United Nations (http://www.fao.org/infoods/infoods/en).

Several steps are involved in calculating nutrient intake (also known as coding or processing). The first is to choose the item in the database that corresponds most closely to the food consumed. If the food consumed is not in the database, a suitable alternative can be chosen by considering the food type, general characteristics and likely nutrient profile. Once the food has been chosen, the nutrient composition of the food quoted in the database is multiplied by the amount of food eaten. To calculate the daily intake for an individual, the contribution of each food is calculated and all the foods for a day summated. If more than one day's data have been collected, it is usual to calculate the average for the number of days recorded. Although it is possible to compute intake by hand, using a calculator and a printed copy of a nutrient database, this is very labour intensive and, in practice, has been superseded by computerisation for most purposes. A number of computerised data entry systems and nutrient calculation programs exist to calculate nutrient intakes (Welch *et al.*, 2001). Prior to purchasing a new entry system, it is important to know the version or food composition database on which it is based.

Dietitians should be aware that the UK food tables are not adequate for estimating salt intake, as the nutrient intakes for recipes or composite dishes do not include salt, and therefore calculations are systematic underestimates.

Estimated food quantities

To obtain quantitative information for nutrients or food groups, actual or estimated food weights are used. For methods using estimated food weights, values also need to be found for the foods described, such as standard units, average portions or household measures. Sources of data are national publications, surveys of weighed dietary assessments, and food manufacturers. Data may also be included in nutrient calculation programs.

Additional sources of nutrients

Proprietary medicines may contain sources of nutrients, and vitamin and mineral supplements can contain considerable amounts of nutrients. Therefore, they should be taken into account when assessing total nutrient intakes (Lentjes *et al.*, 2010). This is particularly important in clinical practice when assessing the likelihood of low or deficient intakes of micronutrients. Current estimates of prevalence of supplement intakes are around 40% in the UK population aged over 40 years (Lentjes *et al.*, 2010).

Measurement error

Measurement error can be defined as the difference between the measured exposure (or measure of dietary assessment) and the true exposure; it is now known that there is measurement error associated with using dietary methods. Measurement error reduces the likelihood that true values have been measured with accuracy, and hence, in nutritional epidemiology, associations between dietary intake and disease outcomes will be affected (Schatzkin & Kipnis, 2004). As the proportion of measurement error increases, the scale of the relationship between diet and disease status will tend towards no relationship. Overall, the effect of measurement error would be to misclassify an individual within a range of intake.

The existence of measurement error also impacts on the interpretation of scientific literature. For instance, it is known that FFQs tend to produce systematically greater estimates of fruit and vegetable intake and of vitamin C intake than recording methods such as 7-day diaries (Dehghan *et al.*, 2007). As a result, fruit and vegetable intake for individuals and populations will be overestimated using an FFQ; more individuals measured with this method will appear to have sufficient intakes than if a record method had been used (Welch *et al.*, 2005). This is an important consideration when deciding upon public health policy and dietary guidelines.

The technique of validation can be used to estimate measurement error. Although full detail of the impact, scale and detection of measurement error is beyond the scope of this chapter, an awareness of the differences between dietary methods and the potential pitfalls when using them is helpful to clinicians in interpreting scientific literature.

Methods of detecting measurement error

There are four major methods of detecting measurement error:

1. Comparison with other diet methods; however, this is not advisable, since individuals report in the same way with all methods, and the errors are correlated (Black & Cole, 2001; Kipnis *et al.*, 2003).
2. Predictor reference methods, such as the Goldberg equations, or percentile cut points to detect energy misreporting and potentially statistically model the effects of misreporting (Stubbs, 2002).
3. Biomarkers (biological markers) in blood or urine, quantitative recovery biomarkers (quantitative estimates of intake over a specific time period) and concentration biomarkers (measure relative concentrations over a distribution) are thought to be independent of errors when measuring intake (Potischman & Freudenheim, 2003). Examples of quantitative markers are urine nitrogen excretion over 24 hours (to estimate protein intake) and energy expenditure measured using the doubly labelled water technique (DLW). Examples of concentration markers are plasma concentrations of n-3 polyunsaturated fatty acids and fish consumption (Welch *et al.*, 2006). Newer methods of identifying biomarkers have been developed recently. These include the use of metabolomic techniques (Brennan, 2016). Metabolomic techniques measure small molecules and the intermediates and products of metabolism. Metabolomics is capable of identifying molecules on metabolic pathways which capture and measure the effects of dietary intake. The metabolome has been measured in biological samples of blood and urine, and newer candidates for nutritional biomarkers identified. A recent study by Playdon *et al.* (2017) found strong associations between healthy eating patterns and biomarkers, identified using metabolomics, in blood.
4. Comparison with disease risk biomarkers, e.g. saturated fat and low-density lipoprotein (LDL) cholesterol (Bingham *et al.*, 2008).

Examples of validation studies are those performed within EPIC Europe and the Observing Protein and Energy Nutrition (OPEN) study in the USA (Kipnis *et al.*, 2003; Slimani *et al.*, 2003).

Although biomarkers are useful in the detection of measurement error, it should be noted that a number of factors influence their interaction with nutrition, e.g. differences in gender or genetics and homeostatic or behavioural influences. Not all associations are linear, e.g. vitamin C concentrations in the blood plateau since additional concentrations are excreted, and smoking impacts on the circulating concentrations of vitamin C.

Sources of measurement error in dietary assessment

There are many sources of measurement error when using dietary assessment. They may occur both during data collection and processing. Systematic bias, interviewer bias, recall bias and social desirability bias have been identified, but there are likely to be other sources of error. Bias can be defined as the modification of a method of measurement by a factor that influences the measurement in one or more directions. Measurement error associated with dietary methods may consist of one or more types of error.

Systematic bias is a systematic mismeasurement of data, and can occur, for instance, if an interviewer consistently fails to use questions to probe for consumption of snacks and additional foods. If systematic bias is identified, it can be overcome by the interviewer training and monitoring interviewers.

The behaviour of interviewers can influence the response of interviewees or clients and introduce interviewer bias. It is important to develop a rapport between interviewers and respondents, and for questions to be asked in an open-ended, neutral manner without value judgements.

Social desirability bias can influence dietary assessment methods as respondents strive to report what they think is required, and not what was actually consumed, e.g. reporting less alcohol consumption or greater consumption of foods with perceived health benefits, such as fish, fruit or vegetables. This is likely to be the cause of misreporting, under-reporting or low-energy reporting, which occurs in certain respondents and can affect clinical practice.

Conclusion

A wide variety of methods exist for measuring dietary intake, and it is essential to understand their advantages and limitations, both for use in clinical practice and when reading and interpreting scientific literature.

Further reading

Cameron ME, Van Staveren WA. (1988) *Manual on Methodology for Food Consumption Studies*. Oxford: Oxford University Press.

Feskanich D, Sielaff BH, Chong K, et al. (1989) Computerized collection and analysis of dietary assessment information. *Comput. Methods Programs Biomed.* 30: 47–57.

Gibson RS. (2005) *Principles of Nutritional Assessment*, 2nd edn. Oxford: Oxford University Press.

Margetts BM, Nelson M. (1997) *Design Concepts in Nutritional Epidemiology*, 2nd edn. Oxford: Oxford University Press.

Pao EM, Cypel YS. (1996) Estimation of dietary assessment. In: Zeigler EH, Filer LJ (eds) *Present Knowledge in Nutrition, 7th edn.* Washington, DC: ILSI Press, pp. 498–507.

Potischman N, Freudenheim JL. (2003) Biomarkers of nutritional exposure and nutritional status: an overview. *J. Nutr.* 133(Suppl 3): 873S–874S.

Thompson FE, Byers T. (1994) Dietary assessment resource manual. *J. Nutr.* 124: 11S.

Willett W. (2012) *Nutritional Epidemiology*, 3rd edn. Oxford: Oxford University Press.

Internet resources

European Food Information Resource (EuroFIR) Network. EuroFIR project website with information on European food composition databases, http://www.eurofir.org

INFOODS Food and Agriculture Organization of the United Nations, http://www.fao.org/infoods/infoods/en

myfood24 – the flagship solution from Dietary Assessment Ltd – is an online tool that was developed to help track, monitor and improve dietary intake, https://www.myfood24.org/web

Public Health England. *McCance and Widdowson's The Composition of Foods*, www.gov.uk/government/publications/composition-of-foods-integrated-dataset-cofid

US Department of Agriculture (USDA). National Nutrient Database for Standard Reference Release 28, https://ndb.nal.usda.gov/ndb

References

Ashfield-Watt PA, Welch AA, Godward S, et al. (2007) Effect of a pilot community intervention on fruit and vegetable intakes: use of FACET (Five-a-day Community Evaluation Tool). *Public Health Nutr.* 10: 671–680.

Automated Self-Administered 24-Hour (ASA24®) (2016). *Dietary Assessment Tool*. Available at https://asa24.nci.nih.gov/researchersite

Bingham S, Luben R, Welch A, *et al.* (2008) Associations between dietary methods and biomarkers, and between fruits and vegetables and risk of ischaemic heart disease, in the EPIC Norfolk Cohort Study. *Int. J. Epidemiol.* 37: 978–987.

Black AE, Cole TJ. (2001) Biased over- or under-reporting is characteristic of individuals whether over time or by different assessment methods. *J. Am. Diet. Assoc.*, 101: 70–80.

Brennan L. (2016) Metabolomics in nutrition research – a powerful window into nutritional metabolism. *Essays Biochem.* 60(5): 451–458.

Cade JE. (2017, Aug) Measuring diet in the 21st century: use of new technologies. *Proc. Nutr. Soc.* 76(3): 276–282.

Cade JE, Burley VJ, Warm DL, *et al.* (2004) Food-frequency questionnaires: a review of their design, validation and utilisation. *Nutr. Res. Rev.* 17: 5–22.

Dehghan M, Akhtar-danesh N, Mcmillan CR, *et al.* (2007) Is plasma vitamin C an appropriate biomarker of vitamin C intake? A systematic review and meta-analysis. *Nutr. J.* 6: 41.

Dietary Assessment Primer, Section Name. (2017) *National Institutes of Health, National Cancer Institute*. Available at https://dietassessmentprimer.cancer.gov. Accessed 1 September 2017.

FSA. (2001) *Food Portion Sizes*. London: The Stationery Office.

FSA/PHE. (2014) *McCance and Widdowson's The Composition of Foods*, 7th edn. Cambridge: Royal Society of Chemistry.

Galante J, Adamska L, Young A, et al. (2016, Feb 28) The acceptability of repeat Internet-based hybrid diet assessment of previous 24-h dietary intake: administration of the Oxford WebQ in UK Biobank. *Br. J. Nutr.* 115(4): 681–686.

Gibson RS. (2005) *Principles of Nutritional Assessment*, 2nd edn. Oxford: Oxford University Press.

Kipnis V, Subar AF, Midthune D, *et al.* (2003) Structure of dietary measurement error: results of the OPEN biomarker study. *Am. J. Epidemiol.* 158: 14–21; discussion 22–26.

Lanigan JA, Wells JC, Lawson MS, *et al.* (2004) Number of days needed to assess energy and nutrient intake in infants and young children between 6 months and 2 years of age. *Eur. J. Clin. Nutr.* 58: 745–750.

Lentjes MA, Bhaniani A, Mulligan AA, *et al.* (2010) Developing a database of vitamin and mineral supplements (ViMiS) for the Norfolk arm of the European Prospective Investigation into Cancer (EPIC-Norfolk). *Public Health Nutr.* 13: 1–13.

Ma Y, Olendzki BC, Pagoto SL., *et al.* (2009) Number of 24-hour diet recalls needed to estimate energy intake. *Ann. Epidemiol.* 19: 553–559.

Mennen LI, Bertrais S, Galan P, *et al.* (2002) The use of computerised 24 h dietary recalls in the French SU.VI.MAX Study: number of recalls required. *Eur. J. Clin. Nutr.* 56: 659–665.

Nelson M, Black AE, Morris JA, et al. (1989) Between- and within-subject variation in nutrient intake from infancy to old age: estimating the number of days required to rank dietary intakes with desired precision. *Am. J. Clin. Nutr.* 50: 155–167.

Nelson M, Atkinson M, Meyer J. (1997) *A Photographic Atlas of Food Portion Sizes*. London: MAFF Publications.

Penn L, Boeing H, Boushey CJ, *et al.* (2010) Assessment of dietary intake: NuGO symposium report. *Genes Nutr.* 5: 205–213.

Playdon MC, Moore SC, Derkach A, et al. (2017, Feb) Identifying biomarkers of dietary patterns by using metabolomics. *Am. J. Clin. Nutr.* 105(2): 450–465. doi: 10.3945/ajcn.116.144501. Epub 2016 Dec 28.

Potischman N, Freudenheim JL. (2003) Biomarkers of nutritional exposure and nutritional status: an overview. *J. Nutr.* 133(Suppl 3): 873S–874S.

Roe L, Strong C, Whiteside C, *et al.* (1994) Dietary intervention in primary care: validity of the DINE method for diet assessment. *Fam. Pract.* 11: 375–381.

Schatzkin A, Kipnis V. (2004) Could exposure assessment problems give us wrong answers to nutrition and cancer questions? *J. Natl. Cancer Inst.* 96: 1564–1565.

Slimani N, Deharveng G, Charrondiere RU, *et al.* (1999) Structure of the standardized computerized 24-h diet recall interview used as reference method in the 22 centers participating in the EPIC project. *European Prospective Investigation into Cancer and Nutrition. Comput. Methods Prog. Biomed.* 58: 251–266.

Slimani N, Bingham S, Runswick S, *et al.* (2003) Group level validation of protein intakes estimated by 24-hour diet recall and dietary questionnaires against 24-hour urinary nitrogen in the European Prospective Investigation into Cancer and Nutrition (EPIC) calibration study. *Cancer Epidemiol. Biomarkers Prev.* 12: 784–795.

Smith AF. (1993) Cognitive psychological issues of relevance to the validity of dietary reports. *Eur. J. Clin. Nutr.* 47(Suppl 2): S6–18.

Stubbs J. (2002) *Detecting and modelling MIS-reporting of food intake in adults.* Available at www.foodbase.org.uk/results.php?f_category_id=&f_report_id=289.

Subar AF, Kirkpatrick SI, Mittl B, *et al.* (2012, Aug) The Automated Self-Administered 24-hour dietary recall (ASA24): a resource for researchers, clinicians, and educators from the National Cancer Institute. *J. Acad. Nutr. Diet.* 112(8): 1134–1137.

Welch AA, McTaggart A, Mulligan AA, *et al.* (2001) DINER (Data Into Nutrients for Epidemiological Research) – a new data-entry program for nutritional analysis in the EPIC-Norfolk cohort and the 7-day diary method. *Public Health Nutr.* 4: 1253–1265.

Welch AA, Luben R, Khaw KT, *et al.* (2005) The CAFE computer program for nutritional analysis of the EPIC-Norfolk food frequency questionnaire and identification of extreme nutrient values. *J. Hum. Nutr. Diet.* 18: 99–116.

Welch AA, Bingham SA, Ive J, *et al.* (2006) Dietary fish intake and plasma phospholipid n-3 polyunsaturated fatty acid concentrations in men and women in the European Prospective Investigation into Cancer-Norfolk United Kingdom cohort. *Am. J. Clin. Nutr.* 84: 1330–1339.

Willett W. (2012) *Nutritional Epidemiology*, 3rd edn. Oxford: Oxford University Press.

SECTION 2

2.4 Food composition tables and databases

Edwige Landais and Michelle Holdsworth

Key points

- Food tables are a vital resource, but to avoid errors from their use, it is essential to understand their strengths and limitations.
- The composition of a particular food can vary as a result of differences in plant and animal genetics, strain and breed variety, farming practices, soil quality, climate, storage conditions and the way in which food has been processed, manufactured or cooked.
- Food tables do not take into account the extent to which a nutrient is absorbed (bioavailability).

Food composition data provide information on the nutritional composition of the edible part of foods, and are available in print (food composition tables) and computerised formats (food composition databases). They are generally used to calculate the food intake of individuals and groups from information gathered during dietary assessment (see Chapter 2.3, Dietary assessment). They are used in different settings, including clinical practice, research, health promotion and the agri-food industry, as shown in Table 2.4.1.

Data in food composition databases come from different sources:

- Original analytical values obtained from chemical analysis of food samples.
- Analytical values from scientific literature or food labels for branded foods.
- Imputed values derived from analytical values of a similar food.
- Calculated values derived from recipes using weight yield and nutrient retention factors.
- Values taken from other tables or databases.
- Presumed values that are assumed to be null.

National food tables

UK food tables

Tables of food composition have been published in the UK since the 1920s, stimulated by concerns over food shortages in the First World War (Church, 2006). They were continued by the pioneering work of McCance and Widdowson, initially conducted under the auspices of the Medical Research Council and subsequently the Ministry of Agriculture, Fisheries and Food (MAFF). In 1987, MAFF, in conjunction with the Royal Society of Chemistry, began the production of a computerised UK National Nutrient Databank (UKNND), from which the fifth edition of *McCance and Widdowson's The Composition of Foods* (Holland *et al.*, 1991a) and a number of detailed supplements were produced. In 2000, responsibility for the maintenance of the UKNND was transferred to the Food Standards Agency (FSA), and in 2016 to the Institute of Food Research (IFR), when it was renamed Food Databanks. The Food Databanks National Capability (FDNC) publishes the tables in book form as *McCance and Widdowson's The Composition of Foods* and electronically as the Composition of Foods Integrated Dataset (CoFID), available at https://www.gov.uk/government/publications/composition-of-foods-integrated-dataset-cofid.

The printed form of the summary edition of *McCance and Widdowson's The Composition of Foods* (Finglas *et al.*, 2015) is widely used; however, it should be appreciated that, while convenient, the single volume edition does not contain the complete set of data available, but only a subset of foods and nutrients. The most comprehensive information is contained within the separately published supplements, as shown in Table 2.4.2, and a complete collection of these should be regarded as the definitive UK food tables. Most of these are now in electronic form and have been integrated into the UKNND (www.food.gov.uk), and are regularly updated as part of a rolling programme of food analysis and analytical reports.

Manual of Dietetic Practice, Sixth Edition. Edited by Joan Gandy.

Companion website: www.manualofdieteticpractice.com

Table 2.4.1 Role of food composition tables

Use	Clinical practice	Health promotion	Research	Agri-food industry
Assessing nutritional status at individual, community and national levels	√	√	√	
Preparing educational materials	√	√		√
Designing therapeutic diets, e.g. hospitals	√		√	
Devising food and nutrition labelling				√
Assessing diet–disease links	√		√	
Developing food products and recipes				√
Monitoring food and nutrient availability		√	√	√
Developing food and nutrient guidelines	√	√	√	√
Monitoring food legislation and safety – consumer protection		√	√	√
Completing missing values in a data set	√	√	√	√

Table 2.4.2 UK food tables and supplements

Single volume summary	
McCance and Widdowson's The Composition of Foods, 7th edition	Finglas *et al.* (2015)
Supplements	
Amino acid composition and fatty acid composition	Paul *et al.* (1980)
Immigrant foods	Tan *et al.* (1985)
Cereals and cereal products	Holland *et al.* (1988)
Milk products and eggs	Holland *et al.* (1989)
Vegetables, herbs and spices	Holland *et al.* (1991b)
Fruit and nuts	Holland *et al.* (1992a)
Vegetable dishes	Holland *et al.* (1992b)
Fish and fish products	Holland *et al.* (1993)
Miscellaneous foods	Chan *et al.* (1994)
Meat, poultry and game	Chan *et al.* (1995)
Meat products and dishes	Chan *et al.* (1996)
Fatty acids	Ministry of Agriculture, Fisheries and Food (1998)
Others	
Foods commonly consumed by South Asians	Judd *et al.* (2000)

Note: Details of the analysis of specific food products and nutrients, e.g. salt in bread, are available at www.food.gov.uk.

A range of nutrient analysis software programmes using the UKNND is available for dietitians and nutritionists (see Chapter 2.3, Dietary assessment). Some less sophisticated nutrient analysis programmes need to be used with caution, particularly those designed for the general publisc or schools, which comprise summarised data derived from main food tables. Data for groups of foods may either be averaged or confined to a few selected options, e.g. data for meat may be confined to a few possible choices from the hundreds cited in the main food tables. Dietary estimates based on such generalised figures can be misleading.

Food tables used outside the UK

In order to be useful and accurate, food tables need to reflect the foods consumed in the food culture in which they are used. Dietary investigations carried out in other parts of the world should use the appropriate local data. Many other countries produce national food composition tables, including several European Union countries, and the first was published in Germany in the 1800s (Church, 2006). The European Food Information Resource project (EuroFIR) initiative was established in 2005 to deliver a comprehensive and validated European databank for nutrients and bioactive compounds for 27 European countries (www.eurofir.org). EuroFIR led to the establishment of a longer-term platform to continue some of these activities through a non-profit international association – EuroFIR AISBL – to support the development and application of food composition data, through international harmonisation. Within the EuroFIR framework, the bioactive constituents of plant-based foods, as well as their biological effects, are combined in a database (Electronic BioActive Substances in Food Information System, or eBASIS, available at http://ebasis.eurofir.org/Default.asp).

The USA also began producing food composition tables in the 1800s and has continued to produce accessible electronic food tables (www.ars.usda.gov). In the late 1970s, the Center for Food Safety and Applied Nutrition (CFSAN) of the US Food and Drug Administration (FDA) developed a standardised system for describing food. This system, called LanguaL (Langua aLimentaria) (www.langual.org), facilitates links to many different food databases and enables data exchange of over 35,000 food products. In the USA, the Department of Agriculture maintains the nutrient database (www.ars.usda.gov).

In 1984, the United Nations University's Food and Nutrition Programme set up the International Network of Food Data Systems (INFOODS), coordinated by the Food and Agriculture Organization (FAO), to improve the quality of food data and also to enable worldwide access. The website of INFOODS (www.fao.org/infoods/

infoods/en/) provides information about all existing food composition tables, some of which are directly accessible through the website.

Derivation of food table data

Before using food table data, it is essential to read the introduction explaining how the values in the tables were derived. This is particularly important if food composition data from more than one source are used alongside standard food table data, e.g. food labelling information, or food tables from other countries, because the definition and expression of the nutrients may not be the same. The factors discussed in the following subsections should be considered when using food composition tables or databases.

Analytical methodology

Different analytical techniques can be used to obtain estimates of the same nutrient. Historically, food analysis consisted of determining the percentage of water, fat, nitrogen and ash (minerals) in a food. Multiplying the percentage of nitrogen by 6.25 derived protein content, as protein is 16% nitrogen on average. While the latter is still widely used, it is now recognised that the amount of nitrogen depends on the protein source (FAO, 2003). Carbohydrate content was estimated by difference, i.e. the percentage of other nutrients was calculated, and carbohydrate was assumed to be the remaining percentage needed to give 100%. This derived figure for carbohydrate included the contribution from dietary fibre or other dietary components.

More recently, chemical analyses methods have become more sophisticated, so different types of sugars (glucose, fructose, galactose, sucrose, maltose, lactose and oligosaccharides) and complex carbohydrates (dextrins, starch and glycogen), amino acids and fatty acids, as well as individual minerals and vitamins, can now be determined. Information on manufactured foods not included in the food tables can increasingly be obtained from food labels or food manufacturers, but much commercial food analysis is still carried out using simpler analytical techniques.

The use of a range of methodologies will result in different estimates of nutrient content. Carbohydrates may be determined as monosaccharide equivalents, actual weights or by difference, as described earlier. Monosaccharide equivalents, the usual form of expression in UK food tables, result in slightly higher estimates of carbohydrate content than when expressed as actual weight, as on most food labels (due to the fact that disaccharides and polysaccharides gain water when hydrolysed). Direct determination of carbohydrates is used in the Food Databanks.

Dietary fibre can be analysed using different methods that give differing estimates. The *McCance and Widdowson* tables and the Food Databank give estimates for non-starch polysaccharides (NSP) based on the Englyst method (Englyst *et al.*, 1994). However, the food industry measures fibre by the AOAC enzymatic gravimetric method, which is now recommended for food labelling purposes. The AOAC method usually gives much higher estimates of fibre content, particularly for cereals, because it includes lignin (or substances measuring as lignin) and resistant starch. The seventh edition of *McCance and Widdowson's The Composition of Foods* (Finglas *et al.*, 2015) includes fibre content of foods measured by both the Englyst and AOAC methods.

Many vitamins are composites of substances with variable degrees of activity and the concentrations will depend on the type of analysis performed. For example, vitamin A may be expressed as retinol and beta-carotene separately, or as retinol equivalents. Different units may also be used (micrograms or International Units, IU). The two components of vitamin A are given separately as retinol (RET) and carotene (CAREQU). Retinol is expressed as the weight of all trans retinol equivalents, i.e. the sum of all trans retinol plus contributions from the other forms after correction to account for their relative activities.

Energy conversion factors used to calculate data

The energy content of food may be measured by bomb calorimetry, but not all food energy can be metabolised; therefore, the conversion factors accounting for this are used to calculate energy yield. Atwater and colleagues derived these factors from meticulous human studies over a century ago (Atwater & Benedict, 1902). It is important to remember that slightly different Atwater factor systems may be used, and the energy content of foods may vary between McCance and Widdowson tables or the Food Databanks and those required for food labelling declarations (Table 2.4.3).

Sampling procedure

Food composition data are derived from a sample of foods and, therefore, their accuracy depends on how representative the sample is. The UK food tables are designed to be as representative as possible. Significant numbers of food samples are purchased from different retail outlets and pooled before analysis. Market share information is used to assess which brands of a particular type of food are included, and recipes are chosen to be as similar as possible to those used in the normal domestic setting. Other sources of food composition data may not be based on such high standards. Details of the samples used in analysis are given for each food item in the tables and database.

Regular data updating

Food composition tables need to be regularly updated for the following reasons:

- New manufactured foods are constantly developed – new manufacturing practices may change the composition of manufactured foods as a result of product reformulation, altered manufacturing processes,

Table 2.4.3 Energy conversion factors (source: Webster-Gandy *et al.* 2012, Table 1.2, p. 11. Reproduced with permission from Oxford University Press)

Nutrient	kcal/g	kJ/g	Comments
Protein	4	17	For food labelling purposes, multiplying the nitrogen content in all foods by 6.25 derives protein content.
			UK food tables use specific conversion factors for different types of foods.
Fat	9	37	The original Atwater factor was 8.9 kcal, but the lower kJ figure is preferable.
Carbohydrate	3.75	16	If carbohydrate is expressed directly or by difference, 4 kcal/g is used, which is the figure used on food labels.
			Values for available carbohydrate are expressed as monosaccharides.
Fibre	2	8	
Polyols (sugar alcohols)	2.4	10	Food labelling uses mean value.
Alcohol (ethanol)	7	29	
Glycerol	4.31	18	Complete metabolism assumed.

fortification and use of nutrients such as beta-carotene or vitamin C as colourings or antioxidants.

- Changes in farming practices can alter the composition of plant and animal products. For example, the fat content and fatty acid profile of meat has changed considerably in the last 30 years due to selective breeding programmes to produce leaner animals, changes in feeding techniques and from modern butchery techniques removing more carcass fat. Development of new crop varieties or changes in fertiliser use can also affect nutritional composition.
- Domestic preparation and cooking practices may change, e.g. vegetables may be steamed rather than boiled, and bread may be made from a domestic bread-making machine.
- New varieties or new sources of supply for raw materials – previously unfamiliar foods are now available in shops, e.g. associated with migrating populations.
- More accurate methods of analysis are developed, e.g. fibre.

The use of old analytical data will considerably increase the likelihood of errors, which will introduce significant errors in even the most detailed dietary assessment. However, in some circumstances, e.g. the analysis of dietary information obtained many years ago, it may be necessary to use composition data that were contemporary at the time in order to obtain realistic estimates of nutrient intake. It is particularly important that those engaged in dietary survey work be aware of the implications of using data from older editions and supplements of *McCance and Widdowson's The Composition of Foods* (Black & Paul, 1999). There are also a number of differences in code numbers between editions of food tables, which can have implications in computerised analysis; a list of current and previous codes is included in the food index to the seventh summary edition of *McCance and Widdowson's The Composition of Foods* (Finglas *et al.*, 2015). It is also important to know which data have been incorporated into nutrient analysis programmes.

Limitations of food composition data

Food tables are an extremely valuable resource, but it is important to understand their limitations and associated problems. Food tables and databases will always have limitations for several reasons, including variability between foods consumed and food table values and bioavailability.

Variability between foods consumed and food table values

Despite careful sampling, the resultant values may be representative of a particular food, but there will still be some variation from foods actually consumed. A number of factors – such as plant or animal species, seasonal changes in feeding practices or growing conditions, or the effects of storage on water content – affect the composition of foods such as meat, milk, eggs or plant crops. Further variability is likely to occur as a result of differences in food manufacture, catering or domestic cooking practices. For example, a lasagne may be a manufactured ready meal, an item prepared by a restaurant or made at home. All will differ in composition, and probably none will exactly match the values given in food tables. In Western diets, comparisons of the nutrient content of diets calculated from food tables and analysed by direct analysis have been shown to range between 2 and 20% (Bingham, 1987). This variability is most likely to occur with micronutrient content due to the following reasons:

- The soil in which a plant was grown, e.g. soil variation can markedly affect selenium content.
- Agricultural practices, e.g. antagonism between soil fertilisation using nitrogen and vitamin C.
- Stage of maturity, e.g. in plant foods, vitamin C content decreases during ripening, whereas carotenoid content increases.
- Duration and conditions of storage before consumption, e.g. water-soluble vitamin content will diminish with time.

- The way the food is cooked, e.g. the potassium content of boiled vegetables will depend on the amount of water used and length of cooking time.
- Use of food fortification in some but not all brands of a particular food, e.g. folate or iron added to breakfast cereals.
- Use of food additives that are also nutrients, e.g. beta-carotene (colour) or vitamin C (antioxidant) may be unexpectedly present in foods such as meat products.

Vitamin C and folic acid naturally vary widely in foods, and both are sensitive to heat and light. In food table analyses, vegetables would usually have been cooked in distilled water and without added salt. This means that the measured content of sodium, chloride and calcium (present in tap water) will be lower than is likely in the domestic setting.

For most dietetic purposes, the importance of any differences between theoretical and actual nutrient composition may be relatively insignificant in the average mixed diet. However, for metabolic studies based on the consumption of very few foods, or where extreme precision is required, duplicates of the actual foods concerned must be prepared for direct laboratory analysis.

Bioavailability

Bioavailability is defined as the proportion of a nutrient that can be absorbed and hence available to the human body. Bioavailability can vary according to several factors:

- Source, e.g. calcium in milk is absorbed more readily than calcium in bread.
- Chemical form, e.g. absorption of haem iron is greater than that of non-haem iron.
- Ease with which the nutrient can be released from the food, e.g. some carbohydrate in fibrous foods cannot be digested and is lost in faeces.
- Presence of factors that inhibit absorption, e.g. phytates in cereal foods can reduce calcium absorption.
- Presence of factors that enhance absorption, e.g. vitamin C enhances absorption of non-haem iron.
- Physiological factors – absorption may be increased in states of nutritional depletion or at times of increased need, e.g. pregnancy.

Bioavailability is most likely to impact on minerals and trace elements such as calcium, magnesium, iron, zinc, copper, manganese and selenium, and vitamins such as folate and B_6. Since these interactions are so variable, UK food tables take no account of bioavailability, and the nutrient content given in the food table is the amount present in the food. The only exception is the allowance made for the reduced activities of the different forms of some vitamins, e.g. 13-cis retinol and retinaldehyde (vitamin A), carotenes other than beta-carotene, and tocopherols and tocotrieols other than alpha-tocopherol (vitamin E). It is important to check if the food composition data nutrient values have been modified to account for bioavailability.

Errors associated with the use of food composition data

Coding errors

In addition to the inherent errors in food table data, additional errors may be introduced into nutrient analysis programmes in the following ways:

- Missing nutrient values in food composition tables may be treated as zero values during calculation, resulting in an underestimation of nutrient intake.
- There may not be a suitable code for the food consumed, or an inappropriate code may be chosen.
- There may be incorrect entry of food code numbers into the computing system.
- Errors can occur in the measurement, recording and estimation of food weights.
- Misclassification can result from a food having different names in different countries or regions within. This is particularly important when working with other nationalities, e.g. in the USA, chips refer to potato crisps rather than fried potatoes as used in the UK.

Interpretation errors based on contribution to the diet

Food tables are useful to help identify good and poor food sources of nutrients, but are not always used appropriately. The values given in tables will identify foods that are particularly concentrated sources of a nutrient, but this does not necessarily mean that a food is an important source of that nutrient in the typical diet. The contribution that a particular food makes to nutrient intake depends on the:

- Concentration of nutrient in the food (content per 100 g) and its bioavailability.
- Amount of the food consumed, i.e. portion size.
- Frequency with which the food is consumed.

For example, parsley is a highly concentrated source of vitamin C, but is unlikely to be a significant dietary source, because it is usually eaten infrequently and in small quantities. In contrast, potatoes are a much less concentrated source of vitamin C, but, because they are a regular feature of many UK diets, they may make a major dietary contribution to vitamin C intake. When giving dietary advice, it is important to remember that, however valuable a food may be as a source of a particularly nutrient, it will make only a small contribution to dietary intake if it is rarely eaten.

Further reading

Greenfield H, Southgate DAT. (2003) *Food Composition Data: Production, Management and Use*, 2nd edn. Rome: FAO.

Klensin JC, Feskanich D, Lin Truswell AS, *et al.* (1989) *Identification of Food Components for INFOODS Data Interchange*. Hong Kong: The United Nations University.

Rand WM, Pennington JAT, Murphy SP, *et al.* (1991) *Compiling Data for Food Composition Data Bases*. Hong Kong: The United Nations University.

Internet resources

EuroFIR Project Website with Information on European Food Composition Databases, http://www.eurofir.org

FAO – INFOODS Information for Nutrient Database Compilers and Suppliers http://www.fao.org/infoods/infoods/en

Food Databanks National Capability, https://fdnc.quadram.ac.uk

USDA Nutrient Data Laboratory, http://www.ars.usda.gov/main/site_main.htm?modecode=80-40-05-25

References

Atwater WO, Benedict FG. (1902) *Experiments on the Metabolism of Matter and Energy in the Human Body, 1898–1900. US Office of Experiment Stations Bulletin No. 109.* Washington, DC: Government Printing Office.

Bingham S. (1987) The dietary assessment of individuals: methods, accuracy, new techniques and recommendations. *Nutr. Abstr. Rev.* 57: 705–742.

Black AE, Paul AA. (1999) McCance & Widdowson's Tables of Food Composition: Origins and Clarification of the Fifth Edition. *J. Hum. Nutr. Diet.* 12: 1–5.

Chan W, Brown J, Buss DH. (1994) *Miscellaneous Foods: Fourth Supplement to The Composition of Foods*, 5th edn. Cambridge: Royal Society of Chemistry/MAFF.

Chan WW, Brown J, Lee SM, *et al.* (1995) *Meat, Poultry and Game: Fifth Supplement to McCance and Widdowson's The Composition of Foods*, 5th edn. Cambridge: Royal Society of Chemistry/MAFF.

Chan W, Brown J, Church SM, et al. (1996) *Meat Products and Dishes: Sixth Supplement to McCance and Widdowson's The Composition of Foods*, 5th edn. Cambridge: Royal Society of Chemistry/MAFF.

Church SM. (2006) The history of food composition databases. *Nutr. Bull.* 31: 15–20.

Englyst HN, Quigley ME, Hudson GJ. (1994) Determination of dietary fibre as non-starch polysaccharides with gas–liquid chromatographic, high-performance liquid chromatographic or spectrophotometric measurement of constituent sugars. *Analyst.* 119: 1497–1509.

Finglas PM, Roe MA, Pinchen HM, *et al.* (2015) *McCance and Widdowson's The Composition of Foods*, 7th summary edn. Cambridge: Royal Society of Chemistry.

Food and Agriculture Organization of the United Nations (FAO). (2003) *Food Energy – Methods of Analysis and Conversion Factors (Technical report).* Rome: FAOUN.

Holland B, Brown J, Buss DH. (1993) *Fish and Fish Products: Third Supplement to the Composition of Foods*, 5th edn. Cambridge: Royal Society of Chemistry/MAFF.

Holland B, Unwin ID, Buss DH. (1988) *Cereals and Cereal Products: Third Supplement to McCance and Widdowson's The Composition of Foods*, 4th edn. Cambridge: Royal Society of Chemistry/MAFF.

Holland B, Unwin ID, Buss DH. (1989) *Milk Products and Eggs: Fourth Supplement to McCance and Widdowson's The Composition of Foods*, 4th edn. Cambridge: Royal Society of Chemistry/MAFF.

Holland B, Welch AA, Unwin ID, *et al.* (1991a) *McCance and Widdowson's The Composition of Foods*, 5th edn. Cambridge: Royal Society of Chemistry/MAFF.

Holland B, Unwin ID, Buss DH. (1991b) *Vegetables, Herbs, and Spices: Fifth Supplement to McCance and Widdowson's The Composition of Foods*, 4th edn. Cambridge: Royal Society of Chemistry/MAFF.

Holland B, Unwin ID, Buss DH. (1992a) *Fruit and Nuts: First Supplement to McCance and Widdowson's The Composition of Foods*, 5th edn. Cambridge: Royal Society of Chemistry/MAFF.

Holland B, Welch A, Buss DH. (1992b) *Vegetable Dishes: Second Supplement to McCance and Widdowson's The Composition of Foods*, 5th edn. Cambridge: Royal Society of Chemistry/MAFF.

Judd PA, Kassam-Khamis T, Thomas JE. (2000) *The Composition and Nutrient Content of Foods Commonly Consumed by South Asians in the UK*. London: The Aga Khan Health Board for the United Kingdom.

Ministry of Agriculture, Fisheries and Food (MAFF). (1998) *Fatty Acids: Seventh Supplement to The Composition of Foods*, 5th edn. Cambridge: Royal Society of Chemistry/MAFF.

Paul AA, Southgate DAT, Russell J. (1980) *Amino Acid Composition (mg per 100g food) and Fatty Acid Composition (g per 100g food): First Supplement to McCance and Widdowson's The Composition of Foods*, 4th edn. London/Cambridge: HMSO/Royal Society of Chemistry.

Tan SP Wenlock RWW, Buss DH. (1985) *Immigrant Foods: Second Supplement to McCance and Widdowson's The Composition of Foods*, 4th edn. London/Cambridge: HMSO/Royal Society of Chemistry.

Webster-Gandy J, Madden A, Holdsworth M. (2012) *Oxford Handbook of Nutrition and Dietetics*, 2nd edn. Oxford: Oxford University Press.

SECTION 3

Nutrition in specific groups

3.1 Women's health

3.1.1 Polycystic ovary syndrome

Yvonne Jeanes

Key points

- Polycystic ovary syndrome (PCOS) presents with a range of symptoms of varying severity.
- Weight management should be the primary therapy in overweight women with PCOS; binge eating behaviour is common in PCOS.
- Dietary modification should aim to improve insulin resistance.
- A patient-centred approach is needed to improve symptoms and reduce the risk of developing diabetes and cardiovascular disease.

Polycystic ovary syndrome (PCOS) is a heterogeneous condition, and women present with one or several of the following symptoms: menstrual irregularity and fertility problems, excess male-pattern hair (hirsutism), male-pattern baldness (alopecia), acne, central adiposity, insulin resistance and depression. Symptoms vary in severity and can change over the lifecycle. PCOS often becomes clinically apparent during adolescence. The diagnostic criteria for PCOS are the presence of two of the following features and exclusion of other endocrine disorders (ESHRE/ASRM, 2004):

- Ovulatory dysfunction – oligo-ovulation leading to oligomenorrhoea (<9 menses/year), or anovulation.
- Androgen excess – clinically (hirsutism, male-pattern alopecia, acne) or biochemically.
- Polycystic ovaries (detected by ultrasound) – several immature follicles (not cysts) around the edge of the ovaries.

Polycystic ovaries (PCO) alone is not diagnostic of PCOS. PCOS can be categorised into the following subgroups (NIH, 2012):

1. Androgen excess and ovulatory dysfunction.
2. Androgen excess and PCO.
3. Ovulatory dysfunction and PCO.
4. Androgen excess, ovulatory dysfunction and PCO.

Women who have androgen excess and ovulatory dysfunction are at the greatest metabolic risk (Bil *et al.*, 2016; Jeanes & Reeves, 2017).

The aetiology of PCOS is complex, with a genetic heritability that is enhanced by environmental factors, especially obesity (Dumesic *et al.*, 2015). Although insulin resistance is not among the diagnostic criteria, both lean and overweight women with PCOS have a form of insulin resistance intrinsic to PCOS (Diamanti-Kandarakis & Dunaif, 2012). Insulin acts directly on the ovary by stimulating androgen production, and reduces the hepatic production of sex hormone–binding globulin (SHBG), resulting in higher free testosterone levels. In combination, hyperinsulinaemia and hyperandrogenemia can disrupt follicle growth, accompanied by menstrual irregularity, anovulatory subfertility and accumulation of immature follicles (Diamanti-Kandarakis & Dunaif, 2012).

Disease consequences

PCOS affects up to 18% of women of reproductive age (March *et al.*, 2010). There is a greater prevalence of obesity (body mass index, BMI >30 kg/m^2) and central obesity as compared to women without PCOS (Lim *et al.*, 2012). Obese women with PCOS are generally more symptomatic and at greater health risk as compared to lean

Manual of Dietetic Practice, Sixth Edition. Edited by Joan Gandy.

Companion website: www.manualofdieteticpractice.com

women with PCOS (Lim *et al.*, 2013). Women with PCOS have a greater risk of developing impaired glucose tolerance (IGT), gestational diabetes and type 2 diabetes mellitus as compared to BMI-matched healthy women. Meta-analyses have reported odds ratios (ORs) of 2.54 for IGT (Moran *et al.*, 2010), 3.43 for gestational diabetes (Qin *et al.*, 2013) and 4.00 for type 2 diabetes mellitus (Moran *et al.*, 2010) (see Chapter 7.12, Diabetes mellitus).

The risk of metabolic syndrome and non-alcoholic hepatic disease (NAFLD) is also higher; meta-analyses reported ORs of 2.20 for metabolic syndrome (Moran *et al.*, 2010) and 3.93 for NAFLD (Ramezani-Binabaj *et al.*, 2014). Women with PCOS have an increased risk of cardiovascular disease (CVD) (Wild *et al.*, 2011) (see Chapter 7.14, Cardiovascular disease). Subsequently, PCOS is significantly associated with an increased risk of coronary heart disease (CHD) (OR 1.44) (Zhao *et al.*, 2016), although there is no increased risk of myocardial infarction. Women with PCOS are at increased risk of endometrial cancer (OR, 2.79); however, the increased risk could be attributed, at least in part, to obesity (Barry *et al.*, 2014).

The symptoms associated with PCOS have been shown to lead to a reduction in health-related quality of life (Jones *et al.*, 2008). Depression and anxiety are common in PCOS (Dokras *et al.*, 2011, 2012). Some studies have shown a higher prevalence of eating disorders in women with PCOS (Morgan *et al.*, 2008; Kerchner *et al.*, 2009). Binge eating behaviours are commonly reported, including in lean women with PCOS (Jeanes *et al.*, 2017). Jeanes et al. (2017) reported similar food cravings in lean women with PCOS and healthy women, and greater food cravings in obese women with PCOS compared with overweight women with PCOS. Although there is a paucity of well-designed studies investigating the eating behaviours of women with PCOS, it is important to consider the psychological impact of PCOS.

Clinical management

Management focuses on treating the symptoms. Lifestyle management to promote weight loss is advocated as the primary therapy in overweight and obese women with PCOS. Weight loss of 5–10% improves many of the associated symptoms (Haqq *et al.*, 2014).

Medical treatments are available for hirsutism, acne and infertility. Metformin is commonly prescribed, as it reduces serum insulin levels in insulin-resistant individuals, and it is also associated with improved pregnancy rates when combined with clomiphene; clomiphene alone is more effective than metformin alone (Tang et al., 2012).

Nutritional consequences

There are no known nutritional consequences specific to PCOS.

Nutritional assessment

Anthropometric measurements include BMI and waist circumference to inform the risk of comorbidities and dietary management. An assessment of dietary habits should also aim to detect any binge eating behaviour (see Chapter 7.10.2, Eating disorders). Many international guidelines recommend screening for IGT and CVD risk factors (Legro *et al.*, 2013; RCOG, 2014).

Nutritional management

Weight loss through dietary restriction and increased physical activity are the primary management strategies for overweight and obese women with PCOS (RCOG, 2014). Studies that have demonstrated the clinical benefit of weight loss in women with PCOS have incorporated a variety of methods to reduce energy intake (Moran *et al.*, 2013). A patient-centred approach that addresses the needs and preferences of patients is important, and behaviour change strategies are recognised as instrumental in weight management (see Chapter 7.13.2, The management of obesity and overweight in adults). A high dropout rate has been reported in lifestyle interventions in infertile overweight/obese women (Mutsaerts *et al.*, 2013). Furthermore, Jeanes *et al.* showed that 40–50% of overweight/obese women with PCOS were not following a diet that would promote weight loss. Barriers to successful dietary and physical activity modification include feeling frustrated and hungry, interference with other responsibilities, adherence difficulty, lack of time and tiredness (Jeanes *et al.*, 2017). The reported hunger may allude to lower meal-stimulated ghrelin levels measured in women with PCOS (Arusoglu *et al.*, 2013); additionally, studies have shown than testosterone stimulates food intake (Asarian & Geary, 2006).

Bariatric surgery results in substantial weight loss and marked improvement of biochemical abnormalities in women with PCOS; a recent meta-analysis reported a reduction in the incidence of PCOS from 45.6 to 6.8% at 12-month follow-up (Skubleny *et al.*, 2016) (see Chapter 13.3, Bariatric surgery). Modifying carbohydrate and fatty acid content of the diet have been proposed as improving insulin sensitivity. Hyperinsulinaemia has a detrimental effect on PCOS symptoms; reducing insulin may therefore be beneficial. Lower glycaemic index (GI) foods or lower glycaemic load (GL) should also be incorporated to additionally reduce risk factors for CVD (see Chapter 7.14.1, General aspects of cardiovascular disease). Greater improvement in insulin sensitivity and regular menses were reported after weight loss with a low dietary GI approach as compared to weight loss through conventional healthy eating (Marsh *et al.*, 2010). Furthermore, Mehrabani *et al.* (2012) reported a reduction in insulin resistance after a hypocaloric, high-protein diet with a lower GL as compared to a conventional hypocaloric healthy-eating intervention. Barr *et al.* (2013) demonstrated an improvement in insulin sensitivity with an isocaloric, reduced GI dietary intervention. These small studies suggest a benefit for promoting lower GI dietary advice to women with PCOS; however, well-controlled studies are needed to improve the evidence base for dietary recommendations.

Dietary saturated fatty acids (SFAs) can influence inflammatory mediators and disrupt insulin signalling (Galgani *et al.*, 2008). Thus, a reduction of total fat intake should focus on lowering SFA intake concurrently with the maintenance of monounsaturated fatty acids and polyunsaturated fatty acids (which do not interrupt metabolism and inflammation to the same extent). Advanced glycation end products (AGEs), pro-inflammatory molecules, are elevated in PCOS (Tantalaki *et al.*, 2014). AGEs derive from endogenous production or can be ingested in high amounts from fast-food. A small study has shown that a 2-month intervention of a low dietary intake of AGEs is associated with improved levels of serum testosterone, oxidative stress and HOMA-IR in PCOS. The role of dietary AGEs as mediators of metabolic and reproductive alterations is an emerging area of dietary modification for PCOS (Tantalaki *et al.*, 2014).

A high proportion of women with PCOS report taking nutrient or herbal supplements, which many felt had a beneficial effect on their symptoms (Jeanes *et al.*, 2009). Vitamin D supplementation has been suggested, as a deficiency has been associated with insulin resistance in women with PCOS, though clinical supplementation studies are inconsistent (He *et al.*, 2015). Several small trials with n-3 fatty acid supplementation indicate beneficial effects on menstrual cyclicity, blood lipids, glucose and insulin levels in women with PCOS, although no effects on reproductive hormones were reported (Nadjarzadeh *et al.*, 2013; Phelan *et al.*, 2011). Chromium picolinate (200–1000 μg/day) may improve insulin sensitivity and ovulation; however, weight loss during the interventions would have influenced the outcomes (Ashoush *et al.*, 2016; Jamilian & Asemi, 2015). A small study reported that cinnamon supplements (1.5 g/day) improved menstrual cyclicity. Cinnamon extract is theorised to improve insulin sensitivity; however, insulin levels were not affected (Kort & Lobo, 2014). Myo-inositol (2 g bds) may improve insulin sensitivity, glucose tolerance, menstrual regularity and ovulation rate; however, well-controlled studies are needed (Facchinetti *et al.*, 2015; Tang *et al.*, 2012).

Consideration of patient-centred immediate goals (improvement of symptoms, fertility, and weight loss) as well as reducing long-term health risks should be incorporated in the dietary management of PCOS. Women who are trying to conceive should also be following a nutritionally adequate diet with folic acid supplements.

Drug–nutrient interactions

Oral contraceptives may negatively impact on insulin sensitivity and dyslipidaemia. Metformin can cause gastrointestinal side effects such as nausea and diarrhoea.

Internet resources

NICE Clinical Knowledge Summary PCOS, cks.nice.org.uk/polycystic-ovary-syndrome#!scenario

PCOS UK, www.pcos-uk.org.uk

Verity (a self-help group for women with PCOS), www.verity-pcos.org.uk

References

Arusoglu G, Koksal G, Cinar N, *et al.* (2013) Basal and meal stimulated ghrelin, PYY, CCK levels and satiety in lean women with polycystic ovary syndrome: effect of low-dose oral contraceptive. *J. Clin. Endocrinol. Metabol.* 98: 4475–4482.

Asarian L, Geary N. (2006) Modulation of appetite by gonadal steroid hormones. *Philos. Trans. R. Soc. Lond. B, Biol. Sci.* 36: 1251–1263.

Ashoush S, Abou-Gamrah A, Bayoumy H, *et al.* (2016) Chromium picolinate reduces insulin resistance in polycystic ovary syndrome: Randomized controlled trial. *J. Obstet. Gynaecol. Res.* 42: 279–285.

Barr S, Reeves S, Sharp K, *et al.* (2013) An isocaloric low glycemic diet improves insulin sensitivity in women with polycystic ovary syndrome. *J. Acad. Nutr. Diet.* 113: 1523–1531.

Barry JA, Azizia MM, Hardiman PJ. (2014) Risk of endometrial, ovarian and breast cancer in women with polycystic ovary syndrome: a systematic review and meta-analysis. *Hum. Reprod. Update.* 20: 748–758.

Bil E, Dilbaz B, Cirik DA, *et al.* (2016) Metabolic syndrome and metabolic risk profile according to polycystic ovary syndrome phenotype. *J. Obstet. Gynaecol. Res.* 42: 837–842.

Diamanti-Kandarakis E, Dunaif A. (2012) Insulin resistance and the polycystic syndrome revisited: an update on mechanisms and implications. *Endocr. Rev.* 33: 981–1030.

Dokras A, Clifton S, Futterweit W, *et al.* (2011) Increased risk for abnormal depression scores in women with polycystic ovary syndrome: a systematic review and meta-analysis. *Obstet. Gynecol.* 117: 145–152.

Dokras A, Clifton S, Futterweit W, *et al.* (2012) Increased prevalence of anxiety symptoms in women with polycystic ovary syndrome: systematic review and meta-analysis. *Fertil. Steril.* 97: 225–230.

Dumesic DA, Oberfield SE, Stener-Victorin E, *et al.* (2015) Scientific statement on the diagnostic criteria, epidemiology, pathophysiology, and molecular genetics of polycystic ovary syndrome. *Endocr. Rev.* 36: 487–525.

ESHRE/ASRM PCOS Consensus Workshop Group. (2004) Revised 2003 consensus on diagnostic criteria and long-term health risks related to polycystic ovary syndrome. *Fertil. Steril.* 81: 19–25.

Facchinetti F, Bizzarri M, Benvenga S, *et al.* (2015) Results from the International Consensus Conference on Myo-inositol and d-chiro-inositol in Obstetrics and Gynecology: the link between metabolic syndrome and PCOS. *Eur. J. Obstet. Gynaecol. Reprod. Biol.* 195: 72–76.

Galgani JE, Uauy RD, Aguirre CA, *et al.* (2008) Effect of the dietary fat quality on insulin sensitivity. *Br. J. Nutr.* 100: 471–479.

Haqq L, McFarlane J, Dieberg G, *et al.* (2014) Effect of lifestyle intervention on the reproductive endocrine profile in women with polycystic ovarian syndrome: a systematic review and meta-analysis. *Endocr. Connect.* 28: 36–46.

He C, Lin Z, Robb SW, *et al.* (2015) Serum vitamin D levels and polycystic ovary syndrome: a systematic review and meta-analysis. *Nutrients* 7: 4555–4577.

Jamilian M, Asemi Z. (2015) Chromium supplementation and the effects on metabolic status in women with polycystic ovary syndrome: a randomized, double-blind, placebo-controlled trial. *Ann. Nutr. Metab.* 67: 42–48.

Jeanes Y, Barr S, Smith K, Hart KH. (2009). Dietary management of women with polycystic ovary syndrome in the United Kingdom: the role of dietitians. *J. Hum. Nutr. Diet.* 22: 551–558.

Jeanes Y, Reeves S. (2017) Metabolic consequences of obesity and insulin resistance in polycystic ovary syndrome; diagnostic and methodological challenges. *Nutr. Res. Rev.* 30: 97–105.

Jeanes Y, Reeves S, Gibson EL, *et al.* (2017) Binge eating behaviours and food cravings in women with polycystic ovary syndrome. *Appetite.* 109: 24–32.

Jones GL, Hall JM, Balen AH, *et al.* (2008) Health-related quality of life measurement in women with polycystic ovary syndrome: a systematic review. *Hum. Reprod. Update* 14: 15–25.

Kerchner A, Lester W, Stuart SP, Dokras A. (2009) Risk of depression and other mental health disorders in women with polycystic ovary syndrome: a longitudinal study. *Fertility and Sterility* 91: 207–212.

Kort DH, Lobo RA. (2014) Preliminary evidence that cinnamon improves menstrual cyclicity in women with polycystic ovary syndrome: a randomized controlled trial. *Am. J. Obstet. Gynacol.* 211: 487–488.

Legro RS, Arslanian SA, Ehrmann DA, *et al.* (2013) Endocrine Society. Diagnosis and treatment of polycystic ovary syndrome: an Endocrine Society clinical practice guideline. *J. Clin. Endocrinol. Metab.* 98: 4565–4592.

Lim SS, Davies MJ, Norman RJ, *et al.* (2012) Overweight, obesity and central obesity in women with polycystic ovary syndrome: a systematic review and meta-analysis. *Hum. Reprod. Update* 18(6): 618–637.

Lim SS, Norman RJ, Davies MJ, *et al.* (2013) The effect of obesity on polycystic ovary syndrome: a systematic review and meta-analysis. *Obes. Rev.* 14(2): 95–109.

March WA, Moore VM, Willson KJ, *et al.* (2010) The prevalence of polycystic ovary syndrome in a community sample assessed under contrasting diagnostic criteria. *Hum. Reprod.* 25: 544–551.

Marsh K, Steinbeck KS, Atkinson FS, *et al.* (2010) Effect of a low glycaemic index compared with a conventional healthy diet on polycystic ovary syndrome. *Am. J. Clin. Nutr.* 92: 83–92.

Mehrabani HH, Salehpour S, Amiri Z. (2012) Beneficial effects of a high-protein, low-glycemic-load hypocaloric diet in overweight and obese women with polycystic ovary syndrome: a randomized controlled intervention study. *J. Am. Coll. Nutr.* 31: 117–125.

Moran LJ, Misso ML, Wild RA, *et al.* (2010) Impaired glucose tolerance, type 2 diabetes and metabolic syndrome in polycystic ovary syndrome: a systematic review and meta-analysis. *Hum. Reprod. Update* 16: 347–363.

Moran LJ, Ko H, Misso M, *et al.* (2013) Dietary composition in the treatment of polycystic ovary syndrome: a systematic review to inform evidence-based guidelines. *J. Acad. Nutr. Diet.* 113: 520–545.

Morgan J, Schotz S, Lacey H, *et al.* (2008) The prevalence of eating disorders in women with facial hirsutism: An epidemiological cohort study. *Int. J. Eat. Disord.* 41: 427–431.

Mutsaerts MA, Kuchenbecker WK, Mol BW, *et al.* (2013) Dropout is a problem in lifestyle intervention programs for overweight and obese infertile women: a systematic review. *Hum. Reprod.* 28: 979–986.

Nadjarzadeh A, Dehghani Firouzabadi R, Vaziri N, *et al.* (2013) The effect of omega-3 supplementation on androgen profile and menstrual status in women with polycystic ovary syndrome: a randomized clinical trial. *Iran J. Reprod. Med.* 11: 665–672.

NIH. (2012) *Evidence-based methodology workshop on polycystic ovary syndrome.* Available at https://prevention.nih.gov/docs/programs/pcos/FinalReport.pdf. Accessed 21 July 2016.

Phelan N, O'Connor A, Tun TK, *et al.* (2011) Hormonal and metabolic effects of polyunsaturated fatty acids in young women with polycystic ovary syndrome: results from a cross-sectional analysis and a randomized, placebo-controlled, crossover trial. *Am. J. Clin. Nutr.* 93: 652–662.

Qin JZ, Pang LH, Li MJ, *et al.* (2013) Obstetric complications in women with polycystic ovary syndrome: a systematic review and meta-analysis. *Reprod. Biol. Endocrinol.* 11: 56.

Ramezani-Binabaj M, Motalebi M, Karimi-Sari H, *et al.* (2014) Are women with polycystic ovarian syndrome at a high risk of non-alcoholic fatty liver disease; a meta-analysis. *Hepat. Mon.* 14: e23235.

Royal College of Obstetricians and Gynaecologists (RCOG). (2014) *Long-term consequences of polycystic ovary syndrome. Green-top Guideline No. 33.* Available at https://www.rcog.org.uk/en/guidelines-research-services/guidelines/gtg33/. Accessed 20 July 2016.

Skubleny D, Switzer NJ, Gill RS, *et al.* (2016) The impact of bariatric surgery on Polycystic Ovary Syndrome: a systematic review and meta-analysis. *Obes. Surg.* 26: 169–176.

Tang T, Lord JM, Norman RJ, *et al.* (2012) Insulin-sensitising drugs (metformin, rosiglitazone, pioglitazone, D-chiroinositol) for women with polycystic ovary syndrome, oligo amenorrhoea and subfertility. *Cochrane Database Syst. Rev.* (5): CD003053.

Tantalaki E, Piperi C, Livadas S, *et al.* (2014) Impact of dietary modification of advanced glycation end products (AGEs) on the hormonal and metabolic profile of women with polycystic ovary syndrome (PCOS). *Hormones.* 13: 65–73.

Wild RA, Rizzo M, Clifton S, *et al.* (2011) Lipid levels in polycystic ovary syndrome: systematic review and meta-analysis. *Fertil. Steril.* 95: 1073–1079.

Zhao L, Zhu Z, Lou H, *et al.* (2016) Polycystic ovary syndrome (PCOS) and the risk of coronary heart disease (CHD): a meta-analysis. *Oncotarget.* 7: 33715–33721.

3.1.2 Premenstrual syndrome

Gaynor Bussell

Key points

- Most women experience premenstrual symptoms; for 8–20%, it is severe.
- Premenstrual symptoms are cyclical and do not occur in anovulatory cycles; it is unrelated to hormonal levels.
- A healthy diet and lifestyle, including avoiding excessive weight gain, can help relieve symptoms.
- Adequate dietary sources of calcium and vitamin D are important. The evidence for the use of supplements is equivocal.

Premenstrual syndrome (PMS) is cyclical and occurs during the luteal phase (1–2 weeks before menstruation); symptoms are relieved by the onset of or during menstruation. Most women experience mild symptoms. However, for 8–20%, its severity can prompt them to seek medical treatment (Chocano-Bedoya *et al.*, 2011); the most severe form, premenstrual dysphoric disorder (PMD), affects 3–8% (Ryu & Kim, 2015).

Symptoms of PMS vary between and within individuals and include mood swings, irritability, increased appetite, carbohydrate and alcohol cravings, breast tenderness, headaches and bloating (Bertone-Johnson *et al.*, 2015). Women with chronic disease, e.g. diabetes, irritable bowel syndrome (IBS) or allergies, may have a low threshold for developing PMS (Altman *et al.*, 2006, Bussell, 1998). Good control of chronic medical conditions may reduce the severity of symptoms (Bussell, 1998).

Aetiology

The cause of PMS is unknown, but it is believed to be due to an increased sensitivity to circulating progesterone and its metabolites (Brown *et al.*, 2009; Imai *et al.*, 2015), plus neurotransmitter abnormalities (Ryu & Kim, 2015). Progesterone production by the corpus luteum of the ovary may provoke symptoms; cyclicity disappears in anovulatory cycles when a corpus luteum is not formed (Imai *et al.*, 2015).

Management

It is difficult to diagnose PMS; the most definitive method is a symptom diary as symptoms will start in the luteal phase and cease at the start of or during menstruation (Samadi *et al.*, 2013; Ugarriza *et al.*, 1998).

There is no universally recognised single treatment for PMS, and women will often use diet, supplements and alternative approaches to relieve symptoms. For mild to moderate symptoms, lifestyle changes and a healthy diet can substantially reduce, if not alleviate, the symptoms (Stewart *et al.*, 1993). For those who are treated with medication (such as anti-depressants and oral contraceptives), the success rate is no greater than 60–70% (Bertone-Johnson *et al.*, 2014), but a healthy lifestyle may make the treatment more successful (Bussell, 1998).

Nutritional management

A healthy diet, regular physical activity, good sleep patterns and stress reduction techniques can help to reduce symptoms (Cheng *et al.*, 2013; Ugarriza *et al.*, 1998). Sustained dietary change is necessary for symptom relief. It was found, in schoolgirls aged 13–19 years, that a dieting behaviour (prevalent in 30% of the sample), increased consumption of junk food and low levels of regular physical activity was associated with increased PMS (Rupa Vani *et al.*, 2013).

Calcium and vitamin D

A diet rich in calcium and vitamin D is associated with a lower incidence of PMS. Lower-fat versions of dairy foods reduce the incidence of PMS (Bertone-Johnson *et al.*, 2005). Calcium (1000 mg/day) and vitamin D (10 μg) taken as supplements may be useful in treating the premenstrual pain and emotional symptoms associated with PMS (Alvir & Thys-Jacobs, 1991; Thys-Jacobs, 1994; Thys-Jacobs *et al.*, 1989). Dietary vitamin D has been shown to reduce the risk of PMS in young women (Bertone-Johnson *et al.*, 2010b). Women with PMS who consumed at least 100 IU/day of vitamin D had a significantly reduced prevalence of PMS as compared to women who consumed less than this amount. Higher blood vitamin D levels may be inversely related to the development of specific menstrual symptoms such as breast tenderness and depression (Bertone-Johnson *et al.*, 2014). There is evidence that a daily supplement of calcium (500 mg) with vitamin B_6 (40 mg) leads to effective control of PMS symptoms (Masoumi *et al.*, 2016).

Magnesium and Iron

Low intake and blood levels of magnesium have been found in PMS sufferers (Posaci *et al.*, 1994; Quaranta *et al.*, 2007). An improvement has been observed in PMS symptoms with magnesium supplementation (Quaranta *et al.*, 2007). However, more recent reviews have concluded that there is little evidence for the effectiveness of magnesium in PMS (Labruzzo *et al.*, 2009; Whelan *et al.*, 2009). A case control study found that a diet providing 22 mg iron daily was linked to 33% decrease in the risk of developing PMS as compared to women who consumed about 10mg (Chocano-Bedoya *et al.*, 2013).

B vitamins

Historically, vitamin B_6 supplements were used to treat PMS, but a pharmacological dose of 50–100 mg was required, and such doses may induce neuropathy (Labruzzo *et al.*, 2009). As a consequence, in the UK, B_6 supplements are only sold in 10 mg ineffective doses. A recent observational study showed that higher intakes of thiamine and riboflavin may reduce the incidence of PMS by 35% (Chocano-Beoya *et al.*, 2011).

Vitamin E, evening primrose oil and essential fatty acids

Vitamin E combined with evening primrose oil has been shown to be effective for premenstrual breast pain (Pruthi *et al.*, 2010). A supplement containing a mixture of essential fatty acids (gamma linolenic acid, linoleic acid, oleic acid) and vitamins (including vitamin E) significantly reduced PMS symptoms, with the 2 g supplement having the greatest effect (Filho *et al.*, 2011). Evening primrose oil was prescribable for PMS due to the presence of gamma linolenic acid. However, many trials were poorly designed and/or showed no reduction in breast pain or other PMS symptoms (Kleijnen, 1994); therefore, it was withdrawn as a prescribable product. Omega 3 fatty acids, at a dose of 2 g daily, has been shown to reduce the psychological symptoms of PMS, including depression and some of the somatic PMS symptoms (Sohrabi *et al.*, 2013).

Fibre

Increasing dietary fibre can help to alleviate the constipation that may occur premenstrually (Bussell, 1998). Appropriate treatment for IBS is helpful in the premenstrual period (Kane *et al.*, 1998).

Alcohol

Alcoholics are prone to PMS (Allen, 1996), and alcohol aggravates the symptoms (Gold *et al.*, 2007). Some PMS sufferers have alcohol cravings premenstrually (Bryant *et al*., 2006); in addition alcohol metabolism may also be impaired (Perry *et al*., 2004).

Soya

A phyto-oestrogen-rich diet has been shown to prolong the follicular phase of the menstrual cycle, thereby reducing the length of the luteal phase (Patisaul & Jefferson, 2010). However, the evidence is equivocal for its use in PMS (Kim *et al*., 2006).

Weight gain

Overweight and obesity is associated with PMS (Bertone-Johnson *et al*., 2010a; Masho *et al*., 2005). Many women report an increase in appetite during the luteal phase (Bryant *et al*., 2006; Tucci *et al*., 2009). Women with PMS have been shown to eat significantly more fat, carbohydrates and simple sugars premenstrually (Cross *et al*., 2001). Conversely, energy expenditure has been shown to increase premenstrually in some women (Henry *et al*., 2003).

SECTION 3

Herbal treatments

Although herbal medicines are used to treat PMS, their effectiveness has not been fully evaluated in randomised controlled trials (Jing *et al*., 2009). Single trials of Jingqianping, *Vitex agnus-castus* (Ambrosini *et al*., 2013), *Ginkgo biloba* and *Crocus sativus* have shown efficacy; however, more trials are needed (Dante & Facchinetti, 2010). Another study found that ginger reduced the symptom scores for PMS, which the authors believed to be due to the inhibition of prostaglandin production (Khayat *et al*., 2014).

Internet resources

National Association for Premenstrual Syndrome, www.pms.org.uk

References

Allen D. (1996) Are alcoholic women more likely to drink premenstrually? *Alcohol*. 31(2): 145–147.

Altman G, Cain KC, Motzer S, *et al*. (2006, Jan–Feb) Increased symptoms in female IBS patients with dysmenorrhea and PMS. Gastroenterol. *Nurs*. 29(1): 4–11.

Alvir JM, Thys-Jacobs S. (1991) Premenstrual and menstrual symptom clusters and response to calcium treatment. *Psychopharmacol. Bull*. 27(2): 145–148.

Ambrosini A, Di Lorenzo C, Coppola G, *et al*. (2013, Mar) Use of *Vitex agnus-castus* in migrainous women with premenstrual syndrome: an open-label clinical observation. *Acta Neurol. Belg*. 113(1): 25–29. doi: 10.1007/s13760-012-0111-4. Epub 2012 Jul 12.

Bertone-Johnson ER, Hankinson SE, Bendich A, *et al*. (2005) Calcium and vitamin D intake and risk of incident premenstrual syndrome. *Arch. Intern. Med*. 165(11): 1246–1252.

Bertone-Johnson ER, Chocano-Bedoya PO, Zagarins SE, *et al*. (2010a, Jul). Dietary vitamin D intake, 25-hydroxyvitamin D3 levels and premenstrual syndrome in a college-aged population. *J. Steroid Biochem. Mol. Biol*. 121(1–2): 434–437.

Bertone-Johnson ER, Hankinson, SE Willett WC, *et al*. (2010b, Nov) Adiposity and the development of premenstrual syndrome. *J. Women's Health (Larchmt)*. 19(11): 1955–1962.doi:10.1089/jwh.2010.2128

Bertone-Johnson ER, Hankinson SE, Forger NG, *et al*. (2014) Plasma 25-hydroxyvitamin D and risk of premenstrual syndrome in a prospective cohort study. *BMC Women's Health*. 14: 56. Published online 2014 Apr 12. doi:10.1186/1472-6874-14-56

Bertone-Johnson *et al*. (2015) Premenstrual syndrome and subsequent risk of hypertension in a prospective study. *Am. J. Epidemiol*. 182 (12):1000–1009.

Brown J, O'Brien PMS, Marjoribanks J, et al. (2009) Selective serotonin reuptake inhibitors for premenstrual syndrome. *Cochrane Database Syst. Rev*. (2): CD001396.

Bryant M, Truesdale KP, Dye L. (2006) Modest changes in dietary intake across the menstrual cycle: implications for food intake research. *Br. J. Nutr*. 96(5): 888–894.

Bussell G. (1998) Pre-menstrual syndrome and diet. *J. Nutr. Environ. Med*. 8: 65–75.

Cheng SH, Shih CC, Yang YK, et al. (2013, Feb) Factors associated with premenstrual syndrome – a survey of new female university students. *Kaohsiung J. Med. Sci*. 29(2): 100–105. doi: 10.1016/j.kjms.2012.08.017

Chocano-Bedoya PO, Manson JE, Hankinson SE, *et al*. (2011) Dietary B vitamin intake and incident premenstrual syndrome. *Am. J. Clin. Nutr*. 93: 1080–1086.

Chocano-Bedoya PO, Manson JE, Hankinson SE, *et al*. (2013, May 15) Intake of selected minerals and risk of premenstrual syndrome. *Am. J. Epidemiol*. 177(10): 1118–1127. doi: 10.1093/aje/kws363.

Cross GB, Marley J, Miles H, *et al*. (2001) Changes in nutrient intake during the menstrual cycle of overweight women with premenstrual syndrome. *Br. J. Nutr*. 85(4): 475–482.

Dante G, Facchinetti F. (2011). Herbal treatments for alleviating premenstrual syndrome: a systematic review. *J. Psychosom. Obstet. Gynecol*. 32(1): 42–51.

Filho R, Lima JC, Pinho N, *et al*. (2011) Essential fatty acids for premenstrual syndrome and their effect on prolactin and total cholesterol levels: a randomized, double blind, placebo-controlled study. *Reprod. Health* 8(1): 2.

Gold EB, Bair Y, Block G, *et al*. (2007) Diet and lifestyle factors associated with premenstrual symptoms in a racially diverse community sample: Study of Women's Health Across the Nation (SWAN). *J. Women's Health (Larchmt.)* 16(5): 641–656.

Henry CJ, Lightowler HJ, Marchini J. (2003) Intra-individual variation in resting metabolic rate during the menstrual cycle. *Br. J. Nutr*. 89(6): 811–817.

Imai A, Ichigo S, Matsunami K, *et al*. (2015) Premenstrual syndrome: management and pathophysiology. *Clin. Exp. Ostet. Gynecol*. 42(2): 123–128.

Jing Z, Yang X, Ismail KMK, *et al*. (2009) Chinese herbal medicine for premenstrual syndrome. *Cochrane Database Syst. Rev*. (1): CD006414.

Kane SV, Sable K, Hanauer SB. (1998) The menstrual cycle and its effect on inflammatory bowel disease and irritable bowel syndrome: a prevalence study. *Am. J. Gastroenterol*. 10: 1867–1872.

Khayat S, Kheirkhan M, Moghadam ZB, *et al*. (2014) Effect of treatment with ginger on the severity of premenstrual syndrome symptoms. *ISRN Obstet. Gynecol*. 792708. Published online 2014 May 4. doi:10.1155/2014/792708.

Kim HW, Kwon MK, Kim NS, *et al*. (2006) Intake of dietary soy isoflavones in relation to perimenstrual symptoms of Korean women living in the USA. *Nurs. Health. Sci*. 8(2): 108–113.

Kleijnen J. (1994) Evening primrose oil. *BMJ* 309: 824–825.

Labruzzo BA, Chasuk R, Kendall S. (2009) Which complementary therapies can help patients with PMS? *J. Fam. Pract*. 58(10): 552–559.

Masho SW, Adera T, South-Paul J. (2005) Obesity as a risk factor for premenstrual syndrome. *J. Psychosom. Obstet. Gynecol*. 26(1): 33–39.

Masoumi SZ, Ataollahi M, Oshvandi K. (2016, Mar) Effect of combined use of calcium and vitamin B6 on premenstrual syndrome symptoms: a randomized clinical trial. *J. Caring Sci.* 5(1): 67–73. doi: 10.15171/jcs.2016.007

Patisaul HB, Jefferson W. (2010) The pros and cons of phytoestrogens. *Front. Neuroendocrinol.* 31(4): 400–419.

Perry BL, Miles D, Burruss K, *et al.* (2004) Premenstrual symptomatology and alcohol consumption in college women. *J. Stud. Alcohol.* 65(4): 464–468.

Posaci C, Erten O, Uren A, *et al.* (1994) Plasma copper, zinc and magnesium levels in patients with premenstrual tension syndrome. *Acta Obstet. Gynecol. Scand.* 73(6): 452–455.

Pruthi S, Wahner-Roedler DL, Torkelson CJ, *et al.* (2010) Vitamin E and evening primrose oil for management of cyclical mastalgia: a randomized pilot study. *Altern. Med. Rev.* 15(1): 59–67.

Quaranta S, Buscaglia MA, Meroni MG, *et al.* (2007) Pilot study of the efficacy and safety of a modified-release magnesium 250 mg tablet (Sincromag) for the treatment of premenstrual syndrome. *Clin. Drug Investig.* 27(1): 51–58.

Rupa Vani K, Veena KS, Subitha L, *et al.* (2013, Nov). Menstrual abnormalities in school going girls – are they related to dietary and exercise pattern? *Clin. Diagn. Res.* 7(11): 2537–2540. Published online 2013 Oct 10. doi: 10.7860/JCDR/2013/6464.3603

Ryu A, Kim T. (2015, Dec) Premenstrual syndrome: a mini review. *Maturitas.* 82(4): 436–440. doi: 10.1016/j.maturitas.2015.08.010. Epub 2015 Aug 28.

Samadi Z, Taghian F, Valiani M. (2013, Jan) The effects of 8 weeks of regular aerobic exercise on the symptoms of premenstrual syndrome in non-athlete girls. *Iran. J. Nurs. Midwifery Res.* 18(1): 14–19.

Sohrabi N, Kashanian M, Ghafoori SS, *et al.* (2013, Jun) Evaluation of the effect of omega-3 fatty acids in the treatment of premenstrual syndrome: 'a pilot trial'. *Complement. Ther. Med.* 21(3):141–146. doi: 10.1016/j.ctim.2012.12.008. Epub 2013 Jan 16.

Stewart AC, Tooley SH, Tooke J, *et al.* (1993) Effect of nutritional programme on premenstrual syndrome and work efficiency. *Complement. Ther. Med.* 1: 68–72.

Thys-Jacobs S. (1994) Alleviation of migraines with therapeutic vitamin D and calcium. *Headache.* 34(10): 590–592.

Thys-Jacobs S, Ceccarelli S, Bierman A, *et al.* (1989) Calcium supplementation in premenstrual syndrome: a randomized crossover trial. *J. Gen. Intern. Med.* 4(3): 183–189.

Tucci SA, Murphy LE, Boyland EJ, *et al.* (2009) [Influence of premenstrual syndrome and oral contraceptive effects on food choice during the follicular and luteal phase of the menstrual cycle]. *Endocrinol. Nutr.* 56(4): 170–175.

Ugarriza DN, Klingner S, O'Brien S. (1998) Premenstrual syndrome: diagnosis and intervention. *Nurse. Pract.* 23(9): 40, 45, 49–52.

Whelan AM, Jurgens TM, Naylor H. (2009). Herbs, vitamins and minerals in the treatment of premenstrual syndrome: a systematic review. *Can. J. Clin. Pharmacol.* 16(3): e407–429.

3.1.3 Menopause

Gaynor Bussell

Key points

- The combination of a healthy diet, keeping active and avoiding weight gain can help alleviate symptoms.
- Some foods such as soya, oily fish, oats, possibly probiotics, and milk products or alternatives can help.
- A Mediterranean diet may offset symptoms.

Menopause occurs when ovulation ceases and oestrogen production decreases, resulting in the cessation of menstruation and bringing about other associated changes. It is a gradual change (perimenopause) that usually happens at an average age of 51 (range 40–58) years. Approximately 75–80% of women suffer menopausal symptoms; 45% find them distressing, while 20–30% find them severe (Hardie *et al.*, 2009). Menopause is self-limiting (usually 2–5 years), although it can extend over a longer period.

The most common menopausal symptoms include hot flushes, night sweats, vaginal dryness, sleep disturbance, mood swings, forgetfulness and lack of concentration (Sussman *et al.*, 2015). Menopausal and postmenopausal women are at increased risk of several conditions, including osteoporosis, hypertension, heart disease and stroke.

Management of associated symptoms and conditions

Weight gain

Lean body mass and metabolic rate decrease during menopause (Hodson *et al.*, 2014), with an associated weight gain of 2–2.5 kg over 3 years (Brończyk-Puzoń *et al.*, 2015). Weight is more likely to be deposited abdominally, thereby increasing the risk of insulin resistance, dyslipidaemia and metabolic syndrome (Mastorakos *et al.*, 2010). Weight gain, especially central adiposity (Raeme, 2008), can exacerbate hot flushes and night sweats (Thurston *et al.*, 2015). Being physically active is associated with fewer menopausal symptoms and may help to reduce central adiposity (Leite *et al.*, 2010; Seo *et al.*, 2010). Higher adherence to a Mediterranean diet is inversely associated with overweight/obesity in perimenopausal and postmenopausal women (Sayón-Orea *et al.*, 2015).

Metabolic syndrome and heart disease

Oestrogen is cardioprotective; by the age of 65 years, the risk of heart disease in women is the same as men. Falling oestrogen levels lead to central adiposity, a risk factor for heart disease and insulin resistance (Llaneza *et al.*, 2010). The incidence of metabolic syndrome increases substantially during perimenopause and leads to an increase in cholesterol and triglycerides, hypertension and risk of diabetes (Polotsky & Polotsky, 2010). Soya-based foods may help improve cholesterol levels (Ma *et al.*, 2013). A Mediterranean diet may be cardioprotective during menopause (Llaneza *et al.*, 2010). Reducing glycaemic load (GL) has been shown to increase HDL cholesterol in postmenopausal women (Shikany *et al.*, 2010). Women with type 2 diabetes tend to have an earlier menopause, and this, together with the diabetes has a synergistic effect on the incidence of cardiovascular disease (Sekhar *et al.*, 2015).

Bone health

Postmenopausal women are at risk of osteoporosis, especially if vitamin D status is low (Cauley, 2015). The rate of bone calcium loss is escalated during menopause (North American Menopause Association, or NAMA, 2010). At-risk menopausal women should be assessed and may need to receive specific dietary counselling (NAMA, 2010). The National Osteoporosis Society (2011) recommends a daily intake of 700 mg of calcium in postmenopausal women, which should be increased to 1000–1200 mg in women with osteoporosis. Women with low serum 25-hydroxyvitamin D (<20 ng/mL) should also receive vitamin D supplements to reduce fracture risk. Vitamin A is associated with an increased risk of osteoporosis; therefore, vitamin A or retinol supplements should be used with caution (Dennehy & Tsourounis, 2010). Weight loss of as little as 5% of body weight is associated with increased bone turnover in postmenopausal women, even when combined with low-impact, weight-bearing exercise (Rector *et al.*, 2009). Weight loss programmes should be combined with high-impact exercise (Engelke *et al.*, 2006) (see Chapter 7.9.1, Osteoporosis).

Cancer

Although oestrogen production decreases during menopause, sex hormone–binding globulin also decreases, leading to a rise in free circulating oestrogen, which increases the risk of developing hormone-sensitive cancers, including breast cancer (see Chapter 7.15.4, Breast cancer). This may be modulated by the increased consumption of brassicas (Fowke *et al.*, 2000) and fibre (Park *et al.*, 2009), and avoiding excess weight gain. Studies show a lower risk of hormone-sensitive breast cancers in postmenopausal women who have consistently consumed a diet rich in soya isoflavones (>42 mg/day) (Magee & Rowland, 2012). There is no increased risk of any cancers when taking a ≤120 mg soya isoflavone supplement for 2 years for bone health (Steinberg *et al.*, 2011). However, women concerned about breast cancer, or women who currently have breast cancer or had it in the past, should discuss with a clinician before taking isoflavones.

Hot flushes

Hot flushes are one of the most common symptoms of menopause, and this can be treated with hormone replacement therapy. Reducing the intake of alcohol, spicy food and caffeine, and losing weight if overweight or obese (Roberts & Hickey, 2016) have been shown to be beneficial. Huang *et al.* (2010) showed that, for every 5 kg lost, there was a 30% improvement in hot flushes (Huang *et al.*, 2010). Exercising regularly to the level of feeling hot and sweaty has also recently been shown to reduce the number and intensity of hot flushes (Bailey *et al.*, 2016). Metabolic health, including insulin resistance and cholesterol level, predict the severity of hot flushes (Thurston *et al.*, 2012).

Hot flushes are less prevalent in countries where soya intake is high, probably owing to soya's high isoflavone content. A 20 mg/day supplement of the potent isoflavone genistein, or consuming 400 mL soya milk or 80 g soya mince a day, may be effective against hot flushes (Taku *et al.*, 2012).

The daily consumption of probiotic bacteria milk and prebiotic fibres may increase the bioavailability of soya isoflavones (Timan *et al.*, 2014); however, more research is needed in this area.

Internet resources

Menopause Exchange, www.menopause-exchange.co.uk
Menopause Matters, www.menopausematters.co.uk
National Osteoporosis Society, www.nos.org.uk

References

Bailey TG, Cable NT, Aziz N, *et al.* (2016) Exercise training reduces the acute physiological severity of post-menopausal hot flushes. *J. Physiol.* 594: 657–667.

Brończyk-Puzoń A, Piecha D, Nowak J, *et al.* (2015) Guidelines for dietary management of menopausal women with simple obesity. *Prz. Menopauzalny.* 14: 48–52.

Cauley JA. (2015) Bone health after menopause. *Curr. Opin. Endocrinol. Diabetes Obes.* 22: 490–494.

Dennehy C, Tsourounis C. (2010) A review of select vitamins and minerals used by postmenopausal women. *Maturitas.* 66: 370–380.

Engelke K, Kemmler W, Lauber D, *et al.* (2006) Exercise maintains bone density at spine and hip EFOPS: a 3-year longitudinal study in early postmenopausal women. *Osteoporos. Int.* 17(1): 133–142.

Fowke JH, Longcope C, Hebert JR. (2000) Brassica vegetable consumption shifts estrogen metabolism in healthy postmenopausal women. *Cancer Epidemiol. Biomarkers Prev.* 9(8): 773–779.

Hardie C, Bain C, Walters M. (2009) Hormone replacement therapy: the risks and benefits of treatment. *J R Coll Physicians Edinb.* 39: 324–326.

Hodson L, Harnden K, Banerjee R, *et al.* (2014) Lower resting and total energy expenditure in postmenopausal compared with premenopausal women matched for abdominal obesity. *J. Nutr. Sci.* 13: 3.

Huang AJ, Subak LL, Wing R, *et al.* (2010) An intensive behavioral weight loss intervention and hot flushes in women. *Arch. Intern. Med.* 170(13): 1161–1167.

Llaneza P, Gonzalez C, Fernandez-Inarrea J, *et al.* (2010). Soy isoflavones, Mediterranean diet, and physical exercise in postmenopausal women with insulin resistance. *Menopause.* 17(2): 372–378.

Leite RD, Prestes J, Pereera GB, *et al.* (2010) Menopause, highlighting the effects of resistance training. *Int. J. Sports Med.* 31(11): 761–767.

Ma D, Taku K, Zhang Y, *et al.* (2013) Serum lipid-improving effect of soyabean β-conglycinin in hyperlipidaemic menopausal women. *Br. J. Nutr.* 110: 1680–1684.

Magee PJ, Rowland I. (2012) Soy products in the management of breast cancer. *Curr. Opin. Clin. Nutr. Metab. Care*. 15: 586–591.

Mastorakos G, Valsamakis G, Paltoglou G, *et al.* (2010) Management of obesity in menopause: diet, exercise, pharmacotherapy and bariatric surgery. *Maturitas*. 65(3): 219–224.

National Osteoporosis Society (NOS). (2011) *All about osteoporosis*. Available at www.nos.org.uk. Accessed 19 July 2016.

North American Menopause Association (NAMA). (2010) Management of osteoporosis in postmenopausal women. *Menopause*. 17(1): 25–54.

Park Y, Brinton LA, Subar AF, *et al.* (2009) Dietary fiber intake and risk of breast cancer in postmenopausal women: the National Institutes of Health–AARP Diet and Health Study. *Am. J. Clin. Nutr.* 90(3): 664–671.

Polotsky HN, Polotsky AJ. (2010) Metabolic implications of menopause. *Semin. Reprod. Med.* 28(5): 426–434.

Raeme NK. (2008) Adiposity and hot flashes: one more tree in the forest. *Menopause*. 15(3): 408–409.

Rector RS, Loethen J, Ruebel M, *et al.* (2009) Serum markers of bone turnover are increased by modest weight loss with or without weight-bearing exercise in overweight premenopausal women. *Appl. Physiol. Nutr. Metab.* 34(5): 933–941.

Roberts H, Hickey M. (2016) Managing the menopause: An update. *Maturitas*. 86:53–58.

Sayón-Orea C, Santiago S, Cuervo M, *et al.* (2015) Adherence to Mediterranean dietary pattern and menopausal symptoms in relation to overweight/obesity in Spanish perimenopausal and postmenopausal women. *Menopause*. 22: 750–757.

Sekhar TV, Medarametla S, Rahman A, *et al.* (2015, Oct) Early menopause in type 2 diabetes – a study from a South Indian Tertiary Care Centre. *J. Clin. Diagn. Res.* 9(10): OC08–OC10.

Seo DI, Jun TW, Park KS, *et al.* (2010) 12 weeks of combined exercise is better than aerobic exercise for increasing growth hormone in middle-aged women. *Int. J. Sport Nutr. Exerc. Metab.* 20(1): 21–26.

Shikany JM, Tinker LF, Neuhouser ML, *et al.* (2010) Association of glycemic load with cardiovascular disease risk factors: the Women's Health Initiative Observational Study. *Nutrition*. 6: 641–647.

Steinberg FM, Murray MJ, Lewis RD, *et al.* (2011) Clinical outcomes of a 2-y soy isoflavone supplementation in menopausal women. *Am. J. Clin. Nutr.* 93(2): 356–367.

Sussman M, Trocio J, Best C, *et al.* (2015) Prevalence of menopausal symptoms among mid-life women: findings from electronic medical records. *BMC Women's Health*.15: 58.

Taku K, Melby MK, Kronenberg F, *et al.* (2012) Extracted or synthesised soybean isoflavones reduce menopausal hot flash frequency and severity: systematic review and meta-analysis of randomized controlled trials. *Menopause*. 19(7): 776–790.

Thurston RC, El Khoudary SR, Sutton-Tyrrell K, *et al.* (2012) Vasomotor symptoms and insulin resistance in the study of women's health across the nation. *J. Clin. Endocrinol. Metab.* 97: 3487–3494.

Thurston RC, Ewing LJ, Low CA, *et al.* (2015) Behavioral weight loss for the management of menopausal hot flashes: a pilot study. *Menopause*. 22: 59–65.

Timan P, Rojanasthien N, Manorot M, *et al.* (2014) Effect of symbiotic fermented milk on oral bioavailability of isoflavones in postnatal women. *Int. J. Food Sci. Nutr.* 65(6): 761–767.

3.2 Preconception and pregnancy

Gail Rees

Key points

- A healthy diet and alcohol avoidance should be advised during the preconception period and pregnancy.
- Supplements of folic acid (usually 400 μg/day) should be taken preconceptually and until the 12th week of pregnancy.
- Being underweight or overweight can affect the outcome of pregnancy.
- A 10 μg supplement of vitamin D should be advised for all women throughout pregnancy and lactation.

Preconception

Body weight and fertility

Low body weight can affect reproductive function by causing hormone imbalances and anovulation; the relative risk of infertility increases in women who are underweight. Obesity also adversely affects ovulation, and obese women have lower natural and assisted fertility rates. Relative rates of infertility gradually increase in women with a BMI greater than 25 kg/m^2 (Homan *et al.*, 2007).

Polycystic ovary syndrome (PCOS) is the most common cause of anovulation, and it is more common in obese women (see Chapter 3.1.1, Polycystic ovary syndrome). High levels of body fat, particularly abdominal adipose tissue, are linked to insulin resistance, and this increases ovarian androgen secretion and abnormal development of follicles. Raised insulin levels also lower the production of sex hormone–binding globulin (SHBG) from the liver, resulting in high free androgen activity. High levels of androgens give rise to amenorrhoea, infertility, hirsutism, acne and alopecia (Ramsay *et al.*, 2006). Weight loss through diet and lifestyle change is the first-line therapy for obese women with PCOS who wish to become pregnant (Balen *et al.*, 2016). A systematic review of the literature on lifestyle changes and PCOS found that lifestyle intervention improves body composition, hyperandrogenism and insulin resistance. However, there was no evidence for the effect of lifestyle interventions on improving glucose tolerance or lipid profiles, and there was no literature assessing clinical reproductive outcomes, quality of life and treatment satisfaction (Moran *et al.*, 2011).

A restrictive diet prior to conception or during pregnancy is not recommended, as this may increase the likelihood of poor micronutrient intakes, which could have an adverse effect on foetal development, maternal nutrient stores and breast milk composition. Therefore, advice should focus on a varied, nutrient-rich diet following healthy eating guidelines, with an active lifestyle to encourage gradual weight loss before conception is attempted.

Male fertility and body weight

Undernutrition and obesity can affect steroid hormone production in men. Obesity in males is associated with reduced insulin sensitivity and decreased testosterone secretion (Pasquali *et al.*, 2007). A meta-analysis by Sermondade *et al.* (2013) found that overweight and obese men had a significantly elevated risk of abnormal sperm count. Obesity is also associated with erectile dysfunction, which may resolve with weight loss (Pasquali *et al.*, 2007).

Alcohol

Female fertility

The relationship between alcohol and female fertility is equivocal. Some studies have shown that alcohol consumption reduces female fertility, and some prospective cohort studies suggest that there is a dose–response relationship between alcohol and infertility. However, a recent prospective cohort study found no effect on fertility with consumption of less than 14 standard servings of alcohol per week (Mikkelsen *et al.*, 2016). However, alcohol is known to be harmful to the foetus, especially

Manual of Dietetic Practice, Sixth Edition. Edited by Joan Gandy.

Companion website: www.manualofdieteticpractice.com

during early pregnancy when the foetus is most susceptible to teratogens (compounds that are harmful to the foetus and cause malformations), and so alcohol is best avoided preconceptually.

Male fertility

A meta-analysis of social and behavioural factors and semen quality in men reviewed 57 cross-sectional studies with 29,914 participants from 26 countries and regions, and concluded that alcohol consumption was a risk factor for lower semen volume (Li *et al.*, 2011).

Folic acid and neural tube defects

The link between folic acid supplementation and a reduction in risk of neural tube defects (NTD) is well established (Czeizel & Dudas, 1992; MRC, 1991). Current advice from the UK Department of Health is to take a supplement of folic acid (400 μg/day) from the time contraception is stopped until the 12th week of pregnancy. To prevent the recurrence of NTDs in the offspring of women or men with an NTD, or for those who have previously had a child with an NTD or have a family history of NTDs, women who may become pregnant should take a daily supplement of 5 mg of folic acid (available on prescription) until the 12th week of pregnancy. Women with diabetes, obesity or coeliac disease, or who are taking medication for epilepsy, are also advised to take 5 mg of folic acid/day.

Despite campaigns to increase awareness, supplement use prior to conception (or prior to neural tube closure) continues to be low, especially in the socially disadvantaged and in ethnic minorities (Brough *et al.*, 2009). Therefore, opportunities to encourage folic acid supplementation prior to conception should be sought, and women should also be advised to consume both naturally rich sources of folate and fortified foods. A good dietary intake is needed throughout pregnancy and lactation as requirements are increased. Women who have not taken folic acid supplements prior to conception should be advised to start immediately and continue until the 12th week of pregnancy. Many countries throughout the world (but not the UK) have introduced mandatory fortification of flour with folic acid. It is estimated that this produces a reduction in NTD incidence of 46% (Blencowe *et al.*, 2010). Table 3.2.1 shows the folic acid content of some foods.

Table 3.2.1 Folic acid content of some foods

Food source (portion size)	Folate per portion (μg)
Broccoli – steamed (85 g)	61
Spinach – boiled (90 g)	73
Baked beans in tomato sauce (135 g)	39
Orange juice (150 g)	27
Wholemeal bread – one slice (36 g)	14
Chicken – roast (100 g)	10
Fortified cereals	
Cornflakes (Tesco) (30 g)	120
Cheerios (Nestle) (30 g)	47
Weetabix, two biscuits (37.5 g)	64

Pregnancy

Basal metabolic rate (BMR) and energy requirements

Energy requirements vary greatly between individuals according to body size and level of activity. During pregnancy, additional energy is needed to support the increase in body tissues of the mother and foetus. Therefore, energy requirements increase due to increases in metabolically active tissues, and the increased energy cost of moving a heavier body (Butte *et al.*, 2004). Hytten and Leitch (1971) calculated theoretical estimates of the components of average pregnancy weight gain. A mean weight gain of 13 kg was calculated (uterus 0.9 kg; breasts 0.4 g; blood 1.2 kg; extracellular fluid 1.2 kg; fat 3.5 kg; plus the products of conception 5.8 kg). It should be remembered that this is a theoretical value and that a wide range of weight gains are associated with a healthy pregnancy.

There are differences in the changes in BMR during pregnancy between women in developed and developing countries. Generally, women in developed countries have been shown to increase BMR, while, in developing countries, BMR decreases early in pregnancy (Prentice *et al.*, 1996). Research also suggests that, while the mean BMR for women in the UK changes little during early pregnancy, some women show increases in BMR at this stage and some show reductions in BMR, making it difficult to recommend an ideal energy intake (Prentice *et al.*, 1989). The UK estimated average requirement for energy intake during pregnancy is therefore unchanged until the third trimester, when there is an increment of 190 kcal (800 kJ)/day, but with the recognition that those who are underweight at the start of pregnancy and those who do not reduce their activity levels may require more (Scientific Advisory Committee for Nutrition (SACN) 2011).

Obesity and weight gain

Maternal obesity is increasing in the UK. In the 19-year period 1989–2007, obesity doubled from 7.6% to 15.6%, and the percentage of women in early pregnancy with a normal-range BMI decreased from 66% to 54% (Heslehurst *et al.*, 2010). Obesity during pregnancy has been associated with many adverse outcomes for the mother, including gestational diabetes, hypertensive disorders, caesarean sections, haemorrhage and wound infections. It is also associated with adverse infant outcomes such as macrosomia, respiratory distress, stillbirth and preterm birth (Knight-Agarwal *et al.*, 2016; Scott-Pillai *et al.*, 2013).

There are currently no UK recommendations for weight gain during pregnancy, as a wide range of weight gain is associated with a healthy pregnancy outcome. However, American guidelines provide guidance for weight gain based on prepregnancy body weight, as shown in

Table 3.2.2 US guidelines for weight gain during pregnancy (Institute of Medicine/National Research Council, 2009)

Body mass index (BMI) category (kg/m^2)	Total weight gain (kg)
Underweight (BMI <18.5)	13–18
Normal weight (BMI 18.5–24.9)	11–16
Overweight (BMI 25–29.9)	7–11
Obese (BMI ≥30)	5–9

Table 3.2.2 (Institute of Medicine/National Research Council, 2009). Gestational weight gain has also been found to predict postpartum weight retention (Nehring *et al.*, 2011). Thus, it is important that excess weight gain be avoided to prevent postpartum obesity and being obese if or when they conceive again. The Royal College of Obstetricians and Gynaecologists (RCOG/CMACE, 2010) have called for research to determine the optimal weight gain during pregnancy for women in different BMI categories.

Current guidance from NICE (2008) in the UK does not include recommendations for routine monitoring of weight gain unless clinical management is likely to be influenced. However, it does recommend that height and weight be measured and recorded for all pregnant women at the first booking clinic (before pregnancy reaches 12 weeks) (NICE, 2010), and that BMI also be calculated. The guidance also states that all obese, pregnant women should be given advice about diet and activity levels, as well as the opportunity for referral to a dietitian (or other trained health professional) for further advice.

Several intervention programmes have been developed to prevent excessive weight gain during pregnancy. A systematic review of randomised controlled trials found that diet or exercise interventions, or both, reduced the risk of excessive gestational weight gain by an average of 20% (Muktabhant *et al.*, 2015), and that diet and exercise interventions combined had beneficial effects in high-risk women, such as lower risk of caesarean delivery and infant macrosomia. However, a recent multicentre UK trial did not show a reduction in the incidence of gestational diabetes or large-for-gestational-age infants (Poston *et al.*, 2015). Table 3.2.3 is a summary of the nutritional requirements during pregnancy (Department of Health (DH), 1991).

Dietary management should ensure that the diet follows general healthy eating principles to provide sufficient micronutrients and protein, with supplementation of folic acid up to the 12th week of pregnancy and vitamin D throughout pregnancy. The diet should avoid those foods thought to be hazardous to the foetus (Table 3.2.4), and weight gain should be controlled by the avoidance of high-energy drinks and snacks, and limiting portion sizes where necessary. In the absence of evidence-based UK guidelines for weight gain, US guidelines may be used if appropriate.

Underweight

It has been estimated in the UK that 5% of pregnant women are underweight (BMI <18.5 kg/m^2) in the first trimester (Heslehurst *et al.*, 2010). Underweight women are at lesser risk of gestational diabetes and pre-eclampsia, but are significantly more at risk of anaemia and of delivering low-birth-weight babies (Scott-Pillai *et al.*, 2013). A dietary assessment should be undertaken to ensure that nutrient requirements are covered, and advice given to ensure that weight gain is appropriate.

Table 3.2.3 Nutritional requirements during pregnancy

Nutrient	Reference nutrient intake	Increment for pregnancy
Protein (g/day)	45	6
Thiamin (mg/day)	0.8	0.1
Riboflavin (mg/day)	1.1	0.3
Niacin (mg/day)	13	No increment
Vitamin B6 (mg/day)	1.2	No increment
Vitamin B12 (μg/day)	1.5	No increment
Folate (μg/day)	200	100
Vitamin C (mg/day)	40	10
Vitamin A (μg/day)	600	100
Vitamin D (μg/day)*	10	No increment
Minerals	Various	No increment

Note: * SACN, 2016.

Table 3.2.4 Food to avoid in pregnancy

Risk	Sources to be avoided
Listeriosis	Mould-ripened soft cheeses, e.g. brie, camembert
	Soft blue vein cheeses, Danish blue
	Unpasteurised cow's, goat's or sheep's milk, or soft cheese made from them
	All types of pâté, including vegetable pâté
Salmonella and other food-borne infections	Raw, undercooked eggs and products containing, e.g. homemade or restaurant-made mayonnaise, mousse, cold soufflés, etc.
	Raw or undercooked meat, poultry
	Raw shellfish
Toxoplasmosis	Unwashed fruit, vegetables and salad
	Cured meats such as salami, Parma ham, pepperoni – unless they are frozen first or cooked before consumption (such as on a pizza)
Vitamin A toxicity	Liver, liver products such as liver pâté, liver sausage, haggis
	Supplements containing retinol, including fish liver oils
Mercury toxicity	Shark, marlin and swordfish
	Limit tuna to a maximum of two tuna steaks a week (140 g cooked) or four cans of tuna a week (140 g drained)
	Maximum of two portions of oily fish per week

Discussion with midwifery colleagues to ensure adequate foetal growth may also be helpful.

Nutritional requirements during pregnancy

Protein

The current UK dietary reference values (DRVs) recommend an increment of 6 g/day of protein during pregnancy. For women aged 19–50 years, this would mean an increase in the reference nutrient intake (RNI) from 45 g/day to 51 g/day. Most women in the UK exceed this amount and so do not need to alter their protein intake.

Fat

There are no recommendations to change the percentage of energy derived from fat during pregnancy. It is assumed that there will be some increment in fat intake as energy needs increase in the third trimester. There has, however, been debate about the requirements for long-chain n-3 fatty acids. Long-chain n-3 fatty acids, particularly docosahexaenoic acid (DHA), are required for brain growth and development of the retina, and so requirements are increased during pregnancy and lactation, but the exact amounts are difficult to quantify. An increase in intake, however, needs to be balanced with advice to moderate oily fish consumption. A recent systematic review has not found evidence to support the use of n-3 supplementation over a range of outcomes including intrauterine growth restriction, preterm birth, gestational diabetes, perinatal mortality, birthweight, infant eye and brain development, and postpartum depression (Saccone *et al.*, 2016). Another systematic review found that fish oil supplementation was associated with reduced risk of preterm delivery and increased birthweight (Chen *et al.*, 2016). However, in countries where fish is more common in the diet, mercury (high levels are associated with nerve damage in the foetus) in blood, placenta and cord blood has exceeded recommended levels, and the levels were highest in those who ate fish more than three times a week (Hsu *et al.*, 2007). Therefore, women who are trying to conceive or who are pregnant should be encouraged to eat oily fish within the guidelines offered by the DH (Table 3.2.4). Fish oil supplements should be avoided during pregnancy due to their high vitamin A content. A pregnancy-specific DHA supplement may be taken if it does not contain retinol.

Vitamins

There are modest increments in the dietary requirement for vitamins, as shown in Table 3.2.3 (DH, 1991). Other than vitamin D and folate, vitamins should be provided by a diet following usual healthy eating guidelines (see also the following sections titled 'Micronutrient supplementation' and 'Healthy Start'). Retinol is teratogenic, and pregnant women will require advice on how to avoid excessive amounts (Table 3.2.4).

Minerals and trace elements

In the UK, there are no recommended increments in mineral or trace element intakes; recommendations for non-pregnant women therefore apply. This is due to physiological changes whereby there is an increased intestinal absorption of minerals. This assumes that there are sufficient minerals in the diet and that the woman has a good prepregnancy nutritional status, so stores can be mobilised. Iron is the mineral most likely to be deficient, and, although there are some savings of iron during pregnancy from the cessation of menstruation, it is sensible to ensure that adequate dietary sources are consumed throughout pregnancy. Haem iron is better absorbed than non-haem iron, and so regular consumption of lean red meat is useful. If meat is not eaten, absorption of iron from vegetable and cereal sources can be improved if consumed with a source of vitamin C and if inhibitors of iron absorption (especially tea) are avoided with meals.

There is increasing evidence that iodine intakes are low in pregnant women in the UK, and mild to moderate iodine deficiency is common (Bath *et al.*, 2013, 2015). Deficiency is associated with adverse child cognitive development. Fish (especially white fish) and dairy products are good sources (although organic milk contains less iodine than conventionally produced milk). Vegans are particularly at risk of low intakes and may need a supplement, but it is not advised to take seaweed or kelp supplements as they can provide excessive amounts. Multivitamins that are formulated for pregnancy and containing 140 ug/day are suitable.

Micronutrient supplementation

Supplementation of some micronutrients is recommended in pregnancy. Folic acid supplementation has been discussed earlier in this chapter.

Vitamin D

SACN (2016) reviewed the DRVs set in 1991 for vitamin D and has now advised an RNI of 10 ug/day of vitamin D for everyone in the general population aged 4 years and over. This RNI also applies to all pregnant and breastfeeding women, who should take a supplement of 10 μg/day to ensure adequacy. Vitamin D insufficiency has been found in pregnant women in some ethnic groups. Brough *et al.* (2010) showed that 70% of women in the first trimester in a diverse ethnic group in London had 25-hydroxy vitamin D below 50 nmol/L, indicating insufficiency. There were significant differences between ethnic groups with 91% of Asian, 85% of African, 71% of Caribbean and 47% of Caucasian women having insufficient vitamin D. Vitamin D is synthesised under the skin from the actions of ultraviolet light, but, in the UK, sunlight is only at the correct wavelength to produce vitamin D in summer. At particular risk are women who cover themselves for religious or cultural reasons or who have limited time outside. Sunscreens also reduce the action of sunlight on the skin. Groups of women that are particularly vulnerable to vitamin D insufficiency include:

- Those of South Asian, African, Caribbean and Middle Eastern origin.
- Those with limited sunlight exposure.

- Those whose diets contain no meat, oily fish, eggs, margarine or breakfast cereal.
- Those with a prepregnancy BMI of >30 kg/m² (obese) have a lower bioavailability of vitamin D as it is sequestered in body fat.

Iron

Iron demands increase in pregnancy, and the mother is put at risk of anaemia by the foetal demands. Historically, all pregnant women were offered supplementation, but increased understanding of the changes in metabolism during pregnancy, such as haemodilution in the mother, has led to changes in routine practice. NICE guidance (2008) recommends that iron supplementation not be routinely offered to pregnant women, and that it is only advised where there is a clinical need. Haemoglobin levels should be measured at the booking appointment and at 28 weeks gestation. Women with haemoglobin levels of <11 g/100 mL at booking or <10.5 g/100 mL at 28 weeks into gestation should be investigated, and iron supplementation offered if indicated. Iron supplementation may result in constipation; appropriate dietary advice should be given.

Multivitamins

Currently, it is not standard advice to recommend universal multivitamin supplementation in the UK. The most recent Cochrane review found that multiple micronutrient supplementation decreased the number of infants born with low birthweight and small for gestational age (Haider & Bhutta, 2017). The studies included in this review were mostly based in low-income and middle-income countries. However, a systematic review of multivitamin use in high-income countries also found a reduction in risk of small-for-gestational-age infants, although a lack of high-quality evidence was noted (Wolf *et al.*, 2017). A placebo-controlled trial carried out in a multiethnic population, did not show any effect of supplementation on mean birthweight or numbers of low-birthweight babies. However, fewer small-for-gestational-age babies were born in the group receiving multi-micronutrient supplementation as compared to the placebo group. This analysis was based on a small number of women who were compliant with taking the supplements (Brough *et al.*, 2010).

A multi-micronutrient supplement specifically manufactured for pregnancy should be considered in all those who are suspected of having an inadequate intake of micronutrients. Appropriate dietary advice should be given, but nutrients are needed quickly in a short time-frame for pregnancy, and dietary changes may take time to adopt. Pregnant teenagers are particularly at risk of inadequate diets and may have additional requirements to support the growth of the mother as well as the foetus. A pregnancy-specific micronutrient supplement should be advised to ensure that it does not contain retinol, and has the required dose of folic acid and suitable amounts of other nutrients for pregnancy. If insufficient calcium is consumed, a calcium supplement may be needed, as calcium is often not present in multi-micronutrient supplements.

Healthy Start

In the UK, the NHS scheme Healthy Start provides vouchers for mothers on low incomes to purchase milk, fresh and frozen fruit and vegetables, or infant formula. Women who are ≥10 weeks pregnant can apply for vouchers at their booking appointment with their midwife and receive them until their child is 4 years old. All teenagers under the age of 18 years are eligible for the scheme even if they or their parents are not on government benefits. Pregnant women and those with children aged 1–4 years receive one voucher each week (currently worth £3.10); two vouchers are given each week for children aged <1 year. To qualify for Healthy Start vouchers, mothers must have a low family income and receive one of the following government benefits:

- Income Support.
- Income-based Jobseeker's Allowance.
- Income-related Employment and Support Allowance.
- Child Tax Credit with a family income of £16,190 / year or less.
- Universal Credit with a family take-home pay of £408 / month or less.

Vitamin tablets containing folic acid (400 μg), vitamin C (70 mg) and vitamin D (10 μg) are available free during pregnancy and until the child is 1 year old under this scheme. Further details can be found at www.healthystart.nhs.uk.

Food safety

During pregnancy, the mother is relatively immunocompromised, and therefore may be more susceptible to infections, including food-borne infections. More care should be taken with food hygiene to avoid infections such as salmonella by ensuring that eggs, meat, poultry and ready meals are thoroughly cooked, and that chilled foods are proper stored. Good kitchen hygiene practices will also help prevent the cross-contamination of cooked food from raw meat and poultry.

Toxoplasmosis

The bacteria *Toxoplasma gondii* can cause severe foetal abnormalities. It can be transmitted by unwashed fruit and vegetables, and is avoided by the careful washing of produce, cleaning kitchen surfaces and washing hands thoroughly. Protective gloves should be worn for gardening and while handling cat litter trays. *Toxoplasma gondii* can also be found in raw meat and unpasteurised milk.

Listeria

Listeria monocytogenes is able to grow at low temperatures and may be present in cook–chill foods, mould-ripened cheeses and pâté. Certain foods should be avoided as a precaution (Table 3.2.4). Listeria infection in pregnancy, although rare, can cause miscarriage, stillbirth and severe illness in the newborn.

SECTION 3

Mercury and polychlorinated biphenyl

The UK Department of Health (DH) advises pregnant and lactating women (and those trying to conceive) to avoid or limit certain oily fish due to mercury and polychlorinated biphenyl (PCB) contamination. These contaminants are present in marine life and subsequently become concentrated up the food chain. Shark, marlin and swordfish should be avoided since a relatively small amount contains sufficient mercury to be potentially neurotoxic to the foetus. Tuna also contains significant amounts of mercury and advice is to limit the amount consumed (Table 3.2.4).

Caffeine

In the UK, DH recommends that pregnant women restrict caffeine intakes to below 200 mg/day. High caffeine intakes have been linked to foetal growth restriction. The Committee on Toxicity (COT, 2008a) reviewed the evidence, including a study by Konje *et al.* (2008), which found a positive association between caffeine intake and increased risk of foetal growth restriction, which was maintained throughout pregnancy. More than 60% of the caffeine consumed during pregnancy in this study was from tea, and only 14% from coffee and 12% from cola. The mean intake of caffeine in this study of 2635 women was 159 mg/day. Exceeding the limit occasionally is not likely to cause problems, because the risks are likely to be very small. There is still the possibility that the association is not causal due to the influence of confounding factors, but a cautious approach is advised. The COT committee also states that there may be a positive association between caffeine intake and miscarriage, but the evidence is unclear.

The amount of caffeine in drinks and foods will vary, depending on the manufacturer and personal preferences. The following examples of drinks and foods contain roughly 200 mg:

- Two mugs of instant coffee (100 mg each).
- One and a half mugs of filter coffee (140 mg each).
- Two to three mugs of tea (75 mg each).
- Five cans of cola (up to 40 mg each).
- Two and a half cans of energy drink (up to 80 mg each).
- Four (50 g) bars of plain chocolate (up to 50 mg each) – milk chocolate contains approximately 50% of the caffeine in plain chocolate.

Alcohol

Current advice from DH (2016) is not to drink alcohol during pregnancy, as this is the safest approach to minimise long-term harm to the infant, and provides a clear and consistent message. Alcohol at any stage of pregnancy can cause foetal alcohol syndrome (FAS) (restricted growth, facial abnormalities, learning and behavioural disorders). There are various degrees of FAS, and, for some women, regularly drinking >1–2 units once or twice a week or episodes of heavier drinking may cause learning and behavioural disorders in babies that may only become more obvious later on in childhood. It is therefore not possible to confirm a level of alcohol consumption that is safe. Results of a systematic review and meta-analysis show that the low-birthweight and small-for-gestational-age risks gradually increase in mothers who consume an average of one or more alcoholic drinks a day. Risks of preterm birth increase by 23% in those who consume three or more drinks per day (Patra *et al.*, 2011).

Peanuts

There is no clear evidence that eating peanuts during pregnancy affects the chances of the infant developing peanut allergy. Results from research in humans are limited, and it is not clear whether the consumption of peanuts during pregnancy increases or decreases the risk of peanut allergy in offspring, or whether there is any effect at all. It is also possible that the effect could differ according to the level of intake. Therefore, current advice is that there is no need to avoid peanuts unless the mother herself is allergic to them (COT, 2008b) (see Chapter 7.11.2, Food hypersensitivity).

Nutrition-related problems

Nausea and vomiting in pregnancy

Nausea and vomiting are common symptoms of pregnancy that usually begin at 4–8 weeks into gestation and last for the first trimester. Although often termed morning sickness, these symptoms can occur at any time of the day and can last all day. Approximately 50–90% of women experience nausea and vomiting, but only a minority experience it after 20 weeks into gestation. Most women manage by keeping well hydrated and by eating an adequate diet, while avoiding foods and smells that precipitate the symptoms. Small, frequent, high-carbohydrate snacks (such as sandwiches and breakfast cereals) and fluids such as milk or fruit juice can help to keep the patient nourished and hydrated. Reassurance can be given that, during the first trimester, energy requirements are not increased, and large hot meals can be avoided if these precipitate vomiting.

A Cochrane review considered several interventions for nausea and vomiting in early pregnancy and found a lack of robust evidence for any interventions. Some studies suggest that the use of ginger might be beneficial, but evidence was not consistent (Matthews *et al.*, 2015). Although not evidence based, the following tips may be beneficial:

- Small frequent snacks – avoid getting very hungry.
- Drink liquids between meals rather than with meals.
- Dry foods may be better tolerated, e.g. dry biscuits, bread, toast and cereal, especially early in the morning.
- Avoid cooking smells and keep rooms well ventilated.
- Avoid high-fat and highly spiced foods.
- Fizzy drinks and ginger-flavoured drinks have anecdotally been reported as helpful.

Hyperemesis gravidarum is a severe form of vomiting which affects less than 1% of pregnant women. It is a serious condition that often requires hospital admission. It is characterised by intractable vomiting and a weight loss of >5% of prepregnancy weight, dehydration, electrolyte imbalances and ketosis. Patients require intravenous rehydration, antiemetics and vitamin supplementation. Thiamin deficiency can occur if vomiting is prolonged, which can result in Wernicke's encephalopathy, and so thiamin administration may be required. Guidance for management is provided by RCOG (2016), although there is currently a lack of robust evidence for any one intervention (Boelig *et al.*, 2016).

Constipation

Constipation is a common problem during pregnancy and is probably caused by changes to gut transit time mediated by the hormonal changes associated with pregnancy. Standard dietary treatment for constipation can be advised, i.e. high-fibre-containing cereals, fruit and vegetables, and ensuring plenty of fluids (see Chapter 7.4.11, Other disorders of the colon and rectum). Faecal bulking agents can be used, and changing the type of iron supplementation may be beneficial.

Heartburn

Heartburn and gastrointestinal reflux are also common problems experienced in pregnancy. Symptoms result from increased abdominal pressure and changes in gut transit time. Symptoms are usually more severe in the final trimester but can start from early pregnancy. Milk-based foods can alleviate the symptoms, and small frequent meals and snacks are sometimes better tolerated that large meals. Some foods such as spicy, fatty or acidic foods and drinks may exacerbate the symptoms. Antacids are commonly prescribed.

Cravings and pica

Pregnant women frequently report cravings for certain foods and food aversions. Common food aversions include tea, coffee and alcohol. There are no reported patterns to the type of foods craved, and no reports that cravings for foods adversely affect the nutritional intake of women. Pica is the craving and consumption of substances other than food, and has been reported worldwide. Substances consumed include earth (geophagy), stones or pebbles (lithophagia), ice (pagophagia) and raw starches (amylophagy). It has been associated with both negative effects on health (e.g. heavy metal poisoning, micronutrient imbalances and transmission of parasites), and positive health effects (e.g. providing micronutrients and relieving gastrointestinal discomfort) (Young *et al.*, 2010). Pica is more common in developing countries than in developed countries. A study of well-nourished Danish women reported an incidence of 0.02% (Mikkelsen *et al.*, 2006).

Internet resources

Committee on Toxicity, http://cot.food.gov.uk/cotstatements
Healthy Start, www.healthystart.nhs.uk

References

Balen AH, Morley LC, Misso M, *et al.* (2016) The management of anovulatory infertility in women with polycystic ovary syndrome: an analysis of the evidence to support the development of global WHO guidance. *Hum. Reprod. Update* 22(6): 687–708.

Bath SC, Steer CD, Golding J, *et al.* (2013) Effect of inadequate iodine status in UK pregnant women on cognitive outcomes in their children: results from the Avon Longitudinal Study of Parents and Children (ALSPAC). *Lancet* 382: 331–337.

Bath SC, Furmidge-Owen VL, Redman CWG, *et al.* (2015) Gestational changes in iodine status in a cohort study of pregnant women from the United Kingdom: season as an effect modifier. *Am. J. Clin. Nutr.* 101: 1180–1187.

Blencowe H, Cousens S, Modell B, *et al.* (2010) Folic acid to reduce neonatal mortality from neural tube disorders. *Int. J. Epidemiol.* 39(Suppl 1): i110–i121.

Boelig RC, Barton SJ, Saccone G, *et al.* (2016) Interventions for treating hyperemesis gravidarum. *Cochrane. Database Syst. Rev.* (5): CD010607. doi: 10.1002/14651858.CD010607.pub2.

Brough L, Rees GA, Crawford MA, *et al.* (2009) Social and ethnic differences in folic acid use preconception and during early pregnancy in the UK: effect on maternal folate status and birth outcome. *J. Hum. Nutr. Diet.* 22(2): 100–107.

Brough L, Rees GA, Crawford MA, *et al.* (2010) Effect of multiple-micronutrient supplementation on maternal nutrient status, infant birth weight and gestational age at birth in a low income multi-ethnic population. *Br. J. Nutr.* 104: 437–445.

Butte NF, Wong WW, Treuth MS, *et al.* (2004) Energy requirements during pregnancy based on total energy expenditure and energy deposition. *Am. J. Clin. Nutr.* 79(6): 1078–1087.

Chen B, Ji X, Zhang L, *et al.* (2016) Fish oil supplementation improves pregnancy outcomes and size of the newborn: a meta-analysis of 21 randomized controlled trials. *J. Matern. Fetal. Neonatal. Med.* 29(12): 2017–2027.

Committee on Toxicity (COT). (2008a) *Statement on the reproductive effects of caffeine. COT Statement.* Available at: https://cot.food.gov.uk/committee/committee-on-toxicity/cotstatements/cotstatementsyrs/cotstatements2008/cot200804. Accessed 24 August 2016.

Committee on Toxicity (COT). (2008b) *Statement on the review of the 1998 COT recommendations on peanut avoidance. COT Statement.* Available at http://cot.food.gov.uk/cotstatements/cotstatementsyrs/cotstatements2008/cot200807peanut. Accessed 24 August 2016.

Czeizel AE, Dudas I. (1992) Prevention of the first occurrence of neural tube defects by peri-conceptional vitamin supplementation. *N. Engl. J. Med.* 327: 1832–1835.

DH. (1991) *Dietary Reference Values for Food Energy and Nutrients for the UK. Report of the Panel on Dietary Reference Values of the Committee on Medical Aspects of Food Policy, 41.* London: HMSO.

DH. (2016) *Alcohol Guidelines Review – Report from the Guidelines development group to the UK Chief Medical Officers.* Available at https://www.gov.uk/government/consultations/health-risks-from-alcohol-new-guidelines. Accessed 16 August 2016.

Haider BA, Bhutta ZA. (2017) Multiple-micronutrient supplementation for women during pregnancy. *Cochrane Database Syst. Rev.* 4: CD004905.

Heslehurst N, Rankin J, Wilkinson JR, *et al.* (2010) A nationally representative study of maternal obesity in England, UK: trends in incidence and demographic inequalities in 619 323 births, 1989–2007. *Int. J. Obes (Lond.)* 34: 420–428.

Homan GF, Davies M, Norman R. (2007) The impact of lifestyle factors on reproductive performance in the general population and those undergoing infertility treatment: a review. *Hum. Reprod. Update* 13: 209–223.

Hsu C-S, Liu P-L, Chien L-C, *et al.* (2007) Mercury concentration and fish consumption in Taiwanese pregnant women. *BJOG* 114: 81–85.

Hytten FE, Leitch I. (1971) *The Physiology of Human Pregnancy*. Oxford: Blackwell Scientific Publications.

Institute of Medicine/National Research Council (Committee to Re-examine IOM Pregnancy Weight Guidelines, Food and Nutrition Board and Board on Children, Youth, and Families). (2009) *Weight Gain During Pregnancy: Reexamining the Guidelines*. Washington, DC: National Academy Press.

Knight-Agarwal CR, Williams LT, Davis D, *et al.* (2016) Association of BMI and interpregnancy BMI change with birth outcomes in an Australian obstetric population: a retrospective cohort study. *BMJ Open* 6: e010667. doi:10.1136/bmjopen-2015-010667

Konje JC, CARE Study Group. (2008) Maternal caffeine intake during pregnancy and risk of foetal growth restriction: a large prospective observational study. *BMJ* 337: a2332.

Li Y, Lin H, Li Y, *et al.* (2011) Association between socio-psycho-behavioral factors and male semen quality: systematic review and meta-analyses. *Fertil. Steril.* 95(1): 116–123.

Matthews A, Haas DM, O'Mathúna DP, et al. (2015) Interventions for nausea and vomiting in early pregnancy. *Cochrane Database Syst. Rev.* 9: CD007575.pub4

Mikkelsen TB, Andersen AM, Olsen SF. (2006) Pica in pregnancy in a privileged population: myth or reality. *Acta Obstet. Gynecol. Scand.* 85(10): 1265–1266.

Mikkelsen EM, Riis AH, Wise LA, *et al.* (2016) Alcohol consumption and fecundability: prospective Danish cohort study. *BMJ* 354: i4262.

Moran LJ, Hutchison SK, Norman RJ, *et al.* (2011) Lifestyle changes in women with polycystic ovary syndrome. *Cochrane Database Syst. Rev.* 7: CD007506.

MRC Vitamin Study Research Group. (1991) Prevention of neural tube defects: results of the MRCs vitamin study. *Lancet* 338: 131–149.

Muktabhant B, Lawrie TA, Lumbiganon P, *et al.* (2015) Diet or exercise, or both, for preventing excessive weight gain in pregnancy. *Cochrane Database Syst. Rev.* (6): CD007145. doi: 10.1002/14651858.CD007145.pub3

Nehring I, Schmoll S, Beyerlein A, et al. (2011) Gestational weight gain and long-term postpartum weight retention: a meta-analysis. *Am. J. Clin. Nutr.* 94: 1225–1231.

NICE. (2008) *Antenatal Care for Uncomplicated Pregnancies. Clinical Guideline no. 62*. London: NICE. Last updated January 2017.

NICE. (2010) *Weight Management Before, During and After Pregnancy. Public Health Guidance 27*. London: NICE.

Pasquali R, Patton L, Gambineri A. (2007) Obesity and infertility. *Curr. Opin. Endocrinol. Diabetes Obes.* 14(6): 482–487.

Patra J, Bakker R, Irving H, *et al.* (2011). Dose–response relationship between alcohol consumption before and during pregnancy and the risks of low birth weight, preterm birth and small for gestational age (SGA) – a systematic review and meta-analyses. *BJOG* 118: 1411–1421.

Poston L, Bell R, Croker H, et al. on behalf of The UPBEAT Trial Consortium. (2015) Effect of a behavioural intervention in obese pregnant women (the UPBEAT study): a multicentre, randomized controlled trial. *Lancet Diabetes Endocrinol.* 3(10): 767–777. 10.1016/S2213-8587(15)00227-2

Prentice AM, Goldberg GR, Davies HL, *et al.* (1989) Energy sparing adaptations in human pregnancy assessed by whole body calorimetry. *Br. J. Nutr.* 62: 5–22.

Prentice AM, Spaaij CJ, Goldberg GR, *et al.* (1996). Energy requirements of pregnant and lactating women. *Eur. J. Clin. Nutr.* 50(Suppl 1): s82–s118.

Ramsay JE, Greer I, Sattar N. (2006) Obesity and reproduction. *BMJ* 333: 1159–1162.

Royal College of Obstetricians and Gynaecologists (RCOG)/CMACE. (2010) *The Management of Women with Obesity in Pregnancy*. London: RCOG. Available at https://www.rcog.org.uk/globalassets/documents/guidelines/cmacercogjointguidelinemanagementwomenobesitypregnancya.pdf Accessed 20Septemebr 2018.

Royal College of Obstetricians and Gynaecologists (RCOG). (2016) *The Management of Nausea and Vomiting of Pregnancy and Hyperemesis Gravidarum. Green-top Guideline No. 69*. London: RCOG. Available at https://www.rcog.org.uk/en/guidelines-research-services/guidelines/management-of-women-with-obesity-in-pregnancy/. Accessed 24 August 2016.

Saccone G, Saccone I, Berghella V. (2016) Omega-3 long-chain polyunsaturated fatty acids and fish oil supplementation during pregnancy: which evidence? *J. Matern. Fetal Neonatal. Med.* 29(15): 2389–2397.

SACN. (2011) *Dietary Reference Values for Energy*. London: TSO.

SACN. (2016) *Vitamin D and Health*. Available at https://www.gov.uk/government/groups/scientific-advisory-committee-on-nutrition. Accessed 17 August 2016.

Scott-Pillai R, Spence D, Cardwell C, *et al.* (2013) The impact of body mass index on maternal and neonatal outcomes: a retrospective study in a UK obstetric population, 2004–2011. *BJOG* 120: 932–939.

Sermondade N, Faure C, Fezeu L, et al. (2013) BMI in relation to sperm count: an updated systematic review and collaborative meta-analysis. *Hum. Reprod. Update* 19: 221–231.

Wolf HT, Hegaard HK, Huusom LD, *et al.* (2017) Multivitamin use and adverse birth outcomes in high-income countries: a systematic review and meta-analysis. *Am. J. Obstet. Gynecol.* 217(4): 404.e1–404.e30.

Young SL, Khalfan SS, Farag TH, *et al.* (2010) Association of pica with anemia and gastrointestinal distress among pregnant women in Zanzibar, *Tanzania. Am. J. Trop. Med. Hyg.* 83(1): 144–151.

3.3 Older adults

Vicki Pout

SECTION 3

Key points

- The older population is diverse, with a wide range of nutritional issues and needs.
- Food has biological, social, psychological and economic aspects that affect the nutritional intake of older people.
- Intakes of energy, protein, vitamin C, vitamin D, folate, iron, zinc and fibre are of most concern.
- Good nutrition contributes to health and the ability to recover from illness, and may improve quality of life and lessen health costs by promoting independence.

There is no standard age for becoming elderly or old; most developed countries take the age when pension benefits can be claimed as the starting point for old age. Although chronological age is used as a marker, it is not synonymous with biological age. In the UK, 65 years is usually taken as old, with age ranges of 65–74, 75–84 and 85+ years. The WHO classifies 45–59 years as middle aged, 60–74 years as elderly, 75–89 years as old and 90+ years as very old. In 2015, an estimated 8.5% of the world's population were aged 65 years or older (WHO, 2015). This is estimated to increase to 12% by 2030, with a global population of those aged 65 years and older of ~1 billion people (United States Census Bureau, 2016).

In 2014, 17.7% of the UK population were aged 65 years and older, and 2.3% were 85 years and older (ONS, 2016). The proportion of people aged over 65 years in the UK increased from 13.8% in 1974 to 17.7% in 2014. This is projected to rise to 24.3% by 2039. There is an ageing of the older population itself. In 1984, 19% of those aged over 65 years were in their 80s, and 2% were ≥90 years and over. By 2014, 22% of those aged over 65 years were in their 80s, with 5% aged 90 years or older (ONS, 2016). In 2012–2014, life expectancy at birth for men in the UK was 79.1 years, and for women 82.8 years; this varies between the home countries (ONS, 2016). This has implications for the provision and management of healthcare and social care resources; 62% of total hospital bed days in England in 2014–2015 were accounted for by older patients (National Audit Office, 2016). As the population ages, there is also a change in the ethnographic make-up. Within minority ethnic groups, there is a trend towards a younger age structure; however, this is changing as the population as a whole grows older.

Over the last 20 years, the range of accommodation available for older people has grown enormously, now encompassing extra care housing, very sheltered housing and assisted living, as well as residential and nursing homes. In 2011, 31% of those aged over 65 years in England and Wales lived alone, and 3.2% lived in a care home (ONS, 2014). It is estimated that approximately 5% of the older UK population live in sheltered housing (Pannell & Blood, 2012).

The ageing process and nutrition

Ageing is a natural process affecting many body systems, as shown in Table 3.3.1.

Anorexia of ageing is seen where appetite and intake are reduced due to age-related changes (Britton & McLaughlin, 2013; Morley, 1997; MacIntosh, *et al.*, 2000). Hunger may be reduced, leading to lower food intake, compounded by early satiety. These factors predispose older people to weight loss and malnutrition.

Food habits and nutritional status

In the UK, the National Diet and Nutrition Survey (NDNS) (PHE, 2014) reported the following intake information for older adults:

- Average daily total energy intake is 1835 kcal for men and 1488 kcal women.
- Mean total fat intake met the recommendation of ≤35% food energy. Saturated fat intake exceeded the recommendation of <11% food energy, but intakes were significantly lower in 2013–2014.
- Fibre intakes were below recommendations.

Manual of Dietetic Practice, Sixth Edition. Edited by Joan Gandy.

Companion website: www.manualofdieteticpractice.com

Table 3.3.1 Effects of ageing on body systems

System	Effects of ageing
Skin	Increased fragility and susceptibility to damage and bruising, elongated wound healing time. Loss of hair, slowing of hair and nail growth. Reduced function of sweat and sebaceous glands. Drier, itchier skin. Reduced vitamin D synthesis. (Farage *et al*., 2009; MacLaughlin & Horlick, 1985; Tobin *et al*., 2017)
Cardiovascular system	Loss of heart muscle with increased fibrous tissue. Decreased cardiac output. Heart rate may decrease. Arrhythmias more common. Aorta becomes thicker and less flexible with increased blood pressure. Baroreceptors less sensitive, which may explain the increase in postural hypotension. (Ferrari *et al*., 2003; Strait & Lakatta, 2012)
Urinary system	Decreased filtration rate. Increased glucose threshold. Impaired renal function and fluid balance. Less concentrated urine. (Andrade & Knight, 2008)
Skeletal system	Osteoporosis, reduced bone density, increased fracture risk. Thinner, more rigid cartilage and connective tissue, making joints less resilient and prone to damage, leading to osteoarthritis and reduced range of movement. Height loss, in part due to curvature and compression of the spine. (Boskey & Coleman, 2010).
Immune system	Impaired T cell function, greater susceptibility to viral infections. (Weiskopf *et al*., 2009).
Digestive system	Reduced swallow function. Decreased motor function and muscle tone predisposing to constipation. Impaired digestive capacity. Increased incidence of diverticular disease, colon polyps, heartburn. (Britton & McLaughlin, 2013; Humbert & Robbins, 2008).
Muscle	Sarcopaenia (decreased muscle strength, power and lean body mass, with increased fat body mass), resulting in decreased functional capacity, frailty and increased risk of falls. (Cruz-Jentoft *et al*., 2014)
Hearing	Hearing loss. Elevated sound threshold. Reduced perception of high frequencies. Intrusion of background noise. Degenerative changes in the inner ear leading to balance impairment. (Liu & Yan, 2007)
Taste and smell	Decreased number of taste buds and loss of taste sensitivity. Reduced saliva production. Reduced number of nasal sensory cells. Reduced olfactory function. (Boyce & Shone, 2006)
Vision	Diminished colour fidelity and peripheral vision. Decreased visual acuity and ability to focus on near objects. Diminished ability to see in dim light and distinguish objects of low contrast. (Britton & McLaughlin, 2013)
Nervous system	Decreased size and mass of the brain, with reduced number and connections of neurones. Slower thought processes and reaction time. Reduced sensitivity to temperature changes and reaction to pressure, possible increased sensitivity to light touch. (Peters, 2006; Wickremaratchi & Llewelyn, 2006)
Respiratory system	Decrease in peak air flow and vital capacity. Weaker respiratory muscles. (Sharma & Goodwin, 2006)
Homeostatic regulation	Reduced ability to maintain homeostasis. (Fedarko, 2011)

SECTION 3

- Women's intake of non-milk extrinsic sugars met recommendations (≤11% of food energy), while that of men exceeded recommendations. Main sources were sugar, preserves, confectionary, soft drinks and fruit juice, and cereal and cereal products (mainly cakes and biscuits).
- 35% of those ≥65 years consumed five or more portions of fruit or vegetables. On average, adults ≥65 years consumed 4.2 portions daily.
- Oily fish intake was below the recommended one portion a week.
- Women ate 57 g per day of red and processed meat, below the current maximum recommendation (70 g); men had a mean intake of 81 g.
- 53% reported drinking alcohol.

More detailed information from the NDNS relating to older people has not been reported since 1998; however, this information is still pertinent and is summarised in Table 3.3.2 (Finch *et al.*, 1998).

Many factors influence dietary intake in older adults, as shown in Table 3.3.3.

Dietary recommendations

Older people are a diverse group with wide-ranging nutritional needs; it is important to consider biological and chronological age when making recommendations. Good nutrition contributes to health and the ability to recover from illness, may lessen the burden of health costs by promoting independence as long as possible and improves overall quality of life (King's Fund Centre, 1992).

Older people should be eating for their health, which may not be the same as healthy eating. People require diets that complement their individual health and nutritional needs. For many, this will be healthy eating, but others may need increased levels of energy or other dietary manipulations. Older people should be encouraged to eat a variety of nutrient-dense foods and maintain an active lifestyle where possible (DH, 1992).

Appetite often declines with age (SACN, 2011), but, other than for energy, most requirements remain at the same levels as for younger adults. The emotional and social aspects of food and the role that food and drink play in life's events should not be underestimated. The impact of illness and disability must be considered, as this can quickly compromise food intake, nutritional status and body weight. Although generally at higher risk of nutrient deficiencies, the older population is diverse, and this may not always be the case. Low intake may not always lead to deficiency, owing to individual variations in requirements or adaptation. Conversely, nutrient intakes may appear adequate, but be inadequate for individuals with higher requirements.

Energy

Older people should be advised to consume enough energy to maintain a healthy body weight. There is only a small age-related decline in energy requirements, mainly due to changes in muscle fat ratios. Energy requirements may be below recommended levels (see Appendix A4), especially if physical activity is limited.

Calcium and vitamin D

Osteoporosis and associated fractures are a major cause of morbidity and mortality in older adults. Over 300,000

Table 3.3.2 Eating habits and nutritional status (Finch *et al.*, 1998)

Free-living	Institutions	All
Lower socioeconomic status correlated with significantly lower intakes of energy, protein, carbohydrate, fibre, some vitamins (especially vitamin C) and minerals	Poor oral health and hygiene as compared to free-living older people. Root decay especially prevalent	Better oral health and number of natural teeth linked with better diet and nutritional status
Heavier than those of the same age 30 years previously, but recorded food energy intake lower	Vitamin D status poor in some, especially in winter	Presence of dental root decay was related to the frequency of intake of high-sugar foods independent of age, gender, social class and region of origin
90% had 7/10 staple items in their home	More likely to consume sugar, preserves, buns, cakes, pastries and cereal-based milk puddings	Biochemical status of most vitamins and minerals adequate for most people
86% visited shops. 55% said food shopping was sometimes done by someone else		Poor folate status in a significant proportion of older people, especially those aged ≥85 years
53% had milk delivered where this was available		Traditional meal pattern of three meals a day plus smaller snacks in between. For some, nutritional contribution from snacks and drinks was considerable
One-third reported taking non-prescribed dietary supplements – most commonly cod liver oil		Most commonly consumed foods were tea, boiled / mashed/ baked potatoes, white bread and biscuits

Note: The intakes of energy, protein, vitamin C, vitamin D, folate, iron, zinc and fibre were of most concern.

Table 3.3.3 Factors associated with dietary intake in older adults

Factor	Description
Food availability	Loss of control over food when shopped for or in care. Lack of nearby supermarkets may restrict food choice if no private transport is available, or if they are unable to use public transport or carry heavy shopping. Lack of help with shopping or food and beverage preparation. Carers may not appreciate the importance of nutrition.
Finances	Low finances and limited budget. Not able to afford nutritionally adequate diet. Supermarkets usually offer best value and special offers on larger-pack sizes of food, which may cost too much or not be able to be stored or used. Concerns about paying bills, e.g. fuel bills in winter.
Cooking	Cooking for self and eating alone. Cooking and living facilities may be inadequate or inaccessible.
Sensory perception	Loss of or altered sense of taste, sight, hearing, smell and thirst.
Health issues	Decreased mobility or physical or mental illness affecting the ability to shop, prepare or consume food, possibly affecting appetite. Chronic or acute pain. Constipation. Confusion or dementia. Drug side effects or interactions may affect appetite, cause taste changes or constipation, or affect absorption of nutrients. May be compounded by polypharmacy. Impaired communication skills, e.g. dementia, loss of hearing or dysphasia. Dysphagia, especially if a modified-texture diet is required. Altered nutritional requirements due to medical conditions.
Food provision	Unfamiliar or culturally inappropriate foods or menu terminology. Repeated investigations or periods of fasting. Poor nutritional content of food. Lack of provision for second helpings. Inappropriate meal times with long gaps when no food or drink is offered.
Lack of interest in food	Poor appetite. Anorexia. Nausea. Depression, cognitive impairment, drowsiness, anxiety. Illness and anxiety. Social isolation.
Inappropriate food	Cultural/religious restrictions. Dietary misconceptions, food myths and incorrect media messages. Unfamiliar foods or menu items. Lack of patient/resident choice and poor menu planning.
Previous experience	Cooking skills, reliance on pre-prepared foods. Education and nutritional knowledge. Personal likes and dislikes. Habit. Fear of complaining about food or asking for food or beverages in case care is compromised.
Mealtime experience	Narrow range of foods eaten. Reluctance to try new foods. Unprotected mealtimes. Poorly served food. Inappropriate portion sizes. Lack of garnishes and condiments. Food served at incorrect temperature or kept warm for long periods. Lack of choice as to whether to join others for meals. Monotonous menus.
Assistance with eating and drinking	Unable to unwrap food. Unable to use cutlery. Inadequate assistance with eating and drinking. Afraid to ask for assistance or may feel they are bothering busy staff. Poor positioning.
Oral problems	Sore or dry mouth. Oral thrush. Ill-fitting dentures. Poor oral hygiene, mouth care or dentition. Reduced number of or no teeth (chewing ability related to number of teeth). Gum disease. Older adults living in care homes more likely to be edentulous and have non-functioning dentition. Untreated dental decay higher in older people, especially among those in care homes (PHE, 2015).

patients present to UK hospitals with fragility fractures every year (NICE, 2012), with most fractures occurring in the wrist, spine or hip (DH, 1998). Calcium, sunlight exposure and dietary vitamin D are important for bone health. A calcium intake of 700 mg/day is recommended. Highest intakes are milk and milk-based foods, white fortified flour products and vegetables (DH, 1998). SACN (2016) recently reviewed data for vitamin D and health (SACN, 2016), and set the recommended nutrient intake (RNI) for vitamin D for the UK population aged ≥4 years at 10μg /d. To protect musculoskeletal health, it was recommended that the serum 25(OH)D concentrations not fall below 25 nmol/L. They advised that everyone should consider a daily supplement of 10 μg vitamin D during autumn and winter. People who rarely expose their skin to the sun (such as those in institutions), who rarely leave their house or who always cover their skin when outside should consider taking a vitamin D supplement all year round. Older people are particularly vulnerable to deficiency owing to less sunlight exposure, reduced efficiency of skin synthesis and poor oily fish consumption.

Vitamin C

An intake of 40 mg/day is recommended (DH, 1991); however, fruit and vegetable consumption may be insufficient to achieve this. This is of particular concern in those individuals who have poor appetites, are frail, dependent on institutional catering or need modified-texture diets. Where supplementation is advised, it should not greatly exceed the RNI.

Vitamin B_{12}

Dietary deficiency is uncommon, and pernicious anaemia is usually caused by absorptive problems. Low intake may be found in those with restricted intakes, e.g. vegetarians or vegans. Attention should also be paid to people with conditions such as Crohn's disease and achlorhydria, or who have had a gastrectomy (Finch *et al.*, 1998).

Iron

The RNI for iron is 8.7 mg/day for those aged >50 years (DH, 1991). A lower intake may be sufficient, especially in post-menopausal women. Intake can be of particular concern where the diet is monotonous or if texture modification is needed. Gastrointestinal blood loss is the most common cause of iron deficiency in older people, which can be caused by a range of factors, including diseases of the genitourinary system, colorectal cancer, anti-inflammatory drugs (e.g. aspirin) or frequent blood tests. In 2010, SACN recommended that emphasis be placed on a healthy, balanced diet, including a variety of iron-containing foods, and that less emphasis be given to the inclusion or avoidance of enhancers or inhibitors of iron absorption.

Zinc

Problems due to low zinc status in the older adult include delayed wound healing and decreased taste acuity (Meunier *et al.*, 2005; Prasad, 1994; Prasad *et al.*, 1992). Intake of zinc can be problematic for those without a varied diet or needing texture modification.

Fluid and hydration

Older people are at greater risk of dehydration, partly due to reduced perception of thirst and the effects of ageing on sodium and water balance (Schols *et al.*, 2009). A loss of body water of 1% can affect physical and cognitive functioning (Mentes, 2006). The prevalence of dehydration varies according to the setting, the methods used to assess dehydration and the definition of dehydration used. Older people are vulnerable to dehydration in all care settings as well as when free-living (Hooper *et al.*, 2015). Common causes of dehydration are shown in Table 3.3.4.

The effects of dehydration can lead to further reduction in fluid intake (Ritz & Berrut, 2005). The effects of dehydration in older adults include:

- Reduced appetite.
- Increased risk of pressure ulcers.
- Poor wound healing.
- Constipation.
- Electrolyte imbalance.
- Falls and fractures.
- Altered cardiac function.
- Unpleasant taste.
- Headaches.
- Drowsiness, confusion.
- Lowered blood pressure.
- Light-headedness / dizziness on standing.
- Urinary tract infections.
- Irritability.

The European Food Safety Agency (EFSA, 2010) recommends total water daily intakes of 2000 mL for women and 2500 mL for men, which includes approximately 20% of water from foods. Adequate fluid intake should be encouraged, and for most this will be 1500–2000 mL daily (EFSA, 2010), equating to six to eight drinks (PHE, 2016). It is important that awareness be promoted that all fluids count. Where poor appetite or nutritional intake is of concern, nourishing fluids should be advised. Fluid intake is of particular concern in individuals who require thickened fluids (Whelan, 2001). Strategies for improving fluid intake include:

- Giving encouragement to maximise intake throughout the day.
- Offering drinks at sessions, e.g. physiotherapy or groups.
- Providing fruit juice and hot drinks at breakfast.
- Training staff on the importance of hydration.
- Ensuring that drinks are available at all times.
- Giving preferred drinks in the preferred receptacle, e.g. cup and saucer, not mug.
- Making drinks attractive, e.g. adding mint, cucumber or citrus fruit; also, ice cubes add additional fluid.
- Giving assistance with drinking.
- Offering a variety of hot and cold drinks.
- Giving a full glass of water with medications.
- Providing drinking aids, e.g. specialist beakers or hydrants.
- Encouraging visitors to drink with older adults.
- Monitoring intake regularly, especially those requiring thickened fluids.

Table 3.3.4 Common causes of dehydration in older adults

Pathological	Ageing	Other
Confusion, unable to ask for a drink, do not recognise thirst, may forget to drink	Altered thirst perception, so do not feel thirsty	Drugs, e.g. diuretics, laxatives, ACE inhibitors, psychotropic medications, polypharmacy
Depression	Increased skin losses due to thinner skin	Fluid restriction, may not always be necessary or reviewed
Drowsiness	Reduced total body water	Institutionalisation, lack of availability of drinks
Decreased mobility or dexterity. Unable to make a drink. Lack of assistance given. Increased dependence on carers for drinks.	Reduced renal function, less concentrated urine	Physical environment, e.g. high room temperature
Conditions affecting fluid requirements or losses, e.g. pyrexia, diarrhoea, exudates, bleeding, vomiting, polyuria		Urinary incontinence or perceived increased micturition after drinking, especially in the evening. Fear of incontinence
Mouth discomfort, e.g. dentition, poor-fitting dentures, sore mouth, coated mouth or tongue		

- Replenishing water jugs frequently.
- Including foods with high water content, e.g. soups, sauces, gravies, jellies, milk puddings, custards, ice creams, lollies.

Physical activity

An active lifestyle should be encouraged, with minimal extended sedentary periods. Activity has health benefits relating to cognitive function, reduction in falls and cardiovascular risk. Exercise can also improve mood and self-esteem, and promote independence. Weight-bearing exercise promotes bone health. Daily activity totalling a weekly minimum of 150 minutes should be aimed for. Muscle-strengthening activities are recommended for at least 2 days a week. Those at risk of falls should carry out activities to improve balance and coordination at least twice a week (DH, 2011).

Nutritional challenges

Some conditions present more frequently with advancing age, such as stroke, dementia, cognitive impairment and osteoporosis. Older people may present with diffuse symptoms such as falls, immobility, incontinence, acute confusion or weight loss, making diagnosis and treatment problematic. There may also be reluctance to visit a GP due to the misconception that disease is a natural part of ageing, or thinking that there is nothing that can or will be done to help. Often, the biggest dietetic challenge is to maintain adequate nutritional intake in the face of multiple factors reducing appetite and food consumption. Conversely, prevalence of obesity in older adults is increasing in all but the very oldest. With improvements in medical treatments, conditions once thought of as affecting younger people are now seen in older adults as they live longer with the condition. For example, in 2015, 34% of people living with diagnosed HIV and receiving care were >50 years (PHE, 2016).

Malnutrition

Malnutrition affects physical and mental functions and the outcome of disease. The effects of malnutrition in older adults is shown in Table 3.3.5.

Factors increasing vulnerability to malnutrition include chronic physical and mental health conditions, recent hospital discharge, social isolation or low income. The prevalence of malnutrition is shown in Table 3.3.6.

Older people at risk of malnutrition have 25% more hospital admissions, 6% more GP visits and 9% more prescriptions than individuals within the normal weight range. For hospitalised patients, those at risk of malnutrition have a significantly longer stay and are more likely to be discharged to a care destination other than their own home (Elia, 2005). Factors affecting malnutrition in older adults are shown in Table 3.3.7.

Davies (1998) identified four types of malnutrition pertinent to older people:

- *Specific malnutrition* – deficiency of a specific nutrient or nutrition-related disease, e.g. scurvy, osteomalacia.
- *Long-standing malnutrition* – often linked with general neglect; clinical appearance of energy and nutrient deficiencies following a period of inadequate intake.
- *Sudden* – marked change in food intake, often after a significant life event, e.g. major fall or bereavement.

Table 3.3.5 Effects of malnutrition (NICE, 2006)

Adverse effect	Consequences
Impaired immune response	Compounded by age-related decrease in immunity
	Increased risk of infection, e.g. pneumonia
	Delayed recovery
Muscle wasting	Decreased muscle strength, increased fatigue, prolonged rehabilitation
	Decreased mobility
	Decreased ability to perform activities of daily living, increased carer burden
	Increased risk of falls and fractures
	Increased risk of heart failure, with wasting of heart muscle compounding age-related decreased cardiac function
Reduced respiratory muscle function	Increased breathing problems, less effective cough mechanism
	Reduced cough pressure
Impaired thermoregulation	Increased risk of hypothermia
Impaired wound healing	Increased risk of pressure ulcers, wound infection and ununited fractures
Psychological effects	Apathy, depression, anorexia, anxiety, fatigue, impaired psychosocial function, low self-esteem
Increased risk of vitamin and other deficiencies	Increased risk of refeeding syndrome
	Increased risk of specific nutrient deficiencies, e.g. iron deficiency anaemia
Overall	Delayed recovery from illness
	Increased mortality

Table 3.3.6 Malnutrition prevalence (BAPEN, 2010)

Group	Malnutrition rate
General population	5% (BMI<20kg/m²)
Free-living older people	14%*
GP and outpatient attendees	18–30%*
Chronic disease	12% underweight
Care homes	16–29% underweight 20–50%*
Hospital admissions – general	15–40%* underweight
Hospital admissions – medical, surgical, elderly and orthopaedic wards	20–60%*

*Using Malnutrition Universal Screening Tool ('MUST').

Table 3.3.7 Factors affecting malnutrition in older adults

Cause of malnutrition	Factors
Altered nutrient requirement	Increased energy requirements, e.g. involuntary movements, pacing, drug–nutrient interactions
Impaired digestion and/or absorption	Drug–nutrient interactions, polypharmacy, bacterial overgrowth, achlorhydria, and problems affecting stomach, intestine, pancreas and liver
Increased nutrient losses	Gastrointestinal losses, e.g. vomiting, diarrhoea, fistulae, stomas. Exudate from wounds or pressure ulcers

- *Recurrent* – barely adequate nutritional status entering a cycle of poor nutrition and repeated episodes of illness.

Common issues

Osteoporosis is common in older people; prevalence increases with age. When assessing an individual nutritionally, their weight and physical activity should be taken into account. Being overweight can impair mobility, leading to increased risk of falls. Being underweight increases risk of falling and consequent fracture.

Dementia and cognitive impairment are important factors in nutritional problems. Individuals may have challenges impacting on their ability to prepare and consume food, and communicate thoughts and feelings related to food. Food is emotive and seen as a vital part of care. When addressing difficulties with eating and drinking, comprehensive and effective communication is needed with persons living with dementia, as well as with their relatives and carers.

The life expectancy of people with learning disabilities (including Down syndrome) has increased with advances in medical care. People with learning disabilities are more likely to develop dementia at an early age. Around 20% of people with a learning disability will develop dementia over the age of 65 years. However, 2% of people with Down syndrome develop dementia in their 30s, rising to >50% of those living over 60 years (Alzheimer's Society, 2015). People with learning disabilities may also experience a more rapid progression of dementia. Care may be hampered by difficulties and delay in diagnosis.

Polypharmacy compounds drug–nutrient interactions or side effects of a single medication. Older people often take a range of medications, including prescribed and over-the-counter medicines, vitamin and mineral supplements, and complementary remedies. It is important to take into account any implications of the medication regimen when performing a dietetic consultation. Common side effects include nausea, dry mouth, altered taste sensation, constipation, diarrhoea and drowsiness.

Care planning

Older people often have multiple comorbidities. The combined effects must be considered when devising nutritional strategies. A checklist for good nutritional care is given in Box 3.3.1.

Free-living and sheltered accommodation

Most older people live in the community. Nutritional intervention usually aims to maintain nutritional status and promote independence for as long as possible to avoid admission to hospitals or other care settings. Care is often provided informally by a relative or carer, or by a paid care package. It is important to ensure that carers be given sufficient information to enable them to provide appropriate nutritional care. Some risk factors for poor nutrition are particularly pertinent to older people living in the community, and should be considered when assessing nutrition in older people (see Table 3.3.8).

Community meals

There are no national standards for nutritional content of community meals. A standard was launched in 2010 (National Association of Care Catering, 2010). Community meals should meet the dietary needs of a variety of groups, from traditional healthy eating, to energy- and nutrient-dense (in small volumes), to modified-texture and therapeutic diets. One meal a day should aim to provide 40–50% of daily nutrient requirements in a realistic volume. There should be sufficient variety to reduce menu fatigue. Some community meals are very low in salt, which can reduce their tastiness; if a meal is not eaten, it provides no nutrition. People should be able to easily choose suitable dishes for their needs.

Community meals may only provide one meal a day, and not always on all 7 days a week. Overall meal, snack and beverage provision must be taken into consideration when working with older people, as well as the need for encouragement and assistance. The human contact involved in delivered hot meals is very important as, for some people, this may be the only contact they have in a day. Delivery staff should be trained to support the older

SECTION 3

Box 3.3.1 Checklist for good nutritional care in older adults

- Ensure people are involved as much as possible with their nutritional care. Follow best practices in decision making if capacity is an issue.
- Ensure the individual's circumstances are fully explored when planning nutritional care.
- Ensure that national regulatory standards for food, fluid and nutritional care are adhered to.
- There is a need for a local healthcare wide strategy for the nutritional care of older people for both malnutrition and obesity.
- Follow local policies for managing the risk of malnutrition and for appropriate prescribing of oral nutritional supplements.
- Regular nutrition screening should occur in all health settings using a validated screening tool. Results and nutritional care plans should be communicated across all care settings. Ensure there is regular monitoring of weight, and food and fluid intake.
- A food-first approach to improving nutritional intake is advised where possible.
- Food should be a highlight of the day.
- In institutional care settings, ensure protected mealtimes are implemented. Give consideration to the timing of meals, appropriate menus, and drink and snack provision.
- Ensure modified-texture meals and thickened fluids are only used when appropriate.
- Raise awareness of the importance of good nutrition and hydration.
- Individualised assistance with eating and drinking should be available, including the provision of specialist aids.
- Set realistic nutritional goals.
- Adequate and effective training on nutritional issues is needed for healthcare and social care staff working with older people. Many health professionals and carers have had very little nutrition training other than education about healthy eating.

Table 3.3.8 Risk factors for poor nutrition in older people living in the community (Davies, 1981)

Theme	Risk factor
Food habits	Less than eight main meals, hot or cold, weekly
	Minimal consumption of milk, fruit and vegetables.
	Wastage of food even when supplied ready-to-eat
	Long periods during the day without food or drink
Physical or mental factors	Depression or loneliness
	Indications of disabilities, including alcohol abuse or dependence
Social	Problems shopping
	Poverty

people to whom they deliver. Some people only order a meal every other day due to the expense. Food is not seen as sufficiently important, as there is a widely held misconception that all people lose weight they get older.

Regulation and monitoring of food and nutritional care in hospitals and other care settings have been strengthened. In England, this is monitored by the Care Quality Commission (CQC, 2008), with Regulation 14 of the Health and Social Care Act (2008) relating to nutrition and hydration needs. Healthcare Inspectorate Wales monitors nutrition through dignity and essential care inspections, while Healthcare Improvement Scotland runs the Improving Nutritional Care programme and lays out guidance for nutritional care in Food, Fluid and Nutritional Care Standards (Health Improvement Scotland, 2014). In Northern Ireland, the Regulation and Quality Improvement Authority has minimum standards for care in nursing homes, residential care and day care settings, including standards for nutrition (Department of Health, Social Services and Public Safety, 2011, 2012a, 2012b, 2015), plus the Promoting Good Nutrition strategy to improve nutritional care of adults (CQC, 2010, 2011).

The CQC published reports looking at dignity and nutrition in hospitals and care homes in England following inspections during 2012 (CQC, 2013a, 2013b). In hospitals where there were problems, the recurrent themes were:

- Not giving the help needed to eat and drink.
- Food and drink consumed not always recorded accurately.
- Not always giving suitable choices of menu.
- Delays in referrals for nutrition or dietetic advice.
- Not giving the opportunity to wash their hands before or after eating.

People living in one in six care homes inspected were not always supported to eat and drink sufficient amounts. In care homes where there were problems, the recurrent themes were:

- The residents were not always given a choice of food or supported to make a choice.
- The residents were not always identified as being at risk of malnutrition or given support to improve nutrition.
- Enough staff was not always available to assist with eating and drinking.

These themes are not new, and have been subjects of high-profile campaigns and media coverage, e.g.

Hungry to be Heard (Age Concern, 2006), Still Hungry to be Heard (Age UK, 2010) and the CARE campaign (Patients Association, 2012).

A positive approach to food and the mealtime experience should be promoted in all healthcare settings (Table 3.3.9). Working with older people will often entail being part of one or more multidisciplinary teams. The makeup of teams vary according to setting, speciality and funding. Good, effective team working can improve the nutritional status of patients, as team members understand the roles that they perform and the contribution they make to nutritional care.

Promoting independence

Many community-based services promote independent living. Providers range from local authorities to private companies and the voluntary sector. The services available in areas differ, as do access routes and eligibility criteria. Much support for older people is provided by family and friends who may be of a similar age to the person they are helping. To provide good nutritional care for older people, it is important to have an understanding of the range of services available in the local area. Table 3.3.10 shows the range of services available in the community setting.

Table 3.3.9 Factors promoting nutritional care

Factor	Comment
Snacks	Snacks should be available between meals. Older adults may rely on snacks if only small meals are managed. Nourishing drinks should be available, e.g. full-fat milky drinks.
Appropriate meals	Dishes, timings and dining arrangements should be appropriate to the population. Routines should be flexible to cope with individual needs. There should be a choice of portion sizes and the provision of seconds. A range of drinks should be available at all times. Meals should be culturally appropriate and meet religious requirements where necessary. The ability to fortify meals should be made available to increase nutritional content, if required.
Assistance	Appropriate assistance with eating and drinking should be available from suitably trained staff. The need for assistance should be assessed on admission and reviewed regularly.
Team work	Nutritional care of patients is the responsibility of the entire health and social team and should be seen as such by all. There should be effective communication among team members, patients and their relatives to ensure consistent messages.
Eating area	Where there is a dining room, it should be comfortable, clean, tidy and have appropriate furniture. Where there is no dining room, bed tables should be cleared and cleaned prior to mealtimes.
Hygiene	People should be given the opportunity to use the toilet and wash their hands prior to meal service. Good oral hygiene should be promoted.
Adaptations	Eating and drinking aids should be available. Modified-texture diets should only be used where this will benefit the patient.

Table 3.3.10 Range of services available in the community setting

Services	Description
Services to prevent hospital admission and/or provide support post-discharge	Social services or private care packages
	Community meals: may be hot meals or delivery of frozen meals
	Rapid response teams to reduce admissions
	Early supported discharge teams providing immediate post-discharge support to reduce readmission
	Intermediate care teams providing rehabilitation at home
	Day hospitals
	Respite care
Local community services	Clubs: retirement, lunch
	Community or day centres
	Cultural and religious activities
Shopping services	Dial-a-ride
	Free supermarket bus
	Internet or telephone shopping and delivery
Voluntary services	Age UK
	Disease specific groups e.g. Alzheimer's Society, Stroke Association and stroke clubs, Parkinson's Society
	Carers UK
	Citizens Advice
	Ex-services groups, e.g. Royal British Legion
	Admiral Nurses – Dementia UK

Further reading

BDA. (2012) *The Nutrition and Hydration Digest: Improving Outcomes through Food and Beverage Services.* www.bda.uk.com/publications/professional/NutritionHydrationDigest.pdf.

British Association of Parenteral and Enteral Nutrition (BAPEN). (2009) *Screening for malnutrition in sheltered housing.* Available at http://www.bapen.org.uk/pdfs/nsw/gnash_exec_summary09.pdf. Accessed 30 June 2017.

Council of Europe Resolution. (2003) *Food and Nutritional Care in Hospitals.* Strasbourg: Council of Europe Publishing.

Crawley H. (2002) *Food drink and dementia. How to help people with dementia to eat well.* www.stir.ac.uk/dsdc.

European Nutrition for Health Alliance. (2006) *Malnutrition among older people in the community: Policy recommendations for change.*

European Society of Parenteral and Enteral Nutrition. (2006) *Nutrition in Ageing: A call to action.*

Gurcharan SR (ed). (2004) *Medical Ethics and the Elderly.* Oxford: Radcliffe Medical Press.

Lennard Jones JE. (2012) *Ethical and Legal Aspects of Clinical Hydration and Nutritional Support.* London: BAPEN.

Malnutrition Task Force. *A review and summary of the impact of malnutrition in older people and the reported costs and benefits of interventions.* Available at http://www.malnutritiontaskforce.org.uk/wp-content/uploads/2014/11/A-review-and-summary-of-the-impact-of-malnutrition-in-older-people-and-the-reported-costs-and-benefits-of-interventions.pdf.

NICE. (2017) *Osteoporosis: assessing the risk of fragility fracture. Clinical Guideline* 146. Available at https://www.nice.org.uk/guidance/cg146. Accessed 30 May 2017.

Office for National Statistics (ONS). (2013) *What Does the 2011 Census Tell Us about Older People?* Available at http://webarchive.nationalarchives.gov.uk/20160105160709/http://www.ons.gov.uk/ons/rel/census/2011-census-analysis/what-does-the-2011-census-tell-us-about-older-people-/what-does-the-2011-census-tell-us-about-older-people--short-story.html. Accessed 30 May 2017.

Office for National Statistics. *Ageing.* Available at https://www.ons.gov.uk/peoplepopulationandcommunity/birthsdeathsandmarriages/ageing.

Scottish Executive National Care Standards. (2007) *Care Home for Older People.*

Voices. (1998) *Eating Well for Older People with Dementia.*

Volkert D, Berner YN, Berry E, *et al.* (2006) ESPEN guidelines on enteral nutrition: geriatrics. *Clin. Nutr.* 25(2): 330–360.

Volkert D, Chourdakis M, Faxen-Irving G, *et al.* (2015) ESPEN guidelines on nutrition in dementia. *Clin. Nutr.* 34(6): 1052–1073.

WHO. (2002) *Keep fit for life: meeting the nutritional needs of older people.* Available at http://apps.who.int/iris/bitstream/10665/42515/1/9241562102.pdf.

Internet Resources

Age UK, www.ageuk.org.uk

British Geriatrics Society, www.bgs.org.uk

Care for Older People Portal, www.knowledge.scot.nhs.uk/home/portals-and-topics/care-for-older-people-portal.aspx

Care Quality Commission Standards of Care, www.cqc.org.uk

Carers UK, www.carersuk.org

Caroline Walker Trust, www.cwt.org.uk

Centre for Policy on Ageing, www.cpa.org.uk

Council of Europe Resolution, www.bapen.org.uk/pdfs/coe_leaflet.pdf.

European Nutrition for Health Alliance, www.european-nutrition.org/publications.cfm.

European Society of Parenteral and Enteral Nutrition, www.espen.org.

Health in Wales: Older People, www.wales.nhs.uk/healthtopics/populations/olderpeople

HSC Knowledge Exchange Northern Ireland: Older People, http://www.knowledge.hscni.net/Topics/Index/47

International Longevity Centre UK, www.ilcuk.org.uk

NHS England Older People, https://www.england.nhs.uk/ourwork/clinical-policy/older-people/

Scottish Executive National Care Standards. www.scotland.gov.uk.

Voices. www.cwt.org.uk.

WHO. *Ageing.* www.who.int/topics/ageing/en/.

References

Age Concern. (2006) *Hungry to be heard. The scandal of malnourished older people in hospital.* Available at http://www.ageuk.org.uk/documents/en-gb/hungry_to_be_heard_inf.pdf?dtrk=true. Accessed 30 June 2017.

Age UK. (2010) *Still hungry to be heard. The scandal people in later life becoming malnourished in hospital.* Available at www.ageuk.org.uk/documents/en-gb/for-professionals/health-and-wellbeing/id9489_still_hungry_to_be_heard_report_28ppa4.pdf?dtrk=true. Accessed 30 May 2017.

Alzheimer's Society. (2015) *Learning disabilities and dementia.* Available at https://www.alzheimers.org.uk/info/20007/types_of_dementia/37/learning_disabilities_and_dementia. Accessed 30 May 2017.

Andrade M, Knight J. (2008) Exploring the anatomy and physiology of ageing part 4 – the renal system. *Nurs. Times* 104(34): 22–23.

Boskey AL, Coleman R. (2010) Ageing and bone. *J. Dent. Res.* 89(12): 1333–1348.

Boyce J, Shone G. (2006). Effects of ageing on smell and taste. *Postgrad. Med. J.* 82(966): 239–241.

British Association of Parenteral and Enteral Nutrition (BAPEN). (2010) Malnutrition Matters: meeting quality standards in nutritional care. Available at http://www.bapen.org.uk/pdfs/nsw/gnash_exec_summary09.pdf. Accessed 30 May 2017.

Britton E, McLaughlin JT. (2013) Ageing and the gut. *Proc. Nutr. Soc.* 72(1): 173–177.

Care Quality Commission (CQC). (2008) Guidance for providers: Regulation 14 of the Health and Social Care Act. Available at http://www.cqc.org.uk/guidance-providers/regulations-enforcement/regulations-service-providers-managers. Accessed 30 May 2017.

Care Quality Commission. (2010) Guidance about compliance. Essential standards of quality and safety. Available at https://services.cqc.org.uk/sites/default/files/gac_-_dec_2011_update.pdf. Accessed 20 September 2018.

Care Quality Commission. (2011) Dignity and Nutrition Inspection Programme. National overview Available at https://www.cqc.org.uk/sites/default/files/documents/20111007_dignity_and_nutrition_inspection_report_final_update.pdf. Accessed 20 September 2018.

Care Quality Commission (CQC). (2013a) *Time to Listen in NHS Hospital: Dignity and Inspection Programme 2012.* Available at https://www.cqc.org.uk/sites/default/files/documents/time_to_listen_-_nhs_hospitals_main_report_tag.pdf. Accessed 30 May 2017.

Care Quality Commission (CQC). (2013b) *Time to Listen in Care Homes: Dignity and Nutrition Inspection Programme 2012.* Available at https://www.cqc.org.uk/sites/default/files/documents/time_to_listen_-_care_homes_main_report_tag.pdf. Accessed 30 May 2017.

Caroline Walker Trust. (2004) *Eating well for older people – practical nutritional guidelines for food in residential and nursing homes and community meals.* Available at http://www.cwt.org.uk/wp-content/uploads/2014/07/OlderPeople.pdf. Accessed 30 May 2017.

Cruz-Jentoft AJ, Landi F, Schneider SM, *et al.* (2014). Prevalence of and interventions for sarcopenia in ageing adults: a systematic review. Report of the International Sarcopenia Initiative (EWGSOP and IWGS). *Age Ageing* 43(6): 748–759.

Davies L. (1981) *Three Score Years … and Then?* London, Oxford: Heinemann Medical Books.

Davies L. (1998) Practical nutrition for the elderly. *Nutr. Rev.* 46: 83–87.

Department of Health, Social Services and Public Safety. (2011) *Residential Care Home Minimum Standards*. Available at https://www.health-ni.gov.uk/sites/default/files/publications/dhssps/care-standards-residential-care-homes.pdf. Accessed 30 June 2017.

Department of Health, Social Services and Public Safety. (2012a) *Day Care Settings Minimum Standards*. Available at https://www.health-ni.gov.uk/sites/default/files/publications/dhssps/care-standards-adult-day-care.pdf. Accessed 30 June 2015.

Department of Health, Social Services and Public Safety. (2012b) Promoting Good Nutrition. A Strategy for Good Nutritional Care for Adults in all Care Settings in Northern Ireland, 2011–2016. Available at https://www.health-ni.gov.uk/sites/default/files/publications/dhssps/promoting-good-nutrition_0.pdf. Accessed 30 June 2017.

Department of Health, Social Services and Public Safety. (2015) Care standards for nursing homes. Available at https://rqia.org.uk/RQIA/media/RQIA/Resources/Standards/nursing_homes_standards_-_april_2015.pdf. Accessed 20September 2018.

DH. (1991) *Dietary Reference Values for Food, Energy and Nutrients for the UK. Report of the Working Group of the Committee on Medical Aspects of Food Policy. Report on Health and Social Subjects 41*. London: HMSO.

DH. (1992) *The Nutrition of Elderly People. Report of the Working Group on the Nutrition of Elderly People of the Committee on Medical Aspects of Food Policy. Report on Health and Social Subjects 43*. London HMSO.

DH. (1998) *Nutrition and Bone Health. Report of the Working Group of the Committee on Medical Aspects of Food Policy. Report on Health and Social Subjects 49*. London: HMSO.

DH. (2011) *Start active, stay active: report on physical activity in the UK*. Available at https://www.gov.uk/government/publications/start-active-stay-active-a-report-on-physical-activity-from-the-four-home-countries-chief-medical-officers. Last accessed 26 May 2017.

Elia M. (2005) *Economic Implications of Malnutrition*. Available at http://www.bapen.org.uk/resources-and-education/publications-and-reports/malnutrition/the-cost-of-disease-related-malnutrition-in-the-uk. Accessed 30 June 2017.

European Food Safety Authority (EFSA). (2010) Scientific opinion on reference values for water. *EFSA J.* 8(3): 1459–1507.

Farage MA, Miller KW, Berardesca E, *et al.* (2009) Clinical implications of aging skin: cutaneous disorders in the elderly. *Am. J. Clin. Dermatol.* 10: 73–86.

Fedarko NS. (2011) The biology of aging and frailty. *Clin. Geriatr. Med.* 27: 27–37.

Ferrari AU, Radaelli A, Centola M. (2003) Invited review: aging and the cardiovascular system. *J. Appl. Physiol.* 95: 2591–2597.

Finch S, Doyle W, Lowe C, *et al.* (1998) *National Diet and Nutrition Survey: People Aged 65 years and Over. Volume 1: Report of the Diet and Nutrition Survey*. London: The Stationery Office.

Health Improvement Scotland. (2014) *Food, fluid and nutritional care standards*. Available at http://www.healthcareimprovementscotland.org/our_work/patient_safety/improving_nutritional_care/nutritional_care_standards.aspx. Accessed 30 May 2017.

Hooper L, Abdelhamid A, Attreed NJ, *et al.* (2015). Clinical symptoms, signs and tests for identification of impending and current water-loss dehydration in older people. *Cochrane Database Syst. Rev.* doi: 10.1002/14651858.CD009647.pub2.

Humbert IA, Robbins J. (2008) Dysphagia in the elderly. *Phys. Med. Rehabil. Clin. N. Am.* 19(4): 853–866.

King's Fund Centre. (1992) *A Positive Approach to Nutrition as Treatment*. London: King's Fund Centre.

Liu X, Yan D. (2007). Ageing and hearing loss. *J. Pathol.* 211: 188–197.

MacIntosh C, Morley JE, Chapman IM. (2000) The anorexia of aging. *Nutrition* 16: 983–995.

MacLaughlin J, Horlick MF. (1985) Ageing decreases the capacity of human skin to produce vitamin D3. *J. Clin. Invest.* 76: 1536–1538.

Meunier N, O'Connor JM, Maiani G. et al. (2005) Importance of zinc in the elderly: the ZENITH study. *Eur. J Clin. Nutr.* 59: S1–S4.

Mentes J. (2006) Oral hydration in older adults. *Am. J. Nurs.* 106: 40–49.

MRC Human Nutrition Research. (2014) *What Do UK Adults Eat?* Available at http://www.mrc-ewl.cam.ac.uk/wp-content/uploads/2014/09/NDNS-summary-Adults.pdf. Accessed 2 September 2018. The publisher is MRC Human Nutrition Research, Cambridge.

Morley JE. (1997) Anorexia of aging: physiologic and pathologic. *Am. J. Clin. Nutr.* 66(4): 760–763.

National Association of Care Catering (2010) *NACC Nutritional Standards for adults*. NACC Faygate, West Sussex UK.

National Audit Office. (2016) *Discharging Older Patients from Hospital*. Available at https://www.nao.org.uk/report/discharging-older-patients-from-hospital. Accessed 30 May 2017.

NICE (2006) Nutrition support for adults: oral nutrition support, enteral tube feeding and parenteral nutrition (CG 32). Available at https://www.nice.org.uk/Guidance/CG32. Accessed 20 September 2018.

NICE (2012) Osteoporosis: assessing the risk of fragility fracture (CG146). Available at https://www.nice.org.uk/guidance/cg146. Accessed 20 September 2018.

Office for National Statistics (ONS). (2014) *Changes in the Older Resident Care Home Population between 2001 and 2011*. Available at http://webarchive.nationalarchives.gov.uk/20160105160709/http://www.ons.gov.uk/ons/dcp171776_373040.pdf. Accessed 30 May 2017.

Office for National Statistics (ONS). (2016) *Estimates of the Very Old (including Centarians), UK: 2002 to 2015*. Available at https://www.ons.gov.uk/peoplepopulationandcommunity/birthsdeathsandmarriages/ageing/bulletins/estimatesoftheveryoldincludingcentenarians/2002to2015. Accessed 30 May 2017.

Pannell J, Blood I. (2012). *Supported Housing for Older People in the UK: An Evidence Review*. York: Joseph Rowntree Foundation.

Patients Association. (2012). *Practices in C.A.R.E review*. Available at https://www.patients-association.org.uk/wp-content/uploads/2014/06/Practices-in-CARE-Review-2012-Final.pdf. Accessed 30 May 2017.

Peters R. (2006) Ageing and the brain. *Postgrad. Med. J.* 82(964): 84–88.

PHE. (2016). *National Diet and Nutrition Survey Results from Years 5 and 6 (combined) of the Rolling Programme (2012/2013–2013/2014)*. Available at https://www.gov.uk/government/uploads/system/uploads/attachment_data/file/551352/NDNS_Y5_6_UK_Main_Text.pdf. Accessed 26 May 2017.

PHE. (2016). *Bulletin 28th July 2016*. Available at www.gov.uk/government/uploads/system/uploads/attachment_data/file/541691/PHE_Bulletin_July_2016.pdf. Accessed 30 June 2017.

PHE. (2015) *What is Known About the Oral Health of Older People in England and Wales? A Review of Oral Health Surveys of Older People*. Available at https://www.gov.uk/government/uploads/system/uploads/attachment_data/file/489756/What_is_known_about_the_oral_health_of_older_people.pdf. Accessed 30 May 2017.

PHE. (2016) *HIV Diagnoses, Late Diagnoses and Numbers Accessing Treatment and Care*. Available at https://www.gov.uk/government/uploads/system/uploads/attachment_data/file/602945/HIV_diagnoses_late_diagnoses_and_numbers_accessing_treatment_and_care.pdf. Accessed 30 May 2017.

PHE. (2016) The Eatwell Guide, https://www.gov.uk/government/publications/the-eatwell-guide. Accessed 20 September 2018

Prasad AS. (1994). Zinc: an overview. *Nutrition* (Burbank, Los Angeles County, Calif.) 11(1 Suppl): 93–99.

Prasad AS, Fitzgerald JT, Hess JW, *et al.* (1992) Zinc deficiency in elderly patients. *Nutrition* 9: 218–224.
Ritz P, Berrut G. (2005) The importance of good hydration for day-to-day health. *Nutr. Rev.* 63(s1): S6–S13.
SACN. (2010) *Iron and Health*. Available at https://www.gov.uk/government/publications/sacn-iron-and-health-report. Accessed 30 May 2017.
SACN. (2011) *Dietary Reference Values for Energy*. Available at https://www.gov.uk/government/uploads/system/uploads/attachment_data/file/339317/SACN_Dietary_Reference_Values_for_Energy.pdf. Accessed 30 May 2017.
SACN. (2016) *Vitamin D and Health*. Available at https://www.gov.uk/government/uploads/system/uploads/attachment_data/file/537616/SACN_Vitamin_D_and_Health_report.pdf. Accessed 30 May 2017.
Schols JMGA, De Groot CPGM, Van Der Cammen TJM, *et al.* (2009) Preventing and treating dehydration in the elderly during periods of illness and warm weather. *J. Nutr. Health Aging* 13: 150–157.
Sharma G, Goodwin J. (2006). Effect of aging on respiratory system physiology and immunology. *Clin. Interv. Aging* 1: 253–260.
Strait JB, Lakatta EG. (2012). Ageing-associated cardiovascular changes and their relationship to heart failure. *Heart Fail. Clin.* 8: 143–164.
Tobin DJ, Veysey EC, Finlay AY. (2017). Ageing and the skin. In: Fillit HM, Rockword K, Young J (eds) *Brocklehurst's Textbook of Geriatric Medicine and Gerontology*, 8th edn. Philadelphia, PA: Elsevier.
United States Census Bureau. (2016) *An Ageing World*. Available at https://www.census.gov/content/dam/Census/library/publications/2016/demo/p95-16-1.pdf. Accessed 30 June 2017. Issued March 2016.
Weiskopf D, Weinberger B, Grubeck-Loebenstein B. (2009) The aging of the immune system. *Transpl. Int.* 22: 1041–1050.
Whelan K. (2001) Inadequate fluid intakes in dysphagic acute stroke. *Clin. Nutr.* 20: 423–428.
WHO. (2015) *World Report on Ageing and Health*. Available at http://www.who.int/ageing/events/world-report-2015-launch/en/. Accessed 30 May 2017.
Wickremaratchi MM, Llewelyn JG. (2006) Effects of ageing on touch. *Postgrad. Med. J.* 82(967): 301–304.

3.4 People in low-income groups

Caroline Bovey, Judith John and Lisa Williams

SECTION 3

Key points

- The relationships between low income, poor health and diet-related inequalities in health are well established.
- There is increasing evidence of people experiencing food poverty and having limited ability to access a healthy, safe and sustainable diet.
- Dietitians should be aware of the social welfare system and take into consideration income levels and their impact when advising on diet.
- Dietitians working in communities are well placed to implement policy and lead local initiatives that can reduce the impact of food poverty and support healthy, affordable and accessible food choices.

While the developed world does not experience the same level of poverty-related malnutrition as the developing world, there are reports that sectors of the population are unable to meet their dietary needs fully. This chapter examines the difficulties that people with low income encounter in relation to accessing an affordable nutritious diet, and explores the inequalities in diet-related ill health. It discusses how countries are trying to measure the size of the problem, the root causes and the ways in which the problems that people experience may be limited through interventions. The main barrier is the income level, whether adequate wages or welfare, but there are initiatives that can help to reduce the impact of low incomes on dietary intake.

Links between low income, diet and health

It is well documented that there is a wide divide in health between the most and least deprived in the UK (Marmot, 2010; ONS, 2014; The Children's Society, 2014). The Marmot Review (2010) recognised the need for ensuring a healthy standard of living for all in order to reduce health inequalities. Besides income, there are health inequalities between people or groups due to social, geographical, biological or other factors, known as the wider determinants of health. These differences can result in people who are the worst off experiencing poorer health and shorter lives (NICE, 2012). While there is improvement in overall life expectancy, and a narrowing of the gap between the most and least deprived, differences in healthy life expectancy (HLE) are still marked. HLE at birth in the most deprived areas was 18.8 years lower for males and 19.3 years lower for females, compared to the least deprived areas (ONS, 2016).

Access to an adequate food supply is the most basic of human needs and rights. People have a right to be adequately nourished to attain and maintain health and dignity (FAO/UN, 1996; Nourish Scotland, 2016; UN General Assembly, 1948, 2014). Money for food is a key flexible item in household budgets, and, in low-income households, the quantity and quality of food purchased and consumed by families is regularly among the first to be sacrificed in times of financial hardship. The Faculty of Public Health (2014) recently stated that '*an affordable, nutritious diet was a pre-requisite for health and that reliance on food aid should not be part of any modern society-wide evidenced based approach to public health policy*'. It highlighted that increasing numbers of UK citizens were not earning enough to meet their most basic nutritional needs, and that families were under pressure to meet rising food prices due to falling or stagnant incomes among low-paid workers. Understanding what constitutes a healthy diet is different from being able to provide the most suitable foods to fulfil that diet, and a range of challenges, including poverty, impact on the food choices that are made.

Poverty is statistically defined in the UK and EU as household income that is below 60% of the national median. This is known as relative income poverty, and moves in line with median income (poverty line). In its Joint Report on Social Inclusion, the European Commission (2014) proposed the following definition

Manual of Dietetic Practice, Sixth Edition. Edited by Joan Gandy.

Companion website: www.manualofdieteticpractice.com

'People are said to be living in poverty if their income and resources are so inadequate as to preclude them from having a standard of living considered acceptable in the society in which they live. Because of their poverty, they may experience multiple disadvantages through unemployment, low income, poor housing, inadequate healthcare and barriers to lifelong learning, culture, sport and recreation. They are often excluded and marginalised from participating in activities (economic, social and cultural) that are the norm for other people, and their access to fundamental rights may be restricted'.

Between 2011 and 2014, almost a third (32.5%) of the UK population experienced poverty at least once (ONS, 2014). About 6.5% of the UK population are said to be living in persistent poverty (ONS, 2016), which equates to 3.9 million individuals experiencing relative low income in the current year, and in at least 2 of the 3 preceding years.

Food purchasing

The Department for Environment, Food and Rural Affairs' (DEFRA) series of Family Food Modules collects detailed quantity and expenditure information on food and drink for both household and eating-out consumption as part of the Integrated Household survey. Energy and nutrient intakes are calculated using standard profiles for each of the 500 types of food. It highlights the compounding effects of falling income and rising food prices over recent years, which reduced food affordability by over 20% for households in the lowest income decile (DEFRA, 2015). Food prices have risen 18% in real terms since 2007, with an above the rate of inflation rise following the economic crash of 2008. Prices reached a peak in 2009, levelled until early 2014, and then fell in real terms by 3.2% in 2015 (DEFRA, 2015), remaining higher than 2007. Influences on price extend beyond basic production costs to include oil and therefore distribution costs and exchange rate pressures, and it is possible that these influences on world markets impact disproportionately on the most vulnerable.

The so-called Age of Austerity has exacerbated trends in class differences (Dowler, 2015), and trends in the percentage of spend on food purchases continue to indicate that low-income households are being hit the hardest, as relative affordability of food products places an increasing burden on the overall budget. Those on low incomes spend a greater proportion of the total household income on food – 15.7% as compared to the national average spend of 11.1% (DEFRA, 2015). For those in the lowest-income households, total food volume purchased has decreased by 8.5%, and spend is up by 23% in total. This seemingly confusing picture is partly explained through one of the range of ways in which households react to food price increases. Trading down by swapping to a more cost-effective brand within the same food category is one coping strategy. The means by which the product is cheaper may be through more basic packaging, a cheaper brand, a lower-quality product or one with a less prestigious provenance (DEFRA, 2015).

Nutritional intakes of people on low income

The impact of low income, food prices and balancing household budgets can have a detrimental effect on nutritional intakes. The Low Income Diet and Nutrition Survey (LIDNS) (Nelson *et al.*, 2007) undertook an in-depth assessment of dietary intakes, food shopping practices, cooking facilities and skills, with the most deprived low-income households, to determine the links between socioeconomic status, dietary intake and current health status. Of the low-income population, 51% reported that they had enough of the kinds of food they wanted to eat. Among those who said that they sometimes or often did not have enough to eat, not having enough money for food was the reason cited most frequently, across all household types (98%). Lack of storage facilities (16%) and lack of transport to get to shops (14%) were also commonly reported themes, illustrating the importance of solutions designed to overcome poverty being multifactorial. About 29% were considered to be living in food-insecure households. Families on a low income reported being unable to afford enough fresh food, such as fruit and vegetables. They were more concerned with staving off hunger, and more likely to favour foods and diets which have a higher satiety value, are cheaper sources of calories and are energy dense, over foods that are nutrient dense and offer protection from (and risk reduction) to disease.

The National Diet and Nutrition Survey (NDNS) (PHE, 2014; 2016) captures intake across groups by equivalised income and grouped into five quintiles, with quintile 5 representing the highest income band. Data affirms that lower income affects household food expenditure, which results in poorer quality diet overall. The reports, do, however, also indicate that few people across all quintiles meet the UK government's recommendations for diet (PHE, 2014; 2016). For macronutrients, there were differences for total energy and protein intakes in women aged 19–64 years, which were significantly lower in quintiles 1–3 than in quintile 5. Findings relating to the quality of the diet were:

- Non-starch polysaccharide (NSP) intakes were significantly lower in the lowest quintile groups as compared to the highest in all age/sex groups, but intakes for all quintiles failed to achieve the population recommendation of 18 g NSP per day. A new recommendation of 30 g fibre per day was set in 2015 based on a broader definition of fibre, which equates to 23 g NSP per day.
- Mean total fruit and vegetable consumption was significantly lower in quintile 1 as compared to quintile 5 in all age/sex groups, with the exception of adults aged 65 years and over.
- Mean consumption of five portions of fruit and vegetables was significantly lower in quintiles 1–3 as compared to quintile 5 for boys aged 11–18 years and adults aged 19–64 years.
- Mean intakes of non-milk extrinsic sugars for adults tended to be higher in the lowest-income quintile as compared to the highest.

- For children of all age groups, mean sugar intakes, and as percentage of energy intake, showed a general increase from quintile 1 to 5; however, all were above the recommended levels.

The greatest differences are seen when comparing micronutrient intakes across quintiles:

- There was a trend of increasing intake from lowest to highest quintile for micronutrients for iron intakes in women aged 9–64 years.
- The proportion of women with iron intakes below the lower reference nutrient intake (LRNI) was higher in the lower quintiles than in quintile 5.
- Mean intake for folate was significantly lower across all age groups and sex in the lower quintiles as compared to the higher.
- For both men and women aged 19–64 years, the mean intake of calcium increased from the lowest to highest quintile, and a substantial proportion of girls aged 11–18 years in all income quintiles had calcium intake values below the LRNI.

Nutritional consequences

Poor diet in adulthood is associated with multiple risk factors for chronic disease. Socially disadvantaged households consume less nutritionally balanced diets and suffer from higher rates of diet-related chronic diseases, such as diabetes, heart disease, obesity and certain cancers, contributing to reduced life expectancy and increased morbidity. There are particularly marked differences in rates of childhood obesity across the social gradient across the UK. Prevalence of obesity in children aged 4–5 years ranged from 12.5% for those in the most deprived areas to 5.5% in the least deprived areas. In year 6 (10–11 years), 26% of children living in the most deprived areas were obese, as compared to 11.7% in the least deprived areas (National Child Measurement Programme England (2016); ONS, 2016). Alongside this is the increased likelihood of overweight and obese tracking into adulthood, and therefore increasing their risk of developing related comorbidities.

Mapping the data onto health outcomes has shown that food insecurity also correlates to a wider range of chronic illnesses. For example, Tarasuk *et al.* (2015) showed that 50% of women in highly food insecure households had suffered from anxiety or mental health disorders, and that the use of health services was much greater among food-insecure people.

The extent of food poverty

The struggle for many people to afford nutritious food is gaining more attention both socially and politically, and has become a subject of policy debate. Much of the concern has arisen because of reports of people needing to access emergency food banks and its recognition of becoming a serious public health problem in high-income countries (Loopstra & Tarasuk, 2013). However, the true extent of food poverty is unclear, as it is not defined clearly or routinely measured. Food poverty is not due to simple causes, but because of the impact of low or falling incomes, as high, or rising, living costs including food prices leads to pressure on household budgets and the inability to afford, or to have access to, quality food to attain adequate nourishment. This is often exacerbated by changes to the social welfare system, which are thought to be driving vulnerable families to use emergency food services (APPG, 2014). It is estimated that more than half a million children in the UK are now living in families that are unable to provide a minimally acceptable diet (Cooper *et al.*, 2014).

There is no single agreed definition of food poverty, and while a number of definitions are relevant that encompass affordability, access and social participation, a definition that is still widely accepted is: '*the inability to acquire or consume an adequate quality or sufficient quantity of food in socially acceptable ways, or the uncertainty that one will be able to do so*' (Dowler *et al.*, 2003). The term household food insecurity is increasingly used to describe the broader phenomenon when people are worried about not having enough food for themselves and their families; however, these terms (food poverty and household food insecurity) are often used interchangeably. The WHO and FAO defines food security as '*when all people, at all times, have access to sufficient, safe and nutritious food to meet their dietary needs and food preferences for an active and healthy life*' (The World Food Summit, 1996). Whichever definition or term is used, it is important to acknowledge that, in the UK, there are significant numbers of the population that are not eating well because they cannot afford to. This has implications for their current health, future health and that of their children.

Data on measuring food insecurity

Information on food insecurity is not collected as part of UK national monitoring surveys; although there are systems to measure food poverty across the devolved nations, these are varied, and use different instruments. Northern Ireland and Wales have used the EU statistics on income and living conditions (EU-SILC) indicators as part of their annual health surveys (Food Research Collaboration *et al.*, 2016). The EU-SILC is a large-scale survey that collects information on income, poverty, social exclusion and living conditions. The standard module, which has been implemented annually in the UK since 2005, includes an indicator of whether a person has a meal with meat, chicken or fish every second day, but this is only one of four food indicators that are routinely measured, and not all countries do so (Carney & Maître, 2012).

There are calls to systematically measure food insecurity on a UK-wide basis as part of existing survey instruments, such as the Health Survey for England (and devolved nation equivalents) or the UK-wide Living Costs and Food Survey, using one of a number of internationally validated tools. This would enable the monitoring of trends over time, and demonstrate the impact of policy interventions (Taylor & Loopstra, 2016). Measurement has become routine in some countries and regions such as the USA, Canada and parts of South and Central America, as well as the Food and Agriculture Organization (FAO) of the United Nations, using validated tools. A recent study by the FAO has measured household food insecurity across 140 countries (FAO, 2016). This used a set of eight questions to ask people about their ability to get enough food in the past year (see Box 3.4.1) (Ballard *et al.*, 2013). The data from the UK showed that 10.1% of people aged 15 years and above were moderately food insecure in 2014. This means they reported experiencing difficulty in securing enough food to eat. Of these people, 4.5% experienced a severe level of food insecurity, typically having gone a whole day without eating because they could not afford enough food (FAO, 2016). This puts the UK in the bottom half of European nations, despite being one of Europe's richer nations however, the small sample size of 1000 people is a limitation.

As part of its obligations under the Sustainable Development Goals (UN, 2016), the UK will need to collect data to adequately report its progress. In particular:

> Goal 2. End hunger, achieve food security and improved nutrition and promote sustainable agriculture. Target #2.1 – *end hunger and ensure access by all people … to safe, nutritious and sufficient food all year round by 2030 (*UN, 2016*)*

This presents an opportunity to introduce a robust measurement which would assist all those whose ambition is to end food insecurity in the UK (The Food Foundation, 2016). Many third-sector organisations use qualitative and quantitative approaches to evidence the difficulties that households face. A number of reports have examined the impact of the recent recession on peoples' ability to access a sufficient, healthy and varied diet, and the strategies that were employed. Affordability (or finance) is also impacted by awareness of what constitutes a healthy diet (related to education, information and skills) and the availability of healthy food in a local area (King *et al.*, 2015).

Box 3.4.1 FAO food insecurity scale

Respondents are asked whether, during the past 12 months:

- You were worried you would run out of food because of a lack of money or other resources?
- You were unable to eat healthy and nutritious food because of a lack of money or other resources?
- You ate only a few kinds of foods because of a lack of money or other resources?
- You had to skip a meal because there was not enough money or other resources to get food?
- You ate less than you thought you should because of a lack of money or other resources?
- Your household ran out of food because of a lack of money or other resources?
- You were hungry but did not eat because there was not enough money or other resources for food?
- You went without eating for a whole day because of a lack of money or other resources?

(Source: Food and Agriculture Organization of the United Nations, 2013; Ballard *et al.*, 2016. Reproduced with permission.)

Affordability

Save the Children (2012), Shelter (2013) and Cooper *et al.* (2014) have reported people cutting back on food and skipping meals because of lack of money and to meet housing costs. Recent research by Barnado's Strategy Unit (2013) also showed that 94% of services reported that food poverty was an issue for the families and young people that they work with, with many referring families and young people to food banks or providing food directly, and providing help with budgeting and cooking classes. The Family Food data shows that food price rises have a strong effect on food shopping for low-income households. Since 2007, the lowest-income households bought less beef, bacon, butter, fish, fruit, tea and biscuits/cakes, but bought more pork, poultry and eggs (DEFRA, 2015). They purchased the least fruit and vegetables at an average of three portions per person in 2014. Fruit and vegetable purchases rise strongly with income, with 52% more being purchased in the highest-income households as compared to the lowest in 2014.

Awareness

The effect of poverty is not always simply about having enough money to afford food. Low-income households often lack physical access to affordable healthy food, the means to cook or sometimes the confidence and necessary skills (Fabian Society, 2015). A lower education level is associated with poorer diet, and the reduction of at home cooking has negatively impacted on the intergenerational transmission of skills (Smith *et al.*, 2014). However, the lack of cooking skills and time allocated to cooking stretches across the income divide (Fabian Society, 2015). The average amount of time spent making the average meal has nearly halved over the last 20 years. In one survey, around two-thirds of respondents said that time pressures had meant they were more likely to consume convenience foods rather than prepare fresh food (Change4Life, 2013).

Parents and professionals have different interpretations of cooking from fresh, and probing is needed to determine what parents really mean. Where parents have a strong desire to act in the best interests of their children, this is often hampered by lack of knowledge and cooking skills. The early stage of parenthood provides an opportunity for nutrition education and developing cooking skills, as parents tend to be more receptive to improving their children's diet (Lovelace & Rabiee-Khan, 2013).

The energy needed to power kitchen appliances such as freezers, microwaves and ovens is a significant cost burden on already squeezed households. The one-off costs of buying new appliances, fixing and replacing them adds a further burden onto budgets. Dowler and Lambie-Mumford (2015) found that people on low income report buying fast food because it requires no cooking. Actions such as travelling to cheaper supermarkets, planning menus, shopping with great care, making use of price promotions and making use of leftover foods demonstrate resourcefulness. Some families buy what is needed for that day or even a single meal, because of having insufficient money to do otherwise.

Availability of affordable healthy food

Limited access to food is also indicative of broader socio-economic inequalities. Areas where food poverty is high are often synonymous with a number of other factors that marginalise people and limit options. The creation of large superstores and out-of-town shopping areas has changed the retail environment to make access to affordable healthy food more challenging for some communities. Superstores are difficult to reach for people on low incomes who have limited transport. People on low incomes in the UK pay higher prices for many essential goods and services than people who are better off. This is known as the poverty premium (Cooper & Dumpleton, 2013). A list of the cheapest available selection of groceries was up to 69% more expensive in some of the poorest areas than in stores belonging to the same chain in wealthier areas (Cooper & Dumpleton, 2013).

Availability of unhealthy food

Takeaway (fast) food outlets primarily offer ready-to-eat, energy-dense foods, which are associated with higher total energy and fat intakes (Lachat *et al.*, 2012). The number of fast food outlets in the UK has risen by around 30,000 to over 90,000 in the last 10 years (The Food Foundation, 2016), with more fast food outlets in deprived areas (Maguire *et al.*, 2015). The Department of Health has acknowledged the importance of public health in local planning policy, and some local authorities have sought to limit the opening of new fast food outlets in certain areas (Public Health England (PHE) *et al.*, 2015). This patchwork of information is revealing, but it does not provide nationally representative data or reflect international best practice in measurement, although it is essential to have qualitative data in addition to robust quantitative data to reflect the lived experiences of people with food insecurity.

Interventions to reduce the impact of food poverty

Many areas have developed food poverty action plans, often as a result of the growing demand for emergency food provision. Use of food banks has been reported to highlight the plight of many people who are using emergency food aid. It is important not to let this distract us from the real underlying issue and chronic long-term situation in which people find themselves in, and also many of whom will not seek or access a food bank. Some areas specifically approach the issue from a rights-based approach and seek to support someone's right to a decent and affordable diet. Sustain's guide on drafting and developing food poverty action plans places actions into three broad categories (Sustain, 2016) (see Table 3.4.1).

Promoting the uptake of Healthy Start Vouchers

Healthy Start is a UK-wide scheme to improve the health of low-income pregnant women and families on benefits and tax credits. It replaced the Welfare Food Scheme in 2006. Those who are eligible receive free vitamins and vouchers worth £3.10 a week that can be spent on plain, fresh or frozen fruits and vegetables, and on milk and infant formula. There is generally a high uptake of the vouchers, but there can be less than 10% of eligible beneficiaries take up the offer of free vitamins (Jessiman *et al.*, 2013). Healthy Start has been seen as reasonably successful with positive indicators of improved outcomes around increased access, uptake and awareness (The Scottish Government, 2015). Women reported that it contributed to them making healthier dietary choices, such as increased quantity and variety of fruit and vegetables purchased. But there are concerns that the vouchers may result in more purchasing of unhealthy food products (Lucas *et al.*, 2013). The evaluation of Healthy Start in Scotland made a number of recommendations, including:

Table 3.4.1 Guide to drafting and developing food action plans (Sustain, 2016)

Taking a preventative approach	Shaping crisis provision	Taking a wider approach
Opportunities for families to develop knowledge and skills, e.g. cooking skills Facilitating access to more affordable, healthier foods, e.g. community hubs, markets, shops and social supermarkets Promoting Healthy Start Vouchers Recognising and supporting the role of food environment in schools and children services year around	Improving signposting, and enhancing information on local preventative support Ensuring support is delivered in a non-stigmatised way Seeking to improve the overall nutritional value of emergency food aid	Using the planning system and business rate relief to shape local areas, e.g. supporting community food growing, local markets and other more affordable fruit and vegetable outlets Limit the spread of unhealthy fast food outlets (particularly near schools

- Eligibility criteria to the scheme could be extended to low-income women in the first weeks of pregnancy and children up to 5 years.
- Voucher value should keep pace with rising food prices.
- More small and local shops, especially in rural areas, should be encouraged to join the scheme in order to increase the scheme's availability, as well as to provide the beneficiaries with access to culturally appropriate foods.
- Increase awareness of the importance of vitamin supplementation (in particular, vitamin D), especially among groups at risk of vitamin deficiency and among front-line health professionals.

Schools

Schools have an important role to play in supporting pupils from lower-income households to eat well. All authorities can ensure maximum uptake of the EU nursery and school milk scheme and free school meals. Universal free school meals have been introduced for years 1, 2 in England and years P1–P3 in Scotland (4–7 years). All Welsh primary schools have access to a free breakfast scheme. Some areas in the UK are developing initiatives to support children and families in need during the summer holiday period. By using public sector assets (schools, catering teams, staff), they provide good-quality meals, sport and nutrition skills education to address household food security, summer holiday learning loss, and social isolation.

Community initiatives

Having the skills, knowledge and confidence to shop for, and prepare, healthy meals can overcome some barriers. Community-based cookery sessions can offer a relaxed environment to learn skills, and these can be delivered by a range of trained practitioners. Community cafes can provide affordable meals in sociable settings in a range of community buildings. They may be set up by volunteers and/or paid staff, and run on a not-for-profit basis. Community gardens enable access to fresh food at low or no cost, in addition to encouraging participants to exercise, develop new skills and make new friends. An example of this is in Belfast, where a large number of such community gardens are functioning (Belfast Food Network, 2015). Community-run food co-ops buy food at affordable prices by ordering in bulk direct from suppliers. Food co-ops can include bag or box schemes, informal groups purchasing produce in bulk to get discounts, fruit and vegetable stalls, food assemblies, mobile stores or a combination of these.

Social supermarkets

Social supermarkets are schemes that enable membership of supermarkets and/or shops selling local, affordable food or surplus at affordable prices. They offer a limited assortment of food and consumer products at a significantly lower consumer price (50–70% less) than regular market prices. The stores' limited assortments consist of surplus products that are supplied free of charge by retailing and manufacturing companies. The products are otherwise unsellable due to short expiry date, surplus product or wrong packaging. They aim to support low-income groups, prevent wastage of food and provide job opportunities.

Low-income issues and dietetic practice

Understanding the complexity of the relationships between social inequality, food, health, and the realities faced by people living constantly on a low income is an important part of the dietitian's competences (UCL Institute of Health Equity, 2013). Dietitians should be aware of the policies and practices impacting on the social and environmental factors that can help support the attainment of an adequate diet. Dietitians can apply the principles of working with local communities around food, including working in partnership with the local community (co-production); designing programmes that tackle the social gradient in health; and taking a life course approach to developing, implementing and evaluating food and health interventions.

Acknowledgement

The Editor acknowledges the prior contribution of Rachel Barton and Diane Talbot.

Further reading

Just Fair Consortium. (2014) *Going Hungry? The Human Right to Food in the UK (Online)*. Available at http://www.just-fair.co.uk/about1-c21gp. Accessed December 2016.

Lambie-Mumford H, O'Connell R. (2015) *Food Poverty and Policy: Evidence Base and Knowledge Gaps*. Sheffield: Sheffield Political Economy Research Institute.

NHS Health Scotland. (2016) *Community Food and Health (Scotland) (Online)*. Available at https://www.communityfoodandhealth.org.uk. Accessed December 2016.

O'Connor N, Farag K, Baines R. (2016) What is food poverty? A conceptual framework. *Brit. Food J.* 118(2): 429–449.

UCL Institute of Health Equity. (2015) *Social Inequalities in the leading Causes of Early Death: A Life Course Approach*. London: UCL.

References

APPG. (2014) *Feeding Britain, A strategy for zero hunger in England, Wales, Scotland and Northern Ireland: the report of the All-party Parliamentary Inquiry into Hunger in the UK*. Available at https://foodpovertyinquiry.files.wordpress.com/2014/12/food-poverty-feeding-britain-final.pdf. Accessed 1 December 2016.

Ballard TJ, Kepple AW, Cafiero C. (2013) *Food insecurity experience scale*. Available at http://www.fao.org/fileadmin/templates/ess/voh/FIES_Technical_Paper_v1.1.pdf. Accessed 21 February 2017.

Barnado's Strategy Unit. (2013) *Families in need of food parcels – the food poverty crisis unwrapped*. Available at http://www.barnardos.org.uk/families_in_need_of_food_parcels_-_2013.pdf. Accessed 1 December 2016.

Belfast Food Network. (2015) *Enough is Enough Report*. Available at http://www.belfastfoodnetwork.org/wp-content/uploads/2016/05/Food-Poverty-Plan-Final.pdf. Accessed 1 December 2016.

Carney C, Maître B. (2012) *Constructing a Food Poverty Indicator for Ireland using the Survey on Income and Living Conditions, Social Inclusion Technical Paper No. 3*. Dublin: Department of Social Protection.

Change for Life (2013) Only one in six mothers cooks from scratch each day. In Fabian Society *A Recipe for Inequality: Why our food system is leaving low-income households behind*. Available at http://foodandpoverty.org.uk/wp-content/uploads/2015/03/ARecipeforInequality_WEB.pdf. (Accessed 26 November 2016).

Cooper N, Dumpleton S. (2013) *Walking the breadline: the scandal of food poverty in 21st-century Britain*. Available at http://policy-practice.oxfam.org.uk/publications/walking-the-breadline-the-scandal-of-food-poverty-in-21st-century-britain-292978. Accessed 4 October 2016.

Cooper N, Purcell S, Jackson R. (2014) *Below the Breadline: The Relentless Rise of Food poverty in Britain, Manchester: Church Action on Poverty, Oxfam, Trussell Trust*. Available at http://policy-practice.oxfam.org.uk/publications/below-the-breadline-the-relentless-rise-of-food-poverty-in-britain-317730. Accessed 26 November 2016.

Department for Environment Food and Rural Affairs (DEFRA). (2015) *Family Food 2014*. York: DEFRA.

Dowler E, Jones C, Finer C. (2003) (eds) *The Welfare of Food: Rights and Responsibilities in a Changing World*. Oxford: Blackwell Publishing, pp. 140–159.

Dowler E. (2012) *The Future of UK Household Security*. London: University of Warwick.

Dowler E, Lambie-Mumford H. (2015) How can households eat in austerity? Challenges for Social Policy in the UK. *Soc. Policy Soc.* 14(3): 417–428.

European Commission. (2014) *Joint report by the Commission and the Council on social inclusion*. Available at http://ec.europa.eu/employment_social/soc-prot/soc-incl/final_joint_inclusion_report_2003_en.pdf. Accessed 30 November 2016.

Fabian Society. (2015) *A recipe for inequality: why our food system is leaving low-income households behind*. Available at http://foodandpoverty.org.uk/wp-content/uploads/2015/03/ARecipeforInequality_WEB.pdf. Accessed 26 November 2016.

Faculty of Public Health. (2014) *Food Poverty and Health: Briefing Paper*. Available at http://www.fph.org.uk/uploads/bs_food_poverty.pdf. Accessed 30 November 2016.

FAO. (2016) *Voices of the Hungry. Technical Report 1*. Available at http://www.fao.org/in-action/voices-of-the-hungry. Accessed 7 December 2016.

FAO/UN. (1996) *Rome declaration on world food security. Available at* http://www.fao.org/docrep/003/w3613e/w3613e00.htm. Accessed 6 December 2016.

Food Research Collaboration, Sustain: The alliance for better food and farming, the Food Foundation, Oxfam, and the Sociology Department of Oxford University. (2016) *Time to count the hungry: The case for a standard measure of household food insecurity in the UK*. Available at http://foodresearch.org.uk/time-to-count-the-hungry-the-case-for-a-standard-measure-of-household-food-insecurity-in-the-uk. Accessed 5 December 2016.

Jessiman T, Cameron A, Wiggins M, *et al.* (2013) A qualitative study of uptake of free vitamins in England. *Arch. Dis. Child.* 98(8): 587–591.

King G, Lee-Woolf C, Kivinen E, *et al.* (2015) *Understanding Food in the Context of Poverty, Economic Insecurity and Social Exclusion*. Brook Lyndhurst for the Food Standards Agency in Northern Ireland.

Lachat C, Nago E, Verstraeten R, et al. (2012) Eating out of home and its association with dietary intake: a systematic review of the evidence. *Obes. Rev.* 13(4): 329–346.

Loopstra R, Tarasuk V. (2013) Severity of household food insecurity is sensitive to change in household income and employment status among low income families. *J. Nutr.* 143: 1316–1323.

Lovelace S, Rabiee-Khan F. (2013) Food choices made by low income households when feeding their pre-school children: a qualitative study. *Matern. Child Nutr.* 11: 870–881.

Lucas P, Jessiman T, Cameron A, *et al.* (2013) *Healthy Start Vouchers Study: The Views and Experiences of Parents, Professionals and Small Retailers in England*. Available at http://www.bristol.ac.uk/media-library/sites/sps/migrated/documents/finalreport2.pdf. Accessed February 2019.

Maguire E, Burgoine T, Monsivais P. (2015) Area deprivation and the food environment over time: A repeated cross-sectional study on takeaway outlet density and supermarket presence in Norfolk, UK, 1990–2008. *Health Place* 33: 142–147.

Marmot M. (2010) *Fair society; healthy lives: strategic review of health inequalities in England post 2010*. Available at https://www.parliament.uk/documents/fair-society-healthy-lives-full-report.pdf. Accessed 21 September 2018.

National Child Measurement Programme England. (2016) *National Statistics 2015–16*. Available at http://content.digital.nhs.uk/catalogue/PUB22269/nati-chil-meas-prog-eng-2015-2016-rep.pdf. Accessed 5 December 2016.

Nelson, M, Ehrens, B, Bates, B *et al.* (2007) *Low Income Diet and Nutrition Survey, vol 1: Summary of key findings*. London: TSO.

NICE. (2012) *Local government briefings: Health inequalities and population health*. Available at https://www.nice.org.uk/advice/lgb4. Accessed 7 December 2016.

Nourish Scotland. (2016) *Report to UN Committee on Economic, Social & Cultural Rights – On the Right to Food*. Available at http://www.nourishscotland.org/nourish-report-to-un-cescr. Accessed 5 December 2016.

Office for National Statistics (ONS). (2014) *Inequality in Healthy Life Expectancy at Birth by National Deciles of Area Deprivation: England, 2009–11*. ONS: England.

Office for National Statistics. (2016) *Healthy life expectancy at birth and age 65 by upper tier local authority and area deprivation: England, 2012 to 2014*. ONS: England.

PHE. (2014) *National diet and nutrition survey: Results from years 1–4 (combined) of the rolling programme (2008/2009–2011/2012)*. Available at https://assets.publishing.service.gov.uk/government/uploads/system/uploads/attachment_data/file/594360/NDNS_Y1_to_4_UK_report_executive_summary_revised_February_2017.pdf. Accessed 21 September 2018.

PHE. (2016) *National diet and nutrition survey: Results from years 5 and 6 (combined) of the rolling programme (2012/2013–2013/2014)*. Available at https://www.gov.uk/government/uploads/system/uploads/attachment_data/file/551352/NDNS_Y5_6_UK_Main_Text.pdf. Accessed 1 November 2016.

Public Health England, Chartered Institute of Environmental Health and Local Government Association. (2015) *Healthy people, healthy places briefing. Obesity and the environment: regulating the growth of fast food outlets*.

Save the Children. (2012) *Child Poverty in 2012: It shouldn't happen here*. Available at http://www.savethechildren.org.uk/resources/online-library/child-poverty-2012-it-shouldnt-happen-here. Accessed 24 October 2016.

Shelter. (2013) *4 out of 10 families cut back on food to stay in their homes*. Available at http://england.shelter.org.uk/news/march_2013/4_out_of_10_families_cut_back_on_food_to_stay_in_their_homes. Accessed 5 December 2016.

Smith, L.P., Ng, S.W. and Popkin, B.M. (2014), "Resistant to the recession: low-income adults. Maintenance of cooking and away from home eating behaviours during times of economic turbulence. *Am. J. Public Health*, 104 (5): 840–846.

Sustain. (2016) *Developing food poverty action plans*. Available at https://www.sustainweb.org/publications/developing_food_poverty_action_plans. Accessed 28 November 2016.

Tarasuk V, Cheng J, de Oliveira C, *et al.* (2015) Association between household food insecurity and annual health care costs. *CMAJ* 187: E429–E436.

Taylor A, Loopstra R. (2016) *Too Poor to Eat, Food Insecurity in the UK: The Food Foundation*. Available at https://foodfoundation.org.uk/wp-content/uploads/2016/07/FoodInsecurityBriefing-May-2016-FINAL.pdf. Accessed 16 March 2018.

The Children's Society. (2014) *Through Young Eyes: The Children's Commission on Poverty*. Available at http://www.childrenssociety.org.uk/sites/default/files/P366%20TCS%20Poverty%20Commission%20Report_LR.pdf. Accessed 1 December 2016.

The Food Foundation. (2016) *Force Fed: Does the Food System Constrict Choices for Typical British Families?* Available at http://foodfoundation.org.uk/wp-content/uploads/2016/07/Force-fed-methods-final.pdf. Accessed 1 December 2016.

The Scottish Government. (2016) *The Healthy Start Scheme: An Evidence Review*. Available at http://www.gov.scot/Resource/0049/00497237.pdf. Accessed 26 November 2016.

The World Food Summit. (1996) *Rome Declaration on World Food Security (Online)*. Available at http://www.fao.org/docrep/003/w3613e/w3613e00.htm. Accessed 7 December 2016.

UN General Assembly. (1948) Universal Declaration of Human Rights, Article 25. Available at http://www.ohchr.org/EN/UDHR/Documents/UDHR_Translations/eng.pdf. Accessed 1 December 2016.

UN General Assembly. (2014) *Report of the special rapporteur on the right to food, Olivier De Schutter*. Available at http://www.srfood.org/images/stories/pdf/officialreports/20140310_finalreport_en.pdf. Accessed 6 December 2016.

UN. (2016) The Sustainable Development Goals (Online). Available at http://www.un.org/sustainabledevelopment/sustainable-development-goals/#. Accessed 7 December 2016.

University College London Institute of Health Equity. (2013) *Working for Health Equity: The Role of Health Professionals*. London. Available at http://www.instituteofhealthequity.org/projects/working-for-health-equity-the-role-of-health-professionals. Accessed 4 October 2016.

3.5 Working with minority ethnic groups

Kirsten Whitehead and Tahira Bashir

Key points

- Populations are becoming more diverse, and dietitians must have a good understanding of the communities they work with.
- Most migrants adopt Western eating habits, while maintaining some traditional eating habits.
- The adoption of unhealthy Western eating patterns and changes in lifestyle have resulted in a rise in chronic diseases among minority ethnic groups.

The aim of this chapter is to introduce considerations that are relevant for working with minority ethnic groups, to provide a short introduction to some of the groups that dietitians are most likely to encounter in the UK and to signpost relevant information about these groups. The UK has a long history of being a multicultural and multiracial society. Migration patterns over the years have been influenced by social and political factors, natural disasters and conflicts across the world, as well as immigration policy. People have come to the UK looking for employment, a better quality of life, to join family members already living here or to escape problems in their country of origin. This means that the countries from which the greatest number of people are migrating changes over time. This is likely to continue over the coming years with ongoing conflicts around the world and the UK's 2016 decision to leave the European Union (Brexit). There are likely to be effects on migration, the staffing and use of the NHS, and cross-border cooperation in relation to health, all potentially impacting on population diversity (McKenna, 2016).

In the UK population census (2011), 87% (55 million people) described themselves as from a white ethnic group, which was a decrease from the previous census in 2001 (Office of National Statistics, or ONS, 2013). The three most common countries of birth of non-UK-born residents were, in descending order, India, Poland and Pakistan. England and Wales have become more ethnically diverse (ONS, 2013), but changes in data collection methods have impacted on the figures, and it has been recommended that more consistent terminology and definitions be used (Marmot, 2010).

In relation to overall proportions of the UK population, in 2011, 13% of the population belonged to a minority ethnic group, and 7% were Asian/Asian British (including Chinese). The remaining were Black/African/Caribbean/Black British (3%), mixed ethnicity (2%) and Gypsy/Traveller/Irish Traveller/other groups (1%) (ONS, 2013). However, these are not evenly distributed geographically. London had the most ethnically diverse population, with high proportions of people of African (7%), Indian (6%) and Caribbean (4.2%) ethnicity. The West Midlands was the next most diverse area, with 4.1% Pakistani, 3.9% Indian and 4.2 % Caribbean ethnicity. Of all people born in the UK, 7.8% are from minority ethnic groups (ONS, 2013). The least diverse area was Wales (ONS, 2012b).

Refugees and asylum seekers may have particularly complex needs. There are many definitions of refugees and asylum seekers, but all consider that the people did not leave their country of origin as a voluntary choice. Most cannot return home due to safety concerns (Bradby *et al.*, 2015). Refugees and asylum seekers may have suffered a variety of physical, mental and emotional traumas, and dietitians should consider what their life experiences were prior to migration, the reasons behind their migration and the circumstances of their life since arriving in their new country (Public Health England (PHE), 2014). These could have a significant impact on nutritional status.

The dietetic workforce needs to be equipped to cater to the needs of this increasingly diverse society (Hickson *et al.*, 2016). As with all service users, dietitians must understand the individuals and their social situations in order to meet the standards of conduct, performance and ethics (Health and Care Professions Council (HCPC), 2016). They should be aware of the minority ethnic groups living in their area of work, but also the history of how, why and when those groups arrived. PHE provides health profiles for populations in particular areas, which include information about ethnicity, social

Manual of Dietetic Practice, Sixth Edition. Edited by Joan Gandy.

Companion website: www.manualofdieteticpractice.com

determinants and health status. These can be accessed at http://fingertips.phe.org.uk/profile/health-profiles.

Health status of minority ethnic groups

It has long been recognised that many people from minority ethnic groups have poorer health than the white British population. These are predominantly non-communicable diseases such as obesity, diabetes, cardiovascular disease and stroke, cancer, as well as mental illness. Lifestyle is highly relevant in the prevention and treatment of these conditions, but they are also strongly influenced by social determinants of health. There is a clear social gradient in health, with those who are of higher social position experiencing better health than those of lower social position (Marmot, 2010). This is thought to be due to the clustering of disadvantages in terms of income, education, housing and other social determinants of health. People from minority ethnic groups are disproportionately affected, and many are disadvantaged.

The 2011 census demonstrated that Pakistani and Bangladeshi women and White Gypsy or Irish Travellers (who were identified for the first time in the 2011 census) suffer the poorest health (Bécares, 2013), which is most pronounced in older age. The Chinese group have consistently reported better health than the white British population. There are significant differences between groups, gender, age and geographical locations, with London having the worst ethnic health inequalities (Bécares, 2013).

NICE (2013) confirmed that people from Asian and other minority ethnic groups are at risk of diabetes and other health conditions related to obesity, but at a lower BMI than the white population, and their needs must be considered in relation to obesity (NICE, 2015) and diabetes (NICE, 2012). Similarly, the need to decrease inequalities and support public health has been highlighted (DH, 2010).

There have been some attempts to better understand the factors influencing health in specific communities, with people from minority ethnic groups who undertake less physical activity and consume poorer diets (August & Sorkin, 2010; Breland *et al.*, 2013) being at greater risk of food insecurity in older age (Deeming, 2011), and being strongly influenced by health beliefs and culture (McEwen *et al.*, 2009). However, there is also evidence of healthcare professionals (HCPs) giving less information to people from minority ethnic groups (Ahmed *et al.*, 2016), and making incorrect assumptions regarding their health beliefs and understanding of health (Grace *et al.*, 2008). There have also been studies that have attempted to deliver culturally appropriate health education, with some positive effects (Attridge *et al.*, 2014). However, these studies are diverse in terms of the minority ethnic group studied and where the research was undertaken. Assumptions cannot be made that the results can be generalised, but the research is part of what will inform understanding of specific communities.

Working with minority ethnic groups

The following section considers aspects that are likely to be relevant for people from a variety of minority ethnic groups and may impact on how and what dietary advice needs to be delivered.

Understanding culture

It is important to avoid making assumptions about people from different minority ethnic groups and to consider that ethnicity is just one part of culture. People may link themselves to a variety of different cultural groups defined by nationality, language, race, age, gender, religion, disability, socioeconomic status, occupation, education, political beliefs or sexuality (Holli & Beto, 2014). Culture may be affected by geographical location or a shared history, which affects behaviours, beliefs and perspectives. It is also dynamic and does not necessarily stay the same (Gable & Herrmann, 2016). Much cultural behaviour may be unconscious, and people may never have questioned it or realised the cultural beliefs that they have. However, culture may have a significant impact on health beliefs and food, and what is considered normal not just the choice of foods but also the social aspects of food behaviour (Gable & Herrmann, 2016). In some cases, culture will link closely with religion, but the two are quite different. Communicating with people from different cultures can therefore be complex, and there is the possibility of miscommunication and misunderstanding (Gable & Herrmann, 2016).

Acculturation

Acculturation is the process of change that people go through so that they become more like people from a different culture. People moving to a new society or cultural group modify their traditions (including their eating habits), attitudes and views on many aspects of daily life to become more like the dominant culture. The extent to which people adapt is highly variable, and may be affected by how long the individual has been in the dominant culture and how old they are, with younger generations being more likely to change. This is particularly likely with food eaten outside the home. Changes in dietary and physical activity habits may lead to a more or less healthy lifestyle, but, for many coming to the UK, their diet becomes less healthy due to the fast food culture, more sedentary lifestyle (Holli & Beto, 2014) and high consumption of products such as sugar-sweetened beverages (Goff *et al.*, 2014).

Cultural competency

There is no one agreed definition of cultural competency but it is about learning to understand and work productively with service users from a range of diverse cultural and social backgrounds (Flying Start NHS, 2017). There may be a need to develop cultural competency, and this has been recognised by the dietetic profession in other countries such as the USA (Hickson *et al.*, 2016).

SECTION 3

Exploring the histories of patients from different backgrounds, particularly when they have recently arrived in a new country, will require sensitivity and excellent communication skills (PHE, 2014). An attitude that is open and respectful towards the cultural aspects of the minority ethnic group is essential. Dietetic practice must incorporate an individual's traditional health beliefs and foods with appropriate recommendations for dietary change. This goes beyond working with an individual and verbal communication, to consider written and other resources used to support interventions, including group education and public health. The wider use of media and technology may give further opportunities for supporting minority ethnic groups.

Many people have a tendency to assume that their own cultural beliefs are the best or the right way to be; this is known as ethnocentrism. This can lead to judging other cultures to be of less value. There may be unconscious bias where service users are treated differently due to some difference, but the HCPs are not aware that they are doing this. Cultural competence education for HCPs is designed to combat this and ensure that service users receive a service that is equitable, effective and relevant. A systematic review of cultural competence education (Horvat *et al.*, 2014) demonstrated a positive improvement in patient care, but with low-quality evidence. This was primarily due to the heterogeneity of interventions, none of which were undertaken in the UK. It is unlikely that pre-registration dietetic education is adequate. Owing to the ongoing changes in population diversity, it is recommended that qualified dietitians undertake cultural competence training, learn to recognise their own biases and develop appropriate strategies to work with different minority ethnic groups (Holli & Beto, 2014).

Literacy

Low literacy levels are common within the UK and should be considered routinely. With minority ethnic groups, dietitians should avoid assuming that someone who speaks English well can also read it. For the non-English-speaking service user, it is also important not to assume that they can read the language that they speak. Indeed, some languages do not have a written form (Holli & Beto, 2014). Information, whether written in English or in the language that an individual speaks, may need to be written very simply and pictures included to illustrate the points being made. Service users may be happy to take written information if they have friends or family who can read it for them, but some may be embarrassed by their lack of ability to read and may try to hide this fact. Careful consideration is required to ensure that information is accessible to service users.

Health beliefs

Western culture holds science in high esteem, and dietitians are trained to work using evidence-based practice. Many other cultures have different food and health beliefs, which may affect how service users view the advice given (Holli & Beto, 2014). Ignoring or not understanding these food and health beliefs can lead to a dietitian suggesting changes that may not make sense or may seem inappropriate to service users. Knowledge about health beliefs is part of the cultural competence that a dietitian must develop.

Aspects of communication

There are many issues that must be considered in relation to communication that can impact on interactions with service users from minority ethnic groups.

Non-verbal communication

Different cultural groups will have different customs, and these too will be influenced by the level of acculturation. These can affect greetings, personal contact, gestures, eye contact, what is considered appropriate personal space and public displays of affection (Holli & Beto, 2014). While a handshake is seen as a normal formal greeting in the UK, this will be highly inappropriate in some cultures, particularly between genders. It is advisable to be guided by the service user and to respond if they offer a hand. Similarly, while eye contact is seen as good communication in Western culture, and lack of it can be disconcerting, direct eye contact may be seen as rude or confrontational in other cultures. Care to avoid making assumptions about what non-verbal communication means is important (Gable & Herrmann, 2016).

Language

The UK has a multicultural and linguistically diverse population. For many people, English is not the primary language spoken at home. With so much diversity, there is vast scope for communication barriers and misunderstandings between English-speaking health professionals and people with no or limited English proficiency. Communicating across language barriers is challenging for all involved (Gable & Herrmann, 2016).

It is important to be clear about what the first language of the service user is. In some countries, e.g. India and Pakistan, many languages are commonly spoken, and there can be regional variations of one language. For those who do speak English, it is advisable to keep checking the level of understanding by asking the service user to explain what they have understood so far. Just asking *'Do you understand?'* is likely to get a positive response, whether the service user understands or not! Speaking clearly and not too fast; avoiding jargon, metaphors and colloquialisms; focusing on one topic at a time; and using visual aids can all be helpful.

It is not just direct translation that may be an issue, but some English words do not have an equivalent in other languages, and so may need to be explained. Similarly, some subject areas that are routine for dietitians are not commonly discussed in other cultures, such as bowel function (Gable & Herrmann, 2016). Being aware of subjects that are taboo or embarrassing to service users can help dietitians to ask questions in a more sensitive way. Explaining the relevance of the information to the medical condition you are working with may be helpful. It may be important to be very clear and specific in certain situations. For example, some cultures have very different views on time-keeping, and service users may not realise that arriving late for an appointment is likely to be a problem, whereas being late is seen as rude in UK culture, but may also mean that an appointment cannot be kept (Gable & Herrmann, 2016).

For those with no, or very limited, English proficiency, it may be appropriate to use interpreters. Family and friends of patients may be used as adequate translators as they are free, may be accessible and readily available; in addition, they know the patients and their problems well. However, there may be issues, e.g. patient confidentiality may be compromised; in addition, patients may be uncomfortable or embarrassed about someone they know discussing sensitive, private matters. Such interpreters may withhold information, especially bad news, or add their own opinion; this may affect patent adherence. Using professional, trained interpreters improves care quality (Kaur *et al.*, 2014).

Religion

Although this is important for many people, for many minority ethnic groups it is central to everyday life. Some minority ethnic groups are highly dominated by one faith, e.g. >90 % of Pakistani people in the UK are Muslims. Conversely, there is a wide range of faiths followed in the Chinese population, including Christianity and Buddhism. Table 3.5.1 provides information on the impact of many common religions on food choice. The Office for National Statistics (www.ons.gov.uk) gives details on which religions are most likely to be observed by which minority ethnic groups. Some religions have little impact on food intake, while others have many rules about foods allowed to be eaten, fasting and where food fits into festivals and celebrations. Observance of festivals is also affected by acculturation, e.g. many service users will celebrate Christmas and Easter even if not of the Christian faith – this may impact on food intake.

Food and minority ethnic groups

The following is a list of questions that dietitians would be advised to have researched prior to working with a specific minority ethnic group:

- What are the traditional foods, and how available and affordable are they locally? Consider each of the food groups in the Eatwell Guide, including commonly eaten foods high in fat and high in sugar, drinks and alcohol consumption.
- Which traditionally eaten foods are healthy/unhealthy? You may need to understand cooking methods and recipes to be able to suggest appropriate adaptations or alternatives. Cooking appliances and methods may be different and may have changed since migration.
- What are the traditional foods that form a normal part of the diet known as? They may have different names.
- How has migration affected food and physical activity behaviours?
- How is life different?
- Which religions are most likely to be followed by this population, and what impact might that have on food and lifestyle? Also consider alcohol consumption, smoking habits and views on physical activity.
- What languages are most likely to be spoken by this group?
- Who makes decisions about the diet at home, e.g. shopping, foods eaten, meal times, different cooking methods and portion size?
- When there is a need to find a healthier alternative, what is acceptable, available and affordable in the local area? Suggest healthier, acceptable Western foods which can also be cheaper. Some traditional foods in the UK may be quite expensive, e.g. tropical fruit and vegetables.
- Are there commonly held health beliefs and/or beliefs about how food and health interact?

When undertaking an assessment with an individual service user, either in consultations or group education, the following may additionally be relevant:

- How much is the service user motivated to make changes, and what support is likely to be received from the family members? Many minority ethnic groups live in extended families. Explore who the service user lives with.
- Identify the barriers to making dietary and lifestyle changes, and how these can be overcome, considering culture-specific factors.
- Ask the service user for more information if you are unsure about any foods or if any clarification is needed. This shows that you are interested in foods that are important to them, and means that you will better understand if adaptation is needed and, if so, how that can be achieved.
- Some tips on considering cultural sensitivity in group education can be found in Avery *et al.* (2016).

Specific minority ethnic groups

The following section covers some specific minority ethnic groups in detail. These groups have been included due to their high prevalence in the UK, the influence of culture/religion on diet and/or their poor health status. It is beyond the scope of this chapter to cover a wider range of groups. See Thaker and Barton (2012) for further information.

South Asian

The South Asian subcontinent, also known as the Indian subcontinent, is the southern region of Asia, which includes Bangladesh, India, Pakistan, Bhutan, Maldives, Nepal and Sri Lanka. The term South Asian defines many ethnic groups with distinctive regions of origin,

Table 3.5.1 Common foods eaten within different religious groups

Food Group	Judaism	Islam	Hinduism	Sikhism	Buddhism	Rastafarianism
Starchy foods	Kosher bread such as matza, cereals, rice, potatoes	Chapatti/roti made from wheat flour or rice flour, bread, couscous, basmati rice, potatoes	Chapatti/roti, bread, puri, potatoes, sweet potatoes, cassava, matoke, rice	Chapatti/roti/paratha, bread, potatoes, rice	Rice, wheat, noodles, corn flour	Brown rice, yam, cassava
Fruit and vegetables	All vegetables All fruit except grapes, which may be restricted	All vegetables, such as lady fingers, okra, bitter melon (karela). All fruit, commonly including mango, starfruit, melon, dates	All vegetables, such as bitter melon (karela), aubergines, spinach All fruit, such as papaya, passion fruit, coconut	All vegetables, such as spinach, aubergines All fruit, commonly including passion fruit, melon	Vegetables such as Chinese cabbage, spinach, leek Fruit, commonly including melon, lychee, bananas.	Fruits and vegetables consumed a lot All vegetables, commonly callaloo, cauliflower All fruit, such as oranges, papaya, coconut, currants
Meat/ chicken	Sheep, cattle, goats, deer are permitted Pig, rabbit are not kosher Chicken, geese, duck, turkey may be eaten	Halal meat only – chicken, mutton, lamb, goat, beef No pork and pork products are permitted	Strict Hindus may be vegetarian Beef is prohibited, whereas less strict Hindus may eat lamb or chicken	Some are vegetarians, but many eat chicken and lamb Strict may not eat pork or beef	Many are vegetarians May eat pork, chicken	Do not eat meat Pork is forbidden
Fish	Fish such as tuna, carp and salmon are permitted Shellfish not permitted	All fish with fins and scales are permitted	Less strict may eat fish	Less strict may eat fish	Fish may be consumed	Fish may be consumed that are less than 30.5 cm Do not eat fish without scales, shellfish
Eggs	Eggs are kosher if from a kosher bird and do not contain blood spots	Eggs are consumed – boiled, fried, omelettes	Very strict do not eat eggs	Very strict do not eat eggs	Eggs may be eaten	Eggs are not eaten
Pulses/ lentils, nuts/ seeds	Variety consumed	Variety consumed such as dals, lentils, chickpeas, split peas	Variety consumed such as dals; nuts and seeds consumed	Variety consumed such as dals, lentils, chickpeas, split peas	Pulses such as mung beans, red beans, seeds and nuts	Variety consumed, such as pigeon peas, butter beans, split peas
Dairy products	Kosher milk – full-fat and semi-skimmed Yoghurt, cheese	Full-fat and semi-skimmed milk and yoghurt; paneer (Indian cheese); lassi drink (sweet or salty)	Full-fat and semi-skimmed milk, yoghurt, paneer, lassi drink (sweet or salty)	Full-fat and semi-skimmed milk, paneer; lassi drink (sweet or salty)	Evaporated milk, full-fat and semi-skimmed milk, soya milk, cheese	Milk from a cow or any other animal is avoided
Fats/oils	Kosher butter and margarine; low-fat varieties are limited	Ghee/butter Groundnut/mustard/olive oil Vegetable oil	Ghee/butter Oils such as sunflower, corn or peanut	Ghee Makhan (home-made butter)	Lard/butter Groundnut (peanut) oil, sesame seed oil	Coconut oil
Beverages	Tea Alcohol	Fruit juices, full-sugar fizzy drinks Tea (traditional tea is made with higher proportion of milk to water) Do not drink alcohol	Full-sugar fizzy drinks, fruit juices, tea Strict do not consume alcohol	Full-sugar fizzy drinks, fruit juices, tea, alcohol	Fizzy drinks, fruit juices, tea, coffee, alcohol	Fruit juices, smoothies and herbal drinks such as tea; avoid alcohol, caffeinated drinks
Desserts	Macaroons, prune hamantaschen (triangular, filled pastry)	Asian sweets such as ladoo, burfi, sevian (milk vermicelli dish), halva, baklava	Asian sweets such as burfi, shrikhand	Asian sweets such as jalebi, ladoo	Fresh fruit, gingered fruit,	Grater cake, toto (small coconut cake), banana fritters
Cooking methods	Meat cannot be eaten with dairy Meat is ritually slaughtered and salted	Permitted animals slaughtered according to Islamic law May use 'Tawa' (griddle) to make chapattis May fry, bake	May use Tawa (griddle) to make chapattis May fry, steam, and bake	May use Tawa (griddle) to make chapattis May fry, bake	May avoid garlic in cooking; dishes are prepared with balance in colours and flavours	Food is organic Ital cooking, which excludes the use of salt, meat (especially pork), preservatives, colouring, flavourings or anything artificial

languages, religions and customs. There are many differences among the countries in their cultural and traditional beliefs and diets, but also many similarities. For many migrant South Asians, reconciling advice on lifestyle behaviour with their own cultural practices is very challenging, particularly regarding dietary change. Unique customs that immigrants have brought with them are a great source of pride and identity, and holding onto these customs is a high priority. A central component of South Asian culture revolves around food and the unique qualities and blend of ingredients, oils and spices that are part of the traditional diet.

For example, the most senior or eldest persons living in the home dominate some extended family households, and the eldest female usually makes dietary decisions. Younger women have expressed difficulties in making healthy dietary changes due to the resistance they encounter from their parents or grandparents (Patel *et al.*, 2012). Migration to the UK can also result in food choices being influenced by the Western diet, especially in the younger generation. This can cause conflict in healthy food choices made from their traditional diet as well as the Western diet.

Religion

Religion is an integral part of the life of South Asians, and each religion has its specific dietary restrictions. The four main religions of South Asians living in the UK are Hinduism, Sikhism, Islam and Buddhism. Table 3.5.1 shows the common foods eaten within different religious groups.

Hinduism

The largest group of British Indians are those of Punjabi origin, accounting for an estimated 45% of the British Indian population in England and Wales, and smaller groups including Gujarati and Malayali communities, with the majority following Hinduism (Chanda & Ghosh, 2013). Depending on the origin of the person, they may speak Gujarati or Hindi, and may also converse in Urdu. The Hindu religion (*Dharma*) is the oldest religion in the world, having existed for over 5000 years. Hinduism is founded on reverence for life, non-violence and a belief in reincarnation. Dietary restrictions were laid down in the Hindu holy book, the Bhagavad Gita.

Dietary restrictions

The Hindu dietary restrictions are as follows:

- Hindus are lacto-vegetarians and believe in Ahimsa, meaning non-violence to all forms of life. They avoid beef, as cows are sacred, and other meat and fish. They do not eat eggs as they are potentially a source of life.
- Animal-derived fats such as dripping or lard are not acceptable, nor are foods that contain animal products, e.g. rennet and gelatine.
- Milk, yoghurt, paneer and butter are consumed because they do not involve killing an animal. Paneer (Indian cheese) and yoghurt are made at home with full-fat milk.
- Cooking with ghee (clarified butter) is believed to sanctify food. Fruit and cooked foods, especially sweet dishes that are offered to the deities in temples (prasad), are made at home with ghee. Ghee and vegetable oils are used in cooking and frying.
- Alcohol is forbidden, but is consumed by some.
- Strict Hindus will be unwilling to eat food unless they are certain that the utensils used in its preparation and service have not been in contact with meat or fish.
- Less strict Hindus may eat lamb, chicken or white fish.

Festivals

There are a number of religious Hindu festivals that may be observed with acts of worship, fasting, offering to deities, feasting, vigil rituals, charity and celebrations with family and friends. Special savoury and sweet dishes are prepared. The dates of the festivals are usually in accordance with the lunar calendar.

- Maha Shivaratri is celebrated to honour Lord Shiva (March) – traditionally, a fast is observed from dawn to dusk, and only pure foods, e.g. milk, fruit, nuts, yoghurt and potatoes, are eaten. Some people will forego all food and have fluids only.
- Ram Navami marks the birthday of Lord Rama (April) – a fast may be observed.
- Janmashtami marks the birthday of Lord Krishna (August) – a fast may be observed.
- Raksha Bandhan marks the special bond between brothers and sisters (August) – the sister will tie a rakhee (wrist band) on her brother, and he in return will give her a gift; a festive meal is prepared.
- Holi is a harvest festival (March) – a bonfire is lit, and foods such as popcorn, dates, coconut and sweets are eaten.
- Navaratri is a festival observed over 9 nights, which celebrates the power of good over evil (October) – some people may fast for all the 9 days. There are special dances held every day.
- Diwali is the festival of lights and signifies the New Year for some Hindu communities (October/November) – it honours Lakshmi, the Goddess of wealth.

Fasting

Some devout Hindus will fast regularly during the week and on religious days; it is mostly a matter of individual preference. The fast will be observed usually for a single day (24 hours), from dawn to dusk, or for several days. Fasting involves willingly abstaining from some or all food, drink or both. Some may have one cooked meal a day or only eat pure foods such as yoghurt and fruit, while others forego all food and may take fluids only.

Sikhism

Most Sikhs in Britain originate from Punjab in India; their mother tongue is Punjabi, but many can also converse in Hindi or Urdu. Sikhism started nearly 300 years ago. Guru Nanak, the first of 10 Sikh Gurus, founded Sikhism; Sikhs believe in one God. The three main principles of Sikhism are:

- Nam Japna – Meditating on God's name (e.g. prayers).
- Kirat Karna – Earning one's living righteously.
- Vand Chhakna – Helping the needy or less fortunate people (i.e. charity).

In 1699, the 10th Guru baptised the Sikhs and ordered the baptised Sikhs to wear five Ks. These are: Kesh (uncut hair), which is kept covered by a turban; Kanga (comb), symbolising cleanliness and order; Kara (steel bangle), symbolising strength and integrity; Kirpan (small sword), symbolising readiness to protect the weak; and Kachhera (underwear shorts), symbolising self-control and chastity. A Sikh gurdwara (place of worship) traditionally serves meals (langar) to anyone at any time, regardless of their caste (class structure determined by birth), religion or class. In the UK, langar is cooked on Saturdays and served after evening prayer.

Dietary restrictions

Sikh dietary restrictions include the following:

- The main food restriction is that Sikhs are not allowed to eat halal or kosher meat. For Sikhs, this is a matter for each individual's conscience. As a group, they are less strict than Hindus and Muslims; however, for each Sikh, the self-imposed restrictions are binding.
- They are unlikely to eat pork, and beef is forbidden, as the cow is considered a sacred animal.
- On the Indian subcontinent, chicken, lamb and sheep are killed by the jatka method (in one stroke); however, this practice is not common in the UK.
- Meat and eggs are included in the diet; however, after the Amrit (baptism) ceremony, individuals will revert to a lacto-vegetarian diet.
- Sikhism has retained many features of Hinduism, e.g. women still follow a lacto-vegetarian diet, even though they cook meat dishes for family members.
- Fasting is forbidden, but many Sikhs still practice this tradition, and women may fast in the same way as Hindus.
- Drinking alcohol, smoking and taking recreational drugs are also prohibited; however, in practice, alcohol consumption by men can sometimes be excessive.

Festivals

There are three main festivals in the Sikh calendar:

- Vaisakhi marks the founding of the khalsa (Sikh community) in 1699 (April) – celebrated with joy and devotion. People attend the gurdwara and offer prayers and eat langar.
- Diwali is the Festival of Light (October/November) – Sikhs celebrated the return of Guro Hargobind by lighting the Golden Temple and this tradition continues today.
- Guru Nanak Gurpurab marks the birth of Guru Nanak, the founder of Sikhism (November) – Sikhs celebrate by reading Guru Granth Sahib, the Sikh holy book. They congregate to sing, pray and eat.

Fasting

Sikhism does not promote fasting, except for medical reasons.

Islam

The South Asian Muslim community in the UK came mainly from Pakistan, Bangladesh and East Africa. However, some Muslims in the UK will have originated from the Middle East, Malaysia, Indonesia, Sri Lanka and Africa. Many Muslims of Asian origin will speak Urdu, Punjabi, Mirpuri or Bengali. Muslims who have come from India or via East Africa may also speak Gujarati, and those from the Middle East may speak Arabic. The religion of Muslims is Islam; the word Islam is an Arabic word meaning submission. All Muslims acknowledge the obligation to signify their submission in terms of the five pillars of Islam. These are:

- *Monotheism* – belief in one God (Allah), and that Mohammed is his true messenger.
- *Prayer* – performed five times a day.
- *Zakat* – giving 2.5% of wealth to the poor and needy annually.
- *Pilgrimage of Hajj* – carried out at least once in a lifetime; Muslims should make a pilgrimage to Mecca if they can afford it.
- *Fasting* – complete abstinence from food and drink from dawn to sunset in the month of Ramadan.

Dietary restrictions

Muslim dietary restrictions laid down in the Holy Quran are:

- Animals to be ritually slaughtered while reciting the name of Allah, and then blood to be allowed to drain (halal meat). Kosher meat may be acceptable.
- All wholesome foods are halal unless it is declared unlawful (haram). Haram foods are:
  - Foods and food products from the pig, and foods containing ingredients or additives derived from the pig; any animal that has not been ritually slaughtered; and any haram source. Strict Muslims will eat from outside the home only if the food served is halal. Halal food is now available in institutions such as schools and hospitals. Ready-made halal frozen foods are produced and sold in shops. Many catering organisations, e.g. restaurants or other eateries, serve halal foods. In practice, this means that a wide range of manufactured foods containing gelatine, animal fats or emulsifiers derived from animal sources will be avoided.
  - Alcohol, including that used in cooking or for medicinal purposes.
- A Muslim might refuse a food if they cannot be sure that it does not contain unlawful ingredients. Similarly, a devout Muslim will be concerned that the dishes used for cooking have not been in contact with unlawful foods.
- Fish is acceptable, provided it has fins and scales. White and oily fish are consumed as a major part of the Bengali Muslim diet.

The Muslim Food Board (UK) produces a regularly updated halal food directory, listing halal-manufactured foods available in the UK.

Festivals

There are two major festivals in the Muslim calendar:

- Eid-al Fitr (little Eid) marks the end of the fasting month of Ramadan, and celebrations are held both in the community and at home. Eid is marked with special prayers, and men may read the prayer at the mosque. Family and friends get together and enjoy celebration food.

- Eid-al Adha (big Eid) commemorates the pilgrimage to Mecca that concludes the Hajj. Eid is marked with prayers in addition to the regular daily prayers, mutual visiting by family and friends, and celebratory meals. Muslims are required to sacrifice a lamb, sheep, cow or goat after Eid-al Adha. During the celebration, this meat is shared among family, friends and the poor. In the UK, Muslims may contribute financially so that an animal is slaughtered by a halal butcher in the UK or abroad and then distributed to the needy.

Fasting

Muslims are required to fast from dawn to sunset during the month of Ramadan, which is the ninth month of the Muslim (lunar) calendar – therefore, the dates change every year. Fasting involves abstinence from all food and drink. It is considered one of the highest forms of worship as it enables people to practise self-discipline, and it helps them to appreciate and share the feelings of the poor and hungry. Muslims should rise just before sunrise (sehri), have a meal similar to breakfast and then break their fast again at sunset (iftari). Feelings of weakness and lethargy can occur because of this abstinence and, to help overcome this, some Muslims rise early and eat a substantial high-carbohydrate, high-fat meal before dawn. Another heavy meal is then taken after sunset.

Elderly people and children under 12 years are exempt from fasting. Women who are pregnant, breastfeeding or menstruating, and people who are ill or travelling during Ramadan, are also exempt, but are expected to compensate by fasting at some other time. Chronically ill people, such as those with diabetes or heart disease, for whom fasting would be physically harmful, are exempt. However, many Muslims still choose to fast, and should be advised accordingly (see Chapter 7.12, Diabetes mellitus). Devout Muslims may also fast once or twice a week in addition to Ramadan (Sarwar & Hamid, 2004).

Meal pattern and social aspects of food

Eating habits among South Asians tend to be similar in many ways. The meal pattern usually consists of three meals and an evening snack. The main meal is usually eaten later (8–9 pm). Traditional breakfast can be tea and flat bread (chapatti, paratha) with a pickle (achaar) or chutney. Foods eaten at lunch and evening meal tend to be similar. They may consist of a staple food such as rice, chapatti with two or three curries (vegetable or lentils/dhal or meat/chicken or fish), and a salad. A small piece of the chapatti is used to scoop up the curry. Cutlery is traditionally not used, and food is usually eaten with the right hand. A variety of fruit can be eaten either as part of a meal or as a snack (Temple & Steyn, 2016).

Most South Asian curries are cooked in vegetable oil, and it can traditionally be used quite liberally. Ghee (clarified butter) can also be used in cooking. Foods such as samosas and pakoras can be deep fried in oil. South Asian cuisine is characterised by the use of herbs and spices. Tea (chai) is consumed throughout the day. The traditional process of making tea is boiling water with tea leaves, along with spices such as cardamom. Sugar is then added, along with milk. Besides tea, other beverages are consumed such as full-sugar fizzy drinks and buttermilk (lassi). Foods such as rice, chapatti flour, oil, fruit and vegetables are traditionally bought in bulk in the UK. Traditional food will be purchased from South Asian supermarkets where possible.

The dietary habits of some ethnic groups living in Europe are likely to become less healthy as individuals increase consumption of processed foods that are energy dense and contain high levels of fat, sugar and salt. Such products often replace healthy dietary components of the native diet, such as fruits, vegetables, nuts and grains. Mixed food habits are emerging mainly among younger people in the second and third generations, most likely due to acculturation and adoption of a Western lifestyle. Age and immigrant generation are the major factors accounting for changes in dietary habits, while income, level of education, dietary laws, religion and food beliefs are also important factors. The risk of chronic disease such as obesity, cardiovascular disease, hypertension and diabetes is reported to be higher in ethnic populations, particularly South Asians (Gilbert & Khokhar, 2008).

Middle Eastern diet

The Middle East is a transcontinental region centred on Western Asia and Egypt. Arabs, Turks, Persians, Kurds and Azers (excluding the Republic of Azerbaijan) constitute the largest ethnic groups in the region by population. The Middle East is very diverse when it comes to religions, many of which originated there. Islam is the largest religion in the Middle East, but Judaism and Christianity are two other major faiths that originated there. The top five languages, in terms of the number of speakers, are Arabic, Hebrew, Persian, Turkish and Kurdish.

Religion

Most of the population practise Islam, although there are different branches and denominations of Islam, each with its own traditions and practices. However, the basic practices of Islam are universal. Restrictions on what Muslims can eat are laid down in the Holy Quran and are regarded as the direct command of Allah, as discussed earlier in text.

Meal pattern and social aspects of food

Traditional Arabic food habits generally consist of three meals a day, with lunch being the main meal. Breakfast may consist of bread with honey or yoghurt. Eggs (baydh) are frequently consumed at meal times, especially breakfast. Lunch may be eaten at about 2–3 pm, and is often the main meal of the day. This is usually a mezze, which is a selection of several dishes. Bread is usually eaten with the main meal or as a starter, with ground chickpeas (hummus), natural yoghurt, cracked wheat and parsley (taboulleh), ground aubergine (baba ghannou) or vine leaves (stuffed with onion, garlic, tomato, rice, herbs and often minced meat – usually lamb). The meal is usually based on starchy foods, particularly rice (roz); this may be boiled, or have meat juices and fat added. Other starchy foods may be specific to particular dishes, such as potatoes, cassava, yam (boiled or fried) and couscous. Vegetables and/or salad are included as part of the main meal. Dressings on salad, with the exception of olive oil, are usually low fat (lemon and garlic). Olive oil may be added liberally to foods such as hummus. A variety of fish, including oily fish (salmon, mackerel and sardines), is consumed, particularly in coastal areas. This is usually shallow fried, but oven baking is becoming more frequent. Chicken and meat can also be a main component of a meal. The evening meal may be consumed late (8–9 pm) and is usually a light meal: bread (flat or sliced, white or brown) and cheese made into a sandwich, or flat traditional bread filled with red or white meat, eaten with cracked wheat, tomato, parsley and a sauce, such as a sesame-based one (sharwama). Meat or vegetables (usually potato, or a dish such as kibbeh) may be eaten. Salad will accompany the meal.

Fruit juices (aasir), water, tea (shay) or Arabic coffee (ground coffee beans brewed with boiling water to which saffron, ginger and cardamom may be added) tend to be the main fluids consumed. Coffee is usually consumed in small cups and accompanied by dates or other snacks. Tea usually has moderate amounts of sugar added to it. Full-sugar carbonated drinks are also consumed. Fruit is usually as a dessert, including dried (dates and figs). Traditional snacks include high-fibre foods, e.g. nuts, dates and fruit. Nuts and seeds are a permanent feature on the table, especially pistachios, walnuts, cashews, sunflower and pumpkin seeds (salted). Sesame seeds are often added to bread and pastries, often with thyme. Sugar (sukkar) and honey (aasat) form the basis of pastries, and are used to sweeten drinks (tea and coffee). The evening meal may be eaten with the family. However, it is common to see many Arabic people eating out with friends and consuming fast foods, similar to those constituting lunch. Alternatively, traditional Arabic foods may be eaten at a restaurant.

The main female, wife or mother, in the household makes decisions regarding the shopping and cooking methods. If there is more than one wife, the first wife of the household will decide about the diet at home. Cooking may be carried out by the main female of the house or by maids. Arabic families may often have maids who do the shopping and cooking (especially in the Middle East). Many of these domestic helpers are from India or Sri Lanka, and they may influence the way food is prepared and cooked. In the UK, women mostly do the cooking; food may be cooked daily (especially if cooks are available) or in bulk. Shallow frying is used frequently for cooking, e.g. for pastries, vegetables such as aubergines, and falafel. Many main dishes use boiling as a cooking method. However, the fat from meats is not removed in this process, and other foods will be added to the dish to make stews. There appears to be healthier, low-fat methods of cooking among the younger generation (Thaker & Barton, 2012).

Although alcohol consumption is prohibited in Islam, its consumption has increased due to availability and peer pressure in the Middle East. It is not uncommon for many Arabic men to drink alcohol at home or socially. It is unusual for Arabic women to drink alcohol. In many Arabic countries, the prevalence of men smoking cigarettes appears to be higher than among women; however, the shisha (waterpipe, hubble-bubble) may be smoked by men and women. It is often seen as a fashionable thing to do, and less stigma is attached to women smoking this. This is now gaining popularity in the West. The shisha is mixed with aromatic herbs (e.g. apple, mango, strawberry, mint or other additives). Smoking aggravates the complications of diabetes and causes hypertension, which is prevalent in many of the Arab countries, and can increase the risk of cancers (Aslam *et al.*, 2014).

Traditionally, foods such as fruit and vegetables are bought in bulk from market stalls; in the UK, traditional foods may not always be available. Arabic foods will be bought from Arabic shops, and other shopping is done from supermarkets. In some countries, multicultural outlets have increased the variety of dishes, including Italian, Chinese and Indian foods, as well as Western fast foods. In the first generation, low-fat and sugar-free foods may not be accepted, but there is greater acceptance for these in the second generation (Chowbey & Harrop, 2016).

African-Caribbean diet

African-Caribbean collectively refers to people who come from the Caribbean but are of African descent. The majority of families of African-Caribbean descent in the UK are from Jamaica and moved to the UK during the 1950s and 1960s. There are now many who are second and third generation, and therefore a high proportion are British. Although English is the first language for most, there may be some in the older generation who speak Creole or Patois.

Religion

Although many African-Caribbean people are Christian, the two main religions that affect dietary practice are Seventh-day Adventism and Rastafarianism.

Seventh-day Adventists

Seventh-day Adventists have a strong belief in the importance of looking after their bodies, by avoiding alcohol, smoking, tea and coffee, and by following a vegetarian diet.

Rastafarianism

Many Rastafarians are vegetarian or vegan; the majority will only eat ital foods, which are foods considered to be in a whole and natural state, with processed or preserved foods excluded.

Meal pattern and social aspects of food

The Caribbean is made up of many islands where food habits and culture are important and different between islands. Dietary practices can vary considerably, and dishes with similar or the same name can contain different ingredients. Acculturation will have a significant impact on this population, with many incorporating typical UK foods and consuming fewer traditional foods (Goff *et al.*, 2014). Traditional dishes can be time consuming to prepare, and are therefore more likely to be eaten at weekends and by older generations. At weekends, there is a tendency towards eating two meals, omitting lunch. Popular cooking methods include stewing, braising, steaming, frying and roasting, and very often involve the use of added fat. Food is highly seasoned, with high amounts of salt used. Desserts are traditionally only eaten on special occasions. For more information on typical Caribbean foods, see Thaker and Barton (2012).

Jewish diet

Israel, the Jewish nation state, is the only country in which Jews make up a majority of the citizens. The largest Jewish community outside of Israel is currently in the USA: other countries include Canada, Argentina and Brazil. The National Equality Panel (2010) showed that the group with the largest median net wealth were Jewish people (Rowlingson, 2012), and they are subsequently not subject to the deprivation common in other minority ethnic groups. In the UK, Jews are British people who are ethnically and/or religiously Jewish. The UK is home to the second largest Jewish population in Europe, and has the fifth largest Jewish community worldwide. English is the primary language spoken, Hebrew is also commonly spoken. Jewish people are very diverse, reflecting differing degrees of acculturation and religious observance of Judaism, an ancient religion.

Dietary restrictions

Jewish people have food customs traditionally associated with their daily lives, holidays and festivals. These are in addition to detailed dietary laws (Kashrut) that date back to the Old Testament and define the selection, preparation and consumption of permitted (kosher) food. Self-discipline and preservation of Jewish spirituality and religious identity underlie these laws, which are as follows:

- Meat and poultry must not be cooked with milk or milk derivatives, or be served at the same meal. Utensils, crockery, pots and pans used for milk and meat must be stored, washed and dried separately.
- All meat and milk products must be bought from a kosher shop bearing a kosher stamp.
- Permitted animals are quadrupeds that chew the cud and have cloven hoofs, such as sheep, goats and cattle. All others, including pigs, are forbidden.
- Poultry such as chicken, duck, goose, turkey and some game birds are permitted. Most others, including birds of prey and ostrich, are forbidden.
- Animals and birds must be slaughtered according to the shechita method. This procedure, considered a painless means of slaughtering an animal, must be carried out by a trained and authorised person, and entails a rapid cut with a sharp knife to sever the jugular vein and carotid artery. The meat must then be salted and soaked in water to remove the blood and render it kosher (permitted).
- Only fish with scales and fins, such as cod, plaice, salmon, tuna, etc., are allowed. Eels, shark, monkfish and all shellfish are forbidden.

The modern orthodox Jew will follow similar rules, but is more integrated with the general population. It is important to establish the level of observance at the time of consultation.

The variety of kosher low-fat, low-sugar dairy foods are limited. During Shabbat and festivals, highly energy-dense foods are served. Shabbat and festival foods from the Ashkenazi tradition (that of families from Eastern Europe and Russia) tend to be of higher energy than traditional Sephardic foods (those of families from Southern Europe, the Middle East and Asia), owing to the different climates where the recipes were developed. A traditional Ashkenazi diet uses large amounts of chicken fat (schmaltz), and may require different dietary modifications from that of the traditional Sephardic diet.

Festivals

Sabbath (Shabbat)

The seventh day of the week is the Sabbath (Shabbat), a day of prayer at the synagogue and of complete rest from work from sundown on Friday to Saturday evening. Writing, operating any electrical equipment, cooking and travelling are among the tasks that are forbidden during the Sabbath and many festivals. All food preparation is done in advance, and large family meals are traditionally eaten.

The New Year (Rosh HaShanah)

The customs and symbols of Rosh HaShanah reflect the holiday's dual emphasis on both happiness and humility. Customs observed include the sounding of the shofar and eating special foods, including round challah, which symbolises the circle of life, and sweet foods for a sweet New Year. This is celebrated on the Hebrew calendar dates in September/October. The Jewish year is based on lunar calculations.

Yom Kippur

Yom Kippur is the Day of Atonement, which is the holiest day of the Jewish calendar. It is on the tenth day of the month of the Tishri in the Jewish calendar. This holiday involves activities such as praying and fasting. Many Jewish people spend time in the synagogue at this time of year. The festival ends on a joyous note, and many Jewish people take part in a festive after-fast meal.

Passover

Passover, which commemorates the exodus of Jews from Egypt, is celebrated for 8 days in early spring (April). No foods made with, or in contact with, wheat, barley, oats or rye (chametz) may be eaten. Unleavened bread (matzah) is eaten in place of normal bread. Cooking and eating utensils that are reserved only for Passover are used.

Fasting

Fasting is for 25 hours and begins on the evening before Yom Kippur. No food or drink is permitted from sunset the evening before to sunset the next day. Unless life or health is concerned, drinking water is not permitted. The idea is that the observer is afflicting the soul to atone for the sins of the past year. Pregnant women, the elderly, children under the age of 9 years and ill persons are exempt from this practice.

Meal pattern and social aspects of food

To avoid any concerns about whether foods are genuinely kosher, some Jews will only shop in a store that exclusively sells kosher food. In the ultra-orthodox Jewish community, a woman runs the house and looks after the children, and the husband goes to work. One of the many laws that exist regarding behaviour is that men and women should not mix together. If a male dietitian is seeing an ultra-orthodox female, she may not want to shake hands or have any contact with him, and may feel uneasy about being in the same room with him, and vice versa.

Polish diet

The Polish population in the UK is the fastest growing minority ethnic group, and, in 2015, in the UK population census, Poland was the most common non-UK country of birth (ONS, 2016). Of the total number of non-UK-born residents in the UK in 2015, 9.7% were born in Poland. Many of the more recent migrants have come for work and are relatively young adults, and subsequently with young families. Common health problems are reported to be related to smoking, excessive alcohol consumption and poor mental health (Coakley, 2011), which is likely to lead to cancer and cardiovascular diseases in later life.

Religion

There are a diversity of religions practised in Poland, but approximately 90% are Roman Catholics who observe varying degree of strictness. Many people celebrate the traditional Christian festivals such as Christmas and Easter with family-based gatherings. Some people will abstain from alcohol or meat during Lent; others may fast on occasions, but there are not set rules about fasting.

Meal pattern and the social aspects of food

Many supermarkets now stock a variety of Polish foods, and there are many Polish shops. Ready-made Polish foods are available and make it easy for many to retain more traditional food habits, but they tend to be high in salt and fat. Some examples of Polish ready-meals are Hunters' stew (bigos, sauerkraut and cabbage stewed with a variety of meats, sausages, bacon and spices), stuffed cabbage parcels (gołabki – cabbage stuffed with rice and pork filling) and meatballs in tomato sauce (pulpety or klopsy). Soups are also popular, often with added cream. Many of the traditional foods take a long time to cook from scratch, making the ready meals an appealing alternative.

The traditional Polish diet contains a lot of meat and sausages, many of which are smoked. A wide variety of fish, many of which are not freely available in the UK, are consumed, also often smoked. Dumplings and pasta shapes, most notably Polish ravioli (pierogi) and kasha (kasza, made from buckwheat, cracked pearl barley or millet, is a popular alternative accompaniment to the main course), and significant amounts of fat, are often added to such foods.

Many types of breads are eaten, and potatoes and rice are commonly consumed. The types of fruit and vegetables consumed in Poland reflect the climate, and many are pickled, which leads to further increase in salt intake (e.g. sauerkraut). Mushrooms and beetroot are widely used. Consumption of sugary foods is also common, including sweetened fruit juice drinks (e.g. Kubuś or Tymbark), honey, fruit compote and soft drinks. For further detail on typical Polish foods, see Thaker and Barton (2012). Although many healthy foods such as fruits, vegetables, starchy foods and fish are consumed, the addition of fat, sugar and salt has a negative impact on the overall dietary balance.

Conclusion

The ethnic and cultural mix of the UK is constantly changing, and there is significant geographical variation. Dietitians must stay informed of the diversity in the locality in which they work. They must be aware of the foods that specific minority ethnic groups traditionally eat, but also consider the social and cultural influences. Above all, as with any patient or patient group, stereotyping and assumptions must be avoided, and individualisation of care plans is essential.

Acknowledgement

The editor acknowledges the prior contribution of Aruna Thaker, Heidi Chan, Ruth Kander, Christina Merryfield and Elzbieta Szymula.

Further reading

Moorley C, Goodfellow B, Corcoran N. (2013) Reaching unreachable groups and crossing cultural barriers. In Corcoran N (ed) *Communicating Health: Strategies for Health Promotion.* London: Sage publications.

Thaker A, Barton A. (2012) *Multicultural Handbook of Food Nutrition and Dietetics.* Oxford: Blackwell Science.

Internet resources

Chinese Health Information Centre, http://chinese-health.org.uk
Chinese National Healthy Living Centre, www.cnhlc.org.uk
Countries and their cultures – United Arab Emirates, www.everyculture.com/To-Z/United-Arab-Emirates.html
Ismaili Nutrition Centre, www.theismaili.org/nutrition
London Beth Din (for kosher food enquiries), www.kosher.org.uk
Muslim Food Board, www.tmfb.net
National Records of Scotland, www.nrscotland.gov.uk
Northern Ireland Statistics and Research Agency, http://www.nisra.gov.uk

Office for National Statistics, www.ons.gov.uk
Seventh-day Adventist Church, www.adventist.org/en/vitality/health
Sikhism Guide, www.sikhismguide.org
South Asian Health, www.nhs.uk/Livewell/SouthAsianhealth/Pages/SouthAsianhealthhub.aspx
South Asian Health Foundation, www.sahf.org.uk
UK census, www.ons.gov.uk/census/2011census/2011ukcensuses

Additional resources

Diabetes UK produces several resources for people with diabetes from minority ethnic groups, and has resources available in different languages (www.diabetes.org.uk).

Local community and religious leaders may be able to help with general information, translation of leaflets and the establishment of contacts with relevant individuals or groups. Local temples and religious establishments or local council offices may be a useful starting point of contact.

Local public health departments may have produced resource material relevant to local minority ethnic groups.

Local voluntary organisations in different areas of the UK run luncheon clubs for local relevant communities.

References

Ahmed NU, Delgado M, Saxena A. (2016) Trends and disparities in the prevalence of physicians counselling on diet and nutrition among the US population, 2000–2011. *Prev. Med.* 89: 70–75.

Aslam HM, Saleem S, German S, *et al.* (2014) Harmful effects of shisha: a literature review. *Int. Arch. Med.* 7: 16.

Attridge M, Creamer J, Ramsden M, *et al.* (2014) Culturally appropriate health education for people in ethnic minority groups with type 2 diabetes mellitus. *Cochrane Database Syst. Rev.* (9): CD006424. doi: 10.1002/14651858.CD006424.pub3

August KJ, Sorkin HD. (2010) Racial/ethnic disparities in exercise and dietary behaviours of middle-aged and older adults. *J. Gen. Intern. Med.* 26(3): 245–250.

Avery AJ, Whitehead KA, Halliday V. (2016) *How to Facilitate Lifestyle Change: Applying Group Education in Healthcare*. Chichester: Wiley Blackwell.

Bécares L. (2013) *Which ethnic groups have the poorest health? Ethnic health inequalities 1991–2011. ESRC Centre on Dynamics of Ethnicity (CoDE)*. Available at http://www.ethnicity.ac.uk/search/?q=poorest+health&site=CoDE&client=CoDE&searchFilter=website. Accessed 27 May 2017.

Bradby H, Humphris R, Newall D, *et al.* (2015) *Public health aspects of migrant health: a review of the evidence on health status for refugees and asylum seekers in the European Region*. Copenhagen: WHO Regional Office for Europe (Health Evidence Network synthesis report 44).

Breland JY, McAndrew M, Gross RL, *et al.* (2013). Challenges to healthy eating for people with diabetes in a low income, minority neighbourhoods. *Diabetes Care.* 36: 2895–2901.

Chanda R, Ghosh S (2013). *The Punjabi Diaspora in the UK: An Overview of Characteristics and Contributions to India (PDF)*. CARIM-India Research Report. Robert Schuman Centre for Advanced Studies, European University Institute, pp. 2–3. Retrieved 22 July 2016.

Chowbey P, Harrop D. (2016) *Healthy eating in UK minority ethnic households: influences and way forward. Discussion Paper*. Race Equality Foundation.

Coakley P. (2011) *Health Needs Assessment of Polish Migrants in Hertfordshire*. Available at https://www.hertfordshire.gov.uk/microsites/jsna/jsna-documents/polish-migrant-jsna-2011.pdf Accessed 11 April 2019.

Deeming C. (2011) Food and nutrition security at risk in later life: evidence from the United Kingdom expenditure and food survey. *J. Soc. Policy.* 40(3): 471–492.

DH. (2010) *Healthy Lives, Healthy People: Our Strategy for Public Health in England*. London: The Stationery Office Limited.

Flying Start NHS. (2017) *Cultural Competence*. Available at https://learn.nes.nhs.scot/735/flying-start-nhs. Accessed February 2019.

Gable J, Herrmann T. (2016) *Counselling Skills for Dietitians*, 3rd edn. Chichester: Wiley Blackwell.

Gilbert PA, Khokhar S. (2008) Changing dietary habits of ethnic groups in Europe and implications for health. *Nutr. Rev.* 66(4): 203–215.

Goff LM, Timbers L, Style H, *et al.* (2014) Dietary intake in Black British adults; an observational assessment of nutritional composition and the role of traditional foods in UK Caribbean and West African diets. *Public Health Nutr.* 18(12): 2191–2201. doi:10.1017/S1368980014002584

Grace C, Begum R, Subhani S, *et al.* (2008) Prevention of type 2 diabetes in British Bangladeshis: qualitative study of community, religious and professional perspectives. *BMJ* 337: a1931. doi:10.1136/bmj.a1931

Health and Care Professions Council. (2016) *Standards of conduct, performance and ethics*. Available at http://www.hcpc-uk.org/aboutregistration/standards/standardsofconductperformanceandethics. Accessed 27 May 2017.

Hickson M, Collinson A, Child J. (2016) *Dietetics: the current context in which we are working and the expected future*. Available at www.bda.uk.com/professional/practice/dietetics_the_current_context_in_which_we_are_working_and_the_expected_future. Accessed 4 March 2017.

Holli BB, Beto JA. (2014). *Nutrition Counseling and Education Skills for Dietetics Professionals*, 6th edn. Baltimore/Philadelphia: Wolters Kluwer/Lippincott Williams and Wilkins.

Horvat L, Horey D, Romios P, *et al.* (2014) Cultural competence education for health professionals. *Cochrane Database Syst. Rev.* (5): CD009405. doi: 10.1002/14651858.CD009405.pub2

Kaur R, Oakley S, Venn P. (2014) Using face-to-face interpreters in healthcare. *Nurs. Times* 110(21): 20–21.

Marmot M. (2010) *Fair society, healthy lives: the Marmot Review: strategic review of health inequalities in England post-2010*. Available at https://www.parliament.uk/documents/fair-society-healthy-lives-full-report.pdf. Accessed date 21 September 2018.

McEwen A, Straus L, Croker H. (2009) Dietary beliefs and behaviour of a UK Somali population. *J. Hum. Nutr. Diet.* 22: 116–121. Doi: 10.1111/j.1365-277X.2008.00939.x

McKenna H. (2016) *Five big issues for health and social care after the Brexit vote*. The Kings Fund, London. Available at www.kingsfund.org.uk/publications/articles/brexit-and-nhs. Accessed 4 March 2017.

Moorley C, Goodfellow B, Corcoran N. (2013) Reaching unreachable groups and crossing cultural barriers. In Corcoran N (ed) *Communicating Health: Strategies for Health Promotion*. London: Sage publications.

National Equality Panel. (2010) An Anatomy of Economic Inequality in the UK. Available at http://eprints.lse.ac.uk/28344/1/CASEreport60.pdf. Accessed 21 September 2018.

NICE PH38. (2012) *Type 2 Diabetes: Prevention in People at High Risk*. Available at https://www.nice.org.uk/guidance/ph38. Accessed 9 June 2017.

NICE PH46. (2013) *BMI: Preventing Ill Health and Premature Death in Black, Asian and Other Minority Ethnic Groups*. Available at https://www.nice.org.uk/guidance/ph46. Accessed 9 June 2017.

NICE CG43. (2015) *Obesity Prevention*. Available at https://www.nice.org.uk/guidance/cg43. Accessed 9 June 2017.

Office of National Statistics (ONS). (2012a) *2011 Census Analysis: Immigration Patterns of Non-UK Born Populations in England and Wales in 2011*. Available at https://www.ons.gov.uk/peoplepopulationandcommunity/populationandmigration/internationalmigration/articles/immigrationpatternsofnonukbornpopulationsinenglandandwalesin2011/2013-12-17. Accessed 27 May 2017.

Office of National Statistics (ONS). (2012b) *Ethnicity and National Identity in England and Wales: 2011*. Available at https://www.ons.gov.uk/peoplepopulationandcommunity/culturalidentity/ethnicity/articles/ethnicityandnationalidentityinenglandandwales/2012-12-11. Accessed 27 May 2017.

Office of National Statistics (ONS). (2013) *2011 Census: Key Statistics and Quick Statistics for Local Authorities in the United Kingdom: Defining characteristics of the UK population on the topics of population, ethnic group and country of birth, health and housing and accommodation*. Available at https://www.ons.gov.uk/peoplepopulationandcommunity/populationandmigration/populationestimates/bulletins/keystatisticsandquickstatisticsforlocalauthoritiesintheunitedkingdom/2013-10-11. Accessed 27 May 2017.

Office for National Statistics (ONS). (2016) Population of the UK by Country of Birth and Nationality: 2015. Available at https://www.ons.gov.uk/peoplepopulationandcommunity/populationandmigration/internationalmigration/bulletins/ukpopulationbycountryofbirthandnationality/august2016. Accessed 27 May 2017.

Patel M, Phillips-Caesar E, Boutin-Foster C. (2012, Oct) Barriers to lifestyle behavioral change in migrant South Asian populations. *J. Immigr. Minor. Health*. 14(5): 774–785.

Public Health England (PHE). (2014) *Assessing new patients from overseas: migrant health guide*. Available at https://www.gov.uk/guidance/assessing-new-patients-from-overseas-migrant-health-guide#checklist-for-new-migrant-patients. Accessed 21 September 2018.

Rowlingson K. (2012) *Wealth Inequality: Key facts – University of Birmingham*. Available at https://www.birmingham.ac.uk/Documents/research/SocialSciences/Key-Facts-Background-Paper-BPCIV.pdf. Accessed 21 September 2018.

Sarwar T, Hamid F. (2004) *Global Nutrition: A Multicultural Resource Pack for Developing Multicultural Dietary Competencies*. London: Brent and Westminster Primary Care Trust.

Temple NJ, Steyn N. (2016) *Community Nutrition for Developing Countries*. Canada: AU Press.

Thaker A, Barton A. (2012) *Multicultural Handbook of Food. Nutrition and Dietetics*. Oxford: Blackwell Science.

3.6 Vegetarianism and vegan diets

Sandra Hood

Key points

- Well-balanced vegetarian and vegan diets are appropriate for all ages and can offer health benefits over non-vegetarian diets.
- A vegetarian and vegan eating pattern is associated with a lower risk of death from ischaemic heart disease and has the potential to be used as a treatment for chronic diseases such as type 2 diabetes, metabolic syndrome, obesity and cardiovascular disease.
- Vegetarians consume widely divergent diets; concerns remain over the possibility of low intakes of vitamin B_{12}, vitamin D, calcium, iodine and n-3 fatty acids in poorly planned diets.

The Vegetarian Society (UK) defines a vegetarian as '*someone who lives on a diet of grains, pulses, legumes, nuts, seeds, vegetables, fruits, fungi, algae, yeast and/or some other non-animal-based foods (e.g. salt) with, or without, dairy products, honey and/or eggs. A vegetarian does not eat foods that consist of, or have been produced with the aid of products consisting of, or created from, any part of the body of a living or dead animal. This includes meat, poultry, fish, shellfish, insects, by-products of slaughter or any food made with processing aids created from these*' (www.vegsoc.org). The Vegan Society (UK) defines veganism as '*a philosophy and way of living which seeks to exclude – as far as is possible and practicable – all forms of exploitation of, and cruelty to, animals for food, clothing or any other purpose … In dietary terms it denotes the practice of dispensing with all products derived wholly or partly from animals*' (www.vegansociety.com). A number of other categories are shown in Table 3.6.1.

Individual consumers may have their own definitions and understandings, which can vary depending on their country of origin, culture, views on animal welfare and other factors. In 2016 (Ispos MORI), there were 1.68 million vegetarians aged 15 years and over in the UK, 3.25% of the population in this age group, including 542,000 vegans (Vegan Society, 2018). This is higher than in the National Diet and Nutrition Survey (NDNS) 2008/9 (Bates, Lennox and Swan (2010). This increase was attributed to ethical concerns and to people choosing a plant-based diet for health reasons and environmental issues. In Europe, around 2–5% of the population is vegetarian; in the USA, 2% of teenagers are vegetarians, with 0.5% of them being vegan (Van Winckel *et al.*, 2011).

Alternatives to foods unacceptable for vegetarians and vegans

There are many alternatives to animal products (Tables 3.6.2 and 3.6.3) that are generally found in supermarkets, with the more unusual items available from health food shops or online shopping.

The labelling of foods as suitable for vegetarians or suitable for vegans has increased and is generally making it easier to identify acceptable products. Problems still exist, e.g. whether eggs used in vegetarian products are free range. It is now mandatory to list allergens in foods including crustaceans, eggs, fish, milk and molluscs (DEFRA & FSA, 2015) (see Chapter 4.5, Food law and labelling).

Reasons for following a vegetarian or vegan diet

Religion

Some religions advocate avoiding animal products, either partially or fully. Vegetarianism is particularly linked with Jainism, where it is mandatory for everyone, and it is not uncommon in other religions, e.g. Hinduism and Buddhism (see Chapter 3.5, Working with minority ethnic groups).

Parental and peer influence

In 1997/1998, one in 10 girls aged 15–18 years reported that they were vegan or vegetarian (Gregory *et al.*, 2000). Support for vegetarian practices from mothers and classmates have been shown to be high, although many adolescents reported finding it difficult to avoid eating

Manual of Dietetic Practice, Sixth Edition. Edited by Joan Gandy.

Companion website: www.manualofdieteticpractice.com

Table 3.6.1 Definitions of vegetarian and vegan diets

	Meat and meat products	Fish, seafood and products	Milk and milk products (including cheese and yoghurt)	Eggs and egg products	Other unacceptable food items	Comments
Vegetarian (Vegetarian Society, UK)	×	×	√ Cheese needs to be animal rennet free	Free-range eggs only		Sometimes referred to as 'lacto-ovo-vegetarian'
Vegan (Vegan Society, UK)	×	×	×	×	Honey, beeswax, some alcohol; all products tested on animals	Many products can have hidden animal ingredients
Lacto-vegetarian	×	×	√ Animal rennet–free cheese	×		
Ovo-vegetarian	×	×	×	Free-range eggs only		
Piscatarian	×	√	√ Cheese needs to be animal rennet free	√		

Table 3.6.2 Alternative foods for vegetarians[1,2,3]

Unacceptable foods	Possible vegetarian alternatives
Meat, fish and poultry, and products including pies, sausages	Nuts, seeds, free-range eggs, dairy products, beans, peas, lentils and peanuts. Quorn[5], soya beans and its products, e.g.[4] tofu, textured vegetable protein (TVP) Cereal-based foods, e.g. bread, pasta, noodles, couscous, quinoa, rice, bulgur wheat, barley, buckwheat, spelt, millet
Meat and fish stocks, soups, gravies	Vegetable stock, yeast extracts, vegetarian gravy mix
Animal fats and fish oils	Trex, Pure, 100% vegetable oils and margarines, vegetarian suet
Fish oils, foods that are n-3 enriched by fish oils	Trex, Pure, Vitalite, 100% vegetable oils and margarines, vegetable suet. Plant sources of n-3 oils, e.g. hempseed, rapeseed and flax/linseed oils; walnuts; and chia seeds
Gelatine[6] and products, including aspic, jelly, marshmallows, jelly-type sweets, gelatine-thickened yoghurts	Agar, carrageenan, pectin and other plant gums. Vegetarian jelly sweets, jellies and yoghurts
Animal-based flavourings, e.g. some brands of Worcester sauce	Yeast extracts, soya sauce, miso, herbs and spices, vegetarian Worcester sauce
Cheese made with animal rennet,[7] including Parmesan, Grana Padano, Gorgonzola	Vegetarian cheese
Animal sources of E numbers: E120 – cochineal/carmine (from crushed insects) E452 – edible bone phosphate (from animal bones) E904 – shellac (derived from lac beetles) Some E numbers may be derived from either plant or animal sources. The Vegetarian Society (UK) provides an online, up-to-date factsheet. E numbers unsuitable for a vegan diet include: E901 – beeswax E913 – lanolin (a wax excreted from sheep skin and extracted from the wool) E1105 – lysozyme (from chicken eggs)	For further information on the origins of E numbers, see www.food-info.net
Eggs from caged hens and products, e.g. quiche	Free-range eggs and products. Egg replacers, e.g. VeganEgg, Ener-G
Alcoholic drinks that have been clarified (fined) using animal-derived products, e.g. chitin[8], gelatine, isinglass[9]. This includes the majority of real ales; bottled naturally conditioned beers; some ciders; and some fortified and unfortified wines	Majority of keg beers and lagers, canned beers Ciders that have been produced without gelatine Majority of organic wines and those produced using non-animal alternatives Majority of spirits and liqueurs. Vegetarian alcoholic drinks

[1] Read labels and ingredients of manufactured products carefully.
[2] Care must be taken in storage and preparation to ensure that the ingredients do not come into contact with animal products.
[3] Vegetarian foods should not be cooked in oils that have been used for frying animal products.
[4] The term 'soya' is used throughout the chapter. *Note*: 'soy' is used in the USA.
[5] Quorn contains free-range egg and is not suitable for vegans.
[6] Gelatine is derived from collagen obtained from animal bones.
[7] Rennet is sourced from the abomasum (fourth stomach) of newly born calves.
[8] Chitin comes from the shells of crustaceans, e.g. crabs, lobsters and shrimps.
[9] Isinglass is extracted from fish swim bladders.

Table 3.6.3 Alternative foods for vegans[1,2,3]

Unacceptable foods	Possible vegan alternatives
Meat, fish and poultry, and products including pies, sausages	Nuts, seeds, beans, peas, lentils and peanuts, and their butters. Soya beans and its products, e.g. textured vegetable protein, tofu Vegan meat substitutes, e.g. vegan sausages, vegan bacon rashers, mock duck Cereal-based foods, e.g. bread, pasta, plain noodles, couscous, quinoa, rice, bulgur wheat, barley, buckwheat, spelt, millet
Eggs and cheese, and products containing them, e.g. some Quorn foods, mayonnaise, quiche, cakes, egg noodles, pesto	Tofu, vegan cheese, vegan mayonnaise, vegan cakes, vegan biscuits, rice noodles, vegan pesto
Meat and fish stocks, soups, gravies	Vegetable stock, yeast extracts, miso
Animal fats and products, e.g. chocolate	Vegan chocolate, carob, 100% vegetable oils, e.g. soya, sunflower, rapeseed, olive, vegetable suet
Fish oils, foods that are n-3 enriched by fish oils	n-3 plant oils, e.g. hempseed, rapeseed and flax/linseed oils, walnuts and chia seeds
Margarines that contain milk products and/or vitamin D_3, ghee	Pure dairy-free spreads, e.g. Vitalite, Pure, Flora Freedom
Gelatine and products, including aspic, jelly, marshmallows, jelly-type sweets, gelatine-thickened yoghurts	Agar-agar, Gelozone, carrageen, pectin, vegan sweets and yoghurts
Animal-based flavourings, e.g. Worcester sauce	Yeast extracts, soya sauce, herbs and spices, vegan Worcester sauce, miso
Animal milks, cheese, yoghurt, cream, ice cream and their products, or products containing whey powder, casein or lactose, e.g. some crisps	Soya-, nut- and cereal-based milks (vitamin- and mineral-fortified products recommended) Soya cheese and alternatives made from nuts and seeds. Nutritional yeast flakes for cheese sauces and adding to savoury dishes Soya yoghurt, desserts, ice cream and other plant alternatives. Non-dairy creams, e.g. soya, nut and rice
E numbers from unacceptable sources	Foods without unacceptable sources of E numbers. See www.food-info.net for useful information about origins of E numbers
Honey, cereal bars containing honey, some breakfast cereals that contain honey/milk/vitamin D_3	Maple syrup, agave nectar, sugar, jams. Vegan cereal bars, pure breakfast cereals not enriched with vitamin D_3 and honey
Alcoholic drinks that have been clarified using animal-derived products, e.g. chitin, gelatine, isinglass. This includes the majority of real ales; bottled, naturally conditioned beers; some ciders; some fortified and unfortified wines	Majority of keg beers and lagers, canned beers, ciders that have been produced without animal-derived products. Majority of organic wines and those produced using non-animal alternatives Majority of spirits and liqueurs

[1] Read labels and ingredients of manufactured products carefully.
[2] Care must be taken in the storage and preparation to ensure that the ingredients do not come into contact with animal products.
[3] Vegan foods should not be cooked in oils that have been used for frying animal products.

meat at home (Trew *et al.*, 2006). There are associations between vegetarianism and anorexia nervosa (Aloufy & Latzer, 2006). However, while being vegetarian does not cause disordered eating, it may camouflage an existing eating disorder.

Animal welfare

Issues concerning animal welfare that may lead to the adoption of a vegetarian or vegan diet include:

- Animal conditions, e.g. restricted space or movement.
- Use of antibiotics and growth promoters to maintain and increase production.
- Intensive breeding and culling programmes.
- Production and killing of animals solely for food (Compassion in World Farming, 2016).

Environmental issues

The resources required for animal food production have a higher environmental impact than those for growing food from plant sources (FAO, 2013). With world food security being an issue, this inefficient use of land may be viewed as unsustainable. In addition, the increased water needs for the production of food from animal sources (as opposed to from plant sources) is also causing concern. The impact on the environment encompasses the following issues:

- Quantity of greenhouse gases produced by animals.
- Damage to ecosystems, the environment and other animals.
- Water contamination.
- Higher carbon footprint.

Health reasons

Vegetarians appear to be more health conscious than non-vegetarians (Bedford & Barr, 2005), and a vegetarian eating pattern is associated with a lower risk of death from ischaemic heart disease (Craig, 2009; Key *et al.*, 2006). Vegetarian diets may be of better quality than omnivore diets, with characteristics typical of a vegan diet (high fruit and vegetable intake, low sodium intake and low intake of saturated fat) having the highest nutritional quality (Clarys *et al.*, 2014). Vegetarians as compared to non-vegetarians have lower:

- Low-density lipoproteins (LDL) cholesterol (Ferdowsian & Barnard, 2009).
- Blood pressure.
- Rates of hypertension.
- Rates of type 2 diabetes (Tonstad *et al.*, 2009; Zaman *et al.*, 2010).
- Risk of metabolic syndrome (Rizzo *et al.*, 2011).
- BMI (Sabate & Wien, 2010; Tonstad *et al.*, 2009).
- Overall cancer rates and risk (Lanou & Svenson, 2010a).

These findings are supported by the Oxford component of the European Prospective Investigation in Cancer and Nutrition (EPIC-Oxford), which included approximately 65,000 participants, of whom 31,000 were non-meat-eaters (Appleby *et al.*, 2002; Davey *et al.*, 2002; Key *et al.*, 2009; Spencer *et al.*, 2003). Bone fracture risk among vegans, vegetarians, meat eaters and fish eaters was similar, i.e. at least 525 mg/day calcium was consumed, (Appleby *et al.*, 2007); normal bone mass has been reported for vegetarians (New, 2004). However, it is acknowledged that there are many factors that may impact on bone health, including other dietary components and lifestyle factors.

Features of a vegetarian diet that may reduce the risk of chronic diseases include lower intakes of saturated fat, and a higher consumption of fruit, vegetables, whole grains, nuts, soya products, fibre, some vitamins and minerals, and phytochemicals (Clarys *et al.*, 2014; Craig, 2010; Craig *et al.*, 2009). The overall antioxidant status is similar between vegetarians and omnivores, but vegetarians have a 15% higher level of plasma carotenoids (Halder *et al.*, 2007). However, it should be noted that vegetarians consume widely divergent diets, and only a well-balanced diet offers potential health benefits (Fraser and Shavlik (2001).

Other lifestyle practices, including physical activity levels, smoking and drinking habits, may also have an impact on the health benefits. Alewaeterers *et al.* (2005) reported that vegetarians smoked less, drank less alcohol and were engaged in more intensive physical activity as compared to a reference population. Dyett *et al.* (2013) also reported that normal BMI, healthy food and lifestyle practices were common among most vegans. In the EPIC-Oxford study, however, such differences in lifestyle factors accounted for <5% of the difference in mean age-adjusted BMI between meat eaters and vegans, whereas differences in macronutrient intake accounted for approximately half of the difference (Spencer *et al.*, 2003).

There have been suggestions that the term vegetarian is not specific and requires fuller clarification, especially in research. People who describe themselves as vegetarian actually occasionally eat meat (Rothgerber, 2014), and Robinson-O'Brien *et al.* (2009) found that approximately one-quarter of those who classified themselves as vegetarians ate chicken. Inconsistencies in definitions may have led to anomalies in findings between studies, such as the differences in the rates of colorectal cancer between vegetarians and other populations (Key *et al.*, 2009; Sanjoaquin *et al.*, 2004) and, as a result, findings might need to be interpreted cautiously (Fraser, 2009).

Compared with other vegetarian diets, vegan diets tend to contain less saturated fat and cholesterol and more dietary fibre, but there is an increased risk of nutritional deficiencies (Craig *et al.*, 2009; Key *et al.*, 2006). Therefore, concern remains over intakes of vitamin B_{12}, vitamin D, calcium and n-3 fatty acids (Pawlak *et al.*, 2014; Tucker, 2014).

Nutritional adequacy of a vegetarian or vegan diet

Protein

Vegetarians and vegans in the UK, Europe and North America consume adequate energy as derived from protein, albeit at lower levels than omnivores (Clarys *et al.*, 2014; Craig *et al.*, 2009). The source of protein is important as this dictates its digestibility. Soya protein can meet needs as effectively as animal protein, whereas, e.g. wheat protein eaten alone may result in reduced efficiency of nitrogen utilisation. Protein requirements may therefore vary depending on food selection. Kniskern and Johnston (2011) have suggested that the dietary reference intake should be increased to 1.0 g/kg (from 0.8 g/kg) when consuming <50% of protein from animal sources. While it was once thought that combinations of plant foods had to be eaten at the same meal to ensure a sufficient intake of amino acids, it is now known that, if energy intake is adequate, and a mixture of plant proteins are eaten over the course of the day, the requirements for essential amino acids will be met (Young & Pellett, 1994).

Fatty acids

The consumption of alpha-linolenic acid (ALA), an n-3 fatty acid obtained from plants, is relatively low in vegetarian and vegan diets as compared to the consumption of n-6 polyunsaturated fatty acids, mainly linoleic acid, from seed oils (Kornsteiner *et al.*, 2008; Sanders, 2009). This results in an unbalanced n-6 to n-3 ratio in vegetarians and vegans, which may inhibit endogenous production of eicosapentaenoic acid (EPA) and docosahexaenoic acid (DHA). Little, if any, EPA and DHA are obtained from a vegetarian or vegan diet (as they are mainly obtained from fish sources, although some spreading fats, soups and sauces have been found to be major sources in vegetarians) (Sanders, 2009; Welch *et al.*, 2010). Studies have shown that tissue levels of n-3 fatty acids are depressed in vegetarians and particularly in vegans, irrespective of the duration of the diet (Kornsteiner *et al.*, 2008; Rosell *et al.*, 2005).

This problem is compounded by an inefficient conversion of ALA by the body to the more active longer-chain metabolites (<5–10% for EPA and 2–5% for DHA) (Davis & Kris-Etherton, 2003). Total n-3 requirements may therefore be higher for vegetarians and vegans than for fish and meat eaters, as they must rely on the conversion of ALA to EPA and DHA (EFSA, 2010). However, Welch *et al.* (2010) found that, although non-fish-eating meat eaters and vegetarians have much lower intakes of EPA and DHA than fish eaters, their n-3 status is higher than would be expected, which suggests a greater conversion of ALA to circulating long-chain n-3 fatty acids in non-fish-eating groups. As yet, there is no documented evidence of adverse effects on health arising from the lower DHA intake in vegetarians.

Nevertheless, optimising intakes of n-3 fatty acids is recommended; the American Dietetic Association (Craig *et al.*, 2009) recommends that '*vegetarians should include good sources of ALA in their diets like flaxseed, walnuts, canola* [rapeseed] *oil and soya. Those with increased requirements of n-3 fatty acids, such as pregnant and lactating women, may benefit from DHA-rich microalgae*'. Other sources of ALA include hemp and chia seeds.

Iron

Vegetarian diets contain mainly non-haem sources of iron, which is less efficiently absorbed than haem iron of animal origin. Vegetarian and vegan diets have generally higher intakes of inhibitors of iron absorption such as phytate, but evidence suggests that the overall effect of enhancers and inhibitors on iron absorption is considerably less than predicted, and does not substantially influence iron status (Scientific Advisory Committee on Nutrition, (SACN) 2010). Soya contains iron mostly in the form of ferritin, which is easily absorbed, despite the presence of phytate; therefore, iron absorption may be higher than previously thought (Lonnerdal *et al.*, 2006). Vegetarians often consume large quantities of non-haem sources of iron such as cereals, legumes, nuts, seeds and fortified foods, and food rich in vitamin C counteract the inhibitory effect that phytates have on the absorption of iron (Gibson *et al.*, 2014; Saunders *et al.*, 2013). SACN (2010) reviewed a number of studies and found that dietary iron intakes of vegetarians are on average similar, or sometimes higher, than those of non-vegetarians although usually within the reference ranges (Haddad *et al.*, 1999).

Zinc

In the EPIC-Oxford study (Davey *et al.*, 2003), vegetarians had lower intakes of zinc than meat eaters (7.67 mg/day versus 9.16 mg/day for women and 8.44 mg/day versus 9.78 mg/day in men), with vegans consuming even lower intakes (7.22 mg/day and 7.99 mg/day for men and women, respectively). Cade *et al.* (2004) confirmed this, a finding consistent with studies in other countries (Tupe & Chiplonkar, 2010).

The effect of phytates and folic acid on zinc bioavailability also causes concern with regards to vegetarian and vegan diets (Craig, 2009; Foster & Samman, 2015; Gibson, 1994; Hunt, 2003). Suitable zinc-rich foods for vegetarians and vegans include legumes, nuts, seeds and soya products; sprouting can increase zinc bioavailability. No evidence has been found for any impact or adverse health effects of lower intakes and biochemical stores on functional immunity (Haddad *et al.*, 1999; Hunt, 2003). Further studies are needed to determine whether physiological adaptations in zinc absorption exist (Foster *et al.*, 2015).

Iodine

The iodine content of most plant foods is variable because it depends on the iodine content of the soil. Foods grown closer to the ocean tend to be higher in iodine. The major animal sources of iodine are dairy products and fish. In the UK, iodine in milk is increased by the use of iodine-fortified cattle feed concentrates. A number of studies have looked at the iodine content of vegetarian and vegan diets, and have found that there is a high potential for deficiency, especially in vegan diets (Leung *et al.*, 2011; Lightowler & Davies, 1998; Sobiecki *et al.*, 2016; Waldmann *et al.*, 2003). However, too much iodine can cause either hypothyroidism or hyperthyroidism. Where iodine-containing foods are consumed, mean iodine intakes can be greatly in excess of the RNI, e.g. if some types of seaweeds are eaten (Lightowler & Davies, 1998). Sea vegetables such as kelp, nori, dulse and alaria can vary in iodine content, and therefore are not reliable sources. The guidance is for vegans not to use seaweed or kelp as an iodine source and to consider a supplement. The adult recommended dietary allowance (RDA) is 150 μg per day, and using a supplement providing 75–100 μg three to four times per week should be adequate but not excessive (Norris & Messina, 2011).

Selenium

Concerns have been raised about the selenium status of non-meat-eaters, as the consumption of red meat is a major determinant of serum selenium (Letsiou *et al.*, 2010). Selenium status in vegetarians (De Bortoli & Cozzolino, 2009; Gibson, 1994) has been found to be adequate. There is, however, insufficient evidence currently to assess the usefulness of biomarkers of selenium status, and whether or not vegetarians and vegans may be selenium deficient could depend on the biomarker chosen (Hoeflich *et al.*, 2010). Cereals, nuts (especially Brazil nuts; three a day will provide approximately 25 μg, around 50% of an adult's RDA) and seeds are all suitable sources of selenium, but the actual content will vary depending on the soil in which they are grown.

Calcium

Calcium intakes of vegetarians are similar to those of meat eaters in both men and women (Cade *et al.*, 2004; Davey *et al.*, 2003). Intakes of calcium by vegans are much lower, with a mean intake of 610 mg/day in men and 582 mg/day in women (Davey *et al.*, 2003), and may fall below the recommended intakes. However, vegan diets are not associated with increased fracture risks if calcium intake meets the UK estimated average requirement of 525 mg/day (Appleby *et al.*, 2007). Calcium-enriched milk alternatives and tofu are excellent sources of bioavailable calcium for vegans alongside kale, okra, pak choi, wholegrain and white bread (fortified with calcium), sesame seeds, tahini, almonds, oranges and dried figs. Some green vegetables such as spinach and Swiss chard are high in calcium, although the calcium is bound to oxalate, and is therefore poorly absorbed. However, the bioavailability of calcium from low-oxalate vegetables such as kale, broccoli, cauliflower and turnip greens can be as high as 50% (Weaver & Plawecki, 1994).

SECTION 3

Vitamin D

The only significant natural sources of vitamin D are fatty fish, eggs from chickens fed vitamin D and mushrooms treated with ultraviolet rays. Vegan sources include fortified foods such as margarine, some breakfast cereals and milk alternatives. Therefore, if exposure to sunlight is limited, there is a potential for all population groups to be at risk of deficiency (SACN, 2016). There are conflicting results with regard to vitamin D status from different populations. No significant difference in serum 25-hydroxyvitamin D status were shown by Chan *et al.* (2009), but the EPIC-Oxford study found that serum 25-hydroxyvitamin D was lower in vegetarians and vegans than in meat eaters (Crowe *et al.*, 2011b). Public health advice is that all people should consider taking a daily supplement containing 10 μg of vitamin D in autumn and winter. Most vitamin D_3 (cholecalciferol) is obtained from foods of animal origin, with the exception of lichen-derived sources, which are suitable for vegans. Vitamin D_2 (ergocalciferol) is obtained from yeast.

Vitamin B_{12} (cobalamin)

Vitamin B_{12} is produced by microorganisms, and is found in substantial amounts only in foods from animals. There are issues with diagnosing vitamin B_{12} deficiency, but low circulating concentrations and low intakes have been recorded in many studies of vegetarians and vegan diets (Pawlak *et al.*, 2014; Sobiecki *et al.*, 2016). Megaloblastic anaemia, a symptom of vitamin B_{12} deficiency, can be masked by high intakes of folic acid, with symptoms only detected at a neurological stage. In the EPIC-Oxford cohort study, folate concentrations were highest among vegans, intermediate among vegetarians and lowest among omnivores (Sobiecki *et al.*, 2016). Vegetarians can obtain vitamin B_{12} from dairy foods or eggs, but the only reliable source for vegans is fortified foods, such as some breakfast cereals, yeast extracts, some plant milks and some soya products. All vegans need to consume fortified foods or take a vitamin B_{12} supplement. It should be noted that there has been confusion between true vitamin B_{12} and inactive analogues. Foods such as fermented soya products, sea vegetables and tofu have all been credited as being a good source of vitamin B_{12}, but they contain inactive analogues.

Vegetarian or vegan diets as treatment for chronic diseases

Weight management

Vegetarians tend to have a lower BMI than non-vegetarians (Appleby *et al.*, 1998; Sabate & Wien, 2010). Vegans tend to have the lowest BMI (Davey *et al.*, 2003; Tonstad *et al.*, 2009), and weight gain over time is lower in vegan and vegetarian diets (Japas *et al.*, 2014; Rosell *et al.*, 2006). The adoption of a nutritionally adequate vegetarian diet has been put forward as a possible approach to treating obesity and weight management (Farmer *et al.*, 2011; Mishra *et al.*, 2013). However, in a randomised clinical trial, Burke *et al.* (2007) found that both vegetarian and non-vegetarian study groups had significant reductions in total energy and fat intakes with reduced weight. Similarly, in the Indian Migration Study (Agrawal *et al.*, 2014), there was no difference in BMI between vegetarians and non-vegetarians. Therefore, while vegetarian and vegan diets are generally effective ways of achieving and maintaining a healthy body weight for many people, focus continues to remain on energy restriction.

Metabolic syndrome and type 2 diabetes

Studies have shown that the prevalence of metabolic syndrome (MetS) and type 2 diabetes is lower in vegetarians than in the general population (Kahleova & Pelikanova, 2015), and that a vegetarian or vegan dietary pattern is an appropriate form of treatment for MetS and type 2 diabetes (Marsh & Brand-Miller, 2011; Sabate & Wein, 2015). From the studies that have demonstrated a significantly lower risk of MetS in vegetarians (Rizzo *et al.*, 2011; Turner McGrievy & Harris, 2014), it is believed that the findings are mainly due to the accompanying weight loss. There were also reduced intakes of saturated fats and high-glycaemic-index foods, and increased intakes of dietary fibre and vegetable protein. Kahleova and Pelikanova (2015) recommended that '*larger clinical trials are needed to confirm the effectiveness and promote the inclusion of vegetarian diets in dietary guidelines for prevention and treatment of type 2 diabetes*'.

Evidence from studies has shown that, rather than the macronutrient composition, the overall quality of the diet is more important in the prevention and management of type 2 diabetes (Ley *et al.*, 2014). With vegetarian and vegan diets being generally high in whole grains, fruits, vegetables, beans and pulses, nuts and seeds, and low in saturated fats and processed foods, they are more consistent with nutritional recommendations for the prevention of type 2 diabetes than omnivorous diets.

Cardiovascular disease

Owing to lower LDL cholesterol concentration in vegetarians and vegans, together with lower BMI and slightly lower systolic blood pressure (Appleby & Key, 2015), it has been suggested that vegetarian and vegan diets could be effective tools in the management of cardiovascular disease (Lanou & Svenson, 2010b). Studies have demonstrated that the lower plasma total cholesterol in vegetarians is primarily due to the reduced LDL cholesterol and a reduction in HDL concentration (Bradbury *et al.*, 2014; Kuchta *et al.*, 2016). This lower total cholesterol concentration is likely to be due to the reduction in saturated fat intake. A meta-analysis and systematic review (Huang *et al.*, 2011) found significantly lower ischemic heart disease mortality in vegetarians as compared to non-vegetarians.

A review by Ferdowsian and Barnard (2009) concluded that plant-based dietary interventions, often in the form of portfolio diets, are effective in lowering plasma cholesterol concentrations to a greater extent than a diet that replaces saturated fat with carbohydrates in the diet. In conjunction with increased exercise, stress management and group support, a vegetarian diet consumed for 1 year was shown to meet key heart health characteristics and reduce risk markers (Marshall *et al.*, 2009).

Other diseases and conditions

Analyses of the risks for several other diseases and conditions have been reported in EPIC-Oxford (Appleby & Key, 2015). The risk of diverticular disease of the colon was 31% lower in vegetarians and 72% lower in vegans as compared to meat eaters, with a strong inverse relationship between dietary fibre intake and diverticular disease (Crowe *et al.*, 2011a). Data from the EPIC-Oxford study also showed that vegetarians and vegans were at lower risk of eye cataract as compared to meat eaters (Appleby *et al.*, 2011). Vegetarians were also found to have a 31% lower risk of kidney stones as compared to those consuming a high-meat diet (Turner *et al.*, 2014).

Dietary considerations for different population groups

Pregnancy and lactation

Well-planned vegetarian and vegan diets are safe for maintaining the health of both mother and child during pregnancy and lactation, but vegan mothers do need to take extra care to ensure an adequate intake of energy and nutrients (British Nutrition Foundation, 2013). Nutrients requiring particular attention include vitamin B_{12}, protein, n-3 fatty acids, iodine (Andersson *et al.*, 2007) and calcium. Supplementation with vitamin D is necessary (as in all pregnancies), as is a reliable source of vitamin B_{12}. Plasma and red blood cell folate concentrations tend to be higher in pregnant vegetarians (probably due to long-term, high-vegetable intakes) than in omnivores. This can reduce the risk of folate deficiency if an adequate vitamin B_{12} supply is ensured (Koebnick *et al.*, 2001); however, folic acid supplements are recommended.

Pregnant vegetarian (and vegan) women are at greater risk of vitamin B_{12} deficiency (Pawlak *et al.*, 2014), and, although it is rare, there have been cases of severe vitamin B_{12} deficiency with neurological damage in the infant as a result (Erdeve *et al.*, 2009; Kocaoglu *et al.*, 2014). An adequate maternal dietary supply of vitamin B_{12} or a daily supplement is essential.

Reference intakes for iron during pregnancy are the same as those for non-pregnant women in the UK (Department of Health, 1991). Iron deficiency anaemia is not uncommon during pregnancy, whether the expectant mother is vegetarian or not.

Vegan diets are generally devoid of pre-formed DHA, and vegetarian diets that include dairy foods and eggs only provide approximately 20 mg/day (Sanders, 2009). Pregnant and lactating vegetarian and vegan women may benefit from DHA-rich supplements. However, there is no strong evidence of adverse effects on health from the lower DHA intake in vegans and vegetarians (Sanders, 2009).

The American Dietetic Association (2009) recommended that pregnant and lactating vegetarians pay attention to the nutritional adequacy of their diets, particularly with regards to vitamin B_{12} and zinc, and be mindful about intakes of iron and folate. Supplements normally advised for pregnant women (400 μg folic acid in the first trimester and 10 μg vitamin D) also apply to vegetarians and vegans. There is currently little evidence as to the adequacy of a vegan diet on birth outcomes in pregnant vegans and few recent studies looking at the long-term effects of a vegan diet on pregnancy.

There is currently no vegan soya formula milk available in the UK. By law, infant formula is fortified with vitamin D, and, at present, this nutrient is obtained from lanolin, which is derived from sheep wool.

Childhood and adolescence

There is sufficient evidence to conclude that the needs of growing children and adolescents can be met by vegetarian and vegan diets that are well balanced and supplemented appropriately (Amit, 2010). A review by Sabate and Wien (2010) of the anthropometry of vegetarian youngsters found conflicting data on the height of vegetarian children, with one study finding that vegetarian children were taller than their omnivorous classmates (Sabate *et al.*, 1991), while another showed that they were shorter (Sabate *et al.*, 1990). One study of predominately vegetarian adolescents showed that they had a significantly lower BMI, waist circumference, total cholesterol to high density lipoprotein (HDL) cholesterol ratio, and LDL cholesterol concentration than their omnivorous classmates (Grant *et al.*, 2008).

There is evidence, however, of inadequate intakes of vitamin D and calcium in vegetarian children aged 2–10 years as compared to omnivores, with subsequent lower levels of biochemical bone turnover markers (Ambroszkiewicz *et al.*, 2007). In a small study, vitamin B_{12} intake was found to be lower in vegetarian preschool children compared with omnivores, although serum vitamin B_{12} concentrations were not affected (Yen *et al.*, 2010). Vitamin A, C and D supplementation is recommended by the UK Department of Health for all children from 6 months to 5 years of age taking less than 500 mL of infant formula, and some are suitable for vegetarians and vegans.

SACN (2010) reported that, in young people aged 4–18 years, there was no association between a vegetarian diet and lower-than-average iron intakes, but that girls aged 15–18 years (whether vegetarian or not) were generally at risk of iron deficiency anaemia; this is also the case for adolescent vegans (Larsson & Johansson, 2002). They also found that the adolescents had dietary intakes below the average requirements for riboflavin, vitamin B_{12}, vitamin D, calcium and selenium.

The Canadian Paediatric Society has issued a position statement on vegetarian diets in children and adolescents (Amit, 2010), and concluded that '*a well-balanced vegetarian diet can provide for the needs of children and adolescents*'. It did, however, raise concerns in the following areas:

- Restrictive vegan diets may cause energy deficits (due to low energy density and bulk), which present challenges in feeding smaller children. The inclusion of soya products, nuts (age appropriate) and nut butters can be useful.
- Due to the lower digestibility of plant proteins, some studies have suggested that protein intake may need to be increased for vegans (an increase of 30–35% for infants up to 2 years of age, 20–30% for 2–6-year-olds, 15–20% for those aged >6 years). Protein sources from different food groups (nuts, seeds, cereals, legumes) need to be encouraged.
- Due to the lower bioavailability of iron and increased needs for iron in children, especially during rapid growth periods, it is prudent to ensure that good sources such as fortified cereals are included and supplementation is considered, particularly in times of higher needs.
- Zinc requirements in vegans may be higher than in omnivores, owing to differences in bioavailability, but additional supplementation is not recommended.
- Iodine supplements may be required.
- Calcium intakes below recommendations have been noted in vegan children, and it is hence essential to ensure an adequate intake of calcium-rich and calcium-fortified foods. Supplementation may be required.
- Adequate sources of alpha-linolenic acid (the precursor of EPA and DHA) are required, and supplements may need to be included in the diets of vegetarian and vegan children.
- Supplementation of vitamin B_{12} or a good intake of fortified foods (at least three servings of vitamin B_{12}-rich foods per day) is essential for vegan children. Infants of vegan mothers are particularly at risk from vitamin B_{12} deficiency.

Public Health England recommends that, in the autumn and winter, a vitamin D supplement should be considered for all children over the age of 5 years, and those who do not get out in the sun, or who always cover their skin, should take a vitamin D supplement throughout the year. The American Dietetic Association (ADA) (Craig *et al.*, 2009) supports these points. Guidelines are available for children being weaned onto a vegetarian diet (Di Genova & Guyda, 2007) that reflect these recommendations. The Vegan Society (UK) (www.vegansociety.com) provides information about the introduction of solid foods for vegan children.

Older adults

In ageing, there is a decreased energy need but increased requirements and/or decreased absorption for some nutrients. This, combined with a smaller appetite and the physical limitations that may increase with age, means that nutrient-dense vegetarian or vegan-acceptable foods should be eaten in line with nutritional requirements (see Chapter 3.3, Older adults). Few studies have looked at the nutritional requirements of elderly vegetarians. Deriemaeker *et al.* (2011) found little difference in dietary intakes, blood parameters and physical characteristics between the institutionalised vegetarian and non-vegetarian elderly. The elderly vegetarians aged well and had good nutrition as compared to elderly omnivores, and the study concluded that '*a vegetarian lifestyle had no negative impact on the health status at older age*'. Vegans and vegetarians who eat limited amounts of dairy products should regularly include a reliable source of vitamin B_{12} in their diet, or consider supplements. An iodine supplement should also be considered along with vitamin D.

Athletes

There is no reason why vegetarian or vegan athletes should perform differently from omnivorous athletes, as long as they are consuming a well-balanced diet; the ADA have concluded that well-planned vegetarian diets are appropriate for athletes (Craig *et al.*, 2009). However, there is no evidence that adopting a vegetarian or vegan diet will improve athletic performance (Fuhrman & Ferreri, 2010). Vegetarian and vegan diets tend to be lower in energy, so thought needs to be given to ensuring an adequate energy intake and meeting protein requirements, but this should not cause any problems unless the diet becomes too bulky. Vegetarian athletes may also be at risk for low intakes of energy, fat, vitamin B_{12}, riboflavin, vitamin D, calcium, iron (particularly in women and during adolescence and pregnancy) and zinc (Rodriguez *et al.*, 2009). There is no current evidence regarding the adequacy of the nutritional intake of vegan athletes (see Chapter 4.3, Sports nutrition).

Acknowledgement

I thank Heather Russell, dietitian at the Vegan Society, and Paul Appleby, statistician and author, for reviewing and commenting on this chapter.

The editor acknowledges the prior contribution of Elaine Gardner.

Internet resources

British Dietetic Association, www.bda.uk.com/foodfacts/vegetarianfoodfacts.pdf
Vegetarian for Life, https://vegetarianforlife.org.uk
Vegan Society (UK), www.vegansociety.com
Vegetarian Society (UK), www.vegsoc.org

References

Agrawal S, Millett CJ, Dhillo PK, *et al.* (2014) Type of vegetarian diet, obesity and diabetes in adult Indian population. *Nutr. J.* 13: 89.

Alewaeterers K, Clarys P, Hebbelinck M, *et al.* (2005) Cross-sectional analysis of BMI and some lifestyle variables in Flemish vegetarians compared with non-vegetarians. *Ergonomics.* 48(11–14): 1433–1444.

Aloufy A, Latzer Y. (2006) [Diet or health – the linkage between vegetarianism and anorexia nervosa]. *Harefuah.* 145(7): 526–531.

Ambroszkiewicz J, Klemarczyk W, Gajewska J, *et al.* (2007) Serum concentration of biochemical bone turnover markers in vegetarian children. *Adv. Med. Sci.* 52: 279–282.

Amit M. (2010) Vegetarian diets in children and adolescents. *Paediatr. Child. Health.* 15(5): 303–308.

Andersson M, De Benoist B, Delange F, *et al.* (2007) Prevention and control of iodine deficiency in pregnant and lactating women and in children less than 2 years old: conclusions and recommendations of the Technical Consultation. *Public Health Nutr.* 10(12A): 1606–1611.

Appleby PN, Allen NE, Key TJ. (2011) Diet, vegetarianism, and cataract risk. *Am. J. Clin. Nutr.* 93: 1128–35.

Appleby PN, Thorogood M. Mann JI, *et al.* (1998) Low body mass index in non-meat eaters: the possible roles of animal fat, dietary fibre and alcohol. *Int. J. Obes. Relat. Metab. Disord.* 22(5): 454–460.

Appleby PN, Davey GK, Key TJ. (2002) Hypertension and blood pressure among meat eaters, fish-eaters, vegetarians and vegans in EPIC-Oxford. *Public Health Nutr.* 5(5): 645–654.

Appleby P, Roddam A, Allen N, *et al.* (2007) Comparative fracture risk in vegetarians and non-vegetarians in EPIC-Oxford. *Eur. J. Clin. Nutr.* 61(12): 1400–1406.

Appleby PN, Key TJ. (2015) The long-term health of vegetarians and vegans. *Proc. Nutr. Soc.* 75: 287–293.

Bates B, Lennox L, Swann G. (2010) *NDNS: Headline results from year 1 of the rolling programme (2008/2009), Department of Health.* London: TSO.

Bedford JL, Barr SI. (2005) Diets and selected lifestyle practices of self-defined adult vegetarians from a population-based sample suggest they are more 'health conscious'. *Int. J. Behav. Nutr. Phys. Act.* 2(1): 4.

Bradbury KE, Cowe FL, Appleby PN, *et al.* (2014) Serum concentrations of cholesterol, apolipoprotein A-I and apolipoprotein B in a total of 1694 meat-eaters, fish-eaters, vegetarians and vegans. *Eur. J. Clin. Nutr.* 68: 178–183.

British Nutrition Foundation. (2015) *Vegetarian and vegan mums-to-be.* Available at https://www.nutrition.org.uk/healthyliving/nutritionforpregnancy/vegetarian.html. Accessed 22 September 2018.

Burke LE, Hudson AG, Warziski MT, *et al.* (2007) Effects of a vegetarian diet and treatment preference on biochemical and dietary variables in overweight and obese adults: a randomised clinical trial. *Am. J. Clin. Nutr.* 86(3): 588–596.

Cade JE, Burley VJ, Greenwood DC, UK Women's Cohort Study Steering Group. (2004) The UK Women's Cohort Study: comparison of vegetarians, fish-eaters and meat-eaters. *Public Health Nutr.* 7(7): 871–878.

Chan J, Jaceldo-Siegl K, Fraser GE. (2009) Serum 25-hydroxyvitamin D status of vegetarians and non vegetarians: the Adventist Health Study 2. *Am. J. Clin. Nutr.* 89(5): 1686S–1692S.

Clarys P, Deliens T, Huybrechts I, *et al.* (2014, Mar) Comparison of nutritional quality of the vegan, vegetarian, semi-vegetarian, pesco-vegetarian and omnivorous diet. *Nutrients.* 6(3): 1318–1332.

Compassion in World Farming. (2016) *Cheap Food Costs Dear.* Available at www.ciwf.org.uk/research/policy-economics/cheap-food-costs-dear/. Accessed 15 November 2016.

Craig WJ. (2009) Health effects of vegan diets. *Am. J. Clin. Nutr.* 89(5): 1627S–1633S.

Craig WJ. (2010) Nutrition concerns and health effects of vegetarian diets. *Nutr. Clin. Pract.* 25: 613–620.

Craig WJ, Mangels AR. (2009) Position of the American Dietetic Association: vegetarian diets. *J. Am. Diet. Assoc.* 109(7): 1266–1282.

Crowe FL, Appleby PN, Allen NE, *et al.* (2011a) Diet and risk of diverticular disease in Oxford cohort of European Prospective Investigation into Cancer and Nutrition (EPIC): prospective study of British vegetarians and non-vegetarians. *BMJ* 343: d4131.

Crowe FL, Steur M, Allen NE, *et al.* (2011b) Plasma concentrations of 25-hydroxyvitamin D in meat eaters, fish eaters, vegetarians and vegans: results from the EPIC-Oxford Study. *Public Health Nutr.* 14(2): 340–346.

Davey G, Allen N, Appleby P, *et al.* (2002). Dietary and lifestyle characteristics of meat-eaters, fish-eaters, vegetarians and vegans. *IARC Sci. Publ.* 156: 113–114.

Davey GK, Spencer EA, Appleby PN *et al.* (2003) EPIC–Oxford: lifestyle characteristics and nutrient intakes in a cohort of 33 883 meat-eaters and 31 546 non meat-eaters in the UK. *Public Health Nutr.* 6:259–268.

Davis BC, Kris-Etherton PM. (2003) Achieving optimal essential fatty acid status in vegetarians: current knowledge and practical implications. *Am. J. Clin. Nutr.* 78(3 Suppl): 640S–646S.

DEFRA, FSA. (2015) *Producing and distributing food – guidance. Food labelling: giving food information to consumers* (27 April 2015). Department of Environment, Food & Rural Affairs and Food Standards Agency.

Deriemaeker P, Aerenhouts D, De Ridder D, *et al.* (2011) Health aspects, nutrition and physical characteristics in matched samples of institutionalised vegetarian and nonvegetarian elderly (>65yrs). *Nutr. Metab.* 8(1): 37.

DH. (1991) *Dietary Reference Values.* London: The Stationery Office.

de Bortoli MC, Cozzolino SM. (2009) Zinc and selenium nutritional status in vegetarians. *Biological Trace Element Research* 127(3): 228–233.

Di Genova T, Guyda H. (2007) Infants and children consuming atypical diets: vegetarianism and macrobiotics. *Paediatr. Child Health.* 12(3): 185–188.

Dyett PA, Sabate J, Haddad E, *et al.* (2013, Aug) Vegan lifestyle behaviors: an exploration of congruence with health-related beliefs and assessed health indices. *Appetite.* 67: 119–124.

EFSA (Expert Food Safety Authority). (2010). Scientific opinion on dietary reference values for fats, including saturated fatty acids, polyunsaturated fatty acids, monounsaturated fatty acids, trans fatty acids, and cholesterol. Panel on Dietetic Products, Nutrition, and Allergies (NDA). *EFSA J.* 8(3): 1461. Available at https://efsa.onlinelibrary.wiley.com/doi/epdf/10.2903/j.efsa.2010.1461. Accessed 22 September 2018.

Erdeve O, Arsan S, Atasay B, *et al.* (2009) A breast-fed newborn with megaloblastic anaemia-treated with vitamin B12 supplementation of the mother. *J. Pediatr. Hematol. Oncol.* 31(10): 763–765.

FAO. (2013) Tackling Climate Change through Livestock. A global assessment of emissions and mitigation opportunities. Food and Agriculture Organization of the United Nations.

Farmer B, Larson BT, Fulgoni VL, *et al.* (2011) A vegetarian dietary pattern as a nutrient-dense approach to weight management: an analysis of the National Health and Nutrition Examination Survey 1999–2004. *J. Am. Diet. Assoc.* 111(6): 819–827.

Ferdowsian HR, Barnard ND. (2009) Effects of plant-based diets on plasma lipids. *Am. J. Cardiol.* 104: 947–956.

Foster M, Herulah UN, Prasad A, *et al.* (2015) Zinc status of vegetarians during pregnancy: a systematic review of observational studies and meta-analysis of zinc intake. *Nutrients* 7: 4512–4525.

Foster M, Samman S. (2015) Vegetarian diets across the lifecycle: impact on zinc intake and status. *Adv. Food Nutr. Res.* 74: 93–131.

Fraser GE. (2009) Vegetarian diets: what do we know of their effects on common chronic diseases? *Am. J. Clin. Nutr.* 89(5): 1607S–1612S.

Fraser GE, Shavlik DJ. (2001) Ten years of life: is it a matter of choice? *Arch. Intern. Med.* 161: 1645–1652.

Fuhrman J, Ferreri DM. (2010) Fueling the vegetarian (vegan) athlete. *Curr. Sports Med. Rep.* 9(4): 233–241.

Gibson RS. (1994) Content and bioavailability of trace elements in vegetarian diets. *Am. J. Clin. Nutr.* 59(5 Suppl): 1223S–1232S.

Gibson RS, Heath AL, Szymiek-Gay EA. (2014) Is iron and zinc nutrition a concern for vegetarian infants and young children in industrialized countries? *Am. J. Clin. Nutr.* 100(1 Suppl): 459S–468S.

Grant R, Bilgin A, Zeuschner C, *et al.* (2008) The relative impact of a vegetable-rich diet on key markers of health in a cohort of Australian adolescents. *Asia Pac. J. Clin. Nutr.* 17: 107–115.

Gregory J, Lowe S, Bates CJ, et al. (2000) *National Diet and Nutrition Survey: Young People Aged 4 to 18 Years. Volume 1: Report of the Diet and Nutrition Survey*. London: TSO.

Haddad EH, Berk LS, Kettering JD, Hubbarb RW, Peters WR. (1999) Dietary intake and biochemical, hematologic and immune status of vegans compared with non vegetarians. *Am. J. Clin. Nutr.* 70 (Suppl): 586S–593S.

Halder S, Rowland IR, Barnett YA, *et al.* (2007) Influence of habitual diet on antioxidant status: a study in a population of vegetarians and omnivores. *Eur. J. Clin. Nutr.* 61(8): 1011–1022.

Hoeflich J, Hollenbach B, Behrends T, *et al.* (2010) The choice of biomarkers determines the selenium status in young German vegans and vegetarians. *Br. J. Nutr.* 104(11): 1601–1604.

Huang CJ, Fan YC, Liu JF, *et al.* (2011) Characteristics and nutrient intake of Taiwanese elderly vegetarians: evidence from a national survey. *Br. J. Nutr.* 106(13): 451–460.

Hunt JR. (2003) Bioavailability of iron, zinc and other trace minerals from vegetarian diets. *Am. J. Clin. Nutr.* 78: 633S–639S.

Japas C, Knutsen S, Dehom S, *et al.* (2014) Body mass index gain between ages 20 and 40 years and lifestyle characteristics of men at ages 40–60 years: the Adventist Health Study 2. *Obes. Res. Clin. Pract.* 8: e549–e557.

Kahleova H, Pelikanova T. (2015) Vegetarian diets in the prevention and treatment of type 2 diabetes. *J. Am. Coll. Nutr.* 34: 448–458.

Key TJ, Appleby PN, Rosell MS. (2006) Health effects of vegetarian and vegan diets. *Proc. Nutr. Soc.* 65(1): 35–41.

Key TJ, Appleby PN, Spencer EA, *et al.* (2009) Cancer incidence in vegetarians: results from the European Prospective Investigation into Cancer and nutrition (EPIC-Oxford). *Am. J. Clin. Nutr.* 89(5): 1620S–1626S.

Kniskern MA, Johnston CS. (2011) Protein dietary reference intakes may be inadequate for vegetarians if low amounts of animal protein are consumed. *Nutrition.* 27(6): 727–730.

Kocaoglu C, Akin F, Caksen H, *et al.* (2014) Cerebral atrophy in a vitamin B_{12}-deficient infant of a vegetarian mother. *J. Health Popul. Nutr.* 32(2): 367–371.

Koebnick C, Heins UA, Hoffmann I, *et al.* (2001) Folate status during pregnancy in women is improved by long-term high vegetable intake compared with the average Western diet. *J. Nutr.* 131(3): 733–739.

Kornsteiner M, Singer I, Elmadfa I. (2008) Very low n-3 long-chain polyunsaturated fatty acid status in Austrian vegetarians and vegans. *Ann. Nutr. Metab.* 52(1): 37–47.

Kuchta A, Ebiedzinska AL, Fijalkowski M, et al. (2016) Impact of plant-based diet on lipid risk factors for atherosclerosis. *Cardiol. J.* 23: 141–148.

Lanou AJ, Svenson B. (2010a) Reduced cancer risk in vegetarians: an analysis of recent reports. *Cancer Manag. Res.* 20: 1–8.

Lanou AJ, Svenson B. (2010b) Vegetarian dietary patterns as a means to achieve reduction in cardiovascular disease and diabetes risk factors. *Curr. Cardiovasc. Risk Rep.* 4: 48–56.

Larsson CL, Johansson GK. (2002) Dietary intake and nutritional status of young vegans and omnivores in Sweden. *Am. J. Clin. Nutr.* 76(1): 100–106.

Letsiou S, Nomikos T, Panagiotakos D, *et al.* (2010) Dietary habits of Greek adults and serum total selenium concentration: the ATTICA study. *Eur. J. Nutr.* 49(8): 465–472.

Leung AM, Lamar A, He X, *et al.* (2011) Iodine status and thyroid function of Boston-area vegetarians and vegans. *J. Clin. Endocrinol. Metab.* 96(8): E1303–1307.

Ley SH, Handy O, Mohan V, *et al.* (2014) Prevention and management of type 2 diabetes: dietary components and nutritional strategies. *Lancet.* 383: 1999–2007

Lightowler HJ, Davies GJ. (1998) Iodine intake and iodine deficiency in vegans as assessed by the duplicate-portion technique and urinary iodine excretion. *Br. J. Nutr.* 80(6): 529–535.

Lonnerdal B, Bryant A, Liu X, *et al.* (2006) Iron absorption from soybean ferritin in nonanemic women. *Am J. Clin. Nutr.* 83(1): 103–107.

Marsh K, Brand-Miller J. (2011) Vegetarian diets and diabetes. *Am. J. Lifestyle Med.* 5: 135–143.

Marshall DA, Walizer EM, Vernalis MN. (2009) Achievement of heart health characteristics through participation in an intensive lifestyle change program (Coronary Artery Reversal Study). *J. Cardiopulm. Rehabil. Prev.* 29(2): 84–94.

Mishra S, Xu J, Agarwal U, *et al.* (2013) A multicenter randomized controlled trial of a plant-based nutrition program to reduce body weight and cardiovascular risk in the corporate setting: the GEICO study. *Eur. J. Clin. Nutr.* 67: 718–724.

New SA. (2004) Do vegetarians have a normal bone mass? *Osteoporos. Int.* 15(9): 679–688.

Norris J, Messina V. (2011) *Vegan for Life*. Boston: Da Capo Press.

Pawlak R, Lester SE, Babatunde T. (2014) The prevalence of cobalamin deficiency among vegetarians assessed by serum vitamin B_{12}: a review of literature. *Eur. J. Clin. Nutr.* 68: 541–548.

Rizzo NS, Sabate J, Jaceldo-Siegl K, *et al.* (2011) Vegetarian dietary patterns are associated with lower risk of metabolic syndrome: the Adventist Health Study 2. *Diabetes Care.* 34: 1225–1227.

Robinson-O'Brien R, Perry CL, Wall MM, *et al.* (2009) Adolescent and young adult vegetarianism: better dietary intake and weight outcomes but increased risk of disordered eating behaviors. *J. Am. Diet. Assoc.* 109(4): 648–655.

Rodriguez NR, DiMarco NM, Langley S.(2009) Position of the American Dietetic Association, Dietitians of Canada, and the American College of Sports Medicine: Nutrition and athletic performance. *J. Am. Diet. Assoc.* 109:509–527.

Rosell MS, Lloyd-Wright Z, Appleby PN, *et al.* (2005) Long-chain n-3 polyunsaturated fatty acids in plasma in British meat-eating, vegetarian and vegan men. *Am. J. Clin. Nutr.* 82(2): 327–334.

Rosell M, Appleby P, Spencer E, *et al.* (2006) Weight gain over 5 years in 21966 meat-eating, fish-eating, vegetarian, and vegan men and women in EPIC-Oxford. *Int. J. Obes. (Lond.)* 30(9): 1389–1396.

Rothgerber H. (2014) A comparison of attitudes toward meat and animals among strict and semi-vegetarians. *Appetite.* 72: 98–105.

Sabate J, Wien M. (2010) Vegetarian diets and childhood obesity prevention. *Am. J. Clin. Nutr.* 91(5): 1525S–1529S.

Sabate J, Linsted KD, Harris RD, *et al.* (1990) Anthropometric parameters of schoolchildren with different life-styles. *Am. J. Dis. Child.* 144: 1159–1163.

Sabate J, Linsted KD, Harris RD, *et al.* (1991) Attained height of lacto-ovo-vegetarian children and adolescents. *Eur. J. Clin. Nutr.* 45: 51–58.

Sabate J, Wein M. (2015) A perspective on vegetarian dietary patterns and risk of metabolic syndrome. *Br. J. Nutr.* 113(S2): S136–S143.

SACN. (2010) *Scientific Advisory Committee on Nutrition: Iron and Health*. London: The Stationery Office.

SACN. (2016) *Scientific Advisory Committee on Nutrition: Vitamin D and Health*. London. The Stationery Office.

Sanders TA. (2009) DHA status of vegetarians. *Prostaglandins Leukot. Essent. Fatty Acids.* 81(2–3): 137–141.

Sanjoaquin MA, Appleby PN, Thorogood M, *et al.* (2004) Nutrition, lifestyle and colorectal cancer incidence: a prospective investigation of 10998 vegetarians and non-vegetarians in the United Kingdom. *Br. J. Cancer* 90: 118–121.

Saunders AV, Craig W, Baimes SK et al. (2013) Iron and vegetarian diets. *Med J Australia* 199(S4):S11–16.

Sobiecki JG, Appleby PN, Bradbury KE, *et al.* (2016) High compliance with dietary recommendations in a cohort of meat eaters, fish eaters, vegetarians, and vegans: results from the European Prospective Investigation into Cancer and Nutrition-Oxford study. *Nutr. Res.* 36(5): 464–477.

Spencer EA, Appleby PN, Davey GK, *et al.* (2003) Diet and body mass index in 38000 EPIC-Oxford meat-eaters, fish-eaters, vegetarians and vegans. *Int. J. Obst. Relat. Metab. Disord.* 27(6): 728–734.

Tonstad S, Butler T, Yan R, *et al.* (2009) Type of vegetarian diet, body weight and prevalence of type 2 diabetes. *Diabetes Care* 32(5): 791–796.

Trew K, Clark C, McCartney G, *et al.* (2006) Adolescents, food choice and vegetarianism. In: Shepherd R, Raats M (eds) *The Psychology of Food Choice*. Wallingford: Cabi Org./Nutrition Society, pp. 247–262.

Tucker KL. (2014) Vegetarian diets and bone status. *Am. J. Clin. Nutr.* 100: 329S–335S.

Tupe R, Chiplonkar SA. (2010) Diet patterns of lactovegetarian adolescent girls: need for devising recipes with high zinc bioavailability. *Nutrition* 26(4): 390–398.

Turner-McGrievy G, Harris M. (2014) Key elements of plant-based diets associated with reduced risk of metabolic syndrome. *Curr. Diab. Rep.* 14(9): 524.

Turner BW, Appleby PN, Reynard JM, *et al.* (2014) Diet and risk of kidney stones in the Oxford cohort of the European Prospective Investigation into Cancer and Nutrition (EPIC). *Eur. J. Epidemiol.* 29: 363–369.

Van Winckel M, Vande Velde S, De Bruyne R, *et al.* (2011) Clinical practice: vegetarian infant and child nutrition. *Eur. J. Pediatr.* 170: 1489–1494.

Vegan Society. (2018) *Find out how many vegans there are in Great Britain*. Available at https://www.vegansociety.com/whats-new/news/find-out-how-many-vegans-are-great-britain. Accessed 16 March 2018.

Waldmann A, Koschizke JW, Leitzmann C, *et al.* (2003) Dietary intakes and lifestyle factors of a vegan population in Germany: results from the German Vegan Study. *Eur. J. Clin. Nutr.* 57: 947–955.

Weaver CM, Plawecki KL. (1994) Dietary calcium, adequacy of a vegetarian diet. *Am. J. Clin. Nutr.* 59(5): 1238S–1241S.

Welch AA, Shakya-Shrestha S, Lentjes MA, *et al.* (2010) Dietary intake and status of n-3 polyunsaturated fatty acids in a population of fish-eating and non-fish-eating meat-eaters, vegetarians, and vegans and the product–precursor ratio [corrected] of alpha-linolenic acid to long-chain polyunsaturated fatty acids: results from the EPIC-Norfolk cohort. *Am. J. Clin. Nutr.* 92(5): 1040–1051.

Yen CE, Yen CH, Cheng CH, *et al.* (2010) Vitamin B-12 status is not associated with plasma homocysteine in parents and their preschool children: lacto-ovo, lacto, and ovo vegetarians and omnivores. *J. Am. Coll. Nutr.* 29(1): 7–13.

Young VR, Pellett PL. (1994) Plant proteins in relation to human protein and amino acid nutrition. *Am. J. Clin. Nutr.* 59(5): 1203S–1212S.

Zaman GS, Zaman FA, Arifullah M. (2010) Comparative risk of type 2 diabetes mellitus among vegetarians and non-vegetarians. *Indian J. Community Med.* 35(3): 441–442.

3.7 People with learning disabilities

Siân O'Shea, Marjory Macleod and Anne Laverty

Key points

- People with learning disabilities (LDs) are nutritionally vulnerable; their needs should be assessed on an individual basis.
- Dietary guidance for clients should be clear and concise, with no more than three key messages or dietary goals at a time.
- Issues of client consent and involvement in the decision-making process must be considered.
- Multidisciplinary and multiagency collaborative working is essential to ensure consistent messages and continuity of care.
- Guidelines for the nutritional management of specific LDs, e.g. Down syndrome and Prader–Willi syndrome (PWS), should be used.

Note: The guidance in this chapter is not applicable to people who have a higher-level autistic spectrum disorder (ASD) such as Asperger's or other specific learning difficulties (SpLD), e.g. attention-deficit disorder (ADD), attention-deficit hyperactive disorder (ADHD), dyslexia, dyscalculia, dyspraxia, and speech and language delay.

Government policy aims to encourage people with learning disabilities (LDs) to access mainstream services (Rutter & Carmichael, 2011). Therefore, healthcare professionals (HCPs), including dietitians, are very likely to encounter people with LDs in general clinics in primary and secondary care. There has also been a major move away from institutionalised care, so that people with LDs are enabled to live within the community, supported by a variety of healthcare and/or social care services as dictated by individual needs.

The health of people with LDs has steadily improved over the last 30 years; however, they still experience a higher burden of ill health and die younger than the general population (Royal College of Nursing, 2013). A significant number of people with LDs living in supported accommodation do not receive a healthy balanced diet (Emerson & Baines, 2011) and have restricted food choices (Koritsas & Iacano, 2016). The training of carers is vitally important to enable these vulnerable people to receive support and nutritional advice applicable to their individual needs. Even though people with LDs have a right to access healthcare services, they are less likely to get some of the evidence-based treatments and checks they need, and more likely to face barriers when accessing services (Black, 2013). Routine health screening for breast cancer, cervical cancer, bowel cancer, men's health screening, etc. are offered to people with LDs, but uptake rates are generally low. To address this issue, people with LDs registered with general practitioners (GPs) are entitled to an annual health check, following which a health action plan will be put in place. As a result of this annual health check, common problems such as obesity, type 2 diabetes and hyperlipidaemia have been highlighted (Robertson *et al.*, 2010).

The range of health needs also includes mental illness, epilepsy, an array of physical and sensory limitations (including impaired sense of touch, temperature, pain, taste and smell), dental disease, heart disease, binge eating disorder, dysphagia, undernutrition, metabolic syndrome and bone disease (Emerson & Baines, 2011; Franssen *et al.*, 2011; Gravestock, 2001; Hsieh *et al.*, 2014; Room *et al.*, 2016).

People with LDs must be enabled, as much as possible, to make informed decisions, and steps must be taken to ensure that this client group has access to both mainstream and specialist services as and when required (Burton *et al.*, 2011). The traditional model of care has changed from the medical to a social model, and staff roles and training now focus on social inclusion, choice, independence and rights (Department of Health (DH), 2010).

Definition of learning disabilities

There is no universally accepted definition for LDs; however, there is general agreement that the term includes a group of lifelong conditions that, as a result of factors occurring prior to birth, at birth, during childhood or up to the age of brain maturity, affect intellectual development (WHO, 2010). The following definition of learning disabilities includes all the requisite dimensions, and is useful for practitioners (WHO, 1992):

Manual of Dietetic Practice, Sixth Edition. Edited by Joan Gandy.

Companion website: www.manualofdieteticpractice.com

- A significant intellectual impairment with an intellectual quotient (IQ) of >2 standard deviations below the general population, i.e. <70 on a recognised IQ test.
- Deficits in social functioning or adaptive behaviour that significantly impact on how well a person's coping skills allow for everyday social demands that present within his or her environment.
- Formal psychological assessments may include the Vineland Adaptive Behaviour Scales and the AAMR Adaptive Behaviour Scales.
- Present before 18 years of age, and are lifelong.

There will be local variations of this definition, and it must be remembered that the use of IQ alone is not sufficient to define this population (Health Inspectorate Wales, 2007).

All children and adults with profound and multiple LDs (PMLDs) need high levels of support with most aspects of daily life. They are among the most marginalised people in society, have some of the highest support needs and are the most reliant on services (Pawlyn & Carnaby, 2009). People with PMLDs:

- Have more than one disability.
- Have a profound LD.
- Have great difficulty communicating.
- May have additional sensory or physical disabilities, complex health needs or mental health difficulties.
- May have behaviours that are challenging.

Whether living at home, with parents, in supported or assisted accommodation, or in residential settings, appropriate support should be available from specialist teams that help clients live an ordinary life within their local communities. The division of what is considered core or specialist is not (or indeed should not be) clear cut, and robust working relationships between teams are essential for the provision of a seamless service for this client group; the dietitian is pivotal to service provision.

People with LDs are more nutritionally vulnerable than the general population for a number of reasons, including the following:

- People with LD have restricted income or poverty.
- People with LD cope with inappropriate or poor living conditions.
- There is poor or limited availability of nutritional food in disadvantaged areas.
- People with LD face difficulties with travel and transport.
- People with LD suffer social isolation.
- People with LD suffer social exclusion.
- Healthcare staff has limited training on LDs.
- People with LD and their carers have limited nutritional knowledge.
- People with LD and their carers have limited budgeting or cooking skills.
- People with LD have reduced abilities to understand and apply health messages, and read or understand food labels.
- People with LD have reduced ability or opportunity to make informed choices.
- People with LD are dependent on others for eating and drinking.

Physiological anomalies, polypharmacy, diagnostic overshadowing, multiple diagnoses and dysphagia are also common in this client group (DH, 2007). Additionally, people with PMLDs are totally dependent on a range of carers, many of whom do not have the knowledge or skills to enable them to provide a well-balanced diet for their clients (Melville *et al.*, 2009). Figure 3.7.1 shows the factors to consider when assessing the needs of LD clients; these will also impact on the given intervention.

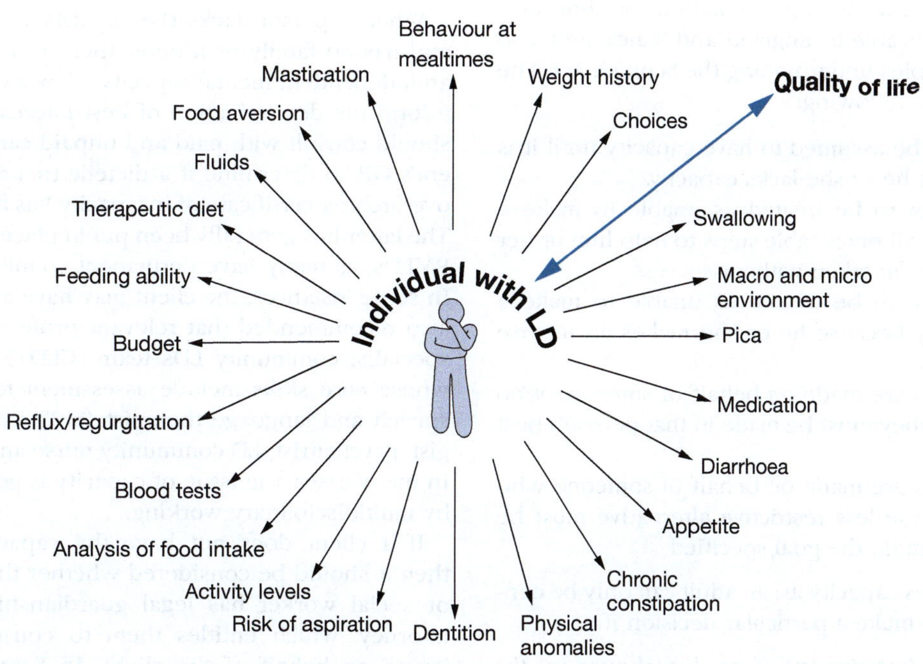

Figure 3.7.1 Factors to consider when assessing nutritional requirements for people with LDs (source: Burton *et al.* (2014), Figure 3.7.1, p. 142. Reproduced with permission from John Wiley & Sons)

Capacity to consent

Consent must always be obtained before dietary interventions. When dealing with the general population, consent is customarily obtained verbally; however, for clients with cognitive impairment, the issue of capacity to consent needs to be explored fully. In determining capacity to consent, it is essential to involve both clients and carers in the assessment and treatment process, and to communicate openly.

Assessments can be carried out without considering whether clients have the ability to give consent to treatment, but their capacity must be determined if treatment is to be given. Determining capacity to consent must always be time and decision specific. A person should not be viewed as unable to make a decision unless all practicable steps to help them do this have been taken without success. This includes employing alternative forms of communication such as symbolised information or signing. Legislation exists to provide a legal framework for decision-making on behalf of adults who lack the capacity to make specific decisions. It also enables adults with the capacity to plan ahead in case of future incapacity. Legislation differs slightly between countries; the relevant legislation for the UK is:

- *Scotland* – The Adults with Incapacity Act (Scottish Parliament, 2000b).
- *England and Wales* – The Mental Capacity Act (MCA) (DH, 2005).
- *Northern Ireland* – Seeking Consent (DHSSPS, 2003).

Relevant excerpts from the legislation are included here as it is core to the care for people with LDs. The Short Reference Guide for Psychologists and Psychiatrists (British Psychological Society, 2007) is recommended as a brief guide to its implementation for clinicians. This guide is applicable to England and Wales, and also reflects the principles underpinning the Scottish Act. The guide includes the following:

- A person must be assumed to have capacity until it is established that he or she lacks capacity.
- A person is not to be treated as unable to make a decision unless all practicable steps to help him or her to do so have been taken without success.
- A person is not to be treated as unable to make a decision merely because he or she makes an unwise decision.
- When decisions are made on behalf of someone who lacks capacity, they must be made in that person's best interests.
- When decisions are made on behalf of someone who lacks capacity, the less restrictive alternative must be considered to attain the goal specified.

The MCA defines capacity as: an adult can only be considered unable to make a particular decision if:

- They have '*an impairment of, or disturbance in, the functioning of the mind or brain*', whether permanent or temporary.

and

- They are unable to undertake any (one or more) of the following steps:
  - Understand the information relevant to the decision.
  - Retain that information (despite use of prompts).
  - Use or weigh that information as part of the process of making the decision.
  - Communicate the decision made (whether by talking, sign language or other means)'.

A functional approach must be taken, so that someone's ability to make a decision is determined by assessing whether he or she can undertake the steps listed in the preceding text. It is not determined by their diagnosis or by the apparent wisdom of their decision. Decision-making capacity is decision and time specific.

The functional approach (best interests)

In considering what is in someone's best interests when making a decision, the person should consider all relevant information, and the following should be taken into account:

- Whether and/or when the person is likely to regain capacity and whether the decision or the act to be undertaken can wait.
- How to encourage and optimise the participation of the person in the decision.
- Past and present wishes, feelings, beliefs and values of the person and any other relevant factors.
- Views of other relevant health, family, carer and social representatives. The decision should be perceived to be in the best interest of the client and not that of the family or carers.

When a person lacks the capacity to make decisions and has no family or friends, there is a duty to appoint an independent mental capacity advocate (IMCA) to help inform the determination of best interests. The dietitian should consult with paid and unpaid carers, and the client's GP, to determine if a dietetic treatment–specific or overarching certificate of incapacity has been completed. The latter has generally been put in place for people with PMLDs, as many have permanent cognitive impairment. In some instances, the client may have an advocate. It is also recommended that relevant professionals from the specialist community LDs team (CLDT) be approached whose core skills include assessment for capacity, e.g. speech and language therapist (SLT), clinical psychologist, psychiatrist, LD community nurse and care manager. In many cases, the issue of capacity is generally decided by multidisciplinary working.

If a client does not have the capacity to consent, then it should be considered whether the carer, relative or social worker has legal guardianship or power of attorney, which entitles them to consent on specific issues on behalf of the client. In Scotland, a welfare guardian may be appointed, who may be granted full or partial powers under the act (Scottish Parliament,

2000a). If there is no welfare guardian, the GP, in consultation with the team, may complete an Adults with Incapacity form, which enables treatments to take place. In emergency situations, the doctor can act without consultation of the team. In Northern Ireland, those close to the incapacitated individual should be involved in the decision-making process (DHSSPS, 2003). In instances where there is no legal guardian, the decision should be reached by consultating all health, family, carer and social representatives. Convening of a multidisciplinary or multiagency meeting is good practice to allow all to participate in decision-making; this must be documented, as well as any decisions made. The key documents for carers on the issue of consent are:

- *Scotland* – Caring and consent: information for carers (NHS Scotland, 2009).
- *England and Wales* – Making Decisions Series of guides for families, friends, carers and professionals (Office of the Public Guardian, 2009).
- *Northern Ireland* – Seeking Consent: Working with people with learning disabilities (DHSSPS, 2003).

Role of advocacy

An advocate enables clients to get their views across, and may be a friend, family member or independently appointed representative following a referral to an advocacy group, service or statute. Anyone can advocate on behalf of an individual, but emotional involvement with the client may make impartiality impossible. The advocate should contribute to the decision-making process on the client's behalf. Where conflict occurs, it should be remembered that the advocate's views, while listened to, have no legal status in relation to consent. In some cases, the advocate's views may conflict with those of others who are involved in the decision-making process. As the client's representative, the advocate should be included in client-specific multidisciplinary or agency meetings to discuss what is perceived to be in the client's best interests.

In England and Wales, statutory IMCAs undergo formal training as stipulated by legislation (DH, 2005) to enable them to assist with decision-making in the best interests of clients who cannot make decisions by themselves or who have no family or friends. In Scotland, a Mental Health Officer may be involved in this decision-making process. In Northern Ireland, the family and carers involved with a client meet with the relevant healthcare and social care professionals to act in the client's best interests.

Ethical issues

It is essential that any concerns raised about the ethical approach of managing a nutritional intervention in any adult with an LD be discussed fully at a multidisciplinary/multiagency meeting. Where appropriate, this should include key family members and an advocate to ensure that all are working in a consistent manner to meet the best interests of the client at all times. All discussions and decisions must be fully documented.

Specific health needs of people with learning disabilities

Clinical syndromes associated with LDs include Down syndrome and Prader–Willi syndrome (PWS).

Down syndrome

Down syndrome, also known as trisomy 21, is the most widely recognised chromosomal disorder and the most common genetic cause of LD. The incidence is approximately 1 in 600–1000 live births, with increasing prevalence rates due to increased life expectancy as the result of advancing medical knowledge and improving care. In addition, later pregnancies are increasingly common, and the incidence of Down syndrome rises with increasing maternal age. There are significant differences between racial and social groups (Shin *et al.*, 2009).

Approximately 12% of neonates with Down syndrome display congenital gastrointestinal anomalies (e.g. Hirschsprung's disease) which require immediate surgical intervention to facilitate nutrition. Congenital heart disease occurs in approximately 40% and may cause faltering growth. Following surgical repair of heart defects, these children's nutritional status will improve. Hypotonia (poor muscle tone), together with a small oral cavity, enlarged tongue and poor suck reflex, can lead to initial feeding difficulties and delayed weaning (see Chapter 3.8.21, Cardiology).

Thyroid dysfunction is more common in people with LDs, with the incidence increasing with age. Hypothyroidism is most frequently reported, but hyperthyroidism can also occur. Thyroid function should be checked at least once every 2 years (Levy *et al.*, 2006), although in many cases this will now be included in the annual health check. Obesity is common, but not inevitable, especially among the female population (Melville *et al.*, 2005). Growth retardation, short stature, hypotonia and a low resting metabolic rate (RMR) may all contribute to the problem. Other factors include poor eating behaviour, excessive energy intake and low exercise levels. Individuals should therefore be encouraged to follow healthy eating guidelines and participate in regular physical activity. People with Down syndrome have an increased incidence of developing type 1 and type 2 diabetes and coeliac disease (Cohen, 2006). Diarrhoea, constipation, abdominal bloating, dyspepsia, mouth ulceration, mood change, arthritis, general fatigue and mild anaemia are common in Down syndrome.

Nutritional management

People with Down syndrome need the same range of nutrients as the general population. Energy intake estimates based on age groups are not appropriate in Down syndrome and need to be tailored to height, weight and physical activity (Murray & Ryan-Krause, 2010). Growth charts have been developed specifically for Down syndrome; standard charts are inappropriate due to developmental delay (Down's Syndrome Medical Interest Group, 2000).

Individuals have been found to be at greater risk of reduced bone mineral density as they age, possibly as a consequence of small stature and sedentary lifestyle (Center *et al.*, 1998). Therefore, a healthy, balanced diet rich in calcium, regular weight-bearing activity, a safe level of sunshine exposure as well as 10 μg vitamin D supplement all year round are recommended.

Dental anomalies include changes in tooth structure, reduced number of teeth and delayed or abnormal eruption; in addition, physical abnormalities of the facial appearance and oral cavity can impact on feeding. Dental disease is common because teeth are more at risk of wear through bruxism (teeth grinding) and decay due to enamel fragility. In addition, gingivitis and oral infections due to mouth breathing can lead to tooth loss and looseness (Hennequin *et al.*, 1999). A healthy, balanced diet that avoids snacks and fizzy drinks can help preserve teeth.

Problems relating to premature ageing with Alzheimer-like changes in the brain have become more apparent as people with Down syndrome are living longer. Between the ages of 40 and 50 years, some individuals display a rapid deterioration in cognitive function. Possible explanations for this include being linked to the extra-genetic material on chromosome 21. Low levels of vitamin E have been found to be associated with dementia in individuals with Down syndrome, but more research is required into the possible effects of supplementation. In order to increase antioxidant intake, a diet rich in fruit, vegetables and oily fish is recommended. Features of rapid ageing in Down syndrome include weight loss, reduction in appetite and problems with chewing and swallowing (Lazenby, 2008). If Alzheimer-like symptoms develop, it is important that steps be taken to ensure adequate nutrition and hydration (see Chapter 7.10.3, Dementias). An individual may lose interest in food, forget to eat or may no longer recognise food or feeding utensils. The following points may help maximise food intake:

- Provide assistance with feeding where appropriate, but maintain independence for as long as possible.
- Small, frequent meals and snacks.
- Offer food that the individual is familiar with; items should be appetising and of appropriate consistency.
- Offer dessert later, rather than presenting it with the main course, as many will reject savoury foods in preference for sweet items.
- Avoid use of patterned plates and table cloths as visual distortion can disguise the food and be off-putting due to sensory overload.
- Avoid external distractions and maintain a peaceful, quiet environment at meal times.
- Avoid food that is too hot or too cold.
- To avoid spillage, do not fill cups, beakers or plates to capacity.
- Use food fortification for extra nutrition.

Most people with Down syndrome live in the community, some with parents or carers, but adults often live independently or semi-independently, and many are able to learn about healthy eating and manage their own diet. A dietitian's role is likely to encompass not only individual assessment but also teaching and educating people with Down syndrome, their parents, carers and other professionals.

Prader–Willi Syndrome

Prader–Willi Syndrome (PWS) is a relatively rare genetically determined neurodevelopment spectrum disorder with symptoms varying in severity and occurrence. It is believed to be caused by dysfunction of the hypothalamus, which controls bodily functions including hunger and satiety, temperature and pain regulation, fluid balance, puberty, emotions and fertility (Lindmark *et al.*, 2010; van Mil *et al.*, 2000a; Vogels *et al.*, 2004; Whittington *et al.*, 2001). The perspective of this condition is changing to that of clients perceiving themselves as being starved rather than over-eating *per se*, the latter being a consequence of the body's reaction to starvation (Holland *et al.*, 2003). It occurs in approximately 1 in 15,000 births, affecting males and females with equal frequency, and all races and ethnicities. This genetic abnormality involves the absence of expression of one or more genes on chromosome 15, and definitive diagnosis is now based on genetic testing and clinical diagnostic criteria (Cassidy *et al.*, 2012).

Clients present with mild to severe LD; verbal skills are often better than functional skills. Obsessional characteristics include food-related hoarding, ritualistic behaviour and an insatiable appetite, which drives the client to seek food (and sometimes fluids), which means they never feel full even after a large meal. This leads to severe hyperphagia, which is driven by a physiological abnormality and is highly resistant to motivational change. PWS is recognised as the most common genetic cause of life-threatening obesity, and up to 25% of obese PWS patients have type 2 diabetes (Butler *et al.*, 2002). Physical characteristics in PWS include:

- Short stature.
- Obesity.
- High vomiting threshold, possibly due to poor muscle tone.
- High pain threshold.
- Poor temperature control – erratic behaviour may occur during very cold or very hot weather.
- Decreased motor skills, hypotonia and poor balance.
- Bowel irregularities.
- Dental abnormalities.
- Abnormally thick and sticky saliva, especially in children.

The approach required in PWS is unique and requires close involvement of the multidisciplinary team (MDT). To work effectively with the client, clear boundaries are required, and due to the nature of the syndrome and the inability to self-regulate, external management of the eating disorder is mandatory. The ethics of this situation have been fully explored in an application submitted for guardianship within the Adults with Incapacity Act (Scotland), to ensure protection of the client (Healy, 2005). Long-term structures and routines in relation to food and behaviours are essential for effective management. This can be seen to conflict with the prevailing healthcare and social care ethics, but too much choice in particular situations can be counterproductive and may result in adverse outcomes. Although people with PWS are capable of making decisions about many areas of their lives, the hypothalamic dysfunction means that they rarely have the capacity to make rational decisions about eating. Even if they can make decisions at one point in time, this may not be the case at other times, particularly in the absence of supervision or environmental restrictions. People with PWS can usually cope with a choice of two food or drink items at one time; more will lead to uncertainty and heightened anxiety, hampering not only decision-making but also general behaviour, and is not recommended. People with PWS do not like sudden change or new experiences; therefore, incremental changes should be made to routines to allow adjustment and acceptance to take place. In order to establish and maintain a successful clinical relationship, the practitioner must give the client:

- Clear expectations and messages – leave no room for misinterpretation.
- Consistent routine and structure that must be followed by everyone.
- Specific feedback.
- Positive reinforcement to help establish new behaviours.
- Avoid confrontation, use eye contact and a gentle manner, and, wherever possible, include the client in decision-making.

A number of appetite suppressants have been tried with mixed results. They are rarely effective in the long term, as they are ineffective in addressing the brain signals that drive the person with PWS to seek food (Whitman, 2016). Treatment using growth hormone which improves growth velocity, and increases lean mass and physical function and ability, has resulted in dramatic benefits (Bridges, 2014; Kuppens *et al.*, 2016; NICE, 2010).

Nutritional management

The obesity associated with PWS is the result of a chronic imbalance between energy intake (due to hyperphagia) and reduced energy expenditure (due to decreased physical activity as a result of hypotonia and reduced metabolic rate). Individuals have a high ratio of body fat to fat-free mass (FFM), where body fat can account for up to 50% of body weight (Butler *et al.*, 2007). Where the appropriate height-to-weight ratio is satisfactory, body fat can account for up to 40% (Schoeller *et al.*, 1988). As metabolic rate is related to FFM, these abnormally high levels of fat result in significantly reduced metabolic rate and, hence, energy requirements. Dietitians must structure weight-reducing plans to reflect this.

Predictive formulae for estimating basal metabolic rate (BMR) in the general adult population have been shown to overestimate BMR in some populations (Ramirez-Zea, 2005; O'Riordan *et al.*, 2010), and this is further distorted in adults with PWS. Additionally, the standard approach to calculating requirements by subtracting 400–1000 kcal for a decrease in energy stores will not necessarily be effective in PWS. Energy requirements in adults with PWS are up to 50% less than those of healthy, age-matched people (Butler *et al.*, 2007; Schoeller *et al.*, 1988; van Mil *et al.*, 2000a). A height-based energy prescription for adults with PWS is a practicable guide, as shown in Table 3.7.1. In predicting the energy requirements from BMR equations, the energy expenditure of physical activity should also be considered. The underdevelopment of muscle and any excess weight limits physical activity. One study in children and adolescents reported a mean physical activity level (PAL) of 1.33 (van Mil *et al.*, 2000b). This is significantly lower than that for obese controls and lower than the PAL of 1.4 previously used in calculating estimated average requirements (EAR) for energy in the UK population (DH, 1991).

The recommended energy intake for adults with PWS is around 800–1200 kcal/day, reducing to 800–1000 kcal/day for weight loss (Gourash & Forster, 2009). At these levels of energy, the diet should be planned using low-energy, nutrient-dense foods to ensure optimal vitamin and mineral intake (Lindmark *et al.*, 2010; Miller *et al.*, 2013). As osteoporosis and low bone mineral density are common in PWS, calcium and vitamin D supplementation should be considered (van Mil *et al.*, 2001).

Adherence to dietary regimens may present many challenges. The dietitian should work closely with the MDT, client and carers to overcome obstacles; this may involve the training of all staff in the management strategies that are required to support PWS clients. All involved must adhere strictly to the prescribed diet, agreed structures and routines, which are required for life and cannot be relaxed even when weight is being maintained.

Clear, straightforward language is required, and the judicious use of terminology, e.g. free fluids will be understood literally by the client, and may result in fluid intoxication. If food-seeking/stealing behaviour is an issue, the team should work together to seek resolutions. Sanctions may be appropriate, but at no time should blame be directed towards the client. The need for rules and routines is inherent in this syndrome (Holland *et al.*, 2003), and can be used advantageously for the positive reinforcement of healthy eating behaviours and regular exercise plans.

Clients with PWS have particular difficulties with short-term memory and in processing spoken information, and tend to display rigid thinking. Forward planning for all changes in routine is therefore an essential component to

Table 3.7.1 Height-based energy prescription for PWS clients aged >16 years (Hoffman *et al.*, 1992)

Outcome to be achieved	Energy/cm height
Weight loss	7–8 kcal (29–33 kJ)
Weight maintenance	10–14 kcal (42–59 kJ)

minimise anxiety and the associated challenging behaviour. Recent evidence suggests the additional concern of subclinical dysphagia, which may contribute to respiratory failure in PWS (Gross *et al.*, 2016). The dietitian plays a pivotal role when working with these clients, as they have the knowledge and skills necessary to guide the management of this disorder.

Other syndromes that cause LDs and their nutritional consequences are shown in Table 3.7.2.

Autism

Autism is a spectrum of lifelong neurodevelopmental disorders with onset noted in early childhood (see Chapter 3.8.6, Autism). Autism is described as: '*A group of disorders characterized by qualitative abnormalities in reciprocal social interactions and in patterns of communication, and by a restricted, stereotyped, repetitive repertoire of interests and activities. These qualitative abnormalities are a pervasive feature of the individual's functioning in all situations*' (ICD 10 & DSM-5). The spectrum ranges from those who are high functioning (often referred as Asperger syndrome) to people who are severely disabled, and may fluctuate over time or in response to changes in circumstances. The ICD classification and DSM-5 also encompass pervasive developmental disorders/not otherwise stated. They all fall under the most widely accepted definition of autism spectrum disorder (Autism Speaks, 2016).

Social and communication skills are affected in 44–52% of LD patients. This affects how patients communicate with and relate to other people, and how they experience the world around them. Prevalence is estimated at 1.1% in the UK (Brugha *et al.*, 2012), with boys five times more likely to be affected than girls. In the majority of cases, causation is unknown. Characterifstics include obsessive desire for order, rigid thinking, inflexibility, reliance on routines, ritualistic behaviour, poor social skills, and visual and sensory perception difficulties. Common comorbidities include attention-deficit hyperactivity disorder (ADHD), food compulsions, food restrictions and gastrointestinal problems. A structured environment, clear boundaries, and rules and routines are essential components to minimise stress. Changes that can be made occur slowly and over a lengthy period.

Nutritional management

Many children with ASD show selective eating and therefore self-limiting diets as a direct result of their disorder (National Autistic Society, 2016). This established eating pattern continues into adulthood and may compromise nutritional status, as the individual may be extremely obsessive, selective and restrictive in food choices. Any alterations in the environment or routine may result in behavioural outbursts or food refusal. Gastrointestinal problems may also affect appetite (Levy *et al.*, 2007a). This is a complex condition that often requires a coordinated multidisciplinary team/multiagency approach. The following professionals may be involved in the community team:

- Behavioural therapist.
- Clinical psychologist.
- Community nurse.
- Consultant psychiatrist.
- Dietitian.
- Occupational therapist.
- Physiotherapist.
- Social worker/care manager.
- SLT – communication.
- SLT – dysphagia.

A detailed nutritional assessment by a specialist dietitian should take place for clients who have selective restricted diets in which food intake and food groups are compromised. There is increasing reporting of nutritional vulnerability in this group; however, the evidence is mixed, with inconsistent results (Marí-Bauset *et al.*, 2015, 2016; Ranjan & Nasser, 2015). The dietitian will advise on any nutritional deficiencies, providing the evidence base for any dietary modifications and offering practical advice on treating deficiencies or implementing dietary modifications. The team can help with guidance on any behavioural and educational techniques (e.g. visual supports or social stories) that may be useful. Recently, cases of night blindness have been reported owing to lack of vitamin A, highlighting the importance of early nutritional assessment (Chui & Watson, 2015).

Common feeding concerns include:

- Difficulty with transition to textures (especially during infancy).
- Increased sensory sensitivity (including oral).
- Difficulty accepting new foods.
- Restricted intake due to colour, texture, packaging and food temperature.
- Decreased selection of food over time.
- Difficulty with changes in meal time environment, e.g. school versus home.
- Difficulty with meal time presentation, e.g. specific plate and cutlery, positioning of food on a plate.
- Continually eating rather than having set meal times.

A large number of therapeutic approaches have been used by parents/carers, such as introducing gluten- and/or casein-free diets (Elder *et al.*, 2006; Millward *et al.*, 2008; Wong & Smith, 2006), with a view that they will improve the client's behaviour or gastrointestinal symptoms. NICE (2012) recommended that exclusion diets (such as gluten, or casein and ketogenic diets), as well as vitamins, minerals and dietary supplements (e.g. vitamin B_6 or Iron), not be used for the treatment of core symptoms of autism. The BDA has produced a professional consensus statement on the dietary management of ASD (Isherwood & Thomas, 2011).

Cerebral palsy

Cerebral palsy (CP) is the most common physical disability in children, and it affects 2–2.5 in 1000 births in the UK (Roebroeck & Stam, 2006) and 3.6 in 1000 births in the USA (Yeargin-Allsop *et al.*, 2008). Known possible causes include oxygen starvation, cerebral bleeding and

Table 3.7.2 Nutritional consequences of other clinical syndromes associated with LDs (adapted from Burton *et al.*, 2009)

Syndrome	Symptoms affecting nutritional status	Nutritional consequences	Issues
Cornelia de Lange syndrome Chromosome 5 abnormality, X chromosome and chromosome 10 responsible for milder form	Low birth weight, delayed growth and stature, developmental delay, cleft palate, gaseous distension May exhibit autistic-like behaviours, including self-injury	Intermittent poor appetite, vomiting, constipation GORD Nutrition intake may be variable, as many behaviours are cyclical	MDT approach required May require a set of nutrition care plans, depending on behaviour and ability to eat and drink
Fragile X syndrome Inhibited mental development, moderate to severe LD Autistic-like behaviour with physical and behavioural features and delayed speech	Need very structured environment, obsessive desire for order and familiarity, poor social skills, rigid thinking, inflexible, cannot cope with change, easily distracted from eating, changed visual perceptions	Nutrition intake may be poor, and is dependent on the degree of food-related obsessive behaviour Need a stable macro-environment (competent staff, pleasant, calm surroundings – no TV or music to detract from meal times), and micro-environment (correct seating, utensils, adherence to eating and drinking guidelines, time)	MDT approach required May require a set of nutrition care plans, depending on behaviour and ability to eat and drink
Klinefelter syndrome Affects males with extra X chromosome. Incidence 1 in 1000 males, 1 in 500 have the extra X syndrome without symptoms of the syndrome	Reduced muscle power and stamina *Note*: most will have a specific learning difficulty, although some may have a degree of LD	Prone to depression, thyroid disease, diabetes, osteoporosis, asthma and heart disease	Difficult to feed, get tired easily Carers need to be patient and persevere with feeding
Rett syndrome Neurodevelopmental disorder characterised by microcephaly, developmental delay, scoliosis, loss of purposeful use of hands, hand flapping, poor muscle tone, gastric abnormalities, seizures and a degree of LD Occurs almost exclusively in girls	Problems with the mechanics of eating Breathing issues, e.g. hyperventilation and breath holding Biting, chewing, swallowing and self-feeding are all affected by very poor muscle tone	Babies have a poor suck reflex and difficulty meeting their requirements, leading to faltering growth Breathing irregularities interrupt feeding Nutritional intake is an issue from birth	Hypotonia with poor food intake necessitates texture modification of food and thickened drinks Difficulties in independent eating as a result of poor hand movements – need to be fed Constipation is very common due to a low intake of fibre and difficulty meeting fluid requirements; may have reduced gut motility
Smith–Magenis syndrome Genetic condition characterised by delayed speech, distinctive facial features, sleep disturbances and behavioural problems, especially self-injurious behaviour Individuals tend to be of short stature and may have scoliosis	Dental agenesis and protruding lower jaw can lead to problems with chewing and the ability to manage textures Feeding difficulties in infancy due to hypotonia causing poor suck reflex and faltering growth There is also evidence of oral sensory motor dysfunction and GORD Many become overweight in teens through to adulthood	Poor oral intake, faltering growth, reluctance to progress to more solid textures Dental problems can necessitate a texture-modified diet Obesity can impact on mobility Behaviour problems can manifest themselves in limited food choices and reluctance to try new foods	Psychological support for challenging behaviours/self-injurious behaviour A healthy, balanced diet and good variety of foods should be encouraged, but may need texture modification, depending on the degree of dental abnormality
Tourette syndrome Neurological disease of unknown origin characterised by chronic muscular tics and vocal tics, and is socially stigmatising Often combined with obsessive compulsive behaviour and ADD	Need very structured environment Obsessive desire for order and familiarity, rigid thinking, inflexible, inability to cope with change, easily distracted from eating, changed visual perceptions Poor social skills	Nutritional intakes are likely to be poor Many clients will have feeding issues	Psychological aspects affect food intake Physical problems affect eating and feeding
Untreated phenylketonuria (PKU) Autosomal recessive genetic condition resulting from a deficiency in the hepatic enzyme phenylalanine hydroxylase Hyperphenylalaninaemia is neurotoxic, and the damage is irreversible	If not treated early, leads to severe intellectual disabilities Challenging behaviours include self-harm and harm to others, food aversions Weight disturbances	Challenging behaviours affect food intake Can present as underweight or overweight	A low phenylalanine diet can improve nutritional status and cognitive abilities in some clients Acceptability may inhibit continuance, and QOL issues need to be addressed before considering implementation of diet Dietetic management depends on symptoms

GORD, gastro-oesophageal reflux disease; MDT, multidisciplinary team; QOL, quality of life; ADD, attention-deficit disorder.

abnormal brain development. Impairment to the immature brain, which can occur before, during or after birth, affects movement, posture and coordination. Depending on the severity of the underlying condition, CP may not become obvious until early childhood. It is a wide-ranging condition and can affect people in many different ways; it is not an LD, although many affected people (but not all) will also have an LD.

CP is not progressive, although some of the effects on the body may become more noticeable, and function may deteriorate with age. There are three types of CP spastic, dyskinetic (also known as athetoid or dystonic) and ataxic, and these generally relate to the part of the brain that has been affected. The effects vary enormously from one person to another, and it is common for an individual to have a combination of two or more types. Some may have this condition so mildly that its effects are barely noticeable, while others may be profoundly affected and require help with many or all aspects of daily life. Many children with CP grow poorly due to the underlying disability, malnutrition, endocrinopathy or poor bone growth (Kuperminc & Stevenson, 2008). Other difficulties and medical conditions that can occur more commonly include:

- Chronic constipation.
- Difficulties in chewing and swallowing, especially with advancing age.
- Epilepsy.
- Gastro-oesophageal reflux disease (GORD).
- LD – mild, moderate or severe.
- Oral dysfunction.
- Vomiting due to gut dysmotility and activated emetic reflex.

Other nutritional considerations in people with learning disabilities

Key nutritional considerations include obesity, underweight, dysphagia, GORD, bone health and *Helicobacter pylori* infection.

Obesity

People with LDs are at greater risk of obesity, up to 59% higher than in the general population (Cartwright *et al.*, 2015). Also, people with mild LD are more likely to become obese than people with more severe LD (Melville *et al.*, 2008; RCN, 2013). Evidence indicates that people with an LD tend to become overweight at an earlier age and stay overweight (Bhaumik *et al.*, 2008; Gale *et al.*, 2009). There are many factors that predispose people with LDs including:

- Attitudes of carers.
- Boredom.
- Communication difficulties.
- Hypothyroidism.
- Lack of knowledge.
- Lack of skills, including literacy.
- Lack of power/control over own life.
- Limited access to exercise.
- Low income.
- Medication (see Table 3.7.3).
- Thyroid disease in Down syndrome.
- Mental illness.
- Misuse of food as rewards or motivators to engage in activities.
- Provision of poor diet.
- Poor self-esteem.
- Sedentary lifestyle.
- Altered body composition leading to lower BMR.

Obesity is less prevalent in adults with PMLDs, but it can occur. Weight maintenance may sometimes be the best outcome, ensuring that the intake is nutritionally sound, which in itself confers positive benefits such as relief from constipation, better mood and generally a better feeling. The impact of medications should not be overlooked as antipsychotic and antidepressant medications may induce undesired and rapid weight gain (Pickrell *et al.*, 2012), as shown in Table 3.7.3. Weight gains of 14 kg in 1 year have been reported (Leslie *et al.*, 2007).

Abdominal obesity can occur if energy requirements are overestimated during gastrostomy feeding. It is important to note that energy requirements for these individuals are often lower than for the general population of comparable weight and height (Fairclough *et al.*, 2008). People with LDs are often dependent on others for menu planning, shopping and cooking. Frequently, carers have little knowledge about healthy eating themselves, and many myths about nutrition get passed on and become part of custom and practice in the care setting. The role of the carers in the prevention of obesity and other lifestyle conditions, as well as in any intervention strategies, should not be overlooked. Their own food beliefs, eating experiences and behaviours are imparted to the client, which places an interesting perspective on client choice (Spanos *et al.*, 2013).

There is little robust evidence describing effective weight loss interventions, whether designed for general use and adapted for people with LDs, or targeted

Table 3.7.3 Weight gain associated with commonly prescribed drugs in LDs (adapted from Leslie *et al.*, 2007. Reproduced with permission from Oxford University Press)

Drug	Indicative condition	Weight change (kg)
Sodium valproate	Bipolar/epilepsy	+1.2–5.8
Lithium	Bipolar/depression	+4.0
Clozapine	Schizophrenia	+4.2–9.9
Olanzapine	Schizophrenia	+2.8–7.1
Risperidone	Psychoses	+2.1–2.3
Ziprasidone	Schizophrenia	−2.7–3.2
Prednisolone	Muscle relaxant	+2
Nortriptyline	Depression	+3.7
Doxepin	Depression	+2.7
Amitriptyline	Depression	+1.7

specifically for people with LDs (Jinks *et al.*, 2011; Spanos *et al.*, 2016). Evidence that people with LDs who are more independent are more likely to be obese (Levy *et al.*, 2006) is contradicted by other studies which suggest that those living in supported accommodation are more likely to be overweight or obese (Moore *et al.*, 2004). Also, Levy *et al.* (2007b) found that those living with their family are more likely to be obese. Therefore, it would seem reasonable that, in all settings, any weight loss intervention must include support and motivation from carers. Lack of diet- and health-related knowledge and competence among care staff can affect the health and well-being of the service users if bad dietary habits and inappropriate lifestyle messages are passed on (Bartley, 2011; Iorizzo & Evans, 2015).

Training programmes on nutrition under the umbrellas of healthcare and social care are becoming more available throughout the UK. Although conventional weight maintenance regimens emphasise on high-fibre diets and high fluid intakes, these are of critical importance in this client group, as some clients have difficulties consuming sufficient fluid. Therefore, encouraging higher intakes of fruit and vegetables, with their naturally high fluid content, may be the preferred option, rather than promoting too much insoluble fibre in the form of wholegrain foods.

In a clinic session, standard pre-appointment processes may need to be adapted; it may be more effective and efficient to telephone the client and/or carer to make the appointment. Also, it should be considered if the appointment needs to be at the beginning or end of a clinic session, to help reduce the client's anxiety levels. Partial booking and similar procedures can be confusing, but if contact by telephone is not feasible, a minimum of (straightforward) words should be used in the appointment letter. To aid attendance, the client/carer should be telephoned and reminded on the working day before the appointment. When consulting in a one-to-one setting, it is essential to consider the points shown in Box 3.7.1.

There is some consensus that multi-component group sessions for clients and carers can be effective, although mainstream programmes may need to be adapted with information in easy-to-read formats and shorter interactive sessions with much reinforcement of key messages (PHE, 2016). Group sessions for adults with LDs aim to enhance the knowledge of various conditions, empowering individuals to take more responsibility for managing their own health problems. Practical cookery sessions encourage people to prepare simple, nutritious dishes in their own homes, reducing dependence on ready meals or fast food (McComb & Gardner, 2016). However, such sessions are time limited, and old habits are often re-established after the group has finished. A means of monitoring is needed to maintain motivation. Box 3.7.2 gives recommendations applicable when consulting in a group setting.

Box 3.7.1 Recommendations for consultation in a one to one setting

- Expect first appointment to focus on getting to know the client and gaining trust.
- Collect information on the client's social and family network, so you know the key people with whom to liaise, i.e. care manager, social worker, day service, college, respite, sitters, family, other healthcare workers currently involved.
- Allow at least 30 minutes per consultation.
- Keep distractions to a minimum.
- Discourage accompanying person (if any) from answering for the client, and, where possible, encourage them to sit behind the client.
- Use straightforward language.
- Pace delivery.
- Ask open questions using no more than two information-carrying words at a time.*
- Count to 10 after each question (if needed) to give the client adequate time to reply.
- Rephrase questions to make sure the client is not just repeating your last word.
- Use visual aids to reinforce the spoken word, such as food models, photographs and symbols.
- Limit any areas for change to a maximum of three.
- Use symbols or photographs, and the fonts Arial, Comic Sans, Univers, Tahoma or Verdana in font size 14 for written communication.
- Obtain the client's consent to send copies of recommendations and any supporting information to the care manager for distribution to day services and respite as appropriate.
- Wherever possible, review with the same accompanying person for consistency.

*An information-carrying word is any word in a sentence that must be understood in order to follow an instruction, e.g. '*Give me the ball*'. The person asking holds out their hand, with only a ball in front of them. The addressee does not have to understand any words, because the person has shown them what they want. This statement has no information-carrying words. If there were to be a ball and a book, and the same question was repeated, the addressee need to know the difference between ball and book. This has one information-carrying word level. Messages can have varying numbers of information-carrying words depending on how they are said and what clues are provided. Close liaison with a SLT is recommended.

Box 3.7.2 Recommendations applicable when consulting in a group setting

- Plan first session solely for getting to know the clients and gaining trust.
- Limit membership to no more than 10 clients; less if sessions involve practical cooking activities.
- Encourage carers to attend, although it is not necessary to exclude any clients who attend without support.
- Two people are needed to facilitate each session.
- Allow a maximum of 2 hours per session, with a break midway.
- Keep to one theme per session.
- Plan a maximum of six sessions, with no more than three key themes for the whole programme.
- Keep distractions to a minimum.
- Discourage accompanying people from answering for the clients.
- Use straightforward language.
- Pace the delivery.
- Ask open questions using no more than two information-carrying words at a time.
- Count to 10 after each question to give the clients adequate time to reply.
- Rephrase questions to make sure the clients are not just repeating the last word.
- Ask clients to repeat tasks given to them.
- Use visual aids and activities such as food models, photographs and symbols to reinforce points.
- Limit any areas for change in individual action plans to a maximum of three.
- Use symbols or photographs, and the fonts Arial, Comic Sans, Univers, Tahoma or Verdana in font size 14 for written communication.
- Make sure that copies of activities, work completed and any supporting information are available in individual take-home files or folders for clients to share with carers.

Monitoring

Regular monitoring is essential for clients with LDs to sustain motivation. Carers should follow the monitoring protocol as advised by the dietitian. Ongoing dietetic review is not necessary, although some adjustments to the timeline in any local pathways should be considered, as the first appointment may be introductory. Once the client and carer have understood the key messages, and actions and targets agreed on, further dietetic reviews may be undertaken at the dietitian's discretion, but with discharge, not ongoing care, in mind.

Practical monitoring issues

For those with poor mobility or balance problems, seated or hoist scales may be necessary. Wheelchair beam or platform scales are available. Changes to the wheelchair will mean that the chair will have to be reweighed. In cases where it is not feasible to weigh a client, global assessment, taking into account fit of clothes and jewellery, can be used as indicators of weight change (Burton *et al.*, 2009).

Body mass index (BMI) must be treated with caution where an individual has altered body composition, as it does not assess fat distribution (SIGN, 2010). Mid-upper-arm circumference and triceps skinfold thickness measurements may be inappropriate (Fairclough *et al.*, 2008) for similar reasons. Targets for BMI in clients with PMLDs should be set at the lower end of the normal range. Achieving a weight loss of 5–10% would be a more appropriate, realistic and achievable goal, irrespective of the degree of obesity, and would confer positive health gains for the individual (DOM UK, 2007; NICE, 2006; SIGN, 2010) (see Chapter 7.13.2, The management of obesity and overweight in adults). The BDA professional consensus statement on weight management for adults with LDs living in the community gives more detailed advice (Burton *et al.*, 2011).

Underweight

Polarisation of weight is common in LD patients, with the incidence of underweight ranging from 14% to 75%, depending on the severity of the LD (Emerson, 2005; Gravestock, 2001). It is not uncommon for severe undernutrition to go unrecognised by support staff and family members, particularly when it has been longstanding Franssen *et al.*, 2011). Underweight is more common in people who are immobile, and unable to feed themselves or tolerate solid foods, or exhibit regurgitation, rumination or chronic vomiting.

For more detailed information, refer to the BDA professional consensus statements on the nutritional care of adults with LDs in care settings (DiMascio *et al.*, 2012) and on home enteral tube feeding for adults with LDs (Fairclough *et al.*, 2008) (see Chapter 6.2, Malnutrition).

Dysphagia

Despite dysphagia being a significant problem in people with LDs, few robust studies have been published. The reported prevalence rate varies from 36% to 73% (Leslie *et al.*, 2009) in inpatient LD populations, and is around 35% in primary care (Wright & Hosweman, 2013). Dysphagia is prevalent in the older adult population (Carrión *et al.*, 2015). Since many more people with LDs are now living into older age, the impact of both risk factors combined should not be underestimated. The range of signs and symptoms of dysphagia in people with LDs include:

- Coughing during, and for up to an hour after, eating and drinking.
- Accumulation of saliva.
- Drooling.
- Choking.
- Food aversion.
- Behaviour changes.
- Rushing food.
- Difficulty in taking medications.

These signs are often attributed to the LD itself and, in many cases, are not investigated; such diagnostic overshadowing is unfortunately a common occurrence in this population (Leslie *et al.*, 2009). During a routine nutritional assessment, the dietitian is in an ideal position to observe the potential signs and symptoms of dysphagia. Insidious onset of symptoms such as unexpected weight loss, taking longer to eat and drink, becoming increasingly selective with food choices and hypersalivation, can be missed or not seen as important by carers or the clients (Burton *et al.*, 2012).

Amylase-resistant thickeners based on guar gum/guar gum–starch combinations have been suggested as beneficial for individuals who hypersalivate, although recent research questions this evidence (Hanson *et al.*, 2012); the best thickener to use will be that preferred by the consumer. The addition of thickener to fluids may lead to an increase in energy intake, resulting in weight gain, which may or may not be advantageous. The dietitian should consider the implications of the additional energy component impact on weight when choosing the type of thickener, as the energy content of thickeners varies. Consideration should also be given to the effect of thickeners on medications, as the bioavailability of certain drugs is reduced. Liaison with local medicines information services is advised. (Cichero *et al.*, 2013) (see Chapter 7.3, Dysphagia).

Review

Oral hygiene is of particular importance in those who eat and drink very little. Reduced stimulation of the oral environment leads to dry mouth (reduced saliva production), increased risk of infection, ulceration and increased build-up of plaque or calculus (tartar). The build-up of plaque and calculus can lead to dental decay owing to the presence of plaque acids, periodontal disease due to plaque toxins and bacteria, and increased risk of aspiration pneumonia (Wales, 2010). Plaque organisms such as *Pseudomonas aeruginosa* and *Klebsiella pneumoniae* are common causal organisms of chest infections (Langmore *et al.*, 1998). Each client will require specific guidelines for oral care based on the vulnerability of his or her airway, the underlying condition and tolerance of routine interventions such as tooth brushing, dental reviews and required treatments. Following risk assessment, oral care plans may include specific proactive and reactive strategies such as positioning for oral care, suitable equipment (e.g. using a small-headed multitufted manual toothbrush or small-headed powered toothbrush), low-foaming toothpaste, need for suction and use of any oral hygiene adjuncts (e.g. prescribed mouthwash). People with LDs who are dependent on others for oral hygiene are at high risk of having poor oral health.

Gastro-oesophageal reflux disease (GORD)

GORD is a common problem in people with LDs, with there being a higher incidence in those with PMLDs. More than 50% of institutionalised people with a moderate to severe LD in the Netherlands were shown to have GORD (Böhmer *et al.*, 1999). Higher incidences have been noted in specific syndromes such as fragile X and Rett syndrome, and in conditions such as CP. People taking antiepileptic medication and those with a history of rumination also display a high incidence of the disease. It is caused by acid from the stomach entering the oesophagus, resulting in heartburn, painful swallowing, vomiting and haematemesis (Crawley, 2007). The pain can be intense, and individuals may not be able to describe what is wrong. This may also contribute to sleep disturbance or challenging behaviour. Many cases are missed, since a single oesophagoscopy and diagnosis requires 24-hour oesophageal pH-metry, which is difficult in this client group. There is justification, therefore, to treat with proton pump inhibitors without prior endoscopy. Recommendations for the management of GORD in clients with LDs include the following:

- Provide small, frequent meals.
- Feed client in an upright position – this may be difficult in those with PMLDs, and advice should be sought from physiotherapists about positioning.
- Feed slowly, and encourage chewing if possible.
- Maintain the client in an upright position for at least 30 minutes after meals.

These recommendations can also be used to assist in the treatment of regurgitation and rumination, which are common. Carers and other key professionals require education and training to understand the rationale for careful feeding and the consequences of not adhering to guidelines.

Helicobacter pylori infection

Helicobacter pylori infection is endemic among the LD population owing to communal living situations, including group homes or shared tenancies, respite homes and attending adult day centres (Clarke *et al.*, 2008; De Schryver *et al.*, 2007). A diagnostic urea breath test is difficult for people to undertake, so other methods such as serological testing or stool sampling are recommended (Scheepers *et al.*, 2000). Infection is associated with peptic ulceration and pain, and can present in people with LDs as nausea, vomiting, general malaise and challenging behaviours when the individual cannot describe the nature of the problem. In extreme circumstances, the first indication of the severity of the problem can be perforation of a gastric ulcer. It has been postulated that the high prevalence of infection with *H. pylori* in people with LDs leads to a higher prevalence of gastric carcinoma. Treatment includes antibiotics and proton pump inhibitors. Reinfection can occur following eradication therapy, and the incidence of this is much higher in people with LDs (Wallace *et al.*, 2002).

Bone health

Vulnerable groups within the community such as those with LDs and epilepsy are at higher risk of osteoporosis and fracture owing to a number of factors (NICE, 2014; Pack & Shane, 2015). These include:

- Higher risk for falls.
- Physical trauma related to the seizures themselves.
- Neurologic disease that underlies the epilepsy (stroke, CP).
- Effects of certain antiepileptic drugs (AEDs) that impair gait stability and alter bone and mineral metabolism.

The AEDs most commonly associated with altered bone and mineral metabolism and decreased bone density are those that induce the cytochrome P450 enzyme system, e.g. phenytoin, primidone, carbamazapine, clonazepam and phenobarbital. There is also a negative association on bone health with sodium valproate. Other risk factors include limited exposure to sunlight, poor diet and low physical activity levels. The following actions are recommended:

- Adults and carers to be given an explanation of bone health and medication (e.g. BDA Food Fact sheet on osteoporosis).
- Serum calcium and alkaline phosphatase measured at baseline and then routinely measured during the health check.
- Adults with a history of fracture, a new fracture and/or a history of prolonged use of AEDs are automatically prescribed vitamin D and calcium supplements. A bone density scan (DXA) may be advised by the consultant.
- Adults receiving vitamin D supplements should have serum 25-hydroxyvitamin D (25(OH)D) levels measured to determine whether vitamin D intake is sufficient to maintain levels within the normal range.

Other factors to consider when working with clients with learning disabilities

Medication

The impact of medication is often overlooked, despite clients with LDs being prescribed a large number of medications to control mood, behaviour and epilepsy on a daily basis as well as required (pro re nata; also known as rescue medication). Some medications, e.g. anticonvulsants and osmotic laxatives, have a direct impact on nutrient absorption. Neuroleptics (antipsychotics) cause pharyngeal weakness and dystonia, while some of the tricyclic antidepressants (e.g. amitriptyline) reduce saliva production, resulting in xerostomia (dry mouth). Medication reviews are important to discuss the impact of new drugs as well as the continued combination of current medications. Medication side effects also include chronic constipation, a frequent problem for people with LDs, which increases the risk of seizure activity. Other medications frequently prescribed for clients with LDs that can impact on nutritional status are shown in Table 3.7.4.

Table 3.7.4 Medications prescribed for clients with LDs that impact on nutritional status (adapted from Burton *et al.*, 2009)

Medication	Nutrition-related side effects
Antiepileptic drugs (AEDs), e.g. phenytoin, primidone, carbamazepine, clonazepam, phenobarbital, sodium valproate	Altered bone and mineral metabolism; decreased bone density
Antipsychotics, e.g. risperidone, aripiprazole	Drowsiness, apathy, confusion, depression Gastrointestinal disturbances, dry mouth, weight gain
Anticonvulsants/antiepileptics, e.g. topiramate, phenytoin	Nausea, vomiting, constipation, diarrhoea, abdominal pain, oedema, appetite changes, confusion, weight gain, dry mouth, weight loss
Antidepressants: tricyclics, amitriptyline	Loss of appetite, constipation, weight gain, dry mouth
Monoamine oxidase inhibitors (MAOIs)	As above plus strict adherence to special diets as certain foods need to be avoided
Selective serotonin reuptake inhibitors (SSRIs), e.g. fluoxetine	Taste disturbance, increased salivation, rhinitis, changes in blood sugars
Anxiolytics, e.g. diazepam	Salivation changes, constipation, diarrhoea, vomiting
Hypnotics, e.g. temazepam	Drowsiness, confusion, gastric irritation
Antimuscarinics, e.g. hyoscine	Constipation, dry mouth, nausea, vomiting
Mood stabilisers, e.g. lithium	Weight gain, excessive thirst, oedema
Laxatives: bulk forming, e.g. methyl cellulose	Flatulence, abdominal distension, gastrointestinal obstruction or impaction
Stimulant, e.g. senna	Diarrhoea, hypokalaemia
Osmotic, e.g. Movicol, lactulose	Long-term use can interfere with the absorption of fat-soluble vitamins, flatulence, abdominal discomfort
Thickeners: starch and gum based	Diarrhoea, constipation, weight gain, interaction with medications

Carers

Carers need to have the skills and knowledge to promote good eating habits and should be encouraged to share good practices with their care teams (Spanos *et al.*, 2013). In some circumstances, there may be a need to address specific issues pertaining to carers, including:

- Varying levels of interest in food and exercise.
- Little or no experience in planning healthy menus or adapting menus to accommodate texture modification.
- Understanding that their clients do not require the same amount of food as they do, and that providing smaller portions is therefore acceptable.
- Bringing their own theories and idiosyncrasies to the meal provision process.
- Perceiving clients as not having fulfilled lives and seeking to redress this in some way using food.
- Using '*it's the client's choice*' as an excuse to provide or allow access to less healthy food from either a nutrient or texture aspect.

Paid carers often struggle to define their role, especially when the issue of choice is so far reaching. Some see their role as protecting the client's long-term health, and so work hard to ensure that healthier choices are made. Others see their role as promoting choice, and that, as long as they enable their client to make a choice, or their client can be seen to be making choices (healthy or unhealthy), they have fulfilled their role. The issue of human rights is also cited and interpreted as people with capacity having the right to make unhealthy choices. Staff need to remember that they have a duty of care to ensure that their client's health needs are met and should endeavour to facilitate informed choices as much as possible. It is important to have an appreciation and understanding of the skills base, values and belief systems of carers and to use this state of reality for training and support. Empowering carers is as important as empowering their clients.

Information

Information needs to be provided in a format that is easily understood, i.e. in an accessible format incorporating a range of techniques, e.g. symbols, photographs, audiovisual aids and Talking Mats™ (see useful resources). With regard to verbal communication, it is important to remember how information is interpreted. Advice may be taken literally, or choice may be limited to a suggestion given, e.g. '*you can have an occasional treat like chocolate*' could be interpreted as '*chocolate is only a treat*'. The term occasional is abstract and subjective, and the same could be said for daily or weekly, or even hourly, depending on the client's understanding of time. Clients should be asked to say in their own words what they understand from the information they have been given. There should be no temptation to use the fact that the client can repeat what has just been said to them as a measure of understanding, as many people with LDs are quite adept at recalling the words most recently spoken to them (termed the 'recency effect') (Kroese *et al.*, 1998).

Bowel function

A standardised way of describing bowel function using the Bristol stool chart is recommended (Lewis & Heaton, 1997). Constipation, in particular, is a frequent problem, and it increases the risk of epileptic seizure activity. However, it often goes unrecognised by carers because it is normal for the client (Cockburn-Wells, 2014). The contributing factors are poor gut motility, chronic inadequate fluid and fibre intake, chronic laxative usage, lack of physical activity and medication side effects. When enteral tube feeding is commenced, there is a risk of faecal impaction and vomiting despite adequate nutrition and fluid. In dysphagia, thickeners have been reported to alter clients' bowel function (diarrhoea or constipation, or both). Bowel function therefore needs to be monitored to prevent complications, and colonisation by *H. pylori* should be considered.

Intractable epilepsy

The ketogenic diet (KD) is a high-fat, moderate-protein, low-carbohydrate diet which is advised on an individual basis. Traditionally, its use has been in paediatrics to treat children and young people with intractable (uncontrolled) epilepsy, as well as Glut 1 dehydrogenase deficiency (Glut 1) and pyruvate dehydrogenase deficiency (PDH). While KD tended to be used for 2 years, there are now many young people carrying on with the diet into adulthood, causing funding issues around transition (Borlot *et al.*, 2016). The modified Atkins diet is now also being used in adults including those with LDs. There has been a significant amount of research in the last 3–4 years looking at KD in brain tumours, especially astrocytomas and gliomas, and other neurological conditions such as Parkinson's disease, Alzheimer's disease and autism (Branco *et al.*, 2016; Martin *et al.*, 2016) (see Chapters 7.6.1 (Parkinson's disease), 7.10.2 (Eating disorders) and 3.8.16 (Neurology and the ketogenic diet).

Quality of life

Any intervention should consider the four principles of medical ethics, i.e. respect for autonomy, beneficence, non-malfeasance and justice (Beauchamp & Childress, 2013), as well as the issue of consent (Burton *et al.*, 2011). It is important to highlight that people with LDs want to be (and should be) seen as equal citizens in their communities and, wherever possible, would prefer to access the same health services as everyone else (Black, 2013; Mencap, 2010). The label learning disability encompasses a wide range of disabilities from mild to profound, and it is important to ensure that choice is available for all. Where it is not possible to meet the specific needs of people with LDs through adapting mainstream services, referral to a local specialist CLDT can be considered. While it is important to appreciate the limitations and expectations of this client group, standard outcome measures used in dietetic practice may not be appropriate. Realistic outcome measures based on thorough assessment of need, ability and quality of life are essential in order to work effectively with, and for, this client group. If the clinical expectations expressed by the professional are not harmonious with the fundamental processes operating within specific genetic syndromes, failure will ensue. It is incumbent on the practitioner to work within the parameters of a specific syndrome such as PWS, or the conditions associated with the LD such as autism, working towards outcomes that are practicable, achievable and, most importantly, meaningful to the client.

It has been recognised for some time that people with LDs can be informative, critical and reliable service users, provided that effective interview methods are employed (Kroese *et al.*, 1998). Closer working partnerships with primary, secondary, tertiary and specialist teams, together with local advocacy groups, could make inclusion a realistic objective for safeguarding health improvements in people with LDs.

Further reading

Dodd K, Turk V, Christmas M. (2010) *Down Syndrome & Dementia – A Resource for Carers and Support Staff*, 2nd edn. Teddington: Down's Syndrome Association.

Gates, B. (ed). (2003) *Learning Disabilities – Toward Inclusion*, 4th edn. London: Churchill Livingstone.

O'Shea S, Macleod M, Laverty A. (2016) Learning disabilities: Prader–Willi syndrome. In: Lawrence J, Douglas P, Gandy J (eds) *Dietetic and Nutrition Case Studies*. West Sussex: Wiley Blackwell, pp. 34–38.

Pawlyn J, Carnaby S. (eds). (2009) *Profound and Multiple Learning Disabilities*. Oxford: Blackwell Publishing.

Peterson JJ, Janz KF, Lowe JB. (2008) Physical activity among adults with intellectual disability living in community settings. *Prev. Med.* 47: 101–106.

Prader–Willi Syndrome Association. (2016a) *Information for Families – Dietary Management and Exercise*. Available at https://www.pwsa.co.uk/information-for-families/dietary-management-and-exercise. Accessed 17 November 2016.

Prader–Willi Syndrome Association. (2016b) About Prader–Willi – Basic Facts. Available at http://www.pwsa.co.uk/information-for-professionals/health. Accessed 17 November 2016.

Thompson J, Pickering S. (eds). (2001) *Meeting the Health Needs of People Who Have a Learning Disability*. Edinburgh: Baillière Tindall.

Internet resources

Abertawe Bro Morgannwg University Health Board for downloadable information sheets in accessible format, www.wales.nhs.uk/sitesplus/863/page/41509

Agored Cymru, https://www.agored.cymru

Autism for Dietitians Masterclass, www.zoeconnor.co.uk

Autismspeaks.org, for information for both professionals and carers, www.autismspeaks.org

Bristol community (LD) dietitians, https://briscomhealth.org.uk/our-services/community-learning-disabilities-team-cldt/

British Dietetic Association, www.bda.uk.com

British Institute of Learning Disabilities, www.bild.org.uk

British Psychological Association, www.bps.org.uk

Caroline Walker Trust Eating Well: Children and Adults with Learning Disabilities, www.cwt.org.uk

Centre for Education & Development: Franchised course – Introduction to mental health, LDs and eating disorders, www.bda.uk.com/ced

Clear Consultancy. For advice and training regarding making information accessible, www.clearforall.co.uk

Color Library Collection – Food. Visual dictionary, www.winslowresources.com

Easy Health – Health information in an easy-to-understand format, www.easyhealth.org.uk

Food and Behaviour Research, www.fabresearch.org

Food, Fitness, Fun! Training pack in weight management for people with LDs www.pavpub.com

Highfield Publications, www.highfield.co.uk

I Can Cook-It! For LD (Public Health Agency, Northern Ireland), http://www.northerntrust.hscni.net/pdf/I_Can_Cook_it_Course_Information_Sheet_2016.pdf

Matthew's Friends – a UK-registered charity specialising in ketogenic diet therapies, http://www.matthewsfriends.org

Mayer-Johnson Special education source materials – symbols, www.mayer-johnson.com

Mencap, www.mencap.org.uk

Mental Capacity Act, Short reference guide for psychologists and psychiatrists, https://www1.bps.org.uk/system/files/Public%20files/Policy/mental_capacity_act_2005_-_short_reference_guide_for_psychologists_and_psychiatrists%20REP47.pdf.

Mental Health Group, www.dietitiansmentalhealthgroup.org.uk

National Autistic Society, www.autism.org.uk

Nutrition and Diet Resources UK, www.ndr-uk.org

PEN: Practice-based Evidence in Nutrition; Dietitians of Canada, www.bda.uk.com/pen. Down Syndrome background.

PMLD LINK. A journal which shares good practice in supporting children and adults with PMLDs, www.pmldlink.org.uk

POMONA Health indicators for people with LDs, www.pomonaproject.org

Qualifications and Credit Framework, www.edexcel.com

Research Autism, www.researchautism.net

Royal Environmental Health Institute Scotland, www.rehis.com

Royal Society for Public Health, www.rsph.org.uk

Scottish Commission for Learning Disabilities (SCLD) for healthy eating resource pack, www.scld.org.uk/healthy-eating-healthy-living-pack

Scottish Intercollegiate Guideline Network, www.sign.ac.uk

SIGN 145 Assessment, diagnosis and clinical interventions, for autism spectrum disorders. https://www.sign.ac.uk/assets/sign145.pdf

Talking Mats™ Communication framework, www.talkingmats.com

Take 5 Multi-component weight management for LD (Spanos *et al.*, 2013), http://onlinelibrary.wiley.com/doi/10.1111/jhn.12051/full

Welsh Government. *Nutrition in community settings: A pathway and resource pack for health and social care professionals, the third sector, care home staff, relatives and carers*. Available at http://gov.wales/topics/health/publications/socialcare/guidance1/nutrition/?lang=en

References

Autism Speaks. (2016) *What is Autism*. Available at https://www.autismspeaks.org/what-autism. Accessed 28 November 2016.

Bartley J. (2011) Promoting healthy eating and weight loss. *Learn. Disabil. Pract.* 14: 12–16.

Beauchamp TL, Childress JF. (2013) *Principles of Biomedical Ethics*, 7th edn. Oxford: Oxford University Press.

Bhaumik S, Watson LM, Thorpe CF, *et al.* (2008) Body mass index in adults with intellectual disability: distribution, association and service implications: a population-based prevalence study. *J. Intellect. Disabil. Res.* 53: 287–298.

Black AE. (2013) *Health inequalities and people with a learning disability*. Available at http://www.niassembly.gov.uk/globalassets/Documents/RaISe/Publications/2013/health/13413.pdf. Accessed 11 November 2016.

Böhmer CJ, Niezen-de Boer MC, Klinkenberg-Knol, E.C. *et al.* (1999) The prevalence of gastroesophageal reflux disease in institutionalized intellectually disabled individuals. *Am. J. Gastroenterol.* 94: 804–810.

Borlot F, Tellez-Zenteno JF, Allen A, *et al.* (2016) Transition from paediatric to adult care for patients with epilepsy: considerations from the adult side. *Neurology* 86(16 Supp): P2006.

Branco AF, Ferreira A, Simões RF, *et al.* (2016) Ketogenic diets: from cancer to mitochondrial diseases and beyond. *Eur. J. Clin. Invest.* 46: 285–298.

Bridges N. (2014) What is the value of growth hormone therapy in Prader–Willi syndrome? *Arch. Dis. Child.* 9: 166–170.

British Psychological Society. (2007) *Mental Capacity Act Short Reference Guide.* Available at www.bps.org.uk. Accessed 23 November 2016.

Brugha T, Cooper SA, McManus S, *et al.* (2012). *Estimating the prevalence of autism spectrum conditions in adults: extending the 2007 Adult Psychiatric Morbidity Survey.* Available at http://content.digital.nhs.uk/catalogue/pub05061/esti-prev-auti-ext-07-psyc-morb-surv-rep.pdf. Accessed 28 November 2016.

Burton S, Cox S, Sandham SM. (2009) Nutrition and hydration. In: Pawlyn J, Carnaby S (eds) *Profound Intellectual and Multiple Disabilities.* Oxford: Blackwell Publishing.

Burton S, Laverty A, Macleod M. People with learning disabilities. In Gandy J (ed). (2014) Manual of Dietetic Practice, 5th Edition.

Burton S, McIntosh P, Jurs A, *et al.* (2011) *Weight management for adults with a learning disability living in the community.* Available at https://matrix.rcn.org.uk/__data/assets/pdf_file/0004/371974/Weight_management_adults_with_learning_disabilities_v1_180311.pdf. Accessed 22 September 2018.

Burton S, Laverty A, Macleod M. (2012) The dietitian's role in the diagnosis and treatment of dysphagia. In: Ekberg O (ed) *Dysphagia, Diagnosis and Treatment.* New York: Springer Verlag.

Butler JV, Whittington JE, Holland AJ, *et al.* (2002) Prevalence of, and risk factors for, physical ill-health in people with Prader–Willi syndrome: a population-based study. *Dev. Med. Child Neurol.* 44: 248–255.

Butler MG, Theodoro MF, Bittel DC, *et al.* (2007) Energy expenditure and physical activity in Prader–Willi syndrome: comparison with obese subjects. *Am. J. Med. Genet. A.* 143: 449–459.

Carrión S, Cabré M, Monteis R, *et al.* (2015) Oropharyngeal dysphagia is a prevalent risk factor for malnutrition in a cohort of older patients admitted with an acute disease to a general hospital. *Clin. Nutr.* 34: 436–442.

Cartwright L, Reid M, Hammersley R, *et al.* (2015) Food choice by people with intellectual disabilities at day centres: a qualitative study. *J. Intellect. Disabil* 19: 103–115.

Cassidy SB, Schwartz S, Miller JL, *et al.* (2012) Prader–Willi syndrome. *Genet Med.* 14: 10–26.

Center J, Beange H, McElduff A. (1998) People with mental retardation have an increased prevalence of osteoporosis: a population study. *Am. J. Ment. Retard.* 103: 19–28.

Chui M, Watson S. (2015) *Xerophthalmia and vitamin A deficiency in an autistic child with a restricted diet.* Available at Casereports.bmj.com/content/2015/bcr-2015-209413.full.pdf. Accessed 27 November 2016.

Cichero JA, Steele C, Duivestein J, *et al.* (2013) The need for international terminology and definitions for texture-modified foods and thickened liquids used in dysphagia management: foundations of a global initiative. *Curr. Phys. Med. Rehabil. Rep* 1: 280–291.

Clarke D, Vemuri M, Gunatilake D, *et al.* (2008) *Helicobacter pylori* infection in five inpatient units for people with intellectual disability and psychiatric disorder. *J. Appl. Res. Intellect. Disabil.* 21: 95–98.

Cockburn-Wells H. (2014) *Managing constipation in adults with severe learning disabilities.* Available at http://journals.rcni.com/doi/pdfplus/10.7748/ldp.17.9.16.e1582. Accessed 27 November 2016.

Cohen WI. (2006) Current dilemmas in Down syndrome clinical care: celiac disease, thyroid disorders and atlanto-axial instability. *Am J Med Genet C Semin Med Genet.* 142: 141–148.

Crawley H. (2007) *Eating Well: Children and Adults with Learning Disabilities.* Available at http://www.cwt.org.uk/wp-content/uploads/2015/02/EWLDGuidelines.pdf. Accessed 10 October 2016.

De Schryver A, Cornelius K, Van Winckel M, *et al.* (2007) The occupational risk of *Helicobacter pylori* infection among workers in institutions for people with intellectual disability. *Occup. Environ. Med.* 65: 587–591.

DH. (1991) *Dietary Reference Values for Food Energy and Nutrients for the United Kingdom. Report 41.* London: TSO.

DH. (2005) *Mental Capacity Act 2005: Code of Practice Department of Constitutional Affairs.* Available at www.dca.gov.uk. Accessed 11 April 2016.

DH. (2007) *Guidance on Services for People with Learning Disabilities and Challenging Behaviour or Mental Health Needs Department of Health.* London: TSO.

DH. (2010) *Valuing People Now: A Three-Year Strategy for People with Learning Disabilities.* London: Department of Health.

DHSSPS. (2003) *Seeking Consent: Working with People with Learning Disabilities.* Scotland. Available at https://www.health-ni.gov.uk/publications/consent-guides-healthcare-professionals. Accessed 27 September 2016.

Dietitians in Obesity Management (DOM) UK. (2007) *The Dietetic Weight Management Intervention for Adults in the One to One Setting – Is it Time for a Radical Rethink?* Birmingham: BDA.

DiMascio F, Hamilton K, Smith L. (2012) *The Nutritional Care of Adults with a Learning Disability in Care Settings.* Available at www.bda.uk.com. Accessed 20 November 2016.

Down's Syndrome Medical Interest Group. (2000) *The UK (2000) Growth Charts.* Available at www.dsmig.org.uk/publications/growthchart.html. Accessed 11 November 2016.

Elder JH, Shanker M, Shuster J, *et al.* (2006) The gluten-free, casein-free diet in autism: Results of a preliminary double blind clinical trial. *J. Autism. Dev. Disord.* 36: 413–420.

Emerson E. (2005) Underweight, obesity and exercise among adults with intellectual disabilities in supported accommodation in Northern England. *J. Intellect. Disabil. Res.* 49: 134–143.

Emerson E, Baines S. (2011) Health inequalities and people with learning disabilities in the UK. *Tizard Learn. Disabil. Rev.* 16: 42–48.

Fairclough J, Burton S, Craven J, *et al.* (2008) *Home Enteral Tube Feeding for Adults with a Learning Disability.* Available at https://www.bda.uk.com/publications/professional/hetf_adults_with_ld Accessed 22 September 2018.

Franssen JL, Maaskant MA, van Schrojenstein Lantman-de Valk HMJ. (2011) Qualitative study of malnutrition in people with intellectual disabilities. *J. Policy Prac. Intellect. Disabil.* 8: 239–246.

Gale L, Naqvi H, Russ L. (2009) Asthma, smoking and BMI in adults with intellectual disabilities: a community-based survey. *J. Intellect. Disabil. Res.* 53: 787–796.

Gourash LM, Forster JL. (2009) *Regulation of Weight in Prader–Willi Syndrome: Theoretical and Practical Considerations.* Available at http://www.pwsausa.org/wp-content/uploads/2016/01/Self-Regulation-in-PWS-by-LG-final-.pdf. Accessed 11 November 2016.

Gravestock S. (2001) Review. Eating disorders in adults with intellectual disability. *J. Intellect. Disabil. Res.* 44: 625–663.

Gross RD, Gisser R, Cherpes G, *et al.* (2016) *Subclinical dysphagia in persons with Prader–Willi syndrome.* Available at NCBI https://www.ncbi.nlm.nih.gov/pubmed/27759943. Accessed 27 November 2016.

Hanson B, O'Leary M, Smith C. (2012) The effect of saliva on the viscosity of thickened drinks. *Dysphagia* 27: 10–19.

Health Inspectorate Wales. (2007) *How Well Does the NHS in Wales Commission and Provide Specialist Learning Disability Services for Young People and Adults?* Caerphilly: Health Inspectorate Wales.

Healy M. (2005) Adults with incapacity and the person with a mild learning disability: the ethical and legal dilemmas posed. *Newsletter for Mental Health Officers in Scotland* 9: 3–4.

Hennequin M, Faulks D, Veyrune J-L, *et al.* (1999) Significance of oral health in persons with Down's syndrome: a literature review. *Dev. Med. Child Neurol.* 41: 275–283.

Hoffman CJ, Aultman D, Pipes P. (1992) A nutrition survey of and recommendations for individuals with PWS who live in group homes. *J. Am. Diet. Assoc.* 92: 823–830.

Holland A, Whittington J, Hinton E. (2003) The paradox of Prader–Willi syndrome: a genetic model of starvation. *Lancet* 362: 989–991.

Hsieh K, Rimmer JH, Heller T. (2014) Obesity and associated factors in adults with intellectual disability. *J. Intellect. Disabil. Res.* 58: 851–863.

Iorizzo H, Evans K. (2015) *Supporting Service Users to Lose Weight*. Available at http://journals.rcni.com/doi/pdfplus/10.7748/ldp.18.4.12.e1618. Accessed 28 November 2016.

Isherwood E, Thomas K. (2011) *Dietary Management of Autism Spectrum Disorder: Professional Consensus Statement*. Available at http://researchautism.net/publications/989/dietary-management-of-autism-spectrum-disorder:-professional-consensus-statement. Accessed 22 November 2016.

Jinks A, Cotton A, Rylance R. (2011) Obesity interventions for people with a learning disability: an integrative literature review. *J. Adv. Nurs.* 67: 460–471.

Koritsas S, Iacano T. (2016) Weight, nutrition, food choice and physical activity in adults with intellectual disability. *J. Intellect. Disabil. Res.* 60: 355–364.

Kroese BS, Gillott A, Atkinson V. (1998) Consumers with intellectual disabilities as service evaluators. *J. Appl. Res. Intellect. Disabil.* 11: 116–128.

Kuperminc MN, Stevenson RD. (2008) Growth and nutrition disorders in children with cerebral palsy. *Dev. Disabil. Res. Rev.* 14: 137–146.

Kuppens RJ, Bakker NE, Siemensma EP, et al. (2016) Beneficial effects of GH in young adults with Prader–Willi syndrome: a 2-year crossover trial. *J. Clin. Endocrinol. Metab.* 101: 4110–4116.

Langmore SE, Terpenning MS, Schork A. (1998) Predictors of aspiration pneumonia. How important is dysphagia? *Dysphagia* 13: 69–81.

Lazenby T. (2008) The impact of aging on eating, drinking, and swallowing function in people with Down's syndrome. *Dysphagia* 23: 88–97.

Leslie P, Crawford H, Wilkinson H. (2009) People with a learning disability and dysphagia: a Cinderella population? *Dysphagia* 24: 103–104.

Leslie WS, Hankey CR, Lean MEJ. (2007) Weight gain as an adverse effect of some commonly prescribed drugs: a systematic review. *QJM* 100: 395–404.

Levy JM, Botuck S, Damiani MR, *et al.* (2006) Medical conditions and healthcare utilization among adults with intellectual disabilities living in group homes in New York City. *J. Policy Pract. Intellect. Disabil.* 3: 195–202.

Levy JM, Botuck S, Rimmerman A. (2007a) Examining outpatient health care utilization among adults with severe or profound intellectual disabilities living in an urban setting: a brief snap shot. *J. Soc. Work Disabil. Rehabil.* 6: 33–45.

Levy SE, Souders MC, Ittenbach RF. (2007b) Relationship of dietary intake to gastrointestinal symptoms in children with ASD spectrum disorders. *Biol. Psychiatry* 61: 492–497.

Lewis SJ, Heaton KW. (1997) Stool form scale as a useful guide to intestinal transit time. *Scand. J. Gastroenterol.* 32: 920–924.

Lindmark M, Trygg K, Giltvedt K, *et al.* (2010) Nutrient intake of young children with Prader–Willi syndrome. *Food Nutr. Res.* 54: doi 10.3402/fnr.v54i0.2112.

Marí-Bauset S, Llopis-González A, Zazpe-García I, *et al.* (2015) Nutritional status of children with autism spectrum disorders (ASDs): a case control study. *J. Autism Dev. Disord.* 45: 203–212.

Marí-Bauset S, Llopis-González A, Zazpe I, *et al.* (2016) Nutritional impact of a gluten-free casein-free diet in children with autism spectrum disorder. *J. Autism Dev. Discord.* 46: 673–684.

Martin K, Jackson CF, Levy RG, *et al.* (2016) *Ketogenic diet and other dietary treatments for epilepsy*. Available at http://www.cochrane.org/CD001903/EPILEPSY_ketogenic-and-other-dietary-treatments-epilepsy. Accessed 28 November 2016.

McComb A, Gardner E. (2016) Public health – learning disabilities. In: Lawrence J, Douglas P, Gandy J (eds) *Dietetic and Nutrition Case Studies*. West Sussex: Wiley Blackwell, pp. 48–51.

Melville CA, Cooper SA, McGrother CW, *et al.* (2005) Obesity in adults with Down syndrome: a case-control study. *J. Intellect. Disabil. Res.* 49: 125–133.

Melville CA, Cooper S, Morrison J. (2008) The prevalence and determinants of obesity in adults with intellectual disability. *J. Appl. Res. Intellect. Disabil.* 21: 425–437.

Melville CA, Hamilton S, Millar S, *et al.* (2009) Carer knowledge and perceptions of healthy lifestyles for adults with intellectual disabilities. *J. Appl. Res. Intellect. Disabil.* 22: 298–306.

Mencap. (2010) *Getting it right: the charter explained (Online)*. Available at https://www.mencap.org.uk/sites/default/files/2016-07/Getting%20it%20Right%20charter.pdf. Accessed 22 September 2018.

Miller JL, Lynn CH, Shuster J, *et al.* (2013) A reduced-energy intake, well-balanced diet improves weight control in children with Prader–Willi syndrome. *J. Hum. Nutr. Diet.* 26: 2–9.

Millward C, Ferriter M, Claver S, *et al.* (2008) Gluten and casein-free diets for autistic spectrum disorder (Cochrane review). *Cochrane Database Syst. Rev.* (2): CD003498.

Moore K, McGillivray J, Illingworth K, *et al.* (2004) An investigation into the incidence of obesity and underweight among adults with an intellectual disability in an Australian sample. *J. Intellec. Dev. Disabil.* 29: 306–318.

Murray J, Ryan-Krause P. (2010) Obesity in children with Down syndrome: Background and recommendations for management. *Pediatr. Nurs.* 36: 314–319.

National Autistic Society. (2016) *Eating & Problems to Look Out For*. Available at http://www.autism.org.uk/about/health/eating.aspx. Accessed 28 November 2016.

NHS Scotland. (2009) Caring and Consent. Available at https://www.nhsinform.scot/media/1302/caring-and-consent-large-print-v3.pdf. Accessed 23 November 2016.

NICE. (2006) *Clinical Guideline 43: Obesity guidance on the prevention, identification, assessment and management of overweight and obesity in adults and children*. London: NICE.

NICE. (2010) *Human Growth Hormone (Somatropin) for the Treatment of Growth Failure in Children*. Available at https://www.nice.org.uk/guidance/ta188. Accessed 11 April 2016.

NICE. (2012) *Autism Spectrum Disorder in Adults: Diagnosis and Management*. Available at https://www.nice.org.uk/guidance/cg142. Accessed 11 November 2016.

NICE. (2014) *Vitamin D: Increasing Supplement Use in At-Risk Groups. NICE Guidelines (PH56) November*. Available at https://www.nice.org.uk/guidance/ph56. Accessed 12 September 2016.

Office of the Public Guardian. (2009) *Making Decisions Series of Guides for Families, Friends, Carers and Professionals*. Available at https://professionals.carers.org/sites/default/files/the-mental-capacity-act-a-guide-for-family-friends-other-unpaid-carers-web-version-2029_0.pdf. Accessed 22 September 2018.

O'Riordan CF, Metcalf BS, Perkins JM, *et al.* (2010) Reliability of energy expenditure prediction equations in the weight management clinic. *J. Hum. Nutr. Diet.* 23: 169–175.

Pack AM, Shane E. (2015) *Antiepileptic Drugs and Bone Disease*. Available at http://www.uptodate.com/contents/antiepileptic-drugs-and-bone-disease. Accessed 11 November 2016.

Pawlyn J, Carnaby S. (ed). (2009) *Profound and Multiple Learning Disabilities*. Oxford: Blackwell Publishing.

Pickrell WO, Lacey AS, Thomas RH, *et al.* (2012) Weight changes associated with antiepileptic drugs. *J. Neurol. Neursurg. Psychiatry*, 84:796–799. Available at http://jnnp.bmj.com/content/84/7/796.full.pdf. Accessed 11 November 2016.

Public Health England (PHE). (2016) *Making reasonable adjustments to obesity and weight management services for people with learning disabilities*. London: PHE.

Ramirez-Zea M. (2005) Validation of three predictive equations for basal metabolic rate in adults. *Public Health Nutr.* 8: 1213–1228.

Ranjan S, Nasser JA. (2015). Nutritional status of individuals with autism spectrum disorders: do we know enough? *Adv. Nutr.* 6: 397–407.

Robertson J, Roberts H, Emerson E. (2011) *The impact of health checks for people with learning disabilities: a systematic review of the evidence*. Available at

Roebroeck ME, Stam HJ. (2006). The epidemiology of cerebral palsy: incidence, impairments and risk factors. *Disabil. Rehabil.* 28: 183–191.

Room B, Timmermans O, Roodbol P. (2016) The prevalence and risk factors of the metabolic syndrome in inpatients with intellectual disability. *J. Intellect. Disabil. Res.* 60: 594–605.

Royal College of Nursing (RCN). (2013) *Meeting the Needs of People with Learning Disabilities*. London: RCN.

Rutter H, Carmichael S. (2011) Health care for people with learning disabilities – how far have we come? The national picture. *Tizard Learn. Disabil. Rev.* 16: 14–17.

Scheepers M, Duff M, Baddeley P, *et al.* (2000) *Helicobacter pylori* and the learning disabled. *Br. J. Gen. Pract.* 50: 813–814.

Schoeller DA, Levitsky LL, Bandini LG, *et al.* (1988). Energy expenditure and body composition in Prader–Willi syndrome. *Metabolism* 37: 115–120.

Scottish Intercollegiate Guideline Network (SIGN). (2010) *SIGN Guideline 115 Management of Obesity*. Available at https://www.sign.ac.uk/sign-115-management-of-obesity.html. Accessed 12 November 2016.

Scottish Parliament. (2000a) *The same as you. A review of services for people with learning disability*. Available at https://www2.gov.scot/resource/doc/1095/0001661.pdf. Accessed 13 September 2016.

Scottish Parliament. (2000b) *Adults with Incapacity (Scotland) Act*. Edinburgh: The Stationery Office.

Shin M, Besser LM, Kucik JE, *et al.* (2009) Prevalence of Down syndrome among children and adolescents in 10 regions of the United States. *Pediatrics* 124: 1565–1571.

Spanos D, Hankey CR, Boyle S. (2013) Carers perspectives of a weight loss intervention for adults with intellectual disabilities and obesity, a qualitative study. *J. Intellect. Disabil. Res.* 57: 90–102.

Spanos D, Hankey CR, Melville CA. (2016) The effectiveness of a weight maintenance intervention for adults with intellectual disabilities and obesity: a single stranded study. *J. Appl. Res. Intellect. Disabil.* 29: 317–329.

van Mil E, Westerterp KR, Gerver, WJ, *et al.* (2000a) Energy expenditure at rest and during sleep in children with Prader–Willi syndrome is explained by body composition. *Am. J. Clin. Nutr.* 71: 752–756.

van Mil E, Westerterp KR, Kester ADM, *et al.* (2000b) Activity related energy expenditure in children and adolescents with PWS. *Int. J. Obes. Relat. Metab. Disord.* 24: 429–434.

van Mil E, Westerterop KR, Gerver WJ, *et al.* (2001) Body composition in Prader–Willi syndrome compared with non-syndromal obesity: relationship to physical activity and growth hormone function. *J. Paediatr.* 139: 708–714.

Vogels A, Van Den Ende J, Keymolen K, *et al.* (2004) Minimum prevalence, birth incidence and cause of death for Prader–Willi syndrome in Flanders. *Eur. J. Hum. Genet.* 12: 238–240.

Wales L. (2010) Providing oral healthcare for patients with a PRG tube. *Dent. Nurs.* 6: 565–568.

Wallace R, Schluter P, Webb P. (2002) Environmental, medical behavioural and disability factors associated with *Helicobacter pylori* infection in adults with intellectual disability. *J. Intellect. Disabil. Res.* 46: 51–60.

Whitman BY. (2016) *Using Medications as a Management Strategy for Persons with PWS*. Available at http://www.pws.org.nz/using-medications-as-a-management-strategy-for-persons-with-pws. Accessed 27 November 2016.

Whittington JE, Holland AJ, Webb T, *et al.* (2001) Population prevalence and estimated birth incidence and mortality rate for people with Prader–Willi syndrome in one UK health region. *J. Med. Genet.* 38: 792–798.

WHO. (1992) *ICD-10 Classification of Mental and Behavioural Disorders: Clinical Depression and Diagnostic Guidelines*. Geneva: World Health Organization.

WHO. (2010) Healthy ageing: adults with intellectual disabilities: summative report. *J. Appl. Res. Intellect. Disabil.* 14: 256–275.

Wong HHL, Smith RG. (2006) Patterns of complementary and alternative medical therapy use in children diagnosed with autism spectrum disorders. *J. Autism Dev. Disord.* 36: 901–909.

Wright D, Howseman T. (2013) *Managing swallowing difficulties in patients with learning disabilities*. Available at http://www.jcn.co.uk/files/downloads/articles/09-2013-learning-disabilities.pdf. Accessed 27 November 2016.

Yeargin-Allsop M, Braun KVN, Doenberg NS, *et al.* (2008) Prevalence of cerebral palsy in 8-year-old children in three areas of the United States in 2002; a multisite collaboration. *Pediatrics* 121: 547–554.

3.8 Paediatric clinical dietetics and childhood nutrition

3.8.1 Introduction

Lisa Cooke and Jacqueline Lowdon

SECTION 3

Key points

- Paediatric dietetics is a medical speciality, and dietitians require postgraduate training.
- Children are not small adults; their physical and medical needs are different from those of adults.
- The nutritional needs for growth must always be considered in addition to any disease-related considerations.

Paediatric dietetics is a medical speciality, and dietitians require postgraduate training to become a specialist paediatric dietitian. Many medical experts view children as small adults, but this a fallacy. Continuous good nutrition during childhood is imperative and lays down the building blocks for a child's future health. Emerging evidence suggests that the child's diet and growth pattern in the first 2 years of life extrapolate to long-term health outcomes (Lanigan & Singhal, 2009; Singhal & Lucas, 2004).

There are 26 children's hospitals in the UK, with many more paediatric tertiary referral centres. Following the recent reorganisation of the health service, tertiary services have reduced in number, becoming more specialised and covering wider geographical areas (McColgan *et al.*, 2016). These specialist centres often manage patient groups on a shared care basis with the local dietitian in the patient's geographical area.

This chapter gives a brief overview of childhood nutrition and paediatric dietetics, discussing the importance of how a child grows and develops, growth monitoring, nutritional assessment, nutritional needs during childhood and the management of clinical diseases and conditions. *Clinical Paediatric Dietetics*, 4th edition (Shaw, 2015), should be consulted for more detailed information and dietetic management. Many of the topics also apply to adults, and further information can be found in the relevant chapters.

Dietetic care must always be supported by specialist paediatric supervision in clinical practice until dietetic competence has been achieved. Paediatric dietetics has a clear career pathway, and the British Dietetic Association (BDA) (www.bda.uk.com) has an active and supportive paediatric group. This group provides a student manual toolkit, so that departments can actively expose student dietitians to the paediatric speciality. As a newly qualified dietitian, or one embarking on a role that involves paediatric medicine, there is a self-directed learning pack that needs to be managed by a paediatric dietetic supervisor with relevant experience. The group produces diet sheets (through Nutrition and Diet Resources UK – www.ndr-uk.org) and position statements, and supports guideline production. It is also actively involved with a master's degree in paediatric dietetics as a distance learning course jointly hosted by Plymouth University and the BDA.

References

Lanigan J, Singhal A. (2009) Early nutrition and long-term health: a practical approach. *Proc. Nutr. Soc.* 68: 422–429.

McColgan M, Winch R, Clark SJ et al. (2016) The changing UK paediatric consultant workforce: report of the Royal College of Paediatrics and Child Health. *Archives of Disease in Childhood* 102:170–173.

Shaw V. (2015) *Clinical Paediatric Dietetics*, 4th edn. Chichester: Wiley.

Singhal A, Lucas A. (2004) Early origins of cardiovascular disease: is there a unifying hypothesis? *Lancet.* 363: 1642–1645.

Manual of Dietetic Practice, Sixth Edition. Edited by Joan Gandy.

Companion website: www.manualofdieteticpractice.com

3.8.2 Growth, nutritional assessment and nutritional requirements

Claire Bullock

The growth of an infant or child is very important, as abnormal growth and development in childhood is associated with morbidity and mortality. Poor growth can be an indicator of underlying disease, poor nutrition, neglect or a combination of these factors. Growth must be regularly and accurately monitored throughout infancy and childhood. Regular monitoring and plotting of weight, height and head circumference on growth charts can help identify whether a child is growing normally or abnormally. Anyone who weighs and measures a child or infant and plots these on a growth chart in the infant's Personal Child Health Record (PCHR; colloquially known as the red book), or *electronic personal child health record* (ePCHR; known as the eRedbook), should be suitably trained. Normal human growth can be divided into two distinctive sections – prenatal growth and postnatal growth.

Prenatal growth

The growth of an infant begins at conception, with the fastest growth period being between conception and birth; this accounts for approximately 30% of eventual height (Tasker *et al.*, 2008). Factors that determine growth during this period include maternal size, maternal nutrition and intrauterine environment. Hormonal factors such as insulin, insulin-like growth factor 2 (IGF-2) and human placental lactogen are important regulators of growth during this period (Tasker *et al.*, 2008).

Postnatal growth

Infancy

Weight

From birth to 24 months, growth is rapid; birthweight doubles in the first 5–6 months and trebles in the first year of life. The rate of growth is largely determined by the nutritional adequacy of the diet. The average weight gain during the first year of life, using the 50th centile for age of the UK–WHO growth charts, is shown in Table 3.8.1. During the second year, a toddler following the 50th centile gains 2.5–2.6 kg (Shaw, 2015).

Table 3.8.1 Average weight gain during the first year of life

Age (months)	Boys (g/week)	Girls (g/week)
1–3	240	210
4–6	130	120
7–9	80	75
10–12	65	60

Linear growth

The length of an infant reflects bone growth and is a better indicator of long-term growth and nutritional adequacy than weight. Expected linear growth is 25 cm during the first year and 12 cm during the second year of life (Thompson, 1998).

Head circumference

Expected rate of growth in head circumference is 1 cm/month in the first year and 2 cm in total for the second year (Thompson, 1998). This reflects the rapid brain growth and development.

Growth velocity

Growth velocity varies, depending on how an infant is being fed. A breastfed infant initially grows at a slower rate than a formula-fed infant.

Childhood

From 2 years until the onset of puberty, the rate of growth is slower and steadier than during infancy. Children gain approximately 2–3 kg in weight and 10 cm in height/year, declining to 6 cm/year until puberty when a further growth spurt occurs. During this period, growth is primarily dependent on the growth hormone (GH), providing that there is adequate nutrition (Tasker *et al.*, 2008).

Puberty

Puberty is defined as the period during which changes occur that are associated with the maturation of the gonads – testes in boys and ovaries in girls. During this period, growth is dependent on the action of GH, testosterone and oestrogen, which induce the characteristic growth spurt of puberty. Puberty starts earlier in females; therefore, they are taller than males between the ages of 10 and 13 years. In males, puberty generally occurs later and at a greater magnitude, resulting in a larger final adult height. On average, puberty usually starts at 10.5 and 12 years in girls and boys, respectively (Tasker *et al.*, 2008). Normal puberty usually occurs gradually over 18 months to 5 years.

General development

Children develop at different rates and stages. For premature infants, developmental age is calculated from the due date rather than date of delivery (DH, 2016). Physical and verbal developmental milestones are monitored. Those relating to food are:

- *11–12 months* – enjoys finger foods.
- *13–15 months* – begins to feed themselves very messily.
- *3–5 years* – uses a knife and fork.

Weaning

The European Society for Paediatric Gastroenterology, Hepatology and Nutrition recommends that weaning begin by 6 months but not before 4 months (17 weeks). Exclusive breastfeeding for about 6 months is desirable and should be continued throughout weaning, particularly in the early stages (Agostoni *et al.*, 2008). DH (1994) recommends that weaning not be delayed beyond 6 months, owing to the increased risk of nutrient and energy deficiencies. Developmental signs that an infant is ready for solids include:

- Putting objects and toys in the mouth.
- Chewing fists.
- Showing interest when others are eating.
- Being hungry between milk feeds or demanding more feeds and taking larger volumes.
- Being able to sit up and support the head.

At around 6 months, infants are generally more accepting of new tastes and textures, and learn to accept them quite quickly (DH, 2016). As weaning is a learning process, infants should be given the opportunity to learn to accept new tastes and textures. Some data suggests that up to 15 positive experiences may be needed for the successful acceptance of a target food (Birch *et al.*, 1987; Wardle *et al.*, 2005). The number of exposures required to reach food acceptance is also age-dependent. During the first year of life, a single positive exposure can lead to the acceptance of the novel item (Birch *et al.*, 1998). Early preferences can affect preferences for foods later in childhood (Beauchamp & Mennella, 2009). Table 3.8.2 shows the developmental stages of weaning, and Table 3.8.3 shows the key stages in the normal development of eating and drinking skills (Coulthard *et al.*, 2009; Northstone *et al.*, 2001; Winstock, 2005). Infants should be offered a variety of foods on a daily basis to provide the required nutrients. Diet alone provides close to, or above, the recommended nutrient intake (RNI) for all vitamins except vitamin D (Bates *et al.*, 2016). Foods high in fat and sugar should not be included in the early weaning diet.

Food neophobia

By 12 months, infants should be eating family foods and be offered a wide range of foods. Food neophobia, when infants become wary of trying new foods, usually peaks at around 18 months. Infants who have a wide variety of family foods by 12 months are usually happy to continue accepting these foods. Between 3 and 5 years, children can develop disgust fears, and may consequently stop eating foods that they previously enjoyed. They often refuse foods that look like something they find disgusting. Children can also develop contamination fears; this often occurs at the same time, and, if a disliked food is put next to a liked food, then the child may refuse both foods (Shaw, 2015).

Nutritional assessment

A nutritional assessment can determine if a child suffers from malnutrition; in developed countries, malnutrition is usually associated with excess weight and inappropriate dietary habits rather than undernutrition. The information required for nutritional assessment should include dietary intake, anthropometric measurements (including height and weight), biochemistry and a clinical assessment that includes a physical examination and medical history.

Dietary intake

The methods for assessing dietary intake in children and young people include 24-hour recall, food frequency questionnaire, dietary history, food diary and weighed food intake. In most cases, it is possible to obtain sufficient information by discussing the children's diet with their parents or carers, and the children themselves, if appropriate. The differences between adults and children include meals and snacks at nursery or school; after-school clubs; bedtime food and drinks; staying with friends and relatives; and, for older children, eating out with friends. Assessing dietary intakes in babies and very

Table 3.8.2 Developmental stages of weaning (source: Shaw (2015). Reproduced with permission from John Wiley & Sons, Ltd.)

Stage	Age guide (months)	Skills to learn	New food textures to introduce
1	6, but not before 4 months (17 weeks) if parents choose to begin earlier	Taking food from a spoon Moving food from the front of the mouth to the back for swallowing Managing thicker purées and mashed food	Smooth purées Mashed foods
2	6–9	Moving lumps around the mouth Chewing lumps Self-feeding using hands and fingers Sipping from a cup	Mashed food with soft lumps Soft finger foods Liquids in a lidded beaker or cup
3	9–12	Chewing minced and chopped food Self-feeding attempts with a spoon	Hard finger foods Minced and chopped family foods

young children can be difficult, particularly if the infant is breastfed. It is possible to calculate how much milk a breastfed baby consumes by weighing the baby before and after each feed over 24 hours. In practice, this is rarely done, as it can cause anxiety. Questions about the length of time the infant feeds for, sleepiness during feeds, frequency of feeds, whether or not the breast is drained and the frequency of wet and dirty nappies are more appropriate and, combined with information about weight gain, can provide information about the likely milk intake. If mothers express breast milk and bottle-feed the baby, the ingested volumes can be easily determined. This would only be appropriate if the mother is returning to work, if the baby is ill and unable to breastfeed, or if the mother is leaving the baby for any length of time. For infants of weaning age, it can be difficult to assess the contribution from food to their overall intake due to the amount that is spat out or smeared around.

Anthropometry

The most widely used measures are weight and height, plus head circumference in infants, which is measured up to 2 years of age. An individual measurement is almost meaningless in isolation as it is impossible to determine whether or not a child is following a satisfactory growth pattern (Michaelsen *et al.*, 2000; Royal College of Nursing (RCN), 2013). Weight and length (or height) measurements should be taken whenever there are concerns about a child's weight gain, growth or development, in addition to routine checks (RCPCH, 2009). Sick infants and children who are hospital inpatients should be weighed at least once a week, and these measurements should be plotted on a centile chart (RCN, 2014).

Growth charts

Growth charts are mathematically created reference curves based on population data to represent the normal genetic growth of healthy children living in a specific environment. There are several growth charts available for use in the UK. The World Health Organization (WHO, 2006) has published Child Growth Standards for infants and children up to the age of 4 years, using data from healthy, full-term infants exclusively breastfed for the first 4 months and partially for a year and weaned at 6 months (De Onis *et al.*, 2004). These growth charts set breastfeeding as the norm. The WHO growth standards are available in centiles, and as Z scores for weight for age, length/height for age, weight/height for age, and body mass index (BMI) for age, for children aged 0–4 years and 4–18 years. In 2007, the UK Department of Health (DH) adopted the WHO growth charts in the UK (DH, 2007) up to 4 years of age, after which the UK1990 charts are used. UK–WHO growth charts should be used for all new births after May 2009 (RCPCH, 2009).

UK–WHO charts

Four versions are available:

- 0–4 years: This should be used for preschool infants and toddlers requiring plotting of growth data in primary or secondary care up to 4 years. It is also suitable for moderately preterm infants (32–36 week gestation). The chart includes a BMI centile lookup and an adult height predictor. These include illustrations and instructions on the interpretation of head circumference (RCPCH, 2013).
- 2–18 years: This is mainly intended to assess the growth of school-age children and young people in primary or secondary care. The chart includes guidance

Table 3.8.3 Key stages in the normal development of eating and drinking skills (Winstock, 2005)

Age (months)	Oral motor skills	Food-related play
0–3	Rhythmical suckle with up and down jaw movements	Sucks well, calm, watches mother
	Sensitive gag reflex	
4–6	Touch of spoon elicits suck	Takes things to mouth
	Spits out food with forward–backward tongue movements	Blows bubbles with saliva
		Pats bottle
6–9	Jaw begins to stabilise	Holds food and toys
	Bites on cup	Desire for some control, messy, plays with food
	Tongue tip up, munching, gag reduces	
9–12	Tongues moves food from side to side	Enjoys playing with food
	Stabilisation of jaw	Can hold a spoon, poor control
	Chewing, closes lips on spoon, spills drink	Squeezes toys and food
12–18	Uses a controlled bite on a biscuit	Pretends to feed self, large teddy or person
	Chews efficiently with rotary tongue and jaw movement	Demands food
18–24	Chews with lips closed	Lifts cup to mouth
	Up and down sucking pattern on cup	Pretends to feed dolls
		Self-feeds, still messy

on the onset and progression of puberty, a BMI centile lookup, an adult height predictor and a mid-parental height comparator. The growth of most children aged less than 4 years should be plotted on the more detailed UK–WHO 0–4-year growth charts. However, children who have been plotted on the NICM chart up to 2 years can transfer onto the 2–18-year chart (RCPCH, 2013).

- Childhood and Puberty Close Monitoring Chart (CPCM) 2–20 years: This is a modification of the main school age chart and is intended for use in children with growth or nutritional problems, and is ideal for use in specialist clinics and special schools (RCPCH, 2013).
- Neonatal and Infant Close Monitoring Chart (NICMC): This is designed for plotting very preterm infants from 23 weeks of gestation, and term infants with early health problems who require close growth monitoring, until 2 years corrected age. This chart features low lines to monitor unusually short or underweight children and the date box system for gestational correction (RCPCH, 2013).

UK1990 charts

These charts were constructed using data from a large number of children in the UK during the late 1980s and describe typical but not necessarily healthy growing children. They are based on formula-fed infants and should be used for children born before May 2009.

Other charts

Charts are available for specific conditions: Down syndrome, Turner syndrome, Williams syndrome and sickle cell disease. Thrive lines are available for assessing faltering growth; separate charts are also available for plotting BMI and head circumference. All charts are gender specific and can be obtained from https://www.rcpch.ac.uk/resources/growth-charts.

Interpretation of centile lines

The UK–WHO growth charts consist of nine centile lines. The 50th centile represents the median for the population, and the 2nd and 98th centiles are two standard deviations (Z scores) above and below the median. The 0.4th centile identifies extremely low measurements, and only (0.4%) optimally growing children will fall in this centile (Wright & Parkinson, 2004).

Plotting on a growth chart

Growth monitoring requires accurate measurements and accurate plotting to see patterns of growth over time. The most common error when plotting growth charts is in calculating an infant's age incorrectly. Age should be calculated in weeks for at least the first 6 months of life, and thereafter in calendar months. If the point marked is within a quarter of a space of the centile line, the infant is described as being 'on the centile'. However, if they are further away, they should be described as being between the two centile lines, e.g. between the 0.4th and the 2nd centile.

Plotting and assessing newborn infants

A baby born after 37 weeks of gestation is considered full term and should be plotted at age 0. The UK–WHO growth charts do not have centile lines for the first 2 weeks after birth, and during this period percentage weight loss should be calculated. All infants tend to lose weight initially and then begin to regain their birthweight between days 3 and 5, and 80% will have regained their birthweight by 2 weeks of age (Wright & Parkinson, 2004). Recovery of birthweight by 2 weeks suggests that feeding is effective and that the child is well (RCPCH, 2009).

Calculating percentage weight loss

Percentage weight loss is the difference between the current weight and the birthweight, expressed as a percentage of the birthweight, i.e.:

$$\text{Amount of weight lost}\,(g) \div \text{birthweight}\,(g) \times 100$$

If babies have a weight loss of ≥10% at or before 2 weeks, they need careful assessment, as this may indicate a possible feeding problem or illness (RCPCH, 2009).

Preterm infants

Preterm charts have been produced using the UK1990 reference data (Cole, 1997). Preterm infants born at or after 32 weeks of gestation should be plotted on the preterm section of the 0–4-year growth chart until they have reached their expected date of delivery (EDD) plus 2 weeks, and then be plotted on the 0–4-year chart using gestational correction. Preterm infants born from 23 weeks of gestation should be plotted on the NICM chart.

Plotting with gestational correction

This should only be used for infants born before 37 weeks and adjusts the plot for the number of weeks an infant is born premature, e.g. infants born at 34 weeks' gestation are 6 weeks premature, and their growth should be corrected by 6 weeks. Measurements are plotted at the child's actual age with a dot, and then a line is drawn back the number of weeks the infant was preterm. This spot is marked with an arrow and shows the child's gestationally corrected centile. Gestational correction should continue until at least 1 year, and until 2 years for infants born before 32 weeks.

Adult height prediction

The UK–WHO 2–18-year charts include an adult height predictor and a parent height comparator. The adult height predictor allows you to estimate the child's adult height based on the current height, but with a regression adjustment to allow for the tendency of very tall and short children to be less extreme in height as adults. This chart does not compare the height of children to that of their parents, and so is more useful for families where one or both parent(s) is/are not the biological parent(s). Eighty percent will have a final adult height within ±6 cm of the predicted adult height (RCPCH, 2015).

Using the parent height comparator gives the mid-parental centile, which is the average adult height centile to be expected for all children of these parents. It incorporates a regression adjustment to allow for the tendency of very tall and short parents to have children with less extreme heights. This means that children of very short or tall parents will have mid-parental centiles nearer to average than might be expected. Comparing the mid-parental centile to the child's current height centile can assess whether the child's growth is proceeding as expected. The larger the discrepancy between the two, the more likely it is that the child has some sort of growth disorder. Most children's height centiles are within ±2 centile spaces of the mid-parental centile, and only 1% will be more than three centile spaces below. Most of these will have no underlying medical condition, but if there are other concerns, a height centile well below the mid-parental centile should be investigated further. A child growing abnormally may still be within mid-parental height range, so any child with obviously abnormal slow growth (e.g. a fall of more than 2 centile spaces) should be investigated whatever their parental heights (RCPCH, 2015).

Growth assessment recommendations

As part of the Healthy Child Programme, children should be routinely assessed to identify the early signs of obesity, and interventions offered from an early stage. The Child Growth Foundation (2012) recommends that infants and children be routinely measured, as shown in Table 3.8.4. If there are concerns, infants and children may be weighed more often, but weighing at intervals too close together is misleading and can cause parental anxiety. Therefore, the recommended frequency of weighing (RCPCH, 2009) is:

- No more than once a month between 2 weeks and 6 months of age.
- Once every 2 months in infants between 6 and 12 months of age.
- Once every 3 months in children over the age of 1 year.

This frequency of weighing should reflect the progressive slowing of weight gain in the first year (Wright *et al.*, 2010). However, in practice, it is common for babies under 6 months to be weighed fortnightly, and those over 6 months monthly if there are concerns about their weight.

Anthropometric measurements

Head circumference

Use a narrow, non-stretch, plastic or disposable paper tape to measure where the head (uncovered) circumference is

Table 3.8.4 Recommended measurements for infants and children (source: Child Growth Foundation, 2012. Reproduced with permission from the Child Growth Foundation, www.childgrowthfoundation.org)

Age	Weight	OFC	Length	BMI	Notes
Birth	X		X or 10 days		Weight: assess malnutrition using 5%/95% thrive line acetates, or if weight/length centiles differ by over 2 centile bands. To resolve any concern: if infant is <6 months, weigh fortnightly; if >6 months, weigh monthly
24–30 hours		X			
5 days	X				
10 days	X		X		OFC: refer ASAP if OFC curve climbs significantly upwards through centile bands. To resolve concern, measure fortnightly
14 days		X			Length: use length predominantly to confirm malnutrition and consider referral (for either slow/excess growth) after three measurements. To resolve concern, measure 3-monthly
6–8 weeks	X	X			
12 weeks	X				
16 weeks	X				
6–8 months	X		X		
12–15 months	X		X	X	
2 years	X		X	X	BMI: Having monitored weight gain/length during infancy, measure both height and weight from approximately 1 year, calculate BMI and refer if indicated. To resolve any concern, calculate BMI 6-monthly and, similarly, refer
3 years	X		X	X	
4 years	X		X	X	
Primary school	X		X	X	BMI: The National Child Measurement Programme (NCMP) measures the height and weight of children in the Reception class (aged 4–5) and year 6 (aged 10–11). Payments for the BMI assessment of all secondary-school-age children of ≥16 years are available under the quality and outcomes framework (QoF)
Year 1					
Year 2	X		X	X	
Year 3	X		X	X	
Year 4	X		X	X	
Year 5	X		X	X	
Year 6	X		X	X	
Secondary school	X		X	X	

OFC, occipitofrontal circumference; BMI, body mass index.

greatest. Three measurements should be made, and the average recorded. UK children have relatively large heads compared with the WHO standard, particularly after 6 months. After 6 weeks, a head circumference below the 2nd centile will only be seen in 1 in 250 children. A head circumference above the 99.6th centile, or crossing upwards through two centile spaces, should only cause concern if there is a continued rise after 6 months, or other signs or symptoms. A number of genetic and acquired conditions will affect head growth, and the measurement of head circumference is not a useful indicator of nutritional status in these conditions (RCPCH, 2009).

Weight

Class III clinical electronic scales with only a metric setting should be used. These should be maintained and calibrated annually (DH, 2010; RCN, 2013). Infants and children under 2 years should be weighed naked on baby scales, to the nearest 10 g (RCN, 2013). Children over 2 years should be weighed in minimal clothing (ideally vest and pants, without shoes) to the nearest 100 g. Older children and adolescents should be weighed without shoes, wearing indoor clothing and with empty pockets. A child who is unable to sit or stand should be weighed in light clothing on a hoist scale (RCN, 2013). If it is not possible to weigh a child, tared weighing should be used: an adult is weighed without their shoes first, and then the undressed child is handed to the adult and the total weight is recorded. The weight of the adult is then subtracted from the total weight to obtain the child's weight (RCN, 2013). Best practice documentation would be to record that a tared weight was required, state who was weighed and show both weights as well as the subtraction result for the child's weight (RCN, 2013).

Length or height

Length is measured in infants and toddlers up to 2 years; height is measured thereafter. Length and height reflect bone growth and are a better indicator of long-term growth and nutritional adequacy than weight. Infants under 2 years should be measured without a nappy or footwear while lying on a length board or mat (RCPCH, 2009). A child's height is usually slightly less than its length due to spinal compression; therefore, the centile lines on the UK–WHO chart shift down slightly at age 2 years to allow for this (RCPCH, 2009). Height is measured using a rigid upright measure with a T piece or a stadiometer, without shoes (RCPCH, 2009). The head should be positioned in the Frankfurt plane, and the ear hole should be lined up with the bottom of the eye socket. If a child over 2 years of age cannot stand, measure length lying down with a Dunmow measure and plot as for height (obtainable from www.healthforallchildren.com).

Weight/height indices

Body mass index

BMI is a useful indicator of fatness and thinness in children from the age of 2 years, when height can be measured with relative accuracy. However, BMI is age dependent and is therefore plotted on centile charts, rather than being read as an absolute number. The 2–18-year growth chart includes a BMI centile look-up and should be used if the weight is above the 75th centile or if the weight and height centiles differ. The child's weight centile is plotted against the height centile, and the corresponding BMI centile is marked on the chart. A child whose weight is average for their height will have a BMI between the 25th and 75th centiles, whatever their height centile. A BMI above the 91st centile suggests overweight; above the 98th centile very overweight (clinically obese) and above the 99.6th centile is severely obese. BMI below the 2nd centile is unusual and may reflect undernutrition, but may simply reflect a small build or low muscle mass (RCPCH, 2015).

Separate BMI charts are available from RCPCH (2013) for use when severe overweight or underweight is a concern, or where there is a need for monitoring. This chart requires calculating and plotting of the BMI. In addition to the usual nine centile lines, the BMI chart displays high lines at +3, +3.33, +3.66 and+4 SD, which can be used to monitor the progress of children in overweight treatment programs. The chart also displays low lines at −4 and −5 SD for those who are severely underweight. Children whose BMI lies below the 0.4th centile are likely to have additional problems and, if not already receiving medical or dietetic attention, should be referred (RCPCH, 2013).

Mid-upper-arm circumference

Mid-upper-arm circumference (MUAC) indicates body fat distribution and can be used to determine malnutrition in children. It can be used as an independent anthropometric assessment tool in determining malnutrition in children aged 6–59 months when compared with the standards developed by WHO (Mei *et al.*, 1997). MUAC may be used for children with renal or liver disease where the presence of fluid overload or ascites makes weight inaccurate. When combined with the triceps skinfold measurement, upper arm muscle and fat stores can be estimated, and these measures correlate well with total body measures of fat mass and fat-free mass (Zemel *et al.*, 1997). MUAC has been correlated to BMI in children (Schweizer & Gerver, 2005), and may also have potential as a simple indicator of overweight and overfatness in children and adolescents (Craig *et al.*, 2014), although further studies are required to confirm this.

Skinfold thickness

Measurement of skinfold thickness can be used to assess nutrition in young infants and older children, but this can be difficult to perform. The process is the same as that for adults, and prediction equations for skinfold thickness are available for children. These measurements are not performed routinely, owing to the distress it can cause children; however, it is used in research, HIV, and renal and liver diseases.

Height age

Height age is the age at which the measured height of the child falls on the 50th centile. Calculation of height age is necessary when determining nutrient requirements for children who are much smaller or taller than their chronological age (Shaw, 2015).

Percentage height for age

Height for age is a measure of linear growth, and a faltering of linear growth is called stunting. Linear growth retardation is generally considered to reflect long-term exposure to nutritional stresses, including an inadequate diet and a high burden of infections, from which catch-up growth is insufficient (Richard *et al.*, 2012). A low height for age reflects a chronic process and is used as an index of chronic undernutrition (WHO, 2003).

Percentage weight for height

Weight for height assesses the appropriateness of a child's weight as compared to its height. It is sensitive to acute nutritional disturbances, and a low weight for height is described as wasting, resulting from weight loss or a failure to gain weight. It can develop rapidly and be reversed rapidly, and is an index of acute undernutrition reflecting severe weight loss, which is often associated with acute starvation and/or severe illness (Michaelsen *et al.*, 2000). Decreased weight for height and height for age are both important risk factors for illness and death during childhood, and changes in weight appear to have a lagged effect on height during early childhood; weight is maintained or regained under periods of nutritional stress at the expense of height (Richard *et al.*, 2012). Both percentage weight for height and percentage height for age are used to classify malnutrition, as shown in Table 3.8.5.

National child measurement programme

All children in the UK in the reception school year (4–5 years) and year 6 (10–11 years) are invited to have their height and weight measured and BMI calculated. Results are sent to parents, which can be of particular benefit, as parents often cannot tell if a child is overweight or obese (Carnell *et al.*, 2005; Jeffery *et al.*, 2005).

Clinical assessment

The two major components of clinical assessment are the medical history and the physical examination. The medical history is similar to that of an adult. In addition, it is usual to obtain information about gestational age and birthweight, infant feeding history (breastfed or formula-fed, age when weaned) and weight trend. Visible signs and symptoms that suggest nutritional deficiencies are the same as in adults. In addition, bone changes owing to vitamin D or calcium deficiency will include craniotabes, parietal and frontal bossing, epiphyseal enlargement and beading of the ribs. A suspected deficiency should be confirmed by biochemical or haematological tests.

Table 3.8.5 Classification of malnutrition using weight for height and height for age (Waterlow, 1972)

Grade of malnutrition	Acute malnutrition (wasting)	Chronic malnutrition (stunting + wasting)
	Weight for height	Height for age
Normal	>90%	>95%
Grade 1 (mild)	80–90%	90–95%
Grade 2 (moderate)	70–80%	85–90%
Grade 3 (severe)	<70%	<80%

Biochemistry and haematology

Laboratory assessment is used primarily to detect subclinical deficiency states, and to confirm a clinical diagnosis. Age-specific normal ranges for biochemical and haematological tests need to be established and used. Table 3.8.6 provides a summary of some biochemical and haematological measurements. Urine is not commonly used for infants and children; a 24-hour urine collection is difficult in babies and children, and the usefulness of a single urine sample for nutritional tests is limited (Shaw, 2015).

Malnutrition screening tools

Malnutrition screening tools have been developed specifically for children admitted to the hospital. The purpose of nutritional screening is to identify patients at high nutritional risk, and it includes anthropometric assessment interpreted within the context of current illness, with the aim of preventing a further decline in nutritional status during hospitalisation (Thomas *et al.*, 2016).

The Nutrition and Hydration Report 2015 (NHS England, 2015) recommends nutritional screening on admission using one of the following nutritional screening tools:

- *STAMP* – the Screening Tool for the Assessment of Malnutrition in Paediatrics; a validated nutritional screening tool for use in hospitalised children aged 2–16 years (McCarthy *et al.*, 2012).
- *PYMS* – the Paediatric Yorkhill Malnutrition Score (PYMS) rates BMI, weight loss, changes in nutritional intake and the predicted effect of the current condition on nutritional status to give a score that reflects the degree of nutritional risk. It can be used in children aged 1–16 years (Gerasimidis *et al.*, 2009).
- *STRONGkids* – consists of a subjective clinical assessment of disease risk, nutritional intake and weight loss for children aged 0–18 years (Hulst *et al.*, 2010).

The absence of a gold standard to define undernutrition and to define nutritional risk in paediatrics has led to different approaches in validating these screening tools. A comparison of STAMP, PYMS and STRONGkids found variations in the identification and classification of malnutrition, as well as poor identification of children who, by anthropometric standards, were malnourished (Chourdakis *et al.*, 2016). Consequently, a consensus has

SECTION 3

Table 3.8.6 Biochemical and haematological tests relating to nutritional status in children (source: adapted from Shaw (2015), Table 1.6, p. 10. Reproduced with permission of John Wiley & Sons, Ltd.)

Nutrient	Test	Normal values in children	Comments
Biochemical tests			
Protein	Total plasma protein	55–80 g/L	Low levels reflect long-term, not acute, depletion
	Albumin	30–45 g/L	
Vitamin B_{12}	Plasma B_{12} value	263–1336 pmol/L	Low levels indicate deficiency
Vitamin C	Plasma ascorbate level	8.8–124 μmol/L	Low levels indicate deficiency
Vitamin A	Plasma retinol level	0.54–1.56 μmol/L	Low levels indicate deficiency
Vitamin D	Plasma 25-hydroxy cholecalciferol level	30–110 nmol/L	Low levels indicate deficiency
Vitamin E	Plasma tocopherol level	α-tocopherol 10.9–28.1 μmol/L	Low levels indicate deficiency
Copper	Plasma level	70–140 μmol/L	Low levels indicate deficiency
Selenium	Plasma level	0.76–1.07 μmol/L	Low levels indicate deficiency
	Glutathione peroxidise activity	>1.77 μmol/L	
Zinc	Plasma level	10–18 μmol/L	Low levels indicate deficiency
Haematology tests			
Folic acid	Plasma folate	7–48 nmol/L	Low levels indicate deficiency
	Red cell folate	429–1749 nmol/L	Low levels indicate deficiency
Haemoglobin	Whole blood	104–140 g/L	Levels <110 g/L indicate iron deficiency
Ferritin	Plasma level	5–70 μg/L	Low levels indicate depletion of iron stores. Ferritin is an acute-phase protein, and it increases during infection

not been reached regarding which screening tool to use for hospitalised children (Huysentruyt *et al.*, 2015).

Nutritional requirements

Infants and children must not be viewed as small adults as they require different nutrients at different levels and a different nutritional balance from adults. The Committee on Medical Aspects of Nutrition (DH, 1991) has established dietary reference values (DRVs) for infants, children and adolescents in the UK. Values have been set for infants fed on formula milks (whose nutrient intakes are dependent on the composition of the feed being offered), but not for breastfed infants, as breast milk is the best form of nutrition for an infant. DRVs are set for normal, healthy individuals. Individual requirements will vary due to age, gender, weight, height, stage of development, body stores, activity levels and genetic factors. Disease process is a further consideration in sick infants and children. It is important to remember to calculate energy requirements and nutrient intakes based on actual weight.

Fluid

Fluid requirements for infants and children are shown in Table 3.8.7. Breastfed babies will regulate fluid intake, and demand feeding will ensure that the infant gets the correct volume of milk and, therefore, nutrients (Shaw, 2015). Ideally, formula-fed infants should be fed on demand, and, for those under 6 months, a fluid intake of 150 mL/kg is required. After 6 months, once an infant has been weaned, fluid requirement drops to 120 mL/kg as food also contains water. After 1 year, thirst will determine how much fluid is taken (Shaw, 2015). In clinical practice, fluid requirements for children over 10 kg are estimated using the equations shown in Table 3.8.8. However, overweight children will require less than the calculated volume per kilogram. For underweight children, fluid requirements should be calculated for the child's actual weight, but they may require increased energy and protein for catch-up growth (Great Ormond Street Hospital, 2014).

Energy

Feeding infants younger than 6 months of age with 150 mL/kg, either with breast milk or formula, will meet their nutritional needs if they do not have raised requirements. Young children continue to have high energy needs, but have a small stomach capacity and often variable appetites (Thompson, 1998). Therefore, they require a nutrient-dense diet to meet needs, although, from 2 years of age, the fat content of their diet can be reduced and lower-fat dairy products can be used, as long as they are thriving, have a good appetite and consume a well-balanced diet. At 5 years, children can use fully skimmed milk if they also meet the preceding criteria. Energy requirements peak during the adolescent years, during their growth spurt. Children with low physical activity levels require less energy. Table 3.8.9

Table 3.8.7 Recommended intakes of fluid and electrolytes for infants and children

Age			RNI			
	Weight (kg)	Fluid (mL/kg)	Sodium		Potassium	
			(mmol/day)	(mmol/kg/day)	(mmol/day)	(mmol/kg/day)
Males						
0–3 months	5.9	150	9	1.5	20	3.4
4–6 months	7.7	150	12	1.6	22	2.8
7–9 months	8.9	120	14	1.6	18	2.0
10–12 months	9.8	120	15	1.5	18	1.8
1–3 years	12.6	90	22	1.7	20	1.6
4–6 years	17.8	80	30	1.7	28	1.6
7–10 years	28.3	60	50	–	50	–
11–14 years	43.1	50	70	–	80	–
15–18 years	64.5	40	70	–	90	–
Females						
0–3 months	5.9	150	9	1.5	20	3.4
4–6 months	7.7	150	12	1.6	22	2.8
7–9 months	8.9	120	14	1.6	18	2.0
10–12 months	9.8	120	15	1.5	18	1.8
1–3 years	12.6	90	22	1.7	20	1.6
4–6 years	17.8	80	30	1.7	28	1.6
7–10 years	28.3	60	50	–	50	–
11–14 years	43.8	50	70	–	80	–
15–18 years	55.5	40	70	–	90	–

RNI, reference nutrient intake (DH, 1991).

Table 3.8.8 Estimation of fluid requirements in children over 10 kg

Body weight (kg)	Estimated fluid requirement
11–20	100 mL/kg for the first 10 kg + 50 mL/kg for the next 10 kg
≥20	100 mL/kg for the first 10 kg + 50 mL/kg for the next 10 kg + 25 mL/kg thereafter

Table 3.8.9 Energy requirements for low physical activity levels in children (FAO/WHO, 1973)

Age	Energy for maintenance and growth as % of total energy expenditure (per kg actual body weight)
<3 months	90
9–12 months	85
2–3 years	77
4–5 years	72
9–10 years	74

gives an approximate guide to the levels of energy intake for maintenance and growth alone, with no allowance for energy for activity. For older children, energy requirements can be estimated by using prediction equations as used in adults.

Energy DRVs are intended only for use in healthy populations, not individuals or groups who require clinical management. Although exclusive breastfeeding is recommended for about the first 6 months of life, it is recognised that infants are fed in a variety of ways. Therefore, separate recommendations have been made for exclusively breastfed infants, breast-milk-substitute-fed infants and those in whom the method of feeding is mixed or unknown (SACN, 2011; particularly tables 14 and 15 in this report).

Protein

High protein intakes in the first 2 years of life may promote overweight and obesity in later life (Agostoni *et al.*, 2008; Michaelsen & Greer, 2014), although more research is needed to establish optimal protein intakes. Formula-fed infants receive on average 0.5g/kg/day more protein than breastfed infants (Michaelsen & Greer, 2014), and the growth of formula-fed infants is known to be faster than that of breastfed infants. Nevertheless, an adequate energy intake is essential at all ages.

SECTION 3

Vitamins and minerals

Vitamin and mineral requirements for healthy children are provided by the DRVs. In disease states, requirements for certain vitamins and minerals will be different for each clinical condition. Due to the risks of vitamin D deficiency in the UK, SACN (2016) recommend:

- A safe intake of 8.5–10 µ/day (340–400 IU) for all infants until 1 year of age, unless they are taking in excess of 500 mL of formula milk per day which is fortified with vitamin D.
- A safe intake of 10 µ/day for children aged 1–4 years.
- A recommended nutrient intake (RNI) of 10 µ/day, throughout the year, for everyone aged ≥4 years.

There was insufficient data to set RNIs for children aged less than 4 years, so safe intakes have been recommended. Vitamin D is free under the Healthy Start scheme for low-income families, either in isolation or as part of a multivitamin/multimineral product such as Abidec, Dalivit, and Ketovite liquid and tablets.

Acknowledgement

The editor acknowledges the prior contribution of Sarah Cawtherley and Claire Conway.

Further reading

Farell E. (2016) *BDA Food Fact Sheet: Complementary Feeding (Weaning)*. Available at www.bda.uk.com/foodfacts.

Great Ormond Street Hospital. (2014) *Great Ormond Street Nutritional Requirements for Children in Health and Disease*, 5th edn. Available at www.gosh.nhs.uk/parents-and-visitors/clinical-support-services/dietetics.

Lawson MS. (2005) Children: nutritional requirements. In: Caballero B, Allen L, Prentice A (eds) *Encyclopedia of Human Nutrition*, 2nd edn. London: Elsevier.

Platt MPW. (2009) Demand weaning: infants' answers to professional dilemmas. *Arch. Dis. Child.* 94: 79–80.

Royal College of Nursing (RCN). (2013) *Standards for the Weighing of Infants, Children and Young People in the Acute Health Care Setting*. London: RCN.

Shaw V. (2015) *Clinical Paediatric Dietetics*, 4th edn. Oxford: John Wiley & Sons, Ltd.

Winstock A. (2005) Eating and Drinking Difficulties in Children. A Guide for Practitioners. Milton Keynes: Speechmark Publishing Ltd.

Internet resources

Child growth foundation, www.childgrowthfoundation.org

European Society for Paediatric Gastroenterology Hepatology and Nutrition (ESPGHAN), http://www.espghan.org

Infant and Toddler Forum, www.infantandtoddlerforum.org

RCPCH Growth Charts, https://www.rcpch.ac.uk/resources/growth-charts

Royal College of Paediatrics & Child Health (RCPCH), www.rcpch.ac.uk

STAMP screening tool, www.stampscreeningtool.org

World Health Organization (WHO) Child Growth Standards, www.who.int/childgrowth/en

References

Agostoni C, Decsi T, Fewtrell M, *et al.* (2008) Complementary feeding: a commentary by the ESPGHAN Committee on Nutrition. *J. Pediatr. Gastroenterol. Nutr.* 46: 99–110.

Bates B, Cox L, Nicholson S, *et al.* (eds). (2016) National Diet and Nutrition Survey Results from Years 5 and 6 (combined) of the Rolling Programme (2012/13–2013/14). London: Public Health England.

Beauchamp GK, Mennella JA. (2009) Early flavor learning and its impact on later feeding behavior. *J. Pediatr. Gastroenterol. Nutr.* 48(Suppl 1): S25–30.

Birch LL, McPhee L, Shoba BC, *et al.* (1987) What kind of exposure reduces children's food neophobia? *Looking vs. tasting. Appetite.* 9(3): 171–178.

Birch LL, Gunder L, Grimm-Thomas K, *et al.* (1998) Infants' consumption of a new food enhances acceptance of similar foods. *Appetite* 30(3): 283–295.

Carnell S, Edwards C, Croker H, *et al.* (2005) Parental perceptions of overweight in 3–5 year olds. *Int. J. Obes. (Lond.)* 29: 353–355.

Child Growth Foundation (CGF). (2012) *Growth Assessment Recommendations*. Milton Keynes: CGF.

Chourdakis M, Hecht C, Gerasimidis K, *et al.* (2016) Malnutrition risk in hospitalized children: use of 3 screening tools in a large European population. *Am. J. Clin. Nutr.* 103: 1301–1310.

Cole TJ. (1997) Growth monitoring with the British 1990 growth reference. *Arch. Dis. Child.* 76(1): 47–49.

Coulthard H, Harris G, Emmett P. (2009) Delayed introduction of lumpy foods to children during the complementary feeding period affects child's food acceptance and feeding at 7 years. *Matern. Child Nutr.* 5: 75–85.

Craig E, Bland R, Ndiranju J, et al. (2014) Use of mid-upper arm circumference for determining overweight and overfatness in children and adolescents. *Arch. Dis. Child.* 99: 763–766.

De Onis M, Garza C, Victora CG, *et al.* (2004) The WHO Multicentre Growth Reference Study: planning, study design and methodology. *Food Nutr. Bull.* 25(1): S15–S26.

DH. (1991) Report on Health and Social Subjects No 41. *Dietary Reference Values for Food Energy and Nutrients for the United Kingdom*. London: The Stationery Office.

DH. (1994) Report on Health and Social Subjects No 45. *Weaning and the Weaning Diet*. London: The Stationery Office.

DH. (2007) *Application of the WHO Growth Standards in the UK*. Department of Health. Available at https://www.gov.uk/government/publications/sacn-application-of-who-growth-standards-in-the-uk.

DH. (2010) Estates and facilities alert: Medical patient weighing scales. Ref: EFA/2010/001. Available at https://www.health-ni.gov.uk/sites/default/files/publications/health/EFA-2010-001A_0.pdf. Accessed 15 October 2018.

DH. (2016) *Birth to Five*. Available at https://www.nhs.uk/start4life/. .

FAO/WHO. (1973) Energy and Protein Requirements: Report of a joint FAO/WHO ad hoc expert committee. FAO Nutrition Meetings Report Series No. 52. WHO Technical Report Series No. 522. Rome and Geneva: FAO/WHO.

Gerasimidis K, Keane O, Macleod I, *et al.* (2009) Criterion validity and interrater reliability of the Paediatric Yorkhill Malnutrition Score. *J. Paediatr. Gastroenterol. Nutr.* 48(Suppl 3): E76.

Great Ormond Street Hospital. (2014) *Great Ormond Street Nutritional Requirements for Children in Health and Disease*, 5th edn. Available at www.gosh.nhs.uk/parents-and-visitors/clinical-support-services/dietetics.Accessed 15 October 2018.

Hulst J, Zwart H, Hop W, *et al.* (2010) Dutch national survey to test the STRONGkids nutritional risk screening tool in hospitalised children. *Clin. Nutr.* 29: 106–111.

Huysentruyt K, Devreker T, Dejonckheere J, *et al.* (2015) Accuracy of Nutritional Screening Tools in assessing the risk of undernutrition in hospitalized children. *J. Pediatr. Gastroenterol. Nutr.* 61(2): 159–166.

Jeffery AN, Voss LD, Metcalf BS, *et al.* (2005) Parents' awareness of overweight in themselves and their children: cross sectional study within a cohort (EarlyBird 21). *BMJ.* 330: 23–24.

McCarthy H, Dixon M, Crabtree I, *et al.* (2012) The development and evaluation of the Screening Tool for the Assessment of Malnutrition in Paediatrics (STAMP©) for use by healthcare staff. *J. Hum. Nutr. Diet.* 25: 311–318.

Mei Z, Grummer-Strawn LM, de Onis M, *et al.* (1997) The development of MUAC-for-age reference data recommended by a WHO expert committee. *WHO Bulletin* 75: 11–18.

Michaelsen KF, Weaver L, Branca F, *et al.* (2000) *Feeding and Nutrition of Infants and Young Children*. WHO Regional Publications, European Series, No 87. Denmark: WHO.

Michaelsen KF, Greer FR. (2014) Protein needs early in life and long-term health. *Am. J. Clin. Nutr.* 99(3): 718S–722S.

National Institute for Clinical Excellence (NICE). (2012) *Nutrition Support in Adults QS24*. Available at www.nice.org.uk/guidance/qs24/chapter/Quality-statement-1-Screening-for-the-risk-of-malnutrition. Accessed 15 October 2018.

NHS England. (2015) *Guidance – Commissioning Excellent Nutrition and Hydration 2015–2018*. Available at www.england.nhs.uk/wp-content/uploads/2015/10/nut-hyd-guid.pdf. Accessed 15 October 2018.

Northstone K, Emmett P, Nethersole F, *et al.* (2001) The effect of age of introduction to lumpy solids on foods eaten and reported feeding difficulties at 6 and 15 months. *J. Hum. Nutr. Diet.* 14: 43–54.

Richard SA, Black RE, Checkley W. (2012) Revisiting the relationship of weight and height in early childhood. *Adv. Nutr.* 3(2): 250–254.

Royal College of Nursing (RCN). (2013) *Standards for the Weighing of Infants, Children and Young People in the Acute Health Care Setting*. London: RCN.

Royal College of Nursing (RCN). (2014) *Malnutrition. What Nurses Working with Children and Young People Need to Know and Do*, 2nd edn. An RCN Position Statement. London: RCN.

Royal College of Paediatrics and Child Health (RCPCH). (2009) UK–WHO Growth Charts – Fact Sheet 6: Plotting and Assessing Infants and Toddlers up to Age 4 Years. Available at https://www.rcpch.ac.uk/resources/growth-charts. Accessed 15 October 2018.

Royal College of Paediatrics and Child Health (RCPCH). (2013) *UK–WHO Growth Charts*. London: RCPCH. Available at https://www.rcpch.ac.uk/resources/growth-charts. Accessed 15 October 2018.

Royal College of Paediatrics and Child Health (RCPCH). (2015) *Fact Sheet: UK 2–18 Years Growth Charts, 2nd edn*. Available at https://www.rcpch.ac.uk/resources/growth-charts

SACN. (2011) *Dietary Reference Values for Energy*. London: The Stationery Office.

SACN. (2016) *Vitamin D and Health*. Available at https://www.gov.uk/government/publications/sacn-vitamin-d-and-health-report. Accessed 15 October 2018.

Schweizer J, Gerver WJ. (2005) Mid-upper arm circumference is a reliable predictor of body-mass index in healthy Dutch children. *J. Pediatr. Gastroenterol. Nutr.* 40: 695.

Shaw V. (2015) *Clinical Paediatric Dietetics*, 4th edn. Oxford: John Wiley & Sons, Ltd.

Tasker R, McClure R, Acerini C. (2008) *Oxford Handbook of Paediatrics*. Oxford: Oxford University Press.

Thomas PC, Marino LV, Williams SA, *et al.* (2016) Outcome of nutritional screening in the acute paediatric setting. *Arch. Dis. Child.* 101(12): 1119–1124.

Thompson JM (ed). (1998) *Nutritional Requirements of Infants and Young Children. Practical Guidelines*. Oxford: Blackwell Science.

Wardle J, Carnell S, Cooke, L. (2005) Parental control over feeding and children's fruit and vegetable intake: how are they related? *J. Am. Diet. Assoc.* 105(2): 227–232.

Waterlow JC. (1972) Classification and definition of protein–calorie malnutrition. *BMJ.* 3: 566–569.

WHO. (2006) Multicentre Growth Reference Study Group. Assessment of differences in linear growth among populations in the WHO Multicentre Growth Reference Study. *Acta Paediatr.* 450 (Suppl): 56–65.

WHO. (2003) *WHO Child Growth Standards*. Available at www.who.int/childgrowth/en. Accessed 15 October 2018.

Winstock A. (2005) *Eating and Drinking Difficulties in Children. A Guide for Practitioners*. Milton Keynes: Speechmark Publishing Ltd.

Wright C, Lakshman R, Emmett P, and Ong K K. (2006) Implications of adopting the WHO 2006 Child growth standard in the UK: two prospective cohort studies. *Arch. Dis. Child.* 93(7): 566–559.

Wright CM, Parkinson KN. (2004) Postnatal weight loss in term infants: what is normal and do growth charts allow for it? *Arch. Dis. Child. Fetal Neonatal Ed.* 89(3): F254–F257.

Wright CM, Williams AF, Elliman D, *et al.* (2010) Using the new UK–WHO growth charts. *BMJ.* 340: 1140.

Zemel BS, Riley EM, Stallings VA. (1997) Evaluation of methodology for nutritional assessment in children: anthropometry, body composition, and energy expenditure. *Annu. Rev. Nutr.* 17: 211–235.

SECTION 3

3.8.3 Growth faltering

Luise V. Marino and Rosan Meyer

Many terms are used interchangeably for growth failure, including malnutrition, faltering growth and undernutrition, but they do not necessarily describe the same level of undernutrition. Although protein–energy malnutrition (PEM) was historically seen as a nutritional deprivation, particularly among children in developing countries, and faltering growth in more affluent societies, it is now acknowledged that both occur in developed and developing countries (Victora *et al.*, 2010). The main difference between PEM and growth faltering is that the latter is a dynamic process of weight/height reduction over time, whereas PEM is a static measurement at a point of time (Olsen *et al.*, 2007; WHO, 2012). Many assessment methods exist to define the dynamic process of faltering growth, including the following (Joosten & Hulst, 2011; Olsen *et al.*, 2007):

- Inadequate growth or weight gain for >1 month in a child under 2 years.
- Weight crossing more than two centiles in >1 month in a child under 2 years.

- Weight loss or no weight gain for >3 months in a child older than 2 years.
- Change in weight for age of>−1 standard deviation (SD) in 3 months for children under 1 year of age on growth charts.
- Change in weight for height of>−1 SD in 3 months for children aged 1 year or older on growth charts.
- Decrease in height velocity of 0.5–1 SD/year at under 4 years and 0.25 SD/year at older than 4 years of age.
- Decrease in height velocity of >2 cm from preceding year during early/mid-puberty.

The most common definition of growth faltering in the UK is weight crossing more than two centiles downwards over 1 month. This would be equal to −0.68 of a Z score, indicating that a child may have weight faltering, but is not yet malnourished according to the WHO definition, e.g. moderate malnutrition using the WHO definition is≤−2 Z scores.

Prevalence

The prevalence of growth faltering among healthy infants in the UK at 6–8 weeks has been reported as 6.1% (McDougall *et al.*, 2009), and it is believed that, in the general infant and toddler population, 5–9% develop growth faltering (Grimberg *et al.*, 2009; McDougall *et al.*, 2009). The prevalence of short stature in the general UK population is reported as being 2.3%. Being short in stature as a result of growth faltering has a more detrimental long-term effect on health than being acutely undernourished. Acute undernutrition has little impact on cognitive development if addressed, as compared to severe and prolonged malnutrition (Rudolf & Logan, 2005; Victora *et al.*, 2010). Most growth faltering occurs between 6 and 18 months (Leroy *et al.*, 2014). In addition, globally, 70% of absolute deficit accumulated in height at 60 months was found to be due to faltering during the first 1000 days (conception to 24 months), but 30% was due to continued increases in deficit in those aged 2–5 years (Leroy *et al.*, 2014).

Chronically ill children have a higher prevalence of growth faltering, ranging from 14% to 24% (Joosten & Hulst, 2011; Pawellek *et al.*, 2008; Pichler *et al.*, 2014); and, in middle income countries such as South Africa and Turkey, it is 34–40% (Groleau *et al.*, 2014). The prevalence of undernutrition within a hospital setting has remained unchanged for 20 years (Sullivan, 2010), although the absolute number of children with malnutrition defined as<−2 z scores is considerably lower at 3.1–7% (Thomas *et al.*, 2016). It is important that dietitians recognise growth faltering early and know how to nutritionally manage the condition.

Children considered to be at a greater nutritional risk include:

- Poorer socioeconomic groups (Panter-Brick *et al.*, 2004).
- Ethnic minorities (Panter-Brick *et al.*, 2004).
- Underlying medical condition (Levy *et al.*, 2009; Staiano, 2003).
- Extreme food fussiness (Haas, 2010; Haas & Maune, 2009).

Growth monitoring

Growth monitoring is essential. There are numerous growth charts, as discussed in Chapter 3.8.2 (Growth, nutritional assessment and nutritional requirements), and it is important that the correct ones be used and the measurements plotted correctly.

Normal growth

Optimal growth is vital, as poor growth impacts on school performance and cognitive development, has been associated with impaired health, and reduces educational and economic performance in adulthood (Dewey & Begum, 2011; Rudolf & Logan, 2005). Poor growth is associated with increased risk of morbidity, mortality and prolonged length of hospital stay (Hecht *et al.*, 2015). Intrauterine growth is the most rapid of all growth; the average birthweight in the UK is 3.3–3.5 kg. Birthweight loss occurs in the first few days of life (up to 10% is physiologically acceptable), and this is more common in exclusively breastfed infants (Cole *et al.*, 2012; de Onis *et al.*, 2004). It can take up to 2 weeks for an infant to regain this weight loss, which is reflected in the UK–WHO growth charts (Cole *et al.*, 2012).

Plotting faltering growth on a growth chart

To identify a child at risk of growth faltering, it is important to review its growth trend. Figure 3.8.1 shows examples of growth curves (which can be applied to length or height and weight); children with the growth curves b or c would be considered to have malnutrition, with Z scores of <2. This can be plotted electronically (www.who.int/growthref/tools/en).

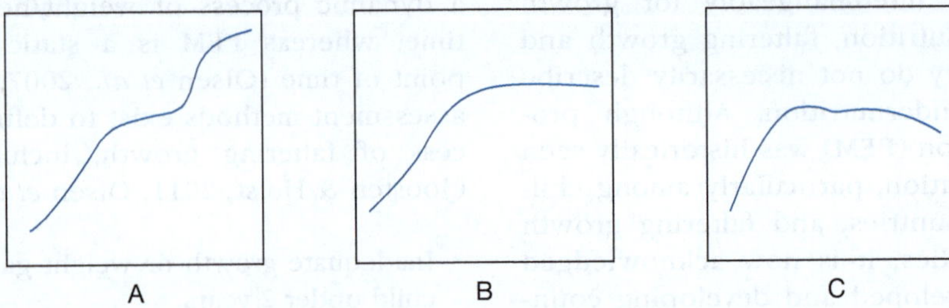

Figure 3.8.1 Examples of growth curves. (A) Growing well; (B) growth faltering; (C) malnutrition (source: WHO, 2009. Reproduced with permission from WHO)

Frequency of monitoring, catch-up growth and follow-up

As would be expected, weight gain is a dietary goal; all children with growth faltering should be followed up, initially monthly (UNICEF, 2005), and, when the child has caught up one to two centiles, or has a weight for height of greater than 90%, or 1 SD increase has been reached, supplementation should be reviewed. At this stage, the child is considered to be nutritionally rehabilitated (Patel *et al.*, 2005).

Acute and chronic growth faltering

It is important to establish if growth faltering is acute or chronic, as this impacts on nutritional management. This can be established by the following (Golden, 2009):

- Acute growth faltering – normal length/height but low weight for height/age. This normally represents an acute event of short duration, e.g. a short episode of illness.
- Chronic growth faltering – short length for age but normal weight for height/length even though underweight for age (e.g. chronic illness such as end-stage renal failure), and represents persistent malnutrition with insufficient macro- and micronutrients to support appropriate growth.
- Acute on chronic growth faltering – short length/height for age but low weight for height/length and underweight for age (e.g. end stage renal failure with a recent lower respiratory tract infection).

Illness-related versus non-illness-related growth faltering

In the past, the terms organic and non-organic growth faltering have been used, but illness-related (medical causes) and non-illness-related faltering growth have been used more recently, which includes socioeconomic, behavioural and environmental factors (Mehta *et al.*, 2013). This better defines the aetiology of faltering growth and recognises the overlap between illness-related and non-illness-related faltering growth (Levy *et al.*, 2009). Ramsay *et al.* (2002) found that a significant number of the children who were classified as non-illness-related growth faltering had subtle neurodevelopmental disorders and pathophysiology (i.e. delayed sucking ability), but were otherwise medically well (Ramsay *et al.*, 2002). It is therefore important not to exclude subtle organic diseases, and to ensure good history-taking practices when establishing the origin of growth faltering.

Illness-related growth faltering

The reasons for poor growth in children with chronic disease is multifactorial and linked to increased requirements, reduced intake and disordered feeding. Children with chronic diseases, e.g. chronic lung disease, cardiac disorders, gastrointestinal disorders and neuromuscular disorders, often have laboured breathing, increased nutrient requirements and/or increased nutrient losses through vomiting and stool losses (Haas & Maune, 2009; Levy *et al.*, 2009; Wiskin *et al.*, 2011).

Non-illness-related growth faltering

Non-illness-related growth faltering relates to poor growth as a result of socioeconomic, behavioural and environment factors (Mehta *et al.*, 2013). This may include a disrupted feeding environment and also neglect. In addition, toddlers are fussy eaters (Jacobi *et al.*, 2003); pickiness narrows the variety of foods consumed by young children (Harding *et al.*, 2010), increasing the risk of being underweight and having nutrient deficiencies (Bowley *et al.*, 2007; Dovey *et al.*, 2008; Ekstein *et al.*, 2010). A degree of neophobia and pickiness is considered to be developmentally appropriate and usually has no impact on growth (Richman *et al.*, 1975; Wright *et al.*, 2007).

Nutritional assessment

Nutritional assessment should include anthropometry, dietary, biochemical and clinical assessment. In addition, it is important to examine a child for signs of acute weight loss by looking at fat distribution. It is important to distinguish between a well thin child who is genetically slender and a child who is growth faltering (UNICEF, 2005). In a child aged under 5 years, there should be a good layer of subcutaneous fat; it is important to consider the following (Figure 3.8.2):

- What do the arms, shoulders, legs and buttocks look like?
- Is there evidence of temporal or facial wasting?
- Are there bracelets of fat around the wrist?
- Are there rolls of fat on the thighs?
- Looking from the side – are there buttocks, or are they flat and sagging?
- Protruding ribs?
- Protruding hips?
- Does the stomach look out of proportion (e.g. distension)?

Iron deficiency anaemia should be considered. In addition to inadequate iron intake, excessive intake of milk (≥600 mL/day) is also associated with low ferritin and haemoglobin levels (Cowin *et al.*, 2001). Pallor is a sign of anaemia and is easiest seen on a child's palm. Compare the colour of skin on your palm to that of the child, grasping the child's hand gently on either side using one hand, but not bending the child's fingers backwards, as this restricts blood flow. If the palm is pale, then there is some evidence of palmar pallor; however, if the child's palm is white, there is severe palmar pallor, and iron treatment should be initiated.

Diet history

A detailed dietary history is invaluable, especially questions relating to feeding and dietary intake. Some

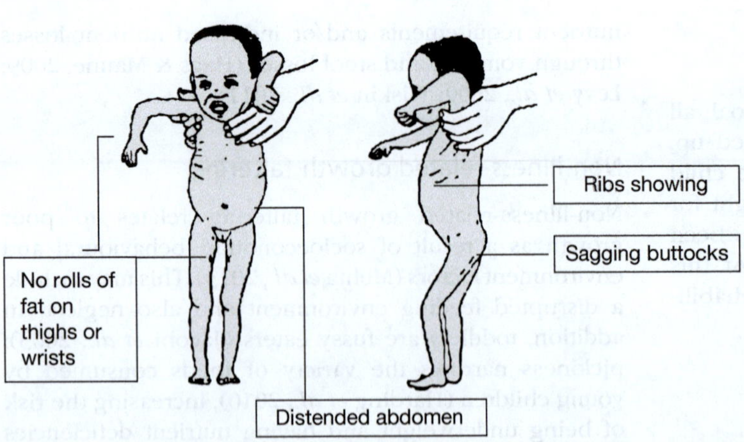

Figure 3.8.2 Appearance of an infant with severe wasting and growth faltering (source: WHO, 2009. Reproduced with permission from WHO)

useful questions to establish dietary and feeding patterns include:

- What type of milk is usually given to the child (include volume and frequency)?
- Are they still breastfed?
- What is the quantity of the main meal eaten? Is it appropriate?
- What is the meal like: Extended? Stressful?
- Did the child eat fish, meat or eggs in the last week, and/or were any foods excluded for religious or dietary reasons?
- Does the family have good access to food?

If the child's food intake is poor, it is important to assess whether the child has anticipatory gagging, vomiting, difficulty swallowing or chewing, poor appetite or frequent loose stools (Kerzner *et al.*, 2015; Levine *et al.*, 2011).

Dietary management

Requirements for catch-up growth

Energy and protein

Ideally validated energy and protein requirements for children with chronic disease and the faltering growth for that population are used. These vary greatly between populations, relating to the pathophysiology of disease, losses and management (De Onis *et al.*, 2010; Suman *et al.*, 2006; Wiskin & Beattie, 2008). Where no guidelines are available, the WHO/FAO/UNO guidelines for energy and protein requirements should be used (Joint WHO/FAO/UNU Expert Consultation, 2007). Protein requirements are based on actual body weight. The focus should be on weight gain and attaining growth with optimal balance between lean and fat mass (73% lean and 27% fat mass) in the accrued tissue (Joint WHO/FAO/UNU Expert Consultation, 2007). Optimal catch-up growth is not only dependent on sufficient energy delivery, but also adequate protein (see Table 3.8.10). An ideal protein–energy (PE) ratio for catch-up growth has been shown to be 8.9–12% (Golden, 2009; Pencharz, 2010). Enriching products with modular additions of fat and carbohydrate alone often results in PE of 4.5–6%, which does not favour optimal catch-up growth in growth faltering infants (Clarke *et al.*, 2007; Pencharz, 2010).

Table 3.8.10 Theoretical energy and protein intake for 5, 10 and 20 g/kg/day catch-up growth

Catch-up growth (g/kg/day)	Protein (g/kg/day)	Energy (kcal/kg/day)	Protein/energy (%)
5	1.82	105	6.9
10	2.82	126	8.9
20	4.82	167	11.5

Table 3.8.11 Rates of weight gain (g/kg/day) required to catch-up

Days	Gender	−1 to 0 z-score	−2 to −1 z score	−2 to 0 z-score
14 days	Male	5.8	5.7	11.4
	Female	6.3	6.1	12.4
20 days	Male	4.1	4.0	8.0
	Female	4.4	4.3	8.7
1 month	Male	2.7	2.6	5.3
	Female	3.0	2.9	5.8

Table 3.8.11 summarises the suggested catch-up rates for children with moderate malnutrition (Golden, 2009). It is recommended that a therapeutic diet for moderate malnutrition should lead to weight gain of 5 g/kg/day, but acknowledges the fact that some children have slower and others faster catch-up.

However, it is important to note that, in this population group, energy requirements are not always increased: attention to micronutrient status may be more important (Wiskin *et al.*, 2016).

Vitamins and minerals

It is important to ensure that children also receive sufficient vitamins and minerals that aid catch-up growth. Insufficient micronutrients, particularly zinc and vitamin A, can lead to suboptimal catch-up growth. Multiple micronutrient supplementation, including vitamins A and D, zinc and iron, is effective in promoting catch-up growth in children under 5 years and should be considered a routine supplement in growth faltering children (Bhaskaram, 2002; Golden, 2009; Ramakrishnan *et al.*, 2009).

Iron

Even mild iron deficiency anaemia (IDA) can have a long-term detrimental influence on mental and psychomotor development (Faldella *et al.*, 2003; Freeman *et al.*, 1998), although there are many confounders, including poverty, maternal education and prematurity (Aggett *et al.*, 2002). The management of IDA through iron-fortified foods or supplementation results in improved growth, although improvements in cognitive outcomes have been harder to define (Domellof, 2010). At-risk children should be encouraged to consume iron-rich foods as part of their daily diet.

Zinc

Zinc supplementation (10 mg/day<6 months; 20 mg/day>6 months) has been shown to significantly reduce morbidity in diarrhoeal disease and pneumonia (Aggarwal *et al.*, 2007; Bajait & Thawani, 2011; Krebs *et al.*, 2014). Zinc supplementation has also been shown to be effective in promoting linear growth (Krebs *et al.*, 2014; Ramakrishnan *et al.*, 2009). Zinc and iron supplementation should be given separately as zinc absorption is affected by iron, although this is seen more strongly with non-haem iron foods, e.g. fruit, vegetables, grains and nuts (Hunt, 2003; Olivares *et al.*, 2007).

Nutritional management of infants and children with faltering growth

This depends on the severity and type of growth faltering (illness-related or non-illness-related). It is important to have good communication skills and start by exploring the circumstances at home, including the child's early feeding history (UNICEF, 2005). Enriched home foods can initially be tried. Food enrichment should be achieved with foods that contain complex food matrix, such as nut butters, rather than just fats or sugar, e.g. cream, or carbohydrate. In more severe faltering growth, energy-dense ready-to-feed formula should be considered (Braegger *et al.*, 2010). Energy-dense, ready-to-feed formulae that deliver energy and protein at an appropriate PE ratio (PER) significantly improve growth and nitrogen status (Clarke *et al.*, 2007). Although it is common practice to increase the nutrient density of standard powdered formulas, attention must be paid to the PER, osmolality and renal solute load (King & Davis, 2010; Pereira-da-Silva *et al.*, 2008; Ziegler & Fomon, 1989).

For the older child, enriching home foods with both energy and protein is the first option; nutritionally complete sip feeds are also appropriate for this population. Wright and Chillingworth (2015) found that energy-dense sip feeds in children with feeding difficulties (with/without faltering growth) suppressed appetite due to energy displacement. The authors cautioned that failure to gain weight on an energy-dense sip feed may be an indication for enteral feeding. Where weight or length gain is not achieved, the nutrition care plan should include, e.g. moving from home-enriched foods to sip feeds and then to enteral tube feeding. However, practicality needs to be considered (Heuschkel *et al.*, 2015).

A time frame for nutrition support should be provided and outcome goals specified. For example, if a child is underweight for age and the target is 1 kg of weight gain, the estimated time to repletion should be calculated. The child's weight gain and growth should then be reviewed, and, if the goal has been achieved, it should be exited from the additional nutritional support. If the goal has not been achieved, further investigation should be undertaken to establish compliance, in addition to quantifying losses, e.g. vomiting or stool. Micronutrient support should also be provided during and following this period.

Psychological aspects of growth faltering

A child's intake can be influenced by parental interactions (Harris, 2010). The factors associated with poor intake may relate to poor appetite regulation (early satiety) (Drewett *et al.*, 2003), sensory hypersensitivity, late introduction of complementary foods and/or oral motor dysfunction. They may also have inherited parental traits of food fussiness, making them more likely to be neophobic and picky, which may impact on weight gain (Harris, 2010).

Behavioural management

Feeding difficulties can have a severe impact on growth, development and behaviour, resulting in significant parental anxiety. There may be no apparent medical cause for the child's extreme fussiness, although parents will often describe early-life feeding difficulties relative to reflux (Rommel *et al.*, 2003), food allergies (Haas, 2010), autism (Volkert & Vaz, 2013) and prematurity (especially gestational age of <34 weeks) (Volkert *et al.*, 2016). Guidelines on feeding difficulties are summarised in Table 3.8.12 (Kerzner *et al.*, 2015).

Feeding skills develop through practise and keen observance, along with developmentally appropriate complementary feeding choices within a responsive feeding environment. Disruption during this period (e.g. owing to illness), adverse reaction to food, or acute or chronic pain (e.g. gastro-oesophageal disease or psychosocial stress) can reinforce the idea that eating food means pain or discomfort, etc., and should therefore be avoided. This can lead to regression of feeding skills, non-acceptance of new foods and/or textures, and altered motivation and feeding practices, leading to parental frustration and anxiety, which is mirrored back to the child.

In children who have been unable to acquire age-appropriate feeding skills, mealtime avoidance strategies are common, e.g. tantrums; volume-limiting eating patterns to avoid pain, discomfort or anxiety; habitual gagging or vomiting; mouth sealing and food refusal; or limited variety of foods consumed (Haas, 2010; Kessler *et al.*, 2010). Feeding difficulties, especially those severe enough to result in growth faltering,

Table 3.8.12 Summary of symptoms for feeding difficulties (Kerzner et al., 2015)

Symptoms	Illness-related red flag signs	Non-illness-related red flag signs
Prolonged mealtimes	Dysphagia	Food fixation (selective, extreme dietary limitations)
Food refusal lasting >1 month	Aspiration	Noxious (forceful and/or persecutory) feeding
Disruptive and stressful mealtimes	Apparent pain with feeding	Abrupt cessation of feeding after a trigger event
Lack of appropriate independent feeding	Vomiting and diarrhoea	Anticipatory gagging
Nocturnal eating in toddler	Developmental delay	Failure to thrive
Distraction to increase intake	Chronic cardiorespiratory symptoms	
Prolonged breastfeeding or bottle-feeding	Growth failure (failure to thrive)	
Failure to advance textures		

are usually managed within a multidisciplinary team involving a physician, dietitian, speech and language therapist, psychologist, nurse, social worker and others (Davis *et al.*, 2009; Harding *et al.*, 2010; Rommel *et al.*, 2003). The management strategy is individualised and dependent on the severity of the type of feeding difficulty and the level of family involvement. Treatment may take the form of individual counselling sessions, group feeding programmes and/or a monitored home programme (Haas, 2010).

Behavioural management aspects in this programme aim to address hypersensitivity issues to texture, smell and taste of food through imaginative and messy play, aimed at promoting sensory integration and building the child's confidence around new food experiences, in addition to practising chewing skills. When trying to address issues related to texture and taste, changes should be implemented slowly and independently of each other, e.g. change one aspect of a meal at a time. It is also imperative to provide support to the parents. Video diaries of mealtimes provide insights into the behavioural patterns of the child and caregiver (Harding *et al.*, 2010). Useful techniques for parents at mealtimes include limiting the length of meal to 30 minutes or less, and reduction in reprimands, coercion and/or coaxing (Harding *et al.*, 2010; Kerzner *et al.*, 2015).

Severe to moderate malnutrition

Products such as F75 and F100, in addition to ready-to-use therapeutic food (RTUF), may be used. The benefit of RTUF over liquid feeds such as F75 and F100, which are reconstituted from powdered milk, is that the high fat content retards microbial growth (WHO, 1999; WHO/UNICEF, 2009). Bacterial contamination of powdered milk feeds is a significant problem and increases the risk of morbidity and mortality (Jalali *et al.*, 2009; Marino *et al.*, 2007).

Where possible, severely malnourished children are managed within a community environment with the aim of reducing the incidence of hospital-acquired infections (Manary *et al.*, 2004; Phuka *et al.*, 2009). Many studies have considered the benefits of RTUF in preventing growth faltering in high-risk communities, in addition to their use in severe acute malnutrition and famine relief settings (Golden, 2009; Isanaka *et al.*, 2015). The benefit of RTUF is high community acceptance, good taste, better catch-up growth, decreased bacterial contamination and no requirement for water (Manary *et al.*, 2004; Phuka *et al.*, 2009).

Internet resources

Growth charts

Cerebral Palsy Growth Charts, http://www.lifeexpectancy.org/articles/GrowthCharts.shtml

UKWHO Growth Charts, www.rcpch.ac.uk/child-health/research-projects/uk-who-growth-charts-early-years/uk-who-growth-charts-early-years

US Centers for Disease Control and Prevention Growth Charts, www.cdc.gov/growthcharts/cdc_charts.htm

WHO Child Growth Standards, www.who.int/childgrowth/standards/en/

References

Aggarwal R, Sentz J, Miller MA. (2007) Role of zinc administration in prevention of childhood diarrhea and respiratory illnesses: a meta-analysis. *Pediatrics.* 119(6): 1120–1130.

Aggett PJ, Agostoni C, Axelsson I, *et al.* (2002) Iron metabolism and requirements in early childhood: do we know enough? a commentary by the ESPGHAN Committee on Nutrition. *J. Pediatr. Gastroenterol. Nutr.* 34(4): 337–345.

Bajait C, Thawani V. (2011) Role of zinc in pediatric diarrhea. *Indian J. Pharmacol.* 43(3): 232–235.

Bhaskaram P. (2002) Micronutrient malnutrition, infection, and immunity: an overview. *Nutr. Rev.* 60(5 Pt 2): S40–S45.

Bowley NA, Pentz-Kluyts MA, Bourne LT, *et al.* (2007) Feeding the 1 to 7-year-old child. A support paper for the South African paediatric food-based dietary guidelines. *Matern. Child Nutr.* 3(4): 281–291.

Braegger C, Decsi T, Dias JA, *et al.* (2010) Practical approach to paediatric enteral nutrition: a comment by the ESPGHAN committee on nutrition. *J. Pediatr. Gastroenterol. Nutr.* 51(1): 110–122.

Clarke SE, Evans S, MacDonald A, *et al.* (2007) Randomized comparison of a nutrient-dense formula with an energy-supplemented formula for infants with faltering growth. *J. Hum. Nutr. Diet.* 20: 329–339.

Cole TJ, Wright CM, Williams AF. (2012) Designing the new UK-WHO growth charts to enhance assessment of growth around birth. *Arch. Dis. Child Fetal Neonatal. Ed.* 97(3): F219–F222.

Cowin I, Emond A, Emmett P. (2001) Association between composition of the diet and haemoglobin and ferritin levels in 18-month-old children. *Eur. J. Clin. Nutr.* 55(4): 278–286.

Davis AM, Bruce AS, Mangiaracina C, *et al.* (2009) Moving from tube to oral feeding in medically fragile nonverbal toddlers. *J. Pediatr. Gastroenterol. Nutr.* 49(2): 233–236.

de Onis M, Onyango AW, Van den Broeck J, *et al.* (2004) Measurement and standardization protocols for anthropometry used in the construction of a new international growth reference. *Food Nutr. Bull.* 25(1 Suppl): S27–S36.

De Onis WB, Meyer R, Desai A, *et al.* (2010) Challenge of predicting resting energy expenditure in children undergoing surgery for congenital heart disease. *Pediatr. Crit. Care Med.* 11(4): 496–501.

Dewey KG, Begum K. (2011) Long-term consequences of stunting in early life. *Matern. Child Nutr.* 7(Suppl 3): 5–18.

Domellof M. (2010) Benefits and harms of iron supplementation in iron-deficient and iron-sufficient children. *Nestle. Nutr. Workshop Ser. Pediatr. Program.* 65: 153–162.

Dovey TM, Staples PA, Gibson EL, *et al.* (2008) Food neophobia and 'picky/fussy' eating in children: a review. *Appetite.* 50 (2–3): 181–193.

Drewett RF, Kasese-Hara M, Wright C. (2003) Feeding behaviour in young children who fail to thrive. *Appetite.* 40(1): 55–60.

Ekstein S, Laniado D, Glick B. (2010) Does picky eating affect weight-for-length measurements in young children? *Clin. Pediatr. (Phila)* 49(3): 217–220.

Faldella G, Corvaglia L, Lanari M, *et al.* (2003) Iron balance and iron nutrition in infancy. *Acta Paediatr. Suppl.* 91(441): 82–85.

Freeman VE, Mulder J, van't Hof MA, *et al.* (1998) A longitudinal study of iron status in children at 12, 24 and 36 months. *Public Health Nutr.* 1(2): 93–100.

Golden MH. (2009) Proposed recommended nutrient densities for moderately malnourished children. *Food Nutr. Bull.* 30(3 Suppl): S267–S342.

Grimberg A, Ramos M, Grundmeier R, *et al.* (2009) Sex-based prevalence of growth faltering in an urban pediatric population. *J. Pediatr.* 154: 567–572.

Groleau V, Thibault M, Doyon M, *et al.* (2014) Malnutrition in hospitalized children: prevalence, impact, and management. *Can. J. Diet. Pract. Res.* 75(1): 29–34.

Haas AM. (2010) Feeding disorders in food allergic children. *Curr. Allergy Asthma Rep.* 10(4): 258–264.

Haas AM, Maune NC. (2009) Clinical presentation of feeding dysfunction in children with eosinophilic gastrointestinal disease. *Immunol. Allergy Clin. North Am.* 29(1): 65–75.

Harding C, Faiman A, Wright J. (2010) Evaluation of an intensive desensitisation, oral tolerance therapy and hunger provocation program for children who have had prolonged periods of tube feeds. *Int. J. Evid. Based Healthc.* 8(4): 268–276.

Harris G. (2010) The psychology behind growth faltering. *Eur. J. Clin. Nutr.* 64(Suppl 1): S14–S16.

Hecht C, Weber M, Grote V, *et al.* (2015) Disease associated malnutrition correlates with length of hospital stay in children. *Clin. Nutr.* 34 (1): 53–59.

Heuschkel RB, Gottrand F, Devarajan K, *et al.* (2015) ESPGHAN position paper on management of percutaneous endoscopic gastrostomy in children and adolescents. *J. Pediatr. Gastroenterol. Nutr.* 60 (1): 131–141.

Hunt JR. (2003) Bioavailability of iron, zinc, and other trace minerals from vegetarian diets. *Am. J. Clin. Nutr.* 78(3 Suppl): 633S–639S.

Isanaka S, Guesdon B, Labar AS, *et al.* (2015) Comparison of clinical characteristics and treatment outcomes of children selected for treatment of severe acute malnutrition using mid upper arm circumference and/or weight-for-height Z-score. *PLoS One.* 10(9): e0137606.

Jacobi C, Agras WS, Bryson S, *et al.* (2003) Behavioral validation, precursors, and concomitants of picky eating in childhood. *J. Am. Acad. Child Adolesc. Psychiatry.* 42(1): 76–84.

Jalali M, Sabzghabaee AM, Badri SS, *et al.* (2009) Bacterial contamination of hospital-prepared enteral tube feeding formulas in Isfahan, *Iran. J. Res. Med. Sci.* 14(3): 149–156.

Joint WHO/FAO/UNU Expert Consultation. (2007) Protein and Amino Acid Requirements in Human Nutrition, World Health Organization, 935.

Joosten KF, Hulst JM. (2011) Malnutrition in pediatric hospital patients: current issues. *Nutrition.* 27(2): 133–137.

Kerzner B, Milano K, MacLean WC Jr, *et al.* (2015) A practical approach to classifying and managing feeding difficulties. *Pediatrics.* 135(2): 344–353.

Kessler DB, Fortune EL, Werner EG, *et al.* (2010) 11-month-old twins with food avoidance. *J. Dev. Behav. Pediatr.* 31(3 Suppl): S112–S116.

King C, Davis T. (2010) Nutritional treatment of infants and children with faltering growth. *Eur. J. Clin. Nutr.* 64(Suppl 1): S11–S13.

Krebs NF, Miller LV, Hambidge KM. (2014) Zinc deficiency in infants and children: a review of its complex and synergistic interactions. *Paediatr. Int. Child Health* 34(4): 279–288.

Leroy JL, Ruel M, Habicht JP, *et al.* (2014) Linear growth deficit continues to accumulate beyond the first 1000 days in low- and middle-income countries: global evidence from 51 national surveys. *J. Nutr.* 144 (9): 1460–1466.

Levine A, Bachar L, Tsangen Z, *et al.* (2011) Screening criteria for diagnosis of infantile feeding disorders as a cause of poor feeding or food refusal. *J. Pediatr. Gastroenterol. Nutr.* 52: 563–568.

Levy Y, Levy A, Zangen T, *et al.* (2009) Diagnostic clues for identification of nonorganic vs organic causes of food refusal and poor feeding. *J. Pediatr. Gastroenterol. Nutr.* 48(3): 355–362.

Manary MJ, Ndkeha MJ, Ashorn P, *et al.* (2004) Home-based therapy for severe malnutrition with ready-to-use food. *Arch. Dis. Child* 89(6): 557–561.

Marino LV, Goddard E, Whitelaw A, *et al.* (2007) Prevalence of bacterial contamination of powdered infant feeds in a hospital environment. *S. Afr. Med. J.* 97(7): 534–537.

McDougall P, Drewitt RF, Hungin APS, *et al.* (2009) The detection of early weight faltering at the 6–8 week check and its association with family factors, feeding and behavioural development. *Arch. Dis. Child* 94: 549–552.

Mehta NM, Corkins MR, Lyman B, *et al.* (2013) Defining pediatric malnutrition: a paradigm shift toward etiology-related definitions. *JPEN J. Parenter. Enteral. Nutr.* 37(4): 460–481.

Olivares M, Pizarro F, Ruz M. (2007) New insights about iron bioavailability inhibition by zinc. *Nutrition.* 23(4): 292–295.

Olsen EM, Peterson J, Skovgaard AM, *et al.* (2007) Failure to thrive: the prevalence and concurrence of anthropometric criteria in a general infant population. *Arch. Dis. Child.* 92: 109–114.

Panter-Brick C, Lunn PG, Goto R, *et al.* (2004) Immunostimulation and growth faltering in UK infants. *Am. J. Hum. Biol.* 16(5): 581–587.

Patel MP, Sandige HL, Ndekha MJ, *et al.* (2005) Supplemental feeding with ready-to-use therapeutic food in Malawian children at risk of malnutrition. *J. Health Popul. Nutr.* 23(4): 351–357.

Pawellek I, Dokoupil K, Koletzko B. (2008) Prevalence of malnutrition in paediatric hospital patients. *Clin. Nutr.* 27(1): 72–76.

Pencharz PB. (2010) Protein and energy requirements for 'optimal' catch-up growth. *Eur. J. Clin. Nutr.* 64(Suppl 1): S5–S7.

Pereira-da-Silva L, Pitta-Gros DM, Virella D, *et al.* (2008) Osmolality of elemental and semi-elemental formulas supplemented with nonprotein energy supplements. *J. Hum. Nutr. Diet.* 21(6): 584–590.

Phuka J, Thakwalakwa C, Maleta K, *et al.* (2009) Supplementary feeding with fortified spread among moderately underweight 6–18-month-old rural Malawian children. *Matern. Child Nutr.* 5(2): 159–170.

Pichler J, Hill SM, Shaw V, *et al.* (2014) Prevalence of undernutrition during hospitalisation in a children's hospital: what happens during admission? *Eur. J. Clin. Nutr.* 68(6): 730–735.

Ramakrishnan U, Nguyen P, Martorell R. (2009) Effects of micronutrients on growth of children under 5 y of age: meta-analyses of single and multiple nutrient interventions. *Am. J. Clin. Nutr.* 89(1): 191–203.

Ramsay M, Gisel EG, McCusker J, *et al.* (2002) Infant sucking ability, non-organic failure to thrive, maternal characteristics, and feeding practices: a prospective cohort study. *Dev. Med. Child Neurol.* 44(6): 405–414.

Richman N, Stevenson JE, Graham PJ. (1975) Prevalence of behaviour problems in 3-year-old children: an epidemiological study in a London borough. *J. Child Psychol. Psychiatry.* 16(4): 277–287.

Rommel N, De Meyer A, Feenstra L, *et al.* (2003) The complexity of feeding problems in 700 infants and young children presenting to a tertiary care institution. *J. Pediatr. Gastroenterol. Nutr.* 37: 75–84.

Rudolf MCJ, Logan S. (2005) What is the long term outcome for children who fail to thrive? *Arch. Dis. Child* 90: 925–931.

Staiano A. (2003) Food refusal in toddlers with chronic disease. *J. Pediatr. Gastroenterol. Nutr.* 37: 225–227.

Sullivan PB. (2010) Malnutrition in hospitalised children. *Arch. Dis. Child* 95(7): 489–490.

Suman OE, Mlcak RP, Chinkes DL. (2006) Resting energy expenditure in severely burned children: analysis of agreement between indirect calorimetry and prediction equations using the Bland–Altman method. *Burns* 32(3): 335–342.

Thomas PC, Marino LV, Williams SA, *et al.* (2016) Outcome of nutritional screening in the acute paediatric setting. *Arch. Dis. Child.* 101(12): 1119–1124. doi:10.1136/archdischild-2016-310484

UNICEF. (2005) *IMCI Integrated Management of Childhood Illness.* Geneva.

UNICEF/WHO/World Bank (2012) Levels & Trends in Malnutrition Available at http://www.who.int/nutgrowthdb/jme_unicef_who_wb.pdf. Accessed 15 October 2018

Victora CG, de Onis M, Hallal PC, *et al.* (2010) Worldwide timing of growth faltering: revisiting implications for interventions. *Pediatrics.* 125(3): e473–e480.

Volkert VM, Vaz PC. (2013) Recent studies on feeding problems in children with autism. *J. Appl. Behavior Analysis* 43(1): 155–159.

Volkert VM, Piazza CC, Ray-Price R. (2016) Further manipulations in response effort or magnitude of an aversive consequence to increase self-feeding in children with feeding disorders. *Behav. Anal. Pract.* 9(2): 103–113.

WHO. (1999) *Management of Severe Malnutrition: A manual for Physicians and other Senior Health Workers.* Geneva: World Health Organisation.

WHO. (2009) *Global Database on Child Growth and Malnutrition: Child Growth Indicators and their Interpretation.* Available at http://www.who.int/nutgrowthdb/en/. Accessed 15 October 2018.

WHO/UNICEF. (2009) WHO Child Growth Standards and the Identification of Severe Acute Malnutrition in Infants and Children A Joint Statement by the World Health Organization and the United Nations Children's Fund. Geneva: WHO.

Wiskin AE, Beattie RM. (2008) Energy requirements in children with inflammatory bowel disease. *J. Pediatr. Gastroenterol. Nutr.* 47(5): 672–673.

Wiskin AE, Haggarty R, Afzal NA, *et al.* (2016) Nutritional perspectives of children with Crohn's disease: a single-centre cohort observation of disease activity, energy expenditure and dietary intake. *Eur. J. Clin. Nutr.* 70(10): 1132–1137.

Wiskin AE, Wootton SA, Hunt TM, *et al.* (2011) Body composition in childhood inflammatory bowel disease. *Clin. Nutr.* 30(1): 112–115.

Wright CM, Parkinson KN, Shipton D. *et al.* (2007) How do toddler eating problems relate to their eating behavior, food preference and growth? *Pediatrics.* 120: e1069–e1075.

Wright CM, Chillingworth A. (2015) The impact of stopping high-energy oral nutritional supplements on eating behaviour and weight gain. *Arch. Dis. Child* 100(11): 1024–1027.

Ziegler EE, Fomon SJ. (1989) Potential renal solute load of infant formulas. *J. Nutr.* 119(12 Suppl): 1785–1788.

3.8.4 Nutritional care of the preterm infant

Heather Norris

The DH (2009) toolkit supports the existing principle that neonatal services should be organised into managed clinical networks with hospitals working as teams to ensure that babies are cared for in appropriate settings. The 23 networks in England are comprised of three types of units:

- Special care units (SCUs).
- Local neonatal units (LNUs).
- Neonatal intensive care units (NICUs).

Not all units have access to a dietitian, but hopefully BAPM recommendations will lead to an increase in (ONS 2016) preterm live birth rate staffing levels (British Association of Perinatal Medicine (BAPM), 2010).

The UNICEF/WHO definition of prematurity is given in Table 3.8.13. In England and Wales, 7.6% of all live births are preterm (ONS, 2016). Preterm infants have missed some, or all, of the third trimester of pregnancy, a period of rapid growth, when nutrient stores are laid down. Consequently, these infants have higher nutritional requirements as compared to term infants. Preterm infants are born with immature organ systems, and establishing enteral feed tolerance can therefore take some time.

Aims of dietetic intervention

The aims of the dietetic intervention are:

- To meet preterm nutritional requirements.
- To promote a postnatal growth rate equivalent to utero-foetal nutrient accretion (~15 g/kg/day).
- To establish enteral feeds as early and as safely as possible.
- To ensure that human milk is used wherever possible.

Methods of feeding preterm infants

Preterm infants are usually fed enterally or parenterally, and transitioned to oral feeding when appropriate.

Table 3.8.13 Definition of prematurity (UNICEF/WHO, 2004)

Extremely preterm	<28 weeks gestation
Preterm	28<32 weeks gestation
Moderate – Late preterm	<37 weeks gestation

Parenteral nutrition

Most babies weighing <1500 g will require parenteral nutrition (PN) to support growth while enteral feeds are being established. BAPM (2016) have produced a framework for practice that encourages widespread use of standardised and concentrated solutions to achieve target nutrition, particularly in the smallest and most vulnerable babies. Guidelines give details of the nutritional requirements for preterm PN (Koletzko *et al.*, 2005; Tsang *et al.*, 2005).

Enteral nutrition

One of the biggest challenges in neonatal dietetics is establishing enteral nutrition while minimising feed-associated risks for developing necrotising enterocolitis (NEC).

Necrotising enterocolitis

This is a potentially life threatening gastrointestinal disease in which the bowel becomes inflamed and damaged to varying extents. Treatment varies from conservative management to extensive bowel resection. No single aetiological factor has been identified, apart from prematurity itself, but up to 95% of cases of NEC occur after enteral feeding has been introduced. Osmolality, rate of feed advancement and choice of milk have historically been questioned. Current research is looking at the role of immunological and genetic factors. Neonatal units with enteral feeding guidelines have a lower incidence of NEC as compared to units without them (Patole & de Klerk, 2005).

Starting and advancing enteral feeds

Feeding guidelines will often categorise babies according to the risk of NEC. Enteral feeds should be started on day 1 of life in stable preterm infants, but a more cautious approach is taken with babies considered to be at high risk. The latter may receive a period of minimal enteral feeding (10–20 mL/kg/day) before feeds are advanced; bigger, less fragile babies start at larger volumes and progress to full feed volumes more quickly. Enteral feeds are given via orogastric or nasogastric (NG) tubes. Bolus is preferred to continuous administration, as this is more physiological and does not affect the length of time it takes to achieve full enteral feeds (Premji & Chessell, 2011). The Speed of Increasing milk Feeds Trial (SIFT, www.npeu.ox.ac.uk/research/sift-242) is looking at the incidence of NEC with feeds advanced at 30 mL/kg vs 18 mL/kg; to date, there is no evidence of a difference. It is yet to be established if the type of milk (breast or formula milk) is significant.

Oral feeding

Babies must be able to coordinate their suck–swallow–breathe pattern before oral feeds are considered (usually ~ 33–36 weeks' gestational age).

Choice of milk

Maternal expressed breast milk (MEBM) is the feed of choice for preterm infants; it confers advantages in terms of neurodevelopmental outcome and immune protection. In addition, preterm infants given MEBM are up to 10 times less likely to develop NEC than those fed exclusively with formula milk (Guy *et al.*, 1997). The high nutritional requirements of preterm infants are not met by MEBM unless fed with large volumes, and, even then, it may not be adequate, depending on the composition. Breast milk fortifier should be added to breast milk to provide adequate protein to meet requirements. Some units routinely add the fortifier when babies reach a certain intake, while others prefer to consider each baby individually.

If MEBM is not available, or contraindicated, donor milk is the second choice, as it has been shown to reduce the risk of NEC and is better tolerated as compared to formula milk. Due to heat treatment, donor milk has reduced immunological components and heat-labile nutrients (Arslanoglu *et al.*, 2013). Fat is also not so well absorbed; therefore, it is used in the short term as a tool for establishing enteral feed tolerance, and babies are then weaned onto preterm formula in order to meet their requirements.

Preterm formula milks are designed to meet the needs of preterm infants if fed at 150 mL/kg/day. Term formula milks are not suitable to meet the needs of preterm infants, and should be avoided. Specialised preterm formulae containing hydrolysed protein and medium-chain triglycerides can be useful – but when there is no preterm equivalent, term formula may be used with careful manipulations, such as supplementation or increasing feed concentration, as necessary.

Preterm enteral nutritional requirements

The full details of enteral nutritional requirements are given by the European Society for Paediatric Gastroenterology Hepatology and Nutrition (ESPGHAN) (Agostoni *et al.*, 2010; Tsang *et al.*, 2005). A summary of selected preterm enteral feeding requirements is shown in Table 3.8.14.

Growth

The most common reason for referral to a dietitian is poor growth. The causes are multifactorial and do not always relate solely to nutrition. Points to consider include:

- Check fluid allowance and consider increasing volume before making feed additions or changing feeds.
- Ensure the working weight is accurate and up to date.
- Make single changes at a time, e.g. increase feed volume before making feed additions such as vitamins/minerals.
- Avoid use of energy supplements such as fat emulsions and glucose polymers, as these add extra energy without increasing the protein and micronutrients needed for growth.

SECTION 3

SECTION 3

Table 3.8.14 Preterm enteral nutritional requirements (Agostoni *et al.*, 2010)

Nutrient	Recommended intake	
	Infant <1 kg	Infant 1–1.8 kg
Fluid (mL/kg/day)	135–200	
Energy (kcal/kg/day)	110–135	
Protein (g/kg/day)	4–4.5	3.5–4
Sodium (mmol/kg/day)	3–5	
Calcium (mmol/kg/day)	3–3.5	
Phosphate (mmol/kg/day)	1.9–2.9	
Vitamin A (μg retinol equivalents/kg/day)	400–1000	
Vitamin D (μg/day)	20–25	
Folic acid (μg/kg/day)	35–100	
Iron (mg/kg/day)	2–3	

Vitamin and mineral supplementation

There are no national guidelines on vitamin and mineral supplementation for preterm infants, and local policy should hence be adhered to. Sodium, phosphate, fat-soluble vitamins, folic acid and iron are often given; zinc and selenium are also required by some infants.

Monitoring

Weight and head circumference should be measured weekly, and length fortnightly. The measurements should be plotted on the UK–WHO low-birthweight growth charts as described in Chapter 3.8.2 (Growth, nutritional assessment and nutritional requirements).

Post-discharge formula

The Advisory Committee on Borderline Substances approves the prescription of post-discharge formula milks for catch-up growth in preterm infants (<35 weeks' gestation at birth) and small-for-gestational-age infants up to 6 months corrected age. However, there is debate about indications for their use (Greer, 2007).

Weaning

Weaning should be considered in preterm infants of 5–8 months uncorrected age to ensure that the sensitive periods for the acceptance of solids are not missed and to allow the development of appropriate feeding skills (King, 2009). A practical guide for parents can be downloaded from the Bliss website (www.bliss.org.uk).

Acknowledgement

The editor acknowledges the prior contribution of Kelly Larmour.

Further reading

Jones E, King C. (2005) *Feeding and Nutrition in the Preterm Infant*. Edinburgh: Elsevier, Churchill Livingstone.

Koletzko B, Poindexter B, Uauy R. (2014) *Nutritional Care of Preterm Infants: Scientific Basis and Practical Guidelines*. Switzerland: Karger.

Internet resources

Bliss – for babies born too soon, too small, too sick, www.bliss.org.uk

British Association for Perinatal Medicine, www.bapm.org

British Dietetic Association, www.bda.uk.com

European Society for Paediatric Gastroenterology, Hepatology, and Nutrition, www.espghan.org

Neonatal Interest Group https://www.bda.uk.com/regionsgroups/groups/paediatric/neonatal/home

Royal College of Paediatrics and Child Health, www.rcpch.ac.uk

References

Agostoni C, Buonocore G, Carnielli VP, *et al.* (2010) Enteral nutrient supply for preterm infants: commentary room the European Society for Paediatric Gastroenterology, Hepatology, and Nutrition Committee on Nutrition. *J. Paediatr. Gastroenterol. Nutr.* 50: 1–9.

Arslanoglu S, Corpeleijn W, ESPGHAN Committee on Nutrition, *et al.* (2013) Donor human milk for preterm infants: current evidence and research directions. *J. Paediatr. Gastroenterol. Nutr.* 57: 535–542.

British Association of Perinatal Medicine (BAPM). (2010) Service Standards for Hospitals Providing Neonatal Care, 3rd edn. Available at https://www.bapm.org/resources/service-standards-hospitals-providing-neonatal-care-3rd-edition-2010?tQSafariFixApplied=true. Accessed 15 October 2018.

Bristish Association of Perinatal Medicine (BAPM). (2016) The Provision of Parenteral Nutrition within Neonatal Services – A Framework for Practice. Available at https://www.bapm.org/resources/provision-parenteral-nutrition-within-neonatal-services-framework-practice-2016?tQSafariFixApplied=true. Accessed 15 October 2018.

DH. (2009) *Toolkit for high quality neonatal services*. Available at http://webarchive.nationalarchives.gov.uk/20130123200735/http://www.dh.gov.uk/en/Publicationsandstatistics/Publications/PublicationsPolicyAndGuidance/DH_107845. Accessed 15 October 2018.

Greer FR. (2007) Post-discharge nutrition: what does the evidence support? *Semin. Perinatol.* 31(2): 89–95.

Guy M, Nicoll A, Lynn R. (eds). (1997) *British Paediatric Surveillance Unit – 11th Annual Report, 1996–1997*. London: Research Division, Royal College of Paediatrics and Child Health.

King C. (2009) An evidence based guide to weaning preterm infants. *Paediatr. Child Health* 19(9): 405–414.

Koletzko B, Goulet O, Hunt J, *et al.* (2005) Guidelines on paediatric parenteral nutrition of the European Society of Paediatric Gastroenterology, Hepatology and Nutrition (ESPGHAN) and the European Society for Clinical Nutrition & Metabolism (ESPEN). *J. Paediatr. Gastroenterol. Nutr.* 41(Suppl 2): S1–87.

ONS (2016) Birth characteristics. Available at www.ons.gov.uk/peoplepopulationandcommunity/birthsdeathsandmarriages/livebirths/datasets/birthcharacteristicsinenglandandwales Accessed 23 November 2016

Patole SK, de Klerk N. (2005) Impact of standardised feeding regimens on incidence of neonatal necrotising enterocolitis: a systematic review and meta-analysis of observational studies. *Arch. Dis. Child. Fetal Neonatal Ed.* 90: F147–F151.

Premji S, Chessell L. (2011) Continuous nasogastric milk feeding versus intermittent bolus milk feeding for premature infants less than 1500 grams. *Cochrane Database Syst. Rev.* 9(11): CD001819.

Tsang R, Uauy R, Koletzko B, *et al.* (2005) *Nutrition of the Preterm Infant: Scientific Basis and Practical Guidelines*, 2nd edn. Cincinnati: Digital Educational Publishing.

United Nations Children's Fund and World Health Organization (UNICEF/WHO). (2004). *Low Birthweight: Country, Regional and Global Estimates*. UNICEF, New York. Available at www.unicef.org/publications/files/low_birthweight_from_EY.pdf. Accessed 19 March 2018.

3.8.5 Community paediatric dietetics

Clare Ewan

Paediatric community dietetics can be entirely based in the community or can cover both acute and community work. For example, in a district general hospital, the paediatric dietitian may cover both acute and community work for general paediatrics. Some posts may cover a particular speciality and be responsible for its caseload both in and out of the hospital. Community paediatrics covers a wide range of work, and paediatric dietitians can be involved in many different activities. These can broadly be divided into clinical work and public health work.

Clinical community dietetics

Clinical community work in paediatrics includes:

- *General dietetic outpatient clinics* – including one-to-one assessments, treatment and education around diet and nutrition specific to the particular child. They can be held in hospital outpatient departments, GP surgeries or health centres.
- *Multidisciplinary clinics* – these are held in a number of places, and can cover a variety of disciplines and conditions, e.g. diabetes clinics (jointly with diabetes specialist nurses and consultants), coeliac clinics (jointly with consultants) and feeding clinics held in hospitals or special schools (jointly with speech and language therapists, community consultants, and other healthcare professionals).
- *Working with staff in child development services*, e.g. involvement in child-centred assessments for children with special needs, in association with consultants and other healthcare professionals; ongoing involvement in multidisciplinary review meetings for children with special needs.
- *Home visiting* – this provides a service for children at home and school.
- *Training for mainstream and special schools* around particular nutritional issues for a child.
- *Home enteral tube feeding services* – services vary; some have a dedicated paediatric dietitian, others have access to a paediatric dietitian.

A smooth transition between acute and community dietetic care is important; therefore, any dietetic plans must be practical and appropriate for the home and school environments. It requires good communication between all members of the team of involved carers and healthcare professionals.

Public health dietetics

Public health work in paediatrics includes:

- Involvement in the development of local nutrition guidelines, e.g. development of weaning guidelines.
- Involvement in wellness programmes, e.g. community food initiatives such as food cafés and cooking skills classes.
- Working with community staff in children's centres and Sure Start facilities to provide information and support around promoting healthy eating for families (see Chapter 3.2, Preconception and pregnancy).
- Working with schools in their delivery of the National Healthy Schools programme, e.g. school meals and packed lunch advice.
- Working with public health nursing teams (health visitors and school nurses) to provide education and training.
- Involvement in the development of local care pathways, e.g. for care of allergy patients and management of medical issues such as constipation.

Working with public health agencies on the development and delivery of weight management programmes (see Chapter 7.13.4, Childhood obesity).

- Working at a strategic level to develop national programmes.

These areas rely on good communication and working between the different teams and agencies to deliver services to benefit their communities (see Chapter 4.2, Public health nutrition).

Internet resources

British Dietetic Association Public Health Specialist Group, www.bda.uk.com/regionsgroups/groups/publichealth

3.8.6 Autism

Emma Mills

Autism, or autistic spectrum disorder (ASD), is a clinically heterogeneous neurodevelopmental condition affecting social skills and communication, often characterised by stereotypic behaviours. The spectrum ranges from individuals who are high functioning (Asperger's) to children with very severe disability. Prevalence is estimated at 5 per 1000, with four times more boys affected than girls. The incidence is increasing partly due to better diagnosis but mostly due to unknown environmental factors that trigger autism in those with a particular genetic susceptibility. Growing evidence suggests that there are significant metabolic and nutritional differences between autistic and neurotypical children, and this knowledge should improve management (Adams *et al.*, 2011). The key features and medical conditions associated with ASD are outlined in Table 3.8.15.

Table 3.8.15 Key features of autistic spectrum disorder

Key feature	Example
Major impairment in social skills/ relationships	No cuddles or signs of affection
	Difficulty making friends
Major impairment in communication	Avoidance of eye contact
	Limited verbalisation
Stereotypic behaviours	Insistence on certain daily rituals
	Repetitive behaviours
	Self-stimulating behaviours (stimming)
Gastrointestinal disturbance	Constipation
	Diarrhoea
	Abdominal bloating and/or pain
	Dysbiosis
	Digestive enzyme deficiency
	Eosinophilic esophagitis
Food hypersensitivity	Non-coeliac gluten sensitivity casein sensitivity
	A1 beta-casein sensitivity
Selective eating	Limited range of acceptable foods
	Hypersensitivity to bitter and sour taste
	Hyposensitivity to sweet and salty taste
	Pica
Sensory processing disorder	Over-responsive or under-responsive
Growth and weight issues	Growth faltering
	Overweight/obesity
Other comorbidities	Epilepsy

Difficulties with communication can make it difficult to understand signs and symptoms, but behaviours that may indicate an underlying illness, pain or discomfort include teeth grinding, frequent clearing of throat/swallowing and covering ears with hands (see Chapter 3.7, People with learning disabilities).

Gastrointestinal disturbance

Gastrointestinal disturbance, especially chronic constipation, is commonly associated with autism and is often related to problem behaviours, disturbed sleep and aggression (Buie *et al.*, 2010). Increased gut permeability, microbiota abnormalities and enzyme insufficiency have been identified in cases of ASD (Hsiao *et al.*, 2013; Luna *et al.*, 2016).

Food hypersensitivity

In addition to increased gut permeability, increased immune reactivity to gluten has been shown in a subset of ASD children (Lau *et al.*, 2013), and reactivity to the cows' milk protein casein, especially the A1 beta-casein, is suggested (Trivedi *et al.*, 2014). Autistic children, especially those with gastrointestinal disturbance, may respond positively to a gluten- and casein-free diet. It is very important to explain to parents the commitment involved in following such a restrictive diet and that an improvement in symptoms may not occur. Symptom score charts should be used to assess each symptom, and telephone or online consultations can be done every 2–4 weeks to support the family. Substituting A1 beta-casein milk (regular cows' milk and dairy) for A2 varieties (a2 cows' milk, goats, ewes and buffalo milk/dairy foods) may improve symptoms without the need for a dairy-free diet in those who are hypersensitive to A1 beta casein.

Selective eating

This is often the biggest concern for parents, and their attitude will influence future progress. Parents should be encouraged to keep mealtimes relaxed and enjoyable, and they need to understand that different strategies are needed for autistic children. It is vital that the diet be assessed for possible deficiencies and to advise accordingly. Sensory processing disorder (SPD), where the sensory aspects of food (taste, texture, smell, colour, consistency) are altered, can be a significant feature of selective eating. If SPD is suspected, then try to expand the range of acceptable foods using food exchanges and chaining (see Chapter 3.7, People with learning disabilities). Over 75% of children with autism have atypical eating behaviour, eat a restricted range of foods and have higher rates of food refusal (Bandini *et al.*, 2010).

Nutritional adequacy

Low levels of calcium, iron, zinc, and vitamins B_3, B_6 and C are linked to autism severity (Adams *et al.*, 2011), and long-term restrictive eating patterns can have serious consequences, including scurvy, vitamin D deficiency, vitamin B deficiencies, permanent blindness (McAbee *et al.*, 2009), optic neuropathy (Pineles *et al.*, 2010) and reduced bone thickness (Hediger *et al.*, 2008). Low levels of the n-3 fatty acids alpha-linolenic acid (ALA), eicosapentaenoic acid (EPA), and docosahexaenoic acid (DHA) are associated with neurodevelopmental disorders and should be addressed through dietary intervention, including supplementation. Unflavoured supplements, e.g. paediatric Seravit (SHS), are often used, although these do not contain fatty acids. Fatty acid supplements that contain EPA and DHA at a combined dose of 500 mg/day are recommended, e.g. NutriAdvanced Eskimo-3 liquid.

Specialist speech and language therapists (SLT) and occupational therapists (OT) are exceptionally useful in helping children with profound SPD to be less orally sensitive and to cope better with the feeding experience.

Growth and weight

Faltering growth can be a problem in some autistic children, but many appear to manage appropriate growth despite eating a limited range of foods. Many older children become overweight due to chronically unbalanced diets. The challenge is to try and improve eating habits as early as possible because, as an adult, personal choice will prevail and intervention will be limited. It is important to note that, even in cases of normal weight or overweight, micronutrient malnutrition is likely to be an issue and should be assessed.

Internet resources

Brain and Body Nutrition, www.brainandbody.co.uk
British Dietetic Association, www.bda.uk.com
Paediatric Autism – a sub-group of the BDA Paediatric Specialist Group
Cultures for Health, www.culturesforhealth.com
Education and Services for People with Autism, www.espa.org.uk
Food and Behaviour Research, www.fabresearch.org
National Autistic Society, www.autism.org.uk
Treating Autism, www.treatingautism.co.uk

Further reading

Pike C. (2015) *Fermented*. London: Kyle Books.
Treating Autism and Autism Treatment Trust. (2014) *Medical Comorbidities in Autism Spectrum Disorders – A Primer for Health Care Professionals and Policy Makers*, 2nd edn. Available at http://nationalautismassociation.org/docs/comorbidities.pdf

References

Adams JB, Audhya T, McDonough-Means S, *et al.* (2011) Nutritional and metabolic status of children with autism vs neurotypical children and the association with autism severity. *Nutr. Metab.* 8: 34.

Bandini LG, Anderson SE, Curtin C, *et al.* (2010) Food selectivity in children with ASD and typically developing children. *J. Pediatr.* 157: 259–264.

Buie T, Campbell DB, Fuch GJ, *et al.* (2010) Evaluation, diagnosis and treatment of gastrointestinal disorders in individuals with ASDs. *Pediatrics.* 125: S1–S18.

Hediger ML, England LJ, Molloy CA, *et al.* (2008) Reduced bone cortical thickness in boys with autism or ASD. *J. Autism Dev. Disord.* 38: 848–856.

Hsiao EY, Mcbride SW, Hsien S, *et al.* (2013, Dec) The microbiota modulates gut physiology and behavioral abnormalities associated with autism. *Cell.* 155(7): 1451–1463.

Lau NM, Green PHR, Taylor AK, *et al.* (2013, Jun) Markers of celiac disease and gluten sensitivity in children with autism. *PLoS One.* 8(6): e66155.

Luna RA, Savidge TC, Williams KC. (2016) The brain–gut–microbiome axis: what role does it play in ASD? *Curr. Dev. Disord. Rep.* 3: 75–81.

McAbee GN, Prieto DM, Kirby J, *et al.* (2009) Permanent visual loss due to dietary vitamin A deficiency in an autistic adolescent. *J. Child Neurol.* 24(10): 1288–1289.

Pineles SL, Avery RA, Liu GT. (2010) Vitamin B12 optic neuropathy in autism. *Pediatrics.* 126(4): 967–970.

Trivedi MS, Shah JS, Al-Mughairy S, *et al.* (2014) Food-derived opioid peptides inhibit cysteine uptake with redox and epigenetic consequences. *J. Nutr. Biochem.* 25(10): 1011–1018.

SECTION 3

3.8.7 Special needs

Clare Ewan

The term special needs covers a wide range of conditions that can be related to congenital problems or acquired injuries. A paediatric dietitian has a role to play in many areas of the care of these children in both the hospital and in the community. The impact on nutrition will vary depending on the condition:

- Lack of, or problems with, physical aspects of feeding.
- Neurodevelopmental delay with a consequent delay in feeding abilities.
- Nutritional requirements that differ from the general paediatric population.
- Diet that needs to be manipulated for treatment and control of the condition.

These children have different nutritional requirements, and there can be wide variations among children with the same condition, e.g. one child with Down syndrome may be able to eat normally, while another may have significant difficulties managing foods within his or her mouth because of tongue thrust (involuntary pushing forward of the tongue). Dietetic needs can change over time, e.g. children with Prader–Willi syndrome frequently have faltering growth and may need tube feeding in their first year of life – whereas, in later life, their unrestricted eating means they are at greater risk of becoming obese.

Cerebral palsy

Cerebral palsy (CP) is a relatively common disorder that often requires paediatric dietetic input. It is a condition in which impairment of the immature brain affects movement, posture and coordination (see Chapter 3.7, People with learning disabilities). Problems in children with CP that affect their feeding and require dietetic support include:

- *Sucking and swallowing problems* leading to poor intake, with consequent faltering growth:
  - Energy supplementation may be needed.
  - Aspiration, with a risk of chest infections, can occur, and therefore food textures may need to be modified or the child may need to be tube-fed.
- *Gastro-oesophageal reflux*:
  - Feeds may need to be thickened.
  - Anti-reflux medication may be prescribed.
  - In severe cases, fundoplication may be performed (see Chapter 3.8.27, General surgery).
- *Faltering growth* – this may be due to a combination of poor intake, and increased requirements due to involuntary movements.
- *Constipation* is common; advice about fluid and food intake may be needed in addition to medication.

Dietetic management

The paediatric dietitian will provide support to families and carers, nursery and school staff, and respite carers. They work with other healthcare professionals in relation to the child's feeding, sometimes in multidisciplinary feeding clinics. These include:

- *Speech and language therapists (SLTs) and occupational therapists* – advise on which types of fluids and foods should be offered to the child, e.g. thickening fluids and/or solids; using special teats (Habermann) or cups (Doidy); and on specific textures of foods to offer.
- *Physiotherapists* – advise on seating and posture that benefit feeding and improve muscle tone.
- *OTs* – advise on adaptations to the child's environment, e.g. seating and cutlery.

Children with special needs are usually measured and plotted on standard or condition-specific growth charts. For many children with special needs, there are challenges around weighing and measuring height. Sitting scales or hoist scales may be used. For children who cannot stand, a supine stadiometer suitable for older children can be used. Lengths can be difficult to obtain in children with scoliosis or contractures, so alternative estimates of linear growth are sometimes used (Spender *et al.*, 1989). Down syndrome–specific growth charts are available in the UK (see Chapter 3.8.2, Growth, nutritional assessment and nutritional requirements). Clinical growth charts for children with CP have been developed in the USA (Brooks *et al.*, 2011).

Other conditions that are classified as special needs and in which paediatric dietitians can be involved include autism, epilepsy, neurological problems (e.g. Parkinson's disease and multiple sclerosis), and inherited metabolic diseases. If a child presents with a rare condition, the charity Contact a Family (www.cafamily.org.uk) may be helpful for parents and healthcare professionals.

Internet resources

Cerebra, www.cerebra.org.uk – A charity that aims to help improve the lives of children with brain-related conditions.

Contact a Family, www.cafamily.org.uk – Information on rare conditions and general advice on long-term conditions.

Dietitians Interested in Special Children (DISC) – A network of UK paediatric dietitians working with children with complex physical needs and learning disabilities, sarahfoster_1@hotmail.com.

Down Syndrome Association, www.downs-syndrome.org.uk.

Down Syndrome Medical Interest Group, www.dsmig.org.uk.

Health for all Children, www.healthforallchildren.co.uk – Growth charts for children with Down syndrome, Turner syndrome, Williams syndrome, Noonan syndrome and homozygous sickle cell disease.

NHS choices, www.nhs.uk/conditions/pregnancy-and-baby/pages/serious-conditions-special-needs.aspx.

SCOPE, www.scope.org.uk – Charity supporting disabled people.

Further reading

Douglas J, Huxham L. (2015) Feeding children with neurodisabilities. In: Shaw V (ed.) *Clinical Paediatric Dietetics*, 4th edn, pp. 774–797. Oxford: Wiley Blackwell.

References

Brooks J, Day S, Shavelle R, *et al.* (2011) Low weight, morbidity and mortality in children with cerebral palsy: new clinical growth charts. *Pediatrics* 128: e299–307.

Spender QW, Cronk CE, Charney EB, *et al.* (1989) Assessment of linear growth of children with cerebral palsy: use of alternative measures to height or length. *Dev. Med. Child Neurol.* 31: 206.

3.8.8 Paediatric general medicine

Laura Sealy

Paediatric general medicine is the initial point of contact for a child's ongoing medical care after consultation with a GP. Children are assessed in an outpatient department or, if an emergency, in a paediatric emergency assessment unit or general ward within a hospital setting. Children can be admitted for a number of reasons but common ones are bronchiolitis, faltering growth and general assessment. Most district general hospitals (DGHs) have a paediatric ward, and this is where many dietitians will have their first experience of working with children. Referrals to the dietitian are made by the consultant, a member of the acute medical team, or by the ward nursing staff after nutritional screening to assess the nutritional risk of the patient.

Care Quality Commission (2014) standards ensure that patients are nutritionally screened within 24 hours of admission and require all patients to be provided with adequate hydration and nutritious, appetising foods to meet their needs. It is imperative to help and encourage those who may require extra support with eating and drinking, and to provide adapted cutlery and closed, lidded cups when needed. These, and other specific measures described in the standard, enable children's hospitals to reduce the risk of poor nutrition and dehydration.

The range of patients seen will differ depending on whether the paediatric dietitian is working in a DGH or a tertiary children's hospital (TCH). The paediatric dietitian working within a DGH will encounter a wide range of scenarios, including food behavioural problems, constipation, breastfeeding advice, weaning advice, toddler diarrhoea, food allergy and intolerances, feeding problems in newborn babies and infants, gastro-oesophageal reflux, growth faltering, type 1 diabetes, obesity, neurological conditions, respiratory diseases and enteral tube feeding. The paediatric dietitian will often share care with a TCH for other specialties, e.g. metabolic diseases and cystic fibrosis, although such conditions may be managed by the TCH. These children may still be admitted to their local DGH, and therefore a good working relationship with the tertiary specialist dietetic team is essential for supporting the care of these children and families. Paediatric dietitians working in TCHs will assess their local acute general patients, including those with all the preceding conditions, through to patients with complex syndromes with feeding difficulties.

A nutritional assessment will be carried out following a trigger from the nutritional screening process or medical referral. This involves translating individual nutritional requirements into practical dietary and feeding plans, to optimise health, growth and development within the parameters of a child's particular condition. It is essential to design a practical plan tailored to the individual, so that families and carers can achieve the desired dietary changes.

Paediatric dietitians will be required to work closely with the multi-disciplinary team to provide advice regarding nutritional assessment and an appropriate working plan for the patient, which will be implemented with the help of nursing staff. Other professionals who may be involved in an acute setting include speech and language therapists, play specialists, food provision staff and specialist nurses.

Upon discharge, it is vital to liaise with health visitors, pharmacists, community children's nurses, social workers, GPs, schools and home enteral tube feeding (HETF) services to provide a safe discharge and continuity of care in the community. Complex discharges are common in general medical or paediatric wards. Some patients have multiagency care, and it is therefore critical to attend multidisciplinary meetings to work effectively with these professionals to provide a safe discharge.

The general medical dietitian will also promote education and training at the ward level to promote awareness on topics such as the effectiveness of nutritional screening, policies around bringing food into the hospital, the accurate use of growth charts, the accurate measuring and recording of anthropometric measurements, discharging a patient home on HETF, the range of nutritional supplements and enteral feeds available and their uses, and improving the awareness of standard operating procedures. General medical paediatric dietetics also entails seeing patients in regular outpatient clinics, both in the hospital and the community. Patients should be seen within 18 weeks of the initial referral date (DH, 2012).

Acknowledgement

The editor acknowledges the prior contribution of Katie Harriman.

References

Care Quality Commission. (2014) *Health and Social Care Act 2008 (Regulated Activities) Regulations: Regulation 14: Meeting nutritional and hydration needs.* Available at https://www.cqc.org.uk/guidance-providers/regulations-enforcement/regulation-14-meeting-nutritional-hydration-needs. Accessed 15 October 2018.

DH. (2012) *Referral to Treatment Waiting Times.* Available at www.dh.gov.uk. Accessed 29 October 2016.

SECTION 3

3.8.9 Paediatric oral nutritional support

Sara Mancell

Children have significantly higher anabolic needs than adults; failure to meet requirements can have long-term impacts on growth and development (Goulet, 2010). When planning oral nutritional support, it is important to be aware of the different settings where children eat. It is often useful to involve extended family members, nurseries or schools in planning. Methods for supporting oral nutrition include:

- Regular meals and snacks.
- Food fortification.
- Energy-dense foods.
- Supplementation.
- Concentrating formula or feed (used primarily for infants on formula milk or older children on specialist powder-based feeds).

Regular meals and snacks

Children should be offered regular meals and snacks to avoid grazing throughout the day. It may help to have set meal and snack times with at least 2 hours in between. It is important to persist with offering snacks at set times even if they are refused, as children may agree to eat these on some of the days if the opportunity is presented. The timing of drinks offered should be considered as many young children find it easier to drink than to eat; it may be better to have drinks after eating.

Food fortification

The nutrient density of a child's usual dietary intake can be increased by adding butter, margarine, oil, double cream, jam, syrup, honey, sugar, peanut butter, skimmed milk powder or cheese (see Chapter 6.3, Oral nutritional support).

Nutrient-dense foods

Nutrient-dense foods can be given to improve the nutritional status of children with faltering growth (Kasese-Hara *et al.*, 2002). It is, however, important that children continue to have a nutritious, balanced diet, especially those who require long-term nutritional support. Examples of nutrient-dense snacks are given in Table 3.8.16.

Supplementation

Ready-made, high-energy infant formulae, oral nutritional supplements (ONS) and modules of individual macronutrients can be used to supplement children's diets.

High-energy infant formula and ONS (oral nutrition supplements)

Liquid high-energy infant formulae contain approximately one-third more energy than standard infant formula, while paediatric ONS contain 1–1.5 kcal/mL. Ready-to-drink products are easy to use, time saving and avoid the risk of reconstitution errors (see Appendix A6).

Supplement modules

Supplement modules based on protein, carbohydrate or fat (see Appendix A6) can be added to foods and drinks. They are useful for achieving precise, tailor-made macronutrient profiles, but care must be taken to maintain the correct balance of nutrients. The protein–energy ratio (PER) is particularly important in pre-weaned infants relying solely on formula. The PER should be 8.9–11.5% for optimal catch-up growth (WHO/FAO/UNU, 2007).

Concentrating formula or feed

Formulae and specialist powder feeds can be concentrated to increase nutrient density. Adding additional powder per 100 mL increases the nutrient density while maintaining the total fluid volume. It is important to be careful when adjusting the concentration of a feed, and this must only be done by an experienced paediatric dietitian.

Cost of oral nutritional support

While ONS products provide a convenient way to increase nutritional intake, compliance may be poor. Nutrient-dense meals and snacks may be preferable and come at a fraction of the price of ONS products (London Procurement Program, 2015). The aim should be to tailor

Table 3.8.16 Examples of nutrient-dense snacks for children

Name	Individual portion size (g)	Energy (kcal/ portion)	Protein (g/ portion)
Sesame snack bar	30	156	3.75
Smooth peanut butter thickly spread on toast	50	200	7.2
Flapjack	34	143	1.9
Oatcakes	30	135	3.3
Alpen strawberry with yoghurt cereal bar	29	120	1.4
Dairylea triangle	16	35	2.1
Babybel cheese	20	61	4.5
Hummus	50	160	3.9
Raisins	42.5	134	1.28
Avocado wedges	80	155	1.5
Greek yoghurt	100	96	9

nutritional support to maximise compliance and, therefore, the effectiveness of treatment.

Internet resources

British National Formulary for Children (BNFC), www.bnfc.org

References

Goulet O. (2010) Growth faltering: setting the scene. *Eur. J. Clin. Nutr.* 64(S1): 2–4.

Joint WHO/FAO/UNU Expert Consultation. (2007) Protein and amino acid requirements in human nutrition. *World Health Organ. Tech. Rep. Ser.* 935: 1–265.

Kasese-Hara M, Wright C, Drewett RF. (2002) Energy compensation in young children who fail to thrive. *J. Child Psychol. Psychiatry.* 43(4): 449–456.

London Procurement Program. (2015) *Paediatric Nutrition Product Pricing.* Available at http://www.lpp.nhs.uk/media/90159/Paediatric-Nutrition-Product-Pricing-121015.pdf. Accessed 20 December 2016.

3.8.10 Paediatric enteral tube nutrition

Gurpreet Sagoo

Enteral nutrition (EN) principles are similar for children and adults (see Chapter 6.4, Enteral nutrition). Children's higher nutrient requirements per kilogram of body weight; metabolic rates and physiological responses; and lower nutritional stores can lead to growth and nutritional problems during key developmental stages. Illness, trauma and surgery increases metabolic demands and can exhaust nutritional reserves. EN via a feeding tube is indicated for infants and children with a fully/partially functioning gastrointestinal tract who are unable to meet their nutritional requirements orally (see Table 3.8.17 for indications). Monitoring of anthropometry, biochemistry and tolerance is essential.

Enteral formulae

Choice of feed depends on age, weight, gut function, dietary restrictions (e.g. allergy or metabolic conditions) and nutritional requirements. A generic guide to feeds is summarised in Table 3.8.18, with further details given in Appendix A6. It may be noted that age and weight parameters will vary between feed suppliers. Due to a European Union Commission Directive (1999/2006), most feeds for children aged over 1 year are nutritionally complete.

Table 3.8.17 Indications for enteral feeding in children (source: adapted from Braegger *et al.*, 2010, Table 2, p. 112. Reproduced with permission from the *Journal of Pediatric Gastroenterology and Nutrition*)

Indication	Examples
Inadequate oral intake due to unsafe swallow or poor suck	Prematurity, neurological disorders (e.g. cerebral palsy), congenital disorders (e.g. tracheo-oesophageal fistula), oncology tumours, trauma and burns
Malabsorption and digestive disorders	Cystic fibrosis, short bowel syndrome, food allergy
Gastrointestinal motility disorders	Gastro-oesophageal reflux, chronic pseudo-obstruction
Increased nutritional requirements and losses	Extensive burns, liver disease, heart disease
Growth failure or chronic malnutrition	Anorexia nervosa, non-organic growth faltering
Disease treatment	Crohn's disease
Metabolic diseases	Type 1 glycogen storage disease

Routes of enteral tube feeding (ETF)

Tubes can be placed in the stomach (gastric) or the jejunum, depending on gastrointestinal function, feeding duration and aspiration risk. The advantages, disadvantages and contraindications for nasogastric (NG), gastrostomy and jejunostomy feeding routes are summarised in Table 3.8.19. The planned procedures/routes should be explained to the child and family. Communication aids can be used, e.g. cartoons, toys, videos, play therapist and specialist literature, as available (GOSH, 2018).

Gastric feeding

Orogastric feeding is primarily used in neonatal units.

Nasogastric feeding

Nasogastric (NG) tubes are often used for short-term feeding (<6–8 weeks) and are considered non-invasive and quick to place. They can be traumatic to place and may be associated with impaired body image in older children. Younger children may experience oral food aversion secondary to NG tube use (Byron, 2007; Mason *et al.*, 2005). Aspiration due to misplacement or dislodgement is a risk, and should therefore be monitored. See Chapter 6.4 (Enteral nutrition) for details on placement checking.

Gastrostomy

This tube is used for longer-term feeding; however, it is indicated in the short term when NG tube placement is not feasible. The most common is percutaneous

Table 3.8.18 Generic guide to paediatric enteral feeds[a]

Age	Weight (kg)	Comments	Type of feed				
			Standard	High energy	Low energy	Fibre	Impaired gut function or allergy
<12 months	Up to 8		Expressed breast milk Pasteurised donor breast milk Standard infant formula[b]	Specialist formula, e.g. Infatrini (Nutricia), Similac (Abbott), SMA High Energy			Hydrolysed or amino acid feeds
1–12 years	8–45	Milk based Premixed, sterile, ready-to-use packs Lactose free Gluten free Nutritionally complete	1 kcal/mL Suitable for most children, promoting adequate fluid intake[c]	1.5 kcal/mL Useful when fluid is restricted	0.75 kcal/mL May be used for children with low energy requirements, e.g. neurological conditions[d] 8–10 years: alternatively, low volumes of adult feeds can be used, but with caution owing to increased protein and micronutrient content[e]	Available ± fibre Fibre may promote improved bowel function[f]	Hydrolysed or amino acid feeds
>12 years	>45	Use feeds designed for 7–12 years if small stature Normal stature – adult feeds *Note*: Caution needed to avoid excessive amounts of protein and micronutrients					Adult elemental feeds introduced gradually due to high osmolality *Note*: Adult partially hydrolysed feeds are not suitable for allergies

[a] See Appendix A6 for details on available paediatric feeds. *Note*: Weight and age parameters will vary depending on the feed company;
[b] See BDA Paediatric Group (2010).
[c] Diamante (2010).
[d] Sullivan *et al*. (2006).
[e] ESPGHAN (2010).
[f] NICE (2010).

Table 3.8.19 Advantages, disadvantages and contraindications of different feeding routes

	Nasogastric feeds	Gastrostomy feeds	Jejunostomy
Advantages	Non-invasive Relatively cheap Placement taught to carer/older child	No need to reinsert Devices can be discrete Less associated oral aversion	Reduced aspiration risk No frequent tube reinsertion
Disadvantages	Nasal and throat irritation/ulceration Irritation to cheek Misplacement while passing tube Easy displacement, need to replace frequently Need to check position frequently Gastric pH affected by milk, medications, etc. Can be difficult to aspirate Aspiration risk Visible Traumatic to place Difficult to unblock Oral aversion and difficulty reinstating oral intake Nausea and vomiting Change in bowel habits – short term only	Can exacerbate GORD May pull at tube Local infection risk Leakage can damage surrounding skin Over-granulation Buried bumper Aspiration risk Can block Nausea and vomiting Change in bowel habits – constipation/diarrhoea Difficulty reinstating oral intake and tube dependency	Tube blockage Easily dislodged Placed with general anaesthetic Nausea and vomiting Bloating Dumping syndrome Continuous feeds only Change in bowel habits – constipation or diarrhoea Difficulty reinstating oral intake
Contraindications	Severe vomiting Intestinal/gastric obstruction Uncontrolled GORD	Gross ascites Severe obesity Clotting abnormalities Ventriculo-peritoneal shunt GI obstruction Severe GORD	Complete intestinal obstruction Clotting abnormalities Gross ascites Severe obesity

GORD, gastro-oesophageal reflux disease.

endoscopic gastrostomy (PEG), but radiologically inserted gastrostomy or surgical placements are also available. They may be replaced for a low-profile skin-level device once the stoma tract is formed, normally after 3 months. However, they are associated with exacerbating gastro-oesophageal reflux disease (GORD); therefore, a fundoplication may be created at the same time as placement (Vernon-Roberts & Sullivan, 2007).

Jejunal feeding

Jejunal feeding is indicated when gastric feeding is not viable, e.g. in gastroparesis, severe GORD, gastric outlet obstruction, etc.

Nasojejunal feeding

These tubes are difficult to place and can migrate into the stomach or higher in the gastrointestinal tract. They are very vulnerable to blocking and are not replaceable at home.

Jejunostomy

Surgical percutaneous endoscopic jejunostomy (PEJ) or jejunal extensions through a PEG (PEG-J) may be indicated in the longer term. Traditionally, feeding has used the continuous provision of a hydrolysed feed. However, polymeric formulae are increasingly being used due to good tolerance (ESPGHAN, 2010). The complications for this type of feeding include dumping syndrome, abdominal pain and diarrhoea, especially if a hyperosmolar feed is used (see Table 3.8.19).

Feed initiation

Feed initiation will depend on the child's clinical status. Infants may commence feeding at 1 mL/hour, while adolescents may tolerate 100 mL/hour or higher. Refeeding risk must be assessed prior to initiation and frequently thereafter.

Feeding methods

The two main methods of feeding are continuous and bolus; bolus feeding has been shown to be more physiologically normal and allows greater mobility. Continuous feeding is often better tolerated in those with GORD, and can be less labour intensive. A combination of both methods can be used.

Overnight feeding

Many community teams no longer use overnight NG feeds, owing to aspiration risks, unless clinically indicated and risk-assessed.

Complications

Complications are similar to those seen in adults, including gastrointestinal disturbances, refeeding risk and potential drug–feed interactions (BAPEN, 2004) (see Chapter 6.4, Enteral nutrition).

Equipment

Pumps, giving sets, pH strips, reservoirs and syringes may be needed. All equipment should be National Patient Safety Agency (NPSA) compliant to avoid confusion between intravenous and enteral equipment.

Home enteral nutrition

Home discharge is a chaotic time for families, and a smooth discharge to the community team is vital. Feed manufacturers provide delivery of feed, plastics and service pumps, and these services are used by most home-fed children (BAPEN, 2010). These services should be initiated prior to the patient's discharge, and training provided to parents/relevant carers. Training should incorporate safety issues, infection control, feeding equipment, practical issues, emergency procedures, and contact details and information on equipment deliveries (Vernon-Roberts, 2009).

Liquidised food via enteral feeding tubes

The BDA promotes the use of licensed, evidence-based, sterile food formulations designed for ETF; however, the use of liquidised food via enteral feeding tubes appears to be increasing, even though it is not supported by best practice guidance. Currently, the BDA does not recommend the use of liquidised food via tubes, owing to the risk of nutritional inadequacy (BDA, 2013). Complications can also include tube blockages and microbial contamination. If fully informed parents/carers wish to use liquidised diets, then the BDA advises that dietitians carry out risk assessments and continue their duty of care and support the family. Further guidance is provided by the BDA position statement (see the following 'Further reading' section).

Acknowledgement

The editor acknowledges the prior contribution of Kate Harris and Sue Williams.

Further reading

Baker SS, Baker RD, Davis AM. (2007) *Pediatric Nutritional Support*. Burlington: Jones and Bartlett Learning.

BDA. (2016). *Policy Statement: Use of liquidised food with Enteral Feeding Tubes*. Available at https://www.bda.uk.com/improvinghealth/healthprofessionals/policy_statements/policystatement_liquidisedfood.

Braegger C, Decsi T, Dias JA, *et al.* (2010) Practical approach to paediatric enteral nutrition: a comment by the ESPGHAN Committee on Nutrition. *J. Paediatr. Gastroenterol. Nutr.* 51(1): 110–122.

Sullivan PB. (2009) *Feeding and Nutrition in Children with Neurodevelopmental Disability*. London: Mac Keith Press.

Internet resources

British Dietetic Association, www.bda.uk.com

Half PINNT for our younger feeders, www.pinnt.com/Half-PINNT.aspx

National Patient Safety Agency Reducing the harm caused by misplaced nasogastric feeding tubes in adults, children and infants (2011), https://www.networks.nhs.uk/nhs-networks/southern-west-midlands-newborn-network/documents/NPSA%20NRLS-1253-Nasogastric%20Alert-08.03.2011-v1.pdf/view

National Patient Safety Alert, www.nhs.npsa.uk

Patients on Intravenous & Nasogastric Nutrition Therapy (PINNT), www.pinnt.com

UK Association for Milk Banking, www.ukamb.org

References

BDA. (2013). *Policy statement: use of liquidised food with enteral feeding tubes*. Available at https://www.bda.uk.com/improvinghealth/healthprofessionals/policystatement_liquidisedfood. Accessed 4 April 2017.

BAPEN. (2004) *Advancing clinical nutrition, drug administration via enteral feeding tubes: a guide for general practitioners and community pharmacists*. Available at www.bapen.org.uk/pdfs/d_and_e/de_gp_guide.pdf. Accessed 4 April 2017.

BAPEN. (2010) *Annual BANS report*. Available at www.bapen.org.uk/pdfs/bans_reports/bans_report_10.pdf. Accessed 4 April 2017.

Braegger C, Decsi T, Dias JA, *et al.* (2010) Practical approach to paediatric enteral nutrition: a comment by the ESPGHAN committee on nutrition. *J. Pediatr. Gastroenterol. Nutr.* 51(1): 110–122.

Byron M. (2007) Interventions with children who are tube-fed. In: Southall A, Schwartz A. (ed) *Feeding Problems in Children*. Oxford: Radcliffe Medical Press.

Diamante A. (2010) Enteral formulas in children: which is the best choice? *Nutr. Ther. Metab.* 28(1): 40–45.

ESPGHAN. (2010) Practical approach to paediatric enteral nutrition. *J. Pediatr. Gastroenterol. Nutr.* 51: 110–122.

European Union Commission Directive. (1999/2006) *Commission directive on dietary foods for special medical purposes (1999/21/EC & 2006/141/EC)*. Available at https://ec.europa.eu/food/sites/food/files/safety/docs/labelling_nutrition-special_groups_food-medical-scf_reports_41_en.pdf. Accessed 6 April 2017.

Great Ormond Street Hospital (GOSH) for Children. (2018) *Nasogastric and orogastric tube management guidelines*. Available at https://www.gosh.nhs.uk/health-professionals/clinical-guidelines/nasogastric-and-orogastric-tube-management. Accessed 6 April 2017.

Mason SJ, Harris G, Blissett J. (2005) Tube feeding in infancy: implications for the development of normal eating and drinking skills. *Dysphagia* 20(1): 46–61.

NICE. (2010) Constipation in children and young people; diagnosis and management of idiopathic childhood constipation in primary and secondary care. Available at www.nice.org.uk/nicemedia/live/12993/48741/48741.pdf. Accessed 4 April 2017.

Sullivan PB, Alder N, Bachlet AM, *et al.* (2006) Gastrostomy feeding in cerebral palsy: too much of a good thing? *Dev. Med. Child Neurol.* 48: 877–882.

Vernon-Roberts A. (2009) The multidisciplinary team and the practicalities of nursing care. In: Sullivan PB (ed) *Feeding and Nutrition in Children with Neurodevelopmental Disability*. London: Mac Keith Press.

Vernon-Roberts A, Sullivan PB. (2007) Fundoplication versus post-operative medication for gastro-oesophageal reflux in children with neurological impairment undergoing gastrostomy. *Cochrane Database Syst. Rev.* (8): CD006151.

3.8.11 Paediatric parenteral nutrition

Jason Beyers

Parenteral nutrition (PN) is only indicated when adequate nutrition cannot be provided by enteral nutrition. Demand varies between institutions and is highest in tertiary care, particularly in neonatology, gastrointestinal surgery, oncology and intensive care. To expedite hospital discharge, home PN is increasing; however, this is dependent on the availability of community services (see Chapter 6.5, Parenteral nutrition). The decision to commence PN should be made as part of an experienced multidisciplinary nutrition support team (NST). Members of the NST should include, as a minimum, a senior paediatrician, pharmacist, nutrition nurse and a dietitian (Agostoni *et al.*, 2005). The dietitian's role is to ensure the child is receiving adequate nutrition to achieve appropriate growth, avoid hyperalimentation and to recommend changes to feeding regimens to optimise feed tolerance. Some indications for PN are listed in Table 3.8.20. If growth is inadequate using enteral nutrition support, PN should be considered for either complementary or full total PN (TPN) support.

Table 3.8.20 Indications for parenteral nutrition in children

Absolute indications	Potential indications
Premature infants	High stoma output
Congenital defects, e.g. gastroschisis	Active inflammatory bowel disease
Short bowel syndrome	Pseudo-obstruction
Necrotising enterocolitis	Intractable vomiting
Malabsorption syndromes	Protracted diarrhoea
Intestinal failure secondary to radiation/cytotoxic therapy	Hypercatabolism
	Postoperative gastrointestinal surgery
	Long periods of nil by mouth

Nutritional requirements

Paediatric PN requirements vary widely within the paediatric population. Guidelines have been developed, however. Nutritional requirements need to be adapted according to the clinical situation, enteral intake and whether catch-up growth, which relates to rapid growth following a period of growth failure, is required.

Energy

Intravenous supply of macronutrients yields greater efficacy than enteral delivery and is approximately 10% less for enteral requirements, due to lack of diet-induced thermogenesis and first-pass losses. It is important to avoid the deleterious effects of hyperalimentation (see Chapter 6.5, Parenteral nutrition) associated with excessive PN energy supply, whether in isolation or in combination with enteral nutrition support, and particularly under critical care support (Fivez *et al.*, 2016). The average daily parenteral energy intakes considered adequate for the majority of children are shown in Table 3.8.21.

Amino acids

The available amino acid preparations for children are Primene, based on the amino acid profile of cord

Table 3.8.21 Energy requirements for parenteral nutrition in children (Koletzko *et al.*, 2005)

Age (year)	kcal/kg/day	kJ/kg/day
Preterm	110–120	460–500
0–1	90–100	380–420
1–7	75–90	315–380
7–12	60–75	275–315
12–18	30–60	125–275

blood, and Vaminolact, based on the profile of breast milk (Grogan, 2007). A minimum of 1.0–1.5 g/kg/day is necessary to prevent negative nitrogen balance; however, higher intakes are required to achieve protein deposition (Koletzko *et al.*, 2005). Many institutions do not account for the potential energy contribution of protein and instead aim to provide protein (expressed as nitrogen) for its biological and physiological roles, excluding it as an energy substrate. The average amino acid requirements are shown in Table 3.8.22.

Lipids

Lipid intake should provide 25–40% of non-protein energy in fully parentally fed children (Grogan, 2007). In the presence of intestinal-failure-associated liver disease (IFALD), this should be reduced to 15–30% (Lacaille *et al.*, 2015). The use of 20% intravenous lipid emulsions (ILEs) are preferred as 10% ILEs contain higher proportions of phospholipids, which have been shown to delay triglyceride clearance (Hojsak *et al.*, 2016). The available range of ILEs contains either soybean oil (Intralipid); soybean oil and coconut oil (Lipofundin); soybean oil and olive oil (ClinOleic); soybean oil, medium-chain triglycerides, olive oil and fish oil (SMOFlipid); or 100% fish oil (Omegaven). ILE-containing fish oils have demonstrated a reversal of the effects precipitating the progression of IFALD in children on long-term PN, but have not demonstrated a reduction in the incidence of cholestasis when compared to 100% soybean-containing ILE (Hojsak *et al.*, 2016). Parenteral lipid intake should be limited to a maximum of 3–4 g/kg/day in infants up to 1 year of age and 2–3 g/kg/day in older children (Koletzko *et al.*, 2005).

Carbohydrates

Dextrose should provide 60–75% of total non-protein energy intake. The type of intravenous (IV) access limits maximum dextrose concentrations of the solution. Central lines can accommodate a safe dextrose concentration of up to 20%, as compared to a maximum of 12% with peripheral lines, which are inserted into smaller veins (Koletzko *et al.*, 2005). The maximum carbohydrate requirements are shown in Table 3.8.23.

Table 3.8.22 Protein requirements for parenteral nutrition in children (Koletzko *et al.*, 2005)

Age	g/kg/day
Preterm infants	1.5–4.0
Term infants	1.5–3.0
Second month to third year	1.0–2.5
Third to 18th year	1.0–2.5

To convert grams of nitrogen (N) to grams of protein, multiply grams of N by 6.25; e.g. 0.17 g N × 6.25 = 1.06 g protein. (*Note*: Some amino acid solutions, e.g. Vaminolact – yield slightly different N-to-protein conversion.)

Table 3.8.23 Maximal parenteral glucose supply for children (Koletzko *et al.*, 2005)

Weight (kg)	g/kg/day
Up to 3	18
3–10	16–18
10–15	12–14
15–20	10–12
20–30	<12
>30	<10

Micronutrients and electrolytes

A review of parenteral vitamin, trace element and electrolyte requirements was published by Koletzko *et al.* (2005). The requirements for vitamins and trace elements are based on standard recommendations, whereas electrolyte requirements are typically based on individual patient requirements adjusted according to serum levels. It is important to be aware that some IV medication and fluid preparations can contribute significant minerals and electrolytes fluctuations, e.g. diuretics can decrease or enhance serum electrolyte levels.

Standard and individually compounded bags

Standardised PN formulations reduce prescribing and compounding time. They can be readily used to commence out-of-hours TPN and should follow the hospital PN guidelines for their initiation and progression for up to 72 hours until the specialist team can review. Due to the wide variations in paediatric nutritional requirements, individualised PN is widely used (Kochevar *et al.*, 2007). Individually compounded bags are based on weight, and are beneficial as macronutrients, micronutrients and volume can easily be tailored to meet specific requirements. Standardised all-in-one bags, usually based on adult requirements, are available for children whose weight is above 30 kg. However, due to the multiple presentations of premix solutions, careful evaluation of the most appropriate bag must be considered.

Complications

Catheter-related sepsis and IFALD are major potential complications of PN. A more detailed account of PN complications can be found in Koletzko *et al.* (2005) and Lacaille *et al.* (2015). Administration of PN by trained staff using the sterile aseptic technique can minimise the risk of catheter-related sepsis (Loveday *et al.*, 2014). Families managing children on HPN are trained to identify early clinical signs of infection and notify the hospital, which will admit the child and assume and treat as a line infection while out ruling other causes. The PN bag is usually disconnected and discarded immediately.

The pathogenesis of IFALD is multifactorial (Bresson *et al.*, 1989; Hojsak *et al.*, 2016; Koletzko *et al*; 2005;

Table 3.8.24 Suggested protocol for monitoring paediatric patients on PN (source: adapted from the Bristol Royal Hospital for Children protocol)

	Prior to initiation	First week	Stable PN
Infusion site		Daily	Daily
Fluid balance	X	Daily	Daily
Glucose		Daily	Only if glucose dose recently increased
Sodium, potassium, urea, creatinine, calcium, phosphate, magnesium	X	Daily	Weekly
Urine sodium, potassium		Weekly	Weekly
Triglycerides[a]		Weekly	Weekly
ALT,[b] AST,[c] ALP,[d] albumin, bilirubin	X	Twice weekly	Weekly
GGT[e]	X	Only repeat if LFT[f] is abnormal	
Acid–base balance		Twice weekly	Weekly
FBC[g]	X	Weekly	Weekly
Ferritin, copper, selenium, manganese, zinc		After 1 month, then every 3 months	
Vitamins A, D, E		After 1 month, then every 3 months	
CRP[h]		After 1 month, then every 3 months	
Weight	X	Daily	Twice weekly
Height/length	X		Monthly
Head circumference (if age <2 years)	X	Weekly	Weekly

[a] Test prior to first PN infusion.
[b] ALT, alanine aminotransferase.
[c] AST, aspartate transaminase.
[d] ALP, alkaline phosphatase.
[e] GGT, gamma-glutamyl transferase.
[f] LFT, liver function test.
[g] FBC, full blood count.
[h] C-reactive protein.

Lacaille *et al.*, 2015). To reduce the risk of IFALD, early consideration of risk factors for the early diagnosis of children, optimisation of early enteral feeding, type of ILE, minimisation of central venous catheter septic events, and medical and surgical strategies (including recognition of small bowel overgrowth) should all be instigated (Lacaille *et al.*, 2015). Cyclical PN can reduce liver dysfunction, which is often given over a 12-hour infusion period on long-term-hospitalised PN or HPN, and is effective in children who can maintain normoglycaemia when off the PN, but is not achievable in premature neonates. ILE sources containing fish oils can reverse IFALD, but not reduce its incidence, suggesting the avoidance of soybean emulsions in long-term PN (Hojsak *et al.*, 2016; Lacaille *et al.*, 2015).

Monitoring

To ensure the PN regimen is suitable for the child's clinical needs and to minimise the risk of complications, it is recommended that an experienced member of the NST conduct regular clinical assessments. A suggested monitoring protocol can be seen in Table 3.8.24. Repeated venepuncture is not advised as children are vulnerable to anaemia. However, each hospital institution will have its own monitoring guidelines specific to the service it provides.

Weaning off parenteral nutrition

It is useful to assess feed tolerance before weaning off PN, especially in infants and toddlers, in order to prevent nutritional and growth deficits. Children who have had an acute episode of intestinal failure may tolerate a rapid reintroduction of enteral and/or oral feeds. In contrast, children with a primary gut diagnosis may require a more gradual reintroduction.

Acknowledgement

The editor acknowledges the prior contribution of Kim Novell.

Internet resources

European Society for Clinical Nutrition and Metabolism (ESPEN), www.espen.org

European Society of Paediatric Gastroenterology, Hepatology and Nutrition (ESPGHAN), www.espghan.org

Half PINNT for our younger feeders, www.pinnt.com/Half-PINNT.aspx

Patients on Intravenous & Nasogastric Nutrition Therapy (PINNT), www.pinnt.com

References

Agostoni C, Axelson I, Colomb V, *et al.* (2005) The need for nutrition support teams in pediatric units: a commentary by the ESPGHAN committee on nutrition. *J. Pediatr. Gastroenterol. Nutr.* 41: 8–11.

Bresson J, Narcy P, Putet G, *et al.* (1989) Energy substrate utilisation in infants receiving total parenteral nutrition with different glucose fat ratios. *Pediatr. Res.* 25(6): 645–648.

Fivez T, KerKlaan D, Mesotten D, *et al.* (2016) Early versus late parenteral nutrition in critically ill children. *N. Engl. J. Med.* 374: 1111–1122.

Grogan J. (2007) Parenteral nutrition. In: Shaw V, Lawson M (ed) *Clinical Paediatric Dietetics*, 3rd edn. Oxford: Blackwell Publishing.

Hojsak I, Colomb V, Braegger C, *et al.* (2016) ESPGHAN committee on nutrition position paper. Intravenous lipid emulsions and risk of hepatotoxicity in infants and children: a systematic review and meta-analysis. *J. Pediatr. Gastroenterol. Nutr.* 62(5): 776–792.

Kochevar M, Guenter P, ASPEN Board of Directors and Task Force on Parenteral Nutrition, *et al.* (2007) ASPEN statement on parenteral nutrition standardization. *JPEN J. Parenter. Enteral. Nutr.* 31(5): 441–488.

Koletzko B, Goulet O, Hunt J, *et al.* (2005) Guidelines on paediatric parenteral nutrition of the European Society of Paediatric Gastroenterology, Hepatology and Nutrition (ESPGHAN) and the European Society for Clinical Nutrition and Metabolism (ESPEN), supported by the European Society of Paediatric Research (ESPR). *J. Pediatr. Gastroenterol. Nutr.* 41: S1–S4.

Lacaille F, Gupte G, Colomb V, *et al.* (2015) Intestinal failure-associated liver disease: a position paper of the ESPGHAN working group of intestinal failure and intestinal transplantation. *J. Pediatr. Gastroenterol. Nutr.* 60(2): 272–283.

Loveday HP, Wilson JA, Pratt RJ, *et al.* (2014) National evidence-based guidelines for preventing healthcare-associated infections in NHS hospitals in England. *J. Hosp. Infect.* 86: S1–S70.

3.8.12 Paediatric gastroenterology

Lauren McVeigh

Infants and children with common gastroenterology disorders are often referred by a GP; complex conditions can warrant referral to a tertiary unit or children's hospital (see Chapter 7.4, Gastrointestinal disorders).

Infants

Reflux

Simple reflux is common in infants. Severe and persistent gastro-oesophageal reflux disease (GORD) can cause vomiting, pain, discomfort and an aversion to feeding. Advice should include holding infants upright after feeding and checking that the flow of milk from the bottle is not too fast. Ensuring that feed volumes are not excessive, and providing smaller, more frequent feeds can be effective. A pre-thickened formula can be used, e.g. SMA Staydown, or a thickener can be added to the regular formula, e.g. Instant Carobel (Cow & Gate). These can be used alongside antireflux medications but not with alginate therapy, e.g. Infant Gaviscon. Thickened feeds may be more difficult for the infant to suck than standard formula and may require a faster-flowing teat. If there is an atopic family history, worsening of symptoms on the introduction of formula or cow's milk protein, or associated diarrhoea or constipation, and in infants whose GORD has not responded to initial management, cow's milk protein intolerance should be considered.

Transient lactose intolerance

Transient lactose intolerance can present following an episode of gastroenteritis, and should not be confused with congenital lactose intolerance. Typically, diarrhoea continues after vomiting has stopped post-gastroenteritis. Loose, watery, acidic stools, often with excessive flatus, are seen. The infant's buttocks can be excoriated and sore, but they are otherwise well and are unlikely to have faltering growth. Treatment is with a lactose-free formula and diet for 6 weeks (MacDonald, 2015) to allow for the return of lactase enzyme activity. The infant should then resume a normal lactose-containing diet. Soya formula should not be used in infants aged under 6 months. In breastfed infants, a maternal dairy-free diet will not affect the lactose content of the breast milk, but if there are no concerns with growth, continuing to breastfeed rather than changing to a lactose-free formula should be encouraged.

Toddlers

Altered stool patterns

Toddlers have variable stool patterns according to their dietary intake, but persistent diarrhoea or constipation can initiate a referral. Toddler diarrhoea is associated with fast food transit which results in undigested in the stool. This diagnosis is made if the child is otherwise well and thriving. The role of diet in treating this is controversial, but any dietary imbalances should be corrected to ensure an age-appropriate quantity of fibre-containing wholegrains, fruit and vegetables, which may have been reduced by parents to try and normalise stools. Limiting fruit juice and squash intake can often help limit symptoms. Constipation is common in toddlers. Ensuring adequate fibre and fluid intake is essential, although there can often be a behavioural component with stool holding and toilet avoidance. Children with chronic constipation who fail to respond to normal treatment should be considered for a cow's milk–free diet (MacDonald, 2015).

Non-IgE-mediated food allergy

Many infants and children with a non-IgE-mediated food allergy present with gastrointestinal symptoms, including vomiting, GORD, constipation, loose and frequent stools, blood and/or mucus in stools, colitis, and faltering growth. The presentation of non-IgE-mediated allergy may develop slowly after hours or days, and reactions typically affect the skin, gastrointestinal tract or lungs. Patients can also present reactions that are both IgE and non-IgE, e.g. eosinophilic oesophagitis, which involves the GI tract (Turnbull *et al.*, 2015). Cow's milk protein allergy is one of the most common food allergies reported, with a prevalence of 2.3% in 1–3-year-olds in the UK, mostly as a non-IgE-mediated allergy (Venter *et al.*, 2008). Typically, it presents soon after initial exposure to cow's milk protein in formula or weaning solids, but also in a lower incidence among exclusively breastfed infants. The prognosis is good, with up to 80–90% of children developing tolerance by 3 years (Venter & Arshad, 2011). See Chapter 3.8.18 (Paediatric food hypersensitivity).

Coeliac disease

Symptoms can include gastrointestinal issues, vomiting, diarrhoea and constipation, along with faltering growth, abdominal distension and poor appetite. Dietary treatment is the same as in adults. However, gluten-free oats should be avoided following diagnosis, and pure, uncontaminated oats should be reintroduced when wellness is achieved, providing symptoms are monitored (Murch *et al.*, 2013). Temporary lactose intolerance may coexist, although it is rarely necessary to exclude lactose unless symptoms persist (see Chapter 7.4.7, Coeliac disease). Annual review is essential and should include:

- Dietary review, including micronutrient intakes – especially iron and calcium.
- Age-appropriate education to allow independence, e.g. parties, eating out, school meals.
- Advice on prescribable gluten-free products (Codex Alimentarius Commission, 1983).
- Monitoring of growth and pubertal assessment.
- Assessment of compliance.

Inflammatory bowel disease

Inflammatory bowel disease (IBD) can present at any age, but more commonly during adolescence (Benchimol *et al.*, 2011). Nutrition is key in the treatment and management of Crohn's disease. Features include raised inflammatory markers, hypoalbuminaemia, loose stools, abdominal pain, nausea, vomiting, weight loss, poor appetite, mouth ulcers, iron deficiency anaemia and delayed puberty. Children can present with significant growth failure (Wiskin *et al.*, 2007); it is also common for dietary restrictions to have been tried before diagnosis, which may have impacted on nutritional status (Rigaud *et al.*, 1994).

In Europe, exclusive enteral nutrition is recommended initially to induce remission in active disease (Beattie *et al.*, 1994; Ruemmele *et al.*, 2014). Elemental feeds were traditionally used, but RCTs have evidenced that the dietary source of protein does not affect efficacy (Grogan *et al.*, 2012; Zachos *et al.*, 2007). Polymeric formulas have been specifically designed for Crohn's disease, e.g. Modulen IBD (Nestlé Nutrition); however, no trials comparing their efficacy with other polymeric feeds have been published. The optimal duration of EEN has not been conclusively evidenced, although 6–8 weeks is most commonly suggested (Whitten *et al.*, 2012). Most children will require 100–120% of EAR for energy. The daily feed volume should be calculated according to requirements, split into six drinks/day and introduced over 2–5 days, depending on tolerance and the risk of refeeding syndrome (BSPGHAN, 2008). Drinks should be taken slowly over 20–30 minutes to prevent osmotic diarrhoea and abdominal cramps. Nasogastric feeding can be used if the child is unable to take sufficient volumes by mouth. Flavourings, chewing gum, mints and flavoured water may aid compliance, but use varies according to local policy. Regular contact and support can also help with compliance. Children with ulcerative colitis have fewer nutritional complications, but may require nutritional support for disease-related malnutrition.

Acknowledgement

The editor acknowledges the prior contribution of Julia Smith.

Further reading

Meyer R., Ventner C. (2015) Food hypersensitivity. In: Shaw V (ed) *Clinical Paediatric Dietetics*, 4th edn. Oxford: Wiley Blackwell.

Internet resources

Children with Crohn's and Colitis, www.cicra.org
Coeliac UK, www.coeliacuk.co.uk
Crohn's and Colitis UK, https://www.crohnsandcolitis.org.uk
Primary Care Society for Gastroenterology, www.pcsg.org.uk

References

Beattie M, Schiffrin EJ, Donnet-Hughes A, *et al.* (1994) Polymeric nutrition as the primary therapy in children with small bowel Crohn's disease. *Aliment. Pharmacol. Ther.* 8: 609–615.

Benchimol EI, Fortinsky KJ, Gozdyra P, *et al.* (2011) Epidemiology of pediatric inflammatory bowel disease: a systematic review of international trends. *Inflamm. Bowel Dis.* 17(1): 423–439.

BSPGHAN. (2008) Guidelines for the management of inflammatory bowel disease (IBD) in children in the United Kingdom. Available at https://bspghan.org.uk/sites/default/files/guidelines/IBDGuidelines.pdf. Accessed 15 October 2018.

Codex Alimentarius Commission. (1983) *Codex Standard for Gluten-Free Foods. Codex standard 118–1981 (revised 2008)*. Codex Alimentarius Commission.

Grogan JL, Casson DH, Terry A, *et al.* (2012). Enteral feeding therapy for newly diagnosed pediatric Crohn's disease: a double-blind randomized controlled trial with two years follow-up. *Inflamm. Bowel Dis.* 18(2): 246–253.

MacDonald S. (2015) Gastroenterology. In: Shaw V (ed) *Clinical Paediatric Dietetics*, 4th edn. Oxford: Wiley-Blackwell Publishing.

Murch S, Jenkins H, Auth M, *et al.* (2013) Joint BSPGHAN and Coeliac UK guidelines for the diagnosis and management of coeliac disease in children. *Arch. Dis. Child.* 98: 806–811.

Rigaud D, Angel LA, Cerf M, *et al.* (1994) Mechanisms of decreased food intake during weight loss in adult Crohn's patients without obvious malabsorption. *Am. J. Clin. Nutr.* 60: 775–781.

Ruemmele F, Veres G, Kolho K, *et al.* (2014) Consensus guidelines of ECCO/ESPGHAN on the medical management of pediatric Crohn's disease. *J. Crohns Colitis* 8: 1179–1207.

Turnbull J, Adams H, Gorard D. (2015) Review article: the diagnosis and management of food allergy and food intolerances. *Aliment. Pharmacol. Ther.* 41: 3–25.

Venter C, Pereira B, Voigt K, *et al.* (2008) Prevalence and cumulative incidence of food hypersensitivity in the first 3 years of life. *Allergy.* 63(3): 354–359.

Venter C, Arshad SH. (2011) Epidemiology of food allergy. *Pediatr. Clin. North Am.* 58(2): 327–349.

Whitten KE, Rogers P, Ooi CY, *et al.* (2012) International survey of enteral nutrition protocols used in children with Crohn's disease. *J. Dig. Dis.* 13(2): 107–112.

Wiskin AE, Wooton SA, Beattie RM. (2007) Nutrition issues in pediatric Crohn's disease. *Nutr. Clin. Pract.* 22(2): 214–222.

Zachos M, Tondeur M, Griffiths A. (2007) Enteral nutritional therapy for induction of remission in Crohn's disease. *Cochrane Database Syst. Rev.* 4: Cd000542.

3.8.13 Cystic fibrosis

Julie Crocker

The majority of infants with cystic fibrosis (CF) are identified through the national screening programme. Diagnosis is confirmed by a sweat test and/or genetic mutation analysis. Most families will be advised of the diagnosis within 3 weeks of their baby's birth; early diagnosis allows treatment to be commenced promptly. One in 10 babies with CF are born with the bowel obstruction meconium ileus. The obstruction may be managed conservatively, but some babies may require urgent surgery to remove the meconium or, in severe cases, an intestinal resection (Patchell, 2015).

Newly diagnosed infants should be seen for dietetic review every 1–2 weeks until treatment is established, malabsorption symptoms are controlled and the infant is thriving. Subsequent follow-up is usually monthly for babies aged up to 1 year, and then every 8 weeks, although more frequent review may be required. Children will either receive full care from a specialist CF centre or shared care within an agreed designated network (Cystic Fibrosis Trust, 2011). A paediatric dietitian is most likely to see children with CF at a multidisciplinary team (MDT) clinic or as an inpatient, particularly during admission for respiratory exacerbations. All children with CF should have an annual assessment, which includes a range of specialist investigations, and a full dietary assessment.

Pancreatic insufficiency

Up to 90% of CF patients will be pancreatic insufficient and will require pancreatic enzyme replacement therapy (PERT). Following diagnosis, measuring the faecal pancreatic elastase assesses pancreatic function. Enteric-coated microspheres is the most common PERT used in infants. Many factors affect the efficacy of PERT; therefore, doses should be advised individually and reassessed regularly, depending on weight gain and symptoms of fat malabsorption.

Nutritional requirements

Energy

The energy requirements of children with CF are variable and generally increase with age and disease severity. Fat malabsorption and increased energy expenditure both increase energy requirements. Therefore, an infant with good absorption control may have normal energy requirements. A teenager with poor respiratory function may have significantly higher energy requirements than expected for age. Many factors may inhibit a child with CF from meeting its increased requirements, including chronic poor appetite, infection-related anorexia, gastro-oesophageal reflux, vomiting, low mood and feeding behaviour problems. Regular review by a dietitian experienced in the management of children with CF is essential. A normal- to high-fat diet should be encouraged (Cystic Fibrosis Trust, 2016).

Micronutrients

In CF, fat-soluble vitamins are usually lost in the stools, and therefore regular vitamin supplements are required. The recommended starting doses are as follows:

- Vitamin A: <1500 IU for infants and 1500–10,000 IU in >1-year age group.
- Vitamin D: 400–2000 IU for infants and 400–5000 IU in >1-year age group.
- Vitamin E: 40–80 IU for infants, 50–150 IU for 1–3-year age group and 150–500 IU for 3-year age group.

Doses should be adjusted in response to serum levels (Cystic Fibrosis Trust, 2016). A diet high in calcium should be encouraged, particularly in adolescence. Calcium supplements may be required if calcium requirements are not met.

Fibre, fluid and electrolytes

Adequate fibre and fluid levels are important as part of a balanced diet to help maintain normal bowel function and prevent constipation. Salt depletion can occur in children with CF with increased sweating and in infancy when dietary intake is normally low. Salt supplementation should be considered, as routinely recommended by some centres. All individuals with CF should be encouraged to eat a diet high in sodium (Cystic Fibrosis Trust, 2016).

Evaluation of growth

Weight and height, and body mass index (BMI) for children over 2 years of age, should be recorded at each clinic visit and plotted on the appropriate growth chart. For children aged 2–18 years, a BMI on or above the 50th percentile is recommended. Children with CF often show delayed puberty, which may lead to an overestimation of malnutrition. Assessment of pubertal stages is therefore important when interpreting growth data.

Feeding

Infants and toddlers

Most infants with CF will thrive on either breast milk or a standard infant formula if malabsorption is controlled. Breastfeeding should be encouraged. High-energy formulae can be useful in infants with poor weight gain. Infants who have had a surgical resection for MI usually require a hydrolysed protein formula. Normal weaning practices are advised with support on modifying pancreatic enzyme doses. If weight gain is poor, advice on food fortification should be given (Cystic Fibrosis Trust, 2016). Feeding behaviour problems such as food refusal and inappropriate parental responses are more common in young children with CF. These issues can result in poor dietary intake and growth, and so should be addressed at an early stage. Joint dietetic and psychology input can be very effective.

School-age children

As children get older, there is an increased likelihood of worsening disease, leading to greater energy requirements. Close monitoring of growth and nutritional status continues to be essential. The need for enzymes can highlight to children with CF that they are different from their peers. This can result in problems of acceptance of their condition and adherence to treatment. Advice should be given to parents on how best to deal with this.

Adolescence

Adolescence is a challenging time in the dietary management of CF. The main growth spurt occurs during this period, and weight gain and growth can decline dramatically. In addition, poor adherence to enzyme, vitamin and nutritional supplementation is common. It is essential to acknowledge what is important to the teenager. Motivational interviewing for goal setting, together with compromise, can be helpful.

Nutrition support

Intervention for poor weight gain should start with improving food and energy intake. The use of dietary supplements, e.g. high-energy sip feeds, may be required. Care should be taken that these are used in addition to current intake, and not as a meal replacement. They may be more useful in the short term, during periods of acute illness, rather than as a long-term intervention. Tube feeding may be required if growth is failing. Families should be involved early in the decision-making process, and their views and individual circumstances taken into account regarding the choice of intervention and timing of feeds. An overnight continuous feed via a gastrostomy is usually the preferred option. Energy-dense feeds are often used to reduce the volume required, and usually provide 30–50% of energy requirements.

Complications

The progressive nature of CF means that complications increase in prevalence as children age and move into adulthood. Complications include diabetes, liver disease, bone disease and distal intestinal obstruction syndrome. Investigations to screen for these complications are carried out during the child's annual review. From 10 years of age, children should have a dual-energy X-ray absorptiometry (DXA) scan to monitor bone density and an oral glucose tolerance test to screen for CF-related diabetes (Cystic Fibrosis Trust, 2016).

Acknowledgement

The editor acknowledges the prior contribution of Alison Coates.

Internet resources

Cystic Fibrosis Trust, www.cftrust.org.uk

References

Cystic Fibrosis Trust. (2011) *Standards for the Clinical Care of Children and Adults with CF in the UK*, 2nd edn. Available at www.cftrust.org.uk. Accessed 26 October 2016.

Cystic Fibrosis Trust. (2016) *Nutritional Management of Cystic Fibrosis*. Available at www.cftrust.org.uk. Accessed 26 October 2016.

Patchell C. (2015) Cystic fibrosis. In: Shaw V. (ed) *Clinical Paediatric Dietetics*, 4th edn. Oxford: Blackwell Publishing.

3.8.14 Paediatric liver disease

Sara Mancell

SECTION 3

Disease process and nutritional consequences

Although a number of aspects of management are similar for adults and children with liver disease, there are some important differences, not least the higher anabolic requirements of children and the need to promote normal growth and development (Leonis & Balistreri, 2008). Management is dependent on whether the liver disease is acute, chronic or metabolic.

Although rare in children, acute liver failure (ALF) is often fatal (Dhawan *et al.*, 2004). The most common causes are acute viral hepatitis, metabolic diseases and toxins, but frequently the cause is not known (Dhawan, 2008). Severe hypoglycaemia may result due to impaired glycogen storage, reduced gluconeogenesis and hyperinsulinism alongside an increased glucose requirement (Cochran & Losek, 2007). This can lead to the breakdown of muscle and fat stores. As the liver's ability to metabolise ammonia is reduced in ALF, hyperammonaemia with associated encephalopathy and cerebral oedema may result (Cochran & Losek, 2007).

Common causes of chronic liver disease (CLD) include biliary atresia, alpha-1-antitrypsin, Alagille syndrome, progressive familial intrahepatic cholestasis, non-alcoholic fatty liver disease, Wilson's disease and intestinal-failure-associated liver disease (Mancell & Kamat, 2015). Malnutrition is one of the most serious problems for children with CLD, and may cause faltering growth, rickets, bleeding and infections (Pawlowska *et al.*, 2007). Malnutrition is associated with increased morbidity and mortality (Ramaccioni *et al.*, 2000).

Inherited metabolic disorders such as tyrosinaemia, fatty acid oxidation disorders, urea cycle defects, glycogen storage disease, galactosaemia and fructosaemia may present as acute liver failure. These disorders require specific dietary treatment (see Chapter 3.8.16, Neurology and the ketogenic diet and Chapter 7.8, Inherited metabolic disorders in adults).

Nutritional assessment

A detailed nutritional assessment is essential in children with liver disease and should be done regularly. The presence of organomegaly and/or ascites may mask the actual body weight, but regular weighing is still essential as they can give an indication of ascites progression. Length/height is a useful long-term measure of chronic malnutrition, while mid-upper-arm circumference and triceps skinfold thickness are sensitive short-term measures, but they are prone to measurement error (Taylor & Dhawan, 2005). Measurement of albumin, immunoglobulins and nitrogen balance are affected by liver function, and are therefore not useful markers of nutritional status (Pawlowska *et al.*, 2007). Fat-soluble vitamins, minerals and trace elements should be monitored to avoid deficiency. Anthropometry, together with biochemistry, clinical features and complications of the disease, dietary intake and social factors should be considered when deciding on the nutritional management of paediatric liver disease.

Nutritional management

Nutritional management depends on whether the presenting condition is acute or chronic.

Acute liver failure

Children are often well nourished if they present immediately after the onset of acute liver failure. The aim is to maintain nutritional status until liver function improves and minimise ALF complications such as hypoglycaemia and hyperammonaemia. Hypoglycaemia is managed by ensuring a constant supply of exogenous glucose (either enterally or intravenously) (Dhawan *et al.*, 2004). Hyperammonaemia is treated with an initial protein restriction (2 g/kg); a prolonged restriction is not recommended as it may increase ammonia due to muscle breakdown (Baker *et al.*, 2007). If an inherited metabolic disorder is suspected, specific diet therapy can be initiated to prevent accumulation of toxic by-products; there is often a delay in starting treatment while the diagnosis is determined.

Chronic liver disease

Malnutrition is common in children with chronic liver disease and may be due to reduced oral intake, malabsorption, increased energy expenditure and metabolic changes, as shown in Table 3.8.25.

Liver transplantation

Tube feeding is typically initiated 3–5 days after transplant. If oral intake was established prior to transplant, a normal diet is usually achieved fairly quickly. Tube feeding may be required for an extended period in children with behavioural feeding difficulties or very poor nutritional status. Parenteral nutrition is considered if there are gastrointestinal complications (e.g. bowel perforation), especially in children who were severely malnourished prior to transplant.

Acknowledgement

The editor acknowledges the prior contribution of Kirsten Tremlett.

Table 3.8.25 Malnutrition in chronic liver disease

Causes of malnutrition	Related factors	Management
Reduced oral intake	Nausea and vomiting Reduced gastric capacity due to organomegaly or ascites Pruritus Oesophageal varices	High-energy, low-volume tube or sip feeds as bolus and/or continuous overnight infusion
Malabsorption	Absent or reduced bile flow Mucosal oedema secondary to portal hypertension	Absent/reduced bile: medium-chain triglycerides and fat-soluble vitamin supplementation Mucosal oedema: hydrolysed protein
Increased energy expenditure	Inflammatory response Increased respiratory effort due to organomegaly or ascites	Energy: 120–150 kcal/kg (infants), 120–160% EAR (children) Protein: 3–4 g/kg
Metabolic changes	Reduced glycogen storage Impaired gluconeogenesis Impaired ammonia breakdown	Preserve lean body mass by avoiding fasting; supplement with branched-chain amino acids; manage hypoglycaemia and hyperammonaemia

References

Baker A, Stevenson R, Dhawan A, *et al.* (2007) Guidelines for nutritional care for infants with cholestatic liver disease before liver transplantation. *Pediatr. Transplant.* 11: 825–834.

Cochran JB, Losek JD. (2007) Acute liver failure in children. *Pediatr. Emerg. Care.* 23: 129–135.

Dhawan A, Cheeseman P, Mieli-Vergani G. (2004) Approaches to acute liver failure in children. *Pediatr. Transplant.* 8: 584–588.

Dhawan A. (2008) Etiology and prognosis of acute liver failure in children. *Liver Transpl.* 14(S2): S80–S84.

Leonis MA, Balistreri WF. (2008) Evaluation and management of end-stage liver disease in children. *Gastroenterology.* 134: 1741–1751.

Mancell S, Kamat D. (2015) Nutritional management of children with liver disease. In: Guandalini S, Dhawan A, Branski D (ed) *Textbook of Pediatric Gastroenterology, Hepatology and Nutrition: A Comprehensive Guide to Practice*. Switzerland: Springer International Publishing, pp. 861–870.

Pawlowska J, Socha P, Socha J. (2007) Nutrition in pediatric patients before liver transplantation. *Rocz. Państ. Zakł. Hig.* 58: 111–118.

Ramaccioni V, Soriano HE, Arumugam R, *et al.* (2000) Nutritional aspects of chronic liver disease and liver transplantation in children. *J. Pediatr. Gastroenterol. Nutr.* 30: 361–367.

Taylor R, Dhawan A. (2005) Assessing nutritional status in children with chronic liver disease. *J. Gastroenterol. Hepatol.* 20: 1817–1824.

3.8.15 Paediatric nephrology

Sarah Trace

In the UK, there are 13 specialist centres for paediatric nephrology, with 10 providing transplantation services. Many children live significant distances away from a renal centre, so will have shared care arrangements at their local hospital. Specialist renal paediatric dietitians can provide training and resources to support local teams. The specialist dietitian has an important role within the MDT; the renal team not only meets the clinical needs of the child, but will also support its social, psychological and educational needs (see Chapter 7.5.1, Renal disorders).

Common presentations

The incidence of acute kidney injury (AKI) is 0.8 per 100,000 of the paediatric population, with the highest incidence in newborns. In children, a common presentation is haemolytic–uraemic syndrome (HUS), associated with *Escherichia coli* infection. AKI may also present secondary to a multifactorial illness in a severely ill child. The incidence of established chronic kidney disease (CKD) requiring renal replacement therapy (RRT) is 5–10 children per million (Singa *et al.*, 2010). Congenital disorders, including congenital anomalies of the kidney and urinary tract and hereditary nephropathies, are responsible for about two-thirds of CKD in developed countries (Harambat *et al.*, 2012).

Nutritional assessment

In addition to the usual considerations during a paediatric nutritional assessment, nutritional care planning for children will depend on the nature and severity of the disease, the resulting biochemical changes and medical management, including RRT methods and fluid status. In CKD, a detailed assessment is complex to perform and needs to be conducted by an experienced renal paediatric dietitian (Royle, 2015). The US National Kidney

Foundation's Kidney Disease Outcomes Quality Initiative Clinical Practice Guideline for Nutrition in Children with CKD is a useful resource (National Kidney Foundation, 2008).

Dietary management

Acute kidney injury

Children with AKI are very ill, frequently unable to eat significantly, highly catabolic and usually require dialysis. Nutritional support is necessary to prevent catabolism and control biochemical disturbances. The choice of support is dependent on intake, and children many require tube feeding. Feed choice and regimen is dependent on the previously described factors and general clinical condition, including the presence of vomiting and/or diarrhoea (Royle, 2015). Fluid restriction makes it very difficult to provide nutritional adequacy, although dialysis allows higher fluid intakes.

Chronic kidney disease

Children with CKD will require specialist renal paediatric dietetic monitoring and advice when the kidney function declines to a glomerular filtration rate (GFR) of 60 mL/min/1.73 m^2 (CKD stage 3) and below. Major feeding difficulties are well recognised in infants and young children with CKD. As with any chronic disease, an infant will struggle with feeding development during repeated periods of illness. Poor growth and weight gain can be major problems in those with advanced disease, and malnutrition is associated with increased mortality (Wong *et al.*, 2002). Dietary restrictions must only be instigated when absolutely necessary. Many infants and children will require tube feeding, but this can be problematic in the very young due to the increased incidence of gastro-oesophageal reflux in CKD (Ruley *et al.*, 1989). As renal function falls, food intake decreases further, as demonstrated by Norman *et al.* (2000). A fall to 85% of the estimated average requirement (EAR) when the GFR was <25 mL/min/1.73 m^2 has been shown (Norman *et al.*, 2000). Uraemia leads to loss of appetite and taste changes (Bellisle *et al.*, 1995). Frequent nausea and vomiting may lead to food refusal, even when the child is well.

Dietary aims

The aim is to optimise nutritional status to promote growth and well-being, while aiding control of biochemical disturbances. There is no evidence that children consume more energy than their EAR, although energy-dense diets and feeds may be needed due to vomiting, or poor or restricted intake. In order to achieve adequate growth, the child's reference nutrient intake (RNI) for protein is the minimum amount that needs to be achieved in non-dialysed children with good appetites. There may be a need to reduce usual protein intake if uraemia is present. However, inadequate protein intakes impact on body composition with a deposition of fat rather than lean tissue (Rees & Shaw, 2007), so care is required. In dialysed children, requirements are determined by RNI, the dialysis method and biochemical assessment (Royle, 2015).

Control of phosphate, calcium, vitamin D and parathyroid hormone levels will help to prevent calcification of the vessels and renal bone disease. Dietary phosphorus intakes usually need to be limited to less than the RNI, although a low-phosphorus diet is difficult to follow and without care may limit protein and micronutrient intake. It is important to concentrate on limiting processed foods that have phosphorus-containing additives. Additional control is usually achieved by phosphate-binding drugs. Fluid and electrolyte requirements depend on disease, biochemical control and RRT. Fluid requirements and restriction or supplementation of sodium and potassium need to be individually tailored. More research is needed to determine other micronutrient requirements. Folic acid, iron and water-soluble vitamins are commonly recommended (Royle, 2015; National Kidney Foundation, 2008; Warady *et al.*, 1994).

Transplantation

Many children will receive a kidney from a live related donor, usually a parent. Immediately following transplant, the child and its family will need advice on basic food safety for a short period while on high doses of immunosuppressant drugs, owing to the increased risk of food poisoning. There can be an increase in appetite due to steroids, so weight gain should be monitored. Long-term aims include the child having a healthy, balanced diet; however, 13% of transplanted children become obese (Hanevold *et al.*, 2005). The importance of healthy eating is stressed due to the high impact of CKD on cardiovascular health (Shroff *et al.*, 2011). A child with CKD has a much higher cardiovascular risk than the healthy age-adjusted population, so the importance of lifelong healthy living is paramount.

References

Bellisle F, Dartois AM, Kleinknecht C, *et al.* (1995) Alteration of the taste for sugar in renal insufficiency: study in the child. *Nephrologie.* 16: 203–208.

Hanevold CD, Ho PL, Talley L, *et al.* (2005) Obesity and renal transplant outcome: a report of the North American pediatric renal transplant cooperative study. *Pediatrics.* 115(2): 352–356.

Harambat J, Van Stralen KJ, Kim JJ, *et al.* (2012) Epidemiology of chronic kidney disease in childhood. *Paediatr. Nephrol.* 27(3): 363–373.

National Kidney Foundation. (2008) Kidney Disease Outcomes Quality Initiative (NKF KDOQI™). *Am. J. Kidney Dis.* 53 (Suppl 2): S1–S124.

Norman LJ, Coleman JE, Macdonald IA, *et al.* (2000) Nutrition and growth in relation to severity of renal disease in children. *Pediatr. Nephrol.* 15: 259–265.

Rees L, Shaw V. (2007) Nutrition in children with CRF and on dialysis. *Pediatr. Nephrol.* 22(10): 1689–1702.

Royle J. (2015) The kidney. In: Shaw V (ed) *Clinical Paediatric Dietetics*, 4th edn. Oxford: Wiley-Blackwell, pp. 242–281.

Ruley EJ, Bock GH, Kerzner B, *et al.* (1989) Feeding disorders and gastroesophageal reflux in infants with chronic renal failure. *Pediatr. Nephrol.* 3(4): 424–429.

Shroff R, Weaver DJ, Mitsnefes MM. (2011) Cardiovascular complications in children with chronic kidney disease. *Nat. Rev. Nephrol.* 7: 642–649.

Singa MD, Castledine D, Van Schalkwyk D, *et al.* (2010) *Demography of UK Paediatric Renal Replacement Therapy Population in 2009. Bristol: UK Renal Registry Bristol.* Available at https://www.renalreg.org/wp-content/uploads/2014/09/Chap05_Renal10_web.pdf. Accessed 30 November 2016.

Warady BA, Kriley M, Uri SA, *et al.* (1994) Vitamin status of infants receiving long-term peritoneal dialysis. *Paediatr. Nephrol.* 8: 354–356.

Wong CS, Hingorani S, Gillen DL, *et al.* (2002) Hypoalbuminemia and risk of death in pediatric patients with end-stage renal disease. *Kidney Int.* 61: 630–637.

3.8.16 Neurology and the ketogenic diet

Camille Newby

Epilepsy is one of the more common neurological disorders in childhood. Epilepsy is defined as a brain disorder in which normal brain function is disrupted by epileptic seizures (Fisher *et al.*, 2005), which is the result of excessive and disorderly neurone activity in the brain (Fisher *et al.*, 2005). There are different types of epileptic seizures, and an individual child may present with a variety of different seizures. Epilepsy is estimated to affect between 260,000 and 416,000 people in England and Wales (NICE, 2012).

Children with epilepsy will be under the care of a specialist paediatric neurology consultant and may also have the support of a clinical epilepsy nurse. The majority of children will have their epilepsy successfully controlled through the use of antiepileptic drugs (NICE, 2012). Children whose seizures do not respond to antiepileptic drugs should be referred to a tertiary care centre for consideration of the use of the ketogenic diet under the care of a specialist paediatric dietitian (NICE, 2012).

Ketogenic diet

In 1921, it was reported that fasting in patients with uncontrolled epilepsy could lead to an improvement in their seizure control (Freeman *et al.*, 2007). During starvation, the body mobilises fat to produce ketone bodies, which can pass through the blood–brain barrier for the brain to use as an alternative energy source. As starvation is not a long-term solution for patients with epilepsy, the ketogenic diet was developed to mimic the metabolic effects of starvation (Freeman *et al.*, 2007). The aim of the high-fat content and limited carbohydrate intake with this diet is to drive the process of ketogenesis, so that ketone bodies will be the body's main source of energy.

The ketogenic diet can be used to treat a range of different types of epilepsy in patients of all ages. It has been noted to be more effective in certain epilepsies, such as severe myoclonic epilepsy of infancy, myoclonic astatic epilepsy and tuberous sclerosis complex (Kossoff *et al.*, 2009). The ketogenic diet is a high-fat diet, with controlled amounts of protein that meet the requirements for growth and a limited amount of carbohydrate. Fat provides 80–90% of the total energy (Zupec-Kania & Zupanc, 2008). Fat is mainly provided from foods, e.g. butter, cream and oil, with enough protein for growth, from poultry, fish and meat, for example. The remaining energy is provided by carbohydrate from fruit and vegetables. Foods high in carbohydrate, e.g. bread, pasta and rice, are often not allowed (Zupec-Kania & Zupanc, 2008). The diet plan is usually based on three to four meals, with snacks if required. There are currently four different types of the ketogenic diet.

Classical ketogenic diet

The classical ketogenic diet is based on long-chain fats and a ratio system of fat to protein and carbohydrate combined. The main ratios used are 4:1 and 3:1; for every 4 or 3 g of fat, there will be 1 g of protein and carbohydrate. The amount of protein is kept to a safe minimum for growth and development, and carbohydrate is limited to achieve the appropriate level of ketosis (Cross *et al.*, 2010). The classical ketogenic diet can be provided to patients who are enterally fed by using the enteral feed Ketocal (Nutricia Metabolics).

Medium-chain triglyceride ketogenic diet

An alternative to the classical ketogenic diet is the medium-chain triglyceride (MCT) ketogenic diet, where MCT is used as a fat source. MCTs are more effective at producing ketone bodies than long-chain triglycerides, allowing more protein and carbohydrate to be consumed, thus improving palatability (Cross *et al.*, 2010).

Modified Atkins diet

The classical and MCT ketogenic diets are very restrictive, and adherence is difficult in older children. A modified Atkins diet (MAD), which is similar to the classical ketogenic diet with a ratio of 1:1, can be successful (Hartman & Vining, 2007). MAD enables the patient to consume more protein and carbohydrate, making the meals more appealing and easier to plan (Kossoff *et al.*, 2009).

Low-glycaemic-index diet

Low-glycaemic-index (GI) treatment was developed following the observation that children on the ketogenic diet tended to have stable blood glucose levels, which may be a reason for its effectiveness (Kossoff *et al.*, 2009). It allows carbohydrate intake of up to 40–60 g/day as long as the carbohydrate integrated into the diet has a GI of <50 (Kossoff *et al.*, 2009).

Monitoring

The ketogenic diet is not balanced and requires close monitoring by a specialist dietitian to ensure sufficient growth and nutritional adequacy. It is important that patients and parents are informed of the adverse effects of the diet, including constipation, vomiting, kidney stones, poor bone mineralisation and poor growth. The diet does not work for everyone, and parents are asked to commit to a trial for 3 months while keeping a seizure diary. This information is used to determine diet effectiveness and the child's quality of life. Typically, a child stays on a ketogenic for 2 years. After 2 years, if the family wants to remain on the diet and the child is not experiencing any adverse effects, this should be supported with continued dietetic follow-up; such diets have been used for up to 12 years (Kossoff *et al.*, 2009).

Discontinuation

The child must be weaned slowly over a 2–3-month period as stopping suddenly can induce life-threatening seizure episodes. The fat to protein and carbohydrate ratio is reduced from 4:1 to 3:1 to 2:1, and once ketosis stops, high-carbohydrate foods can be reintroduced (Kossoff *et al.*, 2009).

Illness

If a child becomes unwell while on the ketogenic diet, the illness must be treated, and this may mean the diet has to stop for a short period of time. If appetite is decreased and meals are not completely eaten, an emergency ketogenic milkshake can be given as a replacement.

Internet resources

International League Against Epilepsy, www.ilae-epilepsy.org
Matthew's Friends (dietary treatments for epilepsy), www.matthewsfriends.org
The Charlie Foundation, www.charliefoundation.org
The Daisy Garland, www.thedaisygarland.org.uk

References

Cross JH, Mclellan A, Neal EG, *et al.* (2010) The ketogenic diet in childhood epilepsy: where are we now? *Arch. Dis. Child.* 95: 550–553.
Fisher RS, van Emde Boas W, Blume W, *et al.* (2005) Epileptic seizures and epilepsy: definitions proposed by the International League Against Epilepsy (ILAE) and the International Bureau for Epilepsy (IBE). *Epilepsia.* 46: 470–472.
Freeman JM, Kossoff EH, Freeman JB, et al. (2007) *The Ketogenic Diet: A Treatment for Children and Others with Epilepsy*, 4th edn. New York: DemosHelth.
Hartman AL, Vining PG. (2007) Clinical aspects of the ketogenic diet. *Epilepsia.* 48: 31–42.
Kossoff EH, Zupec-Kania BA, The International Ketogenic Diet Study Group. (2009) Optimal clinical management of children receiving the ketogenic diet: recommendations of the international ketogenic diet study group. *Epilepsia.* 50: 304–317.
NICE. (2012) The epilepsies: the diagnosis and management of the epilepsies in adults and children in primary and secondary care (CG137). Available at www.nice.org.uk/. Accessed 23 June 2011.
Zupec-Kania B, Zupanc ML. (2008) Long-term management of the ketogenic diet: Seizure monitoring, nutrition, and supplementation. *Epilepsia.* 49(Suppl 8): 23–26.

3.8.17 Inherited metabolic disorders

Katherine Singleton and Barbara Cochrane

There are over 500 known inherited metabolic disorders (IMD) (Burton, 2005), with many being diagnosed in infancy or early childhood. However, with newborn screening, improvements in diagnosis and treatment, children with IMDs are now transitioning into adulthood and require dietary management alongside other lifestyle changes (see Chapter 7.8, Inherited metabolic disorders in adults).

The majority of children with IMD will be seen in a tertiary-level specialist children's hospital, but others may be seen in a local district general hospital (DGH) with shared care arrangements to the specialist centre. A significant proportion will have a disorder that affects the metabolism of lipids, carbohydrates or proteins, and will require specialist dietetic intervention and support as a major part of their ongoing management during their lifetime (Table 3.8.26). The degree of dietary manipulation along with highly specific dietary substitutes will depend on the metabolic disorder.

The IMDs seen most frequently in a DGH are phenylketonuria (PKU) and medium-chain acyl-CoA dehydrogenase deficiency (MCADD). These conditions are diagnosed on a newborn blood spot-screening test (heel prick test), which is carried out on all newborn babies in the UK between 5 and 8 days of age. The aim of the screening is to prevent severe disability or death by commencing appropriate treatment early in the neonatal period. The heel prick test is performed irrespective of feeding times, gestational age or medical condition. In 2015, in England and Wales, newborn screening was expanded to include: maple syrup urine disease (MSUD), homocystinuria (HCU), glutaric aciduria type 1(GA1),

Table 3.8.26 Inherited metabolic disorders affecting carbohydrate, lipid and protein metabolism that require significant dietary treatment

Carbohydrate metabolism disorders	Lipid metabolism disorders	Protein metabolism disorders
Galactosaemia	Medium-chain acyl-CoA dehydrogenase deficiency	Amino acid disorders: Phenylketonuria Maple syrup urine disease Homocystinuria Tyrosinaemia
Glycogen storage diseases	Long-chain acyl-CoA dehydrogenase deficiency	Urea cycle disorders: Ornithine transcarbamylase deficiency Carbamoyl phosphate synthase deficiency Citrullinaemia Argininosuccinic aciduria Arginase deficiency
Fructose-1,6-biphosphatase deficiency	Very-long-chain acyl-CoA dehydrogenase deficiency	Organic acidaemias: Glutaric aciduria type 1 Methylmalonic acidaemia Propionic acidaemia Isovaleric acidaemia
Hereditary fructose intolerance	Multiple acyl-CoA dehydrogenase deficiency Carnitine transporter disorders Peroxisomal disorders Familial hypercholesterolaemia	

and isovaleric acidaemia (IVA); Scotland and North Ireland will expand screening in 2017.

IMDs are rare, one of the commonest being PKU with 1:10,000 live births in the UK (Pollitt *et al.*, 1997), and families can feel very isolated when their child is diagnosed. In addition, many healthcare professionals will have limited knowledge of the complex dietary restrictions required. Charities supporting families with IMDs, such as the National Society for Phenylketonuria (NSPKU) or Children Living with Inherited Metabolic Diseases (CLIMB), are beneficial in providing information and support in the early days following diagnosis. Many patients and parents turn to digital media such as social networking sites for information, but the information available may be out of date, unreliable or not scientifically supported.

Treatment for IMDs is for life, with the paediatric dietitian being an essential member of the metabolic multidisciplinary team, which should also include consultants in metabolic medicine, biochemists, specialist nurses, pharmacists, clinical psychologists and social workers. Even with good metabolic control, the degree of disability is extremely variable, depending on the particular condition and severity of the genetic mutation. Some children will be able to lead a normal life, whereas others will be severely disabled or may die at a young age.

Dietary management

At the time of diagnosis, the paediatric dietitian will be involved to discuss dietary management, prescribe any essential specialist dietary products (e.g. condition-specific formula) and provide written information for the family and carers. This will be followed by regular contact and support at the clinic or via telephone to ensure the child is growing well and adhering to the prescribed dietary plan. Biochemical markers should be monitored to ensure that adjustments are made to the diet in order to maintain good metabolic control.

PKU is a condition easily monitored at home by families, and there is very frequent contact between the dietitian and the family to ensure that phenylalanine levels are optimised to prevent toxicity to the brain. Phenylalanine intake is adjusted in the form of exchanges (50 mg phenylalanine/1 g protein) to maintain levels within the recommended range. The frequency of monitoring varies from weekly to monthly, depending on the child's age and metabolic control.

There are a number of manufacturing companies producing essential dietary supplements and foods that help with adherence to diet. These products will have the specific substrate that cannot be metabolised removed, but will otherwise provide nutritional support for a variety of ages. Low-protein food products include breads, flour, pasta, biscuits and snack items, and savoury mixes.

Emergency regimens

Emergency regimens (ERs) are plans given to patients and their families to prevent decompensation when

SECTION 3

unwell or undergoing periods of fasting, such as planned surgery. Not all IMDs require an emergency regimen. However, they are essential in certain conditions, and, if not used and the patient treated promptly, there is a high risk of metabolic decompensation, encephalopathy or even death. Many patients will carry a copy of their own specifically tailored ER when away from home, and liaising with the patient's metabolic team is also essential.

Treatment for any suspected intercurrent infection is often to stop the usual diet and commence an ER for a period of 24–48 hours. ERs are based on a glucose polymer solution, which provides an exogenous supply of energy and limits the catabolic response that could potentially become toxic. Further details on ERs can be found on the British Inherited Metabolic Diseases Group (BIMDG) website (see Chapter 7.8, Inherited metabolic disorders in adults). If oral intake is not possible, then immediate IV infusion of glucose is required (usually 10% glucose).

Every child requiring an ER will be provided with written information from its dietitian or metabolic consultant, given as part of the management protocol at diagnosis. The ER is updated as the child grows or dietary recommendations change. The concentration of glucose polymer is age dependent and should be reviewed at each clinic appointment to ensure that the parents have the correct concentration, know how to prepare the ER and understand when to use it.

Preparation of ER at home can be inaccurate with incorrect and inappropriate volumes being given (Gokmen-Ozel *et al.*, 2010). One of the specialist manufacturers has developed measured sachets of glucose polymer according to age to help alleviate this problem. Palatability can be improved by adding squash.

Professionals working with IMDs can gain support by becoming members of the BIMDG and the Scientific Society for Inherited Errors of Metabolism (SSIEM). There are patient support groups for specific conditions that dietitians can also use.

Acknowledgement

The editor acknowledges the prior contribution of Diana Webster.

Internet resources

British Inherited Metabolic Diseases Group (BIMDG), www.bimdg.org.uk

Expanded Newborn Screening, www.expandedscreening.org

Galactosaemia Support Group (GSG), www.galactosaemia.org

National Society for Phenylketonuria (NSPKU), www.nspku.org

Scientific Society for Inherited Errors of Metabolism (SSIEM), www.ssiem.org

References

Burton H. (2005) *Metabolic Pathways: Networks of Care*. Cambridge: Public Health Genetics Unit. Available at http://www.phgfoundation.org/documents/69_1135004491.pdf. Accessed 18 February 2019.

Gokmen-Ozel H, Daly A, Davies P, *et al.* (2010) Errors in emergency feeds in inherited metabolic disorders: a randomised controlled trial of three preparation methods. *Arch. Dis. Child.* 95: 776–780.

Pollitt RJ, Green A, McCabe CJ, *et al.* (1997) Neonatal screening for inborn errors of metabolism: cost, yield and outcome. *Health Technol. Assess.* 1: i–202.

3.8.18 Paediatric food hypersensitivity

Rosan Meyer

Food hypersensitivity (FHS) is a term that encompasses both allergies (Immunoglobulin E (IgE)- and non-IgE-mediated) and non-allergic food hypersensitivity (food intolerances) as defined by the European Academy of Allergy and Clinical Immunology (Johansson *et al.*, 2004). Venter *et al.* (2016) recently published 10-year cumulative prevalence and incidence data of food hypersensitivity in the UK, indicating that the prevalence of sensitisation to any allergen was 19.2%. Food challenges were performed to confirm the food hypersensitivity, which indicated cumulative incidence as being 6.8%, while the prevalence was 3.6%. The vast majority of these cases (3.0%) suffered from IgE-mediated food allergy, and only 0.6% had non-IgE-mediated allergies. However, the prevalence of non-IgE-mediated allergy is debatable due to difficulties in recognising symptoms and lack of conclusive diagnostic tools; the prevalence is likely to be higher (Koletzko *et al.*, 2015; Schoemaker *et al.*, 2015). Although food allergy can arise to any food, more than 85% of childhood food allergies are due to milk, egg, peanut, tree nuts, shellfish, fish, wheat, sesame seed and soy (Venter & Meyer, 2010). Prognosis for outgrowing a food allergy remains good; the majority of children outgrow milk, soy and egg allergy, but there has been a shift in acquiring tolerance to later ages. Although recently published data (Schoemaker *et al.*, 2015) on cow's milk protein allergy (CMPA) indicated that, 1 year after diagnosis, 69% of children with non-IgE-mediated and 57% of IgE-mediated CMPA had outgrown their allergy, Skripak *et al.* (2007) indicated that only 19% outgrew their CMPA by age 4 years and 79% by 16 years (Skripak *et al.*, 2007). Allergies to fish, shellfish and nuts are more likely to persist into adult life, although some will be outgrown (Fleischer, 2007; Pascual *et al.*, 2008). Diagnosis involves an allergy-focused history with skin prick or specific IgE testing, diagnostic exclusion diets or food challenges (NICE, 2011; Skypala *et al.*, 2015). Owing to the likelihood of changes in food hypersensitivity status, children will need regular reviews. (See Chapter 7.11.2, Food hypersensitivity, for more information on both testing and food reintroduction.)

Treatment

Although allergen avoidance remains the mainstay treatment, there has been a shift in management, particularly for milk, egg and selective nut allergies. These allergens may not need to be totally avoided if tolerated in baked format; it may be possible to consume milk, eggs and selected nuts with guidance from an experienced allergy dietitian. Baking at high temperature largely destroys the conformational epitopes in cow's milk (Nowak-Wegrzyn *et al.*, 2008) and egg (Leonard *et al.*, 2015). In IgE-mediated allergy, the introduction of baked egg and cow's milk needs to be supervised as severe reactions have been documented (Mehr *et al.*, 2014; Turner *et al.*, 2013), and home introduction should only occur in non-IgE-mediated allergies (Venter *et al.*, 2013). In the past, it was often suggested to avoid all nuts when a child had a diagnosis of allergy to one nut. However, with the emergence of data on nut allergy prevention and component testing, with correct guidance, selective nut eating (nuts a child is not allergic to) is possible (Brough *et al.*, 2015).

Nutritional aspects

The impact of food exclusions can increase the risk of nutritional deficiencies in these children (Flammarion *et al.*, 2011; Meyer *et al.*, 2016). Dietary eliminations that necessitate the avoidance of a whole food group (e.g. cow's milk products), staple food items (e.g. wheat) or multiple foods will have the most impact (Berry *et al.*, 2015; Cho *et al.*, 2011). Children with other coexisting dietary restrictions, e.g. vegetarianism, cultural or religious restrictions, and feeding difficulties, will be at a higher risk of deficiencies as well.

Meyer *et al.* (2015) has recently highlighted that, in food-allergic children, it is not only calcium and vitamin D that may be of concern, and a full nutritional review is therefore recommended. All allergic children should also follow current DH guidelines for vitamin D supplementations. For CMPA, a suitable replacement will be essential where breastfeeding is not available. The following is a summary of guidelines related to the choice of hypoallergenic formula for non-breastfed infants (Fiocchi *et al.*, 2010; Luyt *et al.*, 2014; NICE guidelines, 2011, 2014; Venter *et al.*, 2013):

- Non-breastfed infants and children aged <2 years should be given a suitable infant formula as the main milk replacement:
  - Extensively hydrolysed formulas are suitable for most CMPA infants, but an amino acid formula is suggested if the following conditions exist:
    - Faltering growth/malnutrition.
    - Multiple severe food allergies.
    - Severe non-resolving symptoms on an extensively hydrolysed formula.
    - Anaphylaxis.
    - Severe symptoms while breastfed and not resolving on a maternal elimination diet.
    - Severe gastrointestinal allergies including eosinophilic oesophagitis.
  - Soya infant formula is not recommended for infants aged <6 months (Luyt *et al.*, 2014). Care should also be taken to check for coexisting soya allergy: this is common in non-IgE-mediated allergy (Meyer *et al.*, 2013).
  - When intake of hypoallergenic infant formula is adequate, over-the-counter (OTC) milk substitute may be used for cooking from age 6 months, but not as main milk replacement.
- In children aged >2 years, OTC calcium-enriched milk substitute may be suitable if the child has a good diet (Luyt *et al.*, 2014):
  - Fortified soya, coconut, hemp, oat and nut OTC milk.
  - Rice milk is not recommended in children aged <4.5 years due to its increased arsenic content.
  - Children with CMPA will also react to other mammalian milks (i.e. goat's and sheep's milk); therefore, these milks should not be recommended (Fiocchi *et al.*, 2010).

Dietary management

The main aspects of managing food exclusion are similar to those in adults (see Chapter 7.11.2, Food hypersensitivity). There are additional considerations when managing paediatric food exclusion, which include:

- Other carers, i.e. extended families, nurseries, child minders and schools, may all be involved in food provision and require education and support to safely manage the child's diet while in their care.
- Parties or playgroups – in these situations, food is often readily accessible to children. Advising parents on practical ways of managing these situations is very important.
- Specialist free-from foods can play an important role in maintaining a varied diet while allowing children to eat a similar diet as their peers. Advice on suitable products should be made available to parents, taking into account factors such as cost and nutritional adequacy.

Weaning

Parental anxiety can increase at this time and, in some situations, lead to delayed or restricted weaning. Dietetic advice can help to ensure that infants meet their nutritional needs in addition to developing age-appropriate eating skills. Parents will need to be advised on which foods they can safely introduce to their child's diet; in some situations, testing may support this. While it is important to avoid foods that a child is known or suspected to be sensitive to, there is no evidence supporting delaying weaning (Grimshaw *et al.*, 2013). Early introduction of allergenic foods may prevent the development of further allergies (Fleischer *et al.*, 2016; Perkin *et al.*, 2016).

Adolescence

Older children should be encouraged to become gradually more involved in their dietary management and in the use of emergency medications. As with many chronic conditions, the teenage years may be particularly challenging with regards to compliance, and more input may be required at this stage (Ballmer-Weber, 2015).

Acknowledgement

The editor acknowledges the prior contribution of Sarah Heath.

Further reading

Meyer, R., De Koker, C., Dzubiak, R., *et al.* 2016. The impact of the elimination diet on growth and nutrient intake in children with food protein induced gastrointestinal allergies. *Clin. Transl.*. Allergy, In Press.

Meyer, R., De Koker, C., Dziubak R., *et al.* (2014) Malnutrition in children with food allergies in the UK. *J. Hum. Nutr. Diet.* 27(3): 227–235.

Internet resources

BDA Food Allergy Group, www.bda.uk.com
British Society of Clinical Allergy & Immunology, www.bsaci.org
European Academy of Allergy & Clinical Immunology, http://www.eaaci.org
World Allergy Organization, www.worldallergy.org

References

Ballmer-Weber BK. (2015) Food allergy in adolescence and adulthood. *Chem. Immunol. Allergy*, 101: 51–58.

Berry MJ, Adams J, Voutilainen H, *et al.* (2015) Impact of elimination diets on growth and nutritional status in children with multiple food allergies. *Pediatr. Allergy Immunol.* 26(2): 133–138.

Brough HA, Turner PJ, Wright T, *et al.* (2015) Dietary management of peanut and tree nut allergy: what exactly should patients avoid? *Clin. Exp. Allergy.* 45(5): 859–871.

Cho HN, Hong S, Lee SH, *et al.* (2011) Nutritional status according to sensitized food allergens in children with atopic dermatitis. *Allergy Asthma Immunol. Res.* 3(1): 53–57.

Fiocchi A, Schunemann HJ, Brozek J, *et al.* (2010) Diagnosis and Rationale for Action Against Cow's Milk Allergy (DRACMA): a summary report. *J. Allergy Clin. Immunol.* 126(6): 1119–1128.

Flammarion S, Santos C, Guimber D, *et al.* (2011) Diet and nutritional status of children with food allergies. *Pediatr. Allergy. Immunol.* 22(2): 161–165.

Fleischer DM. (2007) The natural history of peanut and tree nut allergy. *Curr. Allergy Asthma Rep.* 7(3): 175–181.

Fleischer DM, Sicherer S, Greenhawt M, *et al.* (2016). Consensus communication on early peanut introduction and prevention of peanut allergy in high-risk infants. *Pediatr. Dermatol.* 33(1): 103–106.

Grimshaw KE, Maskell J, Oliver EM, *et al.* (2013) Introduction of complementary foods and the relationship to food allergy. *Pediatrics.* 132(6): e1529–e1538.

Johansson SG, Bieber T, Dahl R, *et al.* (2004) Revised nomenclature for allergy for global use: report of the Nomenclature Review Committee of the World Allergy Organization, October 2003. *J. Allergy Clin. Immunol.* 113(5): 832–836.

Koletzko S, Heine RG. (2015) Non-IgE-mediated cow's milk allergy in EuroPrevall. *Allergy.* 70(12): 1679–1680.

Leonard SA, Caubet JC, Kim JS, *et al.* (2015) Baked milk- and egg-containing diet in the management of milk and egg allergy. *J. Allergy Clin. Immunol. Pract.* 3(1): 13–23.

Luyt D, Ball H, Makwana N, *et al.* (2014) BSACI guideline for the diagnosis and management of cow's milk allergy. *Clin. Exp. Allergy* 44(5): 642–672.

Mehr S, Turner PJ, Joshi P, *et al.* (2014) Safety and clinical predictors of reacting to extensively heated cow's milk challenge in cow's milk-allergic children. *Ann. Allergy. Asthma. Immunol.* 113(4): 425–429.

Meyer R, De KC, Dziubak R, *et al.* (2015) A practical approach to vitamin and mineral supplementation in food allergic children. *Clin. Transl. Allergy.* 5: 11.

Meyer R, De Koker C, Dzubiak R, *et al.* (2016) The impact of the elimination diet on growth and nutrient intake in children with food protein induced gastrointestinal allergies. *Clin. Transl. Allergy.* 6: 25.

Meyer R, Fleming C, Dominguez-Ortega G, *et al.* (2013) Manifestations of food protein induced gastrointestinal allergies presenting to a single tertiary paediatric gastroenterology unit. *World Allergy Organ. J.* 6(1): 13.

NICE. (2011) *Diagnosis and assessment of food allergy in children and young people in primary care and community settings.* Available at https://www.nice.org.uk/guidance/cg116/evidence/full-guideline-136470061 Accessed 18 February 2019

NICE. (2014) *Cow's milk protein allergy in children.* NICE: Clinical Knowledge Series, NICE, London.

Nowak-Wegrzyn A, Bloom KA, Sicherer SH, *et al.* (2008). Tolerance to extensively heated milk in children with cow's milk allergy. *J Allergy Clin. Immunol.* 122(2): 342–347, 347.

Pascual CY, Reche M, Fiandor A, *et al.* (2008) Fish allergy in childhood. *Pediatr. Allergy Immunol.* 19(7): 573–579.

Perkin MR, Logan K, Tseng A, *et al.* (2016) Randomized trial of introduction of allergenic foods in breast-fed infants. *N. Engl. J. Med.* 374(18): 1733–1743.

Schoemaker AA, Sprikkelman AB, Grimshaw KE, *et al.* (2015) Incidence and natural history of challenge-proven cow's milk allergy in European children – EuroPrevall birth cohort. *Allergy.* 70(8): 963–972.

Skripak JM, Matsui EC, Mudd K, *et al.* (2007) The natural history of IgE-mediated cow's milk allergy. *J. Allergy Clin. Immunol.* 120(5): 1172–1177.

Skypala IJ, Venter C, Meyer R, *et al.* (2015) The development of a standardised diet history tool to support the diagnosis of food allergy. *Clin. Transl. Allergy.* 5: 7.

Turner PJ, Mehr S, Joshi P, T *et al.* (2013) Safety of food challenges to extensively heated egg in egg-allergic children: a prospective cohort study. *Pediatr. Allergy Immunol.* 24(5): 450–455.

Venter C, Brown T, Shah N, *et al.* (2013) Diagnosis and management of non-IgE-mediated cow's milk allergy in infancy – a UK primary care practical guide. *Clin. Transl. Allergy.* 3(1): 23.

Venter C, Meyer R. (2010) Allergic disease: the challenges of managing food hypersensitivity. *Proc. Nutr. Soc.* 69(1): 11–24.

Venter C, Patil V, Grundy J, *et al.* (2016) Prevalence and cumulative incidence of food hyper-sensitivity in the first 10 years of life. *Pediatr. Allergy Immunol.* 27(5): 452–458.

3.8.19 Paediatric human immunodeficiency virus

Lisa Cooke

There are approximately 1000 children with human immunodeficiency virus (HIV) in the UK (Collaborative HIV Paediatric Study (CHIPS), 2016). The number is declining due to the reduction in transmission rates and the children transitioning into adult services. Most children are of sub-Saharan descent and have acquired the virus from mother-to-child transmission. The majority of children living with HIV in the UK are cared for in three major centres in London: Great Ormond Street Hospital for Sick Children, St Mary's, and St George's. These hospitals form the centres for the hub-and-spoke network of care for children around the rest of the UK (Children's HIV National Network (CHINN)). Smaller numbers of patients are seen within the spoke areas of the network within a defined radius surrounding their locality. Each team should consist of a paediatrician (usually an immunology specialist), specialist nurse, dietitian, psychologist, social worker and pharmacist.

There is still much stigma attached to this condition, and this creates challenges to its management. In the majority of cases, family members also have HIV, and the mothers of these children often carry much guilt from infecting their child. Due to an excellent antenatal screening pathway now in place, there is <1% transmission from mother to child within the UK.

Dietetic management

Since the introduction of highly active antiretroviral therapy (HAART) treatment in the late 1990s, all children, if well managed, should live a full and physically active life. Some of the medications can have gastrointestinal side effects, e.g. nausea. For long-term health and well-being, it is essential that any medication doses be missed as the HIV virus can reactivate. These drugs are continually being manipulated to be one step ahead of the virus, which adapts quickly and becomes resistant to treatment. Dietetic interventions centre on supporting a healthy lifestyle and diet, avoidance of being overweight or underweight, and careful management of lipidaemia.

HIV affects blood cholesterol levels, which are often naturally higher in individuals with the condition. Certain antiretroviral drugs can also raise blood lipid levels. The (paediatric) arm of the BDA group Dietitians Working in HIV/AIDS (DHIVA) called mini-DHIVA – has developed a lipid algorithm to support lipid management. This has been accepted by the Children's HIV Association (CHIVA, www.chiva.org.uk) and is available on their website. Mini-DHIVA has also produced an annual assessment form that all paediatric dietitians working in HIV are encouraged to use with their patients (see www.chiva.org.uk).

Many children are from black and ethnic minority groups, and, due to the high latitude of the UK, vitamin D status is often poor. Levels should be monitored and supplementation prescribed. Prescribing guidelines are available from CHIVE.

The aims of the dietetic intervention are to:

- Monitor growth and development, optimising growth where necessary. Awareness of clinical condition, past medical history, parental heights and current treatment status is necessary to inform the child's predicted growth.
- Measure mid-upper-arm circumference (MUAC) and waist measurement.
- Assess serum lipid levels, CD4% (cell count), renal function, vitamin D levels, blood pressure and insulin levels.
- Assess diet using dietary recall and be guided by the annual assessment form.
- Focus on a cardioprotective-style diet.
- As this is a chronic condition, aim for behavioural change management throughout the child's life.

It is vital that the dietitian be an integrated member of the multidisciplinary team, and be aware of the child's knowledge of his or her condition through close working with this team. Due to the stigma surrounding the condition, it is important that disclosure of the diagnosis be done slowly, age appropriately and fully supported by the parents, within the MDT and supported by all members. Many children will eat a traditional diet at home. Therefore, a good knowledge of sub-Saharan African diets is essential (see Chapter 3.5, Working with minority ethnic groups, and Chapter 7.11.3, Human immunodeficiency virus).

Further reading

Collaborative HIV Paediatric Study (CHIPS). (2011) *Summary data to the end June 2015.*

Internet resources

Children's HIV Association, www.chiva.org.uk

Collaborative HIV Paediatrics Study (CHIPS), http://www.chipscohort.ac.uk

Dietitians working in HIV/AIDS (DHIVA), a group of the BDA, http://dhiva.org.uk

SECTION 3

3.8.20 Paediatric diabetes

Shelley Easter

The incidence of childhood type 1 and type 2 diabetes is increasing (Ma & Chan, 2009). The current estimate of prevalence of type 1 diabetes in children aged 0–15 years in England and Wales is 192.0 per 100,000 (NPDA, 2016). Prevalence figures for children with type 2 diabetes are limited; however, the 2014–2015 NPDA report recorded 533 children and young people aged 5–19 years with this diagnosis.

The DH (2012/2013) guidance document outlines best practices in caring for children with diabetes. A child should be offered four multidisciplinary clinic visits per year, one of which should be an annual review. There should be eight additional support sessions (which can be by phone) of 15 minutes each by any team member. The annual review clinic should include dietary assessment and clinical investigations, including thyroid function – and, from the age of 12 years, retinopathy screening, microalbuminaemia and blood pressure (NICE, 2015).

To ensure that the needs of children and young people with diabetes are met, the MDT based in secondary care should include a paediatrician, diabetes specialist nurse and paediatric dietitian. Access to a psychologist and social worker should be available. Parents of young children should be actively involved, as well as other carers: school, nursery, child minders, etc. (DH, 2001; NICE, 2015; SIGN, 2010; Smart *et al.*, 2014). For each clinic visit, weight and height should be measured and plotted on the appropriate growth chart, in addition to calculating and plotting the BMI. This will help identify normal growth and/or any significant changes in weight as these may reflect changes in glycaemic control (NICE, 2015).

The dietitian's role is to balance the necessity of strict glycaemic control with the family diet and to convert scientific theory about food into practical and sensible advice. The aims of dietetic management are to:

- Provide appropriate energy intake for optimal growth, BMI and health.
- Encourage lifelong healthy eating habits, which preserve social, cultural and psychological well-being.
- Achieve a balance between food intake, requirements and insulin profiles to obtain optimal control.
- Achieve lipid levels in a desirable range.
- Prevent and treat acute complications of diabetes: hypoglycaemia, illness and exercise.
- Reduce the risk of micro- and macro-vascular complications (Smart *et al.*, 2014).

Type 1 diabetes mellitus

There is a preference for intensive insulin regimens, such as multiple daily injections or pump therapy, where education on matching insulin to the desired carbohydrate intake is required. Such regimens allow maximum flexibility in food choices. Individual insulin-to-carbohydrate ratios allow the adjustment of the pre-meal insulin according to the estimated carbohydrate content of the meal or snack. Visual resources can be very useful when educating the family on carbohydrate counting, especially if mathematical skills are not strong or a bolus advisor is not used. *Carbs and Cals* (Cheyette & Balolia, 2016) is a visual guide to carbohydrate and calorie counting, and a useful teaching aid.

Carbohydrate counting education should be offered from diagnosis, and advice on low-glycaemic-index foods is encouraged to optimise glycaemic control (NICE, 2015). To minimise complications, it is now recommended that a HbA1c target level of ≤48 mmol/mol be achieved.

Type 2 diabetes mellitus

Type 2 diabetes is increasingly recognised in children. It is more prevalent in the developed world, where there is an increased prevalence of childhood obesity.

Features associated with the diagnosis are (NICE, 2015; Zeitler *et al.*, 2014):

- Obesity.
- Age >10 years.
- Strong family history of type 2 diabetes.
- Acanthosis nigricans – brown/black velvety hyperpigmentation of the skin.
- High-risk racial or ethnic group.

The aims of nutritional management include the prevention of acute and chronic complications by achieving normoglycaemia, and addressing the child's weight in those with a BMI greater than the 95th percentile and any comorbidities, such as dyslipidaemia. The family should be involved in lifestyle changes, and the parents should be encouraged to act as positive role models. Oral antidiabetic agents may be used to reduce glucose absorption, increase insulin secretion and action, and reduce gluconeogenesis and/or insulin. Regular follow-up with monitoring of weight, glycaemic control and treatment is essential. As per type 1 diabetics, NICE (2015) recommends that the HbA1c target level of ≤48 mmol/mol be achieved to minimise the risk of long-term complications.

Other nutritional considerations

Type 1 diabetes is an autoimmune condition; therefore, there is an increased risk of other autoimmune conditions. Coeliac disease occurs in 0.6–16.4% of children with diabetes (Smart *et al.*, 2014). Annual screening is no longer included in guidance documents (NICE, 2015), but many centres will screen for coeliac disease in the annual review clinic. A gluten-free diet is the only accepted treatment. It is common for those with diabetes who develop coeliac disease not to adhere to the gluten-free diet, as they may be asymptomatic, and dietary manipulation for both disease states is difficult. These children and their families will require additional dietetic support, with realistic, family-centred advice.

Children and young people with type 1 diabetes (particularly young women) have an increased risk of eating disorders. When an eating disorder is identified, joint management involving the diabetes care team and child mental health professionals should be offered (NICE, 2015).

Age-group-specific advice

Infant and toddlers

Breastfeeding to 12 months should be encouraged alongside a healthy weaning diet, which encourages a variety of tastes, colours and textures of foods. Frequent, small meals may promote better glycaemic control, depending on the insulin regimen, and may also avoid food refusal. Insulin pump therapy has been shown to be effective when difficulties arise with food refusal. Parental anxiety is common; consideration of this is a priority when deciding upon the insulin regimen.

Schoolchildren

The diabetes regimen should fit into the school day. Advice should be given on food portion size, healthy food choices, low-fat snacks, reduced-fat dairy products and physical activity to reduce the risk of inappropriate weight gain and cardiovascular disease. Families should be supported with managing, parties and trips away from home. Continuing diabetes nutritional education with the child and family, including problem-solving techniques, may be useful.

Adolescents

Lifestyle advice, support and education targeted towards teenagers are required as they start to take over their diabetes management. Focused surveillance of weight monitoring is also required, as weight loss or poor weight gain may be a sign of insufficient intake, inappropriate insulin administration, disordered eating and/or poor glycaemic control. Careful review of insulin dose, food intake and activity is advisable, and the association between weight loss or failure to gain weight and disordered eating needs to be recognised. Rebellion, binges and erratic eating behaviour may require psychological support and counselling. Going out with peers, parties or holidays, and a healthy lifestyle need to be discussed. Advice on the safe consumption of alcohol and its prolonged glycaemic effect should be discussed, along with advice on increased appetite with alcohol. Careful planning of exercise and sport should be encouraged. Transition from the paediatric service to the adult service should be well planned and involve the young person to ensure it occurs at the right time (NICE, 2015).

Acknowledgement

The editor acknowledges the prior contribution of Natalie Mohamdee.

Further reading

Cheyette C, Balolia Y. (2016) *Carbs & Cals, Carb & Calorie Counter: Count Your Carbs & Calories with Over 1,700 Food & Drink Photos!*, 6th edn. London: Chello publishing.

Hanas R. (2015) *Type 1 Diabetes in Children, Adolescents and Young Adults: How to Become an Expert on Your Own Diabetes*, 6th edn. Somerset: Class Health.

Internet resources

Diabetes and Sport, www.runsweet.com
Diabetes Net, www.diabetesnet.com
Diabetes UK, www.diabetes.org.uk
International Diabetes Federation, www.idf.org
Nutrition and Diet Resources, www.ndr-uk.org
Quality Institute for Self Management and Education & Training, www.qismet.org.uk
SWEET project (Better control in paediatric and adolescent diabetes: working to create centres of reference), www.sweet-project.eu

Insulin pump companies

Accu-chek, www.accu-chek.co.uk
Animas, www.animascorp.co.uk
Medtronic, www.medtronic-diabetes.co.uk
My Life Diabetes Care, www.mylife-diabetescare.co.uk

References

Cheyette C, Balolia Y. (2013) *Carbs & Cals, Carb & Calorie Counter: Count Your Carbs & Calories with Over 1,700 Food & Drink Photos!*, 6th edn. London: Chello Publishing.

DH. (2001) *National Service Framework for Diabetes: Standards*. Available at https://www.gov.uk/government/uploads/system/uploads/attachment_data/file/216212/dh_133585.pdf. Accessed 15 March 2017.

DH. (2012/2013) *Payment by Results Guidance for 2012–2013*. Available at http://webarchive.nationalarchives.gov.uk/20130507170152/https://www.gov.uk/government/uploads/system/uploads/attachment_data/file/151911/dh_126157.pdf.pdf. Accessed 15 March 2017.

Ma R, Chan J. (2009) Diabetes: incidence of childhood type 1 diabetes: a worrying trend. *Nat. Rev. Endocrinol.* 5(10): 529–530.

National Paediatric Diabetes Audit (NPDA). (2016) *National Paediatric Diabetes Audit Report 2014–15 Part 1: Care Processes and Outcomes*. London: Royal College of Paediatrics and Child Health.

NICE. (2015) *Diabetes (type 1 and type 2) in Children and Young People: Diagnosis and Management*. London: NICE. Available at www.nice.org.uk/guidance/NG18. Accessed 17 November 2016.

Scottish Intercollegiate Guidelines Network (SIGN). (2010) *Management of Diabetes, Publication No116*. Edinburgh: SIGN.

Smart C, Annan F, Bruno L, *et al.* (2014) ISPAD clinical practice consensus guidelines 2014 compendium: nutritional management in children and adolescents with diabetes. *Pediatric. Diabetes.* 15(S20): 135–153.

Zeitler P, Fu J, Tandon N, *et al.* (2014) ISPAD clinical practice consensus guidelines 2014 compendium: type 2 diabetes. *Pediatric. Diabetes.* 15(S20): 26–46.

3.8.21 Cardiology

Philippa Wright

Congenital heart disease (CHD) describes defects in the structure of the heart that are present at birth. It affects 1 in every 145 births (www.bhf.org.uk), and there are a number of associated genetic syndromes, e.g. Down syndrome. Children with complex CHD are at increased risk of low birthweight<2.5 kg and being small for gestational age. CHD children are particularly vulnerable to malnutrition due to a combination of severe fluid restriction, inefficient absorption of nutrients and high metabolic demands (Avitzur *et al.*, 2003) (Table 3.8.27). Malnutrition can adversely affect postoperative outcomes and neurodevelopment (Black *et al.*, 2007), and increase the risk of stunting (Marino & Magee, 2015). Children are looked after in designated children's cardiac centres, with shared care arrangements with their local district general hospitals and community, both preoperatively and postoperatively.

Physiology

CHD is defined according to its haemodynamic effects, which fall into two groups: cyanotic and acyanotic. These types of cardiac malformations can have an effect on outcomes regarding growth and nutritional intake. *Cyanosis* refers to a reduced level of oxygen in the blood, and cyanotic lesions have been found to cause the greatest degree of stunting (Jacobs *et al.*, 2000). The acyanotic group of lesions can be further divided into obstructive malformations and left-to-right shunt malformations. These lesions have been observed to affect weight rather than height, especially in the presence of pulmonary hypertension (Mehziri & Drash, 1962; Umansky & Hauck, 1962). In this situation, blood is pumped to the lungs under greater pressure, preventing effective oxygenation. As a result, the heart pumps faster, and the child's breathing increases in an attempt to improve oxygenation. This ultimately increases the child's energy requirements and results in weight loss.

For detailed descriptions of all cardiac lesions, see the British Heart Foundation website (www.bhf.org.uk).

Congestive heart failure

Congestive heart failure (CHF) is the main concern in children with CHD. It occurs when the heart can no

Table 3.8.27 Factors that may influence the development of malnutrition and growth failure in infants with CHD (Nydegger & Bines, 2006)

Causative factors	Physiological impacts
Type and clinical impacts of cardiac disease	Cyanotic versus acyanotic defects
	Shunts
	Congestive heart failure
	Operative status: age at surgery, type of surgery, complications
Disturbances in energy metabolism	Increased energy expenditure
	Cardiac hypertrophy
	Body composition abnormalities
	Increased sympathetic nervous system activity
	Increased haematopoietic tissue
	Increased basal temperature
	Recurrent infections
	Pharmacological agents
Decreased nutritional intake	Anorexia, early satiety
	Pharmacological agents
	Decreased gastric volume caused by hepatomegaly
Disturbances in gastrointestinal function	Malabsorption
	Oedema and chronic hypoxia of the gut
	Interference with drugs
	Compressive hepatomegaly
	Decreased gastric volume
	Increased gastro-oesophageal reflux
Prenatal factors	Chromosomal disorders
	Intrauterine factors
	Birthweight

longer meet metabolic demands. Signs include tachycardia, fatigue on feeding and early satiety, all resulting in growth faltering. Diuretic therapy relieves CHF, but commonly used diuretics can cause sodium, potassium, chloride and calcium losses. While losses can be replaced, it is important to note that persistent hyponatraemia can result in poor growth and must be corrected.

Anaemia can also mimic the signs of CHF; cyanotic children can have higher iron requirements as they have an increased red cell mass. These infants should be screened for iron deficiency using ferritin, red cell indices and total iron-binding saturation, as haemoglobin may be within normal range even though they are iron deficient (Premer & Georgieff, 1999).

Mechanisms of malnutrition in congenital heart disease

Malnutrition can be caused by fluid restriction, poor absorption and fatigue on feeding, causing reduced intake, gastro-oesophageal reflux disease, increased metabolic expenditure, early satiety, anorexia and frequent infections. Energy for growth is diverted to meet increased metabolic demands. Studies give a range of energy requirements from 120 to 170 kcal/kg/day (Ackerman *et al.*, 1998; Barton *et al.*, 1994; Unger *et al.*, 1992; Waterlow, 1992; Yahav *et al.*, 1985). To facilitate weight gain, it is therefore advisable to aim for 110–130 kcal/kg and to increase to 150 kcal/kg if weight gain is not achieved. Protein requirements are 8–11% of energy, 2.6–4 g/kg in infants, and up to 3 g/kg in children older than 1 year (Lawson & Shaw, 2001).

Surgery

After surgery, children will be admitted to the PICU. Postoperative requirements are much lower than previously thought, especially in the immediate postoperative ventilated patient. No difference has been observed between cyanotic and acyanotic lesions; the only statistical difference is for those children requiring cardiopulmonary bypass. The non-bypass group (58.3 kcal/kg) appear to need less energy than the bypass (75 kcal/kg) group. This could be related to inflammatory response to bypass, but further studies are needed (De Wit *et al.*, 2010).

When calculating requirements in the immediately postoperative ventilated cardiac child, it is important to understand the amount of sedation, paralysis and ventilatory support that they are receiving. The Schofield equation is currently recommended for use when calculating postsurgical requirements.

Postoperative weight gain

After discharge from the PICU, the growth-faltering child may need to return to preoperative requirements until catch-up growth has been facilitated. It may be necessary to maintain enhanced energy content feeds and, in some cases, nasogastric or gastrostomy feeds. If fluid is restricted, high-energy formula and/or fortified expressed breast milk will be required. Breast milk can be fortified by adding 3–5% of standard infant powdered formula. If breast milk is not available, then the following high-energy formulae are available:

- SMA High Energy: 91 kcal/100 mL (2 g/100 mL).
- Infatrini/ infatrini peptisorb: 100 kcal/100 mL (2.6 g protein/100 mL).
- Similac High Energy: 101 kcal/100 mL (2.6 g protein/100 mL).

If weight gain is still not achieved after 3–4 g/kg of protein and 150 kcal/kg of energy have been provided, then additional energy can be given through the addition of a glucose and fat polymer. The PER of 9–14% must be preserved (Jackson, 2000; Wharton, 1994). However, the 24-hour urinary sodium balance should be measured if weight continues to falter. As these infants are often fluid restricted, which ultimately impacts on energy intake, it is important to check if an increase of fluids is possible in order to increase nutritional intake.

Feed administration

The method of feed administration is important, and the following steps should be employed, if required, in order to meet the child's dietary requirements for growth or catch-up:

- Offer smaller volumes and more frequent feeds orally.
- Give unfinished feeds via a NG tube if required.
- Give small, frequent bolus feeds via an NG tube.
- Give overnight continuous feeds via an enteral feeding pump in addition to small, frequent daytime feeds (always refer to local policies and guidelines when advising on overnight tube feeding).
- Give feeds continuously over 20 hours via a feeding pump, allowing the gut some time to rest and permitting the pH to return to normal.

Anthropometry

Anthropometric data is essential, and accurate weights, lengths and head circumference must be recorded on growth charts (from the point of referral). Be aware that fluctuating fluid balances can mislead weight records.

Expected weight gain

Expected weight gain values are difficult to achieve in children with CHD; therefore, an average gain of 10–20 g/day would be more appropriate in children under 6 months, and 120–210 g/week in children aged 6–12 months (17–30 g/day) (Forchielli *et al.*, 1994).

Complications

Postoperative complications include the following:

- *Chylothorax* – the accumulation of chyle in the pleural space. Conservative management involves the reduction of long-chain fats (Chan *et al.*, 2005) to <1 g per year of life to a maximum of 5 g/day for 4 weeks.

- *Protein-losing enteropathy* – there is limited evidence regarding specific diet therapy; however, it is suggested that the diet consist of 5–10 g/day of fat and be high in protein, with additional fat replaced with a medium-chain fat source to improve overall energy intake (Shaw & Lawson, 2007).
- *Necrotising enterocolitis (NEC)* – specific lesions and medications (inotropes) may increase the risk of NEC in a child with CHD. Reduced gut perfusion can occur, and the patient will require extremely slow reintroduction of feeds or parenteral nutrition if at risk.

References

Ackerman IL, Karn CA, Denne SC, *et al.* (1998) Total but not resting energy expenditure is increased in infants with ventricular septal defects. *Pediatrics*. 102: 1172–1177.

Avitzur Y, Singer P, Dagan O, *et al.* (2003) Resting energy expenditure in children with cyanotic and noncyanotic congenital heart disease before and after open heart surgery. *J. Parenter. Enteral Nutr.* 27: 47–51.

Barton J, Hindmarsh P, Scrimgeour C, *et al.* (1994) Increased energy expenditure in congenital heart disease. *Arch. Dis. Child.* 70: 5–9.

Black MM, Dubowitz H, Krishnakumar A, *et al.* (2007) Early intervention and recovery among children with failure to thrive: follow up at age 8. *Pediatrics*. 120: 59–69.

Chan E, Russell J, William G, *et al.* (2005) Postoperative chylothorax after cardiothoracic surgery in children. *Ann. Thorac. Surg.* 80: 1864–1871.

De Wit B, Meyer R, Desai A, *et al.* (2010) Challenge of predicting resting energy expenditure in children undergoing surgery for congenital heart disease. *Paediatr. Crit. Care Med.* 11: 496–501.

Forchielli MC, McColl R, Walker WA, *et al.* (1994) Children with congenital heart disease: a nutritional challenge. *Nutr. Rev.* 52(10): 348–353.

Jackson J. (2000) Protein requirements for catch up growth. *Proc. Nutr. Soc.* 49: 507–516.

Jacobs ECJ, Leung MP, Karlberg JP. (2000) Postnatal growth in southern Chinese children with symptomatic congenital heart disease. *J. Paediatr. Endocrinol. Metab.* 11: 195–202.

Lawson M, Shaw V. (2001) *Clinical Paediatric Dietetics*, 2nd edn. Oxford: Blackwell Publishing.

Marino L, Magee A. (2015) A cross-sectional audit of the prevalence of stunting in children attending a regional paediatric cardiology service. *Cardiol. Young* 26: 787–789.

Mehziri A, Drash A. (1962) Growth disturbances in congenital heart disease. *J. Paediatr.* 61: 418–429.

Nydegger A, Bines A. (2006) Energy metabolism in infants with congenital heart disease. *Nutrition* 22: 697–704.

Premer D, Georgieff M. (1999) Nutrition for ill neonates. *NeoReviews* 20(9): e56–e62.

Shaw V, Lawson M. (2007) *Clinical Paediatric Dietetics*, 3rd edn. Oxford: Blackwell.

Umansky R, Hauck AJ. (1962) Factors in the growth of children with patent ductus arteriosus. *Pediatrics*. 30: 540–550.

Unger R, de Kleermaeker M, Giddings S, *et al.* (1992) Calories count: improved weight gain with dietary intervention in congenital heart disease. *Am. J. Dis. Child.* 146: 1078–1084.

Waterlow JC. (1992) *Protein Energy Malnutrition*. London: Edward Arnold, pp. 231–232.

Wharton B. (1994) International recommendations on protein intake in infancy: some points for discussion. *Nestle Workshop Ser.* 33: 67–83.

Yahav J, Avigad S, Frand M, *et al.* (1985) Assessment of intestinal and cardiorespiratory function in children with congenital heart disease on high-calorie formulas. *J. Pediatr. Gastroenterol. Nutr.* 4: 778–785.

3.8.22 Paediatric cancers

Nicola Williams

Approximately 1600 children are diagnosed with cancer in the UK every year. Survival of childhood cancer has more than doubled since the 1960s, with the present survival rate being about 82% (Children's Cancer and Leukaemia Group, 2015). Cancer in children differs from that in adults in terms of the body areas affected and how it responds to treatment. Table 3.8.28 shows the types of cancer seen in children (Cancer Research UK). Depending on the type of cancer diagnosed, treatment will usually comprise of one or more of the following: chemotherapy, surgery, radiotherapy, immunotherapy, and stem cell or bone marrow transplant.

Table 3.8.28 Average number of new cases diagnosed per year in children aged 0–14 years, Great Britain (source: reproduced with permission from Cancer Research UK. http://www.cancerresearchuk.org/sites/default/files/cstream-node/child_inc_iccc_groups_0.pdf.)

Cancer type	Boys	Girls	Children
Leukaemia	262	205	468
Brain, other CNS and intracranial tumours	219	193	412
Lymphomas	115	51	167
Soft-tissue sarcoma	57	41	98
Sympathetic nervous system (SNS) tumours	43	40	83
Renal tumours	38	44	82
Bone sarcoma	35	30	65
Carcinomas and malignant melanoma	25	30	55
Germ cell and gonadal tumours	24	30	55
Retinoblastoma	22	22	44
Hepatic tumours	9	10	18
Other and unspecified cancers	5	3	8

Nutritional implications

Nutrition support is a key part of supportive care for children with cancer to ensure normal growth and development. Children may present malnourished or cachexic at diagnosis; in addition, treatment side effects can impact on nutritional status. It is recognised that good nutrition may reduce treatment complications and

Table 3.8.29 Types of childhood cancers associated with high or low nutritional risk (source: Shaw, 2015, table 21.2, p. 659. Reproduced with permission from John Wiley & Sons, Ltd.)

High nutritional risk	Low nutritional risk
Advanced diseases during initial intense treatment	Acute lymphoblastic leukaemia (ALL) regimen A patients
High-risk neuroblastoma	Non-metastatic solid tumours
Stages III and IV Wilms' tumour	Retinoblastoma
High-risk rhabdomyosarcoma	Hodgkin's disease
Ewing's sarcoma/PNET	Germ cell tumours
Osteosarcoma	Advanced diseases in remission during maintenance treatment
Medulloblastoma/CNS PNET	
B-cell NHL	
AML	
Some acute lymphoblastic leukaemia (ALL) – infants and teenagers, regimen B and C patients, relapsed ALL	
Bone marrow transplant patients – allogeneic, autologous	

infection rates, improve response to intensive anticancer treatments and promote weight gain and growth (NICE, 2005; RCN, 2014; Ward *et al.*, 2015). Table 3.8.29 shows the types of childhood cancers associated with high or low nutritional risk (Shaw, 2015).

Dietetic management

In the UK, there is no specific nutrition screening tool for children with cancer, although a diagnostic tool for malnutrition in these children has been designed for use alongside the Screening Tool for the Assessment of Malnutrition in Paediatrics (STAMP) (McCarthy *et al.*, 2012). For further information, see the Royal College of Nursing (2014).

Nutrition support

Management is determined by nutritional risk of diagnosis, nutritional status, symptoms and anticipated gut function. Symptoms relating to treatment that may impact upon nutritional status include infection, diarrhoea, nausea and vomiting, mucositis, anorexia, xerostomia and constipation. Oral nutritional support may be adequate when nutritional status is stable, but intake is reduced. If nutritional status deteriorates, enteral tube feeding should be started early to prevent further decline in weight and health. Parenteral nutrition is reserved for when gut function is compromised for >5 days. Whole-protein feeds are usually the first choice; however, during treatment that causes severe gastrointestinal toxicity, a hydrolysate or elemental feed is recommended.

Monitoring and follow-up

The child's tolerance to nutritional support may change significantly depending on the type of anticancer therapy it receives. Frequent monitoring of the feeding regimen and anthropometry will ensure that nutritional requirements for normal growth continue to be achieved. As treatment reduces in intensity (called 'maintenance chemotherapy') or is completed, nutritional support can be weaned, with the aim to progress towards a balanced diet.

Internet resources

British Dietetic Association, www.bda.uk.com
British Society of Blood and Bone Marrow Transplantation, http://bsbmt.org
Cancer Research UK, www.cancerresearchuk.org
Children with Cancer UK, www.childrenwithcancer.org.uk
Children's Cancer and Leukaemia Group, www.cclg.org.uk
CLIC Sargent, www.clicsargent.org.uk
International Society of Paediatric Oncology, http://siop-online.org/nutrition-working-group
Macmillan Cancer Support, www.macmillan.org.uk
STAMP screening tool, www.stampscreeningtool.org/stamp.html

References

Cancer Research UK (2009). *Average Number of New Cases Diagnosed per Year, Children (0–14), Great Britain.* Available at http://www.cancerresearchuk.org/sites/default/files/cstream-node/child_inc_iccc_groups_0.pdf. Accessed 22 November.

Children's Cancer and Leukaemia Group. (2015) *Survival Rates.* Available at www.cclg.org.uk/Survival-rates. Accessed 22 November 2016.

McCarthy H, Dixon M, Crabtree I, *et al.* (2012) The development and evaluation of the Screening Tool for the Assessment of Malnutrition in Paediatrics (STAMP©) for use by healthcare staff. *J. Hum. Nutr. Diet.* 25: 311–318.

NICE. (2005) *Improving Outcomes in Children and Young People with Cancer.* London: NICE.

Royal College of Nursing (RCN). (2014) *Nutrition in Children and Young People with Cancer.* RCN Guidance. London: RCN.

Shaw V. (2015) *Clinical Paediatric Dietetics*, 4th edn. Oxford: Blackwell Publishing.

Ward EJ, Henry LM, Friend AJ, *et al.* (2015) Nutritional support in children and young people with cancer undergoing chemotherapy. *Cochrane Database Syst. Rev.* (8): CD003298.

3.8.23 Nutrition support in the critically ill child

Luise V. Marino and Rosan Meyer

Recent advances in anaesthetic and intensive care have improved outcomes in critical illness (Rittirsch *et al.*, 2008). On average, 0.1% of the childhood population in England and Wales is admitted to a PICU per annum; 50% of these are under 1 year of age. The mean stay is 1–2 days (range 1–35 days) (Parslow *et al.*, 2009), although 19% of patients stay for >7 days (PICANET, 2015). Undernutrition is common (Hulst, Joosten *et al.*, 2004), impacting on morbidity, late mortality and length of PICU stay (Bechard *et al.*, 2016; Coss-Bu *et al.*, 2001; Goiburu *et al.*, 2006; Grippa *et al.*, 2016; Marino *et al.*, 2015). It is important to ensure optimal nutritional support from admission to discharge based on anthropometrical and biochemical parameters, clinical assessment and previous dietary intake.

Determining a nutrition care plan

Anthropometry

The rate of acute or chronic malnutrition in PICUs is 18–55% (Bechard *et al.*, 2016). The causes of malnutrition are multifactorial, and include premorbid disease, acute or chronic suboptimal nutritional support, as well as increased protein breakdown and reduced protein synthesis, especially in the acute phase of an illness (Hulst & Joosten, 2006). Every child should have anthropometry measured on admission to calculate its energy and protein requirements; however, due to the clinical condition, this can be challenging (Feferbaum *et al.*, 2009). It is therefore useful to consult the child's growth chart in its personal child health record (PCHR) to ascertain how well the child has been growing. It is quite common practice to estimate the child's weight using the advanced paediatric life support formula ([age + 4] × 2) (Argall *et al.*, 2003). However, Luscombe *et al.* found that this formula significantly underestimates weight, and that the formula [weight = 3(age) + 7] provides better estimation (Luscombe *et al.*, 2011). However, these formulae can never replace actual measurements.

Biochemistry

Biochemical abnormalities are common in critically ill children and may impact on nutritional support. The most important indices to consider include serum urea, glucose, albumin, C-reactive protein, magnesium, calcium, phosphorus, selenium, zinc, manganese and lactate acidosis. It is essential to refer to paediatric ranges as norms (Shaw, 2015), and abnormalities in children will differ from those in adults (Table 3.8.30).

Clinical factors

Critical illness can result in increased glucose synthesis, protein breakdown, fat oxidation and the risk of metabolic derangement (Hulst & Joosten, 2006). A nutritional assessment should take into account these and other factors, in addition to the protein and energy requirements relative to wound healing.

Dietary intake

As compared to adults, children and infants have significantly lower energy stores and need to be able to grow and develop; therefore, they should not have prolonged periods of starvation, e.g. 3–5 days. Nutritional support should be started as soon as possible (Skillman & Wischmeyer, 2008; Skillman & Mehta, 2012). Nutritional guidelines, including feeding protocols and paediatric dietetic care plans, significantly improve nutrition intake in some critically ill children, although they are of limited benefit in children with congenital heart disease. There are many challenges within a PICU setting that impact on the actual delivery of nutrients (Feferbaum *et al.*, 2009; Hulst & Joosten, 2006), such as the following:

- Fluid volume restriction: main barrier to adequate nutrition delivery (Feferbaum *et al.*, 2009).
- Procedural interruptions: account for 11–57% of total interruptions, affecting up to 62% of patients (McClave *et al.*, 1999). Often, feeding rates are not increased to compensate for time lost during the interruption, making it a challenge to achieve nutrition goals (Feferbaum *et al.*, 2009), resulting in energy/protein deficits negatively impacting on weight (Hulst, van Goudoever *et al.*, 2004).
- Interruption due to gastrointestinal intolerance: vomiting, diarrhoea, large gastric residuals and abdominal distension; may occur in up to 57% patients (Hurt & McClave, 2010; Meyer *et al.*, 2009).
- Mechanical problems: nasojejunal tube dislodgement, nasogastric tube blockage and/or enteral feeding pump dysfunction can impact on the amount of feed delivered (Feferbaum *et al.*, 2009).

There is little published data on energy or protein requirements in critically ill children. Table 3.8.31 summarises some recommendations.

Enteral feeding

Type of feed

Ready-to-use paediatric-specific enteral or infant feeds should be used, decreasing the risk of bacterial contamination. The use of energy–nutrient-dense infant formulae

Table 3.8.30 Relevance of biochemical indices in critical illness

Biochemical index	Comment
Serum urea	Indicative of the catabolism/protein breakdown associated with trauma, impaired renal function, dehydration, polyuria or severe sweating impacting on fluid management (Hulst & Joosten, 2006)
	Linked with muscle mass, but not a reliable marker to assess nutritional support
Glucose	Debatable positive impact on outcome, decreasing morbidity and mortality
	Important to monitor, especially in children receiving IV preparations and PN (Skillman & Wischmeyer, 2008)
Albumin	Likely to be low, especially if receiving intravenous saline (McClave *et al.*, 1999)
	Not a good nutritional index, owing to long half-life; a marker of inflammation, intravascular or extravascular fluid shifts and catabolism (Evans *et al.*, 2006)
	Hypoalbuminemia at admission to a PICU is associated with higher 60-day mortality, longer duration of mechanical ventilation and lower probability of ICU discharge; these associations were independent of inflammatory response, clinical severity and nutritional status (Leite *et al.*, 2016)
C-reactive protein (CRP)	Index of the acute phase response, usually measured serially
	Serum prealbumin and CRP are inversely related, e.g. <0.5 mg/mL
	In infants, <0.2 mg/mL is associated with the return of anabolism, with a concomitant rise in prealbumin (van Waardenburg *et al.*, 2009)
Magnesium	Hypomagnesaemia common in critically ill children (Braegger *et al.*, 2010)
Calcium	Strongly associated with hypokalaemia / hypocalcaemia (Hulst & Joosten, 2006)
Phosphorus, selenium, zinc, manganese	Hypophosphataemia (up to 61% of critically ill children) (Santana e Meneses *et al.*, 2009)
	Low serum levels of selenium, zinc and manganese common in critical illnesses (Hulst & Joosten, 2006; Sadoh & Sadoh, 2013); low serum zinc levels are associated with lymphopenia (Heidemann *et al.*, 2013); some children may benefit from supplementation (Wang *et al.*, 2013, 2015)
Lactate acidosis	Common in critically ill children, reflecting hypoperfusion, including diabetic ketoacidosis and septic shock/cardiogenic shock
	Lactic acidosis, base excess and a strong anion gap associated with more risk of death
	A level of >2 mmol/L may be used as a crude proxy for cell function; resolution correlates with survival (Zamberlan *et al.*, 2011)

PN, parenteral nutrition.

are useful in critically ill infants (<1 year) (Evans *et al.*, 2006) where there are fluid restrictions, improving energy and nitrogen balance (van Waardenburg *et al.*, 2009).

Polymeric fibre-containing feeds are appropriate for the majority of critically ill children and are associated with fewer episodes of diarrhoea. A 1 kcal/mL feed will meet the requirements of most children, but, where there is fluid restriction, a 1.5 kcal/mL feed may be more appropriate. A small minority of patients with malabsorption syndromes will require hydrolysed, elemental feeds and/or specialist feeds when indicated (Braegger *et al.*, 2010). It is important to consider micronutrient intake while a child is on PICU. A recent study highlighted that the majority of children did not achieve vitamin and mineral requirements, and, in long-stay patients, this needs to be considered with enteral feeding (Dos Reis Santos *et al.*, 2016).

Initiation of enteral feeds

Most centres aim to start feeds within 12–24 hours of admission (Briassoulis *et al.*, 2001; Meyer *et al.*, 2009), aiming to achieve goal rates as soon as possible using a stepwise approach (Meyer *et al.*, 2009; Zamberlan *et al.*, 2011). Most children tolerate nasogastric tube feeding, but there will be some for whom a nasojejunal feeding tube is indicated (Braegger *et al.*, 2010; Mehta *et al.*, 2009). Although bolus feeding is more physiological, continuous feeds delivered via a volumetric pump may be better tolerated, as they have less impact on clinical indices (Horn & Chaboyer, 2003).

Parenteral Nutrition

Early PN during the first 8 days of admission has not been shown to be beneficial and may increase the risk of infectious morbidity and mortality. However, the mechanisms which may improve clinical outcomes through the withholding of PN during this period need to be further elucidated (Fivez *et al.*, 2016; Mehta, 2016).

Refeeding syndrome

As the prevalence of malnutrition within the PICU population is high, the risk of refeeding syndrome should be considered. When enteral or parenteral nutrition is commenced in children who have not received optimal nutritional support for some time, i.e. ≥3 days, it is important to ensure there is a multidisciplinary approach

Table 3.8.31 Recommendations for energy and protein requirements of critically ill children

	Recommendations
Energy requirements	Schofield equation – without stress addition or activity factor, shown to deliver the closest value to measured REE (Briassoulis *et al.*, 2001; Hulst & Joosten, 2006; Mehta *et al.*, 2009)
	In long-term PICU patients (>7 days), especially where not using muscle relaxants and where there is active physiotherapy, a higher energy intake may be required (van der Kuip *et al.*, 2007)
	Ventilated children can be overfed, especially if liberalising fluid volumes. In particular, children on PN are at risk of being overfed (Fivez *et al.*, 2016). Overfeeding can result in fatty liver, hyperglycaemia, more CO_2 production, increased length of hospital stay (Skillman & Wischmeyer, 2008)
Protein requirements	0–2 years: 2–3 g/kg/day
	2–13 years: 1.5–2 g/kg/day
	13–18 years: 1.5 g/kg/day (Mehta *et al.*, 2009)
	Except in preterm infants, 4 g/kg should not be exceeded, as it increases the risk of hypertonic dehydration and exceeds maximal protein oxidation rates (Klein *et al.*, 1998)
Glucose oxidation rate	The maximal oxidation rate is 5 mg/min/kg/day (7.2 g/kg/day); excessive glucose intake leads to increased risk of hepatic steatosis (fatty liver)/CO_2 production; amounts will vary for critically ill neonates and infants (Koletzko *et al.*, 2005)
Feed composition	10–15% protein energy (Clarke *et al.*, 2007)
	50–55% carbohydrate energy
	35% fat energy (Flaring & Finkel, 2009)
Vitamin requirements	No specific recommendations exist for ventilated patients in PICU
	Many patients require additional supplementation, e.g. premature infants, those undergoing haemofiltration. Blood biochemistry should be monitored (Meyer *et al.*, 2015)

REE, resting energy expenditure.

for determining the risk of refeeding syndrome (Afzal *et al.*, 2002; Byrnes & Stangenes, 2011; Crook *et al.*, 2001; Solomon & Kirby, 1990).

Critically ill children represent a nutritionally vulnerable population who may already be malnourished on admission. Nutritional support in this population group requires attention to detail to ensure that the challenge of meeting nutritional requirements occurs early in their PICU stay, and should focus on achieving equilibrium and not overfeeding or underfeeding.

Internet resources

Paediatric Intensive Care Audit Network (PICANET), www.picanet.org.uk/index.html

References

Afzal NA, Addai S, Fagbemi A, *et al.* (2002) Refeeding syndrome with enteral nutrition in children: a case report, literature review and clinical guidelines. *Clin. Nutr.* 21(6): 515–520.

Argall JA, Wright N, Mackway-Jones K, *et al.* (2003) A comparison of two commonly used methods of weight estimation. *Arch. Dis. Child.* 88(9): 789–790.

Bechard LJ, Duggan C, Touger-Decke R, *et al.* (2016) Nutritional status based on body mass index is associated with morbidity and mortality in mechanically ventilated critically ill children in the PICU. *Crit. Care Med.* 44(8): 1530–1537.

Braegger C, Decsi T, Dias JA, *et al.* (2010) Practical approach to paediatric enteral nutrition: a comment by the ESPGHAN committee on nutrition. *J. Pediatr. Gastroenterol. Nutr.* 51(1): 110–122.

Briassoulis GC, Zavras NJ, Hatzis MD TD. (2001) Effectiveness and safety of a protocol for promotion of early intragastric feeding in critically ill children. *Pediatr. Crit. Care Med.* 2(2): 113–121.

Byrnes MC, Stangenes J. (2011) Refeeding in the ICU: an adult and pediatric problem. *Curr. Opin Clin. Nutr. Metab. Care* 14(2): 186–192.

Clarke SE, Evans S, Macdonald A, *et al.* (2007) Randomized comparison of a nutrient-dense formula with an energy-supplemented formula for infants with faltering growth. *J. Hum. Nutr. Diet.* 20(4): 329–339.

Coss-Bu JA, Klish WJ, Walding D, *et al.* (2001) Energy metabolism, nitrogen balance, and substrate utilization in critically ill children. *Am. J. Clin. Nutr.* 74(5): 664–669.

Crook MA, Hally V, Panteli JV. (2001) The importance of the refeeding syndrome. *Nutrition.* 17(7–8): 632–637.

Dos Reis Santos, M, Leite HP, Luiz Pereira AM. (2016) Factors associated with not meeting the recommendations for micronutrient intake in critically ill children. *Nutrition.* 32(11–12): 1217–1222.

Evans S, Twaissi H, Daly A, *et al.* (2006) Should high-energy infant formula be given at full strength from its first day of usage? *J. Hum. Nutr. Diet.* 19(3): 191–197; quiz 199–201.

Feferbaum R, Delgado AF, Zamberlan P, et al. (2009) Challenges of nutritional assessment in pediatric ICU. *Curr. Opin. Clin. Nutr. Metab. Care* 12(3): 245–250.

Fivez T, Kerklaan D, Mesotten D, *et al.* (2016) Early versus late parenteral nutrition in critically ill children. *N. Engl. J. Med.* 374(12): 1111–1122.

Flaring U, Finkel Y. (2009) Nutritional support to patients within the pediatric intensive setting. *Paediatr. Anaesth.* 19(4): 300–312.

Goiburu ME, Goiburu MM, Bianco H, *et al.* (2006) The impact of malnutrition on morbidity, mortality and length of hospital stay in trauma patients. *Nutr. Hosp.* 21(5): 604–610.

Grippa RB, Silva PS, Barbosa E, *et al.* (2016) Nutritional status as a predictor of duration of mechanical ventilation in critically ill children. *Nutrition.* 33: 91–95.

Heidemann SM, Holubkov R, Meert KL, *et al.* (2013) Baseline serum concentrations of zinc, selenium, and prolactin in critically ill children. *Pediatr. Crit. Care Med.* 14(4): e202–206.

Horn D, Chaboyer W. (2003) Gastric feeding in critically ill children: a randomized controlled trial. *Am. J. Crit. Care.* 12(5): 461–468.

Hulst J, Joosten K, Zimmermann L, *et al.* (2004) Malnutrition in critically ill children: from admission to 6 months after discharge. *Clin. Nutr.* 23(2): 223–232.

Hulst JM, Joosten KF, Tibboel D, *et al.* (2006) Causes and consequences of inadequate substrate supply to pediatric ICU patients. *Curr. Opin. Clin. Nutr. Metab. Care.* 9(3): 297–303.

Hulst JM, van Goudoever JB, Zimmermann LJ, *et al.* (2004) The effect of cumulative energy and protein deficiency on anthropometric parameters in a pediatric ICU population. *Clin. Nutr.* 23(6): 1381–1389.

Hulst JM, van Goudoever JB, Zimmermann LJ, *et al.* (2006) The role of initial monitoring of routine biochemical nutritional markers in critically ill children. *J. Nutr. Biochem.* 17(1): 57–62.

Hurt RT, McClave SA. (2010) Gastric residual volumes in critical illness: what do they really mean? *Crit. Care. Clin.* 26(3): 481–490, viii–ix.

Klein CJ, Stanek GS, Wiles CE 3rd. (1998) Overfeeding macronutrients to critically ill adults: metabolic complications. *J. Am. Diet. Assoc.* 98(7): 795–806.

Koletzko B, Goulet O, Hunt J, *et al.* (2005) 1. Guidelines on Paediatric Parenteral Nutrition of the European Society of Paediatric Gastroenterology, Hepatology and Nutrition (ESPGHAN) and the European Society for Clinical Nutrition and Metabolism (ESPEN), Supported by the European Society of Paediatric Research (ESPR). *J. Pediatr. Gastroenterol. Nutr.* 41(Suppl 2): S1–87.

Leite HP, Rodrigues da Silva AV, de Oliveira Iglesias SB, *et al.* (2016) Serum albumin is an independent predictor of clinical outcomes in critically ill children. *Pediatr. Crit. Care Med.* 17(2): e50–57.

Luscombe MD, Owens BD, Burke D. (2011) Weight estimation in paediatrics: a comparison of the APLS formula and the formula 'weight=3(age)+7'. *Emerg. Med. J.* 28(7): 590–593.

Marino LV, Meyer R. (2015) *The prevalence of malnutrition in a regional paediatric cardiac service and its impact on length of stay following cardiac surgery. Association for European Paediatric and Congenital Cardiology (AEPC).* Prague, Czech Republic.

McClave S, Sexton LK, Spain DA, *et al.* (1999) Enteral tube feeding in the intensive care unit: factors impeding adequate delivery. *Crit. Care Med.* 27(7): 1252–1256.

Mehta NM. (2016) Parenteral nutrition in critically ill children. *N. Engl. J. Med.* 374(12): 1190–1192.

Mehta NM, Compher C, A.S.P.E.N. Board of Directors. (2009) A.S.P.E.N. Clinical guidelines: nutrition support of the critically ill child. *J. Parenter. Enteral. Nutr.* 33(3): 260–276.

Meyer R, Harrison S, Sargent S, *et al.* (2009) The impact of enteral feeding protocols on nutritional support in critically ill children. *J. Hum. Nutr. Diet.* 22(5): 428–436.

Meyer R, Marino L. (2015) *Nutrition in Critically Ill Children*, In Clinical Paediatric Dietetics V Shaw (ed) Oxford: Wiley Blackwell.

Parslow RC, Tasker RC, Draper ES, *et al.* (2009) Epidemiology of critically ill children in England and Wales: incidence, mortality, deprivation and ethnicity. *Arch. Dis. Child.* 94(3): 210–215.

PICANET. (2015) *PICANET Annual Report 2015.* Available at https://www.picanet.org.uk/annual-reporting-and-publications/annual-report-archive/ Accessed 19 February 2019.

Rittirsch D, Flierl MA, Ward PA, *et al.* (2008) Harmful molecular mechanisms in sepsis. *Nat. Rev. Immunol.* 8(10): 776–787.

Sadoh WE, Sadoh AE. (2013) Serum zinc values in children with congenital heart disease. *Afr. Health Sci.* 13(3): 601–606.

Santana e Meneses, JF, Leite HP, de Carvalho WB, *et al.* (2009) Hypophosphatemia in critically ill children: prevalence and associated risk factors. *Pediatr. Crit. Care Med.* 10(2): 234–238.

Shaw V (Ed). (2015) *Clinical Paediatric Dietetics.* Oxford: Blackwell Publishing.

Skillman HE, Mehta NM. (2012) Nutrition therapy in the critically ill child. *Curr. Opin. Crit. Care.* 18(2): 192–198.

Skillman HE, Wischmeyer PE. (2008) Nutrition therapy in critically ill infants and children. *J. Parenter. Enteral. Nutr.* 32(5): 520–534.

Solomon SM, Kirby DF. (1990) The refeeding syndrome: a review. *J. Parenter. Enteral. Nutr.* 14(1): 90–97.

van der Kuip M, de Meer K, Westerterp KR, *et al.* (2007) Physical activity as a determinant of total energy expenditure in critically ill children. *Clin. Nutr.* 26(6): 744–751.

van Waardenburg DA, de Betue CT, Goudoever JB, *et al.* (2009) Critically ill infants benefit from early administration of protein and energy-enriched formula: a randomized controlled trial. *Clin. Nutr.* 28(3): 249–255.

Wang G, Feng X, Yu X, *et al.* (2013) Prognostic value of blood zinc, iron, and copper levels in critically ill children with pediatric risk of mortality score III. *Biol. Trace Elem. Res.* 152(3): 300–304.

Wang G, Wang D, Jiang X, *et al.* (2015) Blood zinc, iron, and copper levels in critically ill neonates. *Biol. Trace Elem. Res.* 164(1): 8–11.

Zamberlan P, Delgado AF, Leone C, *et al.* (2011) Nutrition therapy in a pediatric intensive care unit: indications, monitoring, and complications. *J. Parenter. Enteral. Nutr.* 35(4): 523–529.

3.8.24 Paediatric haematopoietic stem cell and bone marrow transplantation

Laura Sealy

Bone marrow transplantation (BMT), more accurately known as haematopoietic stem cell transplantation (HSCT), is a highly intensive, life-saving therapy, widely used in paediatrics to treat malignant and non-malignant diseases of the bone marrow. High doses of chemotherapy, and sometimes radiotherapy (conditioning regimens), are given to improve the chances of curing the malignant disease, particularly to those with a high risk of relapse. This treatment also destroys the bone marrow, which is then replaced with normally functioning stem cells. However, the resulting toxicities and complications, including severe immune suppression, predispose a child to malnutrition (see Chapter 6.2, Malnutrition). The role of the dietitian is to help optimise nutritional status before, during and after transplant, and thus to minimise the morbidity of the conditioning treatments and complications resulting from the transplant procedure (Ward, 2015).

Transplant procedure

In the UK, there are 16 specialist paediatric units where transplantation is carried out (British Society of Blood and Bone Marrow Transplantation). The main types of transplants are:

- Autologous – child's own marrow or stem cells are frozen (cryopreserved) and returned after treatment with high-dose chemotherapy (stem cell rescue).
- Allogeneic – the child receives donor marrow or stem cells, ideally from a sibling or close relative to enable

SECTION 3

a close tissue type match. This is a more complicated, high-toxicity procedure with a longer recovery period.
- Syngeneic – marrow or stem cells are donated from an identical twin, enabling a perfect genetic match and reduced toxicities.

Prior to admission, stem cells are collected from the bone marrow or peripheral blood, or from umbilical cord blood donation (Lipkin *et al.*, 2005). Following admission, high-dose chemotherapy, with or without total body irradiation (TBI), destroys the remaining cancer cells and the marrow and immune system. The child becomes sick and profoundly immunosuppressed (neutropenic). The stem cells are returned to the child intravenously, and they are isolated for 5–6 weeks to monitor side effects and recovery until they produce new blood cells (engraftment).

Dietary management

The transplant process can cause severe oral and gastrointestinal toxicity. The majority of children require nutritional support (Muscaritoli *et al.*, 2002). Side effects leading to compromised nutritional status include:

- Prolonged anorexia.
- Mucositis.
- Nausea and vomiting.
- Diarrhoea and cramping.
- Malabsorption.
- Bacterial, viral and fungal infections.
- Prolonged taste changes.
- Xerostomia.
- Gastroparesis.
- Acute and chronic graft-versus-host disease (GvHD).
- Hyperglycaemia (as a result of steroid treatment).
- Fatigue.
- Depression.
- Neutropenia (low level or absent neutrophil count).
- Food aversions.

Children may have increased requirements resulting from infection, protein-losing enteropathy, GvHD or veno-occlusive disease of the liver (Kline, 2006). Enteral nutrition via nasogastric, nasojejunal or gastrostomy feeding is preferred using a semi-elemental or elemental feed to protect the gut and aid tolerance during periods of gut toxicity (Ward, 2015). Temporary gastrointestinal failure is common, and, if enteral feeding is not successful, parenteral nutrition is used (Murray & Pindoria, 2009). Advice should be given to minimise the risk of food-borne illness and gastrointestinal infection while the child is immunosuppressed. A low-microbial diet is recommended, and all food must be prepared and cooked safely (Yokoe *et al.*, 2009). The degree and duration of dietary restriction differ between specialist centres.

Acknowledgement

The editor acknowledges the prior contribution of Zoe Hull.

Internet resources

British Dietetic Association, www.bda.uk.com
British Society of Blood and Bone Marrow Transplantation, http://bsbmt.org
Cancer Research UK, www.cancerresearchuk.org
Children with Cancer UK, www.childrenwithcancer.org.uk
Children's Cancer and Leukaemia Group, www.cclg.org.uk
CLIC Sargent, www.clicsargent.org.uk
Macmillan Cancer Support, www.macmillan.org.uk

References

Kline RM. (2006) *Pediatric Haematopoietic Stem Cell Transplantation*. New York: Informa Healthcare USA, Inc.

Lipkin AC, Lenssen P, Dickson BJ. (2005) Nutrition issues in hematopoietic stem cell transplantation: state of the art. *Nutr. Clin. Pract.* 20(4): 423–439.

Murray SM, Pindoria S. (2009) Nutrition Support for Bone Marrow Transplant Patients. The Cochrane Library, Issue 1. Chichester: John Wiley and Sons Ltd.

Muscaritoli M, Grieco G, Capria S, *et al.* (2002) Nutritional and metabolic support in patients undergoing bone marrow transplantation. *Am.J. Clin. Nutr.* 75(2): 183–190.

Ward E. (2015) Childhood cancers. In: Shaw V (ed) *Clinical Paediatric Dietetics*, 4th edn. Oxford: Blackwell Publishing.

Yokoe D, Casper C, Dubberke E, *et al.* (2009) Safe living after hematopoietic stem cell transplantation. *Bone. Marrow. Transplant.* 44: 509–519.

3.8.25 Neurosurgery

Luise V. Marino

Currently, there are 20 centres in the UK that offer children's neurosurgical services, of which only five in England are able to provide access to a full-time consultant paediatric neurosurgeon. The remaining centres rely on adult neurosurgeons to make a specialist assessment of the individual child's needs, which may include surgical intervention (Chumas *et al.*, 2008).

Paediatric neurosurgical services accommodate children with: hydrocephalus undergoing shunt insertion and other related procedures, central nervous system (CNS) tumours, spinal surgery (excluding scoliosis), neurovascular conditions (excluding those related to head injury) and other specialist surgical work, e.g. cerebral abscesses, craniofacial surgery, epilepsy surgery and interventions for CNS malformations, e.g. Budd–Chiari syndrome (Parslow *et al.*, 2005). Emergency management of children with intracranial problems is initiated in the local hospital, whereupon they are transferred to a regional centre for intensive care and management of intracranial problems (including surgical intervention where appropriate) (Tasker *et al.*, 2011).

Severe head injury in children is the highest cause of morbidity and mortality over the age of 1 year (Malakouti *et al.*, 2011). Infants have proportionally more head injuries (Bayreuther *et al.*, 2009; Shi *et al.*, 2009) and increased risk of mortality (Bayreuther *et al.*, 2009). Early nutrition support is recognised as being fundamental to recovery in children with neurological injuries (Malakouti *et al.*, 2011), and early achievement of nutrition goals is associated with shorter length of stay and improved neurological outcomes (Taha *et al.*, 2011). Neurological injuries in children have significant morbid sequelae impacting on short- and long-term memories, in addition to difficulties with executive functioning resulting in attention-deficit disorders, with long-term implications for social, behavioural and cognitive development (Kossoff *et al.*, 2009; Prins, 2008).

Scoring systems and nutrition support

The most common coma scoring system used in children is the modified Child's Glasgow Coma Scale (CGCS) (Kirkham *et al.*, 2008). Children with a CGCS score of ≤12 are likely to require nutrition support via a nasogastric feeding tube, due to either increased risk of aspiration and or dysphagia.

Secondary brain injury

Whilst the primary insult account for some of the early mortality, it is the secondary brain injury, occurring as a result of hypotension, hyperglycaemia and raised intracranial pressure (ICP), which leads to poor outcome. Treatment modalities, including nutrition management, aimed at reducing the incidence of these events have been shown to significantly improve outcome (Sharma *et al.*, 2009).

Nutrition

In order to determine a nutrition care plan for children, a nutrition assessment is essential.

Anthropometry

It is important to consider how well the child has been growing up to the point of admission (see Chapter 3.8.2, Growth, nutritional assessment and nutritional requirements).

Biochemistry

- Glucose – any hyperglycaemia (persistent or episodic) beyond the first 48 hours has been associated with poor outcome (Smith *et al.*, 2011). It is therefore important to ensure that any nutrition support being given does not exceed recommendations.
- Sodium – low-sodium enteral feeds should not be used. Medical management is aimed at maintaining sodium levels at the higher end of normal (usually 145–150 mEq/L), with the aim of reducing ICP as hyponatraemia is detrimental to the brain, resulting in cerebral oedema (Carpenter *et al.*, 2007). However, injudicious use of hypertonic solutions can also result in brain shrinkage, increasing the risk of intracerebral haemorrhage (Patanwala *et al.*, 2010).

Clinical

To understand whether the medical management will impact on the type of nutrition support being provided, it is important to have a basic understanding of the treatment modalities and rationale for their use (Huh & Raghupathi, 2009).

Dietary

Energy and protein

Energy and protein requirements in neurological injury is not well researched. There are some published recommendations, such as the following:

- The Brain Trauma Foundation (2003) proposes providing 130–160% of resting energy expenditure for children with neurological injuries (Malakouti *et al.*, 2011).
- The American Society of Parenteral and Enteral Nutrition (ASPEN) (2009) suggest 2–3 g/kg for 0–2 years of age; 1.5–2 g/kg for 2–13 years of age; and 1.5 g/kg for 13–18 years of age (Mehta & Compher, 2009).

However, other research suggests that energy expenditure in children with TBI has been shown to be no higher than in critically ill children without TBI (Briassoulis *et al.*, 2006), so a similar approach to those used in critically ill children may be more appropriate. In addition, muscle relaxants, sedation, mechanical ventilation and malnutrition lead to a reduction in energy requirements as a result of decreased muscle mass activity (Briassoulis *et al.*, 2000; Vizzini & Aranda-Michel, 2011).

Both overfeeding and underfeeding in neurological injury have negative sequelae, with underfeeding resulting in muscle wasting and weight loss of up to 15% per week (Phillips *et al.*, 1987; Vizzini & Aranda-Michel, 2011), and overfeeding resulting in hyperglycaemia and hepatic steatosis (Vizzini & Aranda-Michel, 2011).

Nutrition support

Nutrition support care plans and review by a paediatric dietitian are associated with early initiation of enteral feeds and increased likelihood of achieving nutrition goals (Malakouti *et al.*, 2012).

Initiation of enteral feeds

Children not fed within 5–7 days have a two- to fourfold increased likelihood of dying (Hartl *et al.*, 2008), as compared to those who are fed within 72 hours (Vizzini

SECTION 3

& Aranda-Michel, 2011). Enteral feeds should be commenced as soon as the child is medically stable (Mehta *et al.*, 2010). Enteral feeding that commenced within 48 h post-injury is associated with better survival, GCS recovery, and outcome among TBI patients, particularly in those with a GCS score of 6–8 (Chiang *et al.*, 2012). For most patients, this is within 4–6 hours post-surgery or post-admission, with the aim of achieving the goal rate within 72 hours (Mehta *et al.*, 2010). However, enteral feeding in neurological injury is not effective in preserving muscle protein, resulting in a negative nitrogen balance and hypoglutaminaemia (Charrueau *et al.*, 2009; Vizzini & Aranda-Michel, 2011). The implementation of feeding protocols may help to achieve nutrition goals (Mehta, 2009; Meyer *et al.*, 2009; Vizzini & Aranda-Michel, 2011).

Children with TBI do not require specialised enteral feeds; however, as bowel motility is often affected by TBI, a fibre-containing feed can be important. Constipation and straining to defecate should be avoided as these increase the risk of raised ICP.

Complications of nasogastric feeding in neurological injury

Complications of particular relevance to children with neurological injury include an increased risk of enteral feeding intolerance, which is correlated with raised ICP and or a low CGCS of ≤8 or less, resulting in delayed gastric emptying (Marino *et al.*, 2003), higher gastric residuals and increased risk of aspiration pneumonitis. Nasojejunal feeds (NJ) should be considered in these children (Vizzini & Aranda-Michel, 2011). Nasogastric and NJ tubes should ideally only be placed for a maximum of 4 weeks, after which a gastrostomy or jejunostomy should be considered, especially in children who remain dysphagic or who have a CGCS of ≤12 (Vizzini & Aranda-Michel, 2011).

Future trends

Nutrition support for children with TBI may, in the future, include the use of acetyl-L-carnitine (Scafidi *et al.*, 2010), n-3 fatty acids (Mills *et al.*, 2011), vitamin E (Aiguo *et al.*, 2010) and ketogenic diets (Prins, 2008; Prins *et al.*, 2005).

References

Aiguo W, Zhe Y, Gomez-Pinilla F. (2010) Vitamin E protects against oxidative damage and learning disability after mild traumatic brain injury in rats. *Neurorehabil. Neural. Repair.* 24: 290–298.

American Society of Parenteral and Enteral Nutrition (ASPEN). (2009) Nutrition support in paediatric critical care. *J. Parenter. Enteral. Nutr.* 33: 260–276.

Bayreuther J, Wagener S, Woodford M, et al. (2009) Paediatric trauma: injury pattern and mortality in the UK. *Arch. Dis. Child Educ. Pract. Ed.* 94: 37–41.

Briassoulis G, Filippou O, Kanariou M, *et al.* (2006) Temporal nutritional and inflammatory changes in children with severe head injury fed a regular or an immune-enhancing diet: a randomized, controlled trial. *Pediatr. Crit. Care Med.* 7: 56–62.

Briassoulis G, Venkataraman S, Thompson AE. (2000) Energy expenditure in critically ill children. *Crit. Care Med.* 28: 1166–1172.

Brain Trauma Foundation. (2003) *Nutrition Guidelines*. Available at http://www.braintrauma.org. Accessed 25 November 2016.

Carpenter J, Weinstein S, Myseros J, et al. (2007) Inadvertent hyponatremia leading to acute cerebral edema and early evidence of herniation. *Neurocrit. Care* 6: 195–199.

Charrueau C, Belabed L, Besson V, *et al.* (2009) Metabolic response and nutritional support in traumatic brain injury: evidence for resistance to renutrition. *J. Neurotrauma.* 26: 1911–1920.

Chiang YH, Chao DP, Chu SF, *et al.* (2012) Early enteral nutrition and clinical outcomes of severe traumatic brain injury patients in acute stage: a multi-center cohort study. *J. Neurotrauma.* 29: 75–80.

Chumas P, Pople I, Mallucci C, *et al.* (2008) British Paediatric Neurosurgery – a time for change? *Br. J. Neurosurg.* 22: 719–728.

Hartl R, Gerber LM, Ni Q, *et al.* (2008) Effect of early nutrition on deaths due to severe traumatic brain injury. *J. Neurosurg.* 109: 50–56.

Huh JW, Raghupathi R. (2009) New concepts in treatment of pediatric traumatic brain injury. *Anesthesiol. Clin.* 27: 213–240.

Kirkham FJ, Newton CR, Whitehouse W. (2008) Paediatric coma scales. *Dev. Med. Child Neurol.* 50: 267–274.

Kossoff EH, Zupec-Kania BA, Rho JM. (2009) Ketogenic diets: an update for child neurologists. *J. Child Neurol.* 24: 979–988.

Malakouti A, Sookplung P, Siriussawakul A, *et al.* (2012) Nutrition support and deficiencies in children with severe traumatic brain injury. *Pediatr. Crit. Care Med.* 13: e18–24.

Marino LV, Kiratu EM, French S, *et al.* (2003) To determine the effect of metoclopramide on gastric emptying in severe head injuries: a prospective, randomized, controlled clinical trial. *Br. J. Neurosurg.* 17: 24–28.

Mehta NM. (2009) Approach to enteral feeding in the PICU. *Nutr. Clin. Pract.* 24: 377–387.

Mehta NM, Compher C. (2009) A.S.P.E.N. Clinical Guidelines: nutrition support of the critically ill child. *J. Parenter. Enteral Nutr.* 33: 260–276.

Mehta NM, Mcaleer D, Hamilton S, *et al.* (2010) Challenges to optimal enteral nutrition in a multidisciplinary pediatric intensive care unit. *J. Parenter. Enteral. Nutr.* 34: 38–45.

Meyer R, Harrison S, Sargent S, *et al.* (2009) The impact of enteral feeding protocols on nutritional support in critically ill children. *J. Hum. Nutr. Diet.* 22: 428–436.

Mills JD, Bailes JE, Sedney CL, *et al.* (2011). Omega-3 fatty acid supplementation and reduction of traumatic axonal injury in a rodent head injury model. *J. Neurosurg.* 114: 77–84.

Parslow RC, Morris KP, Tasker RC, *et al.* (2005) Epidemiology of traumatic brain injury in children receiving intensive care in the UK. *Arch. Dis. Child.* 90: 1182–1187.

Patanwala AE, Amini A, Erstad BL. (2010) Use of hypertonic saline injection in trauma. *Am. J. Health Syst. Pharm.* 67: 1920–1928.

Phillips R, Ott L, Young B, *et al.* (1987) Nutritional support and measured energy expenditure of the child and adolescent with head injury. *J. Neurosurg.* 67: 846–851.

Prins M. (2008) Diet, ketones, and neurotrauma. *Epilepsia.* 49(Suppl 8): 111–113.

Prins ML, Fujima LS, Hovda DA. (2005) Age-dependent reduction of cortical contusion volume by ketones after traumatic brain injury. *J. Neurosci. Res.* 82: 413–420.

Scafidi S, Racz J, Hazelton J, *et al.* (2010) Neuroprotection by acetyl-L-carnitine after traumatic injury to the immature rat brain. *Dev. Neurosci.* 32: 480–487.

Sharma D, Jelacic J, Chennuri R, *et al.* (2009). Incidence and risk factors for perioperative hyperglycemia in children with traumatic brain injury. *Anesth. Analg.* 108: 81–89.

Shi J, Xiang H, Wheeler K, *et al.* (2009) Costs, mortality likelihood and outcomes of hospitalized US children with traumatic brain injuries. *Brain Inj.* 23: 602–611.

Smith RL, Lin JC, Adelson PD, et al. (2011) Relationship between hyperglycemia and outcome in children with severe traumatic brain injury. *Pediatr. Crit. Care. Med.* 3(1): 85–89.

Taha AA, Badr L, Westlake C, *et al.* (2011) Effect of early nutritional support on intensive care unit length of stay and neurological status at discharge in children with severe traumatic brain injury. *J. Neurosci. Nurs.* 43: 291–297.

Tasker RC, Fleming TJ, Young AE, *et al.* (2011) Severe head injury in children: intensive care unit activity and mortality in England and Wales. *Br. J. Neurosurg.* 25: 68–77.

Vizzini A, Aranda-Michel J. (2011) Nutritional support in head injury. *Nutrition* 27: 129–132.

3.8.26 Burns

Jacqueline Lowdon

A burn injury is one of the worst types of trauma. Children who present with burn injuries often have challenging clinical, social and psychological issues. Although significant progress has been made in burn care over the years, it still needs to be delivered as a specialist, multidisciplinary service, due to its complexity and rarity, to achieve the best outcome for the burn-injured child. Over 110 children per day are seen in UK emergency departments with burns (Dunn *et al.*, 2015). Causes and types of burn injuries in children include (Hettiaratchy & Dziewulski, 2004) the following:

- Thermal.
- Chemical.
- Electrical.
- Cold injury.

Rare skin-loss conditions (e.g. vesiculobullous skin disorders and staphylococcal scalded skin syndrome) can also result in significant burn-like wounds and symptoms. In the UK, specialised burn care is organised in tiered care.

Nutritional support

Significant endocrine, metabolic, inflammatory and immune changes occur, resulting in specific nutritional requirements. Therefore, all children admitted with burn injuries are at nutritional risk. Nutritional support is one of the most significant aspects, from resuscitation fluids to the end of rehabilitation. Nutrition support aims to promote optimal wound healing and skin graft take, and maintain normal growth and development and immunological competence.

Calculation of requirements

The extent of skin injury (quantified in terms of the extent of the total body surface area (TBSA) involved and injury depth) and other factors must be considered when assessing requirements:

- Age.
- Sex.
- Weight.
- Height or length.
- Preadmission nutritional state.
- Pre-existing medical condition.
- Special dietary requirements.
- Site of injury.
- Gastrointestinal (GI) function.
- Pyrexia.
- Grafted area.
- Extent of healing.

Minor burn (<10%)

Burn injury in children does not raise the resting energy expenditure (REE) proportionally as much as adults, since children become inactive (Childs, 1994, 1995; Goran *et al.*, 1990). Optimal nutritional state and weight maintenance can normally be achieved by aiming for the EAR for a non-burned child. Children with minor burns are usually encouraged to meet their nutritional requirements orally. However, some children with an injury of <10% may require enteral tube feeding, depending on the site of the burn (e.g. the face), preadmission nutritional status and surgical management (e.g. grafting).

Major burn (≥10%)

In a major burn injury, nasogastric or nasojejunal feeding should be commenced within the first few hours post-injury (McDonald *et al.*, 1991). Very early enteral feeding, within the first 6–12 hours, is associated with improved clinical and biological outcomes (ESPEN, 2013). It reduces the incidence of paralytic ileus, where septic diarrhoea causes paralysis of the ileus muscles, which can occur in severe sepsis. Other benefits include the depletion of stress hormone levels involved in the hypermetabolic response (Herndon & Tompkins, 2004; Mochizuki *et al.*, 1984), increasing immunoglobulin production (Lam *et al.*, 2008), thereby improving immune status and wound healing and reducing the risk of malnutrition and energy deficit (Chiarelli *et al.*, 1990; Venter *et al.*, 2007).

Continuous feeding should be commenced initially and the rate increased slowly, to reach full maintenance within the first 24 hours post-injury (McDonald *et al.*, 1991). Due to the broad spectrum, diarrhoea occurs frequently; this is not usually related to feed osmolality or volume (Thakkar *et al.*, 2005). Feed volume will need to be titrated when oral intake commences, as long as nutritional requirements are still being met. Bolus feeds can be considered once the child starts to eat.

Energy requirements

Energy requirements were thought to increase in a burn injury of ≥10%, and were calculated using formulas such as the Hildreth formula (Hildreth & Carvajal, 1982; Hildreth *et al.*, 1989, 1990, 1993). However, studies have demonstrated that the increase in REE is at its greatest during the first weeks, decreasing progressively thereafter. Also, improvements in burn care have significantly reduced the hypermetabolic response, resulting in reduced nutritional requirements. Indirect calorimetry remains the gold standard for determining energy requirements. In its absence, the Schofield (1985) equation is recommended as an alternative (ESPEN, 2013). However, it may underestimate requirements (Suman *et al.*, 2006), and the calculation should therefore be rounded up. Compared with the Hildreth formula, the results of the Schofield equation appear to be very low. However, ESPEN highlight that burn-injured children are at risk of being overfed, with severe related complications (Burke *et al.*, 1979). Conversely, the risk with the Schofield equation is that it is a fixed equation and does not take into consideration changes over time. Whichever method is used, monitoring is crucial, and the feed regimen should be altered as required.

Protein requirements

Burn-injured children have a higher protein requirement than the RNI. Protein intakes of up to 3 g/kg/day have been reported in children without real advantage. ESPEN (2013) recommended aiming for 1.5–3 g/kg/day.

Type of feed

This should not differ from other critically ill children; polymeric feeds are preferred (Singer *et al.*, 2009). Feed containing dietary fibre is recommended from initiation, as burn-injured patients have a high risk of constipation, owing to fluid movements and the high doses of sedatives and opioids required for frequent analgesia (ESPEN, 2013).

Fluid requirements

All burns units have fluid resuscitation guidelines, and the dietitian will need to work out a feed regimen within this allowance in these guidelines. If the child is pyrexic, an extra 10% for every degree rise in temperature is needed.

Micronutrients

A major burn results in increased micronutrient requirements, owing to the hypermetabolic response, wound healing and exudative losses from open wounds. There are currently no UK paediatric supplement guidelines. However, ESPEN (2013) strongly recommended additional zinc, copper, selenium, and vitamins B_1, C, D and E, with the duration for elevated substitution requirements being determined by the burned surface. Before considering a supplement, the nutritional composition and bioavailability need to be checked in conjunction with biochemical markers.

Parenteral nutrition

Where there is a prolonged paralytic ileus or poor tolerance of enteral feeds, trophic feeds should continue, so that the brush border integrity of the gastrointestinal tract is maintained.

Monitoring

Accurate daily food and fluid charts are essential to monitor and evaluate intake (Vijfhuize *et al.*, 2010). Bowel habits also need to be monitored closely, as this may affect feed tolerance (e.g. analgesia), and being bed bound can result in constipation. Weight should be reviewed when possible. Oedema owing to the initial injury may mask a true weight. Nutritional biochemical markers should be monitored. Burn injuries are dynamic, with changes occurring in the percentage of burn surface area owing to wound healing or degradation. Therefore, nutritional requirements too are likely to change.

Post-discharge

During hospitalisation, the child and family may have been advised about a high-energy, high-protein diet, if oral intake was inadequate, to meet requirements; this needs to be reassessed on discharge.

Internet resources

British Burn Association, https://www.britishburnassociation.org

References

Burke JF, Wolfe RR, Mullany CJ, *et al.* (1979) Glucose requirements following burn injury. *Ann. Surg.* 190: 274–285.

Chiarelli A, Enzi G, Casadei A, *et al.* (1990) Very early nutrition supplementation in burned patients. *Am. J. Clin. Nutr.* 51: 1035–1039.

Childs C. (1994) Studies in children provide a model to re-examine the metabolic response to burn injuries in patients treated by contemporary burn protocol. *Burns.* 20: 291–300.

Childs C. (1995) Feeding the burned patient. Energy requirements, timing and effects of dietary intake. *B J. Intensive Care.* 5: 157–164.

Dunn K, Reade C, Dudley-Southern R, *et al.* (2015) *International Burns Injury Database.* Available at http://www.ibidb.org. Accessed 5 December 2017.

ESPEN. (2013) Nutritional therapy in major burns. *Clin. Nutr.* 32: 497–502.

Goran MI, Peters EJ, Herndon DN, *et al.* (1990) Total energy expenditure in burned children using the doubly labelled water technique. *Am. J. Physiol.* 259: E576–585.

Herndon DN, Tompkins RG. (2004) Support of the metabolic response to burn injury. *Lancet.* 63: 1895–1902.

Hettiaratchy S, Dziewulski P. (2004) ABC of burns: introduction. *BMJ* 328(7452): 1366–1368.

Hildreth MA, Carvajal H. (1982) Caloric requirements in burned children: A simple formula to estimate daily caloric requirements. *J. Burn. Care. Res.* 3(2): 78–80.

Hildreth MA, Herndon DN, Desai MH, *et al.* (1989) Caloric needs of adolescent patients with burns. *J. Burn. Care. Res.* 10(6): 523–526.

Hildreth MA, Herndon DH, Desai MH, *et al.* (1990) Current treatment reduces calories required to maintain weight in paediatric patients with burns. *J. Burn. Care. Res.* 11: 405–409.

Hildreth MA, Herndon DH, Desai MH, *et al.* (1993) Calorific requirements of patients with burns under one year of age. *J. Burn Care Res.* 14: 108–112.

Lam NN, Tien NG, Khoa CM. (2008) Early enteral feeding for burned patients: an effective method which should be encouraged in developing countries. *Burns* 34: 192–196.

McDonald WS, Sharp CW Jr, Deitch EA. (1991) Immediate enteral feeding in burn patients is safe and effective. *Ann. Surg.* 15: 578–579.

Mochizuki H, Trocki O, Dominioni L, *et al.* (1984) Mechanism of prevention of postburn hypermetabolism and catabolism by early enteral feeding. *Ann. Surg.* 200: 297–310.

Singer P, Berger MM, Van den Berghe G, *et al.* (2009) ESPEN guidelines on parenteral nutrition. *Clin. Nutr.* 28: 387–400.

Schofield WN (1985). Predicting basal metabolic rate, new standards and review of previous work. *Hum. Nutr. Clin. Nutr.* 39(Suppl 1): 5–41.

Suman OE, Mlcak RP, Chinkes DL, *et al.* (2006) Resting energy expenditure in severely burned children: analysis of agreement between indirect calorimetry and prediction equations using the Bland–Altman method. *Burns.* 32: 335–342.

Thakkar K, Kien CL, Rosenblatt JI, *et al.* (2005) Diarrhea in severely burned children. *J Parenter. Enteral. Nutr.* 29: 8–11.

Venter M, Rode H, Sive A, *et al.* (2007) Enteral resuscitation and early enteral feeding in children with major burns – effect on McFarlane response to stress. *Burns.* 33: 464–471.

Vijfhuize S, Verburg M, Marino L, *et al.* (2010) An evaluation of nutritional practice in a paediatric burns unit. *S. Afr. Med. J.* 100(6): 383–386.

3.8.27 General surgery

Lynette Forsythe

There are many conditions and surgical procedures that affect a child's feeding ability and require dietetic management including the following.

Oesophageal atresia and tracheo-oesophageal fistula

Oesophageal atresia (OA) is a birth defect in which part of the oesophagus is missing. Tracheo-oesophageal fistula (TOF) is an abnormal connection between the upper part of the oesophagus and the trachea. OA and TOF commonly occur together and are usually repaired at the same time, soon after birth. If the gap in the oesophagus is large, the infant may need to wait a few months for the OA repair to allow the oesophagus to grow. In this case, a gastrostomy tube will be inserted for all feeds (expressed breast milk (EBM) or infant formula).

Narrowing of the oesophagus can happen when scars develop following surgery, making feeding difficult, and the infant may fail to meet their requirements orally. Temporary nasogastric feeding is sometimes needed, followed by an oesophageal dilatation. Weaning is generally started at normal weaning age, although lumpy solids are introduced later, with some foods being more difficult to tolerate. If the repair is delayed, feeding difficulties often occur.

Duodenal atresia

Duodenal atresia occurs in the duodenum and causes blockage. Occasionally, there may not be incomplete atresia, but a partial narrowing (stenosis) instead. Corrective surgery is required, and a transanastomotic tube (TAT) is often inserted down through the baby's nose, into the stomach and through the joint in the duodenum, so that feeds may be started earlier. Some babies will need parenteral nutrition (PN). EBM or infant formula will be slowly introduced and increased as the baby tolerates. Post-surgery, the baby should feed normally.

Congenital diaphragmatic hernia

Diaphragmatic hernias occur when the diaphragm does not form completely, leaving a hole that allows part of the intestine to move into the chest, requiring surgical repair. PN will be commenced, but the baby should successfully wean onto breastfeeding or bottle-feeding. Further dietetic support may be required with nasogastric feeds, owing to vomiting. Some children may develop GORD when they are older.

Gastroschisis and exomphalos

These are abdominal wall defects where corrective surgery is required, and, in some cases, this needs to be a staged repair. The infants are started on PN and then weaned onto feeds. Hydrolysed formulas are often used if EBM is unavailable, especially if the bowel has been handled a lot during surgery. These infants generally can wean onto standard infant formula.

Hirschsprung's disease

Hirschsprung's disease is a disorder of the colon which can lead to severe constipation and intestinal obstruction. Surgery will be required, and may be staged where initially a colostomy is fashioned, and then the stoma will be closed with removal of the non-functioning part of colon, and a pull-through performed where the healthy bowel is connected to the anus to allow faeces to pass. Some children with long-segment Hirschsprung's disease, including small bowel with a stoma in situ, may need dietary manipulation. Children should follow a normal, balanced diet after the pull-through operation.

Ileostomy

Surgical management of necrotising enterocolitis or volvulus may result in an infant having an ileostomy formation. Ileostomy losses above 20 mL/kg/day and increased oral intake may lead to low urinary sodium with a normal serum sodium and inadequate weight gain, needing dietary and medical support.

Short bowel syndrome

Short bowel syndrome (SBS) is defined as intestinal failure secondary to loss of length of the small intestine, often as a result of NEC or congenital gastrointestinal conditions. SBS results in malabsorption, dehydration, fluid and electrolyte imbalances, and failure to thrive. Malabsorption may lead to bacterial overgrowth in the small intestine, especially if the ileocecal valve is resected. PN is required, and enteral feeds of EBM or alternative formula will be started as early as possible. Transition of PN to enteral nutrition is vital to promote optimal intestinal adaptation, to stimulate growth and development, and to minimise the risk of PN-related complications. Careful monitoring of nutritional status and growth velocity on a long-term basis is important.

Fundoplication

Antireflux surgery may be of benefit in confirmed severe GORD where children have been on optimal medical treatment for a long time, when symptoms are not improving, and where faltering growth or impractical feeding regimens are detected. A Nissen fundoplication is most commonly performed where the fundus is wrapped around the lower part of the oesophagus to form a valve between the oesophagus and stomach, such that food and drink are less likely to come back into the oesophagus. After fundoplication, feeds will be recommenced slowly and increased gradually to either the usual regime or according to a new plan that may be more practical. Medical therapy may be reduced or stopped if possible, although the child may still retch with feeds.

Acknowledgement

The editor acknowledges the prior contribution of Shelley Easter.

Further reading

Goulet O, Olieman J, Ksiazyk J, *et al.* (2013) Neonatal short bowel syndrome as a model of intestinal failure: Physiological background for enteral feeding. *Clin. Nutr.* 32(2): 162–171.

NICE. (2015) *Gastro-oesophageal reflux disease: recognition, diagnosis and management in children and young people*. London: https://www.nice.org.uk/guidance/ng1

Petersen D, Shaw V, Johnson T. (2015) Surgery in the gastrointestinal tract. In Shaw V (ed), *Clinical Paediatric Dietetics*. London: John Wiley & Sons Ltd.

Internet resources

Congenital Diaphragmatic Hernia Support Charity, www.cdhuk.org.uk

Hirschsprung's & Motility Disorders Support Network, www.hirschsprungs.info

Trachea-Oesophageal Fistula Support Group, www.tofs.org.uk

SECTION 4

Specific areas of dietetic practice

4.1 Freelance dietetics

Jennette Higgs

Key points

- Freelance practice can be a rewarding career for experienced dietitians, has benefits and risks, and requires careful thought and planning.
- Self-employment has specific legal and financial implications, and professional advice is recommended.
- Constructing a business plan is essential when establishing a new business to assess its viability and monitor its success.
- Professional standards and codes of conduct must be complied with.
- Freelancing is best suited to those with strong self-drive with access to a strong network and support to minimise isolation.

Traditional working patterns are changing, and freelancer numbers have increased by 36% in the 2008–2015 period. In the UK, freelance workers constitute 6% of all employment, with a collective turnover estimated at £120–125 billion (3–4% of total business turnover) (Kitching, 2016). The number of freelance dietitians is increasing. The Freelance Dietitians Group (FDG), a specialist group of the British Dietetic Association (BDA), was formed to support dietitians who are (or are planning to become) freelancers. The following information is intended as guidance only. Professional codes of conduct and legal requirements change, and it is the responsibility of each individual to ensure that these are met. It is recommended that appropriate professional expertise be sought as required.

Becoming a freelance dietitian

For many, the idea of becoming a freelance dietitian is an attractive option. Working freelance usually means becoming self-employed and setting up a small business. However, there are financial, emotional and professional risks involved. Unfortunately, many new small businesses fail in their start-up period. In the UK, half of small businesses fail in the first 4 years (Kitching, 2016); the UK 5-year survival rate for all businesses is 41.4% (ONS, 2016). In order to become successful, there are a number of important issues to address and strategies to develop, which may well fall outside the experience of a previously employed dietitian. There can be a number of reasons for considering the option of becoming a freelance dietitian, however, dietitians need to look honestly at their reasons for considering this freelance option. What are your strengths and weaknesses? Have you got what it takes in terms of motivation, self-confidence and self-discipline?

Implications of becoming self-employed

Before going freelance, it is worth considering what employee benefits may be lost including:

- Financial benefits
  - Regular salary (paid irrespective of whether clients attend for appointments).
  - Annual salary increments, holiday pay, sick pay, maternity/paternity leave.
  - Automatic deductions for national insurance (NI), tax and pension.
  - Professional indemnity insurance.
  - Subsidised canteen, accommodation, car loans, etc.
- Career benefits
  - Recognised career path.
  - Supported continuing professional development (CPD).
  - Paid leave to attend conferences and meetings.
  - Free and ready access to journals and libraries.
  - Immediate support of colleagues and manager for direction/mentoring.
  - Opportunities to work in a range of areas or to specialise.
- Environment
  - Equipment, e.g. desk, chair, computer, printer, telephone, pager, etc.
  - Administrative and secretarial support.
  - Consulting rooms, and booking and appointment services.
  - Diet sheets, resources and equipment, e.g. scales.

Manual of Dietetic Practice, Sixth Edition. Edited by Joan Gandy.

Companion website: www.manualofdieteticpractice.com

Many of these benefits will not be automatically available to the self-employed person. Freelance dietitians must be prepared to take on the uncertainties and expenses associated with working for themselves. The benefits of having the freedom to determine one's own career path must be weighed against the extra time required to manage the business and the uncertainty of where/when the next job will be. Some dietitians may have opportunities to work part-time, alongside being employed, in which case it is essential that all earnings be declared for tax purposes.

A freelance dietitian seldom knows when work will be commissioned, which demands good time management, both in quiet and busy periods. Working freelance may result in working long hours and weekends in order to meet deadlines and, conversely, having unwanted, unpaid free time when contracts and projects have not been won or are scarce. Making effective use of quiet periods and keeping motivated, as well as productive time management and organisation, are essential skills. The nature of freelance work means that a great deal of energy and time needs to be devoted to building and maintaining the business to provide sufficient commissions to equate to a full-time job and salary. Although the number of full-time, freelance dietitians is increasing, many work part-time.

Qualifications and experience

Registration with the Health and Care Professions Council (HCPC) is essential. A minimum of 5 years of supervised, clinical experience is needed for private, clinical practice, as many private medical insurance companies stipulate this as a requirement. A varied dietetic experience after qualification and a broad background is recommended for other areas of freelance work. In addition, other complementary qualifications maybe beneficial for having more flexibility in commissions, e.g. research skills, teaching/presentation skills, sports nutrition, catering, psychology/counselling, marketing, public relations and journalism. If the business includes writing, becoming a member of the Guild of Food Writers or the Guild of Health Writers may be useful. If the business is to offer advice in a particular speciality, the dietitian must have the necessary additional qualifications and experience.

A freelance dietitian must be an all-round business expert, acquiring new skills such as marketing business, tendering procedures, contracts and remuneration proposals for the business to succeed. The most common reason for small-business failure is poor cash flow management (Experian, 2010), and getting advice and training in financial business skills is highly recommended.

Work opportunities

The opportunities are extremely varied, covering a broad spectrum of dietetic practice, as shown in Figure 4.1.1. Some of the common work tasks for freelance dietitians include:

- Writing diet-related articles and books for both the consumer and professional press.
- Media work such as journalism, broadcasting, press releases, scientific or medical briefings, webinars and seminars.
- Resource development.
- Social media activities, including provision of informative dietetic messaging and organising online discussions.
- Consulting in marketing and project management.
- Specialist dietetics, e.g. allergies, child health, obesity and weight management, diabetes, women's or men's health.
- Menu planning, calculations and evaluation.
- Recipe development and analysis.
- Catering, food policies and writing or advising on catering tenders.
- Health claims research for food companies, specifically in relation to the European Nutrition and Health Claims Regulations.
- Sports nutrition/fitness and health advice.
- Health promotion development.
- Project work with schools.
- Workplace nutrition and weight management programmes.

Clients and charges

The fees commanded are likely to vary according to who commissions the work, the scope of services provided and the level of expertise required (see Table 4.1.1). The FDG periodically surveys its members to assess the fees, which can be useful when first setting up as a freelancer. It is appropriate to register with several private medical insurers (PMIs), although each company has its own requirements and specified payment terms. This may mean that the number of consultations or the payment rate may be capped, and the balance of payment may need to be obtained from the clients themselves (see www.freelancedietitians.org for further details).

Planning the business

Setting up a freelance business must be taken seriously. While the professional work may be similar to being employed, the freelance environment is different and demands additional skills and aptitudes to also conduct the financial and business management work. In the early stages, it may be worthwhile asking an experienced freelance dietitian to act as a mentor. In addition to excellent dietetic skills and professionalism, the freelancer also needs to set up a business, and therefore needs to be able to:

- Work independently and unsupported.
- Be fully committed to the project.
- Demonstrate exceptional organisational and multitasking skills.
- Be an ambassador for dietetics and demonstrate an authoritative capability.
- Be proactive, e.g. write a business plan.

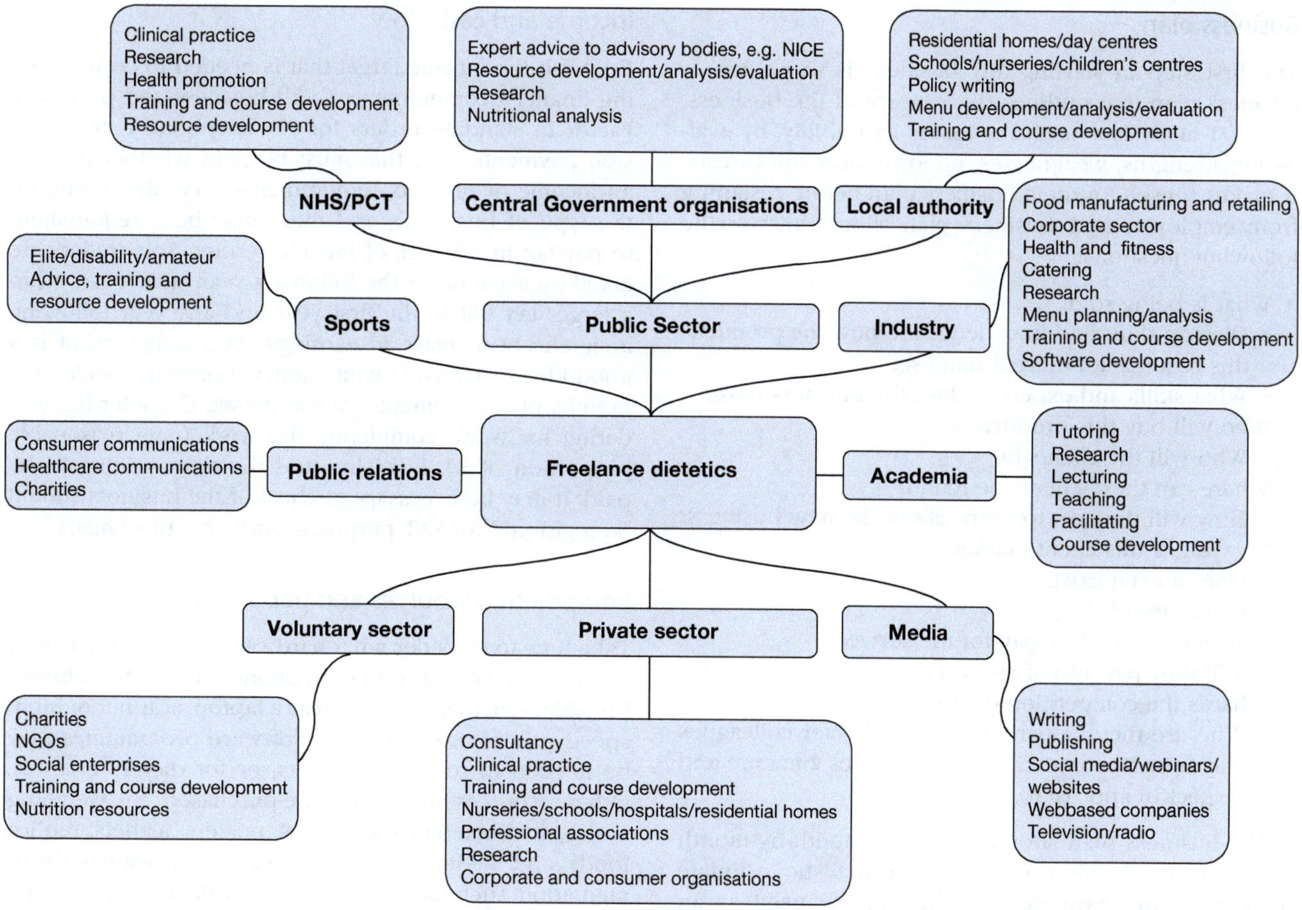

Figure 4.1.1 Work opportunity areas for freelance dietitians (from BDA Freelance Dietitians Group – Where do freelance dietitians work? http://members.bda.uk.com/groups/fdg/files/FDGwheredietitianswork.pdf) [source: The British Dietetic Association 2013. Reproduced with permission of the British Dietetic Association (www.bda.uk.com)]

GP, general practitioner; NHS, National Health Service; NGO, non-government organisation; NICE, National Institute for Health and Care Excellence; PCT, primary care trust.

Table 4.1.1 Examples of clients in the public and private sectors

Public sector	Private sector
GP sessions	Private medical insurance companies, private patients
Hospital clinics	Public relations companies – product promotion and support, brochures, customer leaflets, press releases
Research, e.g. for government bodies/research councils/ universities	Food retailers and manufacturers – strategic advice and support, product development and specifications, customer support, fact sheets, recipe cards, magazine articles, food-labelling checks
Project management for service providers and area teams within the health services	Television, radio and other media – research and consultancy, presenting and expert comment
Expert witness	Publishing companies – newspapers, magazines and books
Education providers, e.g. lecturing, development of programmes and materials	Medical and health charities – advice and creation of support material, project management
	Catering companies – menu analysis and advice; staff nutrition training
	Conference and event organisation or management
	Pharmaceutical companies – technical support

- Cope under stress and pressure.
- Have sufficient funds until work comes in and invoices are settled, which can take 2–4 months.
- Live without the security of a regular salary.
- Take responsibility for tasks previously done by an employer, specifically, taxation, NI payments and pension arrangements.
- Have sufficient experience, confidence and contacts.

SECTION 4

Business plan

The first step in starting any business is to prepare a business plan that outlines the concept of the business. A SWOT analysis is useful to assess its viability, by evaluating strengths, weaknesses, opportunities and threats. It makes sense to write a business plan before resigning from employment. A business plan should answer the following questions:

- What is being sold?
  - Dietetic skills and knowledge are now the products; this requires a different mind-set.
  - What skills and expertise does the business have?
- Who will buy this product?
  - Who will the clients be?
- Where can these clients be found?
  - How will they get to know about the new business?
- How big is this client market?
  - Does it even exist?
  - Can it grow?
- How much will they pay for the services?
  - Will they pay and, if so, when?
- What is the competition doing?
  - Who are the competitors? (*Note*: Former colleagues may now be competitors; this requires a mature and respectful approach).

The business plan should include a month-by-month plan for the coming year, with a realistic estimate of income and expenditure. This can be used as an objective measure of business progress. The plan should be reviewed on a regular basis, so that the business can build on its successes and remain profitable. It should set ambitious but realistic goals within a reasonable time frame. It can be viewed as a starting point and should be reviewed as the business develops. Help in developing a business plan and start-up information can be obtained from the business departments of high street banks and the government organisation Business Link (www.gov.uk/business-support-helpline). Several aspects need to be considered when constructing the business plan.

Type of business

Working practices vary, but the majority of freelance dietitians are self-employed sole traders. There are alternatives to working alone, such as setting up a formal partnership or group practice. Consideration should also be given to forming a limited company. Professional advice should be sought as to which option best suits the individual situation and the needs of each business. All the options will have different financial implications. In addition to doing all the necessary research, talk to people about the business idea, and listen to criticism and negative feedback. It may help to set out the business terms and conditions, including payment terms, confidentiality, ownership of materials and limits of liability.

Income and cash flow

Establish the income target that is needed to cover ongoing financial commitments (both business and personal). Factor in standing orders for NI, telephone rental, pension payments, etc., that must be paid whether there is an income or not. Tax requirements vary (depending on the type of business), and there may be a requirement to pay tax in advance of income receipt. Sole traders are taxed on account for the following year, which can mean a larger tax bill in the first year and any year following a significant increase in earnings. As a safeguard, it is a good idea to set aside contingency monies (consider 4–6 months of requirements) at the outset. Consider the tendering for work, completing the work (or a reasonable proportion of it), invoicing and the time waiting to be paid. It may be necessary to check if the business should be registered for VAT purposes, and what this entails.

Equipment, resources and paperwork

Take time to consider what hardware is needed; it is best to have a dedicated computer, phone line and broadband. Consider whether items such as a laptop, scanner or high-speed printer are essentials. Software programmes may be needed to run spreadsheets, or for dietary analysis. Other resources may need to be purchased, e.g. weighing scales, stadiometers, diet sheets, posters, leaflets, replica foods and audiovisual equipment. Professional documentation such as business cards will be needed, and other paperwork such as invoice templates and contracts need to be developed for the business. While there are many examples to be found on the Internet, professional advice regarding specific content may need to be purchased. Membership of professional organisations, both dietetic and business, is an essential expense that needs to be included.

Office accommodation

Carefully consider whether the business is going to be run from the home or an office. Take advice from experts and consider the advantages and disadvantages of each option.

Working from home

If you intend to work from home, ensure that other household members are in agreement. The business may need to take precedence in order to meet deadlines, and office hours need to be respected by all in the household. Switching off from other activities in the house can be difficult, and it is also easy to be consumed by work and difficult to take breaks, especially if there is an urgent deadline. Establish a proper workspace and schedule adequate rest and relaxation as tiredness will slow work, lead to mistakes and reduce creativity.

If private patients are to be seen from home, it will be necessary to consider aspects such as parking facilities, disabled access, waiting areas, toilet facilities, public liability insurance, personal security and disruption to the family. Use of a domestic residence for business purposes may also have implications in terms of house insurance and council tax. If working from home, then the business (and home address/telephone) may appear on advertising materials and letterheads. Consider privacy and safety, and perhaps opt for a box number address or similar. It is imperative that the business be run with a professional manner and mind set. Assess the visual first impression a client will have when visiting you in your home office, whether face-to-face or virtually, and whether or not it is right for the business.

Renting office space

Having a separate work place can be advantageous for keeping work and private life compartmentalised. It may be more professional to use rented accommodation for consultations rather than at home. There may also be an opportunity to share a receptionist who can take calls or make appointments. Alternatively, there are call centres that can handle your calls and pass on messages by text or email. Suitable premises can include private hospitals, clinics and gyms. It may be worth considering linking up with other professionals, e.g. other dietitians, physiotherapists, etc. It is important to find out what will be included in the rental. Does the room contain a telephone, computer, scales and chairs, or do these need to be provided? Is there safe storage space for equipment allocated within the rental, or does that need to be considered separately? Is the rental per session, week or month? These costs need to be incorporated into the business plan.

Arranging holiday cover

Events such as holidays should be anticipated and strategies developed to minimise their effects on the business, e.g. by informing regular clients that you will be unavailable between certain dates, or arranging with colleagues to provide cover. In this way, the goodwill of the client will be maintained, which is essential for continued business success.

Professional obligations

Registered dietitians must comply with HCPC professional standards and must ensure that the nature of the business, and the way it is conducted and promoted, conforms to these standards (HCPC, 2013, 2016) (see Chapter 1.1, Professional practice). Freelance dietitians working in private practice may take self-referrals. In such cases, dietitians must adhere to a strict code of professional conduct designed to protect the interests of both clients and professionals (BDA, 2017). It is important that freelance dietitians understand the circumstances when medical confirmation, or even formal medical referral, should be obtained for a self-referred patient. Further guidance is available from the FDG.

Setting up a business

A new set of rules and regulations will apply, and a dietitian must think and act as the owner of a business, and not as an employee. For example, a dietitian who sees private patients and keeps patient details on a database will need to register in accordance with the General Data Protection Regulation (GDPR), in force from May 2018 (more information is available from the Information Commissioner's Office, ico.org.uk; there is a small registration fee). It is recommended that independent legal and financial advice be sought to help develop and action the business plan. Some of the issues that may need to be discussed are outlined in the following text.

Banking

At least two business accounts should be opened namely a cheque or current account for day-to-day banking and expenses, and an interest-earning reserve or savings account. Money should be put into this account to pay for tax and NI when it becomes due. Also, given the irregular nature of freelance work, it may be wise to allocate a proportion of earned income to this account to cover quiet periods, or for use during holiday periods or in the event of illness. It is essential that business and personal accounts be kept clearly separate.

Insurance

The types of insurance policies required depend on the professional activities of the business, the type of clients and where the business is being conducted. Careful assessment of the following is required:

- *Additional professional liability insurance* – membership of the BDA includes a certain level of cover. Check the extent of the cover and consider whether circumstances dictate a higher level, or whether this is adequate. *Note*: Some areas of freelance work, although covered by this policy, require notification to the insurance providers to ensure adequate coverage. Additionally, it is advised that a provision for dietetic advice that is not face-to-face, e.g. via the Internet or text, be discussed with the insurance providers.
- *Public liability insurance* – this is an essential requirement of some contracts, but it may also be wise to avail depending on the nature of the business.
- *Additional household insurance* – to protect business hardware.
- *Additional car insurance* – if a car is being used for business purposes, the insurance company must be informed, and the premium may need to be adjusted.
- *Income protection* – this may be needed in case of minor illness or injury during which you are unable to work.
- *Critical illness cover* – this may be recommended in case of serious health problems. This is useful even if

SECTION 4

working part-time, as it could provide money to help with childcare or a partner's expenses during a difficult time.
- Private medical insurance – this may be advantageous as medical treatment can usually be carried out quickly and can be dovetailed with work commitments, thus minimising disruption to earning capacity.

Pension provision

Retirement planning is strongly recommended, and there are tax advantages in doing so. It is a complicated area, and it is important to take proper advice from qualified professionals.

Taxation and national insurance

An accountant should advise on these, and HM Revenue and Customs (HMRC) should be informed as soon as possible after the period of self-employment begins to ensure registration. The HMRC provides fact and advice sheets about all areas relating to taxation and NI.

Taxation

Most self-employed people will complete an annual self-assessment form for the assessment of their tax liabilities. The rules governing the taxation of employed and self-employed people differ in some respects, and HMRC may not regard regular hospital clinic and lecturing commitments as self-employed work. Such details will need to be clarified on an individual basis.

National insurance

Special arrangements apply for self-employed people, and it is essential to get advice on exactly what is required. Currently, Schedule D Class 2 will need to be paid from the outset, preferably by a standing order from the current business account. Class 4 is liable over a certain profit level and is assessed at the annual tax return.

Corporation tax

This is paid by a limited company on overall taxable profits; it is recommended that an accountant be consulted if setting up as a limited company to ensure all regulatory procedures are adhered to.

Setting fees

The rate of fees charged for freelance is important to the profit and sustainability of the business. Charges need to be clearly stated at the outset, and clients need to be clear about what they will be getting for their money. Recommending a fee structure is difficult because of differences in the area of expertise, the client (public or private sector), dietetic experience, the amount of work and time involved, and the degree of difficulty. For individual patients, fees can be set hourly or per therapeutic session (perhaps one of three visits); for private patients or a regular clinic, fees can be calculated per half-day or day, per recipe, or for a one-off lecture or a series of lectures; and for charities or large companies, fees can be calculated for long-term projects, as a retainer, or according to the degree of urgency. Different fees may be necessary according to the region, e.g. fees may be higher in London and South East England. The fees charged must take into account the business set-up and running costs. These overheads include the following:

- The time required to prospect for new business and clients, follow up leads, put together bids and proposals, and attend interviews.
- Taxation, NI, pension, accountant's fees, insurance policies, professional memberships, subscriptions, etc.
- Hardware, e.g. computer, printer, laptop and office furniture.
- Rental of office space, telephone (mobile and landline) and Internet access.
- Website development and hosting.
- Administrative and secretarial help to send out invoices and follow up unpaid invoices.
- Cost of stationery, stamps, printer paper and ink.
- Loss of earnings during holidays or illness, or the costs of providing holiday or sick leave cover.
- Travel costs and travelling time.
- Continuing professional development – costs of journal subscriptions, textbooks and attending meetings, including travelling expenses.
- Other sundry expenses.

Approximately, 40% of the fee charged should be paid into a business reserve or savings account to cover tax, NI, and other expenses, so that money will be available when these are due. This good business habit, together with keeping the invoicing up to date, will help to avoid cash-flow problems. Fees should be competitive and updated annually. Determining charge rates can be difficult, and it is important that a proper rate be charged always, because undercutting fees devalues professional skills. This can undermine the value of both individual expertise and the profession as a whole. It is essential that freelancers not breach competition law by agreeing among themselves what they are going to charge for services, and they must not discuss their fee structure with competitors.

Book keeping

It is essential that records are kept of all income and receipted expenditure. If the business is not too busy or complicated, it might be possible to run accounts on a spreadsheet or simple accounting software. Employing a bookkeeper and/or an accountant with experience may be advantageous, particularly when dealing with HMRC. Invoices need to be sent out regularly to maintain a steady cash flow, and unpaid invoices followed up promptly. Although rare, unpaid debts can arise, so proper invoicing systems need to be in place to help prevent this. If this does happen, there are a number of options available for dealing with non-payment, e.g. invoking the Late Payments Act, the Small Claims Court, or hiring debt collectors.

Contracts

A contract defines the relationship between the business and the client. It needs to reflect and record accurately the joint commercial intentions and visions, so that there are no surprises for the client when an invoice is presented. It can be used as a point of reference to help avoid any disputes, and also as a tool for discussions with regards to further work or time allowance. It should contain case-specific details, such as everyone's designations, dates, payment basis, services to be provided, the boundaries of these services, travelling expenses, time required, etc. To help define the boundaries, it may also be important to detail what is not included. It should also contain legal background details, e.g. terms, responsibilities for defective work, confidentiality and termination of contract. This section may be similar for all work undertaken. A written agreement or contract could be signed before work is started, although a simple exchange of emails setting out the extent, terms and limitations of the work can be sufficient.

Advertising and marketing

Potential clients need to know that the business is operating, who you are and what services are being provided. Advertising products and marketing services is an essential part of the business, but, as a registered dietitian, there are limitations on what can be said, where it can be said and how it is expressed. Generally, it is recommended that advertisements be accurate and restrained; they must not be false, fraudulent, misleading, deceptive, self-laudatory, unfair or sensational. Increasingly, new technologies are being utilised by dietitians to market their services and promote their businesses. Consider establishing a website and registering the business in professional directories or with healthcare providers. It is essential that the right image be communicated via the company name, website, and on headed paper, compliment slips, business cards and leaflets. Ensure that these all reflect what the business is about and what is being marketed. Social media provides an instant and high-profile means to raise awareness; however, it is recommended to always check messaging carefully before going live. Careful consideration of all communications to ensure they remain compliant with regulations and the HCPC code of conduct is essential.

Many jobs are obtained by word-of-mouth from contacts and by reputation. Some may be advertised in professional magazines or on websites. A specialist healthcare employment agency may also be a source of potential work. Ensure that your curriculum vitae is up to date and relevant for each potential client.

Help and support

There is a lot of help available, much of it free, e.g. signing for business support emails from HMRC and government videos, webinars, e-learning, and emails. Local newspapers can be a useful source of information on courses and business networks that can provide help and support. The FDG produces, and continually updates, a series of fact sheets for freelance dietitians on a wide range of topics, including business planning, taxation and accounting for your business, setting up in private practice, and self-referrals. These are an invaluable resource for anyone involved in or contemplating freelance work. Additionally, FDG runs training courses for those new to freelancing.

Maintaining and expanding the business

Getting the business up and running may seem a challenge, but keeping up the momentum is just as important and can be challenging when working alone. It is not easy to look to the future when busy on a daily basis. It is important to maintain a professional approach:

- Keep to deadlines, deliver promptly and always deal with clients in a professional manner.
- Keep up to date with developments in the specified area of practice.
- Pass to other freelance dietitians work that is not within your area of expertise or when there is insufficient time to do the job properly.
- Be proactive – follow up leads and keep in touch with people. Be seen at relevant meetings or present at conferences.
- Consider writing a newsletter for circulation to past and current clients.
- If working from home, dress the part. The freelancer who looks professional will feel more competent when talking to a client on the telephone; and, with the increasing use of video conferencing, this is essential.
- Stay motivated.

Working alone may result in isolation or even boredom, especially after working in a busy department. It is easy to put things off until later, e.g. go shopping rather than follow up client leads. If work does not come in as planned, then there is increased pressure, particularly financial, to succeed. Staying motivated can be one of the most difficult things to do. Making the most of networking opportunities with like-minded colleagues is essential for any freelancer, as knowing that others have the same problems and issues is reassuring, and solutions may become more apparent. The FDG meets regularly and provides such support, in addition to providing essential CPD.

Lack of work

It is possible that there will be times when there is little or no fee-income work. During such periods, consider the following points to make good use of the time:

- Enrol in a course such as media, cookery, food hygiene, advanced computing, web design, etc., and make use of the newly acquired skills, e.g. by writing an article or producing a website.
- Volunteer to be the member of a FDG committee that might be useful and relevant to your business.

- Attend conferences and contact former colleagues.
- Review the business plan and financial matters by ensuring all administrative matters are up to date, e.g. expense receipts.
- Update your curriculum vitae (CV) or the continuing professional development (CPD) portfolio.
- Research a new area of potential work.
- Spend time constructively on social media.

Continuing professional development

Any or all of the range of activities undertaken as a freelance dietitian can be used to provide evidence for CPD. The focus often evolves and changes, and this can be excellent material for the portfolio. The CPD activity could show professional development alongside business development, and evidence could be details from specific examples. It is important to document and evaluate every piece of freelance work and every meeting that is attended. The portfolio should be regularly updated and reviewed to see what has been learned and how this can be extended. This is an intrinsic and necessary part of being a professional.

Acknowledgement

The editor acknowledges the prior contribution of Elaine Gardner.

Internet resources

Federation of Small Businesses, www.fsb.org.uk

Freelance Dietitians Group (FDG), a specialist group of the BDA, www.freelancedietitians.org

Guide to the General Data Protection Regulation, https://ico.org.uk/for-organisations/guide-to-the-general-data-protection-regulation-gdpr

HM Revenue and Customs, www.hmrc.gov.uk

Independent Professional Support body for Contractors, Independents and Freelancers, www.ipse.co.uk

Information Commissioner's Office, https://ico.org.uk

UK government business support, www.gov.uk/business-support-helpline

UK government help for the self-employed, www.gov.uk/government/news/webinars-emails-and-videos-if-youre-self-employed

References

BDA. (2017) *Code of Professional Conduct*. Available at https://www.bda.uk.com/professional/practice/professionalism/code_of_conduct. Accessed 19 February 2019..

European Commission. *EU Register of Nutrition and Health Claims Made on Foods*. Available at http://ec.europa.eu/nuhclaims http://ec.europa.eu/nuhclaims. Accessed 1 June 2016.

Experian. (2010) *Insight Report – Tomorrow's Champions: Finding the Small Business Engines for Economic Growth*. Available at www.experian.co.uk/insight-reports/index.html. Accessed 28 March 2017.

Health & Care Professions Council (HCPC). (2013) *Standards of Proficiency: Dietitians*. London: HCPC. Available at www.hcpc-uk.org/publications/standards/index.asp?id=43

Health & Care Professions Council (HCPC). (2016) *Standards of Conduct Performance and Ethics*. Available at http://www.hcpc-uk.org/aboutregistration/standards/standardsofconductperformanceandethics. Accessed 22 December 2016.

Kitching J. (2016) *Exploring the UK Freelance Workforce in 2015*. *IPSE*. Available at https://www.ipse.co.uk/resource/exploring_the_uk_freelance_workforce_in_2016.html. Accessed 25 September 2018.

Office for National Statistics (ONS). (2016) *Business Demography, UK: 2015*. Change in the number of UK businesses broken down by sector of the economy. Available at https://www.ons.gov.uk/businessindustryandtrade/business/activitysizeandlocation/bulletins/businessdemography/2015. Accessed 22 December 2016.

4.2 Public health nutrition

Kirsten Whitehead and Vanessa Halliday

Key points

- Public health nutrition (PHN) is concerned with promoting physical and mental health and preventing diet-related ill health throughout the population.
- Public health is based on key principles of decreasing inequality, partnership working, empowering communities and developing evidence-based practice.
- Dietitians are part of the public health workforce; the model and process for nutrition and dietetic practice provide a clearly defined structure that is relevant to this field.

SECTION 4

Introduction to Public Health

Public health is defined as the '*the science and art of preventing disease, prolonging life and promoting health through the organised efforts and informed choices of society, organisations, public and private, communities and individuals*' (Wanless, 2004). Public health aims to improve the health of the population and reduce health inequalities by helping people live longer, healthier and more fulfilling lives, while improving the health of the poorest the fastest. It considers the well-being of the population, including mental and physical health, while engendering a sense of control over the way people want to live. Public health focuses on the wider environment by influencing those factors that enable people to make healthier choices. Importantly, public health is about partnership working, involving local and national governments alongside other organisations and stakeholders that contribute to the health and well-being of the population.

A framework for public health policy

At all stages of the lifespan, a range of factors that are within and outside of an individual's control can influence health and well-being. The policy rainbow (Dahlgren & Whitehead, 1991) represents the range, and interrelationship, of factors that influence health (Figure 4.2.1). This model maps non-modifiable individual factors such as gender and age, with social, cultural and environmental factors that can be adapted, expressing them as a series of layers of influence. The relative contribution of each layer to improving health, and the actions required to change each of the influencing factors, has become a framework for the development of public health policy. This model recognises that behaviour change can only take place in a supportive environment. For example, families wanting to maintain a healthy weight will be able to do so more easily in a supportive environment, where food production and retail facilitate access to healthy food at an affordable price, education provides the skills and knowledge to buy and prepare healthy food, employment or benefits provide adequate money, the workplace and schools have food policies in place, and housing is conducive to maintaining a positive family life and healthy food preparation.

Public health systems in the UK

In the UK, the government, along with the devolved administrations of the Northern Ireland Assembly, Scottish Parliament and Welsh Assembly, are responsible for developing public health strategies, legislation and policies. In each of the four countries, there is a specialist public health agency to support the domestic delivery of public health.

England

The Health and Social Care Act (HM Government, 2012) resulted in a reorganisation of the public health system in England. In 2013, Public Health England (PHE) was established as an executive agency sponsored by the Department of Health (DH), with the responsibility for improving health and reducing health inequalities at the local level transferring from the NHS to local authorities.

Manual of Dietetic Practice, Sixth Edition. Edited by Joan Gandy.

Companion website: www.manualofdieteticpractice.com

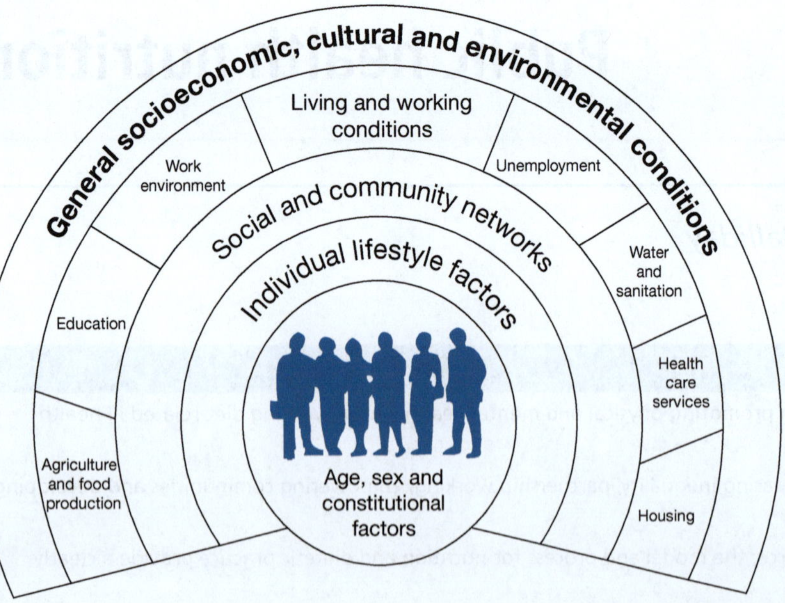

Figure 4.2.1 A social model of health (source: Dahlgren & Whitehead (1991). Reproduced with permission from the Institute for Future Studies, Sweden)

The NHS in England continues to deliver some public health services such as smoking cessation, sexual health, screening and vaccination programmes. Health Education England (HEE) also works with PHE to develop the public health workforce within the NHS and local authority. In England, the four key domains of public health in practice and their objectives (DH, 2012) are as follows:

- Improving the wider determinants of health
  - Objective: To make improvements against wider factors that affect health and well-being, and health inequalities.
- Health improvement
  - Objective: To help people adopt healthy lifestyles, make healthy choices and reduce health inequalities.
- Health protection
  - Objective: To protect the population's health from major incidents and other threats, while reducing health inequalities.
- Healthcare public health and preventing premature death
  - Objective: To reduce the number of people living with preventable ill health and dying prematurely, while reducing the gap between communities.

Northern Ireland

Following reforms to the health and social care system in Northern Ireland, the Public Health Agency was established in 2009. The Public Health Agency works at a regional and local level with four key functions:

- Health and social well-being improvement.
- Health protection.
- Health and social care research and development.
- Supporting public health commissioning and policy development.

Scotland

In Scotland, NHS Health Scotland is the national agency for health improvement and reduction of health inequalities. The role and direction of NHS Scotland in prioritising health inequalities are described in *A Fairer Healthier Scotland Corporate Strategy 2012–2017* (NHS Health Scotland, 2012) and *Strengthening the Function and Re-focussing Action for a Healthier Scotland* (The Scottish Government, 2016). The policy framework focuses on:

- Tackling inequalities in Scottish society.
- Working to ensure children have the best start in life.
- Supporting people to maintain their independence as they age.
- Enabling people to live longer and healthier lives.

Hosted by NHS Health Scotland, the aim of the recently formed Scottish Public Health Network (ScotPHN) is to work on public health priorities and facilitate communication and information exchange across the public health workforce in Scotland.

Wales

Public Health Wales is one of three NHS Trusts in Wales. It provides specialist public health advice and services aimed at protecting and improving health and well-being. It does this, e.g. by providing public health support to the health boards and local authorities in Wales; managing health intelligence and knowledge management services (including the Public Health Wales Observatory); and through the delivery of public health services including health protection, screening programmes and safeguarding. In 2016, the Public Health Outcomes Framework for Wales was published to support the national indicators for Well-being of Future Generation (Wales) Act 2015

Table 4.2.1 Core roles of the public health workforce (adapted from Centre for Workforce Intelligence, 2014; HEE, 2016)

Role	Summary of work
Directors, assistant directors of public health	Provide a management and leadership role in the local authority. Duties are set out in law, often from Acts of Parliament. Must be registered with the UK Public Health Register (PHR), General Medical Council (GMC) or General Dental Council (GDC).
Public health consultants, specialists	Work at a senior strategic or management level, usually in local authorities or public health agencies. Must be registered with the UK PHR, GMC or GDC.
Public health academics	Work in academia, conducting research and teaching in the field of public health.
Public health managers	Experienced and qualified public health staff, usually working in local authorities, managing locally run public health projects and programmes.
Public health scientists	May work in the NHS or public health agencies, often in scientific laboratories that are responsible for analysing samples related to the health of the public.
Intelligence and knowledge professionals	Responsible for the analysis, interpretation and presentation of public health data in organisations such as local authorities and public health agencies.
Public health nurses	Mostly employed in health protection teams within the NHS, local authorities and across public health agencies.
School nurses	Registered nurses or midwives with post-registration specialist training in community public health. Work in schools to support the health and well-being of children and young people.
Health visitors	Registered nurses or midwives with post-registration specialist training in child health. Work as part of the primary healthcare team, supporting new parents and families with pre-school-age children.
Public health practitioners	Key workers involved in all areas of public health, across the public health system. Work often includes the development and implementation of community projects and programmes. Examples of public health practitioner roles include public health nutritionists, health improvement and health protection practitioners.
Environmental health professionals	Usually employed by local authorities, working in line with statutory regulations related to environmental health. For example, investigating outbreaks of foodborne illness or enforcing food hygiene regulations.
Allied health professionals (AHPs)	AHPs can be involved across all four domains of public health: health protection, addressing the wider determinants of health, health improvement and healthcare public health.

(NHS Wales, 2016). The focus of the key outcomes of the framework are:

- Living conditions that support and contribute to health now and for the future.
- Ways of living that improve health.
- Health throughout the life course.

In many other countries, there are public health agencies working to promote and protect the health of their residents. In addition, international agencies, such as the World Health Organisation (WHO), have an important leadership and monitoring role in managing global public health. Examples of relevant international policy documents include Action Plan for the Prevention and Control of Non-communicable Diseases in the WHO European Region 2016–2025 (WHO, 2016a), European Action Plan for Strengthening Public Health Capacities and Services (WHO, 2012a), Global Action Plan for the Prevention and Control of Non-communicable Diseases (WHO, 2013), and Report of the Commission on Ending Obesity (WHO, 2016b).

Public health workforce

The public health workforce is diverse in what it does and the places it works. A recent mapping exercise (Centre for Workforce Intelligence, 2014) suggests that there are 11 core roles within the public health workforce in England (Table 4.2.1), with health visitors, public health practitioners, environmental health workers and school nurses making up the majority of the workforce. Additionally, the Strategy to Develop the Capacity, Impact and Profile of Allied Health Professionals (AHPs) in Public Health 2015–2018 (PHE & AHPF, 2015) clarifies the potential role of AHPs.

Dietitians may be employed in a number of these roles. While the majority will be working in academia or as public health practitioners, some may choose to undertake further training to become a public health consultant. Public health nutritionist roles include the development and evaluation of community nutrition services and programmes; nutrition-related health promotion work, including cook and eat groups; education and training; and contributing to the development and implementation of nutrition-related local policies and strategies. Dietitians working as public health practitioners may work across a broader range of public health matters, such as physical activity or smoking cessation.

Members of the wider workforce, including teachers, urban planners, firemen and directors of finance of health organisations, are also able to influence the health of the population through their roles. Initiatives such as Make Every Contact Count (PHE, 2016), Raising the Issue of Weight (DH, 2006) and Brief Interventions

(Cavill *et al.*, 2011) are examples of how all staff can contribute. All dietitians working within a clinical specialty will be included in this group due to their influence on the wider family or community of the patients that they are working with (PHE & AHPF, 2015). For example, specialist dietitians may be involved in the development of national guidance or position papers, which influence the care of the population of patients with that condition.

Public health nutrition

Public health nutrition (PHN) is concerned with improving the health of the population by focusing on the wider environment to understand and influence the issues that help or hinder people in making healthy food and lifestyle choices. PHN aims to improve the population's health and prevent diet-related illnesses rather than treating the diseases of individual patients.

Nutrition is a major and modifiable determinant of many chronic diseases, and diet can have positive and negative impacts on health throughout life. The Global Burden of Disease Project has informed this understanding using epidemiological data from around the world, analysing the risk factors associated with premature death and disability (Institute for Health Metrics and Evaluation, 2016). In sub-Saharan Africa, childhood and maternal malnutrition remain a leading cause of death, with micronutrient deficiencies including iron deficiency anaemia, iodine, zinc and vitamin A continuing to impact on the health and economic productivity of the population. Although communicable diseases such as malaria, tuberculosis and human immunodeficiency virus remain in many areas of the world, particularly Africa, development and urbanisation in low- and middle-income countries, along with a shift from what was a largely a plant-based diet to one that is more energy-dense and processed, has led to a rapid increase in non-communicable diseases such as obesity, cardiovascular disease and type 2 diabetes. It is these chronic diseases that now contribute the most to premature death and therefore pose the greatest public health burden. Analysis of the 2013 data from the Global Burden of Diseases, Injuries, and Risk Factors Study found that, in England, the combination of behavioural risk factors of suboptimal diet, physical inactivity and a high body mass index contributed the most to disease burden as measured by disability adjusted life years (DALYs) (Newton *et al.*, 2015). Diseases associated with a poor diet are estimated to cost the NHS in the region of £5.8 billion annually (Scarborough *et al.*, 2011). Overall, smoking remains the leading behavioural risk factor for DALYs, with consumption of alcohol also being an important factor.

National food and health policy and guidelines

The following section summarises the main policy documents and stakeholders that have set the direction for public health and PHN in the UK. Since the devolution of powers, it is the responsibility of the national public health agencies to develop and implement public health policies and strategies in their country. For public health dietitians, it is essential to be familiar with the policies and guidelines relevant to the country that they work in.

Healthy Lives, Healthy People: Our Strategy for Public Health in England (HM Government, 2010) set out the UK government's long-term legislation for public health in England. It was part of the reform to the NHS in England introduced in 2010, and builds on the document Equity and Excellence: Liberating the NHS (DH, 2010). The White Paper, and subsequent Health and Social Care Act (HM Government, 2012), include radical changes to how public health is managed in England primarily by transferring the responsibility from the NHS to local government and the creation of PHE. *The Strategic Plan for the Next 4 Years: Better Outcomes by 2020* (2016), published by PHE, outlines the short-term agenda for delivering improvements in public health challenges, such as reducing childhood obesity and increasing physical activity levels.

The following organisations have a strategic role in formulating the PHN policy:

- The DH creates national policies and legislation in England and is responsible for diet, obesity and physical exercise policy through the work of the Health and Wellbeing Directorate. Working with partner agencies such as PHE, their policies and practice on obesity and healthy eating include, e.g.:
    - The Eatwell Guide.
    - Healthy Start.
    - National child measurement programme.
    - Nursery milk.
    - School fruit and vegetable scheme.
    - Workplace health.
- The Scientific Advisory Committee on Nutrition (SACN) is an advisory committee of independent experts that provides advice to PHE and other government agencies and departments. The committee's remit includes advising on the nutrient content of individual foods and diet, and on the nutritional status of people. Recently, the dietary reference values for vitamin D have been revised, culminating in the SACN vitamin D and health report (2016), which outlines new recommendations that everyone over 1 year of age should consume 10 micrograms of vitamin D daily.
- The Food Standards Agency (FSA) is an independent government department set up in 2000 to protect the public's health and consumer interests in relation to food. The FSA is responsible for protecting the public in relation to food safety and food hygiene in England, Northern Ireland and Wales. In England, responsibility for the work around food standards and food labelling policy moved from the FSA to the Department for Food, Environment and Rural Affairs (Defra) in 2010. Food Standards Scotland (FSS) is the public-sector organisation responsible for food safety and food labelling in Scotland.

SECTION 4

- DEFRA is a ministerial department supported by 33 agencies and public bodies responsible for safeguarding the natural environment in England. Their work includes:
  - Animal health and welfare.
  - Environmental protection and pollution control.
  - Food, farming and fisheries, including food labelling.
  - Rural communities and issues.
  - Sustainable development and the green economy.
- The National Institute for Health and Care Excellence (NICE) (England) provides guidance and sets quality standards, based on the best available evidence and knowledge of good practice, to improve people's health and prevent and treat ill health. Within NICE, the Public Health Centre and Social Care Institute are responsible for producing guidance on public health topics, e.g. aspects of health promotion, health protection and service provision. In addition to guidance on more general public health topics such as *Community Engagement: Improving Health and Wellbeing and Reducing Health Inequalities (NG44) (2016)*, recent PHN-related guidance has included *Preventing Excess Weight Gain (NG7)* (2015) and *Weight Management: Lifestyle Services for Overweight or Obese Adults (PH53)* (2014).

National health and nutrition surveys

Measuring the health of the nation, and trends over time, provides information on the state of the public's health that can be used to develop policy, plan services and evaluate the impact of initiatives and interventions. The Health Survey for England began in 1991, randomly sampling information from adults and children who lived in private households in the country. The annual survey includes general questions related to physical and mental health and lifestyle behaviours, in addition to taking measurements such as weight, height and blood pressure. While the Health Survey for England can provide data on the levels of obesity, and fruit and vegetable consumption is monitored every 2 years, it does not include details of dietary intake. In order to understand how diets are changing and to evaluate if healthy eating initiatives are being effective, the National Diet and Nutrition Survey (NDNS) is conducted annually, recruiting between 1000 and 1500 adults and children from across the UK. The NDNS survey includes questions about eating habits, lifestyle behaviours such as physical activity, as well as anthropometric measurements. Participants are also asked to complete a 4-day food and drink diary. Key findings from the 2016 NDNS report (Bates *et al.*, 2016a) identified that 73% of adults (19–64 years) were not meeting the recommended five portions of fruit and vegetables per day, eating on average four portions. Furthermore, in all age groups, the average daily intake of saturated fat exceeded the recommended dietary reference values. Analysis of data from the survey confirms that adults in England continued to exceed the recommended salt intake of 6 g/day (SACN, 2003) by one-third, with women consuming on average 6.8 g/day and men 9.1 g/day (Bates *et al.*, 2016b).

Although only conducted once, the Low Income Diet and Nutrition Survey (LIDNS) provided a comprehensive national overview of the food consumption, nutrient intake and factors influencing the food choice of people living on low incomes. Data were collected between 2003 and 2005 from over 3 500 participants living in the most materially deprived households in the UK. The results suggest that food intake is similar to that of the general population, with fruit and vegetable intakes below the recommended government guidelines and excessive amounts of saturated fat and sugar being consumed. Levels of overweight and obesity were high in both men (62%) and women (63%) (Nelson *et al.*, 2007).

Other national surveys that inform the understanding of health and nutritional intake of adults include the following:

- The Food and You Survey, which is a consumer attitudes survey conducted biennially since 2010. Data collection includes information on eating, cooking and shopping practices, along with behaviours about food safety and dietary restrictions.
- Launched in 2001 following the merger of the National Food Survey (NFS) and Family Expenditure Survey (FES), the Expenditure and Food Survey (EFS) has more recently been renamed the Living Costs and Food Survey (LCFS). Data collection includes information on the household spending on food and drinks for consumption in and out of the home.
- Completed from 2002 to 2008 by each primary care trust, the Primary Care Trust Patient Survey included questions on the fruit and vegetable intake of patients.

As part of the UK government's work to tackle childhood obesity, the National Child Measurement Programme (NCMP) was established in England in 2007. Each year, children aged 4–5 years (reception year) and 10–11 years (year 6) are weighed and measured during the school year, and their BMI centile calculated. The aim of the programme is to inform the local planning and delivery of services for children as well as the gathering of population-level surveillance data allowing trends in growth patterns and obesity to be analysed. Although designed as a surveillance programme, local areas are encouraged to inform parents about a child's weight status and to provide support for achieving healthy lifestyles.

Other national surveys informing the understanding of the health and nutritional intake of children include the following:

- Infant feeding survey, conducted with new mothers every 5 years between 1975 and 2010. The survey focussed on the incidence, prevalence and duration of breastfeeding and infant feeding practices from birth to 9 months.
- TellUs annual survey of children and young people, which includes questions on fruit and vegetable intake and attitudes to the advice they receive on healthy eating.

- School lunch take-up survey, which was commissioned by the Department of Education in 2013/2014 prior to the universal free school meals policy roll out. Previous school meal surveys were conducted by the School Food Trust and the Local Authority Caterers Association, based on data collected by local authorities from primary and secondary schools.

Food choice: Factors to consider when working in public health nutrition practice

In addition to the physiological aspects that affect nutritional requirements and the desire for food, food choice is influenced by individual, social and environmental factors (Shepherd, 1999). At an individual level, gender, age and activity determine our energy and nutritional requirements, with what people choose to eat being adapted through the life course. For some people, physical and mental health conditions such as allergies, diabetes and depression will influence food choice, while moderating food intake in order to control body weight will be important for many. Importantly, life experiences and attitudes also contribute towards food preferences, with factors such as culture, religion and personal values around issues such as animal welfare and the environment influencing what many eat. Social norms and comparisons to friends and family also impact on food choice. Understandably, nutrition education, food literacy, cooking skills and other life commitments all contribute to how these factors affect attitudes to food and what is eaten.

Food marketing and labelling

Marketing and advertising play a critical role in food choice. In the UK, the Committee of Advertising Practice (CAP) maintains the advertising codes that are administered by the Advertising Standards Authority. In relation to food, these standards include, e.g. health claims that refer to how a food or ingredient impacts on health. They also include advertising of food to children, which over recent years has received particular scrutiny. Informed by the WHO recommendations on the marketing of foods and non-alcoholic beverages to children (WHO, 2012b), in the UK, this practice is regulated. Currently, the rules that prohibit the advertisement of foods that are high in fat, sugar and salt during children's programmes are restricted to broadcast media such as TV. In June 2017, this ruling was broadened to incorporate non-broadcast media, including online advertising, for the under-12-year age category.

Information on the nutritional content of foods is available on most packaged foods in the UK and is regulated by legislation from the European Union Food Information for Consumers Regulation (EU FIC). Changes relating to how allergen information is displayed on labels were implemented in 2014. In the UK, historically, back-of-pack nutritional information has been difficult for the consumer to interpret; therefore, front-of-pack (at-a-glance) information labelling has been developed. Two front-of-pack labelling schemes are commonly used in the UK to identify the nutritional content of food. The first is presented in comparison to guideline daily amounts (GDAs), and the second, the colour-coded (traffic light) integrated label. As a guide for consumers, four key nutrients, namely fat, saturated fat, salt and sugar, as well as energy are included (see Chapter 4.5, Food law and labelling). More recently, point-of-purchase information has been expanded to include food purchased in fast food outlets and some restaurant establishments. How this impacts on the behaviour and food choice of the consumer remains uncertain. WHO (2016c) have considered the use of fiscal policies to influence food intake.

Food accessibility and cost

Accessibility to food and the food environment are important aspects of food choice. These should be considered in terms of what shops and supermarkets there are in local communities, as well as transport. The number of local fast food takeaways and restaurants may also influence behaviour. Importantly, ensuring that the food made available in schools and workplace canteens meets healthy eating standards offers huge potential to influence an individual's food choice.

The amount of money available to spend on food plays a significant role in what is eaten. Changes in consumption and attitudes to food have occurred in a period of relative affluence. Food costs in the UK, until the economic downturn in 2008, had been proportionately falling as consumers' disposable income increased. However, between 2007 and 2012, when they reached their peak, food prices rose by 11.5% in real terms, as measured by the Consumer Price Index (Defra, 2016). An increase in the cost of agricultural commodities, along with higher oil prices during these times, led to this above inflation rise in food prices adding substantially to a family's cost of living. As households in the lowest-income groups spend 16% of their disposable income on food (including all foods and non-alcoholic drinks), as compared to those with the highest income spending only 8% (Office for National Statistics, 2010), it is this group that has been most vulnerable to experiencing food insecurity. Until recently, we had started to see a gradual reduction in food prices, albeit in 2015 still at a level 8% higher as compared to 2007. The greatest fall (9.2%) had been seen in butter, margarine and cooking oil, with prices for foods such as bread, meat, milk, eggs, processed foods and alcohol all falling by more than 2% (Defra, 2016).

Food poverty

In times of financial hardship, providing a healthy diet for families is an additional challenge to those living in low-income households and already suffering a disproportionate amount of diet-related ill health. In the UK, it was estimated that, during 2013, over 500,000 people were in need of food aid (Cooper & Dumpleton, 2013). Furthermore, the number of people seeking

SECTION 4

support from food banks has increased dramatically over recent years. These figures suggest an increase in the number of people in the UK experiencing food poverty. However, with no agreed definition or measure of food poverty, determining the incidence is difficult. A report for the FSA in Northern Ireland, Understanding Food in the Context of Poverty, Economic Insecurity and Social Exclusion (King *et al.*, 2015), gave a working definition of *food poverty* thus: '*where constraints are such that it is not possible for individuals or households to consume a nutritionally adequate diet, they could be considered to be in food poverty*'.

Food sustainability

While seasonality of food in the UK was once a significant determinant of choice, nowadays, with international transportation of produce, most items are available throughout the year. However, environmental concerns including the carbon footprint of food, supporting local producers and cost are important for many people when considering the provenance of the food that they purchase. The way that food is grown, processed, stored, distributed, retailed and disposed of has significant economic and environmental impacts. There is increasing recognition that a healthy diet must also be produced in a sustainable way. Definitions of sustainability differ, but generally encompass the three domains of equitable economic development, participatory democratic structures and greater environmental integrity. A popular definition of sustainable development is: development that '*meets the needs of the present without compromising the ability of the future generations to meet their own needs*' (World Commission on Environment and Development, 1987). There is considerable debate about the recommendations for healthy, safe, sustainable, low-environmental-impact food. A sustainable food system has been defined as '*food associated with high levels of well-being, social justice, stewardship and system resilience*' (New Economics Foundation, 2011), a vision that fits well with the holistic approach of public health. It is recognised that '*in terms of the environmental impact of household food consumption, the composition of our diet is more important than how and where food items are produced*' (New Economics Foundation, 2011). There is general agreement on a set of principles that meets the needs for health and the environment, including eating more plant-based foods, eating less meat and processed foods, wasting less food and choosing certified foods where food safety and animal welfare standards are assured.

In 2008, the UK government raised concerns about current food consumption and economic, social and environmental sustainability, and concluded that the way people currently eat is not sustainable for either health or the environment (Strategy Unit, 2008). In particular, it was estimated that 18–20% of greenhouse gas emissions in the UK came from the food chain (Macdiarmid *et al.*, 2011). Changes in food production and food consumption are needed to contribute to the necessary reductions in greenhouse gas emissions. However, reducing food waste and excessive packaging, alongside efficient disposal of waste, are also crucial to reducing the greenhouse gas effect of waste management.

In 2013, 15 million tonnes of food and drink were wasted in the UK food chain (Waste and Resource Action Programme, 2015). The majority (7 million tonnes) was thrown away at a household level, with 3.9 million tonnes coming from the manufacturing process, and just under 3 million tonnes from grocery retail and wholesale. A significant proportion of waste from households is deemed avoidable and due to purchasing, cooking, preparing or serving too much, or because it was not used in time. It has been estimated that the average UK family could save around £480 per year, increasing to £680 for families with children, on food and drink that could have been used but is thrown away (Waste and Resource Action Programme, 2009). The greenhouse gas emissions that this waste food produces is 20 million tonnes; removing this waste is equivalent to the reduction in emissions from taking one in four cars off the roads (Waste and Resource Action Programme, 2009).

Population dietary guidance that takes nutrition, food safety and sustainability of the food supply into account is urgently needed to ensure that consumers receive consistent messages. The public is generally in support of making changes to mitigate climate change; however, when given a list of possible behaviours to achieve this, adopting a lower-impact diet was one they were least likely to try (Defra, 2008). With no current UK government regulatory approach (Priestly, 2016), this will be a challenge for dietitians working in public health in the near future.

SECTION 4

Principles of public health practice

Using and creating the evidence base

All dietetic practice should be based on the best evidence available, and PHN is no exception. There are several journals dedicated to public health or topics that have a public health aspect such as obesity, diabetes and cancer, and many public health topics are covered by NICE guidance. There are also numerous sources of data which help to inform public health work and provide the rationale for working on specific issues in defined populations. These will be discussed further in the following section about assessment.

Additionally, a core function of public health work involves undertaking research. This includes the analysis of population nutritional needs and factors affecting those needs, as well as the evaluation of the effectiveness of public health interventions. It could also include systematic reviews and meta-analysis to collate the evidence and draw conclusions. The public health workforce has a responsibility to work in the way that is the best for the target population and which uses resources effectively. Presenting and publishing results of work undertaken is important, even if the intervention was not successful, as it informs future practice.

Promoting equality and reducing inequality

Inequalities are variations that are not fair or just (Naidoo & Wills, 2016). Tackling inequalities in health outcomes between the most and least disadvantaged people in society remains a significant public health challenge globally. In the UK, there is a social gradient in health, which means that those living in more deprived communities have higher rates of obesity and physical and mental health problems (Marmot, 2010). Life expectancy, as compared to those living in the richest areas, is on average 8 years shorter for men and 7 years shorter for women (Newton *et al.*, 2015). The most effective way to address public health is considered to be one that addresses the wider social determinants of health, such as housing, education, employment and healthcare, so that *'no one should be disadvantaged from achieving their full health potential'* (Whitehead, 2000). Adopting a life course framework by addressing influences from infancy to old age can guide public health approaches that positively impact on the health of the nation. The public health workforce must consider the social determinants of health and the ways to decrease inequalities in health outcomes in whatever work they do.

Partnership working

Partnership working has been described by the WHO (2009) as a collaborative relationship between two or more parties based on trust, equality, and mutual understanding, for the achievement of a specified goal. As public health practice does not happen in isolation, working in partnership with other agencies is essential. In addition to those directly involved in health and public health, such as the NHS and local authorities, the voluntary sector, private sector and the media should be considered.

Partnership working is believed to enhance the coordination of services, avoid duplication or gaps in services, be cost-effective and facilitate the generation of more creative solutions to problems. *Healthy Lives, Healthy People* (HM Government, 2010) suggested that integrated and innovative ways are required to empower people and communities to make healthier choices. Working in partnership, therefore, is not just about other organisations with a public health agenda, but also includes the populations who will benefit from the public health interventions. Target populations need to participate actively in determining the main issues affecting their health and well-being and to be involved in deciding how those issues can be tackled.

Partnerships will vary depending on the type of public health issue. For example, different organisations and populations will be involved when working towards prevention of childhood obesity in the UK as opposed to tackling undernutrition in a developing country. Partnerships also vary in size, vision, focus, resource and the level of community participation. Partnerships are dynamic and will change over time in line with the population needs and concerns. In many cases, working in partnership is a prerequisite to obtaining funding for public health work, so the partnership must form prior to applying for funding. Partnerships can take time to develop, and, in order for them to work well, they need to be equitable; work well as a team; and have a shared vision, good leadership, effective communication channels, and shared resources. Partners need to be committed to working together in order for the benefits to outweigh the costs. In effect, there are risks if a partnership does not function effectively, as well as huge benefits when it does, and the shared accountability is critical.

Community empowerment

Community empowerment is both a principle and the result of public health activity. Public health work aims to empower the community, and individuals within it, to take more ownership, power and control over decisions, events and the use of resources that affect their lives and health. Public health work should be about improving confidence of individuals and communities as well as their ability, or capacity, to achieve the desired outcomes. Active participation of the community in activities relevant to public health is key, but on its own is not enough (Hughes & Margetts, 2011). An empowered community is likely to take more responsibility for challenging and changing the world around them. If empowerment is achieved, then the benefits of an intervention are more likely to be sustained in the long term. There are numerous ways in which empowerment can be achieved, but it is often difficult to measure and evaluate. It can take a long time, and it may be difficult to determine if the intervention itself led to the empowerment, as other factors may be involved. Using qualitative methods such as interviews and focus groups to determine the views of the target population is important to clarify the impact of what has been undertaken (Naidoo & Wills, 2016).

Public health practice

Hughes and Margetts (2011) suggest three core categories of PHN practice: research and analysis, building capacity and intervention management. Public health interventions are diverse, e.g. lobbying for a sugar tax on food, supporting a large employer to develop a healthy food policy for that organisation, campaigning for a health-related change such as the removal of junk food from supermarket checkouts, creating evidence-based resources to support health messages or researching the needs of specific populations. Whatever tasks are undertaken, there will be some aspect of the three core functions incorporated, although the extent of incorporation may differ.

There are many different models and frameworks available to support a systematic approach to developing and implementing public health interventions, and these are described well by Hughes and Margetts (2011). NICE Guideline PH6 (2007) also provides guidance on delivering and evaluating behaviour change interventions for individuals, communities and populations that can help the planning process.

The Model and Process for Nutrition and Dietetic Practice (BDA, 2016) (see Chapter 1.1, Professional practice) provides a clearly defined structure for practice that is also relevant for public health. When working at a population level, there are similarities to clinical practice, but the methods differ. For example, assessing population needs rather than the individual requires different tools and skills.

This section will describe commonly used methods or ways of working in public health that fit with the headings of assessment, identification of nutritional or health need, planning and implementation of an intervention and evaluation. For more detail, see Hughes and Margetts (2011). For health promotion activities, Naidoo and Wills (2016) provide a comprehensive overview. Public health includes health promotion, but is a much broader discipline.

Assessment

There are many different tools which assist those working in public health to understand the population needs and identify appropriate intervention strategies (Naidoo & Wills, 2016). With populations, the identification of a problem and possible intervention(s) is not a one-size-fits-all or off-the-peg activity. A significant amount of time and resource is spent on information gathering that may seem arduous but must be balanced against the intervention costs. These assessment processes are designed to support the development of successful strategies and decrease the chance of inappropriate or ineffective actions. The information gathered is often referred to as public health intelligence. Methods used to support this process include (health) needs assessment, community profiling and asset mapping (not an exhaustive list). All of these are designed to obtain information that supports planning and decision-making. In practice, a combination of approaches is likely to create the best understanding of the population needs (Hughes & Margetts, 2011). Needs assessment and community profiling are seen as downstream or top-down approaches which may be more about identifying health problems from a healthcare perspective, whereas asset mapping comes from the population and is a bottom-up or upstream approach which aims to identify the factors affecting those health problems and is consistent with the preventive approach. Some different assessment methods are described in the following text, followed by a section on identifying sources of useful information.

(Health) Needs assessment (HNA)

HNA is often used in the context of health promotion. It is a systematic process designed to identify the population or community needs, or the gap between existing and desired conditions (Naidoo & Wills, 2016). It is about gathering information that informs the agreement of priorities and resource allocation, leading to health improvement and reduction of inequalities.

The concept of need is widely used but is complex and often not well understood. It should be considered from the viewpoint of all stakeholders, including the population themselves. Felt needs are resources or services that the people in the population want or perceive they need, whereas expressed needs are those they actually demand. Normative needs are those that reflect the professional judgment of what the population needs in comparison with a required standard, i.e. the expert view. Professionals may also compare populations and define comparative needs, i.e. deciding that one population is lacking in comparison with another. HNA is designed to help direct interventions, identify population needs and decrease inequalities (Naidoo & Wills, 2016). For example, a population with higher rates of obesity and diabetes than the national average may need interventions targeted at factors which lead to increased likelihood of obesity, such as high intake of takeaway foods or physical inactivity.

Community profiling

Community profiling is described as the process of collecting and analysing information about the community make-up, health and health needs (Nutland & Cragg, 2015). This will include information such as the age and ethnicity profile of the community; organisational structures; and the social environment, including the economic profile, housing, transport and green areas. These factors can influence, e.g. the physical activity levels and access to healthy food. The provision of health and social services would be considered, and also any local strategies affecting healthy living (Naidoo & Wills, 2016). The resulting community profile may be a written or graphical representation of the information gathered about the characteristics of a geographical location, country, region or local area, or a community (Naidoo & Wills, 2016). In dietetic practice, the community could be a group of people with a specific health problem.

Asset mapping

Asset mapping is often seen as a positive and upstream approach for assessing population needs as it focuses on making an inventory of the assets, capabilities, skills and organisations that are already in the population or community. It is concerned with what the population has as opposed to what they lack. Recognising these assets can promote self-esteem and help to build partnerships between professionals and community members. If there are already skills and other assets available, an intervention may be more sustainable and cost-effective. Community participants may be more motivated and empowered to get involved if they perceive that they have something of value or can contribute. A useful toolkit for asset mapping can be found at http://www.brighterfuturestogether.co.uk/brighter-futures-together-toolkit/map-assets-in-your-community.

Sources of information

There are many different sources of information available to complete assessments, some of which are accessible through library and Internet resources and include

Table 4.2.2 Sources of information

Sources	Information
Sources of population information	Census data (England & Wales), www.ons.gov.uk/census/2011census Office of National Statistics (UK), www.ons.gov.uk
Local authorities	Includes information about a wide range of issues affecting communities, such as care, education, transport, leisure, entertainment, and employment specific to the geographical area.
Public Health England	Health data etc. www.gov.uk/government/organisations/public-health-england
Health profiles	Input postcode to obtain information about that area, including comparison with national data. Helps to identify where a specific population has worse health outcomes than the national average. http://fingertips.phe.org.uk/profile/health-profiles
National surveys	Examples: National Diet and Nutrition Survey, Health Survey for England.
Public Health Observatory	Now part of Public Health England, www.apho.org.uk
Local Government Association	Information on local needs and services http://www.local.gov.uk
Population views	Community surveys, focus groups, patient and public involvement groups, self-help groups for people with diabetes, community groups, public meetings.
Local health trusts	Provide information on what services exist in the area.

a range of national statistics, census data and surveys, as described earlier in this chapter. Some sources can give more localised data that may be relevant for the population, and also put that data into the national context, i.e. find out how this population compares with the national average. There may also be published research that demonstrates how particular problems were tackled earlier, and how successful that was. However, care is needed to avoid making the assumption that your population will respond in the same way. Table 4.2.2 lists some useful sources of information that may help in the assessment process.

In addition to electronic sources, there is huge benefit from meeting people and observing what is actually going on in the community. Public meetings, interviews with community members and other stakeholders, focus groups, observations and community surveys are all possible approaches. Rapid appraisal methods designed to improve community participation can be considered (Tones & Green, 2004). A mix of approaches may give a better insight and allow a more diverse representation of population views. The methods used must consider the literacy, language, age, culture and educational level of the target population in order to make it accessible. All of these approaches require careful planning. For example, a badly designed survey is likely to give erroneous results, which then negatively affect the planned intervention. It is beneficial to work with someone who has expertise in this area, such as a local higher education institute. De Vaus (2002) and Bowling (2009) provide comprehensive information to support good-quality survey design and administration.

For PHN work, it is important to have a good understanding of practical issues such as the accessibility and affordability of healthy food. How practical and feasible is it for this population to move towards a healthier diet? Determining the specific barriers and facilitators to healthy lifestyle choices for a population rather than making assumptions (Pridgeon & Whitehead, 2013) may be worthwhile.

Health and social care trusts may be able to provide information about health-related problems that are impacting the population as well as about service provision and interventions that are ongoing or have happened in the past. It is important to know the history, what worked and what did not (and why).

Other stakeholders will be dependent on the focus of the public health agenda, e.g. healthcare professionals, commissioners and other funding organisations; public health teams; relevant professionals such as teachers, physical activity professionals and social workers; representatives from large employers; community workers and community leaders (may include religious leaders for some communities); food producers and retailers; and those running food banks (not an exhaustive list).

Identification of nutritional or health need

The information gained from the assessment is used to identify the nutritional or health needs and/or the problems that are contributing towards it. It is likely that there are multiple needs and challenges, and that an intervention will have to prioritise the activities believed to have the greatest health impact or tackle the most urgent health problems. The population views will be essential, as targeting what they perceive to be important is more likely to strengthen the partnership and develop community capacity and empowerment. This, in effect, is the same process as negotiating goals with patients based on where they feel they can start behaviour change towards a health-related goal.

There are several well-recognised ways of analysing the information gathered in the assessment process. A determinant analysis examines the factors that contribute to the expression of a health problem. It looks at the causes of the problems, not just what the problems are, and recognises that this is often multi-factorial

(Hughes & Margetts, 2011). It works on the assumption that problems cannot efficiently be addressed without understanding what has caused them, and recognises that most health problems have multiple factors affecting them with negative or positive effects. They are also often interlinked, so it is important to understand the range of potential effects that one change may have.

An analysis of strengths, weaknesses, opportunities and threats (SWOT) is one way to focus and categorise the information gained from the assessment, and this method supports the analysis of the problem and the identification of barriers and facilitators to change. A SWOT analysis should include information not just about the population needs but also on the wider determinants of health.

An alternative approach is to undertake a capacity analysis that identifies what capacity exists in the population, and where the gaps are. This type of analysis can be completed based on the information obtained from asset mapping, rapid appraisal, community engagement and working with stakeholders.

Whichever methods are used, it is important to look at the situation holistically and in partnership with other stakeholders prior to developing your work plan.

Planning and implementation of public health work

This section considers the planning and implementation of a programme of action to address the issue(s) identified from the assessment and identification of nutritional or health needs (analysis). It is the public health equivalent of what plan might be put in place for an individual in a clinical setting. It will also include information on a variety of ways for completing that work, with some examples.

Planning

Public health work is usually a long-term activity, and there will be many tasks that need to be undertaken to achieve the desired outcome. A systematic and logical approach, clearly documented, based on assessment and analysis, and available to all stakeholders, will be required. Using a tool such as a Gantt chart can help with documenting the plan, and can, at a glance, show the timescale for each individual activity being undertaken. Gantt charts can be used for planning, but can also become a working document where the progress of the work is monitored against the plan. More detail on what to include in a Gantt chart or project plan can be found in Hughes and Margetts (2011).

A clear overall aim(s) of what is to be achieved and also more specific objectives are required. Objectives must be specific, measurable, achievable, realistic/relevant, have a time frame (SMART) and relate directly to the overall aim. If objectives are achieved, then the aim should be met. Being realistic with timescales is essential, as activities often take longer to implement than originally thought. There may be short- and/or long-term objectives.

A key decision when planning public health interventions/programmes is what indicators are used to demonstrate success. Public health work often has overall aims that are difficult to measure directly in the short term, such as halting the rise in obesity levels in children or decreasing the number of new incidences of type 2 diabetes. The indicators will show if the planned work has been delivered successfully. Indicators are specific measures chosen to show that an objective has been met. There may be several indicators linked to an objective, and each objective should have at least one indicator (Hughes & Margetts, 2016). The type of indicators, and how that data is to be collected, must be decided upon at the planning stage. In the long term, indicators may measure changes in attitudes, knowledge or behaviour towards the aim, whereas in the short term they may measure if the planned process has been delivered and how well it has been received, e.g. how well the target group engaged with the work, and/or the level of participant satisfaction.

Deciding on what tools will be used to measure indicators is also essential, as they may require resources to be developed. These will feed into the overall evaluation that will be discussed later, but must be planned from the beginning. Involving the target population in this planning stage can help ensure that the measurement tools are appropriate.

Issues such as planning what resources are to be used, where they can be accessed, development time and cost also need to be considered at the beginning of the process. Some suitable resources will be accessible, whereas some may be adapted from other interventions. However, something bespoke may be required to meet the specific population needs. In addition to resource materials, it is important to consider other resources including appropriately skilled people, training, venues, food, travel costs, information technology, communication and stationery.

Implementation

The specific tasks involved in implementation will relate to the type of work being undertaken. This section includes some ways of working in public health that dietitians and public health nutritionists may employ.

Advocacy and lobbying

Advocacy is the process of defending or promoting a cause (Naidoo & Wills, 2016). Many disadvantaged populations do not have the ability or opportunity to make their voice heard, but the public health workforce may be able to provide support. However, it may be that public figures add their voice, which can help bring issues into the public arena and therefore change public opinion. Over time, this can exert pressure on government to change policies. Lobbying is proactive and involves direct action to apply pressure and influence on public officials and governments in relation to the formulation of policies. An example of this is the Junk Free Checkouts campaign, which involved the BDA Obesity Group working in partnership with other organisations in an attempt to have junk food removed from supermarket checkouts, making it easier for parents to avoid buying junk food for their children (see https://www.bda.uk.com/regionsgroups/groups/obesity/junk_free_checkouts).

Public health campaigns

There are many national public health campaigns that often have resources for use at a local level. These include Change4life, Nutrition and Hydration Week and awareness days such as World Diabetes Day. Translating these campaigns to make them relevant, and publicising/using them at a local level, can be an efficient way to utilise resources and promote public health.

Training

There are not enough dietitians to deliver appropriate nutrition messages and care to all members of the population who would benefit; therefore, dietitians train other workers to do this. For example, school nurses are at the forefront of the National Child Measurement Programme and need to be confident and competent at weighing and measuring children, as well as having a motivational approach when discussing weight management with children and families. A joint initiative between the School and Public Health Nurses Association (SAPHNA) and the BDA Public Health Group led to a training programme being developed, evaluated and rolled out to address this issue.

The BDA Work Ready programme (BDA, 2015a) (http://www.bdaworkready.co.uk) is another example of a training programme based on the best evidence available and set up nationally. Dietitians can undergo this accredited training programme, which will equip them with the necessary knowledge, skills and resources to assess the needs of the workforce; work in partnership with relevant stakeholders; and develop, deliver and evaluate work-based nutrition promotion interventions. NICE (LGB2, 2012) specifies that workplaces should provide opportunities for healthy eating. However, most places will need the assistance of a qualified specialist, such as a dietitian, to help make that recommendation a reality. Whereas most dietitians will deliver training, developing a national training programme in partnership with other stakeholders is more efficient in terms of resources and reaches a larger population with consistent messages.

Group education

Group education is a routine part of dietetic practice, e.g. cardiac rehabilitation or structured education for people with diabetes. To be most efficient, education sessions should be designed to be delivered to large numbers of people (the same session delivered on numerous occasions), both the target population and the public health workforce who work with that population. This increases the chance of consistent evidence-based messages being delivered. For a comprehensive overview of how to facilitate lifestyle change via group education, see Avery *et al.* (2016).

Resource development

Developing resources may be necessary for an intervention but may also be a public health intervention in itself. It is time consuming and requires expertise and skills. Before creating anything, it is important to ascertain if appropriate resources already exist. Suitable places to look include the following:

- Public health organisations, e.g. Public Health England.
- Professional organisations, e.g. BDA Fact sheets, BDA Work Ready.
- Charities working with specific health issues, e.g. Coeliac UK, Diabetes UK, British Heart Foundation.
- Campaign related, such as Change4life, Drinkaware, Nutrition and Hydration Week.

For a comprehensive overview of resources for educational activities, see Avery *et al.* (2016). An example of resource development for public health is shown in Table 4.2.3.

Table 4.2.3 The development of the Moving on to Cups leaflet (Public Health Group of the BDA, 2015b)

Process	Rationale/activity
Identification of need	Evidence that UK guidance on introducing a cup to an infant was not being followed.
	Feeding bottles commonly used beyond the appropriate age.
	Inappropriate use of feeding bottles leading to a variety of health issues, affecting large numbers of children across the UK.
	Existing leaflet outdated.
	Therefore, a case for developing a new resource to ensure current evidence-based advice is being communicated to parents.
Review the literature	Published and grey literature systematically searched.
Target group views	Focus group undertaken with Children's Centre managers and parents.
Resource developed	Based on the evidence and target population views.
	Piloted.
	Public-facing leaflet Moving on to Cups produced and sold via the Comic Company.
	Leaflet produced in Welsh.
Sharing information	Journal article (Gardner, 2015)
	BDA policy statement Introducing a Cup to an Infant's Diet (BDA, 2015b).
	Work presented at research symposiums.
	Leaflet publicised at various conferences.
	Leaflet used in training sessions for relevant healthcare staff.

A resource can have a huge impact if such processes are followed and the information is shared extensively.

Policy and guidance development

Health-related policies and guidelines are constantly being developed and reviewed in light of the expanding evidence and changing incidence of health issues. Policies may operate at the global, national and local levels. Few dietitians will be involved at the global level, but there are opportunities for experienced staff to participate at the national level via government ministers or consultations. There are also frequent consultations on NICE guidance that have a nutritional component, and these can be commented on via registered stakeholders such as the BDA. Many national policies are adapted into local delivery programmes for specific population needs, and this is also an area for dietitians to get involved in.

A range of possible public health interventions have been discussed here, but this is by no means all that a dietitian could be involved in. Food and health-related interventions at a local level are likely to be bespoke and include health promotion activities, community development and other ways of engaging with, educating and empowering communities and populations to be able to eat a healthier diet and improve their health and well-being.

Evaluation

Evaluation has been described as '*the systematic examination and assessment of the features of a programme or other intervention in order to produce knowledge that different stakeholders can use for a variety of purposes*' (Rootman *et al.*, 2001). It is essential that evaluation be planned from the beginning. Evaluation requires time, expertise and other resources. Evaluation makes it possible to see what has been achieved, identify strengths and weaknesses, assess acceptability and stakeholder satisfaction, and inform future practice. It is important to consider acceptability, effectiveness, appropriateness, and efficiency, and to ask if the work is promoting equity. In many cases, the assessment will have provided baseline data to compare to. Evaluating the process, using the predetermined indicators, will determine if the plan of work has been adhered to and ascertain the immediate impact.

Evaluation data can be quantitative and/or qualitative, and, in many cases, both will be appropriate. Many of the methods used for assessment can also be used for evaluation, e.g. community surveys, focus groups, rapid appraisal and interviews. The same considerations in relation to what is appropriate for the population will apply. More detailed information on evaluation of training and education can be found in Avery *et al.* (2016), and on evaluation generally in Naidoo and Wills (2016).

Dissemination of results

It is important to share learning from work that is completed, even if the objectives are not fully met. Many people lack confidence in this area, but sharing results is essential for a variety of reasons, including developing the evidence base and informing future practice. In most cases, report writing for the stakeholders and funders is a routine requirement, but results should also be shared with the target population as well as wider audiences. The Council for Allied Health Professions Research (https://cahpr.csp.org.uk) provides a wide range of useful information, including guidance on how to prepare posters, run a journal club and get research published (see Chapter 1.1, Professional practice). Dietitians should be key contributors to developing the evidence base for public health. It may be easier to start with smaller audiences and contribute to newsletters or ezines, share work at a branch or specialist group meeting, and submit abstracts to the BDA research symposium or other conferences, before moving on to full-scale research articles. A good way to start is by working in partnership with colleagues to complete reports. It is important to remember that it is not just dietitians who will be interested in the findings but also others working in public health.

Public health strategies

There are many national PHN strategies that dietitians can be involved in. The following tables highlight key recommendations and initiatives and are split into stages of life. Table 4.2.4 includes initiatives targeted at maternal health and early years, Table 4.2.5 focuses on school-aged children, and Table 4.2.6 identifies initiatives that are relevant throughout the life course. This is not a complete list, but gives some indications of what PHN interventions and initiatives are ongoing which may link with work at a local level. In many cases, dietitians will be promoting or raising awareness of policy and initiatives, and training others on how to address or deliver them at a local level. They may also be actively facilitating the implementation of policy in partnership with other stakeholders, and may use the resources to support local education and training events.

Continuous professional development in public health

There are many opportunities available to develop public health knowledge and skills, whether it is through day-to-day work or in a more structured and formal way.

Shadowing

A lot can be learned by shadowing experienced colleagues and observing the work that they are involved in. There are many people and organisations from all sectors involved in public health, including the local authorities. Although professional background may be different, much of the knowledge and many of the public health skills will be transferable and can be applied in a variety of situations. Dietitians may benefit from learning about the nutrition-related roles that different people and organisations have. They may also gain understanding of the challenges and difficulties that they may face, and about how these may be overcome. Looking further than an individual professional role towards the initiatives

Table 4.2.4 Recommendations and initiatives targeted at maternal health and the early years

Recommendation/initiative	Target population	Examples of implementation
Folic acid Women should take a folic acid supplement (400 µg/day) prior to and up to 12 weeks after conception (SACN, 2006) to minimise the risks of neural tube defects	Pregnant women and those planning to conceive	Health centres provide maternal Healthy Start vitamins to eligible women Products such as pregnancy-testing kits include information on the importance of supplementation
Vitamin D supplementation Vitamin D supplement (10 µg/day) should be taken during pregnancy and while breastfeeding to reduce the risks of the baby developing rickets (SACN, 2016)	Pregnant and breastfeeding women	Health centres provide maternal Healthy Start vitamins to eligible women Midwives provide women with information and advice on the benefits of taking vitamin D and the availability of supplements on prescription
Breastfeeding Exclusive breastfeeding up to 6 months of age (DH, 2003) Increasing extended breastfeeding rates	Pregnant and breastfeeding women	Maternity hospitals provide structured programmes to support breastfeeding Breastfeeding peer support programmes are developed
Healthy Start Healthy Start is a UK-wide government scheme to improve the health of low-income pregnant women and families (https://www.healthystart.nhs.uk/for-health-professionals)	Pregnant women and parents of children aged under 4 years on benefits and tax credits	Health centres and professionals provide free vouchers to eligible families every week to spend on milk, fresh and frozen fruit and vegetables, and infant formula milk Health centres and professionals provide free maternal Healthy Start vitamins (folic acid, vitamins C and D), and Healthy Start vitamin drops (vitamins A, C and D) to children Supporting the appropriate introduction of solids
Children's centres Children's centres provide a variety of advice and support for parents and carers. Children's centres should be developed in line with the needs of the local community; therefore, each children's centre is unique	Pregnant women and families with preschool children	Core services provided include: Child and family health services, such as breastfeeding support Childcare and early learning Advice on parenting, local childcare and specialist services for families, such as speech and language therapy, healthy eating advice or help with managing money Advice on finding work or training opportunities, signposting to the local Jobcentre and training providers
Food and drink guidelines for early years Voluntary food and drink guidelines for early years settings in England, published by the School Food Trust (SFT, 2012), include recommendations about what types of foods and portion sizes are appropriate to meet a child's nutritional needs (http://childrensfoodtrust.org.uk/wp/childrens-food-trust/early-years/)	Children under 5 years attending early years settings	Development of the online learning network about providing healthy children's food (http://childrensfoodtrust.org.uk/wp/childrens-food-trust/schools/training-for-schools)
Nursery Milk Scheme In England, and on behalf of the devolved administrations in Scotland and Wales, the DH administers the Nursery Milk Scheme (https://www.nurserymilk.co.uk/about-nursery-milk-scheme)	Children under 5 years attending childcare	189 mL (1/3 pint) of milk given free of charge for each day the child attends registered day-care facilities (including childminders) for 2 hours or more
The Healthy Child Programme The Healthy Child Programme (DH, 2009) is the early intervention and prevention programme that begins in pregnancy and continues through childhood. It offers every family a programme of screening tests, immunisations, development reviews, information, and guidance to support parenting and healthy choices	Pregnant women and families with children aged under 5 years	Health visitor visits homes and conducts reviews to advise parents on healthy start issues and local services Tackling obesity through the Healthy Child Programme (Rudolf, 2009) provides supporting evidence, a framework for action, and resources for practitioners who are working with families with preschool children Healthy Child Programme e-learning resources for healthcare professionals (available at http://www.e-lfh.org.uk/programmes/healthy-child-programme)
Start4life Start4life is part of the Change4life social marketing campaign to support families in achieving behaviour change for a healthier life (https://www.nhs.uk/start4life)	Pregnant women and new parents	Start4life campaign resources, e.g. posters and leaflets (available at https://campaignresources.phe.gov.uk/resources/campaigns/2-start-4-life/resources) Weekly email and text messaging advice to support healthy living

Table 4.2.5 Recommendations and initiatives targeted at school-aged children

Recommendation/initiative	Target population	Examples of implementation
National Child Measurement Programme (NCMP, England) The NCMP, established in 2007, is part of the UK government's work programme on childhood obesity. It is operated jointly by the DH and the Department for Education (https://www.gov.uk/government/collections/national-child-measurement-programme)	School children aged 4–5 years (reception year) and 10–11 years (year 6)	Annually, at school, children have their height and weight measured. This information is then used to inform planning and delivery of local children's services and to collect data on a population level, allowing for analysis of trends in obesity
School Fruit and Vegetable Scheme The DH's 'School Fruit and Vegetable Scheme' was introduced in 2004 as part of wider efforts to increase people's fruit and vegetable intake to a healthy five-a-day target (http://webarchive.nationalarchives.gov.uk/+/www.dh.gov.uk/en/Publichealth/Healthimprovement/FiveADay/FiveADaygeneralinformation/DH_4002149)	School children aged 4–6 years in England	Children in state schools in England receive a free piece of fruit or vegetable each school day
The School Food Plan and School Food Standards The School Food Plan was launched by the Department of Education in 2013 with the aim of improving food in schools (http://www.schoolfoodplan.com/the-plan)	School-age children in the UK	Development of a school food standards poster (http://whatworkswell.schoolfoodplan.com/articles/view/372) Resources to improve the dining room experience (http://whatworkswell.schoolfoodplan.com/articles/category/2/the-lunchtime-experience)
Universal Infant Free School Meals (UIFSM) In September 2014, UIFSM was rolled out across England with the aim of improving the nutritional quality of food that children eat (https://www.gov.uk/guidance/universal-infant-free-school-meals-guide-for-schools-and-local-authorities)	School children aged 4–7 years (reception, year 1 and 2)	Children attending a state-funded school are provided with a free school meal UIFSM resources (http://thegreatschoollunch.co.uk/resources/uifsm-free-resources-for-you)
Free School Meals In England and Wales, free school meals are available to children from families in receipt of benefits and tax credit	Nursery and school-age children from low-income families	Children attending a state-funded school are provided with a free school meal
The School Milk Scheme The aim of the European Union – funded school milk subsidy scheme is to encourage children to drink milk and to develop a lasting habit of consuming milk (https://www.gov.uk/topic/farming-food-grants-payments/school-milk-scheme)	School-age children	Milk is distributed to children as a mid–morning or afternoon drink or to drink with a meal (not used in the preparation of meals)
Sugar reduction plan In 2015, recommendations regarding the contribution that sugar should provide towards total energy in our diets were changed from 10% to 5% (SACN, 2015). The *Childhood obesity: plan for action* (DH, 2016b) outlines several initiatives, including those that aim to reduce sugar intake	Food industry	From 2018, a levy was imposed on the soft drinks industry, to be charged on producers of sugar-containing soft drinks with total sugar content of ≥5 g of sugar per 100 mL By 2020, a 20% reduction in sugar should be effected across a range of products (with a 5% reduction in year 1). Products included will be those that contribute substantially to the sugar intake in children's diets Dietitians can check to confirm that there are no harmful effects of these changes on the overall diet

Table 4.2.6 Recommendations and initiatives targeted throughout the life course

Recommendations/initiatives	Target population	Examples of implementation
Change4life A social marketing campaign in England and Wales, designed to help families make behaviour change and adopt a healthier lifestyle to prevent obesity (http://www.nhs.uk/change4life/Pages/change-for-life.aspx)	Adults and families	Previous campaigns have included Swap it, don't stop it, Let's dance with Change4Life and Change4Life BME Activity
The Food for Life partnership This focuses on transforming food culture (http://www.foodforlife.org.uk/about-us/transforming-food-culture)	Schools, hospitals, care homes, communities	'Food for life' school awards for schools that demonstrate good practice around school meals and food education Resources for hospitals to support NHS staff health and well-being
Public Health Responsibility Deal (England) The responsibility deal is a voluntary agreement between businesses and the government to improve public health (https://responsibilitydeal.dh.gov.uk)	Businesses and the food industry	Four networks: Alcohol network; Food network; Health at work network; Physical activity network The food network has pledged to encourage the food industry and caterers to remove *trans*-fatty acids from foods, reduce salt and energy content, increase fruit and vegetable content, and label energy at point of purchase

and interventions themselves can provide insight into different aspects of public health practice.

Mentoring

Dietitians new to public health may benefit from being mentored, i.e. having a more experienced colleague (not necessarily a dietitian) to share ideas with, and to obtain advice and career direction. It needs to be someone reasonably accessible (although this does not have to be face to face), and who is prepared to give you some time on a regular basis. Often, dietitians in public health are quite isolated professionally and may not have a dietetic professional lead in their workplace, so a mentor may be very helpful.

Public health networks

Public health networks can be a very good way to interact with others with similar roles, identify people who it may be useful to shadow, find a mentor, share experiences and access training opportunities.

Public health specialist group of the BDA

The BDA specialist group for dietitians interested in public health works to improve and protect the health of the population through good nutrition. The aim of the group is to become a significant and well-recognised professional voice in public health across the UK. The group acts as a support for members and has links with other appropriate organisations. A key area of work involves coordinating the contribution to consultations related to PHN. The discussion forum and training events are good starting points for learning more about what dietitians are doing in this specialist area. The group has supported the development of an online public health course, hosted on the BDA web page, which offers practical information and activities to support dietitians to understand where public health fits into their work and how to develop their skills and knowledge. There are opportunities for group members to get involved in specific tasks and finish activities which can build skills and knowledge.

Local and regional networks

There are active networks in different regions and in the devolved countries. PHE have regional offices and run local networks where public health practitioners can meet, present their work, share ideas and/or have workshops on subjects specific to their needs. Details of regional contacts are available at www.gov.uk/government/organisations/public-health-england.

Public health training

The level and type of training required will depend on the requirements of the role and the dietitian's career aspirations. Many dietitians want to develop their skills in specific areas, while other wish to have their skills recognised and obtain formal qualifications or formal recognition. Many organisations provide training/educational events that may be valuable, depending on individual needs. Educational opportunities are listed in Table 4.2.7; the list is not exhaustive. It is also important to recognise some of the key skills for public health work and access training in those areas, e.g. group facilitation, communication skills, research skills and evaluation methods.

Recognition for public health expertise

Registered nutritionist

Registered dietitians with a minimum of 3 years of public health experience can apply to become a registered nutritionist via the Association for Nutrition (http://www.associationfornutrition.org). This demonstrates that public

Table 4.2.7 Educational opportunities

Organisation	Learning opportunities and events
The Nutrition Society (www.nutritionsociety.org)	Regular conferences and training events, including a student conference
	Student members are offered reduced attendance fees
	Scottish and Irish sections make events more accessible and locally relevant
Royal Society of Public Health (www.rsph.org.uk)	Provide courses on food safety and nutrition, mental health, health improvement and many other subjects
	Deliver bespoke training courses to local organisations
BDA	Join the public health specialist group and get involved
	Check the conferences as public health is often included
	The annual research symposium includes a public health stream – opportunities to present and discuss own work and learn about other PH dietitians' work
	Access the online module
	Become a BDA public health champion
Public Health England	Regional workshops and networking events
	National conferences
Faculty of Public Health (www.fph.org.uk)	Associates (no fees) have access to information and updates and access to events
The UK body that sets the standards for consultants in public health. (*Note*: The organisation is not just for doctors)	Annual conference and exhibition
	Quarterly newsletters
Universities – postgraduate courses	Master's modules, postgraduate certificates, diplomas or master's degrees
	Relevant subjects include public health, PHN or specific health or lifestyle issues that are public health problems, e.g. child health, obesity, physical activity
	Part-time course, some distance-learning options and open online courses are available

health is a specialism of dietetics, and that, although all dietitians can undertake some public health work within their roles, experience and postgraduate training is required to specialise in this area.

UK Public Health Register (UKPHR)

The UKPHR is an independent regulator that provides professional regulation to public health specialists and public health practitioners, most dietitians and would-be practitioners (see Table 4.2.1). The UKPHR gives guidance on what would be suitable evidence for CPD in order to be registered but do not provide CPD itself. They validate regional training schemes to support registration.

There are many options for improving knowledge and qualifications in public health and for getting involved. As public health is a very dynamic area and changes in policy, guidance and organisational structures occur regularly, keeping up to date is extremely important and CPD essential.

Acknowledgement

The editor acknowledges the prior contribution of Alison Nelson.

Further reading

Hughes R, Margetts B. (2011) *Practical Public Health Nutrition*. Chichester: Wiley-Blackwell.

Public Health Specialist Group of the British Dietetic Association. (2015) Moving on to Cups. Available at http://www.comiccompany.co.uk/?category=2&collection=359. Accessed 10 January 2017.

Internet resources

Association for Nutrition, www.associationfornutrition.org

Children's Food Trust, www.childrensfoodtrust.org.uk

Department for Environment, Food and Rural Affairs (Defra), www.gov.uk/government/organisations/department-for-environment-food-rural-affairs

Faculty of Public Health, www.fph.org.uk

Food Standards Agency, www.food.gov.uk

Food Standards Scotland, www.foodstandards.gov.scot

Global Burden of Diseases, Injuries, and Risk Factors Study, www.healthdata.org/gbd

Health Education England, https://hee.nhs.uk

Love Food Hate Waste, www.lovefoodhatewaste.com

NHS Health Scotland, www.healthscotland.com

Outcomes Framework Scotland (2015), www.healthscotland.com/OFHI/index.html

Public Health Agency (Northern Ireland), www.publichealth.hscni.net

Public Health England, www.gov.uk/government/organisations/public-health-england

Public Health Outcomes Framework (2016–2019) at a glance document (England), www.gov.uk/government/uploads/system/uploads/attachment_data/file/520457/At_a_glance.pdf

Public Health Outcomes Framework (2016) Wales, http://gov.wales/docs/phhs/publications/160329frameworken.pdf

Public Health Wales, www.publichealthwales.wales.nhs.uk

Public Health Wales Observatory, www.wales.nhs.uk/sitesplus/922/home

Royal Society of Public Health, www.rsph.org.uk

Scottish Public Health Network (ScotPHN), http://www.scotphn.net
The Institute of Health Equity, www.instituteofhealthequity.org
UK Public Health Register, www.ukphr.org

References

Avery A, Whitehead K, Halliday V. (2016) *How to Facilitate Lifestyle Change: Applying Group Education in Healthcare*. Chichester: Wiley-Blackwell.

Bates B, Cox L, Nicholson S, *et al.* (2016a) *National Diet and Nutrition Survey: results from years 5 and 6 (combined) of the rolling programme (2012/2013–2013/2014) (online)*. Available at https://www.gov.uk/government/uploads/system/uploads/attachment_data/file/551352/NDNS_Y5_6_UK_Main_Text.pdf. Accessed 10 January 2017.

Bates B, Cox L, Maplethorpe N, et al. (2016b) *National Diet and Nutrition Survey: assessment of dietary sodium (19 to 64 years) in England, 2014*. Available at https://www.food.gov.uk/sites/default/files/nisodium_0.pdf. Accessed 10 January 2017.

BDA. (2015a) *Supporting Healthier Working Lives Through Dietitian-Led Wellness Initiatives*. Available at http://www.bdaworkready.co.uk. Accessed 10 January 2017.

BDA. (2015b) *Introducing a Cup to an Infant's Diet*. Available at https://www.bda.uk.com/improvinghealth/healthprofessionals/introducing_a_cup_to_an_infants_diet. Accessed 10 January 2017.

BDA. (2016) *Model and Process of Nutrition and Dietetic Practice*. Available at www.bda.uk.com/publications/professional/model_and_process_for_nutrition_and_dietetic_practice_. Accessed 10 January 2017.

Bowling A. (2009) *Research Methods in Health: Investigating Health and Health Services*, 3rd edn. Maidenhead: Open University Press.

Cavill N, Hillsdon M, Anstiss T. (2011) *Brief Interventions for Weight Management*. Oxford: National Obesity Observatory.

Cavill N, Roberts K, Ells L. (2015) *Evaluation of Weight Management, Physical Activity and Dietary Interventions: An Introductory Guide*. Oxford: Public Health England.

Centre for Workforce Intelligence. (2014) *Mapping the Core Public Health Workforce (Online)*. Available at http://www.cfwi.org.uk/publications/mapping-the-core-public-health-workforce/. Accessed 10 January 2017.

Cooper N, Dumpleton S. (2013) *Walking the Breadline: the Scandal of Food Poverty in 21st Century Britain (online)*. Available at http://www.church-poverty.org.uk/news/pressroom/resources/reports/walkingthebreadlinefile/view. Accessed 10 January 2017.

Dahlgren G, Whitehead M. (1991) *Policies and Strategies to Promote Social Equity in Health*. Stockholm: Institute for Futures Studies.

Defra. (2008) *A Framework for Pro-environmental Behaviours*. Available at www.defra.gov.uk/publications/files/pb13574-behaviours-report-080110.pdf. Accessed 10 January 2017.

Defra. (2016) *Food Statistics Pocketbook 2015 in Year Update*. Available at https://www.gov.uk/government/uploads/system/uploads/attachment_data/file/526395/foodpocketbook-2015update-26may16.pdf. Accessed 10 January 2017.

de Vaus D. (2002) *Surveys in Social Research*, 5th edn. London: Routledge.

DH. (2003) Infant feeding recommendation. Available at http://webarchive.nationalarchives.gov.uk/20130315211757/http://www.dh.gov.uk/prod_consum_dh/groups/dh_digitalassets/@dh/@en/documents/digitalasset/dh_4096999.pdf. Accessed 25 September 2018.

DH. (2006) The pathway for the management of overweight and obesity: Raising the issue of weight tool. Available at http://www.htmc.co.uk/resource/data/htmc1/docs/Care%20pathway%20for%20the%20management%20of%20overweight%20and%20obesity.pdf. Accessed 24 September 2018.

DH. (2009) *Healthy Child Programme Pregnancy and the First Five Year of Life*. Available at https://www.gov.uk/government/uploads/system/uploads/attachment_data/file/167998/Health_Child_Programme.pdf. Accessed 10 January 2017.

DH. (2010) *Equity and Excellence: Liberating the NHS*. Available at https://www.gov.uk/government/uploads/system/uploads/attachment_data/file/213823/dh_117794.pdf. Accessed 10 January 2017.

DH. (2012) *The Public Health Outcomes Framework for England, 2013–2016*. Available at https://www.gov.uk/government/uploads/system/uploads/attachment_data/file/216159/dh_132362.pdf. Accessed 10 January 2017.

DH. (2016a) *Vitamin D – Advice on Supplements for At-risk Groups*. Available at https://www.gov.uk/government/publications/vitamin-d-advice-on-supplements-for-at-risk-groups. Accessed 10 January 2017.

DH. (2016b) *Childhood Obesity: A Plan for Action*. Available at https://www.gov.uk/government/uploads/system/uploads/attachment_data/file/546588/Childhood_obesity_2016__2__acc.pdf. Accessed 10 January 2017.

Gardner E. (2015) Best practice in infancy: moving onto cups. *J. Fam. Health Care* 25(2).

Health Education England (HEE). (2016) *Public Health Roles*. Available at https://www.healthcareers.nhs.uk/explore-roles/public-health. Accessed 10 January 2017.

HM Government. (2010) *Healthy Lives, Healthy People: Our Strategy for Public Health in England*. Available at https://www.gov.uk/government/uploads/system/uploads/attachment_data/file/216096/dh_127424.pdf. Accessed 10 January 2017.

HM Government. (2012) *Health and Social Care Act 2012 Chapter 7*. Available at http://www.legislation.gov.uk/ukpga/2012/7/contents/enacted. Accessed 10 January 2017.

Hughes R, Margetts B. (2011) *Practical Public Health Nutrition*. Chichester: Wiley-Blackwell.

Institute for Health Metrics and Evaluation. (2016) *Global Burden of Disease (GBD) (Online)*. Available at http://www.healthdata.org/gbd. Accessed 10 January 2017.

King G, Lee-Woolf C, Kivinen E, *et al.* (Brook Lyndhurst) (2015) *Understanding Food in the Context of Poverty, Economic Insecurity and Social Exclusion*. Brook Lyndhurst for the Food Standards Agency in Northern Ireland.

Macdiarmid J, Kyle J, Horgan G, *et al.* (2011) Livewell: A Balance of Healthy and Sustainable Food Choices. Available at http://assets.wwf.org.uk/downloads/livewell_report_jan11.pdf. Accessed 10 January 2017.

Marmot M. (2010) *Fair Society Healthy Lives 'The Marmot Review'*. Available at http://www.instituteofhealthequity.org/. Accessed 10 January 2017.

Naidoo J, Wills J. (2016) *Foundations for Health Promotion*, 4th edn. London: Elsevier.

Nelson M, Erens B, Bates B, *et al.* (2007) *Low Income Diet and Nutrition Survey Summary of Key Findings*. Available at https://www.researchgate.net/publication/237525227_Low_income_diet_and_nutrition_survey. Accessed 10 January 2017.

New Economics Foundation (NEF). (2011) *Re-framing the Great Food Debate: The Case for Sustainable Food (Online)*. Available at https://www.food4families.org.uk/userfiles/resources/nef-re-framingthegreatfooddebate-thecaseforsustainablefood.pdf. Accessed 10 January 2017.

Newton JN, Briggs AD, Murray CJ, et al. (2015) Changes in health in England, with analysis by English regions and areas of deprivation, 1990–2013: a systematic analysis for the Global Burden of Disease Study 2013. *Lancet*. 386: 2257–2274.

NHS Health Scotland. (2012) *A Fairer Healthier Scotland Corporate Strategy 2012–2017*. Available at http://www.healthscotland.com/uploads/documents/5792-CorporateStrategy.pdf. Accessed 10 January 2017.

NHS Wales. (2016) *Measuring the Health and Well-being of a Nation: Public Health Outcomes Framework for Wales*. Available

SECTION 4

at http://gov.wales/docs/phhs/publications/160329frameworken.pdf. Accessed 10 January 2017.

NICE. (2007) *Public Health Programme Guidance No.6, Behaviour Change at Population, Community and Individual Levels*. London: NICE.

NICE. (2012) *LGB2, Workplace Health*. Available at https://www.nice.org.uk/advice/lgb2/chapter/introduction. Accessed 10 January 2017.

NICE. (2014) *Weight Management: Lifestyle Services for Overweight or Obese Adults (PH53)*. Available at https://www.nice.org.uk/guidance/ph53. Accessed 10 January 2017.

NICE. (2015) *Preventing Excess Weight Gain (NG7)*. Available at https://www.nice.org.uk/guidance/ng7.

NICE. (2016) Community Engagement: Improving Health and Wellbeing and Reducing Health Inequalities (NG44). Available at https://www.nice.org.uk/guidance/ng44. Accessed 10 January 2017.

Nutland W, Cragg L. (eds) (2015) *Health Promotion Practice*, 2nd edn. Maidenhead: McGraw-Hill Education/Open University Press.

Office for National Statistics (ONS). (2010) *A Report on the 2009 Living Costs and Food Survey*. Newport: Office for National Statistics.

PHE. (2016) *The Strategic Plan for the Next Four Years: Better Outcomes by 2020*. Available at https://www.gov.uk/government/uploads/system/uploads/attachment_data/file/516985/PHE_Strategic_plan_2016.pdf. Accessed 10 January 2017.

PHE and Allied Health Professionals Federation. (2015) A strategy to develop the capacity, impact and profile of allied health professionals in public health 2015–2018. Strategy from the Allied Health Professionals Federation supported by Public Health England. Available at http://www.ahpf.org.uk/files/AHP%20Public%20Health%20Strategy.pdf. Accessed 10 January 2017.

PHE, NHS England and Health Education England with the Support of Partner Organisations. (2016) *Making Every Contact Count (MECC): Consensus Statement*. Available at https://www.gov.uk/government/uploads/system/uploads/attachment_data/file/515949/Making_Every_Contact_Count_Consensus_Statement.pdf. Accessed 10 January 2017.

Pridgeon A, Whitehead K. (2013) A qualitative study to investigate the drivers and barriers to healthy eating in two public sector workplaces. *J. Hum. Nutr. Diet.* 26(1): 85–95.

Priestly S. (2016) *Food Waste: House of Commons Library Briefing Paper Number CBP07552*. Available at http://researchbriefings.parliament.uk/ResearchBriefing/Summary/CBP-7552. Accessed 10 January 2017.

Rootman I, Goodstadt M, Hyndman B, *et al.* (eds) (2001) *Evaluation in Health Promotion: Principles and Perspectives*. WHO, Denmark. Available at http://www.euro.who.int/__data/assets/pdf_file/0007/108934/E73455.pdf. Accessed 10 January 2017.

Rudolf M. (2009) Tackling obesity through the Healthy Child programme Available at www.nooo.org.uk. Accessed 24 September.

SACN. (2003) *SACN Salt and Health Report*. Available at https://www.gov.uk/government/publications/sacn-salt-and-health-report. Accessed 10 January 2017.

SACN. (2006) *Folate and Disease Prevention*. Available at https://www.gov.uk/government/uploads/system/uploads/attachment_data/file/338892/SACN_Folate_and_Disease_Prevention_Report.pdf. Accessed 10 January 2017.

SACN. (2015a) *Vitamin D and Health Report*. Available at https://www.gov.uk/government/uploads/system/uploads/attachment_data/file/537616/SACN_Vitamin_D_and_Health_report.pdf. Accessed 10 January 2017.

SACN. (2015b) *Carbohydrate and Health*. Available at https://www.gov.uk/government/uploads/system/uploads/attachment_data/file/445503/SACN_Carbohydrates_and_Health.pdf. Accessed 10 January 2017.

SACN Vitamin D and health Available at https://assets.publishing.service.gov.uk/government/uploads/system/uploads/attachment_data/file/537616/SACN_Vitamin_D_and_Health_report.pdf. Accessed 25 September 2018.

Scarborough P, Bhatnagar P, Wickramasinghe KK, *et al.* (2011) The economic burden of ill health due to diet, physical inactivity, smoking, alcohol and obesity in the UK: an update to 2006–2007 NHS costs. *J. Public Health (Oxf)*. 33(4): 527–535.

Scottish Government. (2016) *Strengthening the function and re-focussing action for a healthier Scotland: 2015 review of public health in Scotland*. Edinburgh: The Scottish Government.

Shepherd R. (1999) Social determinants of food choice. *Pro. Nutr. Soc.* 58(4): 807–812.

Standards for your school http://childrensfoodtrust.org.uk/wp/childrens-food-trust/schools/school-food-standards/standards-for-your-school-food/ Accessed 24 September 2018

Strategy Unit. (2008) *Food Matters Towards a Strategy for the 21st Century*. London: Cabinet Office.

Tones K, Green J. (2004) *Health Promotion: Planning and Strategies*. London: Sage Publications.

Wanless D. (2004) *Securing Good Health for the Whole Population: Final Report*. London: Department of Health.

Waste and Resource Action Programme (WRAP). (2009) *Household Food and Drink Waste in the UK*. Available at http://www.wrap.org.uk/retail_supply_chain/research_tools/research/report_household.html. Accessed 10 January 2017.

Waste and Resource Action Programme (WRAP). (2015) *Estimates of food and packaging waste in the UK grocery, retail and hospitality supply chains*. Available at http://www.wrap.org.uk/sites/files/wrap/UK%20Estimates%20October%2015%20%28FINAL%29_0.pdf. Accessed 10 January 2017.

Whitehead M. (2000) *The concepts and principles of equity and health, WHO*. Available at http://salud.ciee.flacso.org.ar/flacso/optativas/equity_and_health.pdf. Accessed 25 September 2018.

WHO. (2009) *Building a Working Definition of Partnership: African Partnerships for Patient Safety (APPS)*. Available at http://www.who.int/patientsafety/implementation/apps/resources/defining_partnerships-apps.pdf?ua=1. Accessed 10 January 2017.

WHO. (2012a) *European action plan for strengthening public health capacities and services*. Copenhagen: WHO.

WHO. (2012b) *A framework for implementing the set of recommendations on the marketing of foods and non-alcoholic beverages to children*. Available at http://apps.who.int/iris/bitstream/10665/80148/1/9789241503242_eng.pdf?ua=1. Accessed 10 January 2017.

WHO. (2013) *Global Action Plan for the Prevention and Control of Non-Communicable Diseases*. Available at http://www.who.int/nmh/events/ncd_action_plan/en/. Accessed 10 January 2017.

WHO. (2016a) *Action Plan for the Prevention and Control of Non-communicable Diseases in the WHO European Region 2016–2025*. Copenhagen: WHO. Available at http://www.euro.who.int/__data/assets/pdf_file/0008/346328/NCD-ActionPlan-GB.pdf?ua=1. Accessed 20 December 2017.

WHO. (2016b) *Report of the Commission on Ending Childhood Obesity*. Available at http://apps.who.int/iris/bitstream/10665/204176/1/9789241510066_eng.pdf?ua=1. Accessed 10 January 2017.

WHO. (2016c) *Fiscal Policies for Diet and Prevention of Non-communicable Diseases*, Geneva: WHO. Available at http://apps.who.int/iris/bitstream/10665/250131/1/9789241511247-eng.pdf?ua=1. Accessed 10 January 2017.

World Commission on Environment and Development (WCED). (1987) *Our Common Future*. Available at http://www.un-documents.net/our-common-future.pdf. Accessed 10 January 2017.

4.3 Sports nutrition

Louise Sutton

Key points

- Energy and macronutrient needs, particularly carbohydrate and protein, must be met during training and competition to maintain body mass, recover energy stores and provide adequate protein for tissue growth and repair.
- Fat intake should contribute appropriately to energy demands within the context of weight management as appropriate to individual and sports requirements.
- Good hydration practices are important to health and optimal performance in sports.
- Micronutrients of key concern include iron, calcium and vitamin D.
- Individualised nutrition plans subsequent to comprehensive nutritional assessment will benefit all athletes, but particularly elite performers in whom nutrition goals and requirements will not be static and will warrant a periodised approach.

Sports nutrition remains an emerging and dynamic discipline within the fields of sports science and dietetic practice. Individuals participate in sports at different levels and for different reasons, but all athletes, whatever their level, can benefit from making good food choices that support consistent training, maximise performance and maintain good health.

Athletes, especially elite athletes, have widely accepted the need for well-designed systematic training programmes, but have seemingly been slower to adopt well-planned dietary strategies. This is changing, with coaches and athletes now clearly recognising that unbalanced and inadequate nutritional intakes can lead to poor training and competition performance, lethargy, increased risk of injury and illness, and unfavourable gains or losses in body mass. This has led to the recognition that nutrition support needs to be periodised, meeting the needs of daily training programmes within different phases of training and competitive cycles.

Appropriate selection of foods and fluids, timing of intake, and supplement choice, where appropriate, will benefit both health and performance. Nutrition is likely to have its biggest impact on performance by supporting athletes to train consistently and effectively to produce the desired adaptations in response to training. Both recreational and elite athletes will benefit from sound nutritional practices, while individualised nutrition direction and advice, subsequent to a comprehensive nutritional assessment, that takes account of the specificity of the sport/event, performance goals, practical challenges, food preferences and weight management targets, will particularly benefit elite performers. Due to the diversity of sporting activities and levels of performance, it is beyond the scope of this short chapter to provide detailed guidelines for every sport. However, the following are some generic sports nutrition principles applicable to all athletes:

- Energy and macronutrient needs, particularly carbohydrate and protein, must be met during training and competition to maintain body mass, recover energy stores and provide adequate protein for tissue growth and repair.
- Fat intake should contribute appropriately to energy demands within the context of weight management and be adequate to supply essential fatty acids and fat-soluble vitamins.
- Micronutrient intakes should at least match the requirements for the population as a whole.
- Commence exercise euhydrated and drink enough fluid during and after exercise to balance fluid losses through a customised approach.

Adequate amounts of food and fluid consumed before, during and after exercise will help maintain blood glucose during exercise, maximise performance and speed up recovery post-exercise. The International Olympic Committee (IOC, 2010) advises athletes to adopt specific nutritional strategies before, during and after training and competition to maximise performance. Evidence-based guidelines, such as those produced by

Manual of Dietetic Practice, Sixth Edition. Edited by Joan Gandy.

Companion website: www.manualofdieteticpractice.com

the American College of Sports Medicine (ACSM, 2016), are available on the amount, composition and timing of food intake, and athletes are advised of the benefits of seeking qualified guidance to formulate sport-specific nutritional strategies, such as dietetic and nutrition practitioners registered with the Sport and Exercise Nutrition Register (SENr).

Energy metabolism during exercise

Energy is largely stored in the body as glycogen and fat. The body stores an average of 375–475 g of glycogen, up to a maximum of approximately 600 g in muscle and a further 100 g in the liver. This is sufficient to run about 20 miles. The body's reserves of fat for all practical purposes are unlimited, even in the leanest of athletes. A third fuel is phosphocreatine; very small amounts of this are stored in the muscle, sufficient to run for 5–6 seconds.

During exercise, the working muscles convert stored energy into kinetic energy to fuel movement. The energy needs of the muscles are covered by accelerating the rate of adenosine triphosphate (ATP) resynthesis to match the rate at which ATP is utilised. ATP is produced when muscle cells metabolise carbohydrate and fatty acids in the presence of oxygen; this is aerobic metabolism. It can also be produced without the presence of oxygen, but during anaerobic metabolism only carbohydrate can be utilised. Therefore, the two main fuels for muscle metabolism are carbohydrate and fat. Fatigue often coincides with depletion of the carbohydrate reserves.

Energy requirements and availability

Energy expenditure due to physical activity generally accounts for 25–35% of daily energy turnover, but can account for as much as 75% during intense training of long duration. Energy intakes can therefore vary from 1500 kcal/day for young female gymnasts to 6000–7000 kcal/day for competitive cyclists riding multiday stage races such as the Tour de France. In sports where a specific body image or size is required, e.g. bodybuilding and ballet, or where a sport requires athletes to compete in a weight category, such as boxing or lightweight rowing, athletes may be required to restrict energy intake to lose weight or maintain a particular body composition.

Female athletes who follow intensive training programmes while restricting energy intake may experience other related problems, such as menstrual dysfunction, decreased bone density and iron deficiency anaemia. Lower energy intakes may also be associated with micronutrient intakes below recommended values.

Beyond the usual factors that affect energy requirements, energy expenditure for different sports is largely dependent on the duration, frequency and intensity of activity, and the prior nutritional status of the athlete. Meeting energy requirements should be the main nutritional concern for athletes. During periods of high-intensity and/or high-duration training, athletes need to consume adequate energy to maintain health, body weight and composition, and to maximise training effects. Low energy intake or availability can result in losses of lean mass, loss or failure to gain bone density, disturbance in menstrual function, increased risk of injury, illness and fatigue, and delayed recovery from training and competition. Inadequate energy intake relative to energy expenditure has the potential to compromise performance and counteract the benefits of training. Losses in lean tissue as a result of inadequate energy intake can result in losses in strength and endurance, as well as compromised musculoskeletal, endocrine and immune function, in addition to poor overall nutrient intakes. Most athletes will have a weight management concern, whether this is gains in lean mass, losses in fat mass or achievement of weight maintenance during intense training blocks. As such, energy requirements and budgets may need to be considered alongside sensible body weight and composition targets, and should be individualised and periodised.

The concept of energy availability, i.e. the amount of energy available to perform all other functions after exercise training expenditure is subtracted, is defined as dietary intake minus energy expenditure normalised to fat-free mass (FFM). It has been proposed that 30 kcal/kg of FFM/day might be the lower threshold of energy availability for women. The IOC (2010) advises that low energy availability be avoided and dieting discouraged, and that athletes at risk of disordered eating patterns and reproductive disorders be referred promptly to relevant health professionals for evaluation and treatment.

Macronutrient requirements for sport

Essentially, athletes do not need to eat substantially differently from the recommended diet for the general population; however, for athletes there has been a shift away from using percentage recommendations for carbohydrate and protein intake goals in favour of prescriptions relative to body weight. This allows for recommendations to be scaled to the vast range in the body sizes of athletes. Even so, such prescription requires careful monitoring and evaluation alongside consideration of the importance of nutrient intake timing and weight management goals to optimise training performance and adaptation.

Role of carbohydrate in training and recovery

It is important to appreciate that, whatever exercise is performed, some carbohydrate will always be used. The longer or harder the exercise, the greater the demands placed on carbohydrate stores to maintain the desired rate of ATP resynthesis. Consequently, without adequate muscle glycogen as a reserve, the ability to perform high levels of work is markedly impaired.

Muscle glycogen becomes totally depleted after 2–3 hours of continuous exercise at intensities of 60–80% maximal oxygen uptake (VO_2 max). Severe depletion can also be achieved after only 15–30 minutes of exercise at intensities of 90–130% VO_2 max when intervals of 1–5 minutes of exercise followed by rest are repeated.

This type of short, intermittent, high-intensity exercise is a pattern found typically in many individual and team sports, such as football, hockey and tennis, and demonstrates the importance of carbohydrate as a fuel for all types of sport, and not just endurance sports. Athletes who train and compete regularly need to ensure adequate carbohydrate consumption if they are to avoid residual fatigue and poor performance.

Glycogen is restored at a rate of about 5%/hour. After exhaustive exercise, up to and beyond 20 hours may be needed to fully replenish stores. During the first 2 hours after exercise, muscle glycogen resynthesis proceeds at a slightly higher rate of 7%/hour, making it important that athletes consume carbohydrate during this time. If glycogen reserves are low, the point at which glycogen becomes limiting may be attained more rapidly. If the process of incomplete refuelling continues, there is a progressive depletion of glycogen stores within the working muscles, resulting in a feeling of continual lethargy. The quality and quantity of training will be impaired, leading to a decrease in overall performance. There is also the potential for blood sugar levels to fall during training, affecting brain function, concentration and coordination, and resulting in an increased injury risk.

Carbohydrate recommendations

The guidelines from ACSM (2016) are summarised in Table 4.3.1. These guidelines need to be personalised and periodised to take account of total energy needs, specific training demands and feedback on performance. Sufficient foods containing carbohydrate should be consumed on a regular basis to maintain glycogen levels. In most cases, nutrient-rich starchy foods are the best choice; however, athletes may also need to include sugary sources of carbohydrate, such as sweets, jam or sugar, or sports food such as drinks, bars and gels, to meet high overall energy requirements within the context of achieving an overall balanced intake.

Training versus competition

Different sports operate in different time frames for training and competition, and therefore require distinctive energy and carbohydrate intakes. Generally, endurance athletes such as long-distance runners or cyclists and triathletes will train and compete for long periods. Sprinters will compete over very short periods but train for longer periods, and multi-sprint sports such as rugby, football or netball require training and competition over 1–2 hours, but have periods of relative inactivity within that time period. Each sport will have complex training programmes, including strength and conditioning, endurance, speed and skills specific elements. When assessing requirements before, during and after training, it is important to remember that each training session will affect nutritional requirements differently.

Table 4.3.1 Carbohydrate requirements for fuelling and recovery (ACSM, 2016)

Type of training	Carbohydrate targets (g/kg body weight/day)
Light (low-intensity or skill-based training)	3–5
Moderate (~1 hour per day)	5–7
High (endurance programmes 1–3 hour per day of moderate to high intensity)	6–10
Very high (extreme programmes (4–5+ hour per day of moderate to high intensity)	8–12

Prior to exercise

The timing of carbohydrate intake in relation to training can be manipulated to promote or reduce carbohydrate availability. In most cases, to support performance, athletes should aim to begin every bout of training and competition fully recovered, with glycogen stores that are adequate to cope with the workload to be undertaken. This may be more difficult to achieve for athletes with multiple bouts of training and/or competition in a day. Eating a meal rich in carbohydrate 3–4 hours prior to exercise increases glycogen stores in the muscles and liver. The quantities of carbohydrate that are appropriate at this time will vary according to the sport, the athlete, and their prior nutritional status and overall daily needs.

Endurance events require optimal glycogen stores to maximise performance. The traditional carbohydrate loading method popular during the late 1960s and 1970s is no longer used, having been replaced with a tapering of training and an increase in carbohydrate intake over the 3–5 days prior to competition. Subsequent increases in glycogen stores not only benefit the endurance athlete but also may help in sports situations where competition may last for several days. Commencing competition with high glycogen stores may assist in offsetting progressive depletion with each bout of competition. A possible disadvantage of increasing glycogen stores is the commensurate increase in body weight through the associated storage of water with glycogen. This may be an important consideration where an athlete competes in a weight-category sport such as judo or in events covering significant distance, e.g. marathon running.

Training with low carbohydrate availability may be incorporated into the training plans of endurance athletes to enhance the training stimulus or adaptive response. This may be deliberately achieved by reducing total carbohydrate intake or by manipulating intake related to specific sessions, such as training in a fasted state, or undertaking subsequent sessions without sufficient refuelling, but should be carefully monitored and evaluated.

During exercise

The consumption of carbohydrate during competitions of long duration or between bouts of intermittent competition will enhance performance. Muscle glycogen stores and the availability of carbohydrate during exercise are major determinants of endurance performance. The delivery of carbohydrate during exercise becomes more significant when muscle glycogen stores are low at the onset of exercise.

During exercise, the ingestion of carbohydrate is often limited to that which can be taken in fluid form. If exercise duration continues beyond 1 hour, it is recommended that carbohydrates be ingested at a rate of 30–60 g/hour to maintain the oxidation of carbohydrates and delay fatigue. Mixing different forms of carbohydrate has been shown to increase carbohydrate oxidation up to 90 g/hour, which may be required to optimise performance in events lasting >2.5–3 hours.

Athletes are advised to practice consuming carbohydrate during training and to develop individual strategies, making use of sports foods and drinks containing carbohydrate combinations that will allow for maximal absorption from the gut with minimal gastrointestinal disturbance. In competition, the opportunity to consume foods and fluids will be dictated by the rules and nature of the sport. Some athletes may benefit from the newer concept of carbohydrate mouth rinsing where frequent exposure to carbohydrate in the mouth and oral cavity appears to be effective in stimulating the brain and central nervous system to enhanced perceptions of well-being and increased pacing strategies.

Post-exercise

To facilitate rapid recovery, athletes should aim to consume carbohydrate at the rate of 1.0–1.2 g/kg body weight per hour within 30 minutes and again every 2 hours for 4–6 hours for adequate replacement of glycogen stores. Adequate refuelling is particularly important when there are 8 hours or less before the next training or competition bout. The addition of protein may have additional benefits in enhancing both muscle protein and glycogen synthesis. Many athletes find solid food immediately after exercise unpalatable, and therefore drinks containing carbohydrate may be useful. Foods with a high glycaemic index are generally thought to be beneficial during this initial post-exercise period.

Protein

Regular exercise has been shown to increase protein needs. With regards to resistance training, muscle protein synthesis appears to be upregulated for at least 24 hours after the exercise bout, with increased sensitivity to protein intake over this period. Athletes should consume daily amounts greater that those recommended for the general population, but a varied diet that meets energy requirements will often provide a protein intake in excess of requirements. Recent recommendations emphasise the importance not only of quantity but also well-timed protein intake to maximise metabolic adaptation to training. While further research is required to distil recommendations in terms of protein quality, timing, and quantity and value of protein supplementation, specifically where individual amino acids may be concerned, the current consensus evidence suggests that athletes require 1.2–2.0 g of protein/kg body weight/day, with higher intakes indicated for periods of intensified training or where energy restriction is required.

The high energy intakes typical of athletes make these recommendations generally easy to attain without dietary manipulation. Intake goals should be achieved by adopting strategies that allow for a regular spread of moderate amounts of high-quality protein throughout the day and following intense workouts in quantities of 15–25 g (0.25–0.3 g/kg body weight) to aid the repair of damaged tissue and long-term maintenance or gain of muscle mass. Dairy proteins appear to be a useful choice post-exercise, primarily due to leucine content. Athletes with restricted energy intake may require dietary manipulation to achieve their protein requirements. Those who are vegetarian, and particularly vegans, may also need some guidance to ensure adequate protein intake, particularly if also consuming low-energy diets. The consumption of adequate energy, particularly from carbohydrate, is important to protein metabolism to ensure amino acids are spared for protein synthesis.

Fat

Fat is a source of energy, fat-soluble vitamins and essential fatty acids, and it is an important nutrient in the diet of athletes. However, there is no need to supplement the normal diet with additional fat; intakes of >30% of total energy are likely to indicate an inadequate intake of carbohydrate. In addition, intakes of <20% of total energy do not appear to benefit performance. Athletes should aim to avoid excessive amounts of fat in the diet, and would normally be encouraged to look to lower-fat versions of foods where appropriate, unless they have exceptionally high overall energy requirements. While many athletes are familiar with the concepts around the need for carbohydrate in the diet, the issue of including adequate and appropriately healthy fats may not always be fully understood. High-fat/restricted-carbohydrate diets have received recent attention; however, claims that they provide a benefit to performance in elite athletes are yet to be substantiated by the research literature.

Fluid balance

Considerable care should be taken by all athletes to ensure adequate hydration before, during and after exercise to avoid thermal distress. Dehydration can increase perception effort and compromise performance, particularly in hot and high-altitude conditions, and may also impair cognitive performance. Sweat rates for any given activity, and therefore fluid losses, will vary according to ambient temperature, humidity, body mass, genetics, state of heat acclimatisation, metabolic efficiency and even clothing. Sweat rates can range from as little as 0.3 L/hour to typically maximum rates of 2–3 L/hour. It is important to recognise that large inter-individual variation in sweat losses can occur even when the same or similar exercise is carried out in the same conditions.

Where sweat losses greatly exceed replacement, the circulatory system is unable to cope, and skin blood flow slows. This is accompanied by a reduction in sweating and the ability to lose heat; thus, body temperature will rise, with potentially fatal consequences. Although sweating is a very effective way of losing heat, care must be taken to ensure that this process is not impaired through dehydration.

The addition of sodium to sports drinks aids the absorption of water and thus the process of rehydration. Further, this sodium prevents a drop in plasma sodium concentration and plasma osmolality that would occur during exercise with the ingestion of large volumes of plain water. A drop in plasma sodium concentration and plasma osmolality would result in diuresis, with an accompanying decline in desire to drink, resulting in a lower fluid consumption. Athletes participating in endurance events, particularly ultra-endurance events, can be at risk of hyponatraemia if they drink copious amounts of plain water; this is most often reported in the non-elite.

Fluid intake

Hydration strategies should be individualised, the ideal strategy covering the athlete's daily fluid requirements plus additional requirements of each bout of training or competition. As acute changes in body mass generally reflect shifts in body water, assuming the athlete is in energy balance, the daily hydration status can be estimated by monitoring early morning body mass measured on waking and after voiding. Drinks used for exercise lasting more than an hour, or sports that stimulate heavy sodium losses through sweating, should include sodium. There is a range of commercial sports drinks available that athletes can use around training and competition. These contain carbohydrate and electrolytes at levels that will be acceptable for use before, during and after most sports; these will typically be labelled as isotonic. Hypertonic drinks contain more carbohydrate and may be useful where the focus is on refuelling. Where rehydration is a priority, hypotonic drinks may be beneficial where the carbohydrate content is low and sodium content higher. Emphasis should be placed on good oral hygiene when using sports drinks.

Prior to exercise

Euhydration should be strived for prior to training or competition. This can be achieved by:

- Constantly being aware of fluid status, and maintaining good fluid intake at all times.
- Drinking 5–10 mL/kg body mass of water or sports drink 2–4 hours before exercise to achieve urine that is pale-yellow in colour while providing sufficient time for any excess fluid consumed to be voided.

Markers of urine osmolality, specific gravity and colour can be used as a guide to euhydration.

During exercise

The achievement of fluid balance during exercise is not always possible as a result of maximal sweat rates exceeding maximal gastric emptying. The aim of drinking during exercise is to limit dehydration to <2% of body mass. The amount and rate of fluid replacement achieved will be dependent on individual sweat rate, exercise duration and intensity, and opportunities to consume fluids. The use of beverages containing carbohydrate and electrolytes can help to maintain fluid and electrolyte balance, especially during the performance of endurance exercise. Regular assessment of pre to post-exercise body weight can assist in determining sweat rates and customising individual hydration programmes. Without the presence of other factors that alter body mass during exercise, such as sizable loss of substrate, which may occur during very prolonged exercise, a loss of 1 kg body weight represents approximately 1 L sweat loss.

When exercise lasts less than an hour and temperatures are not high, fluid may not be needed during the exercise period. However, when exercise is of long duration or results in excessive sweating, it is advisable to drink during the exercise period. In such cases, hydration strategies during exercise should aim to:

- Ensure individualised hydration plans based on the knowledge of sweat rates, and match fluid losses through sweat with fluid intake, but typically intakes of 0.4–0.8 L/h are achievable.
- Minimise body weight losses to 1–2%, especially in hot and humid conditions.
- Use palatable drinks as the presence of flavour in a drink may increase voluntary fluid intake.
- Use training sessions to practice drinking during exercise.

Post-exercise

Athletes will complete most exercise bouts with some degree of dehydration. The volume of fluid consumed following exercise needs to replace that lost as sweat, but should also take account of the ongoing sweat losses during the immediate recovery period. Therefore, fluid intake during this period should exceed losses, with athletes aiming to consume ~125–150% of fluid deficit, i.e. for every litre lost, 1.25–1.5 L should be drunk. Strategies implemented following exercise should ensure that:

- Rehydration starts immediately, particularly when repeated bouts of exercise must be performed.
- Sweat rates calculated from before and after weighing are taken into account.
- Athletes carry their own supply of fluid in their kit bags.
- Drinks contain some sodium to assist rehydration by stimulating thirst.
- Drinks contain some carbohydrate to help replace energy needs where appropriate.

Other considerations

Weight control

In most cases, the aim of a weight loss diet for an athlete is to decrease body fat stores without affecting glycogen, water or lean body mass content. The diet must contain sufficient carbohydrate to restock glycogen stores between each bout of training. It will need to be low in fat and may require a proportionately high protein content, in addition to providing all essential nutrients in a total energy intake that will achieve the desired weight loss over a sensible period.

If loss of performance due to dehydration and glycogen depletion is to be avoided, rapid weight loss by dietary or non-dietary methods should be discouraged. Where weight loss is a long-term goal, well-planned weight reduction programmes are essential if athletes are to maintain training and not impair performance and health. An individualised diet and training prescription should consider goals, present training demands and nutrition practices, and previous weight loss approaches, but creating an energy deficient of ~250–500 kcal/day is a sound practical strategy, with or without slight increases in energy expenditure.

Where weight gain is required, the athlete will want to increase lean body mass rather than body fat content. Muscle mass is determined by training effect and adaptation. Advice for the athlete desiring weight gain is to ensure an adequate overall diet with a high proportion of carbohydrate and adequate protein that achieves ~500 kcal/day positive energy balance. A conscious effort may be required to increase food intake. Meals should not be missed, and high-carbohydrate snacks should be consumed between meals as appropriate.

Micronutrients

Careful selection of nutrient-dense foods should reduce the risk of micronutrient deficiencies; however, the micronutrients commonly found to be of concern in the diets of athletes are vitamin D, calcium and iron. The IOC (2010) warns that athletes should be particularly aware of their needs for these nutrients, but that the use of large amounts through supplementation may be harmful.

Supplementation should not compensate for poor food choices, but may provide a short-term option when food intake or choice is restricted due to constant travel, giving rise to limited food choice, or restriction of food intake to maintain low body weight. Single nutrient supplementation may be necessary for specific medical or nutritional purpose, e.g. iron supplementation to correct anaemia. Female athletes with amenorrhoea or dysmenorrhoea have an increased risk of developing osteoporosis due to reduced levels of oestrogen. Improved calcium intakes are particularly important in athletes with low bone density, menstrual irregularities and low calcium intakes, since stress fractures are particularly common in this group of athletes.

Athletes who run the greatest risk of poor micronutrient status are those who restrict energy intake; who undertake severe weight loss practices; who eliminate, through choice or need, one or more food groups; or who repeatedly consume unbalanced low-nutrient-density diets. Theories are emerging that supplemental dietary antioxidants may reduce the oxidative stress and skeletal muscle damage associated with strenuous exercise, but athletes are advised to maintain an adequate intake through good nutrition.

Supplementation

Athletes should be counselled about the appropriate use of sports foods and nutritional ergogenic aids. Sports dietitians and registered sports and exercise nutritionists need to constantly update their knowledge in this area. The manufacture, processing, labelling and marketing of these products is poorly regulated, with variable quality control. The vast array of available products make convincing claims including better recovery, increased strength and size, loss of body fat and enhanced immune function. As such, it is easy to appreciate the attraction of such products for the athlete.

The list of supplements is exhaustive, but they can essentially be broken down into two main categories:

1. Nutrient supplements or sports foods, which can be used to assist athletes in meeting their overall nutritional needs. This might be by way of providing a practical alternative to food, or by helping to meet their higher-than-average requirements for nutrients, particularly carbohydrate and protein.
2. Ergogenic aids, which are assumed to enhance performance above and beyond what is normally expected. Nutritional ergogenic aids generally aim to enhance performance through effects on energy, body composition and alertness.

Nutrient supplements and sports foods

Nutrient supplements can assist athletes to achieve optimal nutritional requirements. These products include sports drinks, gels and bars, liquid meal and protein supplements, carbohydrate powders, and multivitamin and mineral supplements. Athletes may find these products useful in helping them to meet their nutritional goals during particularly demanding periods of training and competition.

The key question with nutrient supplements and sports foods is knowing how and when to use them to maximum benefit to support the attainment of nutrition goals. If used appropriately, they can play a role in assisting athletes to train and compete at their best, but the support of a sports dietitian or registered sports and exercise nutritionist may be required to develop optimum nutritional strategies where these products feature. They are generally more expensive than similar everyday food items, but, in some circumstances, the extra expense and convenience may be worth it.

Nutritional ergogenic aids

There is scientific support for performance enhancement with some supplements such as creatine and caffeine, with beetroot juice gaining evidence from an ergogenic effect. Other products such as colostrum and beta-hydroxy-beta-methylbutyrate (HBM) are still under scientific scrutiny to assess their benefits or practical uses. Creatine phosphate is used as a fuel source in the first few seconds of a sprint. Creatine supplementation can increase muscle creatine phosphate levels, and as such may assist athletes to recover more quickly between repeated bouts of high-intensity effort. It may also lead to increases in muscle bulk. Caffeine is a central nervous system stimulant commonly available in a wide range of foods and beverages. Several studies have shown a performance-enhancing effect for caffeine during exercise of varying intensities and duration. Sensitivity to caffeine varies between individuals, and overconsumption can produce a range of side effects, such as insomnia, headache, abdominal discomfort, impaired coordination and muscle tremors, all of which can have a negative impact on training and competition performance. The mild diuretic effect of caffeine may need to be considered when exercising for prolonged duration or in hot and humid conditions.

Beetroot juice is rich in nitrate. Following ingestion, nitrate is converted to nitrite and stored and circulated in the blood. In situations of low oxygen availability, nitrite can be converted into nitric oxide, which is known to have a number of roles in vascular and metabolic control. Nitrate supplementation reduces the oxygen cost of submaximal exercise, and can, in some situations, enhance exercise tolerance and performance. Research is at an early stage, and the precise conditions in which nitrate may be ergogenic have yet to be fully established. Currently, there is more evidence of greater performance improvements in recreationally active individuals than elite athletes. Likely side effects include mild gut discomfort and pink-coloured urine and stools, both of which are harmless.

Points to consider

Athletes considering the use of a supplement should ensure that it is legal; is backed by sound scientific reason and has sound guidelines for its use; and can be obtained through a reliable source. Indiscriminate use of supplements is unwise. Before deciding to use any supplement, athletes should be cautioned to undertake a cost–benefit analysis in terms of the potential performance benefits weighed against the costs, not only in terms of finance but also the adverse effects on health and performance and the likelihood of contamination with banned or other undesirable substances.

Contaminated supplements have often been blamed for athletes testing positive for a banned substance, with subsequent claims that the prohibited substance was not declared in the product list of ingredients. With the inception of the World Anti-Doping Code (World Anti-Doping Agency, 2009) and the implications of strict liability, athletes are strictly held responsible for any prohibited substance found in their system. As such, athletes are strongly advised to be cautious and vigilant about the use of any supplement, and to consider that diet, lifestyle and training should all be optimised before turning to supplements to rectify any shortfall in performance potential. Generally, products manufactured in the food and pharmaceutical industries are safer, as standards are more rigorous. If in doubt, athletes should consider asking the manufacturer for a written declaration that the product only contains what is stated on the label, and check carefully where ingredients are sourced from and how and where the product is packaged. The SENr (2016) has published a position statement on Supplement use in Sport. This provides athlete support personnel, such as the registered dietitian or sports and exercise nutritionist, with a guide to appropriately assess the need for supplementation, assess the risk of supplementation, understand the consequences of taking supplements from an anti-doping perspective, and provide practical guidelines and tools for their safe usage.

UK Anti-Doping has responsibility for ensuring that sports bodies in the UK are compliant with the World Anti-Doping Code through the implementation and management of the UK National Anti-Doping Policy. Athletes are advised to be vigilant in choosing to use any supplement. No guarantee can be given that any particular supplement is free from prohibited substances. A number of initiatives to support athletes have been created globally to identify whether a prohibited substance can be identified in a supplement. In the UK, HFL Sports Science has taken the lead to create a scheme to support athletes in assessing the risk of supplement use. The Informed Sport programme is designed to evaluate the integrity of supplement manufacturing processes, and to screen supplements and ingredients for the presence of prohibited substances that are cited on the World Anti-Doping Code prohibited list. This list is annually updated. Further information can be found at www.informed-sport.com.

Practical issues

Athletes will benefit from the guidance of qualified professionals who can advise on individual energy, nutrient and fluid needs to develop sport-specific nutritional strategies for training, competition and recovery. To achieve this, they may need very practical advice concerning shopping, food preparation and cooking to meet their requirements. On a practical level, one of the greatest difficulties facing the athlete is simply finding time for food while coping with training, travel, competition and employment or education.

Nutritional needs for special populations (including children and young athletes) and those with special needs (e.g. athletes with diabetes, gastrointestinal disorders and disabilities) are beyond the scope of this chapter, but are discussed in detail in Burke and Deakin (2015).

Further reading

Burke LM, Deakin V. (eds). (2015) *Clinical Sports Nutrition*, 5th edn. Sydney, Australia: McGraw Hill Education.

International Olympic Committee (IOC). (2011) IOC consensus statement on sports nutrition 2010. *J. Sports Sci.* 29(S1): S3–4.

Jeukendrup A. (2010) *From Lab to Kitchen*. UK: Meyer & Meyer.

Jeukendrup A, Gleeson M. (2010) *Sports Nutrition. An Introduction to Energy Production and Performance*, 2nd edn. Human Kinetics. Champaign, IL, USA.

Joint Position Statement of the American Dietetic Association, Dietitians of Canada, and the American College of Sports Medicine. (2016) Nutrition and athletic performance. *Med. Sci. Sports Exerc.* 48(3): 543–568.

Mountjoy M, Sundgot-Borgen J, Burke L, *et al.* (2014) The IOC consensus statement: beyond the Female Athlete Triad – Relative Energy Deficiency in Sport (RED-S). *Br. J. Sports Med.* 48: 491–497.

Journals

British Journal of Sports Medicine
International Journal of Sport Nutrition & Exercise Metabolism
Journal of Sport Sciences
Medicine & Science in Sport & Exercise

Internet resources

American https://www.acsm.org/acsm-positions-policy
Australian Institute of Sport, www.ausport.gov.au/ais/nutrition
Informed Sport Programme, www.informed-sport.com
Sport and Exercise Nutrition Register, www.senr.org.uk
UK Anti-Doping, www.ukad.org.uk
UK Sport, www.uksport.gov.uk
World Anti-Doping Agency, www.wada-ama.org

Position papers and references

Burke LM, Deakin V. (eds). (2015) *Clinical Sports Nutrition*, 4th edn. Sydney, Australia: McGraw Hill Education.

Joint Position Statement of the American Dietetic Association, Dietitians of Canada, and the American College of Sports Medicine. (2016) Nutrition and athletic performance. *Med. Sci. Sports Exerc.* 48(3): 543–568.

International Olympic Committee (IOC). (2010) *IOC Consensus Statement on Sports Nutrition*. Available at www.olympic.org. https://stillmed.olympic.org/Documents/Reports/EN/CONSENSUS-FINAL-v8-en.pdf. Accessed 8 October 2018.

World Anti-Doping Agency. (2009) *World Anti-Doping Code*. Available at www.wada-ama.org. Accessed 15 November 2016.

4.4 Food service

4.4.1 Food service in hospitals and institutions

Lauren Bowen, Joana Jardim, Lisa Baker and Sarah Wallis

Key points

- Promoting excellent food and beverage services is everyone's responsibility: those involved in its planning, delivery and execution need to work closely together to ensure that a patient-centred meal provision is promoted. Dietitians are fundamental to this process.
- Food and beverages services are governed by standards and legislations, ensuring that menus are not only nutritionally adequate but can also cater to a range of special and therapeutic diets, and cultural and religious needs.
- The focus on health and well-being is significant for food and beverages served to staff and visitors.

SECTION 4

Hospitals

Hospital food standards

The Hospital Food Standards Panel was established to examine existing standards in healthcare and to recommend those that should be applied and monitored. Over 90 potential standards were considered, but only five were identified as those that would induce the biggest improvement in the nutrition and hydration care of patients, staff and visitors (Department of Health (DH), 2014). The standards are legally binding under the NHS standard contract service conditions for hospitals (SC 19 Food Standards) (NHS England, 2016a). The required hospital standards are described in the following text.

For patients

The 10 key characteristics of good nutrition and hydration care

The 10 key characteristics were originally based on the Council of Europe Resolution on Food and Nutritional Care in Hospitals (CoE, 2003). This contained over 100 recommendations and were summarised by the Council of Europe Alliance into 10 key characteristics. In 2015, NHS England reviewed the Council of Europe's 10 key characteristics (NHS England, 2015). These characteristics include the screening and delivery of safe, appropriate food and drink by all care providers within a local nutrition and hydration policy.

The Nutrition and Hydration Digest

The Nutrition and Hydration Digest (BDA, 2017b) sets out comprehensive standards for use in food services, providing details on requirements for nutrition, menus, coding and analysis.

Malnutrition Universal Screening Tool (or equivalent validated nutrition screening tools)

The Malnutrition Universal Screening Tool ('MUST') is a five-step screening tool to identify adults who are malnourished, at risk of malnutrition (undernutrition) or obese. It includes guidelines which can support the development of a care plan and is used in hospitals and care homes (BAPEN, 2016).

For staff and visitor catering

Healthier and more sustainable catering: Nutrition principles

Healthier and More Sustainable Catering: Nutrition Principles (PHE, 2017) outlines how NHS catering providers can ensure that the food they provide allows the population that it is catering for to meet its dietary requirements for each meal part.

Healthier eating for the whole hospital community

Healthier eating for staff and visitors is receiving an increasing amount of attention. The impact of obesity on the NHS has been highlighted by NHS employers,

Manual of Dietetic Practice, Sixth Edition. Edited by Joan Gandy.

Companion website: www.manualofdieteticpractice.com

who have, using an obesity infographic, urged staff to be healthier and physically active (NHS Employers, 2015). Of the 1.2 million NHS employees, it is estimated that around 300,000 would be classified as obese, and 400,000 as overweight (DH, 2009). Many hospital staff rely on food provided by their workplace for a large proportion of their daily energy and nutrient intake (DH, 2014). Food services have an obligation to staff well-being and need to consider the suitability of choices 24 hours a day.

Commissioning for Quality and Innovation (CQUIN) is a payments framework that encourages care providers to continually develop how care is delivered to improve experience and outcomes for all. The importance of health and well-being within the NHS was recognised when NHS England launched a national CQUIN titled Healthy Food for NHS Staff, Visitors and Patients. The purpose of this national CQUIN was to create a change in organisational behaviour and culture towards the food and drinks sold on NHS premises (NHS England, 2016b).

In 2017, NHS England announced that it would also be introducing a voluntary sales reduction scheme to reduce the amount of sugar-sweetened beverages (SSB) sold on NHS premises. NHS England have stated that non-compliance may result in an outright ban of SSB being considered (NHS England, 2017).

For all catering

Government buying standards for food and catering services

The government has produced buying standards to help food and beverage services achieve sustainable standards (DEFRA, 2015). Food services have a responsibility to promote sustainable practice, looking at benefits to both society and the economy. This includes factors such as food miles, sourcing local produce if possible, buying fish from sustainable stock, considering seasonal food and ensuring meat is obtained with animal welfare assurance. Ethically sourced products such as coffee, tea and chocolate may also be considered. Menus should be planned with sustainability in mind, but must provide good nutritional value for money.

Sustainable procurement also impacts on the environment and needs discussion. How much energy is used to prepare and cook meals? How much water and energy is consumed when cleaning crockery, equipment and utensils? Where does food waste go? Could the food be safely recycled or used for animal food?

Hospital food and drink strategy

With these five hospital food standards in mind, under the NHS standard contract (NHS England, 2016a), every hospital must develop and maintain a food and drink strategy, addressing the following issues:

- The nutrition and hydration needs of patients.
- Healthier eating for the whole hospital community, especially staff.
- Sustainable procurement of food and catering services (DH, 2014); a toolkit was developed to support this (DH, 2016).

A recent report has shown good progress, with over half of NHS hospitals now fully compliant with the standards, and over 90% of hospitals have confirmed that they are working towards meeting them (DH, 2017b).

The hospital nutrition steering committee

The British Association of Parenteral and Enteral Nutrition (BAPEN) recommends that each hospital have a nutrition steering committee to oversee and advise on all aspects of nutrition. It should be a multi-disciplinary team and have representatives from across the organisation, such as nurses, pharmacists, consultants from medicine and surgery, caterers and dietitians. The committee could be split into smaller working parties, as its remit is vast, covering many nutritional interventions from parenteral nutrition to overseeing the successful implementation of the hospital's food and drink strategy. The steering committee would focus on the 11 key aspects of good nutritional practice in the care setting; these include: screening tools and pathways, audit and education to staff, and the overseeing of commercial food outlets on the hospital premises (BAPEN, 2012a).

Patient-led assessments of the care environment (PLACE)

PLACE assessments involve local people (patient assessors) going into hospitals as part of teams to assess (through observation and survey) how the environment supports the provision of clinical care. PLACE evaluates privacy and dignity, food and hydration, cleanliness and general building maintenance, and, more recently, the extent to which the environment is able to support the care of those with dementia and/or disabilities (DH, 2017a).

Care homes

While excellent nutritional care systems and processes in care homes is essential to ensure that residents are provided with a food service that meets their individual needs, there are a limited number of standards that this sector is required to meet. Nutritional care is examined during CQC inspections (CQC, 2015, 2017) when care homes are required to demonstrate how people are supported to eat and drink enough to maintain a balanced diet. A number of prompts are offered, including how people can be involved in making decisions about what they eat and drink, whether they enjoy the food services, and how specific dietary needs are met. The DH (2003) has published national minimum standards for care homes. The outcome relating to meals and mealtimes states that '*service users receive a wholesome, appealing, balanced diet in pleasing surroundings at times convenient to them*', and is supported by a list of standards.

Other tools that are widely used in care homes to support the provision of nutritional care include 'MUST' (BAPEN, 2016) and the dysphagia diet food texture descriptors (NPSA, 2012). Use of these tools should be encouraged where they are not embedded into practice. A commonly used good practice guide is the National Association of Care Catering's (NACC) Nutritional

Standards for Adults (NACC, 2014), providing a greater level of detail about the meals and menus that should be provided within care homes.

The role of the catering dietitian within food services

The catering dietitian plays a crucial role in the provision of an excellent food and beverage service for patients and residents in care homes, ensuring that all procedures are in place to deliver exceptional nutrition and hydration.

This role involves working as part of a multidisciplinary team alongside nurses, speech and language therapists, clinical dietitians, catering managers, back-of-house (chefs, catering assistants) staff, and front-of-house (host/hostess) catering staff. The catering dietitian is the link between clinical staff and non-clinical staff, supporting the communication between different departments.

Where catering dietitians work in a hospital or care setting, or for organisations such as contract caterers, they generally undertake a non-clinical role and do not give therapeutic advice to patients on an individual basis. However, the decisions they make impact on nutritional care and the clinical outcomes of a wide range of patient groups, so it is important that they have a good understanding of general and therapeutic dietary needs. Catering dietitians can also improve the health of staff and visitors by becoming involved in healthy workplace initiatives.

How do clinical dietitians fit into food services?

Clinical or catering liaison dietitians (clinical dietitians who usually works for the hospital with a proportion of their working time dedicated to food services) also contribute to excellent food and beverage services. They provide clinical advice on special diets and nutritional requirements for patients or residents, and get involved in planning menus at a local level. They play a crucial role in making sure the food and beverages provided are the most adequate in terms of quality and nutrition, and also satisfy the nutritional needs of different patient and resident groups (BDA, 2017a).

Guidance and legislation

The latest guidance and legislation in the UK can be seen in Table 4.4.1. Refer to Wilson (2014) for a more comprehensive review of guidance and opinion on food service in the UK since 1990.

Prevalence of malnutrition

Malnutrition affects 25% of adults admitted to hospital (BAPEN, 2012b) and 35% of individuals admitted to care homes (Wise, 2015). If we consider the number of patients at risk of becoming malnourished due to reduced intake or increased nutritional requirements, this number is likely to be an underestimate (see Chapter 6.2, Malnutrition). However, as levels of obesity in society rise, this will also be reflected in the hospital setting (NHS Digital, 2016).

Food and beverage services

Nutrition and hydration are vital parts of a patient's or resident's care in hospitals and care homes. Eating well helps fight infection, replace lost nutrients, prevent weight loss and provide the energy to recover. Fluid intake is also important to ensure hydration and improved well-being (BAPEN, 2010; Carter, 2015). The food and beverages provided are only a part of this. Food services can prepare the best-quality, nutritious and suitable food – but, if the delivery and service of this food is poor, then they have failed. Well-trained ward staff can ensure that the environment is conducive to eating; that patients or residents are ready; that appropriate equipment is available; and that the food is well presented and individuals are encouraged.

Nutritional content

Menus must cater to a wide range of patients and residents in terms of choice and requirements. A paradox exists around food service in hospitals and care homes; there are patients who, due to their clinical conditions, will require a diet that is high in energy and/or protein, and there are also patients who may require a diet lower in fat, salt and sugar. Patient menus must be able to accommodate both ends of this nutritional spectrum (BDA, 2017a). The nutrient standards for adults in care settings are shown in Table 4.4.2.

Standard menus must meet the needs of the nutritionally well and the nutritionally vulnerable. They should be planned using the Day Parts model (BDA, 2017a), where a whole day's menu is separated into daily eating events, including breakfast, midday and evening meals, milk for beverages, and snacks reflecting the contribution of energy and protein over the whole day to provide an adequate overall intake.

Menu planning

Successful menu planning reflects the needs of short- and long-stay patients as well as differing patient groups, including (but not limited to) paediatrics, renal, elderly and mental health patients. It is important that menus be designed using a multidisciplinary approach. Stakeholders such as dietitians, speech and language therapists, nursing staff, caterers and patient or resident representatives should have input into the content. Each person brings different skills and knowledge, which contribute to a well-planned menu for a diverse patient population. Menus must not only meet nutritional requirements but also budgetary constraints; the food services team will also need to confirm that there is adequate, working equipment, appropriate storage (dry stores, chillers and freezers), kitchen space and skilled staff to implement the menu.

Table 4.4.1 Guidance and legislation relating to food services

Year	Organisation and report title	Main points
2011	European Parliament *EU Regulation 1169/2011 on the provision of food information to consumers*	Consolidates general food and nutrition labelling requirements into a single regulation Requires pre-packed items to provide mandatory information on back-of-pack Stipulates how pre-packaged foods must display their allergen information For food served loose, information as to whether the meals contain any of the 14 allergens must be made available
2012	National Patient Safety Agency Dysphagia Expert Reference Group *Dysphagia Diet Food Texture Descriptors*	Defines textures of food for the management of dysphagia at a national level
2013	Hospital Caterers Association *A Good Practice Guide to ward-level services*	A manual for delivering excellence in food and beverage services
2014	British Dietetic Association *Allergen Toolkit for Healthcare Catering*	Steps that must be taken in order to comply with the allergen requirements of EU FIC[a] Outlines how to implement an effective allergen management program, train staff in food allergen risks and how to communicate accurate and consistent information on the allergens in your food
2014	DH *The Hospital Food Standards Panel's Report on Standards for Food and Drink in NHS Hospitals*	Identifies the legally binding standards for food and drink in the NHS
2014	National Association of Care Catering *Nutritional Standards for Adults*	Details the nutritional standards that meals and menus should provide within care homes
2015	British Dietetic Association Food Services Specialist Group *The Nutrition and Hydration Digest: Compliance Checklist*	A tool for hospitals to assess their compliance to the *Nutrition and Hydration Digest*
2016	British Dietetic Association Food Services Specialist Group *Nutrition Toolkit for Healthcare Catering*	Outlines steps that must be taken in order to comply with the nutrition labelling requirements of EU FIC[a] Key requirements expressed as a simple flowchart
2016	The International Dysphagia Diet Standardisation Initiative (IDDSI) *The IDDSI Framework and Descriptors*	International standardised terminology and descriptors for dysphagia diets that meet the needs of individuals with dysphagia across all age spans, care settings, and cultures
2017	British Dietetic Association *The Nutrition and Hydration Digest: Improving Outcomes through Food and Beverage Services, 2nd edition*	A comprehensive source of standards, coding, guidance and good practice for dietitians, other allied health professionals and caterers

[a] EU FIC, European Union Food Information to Consumers Regulation.

Table 4.4.2 Nutrient standards (BDA, 2017a). Reproduced with permission from the BDA Food Services Specialist Group

Nutrient (/day)	Nutritionally well	Nutritionally vulnerable	Provided
Energy (kcal)	1840–2772		Daily
Protein (g)	56[a]	66–83	Daily

[a] For females of the same age bracket, the RNI is 45 g.

Menu content

In line with legislation (BDA, 2017a; DH, 2014) and local nutrition policies, menus must include sufficient choice of healthier eating, higher-energy, vegetarian and softer options. They must reflect the needs of the patient population, recognising religious, cultural, personal and lifestyle considerations, as well as therapeutic needs and variable appetites. Menus should be based on the Eatwell Guide (PHE, 2016) to ensure that all nutrients are included.

Menu design and structure

À la carte

An à la carte menu offers the same set of extended choices for both lunch and supper each day, which may help patients select a choice they will really enjoy. This style of menu can cause issues with menu fatigue for very-long-stay patients or residents, as they can often exhaust the selection.

Cyclical

A cyclical or cycle menu offers different choices for both lunch and supper each day, ranging from 1–4 weeks in length. This style of menu is often used for long-stay patients/residents (e.g. mental health) or care homes, where it is important to offer variety each day. It can be repetitive over the cycle in terms of choice if not well planned.

A standard menu structure for both of these styles is shown in The Nutrition and Hydration Digest (BDA, 2017b).

Food composition

Before planning a menu, it is essential to establish what ingredients, food products or dishes are available. Procurement processes must ensure that all food safety and industry legislation is followed (FSA, 2017). The agreements with suppliers will ensure safety and integrity of the food provided (HCA, 2013). Specifications will be agreed to, and information such as quality, assurance of source, nutrition and allergens must be available. Standard recipes must be planned, analysed and followed, as they offer a method of control (BDA, 2017a). Thought needs to be given to the food-related PLACE questions and the details within these, such as the amount of cereals served and which condiments are available (DH, 2017). PLACE offers a benchmark into how food services can be improved; it should not be thought of as a tick box activity, but rather as a way to ensure that your food services are excellent.

How to plan a menu

Menu planning is easiest when approached in a very practical paper-and-pencil style. Using paper means you can move the weeks around to easily make sure Sunday supper (week 2) does not clash with Monday lunch (week 1), for example using a Microsoft Excel spreadsheet, you can plan the menu across a landscape file to ensure issues such as bland colour and repetition are avoided.

Consider all main meat or fish dishes first, e.g. beef, lamb, chicken, pork, and fish, and then repeat mixing the order slightly. Plan roast dinners (usually Sunday) and fish dishes (usually Friday). Allow for regional dishes, e.g. Cornish pasty, Bakewell tart and include both modern- and traditional (comfort) style choices as relevant to the population group.

Plan vegetarian main dishes, ensuring adequate variety of protein sources, e.g. cheese, eggs, lentils and pulse-based selections. Add carbohydrate and vegetables next to suit the main meal choices, ensuring no meal-to-meal and day-to-day repetition, and considering softer options as well. Finally, plan salads and sandwiches, starters and desserts. Ensure that soups do not clash with the vegetarian main or vegetable choices, e.g. do not plan vegetable soup with vegetable casserole. Table 4.4.3 gives an example of one meal on a cyclical menu.

Table 4.4.3 Example of a menu plan – Week 1, Monday Lunch

Week 1 Lunch	Monday	Dietary coding
Starters	Nourishing leek and potato soup	E S V
	Fruit juice	H S V
Main 1	Beef casserole	H S
Main 2	Breaded fish	E
Vegetarian main	Vegetable lasagne	E S V
Carbohydrate 1 (one soft)	Mashed potato	H S V
Carbohydrate 2	Chips	E V
Vegetable 1 (one soft)	Carrots	H S V
Vegetable 2	Mushy peas	E V
Salads	Ham	H
Served with bread roll, sunflower spread/butter, fresh salad	Three bean	H V
Sandwiches	Chicken mayonnaise	E
White or wholemeal bread	Cream cheese	E S V
Jacket potatoes	Tuna mayonnaise	E
Served with sunflower spread/butter and fresh side salad	Baked beans	H V
	Cheddar cheese	E V
Dessert 1	Chocolate sponge and custard	E S V
Dessert 2	Rice pudding	H S V
Dessert 3	Fresh fruit – banana	H S V
Dessert 4	Full-fat creamy yoghurt	S V
Dessert 5	Cheese and biscuits	V

In the planning stages, dietitians will take both a qualitative and quantitative approach to the menu in development. They will ensure that the menu offers adequate choice and variety in terms of types of dishes, e.g. different protein bases (meat, fish, chicken, beans, pulses); different styles of cooking (casseroles, roasts, stews, plain meats, pies); different carbohydrate and vegetable accompaniments; textures and colours; and, of course, the nutritional content of each item planned on the menu to support the key requirements for coding. A qualitative menu assessment checklist can be found in The Nutrition and Hydration Digest (BDA, 2017b).

Menu capacity

The dietitian will complete a final analysis to ensure the menu meets the nutritional parameters as required by legislation using the minimum/maximum method (outlined in The Nutrition and Hydration Digest; see BDA, 2017b), which assesses energy and protein as the main nutrient markers.

Dietary coding

Once nutritionally analysed, a menu can be dietary coded. Coding should be kept to a minimum, as too many codes on a menu can be confusing. Dietary coding is provided for guidance for the patient, and the main codes recommended are healthier eating (H or ♥), higher energy (E or ↑), softer (easier to chew) (S), and vegetarian (lacto-ovo) (V) (BDA, 2017a).

Menu implementation

The menu will then be ready to be implemented, and must be reviewed in terms of acceptability and quality through patient satisfaction surveys, audits and monitoring of food waste. The menu must also be acceptable to the food services team in terms of practicality around production, labour, logistics, waste, and, of course, cost.

Menu review

It is good practice to monitor the meals offered on the menu, reviewing and refreshing menus twice a year to include seasonal and varied choices such as lighter dishes for summer, heavier dishes for winter, and seasonal fruit and vegetables. Refreshing choice (e.g. sandwich fillings) will ensure variety, particularly for patients and residents who are long stay or frequent re-admissions. Using information from surveys and PLACE assessments (DH, 2017a), and involving both the multidisciplinary team and patients, will support change where it appears necessary.

Snacks and 24-hour catering

The menu-planning team must consider all food and beverages offered to patients and residents. A variety of snacks, such as biscuits, cakes, fruit or sandwiches, need to cater for the nutritionally well and nutritionally vulnerable. A minimum of two snacks per day is recommended (BDA, 2017a). Out-of-hours food services for a patient who has missed a meal, returned to the ward after a procedure, or is newly admitted also needs consideration. This could be a cold snack box-style option or a hot choice, again ensuring choice for therapeutic or special diets where possible. The logistics of ensuring the patient gets a safe and nutritious meal must also be considered.

Beverages

A selection of beverages – including tea, coffee, milk-based drinks, water, fruit juices, and cordials – should be readily available 24 hours a day, and a minimum of seven beverages must be offered to patients throughout the day, including in-between meals (HCA, 2013).

Therapeutic and special diet menus

It is important for ward staff to identify patients who have a clinical need for a therapeutic or special diet menu, such as those with coeliac disease, lactose intolerance, low sodium or low potassium requirements, neutropenic diets, and allergies, as well as those requiring cultural or religious choices. This need should be communicated to food service staff to ensure that the patient is provided with suitable, safe food and drinks. A summary of the diets likely to be required in the healthcare setting can be seen in Table 4.4.4. Food services must cater for those with specialist needs. Meals may need to be made to order by a diet chef or purchased in already prepared form from an external manufacturer. Regular training of chefs and food service staff is key to ensuring safety and consistency in meal preparation. Standard recipes and procedures must be followed along with any specific guidelines from the dietitian. Food services should be monitored to ensure they are following the agreed procedures. Food service staff will be able to advise patients if any of the 14 main allergens are present (BDA, 2014).

Designing flexible menus that are focused on group needs, such as finger food menus for dementia patients

Table 4.4.4 Summary of diets in the healthcare setting

Diet type	Summary
Standard diets	Meet the nutritional needs of the majority of the population, and should use dietary codes to communicate key information to this core group of patients.
Modified-texture diets	Meet the Dysphagia Diet Food Texture Descriptors (NPSA, 2012) needed for those with oropharyngeal dysphagia. A set of guidelines has been produced by the International Dysphagia Diet Standardisation Initiative (IDDSI, 2016). It has been recommended that the UK adopt IDDSI in place of the current standards, and both the BDA and Royal College of Speech and Language Therapists are planning for these to be introduced by April 2019.
Religious, cultural, personal and lifestyle considerations	Meet cultural or religious choices, including vegan and personal preferences Some meals, e.g. halal and kosher, are purchased in as they are prepared in specially approved kitchens. This ensures authenticity and acceptability for patients.
Therapeutic diets	Specific menus and/or foods are prescribed by the dietitian as part of the treatment for a medical condition, e.g. low-potassium meals for renal patients, or gluten-free foods for patients with coeliac disease.
Test or investigation diets	Temporary diets to be followed prior to surgery, e.g. low fat before a cholecystectomy.
Specific patient groups	Increasingly, hospitals are providing menu options for specific patient groups, such as maternity and oncology patients.

or paediatric menus, is critical to improving the nutrition and hydration of end users. Ensuring accessibility to appropriate crockery and cutlery is essential for anyone who requires this, such as two-handed beakers, plate lips and left-handed cutlery. Braille menus for visually impaired patients or menus translated into different languages appropriate to the local population are also readily in use. This should encourage an improved patient experience and support better nutrition and hydration for the patient or resident.

Food service systems

There are a number of systems that can be adopted in order to provide food to end users (Tables 4.4.5, 4.4.6 and 4.4.7). Food may be cooked on site from fresh, raw ingredients, or bought in already cooked, in either a chilled or frozen format to be reheated (regenerated) when required. It is difficult to establish how many hospitals cook fresh, as they often use hybrid systems, e.g. a hospital might cook fresh for the majority of patients but may buy in frozen, prepared, modified-texture meals. Anecdotal evidence estimates that 40% of hospitals use a cook/chill or cook/freeze system, while 60% cook freshly.

Kitchens and food safety

Space in both the main and ward kitchens will be of consideration in the type of food service system implemented. Space is not always readily available, so some healthcare settings use a combination of systems. Some hospitals have diet bay areas where trained diet chefs can cook to order. Others do not, and may have to buy meals in. Food safety and the handling of food must comply with all food safety legislation (FSA, 2017), and healthcare establishments will develop their own policies to achieve this (HCA, 2013).

Table 4.4.5 Food service systems – preparation and storage

System of food preparation and storage	Benefits	Concerns
Cook fresh		
Food is prepared and cooked on site in a traditional manner, distributed at the appropriate temperature, either plated or in bulk	Flexibility – recipes can be adapted quickly to meet unusual requirements Food preparation skills maintained on site Traditional and regional variability	Depends on a well-trained and skilled workforce Production facilities are expensive to maintain and take up a lot of space
Cook chill		
Food is cooked, quickly blast-chilled and stored at a controlled temperature for up to 5 days. It is then reheated (regenerated) and made ready for service. It is possible to include a combination of fresh/raw ingredients or partially/fully cooked ingredients which can be cooked using steam and pressure technology	Labour saving Cost-effective Reduces hot holding time of food, enhancing nutritional value and quality Can increase the variety of food available on the menu; however, depends on storage space	Regeneration must be done skilfully to optimise food quality and safety Some dishes are not suitable for this type of service (e.g. puff pastry dishes) Less flexible service and increased dependence on outside supplier if no production facilities are maintained on site Can be wasteful, as meal requirements must be estimated and order placed in advance. Regenerated meals cannot be re-used
Cook freeze		
Food is cooked, quickly blast-frozen and stored until required (up to 12 months). Frozen food can be distributed, and then reheated (regenerated) and made ready for service	As per cook chill Increased shelf life makes distribution logistics easier Less waste, as the food can be taken from freezer on the day the meal is required	As per cook chill Energy costs associated with freezing, storage and regeneration Need enough freezer space storage
Cook chill or freeze plated		
A variation of cook chill/cook freeze, where the food is plated, packed and sealed in a container. There are various types of packaging possible (e.g. packaging with a valve, which allows steam pressure cooking; or easy-opening packaging that allows food to be presented on a plate to the patient in a consistent way) The whole package is reheated (regenerated) in an oven or microwave	As per cook chill/cook freeze Allows patient choice at short notice, e.g. out of hours	As per cook chill/cook freeze

Table 4.4.6 Food service systems – distribution to the wards

Method	Benefits	Concerns
Plated service		
Food is plated centrally and distributed, or sent directly to the ward as individually packaged meals for reheating and plating at ward level	Good portion control Food safety risks contained in one area Fewer staff required on the ward Reduced food waste Efficient service	Difficult to maintain food temperature and quality during distribution (centrally plated only) Kitchen staff do not know who they are serving/reduced flexibility (centrally plated only)
Bulk food service (multi-portion)		
Food is distributed in containers and plated at ward level	Food choice takes place at bedside or point of service Food temperature and quality easier to maintain during distribution Flexibility in terms of garnishing the food and portion sizes Ward food service staff get to know the patients	More space required at ward level More food-handling risks at ward level Portion control more complex; however, portion sizes are more flexible More staff required at ward level to support an efficient service

Table 4.4.7 Food service systems – food service at ward or dining area

Method	Benefits	Concerns
Tray service		
Food is assembled on a tray and eaten at the bedside or in bed	No communal ward areas needed Tight control of therapeutic and special diets May be preferred by patients with eating difficulties (improved dignity) Privacy Suitable for bedbound patients	Second helpings more difficult to provide Lack of social interaction Assistance might be required with packaging If whole meal is served, parts of it may go cold
Trolley-style service		
Service users choose their meal at the trolley and can eat either at the bedside or/in a communal dining area, e.g. long-stay patients	Flexibility of service; food choice and portion size available at point of service Possibility of social interactions	More food service equipment needed at ward level Patients need to be mobile
Dining area service		
Service users eat together in a dining area, e.g. care home residents	As per trolley-style service Mealtimes become an occasion, and can be used as a rehabilitative activity	Requires a degree of independence or increased staffing Communal dining area needed

Budget

New standards and legislation such as the Hospital Food Standards Report (DH, 2014) and PLACE (DH, 2017a) have put hospitals under increased pressure to provide nutritious, environmentally sustainable food within financial targets and local cost improvement programmes. On average, the cost of feeding one in-patient per day in a general acute hospital is £11.07 (HSCIC, 2017). However, the amount of money that institutions have per head per day at their disposal varies greatly, and studies have shown that there is no direct link between the quality of food and the cost to the institution (DH, 2012).

Paper and electronic meal ordering

Orders can be taken on a paper menu card by the patient or ward staff. In some cases, this system of meal ordering may need to be done a day in advance, as it can be a lengthy process to collate all the information needed prior to food production. The use of technology has many advantages. Both hospitals and care homes are increasingly adopting electronic meal-ordering systems that allow ordering to be completed at the patient's bedside on a mobile device by a member of staff, closer to the service time. Patients will still need to see what is on offer, information that could be available on the hospital's Internet pages, a booklet menu at the bed side, or a poster on the wall.

The collated orders are electronically transferred to the main kitchen; food is then prepared and distributed to the wards as needed. Information is stored centrally, making it much easier to track food or meals. This is important for ward changes, new admissions and discharges. It also takes into consideration food allergies and special diets, which enhances patient safety. As a management tool, it supports closer control of costs and food waste.

Food waste

Food waste is indicative of both clinical and economic costs; a meal uneaten has no nutritional value (BDA, 2017a), and is just as expensive to produce as a meal that is eaten. Tackling food waste was identified by 83% of caterers as a priority at their trusts (CSC, 2016), and dietitians can take a pro-active role in monitoring this area. Managing Food Waste in the NHS states a target level of 10% plate waste (DH, 2005). Although evidence on current levels of hospital plate waste is limited, studies suggest that it may be upwards of 14% (DH, 2015). According to 57% of caterers, the biggest source of food waste was bulk trolley waste, when patients chose not to take their original choice, and 69% stated that ordering too far in advance was the biggest cause (CSC, 2016).

Kitchen-generated waste

Purchased food and ingredients must meet agreed standards. Strict stock management and rotation, the checking of freezer and fridge temperatures, and the use of lists and date stickers are simple methods to ensure minimal loss in the kitchen. Flexibility in the use of food not needed for patients in the hospital restaurants can help reduce waste, provided health and safety guidelines are adhered to.

Ward-generated waste

It is important to distinguish between trolley waste (food that is left over after the meal service) and plate waste (which indicates that the patient was unable to consume part or all of the meal). The reasons for this are important to the clinical staff and the food service department to ensure that patients enjoy their mealtime experience. Plate waste may indicate poor appetite or inadequate encouragement or support, but it may also highlight possible problems with the food itself, e.g. taste, temperature, quality, choice or presentation. Monitoring and analysing waste is important to understand if the food service system in place is working well, and if the menus are suitable for the patients or residents.

Initiatives to improve the patient experience

Many hospitals have implemented a protected mealtime policy to prevent unnecessary interruptions during the meal service. The use of a coloured tray may indicate to ward staff that a particular patient needs support with the meal. Patients who are able to mobilise to a dining table with other patients may well enjoy their meal and eat more. Ultimately, it is essential that patients reach their chosen meals which are nutritionally appropriate for them, plated in an appetising manner, and support provided to enable them to eat in a favourable environment. Volunteers or mealtime companions may facilitate this to a greater degree (WRAP, 2016). These initiatives need co-operation and good communication from all clinical and ward staff to be successful, and the dietitian can play a key role in training around this.

Audit

Audit should be built into each hospital's individualised food and drink strategy. Clear objectives and outcomes from both patient and food service perspectives should be linked to national standards, and the audit loop closed, ensuring that food services play a full role in the nutritional support of patients. Audit for all healthcare settings can be based around CQC inspection areas to ensure that nutrition standards are achieved (CQC, 2015).

Social media

Social media is a fast-growing communication method; 37% of the global population use social media (Weare-social, 2017). Twitter, Facebook, Pinterest and Instagram are well-known examples of social media platforms that are used regularly by the food industry and the NHS to promote their work. However, for any organisation, exposing itself to the social media world is not risk free, as it allows disgruntled customers to air their views very quickly to a large listener base. In particular, emotive subjects such as hospital food result in bad news generating much interest, particularly by newspaper and TV shows. This has resulted in most large organisations investing in a dedicated social media team who ensure that any negative comments are quickly rectified.

Promoting food services in healthcare

Providing safe, nutritious, appetising and tasty food in the healthcare setting is a challenge. The reasons for this are multifactorial but include reduced budgets, space/equipment restraints and a diverse patient group. However, in recent years, there have been great improvements in healthcare food provision, brought about by numerous factors, including new legislation and guidelines; a better understanding of challenges; and a sense of the catering, clinical and dietetic teams working together in an increasingly united way. It is important to highlight best practice and take opportunities to promote excellent and effective food and beverage services wherever possible.

Acknowledgement

The editor acknowledges the prior contribution of Richard Wilson.

Internet resources

British Dietetic Association Food Services Specialist Group, www.bda.uk.com/regionsgroups/groups/foodservices/home
Hospital Caterers Association, www.hospitalcaterers.org
National Association of Care Catering, www.thenacc.co.uk

References

BDA. (2014) *Allergen Toolkit for Healthcare Catering*. Available at https://www.bda.uk.com/publications/professional/food_allergen_toolkit_food_counts. Accessed 24 April 2017.

BDA. (2017a) *Impact of Dietetic Services on Food Service, Food Provision and Food Quality*. Available at https://www.bda.uk.com/improvinghealth/healthprofessionals/food_service_provision. Accessed 16 March 2018.

BDA. (2017b) *The Nutrition and Hydration Digest: Improving Outcomes through Food and Beverage Services*, 2nd edn. Available at https://www.bda.uk.com/publications/professional/NutritionHydrationDigest.pdf. Accessed 22 November 2017.

British Association of Parenteral and Enteral Nutrition (BAPEN). (2010) *Malnutrition Matters, Meeting Quality Standards in Nutritional Care*. [Online] Available at http://www.bapen.org.uk/pdfs/toolkit-for-commissioners.pdf. Accessed 24 April 2017.

British Association of Parenteral and Enteral Nutrition (BAPEN). (2012a) *The Hospital Nutrition Steering Committee*. Available at http://www.bapen.org.uk/resources-and-education/tools/ofnosh/nutrition-services?showall=1. Accessed 24 April 2017.

British Association of Parenteral and Enteral Nutrition (BAPEN). (2012b) *Nutrition Screening Survey in the UK and Republic of Ireland in 2011. Hospitals, Care Homes and Mental Health Units*. Available at http://www.bapen.org.uk/pdfs/nsw/nsw-2011-report.pdf. Accessed 24 April 2017.

British Association of Parenteral and Enteral Nutrition (BAPEN). (2016) *Malnutrition Universal Screening Tool (MUST)*. Available at http://www.bapen.org.uk/screening-and-must/must/must-toolkit. Accessed 22 November 2017.

Care Quality Commission (CQC). (2015) *Guidance for Providers on Meeting the Regulations*. Available at http://www.cqc.org.uk/sites/default/files/20150324_guidance_providers_meeting_regulations_01.pdf. Accessed 22 November 2017.

Care Quality Commission (CQC). (2017) *Regulation 14 Meeting Nutritional and Hydration Needs*. Available: at http://www.cqc.org.uk/content/regulation-14-meeting-nutritional-and-hydration-needs. Accessed 22 November 2017.

Carter L. (2015) The importance of maintaining good hydration in older people. Nursing in Practice (85). Available at https://www.nursinginpractice.com/article/importance-maintaining-good-hydration-older-people. Accessed 9 October 2018.

Cost Sector Catering (CSC). (2016) *Hospital caterers blame food waste on advanced meal ordering: April 2016*. Available at http://costsectorcatering.co.uk/hospital-caterers-blame-food-waste-advanced-meal-ordering. Accessed 24 April 2017.

Council of Europe Resolution (CoE). (2003) *Food and Nutritional Care in Hospitals: How to Prevent Under-Nutrition – Report and Recommendations of the Committee of Experts on Nutrition, Food Safety and Consumer Protection*. Strasbourg: Council of Europe Publishing.

Department for Environment, Food and Rural Affairs (Defra). (2015) *The Government Buying Standards for Food and Catering Services*. Available at https://www.gov.uk/government/uploads/system/uploads/attachment_data/file/418072/gbs-food-catering-march2015.pdf. Accessed 22 November 2017.

DH. (2003) *Care Homes for Older People, National Minimum Standards*. Available at http://www.dignityincare.org.uk/_library/resources/dignity/csipcomment/csci_national_minimum_standards.pdf. Accessed 24 April 2017.

DH. (2005) *Managing Food Waste in the NHS*. Available at https://www.2degreesnetwork.com/groups/2degrees-community/resources/dept-health-managing-food-waste-nhs/. Accessed 24 April 2017.

DH. (2009) *Healthy Weight, Healthy Lives: One Year On*. Available at http://webarchive.nationalarchives.gov.uk/20100407220245/http://www.dh.gov.uk/prod_consum_dh/groups/dh_digitalassets/documents/digitalasset/dh_097623.pdf. Accessed 24 April 2017.

DH. (2012) *NHS spends more on hospital food but significant variation remains*. Available at https://www.gov.uk/government/news/nhs-spends-more-on-hospital-food-but-significant-variation-remains. Accessed 24 April 2017.

DH. (2014) *The Hospital Food Standards Panel's report on standards for food and drink in NHS hospitals*. Available at https://www.gov.uk/government/uploads/system/uploads/attachment_data/file/523049/Hospital_Food_Panel_May_2016.pdf. Accessed 24 April 2017.

DH. (2015) *Hospital Food Standards Panel – Summary Cost Benefit Analysis*. Available at https://www.gov.uk/government/uploads/system/uploads/attachment_data/file/399349/hospital-food-cb-analysis.pdf. Accessed 24 April 2017.

DH. (2016) *A toolkit to support the development of a hospital food and drink strategy*. Available at https://www.gov.uk/government/uploads/system/uploads/attachment_data/file/499745/Toolkit_Feb_16.pdf. Accessed 24 April 2017.

DH. (2017a) *Patient-Led Assessments of the Care Environment (PLACE) – NHS England*. Available at http://www.digital.nhs.uk/catalogue/PUB30055. Accessed 22 November 2017.

DH. (2017b) *Compliance with Hospital Food Standards in the NHS*. Available at https://www.gov.uk/government/uploads/system/uploads/attachment_data/file/586490/HFSP_Report.pdf. Accessed 22 November 2017.

FSA. (2017) *General Food Law*. Available at https://www.food.gov.uk/enforcement/regulation/foodlaw. Accessed 22 November 2017.

Health and Social Care Information Centre (HSCIC). (2017) *Hospital Estates and Facilities Statistics (ERIC Returns)*. Available at http://hefs.hscic.gov.uk/DataFiles.asp. Accessed 22 November 2017.

Hospital Caterers Association (HCA). (2013) *A Good Practice Guide to Ward Level Services*. Available at http://www.hospitalcaterers.org/publications/. Accessed 24 April 2017.

National Association of Care Catering (NACC). (2014) *Nutritional Standards for Adults*. Available at http://www.thenacc.co.uk/shop/category/Good+Practice+Guides. Accessed 24 April 2017.

National Patient Safety Agency (NPSA). (2012) *Dysphagia Diet Food Texture Descriptors*. Available at https://docs.google.com/a/nihr.ac.uk/viewer?a=v&pid=sites&srcid=bmloci5hYy51a3xkeXNwaGFnaWEtdG9vbGtpdHxneDo1MzRlODJjZTQ0NWQyYjhh. Accessed 24 April 2017.

NHS Employers. (2015) *Obesity and the Impact on the NHS: Infographic*. Available at http://www.nhsemployers.org/case-studies-and-resources/2015/01/obesity-and-the-impact-on-the-nhs-infographic. Accessed 24 April 2017.

NHS England. (2015) *10 Key Characteristics of Good Nutrition and Hydration Care*. Available at https://www.england.nhs.uk/commissioning/nut-hyd/10-key-characteristics/. Accessed 24 April 2017.

NHS England. (2016a) *2017/19 NHS Standard Contract*. Available at https://www.england.nhs.uk/nhs-standard-contract/17-18/. Accessed 22 November 2017.

NHS England. (2016b) *2016/17 CQUIN*. Available at https://www.england.nhs.uk/nhs-standard-contract/cquin/cquin-16-17/. Accessed at 24 April 2017.

NHS England. (2017) *Action to reduce sales of sugar-sweetened beverages on NHS premises*. Available at https://www.england.nhs.uk/wp-content/uploads/2017/04/sugar-action-doc.pdf. Accessed 2 September 2017.

NHS Digital (2016) Health survey for England. Available at https://digital.nhs.uk/data-and-information/publications/statistical/health-survey-for-england/health-survey-for-england-2016. Accessed 9 October 2018.

PHE. (2017) *Healthier and More Sustainable Catering: Nutrition Principles*. Available at https://www.gov.uk/government/uploads/system/uploads/attachment_data/file/595126/Healthier_and_more_suistainable_nutrition_principles.pdf. Accessed 24 April 2017.

The International Dysphagia Diet Standardisation Initiative (IDDSI). (2016) *The IDDSI Framework and Descriptors*. Available at http://iddsi.org/framework/. Accessed 23 November 2017.

The Waste and Resources Action Programme (WRAP). (2016) *Preventing Waste in the Healthcare Sector*. Available at http://www.wrap.org.uk/content/preventing-waste-healthcare-sector. Accessed 24 April 2017.

Wearesocial. (2017) *Digital in 2017: Global Overview*. Available at https://wearesocial.com/uk/special-reports/digital-in-2017-global-overview. Accessed 23 November 2017.

Wilson R. (2014) Food service: Hospitals and institutions. In: Gandy J (ed) *Manual of Dietetic Practice*, 5th edn. Chichester UK: Wiley Blackwell.

Wise J. (2015) Patients admitted to hospital from care homes are at higher risk of dehydration, study finds. *BMJ* 2015; 350:h249.

4.4.2 Prisons

Laura Rowe

Key points

- The institution provides, depending on the category of prison, all food and drink, apart from some snacks and soft drinks.
- The prison governor has responsibility for catering and enforcing Ministry of Justice instructions.
- Food plays a key role in the physical, mental and emotional well-being of prisoners.
- Prison populations are at risk of obesity and associated health risks.

SECTION 4

Unlike other institutions, prisons provide all the food and drink, apart from some snacks and soft drinks, consumed by prisoners. Generally, prisoners can purchase additional snacks and drinks from the canteen. The primary objective of prison catering is '… *to provide a varied and healthy menu which takes account of prisoners' preferences whilst maintaining compliance with all relevant food safety legislation*' (Department of Justice Northern Ireland, 1995). Since 1994, the prison population has risen by approximately 41,000, to around 85,000 in 2016 (Ministry of Justice, 2016).

Meal provision and dietary quality

The quality and quantity of food available in prison has a significant impact on prisoners' quality of life, health and behaviour. Food is key to the physical, mental and emotional well-being of prisoners. Mealtimes represent a focal point of the day in prison, breaking the monotony of prison life (HM Inspectorate of Prisons, 2016). In the UK, Instruction PS44/2210 (Ministry of Justice, 2010) details prison catering services. All prisons use a preselected, multichoice, cyclical menu for lunch and evening meal, which covers a minimum 4-week cycle. Prison rule 24 requires the provision of three meals per day, but the daily energy intakes from meals are not stipulated. It has been noted that young offenders, who generally have a greater energy requirement, are not offered larger portions to account for this (HM Inspectorate of Prisons, 2016). The average daily allowance for food is £2.02 per day, increased from £1.87 in 2006 (National Offender Management Service, 2015).

The Ministry of Justice (2010) instruction on catering states that '… *food provided shall be wholesome, nutritious, well prepared and served, reasonably varied and sufficient in quality*'. The NAO report found that food served to prisoners was in line with national recommendations as given in the Balance of Good Health, which has been superseded by the Eatwell Guide (see Chapter 2.1, Dietary reference values and food-based dietary guidelines). A recent report from the HM Inspectorate of Prisons (2016) reviewed food provision in prisons and found that the food served was of a reasonable quality and quantity; however, prisoner feedback was that the food was generally poor. Almost all the inspected establishments offered menus that catered for religious and other dietary requirements; however, choice was usually very restricted. In line with previous reports, early mealtimes continue to be a problem, with lunches being served as early at 11.10 am and evening meals at 4.15 pm; this can cause challenges for prisoners requiring medications at mealtimes. At most prisons, snacks items were available to purchase, but the majority of these were high in fat, sugar and salt. Servery supervision was also a concern, with bullying, favouritism in portion sizes, and food running out being some of the problems. The report recommended to the National Offender Management Service that minimal nutritional values should be set out and that meal times should be re-arranged to reflect social norms out of prison (HM Inspectorate of Prisons, 2016).

The prison governor has the overall responsibility for catering standards, and the kitchens are inspected daily by the prison governor or an assistant. The catering manager at each prison is responsible for implementing standards. Her Majesty's Inspectorate of Prisons and the Independent Monitoring Board are responsible for monitoring all aspects of prison life, including catering. The prison authorities also recognise that appropriate support for prisoners around healthy eating education is important during the rehabilitation and re-integration phases (HM Inspectorate of Prisons, 2016).

Non-communicable diseases

Offenders are drawn from a population with significantly raised risk of developing a range of non-communicable diseases (NCDs) such as obesity, cardiovascular disease (CVD), diabetes and cancer. Conditions requiring self-care are challenging to manage in a prison setting; however, conversely, for prisoners with a previously chaotic lifestyle, prison may allow them to adopt health-promoting activities. Prison-based health assessments should include discussions about healthy diets and healthier food options available in the prison (NICE, 2016).

A systematic review (Herbert *et al.*, 2012) showed an increase in some risk factors for NCDs; female prisoners were more likely than men to be overweight or obese. UK prisoners were less physically active than the general population. Plugge *et al.* (2009) surveyed CVD risk factors in female prisoners in the UK and found that 30% were obese, 86% did not eat five or more pieces of fruit and vegetables per day, 85% smoked and 87% were insufficiently active. The authors repeated the survey a month into the women's sentences and found few improvements in risk factors.

There is an absence of robust, systematic, healthy lifestyle education for prisoners, which was previously highlighted by Plugge *et al.* (2009). This is despite the NAO (2006) report recommending that the Prison Service should raise awareness of healthy eating by educating prisoners, using posters and actively promoting healthy eating on a regular basis. Throughout Europe and North America, there are examples of prison-food-related interventions, including nutrition education, gardening and healthy choices in the shop, and cookery lessons (WHO, 2015). Wide-scale programmes exist in the USA, e.g. the WISEWOMAN programme, which provides heart disease screening and interventions in women's prisons (Khavjou *et al.*, 2007). It has helped identify undiagnosed hypertension and dyslipidaemia, and offers interventions to improve health.

Dietetic practice in prisons and with prisoners

Given the rising levels of nutrition-related diseases, it is likely that dietitians will increasingly be asked to advise prisons or prisoners (either in prisons or hospitals). Currently, there is no guidance for dietitians working in prisons on how to deal with situations such as patients in restraints, lack of privacy and the prison regimen. The British Medical Association (2009) provides guidance on the medical care for prisoners that dietitians may find useful. The guidance states the following:

- Detained prisoners must have the same standards of care as the rest of society, including respect for patient dignity and privacy.
- To determine the degree of supervision required, risk assessment must be carried out prior to a prisoner going into hospital. Risk assessment includes: the prisoner's condition, any medical objection to the use of restraints, nature of the prisoner's offence, security of the consulting room and risk of violence to self or others.
- Where escape is unlikely, escort and bed watch by one prison officer, without restraints, is sufficient.
- Hospitals should be informed in advance about the levels of escort and restraint envisaged, and hospital staff should have the opportunity to discuss when the level of restraint is clinically unacceptable.

More recently, prisons are increasingly using telemedicine for consultations between prisoners and healthcare professionals, including dietitians.

Nutrition and behaviour

The relationship between nutrition and criminal or delinquent behaviour is receiving increasing attention; however, evidence remains sparse. Benton (2007) reviewed the evidence for a relationship between diet and antisocial, violent and criminal behaviour. A meta-analysis showed that elimination diets reduced hyperactivity-related symptoms and that polyunsaturated fatty acid supplementation decreased violence in children. Vitamin and mineral supplements reduced antisocial behaviour, and aggression was linked to low blood glucose levels in adults. Benton (2007) concluded that the reactions to foods were inconsistent and not observed in all participants. There is clearly a need for more well-designed research in this area.

Acknowledgement

The editor acknowledges the prior contribution of Joan Gandy.

Further reading

Cross M, MacDonald B. (2009) *Nutrition in Institutions*. Oxford: Wiley Blackwell.

WHO. (2015) *Food systems in correctional settings*. Available at http://www.euro.who.int/__data/assets/pdf_file/0006/292965/Food-systems-correctional-settings-literature-review-case-study.pdf?ua=1. Accessed 5 October 2016.

Internet resources

Department of Justice Northern Ireland, www.dojni.gov.uk/catering
Inside Time (national newspaper for prisoners), www.insidetime.org
Ministry of Justice, www.justice.gov.uk
National Audit Office, www.nao.org.uk
Vegan Prisoners Support Group, www.vpsg.org

References

Benton D. (2007) The impact of diet on anti-social, violent and criminal behaviour. *Neurosci. Biobehav. Rev.* 31: 752–774.

Department of Justice Northern Ireland. (1995) *Catering*. Available at www.dojni.gov.uk/catering. Accessed 8 March 2013.

Herbert K, Plugge E, Foster C, *et al.* (2012) Prevalence of risk factors for non-communicable diseases in prison populations worldwide: a systematic review. *Lancet* 379: 1975–1982.

HM Inspectorate of Prisons (2016, July). *Life in Prison: Food Report*. Available at https://www.justiceinspectorates.gov.uk/hmiprisons/wp-content/uploads/sites/4/2016/09/Life-in-prison-Food-Web-2016.pdf. Accessed 9 October 2018.

Khavjou OA, Clarke J, Hofeldt RM, *et al.* (2007) A captive audience: bringing the WISEWOMAN program to South Dakota prisoners. *Women's Health Issues*. 17: 193–201.

Ministry of Justice. (2010) *Instruction PS44/2210: Catering – Meals for Prisoners*. Available at www.justice.gov.uk/offenders/psis. Accessed 8 March 2013.

Ministry of Justice. (2016) *Prison Population Figures*. Available at www.gov.uk/government/statistics/prison-population-figures-2016. Accessed 16 September 2016.

National Audit Office (NAO). (2006) *HM Prison Service – Serving Time: Prisoner Diet and Exercise*. Available at https://www.nao.org.uk/report/serving-time-prisoner-diet-and-exercise/. Accessed 9 October 2018.

National Offender Management Service. (2015) *Freedom of Information Request*. Available at www.gov.uk/government/uploads/system/uploads/attachment_data/file/438939/daily-food-allowance-per-prisoner.doc. Accessed 5 October 2016.

NICE. (2016) *Physical Health of People in Prison Guideline*. Available at www.nice.org.uk/guidance/GID-CGWAVE0729/documents/short-version-of-draft-guideline-2. Accessed 5 October 2015.

Plugge EH, Foster CE, Yudkin PL, *et al.* (2009) Cardiovascular disease risk factors and women prisoners in the UK: the impact of imprisonment. *Health Promot. Int.* 24: 334–343.

4.4.3 Armed Forces

Paula Wood

SECTION 4

Key points

- A Ministry of Defence (MOD) contractor is responsible for the procurement, management, storage and distribution of food worldwide.
- The UK Armed Forces have military chefs whose primary role is food supply and provision on deployments.
- Military personnel are provided with nutrition education throughout their careers to help optimise their health and physical and cognitive performance.

The MOD has a duty of care to supply all recruits and serving members of the Armed Forces with appropriate nutrition to support their health and well-being. Food is supplied worldwide to personnel to ensure these requirements are met. Defence Equipment and Support (a bespoke training entity of MOD) is responsible for food supply and has contracted a supplier to deliver this. The Defence Catering Manual Joint Service Publication 456 covers every aspect of food provision (Ministry of Defence, 2016). Contractors must conform to a quality standard and supply products that provide choice and meet the healthy eating policy.

In military establishments, the Pay as You Dine (PAYD) system provides catering for non-operational food service; it is not used in military recruit and officer cadet training establishments or in the operational context. This system replaced the daily food charge, which was deducted from service personnel's salary regardless of whether food was taken or not. The system provides three core meals, and personnel only pay for food taken; they also have access to other foods. The core meals must provide at least six items at breakfast and lunch, and provide a three-course dinner. Some bases provide cooking facilities, enabling those that live there to self-cater; many personnel do not live on base.

The MOD developed the Military Dietary Reference Values (2008), followed by further recommendations for energy requirements for military personnel in an SACN statement (2016). These provide guidance on the macro- and micronutrient requirements for adults and adolescents who are operational, non-operational or undergoing training. The MOD has been proactive in developing nutrition and hydration guidance. It emphasises how appropriate nutrition and hydration will optimise physical and cognitive performance, reduce the risk of injury, promote quick recovery from arduous physical activity and maintain fitness and health. There are a number of guides available to recruits and trained personnel, including: Commanders' Guide – Nutrition for Health and Performance (Messer *et al.*, 2005), The Armed Forces Personal Guide to Nutrition (Casey & Wood, 2006), Commanders' Guide – Fluid Intake during Military Operations in the Heat (Nevola *et al.*, 2005) and Food for Thought DVD (DFS IPT, 2007).

The Armed Forces Nutrition Advisory Service offers advice and information on nutrition, diet and military feeding; this is only available to UK military personnel and MOD civil servants. Unlike the USA and Canada, there is no capacity for dietitians to be members of the Armed Forces in a dietetic role. A small number of dietitians are employed directly by MOD research establishments and healthcare providers. Other dietitians work in liaison with military medical services, e.g. Royal Centre for Defence Medicine, Birmingham.

Operational Ration Packs (ORPs)

Personnel are issued with individual 24-hour ORP when they are deployed on operations. The ORP is designed to be a sole source of nutrition over this period of time; field-catering facilities are provided as soon as is practicable. There are a number of ORPs available for specific operations (e.g. cold climate, jungle and patrol), and for cultural dietary requirements (e.g. vegetarian, kosher and halal). The 10-man ORP is designed to be used by military chefs in the field kitchen.

Acknowledgement

The editor acknowledges the prior contribution of Joan Gandy.

Further reading

Research and Technology Organisation, North Atlantic Treaty Organisation. (2010) Final Report of RTO Task Group RTG-154: Nutrition Science and Food Standards for Military Operations. *RTO-TR-HFM-154, AC/323(HFM-154)TP/291*. Available at https://www.sto.nato.int/publications/.../RTO-TR-HFM-154/$$TR-HFM-154-ALL.pdf. Last accessed 26 June 2016.

References

Casey A, Wood P. (2006) *The Armed Forces Personal Guide to Nutrition*. UK: Expert Panel on Armed Forces Feeding.

Casey S. (2008) *Military Dietary Reference Values*. Farnborough, UK: QinetiQ Ltd.

Defence Food Services Integrated Project Team (DFS IPT). (2007) *Food for Thought (DVD)*. British Defence Film Library No. C5117/06.

Messer P, Owen G, Casey A. (2005) *Commanders' Guide – Nutrition for Health and Performance*. UK: Expert Panel on Armed Forces Feeding.

Ministry of Defence. (2016) The Defence Catering Manual JSP 456. Available at https://www.gov.uk/government/collections/defence-catering-manual-jsp-456. Last accessed 26 June 2016.

Nevola VR, Staerck J, Harrison M. (2005) *Commanders' Guide – Fluid Intake during Military Operations in the Heat*. UK: Expert Panel on Armed Forces Feeding.

SACN. (2016) *Statement on Military Dietary Reference Values for Energy*. Available at https://www.gov.uk/government/uploads/system/uploads/attachment_data/file/583321/SACN_military_DRVs_for_energy_position_statement.pdf. Last accessed February 2018.

4.5 Food law and labelling

Fionna Page and Ruth Birt

Key points

- Many UK laws relating to food, e.g. labelling, additives and claims, are of European Union (EU) origin.
- The Food Standards Agency (FSA) is responsible for food safety and food hygiene across the UK.
- Responsibilities for food labelling are split between the FSA, the Department of Health and the Department for Environment, Food and Rural Affairs (Defra).
- How the EU rules affect food law and labelling in the UK in the future will depend on the changes to the UK's membership in the EU.

SECTION 4

History of food legislation in the UK

After years of attempts at food regulation since 1266, the Food and Drugs Act 1938 was the first to combine specific food legislation with public health measures; at this time, food poisoning became notifiable across the UK. The act introduced controls for new areas such as misleading labelling and advertising, and powers were introduced to regulate the composition and labelling of foods, as well as on the sanitary conditions of food on sale for human consumption. The act was suspended for the duration of World War 2; however, owing to concerns about food substitutes being passed off as originals and insufficient nutrition being provided to ensure a staple diet to keep people fit and healthy, emergency powers were introduced. In 1955, a consolidating Food and Drug Act came into being, which was to remain the basis for food legislation until general legislation covering the composition, labelling, hygiene and safety of food in the UK was introduced in 1984 with the Food Act (the Medicines Act superseded the drug aspect in 1968). However, during the 1980s, there was a general increase in the number of reported cases of food poisoning, and a number of well-publicised food scares linked to *Salmonella* infection in raw eggs, *Listeria* contamination in foods such as soft cheeses and pâtés (believed to increase the number of miscarriages and stillbirths), and an outbreak of botulism caused by hazelnut yoghurt. In July 1989, the government announced far-reaching proposals to change the law in a white paper titled *Food Safety – Protecting the Consumer*. As a result, food legislation underwent its first major review since the 1940s, culminating in the Food Safety Act 1990.

In the UK, there is now an extensive array of legislation, codes of practice and guidance covering the whole area of food from production to distribution, packing, labelling and sale, and these may be of UK origin or be influenced or driven by European or international standards.

International food legislation

Since food is both imported into and exported from the UK, legislation on the standards of composition and labelling must be compatible with, and, in some instances, comply with, international standards.

The European Union

Membership in the European Union (EU) has meant that the UK has been required to implement European Commission (EC) regulations and directives, and this has been a major influence on UK food legislation. The implications of the UK leaving the EU and its impact on food law and labelling are not yet clear.

Codex Alimentarius Commission

Codex, as it is usually known, has a fundamental mandate to develop international standards and norms for consumer health protection and fair practices in the food trade. It is comprised of two United Nation bodies, the Food and Agriculture Organization and the World Health Organization, and has a wide membership of the majority of developing and developed countries. Codex recommendations have no statutory force, but members

Manual of Dietetic Practice, Sixth Edition. Edited by Joan Gandy.

Companion website: www.manualofdieteticpractice.com

are encouraged to apply its norms to the widest extent possible as a basis for domestic regulation and international trade. In general, Codex standards are incorporated into European, and hence UK, legislation, and, in recent years, have been important in the resolution of trade disputes across continents.

Current UK food legislation

An understanding of the different types of legislation gives an insight into how and when food legislation becomes effective in the UK. Since the UK is a currently a member of the EU, all EU regulations and directives must be implemented in the UK regulatory system. This is possible under the Food Safety Act 1990 (classed as primary legislation), which not only provides the framework for all domestic food legislation, but also the powers to make secondary legislation to implement EU laws. This may change over time due to changes in the UK's membership in the EU.

Regulations and directives

EC Regulations are effective in all member states as soon as the EC Council adopts them. EC Directives, on the other hand, do not become effective until they are written into a country's own legislation and, in the UK, they are actually also called regulations. For example, to allow for enforcement and execution of the EU Novel Foods Regulation, EC 258/97, the UK had to introduce its own regulations, called The Novel Foods and Novel Food Ingredients Regulations 1997 (SI 1997/1335). European legislation is denoted by EC, followed by the number (in this case, 258) and the year of publication. The UK regulation is denoted by SI (for statutory instrument), the year of publication and the number (in this case, 1335). These unique identifying numbers are important for citing the correct piece of legislation.

Most of the key provisions in food law are contained in legislation that sets out the specific details governing matters, such as the following:

- Food labelling.
- Food hygiene.
- Animal, meat and meat products, e.g. those concerned with the examination for residues and maximum residue limits.
- Registration of food premises.
- Regulations on milk and dairies.
- Food composition.
- Use of food additives.
- Use of food-packaging materials.

Regulations are kept under review and are subject to change (in the form of amendments), either as a result of review or in order to harmonise food law within the EU. Some important regulations are those concerning labelling, sweeteners, colours, flavouring, miscellaneous food additives and organic foods. In addition to these general (horizontal) regulations that apply across food categories, there are specific (vertical) regulations applying to the composition of specific foods, such as bread and flour, chocolate and chocolate products, milk and soft drinks. There are also specific hygiene regulations relating to the production of milk, meat and other animal products.

Previously, certain specialist categories of foods for particular nutritional uses (dietetic foods) had specific compositional and labelling rules as laid down in the European PARNUTS Directive 2009/39/EC. This was fully repealed in July 2016, with some categories now being governed by general food law, e.g. sports foods. A framework for certain specialist foods has been retained as the regulation on *Foods for Specific Groups* (Regulation (EU) No. 609/2013). These include foods intended for infants and young children (infant formulae, follow-on formulae and weaning foods); foods for special medical purposes (FSMPs), such as sip and tube feeds, among others; and total diet replacement for weight control. Individual EU-delegated regulations have been published for infant and follow-on formulae (Regulation (EU) No. 2016/127), FSMPs (Regulation (EU) No. 2016/128) and total diet replacement products for weight control (Regulation (EU) No. 2017/1798); these stipulate specific compositional and information requirements. The updated delegated regulation on weaning foods (*Processed Cereal Based Foods and other Baby Foods*) is not expected until 2019/2020, as the EC has issued a mandate to the European Food Safety Authority (EFSA) to consider if any update on the age of introduction of such foods is necessary. The EC will be considering those products currently on the market, and individual dietary guidelines, before confirming if there is any need to change current compositional guidelines.

Gluten-free foods are now legislated under Regulation (EU) No. 1169/2011 on *Food Information to Consumers*, but the rules and gluten levels for the use of the terms *gluten-free* and *very low gluten* from earlier EU-harmonised rules have been retained, as follows:

- *Gluten free* – the gluten content of foods bearing this claim must not exceed 20 ppm.
- *Very low gluten* – the gluten content of foods bearing this claim must not exceed 100 ppm (only foods with cereal ingredients that have been specially processed to remove the gluten may make this claim).

The Food Safety Act

The Food Safety Act (1990) is the main piece of UK legislation on food safety and consumer protection in Great Britain (GB); a separate but similar law applies in Northern Ireland. The act provides the framework for UK food law but does not, in itself, contain the specific rules governing matters such as the safety, quality, and description or labelling of food. These details are set out in regulations and orders (classed as secondary legislation) made under the act. Codes of practice can also be issued under Section 40 of the Food Safety Act 1990. These are documents issued by ministers for the guidance of food authorities, the provisions for which can be enforced by direction and court order.

The aims of the Food Safety Act are to:

- Ensure that all food produced for sale is safe to eat, meets quality expectations and is not misleadingly presented.
- Provide legal powers and penalties.
- Enable the UK to fulfil its responsibilities in the EC.
- Keep pace with technological change.

The Food Safety Act (1990) has four main parts: preliminary; main provisions; administration and enforcement; and miscellaneous and supplemental.

Part I: Preliminary

This sets out the full scope of the act and the responsibilities for those involved in enforcing it. It covers the whole of GB and provides for regulations covering all aspects of food production, processing and selling, from the farm to the retailer. Its definitions of food have been widened to include slimming aids, dietary supplements and tap water, and premises now include most Crown properties, ships and aircraft. The act also sets out the principle that local authorities are responsible for enforcing most aspects of food law.

Part II: Main provisions

The main provisions of the act, namely food safety, consumer protection, regulation-making powers and defences, are covered in this part of the act.

Offences

The main offences under the Food Safety Act are:

- Selling, or possessing for sale, food that does not comply with food safety requirements.
- Rendering food injurious to health.
- Selling, to the purchaser's prejudice, food that is not of the nature, substance or quality demanded.
- Falsely or misleadingly describing or presenting food.

Food safety requirements apply to food throughout the food chain, and not just that for retail sale. Food is injurious to health if it could harm part of the population either in the short term, e.g. cause food poisoning, or long term, e.g. contaminated with lead. *Not of the nature or substance demanded* means that it is illegal to sell cod described as 'haddock', or cola instead of 'diet cola'. A purchaser can range from a customer at a shop to one supplier buying from another. *Falsely or misleadingly described or presented* applies to written statements or pictorial representations which are untrue. Additional constraints are also laid down in food labelling regulations.

Defences

One significant aspect of food legislation introduced under the 1990 act was that due diligence became grounds for defence. Thus, for example, a retailer who unwittingly sold a contaminated food would not be guilty if it could be shown that the contamination occurred at an earlier stage in the supply chain and that the retailer could not have known that the product was unfit for sale. In practice, this means that the onus is on the food industry and food importers to supply safe food, and this is considered to be a far-reaching and important aspect of the act.

Novel foods

The act also contains powers to make regulations covering the sale of novel foods, i.e. those that are new or have only been rarely eaten in this country. Another significant piece of legislation then introduced was the EU Regulation (EC) No 258/97 concerning novel foods and novel food ingredients, which applies to the placing of novel foods or ingredients onto the EU market that have not previously been used for human consumption to a significant degree. Detailed rules for the authorisation of novel foods, ingredients and processes were laid down, including the introduction of a means of mandatory notification for foods or ingredients containing, consisting of, or produced from genetically modified organisms (GMOs), subsequently updated over the years. Regulation EC No 258/97 and updates will soon be repealed and replaced by Regulation (EU) 2015/2283, which has been introduced to simplify the current authorisation procedure and to take account of recent developments in EU law and technological progress. It will introduce a centralised risk assessment process performed by EFSA.

Part III: Administration and enforcement

This lays down procedures for the sampling and analysis of products, powers of entry, obstruction and enforcement. It also deals with the legal aspects of prosecution and appeal procedures.

Part IV: Miscellaneous and supplemental

This covers the issuing of codes of practice to food authorities on the execution and enforcement of legislation, and directions on the specific steps to be taken to comply with a code. Other details pertain to the areas of coverage of the act and the other aspects of its implementation.

Other food-related UK legislation

Several other Acts of Parliament, and their subsidiary regulations, also impact in various ways on the provision, sale or safety of food. It was the Food Standards Act 1999 that set up the Food Standards Agency (FSA) and transferred functions and powers relating to food standards and safety to it. The FSA is an independent government department which provides advice and information to the public and government on food safety from farm to fork. It also protects consumers through effective food enforcement and monitoring. The FSA is accountable to parliament through health ministers, and to the devolved administrations in Scotland, Wales and Northern Ireland for its activities within their areas. The FSA obtains independent expert advice from its scientific advisory committees, and commissions research to support its functions.

European legislation on general food safety is contained in the General Food Law Regulation (EC) 178/2002, which introduced many key procedures for food safety matters, including the establishment of EFSA. In the UK, the General Food Regulations 2004 No 3279 (and amendments) provides for the enforcement of certain provisions of Regulation (EC) 178/2002 (including imposing penalties), and amends the Food Safety Act 1990 to bring it in line with Regulation (EC) 178/2002. Similar legislation applies in Northern Ireland.

An excellent guide to food law is supplied by the FSA as The Food Law Guide (www.food.gov.uk). It covers legislation in effect in England, Wales and Northern Ireland. The Food Standards Scotland (www.foodstandards.gov.scot) also has useful information. Food Standards Scotland (FSS) is the public sector food body for Scotland, launched on 1 April 2015, taking over the responsibilities previously carried out in Scotland by the FSA, with an increased role in regards to healthy eating. The FSS has been established to provide independent information and advice on food safety and standards, nutrition, and labelling to consumers in Scotland.

Law enforcement

The FSA works with enforcement officers to ensure that food (and feed) law is applied across the entire food chain as a result of its statutory powers to strengthen enforcement of food standards, and to ensure that national objectives are delivered. The responsibilities of all the enforcement authorities in the UK are set out, and agreements are in place that provide a structure to the FSA's supervision of local authority enforcement work.

The Food Law Codes of Practice for each of the four countries in the UK set out the way local authorities should apply food law, and how they should work with food businesses. The FSA (and FSS) provides guidance on specific regulations that are relevant to enforcement officers and food businesses to ensure that the law is clear. The Local Government Association (LGA) provides one link between local food enforcement in England and Wales, and the central government, giving advice and guidance to local authorities.

Local enforcement officers have wide powers to inspect any stage of the production, manufacturing, distribution, and retail chain, and have a responsibility to investigate any food complaints passed on to them by consumers. Food premises are inspected at a frequency dependent on risk. The frequency of physical inspections can vary from once every 6–24 months. Enforcement officers also have the power to take samples of food for testing to ensure compliance with food legislation, as well as the powers to take action against food premises that do not comply with the food law. This enforcement action can range from issuing warnings and improvement or prohibition notices, to instigating prosecutions. The courts can inflict heavy penalties for non-compliance, including the closure of a business where conditions are particularly bad.

Food labelling

Food labels are the principal method by which consumers get information about their food. Labels must be accurate and must not mislead, so that consumers can make informed choices about the food they buy. From October 2010, the responsibility for food labelling was divided between three government departments in the UK, as illustrated in Figure 4.5.1. The FSA leads on food safety–related labelling. Nutrition labelling sits with the Department of Health (DH) to help towards a consistent approach to nutrition policy. Other areas of non-safety-related food labelling are the responsibility of the Defra, whose role also includes coordination of labelling policy across government. It should be noted that responsibilities for food labelling differ across the UK home countries.

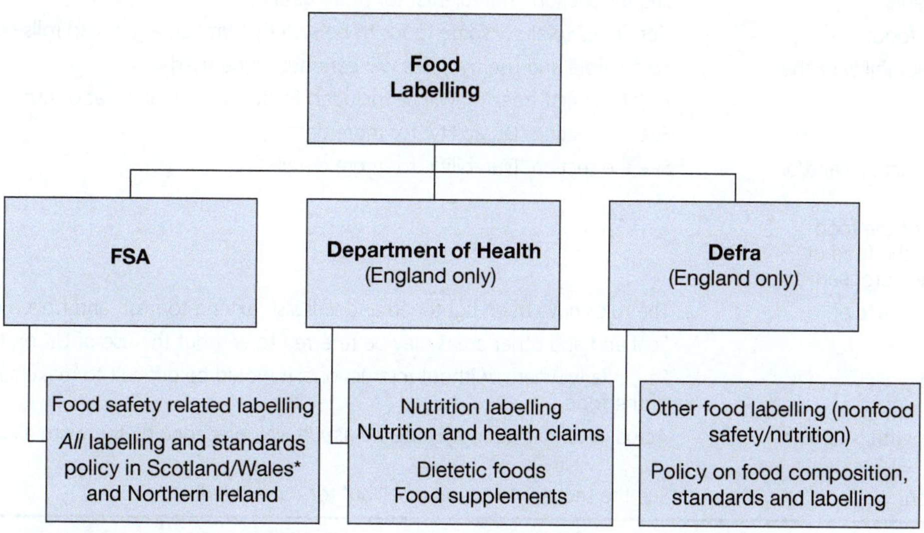

Figure 4.5.1 Responsibility for food labelling in the UK
*Except responsibility for nutrition labelling which lies with the Welsh Assembly Government

Labelling regulations

Food information regulation (FIR)

Food labelling in the UK is principally controlled by the Food Information for Consumers Regulation No. 1169/2011 (FIR). The general principle of FIR is primarily to provide a basis for consumers to make informed choices about the food they consume, and to prevent misleading practices. It also prohibits claims that foods prevent, treat or cure human disease; the so-called medicinal claims.

The legislation includes rules on nutrition labelling, provision of allergen information, labelling clarity, added caffeine in foods and high-caffeine drinks, country-of-origin labelling, the labelling of water content of some meat and fish products, and voluntary calorie labelling on alcoholic drinks. The FIR requires that all foods intended for the final consumer, including foods supplied to or delivered by mass caterers (subject to certain exceptions), be marked or labelled with the mandatory food information as shown in Table 4.5.1. Nutrition labelling is now mandatory on most prepacked foods.

Additional mandatory information is required on some foods, e.g. foods packaged in certain gases, foods containing sweeteners, certain frozen meat and fish products, and foods containing liquorice. Drinks high in caffeine (>150 mg/L), other than those based on tea or coffee or their extracts, will need to show the caffeine content in milligram per 100 mL and carry the warning *High caffeine content – Not recommended for children or pregnant or breastfeeding women*. Foods with added caffeine will need to carry the warning *Contains caffeine – Not recommended for children or pregnant women* and also show the caffeine content.

The FIR specifies that food information should be available, easily accessible and visible, and, where appropriate, indelible, and also places special emphasis on the legibility of the mandatory information on food labels and specifies a minimum font size of 1.2 mm (0.9 mm for small packages).

Product name

A clear description of the product is required, e.g. Pilchards in tomato sauce. If the product has a non-descriptive brand name, e.g. Marmite, some indication of its nature must be given, e.g. Yeast extract. The name must also indicate if the product has undergone any

Table 4.5.1 Mandatory information on food labels as required by FIR

Mandatory food information	Notes[a]
Food name	A legal name, customary name or descriptive name must be used See the section 'Product name' for examples
List of ingredients	Must include all the ingredients in the food in descending order of weight (an ingredient list or certain ingredients can be omitted in some circumstances) Annexes to the regulation give detailed rules for listing ingredients by weight, names of ingredients, food additives, enzymes and flavourings, and compound ingredients
Ingredients or processing aids causing allergies or intolerances	Annex II of the regulation lists the substances or products causing allergies or intolerances that must be indicated in the list of ingredients and given special emphasis, e.g. using bold font The rules will extend to foods sold loose and foods sold by caterers
Quantity of ingredients	See the section 'Ingredients' for more detail
Net quantity of the food	Continues to allow some foods to be sold by number, e.g. bread rolls or eggs
Date of minimum durability or the use-by date	Best before and use by dates will continue to be used A date of first freezing will be included for foods such as meat or fish See the section 'Durability' for more detail
Special storage instructions and/or conditions of use	See the section 'Durability' for more detail
Name and address of the food operator marketing the food or importing it into the European Union	
Country of origin or place of provenance	The rules have been tightened and will also extend to fresh and frozen meat Scotland and other areas may be referred to without the use of UK on the label
Instructions for use	Particularly where, without instructions, it would be difficult to make appropriate use of the food
For alcoholic drinks with >1.2% by volume of alcohol	Actual alcoholic strength labelled as X% vol, preceded by the word alcohol or alc
Nutrition declaration	See the section 'Nutrition labelling' for more detail

[a]Refer to Regulation (EU) No1168/2011 and relevant annexes for full details.

form of processing, e.g. UHT milk or Smoked mackerel. Descriptions must also not be misleading; if a product is described as raspberry yogurt, then it must contain raspberries, not just raspberry flavouring. Some foods have customary names, e.g. cream crackers, which do not contain cream but the name is considered to be sufficiently familiar not to be misleading. Other foods have prescribed names with strict rules governing their use, e.g. margarine must contain 80% fat; if the product contains less than this, it must be called something else, such as a spread.

Ingredients

These are given in descending order of content; hence, for instance, if water is the first item listed, then water is the most abundant ingredient. In the past, food ingredient lists only provided a limited guide to food quality, e.g. whether a hamburger contains cereal filler as well as meat. In 2000, this was strengthened by the EC requirement for Quantitative Ingredients Declaration (QUID). Most food products now must state the quantity of any ingredients that:

- Appear in the name of a food or are usually associated with that name by consumers.
- Are emphasised on the label in words, pictures or graphics.
- Are essential to characterise the food and to distinguish it from products with which it might be confused because of its name or appearance.

Declarations must appear in, or next to, the name of the food, or in the ingredients list, and must be shown as a percentage (based on the amount of the ingredient used at the manufacturing stage). The aim is to help the consumer compare the quality of similar foods by being able to see how much ham and mushroom are present in a ham and mushroom pizza or pork in pork sausages.

Allergens

In the past, substances that were part of a compound ingredient comprising <25% of the finished product did not have to be itemised separately. This meant that potentially allergenic substances, such as small amounts of milk, wheat or gluten, did not appear in the ingredient list, making it difficult for individuals to avoid potentially allergenic substances. New food labelling regulations, implementing a 2003 EU directive, came into force in the UK at the end of 2005. One of the main purposes of the changes was to remove the 25% rule and to ensure that all allergenic ingredients, as defined in the directive, are included in ingredient lists (see Chapter 7.11.2, Food hypersensitivity). The 14 allergenic food ingredients, and derivatives, that must be declared are listed in the following:

- Cereals containing gluten.
- Crustaceans.
- Eggs.
- Fish.
- Peanuts.
- Soyabeans.
- Milk (including lactose).
- Nuts (from trees).
- Celery.
- Mustard.
- Sesame seeds.
- Sulphur dioxide >10 ppm.
- Lupin.

Highly processed ingredients derived from these allergens are exempt if they no longer contain allergenic proteins. These rules apply to all foods, including prepacked foods, food sold loose and foods sold in health food shops or catering establishments.

Durability

This must be indicated either by a *use by* or *best before* date, and there is an important difference between the two. Highly perishable fresh foods, e.g. dairy products, must have a *use by* date, and after this time it should be assumed that the food is no longer safe to eat. To minimise the risk of food poisoning, use by dates should be strictly observed. The *best before* date applies to foods with a shelf life of weeks, months or even years, e.g. breakfast cereals or canned foods. After this date, there may be some deterioration in the quality of the texture and flavour of the product, but the food will not necessarily be unsafe to eat. If any special storage conditions such as refrigeration are necessary, these must be shown close to the 'use by' or 'best before' date.

Food additives and E numbers

A food additive is defined as any substance not normally consumed as a food by itself and not normally used as a typical ingredient in a food, but which is intentionally added to a food for functional purposes. Types of food additives are preservatives, antioxidants, emulsifiers and stabilisers, colours, sweeteners, flavour enhancers and flavourings. The safety of food additives is rigorously tested and periodically reassessed. The FSA is the responsible authority in the UK for giving advice on the safety of additives. At the EU level, all additives currently allowed have been evaluated by the EFSA, or its predecessor, the Scientific Committee for Foods (SCF), and given an E number.

It is perhaps ironic that the E number classification system, originally intended as a way of providing assurance that an additive's safety had been evaluated, came to be regarded by the general public as a symbol of undesirable food. As a result of the bad image associated with E numbers, food manufacturers are increasingly declaring additives in ingredients lists by their chemical name rather than their E serial number (a permitted option under food labelling legislation). From a dietetic viewpoint, this can make it more difficult for any client who may need to avoid particular additives, as they now have to memorise complex chemical names rather than simple numbers. The E number classification system and a list of food additives are given on the FSA website at https://www.food.gov.uk/business-guidance/eu-approved-additives-and-e-numbers.

FIR determines the way in which additives present in foods are declared on food labels. Those used as ingredients in prepackaged foods must be listed in an ingredients list by the appropriate category name of the function, e.g. preservative. This must be followed by their specific name, e.g. sulphur dioxide, or E number, e.g. E220. If an additive has more than one function, e.g. emulsifier and thickener, the category name that describes its principal function should be used.

Flavourings are slightly different because there are so many of them, and they are harder to categorise. They may therefore be declared by the term 'flavourings', while natural flavourings may be declared if in line with the provisions of the EU definitions introduced in 2008.

Foods containing artificial sweeteners require a declaration that the food contains sweeteners or, if sugars (any added mono- or disaccharide) are also present, a declaration of sweeteners and sugars. There are additional labelling requirements for foods containing aspartame (stating that it is a source of phenylalanine) and polyols (excessive consumption of which may have a laxative effect).

Consumer attitude to additives

Many consumers view the presence of additives in foods with great suspicion, believing them to be undesirable in principle, synthetic in nature and a common cause of allergies. However, many of these anxieties are misplaced. Food additives fulfil a useful purpose in retarding microbial spoilage, prolonging shelf life, and improving taste, colour and texture. Many food additives are natural or nature-identical substances, or even nutrients such as beta-carotene (used as a food colour) or vitamin C (used as an antioxidant). While some people can react to certain additives, this type of food intolerance is relatively rare (see Chapter 7.11.2, Food hypersensitivity).

The food industry has responded to consumer concerns by carefully assessing the necessity for additives and reducing the level of usage as much as possible, particularly the use of azo food dyes in soft drinks and sweets, and substituting synthetic compounds with more natural alternatives. An interesting development came from the FSA recommendations to government ministers for a ban on the use of certain colours after a study that looked into the effects of six colours and their effect on children's behaviour. The colours are tartrazine (E102), quinoline yellow (E104), sunset yellow (E110), carmoisine (E122), ponceau 4R (E124) and allura red (E129) (McCann *et al.*, 2007). Over the past few years, the FSA has worked with the UK food industry to voluntarily remove these six colours from food and drink, and to make this information available to consumers. A mandatory warning laid down in EU legislation will make it easier for people to choose products that are free from these colours. Legislation was introduced in 2010 that all food placed on the market containing any of these six colours should carry additional label information that 'consumption may have an adverse effect on activity and attention in children'.

Nutrition labelling

FIR lays down a prescribed format for the nutrition labelling of foods and specific requirements for the content, calculation, expression and presentation of the nutrition declaration. Up until 2016, nutrition labelling was voluntary, except where a nutrition or health claim was made. Nutrition labelling is now mandatory for the majority of foods. Table 4.5.2 shows the format for the nutrition declaration. A declaration for energy and each of the nutrients shown in bold is mandatory and can voluntarily be supplemented with an indication of the amounts of monounsaturates, polyunsaturates, polyols, starch, fibre, and vitamins and minerals.

Salt is included in place of sodium to aid consumer understanding. Values should be expressed per 100 g or per 100 mL, and there are options for presenting the nutrition declaration on a per-portion basis or per consumption unit in certain circumstances, provided that the portion or the unit used is quantified on the label and that the number of portions or units contained in the package is stated. The FIR gives the option to express the energy value, fat, saturates, carbohydrate, sugars, protein and salt as a percentage of the reference intakes (Table 4.5.3).

The rules governing the labelling of vitamins and minerals are more complex. The content of these nutrients can only be declared if a food will provide a significant amount of the nutrient reference values (NRVs) as listed in the annex of the regulation (Table 4.5.4). This is defined as 7.5% of the NRV supplied by 100 mL for beverages; 15% of the NRV supplied by 100 g or 100 mL for products

Table 4.5.2 Food Information Regulation (FIR) nutrition declarations[a]

Energy (kJ/kcal)
Fat (g)
Of which
– saturates (g)
– monounsaturates (g)
– polyunsaturates (g)
Carbohydrate (g)
Of which (g)
– sugars (g)
– polyols (g)
– starch (g)
Fibre (g)
Protein (g)
Salt (g)
Vitamins and minerals[b]

[a] These rules do not apply to food supplements or natural mineral waters.
[b] Units are specified in the Annex of the Regulation.

Table 4.5.3 FIR reference intakes for energy and selected nutrients other than vitamins and minerals (adults)

Energy or nutrient	Reference intake
Energy (kcal)	2000 (8400 kJ)
Total fat (g)	70
Saturates (g)	20
Carbohydrate (g)	260
Sugars (g)	90
Protein (g)	50
Salt (g)	6
Sodium (g)	–
Dietary fibre (AOAC) (g)	–

Table 4.5.4 Nutrient reference values (NRVs)

Nutrient	NRV
Vitamin A (μg)	800
Vitamin D (μg)	5
Vitamin E (mg)	12
Vitamin K (μg)	75
Vitamin C (mg)	80
Thiamine (mg)	1.1
Riboflavin (mg)	1.4
Niacin (mg)	16
Vitamin B_6 (mg)	1.4
Folic acid (μg)	200
Vitamin B_{12}(μg)	2.5
Biotin (μg)	50
Pantothenic acid (mg)	6
Potassium (mg)	2000
Chloride (mg)	800
Calcium (mg)	800
Phosphorous (mg)	700
Magnesium (mg)	375
Iron (mg)	14
Zinc (mg)	10
Copper (mg)	1
Manganese (mg)	2
Fluoride (mg)	3.5
Selenium (μg)	55
Chromium (μg)	40
Molybdenum (μg)	50
Iodine (μg)	150

other than beverages; and 15% of the NRV per portion if the package contains only a single portion. The EC has committed to look at the issue of trans fats and may, in due course, introduce legislative proposals for the labelling of trans fats on foods. A report published in 2015 by the EC concluded that setting a legal limit for industrial trans fatty acid content in foods would be the most effective measure for public health, consumer protection and maintaining market access across Europe. However, a public consultation and impact assessment will need to be completed before rules can be agreed and put in place. The relevance of this to the UK will depend on the outcome of negotiations to leave the EU.

Table 4.5.5 FIR reference intakes for energy and selected nutrients other than vitamins and minerals (adults)

Nutrient	Energy value	
	kJ/g	kcal/g
Carbohydrate (except polyols)	17	4
Polyols	10	2.4
Protein	17	4
Fat	37	9
Salatrims[a]	25	6
Alcohol (ethanol)	29	7
Organic acid	13	3
Fibre	8	2
Erythritol	0	0

[a] Short-chain and long-chain acyl triglyceride molecule.

Issues relevant to nutrition labelling in the UK

Some aspects of nutrition labelling information that should be noted are listed in the following:

- *Energy* – for nutrition labelling purposes, energy content is derived using a conversion factor of 4 kcal/g for carbohydrate and sugars, rather than 3.75 kcal/g used by standard UK food tables. The energy content declared on food labels will therefore be slightly higher than food table values. The FIR also includes additional conversion factors for the calculation of energy values for labelling purposes (Table 4.5.5). *Note*: Fibre now has a conversion factor of 8 kJ/g or 2 kcal/g.
- *Fibre* – a new definition of fibre was introduced in 2008, which expanded the previous definition to include carbohydrate polymers with three or more monomeric units, which are neither digested nor absorbed in the human small intestine. The Association of Official Analytical Chemists (AOAC) method for analysis of fibre should be used. However, UK food tables mainly give dietary fibre (non-starch polysaccharide) values using the Englyst method and the AOAC method only for a very limited number of foods.
- *Salt* – the FIR stipulates that salt in grams be declared to aid consumer understanding. UK food tables provide sodium content in milligrams.
- *Accuracy* – nutrition information on food labels is mainly estimated using published data on food composition, as the alternative laboratory analysis is

SECTION 4

expensive for food manufacturers and is prone to sampling errors, especially for non-homogeneous foodstuffs. There will therefore be some variability between the declared values and those determined by analysis of a sample of the foodstuff. An acceptable margin for error is not specified by law and should reflect the type of foodstuff. For example, a foodstuff consisting of chunks of meat and vegetables in a sauce will be inherently more variable than a homogenous foodstuff such as chocolate, and this must be reflected in the acceptable margin for error.

- *NRVs* – the NRVs for vitamins and minerals, against which the amounts in food are compared in the nutrition panel, are a set of adult data produced specifically for labelling purposes.
- *Front-of-pack labelling (FoP) and %RI* – Table 4.5.2 shows what is known as the back-of-pack nutrition declaration. In the UK, manufacturers have been using FoP labelling for several years, and several different presentations have emerged. The FIR allows the option to continue to voluntarily repeat FoP information on nutrients of importance to public health (energy value or energy value plus fat, saturates, sugars and salts). In 2013, DH provided guidance for businesses on developing FoP nutrition labelling which includes details on how to include information on %RI and colour coding. Examples are shown in Figures 4.5.2 and 4.5.3.

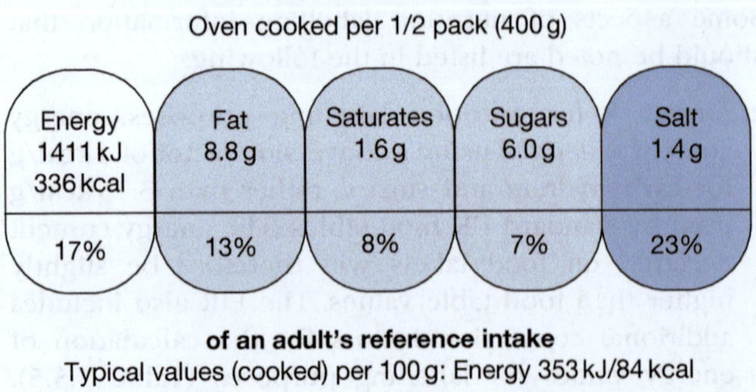

Figure 4.5.2 Example of front-of-pack label for a food product (contains public sector information licensed under the Open Government Licence v3.0; adapted from DH, 2013)

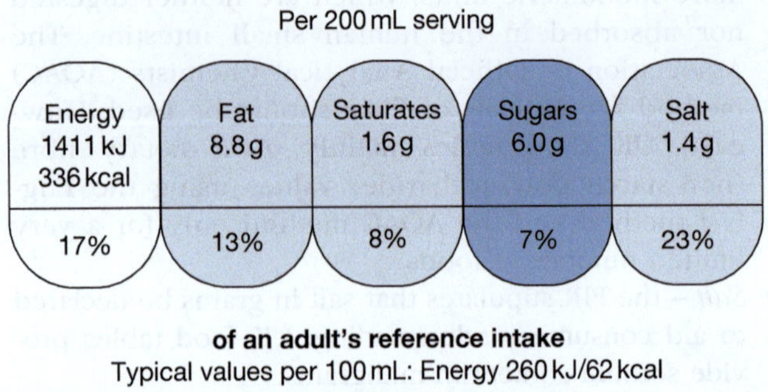

Figure 4.5.3 Example of front-of-pack label for a drink product (contains public sector information licensed under the Open Government Licence v3.0; adapted from DH, 2013)

Nutrition and health claims

Nutrition and health claims can be a useful way of conveying information to consumers to help them choose foods with particular nutritional features and health benefits. However, people need to be able to do so without being misled. In December 2006, Regulation No 1924/2006 on nutrition and health claims made on foods was published with the aim of protecting consumers from false or misleading claims, in addition to harmonising the legislation on claims across the EC to facilitate trade. It applies to nutrition and health claims made in commercial communications to the final consumer, including claims made in the labelling, presentation and advertising of food. It also applies to foods supplied to restaurants, hospitals, schools and other mass caterers. The legislation defines what is meant by a claim, and defines the different type of claims (Table 4.5.6).

The regulation is complex and sets out many requirements for the authorisation and use of nutrition and health claims. In 2011, DH issued an extensive guidance document giving regulatory and best practice advice on how to comply with the regulation (DH, 2011). It covers the whole of the UK. Along with the regulation itself, DH guidance document is essential reading for anyone involved in this area. The regulation sets out general principles for all claims and

Table 4.5.6 Key definitions included in Regulation 1924/2006 on nutrition and health claims made on foods

Term	Definition
Claim	A claim is defined as *'any message or representation, which is not mandatory under Community legislation or national legislation, including pictorial, graphic or symbolic representation, in any form, which states, suggests or implies that a food has particular characteristics'*
Nutrition claim	Any claim that states, suggests or implies that a food has particular beneficial nutritional properties due to the energy that it: 1. provides 2. provides at a reduced or increased rate 3. or does not provide and/or the nutrients or other substances that it: 1. contains 2. contains in reduced or increased proportions 3. or does not contain
Health claim	Any claim that states, suggests or implies that a relationship exists between a food category, a food or one of its constituents and health
Reduction of disease risk claim	Any claim that states, suggests or implies that the consumption of a food category, a food or one of its constituents significantly reduces a risk factor in the development of a human disease

further specific conditions for nutrition and health claims, which include the following:

- Claims *must not*: be false, ambiguous or misleading; suggest that a balanced and varied diet cannot provide appropriate quantities of nutrients; encourage or condone excess consumption of a food; or refer to changes in bodily functions that could exploit fear in the consumer.
- Claims must be based on generally accepted scientific data and be well understood by the average consumer.
- In most cases, if a claim is made, nutrition labelling is mandatory.
- Only nutrition claims listed in the annex to the regulation are permitted, and only if they meet the conditions of use stipulated for that claim (Table 4.5.7).

Table 4.5.7 Nutrition claims and conditions applying to them as listed in the Annex of Regulation 1924/2006 on nutrition and health claims made on foods

Claim	Condition
Low energy	No >40 kcal (170 kJ)/100 g or 20 kcal (80 kJ)/100 mL
Energy reduced	At least 30% reduction
Energy free	No >4 kcal (17 kJ)/100 mL
Low fat	No >3 g of fat/100 g or 1.5 g/100 mL (1.8 g for semi-skimmed milk)
Fat free	No >0.5 g fat/100 g or 100 m; 'X% fat free' prohibited
Low saturated fat	No >1.5 g/100 g or 0.75 g/10 mL; no >10% of energy
Saturated fat free	No >0.1 g/100 g or 100 mL
Low sugars	No >5 g/100 g or 2.5 g/100 mL
Sugar free	No >0.5 g/100 g or 100 mL
With no added sugars	No added mono- or di-saccharides or any other food used for its sweetening properties; if sugars naturally present, the label should include 'CONTAINS NATURALLY OCCURRING SUGARS'
Low sodium/salt	No >0.12 g of sodium (or the equivalent value for salt)/100 g or 100 mL; note that the rules for waters differ
Very low sodium/salt	No >0.04 g of sodium (or the equivalent value for salt)/100 g or 100 mL; note not permitted for waters
Sodium or salt free	No >0.005 g of sodium (or the equivalent value for salt)/100 g or 100 mL
No added sodium/salt	Does not contain any added sodium/salt or any other ingredient containing added sodium/salt, and contains no more than 0.12 g sodium, or the equivalent value for salt, per 100 g or 100 mL
Source of fibre	At least 3 g/100 g or 1.5 g/100 kcal
High fibre	At least 6 g/100 g or 3 g/100 kcal
Source of protein	At least 12% of energy
High protein	At least 20% of energy
Source of (named vitamin/s and/ or mineral/s)	Significant amount (15% NRV/100 g)
High (named vitamin/s and/or mineral/s)	At least twice the value of 'source of' (30% NRV/100 g)
Contains (name of nutrient or other substance)	For vitamins and minerals, same level as 'source of'; Article 5 of particular importance for claims relating to other substances and nutrients
Increased (name of nutrient)	Meets requirements for 'source of' and at least 30% more than a similar product
Reduced (name of nutrient)	At least 30% less than a similar product; for micronutrients: 10% difference in reference values; for sodium (or the equivalent value for salt): 25% difference; other rules apply for 'reduced saturated fat' and reduced sugars'
Light/lite	As 'reduced'
Natural/naturally	Prefix 'natural/naturally' may be used where food naturally meets the conditions for nutrition claims
Source of n-3 fatty acids	At least 0.3 g of alpha-linolenic acid/100 g and 100 kcal, or at least 40 mg of EPA and DHA/100 g and 100 kcal
High n-3 fatty acids	At least 0.6 g of alpha-linolenic acid/100 g and 100 kcal, or at least 80 mg of EPA and DHA/100 g and 100 kcal
High monounsaturated fat	>20% energy; at least 45% fatty acids present derived from monounsaturated fat
High polyunsaturated	>20% energy; at least 45% of fatty acids present derived from polyunsaturated fat
High unsaturated fat	>20% energy; at least 70% of fatty acids derived from unsaturated fat

See http://ec.europa.eu/nuhclaims for a full, up-to-date list of nutrition claims and conditions.

SECTION 4

Table 4.5.8 Examples of authorised health claims listed in the EU Register on nutrition and health claims

Claim type	Nutrient, substance, food or food category	Claim	Conditions of use of the claim
Function health claim – Article 13(1)	Calcium	Calcium is needed for the maintenance of normal bones	The claim may be used only for food which is at least a source of calcium as referred to in the claim 'SOURCE OF [NAME OF VITAMIN/S] AND/OR [NAME OF MINERAL/S]', as listed in the Annex to Regulation (EC) No 1924/2006
Disease risk reduction claim – Article 14(1)(a)	Oat beta-glucan	Oat beta-glucan has been shown to lower/reduce blood cholesterol; high cholesterol is a risk factor in the development of coronary heart disease	Information shall be given to the consumer that the beneficial effect is obtained with a daily intake of 3 g of oat beta-glucan; the claim can be used for foods that provide at least 1 g of oat beta-glucan per quantified portion
Children's development and health claim – Article 14(1)(b)	Vitamin D	Vitamin D is needed for normal growth and development of bone in children	The claim can be used only for food that is at least a source of vitamin D as referred to in the claim 'SOURCE OF [NAME OF VITAMIN/S] AND/OR [NAME OF MINERAL/S]', as listed in the Annex to Regulation 1924/2006

See http://ec.europa.eu/nuhclaims/ for a full, up-to-date list of authorised and non-authorised health claims.

- Only authorised health claims included in the EU Register can be used on food, and claims must meet the conditions of use (see Table 4.5.8 for examples of authorised claims).
- Claims must not be made on alcoholic beverages containing >1.2% by volume of alcohol (see regulation for limited exceptions).
- Health claims not permitted include those that suggest that health could be affected by not consuming the food, or those that make reference to the amount or rate of weight loss.
- Health claims that make reference to recommendations of individual doctors or health professionals are not allowed on food labelling. This is covered by Article 12(c) within the regulation, and is explained in more detail within the DH guidance document. However, there is still debate about what is permitted. The British Dietetic Association (BDA) has been active on this topic and can provide an update for anyone concerned about the issue.
- Nutrient profiles (restrictions on the use of claims on certain foods or categories of foods based on their nutritional composition) have still not been adopted, and are the subject of much debate.

Health claims require authorisation under the regulation. The Panel on Dietetic Products, Nutrition and Allergies (NDA) of the EFSA is responsible for scrutinising the scientific substantiation for health claims submitted by food business operators. Specific rules apply for claims regarding disease risk reduction and for those that refer to children's health and development. ESFA's opinions inform EC decisions about whether a claim will be included in the EU Register. Claims that a food can treat, prevent or cure (medicinal claims) continue to be prohibited.

Addition of nutrients

In December 2006, Regulation (EC) 1925/2006 on the addition of vitamins and minerals and certain other substances to foods was published to provide the same rules throughout the EC. Other substances are those, other than vitamins and minerals, which have a physiological effect. The regulation prohibits their addition to unprocessed foods such as fruit, vegetables, meat, poultry and fish, and to beverages containing >1.2% by volume of alcohol. It includes lists of the vitamins and minerals that may be added to foods and the form in which they may be added.

Further reading

Thompson K. (1996) *The Law of Food and Drink*. Kent: Shaw & Sons.

Internet resources

British Specialist Nutrition Association Ltd. (BSNA), www.bsna.co.uk
Department for Environment Food and Rural Affairs (Defra), www.defra.gov.uk
DH, www.dh.gov.uk
European Commission (EC) Register of nutrition and health claims made on foods, http://ec.europa.eu/nuhclaims
European Food Safety Authority (EFSA), www.efsa.europa.eu
Food Standards Agency (FSA) for England, Northern Ireland and Wales, www.food.gov.uk
Food Standards Agency Scotland, www.foodstandards.gov.scot
Food Standards Agency Wales, www.food.gov.uk/wales
Institute of Grocery Distribution (IGD), www.igd.com
The Stationery Office (TSO), www.tsonline.co.uk

References

DH. (2011) *Nutrition and health claims. Guidance to compliance with Regulation (EC) 1924/2006 on nutrition and health claims made on foods*. Available at https://www.gov.uk/government/

uploads/system/uploads/attachment_data/file/204320/Nutrition_and_health_claims_guidance_November_2011.pdf. Accessed 6 October 2016.

DH. (2013) *Guide to creating a front of pack (FoP) nutrition label for pre-packed products sold through retail outlets.* Available at https://www.gov.uk/government/uploads/system/uploads/attachment_data/file/300886/2902158_FoP_Nutrition_2014.pdf. Accessed 6 October 2016.

EU Regulation (EC). (2006) *1924/2006 of the European Parliament and of the Council of 20 December 2006 on nutrition and health claims made on foods. O.J. L12, 18.1.2007, 3-18.* Available at http://ec.europa.eu/nuhclaims. Accessed 25 October 2012.

EU Regulation (EC). (2011) *1169/2011 of the European Parliament and of the Council of 25 October 2011 on the provision of food information to consumers. O.J. L304, 22.11.11, 18-61.* Available at http://eur-lex.europa.eu/LexUriServ/LexUriServ.do?uri=OJ%3AL%3A2011%3A304%3A0018%3A0063%3AEN%3APDF. Accessed 6 October 2016.

McCann D, Barrett A, Cooper A, *et al.* (2007) Food additives and hyperactive behaviour in 3-year-old and 8/9-year-old children in the community: a randomised, double-blinded, placebo-controlled trial. *Lancet* 370: 1560–1567.

The Food Safety Act. (1990) *Chapter 16.* Available at http://www.legislation.gov.uk./ukpga/1990/16/contents. Accessed 6 October 2016.

SECTION 5

Other topics related to practice

5.1 Genetics and nutritional genomics

Kevin Whelan and Sherly X. Li

Key points

- Dietitians should be able to recognise modes of inheritance, gather and use multigenerational family history, and communicate genetic information relevant to their area of work.
- Modes of inheritance vary for single-gene conditions and chromosomal conditions, but patterns can be detected that enable traits to be detected and risk to be estimated.
- Nutritional genomics is the investigation or application of the interaction between genetics, diet and nutrition, and consists of nutrigenomics (how diet and nutrients affect gene expression) and *nutrigenetics* (how genetic variation modifies an individual's response to diet and nutrients).

Genetics

Diet plays a role in the treatment of many conditions that have a genetic component, e.g. phenylketonuria (PKU), cystic fibrosis and familial hypercholesterolaemia. Technological advances enable better understanding of these conditions as well as the discovery of the genetic basis for an increasing number of other conditions. Such advances allow the development of new therapies, including, in many instances, dietary manipulation. To ensure that patients have access to genetic advances, now and in the future, dietitians must be able to conduct a number of genetic-based activities. Examples of such activities include recognising modes of inheritance in families, gathering multigenerational family history information to draw a family tree (pedigree) and communicating genetic information to individuals, families and healthcare staff (Skills for Health/NGEDC, 2007).

Recognising a mode of inheritance

Genes are short sections of deoxyribonucleic acid (DNA) that code for the production of a specific protein. DNA consists of a series of nucleotide molecules bound in a long double-helical structure. Nucleotides consist of a five-carbon sugar unit bound to at least one phosphate group and one of four potential bases; adenine, guanine, thymine or cytosine. The order of these four nucleotide bases on the DNA is the code responsible for defining the order of amino acids during protein synthesis.

Proteins have a wide range of functions, including transport (e.g. haemoglobin), structure (e.g. actin and myosin) and metabolism (e.g. enzymes such as lipase). Genes come in pairs, called an allele (one from each parent), and are located on chromosomes. In a gene, both alleles can be the same (homozygous) or they can be different (heterozygous). A mutation in a single gene, or a pair of genes (allele), can result in the absence or inadequate amounts of the protein that the gene codes for, or synthesis of a malformed protein that does not function properly. This can cause disorders such as sickle cell disease, muscular dystrophy or cystic fibrosis, and these can be passed on to future generations via meiosis and fertilisation.

Being able to recognise the mode of inheritance of a particular mutation, and hence a condition, enables the dietitian to give dietary advice to the individual and their families appropriately (e.g. cholesterol-lowering advice in familial hypercholesterolaemia), and also to explain the process if patients ask about the genetic basis of their condition. There are several modes of inheritance, and these are explained in the following text. Table 5.1.1 summarises some of the different conditions that result from the different modes of inheritance, along with an example pedigree for each.

Single-gene conditions

Single-gene conditions are individually rare, but their high recurrence in affected families means that it is important for people with these conditions to be

Manual of Dietetic Practice, Sixth Edition. Edited by Joan Gandy.

Companion website: www.manualofdieteticpractice.com

Table 5.1.1 Examples of inheritable conditions with different modes of inheritance (source: reproduced with permission from the NHS National Genetics Education and Development Centre)

Type of inheritance	Example conditions	Clinical features of inheritance	Probability of having a child with the condition	Example family tree
Single gene: autosomal dominant	Familial hypercholesterolaemia (FH) Adult polycystic kidney disease Huntington's disease	Males and females are affected in equal proportions The condition is seen in multiple generations All forms of inheritance are observed, e.g. male to male, female to male, etc.	One in two, where one parent is affected 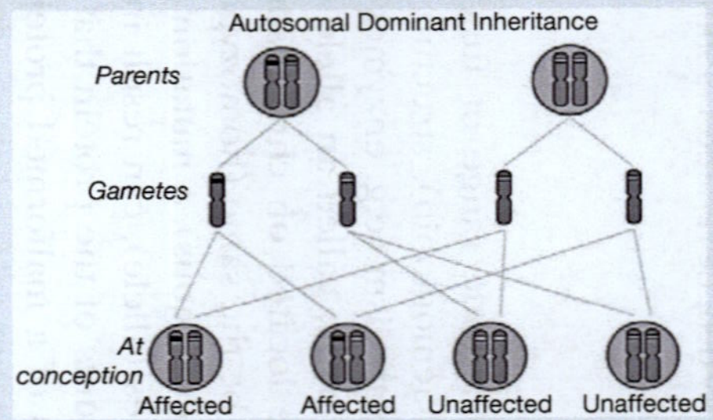	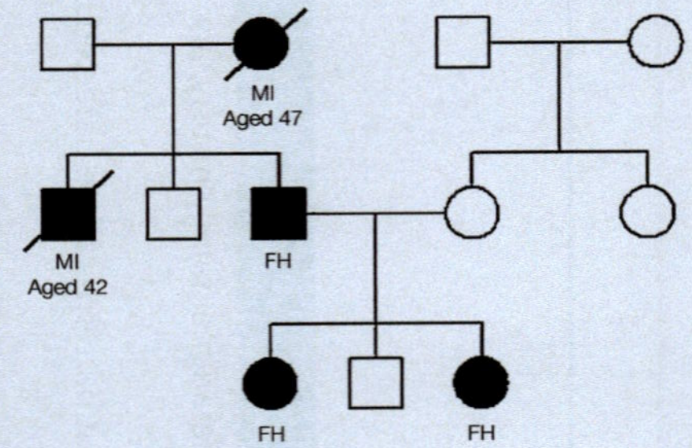
Single gene: autosomal recessive	Cystic fibrosis MCADD Haemochromatosis Phenylketonuria	Males and females are affected in equal proportions Affected individuals are usually in a single sibship in one generation Parents of an affected individual will both be carriers for the condition	One in four, where both parents are carriers 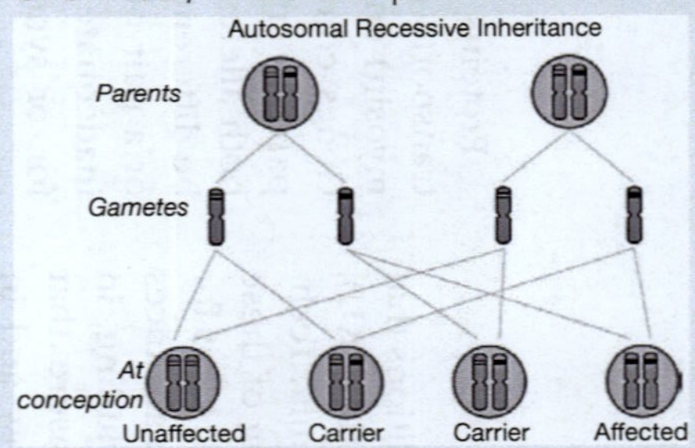	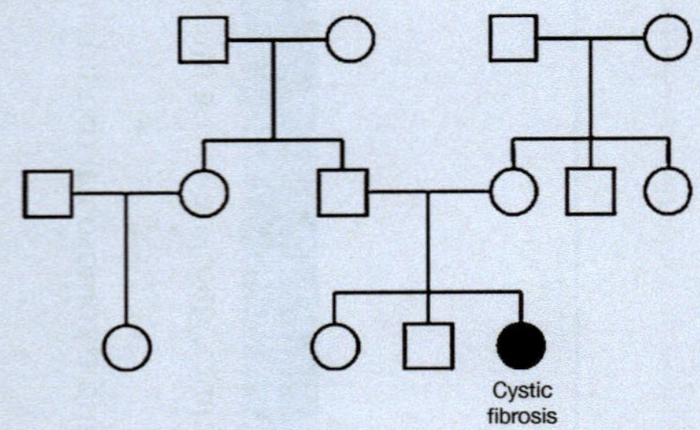
Single gene: X-linked recessive	Adrenoleukodystrophy Duchenne muscular dystrophy Haemophilia	Males are affected almost exclusively The mutation is transmitted through female carriers to their sons Affected males cannot transmit the condition to their sons	One in two in males, where the mother is a carrier 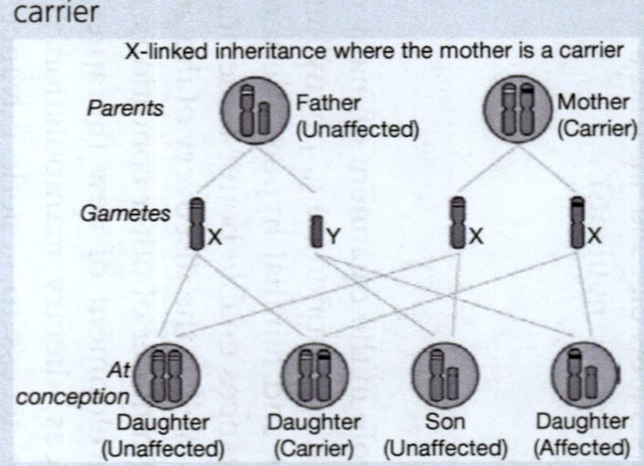	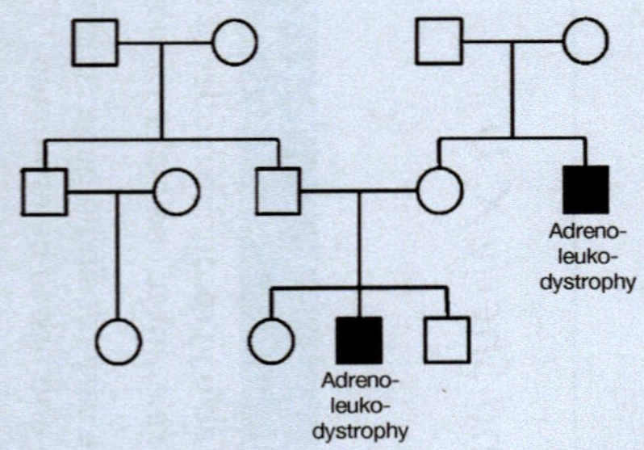

Type of inheritance	Example conditions	Clinical features of inheritance	Probability of having a child with the condition	Example family tree
Chromosomal	Down syndrome	A higher number of miscarriages in a family than would be expected The presence of congenital anomalies, dysmorphic features, intellectual disability and developmental delay	This varies widely, depending on the nature of the chromosomal condition	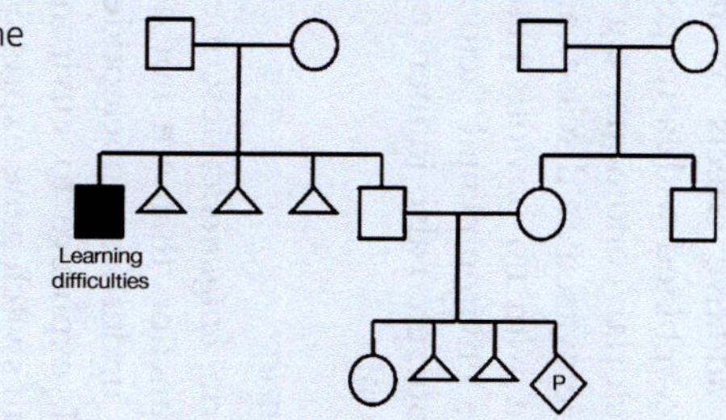
Multifactorial	Coronary artery disease Diabetes mellitus Obesity	There is no clear pattern of inheritance in the family	Difficult to calculate due to the interaction of genetic and environmental factors Probabilities can be calculated using tables of empiric risk Recurrence risk increases as the number with the condition in the family increases Recurrence risk increases if the condition in the family is severe Recurrence risk increases the more closely related an individual is to an affected person, e.g. higher risk for first-degree relatives than second-degree relatives	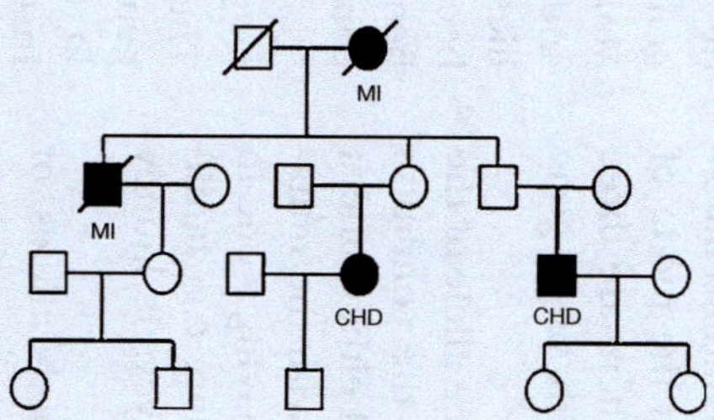

MCADD, medium-chain acyl-CoA dehydrogenase deficiency.

identified and supported. Single-gene conditions are caused by a mutation in one particular gene or pair of alleles that significantly affects the production or function of its resulting protein. The probability of children inheriting a single-gene condition depends on the mode of inheritance exhibited by the condition. There are three main modes of inheritance associated with single-gene conditions.

In autosomal dominant conditions, if one allele of the gene has a mutation, it is sufficient for the condition to be present. At conception, a child will either inherit the usual copy of the gene or the gene with the mutation from the affected parent, therefore, having a one in two probability of inheriting the condition, e.g. familial hypercholesterolaemia and adult polycystic kidney disease.

In autosomal recessive conditions, both alleles of the gene need to have a mutation for the condition to occur, and therefore a mutated gene is inherited from both parents. When both parents are carriers for the condition (i.e. they each have only one gene with a mutation, so are not affected by the condition), they have a one in four probability of having a child who does not inherit a mutation from either parent, a one in two probability of having a child who is a carrier (but is not affected by the condition) and a one in four probability of having a child who has the condition, e.g. cystic fibrosis, PKU, medium-chain acyl-CoA dehydrogenase deficiency (MCADD) and hereditary haemochromotosis.

X-linked recessive conditions are caused by gene mutations on the X chromosome. Males have one X chromosome (XY), and females have two X chromosomes (XX). Therefore, in X-linked recessive conditions, males are affected almost exclusively, as the gene mutation only needs to be present on their one X chromosome, whereas females are usually unaffected, as they have the usual copy of the gene on their other X chromosome. For a mother who is a carrier for an X-linked condition, sons have a one in two probability of inheriting the condition and daughters have a one in two chance of being a carrier. For a father who is affected by an X-linked condition, all sons will be unaffected and all daughters will be carriers, e.g. adrenoleukodystrophy.

Chromosomal conditions

Chromosomal conditions are caused by alterations in gene dosage, usually due to changes in the number of copies of genes. They are caused by unusual events during meiosis that results in cells with extra chromosomes (more than two copies), too few chromosomes (fewer than two copies) or chromosomes containing the incorrect amount of DNA. For example, Down syndrome is caused by the presence of an extra copy of chromosome 21 (three copies in total (trisomy)). While chromosomal conditions are usually one-off events, some can be inherited and may be indicated within a family by recurrent miscarriages and clustering of individuals with learning difficulties.

Multifactorial or common complex conditions

The majority of conditions develop due to the interplay of multiple factors. Multifactorial conditions are caused by the additive effects of minor alterations in many genes, combined with a range of environmental factors. Multifactorial conditions, e.g. type 2 diabetes, obesity and cardiovascular disease, are seen to cluster in families but with no obvious pattern of inheritance, partly because environmental factors (diet, exercise, smoking behaviour, etc.) also influence the risk of developing the condition.

Epigenetics

The term *epigenetic* describes heritable influences on gene function that are not accompanied by alteration in the underlying nucleotide sequence on the DNA. Instead, exposure to environmental factors (including diet) can switch gene expression on or off, and alter how easy it is for the DNA to be transcribed in order to start the pathway of protein production. Examples of epigenetic changes include altered levels of methylation of the DNA, histone modification and RNA-associated silencing. This may increase the risk of certain diseases. Epigenetic changes can be passed on to offspring and influence their susceptibility to developing those disorders.

Somatic mutations (cancer)

Cancers can be caused by gene mutations. A person can inherit a cancer risk gene from a parent, which is then present in all cells, including the germ cells (reproductive cells, i.e. egg and sperm). Therefore, this gene mutation can be inherited, resulting in a family with an inherited cancer syndrome. The gene *BRCA1* is expressed in breast tissue and produces the breast cancer type 1 susceptibility protein, which is involved in repairing faulty DNA. People with this mutation therefore have an impaired ability to repair faulty DNA, and as a result are at greater risk of breast cancer. It is important that individuals with the *BRCA1* mutation from families with inherited cancer syndrome be identified, so that they can be offered genetic testing, increased screening and appropriate clinical management.

However, some cancers are not genetically inherited. Some cancers result from the accumulation of new gene mutations in somatic cells during the lifetime of that person, leading to uncontrolled cell division and growth. As these alterations are not present in the germ cells (egg, sperm), they are not usually passed on to children.

Genetics in clinical dietetic practice

Gathering and using multigenerational family history and family tree

Gathering a multigenerational family history can be useful to healthcare professionals, including dietitians, because it can enable identification of other affected family members and can be used to predict the probability that the condition may be passed on to offspring. Patients with a condition with a genetic component may ask dietitians about the risk of their children also developing the condition. Thus, dietitians must identify the patients in whom taking a family history is an important part of the assessment process.

It is recommended that a genetic family history be gathered and drawn in a particular way to make interpretation easier, as well as to facilitate the sharing of the resultant pedigree with other healthcare professionals. Figure 5.1.1 shows the symbols that are used to draw a pedigree. It also shows the specific order that is recommended for collecting a family history to enable drawing a pedigree, e.g. it is best to ask about and draw the history of the relatives in box 1 before those in box 2, etc. The completed three-generation family history should be dated and signed by the healthcare professional who recorded it.

Genetic family history information is confidential; recording relevant information (conditions, cause of death, etc.) in a family is permissible without the explicit consent of all those shown on the pedigree, as long as it is necessary to do so for health purposes. Many individuals expressly state that they want the family history information to be available to other family members and professionals to assist in diagnosis and care, and this consent should be obtained and recorded.

Communicating genetic information

Dietitians may be asked by patients and their families to explain genetic concepts and diagnoses, and must therefore have a thorough understanding of the issues surrounding the communication of information of this nature. The amount of information given at any one time needs to be tailored to the preferences and needs of the individual (Burke *et al.*, 2007). If patients are dealing with complex emotions that can accompany a diagnosis, e.g. guilt and blame, they may not be able to actively hear, understand and process a great deal of information. The information should be non-directive and non-judgemental. It is important to be sensitive to the emotional impact of the genetic information on the patients and their wider families. Simple, non-emotive language is preferable, e.g. *altered gene* is preferable to *gene mutation*, and *risk* should be replaced by *chance*. Patients may ask to be referred to reliable sources of genetic information, including the Internet, support groups and written materials (Burke *et al.*, 2007).

Mendelian randomisation as a research tool

Mendelian randomisation is a statistical tool used to study causal relationships between risk factors (e.g. alcohol intake) and outcomes (e.g. cardiovascular disease) by using genes (e.g. a genetic variant within the alcohol dehydrogenase 1B gene) as a proxy for the risk factor of interest (Holmes *et al.*, 2014). It is still a developing method, but may be helpful in addressing some of the limitations of observational research and for studying dietary factors that are difficult to examine in a randomised controlled trial (e.g. dietary interventions that require long duration of exposure or where randomised controlled trials are unethical) (Haycock *et al.*, 2016).

Nutritional genomics

Nutritional genomics is the investigation or application of the interaction between genetics, genomics, diet, nutrition and other environmental factors, specifically in relation to the maintenance of health and the prevention or treatment of disease. Some definitions of nutritional genomics are even broader and include the application of genomic technologies to the study of nutritional sciences and food technology (Brown & van der Ouderaa, 2007). In light of this, the importance of nutritional genomics to all aspects of dietetic practice, both now and in the future, is undeniable.

Broadly speaking, nutritional genomics consists of two distinct areas, nutrigenomics and nutrigenetics. Nutrigenomics relates to how diet and nutrients affect gene expression and subsequent protein translation, and therefore metabolism, physiological function and health. In contrast, nutrigenetics (also known as the study of gene–diet interactions) relates to how genetic variation within an individual modifies that person's response to diet and nutrients, and therefore ultimately health or disease. Taken together, they can be viewed as two parallel themes that run in opposite directions, one relating to how diet influences gene expression (nutrigenomics) and the other to how genes influence the response to different diets (nutrigenetics) (Brown & van der Ouderaa, 2007).

In the future, nutritional genomics may revolutionise healthcare, and therefore the way in which dietitians practice, owing to its potential to:

1. Optimise targeting dietary interventions to people most likely to respond well to them;
2. Improve the cost and health effectiveness of existing preventive and treatment paradigms;
3. Reduce unnecessary adverse consequences of dietary interventions;
4. Increase patient adherence to health practitioners' recommendations; and
5. Identify novel dietary interventions that are beneficial only in a defined genetic subgroup of the population (Franks *et al.*, 2013).

In many areas, dietitians already personalise advice by providing evidence-based dietary counselling to people with genetic disorders. However, this advice is largely based on a cluster of symptoms, clinical diagnosis and personal dietary preferences, rather than on the patient's genetic profile *per se*. For multifactorial chronic diseases, e.g. obesity, diabetes and cardiovascular disease, the science of nutritional genomics may lead to genetics-based personalised nutritional recommendations, e.g. reducing saturated fat intake only in those with a specific genotype (Lovegrove & Gitau, 2008). However, this science awaits further development before it can be integrated into dietetic practice (Camp & Trujilo, 2014).

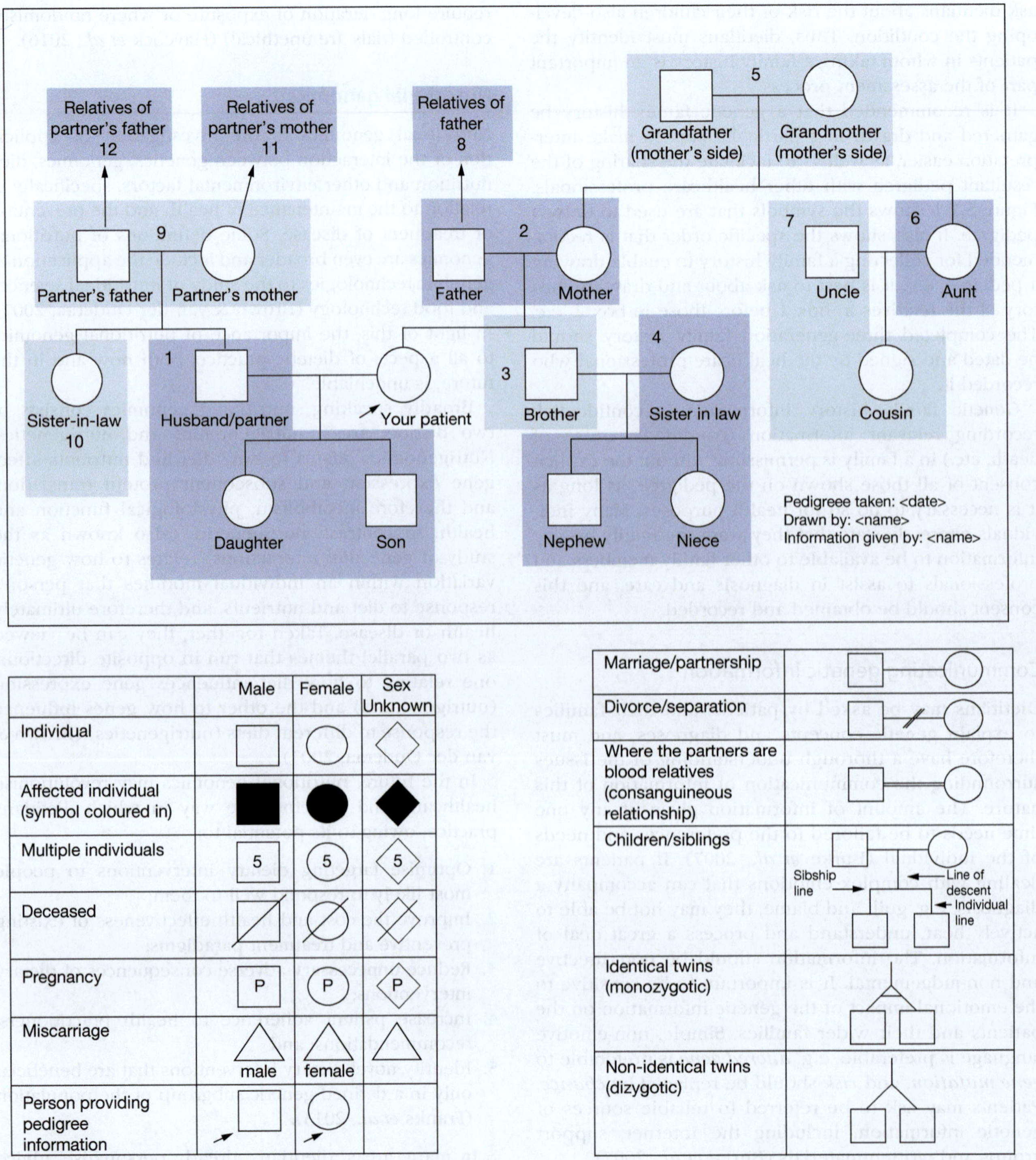

Key Information

For each key person, record under the pedigree symbol the following information as appropriate:

- Name
- Date of birth (DOBs are preferable to current ages or estimates)
- Relevant symbols and/or diagnoses and age at diagnoses (if known)
- Cause of death and age at death (if known)

Figure 5.1.1 Stepwise approach to drawing a family pedigree (source: Reproduced with permission from the NHS National Genetics Education and Development Centre)

Current evidence for nutritional genomics

There is emerging evidence for the role of nutrigenetics (the influence of genetic variation on response to diet and nutrients) in cardiometabolic diseases (e.g. obesity, diabetes and cardiovascular disease). The effect of dietary fat on cardiovascular risk factors has been extensively studied in large populations. However, there is wide variation in the effectiveness of altering fat intake to reduce cardiovascular disease, which is often accounted for by variations in dietary adherence between individuals. However, genotype may influence response to intake of polyunsaturated fats (PUFA). For example, in a study of middle-aged individuals of European descent with metabolic syndrome, participants were allocated to one of four isocaloric diets differing in total quantity or quality of fat and lasting 12 weeks. Among those who increased their PUFA intake (measured as an increase in the proportion of blood n-3 PUFA), there was a raised concentration of apo CII among those carrying the *E2* allele for the apolipoprotein E (*apoE*) gene, as opposed to a reduction in apo CII in those with the *E3/E3* genotype and no effect in *E4* carriers (Fallaize *et al.*, 2017). Apo CII regulates blood lipids and helps to reduce circulating triglycerides, a risk factor for cardiovascular disease.

ApoE is a protein that facilitates the clearance of chylomicrons and very-low-density lipoproteins from the bloodstream. The gene encoding *apoE* can have natural variations (polymorphisms) comprising three common versions (ε2, ε3, ε4). As humans carry two alleles (one from each parent), there are several different permutations. Therefore, humans can have one of three possible homozygous genotypes (ε2/2, ε3/3, ε4/4) or three heterozygous genotypes (ε2/3, ε2/4, ε3/4). The most common allele is ε3, followed by ε4 and ε2. A meta-analysis has indicated that people with an ε2 allele (e.g. ε2/2, ε2/3) have a reduced risk of coronary heart disease, whereas people with an ε4 allele (e.g. ε4/4, ε3/4) have an increased risk of coronary heart disease (Bennet *et al.*, 2007) (Table 5.1.2).

In a trial comparing a low-fat diet with a high-saturated-fat diet supplemented with DHA, participants on the latter diet showed a significantly greater triglyceride-lowering effect. This effect was larger among *E4* carriers (30% lower triglyceride levels than those on the low-fat diet) as compared to those possessing the *E3/E3* genotype (only 17% lower than those on the low-fat diet) (Carvalho-Wells *et al.*, 2012). Large randomised controlled trials are required before widespread application of this evidence is possible in dietetic practice. However, these data highlight the possibility that patients with hyperlipidaemia might one day be screened for their *apoE* gene, in order that they might be targeted with intensive dietary counselling according to their genotype.

Table 5.1.2 Association between *apoE* polymorphisms, coronary risk and diet

Allele	Allele frequency (Bennet *et al.*, 2007)	Coronary risk[a] odds ratio (95% CI)	Impact of high-saturated-fat diet plus DHA versus low-fat diet on triglyceride levels (Carvalho-Wells *et al.*, 2012)
ε2	0.07	0.80 (0.70–0.90)	Not measured
ε3	0.82	1.00	17% lower
ε4	0.11	1.06 (0.99–1.13)	30% lower

[a]Compared with ε3/ε3 (Bennet *et al.*, 2007).

Another area for the application of nutrigenetics in cardiovascular disease is in relation to the gene coding for the enzyme methylene tetrahydrofolate reductase (*MTHFR*). This enzyme is involved in folate metabolism, and therefore regulates plasma concentrations of homocysteine, which at high levels are a risk factor for cardiovascular disease. A common polymorphism can occur to one specific nucleotide base of the *MTHFR* gene (and hence it is called a single-nucleotide polymorphism, or SNP). This SNP occurs at nucleotide position 677 and involves a cytosine (C) base being replaced by a thymine (T) base; hence, it is described as *MTHFR* 677C>T. Most people have the CC genotype, whereas those with an affected T allele (CT or TT genotypes) can still produce the MTHFR enzyme, but its activity is reduced.

People with this SNP have less efficient folate metabolism and an approximately 20% higher plasma homocysteine concentration than those who do not (Jacques *et al.*, 1996). This may explain why people who are homozygous for this SNP (TT) have a 16% higher chance of developing coronary heart disease as compared to people who are homozygous wild type (CC) (Klerk *et al.*, 2002).

Dietary intervention with folate supplementation reduces homocysteine concentrations, particularly in those with the *MTHFR* TT genotype. For example, in a large meta-analysis of observational studies, the effect of *MTHFR* 677C→T on homocysteine was reduced with increasing folate availability (according to folate fortification policy) (Holmes *et al.*, 2011). Nutrigenetic testing for the *MTHFR* C677T (TT) polymorphism might enable targeted folate supplementation in those most likely to respond. However, a meta-analysis of trials for homocysteine-lowering interventions (e.g. folate supplementation) did not identify the same reduction in stroke among those with the *MTHFR* 677C→T variant (Holmes *et al.*, 2011). Another meta-analysis indicated that, although folate supplementation resulted in a 25% reduction in homocysteine concentrations, this did not have an effect on cardiovascular events, cancer or 5-year mortality (Clarke *et al.*, 2010), raising the possibility that elevated plasma homocysteine is a marker of risk rather than a risk itself.

Barriers to nutritional genomics in practice

In the future, nutritional genomics could have a major impact on dietetic practice, offering the potential for targeted dietary interventions based on the understanding of an individual's genotype (personalised nutrition). However, research to support its application is currently in its infancy because of inconsistencies between studies' findings lending to challenges in its interpretation (Camp & Trujilo, 2014; Li *et al.*, 2017). Replicated findings from larger-scale studies, including dietary interventions, to demonstrate nutritional, metabolic and clinical benefits are required.

A commonly asked question is whether disclosure of genetic risk information may motivate some people in adopting healthy behaviours and subsequently improve health outcomes. The hypothesis that genetic risk information has personal salience and is a potent motivator for behaviour change is supported by the Health Belief Model. However, reviews summarising studies examining this have confirmed that it does not have greater benefits in changing dietary behaviour or clinical outcomes such as weight, as compared to non-genetic risk information (Hollands *et al.*, 2016; Li *et al.*, 2016). A large, European-wide, Internet-based trial on personalised nutrition (Food4Me) found that any form of personalisation (i.e. according to participant's intake; anthropometric or biochemical marker/s; or by genetic information) results in a greater level of healthy eating, as compared to those given conventional, non-personalised, dietary advice (Celis-Morales *et al.*, 2017). This suggests that the process of personalisation (i.e. tailoring advice), rather than the tool used to convey personalisation (e.g. genes), is more important in promoting dietary behaviour change. The potential for ethical, legal and social issues associated with research and practice in genetics and nutritional genomics is emerging. These include how genetic information is analysed, stored and used, particularly in relation to confidentiality, and the avoidance of *genetic discrimination* by those interested in an individual's risk of disease, e.g. health insurers and employers (Reilly & Debusk, 2008).

Finally, studies have shown that dietitians have positive attitudes towards genetics and nutritional genomics, but many have too limited knowledge and confidence to enable them to be involved (Collins *et al.*, 2013; Li *et al.*, 2014; Whelan *et al.*, 2008). Although there is currently limited evidence to support nutritional genomic interventions, dietitians must clearly be competent and skilled to be able to act upon new research evidence as and when it is published.

Acknowledgement

The editor acknowledges the prior contribution of Joanna Instone.

Further reading

DeBusk RM, Fogarty CP, Ordovas JM, Kornman KS. (2005) Nutritional genomics in practice: where do we begin? *J. Am. Diet. Assoc.* 105: 589–598.

Li SX, Lovegrove JA. (2016) Genetics and hyperlipidaemia. In: Lawrence J, Douglas P, Gandy J (eds) *Dietetic and Nutrition Case Studies*. UK: Wiley, pp. 55–58.

Stover PJ, Caudill MA. (2008) Genetic and epigenetic contributions to human nutrition and health: managing genome–diet interactions. *J. Am. Diet. Assoc.* 108: 1480–1487.

Internet resources

Genomics education programme https://www.genomicseducation.hee.nhs.uk/

National Genetics Education and Development Centre, www.geneticseducation.nhs.uk/index.aspx

Nutrigenomics Organisation (NuGO), www.nugo.org

Practice-based Evidence in Nutrition (PEN) Knowledge pathway on nutritional genomics, https://www.pennutrition.com/index.aspx

References

Bennet AM, Di Angelantonio E, Ye Z, *et al.* (2007) Association of apolipoprotein E genotypes with lipid levels and coronary risk. *JAMA* 298: 1300–1311.

Brown L, van der Ouderaa F. (2007) Nutritional genomics: food industry applications from farm to fork. *Br. J. Nutr.* 97: 1027–1035.

Burke S, Bennett C, Bedward J, *et al.* (2007) *The Experiences and Preferences of People Receiving Genetic Information from Healthcare Professionals*. Birmingham: National Genetics Education and Development Centre.

Camp KM, Trujillo E. (2014) Position of the Academy of Nutrition and Dietetics: nutritional genomics. *J. Acad. Nutr. Diet.* 114(2): 299–312.

Carvalho-Wells AL, Jackson KG, Locyer S, *et al.* (2012) APOE genotype influences triglyceride and C-reactive protein responses to altered dietary fat intake in UK adults. *Am. J. Clin. Nutr.* 96(6): 1447–1453.

Celis-Morales C, Livingstone KM, Marsaux CFM, *et al.* (2017) Effect of personalized nutrition on health-related behaviour change: evidence from the Food4me European randomized controlled trial. *Int. J. Epidemiol.* 46(2): 578–588.

Clarke R, Halsey J, Lewington S, *et al.*, B-Vitamin Treatment Trialists' Collaboration. (2010) Effects of lowering homocysteine levels with B vitamins on cardiovascular disease, cancer, and cause-specific mortality: meta-analysis of 8 randomized trials involving 37485 individuals. *Arch. Intern. Med.* 170: 1622–1631.

Collins J, Bertrand B, Hayes V, *et al.* (2013) The application of genetics and nutritional genomics in practice: an international survey of knowledge, involvement and confidence among dietitians in the US, Australia and the UK. *Genes Nutr.* 8(6): 523–533.

Fallaize R, Carvalho-Wells AL, Tierney AC, *et al.* (2017) APOE genotype influences insulin resistance, apolipoprotein CII and CIII according to plasma fatty acid profile in the Metabolic Syndrome. *Sci. Rep.* 7(1): 6274. doi: 10.1038/s41598-017-05802-2.

Franks PW, Pearson E, Florez JC. (2013) Gene–environment and gene–treatment interactions in type 2 diabetes: progress, pitfalls, and prospects. *Diabetes Care*. 36: 1413–1421.

Haycock PC, Burgess S, Wade KH, *et al.* (2016) Best (but oft-forgotten) practices: the design, analysis, and interpretation of Mendelian randomization studies. *Am. J. Clin. Nutr.* 103(4): 965–978.

Hollands GJ, French DP, Griffen SJ, *et al.* (2016) The impact of communicating genetic risks of disease on risk- reducing health behaviour: systematic review with meta-analysis. *BMJ* 352(1102): doi: 10.1136/bmj.i1102

Holmes MV, Dale CE, Zuccolo L, *et al.* (2014) Association between alcohol and cardiovascular disease: Mendelian randomisation analysis based on individual participant data. *BMJ* 349: g4164.

Holmes MV, Newcombe P, Hubacek JA, *et al.* (2011) Effect modification by population dietary folate on the association between MTHFR genotype, homocysteine, and stroke risk: a meta-analysis of genetic studies and randomised trials. *Lancet* 378(9791): 584–594.

Jacques PF, Bostom AG, Williams RR, *et al.* (1996) Relation between folate status, a common mutation in methylene tetrahydrofolate reductase, and plasma homocysteine concentrations. *Circulation* 93: 7–9.

Klerk M, Verhoef P, Clarke R, *et al.*, MTHFR Studies Collaboration Group. (2002) MTHFR 677C-->T polymorphism and risk of coronary heart disease: a meta-analysis. *JAMA* 288: 2023–2031.

Li SX, Collins J, Lawson S, *et al.* (2014) A preliminary qualitative exploration of dietitians' engagement with genetics and nutritional genomics: perspectives from international leaders. *J. Allied Health* 43(4): 221–228.

Li SX, Imamura F, Ye Z, *et al.*, EPIC-InterAct Consortium. (2017) Interaction between genes and macronutrient intake on the risk of developing type 2 diabetes: systematic review and findings from EPIC-InterAct. *Am. J. Clin. Nutr.* 106(1): 263–275.

Li SX, Ye Z, Whelan K, *et al.* (2016) The effect of communicating the genetic risk of cardiometabolic disorders on motivation and actual engagement in preventative lifestyle modification and clinical outcome: a systematic review and meta-analysis of randomised controlled trials. *Br. J. Nutr.* 116(5): 924–934.

Lovegrove JA, Gitau R. (2008) Personalized nutrition for the prevention of cardiovascular disease: a future perspective. *J. Hum. Nutr. Diet.* 21: 306–316.

Reilly PR, Debusk RM. (2008) Ethical and legal issues in nutritional genomics. *J. Am. Diet. Assoc.* 108: 36–40.

Skills for Health/NGEDC. (2007) *Enhancing patient care by integrating genetics in clinical practice: UK workforce competencies for genetics in clinical practice for non-genetics healthcare staff.* Birmingham: National Genetics Education and Development Centre.

Whelan K, McCarthy S, Pufulete M. (2008) Genetics and diet–gene interactions: involvement, confidence and knowledge of dietitians. *Br. J. Nutr.* 99: 23–28.

SECTION 5

5.2 Functional foods

Lisa Ryan

Key points

- Functional foods, when consumed regularly as part of the usual diet, have a specific health beneficial effect beyond their basic nutritional value.
- The beneficial health effects are due to the presence of a variety of bioactive components that elicit their effects via a number of different mechanisms.
- Functional foods encompass a very broad range of products, including infant formulas, medical foods, performance foods, probiotics and foods designed to deliver specialised nutrients and non-nutrients.
- In Europe, the assessment of the scientific evidence to support health claims is the responsibility of the European Food Safety Authority (EFSA).

Certain foods and food ingredients are being studied for their roles in preventing and treating chronic diseases, and for their benefits in slowing the ageing process and affecting mood and performance. These foods, known as functional foods, have the potential to promote better health and well-being, thereby helping to reduce the risk of chronic disease and to improve specific health functions.

The concept of functional foods first emerged in Japan as a result of escalating healthcare costs. As the concept of functional foods grew, the Japanese government promoted the idea of functional foods as a possible way of improving the health of their ageing population. In 1991, the Japanese renamed functional foods as foods for specified health use (FOSHU), and defined them as '*processed foods containing ingredients that aid specific bodily functions in addition to being nutritious*'. A regulatory system was established to approve such foods and to evaluate the scientific justification of claims. In Japan, FOSHU foods bear a seal of approval from the Ministry of Health and Welfare, making them easily recognisable to the consumer (Arai, 1996). The area of functional foods is expanding and now represents one of the most dynamic growth categories to have emerged from food science and nutrition.

In contrast to Japan, no legal definitions are available in either the USA or Europe for functional foods. However, they may be broadly defined as '*foods similar in appearance to conventional foods that are consumed as part of a normal diet and have demonstrated physiological benefits and/or reduce the risk of chronic disease beyond basic nutritional functions*' (Clydesdale, 1997). A functional food may be:

- A natural food.
- A food to which a component has been added.
- A food from which a component has been removed.
- A food where one or more components have been modified.
- A food in which the bioavailability has been modified.
- Any combination of the above.

Functional foods may be classified according to the type of food (Table 5.2.1) or bioactive ingredient (Table 5.2.2) used.

Table 5.2.1 Categories of functional foods (source: Arvanitoyannis & Van Houwelingen-Koukaliaroglou, 2005. Reproduced with permission of Taylor & Francis)

Category	Example
Basic foods	Tomatoes (rich in natural antioxidant lycopene)
Processed foods	Oat bran cereal
Processed food with added ingredients	Calcium-enriched fruit juice
Foods enhanced to have functional component	Oat bran with higher levels of beta-glucan
Isolated, purified preparations of active food ingredients	Soya isoflavones

Manual of Dietetic Practice, Sixth Edition. Edited by Joan Gandy.

Companion website: www.manualofdieteticpractice.com

Table 5.2.2 Examples of bioactive functional food ingredients

Functional ingredient	Food source	Potential effect on health
Anthocyanins	Strawberries, blueberries, blackberries	Protect against age-related cognitive decline; increase insulin sensitivity
Beta-glucan	Oats	Lowers blood cholesterol
		Reduces the postprandial glycaemic response
		Aids weight control
Conjugated linoleic acid (CLA)	Cheese, meat products	Improves body fat composition
		Enhances immune system
		Reduces risk of cancer
Epigallocatechin gallate (catechin)	Green tea	Increased thermogenesis and fat oxidation
Flavonoids	Tea, fruit, vegetables	Neutralise free radicals
		Reduce risk of cancer
Lycopene (carotenoid)	Tomatoes	Reduces risk of prostate cancer
Medium-chain triacylglycerols (MCTs)	Coconut oil, palm kernel oil	Increased thermogenesis and fat oxidation; decreased fat deposition
n-3 Fatty acids (ALA/EPA/DHA)	Salmon and fish oils	Reduce risk of cardiovascular disease
		May improve mental and visual functions
Phytoestrogens, e.g. isoflavones	Soya beans and soya-based foods	Alleviate symptoms associated with menopause
		Protect against heart disease and some cancers
		Lower LDL and total cholesterol
		Improve bone mineral density
Plant sterols/stanols/stanol esters	Corn, soya, wheat, wood oils	Reduce the absorption of cholesterol in the body
		Lower blood cholesterol levels (total and LDL cholesterol by ~10%)
		Note: May interfere with the absorption of other fat-soluble components from the diet; data on effects of long-term consumption at levels >3 g/day are limited
Prebiotics, e.g. inulin, fructooligosaccharides	Jerusalem artichokes, shallots, onion powder	Stimulate the growth of certain bacteria in the colon
		Improve quality of intestinal microflora; gastrointestinal health
Probiotics, e.g. *Lactobacillus acidophilus*	Yoghurt and other dairy products	Improve quality of intestinal microflora; gastrointestinal health
Resveratrol	Red wine	Beneficial effects on CVD function

LDL, low-density lipoprotein.

Ingredients

A food is said to be functional if it contains a food component (nutrient or non-nutrient) that affects one or more targeted functions in the body in a positive way. They are similar in appearance, smell and taste to a conventional food and are consumed as part of the usual diet. Functional foods represent an increasingly diverse collection of foods, e.g. infant formulas, medical foods, performance foods, probiotics and foods designed to deliver specialised nutrients and components (such as fibre, vitamins, minerals, antioxidants, prebiotics, dairy proteins, soya proteins, fats and oils). The beneficial health effects are due to the presence of a variety of bioactive components that elicit their effects via several different mechanisms. These substances (bioactives) often originate from plant sources, but some are derived from animals and microorganisms (Table 5.2.2).

There are several different steps involved in determining the potential role of functional ingredients in disease prevention, such as identifying the following:

- Rate and extent of absorption, including enterohepatic circulation.
- Metabolic conversions of compounds in intestinal and liver cells/tissues.
- Binding serum proteins.
- Plasma levels of aglycones and conjugates.
- Urinary excretion.
- Molecular modes of action.

Regulation

The effects of functional foods on health must be scientifically proven before claims can be made for a food (see Chapter 4.5, Food law and labelling). Some bioactives have regulatory approval and are already available in the marketplace; however, they are relatively few in number. In Europe, the assessment of the scientific evidence to support health claims is the responsibility of EFSA, which evaluates claims under articles 13 (general function claims) and 14 (disease claims) of the 2007 European Union regulation EC no. 1924/2006. When assessing the evidence, EFSA considers the extent to which:

1. The food/constituent is defined and characterised.
2. The claimed effect is defined and is a beneficial physiological effect.
3. A cause-and-effect relationship is established between the consumption of the food/constituent and the claimed effect (for the target group under the proposed conditions of use).

Scientific substantiation requires a favourable outcome to all three questions.In the USA, the Food and Drug Administration (FDA) evaluates claims for food and dietary supplements in three different categories:

- Health claims to describe a relationship between a food substance (a food, food component, or dietary supplement ingredient) and reduced risk of a disease or health-related condition.
- Nutrient content claims that characterise the level of a nutrient in a food.
- Structure/function claims that may describe the role of a nutrient or dietary ingredient intended to affect the normal structure or function of the human body, e.g. *calcium builds strong bones*. In addition, they may characterise the means by which a nutrient or dietary ingredient acts to maintain such structure or function, e.g. *fibre maintains bowel regularity* or *antioxidants maintain cell integrity*.

Functional food ingredients

It is known that patterns of food consumption play an important role in the development of chronic diseases such as cardiovascular disease (CVD), type 2 diabetes, osteoporosis, certain cancers, obesity and cognitive decline. The inclusion of functional food ingredients in the diet may make it possible to modulate several identified major risk factors for chronic disease, and thus may be of great importance for health.

Plant sterols/stanols

Plant sterols (phytosterols) are naturally occurring components of plant wall membranes and are found in small amounts in many grains, vegetables, fruits, legumes, nuts and seeds. They resemble cholesterol in function and structure, differing in the composition of their side chain (the cholesterol side chain is comprised of eight carbon atoms, whereas most phytosterol side chains contain 9–10 carbon atoms). Over 40 plant sterols have been identified to date; however, the three most abundant plant sterols are sitosterol, campesterol and stigmasterol. The term phytosterols is often used in a generic sense to encompass both plant sterols and stanols. Stanols are saturated derivatives of sterols and are less abundant in nature than sterols, but are more commonly used in functional food products. To improve their solubility, phytosterols are often combined with a fatty acid ester to produce plant sterol and stanol esters. Plants sterols and stanols reduce total and LDL cholesterol in humans with mild to moderate hypercholesterolaemia. Phytosterols reduce the absorption of cholesterol by competing for incorporation into mixed micelles and also inhibit the reabsorption of endogenous cholesterol. Therefore, when phytosterols are part of the regular diet, they have an overall lowering effect on serum cholesterol concentrations (Richelle *et al.*, 2004). The average daily diet contains approximately 0.25 g of plant sterols, although this may be twice as high in a vegetarian diet. Phytosterols at doses of approximately 2–2.5 g per day are required to lower LDL cholesterol (Ellegard *et al.*, 2007; Moruisi *et al.*, 2006). Dairy spreads fortified with phytosterols (~2 g/ daily portion) have been developed as functional foods. The added phytosterols in fortified dairy spreads have been shown to reduce the absorption of cholesterol in the gut (both dietary and endogenous) and to lower blood LDL cholesterol by ~7–10.5% in both men and women (EFSA, 2009). The results of a number of clinical intervention trials suggest that a 10% reduction in LDL cholesterol induced by medication or dietary modification could decrease the risk of coronary heart disease by approximately 20%. The effect of long-term use of foods enriched with plant sterols or stanols on cardiovascular disease risk is not known.

β-glucans

β-glucan is a soluble dietary fibre found in cereals such as barley and oats. Other cereals (sorghum, wheat, maize and rye) also contain some β-glucan, but in much lower amounts. Non-cereal sources include certain types of seaweed and different species of mushrooms including reishi, shiitake and maitake. Structurally, β-glucans are a heterogeneous group of non-starch polysaccharides consisting of D-glucose monomers linked by β-glycosidic bonds. β-glucans from different cereals vary in the ratio of β-(1->4): β-(1->3) linkages. The source, structure and molecular weight of different β-glucans can have important implications for physiological function (Lazaridou & Biliaderis, 2007). There is considerable growing interest in the potential role that β-glucans can play in protecting against coronary heart disease (CHD). In addition to the known hypocholesterolaemic properties of β-glucans in increasing the viscosity of the digesta and providing fermentable matter for colonic microflora, consumption of β-glucans is also associated with increased bile acid excretion and upregulation of 7 β-hydrolase, an enzyme involved in cholesterol elimination from the body (Yang *et al.*, 2003). Oat breakfast cereals enriched with oat β-glucan at doses of at least 3 g/day have shown a significant decrease in LDL cholesterol concentrations and are readily available as functional foods with accepted health claims in a number of countries (EFSA, 2010).

Polyphenols

The Mediterranean Paradox has questioned how a diet that is high in saturated fat with regular consumption of red wine could be protective against CHD. Part of the explanation for this paradox is thought to be the presence of polyphenols (most notably resveratrol) in red wine. Polyphenols are a group of biologically active compounds found ubiquitously in plants. They are comprised of four main groups: phenolic acids, flavonoids, stilbenes and lignans, and are found abundantly in foods such as fruits and vegetables, and also from sources such as dark chocolate, tea and wine. Resveratrol has been shown to induce vasorelaxation through the activation or increased generation of nitric oxide. This mechanism, as well as the ability to protect against LDL oxidation and platelet aggregation, is one of the proposed reasons behind the cardioprotective effects of red wine polyphenols.

Tea is also rich in a number of different polyphenols, particularly flavonoids. Both green tea and black tea come from the leaves of the plant *Camellia sinensis*; however, the processing that the leaves undergo to make the final tea is different. The leaves for black tea are fully oxidised, while those for green teas are lightly steamed before being dried. Black and green tea contain similar amounts of total flavonoids; however, they differ in their chemical structure. Green tea contains more of the simple flavonoids called catechins, while the oxidation that the leaves undergo to make black tea converts these simple flavonoids to more complex varieties called theaflavins and thearubigins. A Cochrane review by Hartley *et al.* (2013) concluded that the evidence is promising to suggest that green and black tea have a positive impact on blood pressure, blood lipids and overall cardiovascular risk reduction. Extracts rich in bioactives from tea could therefore be incorporated as functional food ingredients. Flavonoids from tea have also been investigated for their potential role in protecting against cognitive decline.

Medium-chain triacylglycerols

Medium-chain triacylglycerols (MCTs) typically contain fatty acids with chain lengths ≤ 12 carbon atoms and are processed very differently from long-chain triacylglycerols (LCTs) in the body. Due to their chain length, MCTs can be absorbed into the gastrointestinal tract and transported to the liver via portal circulation without incorporation into chylomicrons. As a result, MCTs are oxidised to a greater extent than LCTs, and therefore are primarily used as a source of energy and have less opportunity to be deposited as adipose tissue. This has led to a considerable number of studies investigating the effect of MCTs, typically found in coconut oil and palm kernel oil, as potential functional ingredients for weight loss. Studies in animals have consistently shown that rats have less adipose tissue when fed MCTs as compared to LCTs.

Human studies have shown that MCTs increase fat oxidation and postprandial thermogenesis as compared to LCTs, and that diets rich in MCTs can increase satiety and reduce food intake as compared to diets rich in LCTs (Clegg *et al.*, 2013). Many of the studies in this area have been acute postprandial investigations. However, St-Onge *et al.* (2003) investigated the effect of long-term consumption (4 weeks) of MCTs as compared to LCTs on energy expenditure, substrate oxidation and body composition in obese women. They demonstrated that meals supplemented with MCTs significantly enhanced energy expenditure and fat oxidation as compared to LCT-enriched meals, suggesting that long-term usage of MCTs may result in weight loss via enhanced energy expenditure in women.

Phytoestrogens

Phytoestrogens are plant-derived oestrogens that can interact with oestrogen receptors (ERα and ERβ) and mimic the action of oestrogen in the human body. They can have agonist and/or antagonist effects on oestrogen receptors. There are three main classes of phytoestrogens – isoflavones, lignans and coumestans. Soya beans are the most widely used dietary source of phytoestrogens, and they are particularly rich in the isoflavones genistein and daidzein, although the levels of these isoflavones vary greatly, depending on the growing conditions, source, and extraction and processing methods of the soya bean.

Epidemiological studies have consistently shown a lower incidence of fractures in Asian women as compared to Caucasian women, which has often been attributed to the higher isoflavone intake in these regions (Lagari & Levis, 2010). Since phytoestrogens interact with oestrogen receptors, it has been hypothesised that they may have an effect on bone health and may be of importance as functional dietary aids to reducing postmenopausal bone loss. This has led to extensive investigation of the use of isoflavones to help reduce menopausal symptoms and the risk of osteoporosis. The results from in vitro studies have shown that soya isoflavones can positively impact on bone health by inhibiting bone resorption and stimulating bone formation. Findings from investigations in animals suggest that the role of isoflavones in bone health may be in prevention rather than as therapeutic aids.

To date, the research in humans has yielded conflicting results. It is clear that phytoestrogens can be protective; however, short-term intake is unlikely to yield beneficial results. Nevertheless, intervention studies have shown a reduced rate of bone turnover and an increase in bone density following supplementation with phytoestrogens (generally a combination of genistein and daidzein) (Cornwell *et al.*, 2004). Castelo-Branco and Soveral (2013) have suggested that the effect of soya isoflavones on bone mineral density is mediated by eqoul production (equol producers seem to have a more positive response to isoflavone supplementation), reproductive status (the perimenopausal period is the best stage to intervene for prevention of bone loss), dose, supplement type and length of duration.

Omega-3 fatty acids

Omega-3 fatty acids are polyunsaturated fatty acids found in various plants and marine life. Longer-chain derivatives such as eicosapentaenoic acid (EPA) and docosahexaenoic acid (DHA) seem to be consistently associated with health benefits. n-3 fatty acids have been shown to decrease blood pressure, reduce inflammatory processes (often seen in CVD) and have a positive effect on fatty acids. Plants typically contain the parent n-3 fatty acid, α-linolenic acid (ALA), which is essential in humans, as it cannot be synthesised endogenously. Although the longer-chain n-3 derivatives can be formed from ALA, research suggests that this is an inefficient process (Brenna *et al.*, 2009). Furthermore, n-6 fatty acids compete with n-3 fatty acids for metabolising enzymes. Therefore, an excess of n-6 fatty acids in the diet, as is typical of many Western diets, will favour the production of longer-chain n-6 family derivatives. The main dietary source of EPA and DHA is oil-rich fish.

It has been suggested that n-3 fatty acids may be important for cognitive health, given that they are a major structural component of brain tissue, their antioxidant properties and also their importance in reducing the risk of vascular complications (Ammann *et al.*, 2013). Indeed, reduced levels of n-3 fatty acids have been identified in areas of the aged brain that are important for cognitive function. DHA is an important component of neuronal membranes, and both EPA and DHA have been shown to play a protective role in preventing cognitive impairment by enhancing neuronal function and decreasing inflammation, oxidation and cell death. Patients suffering from Alzheimer's disease have decreased levels of serum, brain and neuronal DHA as compared to healthy controls (Robinson *et al.*, 2010).

The exact role of the n-3 fatty acids in cognitive health remains unclear, but DHA has a potential role in neuronal transmission, brain glucose uptake, and learning and memory, and ALA and EPA may provide a limited amount of substrate for conversion to DHA, as well as complementary roles in ketogenesis and supplying energy to the brain (Freemantle *et al.*, 2006). Further potential roles of DHA in relation to reducing the risk of dementia are summarised in a review by Cole *et al.* (2009), who also highlight that the effects of DHA may require adequate amounts of accompanying antioxidants such as vitamin E and C.

Future perspectives

Several the most prevalent diseases in men and women – such as cardiovascular disease, cancer, obesity, osteoporosis and cognitive decline – are affected by diet and lifestyle. To date, a variety of bioactive ingredients have been identified that confer a range of health benefits and may play an important role in health. Research has shown that a good quality diet may not be sufficient. The consumption of functional food ingredients may therefore have the potential to prevent the development and/or slow the progression of a number of chronic diseases. Although this is a vibrant and very exciting area of research, more evidence is required from well-controlled human studies to prove the efficacy of functional foods.

References

Ammann EM, Pottala JV, Harris WS, *et al.* (2013) Omega-3 fatty acids and domain-specific cognitive aging: secondary analyses of data from WHISCA. *Neurology* 81(17): 1484–1491.

Arai S. (1996) Studies of functional foods in Japan – state of the art. *Biosci. Biotechnol. Biochem.* 60: 9–15.

Arvanitoyannis IS, Van Houwelingen-Koukaliaroglou M. (2005) Functional foods: a survey of health claims, pros and cons, and current legislation. *Crit. Rev. Food Sci. Nutr.* 45: 385–404.

Brenna JT, Salem N Jr, Sinclair AJ, *et al.* (2009) α-Linolenic acid supplementation and conversion to n-3 long-chain polyunsaturated fatty acids in humans. *Prostaglandins Leukot. Esssent. Fatty Acids* 80: 85–91.

Castelo-Branco C, Soveral I. (2013) Phytoestrogens and bone health at different reproductive stages. *Gynecol. Endocrinol.* 29(8): 735–743.

Clegg ME, Golsorkhi M, Henry CJ. (2013) Combined medium-chain triglyceride and chilli feeding increases diet-induced thermogenesis in normal-weight humans. *Eur. J. Nutr.* 52: 1579–1585.

Clydesdale FM. (1997) A proposal for the establishment of scientific criteria for health claims for functional foods. *Nutr. Rev.* 55: 413–422.

Cole GM, Ma QL, Frautschy SA. (2009) Omega-3 fatty acids and dementia. *Prostaglandins Leukot. Essent. Fatty Acids* 81(2–3): 213–221.

Cornwell T, Cohick W, Raskin I. (2004) Dietary phytoestrogens and health. *Phytochemistry* 65: 995–1016.

EFSA. (2009) Scientific opinion on plant sterols and plant stanols on blood LDL-cholesterol. *EFSA J.* 1175: 1–9.

EFSA. (2010) Scientific opinion on the substantiation of a health claim related to oat beta-glucan and lowering blood cholesterol and reduced risk of (coronary) heart disease pursuant to Article 14 of Regulation (EC) No 1924/2006. *EFSA J.* 8(12): 1885, 1–15.

Ellegard LH, Andersson SW, Normen AL, *et al.* (2007) Dietary plant sterols and cholesterol metabolism. *Nutr. Rev.* 65(1): 39–45.

Freemantle E, Vandal M, Tremblay-Mercier J, *et al.* (2006) Omega-3 fatty acids, energy substrates, and brain function during aging. *Prostaglandins Leukot. Essent. Fatty Acids* 75(3): 213–220.

Hartley L, Flowers N, Holmes J, Clarke A, Stranges S, Hooper L, Rees K. (2013) Green and black tea for the primary prevention of cardiovascular disease. *Cochrane Database Syst. Rev. 2013 Jun* 18(6):CD009934.

Lagari C, Levis S. (2010) Phytoestrogens and bone health. *Curr. Opin. Endocrinol. Diabetes Obes.* 17: 546–553.

Lazaridou A, Biliaderis CG. (2007) Molecular aspects of cereal *β*-glucan functionality: physical properties, technological applications and physiological effects. *J. Cereal Sci.* 46: 101–118.

Moruisi KG, Oosthuizen W, Opperman AM. (2006) Phytosterols/stanols lower cholesterol concentrations in familial hypercholesterolemic subjects: a systematic review with meta-analysis. *J. Am. Coll. Nutr.* 25(1): 41–48.

Richelle M, Enslen M, Hager C, *et al.* (2004) Both free and esterified plant sterols reduce cholesterol absorption and the bioavailability of beta-carotene and alpha-tocopherol in normocholesterolemic humans. *Am. J. Clin. Nutr.* 80(1): 171–177.

Robinson JG, Ijioma N, Harris W. (2010) Omega-3 fatty acids and cognitive function in women. *Womens Health (Lond).* 6(1): 119–134.

St-Onge MP, Bourque C, Jones PJH, *et al.* (2003) Medium- versus long-chain triglycerides for 27 days increases fat oxidation and energy expenditure without resulting in changes in body composition in overweight women. *Int. J. Obes. Relat Metab Disord.* 27: 95–102

Yang JL, Kim YH, Lee HS, *et al.* (2003) Barley beta-glucan lowers serum cholesterol based on the up-regulation of cholesterol 7 alpha-hydroxylase activity and mRNA abundance in cholesterol-fed rats. *J. Nutr. Sci. Vitaminol. (Tokyo).* 49(6): 381–387.

5.3 Medicines management

Najia Qureshi and Joan Gandy

Key points

- Advanced dietetic practitioners, with appropriate training, can now have supplementary prescribing rights.
- Nutrition can affect the therapeutic action of many drugs by influencing drug absorption, metabolism and excretion.
- The action and/or side effects of drugs may result in marked changes in food intake. Drugs can also impair nutrient absorption or metabolism, or increase nutrient excretion.
- Information about therapeutic drug use, including over-the-counter medicines, herbs, alcohol consumption and tobacco use, should be obtained during a nutritional assessment.

There is a close relationship between medicine and food for many conditions such as diabetes, renal disease, gastrointestinal disorders and malnutrition, and dietitians have always considered food–drug interactions in their practice. Dietetic intervention is fundamental to the effective management of long-term conditions such as diabetes, renal disease, gastrointestinal disorders, cystic fibrosis and cancer. As people live longer with increasingly complex and multiple long-term conditions, dietitians have the potential to significantly improve the quality of care that patients with nutritional needs receive, through timely access to medicines.

The British National Formulary (BNF) is used as a quick reference tool which aims to provide prescribers, pharmacists and other healthcare professionals with sound up-to-date information about the use of medicines. It includes key information on the selection, prescribing, dispensing and administration of medicines.

Prescription-only medicines

Prescription-only medicines (POMs) need a prescription issued by a GP or other suitably qualified healthcare professional, including advanced practice nurses, pharmacists, physiotherapists, radiographers, chiropodists and podiatrists, and dietitians; they include medicines such as insulin, phosphate binders, parenteral nutrition, etc.

Nutrition borderline substances

In certain conditions, some foods may be considered as drugs. The Advisory Committee on Borderline Substances (ACBS) recommends products to be included in the BNF on the basis that they may be regarded as drugs for the management of specified conditions, e.g. oral nutritional supplements, nutrition products for metabolic diseases, and gluten-free products. Patient access to any nutrition borderline substances (NBSs) is complex and strictly governed. Dietitians are able to advise on these medicines, but only within the scope of their practice, training and education. Patients can obtain the medicines they need, at NHS expense, through a variety of different mechanisms:

- Prescription to be taken to a pharmacy for dispensing.
- Supply of a short course of medicine, or direct administration, e.g. injection.
- Local arrangements for the management of NBS.

All registered dietitians are able to manage NBS within their scope of practice. However, only those dietitians who have met the entry criteria and successfully completed an HCPC-approved postgraduate course in prescribing can use supplementary prescribing rights.

Prescribing frameworks

There are two frameworks that can be used by advanced practitioners to prescribe medicines for their patients; supplementary and independent prescribing.

Supplementary prescribing

A supplementary prescriber forms a voluntary prescribing partnership with an independent prescriber (usually

Manual of Dietetic Practice, Sixth Edition. Edited by Joan Gandy.

Companion website: www.manualofdieteticpractice.com

a doctor), to implement an agreed patient-specific clinical management plan (CMP) with the patient's agreement. Supplementary prescribing is intended for ongoing care (DH, 2005).

Independent prescribing

An independent prescriber is a practitioner responsible and accountable for the assessment of patients with undiagnosed and diagnosed conditions and for decisions about the clinical management, including the prescription of medicines.

The dietetic profession was granted supplementary prescribing rights in 2016. This gave trained, advanced dietitians the ability to provide their patients with a prescription for the medicines they require, in the correct dosage, when they needed it, and without the need for a further appointment with the doctor/GP just to obtain the prescription. Advanced dietitians who undertake roles within multi-disciplinary teams are required to undertake postgraduate-level education and training in order to become supplementary prescribers. A dietitian's HCPC registration is then annotated to identify this qualification. It should be noted that dietitians are currently not able to practice as independent prescribers.

Case examples

Advanced dietitian working in chronic kidney disease

Renal consultants refer patients to an advanced dietitian as the most appropriate healthcare professional to assess the patient's diet and advise on the optimum phosphate binder medication and dosage in relation to this. Poor phosphate management results in a higher risk of fractures in weakened bones and a hardening of the blood vessels (cardiovascular disease), leading to heart failure. With supplementary prescribing rights, the advanced dietitian is able to advise the patient on the diet, and supply the patient with a more tailored and timely prescription against an agreed CMP, for dispensing at a local pharmacy without the need to refer back to a prescribing physician. This saves hospital/GP appointments, reduces the patient pathway and improves the patient experience of coordinated seamless management.

Advanced nutrition support dietitian

Patients with intestinal failure (IF) who do not have adequate bowel function to absorb enough fluid and nutrition rely on parenteral nutrition (PN). Many patients will only require PN until the medical condition can be resolved, while others will require PN at home for life. The advanced nutrition support dietitian completes a clinical and nutritional assessment; calculates the nutritional requirements including fluid, energy, nitrogen, electrolytes and duration of infusion; and, according to the patient's biochemistry, requests a prescription for PN to be made up in a pharmacy compounding unit. The dietitian usually needs to access a doctor to generate the prescription advised by the dietitian. Getting the PN prescription signed is frequently a time-limiting step to making the changes required, which can put the patient at risk of metabolic complications including malnutrition, dehydration/fluid overload and electrolyte abnormalities, and deterioration in liver function. The advanced dietitian with supplementary prescribing rights will develop a CMP with the independent prescriber on diagnosis, enabling patients to receive the correctly formulated PN for their needs, without unnecessary delay in commencement and adjustment of PN.

Drug–nutrient interactions

There are many interactions between drugs and both macronutrients and micronutrients. Drugs and nutrients are absorbed from similar sites and metabolised and excreted in similar ways. Therefore, just as a drug can interfere with the action of another, some drugs may interfere with the action of a nutrient, or vice versa. It is essential that dietitians have knowledge of these interactions and alert medical personnel to possible problems they may not be aware of (Boullata & Hudson, 2012). Prescribed drugs are likely to have the greatest nutritional implications, since they are the most powerful or high-dose forms of medication. However, it is important to consider that people often self-administer other types of preparations with pharmacological effects and nutritional implications. These include:

- Over-the-counter drugs, e.g. analgesics, indigestion remedies, laxatives.
- Herbal remedies, including Chinese herbal remedies (see Chapter 5.4, Alternative and complementary therapies).
- Nutritional supplements, e.g. fish oil capsules, large doses of vitamins.
- Alcohol.
- Tobacco.
- Illegal substances.

Drug abuse can cause many nutritional problems, both directly from the effects of the drug itself and indirectly from the poor dietary habits and living conditions often associated with it. Drug–nutrient interactions can be broadly categorised into:

- Effect of nutrition on drugs – the influence of nutritional factors on drug absorption, action and effectiveness.
- Effect of drugs on nutrition – the influence of drugs on nutritional intake, metabolism, excretion and requirements.

Classes of drugs that are most likely to have nutritional implications are shown in Table 5.3.1. Many drugs used in the treatment of mental illness have drug–nutrient interactions, and these are summarised in detail in Table 7.10.6 (see Chapter 7.10.1, Nutrition and mental health). Cytotoxic chemotherapy drugs are also known to have effects on nutritional status, and these are discussed further in Chapter 7.15 (Cancer). This chapter gives an overview of the subject with examples; it is not

Table 5.3.1 Examples of drugs that are most likely to have nutritional implications

Class of drug	Possible nutritional implications
Amphetamines	Increased appetite
Antacids	Can bind with minerals such as phosphorus, magnesium, iron, and zinc, and reduce their absorption
	Antacids raise gastric pH, which may also impair the absorption of some trace elements, especially vitamin B_{12}, which requires acid conditions for its release from dietary protein
Antibiotics	Anorexia
	Altered gut flora and diarrhoea
	Tetracycline forms complexes with calcium (in foods or mineral supplements), reducing the absorption of both
Anticoagulants	Warfarin action is impaired by vitamin K
Anticonvulsants	Interfere with folate metabolism
	Interfere with vitamin D metabolism
Antidepressants	Anorexia
	MAOI type A usage necessitates avoidance of tyramine[a]
Antihyperlipidaemics	Clofibrate and cholestyramine can result in malabsorption, especially of minerals and fat-soluble vitamins
Antipsychotics	Some types markedly increase appetite[a]
Antirheumatics	Methotrexate inhibits folate metabolism
	Penicillamine reduces absorption of iron and zinc
Corticosteroids	Anabolic effects and weight gain
	Glucose intolerance
Cytotoxic (anticancer) drugs	Anorexia
	Taste changes
	Sore and painful mouth and tongue
	Nausea, vomiting and diarrhoea
	Damage to intestinal villi
	Interfere with folate metabolism (especially methotrexate)
	Reduce thiamine status
Dopaminergic drugs (used in Parkinsonism)	Levodopa causes nausea and vomiting if taken on an empty stomach
	Levodopa absorption is inhibited by iron supplements
	Levodopa can be inhibited by B_6 supplements
Diuretics	Thiazide and loop diuretics can cause excessive urinary loss of potassium, calcium, zinc and water-soluble vitamins
	Dehydration
Hypoglycaemics	Action has to be balanced against carbohydrate intake
	Alcohol can potentiate their action
	Chlorpropamide can react with alcohol and cause facial flushing
Laxatives	Reduced absorption of nutrients (liquid paraffin)
Mood stabilisers	Lithium action is affected by dietary sodium[a]
Non-steroidal anti-inflammatory drugs (NSAIDs)	Gastric irritation and risk of bleeding if taken on an empty stomach
	Aspirin increases vitamin C excretion
Oral contraceptives	Affect glucose and lipid metabolism
	Can cause weight gain

[a] See Chapter 7.10.1 Nutrition and mental health; MAOI, monoamine oxidase inhibitors.

definitive, and the titles listed in the resources section of this chapter should be consulted for further detail.

Effects of nutrition on drugs

The metabolism of a drug may involve the following stages, any of which can be influenced by nutrition:

- Transport from the gut lumen to intestinal enterocytes (if the drug is taken orally), sometimes followed by presystemic metabolism prior to absorption into the blood.
- Transport in the blood, usually bound to plasma proteins.
- Deactivation by a two-stage metabolic process:

- Oxidation by microsomal enzyme systems, involving reduced nicotinamide adenine dinucleotide (NADPH) and cytochrome P450, predominantly in the liver but also in other organs, including the lungs and small intestine.
- Conjugation with glucuronic acid, sulphate or glycine.
- Excretion of the conjugate in urine or bile.

Table 5.3.2 gives examples of drug–nutrient interactions that affect drug absorption, metabolism or excretion. It may be noted that this list is not exhaustive; Stockley's Drug Interactions or the British National Formulary should be consulted for further information.

Table 5.3.2 Examples of drug–nutrient interactions affecting absorption, metabolism and excretion of drugs (adapted from Webster-Gandy *et al*., 2011, tables 38.1, and 38.2 pp. 738–740. Reproduced with permission from Oxford University Press)

Drug or class of drug	Food and/or nutrient	Effect of interaction and advice
Absorption		
Bismuth Flucloxacillin Phenoxymethylpenicillin Rifampicin	Presence of food in the stomach	Absorption delayed and reduced Advise to take on an empty stomach or 1 hour before food
Ciprofloxacin Norfloxacin Tetracyclines	Milk and dairy products	Absorption reduced Advise to leave 2-hour gap between drug and dairy consumption
Theophylline	High-protein diet	Bioavailability reduced by high-protein diets
	High-carbohydrate diet	Bioavailability increased by high-carbohydrate diets
Ciprofloxacin Digoxin Phenytoin Rifampicin Tetracycline Theophylline	Enteral feeds	Absorption reduced Leave time gap between giving medication and enteral feed
Metabolism		
Amiodarone Buspirone Calcium channel blockers Carbamazepine Ciclosporin Colchicine Corticosteroids Coumarins Digoxin Fexofenadine Simvastatin	Grapefruit juice	Metabolism of drug altered due to liver enzyme, cytochrome P450, stimulation Advise to follow manufacturer's instructions
Warfarin	Large amounts of Brussel sprouts, green vegetables, cabbage, lettuce, green tea, excess quantities of ice cream, avocado, mango	Drug metabolism increased and anticoagulant effect of warfarin decreased Anticoagulant effect of warfarin increased *Note*: A fatal incident reported
	Cranberry juice	Anticoagulant effect of warfarin increased
	High doses of vitamin E	
Levodopa, phenobarbital, phenytoin	Vitamin B_6 (pyridoxine)	Effects of levodopa reduced by concurrent supplementation of pyridoxine Advise to avoid vitamin B_6
Excretion		
Lithium	Salt (sodium)	Excretion affected by increased and decreased salt intake Advise to keep sodium intake constant once stabilised on lithium

Drug absorption

The pharmacological effect of an orally administered drug depends on the rate and extent to which it is absorbed from the gastrointestinal tract. This can be delayed or enhanced by the presence or absence of food. The presence of food in the stomach and proximal intestine may reduce drug absorption as a result of the following:

- Delayed gastric emptying.
- Altered gastrointestinal pH.
- Competition for binding sites with nutrients.
- Chelation of drugs by food cations, e.g. tetracyclines chelate calcium ions present in milk and dairy products, resulting in reduced absorption of both calcium and antibiotic.
- Dietary fats impeding the absorption of hydrophilic drugs.

Some drugs must therefore be taken on an empty stomach in order to maximise their rate of absorption and therapeutic effect. Conversely, others must be taken with food to achieve a slower, more sustained rate of absorption or to minimise side effects such as gastric irritation, e.g. aspirin and other non-steroidal anti-inflammatory drugs (NSAIDs). Medicines should be taken with water, since drinks such as fruit juice, tea and coffee can alter the drug's pH balance and therefore its properties.

Drug transport

Many drugs are transported in blood bound to plasma proteins. Severe malnutrition, or diseases such as liver disease affecting the synthesis of plasma proteins, may reduce the body's ability to transport drugs, and hence impair their effectiveness.

Drug metabolism

Factors that affect the deactivation or conjugation of a drug can alter its pharmacological or toxic effects. Periods of short-term starvation or prolonged periods of nutritional inadequacy can influence the effectiveness or safety of drugs. The amount of a drug required to produce a certain pharmacological effect is determined by body weight. Sudden reduction in weight or dehydration may therefore result in overdose. Undernutrition also reduces the activity of microsomal drug-metabolising enzymes, and this can either diminish a drug's effectiveness (by reducing the rate of synthesis of an active metabolite) or enhance its toxicity (by reducing the rate of its excretion) (Dickerson, 1988). In addition, the metabolism of drugs is affected by the amount of water in the body, and this can be perturbed by dehydration or oedema, including that associated with kwashiorkor (protein energy malnutrition) (Oshikoya & Senbanjo, 2009). Some drugs are fat soluble, e.g. barbiturates; therefore, their metabolism will be affected by both decreased and increased levels of adipose-tissue-associated fat. The effects of obesity on drug metabolism vary, depending on the pathway by which they are metabolised (Brill *et al.*, 2012). Obviously, decreased or increased clearance rates may lead to potentially impaired drug action or increased possibility of side effects. Doses may need to be adjusted, as some are based on ideal body weight rather than actual body weight, e.g. anaesthesia.

It is important to consider that drug–nutrient interactions may be variable, with some individuals being more susceptible than others. An example of this is the interaction between grapefruit juice and simvastatin that results in increased levels of the circulating drug, which has the potential to increase side effects. However, there is debate as to whether or not this potential effect outweighs the potential beneficial effect of simvastatin on cholesterol levels (Backman & Bakhai, 2013; Pirmohamed, 2013).

Drug excretion

Urinary acidity affects drug reabsorption from the renal tubules. Supplemental intakes of nutrients that increase urinary acidity, e.g. large amounts of vitamin C, can decrease the excretion of salicylate drugs such as aspirin.

Potentially serious interactions

The following interactions have the potential to lead to serious events:

- Warfarin and vitamin K–containing foods.
- Warfarin and cranberry juice.
- Grapefruit juice and fexofenadine or ciclosporin.
- Angiotensin-converting enzyme (ACE) inhibitors or angiotensin II receptor antagonists and potassium supplements or salt substitutes – these drugs may cause potassium retention, which may be exacerbated by potassium supplements and potassium-containing salt substitutes, resulting in hyperkalaemia.
- Monoamine oxidase inhibitors (MAOIs) and tyramine – patients taking MAOIs (e.g. phenelzine and moclobemide) should avoid tyramine-containing foods (e.g. mature cheese, yeast extracts, soya bean products, pickled herring, red wine), as these may cause a dramatic increase in blood pressure and palpitations.
- Isotretinoin and vitamin A – isotretinoin is a retinoid used for the treatment of acne. Due to the risk of vitamin A toxicity, it should not be used with vitamin A supplements.

Effects of drugs on nutrition

Drugs may affect food intake or the absorption, metabolism or excretion of nutrients. This may have implications in terms of food choice and/or nutritional requirements.

Food intake

Food intake may be reduced as a result of drugs that have the following effects:

- Anorexia – either as a direct effect of the drug on appetite, e.g. cytotoxic chemotherapy drugs, or as a result of side effects such as drowsiness or lethargy, e.g. tranquillisers.

- Cause nausea and vomiting – this is a common side effect of many drugs.
- Gastrointestinal tract effects, e.g. NSAIDs often cause gastric irritation and should be taken with, or after, food. Other drugs may cause bloating or early satiety. Chronic abdominal pain or diarrhoea may reduce the desire to eat.
- Taste changes – many drugs (e.g. cytotoxic chemotherapy drugs) make food taste bland (ageusia) or change taste perception (dysgeusia). Many patients receiving some cytotoxic drugs report a metallic taste, often associated with protein consumption.
- Dry mouth (xerostomia) – lack of saliva makes it difficult to masticate and swallow food, especially those of a dry or fibrous consistency.
- Sore or painful mouth (mucositis) or tongue (glossitis) – these are common side effects of chemotherapy that can significantly impair food intake.
- Impaired memory or confusion – people may forget to eat.

Drugs may also increase food intake and weight gain if they stimulate appetite or induce cravings. Corticosteroids, insulin and some psychotropic drugs are known to have either or both these effects (see Chapter 7.10.1, Nutrition and mental health).

Nutrient absorption

Absorption can be impaired as a result of:

- Formation of insoluble complexes – many drugs can chelate with minerals and trace elements, e.g. penicillamine (sometimes used in the treatment of rheumatoid arthritis) chelates zinc; cholestyramine binds with iron; and antacids may bind with phosphorus.
- Competition for binding sites, e.g. salicylates (aspirin) compete with vitamin C; and sulphasalazine, used in the treatment of arthritis, impairs folate absorption.
- Damage to the absorptive surface of the intestinal mucosa – cytotoxic chemotherapy can cause villous atrophy, resulting in malabsorption.
- Binding of bile acids – fat-soluble vitamin absorption will be impaired by bile-salt-binding drugs such as cholestyramine.
- Lipase inhibitors that reduce fat absorption and are used to aid weight loss, e.g. orlistat, may impair absorption of fat-soluble vitamins.
- Increased intestinal motility – drugs that cause diarrhoea or stimulate peristaltic activity, e.g. senna or phenolphthalein laxatives, may result in nutrient losses.

Nutrient metabolism

Some drugs may affect lipid or glucose metabolism. The following drugs may result in dyslipidaemia:

- Beta blockers.
- Corticosteroids.
- Thiazide diuretics.
- Anabolic steroids.
- Some anti-HIV drugs.
- Retinoids.
- Combined oral contraceptives.

Drugs that may affect glucose tolerance, apart from those used to manage diabetes, include thiazide diuretics and corticosteroids.

Micronutrient metabolism

Micronutrients are cofactors and coenzymes in many metabolic pathways, including those that metabolise drugs. Increased activity of these pathways as a result of drug metabolism may increase micronutrient requirements. Drugs can also compete with, or inhibit, the metabolic conversion of some micronutrients to their active metabolites, particularly folate. Some medicines may require nutritional supplements to prevent detrimental effects. These include:

- Corticosteroids – long-term oral use or high inhaled doses are risk factors for osteoporosis; therefore, calcium supplements are needed.
- Methotrexate – a folate antagonist, so a folate supplement (5 mg/day) is needed to prevent deficiency. It is used in rheumatoid arthritis and in cancer chemotherapy.
- Isoniazid – an antibiotic used in the treatment of tuberculosis; may have an antipyridoxine effect, and a 10 mg/day supplement of pyridoxine is recommended.
- Antiepileptic drugs in pregnancy – many are associated with birth defects; 5 mg/day of folate should be prescribed, as women with epilepsy are more likely to have low folate levels.
- Some cytotoxic antibiotics, imidazole, antifungal agents and anticonvulsants (e.g. phenytoin, phenobarbitone and primidone) impair vitamin D metabolism by inhibiting the conversion of 25-hydroxyvitamin D to the active form 1,25-dihydroxyvitamin D, with consequent disturbances in calcium metabolism and adverse effects on bone (Expert Group on Vitamins and Minerals, 2003).

Drugs may also affect the metabolism of dietary components. Type A monoamine oxidase inhibitors (MAOI A) exert their antidepressant effect by inhibiting the breakdown of endogenously produced amine neurotransmitters. However, they also inhibit the breakdown of dietary amines such as tyramine, which, if allowed to accumulate, can produce a dangerous rise in blood pressure. Patients on these drugs, therefore, must avoid dietary sources of tyramine and other vasoactive amines (see Chapter 7.10.1, Nutrition and mental health).

Nutrient excretion

In addition to their intended increase in sodium excretion, diuretic drugs can also result in enhanced losses of other elements such as potassium, calcium, magnesium and zinc. Tetracycline increases the urinary excretion of vitamin C.

SECTION 5

Clinical significance of drug–nutrient interactions

It is important to remember that poor nutritional status can impair drug metabolism, and that drug treatment can have a detrimental effect on nutritional status. However, not all drug–nutrient interactions are clinically significant. In many instances, any losses in nutrient availability or drug action will be small and may be of short duration. Drugs that are most likely to have dietetic implications are those that:

- Have a narrow range between therapeutic effect and toxicity, e.g. lithium and anticoagulants.
- Need to be taken for a prolonged period of time.
- Have implications in terms of the timing of food intake (habitual meal pattern may need to be adjusted).
- Necessitate dietary restrictions or regulation (food choice may need to be altered).
- Have side effects that impact on appetite or gastrointestinal function.
- Directly compete with a nutrient, e.g. vitamin K and warfarin.

Factors that increase the risk from drug–nutrient interactions include:

- Presence of gastrointestinal, liver and/or renal function.
- A nutritionally compromised state due to poor diet, alcoholism or disease.
- Recent weight loss.
- Dehydration.
- Multiple drug therapy.
- Prolonged drug therapy.

Many of these factors are likely to coexist in older adults. In addition, the physiological changes that occur with age such as a decrease in fat-free mass and body water, decreased plasma protein concentration, and general decline in renal and liver function mean that the risk of adverse drug reactions is much higher (Klotz, 2009; Szabolcs *et al.*, 2017). For this reason, it is a requirement that drug data sheets provide details of suitable dosages for elderly people.

Elderly people are also more likely to be given the types of drugs that have powerful effects and are more likely to impact on nutrition, e.g. anti-Parkinson's drugs. Diminished salivation in the elderly may make it more difficult to swallow tablets, and oesophageal motility disorders lead to bulky drugs sticking in the oesophageal mucosa. Other problems such as failing memory, poor hearing and vision, and difficulty with opening containers may mean that drug regimens are not followed correctly, particularly if they are complex. Drug usage is therefore an important consideration in the dietary assessment of elderly people.

Due to the nature of nutrients in enteral tube feeds, drug–nutrient interaction potential is increased. Drugs in liquid form may interact with constituents of the feed preparation, thereby altering their bioavailability and requiring dose adjustment, e.g. digoxin. There are clinically significant interactions between enteral feeds and phenytoin, theophylline, digoxin, ciprofloxacin, tetracyclines and rifampicin.

Alcohol and drugs

It is important to always assess alcohol intake as part of a nutritional assessment, in part because it can affect drug–nutrient interactions. It may enhance the action of many drugs acting on the brain, e.g. antidepressants, benzodiazepines and antiepileptic drugs, leading to impaired mental ability and increased sedation. It is a misconception that all antibiotics interact with alcohol; however, there are significant interactions with metronidazole and tinidazole, leading to nausea, vomiting and flushing. Even small amounts of alcohol consumed with disulfiram (used to treat alcohol dependence) cause facial flushing, tachycardia, giddiness, hypotension and potential collapse. Large changes in alcohol consumption will affect the anticoagulant effect of warfarin. It may be noted that some mouthwashes contain sufficient alcohol to cause this reaction.

Specific drug–nutrient interactions are discussed in the chapters in Section 7.

Further reading

Boullata JI, Armenti VT (eds) (2009) *Handbook of Drug–Nutrient Interactions*. New York: Humana Press.

Expert Group on Vitamins and Minerals. (2003) *Safe Upper Levels for Vitamins and Minerals*. London: Food Standards Agency. Available at http://cot.food.gov.uk/cotreports/cotjointreps/evmreport/. Accessed 10 March 2013.

Preston CL. (2017) *Stockley's Drug Interactions*, 13th edn. London: Pharmaceutical Press.

Internet resources

Advisory Committee on Borderline Substances, www.gov.uk/government/groups/advisory-committee-on-borderline-substances

BNF Interactions checker, https://bnf.nice.org.uk/interaction/

British National Formulary (BNF), www.bnf.org

Medicines and Healthcare Products Regulatory Agency (MHRA), www.mhra.gov.uk

Medscape Drug Interaction Checker (*Note*: This is USA-based, and drug names may therefore vary), http://reference.medscape.com/drug-interactionchecker

Monthly Index of Medical Specialties (MIMS), www.mims.co.uk

UKMi National Medicines Information for Healthcare Professionals, www.ukmi.nhs.uk

References

Backman WD, Bakhai A. (2013) Drug–grapefruit juice interactions. *BMJ Rapid Response*. Available at www.bmj.com/content/346/bmj.f1/rr/627070. Accessed 27 September 2017.

Boullata JI, Hudson LM. (2012) Drug–nutrient interactions: a broad view with implications for practice. *J. Acad. Nutr. Diet.* 112: 506–517.

Brill ME, Jeroen D, van Rongen A, *et al.* (2012) Impact of obesity on drug metabolism and elimination in adults and children. *Clin Pharmacokinet.* 51: 277–304.

DH. (2005) *Supplementary Prescribing by Nurses, Pharmacists, Chiropodists/Podiatrists, Physiotherapists and Radiographers within the NHS in England: A Guide for Implementation*. DH, London

Dickerson JWT. (1988) The interrelationships of nutrition and drugs. In: Dickerson JWT, Lee HA (eds) *Nutrition and the Clinical Management of Disease*, 2nd edn. London: Edward Arnold, pp. 392–421.

Expert Group on Vitamins and Minerals (EVM). (2003) *Safe Upper Levels for Vitamins and Minerals*. London: Food Safety Agency. Available at http://cot.food.gov.uk/cotreports/cotjointreps/evmreport. Accessed 27 September 2017.

Klotz U. (2009) Pharmacokinetics and drug metabolism in the elderly. *Drug Metab. Rev.* 41(2): 67–76.

Oshikoya KA, Senbanjo IO. (2009) Pathophysiological changes that affect drug disposition in protein energy malnourished children. *Nutr. Metab. (Lond).* 6: 50.

Pirmohamed M. (2013) Drug–grapefruit juice interactions. *BMJ* 346: f1.

Szabolcs P, Navis G, de Borst MH, *et al.* (2017) Public health relevance of drug–nutrition interactions. *Eur. J. Nutr.* 56: S23–S36.

Webster-Gandy J, Madden A, Holdsworth M. (2011) *Oxford Handbook of Nutrition & Dietetics*, 2nd edn. Oxford: Oxford University Press.

5.4 Alternative and complementary therapies

Joan Gandy

Key points

- Complementary therapies are used alongside conventional treatment; alternative therapies are used instead of conventional treatment or advice.
- Herbal remedies have potent effects and many interact with conventional drugs.
- Dietitians should ask about the use of CAM, especially dietary supplements, during a nutritional assessment to assess the likely impact on nutrient intake and conventional treatments.

The use of complementary medicine therapies (which includes the use of supplements) and alternative therapies (CAM) is increasing. In 2010, it was estimated that the prevalence of CAM use in England in the previous 12 months was 26%; lifetime use was estimated at 44% (Hunt *et al.*, 2010). Its use was common among people taking prescription medicines. Therefore, it is essential that dietitians be aware of CAM's efficacy, potential risks and benefits. Dietitians should enquire about their use in all nutritional assessment and be able to advise on their efficacy and safety to enable clients to make informed choices. The Cochrane collaboration (Mannheimer & Berman, 2008) describes CAM as '*a broad domain of healing resources that encompasses all health systems, modalities, and practices and their accompanying theories and beliefs, other than those intrinsic to the politically dominant health system of a particular society or culture in a given historical period. … Boundaries within CAM and between the CAM domain and that of the dominant system are not always sharp or fixed*'.

There is a fundamental difference between complementary and alternative therapies, which are described by the US National Center for Complementary and Alternative Medicine (NCCAM, 2016):

- 'If a non-mainstream practice is used together with conventional medicine, it's considered complementary'.
- 'If a non-mainstream practice is used in place of conventional medicine, it's considered alternative'.

In addition, NCCAM defines integrative (integrated) medicine as '*the combination of conventional medicine and CAM whose safety and effectiveness are supported by some high-quality evidence*'.

There are many forms of CAM, and it is not possible to provide a definitive list. In 2011, Weiland *et al.* developed an operational classification of CAM for the Cochrane Collaboration. A full list of the CAM therapies included in this classification can be found at http://cam.cochrane.org/operational-definition-complementary-medicine. This classification forms the basis of search terms within the Cochrane Collaboration. As micronutrients are used routinely in conventional medicine, the following treatments are not considered as CAM:

- Vitamins and other supplements that are administered parenterally in hospital settings.
- Dietary supplementation for treatment or prevention of medically diagnosed deficiency states or disorders.
- Vitamin or mineral supplements for preventing or treating disease in countries where vitamin or mineral deficiency is widespread.

In the UK, most CAM practitioners work in private practice; however, some CAM therapies are offered in the NHS. This is controversial; however, the use of a limited number of CAM therapies are supported by NICE for use in the NHS, e.g. the Alexander technique for Parkinson's disease.

When enquiring about the use of CAM, it is important that dietitians be respectful of the reasons for their use as these may be cultural or religious, e.g. Ayurveda is commonly used in India. The reasons people use CAM therapies are complex and include the following (Hollander & Mechanick, 2008):

- People feel that symptoms, especially fatigue and chronic pain, are not adequately addressed by conventional practitioners.

SECTION 5

Manual of Dietetic Practice, Sixth Edition. Edited by Joan Gandy.

Companion website: www.manualofdieteticpractice.com

- Some prefer to use natural products, as they believe these are safer than manmade products such as medicines.
- Some are misled by claims of dramatic improvements in health and cures.
- Many consumers are confused by the often-spurious scientific claims of some treatments.
- Terminally ill people and carers who have exhausted conventional treatment may seek further treatments outside conventional medicine.

Dietitians must be aware of the significance of the use of CAM, since, while some are innocuous, there are potential problems with some treatments. These therapies are particularly popular in some clinical areas, e.g. multiple sclerosis and cancer, and dietitians specialising in these areas must be conversant with them and any potential problems (see Chapter 7.6.4, Multiple sclerosis and Chapter 7.15.1, General aspects of cancer). These problems include:

- Lack of nutritional expertise of the practitioner, including ignorance of biochemistry and physiology (see the section 'Professional regulation' later in this chapter).
- Diagnosis of a non-existent nutritional problem, especially deficiencies. Such deficiencies may be misdiagnosed by the use of tests that have little validity, e.g. hair analysis (Ernst, 2001). Other methods are used that have no credibility or scientific basis, e.g. kinesiology and Vega (electrodermal) testing. Laboratory tests for micronutrients are reviewed by Bender (2009).
- Lack of informed guidance – people may obtain information from less reliable resources such as some Internet sites. Schmidt and Ernst (2004) found that many websites endorsed unproven therapies and that a significant proportion of them were giving advice that could be detrimental. They considered that some raised serious concern as they overtly discouraged patients from using conventional therapy.
- Some therapies may do harm – elimination diets may be recommended without an in-depth understanding of nutrition, resulting in deficiencies (see Chapter 7.11.2, Food hypersensitivity). Some alternative therapists advocate stopping conventional treatments, which can have potentially harmful consequences, e.g. advising a type 1 diabetic to stop insulin treatment. Other therapies such as Chinese herbs may cause serious drug interactions.

Some patients, their family or carers may have particularly strong beliefs about the use of CAM therapies, and this requires careful consideration. Dietitians should explore with clients and/or carers the reasons for CAM use, offering appropriate advice and presenting the evidence base as appropriate.

Professional regulation

Unlike medicine, nursing and the allied health professions, CAM practitioners are poorly, if at all, regulated, and there is usually no minimum level of knowledge of expertise. While there are professional bodies for some CAM therapies, e.g. the British Acupuncture Council, these are often self-regulatory, and the titles are unprotected. In addition, unregulated practitioners will not necessarily be covered by professional indemnity insurance, and therefore they practice without this protection for themselves and their patients (consumers).

Within the field of nutrition, only the title dietitian (or dietician) is protected by law; anyone using the title of dietitian must be registered with the Health and Care Professions Council (HCPC) (see Chapter 1.1, Professional practice). Someone using this title without registration is liable to persecution. The titles nutritionist and nutrition therapist are not protected; therefore, these can be used without formal qualifications (British Dietetic Association (BDA), 2014). However, many nutritionists are registered with the Association for Nutrition (AfN), which has proficiency and competency criteria, and promotes continuing professional development (CPD) and safe conduct. Similar to the HCPC, the AfN requires registrants to maintain their knowledge and expertise through CPD. Only nutritionists registered with the AfN can use the title registered nutritionist. The AfN is working towards making the title nutritionist protected. Nutrition therapists are not required to be registered, although they do have a professional body (the British Association for Applied Nutrition and Nutritional Therapy). The differences between dietitians, nutritionists and nutrition therapists are discussed further by the BDA (2014).

Nutritional supplements

Nutritional supplements are taken orally as capsules, pills, liquids or powders, and in addition to food (Webb, 2006). Supplements may include essential nutrients, e.g. minerals, vitamins and fatty acids, that may usually be in the diet and/or have well-established functions in the body, e.g. creatine. Alternatively, they may be plant extracts, e.g. garlic. In 2008, one-third of adults in the UK reported taking supplements on most days (Food Standards Agency (FSA), 2008). The three most popular supplements were multivitamins (36%), cod liver oil (35%) and vitamin C (35%). The use of dietary supplements is increasing in many developed countries, including the UK (NHS & BAZIAN, 2011) and the USA (Gahche *et al.*, 2011); over 50% of people surveyed in the USA reported using dietary supplements.

Supplement usage is not necessarily undesirable; fish oils are beneficial for cardiovascular health, and people who do not eat oily fish may benefit from taking them as supplements. Folic acid supplementation is recommended for women for the first 12 weeks of pregnancy. There are many circumstances in which vitamin and mineral supplementation may be either necessary or a sensible precaution, including the following:

- People with an identified vitamin or mineral deficiency, e.g. iron.
- People with increased physiological needs, e.g. pregnant women, infants and children.

- People with increased nutrient losses as a result of gastrointestinal disease or resection, other disorders or side effects of drug treatment.
- People with poor appetite, eating or swallowing difficulties due to illness.
- Elderly people, especially those in residential care or with poor wound healing.
- People on either prescribed or self-imposed restrictive diets.
- People at high risk of disorders such as osteoporosis or rickets.

There is evidence to suggest that many of those who take vitamin and/or mineral supplements are the least likely to need them (Cade *et al.*, 2004). The National Diet and Nutrition Survey showed that supplement users often had a higher micronutrient intake from food sources alone than non-supplement users (Henderson *et al.*, 2003). Conversely, people who might benefit from certain supplements may not be taking them. The majority of women of child-bearing age do not consume sufficient folate to provide protection against neural tube defects in the event of planned or unplanned pregnancy (Henderson *et al.*, 2003).

The reasons given for supplement usage vary. In general, people choose to take multivitamin and mineral products in the belief that they will boost energy, reduce the effects of ageing, cut the risk of disease such as cancer, extend life or treat specific conditions, e.g. arthritis (FSA, 2008). The marketing of dietary supplements will undoubtedly affect the decision to take dietary supplements, especially for those aimed at particular groups of people, e.g. the elderly. Supplements of single nutrients tend to be chosen for more specific reasons and to prevent or treat a particular condition or symptom (Neuhouser *et al.*, 1999).

Problems associated with supplement use

While use of some supplements is based on sound evidence of efficacy, e.g. folate in pregnancy to prevent neural tube defects, use of others is based on more dubious claims or misinformation (Satia-Abouta *et al.*, 2003). For example, enzymes present in some supplements cannot be of any benefit as they will be denatured as soon as they come into contact with stomach acid and rendered ineffective. Some trace elements available in supplements are not essential for human nutrition (Expert Group on Vitamins and Minerals (EVM), 2003).

Safety

The report by the EVM (2003) highlighted the fact that remarkably little is known about the requirements, mode of action, bioavailability and toxicity of many micronutrients. It attempted to determine safe upper levels, but, in many cases, there was insufficient data to assess the nutritional and toxicological implications. There was a lack of well-designed, large, comparative human studies of significant duration at different levels of intake and with adequate assessment of possible adverse effects. There was even less information on potentially vulnerable groups, e.g. children or the elderly. The toxicity of some nutrients has only been evaluated in animals, and their relevance to humans is uncertain. The EVM set safe upper levels for eight vitamins and minerals; for another 22, the data were limited, and only possible guidance levels were set. Neither safe nor guidance levels could be set for three others.

The EVM report concluded that, while current intakes of most vitamins and minerals are not harmful, several may have temporary side effects if taken in high doses. Others may have irreversible adverse effects if taken in large amounts over long periods of time (Table 5.4.1). Concerns over possible risks from prolonged high intakes of vitamin A were also highlighted and, following further review, the Scientific Advisory Committee on Nutrition (SACN) (2005) recommended that people who consume liver (the main dietary source of vitamin A) more than once a week, or older adults who are at risk of osteoporosis, should be cautious about taking retinol-containing supplements. Women who are, or may become, pregnant are advised to avoid vitamin A supplements.

Overdosage

Overdosage with vitamins and minerals can occur as a result of taking a preparation that provides many times the reference nutrient intake (RNI) for a nutrient in the belief that it will have more therapeutic benefits. However, inadvertent overdosing may occur as a result of the following:

- Taking inappropriate combinations of supplements. For example, people may take a multivitamin preparation for bone and joint along with a healthy heart supplement, unaware that each contains more than the RNI for vitamins A and D.
- The vitamin content of some supplements may be significantly higher than the amount stated to be present to allow for natural deterioration during the shelf life of the product (EVM, 2003). This is particularly likely to be the case with supplements containing vitamins A, D and E, which are prone to oxidation.

Fat-soluble vitamins are stored in the body, and the risks associated with prolonged high intakes, particularly from vitamins A and D, are well documented. The risk of overdosage from water-soluble vitamins is much less as excessive intakes are usually excreted in the urine. However, the risks are not negligible; irreversible neurological damage can occur following excessive intakes of vitamin B_6. Excessive intakes of some minerals and trace elements (especially iron, copper, fluorine and sodium) can be directly toxic. The threshold between safe upper limits and toxicity may be small in some cases.

Interactions

Although overt toxicity is rare, the long-term consequences of excessive high intakes of some vitamins and minerals may be significant. High intake of one, e.g. iron, can impair absorption of another, e.g. zinc, and cause

Table 5.4.1 Possible adverse effects of vitamin and mineral supplements (EVM, 2003; FSA, 2008)

Nutrient	Possible adverse effects
Beta-carotene	Long-term intake of >7 mg/day may increase the risk of lung cancer
	Supplements should not be taken by people who smoke
Nicotinic acid	50-mg doses can cause skin flushing and other reversible side effects such as gastrointestinal disturbances
	Prolonged intake of higher doses may cause liver dysfunction
	It is recommended that supplemental intakes not exceed 17 mg/day
Vitamin A	Excessive intake is teratogenic and may also cause irreversible bone and liver damage
	Retinol-containing supplements should be avoided by people who consume liver more than once a week, or older adults at risk of osteoporosis
	Pregnant women should avoid taking supplements
Vitamin C	>1000 mg/day may cause abdominal pain and/or diarrhoea
Vitamin B_6	>200 mg/day may cause irreversible neurological damage
	It is recommended that supplementary intakes not exceed 10 mg/day
Calcium	>1500 mg/day may cause abdominal pain and/or diarrhoea
Iron	>17 mg/day may cause constipation, nausea and abdominal pain
Magnesium	>400 mg/day may cause osmotic diarrhoea
Manganese	Neurotoxic at high levels of intake
	It is recommended that supplemental intakes not exceed 4 mg/day; and, in older adults, not exceed 0.5 mg/day
Nickel	Nickel-containing products may cause a skin rash in sensitive individuals
Phosphorus	>250 mg/day may cause mild stomach upset in sensitive individuals; long-term excessive intake may be detrimental to bone health
Zinc	High intakes impair absorption of iron and copper and may also have gastrointestinal side effects; it is recommended that supplemental intakes not exceed 25 mg/day

a deficiency. Interactions are particularly likely between elements that are close to each other in the periodic table, e.g. iron, copper, manganese, zinc and chromium (EVM, 2003). Antioxidants also function as part of a coordinated biochemical chain of defence against free radicals; high doses of a single antioxidant supplement such as vitamin E could disturb the antioxidant and pro-oxidant balance and lead to potential risks (Opara, 2002).

Supplemental intakes of some micronutrients can also interact with medicinal drugs, e.g. vitamin B_6 can reduce the therapeutic effect of levodopa (used to treat Parkinson's disease) and interact with other drugs such as isoniazid, theophylline and phenobarbitone (see Chapter 5.3, Medicines management). It is easy to cause nutritional imbalances by the use of supplements, whereas it is very difficult to do so by consuming food. In order to avoid the potential risks, the use of isolated supplements, particularly in high doses, should therefore be avoided other than in cases of clear clinical need.

Of more concern are the findings that some of these supplements may be associated with long-term risks. A meta-analysis of seven large randomised trials showed a small but significant increase in all-cause mortality and cardiovascular death with beta-carotene therapy (Vivekananthan *et al.*, 2003). Supplemental intakes of beta-carotene may increase the risk of lung cancer in people with a history of smoking (Albanes *et al.*, 1996; EVM, 2003; Omenn *et al.*, 1996). Supplemental intakes of vitamin E in excess of 400 IU/day (268 mg/day) may be associated with premature mortality (Miller *et al.*, 2005). Many consumers of megadoses of micronutrients are aware of the potential of overdose but continue to take large doses of supplements (FSA, 2008).

Regulation of supplements

The EU Food Supplements Directive (EC 46/2002) outlines a framework for certain classes of food supplements. It regulates and guarantees the legal status of these classes of supplements within the UK and throughout Europe. Vitamin and mineral supplements must be safe and appropriately labelled to enable consumers to make informed choices (see Chapter 4.5, Food law and labelling). More information on the classification of supplements as food or medicine can be found at the Government Chemist website (www governmentchemist.org.uk).

Herbal medicine

Herbal medicine is based on the use of plants or plant extracts to treat disease. Herbal remedies are one of the most powerful forms of complementary therapies, and there are considerable risks from their inappropriate use. In the UK, the main systems of herbal medicine practised are Western and Chinese. Western herbal medicine is largely, although not exclusively, based on the use of plants native to Britain, Europe and North America. Chinese herbal medicine is part of traditional Chinese medicine (TCM), which may include other CAM therapies, e.g. acupuncture. Other forms of herbal medicine include Ayurveda and Tibetan. Practitioners prescribe herb mixtures based on an individual's symptoms and condition. People can also purchase over-the-counter herbal remedies from retail outlets or via the Internet.

Problems associated with their use

Herbal medicines are often assumed to be safe as they are natural products. However, herbal remedies can be associated with problems including:

- Potency – herbal remedies contain potent pharmacological ingredients that can have similar effects as many conventional drugs. Many conventional drugs have been developed following observations of the effects of certain plants, e.g. salicylic acid is found in willow bark, and its salts (salicylates) are manufactured as analgesics, e.g. aspirin.
- Interactions – herbal ingredients can interact with other herbs, conventional drugs and nutrients in foods (Table 5.4.2).
- Purity – herbal medicines made to poor standards may be a health risk. Poor manufacturing practices in some countries have resulted in contamination with heavy metals or toxic herbs, posing a significant risk to health (Goudie & Kaye, 2001). Inadequate labelling or batch-to-batch variation in ingredient types, levels of active substance and proportions can lead to herbal medicines being used incorrectly (Dunning, 2004).

Some herbal products sold in the UK must be licensed like other medicines, but many over-the-counter products are exempt. The Medicines and Healthcare Products Regulatory Agency (MHRA) has a traditional herbal medicines registration scheme to ensure that unlicensed over-the-counter traditional herbal medicines meet assured standards of safety, quality and patient information. In the UK, suspected adverse reactions to both licensed and unlicensed herbal preparations can be reported using the yellow card system. The MHRA also issues alerts about cases of poisoning and adverse reactions.

Herbal remedies such as feverfew, golden seal, juniper, mistletoe, nutmeg, rosemary and sage are contraindicated in pregnancy due to the increased risk of miscarriage. No herbal preparation should be taken during the first 3 months of pregnancy.

Common herb–drug interactions

The number and availability of herbs as supplements and as complementary therapy are increasing, leading to increased potential for herb–drug interactions. It is important to assess herb intake during a nutritional assessment since, similar to conventional drugs, they have the potential to enhance or reduce drug action.

Table 5.4.2 Most common herb–drug interactions (source: Webster-Gandy *et al.*, 2012, table 38.5, p. 744. Reproduced by permission from Oxford University Press)[a]

Herb	Interacts with	Comment
St John's wort	Antidepressants	Drug plasma concentration reduced, leading to reduced therapeutic effect
	Antivirals: HIV protease inhibitors (atazanavir, indinavir, nelfinavir, ritonavir, saquinavir)	Reduced therapeutic effect
	HIV non-nucleoside reverse transcriptase inhibitors (efavirenz, nevirapine)	Reduced therapeutic effect
	Anticonvulsants (carbamazepine, phenobarbital, phenytoin)	Reduced control of seizures
	Ciclosporin, tacrolimus	Increased risk of transplant rejection
	Digoxin	Reduced therapeutic effect
	Oral combined contraceptives, oestrogen-containing patches and vaginal rings	Reduced therapeutic effect
	Voriconazole	Reduced therapeutic effect
	Theophylline	Reduced asthma control
	Warfarin	Reduced anticoagulant effect
	SSRIs (fluoxetine, paroxetine, sertraline)	Increased serotonergic effects
	Triptans (sumatriptan, naratriptan, rizatriptan, zolmitriptan)	Reduced therapeutic effect
Ginkgo biloba	Anticoagulant (warfarin)	Increased risk of bleeding
	Antiplatelet (aspirin)	
Ginseng	Anticoagulant (warfarin)	Increased risk of bleeding
Dong quai	Anticoagulant (warfarin)	Increased risk of bleeding
Echinacea	Immunosuppressant	Possible immune stimulation
Saw palmetto	Anticoagulant (warfarin)	Altered anticoagulation

[a]This list is not exhaustive. *Stockley's Drug Interactions* or *British National Formulary* should be consulted for further details.
SSRI, selective serotonin reuptake inhibitor.

Examples of common herb–drug interactions are shown in Table 5.4.2. St John's wort (*Hypericum perforatum*) is commonly used as an antidepressant. However, it induces liver enzymes and reduces the effect of several drugs; a physician or pharmacist should be consulted before concomitant use.

Evidence base for CAM therapies

Dietetics is an evidence-based practice, and dietitians, like other regulated healthcare professionals, have a responsibility to use the best possible practice (see Chapter 1.1, Professional practice). It is therefore reasonable to expect the same level of rigour for all therapies, including CAM (Lewith *et al.*, 2000). There are innate difficulties in conducting this research as funding and support may not be available, and there is resistance from some CAM therapists who question the salience of conventional methods of assessment (Jackson & Scambler, 2007). Perhaps for these reasons, the available evidence is often from studies conducted in small groups of subjects. In addition, studies may not be well constructed. This limits the ability to produce high-level evidence such as systematic reviews and meta-analyses. However, some high-level evidence for the efficacy and safety of CAM is available. For example, Posadzki *et al.* (2012) recently published a systematic review of published case reports and case series on the adverse effects of homeopathy.

As a result of the increasing use of CAM in the USA, the National Institute of Health has established the National Center for Complementary and Alternative Medicine (NCCAM) with the mission '*… to define, through rigorous scientific investigation, the usefulness and safety of complementary and alternative medicine interventions and their roles in improving health and health care*'. It funds research and produces publications and guidelines on CAM for healthcare professionals and the public.

Dietitians should look for and critically appraise the evidence for CAM as they would conventional medicine (see the section 'Evidence-based practice' in Chapter 1.1). The Cochrane Collaboration is a reliable source of evidence, and reviews are available on many topics, e.g. aromatherapy for dementia.

While it is understandable that people with incurable or chronic conditions may use CAM, its use should be underpinned by evidence of efficacy and safety. However, when there is no risk to the client, the potential placebo effect should be considered, although vulnerable patients must not be given false hope or have necessary treatments delayed. Ultimately, the patient is responsible for making the decision to follow a complementary or alternative dietary regimen. However, it is the responsibility of the dietitian to ensure that the patient has been given sufficient scientifically based information on which to base that decision.

Further reading

Ernst E. (2008) *Oxford Handbook of Complementary Medicine*. Oxford: Oxford University Press.

Expert Group on Vitamins and Minerals (EVM). (2003) *Safe Upper Levels for Vitamins and Minerals*. London: FSA. Available at https://cot.food.gov.uk/sites/default/files/vitmin2003.pdf.

Webb G. (2006) *Dietary Supplements and Functional Foods*. Oxford: Blackwell Publishing.

Webb GP. (2011) *Dietary Supplements and Functional Foods*, 2nd edn. Oxford: Wiley-Blackwell.

Wieland LS, Manheimer E, Berman BM. (2011) Development and classification of an operational definition of complementary and alternative medicine for the Cochrane Collaboration. *Altern. Ther. Health Med.* 17(2): 50–59.

Internet resources

Cochrane Complementary Medicine, http://cam.cochrane.org

Consumer Lab, www.consumerlab.com

European Medicines Agency (Search for herbal medicines for human use), www.ema.europa.eu

Government Chemist (UK), www.governmentchemist.org.uk

Health and Food Supplements Information Service, www.hsis.org

Medicines and Healthcare Products Regulatory Agency, www.mhra.gov.uk

National Center for Complementary and Alternative Medicine, http://nccam.nih.gov

Natural Medicines, https://naturalmedicines.therapeuticresearch.com

Office of Dietary Supplements (National Institute for Health, USA), https://ods.od.nih.gov

PEN – Practice-based evidence in Nutrition, www.pennutrition.com

References

Albanes D, Heinonen OP, Taylor PR, *et al.* (1996) Alpha-tocopherol and beta-carotene supplements and lung cancer incidence in the alpha-tocopherol, beta-carotene (ATBC) cancer prevention study: effects of base-line characteristics and study compliance. *J. Natl. Cancer Inst.* 88(21): 1560–1570.

BDA. (2014) *Dietitian, nutritionist, nutritional therapist or diet expert? A comprehensive guide to roles and functions*. Available at https://www.bda.uk.com/publications/dietitian_nutritionist.pdf. Accessed 10 October 2018.

Bender DA. (2009) *Nutritional Biochemistry of the Vitamins*, 2nd edn. Cambridge: Cambridge University Press.

Cade JE, Burley VJ, Greenwood DC. (2004) The UK Women's Cohort Study: comparison of vegetarians, fish-eaters and meat-eaters. *Public Health Nutr.* 7(7): 871–878.

Dunning T. (2004) Complementary therapies: considerations for diabetes care. *Pract. Diabetes Int.* 21(3): 118–125.

Ernst E (ed). (2001) *The Desktop Guide to Complementary and Alternative Medicine – An Evidence-Based Approach*. Edinburgh: Mosby.

Expert Group on Vitamins and Minerals (EVM). (2003) *Safe Upper Levels for Vitamins and Minerals*. London: Food Standards Agency. Available at https://cot.food.gov.uk/sites/default/files/vitmin2003.pdf. Accessed 19 January 2018.

FSA. (2008) *Consumer Consumption of Vitamin and Mineral Food Supplements*. London: TSO.

Gahche J, Bailey R, Burt V, *et al.* (2011, April) Dietary supplement use among U.S. adults has increased since NHANES III (1988–1994). *NCHS Data Brief* (61): 1–8.

Goudie A, Kaye JM. (2001) Contaminated medication precipitating hypoglycaemia. *Med. J. Aust.* 175(5): 256–257.

Henderson L, Irving K, Gregory J, *et al.* (2003) *National Diet and Nutrition Survey: Adults Aged 19 to 64 Years. Volume 3: Vitamin and Mineral Intake and Urinary Analytes*. London: The Stationery Office.

Hollander JM, Mechanick JI. (2008) Complementary and alternative medicine and the management of the metabolic syndrome. *J. Am. Diet. Assoc.* 108(3): 495–509.

Hunt KJ, Coelho HF, Wider B, *et al.* (2010) Complementary and alternative medicine use in England: results from a national survey. *Int. J. Clin. Pract.* 64: 1496–4502.

Jackson S, Scambler G. (2007) Perceptions of evidence-based medicine: traditional acupuncturists in the UK and resistance to biomedical modes of evaluation. *Sociol. Health Illn.* 29: 412–429.

Lewith GT, Ernst E, Mills S, *et al.* (2000) Complementary medicine must be research led and evidence based. *BMJ* 320: 188.2.

Mannheimer B, Berman B. (2008) *Cochrane complementary medicine field. About the Cochrane Collaboration (Fields), Issue 2.* Available at http://www.mrw.interscience.wiley.com/cochrane/clabout/articles/CE000052/frame.html. Accessed 11 March 2013.

Medicines and Healthcare Products Regulatory Agency (MHRA). (2013) *Toxic Poisoning Alert for Online Chinese Medicines.*

Miller ER 3rd, Pastor-Barriuso R, Dalal D, *et al.* (2005) Meta-analysis: high-dosage vitamin E supplementation may increase all-cause mortality. *Ann. Intern. Med.* 142(1): 37–46.

National Center for Complementary and Alternative Medicine (NCCAM). (2016) *Complementary, Alternative, or Integrative Health: What's in a Name?* Available at https://nccih.nih.gov/health/integrative-health#cvsa. Accessed 19 January 2018.

Neuhouser ML, Patterson RE, Levy L. (1999) Motivations for using vitamin and mineral supplements. *J. Am. Diet. Assoc.* 99(7): 851–854.

NHS & BAZIAN. (2011) *Supplements – Who Needs Them?* Available at www.nhs.uk/news/2011/05May/Documents/BtH_supplements.pdf. Accessed 11 March 2013.

Omenn GS, Goodman G, Thornquist M, *et al.* (1996) Chemoprevention of lung cancer: the beta-Carotene and Retinol Efficacy Trial (CARET) in high-risk smokers and asbestos-exposed workers. *IARC Sci. Publ.* 136: 67–85.

Opara EC. (2002) Oxidative stress, micronutrients, diabetes mellitus and its complications. *J. R. Soc. Promot. Health* 122: 28–34.

Posadzki P, Alotaibi A, Ernst E. (2012) Adverse effects of homeopathy: A systematic review of published case reports and case series. *Int. J. Clin. Pract.* 66(12): 1178–1188.

SACN. (2005) *Review of Dietary Advice on Vitamin A.* London: The Stationery Office. Available at https://assets.publishing.service.gov.uk/government/uploads/system/uploads/attachment_data/file/338853/SACN_Review_of_Dietary_Advice_on_Vitamin_A.pdf. Accessed 10 October 2018.

Satia-Abouta J, Kristal AR, Patterson RE, *et al.* (2003) Dietary supplement use and medical conditions: the VITAL study. *Am. J. Prev. Med.* 24(1): 43–51.

Schmidt K, Ernst E (2001) Assessing websites on complementary and alternative medicine for cancer. *Ann Oncol.* 15(5): 733–742.

Vivekananthan DP, Penn MS, Sapp SK, *et al.* (2003) Use of antioxidant vitamins for the prevention of cardiovascular disease: meta-analysis of randomised trials. *Lancet* 361: 2017–2023.

Webster-Gandy J, Madden A, Holdsworth M. (2012) *Oxford Handbook of Nutrition & Dietetics*, 2nd edn. Oxford: Oxford University Press.

PART 2
Clinical dietetic practice

SECTION 6

Nutrition support

6.1 Nutritional requirements in clinical practice

C. Elizabeth Weekes

Key points

- The determination of nutritional requirements requires a significant element of clinical judgment.
- Irrespective of the method used, requirement calculations should be interpreted with care and used only as a starting point.
- The requirements for a number of nutrients in illness and injury have yet to be established.

The aim of devising a nutritional prescription is to provide patients with their complete requirements either via a single route or any combination of oral, enteral or parenteral nutrition, while avoiding the known complications associated with both underfeeding and overfeeding (ASPEN, 2002; NICE, 2006). The estimation of nutritional requirements is an important part of patient assessment, yet no single, validated method for estimating requirements exists, and the evidence-base for all prediction methods currently in use is poor (Reeves & Capra, 2003). Practitioners need, therefore, to exercise a considerable degree of clinical judgment when determining the nutritional requirements of an individual.

All prescriptions for nutritional support should take account of the patient's needs for energy, protein, fluid, electrolytes, micronutrients and fibre (NICE, 2006). However, a number of factors complicate the determination of nutritional requirements in clinical practice (see Table 6.1.1) and should be considered prior to estimating the requirements of an individual. Even within a single disease, individual variation (e.g. due to age, co-morbidities, nutritional status, response to surgery or treatment) may make prognosis unpredictable. Furthermore, illness or injury does not have a consistent effect on energy expenditure, and this is also likely to be the case for other nutrients. Different treatment modalities, e.g. surgery, chemotherapy or pharmacological agents, may influence requirements in different ways, and the same treatment may have very different effects in individuals with the same disease. These differences in response to treatment may be due at least in part to genetic predispositions and environmental influences. The measurement and assay techniques used to assess nutrient status and determine nutritional requirements are not always fully described in the literature and may differ between studies (equipment, timing, protocols etc.), thus making comparisons difficult. Furthermore, older studies may not be relevant to current practice due to advances in diagnostic procedures and management strategies, e.g. the advent in the late 1990s of highly active antiretroviral therapy (HAART) for the treatment of HIV infection. Irrespective of the route and likely duration, the aims and objectives of nutritional support should be clearly defined and documented at baseline, reviewed at each stage of the patient's illness and nutritional support amended accordingly, e.g. minimising losses in acute illness, nutritional repletion in the recovery phase (NICE, 2006).

Energy

Basal metabolic rate and total energy expenditure

In healthy individuals, total energy expenditure (TEE) comprises basal metabolic rate (BMR), dietary-induced thermogenesis (DIT) (i.e. energy expended in the digestion, absorption and transport of nutrients), and physical activity (see Figure 6.1.1). Basal metabolic rate (BMR), i.e. the metabolic activity required to maintain life, comprises approximately 60% of TEE, and, in any individual, measured BMR is highly reproducible. The conditions essential for the measurement of BMR are:

- Post-absorptive (12-hour fast).
- Lying still at physical and mental rest (but not asleep).
- Thermo-neutral environment (27–29 °C).
- No stimulants such as tea, coffee or nicotine in the previous 12 hours.
- No heavy physical activity during the previous day.
- Validation gases must be calibrated to ensure measurements are accurate and reliable.
- Steady-state must be established, i.e. <10% difference in minute-to-minute oxygen (VO_2) and carbon dioxide (VCO_2) volume measurements over 5 minutes.

Manual of Dietetic Practice, Sixth Edition. Edited by Joan Gandy.

Companion website: www.manualofdieteticpractice.com

Table 6.1.1 Factors affecting nutritional requirements in illness and injury

Nutritional requirements	Factors
Basal requirements	Age
	Sex
	Body weight
	Body composition (proportions of fat and muscle mass)
	Previous and current nutritional intake
	Ambient temperature
Goals of treatment	Diagnosis
	Prognosis
	Likely duration of nutritional support
Disease effects	Metabolic state (e.g. catabolic, normobolic or anabolic)
	Severity of illness
	Inflammatory response
	Gastrointestinal function
	Medical interventions (e.g. mechanical ventilation, radiotherapy, chemotherapy, hormone treatment or transplantation)
	Surgery
	Pharmacological interventions, e.g. sedation, oral steroid therapy
	Pain
	Psychological state
Activity	Mobility status, e.g. bed-bound, mobile on ward
	Level of consciousness
	Neuromuscular function

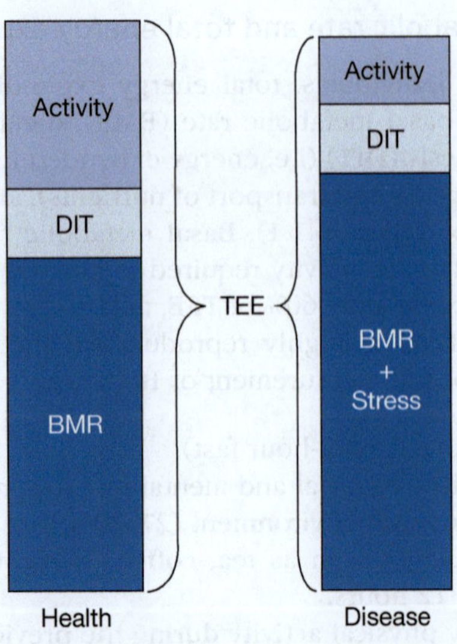

Figure 6.1.1 Energy expenditure in health and disease (source: The British Dietetic Association, 2013. Reproduced with permission from The British Dietetic Association, www.bda.uk.com)

If any of these criteria are not met, then the measurement is defined as resting energy expenditure (REE) or resting metabolic rate (RMR). The most accurate method for measuring energy expenditure is indirect calorimetry (Branson & Johannigman, 2004). However, in the clinical situation, it is rarely possible to measure BMR, owing to the exacting requirements listed earlier. Therefore, in sick or injured subjects, REE will comprise BMR plus the effect of any metabolic response to injury or disease. If the patient has not fasted, the REE measurement may also include some proportion of DIT. In some patients, such as those with involuntary movements due to neuromuscular dysfunction, an element of physical activity may also be included during measurements of REE. Conversely, if measurement conditions are strictly controlled, REE may not equate to total energy requirements, since neither activity nor DIT will be accounted for.

A large number of BMR prediction equations exist, although the most commonly cited are Harris-Benedict (Harris & Benedict, 1919) and Schofield (Schofield, 1985). More recently, the Henry (Oxford) equations (Henry, 2005) have been evaluated (Ramirez-Zea, 2005; SACN, 2011) and recommended as the most rigorously tested and applicable to modern healthy populations. The Henry equations were derived from a database of 10,552 BMR values in studies conducted from 1914 to 2005, including a larger cohort of elderly subjects than in previous databases. Only studies where conditions met strict criteria for BMR measurements were included. The vast majority of clinical studies compare measured energy expenditure with the Harris–Benedict equations, and only a small proportion compare with other equations.

Inflammatory state

In sick or injured individuals, TEE is influenced by many factors, and, in any individual patient, it may be lower, similar to or, in rare cases, higher than requirements in healthy populations (see Figure 6.1.1). In the majority of chronic conditions, BMR is usually normal or may be slightly increased. Since any metabolic-stress-induced increase in BMR is often accompanied by a decrease in physical activity, TEE in chronically ill individuals is usually normal or decreased (Kulstad & Schoeller, 2007; SACN, 2011).

Acute illness increases BMR above that predicted for healthy individuals of the same age and weight, usually by 0–40%, and, very rarely, up to 100%. Both the magnitude and duration of the increase are dependent on the presence of an inflammatory response, and thus assessment of patients' inflammatory states may assist in the determination of their energy requirements. To avoid the risk of overfeeding in acutely ill individuals, it might be prudent to include a stress factor in any estimate of energy requirements only while there is biochemical and clinical evidence of an inflammatory response, e.g. elevated C-reactive protein or white cell count, low serum albumin, poor appetite or oedema.

In the presence of an inflammatory response, weight gain and other clinical benefits are unlikely to be achieved with nutritional support alone (Streat *et al.*, 1987), and the goal of nutritional support is usually to minimise losses while the patient is in this state. Aggressive nutritional support should only be considered when the patient is more able to utilise the nutrients provided, i.e.

during recovery (anabolic phase). A patient is likely to be moving into the recovery phase as oedema resolves and the parameters listed earlier return to the normal range.

Physical activity

Individuals requiring nutrition support range from paralysed and sedated, critically ill patients to fully mobile patients on the ward or in the community. To date, however, there is a relative lack of research on the effects of illness and injury on physical activity levels (Elia, 2005), although a recent report concluded that acute illness is usually accompanied by a decrease in physical activity that compensates for any increase in BMR (SACN, 2011). The energy expended in physical activity is lowest in the sickest patients, with sedated, ventilated patients usually expending <10% above BMR in physical activity. This can be highly variable, however, especially in agitated patients (Frankenfield, 2006). In hospitalised individuals, it is reasonable to assume that physical activity will be lower than habitual levels. For example, in pre-operative patients, activity accounts for 20% above BMR, while physical activity may decrease post-operatively to 5% BMR in the first few days, increasing to 15% BMR by days 9–12 (Kinney *et al.*, 1968).

While it might be expected that physical activity will be increased in patients receiving active physiotherapy, moving painful or damaged limbs, or in those with abnormal neuromuscular function, this may not result in increased TEE as the patient compensates by resting or sleeping. For example, in patients with involuntary movements due to Parkinson's disease, TEE was not found to be increased due to a reduction in the energy expended in voluntary physical activity (Toth *et al.*, 1997).

As patients recover from illness, or once they are discharged from hospital, the component of TEE that is most likely to change is the physical activity level, assuming there have been no effects on neurological or muscular function. In the community, some patients receiving nutritional support, irrespective of feeding route, may have similar activity levels as healthy individuals, whereas house-bound or nursing-home patients are likely to have physical activity levels similar to hospital patients. In the determination of energy requirements, regular assessment of habitual activity is important; however, the best method for assessing physical activity levels objectively in clinical practice has yet to be determined (Frankenfield & Ashcraft, 2011). Multiplication factors for physical activity do exist (Taylor, 2007), but are as variable and open to misinterpretation as stress factors, and thus a considerable degree of clinical judgement is required in their use.

Dietary-induced thermogenesis (DIT)

Dietary-induced thermogenesis (DIT) usually accounts for 8–10% of TEE, and, in healthy individuals, the main determinant of DIT is the energy content of the food, followed by the protein fraction (Benedict & Carpenter, 1918). The effects of injury and sepsis on DIT are unclear, although evidence suggests the effects are similar to those in healthy individuals (Westerterp, 2004). While differences in DIT might be expected when comparing the parenteral with the enteral route, studies have so far failed to show a significant difference (Stokes & Hill, 1993). When enteral feed is given as a bolus, the effect on DIT is similar to that observed with food, i.e. an increase in TEE of 8–10% occurs. In contrast, the continuous infusion of nutrients does not significantly increase REE over fasting level (Heymsfield *et al.*, 1987). In the determination of energy requirements, there is rarely a need to make a separate adjustment for DIT, as most prediction equations were derived from data collected from subjects who were receiving nutritional support during metabolic measurements. The effects of DIT are therefore already included in the equation.

Prediction methods

The most accurate methods for determining energy requirements are calorimetry and the doubly labelled water technique; however, these methods are generally too expensive and impractical for routine clinical use (Branson & Johannigman, 2004). In clinical practice, therefore, energy requirements are usually estimated using published prediction methods. Three main methods for estimating energy requirements exist, all of which use some combination of body weight, age or sex. The factorial method involves estimating BMR from prediction equations and then adding factors for metabolic stress, physical activity and DIT (e.g. Taylor, 2007; PENG, 2011). An alternative method has been proposed by other organisations (ASPEN, 2002; NICE, 2006) where requirements are based on energy values per kg body weight, adjusted for particular purposes, e.g. 25–30 kcal/kg body weight for bedridden patients (Table 6.1.2). A number of disease-specific regression equations have been derived, in particular for critical care (Frankenfield *et al.*, 2005) and burns (Ireton-Jones *et al.*, 1992).

All three methods are open to criticism, e.g. the current PENG (2011) guidelines involve calculating BMR using the Henry equations (Henry, 2005) and adding a factor (0–60%) to take account of metabolic stress, and adding another factor (10–25%) to take account of activity and diet-induced thermogenesis (DIT). All these steps have the potential to introduce error. All BMR prediction equations were derived for use in healthy populations, and their use in sick individuals could therefore be open to criticism. Furthermore, the data used to derive the stress factors is unclear, and there is considerable scope for misinterpretation by inexperienced practitioners. While there is a lack of evidence to support this method, the approach is easy to use and takes account of the main factors that impact on an individual's energy requirements, i.e. weight, age, gender, physical activity level and dietary-induced thermogenesis.

While easy to use and based on the parameter with the greatest influence on BMR, the second method (kcal/kg body weight) does not account for changes in energy expenditure with age, gender or metabolic state, and it is

Table 6.1.2 Guidelines for estimating nutritional requirements in stable patients

Energy (Per kg per day)	Protein (Per kg per day)	Micronutrients
25–35 kcal (105–147 kJ) (NICE, 2006)[a]	0.8–1.5 g (NICE, 2006)[a]	Provision of adequate electrolytes, minerals, micronutrients (allowing for any pre-existing deficits, excessive losses or increased demands) and fibre if appropriate (NICE, 2006)[a]
20–35 kcal (84–147 kJ) (ASPEN, 2002)[b]	0.8–2.0 g (ASPEN, 2002)[b]	Recommendations are made for specific nutrients based on route of administration. For enteral nutrition, recommendations are based on the RDA/AI levels, and for parenteral nutrition, recommendations were made on the assumption that patients had increased requirements (ASPEN, 2002)[b]

[a]For patients who are not severely ill or injured, nor at risk of re-feeding syndrome; [b]for unstressed adult patients with adequate organ function; RDA = recommended daily allowance; AI = adequate intake.

unclear for people who are obese whether requirements should be calculated using actual or ideal body weight. Their applicability for depleted individuals has also been questioned. Similarly, there are no defined criteria for when to use 20, 25, 30 or 35 kcal/kg/day.

Disease-specific equations are based on physiological variables that may change considerably over a short period of time, e.g. body temperature, heart rate and minute ventilation. While they may be more accurate in the specific population for which they were derived, these equations too are open to similar criticisms regarding validity, and currently there are no indications on how frequently requirements should be reviewed and amended in the light of any changes in these variables. Furthermore, it is yet to be determined if amending feeding regimens in response to changes in physiological variables results in beneficial outcomes.

The data used to derive all prediction methods is difficult to locate, and not one of the methods described in the preceding text has been fully validated (Reeves & Capra, 2003). Furthermore, while prediction methods may provide adequate estimates of requirements for groups of patients, they all have a poor predictive value for individuals. Regardless of the method used, all estimates of energy requirements should be interpreted with care and used as a starting point only. Since any one of a number of factors might vary during a patient's illness and recovery, requirements should be reviewed and re-calculated regularly to avoid either underfeeding or overfeeding (NICE, 2006). The importance of monitoring cannot be too highly emphasised.

Protein (Nitrogen)

In clinical practice, the determination of protein (nitrogen) requirements is complicated by the fact that protein homeostasis is in a state of constant flux. In the healthy individual, protein requirements are dependent to a varying degree on a number of factors, including recent and long-term protein and energy intakes, physical activity and the quality of the protein consumed (Calloway & Spector, 1955). A chronic lack of protein (and energy) results in the body adapting to starvation in order to preserve body protein stores. In illness or injury, determination of protein requirements is further complicated by the metabolic state of the patient and the presence or absence of an inflammatory response. The maintenance of nitrogen balance depends on long-term and recent nitrogen and energy intakes and clinical state in injury or illness. As a result, it is very difficult to predict requirements in any one individual at any particular time.

In severe chronic illness, such as cancer, chronic respiratory failure or cardiac failure, the presence of cachexia may further complicate the picture (see Chapter 7.15.9, Cancer cachexia). Cachexia results in severe and specific loss of skeletal muscle mass, with relative preservation of visceral protein, as the body re-prioritises protein metabolism away from the peripheral tissues and towards the liver. This preferential loss of skeletal muscle mass occurs even during periods of poor dietary intake. In the short term, this response may be beneficial as protein stores are liberated to mount the immune response and promote healing. However, in the longer term, or if the loss of muscle mass is excessive, this is detrimental to the patient (WHO/FAO/UNU, 2007).

A recent systematic review concluded that a prescription consisting of 1.0–1.2 g protein/kg body weight/day is likely to provide sufficient protein for the majority of hospitalised patients (Ferrie *et al.*, 2013). In those who are metabolically stressed, however, requirements may be higher, although current recommendations suggest that provision of more than 1.5–2.0 g protein/kg/day is unlikely to be beneficial in terms of clinical outcome, and may indeed be detrimental, particularly in patients who have had a prolonged period of poor intake and are therefore at risk of re-feeding syndrome (NICE, 2006).

The largest nitrogen losses have been documented in sepsis, major trauma and burns (Ferrie *et al.*, 2013). In these conditions, nitrogen balance is almost impossible to achieve in the early catabolic phase post-injury, and currently there appears to be little to gain from providing nitrogen in excess of 1.5 g protein/kg body weight in the critically ill (NICE, 2006), although this is open to debate (Frankenfield, 2006).

In the past, guidelines for dietary protein have advised a similar intake for all adults, regardless of age. Evidence suggests, however, that older people may

SECTION 6

require a higher protein intake than younger adults (Bauer *et al.*, 2013). This may be due in part to a declining anabolic response to protein intake in older people and to the fact that older people consume less protein than those who are younger (Kurpad & Vaz, 2000). In illness or following injury, older people may need to consume more protein to offset the impact of catabolism and/or the inflammatory response. The PROT-AGE guidelines (Bauer *et al.*, 2013) make recommendations for protein intake levels in older patients with specific diseases. The authors conclude that older adults who have an acute or chronic disease need more dietary protein (i.e. 1.2–1.5 g/kg body weight/day) than younger people, and older people with severe illness or injury or with severe malnutrition may need as much as 2.0 g/kg body weight/day. Older people with severe kidney disease who are not on dialysis are an exception to these recommendations. It must be recognised, however, that the evidence base for protein requirements in many clinical conditions in older people is lacking, and the PROT-AGE group did not conduct a systematic review in the preparation of their guidelines.

The repletion of protein stores is most likely to be effective once a patient is in the recovery (anabolic) phase, is able to mobilise, and when adequate amounts of energy are also provided (WHO/FAO/UNU, 2007).

Fluid

In health, fluid requirements are 25–35 mL/kg body weight. This is approximately 2000–3000 mL for individuals within the normal range for body mass index (BMI). The metabolic response to acute illness and injury results in changes in fluid and electrolyte balance, such that water and sodium are retained avidly. This often results in oedema in the early days of illness that may take up to 10 days to return to normal, or longer in the presence of sepsis or other complications. Recovery is accompanied by a return of the capacity to excrete any excess salt and water acquired during the acute phase.

In post-surgical patients, there is evidence that poor fluid management (usually administration of excess fluid sodium and chloride) is a common cause of oedema, prolonged ileus and other complications, and has an adverse effect on patient outcome (Lobo *et al.*, 2006). Patients are, therefore, extremely susceptible to errors in fluid prescription early after injury or surgery. The NICE (2013) guidelines provide recommendations for the safe use of intravenous therapy in hospitalised adults, and focus on assessment and monitoring as well as providing algorithms for fluid resuscitation, routine maintenance, and replacement and redistribution. The guideline committee recommends that food and fluids be provided orally or enterally, and that intravenous infusions be discontinued as soon as possible. In disease or following surgery, estimates of fluid requirements should take into account any losses resulting from pyrexia, drains, diarrhoea, burns, stomas and fistulae (see Figure 6.1.2), and all sources of fluids should be considered (including fluids given with some intravenous drugs) to minimise the risks of over-hydration, especially in patients receiving enteral or parenteral nutrition.

There is currently insufficient evidence to provide guidelines on sodium and fluid requirements in very thin or obese individuals, and therefore patients at the extremes of BMI should be monitored closely for signs of over-hydration or under-hydration, and fluid prescriptions adjusted accordingly.

Micronutrients

In the presence of illness or injury, micronutrient deficiencies may occur for a variety of reasons although blood measurements may not be reliable markers of micronutrient status (Shenkin, 2000):

- Inadequate (or imbalanced) intake.
- Increased metabolic rate and increased number of biochemical reactions.
- Adverse effects of treatment.
- Increased oxidative stress.
- Losses from fistulae, burns, diarrhoea, dialysis.

The effects of micronutrient deficiency are non-specific and insidious (e.g. muscle weakness, anorexia, depression), and are commonly associated with acute and chronic illness. Suboptimal levels may impair function before signs of deficiency become evident, and micronutrient deficiencies may therefore go undiagnosed in the presence of illness or injury.

In the absence of an adequate evidence base, recent guidelines for the provision of micronutrients to patients with acute or chronic illness (Arends *et al.*, 2006) are non-specific, in that they state that provision should be based on recommended daily allowance (RDA)/adequate intake (AI) levels (Table 6.1.2). While recognising that RDA/AI levels are recommended for healthy populations rather than sick individuals, in the absence of evidence, this pragmatic approach would appear to be justified. In some patients with long-term chronic conditions (e.g. cancer, multiple sclerosis, rheumatoid arthritis), excess micronutrient intake may be of concern, particularly in those utilising a number of non-prescription supplements. During assessment, the potential adverse effects of self-dosing of alternative medicines and/or vitamin and mineral supplements should always be considered.

With regard to nutritional support, most standard oral nutritional supplements and enteral feeds contain sufficient minerals and electrolytes to meet daily requirements for sodium, potassium, magnesium and phosphate (NICE, 2006), but only if the patient is receiving enough of the feed to meet all their energy needs. Since many patients are either receiving less than full nutrition from these products or have pre-existing deficits, high losses or increased demands, additional provision may be required. However, care is needed to avoid excessive provision in some patients, e.g. those with renal or liver impairment. Some specialised feeds are designed specifically to provide adequate electrolytes, vitamins and minerals in lower-energy provision, for patients with low total energy needs.

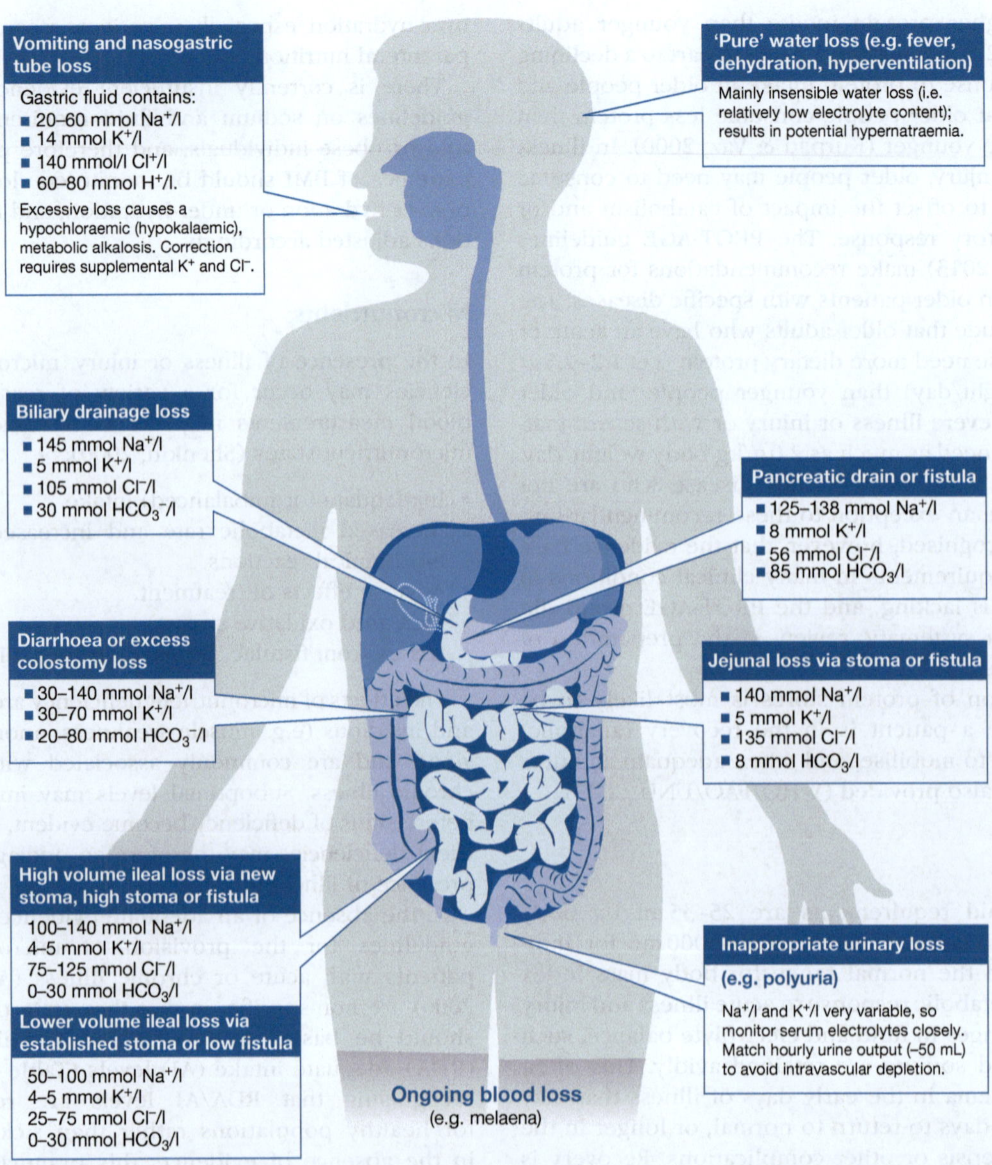

Figure 6.1.2 Ongoing fluid losses (© NICE, 2013 Diagram of Ongoing Loss. Available from https://www.nice.org.uk/guidance/cg174/resources/diagram-of-ongoing-losses-191664109. All rights reserved)

Pre-mixed parenteral nutrition bags contain very variable amounts of electrolytes and minerals, and care is needed to avoid giving PN with either inadequate or excessive electrolyte and/or mineral content (NICE, 2006). As with electrolytes and minerals, most standard oral and enteral feeds contain enough vitamins and trace elements to ensure that needs are met if patients are taking enough feed to meet their daily energy needs. However, when this is not the case, further balanced micronutrient supplementation may be required, especially in those with pre-existing deficits, poor absorption, increased demands or high losses (NICE, 2006). Premixed PN bags invariably contain inadequate levels of some micronutrients, and therefore need additions to be made prior to administration. The provision of PN without adequate micronutrient content must be avoided.

Special considerations

Estimating energy and protein requirements in obese patients

The factor that has the greatest influence on BMR is actual body weight (Horgan & Stubbs, 2003). However, some clinicians have recommended the use of adjusted weights to calculate BMR from prediction equations in subjects at the extremes of BMI. Regardless of BMI, rapid weight loss is associated with increased complications and poor outcome in hospitalised patients (NICE, 2006), and weight loss should therefore not be a nutritional goal during acute illness or following injury, even in the obese. Figure 6.1.3 shows how changes in weight and body composition affect BMR. The excess body weight in obese individuals largely comprises tissue with a low metabolic rate, and some clinicians have

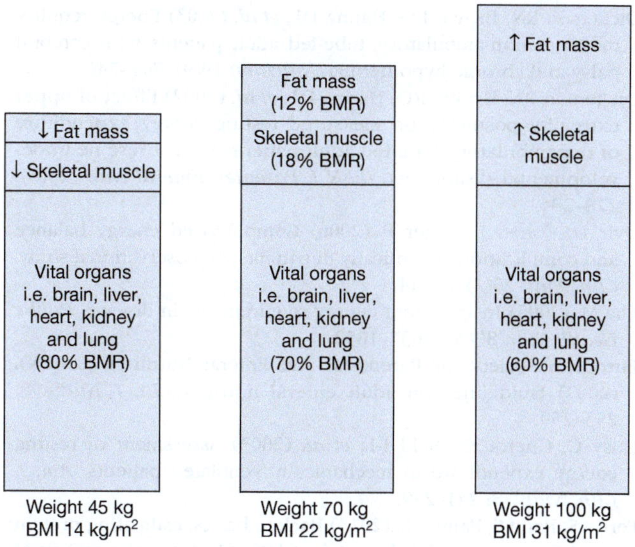

Figure 6.1.3 Effects of changes in body composition on basal metabolic rate (BMR)

therefore recommended adjusting weight downwards to calculate BMR, e.g. 25% adjusted weight = actual body weight × 0.25 + ideal body weight (Ireton-Jones, 2005). Other authors, however, recommend the use of actual body weight (Krenitsky, 2005), since BMR prediction equations were derived from data on individuals across the range of BMI, and actual rather than adjusted body weight was used to develop the equations. As there is no good evidence to support the use of adjusted body weight or specific cut-offs, clinical judgment is required to minimise the risks of overestimating or underestimating energy requirements in obese individuals (BMI > 30 kg/m^2). In clinical practice, actual body weight should be used to estimate BMR in obese individuals (Frankenfield & Ashcraft, 2011), but the assignment of stress factors should be undertaken with caution (PENG, 2011). Alternatively, energy requirements can be calculated using 19–21 kcal/kg actual body weight (Glynn *et al.*, 1999). However, it may be beneficial in some conditions (e.g. cancer of the breast and prostate) to aim for weight loss once a full recovery has been made in order to aid mobility and reduce the risk of recurrence (World Cancer Research Fund, 2007).

Protein

Since protein requirements are, to a large extent, determined by lean body mass, there is an argument for using an adjustment to the actual body weight to calculate protein requirements in obese patients, or to use ideal rather than actual body weight, although original work relating to this suggestion is difficult to locate.

Re-feeding syndrome

There are several published regimens for managing patients at risk of re-feeding syndrome. The lack of randomised controlled trials in this area, however, means that management is based on consensus and expert opinion rather than evidence (Khan *et al.*, 2011). Irrespective of which regimen is employed, the common principles are to prevent re-feeding syndrome by cautious re-introduction of energy and correction of biochemical abnormalities. While some authors recommend the correction of biochemical abnormalities prior to the introduction of energy and other macronutrients (Crook *et al.*, 2001), others recommend that both can occur in tandem without deleterious effects to the patient (NICE, 2006). There are currently no published randomised trial data to support either view. It is likely that the problems associated with re-feeding are less likely to arise with oral nutrition support, since starvation is usually accompanied by a loss of appetite. However, care should be taken in the prescription of oral nutrition supplements, particularly in the area of eating disorders (NICE, 2006). Underweight individuals tend to lose muscle and fat stores while preserving tissues with a high metabolic rate, i.e. brain, liver, heart and kidney. On a body weight basis, their metabolic rate is about 25% higher than in normal-weight individuals, and some clinicians have used this as a rationale to use ideal or usual body weight instead of actual body weight when calculating BMR. For a full discussion on the management of severely depleted individuals, please see a report recently published by the Royal College of Psychiatrists and the Royal College of Physicians (MARSIPAN, 2010) (also see Chapter 6.4 in this book, Enteral nutrition).

Estimating requirements for patients with abnormal fluid status

Oedema and ascites increase body weight without increasing metabolically active tissue. In the presence of over-hydration, therefore, dry weight should be measured after paracentesis, drainage of ascites or dialysis, and used to calculate BMR. In those patients where excess fluid cannot be removed, consider using the last recorded weight prior to developing ascites or oedema, or estimating dry weight using the following equation:

$$\text{Estimated dry weight} = \text{actual body weight} - (\text{weight of ascites} + \text{weight of oedema})$$

Estimating energy requirements for critically ill patients

In comparison with other clinical populations, there are considerably more studies measuring the energy expenditure of critically ill patients. The evidence-base for protein provision in critically ill patients is more limited, however, and there is even lesser evidence for micronutrient provision.

Reported energy requirements for Intensive Therapy Unit (critical care) (ITU) patients vary considerably, in part owing to the heterogeneity of the different ITU populations studied, and also due to differences in definitions of critical illness and/or the presence of sepsis. In addition to the factors that affect energy expenditure in general (e.g. age, gender and weight), the determination of energy requirements in ITU patients is complicated by a number of additional metabolic and management factors including hyperglycaemia, the presence or absence of sedation, ventilation mode, and/or the fraction of inspired oxygen. In the ITU setting, the estimation of an individual patient's energy requirements can be particularly challenging.

In bed-bound, artificially ventilated patients, BMR is frequently increased. However, TEE is not usually elevated, mainly because of minimal physical activity and/or sedation (SACN, 2011). In the most acutely ill patients (e.g. severe burns), however, TEE may be transiently elevated above normal (Bessey & Wilmore, 1988). For a full discussion of nutritional requirements in critically ill patients, see Chapter 7.17.1 in this book, Critical care.

References

ASPEN Board of Directors and the Clinical Guidelines Task Force. (2002) Guidelines for the use of parenteral and enteral nutrition in adult and paediatric patients. *JPEN J. Parenter. Enteral Nutr.* 26(1 Suppl): 1SA–138SA.

Arends J, Bodoky G, Bozzetti F, *et al.* (2006) ESPEN guidelines on enteral nutrition: non-surgical oncology. *Clin. Nutr.* 25: 245–259.

Bandini LG, Puelzl-Quinn H, Morelli JA, *et al.* (1995) Estimation of energy requirements in persons with severe central nervous system impairment. *J. Pediatr.* 126(5 Pt 1): 828–832.

Bauer JM, Biolo G, Cedeholm T *et al.* (2013) Evidence-based Recommendations for Optimal Dietary Protein Intake in Older People: A Position Paper From the PROT-AGE Study Group. *J. Am. Medical Directors Association* 14(8): 542–559.

Benedict FG, Carpenter TM. (1918) *Food Ingestion and Energy Transformation with Special Reference to the Stimulating Effects of Nutrients*. Pub. No. 261. Carnegie Institution of Washington.

Bessey PQ, Wilmore DW. (1988) The burned patient. In *Nutrition and Metabolism in Patient Care*. London: W.B. Saunders, pp. 672–700.

Boullata J, Williams J, Cottrell F, *et al.* (2007) Accurate determination of energy needs in hospitalized patients. *J. Am. Diet. Assoc.* 107: 393–401.

Brandi LS, Bertolini R, Santini L, *et al.* (1999) Effects of ventilator resetting on indirect calorimetry measurement in the critically ill surgical patient. *Crit. Care Med.* 27(3): 531–539.

Branson RD, Johannigman JA. (2004) The measurement of energy expenditure. *Nutrition in Clinical Practice* 19:622–636.

British Artificial Nutrition Survey. (2010) *Artificial Nutrition Support in the UK 2000–2009*. Redditch, Worcs: The British Association for Parenteral and Enteral Nutrition (ISBN: 978-1-899467-61-7).

Burge JC, Goon A, Choban PS, *et al.* (1994) Efficacy of hypocaloric total parenteral nutrition in hospitalized obese patients: A prospective, double-blind randomised trial. *JPEN J. Parenter. Enteral Nutr.* 18(3): 203–207.

Calloway DH, Spector H. (1955) Nitrogen utilization during caloric restriction. II. The effect of variation in nitrogen intake. *J. Nutr.* 56(4): 545–554.

Choban PS, Burge JC, Scales D, *et al.* (1997) Hypoenergetic nutrition support in hospitalized obese patients: a simplified method for clinical application. *Am. J. Clin. Nutr.* 66(546): 550.

Committee on the Medical Aspects of Food (COMA). (1991) *Dietary Reference Values for Food Energy and Nutrients for the United Kingdom*. London: Department of Health, HMSO, 41.

Crook MA, Hally V, Panteli JV. (2001) The importance of the refeeding syndrome. *Nutrition* 17(7–8): 632–637.

Dickerson RN, Brown RO, Gervasio JG, *et al.* (1999) Measured energy expenditure of tube-fed patients with severe neurodevelopmental disabilities. *J. Am. Coll. Nutr.* 18(1): 61–68.

Dickerson RN, Brown RO, Hanna DL, *et al.* (2003) Energy requirements of non-ambulatory, tube-fed adult patients with cerebral palsy and chronic hypothermia. *Nutrition* 19(9): 741–746.

Dickerson RN, Brown RO, Hanna DL, *et al.* (2002) Effect of upper extremity posturing on measured resting energy expenditure of nonambulatory tube-fed adult patients with severe neurodevelopmental disabilities. *JPEN J. Parenter. Enteral Nutr.* 26(5): 278–284.

Dvir D, Cohen J, Singer P. (2006) Computerized energy balance and complications in critically ill patients: an observational study. *Clin. Nutr.* 25(1): 37–44.

Elia M. (2005) Insights into energy requirements in disease. *Public Health Nutr.* 8(7A): 1037–1052.

European Society for Parenteral and Enteral Nutrition (ESPEN). (2007) Guidelines on adult enteral nutrition. *Br. J. Nutr.* 98: 253–259.

Faisy C, Guerot E, Diehl J-L, *et al.* (2003) Assessment of resting energy expenditure in mechanically ventilated patients. *Am. J. Clin. Nutr.* 78: 241–249.

Ferrie S, Rand S, Palmer S. (2013) Back to basics: estimating protein requirements for adult hospital patients. A systematic review of randomised controlled trials. *Food Nutr. Sci.* 4: 201–214. 10.4236/fns.2013.42028

Frankenfield D. (2006) Energy expenditure and protein requirements after traumatic injury. *Nutrition in Clinical Practice* 21(5): 430–437.

Frankenfield DC, Roth-Yousy L, Compher C. (2005) Comparison of predictive equations for resting metabolic rate in healthy nonobese and obese adults: a systematic review. *J. Am. Diet. Assoc.* 105(5): 775–789.

Frankenfield DC, Ashcraft CM. (2011) Estimating energy needs in nutrition support patients. *JPEN J. Parenter. Enteral Nutr.* 35(5): 563–570.

Glynn CC, Greene GW, Winkler MF, *et al.* (1999) Predictive versus measured energy expenditure using limits of agreement analysis in hospitalised, obese patients. *JPEN J. Parenter. Enteral Nutr.* 23:147–154.

Harris JA, Benedict FG. (1919) *Biometric Studies of Basal Metabolism in Man*. Washington DC: Carnegie Institute of Washington, Publication No. 297.

Henry CJK. (2005) Basal metabolic rate studies in humans: measurement and development of new equations. *Public Health Nutr.* 8(7A): 1133–1152.

Heymsfield SB, Casper K, Funfar J. (1987) Physiologic response and clinical implications of nutrition support. *Am. J. Cardiology* 60(12): 75G–81G.

Horgan GW, Stubbs J. (2003) Predicting basal metabolic rate in the obese is difficult. *Eur. J. Clin. Nutr.* 57(2): 335–340.

Ibrahim EH, Mehringer L, Prentice D, *et al.* (2002) Early versus late enteral feeding of mechanically ventilated patients: results of a clinical trial. *JPEN J. Parenter. Enteral Nutr.* 26(3): 174–181.

Ireton-Jones CS, Turner WW, Liepa GU, *et al.* (1992) Equations for the estimation of energy expenditure in patients with burns with special reference to ventilatory status. *J. Burn Care Rehabil.* 13: 330–333.

Ireton-Jones CS, Jones JD. (2002) Improved equations for predicting energy expenditure in patients: the Ireton-Jones equations. *Nutr. Clin. Pract.* 17(1): 29–31.

Ireton-Jones CS. (2005) Adjusted body weight, con: why adjust body weight in energy-expenditure calculations? *Nutr. Clin. Pract.* 20: 474–479.

Johnson RK, Hildreth HG, Contompasis SH, *et al.* (1997) Total energy expenditure in adults with cerebral palsy as assessed by doubly labeled water. *J. Am. Diet. Assoc.* 97(9): 966–970.

Kan MN, Chang HH, Sheu WF, *et al.* (2003) Estimation of energy requirements for mechanically ventilated, critically ill patients using nutritional status. *Crit. Care.* 7(5): R108–R115.

Khan LUR, Ahmed J, Khan S, *et al.* (2011) Refeeding syndrome: a literature review. *Gastroenterol. Res. Pract.* Article ID 410971.

Kinney JM, Long CL, Gump FE, Duke JH Jr. (1968) Tissue composition of weight loss in surgical patients. I. Elective operation. *Annals of Surgery* 168(3): 459–474.

Krenitsky J. (2005) Adjusted body weight, pro: evidence to support the use of adjusted body weight in calculating calorie requirements. *Nutr. Clin. Pract.* 20: 468–473.

Krishnan JA, Parce PB, Martinez A, *et al.* (2003) Caloric intake in medical ICU patients: consistency of care with guidelines and relationship to clinical outcomes. *Chest.* 124: 297–305.

Kulstad R, Schoeller DA. (2007). The energetic of wasting diseases. *Curr. Opin. Clin. Nutr. Metab. Care.*10(4): 488–493.

Kurpad AV, Vaz M. (2000) Protein and amino acid requirements in the elderly. *Eur. J. Clin. Nutr.* 54: S131–S142.

Lobo DN, Macafee DAL, Allison SP. (2006) How perioperative fluid balance influences postoperative outcomes. *Best Pract. Res. Clin. Anaesthesiol.* 20(3): 439–455.

McCrory MA, Kim HR, Wright NC, *et al.* (1998) Energy expenditure, physical activity, and body composition of ambulatory adults with hereditary neuromuscular disease. *Am. J. Clin. Nutr.* 67: 1162–1169.

Martin MM, Doig GS, Heyland DK, *et al.* (2004) Multicentre, cluster-randomized clinical trial of algorithms for critical-care enteral and parenteral therapy (ACCEPT). *CMAJ.* 170(2): 197–204.

Mehanna HM, Moledina J, Travis J. (2008) Refeeding syndrome: what it is, and how to prevent and treat it. *BMJ.* 336(7659): 1495–1498.

Miller MD, Daniels LA, Bannerman E, *et al.* (2005) Resting energy expenditure measured longitudinally following hip fracture compared to predictive equations: is an injury adjustment required? *Br. J. Nutr.* 94(6): 976–982.

NICE. (2006) *Nutrition support in adults: Oral nutrition support, enteral tube feeding and parenteral nutrition. Clinical Guideline* 32. Available at https://www.nice.org.uk/guidance/cg32. Accessed 4 October 2017.

NICE. (2013) Intravenous fluid therapy in adults in hospital. Clinical guideline [CG174]. Available at https://www.nice.org.uk/Guidance/CG174. Accessed 10 October 2018.

NICE. (2017) *Intravenous fluid therapy in adults in hospital Clinical guideline [CG174].* Available at https://www.nice.org.uk/guidance/cg174. Accessed 1 October 2017.

Patino JF, de Pimiento SE, Vergara A, *et al.* (1999) Hypocaloric support in the critically ill. *World J. Surg.* 23(6): 553–559.

Ramirez-Zea M. (2005). Validation of three predictive equations for basal metabolic rate in adults. *Public Health Nutr.* 8(7A): 1213–1228.

Reeves MM, Capra S. (2003) Predicting energy requirements in the clinical setting: are current methods evidence based? *Nutr. Rev.* 61(4): 143–151.

Royal College of Psychiatrists and the Royal College of Physicians. (2010) Report from the MARSIPAN group. MARSIPAN: Management of Really Sick Patients with Anorexia Nervosa. College Report CR162.

SACN. (2011). *Dietary Recommendations for Energy.* Available at https://www.gov.uk/government/uploads/system/uploads/attachment_data/file/339317/SACN_Dietary_Reference_Values_for_Energy.pdf. Accessed 4 October 2017.

Schofield WN. (1985). Predicting basal metabolic rate, new standards and review of previous work. *Hum. Nutr. Clin. Nutr.* 39: 5–41.

Shenkin A. (2000) Micronutrients in the severely-injured patient. *Proc. Nutr. Soc.* 59: 451–456.

Stanga Z, Brunner A, Leuenberger M, *et al.* (2008) Nutrition in clinical practice – the refeeding syndrome: illustrative cases and guidelines for prevention and treatment. *Eur. J. Clin. Nutr.* 62(6): 687–694.

Stokes MA, Hill GL. (1993) Total energy expenditure in patients with Crohn's disease: measurement by the combined body scan technique. *J. Parenter. Enteral Nutr.* 17(1): 3–7.

Streat SJ, Beddoe AH, Hill GL. (1987) Aggressive nutritional support does not prevent protein loss despite fat gain in septic intensive care patients. *J. Trauma* 27: 262–266.

Swinamer DL, Grace MG, Hamilton SM, *et al.* (1990) Predictive equation for assessing energy expenditure in mechanically ventilated critically ill patients. *Crit. Care Med.* 18: 657–661.

Taylor SJ. (2007) *Energy and Nitrogen Requirements in Disease States.* London: Smith-Gordon.

Todorovic V, Micklewright A, On behalf of the Parenteral and Enteral Nutrition Group of the British Dietetic Association (PENG). (2011) *A Pocket Guide to Clinical Nutrition.* Birmingham: BDA.

Toth MJ, Fishman PS, Poehlman ET. (1997) Free-living daily energy expenditure in patients with Parkinson's disease. *Neurology.* 48(1): 88–91.

Villet S, Chiolero RL, Bollmann MD, *et al.* (2005) Negative impact of hypocaloric feeding and energy balance on clinical outcome in ICU patients. *Clin. Nutr.* 24(4): 502–509.

Weekes CE. (2007) Controversies in the determination of energy requirements. *Proc. Nutr. Soc.* 66: 367–377.

Weekes CE. (2011) Nutritional requirements in cancer. In: Shaw C (ed) *Nutrition and Cancer.* UK: Blackwell Publishing Ltd.

Westerterp KR. (2004) Diet induced thermogenesis. *Nutr. Metab. (Lond).* 1(1): 5.

Westerterp KR. (2017) Doubly labelled water assessment of energy expenditure: principle, practice, and promise. *Eur. J. App. Physiol.* 117: 1277–1285. doi 10.1007/s00421-017-3641-x.

WHO/FAO/UNU Expert Consultation. (2007) Protein and amino acid requirements in human nutrition, Joint WHO/FAO/UNU Expert Consultation, *World Health Organization Technical Report Series 935*, World Health Organization.

World Cancer Research Fund. (2018) *Food, Nutrition, Physical Activity, and the Prevention of Cancer: A Global Perspective.* Washington DC: AICR. Available at www. https://www.wcrf.org/dietandcancer. Accessed 10 October 2018.

Zauner A, Schneeweiss B, Kneidinger N, *et al.* (2006) Weight-adjusted resting energy expenditure is not constant in critically ill patients. *Intensive Care Med.* 32(3): 428–443.

6.2 Malnutrition

Rebecca Stratton

Key points

- Malnutrition adversely affects physical and psychological health, and impairs recovery from disease, increasing mortality, complications, hospital stay and use of other healthcare resources.
- Malnutrition is common and costly, but is often unrecognised and untreated.
- Routine and regular screening – using a quick, simple-to-use, valid, evidence-based tool with a care plan – is recommended to improve the detection and treatment of malnutrition.
- Treatment should be undertaken promptly with appropriate nutritional support; energy, protein and other nutrients, including micronutrients, should be considered.

Malnutrition can be defined as *'a state of nutrition in which a deficiency or excess (or imbalance) of energy, protein and other nutrients causes measurable adverse effects on tissue/body form (body shape, size, composition), body function and clinical outcome'* (Elia, 2000, p. 2). Malnutrition is a broad term that includes not only protein energy malnutrition (both over- and undernutrition), but malnutrition of other nutrients, such as micronutrients. The adverse effects of malnutrition will mostly respond to nutritional treatment. This chapter concentrates on protein energy malnutrition (described here as malnutrition).

Prevalence of malnutrition and at-risk groups

Malnutrition is common, and is a major clinical and public health problem in the UK (Elia, 2000; Elia & Russell, 2009). At any given point in time, >3 million people in the UK are malnourished, with most (~93%) living in the community (Elia & Russell, 2009). Although malnutrition among people in hospitals was identified over three decades ago (Bistrian *et al.*, 1974; Hill *et al.*, 1977), it remains a common and often unrecognised problem (Elia, 2003; Stratton *et al.*, 2003). The British Association for Parenteral and Enteral Nutrition (BAPEN) national screening weeks have shown that approximately one-third of hospital admissions are at risk of malnutrition (Russell & Elia, 2014). Smaller surveys in hospitalised infants and children also suggest that malnutrition is common (Gerasimidis *et al.*, 2011; Pichler *et al.*, 2014; Stratton *et al.*, 2003).

The prevalence of malnutrition depends on the criteria used to define it and varies with age, the associated clinical condition and the type of treatments (including surgery) being undertaken. The frequency of malnutrition, and the risk of developing malnutrition, is typically highest in:

- Infants, young children and the elderly.
- Patients with gastrointestinal, respiratory or renal disease, and malignancy.
- Those with multiple comorbidities, including the critically ill.
- Individuals undergoing complex surgery, transplantation or burns treatment.

Once in hospital, deterioration in nutritional status often occurs unless action is taken to prevent it. Between 30 and 90% of adults and children lose weight while in hospital (Stratton *et al.*, 2003). This is partly because malnutrition is often unrecognised and untreated, frequently going undetected. Measurement and documentation of important nutritional information, including body mass index (BMI), unintentional weight loss and recent food intake, in hospital inpatients, outpatients and in many other care settings, are often lacking (Cawood *et al.*, 2008; Elia, 2000; Volkert *et al.*, 2010). This is partly due to the absence of formal screening programmes that link the recognition of malnutrition with treatment plans.

At any point in time, only about 2% of the >3 million adults at risk of malnutrition are in hospital, with 5% in care homes and the remainder in the community (2–3%

SECTION 6

Manual of Dietetic Practice, Sixth Edition. Edited by Joan Gandy.

Companion website: www.manualofdieteticpractice.com

in sheltered housing) (Elia *et al.*, 2010). Surveys suggest that 15–30% outpatients, 5–23% patients visiting a general practitioner (GP), 25% patients receiving district nursing care, 30–40% care home residents and 10–14% of individuals in sheltered housing are at risk of malnutrition (Elia *et al.*, 2015). The elderly is a group at particular risk, as suggested by a secondary analysis of a national survey, which found that 12% free-living and 21% institutionalised elderly are at risk of malnutrition, and that geographical inequalities exist (higher rates of malnutrition in the north than in the south of England) (Elia & Stratton, 2005). In addition, malnutrition is more common in those from more deprived areas (Collins *et al.*, 2016; Stratton & Elia, 2006). In community settings, as in hospitals, malnutrition is often undetected and untreated (Cawood *et al.*, 2008; Volkert *et al.*, 2010). An increasingly ageing population, the ongoing pressure on healthcare and social care resources, and the community-led NHS structure mean that a greater proportion of sick and debilitated individuals are cared for outside the hospital, with services commissioned by GP-led clinical commissioning groups (NHS Five Year Forward View, 2014). Sustainability and transformation plans (STPs) are now being implemented in local geographic areas to transform health and care outcomes delivered by NHS providers, CCGs, local authorities and care services, but their impact on malnutrition and nutritional care services has yet to be seen.

Causes of malnutrition

In the UK, the primary cause of malnutrition is disease, hence the term disease-related malnutrition. Other causes include poverty and deprivation, and behavioural problems in children. Disease-related malnutrition arises when nutritional intake does not meet nutritional needs because of decreased dietary intake, increased nutritional requirements or an impaired ability to absorb or utilise nutrients. Insufficient dietary intake is the main reason for malnutrition developing and progressing, and there are many factors that limit nutritional intake (see Figure 6.2.1). Broadly, these factors can be divided into two types:

- Disease-related factors that reduce intake despite availability of food.
- Other factors such as inadequate availability, quality or presentation of foods that reduce intake.

Numerous studies across many different diagnostic groups have documented energy, protein and micronutrient intakes to be insufficient to meet nutritional requirements, particularly in institutionalised patients. Also, studies have shown that food in institutions (hospitals, care homes) is often not consumed and is therefore wasted, sometimes because catering practices do not meet the needs of the sick (see Chapter 4.4.1, Food service). Nutritional support (oral nutritional

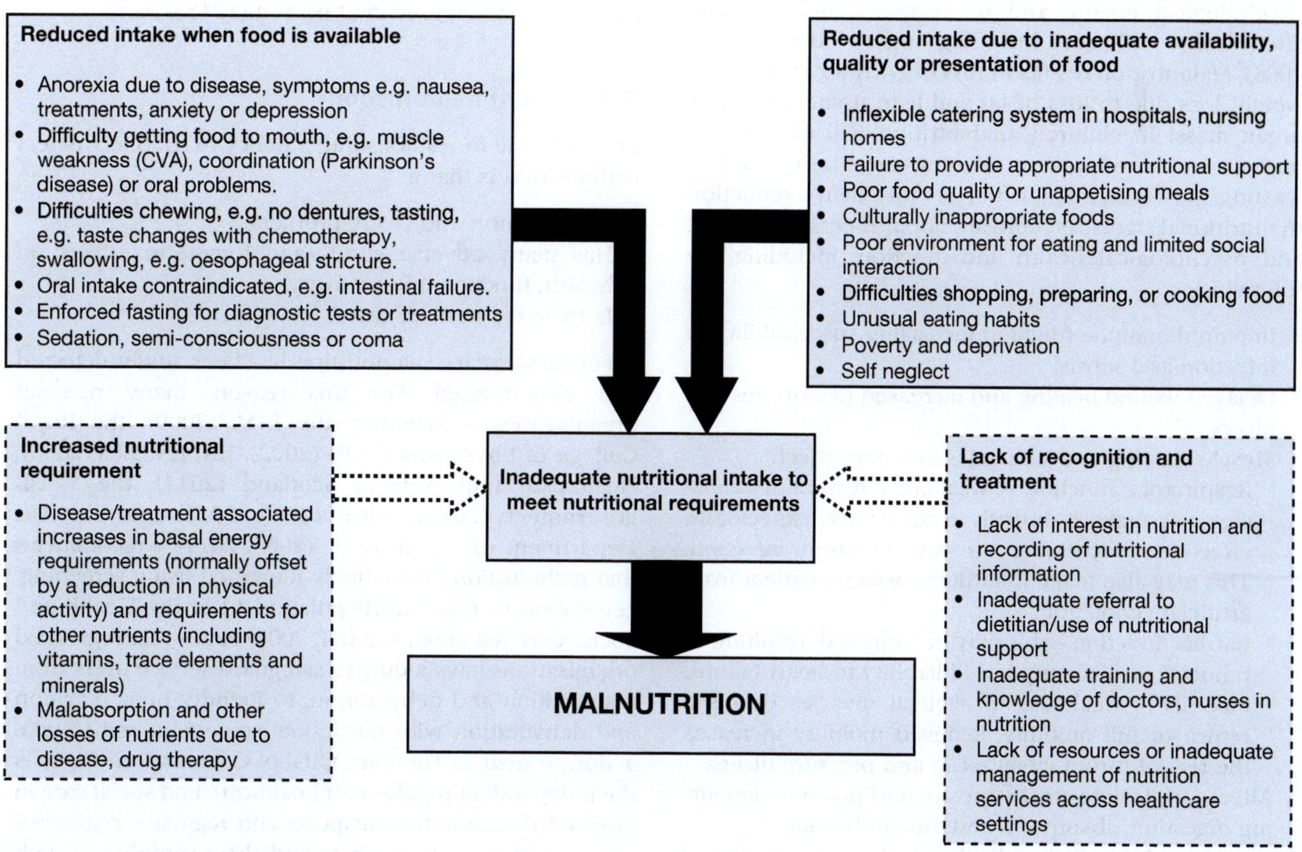

Figure 6.2.1 Causes of malnutrition

supplements, enteral tube feeding, parenteral nutrition) is often not used early enough or frequently enough to prevent or treat malnutrition, despite a large and growing evidence base that indicates the benefits of nutritional support if used appropriately. This is increasingly an issue as current economic constraints mean budget holders may choose to withhold prescribed nutritional care, failing to recognise that greater costs result when leaving malnutrition untreated (increased costly hospital admissions and complications such as infections and pressure ulcers) (Elia *et al.*, 2015).

Malnutrition may also arise if total requirements for energy and nutrients are increased with disease, after trauma and surgery, and with some treatments, e.g. drug therapy and chemotherapy. Increments in basal energy metabolism occur in a number of disease states, post-operatively and in sepsis and burns patients. However, in many cases, this is offset by reductions in physical activity (Gibney *et al.*, 1997; Jebb, 1997), so that total energy expenditure is not substantially increased (see Chapter 6.1, Nutritional requirements in clinical practice). Increased nutrient losses and inability to absorb nutrients also elevate requirements, increasing the risk of malnutrition developing.

Consequences of malnutrition

Malnutrition has a diversity of effects, influencing every system of the body. It has many adverse consequences on body structure and function, physical and psychological health, and on recovery and outcome after disease and injury, including surgery (Stratton *et al.*, 2003). Malnutrition results in loss of body structure, with weight loss due to loss of fat and lean tissue, including organ mass. In children, malnutrition will also impair growth and development, leading to stunting and/or wasting. However, malnutrition is more than a reduction in nutritional status, as there are impairments in physical and psychological health and function, including the following:

- Impaired immune function increasing susceptibility to infection and sepsis.
- Delayed wound healing and increased risk of pressure ulcers.
- Muscle wasting and weakness that may affect:
  - Respiratory function – weakened respiratory muscles may make it difficult to cough and expectorate effectively, increasing the risk of chest infection. This may also make it harder to wean a patient from artificial ventilation.
  - Cardiac function – this may be impaired, resulting in reduced cardiac output and liability to heart failure.
  - Mobility – weakness of skeletal muscles delays a return to full mobility. Reduced mobility increases the risk of thromboembolism and pressure ulcers.
- Altered gastrointestinal structure and function, impairing digestion, absorption and the gut barrier.
- Apathy and depression, leading to loss of morale and reduced will to recover.
- General sense of weakness and illness, which impairs appetite and physical ability to eat, and hence tends to perpetuate and worsen the state of malnutrition.
- Adverse effects on learning and behaviour in children, with potential long-term deficits in cognition.
- Poor libido, fertility, pregnancy outcome and mother–child interactions.

These physical and psychological consequences of malnutrition increase susceptibility to disease, impair clinical outcome and increase healthcare use and costs. Individuals identified as being at risk of malnutrition have:

- Increased risk of mortality and complications during and after hospitalisation.
- Longer hospital stays and greater hospital costs.
- Greater requirement for healthcare post-discharge.
- Increased risk of admission to hospital and more visits to the GP.

Consequently, increased use of healthcare resources means malnutrition is very expensive. A recent report estimated that the annual expenditure owing to malnutrition in England (in adults and children) was £19.6 billion (approximately 15% of the total expenditure on healthcare and social care) (Elia *et al.*, 2015). Most of the expenditure was due to healthcare rather than social care, and from secondary (hospital) care rather than primary care of adults (mostly older adults), rather than in children. The healthcare cost of a malnourished patient (£7408 per year) is more than three times greater than that of a non-malnourished person (£2155/year).

Detection of malnutrition

The rationale for establishing a policy to routinely detect malnutrition is that it:

- Is a common and costly problem.
- Has many adverse short- and long-term effects on health, function and recovery.
- Is treatable in most cases.

For many years, malnutrition has been under-detected and undertreated. For this reason, many national organisations – including the BDA (2009), the Royal College of Physicians (RCP) (2002), BAPEN (Elia, 2003), Healthcare Improvement Scotland (2014), the Welsh government (2013), NICE (2006, 2012) and the UK Department of Health (DH) (2008, 2014) – recommend that malnutrition be routinely identified using screening. Legislation in England (Regulation 14 of the Health and Social Care Act 2008; see DH, 2008) states that registered organisations have a duty to safeguard service users from malnutrition and dehydration, to identify poor nutrition and dehydration with nutritional screening, and to take action to treat it. The Care Quality Commission (CQC) is the independent regulator of healthcare and social care in England that monitors, inspects and regulates registered care-providing organisations and their compliance with this aspect of the law.

It has also been suggested that obesity should be routinely identified, ideally using the same screening procedure (Elia, 2003). Obesity has many health risks (see Chapter 7.13.1, General aspects and prevention of obesity), but its treatment should not generally be undertaken in those who are acutely unwell. Such patients may still be at risk of malnutrition due to weight loss or limited dietary intake (e.g. nil by mouth post-stroke), and should be treated accordingly.

Screening

Screening is a rapid, simple and general procedure, often carried out at first contact with an individual, to detect those with significant risk of malnutrition, so that action plans for monitoring and/or treatment can be implemented. Some individuals may need help or advice with eating and drinking; others may need special diets and a referral to a dietitian for expert advice. Screening should be routinely and regularly undertaken in hospitals, nursing and residential care, and in other primary care settings, e.g. patients seen by district nurses, at-risk groups or newly registered patients in GP practices. The frequency of screening and any associated monitoring and treatment will depend on the patient group, the healthcare setting and the resources available.

Screening is a multidisciplinary responsibility and can be undertaken by nurses, doctors, dietitians or other healthcare professionals. Screening, using a test or tool, should be part of a screening programme that includes a full range of activities from identification of risk with the tool, to diagnosis and treatments. Screening can precede nutritional assessment, which is a more in-depth and specific evaluation of those individuals at risk, and is typically undertaken by a dietitian (see Chapter 2.2, Assessment of nutritional status). Nutritional assessment may be required in the case of serious nutritional problems, to identify micronutrient status or to undertake other detailed dietary investigations. Although dietitians have the expertise, it is neither practical nor cost-effective for them to assess the nutritional status of every patient admitted to hospital, and they are unlikely to come into direct contact with many of those at risk in the community (often only after problems have arisen). Therefore, identification of people with, or at risk of, malnutrition requires a locally agreed policy and the assistance of other health professionals.

There are many screening tools in use in clinical practice, but it is important to use a tool that meets the important characteristics listed in Table 6.2.1. A screening tool for malnutrition should attempt to establish the following in the most objective way possible:

- Chronic protein energy status, e.g. BMI, weight for height, weight and height for age.
- Any recent changes in protein energy status, e.g. weight loss, inadequate dietary intake.
- Any likely future changes in protein energy status, e.g. likelihood of inadequate dietary intake and weight loss.

When objective measures are not feasible (e.g. in an acutely unwell, bed-bound individual), or there is concern about their interpretation (e.g. oedema), alternative measures should be considered. As part of the screening programme, the underlying cause of changes in nutritional status (e.g. disease or condition, psychosocial issues and behavioural problems) should also be established and treated if appropriate (e.g. for those who are terminally ill, active treatment may not be undertaken). Although there are many factors that increase

Table 6.2.1 Important characteristics of a screening tool for malnutrition

Characteristic	Attributes
Practical	Quick and easy to complete and to understand
	Has a range of alternative measures for when weight or height cannot be measured
Universal	Can be used in all adults of all ages (including the elderly), including the sick and healthy; is applicable across different care settings (hospital, GP practice, nursing home, free living); allows continuity of care
	Can be used for public health purposes
Reliable	Good reproducibility between users
	Good internal reliability
Valid	Content, face, internal, concurrent and predictive validity
Evidence based and independently peer-reviewed	
Linked to a care plan for treatment	Facilitates nursing and other staff initiating appropriate monitoring or treatment and referral to the dietitian or nutrition support team
Developed by a multidisciplinary group for use by all healthcare professionals	
Acceptable to patients and healthcare professionals	

an individual's risk of malnutrition, e.g. gastrointestinal symptoms, metabolic stress and pressure ulcers, they do so by affecting the adequacy of nutritional intake relative to an individual's nutritional needs. In most cases, nutritional intake is reduced, nutritional needs are not met and the result is that weight is lost. Therefore, a screening tool is able to assess the risk of malnutrition simply by identifying chronic protein energy status (e.g. BMI in adults), and previous and predicted recent changes in status (e.g. weight loss and reduced dietary intake). Thus, screening can reflect aspects of an individual's nutritional status, encompassing:

- Past, e.g. unintentional weight loss and lack of nutritional intake.
- Present, e.g. BMI.
- Future, e.g. potential for lack of nutritional intake and weight loss.

The past can be most easily assessed using unintended weight loss over a defined time scale, e.g. 3 months. This is assessed in terms of the extent of unintentional body weight loss, ideally as a percentage of usual body weight, e.g. >10% of weight lost in 3 months. A period of 3–6 months is the most common timeframe over which to assess weight loss, although it can be a shorter (e.g. 1 week) or longer (e.g. 1 year) time interval. Weight loss is also a marker for inadequacy of nutritional intake. No nutritional intake for >5 days (without disease) equates to a weight loss of 5–10% (Elia, 2003). Detailed dietary history is not taken as part of screening since it is time consuming and requires a nutritional expert, e.g. dietitian, to undertake (screening is not usually undertaken by dietitians). Detailed dietary information may be obtained as part of nutritional assessment.

The present or current status of an individual can be objectively identified using BMI. This is a simple and reproducible index that reflects body composition and function. A BMI of <20 kg/m² is considered to be underweight, and a BMI of <18.5 kg/m² as severely underweight. Individuals with a BMI of >30 kg/m² are considered obese. These are nationally recognised and accepted cut-offs for BMI, and they are based on the loss of physiological function and well-being, and increased clinical risk as BMI decreases. They are consistently recommended for all adults, including elderly people. However, these cut-offs denote only risk of malnutrition, as some individuals may be constitutionally thin, fit and well despite having a low BMI.

When screening for the risk of malnutrition, particularly in the acute setting, a consideration of the future likelihood of deterioration in nutritional status (poor, inadequate nutritional intake leading to weight loss) is needed. For example, a free-living individual suffers a stroke and is admitted to hospital, unable to swallow and eat. Despite having a desirable BMI and no history of weight loss, patients are at risk of malnutrition as they will be unable to eat for >5 days. During this timeframe, even an individual without disease or injury would lose 5–10% of body weight, feel unwell and lose muscle mass (Elia, 2003). Similarly, those who suffer severe injury are unconscious and have intestinal failure, and many others with severe, acute illness are at risk of malnutrition due to a prolonged inability to eat or drink. These individuals will usually require nutritional assessment by a dietitian or nutrition support team, and the provision of artificial nutritional support.

Similar principles apply to screening for malnutrition in paediatrics, although there is more complexity, as consideration of growth and development is required. Anthropometric measurements have been widely used to screen for malnutrition in children. These include weight for age, height for age, BMI for age, weight for height and mid-upper-arm circumference (see Chapter 3.8.2, Growth, nutritional assessment and nutritional requirements). The WHO charts for children (aged 0–4 years) are purported to reflect optimal growth in children of all ethnic groups because of the striking similarities in results obtained from the countries that contributed data (Wright *et al.*, 2010). The charts are based on anthropometric measurements obtained from children who were breastfed for about 6 months by relatively affluent, non-smoking mothers who experienced a healthy pregnancy. The charts, which have separate sections for preterm babies, infants aged 0–1 years and older children, have been widely adopted in the UK and other countries. Establishing the most appropriate cut-off points for unintentional weight change in children of different ages can be difficult because growth rates vary considerably with age. In contrast to adults, where weight maintenance is considered to be normal, failure to increase weight over even a short period of time, e.g. 1 month, in a rapidly growing child may represent substantial growth failure, and a 5% weight loss over the same period can be of serious concern. In clinical practice, rapid changes in weight, dietary intake and disease-related factors might all need to be taken into account. A variety of screening tools have been developed for use in children (mostly in hospital settings), such as Paediatric Yorkhill Malnutrition Score (PYMS), Screening Tool for Risk on Nutritional Status and Growth (STRONGkids), and Screening Tool for the Assessment of Malnutrition in Paediatrics (STAMP). Nevertheless, a universally accepted tool is lacking (Chourdakis *et al.*, 2016), and discrepancies exist between the currently available tools as they incorporate different criteria to detect malnutrition (see Chapter 3.8.2, Growth, nutritional assessment and nutritional requirements).

Individuals with other nutritional concerns or problems may need to be referred to a dietitian for more detailed evaluation of the extent or risk of nutritional depletion (Chapter 2.2, Assessment of nutritional status). Particular attention should be paid to the aspects shown in Table 6.2.2. The nature and extent of these problems will determine the way malnutrition is managed or averted. All individuals requiring detailed nutritional assessment and artificial nutritional support need to be referred to a dietitian or nutrition support team (see Chapter 6.3, Oral nutritional support and Chapter 6.4, Parenteral nutrition).

Table 6.2.2 Aspects relating to malnutrition to be considered in nutrition assessment

Aspects	Description
Dietary aspects	Adequacy of current intake
	Recent changes in food intake
	Appetite Existence of factors likely to impair food intake
Clinical aspects	Presence of factors likely to increase nutrient requirements
	Presence of factors likely to increase nutrient losses
	Acute or chronic disease affecting the gastrointestinal tract
	Use of drugs and other treatments affecting food intake or nutrient utilisation
Physical aspects	Signs of muscle wasting, emaciation or oedema
	Presence of pressure ulcers (stages I–IV) or other wounds (see Chapter 7.17.6, Wound healing, tissue viability and pressure sores)
Anthropometric aspects	Degree and rapidity of any unintended weight loss BMI, growth (in infants and children)
	Evidence of muscle wasting, e.g. reduced mid-arm muscle circumference or grip strength
Psychosocial aspects	Depression, anxiety or apathy
	Social isolation
	Poverty

Setting up a screening programme

To facilitate a screening programme, which includes routine screening, monitoring, assessment and treatment plans, and which may include referral to a dietitian, the following are suggested:

- Establish a policy locally that ensures that screening is undertaken and repeated as appropriate (specifying areas, if any, that are exempt from routine screening).
- Agree on the screening tool to be used locally and the resources available for a screening programme across healthcare settings.
- Devise locally agreed care plans for monitoring and treating those identified by screening.
- Ensure equipment required for screening, e.g. weighing scales, stadiometers/length boards, tape measures and callipers, is available and regularly calibrated as appropriate.
- Establish the criteria for those requiring more detailed nutritional assessment and dietetic referral (this will vary locally depending on the resources available).
- Set up systems for the documentation of the results of screening, monitoring and treatment.
- Regularly audit the efficacy of the screening programme.

Malnutrition Universal Screening Tool ('MUST')

Although there are several screening tools available for adults, the Malnutrition Universal Screening Tool ('MUST') is mentioned here as an example because it meets all the key characteristics outlined in Table 6.2.1. 'MUST' was developed by the Malnutrition Advisory Group, a multidisciplinary group of the BAPEN, and it is supported by the BDA, the Royal College of Nursing, the Registered Nursing Homes Association and the RCP (England). 'MUST' is also recommended in Scotland and Wales (Healthcare Improvement Scotland, 2014; Welsh Government, 2013). NICE Clinical Guidelines and Quality Standards (CG32 2006, QS24 2012) also recommend the use of 'MUST'. The tool has been extensively peer-reviewed by many national organisations and independent healthcare practitioners for use in clinical settings and for public health.

'MUST' (see Figure 6.2.2) is an evidence-based tool (Elia, 2003) that has been designed to help identify adults who are at risk of malnutrition, as well as those who are obese. It has not been designed to detect poor vitamin and mineral status. 'MUST' involves the identification of chronic protein energy status (BMI), change in status (unintentional weight loss) and the presence of an acute disease resulting in, or likely to result in, no dietary intake for >5 days. It has been developed for use in all adults, including the elderly, the sick and healthy free-living individuals, and those in healthcare i.e.:

- Hospital wards.
- Outpatient clinics.
- General practice.
- Community settings, e.g. patients receiving care at home, in care homes or sheltered housing.
- Public health.

'MUST' can be applied to all types of adult patients, is easy and rapid to use, and can be used by multidisciplinary teams; it is reproducible, internally consistent and valid. It can be used in situations where weight or height cannot be measured, providing a range of alternatives, including reported or documented measurements, other surrogate measures, subjective criteria and clinical judgement. The tool categorises individuals into low, medium and high risk of malnutrition, and identifies the obese. 'MUST' provides guidelines for care plans, which should be modified to suit local policy and resources.

Practicalities

'MUST' is a five-step screening tool which includes simple management guidelines that can be used to develop a care plan. The steps are shown in Figure 6.2.2, and are listed in the following text:

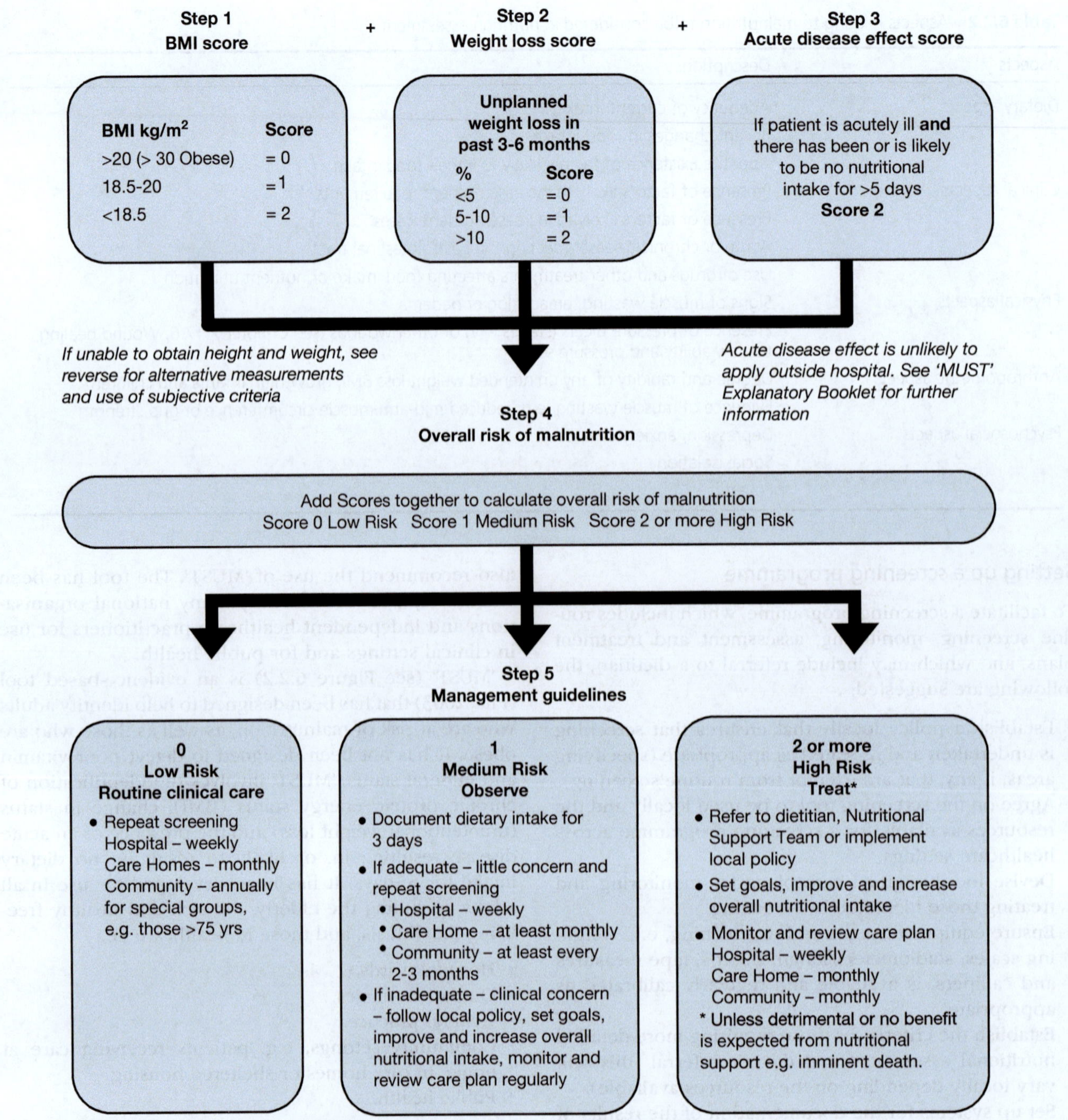

Figure 6.2.2 Malnutrition Universal Screening Tool 'MUST'. Source: British Association for Parenteral and Enteral Nutrition (BAPEN) 2013. Reproduced with permission of the British Association for Parenteral and Enteral Nutrition, www.bapen.org.uk.

Step 1

Measure height and weight to calculate BMI and a BMI score. If unable to measure weight and/or height, use alternative procedures:

- Recently documented or self-reported height and weight (if reliable and realistic).
- If an individual is unable to report his or her height, use a surrogate measure to estimate height, e.g. ulna length (see Appendix A3) or knee height.
- If weight and height cannot be obtained, use mid-upper-arm circumference (MUAC) to estimate BMI. If MUAC is <23.5 cm, BMI is likely to be <20 kg/m^2. If MUAC is >32.0 cm, BMI is likely to be >30 kg/m^2.

Step 2

Note the percentage unplanned weight loss and give a weight loss score. If recent weight loss cannot be calculated:

- Use self-reported weight loss (if reliable and realistic).
- Changes in MUAC can also be used as an approximate indication of weight loss, e.g. a 10% reduction in MUAC suggests a weight loss of 10%.

Step 3

Establish if there is an acute disease effect and score (for patients who are acutely ill and for whom there has been or is likely to be no nutritional intake for >5 days – unlikely to apply outside of hospital).

Step 4

Add scores from steps 1–3 to obtain the overall risk of malnutrition.

Step 5

Use management guidelines and local policy to develop appropriate care plans. If BMI or weight loss (steps 1 and 2) cannot be obtained, the following criteria can assist in the professional judgement of whether an individual is at risk of malnutrition (medium and high risk) or not (low risk):

- BMI – obtain a clinical impression of whether the individual is very thin (obvious wasting)/thin, or is of acceptable weight, overweight or obese.
- Unplanned weight loss – obtain a clinical impression of whether the individual has lost weight. Have clothes and/or jewellery become loose fitting? Is there a history of decreased food intake, reduced appetite or swallowing problems over the past 3–6 months? Is there evidence of underlying disease, psychosocial problems or physical disabilities that are likely to cause weight loss?

Care should be taken when interpreting BMI or percentage weight loss in individuals with fluid disturbances, plaster casts, amputations and critical illness, and in pregnant or lactating women (Elia, 2003). For more information on undertaking 'MUST', charts to calculate BMI and weight loss scores, electronic applications, use of alternative measures, and screening individuals in whom extra care in interpretation is needed, see Elia (2003), as well as www.bapen.org.uk.

Self-screening with 'MUST'

A patient-friendly version of 'MUST' has been developed for adults to screen themselves for malnutrition, or for a carer to screen a relative, where appropriate. Self-screening in outpatients has been shown to be reproducible, to have good concurrent validity with healthcare professional screening, and to be easy for a wide variety of individuals to complete and predict patient outcome (Cawood *et al.*, 2012; McGurk *et al.*, 2013). Further information can be found on www.bapen.org.uk. Decisions are needed locally on how best to implement self-screening within different care settings appropriately (e.g. in outpatients, sheltered housing, general practice etc.) as part of the overall management of malnutrition.

Benefits of implementing a screening programme

Considering the enormous costs of disease-related malnutrition, a condition that is largely treatable, prompt identification with screening, followed by the most appropriate, effective, evidence-based treatment is recommended (Elia, 2003; Elia *et al.*, 2005; NICE, 2006). NICE recently released a summary of which sets of NICE clinical guidelines produced the greatest cost savings (accessed December 2016). The guideline on nutritional support (in the form of oral nutritional support, tube feeding and parenteral nutrition) was in the top two. Specifically, NICE suggest that improving systematic screening, assessment and treatment of malnourished patients (NICE CG32 guideline) could lead to an estimated cost saving of £72,800 per 100,000 individuals. NICE makes the following suggestion: '*If this guidance* [CG32] *were fully implemented and resulted in better nourished patients, then this would lead to reduced complications such as secondary chest infections, pressure ulcers, wound abscesses and cardiac failure. Conservative estimates of reduced admissions and reduced length of stay for admitted patients, as well as reduced demand for GP and outpatient appointments, indicate that significant savings are possible*' (NICE, 2016).

Pragmatic programmes of screening implementation (using 'MUST') in care homes have highlighted some such benefits (Baggaley *et al.*, 2013; Cawood *et al.*, 2009). Programmes involving education and training on malnutrition; screening and treatment using the framework of 'MUST'; locally agreed care plans; and monitoring improved the documentation of nutritional status, the proportion of residents screened, and the use of appropriate care plans. After the implementation of the screening programme, a reduction in the number and duration of hospital admissions was observed, associated with a significant cost saving. Similar improvements in nutritional care and outcome have been observed in other settings, e.g. hospital wards, where screening has been implemented (Kruizenga *et al.*, 2005; Rypkema *et al.*, 2003).

Treatment of malnutrition

Following the identification of patients at risk of malnutrition with screening, there is a need to implement evidence-based treatments. Nutritional treatment of malnutrition (often termed nutritional support) can encompass modification of the diet (dietary fortification), dietetic counselling, use of oral nutritional supplements (single and multinutrient supplements), enteral tube feeding, parenteral nutrition and combinations of these therapies (Figure 6.2.3). The nutritional treatment of malnutrition should be undertaken alongside management of the underlying causes of malnutrition, e.g. disease, symptoms associated with disease and its treatment, and psychosocial problems.

The best strategy for treating malnutrition should be devised for the individual patient, while considering several factors. First, the type of nutritional treatment chosen will depend on whether the individuals are safely and physically able to eat and drink. If they are, consideration is needed of the likely adequacy of intake, which may be severely compromised by anorexia, other side effects of disease, and any modifications required, e.g. texture, composition (see later). In addition to the diet, oral nutritional supplements and feeding via tube may be required. If the individual is not safely able to eat and drink, and oral intake is contraindicated, non-oral means of feeding are required (enteral tube feeding). If feeding into the gastrointestinal tract is contraindicated, then intravenous feeding (parenteral nutrition) is considered (see Chapters 6.3, Oral nutrition support, Chapter 6.4, Enteral nutrition and Chapter 6.5, Parenteral nutrition). For some patients, combinations of treatments will be required.

Second, the method of nutritional support chosen may vary depending on whether an individual will require short- or long-term support, if they are acutely or chronically ill, and if they are in hospital or in the community. In the community, the ability of individuals and their carers/parents to manage nutritional support (e.g. for the very young and old) and their preferences regarding feeding methods need to be considered. Nutritional treatments may need to be modified (in texture, composition, consistency and quantity) if there are symptoms (e.g. nausea, swallowing problems, severe anorexia, electrolyte disturbances, etc.) associated with the disease or its treatment (see Chapter 7.3, Dysphagia). Deficiencies of micronutrients (e.g. vitamins, minerals and trace elements) frequently coexist (Elia & Stratton, 2005; Finch *et al.*, 1998). Nutritional treatment of malnutrition should consider the provision of micronutrients in addition to energy and protein. All micronutrient deficiencies should be corrected.

Active nutritional treatment may not be considered appropriate in terminally ill or dying patients. For more

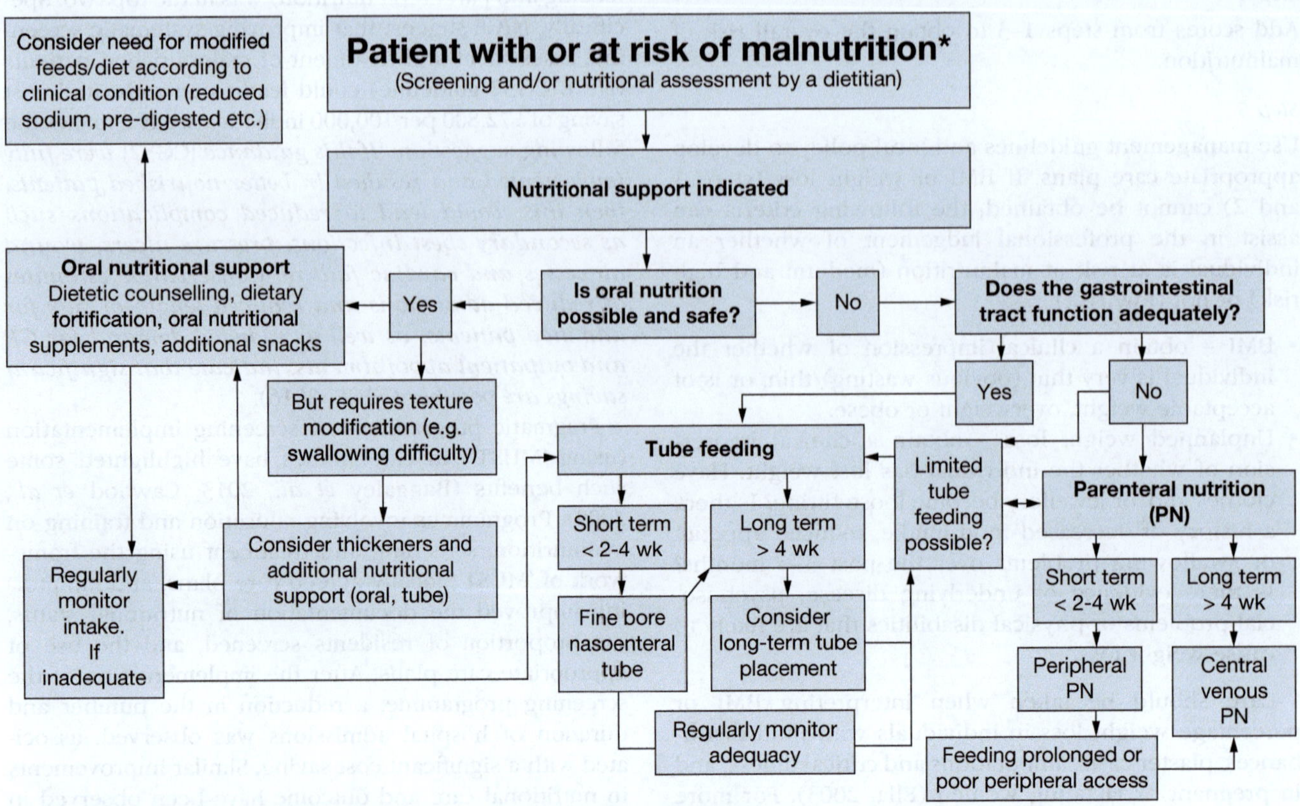

* For all patients, treat underlying conditions, ensure help with feeding and help/advice on special diets as required (gluten free, low sodium, diabetic, texture modification).

Figure 6.2.3 Algorithm for the treatment of malnutrition

information on the ethics of withholding or withdrawing feeding, see Lennard-Jones (1998), as well as Chapter 7.16 (Palliative and end-of-life care) in this book. Once the extent of the shortfall between an individual's nutritional requirements and his or her current or anticipated dietary intake (which could be from food and drink, or may be nothing if intake is contraindicated) has been estimated, the types and quantities of nutritional support can be chosen. Most individuals with malnutrition, both in hospital and in the community, can be managed orally with diet and supplementation. The choices about which form of treatment to use will largely depend on the needs of the individual patient, although local policy and resources need also to be considered. These needs may change during the course of treatment, and so regular monitoring and changes to the types of nutritional support used are required.

Practical pathways for managing malnutrition in the community, including malnutrition in some specific patient groups (e.g. chronic obstructive pulmonary disease, lung cancer), provide further guidance on identifying malnutrition and first-line nutritional support (www.malnutritionpathway.co.uk).

Monitoring progress

With nutritionally compromised individuals, it is essential that their condition and the effectiveness of the nutritional support strategy be reviewed at regular intervals. Nutritional support should not be prescribed or provided indefinitely, and goals for treatment should be set and monitored. As a result of monitoring, the type or level of nutritional support may need to be adjusted, dietary guidance amended or reinforced, and new goals set. Monitoring may include assessments of the following:

- Weight loss, stabilisation or gain (may repeat screening), and growth.
- Body composition (e.g. muscle mass) and function (e.g. strength, ability to walk and quality of life).
- Changes in nutritional (and fluid) intake – quantity, type, variety. Weight change can be a marker of the adequacy of nutritional intake.
- Effectiveness of remedial suggestions (e.g. change in drug therapy or texture of foods) for alleviating problems with food intake.
- Bowel function, fluid and electrolyte balance, swallowing function, skin condition, or other symptoms indicative of malnutrition and micronutrient status.
- Compliance with nutritional support.

The frequency of monitoring will depend on the following:

- Severity of malnutrition.
- Clinical condition of the individuals (stable, deteriorating, improving) and their age.
- Type of nutritional support being used, e.g. patients receiving artificial nutrition may need daily monitoring.
- Setting of an individual (hospital, nursing home, home).
- Resources available for follow-up and monitoring.

Acknowledgement

The editor acknowledges the prior contribution of Marinos Elia.

Further reading

Elia M. (2003) *Screening for Malnutrition: A Multidisciplinary Responsibility. Development and use of the Malnutrition Universal Screening Tool ('MUST') for Adults*. Redditch: BAPEN.

Elia M, Malnutrition Action Group of BAPEN (Evans E, Russell C, Stratton R, Todorovic V) and Malnutrition Group of NIHR BRC (Nutrition) Southampton (Jackson A, Smith T, Stratton R, Stroud M, Wootton S). (2015) *The cost of malnutrition in England and the potential cost savings from nutritional interventions*. NIHR/BAPEN.

NICE. (2006, 2012) *Nutrition Support in Adults. Clinical Guideline 32 and Quality Standard 24*. London: NICE.

Stratton RJ, Green CJ, Elia M. (2003) *Disease-Related Malnutrition: An Evidence Based Approach to Treatment*. Oxford: CABI Publishing.

Internet resources

Care Quality Commission, www.cqc.org.uk

NICE Clinical Guidance Nutrition support for adults: oral nutrition support, enteral tube feeding and parenteral nutrition CG32. www.nice.org.uk/Guidance/CG32

NICE Nutrition support in adults QS24, www.nice.org.uk/Guidance/QS24

Malnutrition pathway, www.malnutritionpathway.co.uk

'MUST': Further supporting information about 'MUST', the tool, and self-screening can be downloaded from www.bapen.org.uk

References

Baggaley E, Wincup L, Ashman KE, *et al.* (2013) Effectiveness of implementing a nurse led policy for the management of malnutrition. *Clin. Nutr.* 32: S231.

Bistrian BR, Blackburn GL, Hallowell E, *et al.* (1974) Protein status of general surgical patients. *JAMA* 230: 858–860.

BDA. (2009) *A Framework for Screening for Malnutrition*. Birmingham: BDA.

Cawood AL, Smith A, Dalrymple-Smith J, *et al.* (2008) Prevalence of malnutrition and use of nutritional support in Peterborough Primary Care Trust. *J. Hum. Nutr. Diet.* 21: 384.

Cawood AL, Smith A, Pickles S, *et al.* (2009) Effectiveness of implementing MUST into care homes within Peterborough Primary Care Trust, England. *Clin. Nutr.* 4: 81.

Cawood AL, Elia M, Sharp SK, *et al.* (2012) Malnutrition self-screening by using MUST in hospital outpatients: validity, reliability, and ease of use. *Am. J. Clin. Nutr.* 96: 1000–1007

Chourdakis M, Hecht C, Gerasimidis K, *et al.* (2016) Malnutrition risk in hospitalized children: use of 3 screening tools in a large European population. *Am. J. Clin. Nutr.* 103: 1301–1310.

Collins P, Elia M, Kurukulaaratchy RJ, *et al.* (2016) The influence of deprivation on malnutrition risk in outpatients with chronic obstructive pulmonary disease (COPD). *Clin. Nutr.* DOI: 10.1016/j.clnu.2016.11.005

DH. (2008) *Heath and Social Care Act*. London: DH.

DH. (2014) *The Hospital Food Standards Panel's Report on Standards for Food and Drink in NHS Hospitals*. London: DH

Elia M. (2000) *Guidelines for Detection and Management of Malnutrition*. Maidenhead: Malnutrition Advisory Group, Standing Committee of BAPEN.

Elia M. (2003) *Screening for Malnutrition: A Multidisciplinary Responsibility. Development and Use of the Malnutrition Universal Screening Tool ('MUST') for Adults*. Redditch: BAPEN.

Elia M, Russell CA. (2009) *Combating Malnutrition: Recommendations for Action*. Redditch: BAPEN.

Elia M, Stratton RJ. (2005) Geographical inequalities in nutrient status and risk of malnutrition among English people aged 65 years and over. *Nutrition*. 21: 1100–1106.

Elia M, Zellipour L, Stratton RJ. (2005) To screen or not to screen for adult malnutrition. *Clin. Nutr.* 24: 867–884.

Elia M, Russell CA, Stratton RJ. (2010) Malnutrition in the UK: policies to address the problem. *Proc. Nutr. Soc.* 69: 470–476.

Elia M, Evans E, Russell C, *et al.* (2015) *The cost of malnutrition in England and potential cost savings from nutritional interventions.* NIHR Southampton Biomedical Research Centre and BAPEN.

Finch S, Doyle W, Lowe C, *et al.* (1998) *National Diet and Nutrition Survey: People Aged 65 Years and Over, 1: Report of the Diet and Nutrition Survey*. London: The Stationery Office.

Gerasimidis K, Keane O, Macleod I, *et al.* (2010) A four-stage evaluation of the Paediatric Yorkhill Malnutrition Score in a tertiary paediatric hospital and a district general hospital. *Br. J. Nutr.* 104: 751–756.

Gerasimidis K, Macleod I, Maclean A, *et al.* (2011) Performance of the novel Paediatric Yorkhill Malnutrition Score (PYMS) in hospital practice. *Clin. Nutr.* 30: 430–435.

Gibney E, Elia M, Jebb SA, *et al.* (1997) Total energy expenditure in patients with small-cell lung cancer: results of a validated study using the bicarbonate-urea method. *Metabolism*. 46: 1412–1417.

Healthcare Improvement Scotland. (2014) *Food, Fluid and Nutritional Care Standards*. Edinburgh: Healthcare Improvement Scotland.

Hill GL, Blackett RL, Pickford I, *et al.* (1977) Malnutrition in surgical patients: an unrecognised problem. *Lancet*. 1: 689–692.

Jebb SA. (1997) Energy metabolism in cancer and human immunodeficiency virus infection. *Proc. Nutr. Soc.* 56: 763–775.

Kruizenga HM, Van Tulder MW, Seidell JC, *et al.* (2005) Effectiveness and cost-effectiveness of early screening and treatment of malnourished patients. *Am. J. Clin. Nutr.* 82: 1082–1089.

Lennard-Jones JEB. (1998) *Ethical and Legal Aspects of Clinical Hydration and Nutritional Support*. Maidenhead: BAPEN.

McGurk P, Jackson JM, Elia M. (2013) Rapid and reliable self-screening for nutritional risk in hospital outpatients using an electronic system. *Nutrition*. 29(4): 693–696.

NICE. (2006) *Nutrition Support in Adults: Oral Nutrition Support, Enteral Tube Feeding and Parenteral Nutrition. Clinical Guideline 32*. London: NICE

NICE. (2012) *Nutrition Support in Adults. Quality Standard 24*. London: NICE.

NHS. (2014) *Five Year Forward View*. London: NHS.

Pichler J, Hill SM, Shaw V, *et al.* (2014) Prevalence of undernutrition during hospitalisation in a children's hospital: what happens during admission? *Eur. J. Clin. Nutr.* 68: 730–735.

Royal College of Physicians (RCP). (2002) *Nutrition and Patients. A Doctor's Responsibility. Report of a working party of the Royal College of Physicians*. London: RCP.

Russell CA, Elia M. (2014) *Nutrition Screening Surveys in hospitals in the UK 2007–2011. A report based on the amalgamated data from the four Nutrition Screening Week surveys undertaken by BAPEN in 2007, 2008, 2010 and 2011*. Redditch: BAPEN.

Rypkema G, Adang E, Dicke H, *et al.* (2003) Cost-effectiveness of an interdisciplinary intervention in geriatric inpatients to prevent malnutrition. *J. Nutr. Health Aging* 8: 122–127.

Stratton RJ, Elia M. (2006) Deprivation linked to malnutrition risk and mortality in hospital. *Br. J. Nutr.* 96: 870–876.

Stratton RJ, Green CJ, Elia M. (2003) *Disease-Related Malnutrition: An Evidence Based Approach to Treatment*. Oxford: CABI Publishing.

Volkert D, Saeglitz C, Gueldenzoph H, *et al.* (2010) Undiagnosed malnutrition and nutrition-related problems in geriatric patients. *J. Nutr. Health Aging*. 14: 387–392.

Welsh Government. (2013) *Nutrition in community settings. A pathway and resource pack for health and social care professionals, the third sector, care home staff, relatives and carers*. Cardiff: Welsh Government.

Wright CM, Williams AF, Elliman D, *et al.* (2010) Using the new UK–WHO growth charts. *BMJ* 340: c1140.

6.3 Oral nutritional support

Abbie Cawood
Additional contributor: Rebecca Stratton

Key points

- The role of the dietitian is to provide evidence-based advice on the most appropriate oral nutritional support for patients, and tailor dietary advice to their needs.
- Oral nutritional support aims to improve the nutritional intake of macronutrients and micronutrients; approaches include fortified foods, snacks, nourishing drinks and oral nutritional supplements (ONS).
- Dietary strategies improve intake, weight and body composition, and can have some benefits on functional outcomes, but clinical efficacy has not been fully assessed.
- ONS has been shown to improve intake, weight, and body composition, with other clinical and economic benefits, e.g. improved function, reduced complications and readmissions to hospital.
- All patients receiving oral nutritional support should be monitored regularly against the goals of the intervention.

Oral nutritional support is a collective term used to describe the nutritional options available via the oral route, to manage people who have been identified as malnourished or at risk of malnutrition (see Chapter 6.2, Malnutrition). Oral nutritional support should consider macronutrients (energy, carbohydrate protein, fat) and micronutrients (NICE, 2006a). Oral nutritional support options include any of the following methods to improve nutritional intake, as defined by NICE (2006a):

- Fortified foods with protein, carbohydrate and/or fat plus vitamins and minerals.
- Snacks.
- Altered meal patterns, practical help with eating.
- Oral nutritional supplements (ONS).
- Provision of dietary advice – including all the preceding points, and tailoring counselling to the patient's clinical, nutritional, social and psychological needs.

Who should receive oral nutritional support?

Oral nutritional support should be considered for patients with inadequate food and fluid intakes to meet requirements, unless they cannot swallow safely, have inadequate gastrointestinal function or if no benefit is anticipated, e.g. end-of-life care (NICE, 2006a) (see Chapter 7.16, Palliative and end-of-life care). For other nutritional support options, see Chapter 6.4 Enteral nutrition and Chapter 6.5, Parenteral nutrition. Healthcare professionals should consider oral nutritional support to improve nutritional intake in people who can swallow safely and are malnourished or at risk of malnutrition (NICE, 2006a) (see Chapter 6.2, Malnutrition). This is an 'A grade' recommendation in the NICE CG32 Nutritional Support in Adults (2006a), which is the highest classification of recommendations based on the highest level of evidence. NICE reviewed the evidence in 2014 and 2017 and found nothing to affect the recommendations. Other national bodies also highlight the need for nutritional management including:

- Care Quality Commission (2015), as part of the Health and Social Care Act, which states that people must have their nutritional needs assessed, and that food must be provided to meet those needs; this includes prescribed nutritional supplements.
- Department of Health (2010) Essence of Care Framework similarly highlights that nutritional support should be considered for people who are at risk of malnutrition or who are malnourished.
- Statement 2 of NICE Quality Standard 24 states that people who are malnourished or at risk of malnutrition should have a management care plan that aims to meet their nutritional requirements (NICE, 2012).
- British Dietetic Association (BDA, 2012) – Policy Statement: The care of nutritionally vulnerable adults in community and all health and care settings.

Manual of Dietetic Practice, Sixth Edition. Edited by Joan Gandy.

Companion website: www.manualofdieteticpractice.com

Role of the dietitian in oral nutritional support

The role of the dietitian is to provide evidence-based advice on the most appropriate oral nutritional support option for the patient. The dietitian provides tailored dietary advice according to the patient's disease, symptoms and treatment regimen, while considering the patient's social, physical, psychological, clinical and nutritional needs. Advice may be given on dietary fortification (in addition to the encouragement to eat), food choice and preparation, and how to overcome anorexia or specific difficulties with eating, perhaps due to side effects or symptoms associated with a disease or its treatment. Dietary strategies encompass food fortification, i.e. extra snacks and nourishing drinks that can be used on their own or in combination with other nutritional support strategies such as ONS and artificial nutrition. Individual patient needs should always be taken into consideration; dietary strategies alone may be adequate for some patients, whereas, for others, ONS may be the most clinically effective option and should not be delayed.

The effectiveness of dietary advice will depend on many factors, including the method of counselling used, content and form of the advice given, and the patients themselves. The efficacy of dietary advice may be limited in the very sick, those with poor consciousness or limited comprehension, and when there are possible time constraints in acute settings. In all settings, dietitians can provide invaluable encouragement and advice (both verbal and written) in the treatment of malnutrition and in the nutritional management of many complex disease states. However, dietetic services can sometimes be sparse, which means dietitians are unable to oversee the management of every individual who needs nutritional support. Therefore, dietitians have an important role as educators of medical, social care and nursing staff, particularly in the primary and social care sectors, regarding measures that can be taken to improve oral intake. There are several examples of evidence-based pathways that have been developed nationally to improve the use of oral nutritional support, and specifically ONS. These can be used by dietitians to support the development of local guidelines for other healthcare professionals to follow, e.g. managing adult malnutrition in the community (www.malnutritionpathway.co.uk).

Oral nutritional support strategies to improve nutritional intake

There are several oral nutritional support strategies available, as shown in Figure 6.3.1.

Fortified food

The aim of food fortification should be to increase the nutrient density, and not the actual amount of food consumed. In practice, food fortification, primarily with the addition of energy-rich foods, mostly results in increasing energy intakes. Food fortification practices include the following:

- Fortifying milk by adding four tablespoons of skimmed milk powder to 1 pint of milk. This can then be used throughout the day in drinks, on cereals, or for custard, milk puddings, etc.
- Adding grated cheese to soup, savoury dishes and mashed potato.
- Adding double cream to soup, mashed potato, sauces or desserts.
- Adding butter or oil to vegetables, pasta and scrambled egg, and during cooking.
- Adding jam, syrup or honey to breakfast cereals, milk puddings or other desserts.
- Adding sugar to foods or drinks.
- Avoidance of low-fat, low-sugar and diet foods and drinks.

However, NICE (2006a) stated that care should be taken when using dietary fortification in isolation, as this approach tends to supplement energy but not other nutrients. Ideally, patients should be encouraged to fortify their diets with foods that are energy and nutrient dense.

The use of food fortification may be an attractive option for patients with anorexia, as the quantity and volume of food consumed does not increase and familiar food ingredients are used. However, dietary fortification may alter the sensory properties of foods, which may or may not be desirable for individual patients. Fortification using high-fat foods (especially those with a high saturated fat content, such as butter, cream and hard cheese) may not be desirable for some patients, e.g. those with high cholesterol levels. There may also be practical difficulties on busy hospital wards or if patients are physically (e.g. disability or fatigue) or mentally unable or unwilling to modify their diets at home without help, thereby reducing compliance. For all patients, the costs of this approach need to be considered, along with issues of purchasing, preparation and storage. Thought should also be given to dietary recommendations that other family members may be following, and which may conflict with the strategies for managing malnutrition, e.g. weight-reducing advice for the management of obesity.

Snacks

Additional food items in the form of snacks can be used in the treatment of malnutrition with the aim of increasing nutritional intake. As with food fortification, consideration should be given to improving energy, protein and micronutrient intakes. Compliance with such a strategy may be good, as snacks are familiar and generally well liked. Examples include cake or malt loaf, yoghurt, custard, toasted crumpets or teacakes with butter, and cheese and crackers. It may also be helpful to recommend eating small amounts of food as snacks throughout the day. Snacks may not be effective in patients with anorexia who may be unable to eat more food, or in patients with physical difficulties with eating (chewing, swallowing). For free-living patients, there are also cost considerations and issues of purchase, preparation and storage.

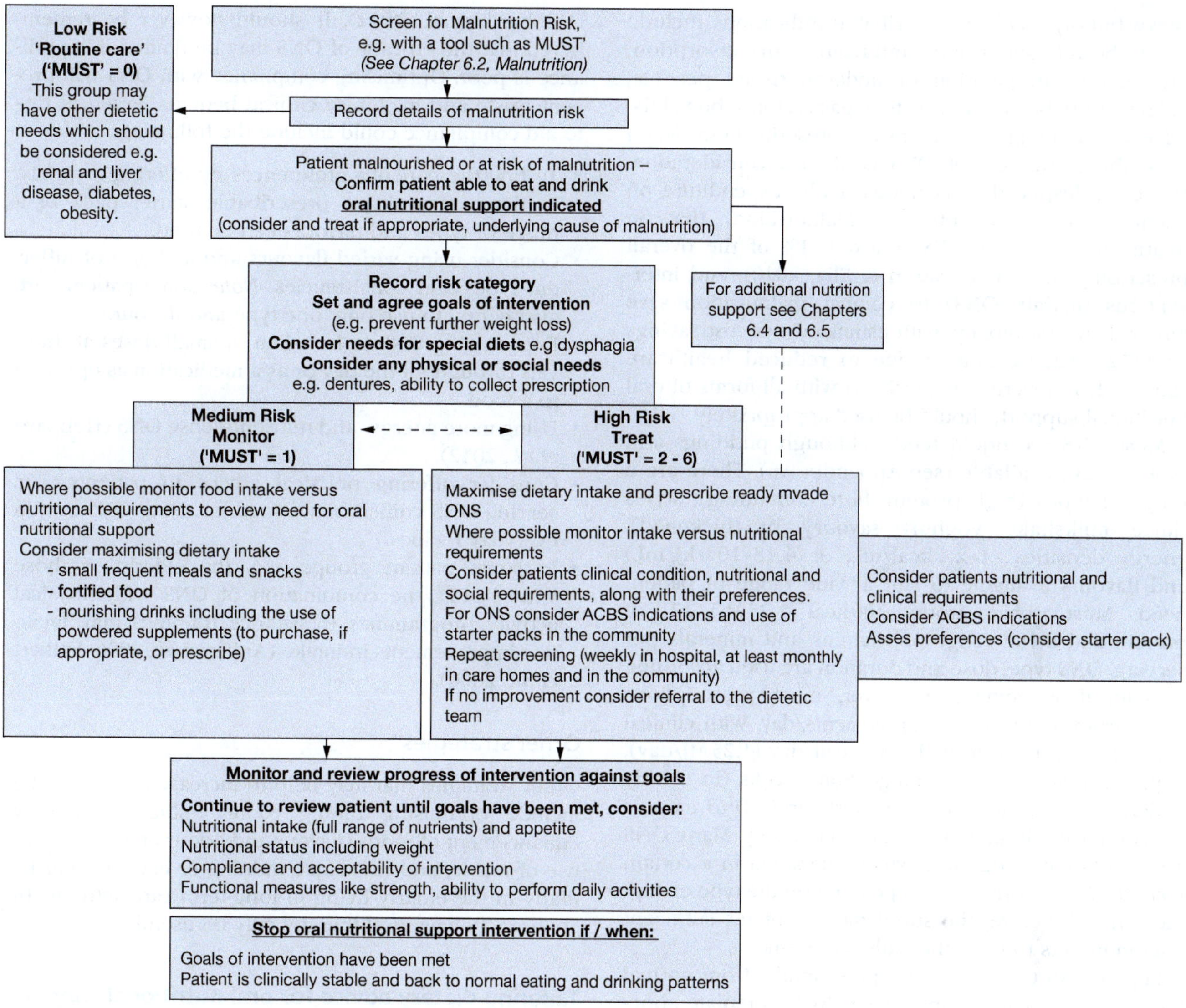

Figure 6.3.1 Algorithm for oral nutrition support in the management of malnutrition

Nourishing drinks

As far as possible, patients should be encouraged to consume drinks that are better sources of nourishment than just tea, coffee or water. Liquids tend to be less satiating than solid foods, so can be a good option to increase the nutritional intake in patients with very poor appetites. Depending on individual patients and their clinical conditions, suitable suggestions include the following:

- Milky drinks, e.g. cocoa, drinking chocolate, malted milk drinks, milkshakes, and coffee made with either full-fat milk, fortified milk, or calcium-enriched alternatives.
- Soup (especially condensed or 'cream of' varieties).
- Fruit juices or smoothies (or drinks enriched with micronutrients).
- Powdered supplements that can be made up with water or milk, e.g. Complan and Meritene; these can be purchased, although some are available on prescription.

Oral nutritional supplements (ONS)

ONS, sometimes referred to as sip feeds, typically contain a mix of macronutrients (protein, carbohydrate and fat) and micronutrients (vitamins, minerals and trace elements). As with tube feeds, ONS are foods for special medical purposes (FSMPs), and as such are regulated under the Foods for Specific Groups Regulation 609/2013 and the Food Information for Consumers Regulation 1169/2011. These regulations define and categorise the products, give compositional guidelines and set out labelling requirements. These products are specially formulated, intended for the dietary management of patients who are unable to meet their nutritional needs through diet alone, and should be used under medical supervision. ONS can be prescribed in the community (BMJ Group and the Royal Pharmaceutical Society of Great Britain, 2011) for the management of disease-related malnutrition. Prescribing details can be found in the British National Formulary (BNF) section 9.4.2

(www.bnf.org). Other prescribable indications include short bowel syndrome, intractable malabsorption, preoperative preparation of undernourished patients, inflammatory bowel disease, total gastrectomy, bowel fistulae and dysphagia; dietitians can prescribe ONS. When prescribing, the cost of ONS is often a consideration. However, despite the enormous public expenditure on malnutrition (see Chapter 6.2, Malnutrition), that on treatments including ONS is low (~1% of the overall prescribing budget) (Stratton & Elia, 2010), and interventions (mainly ONS) to combat malnutrition save rather than cost money, with estimated net cost savings of £172.2–£229.2 million due to reduced healthcare (Elia, 2015). Nevertheless, ONS, as with all forms of oral nutritional support, should be used appropriately.

Most ONS are liquid feeds, although puddings and powders are available (see Appendix A6). There are a range of types (high protein, fibre containing), styles (juice, milkshake, yoghurt, savoury, pre-thickened), energy densities (1–2.4 kcal/mL, or 4.18–10.0 kJ/mL) and flavours available to suit a wide range of patient needs. Most provide around 300 kcal (1.25 MJ), 12 g of protein and a full range of vitamins and minerals per serving. ONS type, dose and duration are used according to clinical judgement. However, most prescriptions range from one to three supplements/day, with clinical benefits typically seen with >300 kcal/day (1.25 MJ/day). Supplementation periods range from weeks (in elderly patients who are acutely ill or post-surgical) to months for chronically ill patients in the community. Many ONS are nutritionally complete when consumed in a certain volume (2–7 servings/day, depending on the type of supplement); therefore, the supplement contains sufficient micronutrients to meet the daily requirements.

Liquid ONS tend not to suppress intake from normal food, and, in some groups, may help to stimulate appetite (NICE, 2006a; Stratton & Elia, 2007). ONS should not replace the provision of good food or nutritional care (including help with feeding and meal provision) in hospitals and care homes, or in a person's own home. Patients likely to benefit from ONS across both hospital and community settings include acutely ill hospitalised patients (especially the elderly, and hip fracture and gastrointestinal surgical patients); malnourished patients recently discharged from hospital; and those with chronic conditions such as cancer, chronic obstructive pulmonary disease (COPD), neurological conditions, and renal and liver disease (NICE, 2006a; Stratton & Elia, 2007). ONS are also used before and after surgery and perioperatively, as part of the nationally recognised Enhanced Recovery After Surgery (ERAS) programme to improve outcomes after surgery, reduce complications, and promote early discharge of patients (see Chapter 7.17.5, Surgery). Suitability of ONS for specific ethnic groups, people with allergies, vegans and those with other special requirements should always be checked.

Patients find ONS an acceptable form of nutritional support (NICE, 2006a), and compliance with ready-made ONS has been shown to be good (78% of prescribed volume consumed), although this varies across settings (Hubbard *et al.*, 2012). It should however be remembered that the efficacy of ONS may be limited if compliance is poor. Optimising compliance with ONS will prevent waste and maximise clinical benefits. Practical tips to aid compliance could include the following:

- Testing the patient's preferences by offering a variety. In the community, a prescribable starter pack of a range of types and flavours can be tried.
- Consider using varied flavours and a choice of different types and consistencies. *Note*: Some patients are also happy to use only one type and flavour.
- Encouraging ONS to be taken in small doses at intervals throughout the day or as a medication as opposed to a food.
- Using more energy- and nutrient-dense ONS (Hubbard *et al.*, 2012).
- Consider offering practical advice to patients, e.g. serving ONS chilled or warmed, or using ONS within everyday recipes.
- In some patient groups, e.g. the elderly or those with COPD, the combination of ONS with physical activity programmes (resistance training) may facilitate improvements in intake (Anker *et al.*, 2006; Volkert *et al.*, 2006).

Other strategies

Other strategies that may help to increase dietary intake include optimising dining room ambience, sensory enhancement of foods (flavour and odour enhancement), use of music, and resistance training or exercise, particularly in the elderly living in long-term care settings. In children, behavioural therapy may be useful.

Tailoring dietary advice for oral nutritional support (including practical considerations)

Many factors can impair nutritional intake, with the main factors being disease and its treatment (Stratton *et al.*, 2003). Whenever possible, the underlying cause impairing intake should be identified and addressed. In addition to disease, other factors include social, functional, physical, mechanical and environmental issues; these differ depending on where the patient resides (own home, care home, hospital, living alone, etc.). Considerations when tailoring dietary advice for oral nutritional support may include the following:

- Effect of the disease or its management (treatment, surgery), e.g. side effects such as nausea and vomiting, taste changes, dry or painful mouth, and the need for modified texture.
- Ability to shop (physical, financial) or collect prescriptions.
- Ability to prepare food or the need for assistance with eating.
- Dentition, loss of appetite, fatigue, and early satiety, e.g. stomach resection, abdominal tumours or ascites often result in people feeling full when consuming a small quantity of food.

In addition to advising on the most suitable form of oral nutritional support, dietary advice can also be tailored and personalised for each individual patient. Some of the practical suggestions discussed in following text may be of help.

Social and functional considerations

These will include factors such as the ability to shop, collect prescriptions or prepare food. Useful strategies include the following:

- Encourage patients to ask for and accept help from neighbours and friends.
- Encourage patients to make use of local support services, e.g. social services, home help, meals on wheels and day care facilities, which can provide practical help in terms of shopping, cooking or meal provision, and perhaps lessen the social isolation of those who live alone.
- If the patient has limited functional ability and/or no carer or home support, consider readymade meals, snacks, drinks and ONS as appropriate.
- Encourage the use of a pharmacy delivery service if ONS are prescribed.

Physical considerations

Physical considerations include poor appetite, tiredness and early satiety, which may be addressed by considering the following:

- Increase energy and nutrient density and/or decrease amount or volume of food or supplement.
- Offer a smaller portion size and avoid overwhelming platefuls of food (little and often).
- Advise light physical exercise which may improve appetite, e.g. a short walk.
- A small amount of alcohol before or with a meal (if allowed) can stimulate appetite.
- Try spreading meals and snacks throughout the day or try nourishing drinks.
- Consider eating when appetite is best.
- Make use of convenient, simple-to-prepare foods or meals.
- Choose foods that are particularly fancied, regardless of the time of day.
- Avoid strong cooking smells that could be off-putting.
- Take time to eat and relax after meals or between courses.
- Avoid filling up with large volumes of liquid before, during or after meals.
- Some patients (particularly those with early satiety) may find that fatty, greasy or rich foods exacerbate their feelings of fullness and would benefit from avoiding these.
- If appetite is poor, e.g. in acute illness or the post-operative period, patients may find nourishing drinks and ONS less satiating than additional food stuffs.

Specific symptoms related to illness or treatment side effects

Nausea and vomiting

Nausea and vomiting can occur for several reasons; they are a consequence of many disease states and a common side effect of treatments, e.g. chemotherapy. If nausea and vomiting are severe and food cannot be taken at all, hydration is the first priority. Antiemetics and additional nutritional support can be considered. Useful strategies include the following:

- Make use of times when the feeling of nausea is less to eat or prepare foods. Eat anything that is fancied when it is wanted.
- Avoid cooking smells or letting smells linger in the house. Ask someone else to cook, or make use of convenience foods (e.g. readymade foods, drinks, snacks and supplements) that create little smell.
- Avoid fatty and fried foods.
- Avoid drinks with meals and serve food relatively dry (unless on a modified consistency diet).
- Sipping drinks and ONS through a straw may be helpful (less likely to detect odour of fluid, resulting in lower taste sensitivity).
- Cold foods (e.g. cold meat, cheese and sandwiches) may be better tolerated than hot foods, as they have less smell.
- Savoury foods and drinks may be more acceptable than sweet-tasting items.
- Ginger-flavoured drinks and foods may be helpful, e.g. ginger ale, ginger beer, ginger biscuits and ginger tea.
- Early-morning nausea may be alleviated by dry carbohydrate-based foods such as unbuttered toast, cream crackers and plain biscuits.
- Eating or drinking something as soon after vomiting as possible. Ice lollies/ice cubes can clear the mouth.
- Avoid lying down after eating.

Taste problems

Some people are born with taste disorders, but most develop after an illness or injury. People may experience a reduced ability to taste (hypogeusia), an inability to taste (ageusia) or a distorted or altered ability to taste (dysgeusia); many taste disorders are linked to smell disorders. Causes of taste problems include the following:

- Upper-respiratory and middle-ear infections.
- Radiation therapy for cancers of the head and neck.
- Medications, including some antibiotics and antihistamines.
- Head injury.
- Some ear, nose and throat surgeries.
- Poor oral hygiene and dental problems.

Useful strategies include the following:

- Prepare foods with a variety of colours and textures.
- Use aromatic herbs and spices to add more flavour.
- Avoid combination dishes such as casseroles that can hide individual flavours and dilute taste.

- Allow hot food to cool a little before consumption; high temperatures can accentuate unpleasant taste sensations.
- If meat tastes unpleasant, try alternatives such as fish, eggs, cheese and dairy products. Cold meats may taste better than hot meats. Marinades and sauces can also be helpful.
- Use sharp-tasting foods and drinks that are refreshing, e.g. fresh fruit, boiled sweets, mints, lemonade, fruit juice and tonic water.
- If using ONS, consider more tart flavours or a different style, e.g. juice and yoghurt.

Specific taste problems

- Bitterness – avoid foods sweetened with saccharine which can exacerbate this sensation.
- Metallic – gargle with lemon juice in water before eating; use plastic cutlery.
- Sweetness – can be offset by adding lemon juice or diluting drinks with soda or mineral water. Adding spices such as ginger, nutmeg or cinnamon to desserts and puddings may reduce the sensation of sweetness.
- Saltiness – avoid salt and salty foods or accompaniments, e.g. salted nuts or crisps, packet soups, gravy, sauces, bacon, ham, and other types of preserved or canned meat. Adding a pinch of sugar to some foods before serving may be useful.

Dry mouth (xerostomia)

This is a common consequence of damage to the salivary glands, usually as a result of surgery or radiotherapy to the head and neck region. The resulting lack, or even absence, of saliva makes mastication and swallowing difficult. Lack of saliva can predispose to tooth decay, and hence good oral hygiene should be encouraged in all patients. Artificial saliva sprays, gels or salivary-stimulant pastilles are prescribable for dry mouth associated with radiotherapy or other conditions.

Useful strategies include the following:

- Moisten meals with gravy, sauces, butter, cream or evaporated milk.
- Avoid very dry hard foods, e.g. biscuits, crackers or toast.
- Sip drinks frequently, particularly with meals.
- Suck items that help stimulate saliva flow, e.g. boiled sweets, fruit pastilles, pineapple chunks, grapefruit segments and ice cubes (perhaps flavoured with lemon juice or made from fruit juice); avoid in patients who have a sore mouth.
- Choose sharp-tasting foods, e.g. lemon-flavoured foods, grapefruit, gooseberry or rhubarb; avoid in patients with sore mouths.

Sore or painful mouth

This may result from infection, inflammation or ulceration of the oral areas, making eating painful and difficult. Stomatitis (inflammation of the mucous lining of the mouth, e.g. cheeks, gums, tongue, roof or floor of mouth) and mucositis (painful inflammation and ulceration of the gastrointestinal tract, including the mouth) may follow radiotherapy in the head and neck area, or as a side effect of some chemotherapy drugs. It is important to ensure that patients are receiving effective pain control at appropriate times to avoid compromising food intake more than is necessary. Appropriate mouth care should be undertaken. Useful strategies include the following:

- Eat soft, moist foods by adding sauces, gravy, custard, etc. Some foods may be easier to eat if they are mashed or liquidised.
- Avoid very dry or rough-textured foods, e.g. toast, raw vegetables, cereal bars or crisps.
- Avoid foods and drinks at extremes of temperature that can exacerbate pain.
- Avoid salty or highly spiced foods, e.g. salted crackers, salted nuts, crisps, pepper, chilli, curry powder and soya sauce.
- Avoid tart beverages, e.g. pure orange juice and grapefruit juice.
- Use ice lollies, ice cubes or frozen ONS for a soothing effect.

Swallowing difficulties (dysphagia)

Swallowing difficulties may seriously compromise nutritional intake, and it is important that dysphagia be properly assessed and managed. Improving nutritional intake in patients with dysphagia can be achieved with oral nutritional support. Dysphagia is a prescribable indication for ONS; a variety of thickeners and pre-thickened ONS (stage 1–3) are available. Tube feeds may be necessary if the swallowing difficulty severely limits or prevents safe oral intake (see Chapter 7.3, Dysphagia).

Summary of the evidence for oral nutritional support strategies

Dietary fortification

Trials in institutions (including hospitals) have shown that dietary fortification, using food items (e.g. cream) and glucose polymers, can significantly increase energy intakes (e.g. Barton *et al.*, 2000; Gall *et al.*, 1998; Odlund-Olin *et al.*, 2003). However, these trials do not assess patient outcomes or the cost-effectiveness of this approach. The addition of food snacks can increase energy (Turic *et al.*, 1999; Simmons *et al.*, 2010) and protein intakes (Smoliner *et al.*, 2008) in nursing home residents and children with cystic fibrosis (Hanning *et al.*, 1993). There are relatively few studies with data on outcomes (functional or clinical) or the cost-effectiveness of these strategies, and findings are inconsistent (Baldwin & Weekes 2012; Kimber *et al.*, 2015). For some patient groups, food snacks may be less effective at improving nutritional intakes than liquid ONS (e.g. Turic *et al.*, 1999; Stratton *et al.*, 2006). Dietary advice (tailored advice from a dietitian) may lead to improvements in weight, body composition and quality of life in some patient groups (COPD, cancer) (Baldwin & Weekes, 2011; Ravasco *et al.*, 2005; Weekes *et al.*, 2009). However, the impact of dietary strategies on clinical outcome and healthcare costs in most patient groups and settings has not been fully addressed in well-designed randomised controlled trials, and is a research priority.

Oral nutrition supplements

There is a large evidence base for ONS in different patient groups, in both hospital and community settings. Current evidence from systematic reviews and meta-analyses (Avenell & Handol, 2010; Baldwin & Weekes, 2011; Cawood *et al.*, 2012; Collins *et al.*, 2012; Elia *et al.*, 2005, 2006; Koretz *et al.*, 2007; Milne *et al.*, 2006, 2009; NICE, 2006a; Potter *et al.*, 1998; Stratton *et al.*, 2003, 2005; Stratton & Elia, 2007) suggest that total nutritional intake is significantly improved by ONS in most patient groups in hospital and community settings. In the community, improvements in intake are more likely in those who are underweight (BMI <20 kg/m^2). Food intake tends not to be reduced.

Improvements in body weight and composition (and growth in children) occur with supplementation. ONS tend to attenuate weight loss in the acutely ill hospitalised patient, and significantly increase weight gain in chronically ill community patients, with weight gain being more likely in those who are underweight (BMI <20 kg/m^2) and have recently lost weight. Improvements in weight in the acutely ill who consume ONS are related to improvements in physical function. Functional improvements, which vary according to the patient group, can occur with supplementation. These include increased muscle strength, quality of life, walking distances, activities of daily living, immunological benefits, reduced fatigue and improved wound healing. In those with chronic disease, improvements in function are more likely in those who are underweight (BMI <20 kg/m^2) and who gain weight with supplementation.

Systematic reviews and meta-analyses indicate fewer complications such as infections and pressure ulcers with ONS. These can also prevent pressure ulcers in at-risk groups. Reductions in mortality have been consistently shown with ONS versus routine care in acutely ill, hospitalised and elderly patients with a range of conditions.

ONS can reduce hospital stay length and the number of hospital admissions and readmissions (Stratton *et al.*, 2013), with potential cost savings. Cost analysis indicates that intervention with ONS can reduce healthcare costs and be cost-effective in those at risk of malnutrition across hospital and community settings, showing that the investments to implement better nutritional care is more than offset by the returns (Cawood *et al.*, 2010; Elia *et al.*, 2016a, 2016b; NICE, 2006b). Cost-effectiveness analyses take into account the benefits of the intervention balanced against the costs of the intervention, including the use of healthcare professional resources, e.g. review and monitoring.

Monitoring of oral nutritional support strategies

Specific targets or goals of oral nutritional support that are appropriate for the individual patient, which may vary depending on disease and setting of the patient, should be recorded. These could include the following:

- Measures of energy and nutritional intake.
- Appetite.
- Nutritional status.
- Anthropometric measurements (weight, BMI, mid-arm-muscle circumference, triceps skinfold thickness).
- Functional measures, e.g. strength using hand grip dynamometry.
- Clinically relevant outcomes, e.g. pressure ulcer size, infection, quality of life, daily activities.

Regular monitoring of patients receiving oral nutritional support should be undertaken to:

- Assess compliance and acceptability.
- Monitor effectiveness against goals.
- Encourage compliance where appropriate.
- Assess whether current strategy is still required or if other forms of nutritional support, e.g. tube feeding, are warranted.
- Monitor changes in clinical and nutritional status.

Patients receiving oral nutritional support in the community should be monitored every 3–6 months, or more frequently if there is any change in clinical condition (NICE, 2006a). Patients receiving oral nutritional support in the hospital setting should be monitored daily initially, reducing to twice weekly when stable (NICE, 2006a).

Discontinuation strategy

Oral nutritional support should be stopped when the patient is established on adequate oral intake from normal food, or when the decision is made to feed solely via another route, e.g. enteral or parenteral nutrition.

Further reading

Gibney M, Elia M, Ljunggvist O, *et al.* (2005) *Clinical Nutrition (The Nutrition Society Textbook)*. Oxford: Wiley Blackwell.
Sobotka L. (2011) *Basics in Clinical Nutrition*, 4th edn. Prague: Galen.

Internet resources

British National Formulary (BNF) section 9.4.2, www.bnf.org
Lung cancer nutrition, http://lungcancernutrition.com
Malnutrition pathway, www.malnutritionpathway.co.ukMalnutrition pathway for COPD, https://staging.malnutritionpathway.co.uk/copd
NICE (2006 (updated 2017)) Guideline CG32 Nutrition support in adults, http://guidance.nice.org.uk/CG32/NiceGuidance/pdf/English

References

Anker SD, John M, Pedersen PU, *et al.* (2006) ESPEN guidelines on enteral nutrition: cardiology and pulmonology. *Clin. Nutr.* 25: 311–318.

Avenell A, Handol HH. (2010) Nutritional supplementations for hip fracture aftercare in older people (review). *Cochrane Database Syst. Rev.* 1: CD001880.

Baldwin C, Weekes CE. (2011) Dietary advice with or without oral nutritional supplements for disease related malnutrition in adults. *Cochrane Database Syst. Rev.* 9: CD002008.

Baldwin C, Weekes CE. (2012) Dietary counselling with or without oral nutritional supplements in the management of malnourished patients: a systematic review and meta-analysis of randomised controlled trials. *J. Hum. Nutr. Diet.* 25: 411–426.

Barton AD, Beigg CL, Macdonald IA, *et al.* (2000) A recipe for improving food intakes in elderly hospitalized patients. *Clin. Nutr.* 19: 451–454.

BMJ Group and the Royal Pharmaceutical Society of Great Britain. (2016) *British National Formulary*. London: BMJ Group.

British Dietetic Association (BDA). (2012) *Policy Statement: The care of nutritionally vulnerable adults in community and all health and care settings.* Available at https://www.bda.uk.com/improvinghealth/healthprofessionals/malnutritionpolicy. Accessed 12 January 2017.

Care Quality Commission (CQC) Regulation 14: (2015) *Meeting nutritional and hydration needs* (last updated 13 February 2015). Available at http://www.cqc.org.uk/content/regulation-14-meeting-nutritional-and-hydration-needs. Accessed 12 January 2017.

Cawood AL, Green C, Stratton RJ. (2010) The budget impact of using oral nutritional supplements in older community patients at high risk of malnutrition in England. *Proc. Nutr. Soc.* 69(OCE7): E544.

Cawood AL, Elia M, Stratton RJ. (2012) Systematic review and meta-analysis of the effects of high protein oral nutritional supplements. *Aging Res. Rev.* 11(2): 278–296.

Collins PF, Stratton RJ, Elia M. (2012) Nutritional support in chronic obstructive pulmonary disease (COPD): a systematic review and meta-analysis. *Am. J. Clin. Nutr.* 95(6): 1385–1395.

DH. (2010) *Essence of Care 2010. Benchmarks for Food and Drink.* London: The Stationery Office.

Elia M. (2015) *The cost of malnutrition in England and potential cost savings from nutritional interventions.* Available at http://www.bapen.org.uk/pdfs/economic-report-full.pdf. Accessed 11 October 2018.

Elia M, Ceriello A, Laube H, *et al.* (2005) Enteral nutritional support and use of diabetes-specific formulas for patients with diabetes: a systematic review and meta-analysis. *Diabetes Care.* 28: 2267–2279.

Elia M, Van Bokhorst-de Van der Schueren M, Garvey J, et al. (2006) Enteral (oral or tube administration) nutritional support and eicosapentaenoic acid in patients with cancer: A systematic review. *International Journal of Oncology* 28: 5–23.

Elia M, Normand C, Laviano A, *et al.* (2016a) A systematic review of the cost and cost effectiveness of using standard oral nutritional supplements in community and care home settings. *Clin. Nutr.* 35(1): 125–137.

Elia M, Normand C, Norman K, *et al.* (2016b) A systematic review of the cost and cost effectiveness of using standard oral nutritional supplements in the hospital setting. *Clin. Nutr.* 35(2): 370–380.

Foods for Specific Groups. (2013) Regulation (EU) No 609/2013 of the European Parliament and of the Council of 12 June 2013 on food intended for infants and young children, food for special medical purposes, and total diet replacement for weight control. *Off. J. Eur. Union* L181: 35–56.

Food Information for Consumers. (2011) Regulation (EU) No 1169/2011 of the European Parliament and of the council of 25 October 2011 on the provision of food information to consumers. *Off. J. Eur. Union* L304: 18–62.

Gall MJ, Grimble GK, Reeve NJ, *et al.* (1998) Effect of providing fortified meals and between-meal snacks on energy and protein intake of hospital patients. *Clin. Nutr.* 17: 259–264.

Hanning RM, Blinkie CJR, Bar-Or O, *et al.* (1993) Relationships among nutritional status and skeletal and respiratory muscle function in cystic fibrosis: does early dietary supplementation make a difference? *Am. J. Clin. Nutr.* 57: 580–587.

Hubbard GP, Elia M, Holdoway A, *et al.* (2012) A systematic review of compliance to oral nutritional supplements. *Clin. Nutr.* 31: 293–312.

Kimber K, Gibbs M, Weekes C, *et al.* (2015) Supportive interventions for enhancing dietary intake in malnourished or nutritionally at risk adults: a systematic review of nonrandomised studies. *J. Hum. Nutr. Diet.* 28(6): 517–545.

Koretz R, Avenell A, Lipman T, *et al.* (2007) Does enteral nutrition affect clinical outcomes? A systematic review of the randomized trials. *Am. J. Gastroenterol.* 102(2): 412–429.

Milne AC, Avenell A, Potter J. (2006) Meta-analysis: protein and energy supplementation in older people. *Ann. Inter. Med.* 144: 37–48.

Milne AC, Potter J, Vivanti A, *et al.* (2009) Protein and energy supplementation in elderly people at risk from malnutrition. *Cochrane Database Syst. Rev.* 2: CD003288.

NICE. (2006a) *Nutrition Support in Adults. Oral Nutrition Support, Enteral Tube Feeding and Parenteral Nutrition. Clinical Guideline 32.* London: NICE.

NICE. (2006b) *Nutrition Support in Adults. Oral Nutrition Support, Enteral Tube Feeding and Parenteral Nutrition. Costing Report.* London: NICE.

NICE. (2012) *Nutrition Support in Adults. NICE quality standard QS24.* Available at https://www.nice.org.uk/guidance/qs24.

Odlund-Olin A, Armyr I, Soop M, *et al.* (2003) Energy enriched meals improve energy intake in elderly residents in a nursing home. *Clin. Nutr.* 22(2): 125–131.

Potter J, Langhorne P, Roberts M. (1998) Routine protein energy supplementation in adults: systematic review. *BMJ* 317: 495–501.

Ravasco P, Monteiro-Grillo I, Marques Vidal P, *et al.* (2005) Impact of nutrition on outcome: a prospective randomized controlled trial in patients with head and neck cancer undergoing radiotherapy. *Head Neck.* 27(8): 659–668.

Simmons SF, Zhuo X, Keeler E. (2010) Cost-effectiveness of nutrition interventions in nursing home residents: a pilot intervention. *J. Nutr. Health. Aging.* 14: 367–372.

Smoliner C, Norman K, Scheufele R, Hartig W, Pirlich M, Lochs H. (2008) Effects of food fortification on nutritional and functional status in frail elderly nursing home residents at risk of malnutrition. *Nutrition* 24: 1139–1144.

Stratton RJ, Elia M. (2007) A review of reviews: A new look at the evidence for oral nutritional supplements in clinical practice. *Clin. Nutr. Suppl.* 2: 5–23.

Stratton RJ, Elia M. (2010) Encouraging appropriate, evidence-based use of oral nutritional supplements. *Proc. Nutr. Soc.* 69(4): 477–487.

Stratton RJ, Green CJ, Elia M. (2003) *Disease-Related Malnutrition: An Evidence Based Approach to Treatment.* Oxford: CABI Publishing.

Stratton RJ, Ek A-C, Engfer M, *et al.* (2005) Enteral nutritional support in prevention and treatment of pressure ulcers: a systematic review and meta-analysis. *Ageing Res. Rev.* 4: 422–450.

Stratton RJ, Bowyer G, Elia M. (2006) Food snacks or liquid oral nutritional supplements as a first line treatment for malnutrition in post-operative patients. *Proc. Nutr. Soc.* 65: 4A.

Stratton RJ, Hebuterne X, Elia M. (2013) A systematic review and meta-analysis of the impact of oral nutritional supplements on hospital readmissions. *Ageing Res. Rev.* 12(4): 884–897.

Turic A, Gordon KL, Craig LD, *et al.* (1999) Nutrition supplementation enables elderly residents of long-term-care facilities to meet or exceed RDAs without displacing energy or nutrient intakes from meals. *J. Am. Diet. Assoc.* 98: 1457–1459.

Volkert D, Berner YN, Berry E, *et al.* (2006) ESPEN Guidelines on Enteral Nutrition: Geriatrics. *Clin. Nutr.* 25(2): 330–360.

Weekes CE, Emery PW, Elia M. (2009) Dietary counselling and food fortification in stable COPD: a randomised trial. *Thorax.* 64(4): 326–331.

6.4 Enteral nutrition

Sarah Armer, Rhys White and Helen McNair

Key points

- The decision to start feeding should consider the ethics of individual patient circumstances, the requirement to do no harm and the potential improvement in quality of life.
- The route of feeding and feeding regimen, including timing and type of feed, should be decided on an individual basis, taking into account clinical indications, treatment plan and nutritional status.
- Effective monitoring will help to ensure that nutritional support is provided safely, complications are detected early and treated effectively, and nutritional objectives are met and/or reviewed.
- Patients going home on enteral feeding should have an individual discharge plan.

Enteral tube feeding (ETF) is a widely used method for ensuring adequate nutrition in patients who have a functioning gastrointestinal tract but are unable to maintain an adequate or safe oral intake. Enteral feeding (EF) in both the hospital and community setting is becoming increasingly common, as a range of access and delivery methods have been successfully established. Prior to initiating ETF, ethics and consent should be considered (British Society of Gastroenterology (BSG), 1999), in addition to practical issues such as discharge planning, training and support in the community. Dietitians are uniquely placed to provide guidance and recommendations regarding nutritional support, and play a key role within the multidisciplinary team (MDT) in the treatment of patients requiring EF (American Dietetic Association, 1997).

Indications for enteral nutrition

EF is indicated when oral intake is insufficient or unsafe (NICE, 2006), and is the preferred option whenever a patient's gastrointestinal tract is accessible and functioning (Stroud *et al.*, 2003). It is most commonly used in patients with the following features or disorders (NICE, 2006):

- Unconscious patients.
- Neuromuscular swallowing disorders, e.g. stroke.
- Physiological anorexia.
- Upper-gastrointestinal obstruction, e.g. head and neck tumours.
- Gastrointestinal dysfunction or malabsorption, e.g. pancreatitis, gastrointestinal dysmotility.
- Increased nutritional requirements.
- Psychological problems.
- Specific treatment, e.g. Crohn's disease.

Several factors need to be considered when deciding to initiate ETF. These include the risks and benefits of ET placement, the most appropriate method of tube placement and selection of the most suitable feeding tube. The decision should be made following a multidisciplinary discussion, and the views and wishes of the patients and/or their families or carers should be considered. A decision to enterally feed a patient may also be influenced by the future treatments required, e.g. surgery or radiotherapy. Nutritional support should be tailored to the clinical state and the perceived best outcome for the patient (see Chapter 2.2, Assessment of nutritional status and Chapter 6.1, Nutritional requirements in clinical practice).

Ethical considerations

Ethical issues should always be considered before initiating ETF, and consent must be obtained if a patient has the mental capacity. Consent and ethics must be considered before nasogastric (NG) tube placement. Even when only short-term nutritional support is thought to be necessary, informed consent should be obtained (if possible), and ethical issues should be considered (RCP & BSG, 2010). Ideally, a multidisciplinary nutrition support team (NST)

Manual of Dietetic Practice, Sixth Edition. Edited by Joan Gandy.

Companion website: www.manualofdieteticpractice.com

should be available to assess patients. The team is ideally placed to communicate with patients, carers and the referring team regarding appropriate feeding options. A well-functioning NST can reduce the number of inappropriate gastrostomy placements (Abuksis *et al.*, 2004; Sanders *et al.*, 2002). In the absence of a formal NST, e.g. in community settings, an MDT meeting should be held involving the patient, family, relevant care staff, dietitian and any other relevant health professionals to discuss the instigation of EF.

When making a decision regarding EF, it is essential to first establish the indication for nutritional intervention, treatment goal, and the will and consent of each individual patient (Druml *et al.*, 2016). While offering adequate food and water to patients is a basic duty of care, artificial nutritional support (both enteral and parenteral) is regarded as a medical treatment. Any previous relevant opinions of the patient must be taken into account. Under the Mental Capacity Act (2005), the medical team is required to obtain the view of the family and carers. Patients may have conferred a Lasting Power of Attorney (LPA), giving someone else the authority to make decisions about their health and personal welfare. The Royal College of Physicians (RCP) and the British Society of Gastroenterology (BSG) (2010) have provided a comprehensive overview of the legal position regarding the withholding and withdrawing of life-prolonging medical treatment, including nutritional support (see Chapter 1.1, Professional practice and Chapter 7.16, Palliative and end-of-life care). The treating physician is responsible for making the final decision and is ultimately accountable. In cases where the benefits of nutritional support are uncertain, a time-limited trial can be undertaken with clearly agreed objectives. Open communication with family members, carers and the MDT is essential.

The issue of whether to continue feeding severely ill patients who have a poor prognosis is less clear; nutritional care should always be considered on an individual basis. The decision to withdraw artificial nutrition support should be considered on a case-by-case basis. The overall benefit to the patient, including the purpose of nutritional intervention, risks, and the significance of nutrition in the latter stages of life should be considered (Druml *et al.*, 2016).

Routes of enteral feeding

EF is preferable to parenteral nutrition (PN) when the gut is accessible and has adequate absorptive capacity, as it is more physiological and cheaper (Stroud *et al.*, 2003). Only a few patients cannot receive some form of EF. The route of EF is decided on an individual basis according to the clinical indications, treatment plan and nutritional state. It may be delivered:

- Directly into the stomach (gastric feeding) via orogastric, NG, gastrostomy or oesophagostomy tube.
- After the stomach (post-pyloric feeding) via nasoduodenal or nasojejunal tube, gastrojejunostomy or jejunostomy.

Gastric feeding routes

Nasogastric feeding

This is usually used for short-term nutritional support (<6 weeks), or in the longer term when other options such as gastrostomy feeding are contraindicated or inappropriate (Stroud *et al.*, 2003). Each patient should have individual nutritional risk assessment carried out prior to passing an NG tube (NGT), and managing healthcare professionals (HCPs) should ensure that recommendations to reduce the harm caused by misplaced NGTs are followed (National Patient Safety Agency, or NPSA, 2005, 2011).

A fine-bore NGT, usually made from polyvinyl chloride (PVC), polyurethane (PU) or silicone, is inserted through the nose and into the stomach. PVC tubes are suitable for short-term feeding (<10 days), and are usually rigid and wide-bore (10–18 FG; French gauge). The complications associated with wide-bore tubes are well known (nasal erosion, oesophageal ulceration), but they should be considered in patients at high risk of pulmonary aspiration, with conversion to a fine-bore tube once successful gastric emptying is established. More expensive and durable PU tubes are more suitable for longer-term use. Fine-bore feeding tubes are usually of 6–9 FG. Tubes must be radio-opaque throughout their length and have visible markings to ensure accurate identification and documentation of position (NPSA, 2011).

Other methods of gastric placement are:

- Orogastric – used in head injury patients or in those with facial trauma.
- Cervical pharyngostomy, oesphagostomy and stomagastric tubes – used in head and neck cancer patients.

Confirmation of gastric tube placement

It is vital to establish that the tube tip is positioned in the stomach (and not in the lungs) before each feeding episode, before flushing with water or medication, and if there is any doubt about tube's position. Deaths resulting from the misplacement of NG tubes have been reported (NPSA, 2005, 2011). The following methods for confirming NG tube placement are recommended (NPSA, 2005, 2011):

- *Stomach aspirate pH* – aspirate stomach contents, and check that it is acidic, pH ≤ 5.5, using CE-marked pH indicator strips or paper (pH ≤ 5 on paper that does not have ½ markings). If the patient is on continuous feeding or receiving drugs such as antacids (including proton pump inhibitors), the pH may be >5.5. If feed is present, pH should be rechecked up to 1 hour after feeding. If antacids are used, the timing of their consumption may need to be reviewed.
- *X ray confirmation* – this should only be undertaken if there is doubt about the position of the tube or difficulty in obtaining aspirate. An X ray only confirms the position of the NG tube tip at the time of the X ray, and, as the tip may become dislodged following the X ray, further confirmation of gastric pH will be required.

It is important that nothing be administered via the NGT until gastric placement is confirmed; internal stylets/guidewires should not be lubricated before gastric placement is confirmed (NPSA, 2012).

Alternative methods for placing and confirming nasogastric tube position

Electromagnetic sensing devices permit real- time tracking of feeding tube position during placement, e.g. Cortrak 2 Enteral Access System™ (Corpak Medsystems). This device has been shown to successfully place and confirm the position of gastric tubes (Taylor *et al.*, 2014). However, NHS England (2013) recommends that HCPs perform pH or X ray testing to confirm correct placement of NGTs after initial insertion, even when using placement devices.

Feeding tubes with specialist technology that incorporates an integrated real-time imaging system (IRIS) have been developed (Coviden Commercial Ltd). A 3 mm camera visually aids tube placement by enabling clinicians to identify anatomical markers during the placement. The feeding tube is connected to a small touchscreen console via an interface cable. However, clinical studies evaluating its use and cost-effectiveness are needed.

Gastrostomy feeding

A gastrostomy is the creation of an artificial tract between the stomach and the abdominal surface, and is commonly used for long-term enteral support. A gastrostomy can be placed endoscopically (percutaneous endoscopic gastrostomy, or PEG), surgically or radiologically (radiologically inserted gastrostomy, or RIG). The terms PEG and RIG describe the actual procedure; however, the remaining gastrostomy tube often continues to be referred to as a PEG or RIG, which can lead to confusion, given that some gastrostomy tubes can be inserted endoscopically or radiologically. It is important that dietitians understand the differences between the types of tubes and the correct terminology to describe them.

To provide appropriate and safe management of a gastrostomy tube, information regarding when the tube was inserted and how it is retained is important and helps to reduce the risk of complications. Prior to the placement of a gastrostomy tube, a full nutrition assessment should be conducted and the ability to manage the tube confirmed. Placement of a gastrostomy is a consented procedure; patients should have the full risks and benefits of placing the tube explained prior to consenting (Westaby *et al.*, 2010). Tubes specifically designed for gastrostomy use should be used and have an ENFit connector.

Percutaneous endoscopic placement

A PEG is placed under direct visualisation using an endoscope. Transillumination of the abdominal wall identifies the appropriate site for insertion. An incision is made into the stomach and a loop of thread introduced. The thread is grasped internally and pulled up to the mouth using the endoscope. A gastrostomy tube is attached to the thread, pulled down through the oesophagus, and pulled into the stomach and through the abdominal wall to lie with its internal bumper against the gastric mucosa. A flange and clamp are fitted externally. Endoscopic tubes can also be placed using gastropexy and a direct puncture tube insertion. The tube is inserted directly into the stomach through an external puncture, and the stomach is sutured to the abdominal wall until the stoma tract matures. This negates the need for a tube to be pulled through the mouth and oesophagus if there is an obstruction. The advantages of using a PEG include the following:

- Performed as a day care procedure, reducing costs as compared to other placement methods.
- High success rate.
- Fast, <20 minutes.
- General anaesthetic not required routinely.
- Low incidence of complications.

The contraindications and other considerations with PEG placement include the following:

- Severe obesity.
- Portal hypertension or gastric varices.
- Coagulation abnormalities.
- Active gastric ulceration or malignancy.
- Total or partial gastrectomy.
- Ascites.
- Peritoneal dialysis.
- Oesophageal or gastric tumours that prevent passage of an endoscope.
- Oropharyngeal or oesophageal carcinoma – placement of a PEG tube using the standard pull-through technique is associated with a small risk of tumour implantation at the skin site (Cappell, 2007). To reduce this risk, particularly in patients for whom cancer therapy is of curative intent, gastrostomy placement should be achieved by a direct gastric puncture technique (Foster *et al.*, 2007).
- Chronic progressive neurological and neuromuscular disorders, e.g. motor neurone disease. There may be an increased risk associated due to the use of sedation, as patients have a degree of respiratory compromise. There is some evidence to suggest that radiologically placed tubes may confer a survival benefit in these patients, as it avoids the risk of sedation (Shaw *et al.*, 2006).

Removal and replacement of a percutaneous endoscopic gastrostomy tube

Tubes with compressible or deflatable internal bumpers are traction-removable, and therefore help avoid the need for a further endoscopy. Non-traction-removable tubes will require endoscopic removal following the manufacturer's instructions. Removal is performed by cutting the tube and allowing the internal bumper to pass through the gastrointestinal tract naturally. A risk assessment and appropriate patient follow-up is recommended, given the risk of bowel obstruction, perforation and possible death (MHRA, 2012).

There are two types of bedside replacement gastrostomy tubes:

- *A balloon-retained gastrostomy device* – a balloon is inflated internally with sterile water or saline to hold the tip of the feeding tube against the gastric wall following percutaneous insertion. These tubes usually have a length of tube externally, but low-profile tubes, or buttons, are also available which are flush to the skin and therefore more discreet.
- *A flexible bumper-retained gastrostomy device* – held in place by either a flexible internal cage-like bumper or an internal bolster that is deployed by cutting an external suture.

Radiological placement

Gastrostomy tubes can also be placed radiologically. A nasogastric or orogastric tube is required to dilate the stomach with air, and, under X ray guidance, gastropexy sutures are inserted to anchor the stomach to the anterior abdominal wall. A gastrostomy is inserted and its position confirmed in the stomach. Balloon gastrostomies or 'pig tail' tubes are most commonly used. Disc or bumper-retained gastrostomies can also be placed radiologically using the pull-through technique as described. Tubes inserted using this technique are sometimes referred to as a per-oral image-guided gastrostomy (PIGG), and have the advantage of not requiring gastropexy and allowing the insertion of a lower maintenance tube, i.e. bumper/disc retained. However, they are technically more difficult to insert radiologically than endoscopically.

The advantages of RIG placement include:

- Very low risk of tumour seeding from head and neck tumours with direct puncture method as no endoscope required.
- Sedation not required.
- Clear picture of anatomy allows tube placement in difficult patients where endoscopic placement may have been unsuccessful.

Surgical placement

Surgically inserted gastrostomies are becoming less common with the increasing use of PEGs and RIGs. Surgically placed gastrostomies require a mini laparotomy and general anaesthetic. When a gastrostomy is inserted surgically, it requires a purse string suture around the gastrostomy tube in the stomach wall to keep it in place.

Post-insertion instructions

It is safe to commence feeding 4 hours after PEG insertion (NICE, 2006), although local policy may vary. There is no clear consensus on when it is safe to first use a newly inserted RIG for feeding; some centres feed after 4 hours and others wait 24 hours. Potential complications include peritonitis, infection, bowel perforation, haemorrhage and aspiration pneumonia). Prompt recognition of complications with early action reduces the risk of serious harm or death. The NPSA (2010) recommends that:

- Local protocols specify the observations to be taken in the immediate recovery period.
- Medical notes be marked with a high-visibility sticker, warning of possible complications and necessary action.
- Where patients are discharged within 72 hours, equivalent warnings should be communicated to the GP, community nurses, care home nurses, as well as to the patient and/or carers.

Post-pyloric feeding routes

Nasoduodenal or nasojejunal feeding

A feeding route bypassing the stomach overcomes the problem of gastroparesis and subsequent aspiration risk. In patients with high gastric aspirates, the small bowel may be working normally. Tubes can be placed endoscopically under X ray guidance or at the bedside. The risk of aspiration is reduced most significantly when the feeding tube is inserted beyond the ligament of Treitz, i.e. intrajejunal placement (Heyland *et al.*, 2001). Tubes incorporating a lumen for gastric aspiration are also available.

The techniques for bedside placement of nasojejunal tube using different patient positions and prokinetic agents have varying rates of success. Self-advancing PU tubes, e.g. Tiger 2™ Tube (Cook Medical, USA), have unique alternating cilia-like flaps that allow peristalsis to pull the tube into the small bowel more effectively than standard bedside placements. Endoscopic placement is time-consuming and costly, and may not be easily accessible to intensive care patients. A newer bedside technique using a transnasal endoscope for placing nasojejunal tubes has shown promising results, but requires further evaluation (Zick *et al.*, 2011). As with gastric placement, Cortrak 2® has also been demonstrated to be reliable in ascertaining post-pyloric tube placement (Powers *et al.*, 2011; Rao *et al.*, 2009).

Gastrojejunostomy

Post-pyloric feeding access can be obtained in patients with established gastrostomy access by the insertion of an extension device which threads through the existing gastrostomy lumen into the jejunum. A dedicated gastrojejunostomy combination must be used, as most basic gastrostomies cannot house jejunal extensions. Direct puncture techniques can also be used to place gastrojejunal tubes under X ray guidance. These tubes have a gastric internal retention device that can be either a balloon or disc-like bumper.

Jejunostomy

Jejunostomies create a stoma tract between the jejunum and the abdominal surface, and can be placed surgically or radiologically. A jejunostomy is often inserted when major gastrointestinal or hepatobiliary surgery necessitates post-pyloric feeding. It is not, however, without complications, and the optimal route of feeding after upper gastrointestinal surgery is yet to be determined (Weijs *et al.*, 2015). A feeding jejunostomy should be considered if gastric feeding has failed, and may provide a useful route that avoids PN. There is no internal retention device, so these tubes must be secured externally.

The tubes usually directly puncture the jejunum, although some are designed to be tunnelled under the skin and are held in place using a cuff under the skin surface.

A whole-protein feed should be well tolerated in jejunostomy feeding. However, if there is pancreatic or biliary insufficiency, or if the jejunostomy has been sited in the lower small bowel, a peptide-based or elemental feed may be indicated. Feed usually commences at a low volume and is increased slowly until the optimum feeding rate is achieved. Continuous feeding over 24 hours may prevent tube blockage. Jejunostomy tubes often have a thin diameter, e.g. 9 FR, and regular flushing of the tube with water may therefore be necessary to prevent blockage.

Enteral feed delivery

A feeding regimen should be documented in the patient's care plan for nursing staff, or for patients/carers to refer to if home EF takes place. The regimen should include the feed, feeding times, drip rate and additional fluid requirements. Timings should include feed breaks to encompass the psychosocial aspects of feeding, together with the influence on other clinical interventions, e.g. physiotherapy and drug–nutrient interactions. Patients wishing to pump feed at home overnight when they are alone or unsupervised should have the risks explained to them, and this should be documented in their care plan, as some local policies may advise against this.

It is usual to start feeding at no more than 50% feed requirements to ensure metabolic and gastrointestinal tolerance to the feed (NICE, 2006). Drip rates can then be increased at regular intervals until the maximum desired drip rate is achieved. Guidance for feeding patients at risk of refeeding syndrome is covered under 'Refeeding syndrome' section.

Bolus feeding

Bolus feeding is the delivery of approximately 100–400 mL of feed over 10–30-minutes. Administration is usually by syringe, using the syringe barrel as a funnel to allow the feed to infuse using gravity or using the plunger. Bolus feeding can also be provided via a feeding pump, although it is important to be aware of the maximum drip rate that the feed pump can achieve. The tube should be flushed before and after delivery of the feed bolus. Bolus feeding regimens are advantageous, in that they are more physiologically normal, can allow greater flexibility for the patient as they fit with normal eating patterns, and may be preferable for those who do not wish to be restricted by feeding equipment for several hours a day. Bolus feeding may also be the regimen of choice for patients who interfere with tubing and feeding equipment during continuous feeding. Patient positioning should also be considered; it is advisable for patients to remain in a semi-upright position during and for 1 hour after feeding (Metheny *et al.*, 2006).

Continuous feeding

Continuous feeding usually requires a pump and feeding set for administration, and, if ready-to-hang formulae are not used, a feed reservoir. Continuous feeding usually refers to feeding at rates of 50–200 mL/hour over 16–20 hours, although 24-hour feeding is standard practice in critical care for patients on sliding scale insulin. A rest period of at least 90 minutes is needed as it allows gastric pH to fall sufficiently to promote antibacterial conditions in the stomach (Bonten *et al.*, 1994). A longer planned rest period allows more flexibility, e.g. to catch up if feeding has been interrupted during the day, or to allow sufficient time for therapy. A rest period can provide an overnight break for those without urinary catheterisation and in those who may otherwise experience nocturia and interrupted sleep. Alternatively, a rest period can be given during the day, so that the patient is unencumbered by EF equipment, and to promote intake of oral diet if appropriate.

Continuous feeding is usually the feeding method of choice for patients who are fed via a post-pyloric route; however, bolus feeding is not contraindicated for these patients and can be used if tolerated. In deciding whether continuous and/or bolus feeding would be most appropriate, patient preference, risk of tube dislodgement and mobility of the patient should be considered (NICE, 2006).

In patients at risk of pulmonary aspiration, regular aspiration of the NG tube is routinely undertaken to assess adequacy of gastric emptying. However, there is little evidence to support the conventional use of measuring gastric residual volumes (GRVs). Instead, it is suggested to monitor trends to identify any gradual increase in GRVs; interpretation of these results should be modified so as not to interrupt the delivery of EF (Hurt & McClave, 2010). GRVs up to 500 mL are not associated with adverse outcomes, and this value can be recommended as a normal limit (*Montejo et al.*, 2010) (see Chapter 7.17.1, Critical care).

Enteral feed formulae

EF formulae can be categorised into whole-protein (polymeric) feeds, including disease-specific feeds, and elemental or peptide feeds (see Table 6.4.1). A summary of EF products currently available in the UK can be found in Appendix A6.

Whole-protein (polymeric) feeds

These require an intact gut for their digestion and absorption. The constituents of whole-protein feeds are as follows:

- *Protein* – usually milk or hydrolysed casein, although a soya protein formula is available for those with milk protein intolerance.
- *Carbohydrate* – usually maltodextrin, glucose, sucrose or corn syrup solids.

Table 6.4.1 Condition-specific feeds

Type of feed	Comment
Renal feeds	Suitable for patients on electrolyte and fluid restrictions. Similar or lower protein–energy ratio as compared to standard feeds. Energy-dense versions for fluid restriction are available, with subtle modification of other nutrients, e.g. higher water-soluble vitamin content to allow for intradialytic losses.
Low-sodium feeds	Standard feeds with a sodium content reduced to 10–15 mmol/L. Clinical hypernatraemia is often secondary to dehydration, so the use of a standard feed (providing 35–40 mmol Na/L) provides less sodium than plasma levels. Low-sodium feeds may be beneficial for patients with ascites (liver disease).
Respiratory feeds	Contain a higher percentage of energy content from fat, which reduces the amount of carbon dioxide produced from feed metabolism – may be useful in patients with respiratory failure. However, evidence of the benefit of these feeds is limited, and avoidance of overfeeding is as clinically significant as the choice of feed in respiratory failure (Malone, 1997).
Immune feeds	Contain variable amounts of specific amino acids or fats, together with altered levels of specific micronutrients that have an attributed immune benefit, e.g. glutamine, arginine, dietary nucleotides, fish oils, β-carotene and fructo-oligosaccharides. More expensive than standard feeds. Evidence that they may benefit some surgical patients (Waitzberg *et al.*, 2006).
Elemental/peptide feeds	Provide nitrogen in the form of free amino acids or peptides. Indicated in the presence of severe maldigestion or malabsorption. With severe gut impairment, a predigested formula may be indicated. Appropriate use of these feeds may reduce the requirement for PN (Hamaoui *et al.*, 1990). No clinical benefit in using peptide feed rather than whole-protein feed in patients with Crohn's disease (Zachos *et al.*, 2006).

- *Dietary fibre* – various feeds are available containing added soluble and insoluble fibres. Insoluble fibre has most effect on gut barrier function, while soluble fibre can increase short-chain fatty acid production (Silk, 1993). Therefore, a mixed fibre source (as is found in most commercially available feeds) is advised. Elia *et al.* (2008) suggest that fibre-supplemented enteral formulae have important physiological effects and clinical benefits, and may help to reduce the incidence of diarrhoea.
- *Fat* – usually a vegetable oil derivative, although many feed companies are now re-blending fats to alter the ratio of n-3 to n-6 polyunsaturated fatty acids (PUFAs) and increase the monounsaturated fat content. n-3 PUFAs may be provided by the use of canola or rapeseed oil, or by fish oils to provide direct sources of eicosapentaenoic acid (EPA) and docosahexaenoic acid (DHA). Provision of n-3 PUFAs can downregulate the inflammatory response by reducing arachidonic acid (n-6 PUFA) metabolites, but the mechanism to convert n-3 PUFAs to the active EPA and DHA is impaired in the severely ill.
- *Vitamins, minerals and electrolytes* – in the UK, all EFs provide 100% of the recommended nutrient intake for micronutrients (excluding electrolytes) in a specified volume of feed (usually 1–1.8 L of standard EF). Current levels of micronutrients must comply with the European Union (2013) regulation food intended for infants and young children, food for special medical purposes, and total diet replacement for weight control (Regulation 609/2013).

Types of whole-protein feeds can be categorised as:

- *Standard adult formulae* – provide 1 kcal/mL (4.18 kJ/mL) and are suitable for the majority of patients; available with and without fibre.
- *High-energy adult formulae* – provide 1.2–2.4 kcal/mL (5.02–10.03 kJ/mL) and are useful for patients on fluid restriction or with increased nutritional requirements, e.g. burns patients. The electrolyte and protein content of these feeds are variable. Fibre-containing, energy-dense feeds are also available, but only up to energy densities of 2 kcal/mL.
- *Low-energy formulae* – provide 1–1.2 kcal/mL (4.18–5.02 kJ/mL) and 1000 mL of these usually meets the nutritional needs of patients with low energy and/or fluid requirements, e.g. elderly bed-bound patients.
- *Disease-specific enteral formulae* – a variety of EFs are provided for a variety of conditions. However, dietitians should consider the use of specific products within the context of the patient's clinical status, and not take the manufacturer's recommended client group as the sole indication for use. A brief overview of some disease-specific feeds is given in Table 6.4.1.

Liquidised food

There has been an increasing trend in patients wishing to administer liquidised food rather than sterile, prescribed feeds via their feeding tubes. This is not currently recommended due to concerns regarding the nutritional adequacy of the food, and the increased risk of tube blockage and gastric infection, particularly in those who are immunocompromised or jejunally fed. Some patients wish to proceed with this type of feeding, despite being fully aware of the associated risks. In these circumstances, dietitians have a responsibility to ensure that patients have all the necessary information to make a fully informed choice, and to continue to support patients in the decision they have made. Dietitians should ensure that a risk assessment is completed, and may consider seeking additional support from the local risk management team. The outcome of this process, in addition to the patient's reasons for choosing to feed in this way, should be documented. Further information and resources can be found on the Parenteral and Enteral Nutrition Group (PENG) website (www.peng.org.uk).

Drug–nutrient interactions

EF may interfere with the dosage, presentation and action of many drugs. Crushing oral preparations to pass down a tube may compromise their activity, cause tube occlusion and has the potential to cause fatality, particularly if slow-release preparations are used. Some medications are not available in liquid form; therefore, alternative formulations or preparations should be sought. Drugs should not be added to the feed infusion, as this may alter the stability of the medication and introduce a potential route of contamination into the EF. Liaison with a pharmacist will ensure optimal EF and drug administration. A practical guide to the administration of drugs during EF can be found on the BAPEN website (www.BAPEN.org.uk).

Common drugs such as phenytoin, ciprofloxacin, tetracyclines, penicillin, sucralfate and theophylline bind to the feed and/or have altered absorption kinetics, so should be administered during a rest period. Other drugs that can affect/be affected by EFs are digoxin, carbamazepine and antacids. For further reading, see Bradnam and White (2015), and Chapter 5.3 (Medicines management).

Enteral feeding monitoring

The main objectives of monitoring nutritional support are to ensure that it is provided safely, complications are detected early and treated effectively, and nutritional objectives are met and/or reviewed, thereby ensuring the effectiveness of the nutritional intervention. Close liaison with colleagues, patients and carers is vital when initiating and monitoring EF (NICE, 2006), and all have a role to play in the monitoring process. For example, in the community, the patient and/or carer may be responsible for most of the monitoring. In hospital settings, dietitians will not be directly responsible for performing all of the monitoring, but it is their responsibility, in conjunction with the wider MDT and the patients, to agree to an appropriate monitoring plan and to review the results. Table 6.4.2 details the range of parameters that should be considered for monitoring of nutritional support (NICE, 2006).

The frequency and choice of monitoring is dependent on many variables, including the nature and severity of the underlying disease state, whether previous results were abnormal, the type of nutritional support used, the tolerance of nutritional support, the nutritional care setting and the expected duration of the nutritional support (NICE, 2006). Monitoring frequency may need to be more intense at the start of treatment, but should continue throughout the episode of care. Monitoring should be interpreted with caution, as a full understanding of the meaning of a result is needed before any changes are made. There is no one test that will measure nutritional status, and therefore a combination of clinical and laboratory results should be used. Additional guidance on monitoring patients on EF can be found in Micklewright and Todorovic (2011) and NICE (2006).

Complications of enteral feeding

Refeeding syndrome

Refeeding syndrome (RFS) is a group of clinical symptoms and biochemical shifts that can occur in malnourished or starved individuals upon the reintroduction of nutrition. There is no universally accepted definition or diagnostic criteria for RFS. This limits effective research into its management, and therefore it remains poorly understood by clinicians. Nutritional treatment of patients at risk of RFS should be provided by HCPs with adequate training in nutrition support (NICE, 2006).

During starvation, the body conserves energy, including a reduced action of cellular pumps. Electrolytes are able to leak across cell membranes into the plasma and are renally excreted, leading to whole-body deficits. Once glycogen stores have been exhausted, energy metabolism switches to fat and the production of ketone bodies. The reintroduction of nutrition elicits the following metabolic changes:

- Carbohydrate results in increased insulin secretion, leading to cellular re-uptake of glucose, phosphate, magnesium and potassium, with a simultaneous fall in serum levels. These biochemical abnormalities can result in a spectrum of presentations, from fluid retention to cardiac arrhythmias, respiratory insufficiency and, ultimately, death.
- Reactivation of the sodium/potassium membrane pump leads to further movement of K^+ into cells, with a simultaneous movement of sodium and fluid out of the cells into the extracellular space.
- Reduced renal function impairs the ability to excrete this influx of sodium and water; this leads to fluid overload and oedema.
- Thiamine demand and utilisation is increased upon the reintroduction of glucose, owing to its role as a co-factor for carbohydrate metabolism. Deficiency can result in Wernicke–Korsakoff encephalopathy.

At-risk patients are those who have had very little or no food intake for >5 days, especially if already undernourished (BMI <20 kg/m^2); or those who have unintentional

Table 6.4.2 Monitoring of patients receiving enteral feeding

Monitoring parameter	Examples of monitoring	Rationale
Nutritional intake	Food charts, fluid charts, patient reporting	Compare prescribed with actual volume of feed delivered. Facilitate transition between different forms of nutritional support. Prevent over-hydration and under-hydration. Take account of energy and electrolyte content of IV/enteral fluid. Infusions.
Anthropometry	Weight, BMI, mid-upper-arm circumference, triceps skinfold thickness, hand grip dynamometry	Monitor nutritional status changes. Ensure nutritional objectives are met.
Clinical chemistry	Biochemistry, haematology	Aids interpretation of hydration status, metabolic stress, specific nutrient deficiencies and metabolic abnormalities.
Clinical condition	Consciousness, swallow status, temperature	Observe changes which may affect nutritional requirements and most appropriate route of access. Ensure that the type of nutritional support provided remains appropriate. Monitor for infection.
Medications prescribed	Drug charts	To be aware of side effects that may affect tolerance of ETF, e.g. nausea/altered bowel habit. To be aware of possible drug–nutrient interactions. To be aware of drugs that may affect timing of ETF. Ensure that drugs are in appropriate form for administration via feeding tube. Reduce incidence of tube blockage. To be aware of the importance of adequate flushing of tubes before and after administration of medication. To be aware of medication that may contribute to energy intake, e.g. propofol.
Gastrointestinal tolerance	Stool charts, gastric residual volumes	Monitor bowel function and feed tolerance. Assess gastric emptying, and therefore determine the appropriateness of gastric feeding.
Feeding device	Observe position and condition of feeding tube and the site of tube insertion	Ensure appropriate position of feeding tube. Monitor for signs of infection and/or irritation. Check for leaks and cracks in tube.
Nutritional goals and outcomes	Dependent on specific goals set, but likely to include a measure of nutritional intake and nutritional status	Ensure progress towards agreed objectives. Ensure clinical effectiveness of dietetic intervention. Ensure objectives remain realistic and achievable. Ensure that nutritional interventions remain appropriate to the overall care of patients.

weight loss of >5% within the last 3–6 months NICE (2006). High-risk patients are those with any one of the following:

- BMI <16 kg/m².
- Unintentional weight loss of >15% within the last 3–6 months.
- Very little or no nutrition for >10 days.
- Low levels of potassium, magnesium or phosphate prior to feeding.

Patients with two or more of the following are also considered to be at high risk:

- BMI <18.5 kg/m².
- Unintentional weight loss of >10% within the last 3–6 months.
- Very little or no nutrition for >5 days.
- Some drugs, including insulin, chemotherapy, antacids or diuretics, or alcohol abuse.

It is important to note that patients with normal levels of potassium, magnesium and phosphate prior to the commencement of feed can still be at risk of RFS (Marinella, 2004; NICE, 2006). RFS can occur in patients fed orally, enterally or parenterally; it is less likely to occur in those fed orally (Fung & Rimmer, 2005), since starvation is usually accompanied by a reduction in appetite. However, care should be taken when prescribing oral nutritional supplements.

There are several guidelines available for the management of RFS (Khan *et al.*, 2011; NICE, 2006; Royal College of Psychiatrists, 2014; Stanga *et al.*, 2008). Current evidence indicates that the most effective management of refeeding syndrome may differ across different clinical conditions (Doig *et al.*, 2015; Garber *et al.*, 2016). The most widely reported guidelines are those from NICE (2006), which make the following recommendations:

- *At-risk patients:*
  - Introduce feeding at a maximum of 50% of total energy requirements for the first 2 days, increasing to full requirements if no biochemical abnormalities are detected.
  - Meet full requirements for fluid, electrolytes, vitamins and minerals from day 1 of feeding.
- *High-risk patients:*
  - Consider starting nutrition at a maximum 10 kcal/kg and increase slowly to meet full requirements by 4–7 days. Any increase in feed should be dependent on trends in biochemistry.
  - Potassium, magnesium and phosphate supplementation should be given from the outset (unless blood levels are already high).
  - Give thiamine and a multivitamin.
  - Restore circulatory volume and monitor fluid balance closely.
  - Monitor appropriate biochemistry, including potassium, phosphate and magnesium.
  - In extreme cases (e.g. BMI <14 kg/m^2, very little or no nutrition for >15 days, or prefeeding hypokalaemia, hypophosphataemia or hypomagnesaemia), consider starting feed at 5 kcal/kg (21 kJ/mL).

A UK survey regarding attitudes towards the NICE guidelines found that approximately one-third of clinicians found them excessively cautious (De Silva *et al.*, 2008), with another survey of practice finding that starting at 20 kcal/kg was common, increasing to full requirements over 3–4 days (Wagstaff, 2011).

Some guidelines recommend higher feeding thresholds than NICE, and suggest that limiting carbohydrate provision to less than 50% of energy intake may limit refeeding syndrome (Culkin & White, 2017). Close communication with the medical team is crucial to prevent and recognise RFS. A clear plan should be formulated to ensure that all team members are aware of their roles and responsibilities in close monitoring and treatment.

Aspiration

Aspiration risk for gastrostomy feeding is the same as for NG feeding, and can occur without any obvious signs of vomiting or regurgitation. Gastroparesis may be a result of disease management, starvation, or nerve damage, e.g. diabetic neuropathy (see Chapter 7.4.4, Gastroparesis). Regurgitation of stomach contents and aspiration into the lungs can cause asphyxia; even small amounts increase the risk of pneumonia. The aspiration risk has traditionally been assumed to increase with residual volumes of 200 mL or above (McClave *et al.*, 1992); however, more recent evidence suggests that a value of 500 mL can be recommended as a normal limit for GRVs (Montejo *et al.*, 2010) (see Chapter 7.17.1, Critical care). Failure to establish gastric emptying is not a reason for immediate PN support, and post-pyloric feeding should be considered before this option. Prokinetic agents such as metoclopramide and domperidone are not recommended for the long-term treatment of gastro-oesophageal reflux disease, owing to the risks of these medications outweighing the benefits (EMA, 2013, 2014).

If aspiration is a risk, the following actions may be taken:

- Elevate the head and upper body to at least 30°, and maintain this position during and for 1 hour after feeding.
- Consider a post-pyloric feeding route – jejunostomy feeding with aspiration of gastric contents by an NG tube is the only safe way to prevent feed aspiration (Elpern, 1997).

Other risk factors associated with the development of aspiration pneumonia include advancing age, poor oral hygiene, impaired consciousness and sedative medications (Loeb *et al.*, 2003).

Diarrhoea

Diarrhoea is common in enterally fed patients, but is rarely attributable to the EF (Bowling & Silk, 1998), although it may be attributed to the feeding mechanism. Prolonged use of antibiotics results in *Clostridium difficile* overgrowth, and subsequent diarrhoea (Bliss *et al.*, 1998). Enteral administration of magnesium or electrolytes can cause osmotic diarrhoea. Osmolality of the feed is rarely a concern, and feed dilution exacerbates the problem. Management of diarrhoea in enterally fed patients should include the following steps:

- Obtain a stool sample to exclude pathogenic bacteria overgrowth.
- Review the need for, and choice of, antibiotic.
- Ensure adequate hydration – additional fluid may be required as a result of increased losses.
- Reduction in infusion rate of post-pyloric feed.
- Use of a peptide feed if malabsorption is suspected.
- Bile acid sequestrants, e.g. cholestyramine, if bile salt diarrhoea is suspected.
- Review medications (drugs in a sorbitol syrup containing ≥15 g of sorbitol can have a laxative effect).
- Consider a fibre-containing feed; fibre helps minimise diarrhoea in enterally fed patients, particularly in those who are not critically ill (Kamarul Zaman *et al.*, 2015).
- Current evidence to support probiotic use in the management of diarrhoea in critically ill enterally fed patients remains unclear (Jack *et al.*, 2010).

Tube blockage

The small internal diameter of fine-bore tubes increases the risk of occlusion. The most common cause is coagulation of feed by drug syrups and suspensions, combined with inadequate tube flushing, or obstruction by particles of crushed oral medications. Tube occlusion risk can be minimised by:

- Flushing the tube regularly with water.
- Flushing the tube with water during and following drug administration.

- Giving medicines individually, rather than together, to avoid precipitation from drug interactions.
- Using drugs in syrup or dispersible form, rather than as crushed tablets.

Consideration should be given to the type of water used to flush EF tubes. For gastric tubes, the choice is tap, cooled, boiled, or sterile water, but a risk assessment should be undertaken as the choice may be different in the hospital and the patient's home. For post-pyloric feeding, sterile water should be used; it is important to take into consideration that, once the container has been opened, it is no longer sterile. Flushing with warm water should be tried initially to unblock a tube, along with manipulation of the tube. Soda water and sodium bicarbonate can also be effective in clearing a blockage. Cola, pineapple juice and lemonade should not be used, as the acidity may contribute to occlusion by denaturing the proteins in the EF (Beckwith *et al.*, 2004). Pancreatic enzymes are effective, and can unblock a feeding tube blocked with feed within 10–20 minutes (Marcaud & Stegall, 1990); other agents are commercially available. Although gastrostomy tubes are larger in size, blockages can still occur, and therefore measures to minimise risk should still be taken.

Microbiological contamination of feed

EFs provide an ideal growth medium for microbial contamination, but low counts of non-pathogenic bacteria are clinically unimportant. Bacterial growth within the feed can be minimised through the following steps:

- Using commercially prepackaged, sterile, ready-to-hang feeds (Beattie & Anderton, 1999, 2001). Modular feeds carry a greater risk of microbiological contamination.
- Limiting the hanging time of the feed to a maximum of 24 hours, or 4 hours for non-sterile feeds (Payne-James *et al.*, 1992).
- Replacement of reservoir and giving set daily.
- Filling the feeding reservoir with feed for up to 24 hours, rather than 4 hours (Patchell *et al.*, 1998).
- Hygienic handling of systems and adequate hand hygiene (Lee & Hodgkiss, 1999).
- Ensuring that systems marked as 'single use' are used only once.
- Ensuring that reusable equipment for single-patient use (e.g. syringes, NG tubes and guide wires) are cleaned, labelled and stored appropriately in accordance with local policy.

Additional care should be taken with jejunal feeds in patients with achlorhydria and immunosuppressed patients as their lack of gastric acidity and impaired immune function, respectively, may increase infection risk.

Accidental tube removal

Feeding tubes can become dislodged or may be removed accidentally. NG tubes should be removed completely and repassed (with the same tube and original guide wire if single-patient use), and position reconfirmed. If a gastrostomy tube is accidentally removed, prompt replacement is required to preserve the stoma tract, which can start to heal immediately. Balloon replacement tubes can be used, and a spare tube should be routinely supplied to the patient in case of such circumstances. Where there is no spare tube available, a Foley catheter can be used to maintain the tract until an appropriate feeding tube is reinserted. This is generally discouraged; however, if a Foley catheter is used to preserve the tract, it must not be used for feeding, and end users should be made aware of the potential risks of its use in this way (MHRA, 2010). Stoma plugs are now commercially available, designed solely to preserve the stoma tract in cases of accidental tube removal. It is essential that patients and carers be aware of what to do if the feeding tube becomes dislodged or is removed. Adequate training and education should be provided for patients, carers and professionals.

Stoma site problems

Stoma site complications include leakage, exit-site infections, pneumoperitoneum, intra-abdominal abscesses, necrotising fasciitis, problems with self-care secondary to poor placement, and infection, which can be potentially fatal (Hanlon, 1998). Overgranulation is also a common stoma site problem, but this can generally be reduced by correctly positioning the external fixation device (Best, 2004). Minor complications can usually be managed without admission to hospital; a swab of the site may be useful to rule out infection. Thorough hand hygiene and avoiding unnecessary dressings around the stoma site can help minimise the risk of such problems, as can good training for patients and carers regarding tube care. Regular assessment of the stoma site should be integrated into the monitoring protocols. A specialist EF nurse can advise regarding treatment for minor gastrostomy-related complications, and this service is often supplied as part of the EF contract for hospitals and community settings.

Buried bumper syndrome

Buried bumper syndrome (BBS) occurs when the gastric mucosa grows over the internal bumper of the gastrostomy tube, resulting in migration through, or into, the abdominal wall. This can result in mechanical feed delivery failure, pain, peritonitis and even death. BBS can be prevented by ensuring that the tube is measured and fitted correctly, and regularly introduced into the stomach and rotated. Should BBS occur, the tube must be removed endoscopically or surgically.

Enteral feeding equipment

The equipment required for ETF depends on the method used. Bolus feeding requires syringes for fluid and feed delivery. Continuous feeding requires a pump, giving sets, syringes and possibly feeding reservoirs if a modular feed or extra water is being administered via the pump. Pumps can be used for ambulatory feeding with the addition of a backpack or carry case, which can usually be obtained through the EF supplier. Large syringes are used for water flushes and administration of feed; the smaller syringes are used for more accurate measurement and administration of medicines. The International Organisation for Standardisation (ISO) has developed a new global standard for all EF connectors called ENFit, which was phased in from 2015 to reduce the risk of misconnections and improve patient safety.

Weaning

Although many patients will rely on EF as their sole source of nutrition for life, some may be able to resume oral feeding. Once oral feeding has been deemed safe to recommence, EF can be continued in conjunction with an oral diet during the transitional period. The feeding rate or bolus size can be increased to allow a longer rest period, and a higher-energy feed can be used or the feed can be reduced to provide <100% of estimated requirements. Bolus feeding or overnight feeding can be useful in ensuring that nutritional requirements are met while encouraging daytime oral intake during the transitional period. Care should be taken to ensure that patients do not become dehydrated during the weaning process; additional fluid boluses can help to minimise this risk.

Home enteral feeding

Home enteral feeding (HEF) is an expanding area of nutritional support (BAPEN, 2010). The majority of HEF patients have had a stroke, head and neck cancer, or a degenerative disorder, e.g. motor neurone disease (BAPEN, 2011). In recent years, there has been a slight decrease in the number of patients reportedly commencing HEF due to swallowing problems, and a slight increase in those commencing HEF to improve nutritional status (BAPEN, 2011). The dietitian's role in the discharge into the community of patients on nutritional support is integral to the process. Local policies and procedures should be in place for training, discharge planning and monitoring of the patient (Elia, 1994). Pressure on hospital beds often leads to early discharge, and it is therefore important that patients be reviewed regularly during the initial period to ensure that optimal nutritional support is achieved, and that plans for discharge be made in an appropriate and timely manner.

EFs prescribed in the community are available on prescription, but the feeding equipment is usually financed by primary care, depending on contractual agreements. Determination of who pays for the equipment must be confirmed before the patient is discharged. Most UK feed companies provide training, delivery of feeds and equipment, and servicing of pumps to community patients.

Timely and effective communication is necessary to ensure that a patient is discharged safely on HEF. The discharge planning process should take into account the knowledge, skills and support network of those who will be responsible for caring for the tube and setting up the feed once the patient is home. The patient and family are usually encouraged to manage these themselves, with adequate training and support provided pre- and post-discharge. However, if this is not possible, the responsibility may fall to district nursing teams. Many patients are discharged to nursing homes; therefore, adequate and regular training for care staff should be arranged. The feeding regimen may be altered for discharge to best fit with usual home routines and patient/carer preferences. Table 6.4.3 outlines the steps in discharge planning and the dietitian's roles and responsibilities.

The role of the HEF dietitian involves the physical, biochemical and anthropometrical monitoring of patients, and addressing the impact of this potentially life-changing intervention. Quality-of-life issues should

Table 6.4.3 Discharge planning for patients receiving HEF

Stage of discharge planning	Dietitian's role and responsibility
Decision made to insert feeding tube	Part of the MDT; can offer advice regarding what EF will entail to ensure patients/carers make an informed decision.
Decision made to discharge home	Inform HEF dietitian.
	Ensure patient and carers are appropriately trained to use the feeding pump and to care for the tube.
	Provide written information and contact details.
	Involve other services if required, e.g. district nurse.
	Ensure feeding regimen is suitable for home.
On discharge	Ensure patient is discharged with sufficient supply of feed and equipment until repeat prescription and delivery have been confirmed.
	Order supplies, request feed prescription from GP and arrange ongoing delivery of feed and equipment.
	Handover to HEF dietitian.
Post-discharge	Ensure patient and carers are familiar with management of tube and administration of feed.
	Ensure patient has all necessary equipment.
	Monitor nutritional support intervention and provide a follow-up plan.

be examined to ensure that the feeding regimen is acceptable and suitable for the individual. Patient support groups, such as Patients on Intravenous and Nasogastric Therapy (PINNT), may be useful. Some HEF dietitians also take on the extended role of replacing balloon replacement gastrostomies and NG tubes, and this can help prevent unnecessary hospital admissions, reduce the burden on the acute setting and enable feeding to continue with minimum disruption.

Further reading

Bradnam V, White R, on behalf of the British Pharmaceutical Nutrition Group. (2011) *Handbook of Drug Administration via Enteral Feeding Tubes*, 2nd edn. London: Pharmaceutical Press.

Micklewright A, Todorovic V (eds) and the Parenteral and Enteral Nutrition Group of the British Dietetic Association (PENG). (2011) *A Pocket Guide to Clinical Nutrition*, 4th edn. PEN Group Publications.

NICE. (2006) *Nutrition Support in Adults. Clinical Guideline 32.* London: NICE.

Stroud M, Duncan H, Nightingale J, British Society of Gastroenterology. (2003) Guidelines for enteral feeding in adult hospital patients. *Gut* 52(7): vii1–vii12.

Westaby D, Young A, O'Toole P, *et al.* (2010) The provision of a percutaneously placed ETF service. *Gut* 59: 1592–1605.

Internet resources

American Society for Parenteral and Enteral Nutrition (ASPEN), www.nutritioncare.org

British Association for Parenteral and Enteral Nutrition (BAPEN), www.bapen.org.uk

European Society for Clinical Nutrition and Metabolism (ESPEN), www.espen.org

Parenteral and Enteral Nutrition Group of the British Dietetic Association (PENG), www.peng.org.uk

Patients on Intravenous and Nasogastric Nutrition Therapy (PINNT), www.pinnt.com

References

Abuksis G, Mor M, Plaut S, *et al.* (2004) Outcome of percutaneous endoscopic gastrostomy (PEG): comparison of two policies in a 4-year experience. *Clin. Nutr.* 23(3): 341–346.

American Dietetic Association (ADA). (1997) Position paper. The role of registered dietitians in enteral and parenteral nutrition support. *J. Am. Diet. Assoc.* 97: 302–304.

Beattie TK, Anderton DA. (1999) Microbial evaluation of four enteral feeding systems which have deliberately been subjected to faulty handling procedures. *J. Hosp. Infect.* 42: 11–20.

Beattie TK, Anderton DA. (2001) Decanting versus sterile pre-filled nutrient containers – the microbial risks in enteral feeding. *Int. J. Environ. Health Res.* 11(1): 81–93.

Beckwith MC, Feddema SS, Barton RG. (2004) A guide to drug therapy in patients with enteral feeding tubes: dosage form selection and administration methods. *Hosp. Pharm.* 39: 225–237.

Best C. (2004) The correct positioning and role of an external fixation device on a PEG. *Nurs. Times* 100: 18–50.

Bliss DZ, Johnson S, Savik K, *et al.* (1998) Acquisition of *Clostridium difficile* and *Clostridium difficile*-associated diarrhoea in hospitalised patients receiving tube feeding. *Ann. Inter. Med.* 129: 1012–1019.

Bonten MJM, Gaillard CA, van Tiel FH, *et al.* (1994) Continuous enteral feeding counteracts preventive measures for gastric colonisation in intensive care unit patients. *Crit. Care Med.* 22: 939–944.

Bowling TE, Silk DBA. (1998) Colonic responses to enteral tube feeding. *Gut* 42: 147–151.

Bradnam V, White R, on behalf of the British Pharmaceutical Nutrition Group. (2015) *Handbook of Drug Administration via Enteral Feeding Tubes*, 3rd edn. London: Pharmaceutical Press.

British Association for Parenteral and Enteral Nutrition (BAPEN). (2010) Artificial Nutrition Support in the UK 2000–2009. A Report by the British Artificial Nutrition Survey (BANS), a committee of BAPEN (The British Association for Parenteral and Enteral Nutrition). Available at https://www.bapen.org.uk/pdfs/bans_reports/bans_report_10.pdf. Accessed 11 October 2018.

British Association for Parenteral and Enteral Nutrition (BAPEN). (2011) Artificial Nutrition Support in the UK 2000–2010 A Report by the British Artificial Nutrition Survey (BANS), a committee of BAPEN (The British Association for Parenteral and Enteral Nutrition). Available at www.bapen.org.uk. Accessed 12 May 2016.

British Society of Gastroenterology (BSG). (1999) *Guidelines for Informed Consent for Endoscopic Procedures.* London: BSG.

Cappell MS. (2007) Risk factors and risk reduction of malignant seeding of the percutaneous endoscopic gastrostomy track from pharyngoesophageal malignancy: a review of all 44 known reported cases. *Am. J. Gastroenterol.* 102: 1307–1311.

Culkin A, White R. (2017) Refeeding syndrome. In: Micklewright A, Todorovic V and the Parenteral and Enteral Nutrition Group of the British Dietetic Association (PENG) (eds) *A Pocket Guide to Clinical Nutrition*. Birmingham: PEN Group Publications.

De Silva A, Smith T, Stroud M. (2008) NICE on refeeding syndrome: attitudes to NICE guidance on refeeding syndrome. *BMJ* 337(7661): 67.

Doig G, Simpson F, Heighes P, *et al.* (2015) Restricted versus continued standard caloric intake during the management of refeeding syndrome in critically ill adults: a randomised, parallel-group, multicenter, single-blind controlled trial. *Lancet Respir. Med.* 3, 943–952.

Druml C, Ballmer PE, Druml W, et al. (2016) ESPEN guideline on ethical aspects of artificial nutrition and hydration. *Clin. Nutr.* 35: 545–556.

Elpern EH. (1997) Pulmonary aspiration in hospitalized adults. *Nutr. Clin. Pract.* 12: 5–13.

Elia M (ed). (1994) Enteral and Parenteral Nutrition in the Community. *BAPEN Working Party Report.* Maidenhead: BAPEN.

Elia M, Engfer MB, Green CJ, *et al.* (2008) Systematic review and meta-analysis: the clinical and physiological effects of fibre-containing enteral formulae. *Aliment. Pharmacol. Ther.* 27: 120–145.

European Medicines Agency (EMA). (2013) *European Medicines Agency recommends changes to the use of metoclopramide*. Available at https://www.ema.europa.eu/documents/press-release/european-medicines-agency-recommends-changes-use-metoclopramide_en.pdf. Accessed 11 October 2015.

European Medicines Agency (EMA). (2014) *CMDh confirms recommendations on restricting use of domperidone-containing medicines. European Medicines Agency*. Available at https://www.ema.europa.eu/news/cmdh-confirms-recommendations-restricting-use-domperidone-containing-medicines. Accessed 11 October 2018.

European Union (EU). (2013) Regulation (EU) No 609/2013 of the European Parliament and of the Council of 12 June 2013 on food intended for infants and young children, food for special medical purposes, and total diet replacement for weight control and repealing Council Directive 92/52/EEC, Commission Directives 96/8/EC, 1999/21/EC, 2006/125/EC and 2006/141/EC, Directive 2009/39/EC of the European Parliament and of the Council and Commission Regulations (EC) No 41/2009 and (EC) No 953/2009. *Off. J. Eur. Union* L181/35.

Foster JM, Filocamo P, Nava H, *et al.* (2007) The introducer technique is the optimal method for placing percutaneous endoscopic gastrostomy tubes in head and neck cancer patients. *Surg. Endosc.* 21: 897–901.

Fung AT, Rimmer J. (2005) Hypophosphataemia secondary to Oral Refeeding Syndrome in a patient with long-term alcohol misuse. *Med. J. Aust.* 183(6): 324–326.

Garber A, Sawyer S, Golden N, *et al.* (2016) A systematic review of approaches to refeeding in patients with anorexia nervosa. *Int. J. Eat. Disord.* 49: 293–310.

Hamaoui E, Lefkowitz R, Olender L, *et al.* (1990) Enteral nutrition in the early postoperative period: a new semi-elemental formula versus total parenteral nutrition. *JPEN J. Parenter. Enteral Nutr.* 14: 501–507.

Hanlon MD. (1998) Preplacement marking for optimal gastrostomy and jejunostomy tube site locations to decrease complications and promote self-care. *Nutr. Clin. Pract.* 13: 167–171.

Heyland DK, Drover JW, MacDonald S, *et al.* (2001) Effect of post-pyloric feeding on gastroesophageal regurgitation and pulmonary microaspiration: results of a randomized control trial. *Crit. Care Med.* 29: 1495–1501.

Hurt RT, McClave SA. (2010) Gastric residual volumes in critical illness: what do they really mean? *Crit. Care Clin.* 26(3): 481–490.

Jack L, Coyer F, Courtney M, *et al.* (2010) Probiotics and diarrhoea management in enterally tube fed critically ill patients – what is the current evidence? *Intensive Crit. Care Nurs.* 26(6): 314–326.

Kamarul Zaman M, Chin, K, Rai V, *et al.* (2015) Fibre and prebiotic supplementation in enteral nutrition: a systematic review and meta analysis. *World J. Gastroenterol.* 21(17): 5372–5381.

Khan L, Ahmed J, Khan S, *et al.* (2011) Refeeding syndrome: a literature review. *Gastroenterol. Res. Pract.*, Article ID 410971

Lee CH, Hodgkiss IJ. (1999) The effect of poor handling procedures on enteral feeding systems in Hong Kong. *J. Hosp. Infect.* 42: 119–123.

Loeb MB, Becker M, Eady A, *et al.* (2003) Interventions to prevent aspiration pneumonia in older adults: A systematic review. *J. Am. Geriat. Soc.* 51(7): 1018–1022.

Malone AM. (1997) Is a pulmonary enteral formula warranted for patients with pulmonary dysfunction? *Nutr. Clin. Prac.* 12: 168–171.

Marcaud SP, Stegall KS. (1990) Unclogging feeding tubes with pancreatic enzyme. *JPEN J. Parenter. Enteral Nutr.* 14: 198–200.

Marinella MA. (2004) Refeeding syndrome: implications for the inpatient rehabilitation unit. *Am. J. Phys. Med. Rehabil.* 83: 65–68.

McClave SA, Snider HL, Lowen CC, *et al.* (1992) Use of residual volume as a marker for enteral feeding intolerance: prospective blinded comparison with physical examination and radiographic findings. *JPEN J. Parenter. Enteral Nutr.* 16: 99–105.

Medicines and Healthcare products Regulatory Body (MHRA). (2010) *Users should avoid (if possible) off label use of medical devices, the modification of medical devices and the use of non CE-marked medical devices in clinical settings (MDA/2010/001).* London, MHRA.

Medicines and Healthcare products Regulatory Body (MHRA). (2012) One liners issued April 2012. Available at http://webarchive.nationalarchives.gov.uk/20141205150130/http://www.mhra.gov.uk/home/groups/dts-bs/documents/publication/con149727.pdf. Accessed 4 August 2016.

Metheny NA, Clouse RE, Chang YH, *et al.* (2006) Tracheobronchial aspiration of gastric contents in critically ill tube fed patients: frequency, outcomes, and risk factors. *Crit. Care. Med.* 34(4): 1007–1015.

Micklewright A, Todorovic V (eds). and the Parenteral and Enteral Nutrition Group of the British Dietetic Association (PENG). (2011) *A Pocket Guide to Clinical Nutrition.* Birmingham: PEN Group Publications.

Montejo JC, Minambres E, Bordeje L, *et al.* (2010) Gastric residual volume during enteral nutrition in ICU patients: the REGANE study. *Intensive Care Med.* 36(8): 1386–1393.

National Patient Safety Agency (NPSA). (2005) *Reducing the Harm caused by Misplaced Nasogastric Feeding Tubes. Patient Safety Alert 05.* London: NPSA.

National Patient Safety Agency (NPSA). (2010) *Early Detection of Complications after Gastrostomy. Rapid Response Report NPSA/2010/RRR010.* London: NPSA.

National Patient Safety Agency (NPSA). (2011) *Reducing the Harm Caused by Misplaced Nasogastric Feeding Tubes in Adults, Children and Infants. Patient Safety Alert 002.* London: NPSA.

National Patient Safety Agency (NPSA). (2012) *Harm from Flushing of Nasogastric Tubes before Confirmation of Placement. NPSA/2012/RRR001.* London: NPSA.

NHS England. (2013) *Patient Safety Alert. Stage One: Warning. Placement devices for nasogastric tube insertion. DO NOT Replace Initial Position Checks. NHS/PSA/W/2013/001.* London: NHS England.

NICE. (2006) *Nutrition Support in Adults. Clinical Guideline 32.* Available at https://www.nice.org.uk/guidance/cg32 Accessed 21 February 2019.

Patchell CJ, Anderton DA, Holden C, *et al.* (1998) Reducing bacterial contamination of enteral feeds. *Arch. Dis. Child.* 78: 166–168.

Payne-James JJ, Bray J, Rana S, *et al.* (1992) Retrograde (ascending) bacterial contamination of enteral diet administration systems. *JPEN J. Parenter. Enteral Nutr.* 16: 369–373.

Powers J, Luebbehusen M, Spitzer T, *et al.* (2011) Verification of an electromagnetic placement device compared with abdominal radiograph to predict accuracy of feeding tube placement. *JPEN J. Parenter. Enteral Nutr.* 35: 535–539.

Rao MM, Kallam R, Arsalanizadeh R, Gatt M, MacFie J. (2009) Placing of enteral feeding tubes by the bedside using an electromagnetic sensing device. *Br. J. Intensive Care* 19: 54–59.

Royal College of Physicians (RCP) and British Society of Gastroenterology (BSG). (2010) *Oral Feeding Difficulties and Dilemmas: A Guide to Practical Care Particularly Towards the End of Life.* London: Royal College of Physicians.

Royal College of Psychiatrists. (2014) *MARSIPAN: Management of Really Sick Patients with Anorexia Nervosa*, 2nd edn. London, UK: Report CR189 Royal College of Psychiatrists.

Sanders DS, Carter MJ, D'Silva J, *et al.* (2002) Percutaneous endoscopic gastrostomy: a prospective audit of the impact of guidelines in 2 district general hospitals in the United Kingdom. *Am. J. Gastroenterol.* 97: 2239–2245.

Shaw AS, Ampong MA, Rio A, *et al.* (2006) Survival of patients with ALS following institution of enteral feeding is related to preprocedure oximetry: a retrospective review of 98 patients in a single centre. *Amyotroph. Lateral Scler.* 7: 16–21.

Silk DBA. (1993) Fibre and enteral nutrition. *Clin. Nutr.* 12(1): 106–113.

Stanga Z, Brunner A, Leuenberger M, *et al.* (2008) Nutrition in clinical practice – the refeeding syndrome: illustrative cases and guidelines for prevention and treatment. *Eur. J. Clin. Nutr.* 62: 687–694.

Stroud M, Duncan H, Nightingale J, British Society of Gastroenterology. (2003) Guidelines for enteral feeding in adult hospital patients. *Gut* 52(7): vii1–vii12.

Taylor S, Allan K, McWilliam H, *et al.* (2014) Confirming nasogastric tube position: electromagnetic tracking. *Br. J. Nurs.* 23: 354–358.

Wagstaff G. (2011) Dietetic practice in refeeding syndrome. *J. Hum. Nutr. Diet.* 24: 505–515.

Waitzberg DL, Saito H, Plank LD et al., (2006) Postsurgical infections are reduced with specialized nutrition support. *World J. Surgery* 30:1592–1604.

Weijs T, Berkelmans G, Nieuwenhuijzen G, *et al.* (2015) Routes for early enteral nutrition after esophagectomy: a systematic review. *Clin. Nutr.* 34: 1–6.

Westaby D, Young A, O'Toole P, *et al.* (2010) The provision of a percutaneously placed enteral tube feeding service. *Gut* 59: 1592–1605.

Zachos M, Tondeur M, Griffiths AM. (2006) Enteral nutritional therapy for induction of remission in Crohn's disease (Review). *Cochrane Database Syst. Rev.* 1: CD000542.

Zick G, Frerichs A, Ahrens M, *et al.* (2011) A new technique for bedside placement of enteral feeding tubes: a prospective cohort study. *Crit. Care* 15: R8.

6.5 Parenteral nutrition

Melanie Baker and Lynn Harbottle

Key points

- Parenteral nutrition (PN) should only be used when the enteral route is inaccessible or inadequate.
- PN can be given peripherally or centrally, depending on the predicted duration, availability of venous access and nutritional requirements.
- Electrolytes and micronutrients must be included to meet individual nutritional requirements.
- Detailed pre-feeding assessment and close monitoring for metabolic, infectious or mechanical complications is essential.
- Nutrition teams have an important role in ensuring quality control around the initiation, supply, monitoring and auditing of PN practice and outcomes.

Parenteral nutrition (PN) encompasses the delivery of all nutrients, electrolytes and fluid directly into a central or peripheral vein. It provides nutritional support when the gastrointestinal tract is deemed unsafe or inaccessible, or if absorption via enteral or oral feeding is inadequate to meet full nutritional requirements (NICE, 2006). Although PN is an essential and potentially life-saving therapy, it is expensive and may be associated with a high risk of serious and, occasionally, life-threatening complications, including line infections, micronutrient deficits, electrolyte disturbances, liver dysfunction, hyperglycaemia, hyperlipidaemia and cardiac failure (Austin & Stroud, 2007). Many of the complications associated with PN, highlighted in early research, may have been due to inappropriate use, inadequate line care, unbalanced formulations and significant overfeeding (Koretz *et al.*, 2001). To reduce complications, it is vital that PN be administered appropriately and monitored closely.

The British Association for Parenteral and Enteral Nutrition (BAPEN) and NICE have repeatedly recommended that patients on PN be managed by multidisciplinary nutrition support teams (NSTs) with appropriate expertise. Such teams have been shown to improve patient outcomes (Hvas *et al.*, 2014) and deliver cost savings (Kennedy & Nightingale, 2005). Despite this, a National Confidential Enquiry into Patient Outcome and Death (NCEPOD) report in 2010 indicated that only 60% of UK hospitals had established nutrition teams. Metabolic complications were reported in 40% of patients. NCEPOD also noted unnecessary delays in recognising the need for and instituting PN, deficiencies in assessment and monitoring, inappropriate fluid administration and poor documentation of nutritional issues. They recommended that all hospitals have PN proformas to ensure a robust assessment, including indications, treatment goals, risk and precautions taken against refeeding syndrome and clinical monitoring. In addition, they recommended dedicated catheter insertion services, better education for clinical staff and that PN should not usually be started outside normal working hours.

Indications

Clinical indications

PN should only be used when nutritional needs cannot be fully met by the oral/enteral routes. Assessment of gastrointestinal function is required, ideally undertaken by an NST. Advances in enteral nutrition (EN) delivery techniques, particularly the use of post-pyloric feeding tubes, have reduced the need to give PN, e.g. surgical jejunostomy feeding after upper gastrointestinal tract surgery (Wheble *et al.*, 2012), and EN is now used in clinical conditions for which PN was previously favoured, e.g. acute pancreatitis (Tenner *et al.*, 2013). Indications for short–medium-term PN (<14–28 days) include:

- Major gastrointestinal surgery – where there is no suitable EN access or it is contraindicated, e.g. intra-abdominal sepsis or perforation.

Manual of Dietetic Practice, Sixth Edition. Edited by Joan Gandy.

Companion website: www.manualofdieteticpractice.com

- Enterocutaneous fistulae – where position, volume or sepsis prevent enteral feeding.
- Gastrointestinal obstruction – where enteral access is not possible.
- Prolonged postoperative ileus.
- Severe malabsorption.
- Severe mucositis following chemotherapy.
- Multiorgan failure causing impaired tolerance to full enteral feeding.

Intestinal failure (IF) is often short term and self-limiting (see Chapter 7.4.9, Intestinal failure and intestinal resection), but more prolonged IF may result in patients remaining PN dependent for months or even permanently (Bozzetti *et al.*, 2014). This may occur in:

- Short bowel syndrome – resulting from Crohn's disease, intestinal ischaemia, surgical complications.
- Motility disorders.
- Chronic malabsorption.
- Radiation enteritis.

Nutritional indications

PN should be considered in those who are malnourished (body mass index, or BMI <18.5 kg/m², or >10% unintentional recent weight loss, or BMI <20 kg/m² and >5% unintentional recent weight loss) or are at risk of becoming so and who fit the clinical indications (NICE, 2006). It is not generally indicated in previously well-nourished patients (BMI >20 kg/m² and <5% recent weight loss) exposed to short periods (up to 5 days) of inadequate nutrition.

Ethical considerations

PN may not be appropriate if it prolongs survival without an improved quality of life, e.g. metastatic bowel obstruction due to advanced disease. ESPEN recommends that long-term PN be offered in those with IF due to incurable disease; if EN is insufficient, the expected survival due to tumour progression is longer than 2–3 months, and it is expected that PN can stabilise or improve performance status and quality of life (Bozzetti *et al.*, 2009). The ethical aspects of feeding should be considered before treatment is commenced, and reviewed on a regular basis (Shang *et al.*, 2006).

Treatment goals

A thorough assessment should consider goals of therapy from the outset. The overall aim should be that gastrointestinal function would recover to facilitate adequate oral/enteral feeding, although a prolonged period of PN may be required for gastrointestinal adaptation or if further surgery is required to restore gut integrity and function.

Nutrition assessment

Prior to initiating PN, a detailed nutritional assessment should be undertaken, including lean and fat mass, baseline biochemistry and hydration status, and refeeding risk (based on period of starvation, BMI, percentage weight loss and electrolyte levels) (NICE, 2006). See Table 6.5.1 for more details on the baseline assessment.

Table 6.5.1 Baseline assessment of a patient requiring parenteral nutrition

Parameter	Rationale
Indication for PN	To ensure appropriateness of treatment and why EN is not appropriate.
Goal and expected duration of treatment	Determined by considering the overall clinical picture and patient prognosis.
Access route for administration	To ensure PN is given via an appropriate route to establish whether central/peripheral PN will best meet requirements, and to reduce the risk of complications.
Nutritional assessment, i.e. weight, percentage weight loss, body mass index, anthropometry	Assessment of nutritional status, fluid balance and refeeding risk.
Previous nutritional intake	To predict the risk of refeeding syndrome when PN begins.
Clinical status – appearance, blood pressure, temperature	General condition, fluid balance, presence of infection (will affect requirements).
Drug therapy	Fluid/electrolyte content of concurrent treatment, e.g. IV fluids/medications; whether the patient is on appropriate medication to promote gut function.
Hydration status (fluid balance charts)	Fluid balance, additional gastrointestinal losses to be replaced, e.g. vomit, fistula, drain output.
Urea and creatinine	Fluid balance, renal function.
Electrolytes – sodium, potassium, calcium, phosphate, magnesium	Fluid balance, electrolyte status, refeeding risk.
Full blood count and C-reactive protein	Presence of infection and anaemia.
Albumin	Used in combination with inflammatory markers to assess catabolic state.
Coagulation parameters	Before insertion of line.

Routes of administration

PN may be administered via a central or peripheral vein, according to the condition and availability of vascular supply, nutritional requirements and anticipated PN duration.

Peripheral access routes

Peripheral catheters, normally sited in a superficial vein in the hand or forearm, may be suitable for short-term peripheral parenteral nutrition (PPN) of less than 14 days. PPN can be given via either:

- A cannula (venflon), where the smallest gauge possible should be used to allow dilution of the PN solution in the vein.
- Midline catheter, extending 10–15 cm from the insertion point at the antecubital fossa (elbow) in either the basilic or cephalic vein (Figure 6.5.1).

PPN avoids the clinical risks and costs of central venous catheters (Pittiruti *et al.*, 2009), but patients must have good peripheral venous access. Thrombophlebitis is a common problem that may be minimised by rotating the insertion site (in the case of a venflona) and by avoiding high-osmolality PN regimens (Anderson *et al.*, 2003). Specifically designed PPN solutions are available, but there are limits to the electrolyte additions that can be made, particularly potassium; PPN is therefore not suitable for patients with high requirements or those requiring a fluid restriction.

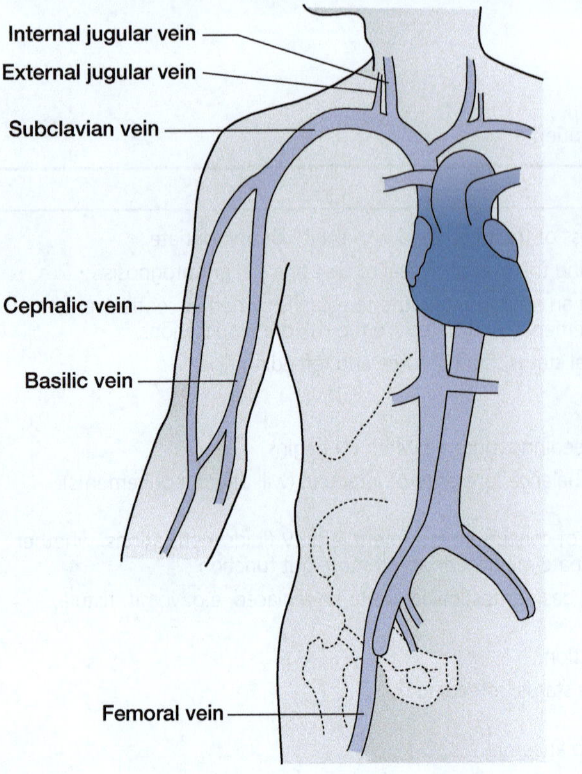

Figure 6.5.1 Access routes for parenteral nutrition (source: Dougherty & Lamb (2008); figure 10.1, p. 263. Reproduced with permission from Blackwell Publishing)

Central Access Routes

Central venous catheters (CVCs) may be placed in the jugular (neck), subclavian (chest) or femoral (groin) veins (see Figure 6.5.1). Jugular lines are easy to access but can be difficult to secure and uncomfortable. Femoral veins may increase the risk of infection due to the proximity of urine, stoma or fistulae. Guidelines for CVC management encompass insertion and subsequent care (Loveday *et al.*, 2014; Pittiruti *et al.*, 2009). Confirmation of the correct placement, tip position and the absence of insertion-related complications should be ascertained before feeding is commenced. A variety of CVCs are available for PN:

- Short-term single or multi-lumen, non-tunnelled catheters. Multi-lumen catheters may contain two to five separate lumens, where one lumen should be dedicated solely for PN use.
- Single- or multi-lumen tunnelled lines where the skin entry point is away from entry into the vein.
- Peripherally inserted central catheters (PICCs), normally inserted at the elbow (antecubital fossa), with the end advanced into a central vein.
- Implantable devices (ports); the port, attached to a catheter, sits under the skin and is accessed by piercing the skin with a needle.

A CVC should be used with the minimum number of lumens essential for the management of the patient (Loveday *et al.*, 2014). PICC are recommended for short-medium-term use, however, they can limit arm movement and can be prone to occlusion or kinking (Cowl *et al.*, 2000). For long-term feeding, a tunnelled CVC or implantable port are recommended (Pittiruti *et al.*, 2009).

Administration

To reduce infection, PN bags should only be administered by healthcare professionals, patients or carers who are assessed as competent and adhere to policies that prevent catheter-related blood stream infections (Loveday *et al.*, 2014). Most PN is administered continuously over 24 hours, but cyclical infusion may have physiological and psychological advantages, can reduce thrombophlebitis in PPN and is recommended by bodies such as NICE (2006) once the patient is biochemically stable.

Formulations

PN regimens should be formulated after the assessment of individual patient requirements. Although this usually involves a dietitian, only doctors could prescribe PN bags until recently. However, in 2016, dietitians achieved supplementary prescribing status, thereby facilitating greater autonomy. It is anticipated that this will lead to more efficient and cost-effective inpatient and home PN (HPN) patient management, and that it will contribute to improved clinical outcomes.

Various PN regimens are available, and local decision-making will depend on pharmacy compounding facilities, contractual arrangements and the need for specialist feeds to suit specific patient populations, e.g. renal. The main forms of PN regimen are:

- Ready-made, multi-chamber, all in one (AIO) bags, containing carbohydrate, amino acids and fat sources in separate chambers, with or without electrolytes, to be mixed just before use. These have a long shelf life before they are mixed, but do not contain micronutrients and are not recommended unless vitamins and trace elements are added (NICE, 2006). Depending on pharmacy compounding facilities, it may be possible to make additional electrolyte additions if required.
- Tailored bespoke bags are made specifically to an individual's requirements but require adequately resourced aseptic unit facilities.

Stability is affected by the volume, proportion and formulation of different constituents. Therefore, the final volume or electrolyte content may not achieve estimated requirements, and all formulation requests should be discussed with the pharmacist. Bags with all additions should be made under full pharmacy aseptic conditions, with no subsequent tampering that might increase infection risk or compromise stability. A range of multi-chamber bags should be stocked (to suit low and high electrolyte requirements), with bespoke bags available for those patients with specific needs not met by the AIO range.

Constituents

Macronutrients

Energy and protein requirements should be estimated by standard methods (Chapter 6.1, Nutritional requirements in clinical practice). In AIO regimens, the amount and percentage of macronutrients is fixed, whereas tailored regimens offer flexibility to modify the proportions of fat, carbohydrates and amino acids, and may hence be indicated in specific circumstances, e.g. reduced fat content required to minimise hepatobiliary complications in long-term PN.

Protein

Protein is supplied as a balanced mixture of crystalline amino acids, or dipeptides for the less soluble heat-labile amino acids. The optimal PN amino acid profile remains unclear. Standard AIO formulations provide 5–18 g nitrogen. It may be possible to exceed this amount in tailored regimens, depending on stability limits. Glutamine is not present in most commercially available amino acid solutions due to its instability. However, it can be added to a PN bag with other additions prior to administration.

Fat

PN lipid emulsions offer an energy-dense isotonic alternative to dextrose and normally provide <50% of non-nitrogen energy needs. Typical PN regimens provide 400–1000 kcal/day. The first commercially available solutions contained long-chain triglycerides (LCTs) from soya bean oils, rich in n-6 polyunsaturated fatty acids (PUFA). Lipid emulsions contain essential fatty acids (EFA) which maintain cell membrane integrity and immune function. In long-term totally-PN-fed patients, it is recommended that a minimal supply of 1 g/kg/week be given to prevent EFA deficiency (Pironi *et al.*, 2016). The high n-6 content of soya bean lipid may have adverse effects on immune function, particularly in critically ill patients (Furukawa *et al.*, 1999), and excessive amounts have been implicated in hypertriglyceridaemia and hepatobiliary disease. To prevent intestinal-failure-related liver disease in long-term PN-fed patients, soya bean lipid amounts should be less than 1 g/kg/day (Pironi *et al.*, 2016). Newer formulations contain mixtures of lipid sources in various combinations, e.g. monounsaturated from olive oil, medium-chain triglycerides (MCTs) from coconut oil and n-3 PUFA from fish oil. These have been shown to offer clinical benefits over soya-bean-oil-based solutions. However, studies are based on small numbers in diverse clinical situations, and the optimal lipid profile for different conditions remains unclear (Calder *et al.*, 2015).

Carbohydrate

Glucose is available in concentrations of 5–70%, and typical PN regimens provide 400–1200 kcal/day. To avoid excessive amounts, a maximum glucose oxidation rate (GOR) of 4–7 mg/kg/min has been suggested (Burke *et al.*, 1979). If a balance of both lipid and carbohydrate is given, this should not be exceeded.

Electrolytes

The electrolyte content of PN should be based on individual patient requirements, including additional amounts to cover losses (fistula, vomit, refeeding risk) or reductions (renal impairment, fluid overload). Recommendations for electrolyte requirements given intravenously differ from oral and enteral routes. When determining PN electrolyte content, it is important to consider the contribution from intravenous infusions and medications and to discuss with the medical team whether these will continue once PN starts.

Electrolyte additions should be modified according to serum trends rather than single levels (see Table 6.5.2). If PN electrolyte additions cannot meet requirements, supplementary electrolytes may need to be infused separately.

Micronutrients

Vitamins and trace elements should always be included in PN prescriptions. They are normally provided by standard vitamin and trace element solutions devised for PN. However, these may be inadequate to replete body stores, and, in severe malnutrition or metabolic stress, additional amounts may be needed. As intravenous administration bypasses the normal process of selective absorption and liver processing, this may increase the risk of overdosage of some micronutrients (Buchman *et al.*, 2009). There should be local policies in place regarding the measurement and interpretation of micronutrient results, recommended frequency of testing and appropriate supplementation, as PN additions (if possible) or separately.

Table 6.5.2 Adjustments of parenteral nutrition formulations in response to monitoring

Electrolyte	Standard requirement[a] (not considering replacement of additional losses)	Usual level of adjustment[b]	Changes unlikely to be clinically significant[b]
Sodium	1.0–1.5 mmol/kg	Multiples of 40 mmol/day	±10–20 mmol
Potassium	1.0–1.5 mmol/kg	Multiples of 20 mmol/day	±5–10 mmol
Magnesium	0.1–0.2 mmol/kg	5–10 mmol/day	0–5 mmol
Calcium	0.1–0.15 mmol/kg	2.5–5 mmol/day	0–2.5 mmol
Phosphate	0.3–0.5 mmol/kg	10 mmol/day	0–5 mmol

[a] Elia (1990);
[b] Austin and Stroud (2007).

Fluid

Individual fluid requirements should be calculated in the usual way (see Chapter 6.6, Fluids and electrolytes). PN regimens commonly provide 2000–3500 mL/day. Lower and higher volumes are available, but stability issues may affect macronutrient and electrolyte contents. PN volume should always be recorded and considered when determining IV fluid requirements to prevent excess fluid delivery and clinical overload, a significant problem noted by NCEPOD (2010). Consideration should also be given to the sodium content of the fluid used (Powell-Tuck *et al.*, 2011).

Initiating Parenteral Nutrition

It is recommended that initial PN regimens aim for approximately 50% of energy requirements, unless the patient is considered to be at risk of re-feeding syndrome. In those assessed as high risk, lower initial energy intakes of 5–10 kcal/kg/day are recommended (NICE, 2006), although it may be more appropriate physiologically to restrict carbohydrate rather than total energy provision. To minimise refeeding problems, it is also vital that electrolytes and micronutrients are administered from the outset of feeding, and that serum electrolytes are monitored and proactively supplemented. As thiamin requirements are increased to support carbohydrate metabolism in the refeeding phase, additional IV B vitamin supplementation is required immediately prior to PN administration and for the first 3–10 days (depending on refeeding risk).

Monitoring

Monitoring of clinical state, nutritional requirements, anthropometry, biochemistry and line integrity is essential. Daily biochemical monitoring should generally be undertaken for the first 3 days and until levels normalise. The range and frequency of monitoring will then depend on the nature and severity of illness, degree of malnutrition and length of time on PN. Cardiac monitoring is recommended for any patients at extremely high risk of refeeding syndrome and those with pre-existing cardiac arrhythmias (Austin & Stroud, 2007).

Complications

Metabolic complications

Adaptive reductions in cellular activity and organ function in starvation are accompanied by intracellular micronutrient, mineral and electrolyte losses (Stanga *et al.*, 2008). Upon re-feeding, the greater the carbohydrate load (with associated insulin response), the more significant the cellular re-uptake and falls in serum electrolytes. Retention of sodium and fluid, hypokalaemia, hypophosphataemia and hypomagnesaemia (due to rapid intracellular uptake of potassium, phosphate and magnesium for cellular recovery and metabolic activity) may then ensue. Thiamin depletion due to increased metabolic activity and glucose and lipid metabolic abnormalities may also occur. These complications may lead to oedema, cardiac overload and failure, respiratory problems, liver function abnormalities, gastro-intestinal problems and potentially death (Crook, 2001; Stanga *et al.*, 2008; Tomlin *et al.*, 2007).

Refeeding problems may present a greater risk in PN as it bypasses the enteral route, which limits the tolerance and absorption of nutrients. NCEPOD (2010) reported a PN metabolic complication rate of 39%, with hypophosphataemia being the most commonly recorded problem. The relative incidence of refeeding syndrome in PN, rather than oral or enterally fed patients, is not known, but it has been reported that hypophosphataemia is less common in high-risk PN-fed patients than in those on nasogastric feeds (Zeki *et al.*, 2011). Table 6.5.3 provides details of potential metabolic complications, possible causes and risk reduction guidance.

Mechanical complications

Insertion-related complications include insertion failure, pneumothorax or haemothorax, thrombosis, cardiac arrhythmias and nerve injury (Bowling, 2004). Longer-term complications include thrombus, catheter-occlusion or fracture.

Infectious complications

CVC-related infections may originate from endogenous skin flora (most common), contamination of the catheter

Table 6.5.3 Potential metabolic complications of parenteral nutrition

Complication	Possible causes	Prevention
Over-hydration, oedema	Provision of excessive or inappropriate fluid/sodium.	Detailed assessment of patient needs, including losses. Consider other concurrent sources of fluid prior to deciding on PN volume.
Hyperglycaemia	Excessive provision of glucose. Severe metabolic stress. Inappropriate insulin treatment.	Glucose oxidation rate should not be exceeded. Blood glucose should be regularly monitored. Insulin should be provided if required.
Electrolyte abnormalities, including refeeding syndrome	Inadequate electrolytes or excessive glucose, especially initially.	Detailed assessment and monitoring. Proactive supplementation according to local guidance and clinical advice.
Deranged liver function tests	Common in patients given PN, but feed is rarely the main cause (Culkin & Gabe, 2010).	Exclude sepsis, medication, underlying liver disease. Review total energy to avoid overfeeding. Consider type of fat given. Consider cyclical feeding.
Hypertriglyceridaemia	Metabolic capacity of the liver to clear fat is exceeded.	Avoid excessive lipid provision Monitor Reduce or occasionally remove lipid from PN (Llop *et al.*, 2003).

hub or contamination of the CVC from a distant site. Catheter-related sepsis is a serious concern and requires immediate treatment according to local policies. It can be prevented by strict adherence to aseptic techniques, only experienced staff being permitted to handle PN lines, using closed systems, and using dedicated lines where possible (Loveday *et al.*, 2014).

Weaning from parenteral nutrition

PN should never be stopped abruptly as rebound hypoglycaemia can occur. As IF resolves, oral or enteral nutrition should be reintroduced, accompanied by a reduction in PN infusion rate, avoiding fluid overload, overfeeding and electrolyte imbalances. This can be achieved by slowing the infusion rate or by compounding a series of individually modified bags. Supplementary PN should not impair appetite (Reifen *et al.*, 1999), although many PN patients express early satiety and may be anxious about increasing oral intake, particularly after a prolonged period of gut rest, and may need appropriate support and advice.

Home parenteral nutrition

Home parenteral nutrition (HPN) is indicated in permanent IF, or if a prolonged period of PN is required prior to further surgery to restore gastrointestinal function. Patients should be referred to specialist centres with experience in managing longer-term considerations such as hepatobiliary, metabolic and nutritional complications (e.g. micronutrient status), venous access issues and management of the underlying IF (Nightingale, 2003).

Regimens may differ significantly from inpatient regimens in terms of their composition and frequency, based on variable nutritional needs and activity levels. Infusions are commonly administered overnight to allow increased mobility during the day. To avoid hepatobiliary complications, total energy or lipid content may be reduced, and some fat-free bags may be indicated. Provided that fluid balance is maintained, some patients may not require daily feeds.

Further reading

Austin P, Stroud M. (2007) *Prescribing Adult Intravenous Nutrition*. London: Pharmaceutical Press.

Bowling T. (2004) *Nutritional Support for Adults and Children: A Handbook for Hospital Practice*. Oxford: Radcliffe Medical Press.

Micklewright A, Todorovic V. (2005) *A Pocket Guide to Clinical Nutrition*. Birmingham: PEN Group Publications.

Internet resources

British Association for Parenteral & Enteral Nutrition (BAPEN), www.bapen.org.uk

National Confidential Enquiry into Patient Outcome and Death, www.ncepod.org.uk

Parenteral and Enteral Nutrition Group (PENG) of the British Dietetic Association, www.peng.org.uk

Patients on Intravenous & Nasogastric Nutrition Therapy (PINNT), www.pinnt.com

References

Anderson ADG, Palmer D, Macfie F. (2003) Peripheral parenteral nutrition. *Br. J. Surg*. 90(9): 1048–1054.

Austin P, Stroud M. (2007) *Prescribing Adult Intravenous Nutrition*. London: Pharmaceutical Press.

Bowling T. (2004) *Nutritional Support for Adults and Children: A Handbook for Hospital Practice*. Oxford: Radcliffe Medical Press.

Bozzetti F, Arends J, Lundholm K, *et al.* (2009) ESPEN Guidelines on Parenteral Nutrition: non-surgical oncology. *Clin. Nutr.* 28: 445–454.

Bozzetti F, Staun M, Van Gossum A. (2014) *Home Parenteral Nutrition*. Wallingfrod, Oxfordshire: CABI.

Buchman AL, Howard LJ, Guenter P, *et al.* (2009) Micronutrients in parenteral nutrition: too little or too much? The past, present and recommendations for the future. *Gastroenterology* 137: S1–S6

Burke JF, Wolfe RR, Mullany CJ, *et al.* (1979) Glucose requirements following burn injury. Parameters of optimal glucose infusion and possible hepatic and respiratory abnormalities following excessive glucose intake. *Ann. Surg.* 190(3): 274–285.

Calder PC, Waitzberg DL, Kolezkko B (ed). (2015) *Intravenous Lipid Emulsions. World Rev. Nutr.* Karger Publishing. (doi:10.1159/000367703).

Cowl CT, Weinstock JV, Al Jurf A, *et al.* (2000) Complications and cost associated with parenteral nutrition delivered to hospitalised patients through either subclavian or peripherally-inserted central catheters. *Clin. Nutr.* 19(4): 237–243.

Crook MA, Hally V, Panteli JV. (2001) The importance of the refeeding syndrome. *Nutrition* 17(7–8): 632–637.

Culkin A, Gabe SM. (2010) Abnormal liver function tests in the parenteral nutrition fed patient. *Frontline. Gastroenterol.* 1: 98–104.

Dougherty L, Lamb J. (eds), *Intravenous Therapy in Nursing Practice.* Oxford: Blackwell.

Elia M. (1990) Artificial nutrition support. *Med. Int.* 82: 3392–3396.

Furukawa K, Tashiro T, Yamamori H, *et al.* (1999) Effects of soybean oil emulsion and eicosapentaenoic acid on stress response and immune function after a severely stressful operation. *Ann. Surg.* 229: 255–261.

Hvas CL, Farrer K, Donaldson E, *et al.* (2014) Quality and safety impact on the provision of parenteral nutrition through introduction of a nutrition support team. *Eur. J. Clin. Nutr.* 68: 1294–1299.

Kennedy JF, Nightingale JMD. (2005) Cost savings of an adult hospital nutrition support team. *Nutrition* 21(11): 1127–1133.

Koretz RL, Lipman TO, Klein S. (2001) AGA technical review on parenteral nutrition. *Gastroenterology* 121(4): 970–1001.

Llop J, Sabin P, Garaw M, *et al.* (2003) The importance of clinical factors in parenteral nutrition associated hypertriglyceridemia. *Clin. Nutr.* 22(6): 577–583.

Loveday HP, Wilson JA, Pratt RJ, *et al.* (2014) EPIC3: National evidence-based guidelines for preventing healthcare-associated infections in NHS hospitals in England. *J. Hosp. Infect.* 86(1): S1–S70.

National Confidential Enquiry into Patient Outcome and Death (NCEPOD). (2010) *A mixed bag. An enquiry into the care of hospital patients receiving parenteral nutrition*. Available at https://www.ncepod.org.uk/2010pn.html. Accessed 9 August 2013.

NICE. (2006) *Nutrition Support in Adults. Clinical Guideline 32.* Available at https://www.nice.org.uk/guidance/cg32 Accessed 21 February 2019.

Nightingale JM. (2003) Hepatobiliary, renal and bone complications of intestinal failure. *Best Pract. Res. Clin. Gastroenterol.* 17(6): 907–929.

Pittiruti M, Hamilton H, Biffi R, *et al.* (2009) ESPEN guidelines on parenteral nutrition: central venous catheters (access, care, diagnosis and therapy of complications). *Clin. Nutr.* 28: 365–377.

Pironi L, Arends J, Bozzetti F, et al. (2016) ESPEN guidelines on chronic intestinal failure in adults. *Clin. Nutr.* 35: 247–307.

Powell-Tuck J, Gosling P, Lobo DN, et al. (2011). British Consensus Guidelines on Intravenous Fluid Therapy for Adult Surgical Patients GIFTASUP. Available at http://www.bapen.org.uk/pdfs/bapen_pubs/giftasup.pdf. Accessed online 20 July 2011.

Reifen R, Khoshoo V, Dinari G. (1999) Effect of parenteral nutrition on oral intake. *J. Pediatr. Endocrinol. Metab.* 12: 203–205.

Shang E, Weiss C, Post S, *et al.* (2006) The influence of early supplementation of parenteral nutrition on quality of life and body composition in patients with advanced cancer. *JPEN J. Parenter. Enteral. Nutr.* 30: 222–230.

Stanga Z, Brunner A, Leuenberger M, *et al.* (2008) Nutrition in Clinical Practice – the refeeding syndrome: illustrative cases and guidelines for prevention and treatment. *Eur. J. Clin. Nutr.* 62: 687–694.

Tenner S, Baillie J, DeWitt J, *et al.* (2013) American College of Gastroenterology guideline: management of acute pancreatitis. *Am. J. Gastroenterol.* 108: 1400–1415.

Tomlin G, O'Connor M, Dehavillande J, *et al.* (2007) Guidelines for the Prevention and Management of the Re-feeding Syndrome. Oxford: Radcliffe Hospitals.

Wheble GAC, Knight WR, Khan OA. (2012) Enteral vs total parenteral nutrition following major upper gastrointestinal surgery. *Int. J. Surg.* 10(4): 194–197.

Zeki S, Culkin A, Gabe SM, *et al.* (2011) Refeeding hypophosphataemia is more common in enteral than parenteral feeding in adult patients. *Clin. Nutr.* 30(3): 365–368.

6.6 Fluids and electrolytes

Rebecca Lindstrom Sowman and Claudia Rueb

Key points

- Water is essential for survival and has many functions in the body.
- Regulation of body fluid is under tight homeostatic control; maintenance of fluid balance is an important aspect of dietetic management.
- Disorders of electrolyte and water balance are common in clinical practice, particularly as a result of surgery, trauma, disease and drug therapy.
- Managing fluids and electrolytes is complex and can be challenging; it requires extensive knowledge and experience, usually from a lead clinician.

Humans can survive for several weeks without food, but cannot withstand water deprivation for more than a few days. Water has many vital functions in the body, including:

- As a solvent for ions and molecules.
- As a transport medium, especially for the excretion of osmotically active solutes such as urea and salts.
- As a lubricant.
- In temperature regulation.

Body fluids

Water is the most abundant body fluid and accounts for approximately 60% total body weight in men and 50% in women. Lean body tissue has a high water content of 75%, in contrast to 10% in adipose tissue. In obese patients, lean body weight should be used to determine total body water (TBW).

Body fluid compartments

Total body water has two main compartments: intracellular fluid (ICF, 67%) within the cells, and extracellular fluid (ECF, 33%) outside the cells. Extracellular fluid is further subdivided into interstitial fluid, which includes the fluid surrounding the cells and the fluid of the lymphatic system, and intravascular fluid, the fluid portion of the blood (plasma volume) (see Figure 6.6.1).

Movement and regulation of fluids

A number of processes determine the movement of water and other substances between body fluid compartments. Cell membranes can be permeable, semi-permeable or impermeable to certain molecules, and act as an effective barrier between the cell and interstitial fluid by controlling the exchange of solutes and water. The movement of water across semi-permeable membranes is known as osmosis; water moves into an area of higher solute concentration to achieve equilibrium.

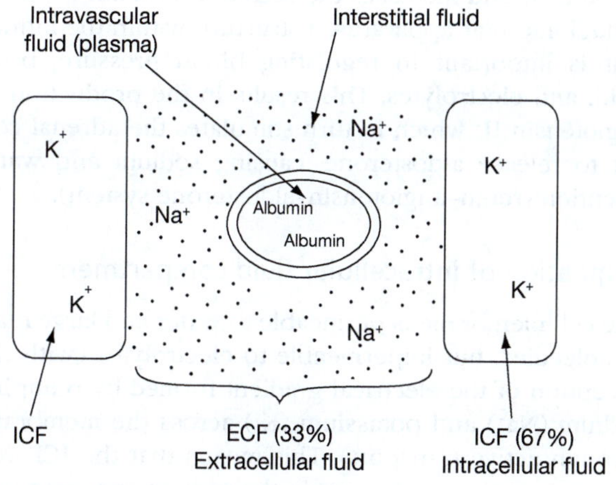

Figure 6.6.1 Body fluid compartments

Manual of Dietetic Practice, Sixth Edition. Edited by Joan Gandy.

Companion website: www.manualofdieteticpractice.com

Osmotic pressure of a solution is the pressure by which water is drawn into it through the semi-permeable membrane, and is often used to express the concentration of the solution (the more solutes, the greater its osmotic pressure). Each fluid compartment contains one principle solute that determines the osmotic pressure. The effective osmotic pressure of a solution is also known as tonicity, and is maintained by the following factors:

- Potassium retains water in the intracellular space.
- Sodium retains water in the extracellular space.
- Plasma proteins retain water in the intravascular space; albumin is the most important plasma protein in maintaining oncotic pressure. Oncotic pressure is the osmotic pressure of a solution with colloids (proteins) as the main solute.

Regulation of extracellular fluid compartment

The volume of the ECF is controlled by the sodium content, and homeostatic mechanisms are directed at controlling the retention or excretion of sodium. Sodium homeostasis depends on renal excretion. An increased intake in sodium leads to a higher ECF osmolarity, which triggers thirst and the release of antidiuretic hormone (ADH) (vasopressin). The presence of ADH leads to the passive reabsorption of water by the kidneys and allows osmolarity to return to normal by increasing the ECF volume. This in turn triggers a different pathway to stimulate sodium and water loss, and the ECF will return back to normal. Altered ECF (changes in blood volume and subsequently blood pressure) can be detected by volume receptors in the large veins and atrium of the heart. The volume receptors trigger a pathway that affects ADH release and regulates the kidneys' production of urine. The kidneys also play a significant role in controlling the ECF volume. A reduction in blood pressure reduces renal blood flow and increases the secretion of renin from the juxtaglomerular apparatus, a structure within the kidney that is important in regulating blood pressure, body fluid, and electrolytes. This results in the production of angiotensin II, which in turn stimulates the adrenal cortex to release aldosterone, causing sodium and water retention (renin–angiotensin–aldosterone system).

Regulation of intracellular fluid compartment

The cell membrane is permeable to water and large macromolecules, but impermeable to electrolytes (with the exception of the electrical gradient formed by pumping sodium (Na^+) and potassium (K^+) across the membrane through active transport). This means that the ICF volume is sensitive to changes in the sodium concentration of the ECF. A high ECF sodium concentration will result in water moving out of the cells by osmosis, causing cells to shrink; with low ECF sodium concentration, water will move into the cells, and they swell. Cell function can be impaired as a result of the change in cell volume, and the brain in particular can be affected by swelling. Maintaining extracellular fluid osmolarity is therefore paramount.

Fluid balance

Water homeostasis is dependent on the control of water intake and water output, and is regulated on three levels:

- Gastrointestinal tract – fluids and electrolytes are produced and mostly reabsorbed along the GI tract.
- Kidneys – sodium and water excretion is largely regulated via ADH.
- Renin–angiotensin–aldosterone system – this regulates sodium excretion and blood pressure.

If any of these systems fail or begin to fail, fluid and electrolyte imbalances may occur.

Disorders of sodium and water balance

Disorders of sodium (and other electrolytes) and water balance are a common occurrence in clinical practice, particularly as a result of surgery, trauma, disease and drug therapy. Appropriate treatment to correct any disorder needs to be based on a careful physical examination and interpretation of both serum and urine biochemistry. Any disorders of sodium and water balance will be reflected in the serum sodium concentration.

Sodium deficit

Sodium cannot be lost from the body without water. A sodium deficit may occur as a result of gastrointestinal losses, e.g. diarrhoea, diuretic therapy, Addison's disease, diabetic ketoacidosis, ascites and chronic kidney disease. The result is a decrease in the ECF volume, with associated hypertension and tachycardia. If the sodium deficit is severe, there is a risk of circulatory failure and renal failure, although ICF levels are unaffected. In the case of a sodium deficit, it is the total amount of ECF sodium that is important. There may be little change in the serum sodium concentration as water loss may increase as a compensatory effect. Sodium deficiency is normally treated with intravenous infusion of 0.9% sodium chloride.

Sodium excess

This can be the result of reduced sodium excretion, e.g. renal sodium retention secondary to kidney disease, primary or secondary aldosteronism; another cause can be the intravenous administration of sodium bicarbonate to correct metabolic acidosis in the clinical setting; or large volumes of 0.9% saline where there are hypotonic losses such as in diabetes mellitus. Sodium retention leads to expansion of the ECF volume where oedema and hypertension may be present. Increased serum sodium may stimulate thirst.

Water deficit

Water deficit usually results from an inadequate intake, often due to the inability to drink, inadequate intravenous fluid or excessive loss. Thirst and oliguria with highly concentrated urine will normally be present.

There is less effect on the ECF volume than from the loss of a similar volume of isotonic fluid; hypernatraemia is usually present.

Water excess

This is usually caused by either impaired water excretion, e.g. inappropriate (increased ADH secretion or renal failure) or excessive water intake, usually in association with impaired excretion. If severe, cerebral overhydration and oedema can occur; hyponatraemia is usually present.

Sodium

Sodium (Na^+) is the principal extracellular cation and controls the volume of the extracellular fluid in the body. The average dietary sodium intake in the UK is 8.1 g/day (138 mmol/day). A small amount of sodium is lost via sweat and faeces; the majority is excreted via the kidneys. Urinary sodium levels usually reflect dietary sodium intake, unless there are significant extrarenal losses such as diarrhoea or vomiting.

Hyponatraemia

Hyponatraemia is defined as a serum sodium level of <135 mmol/L. Risk factors include increasing age, lower body weight, thiazide and thiazide-like diuretics, hypotonic intravenous fluids and surgery.

Symptoms

Clinical manifestations of moderate hyponatraemia (serum sodium 125–129 mmol/L) can be nausea, headache and confusion. Severe hyponatraemia (serum sodium level <125 mmol/L) is associated with vomiting, agitation, psychosis and seizures.

Diagnosis and management

The main cause of hyponatraemia is an imbalance between extracellular water and sodium, where water is in excess as opposed to sodium. In order to treat this condition successfully, it is helpful to understand the aetiology of hyponatraemia. Serum osmolality (serum tonicity) describes the amount of chemicals dissolved in the liquid component (serum) of the blood, including sodium, chloride, bicarbonate, protein and glucose, and is used as a first step to categorise hyponatraemia. If a measurement is not available, serum osmolality can be estimated as $2 \times (Na^+ + K^+) + urea + glucose$ (mmol/L).

For example $2 \times (Na^+\ 136 + K^+\ 4.2) + urea\ 5.0 + glucose\ 4.1 = 287$ mmol/kg H_2O.

Normal serum osmolality is 275–290 mmol/kg H_2O, but reference ranges vary slightly.

Hyponatraemia can be classified as:

- Hypertonic hyponatraemia: serum osmolality >290 mmol/kg H_2O.
  - High serum tonicity, e.g. hyperglycaemia.
- Isotonic hyponatraemia: serum osmolality 275–290 mmol/kg H_2O.
  - Normal serum tonicity, caused by hyperlipidaemia, hyperproteinaemia.
- Hypotonic hyponatraemia: serum osmolality <275 mmol/kg H_2O.
  - Low serum tonicity.

Hypotonic hyponatraemia can occur with decreased, normal or increased existing sodium stores (i.e. hypovolaemic, euvolaemic and hypervolaemic hyponatraemia, respectively) (see Table 6.6.1).

Management of non-hypotonic hyponatraemia

This focuses on the underlying disorder rather than the hyponatraemia itself.

Management of hypotonic hyponatraemia

Treating patients with euvolaemic and hypervolaemic hyponatraemia successfully means eliminating the underlying cause as well as restricting water. In symptomatic hyponatraemia, the use of hypertonic saline

Table 6.6.1 Hypotonic hyponatraemia

States of hypotonic hyponatraemia	Changes in water and/or sodium	Underlying cause
Hypovolaemia	Loss of water and sodium	Renal: urinary sodium >20 mmol/L • Thiazide diuretics, salt-wasting nephropathy • Ketonuria, adrenal insufficiency
		Extrarenal: urinary sodium <20 mmol/L • Gastrointestinal losses • Excessive sweating, blood loss
Euvolaemia	Increase in water	Hypothyroidism, polydipsia
		SIADH, post-operative state
Hypervolaemia	Increase in sodium and water	Urinary sodium >20 mmol/L • Renal failure
		Urinary sodium <20 mmol/L • Disorders associated with oedema (e.g. congestive cardiac failure, liver cirrhosis, nephrotic syndrome)

SIADH, syndrome of inappropriate secretion of antidiuretic hormone.

SECTION 6

(e.g. 3% NaCl) may be necessary to achieve a satisfactory increase in sodium, and furosemide is often used in combination to limit treatment-induced expansion of extracellular fluid volume. Most patients with hypovolaemic hyponatraemia can be treated successfully with isotonic saline (0.9% NaCl). Correction of serum sodium levels should not exceed 8–10 mmol/L per 24 hours to prevent irreversible brain damage.

Hypernatraemia

Hypernatraemia is defined as a serum sodium level of >145 mmol/L. Patients at risk of developing an elevated serum sodium level are those with a decreased ability to recognise thirst, or those with reduced access to water. This includes infants, the elderly and patients with altered cognitive function or mental status.

Symptoms

Clinical manifestations of moderate hypernatraemia (serum sodium of 151–160 mmol/L) include excessive thirst, anorexia, insomnia and muscle twitching, while severe hypernatraemia (serum sodium level >160 mmol/L) is associated with altered mental status, irritability, seizures and coma.

Diagnosis and management

The main cause of hypernatraemia is an imbalance between extracellular water and sodium, with an excess of sodium. Hypernatraemia can occur with decreased, normal or increased total body sodium (i.e. hypovolaemic, euvolaemic and hypervolaemic hypernatraemia, respectively). In order to treat this condition successfully, it is helpful to understand the aetiology of hypernatraemia (see Table 6.6.2). Treating hypernatraemia successfully means eliminating the underlying cause as well as correcting the lack of water.

When replacing water, fluids should ideally be given orally or enterally via a feeding tube. If there is no enteral access available, fluids should be administered intravenously. Infusates should be hypotonic (e.g. 5% glucose and 0.45% NaCl), and serum sodium levels should not be corrected by >10 mmol/L per 24 hours to avoid cerebral oedema and convulsions.

Potassium

Potassium (K^+) is the principal intracellular cation in contrast to sodium, which is the major extracellular cation. The sodium–potassium ATPase pump in the cell membrane maintains the difference in distribution of the two cations by pumping three sodium ions out of cells in exchange for two potassium ions. The ratio of the potassium concentrations in the extracellular fluids and in the cells is the main determinant of the resting membrane potential, which is essential for normal muscle and neural function. Both hypo- and hyperkalaemia can therefore cause muscle paralysis and potentially fatal cardiac arrhythmias.

Hypokalaemia

A range of clinical conditions can result in hypokalaemia, which may occur with or without potassium loss. It is generally defined as a serum potassium level of <3.5 mmol/L. In case of potassium depletion, the kidney can significantly reduce potassium excretion; insufficient intake is therefore rarely the sole cause for hypokalaemia. Its causes include:

- Hypokalaemia without potassium loss:
  - Alkalosis (results in the movement of K^+ into cells in exchange for an equimolar number of H^+).
  - Insulin excess (drives K^+ into cells, may be more noticeable during the treatment of diabetic ketoacidosis (DKA) or nonketotic hyperglycaemia).
  - Increased cellular uptake (e.g. treatment of megaloblastic anaemia).
  - Refeeding syndrome.
  - Elevated beta2-adrenergic activity (catecholamines regulate potassium entry into cells by increasing the activity of the sodium–potassium ATPase pump).
- Hypokalaemia with potassium loss:
  - Gastrointestinal loss – vomiting, diarrhoea, laxatives.
  - Excess alcohol.

Table 6.6.2 Identifying cause and management of hypernatraemia

States of hypernatraemia	Changes in water and/or sodium	Underlying cause
Hypovolaemia	Loss of water and sodium	Renal: >20 mmol/L urinary sodium • Renal failure • Diuretics Extrarenal: <20 mmol/L urinary sodium • Gastrointestinal losses • Excessive sweating, fever • Burns
Euvolaemia	Loss of water	Diabetes insipidus
Hypervolaemia	Increase in sodium	Cushing's syndrome Primary hyperaldosteronism Excess administration of sodium-containing IV fluids

- Urinary loss – primary aldosteronism, type 1 and 2 renal tubular acidosis, diuretics, corticosteroids, leukaemia, hypomagnesaemia, polyuria, excess intake of liquorice.

Management

The immediate goal of treatment is to raise serum potassium to a safe level and for the underlying cause to be identified and treated. The amount of potassium required depends on the severity of hypokalaemia, clinical situation, renal function and if the cause of hypokalaemia has been addressed. In mild to moderate hypokalaemia, potassium can often be given orally, but may result in gastrointestinal side effects, e.g. nausea, vomiting and diarrhoea. Potassium is often administered intravenously as potassium chloride (KCl) in a controlled manner to reduce the risk of hyperkalaemia.

Hyperkalaemia

Acute, severe hyperkalaemia requires urgent treatment. The threshold for emergency treatment varies, but most guidelines recommend that emergency treatment be given if the serum potassium is ≥6.5 mmol/L with or without ECG changes. Hyperkalaemia occurs in a variety of clinical settings, but is usually a result of renal failure. Dietary-induced hyperkalaemia generally involves concurrent renal insufficiency. Causes of hyperkalaemia include:

- Increased potassium release from cells:
  - Insulin deficiency – DKA, hyperosmolar / hyperglycaemic state.
  - Metabolic acidosis.
  - Pseudohyperkalaemia, e.g. release of intracellular K^+ during phlebotomy.
  - Catabolic states, e.g. tumour lysis syndrome and rhabdomyolysis (recent history of muscle damage relating to seizures, ischaemia, exercise, trauma or medications such as statins, etc.).
  - Drug related (e.g. beta blockers, digoxin and suxamethonium).
  - Hyperkalaemic periodic paralysis.
- Reduced urinary potassium excretion:
  - Acute and chronic kidney disease.
  - Hypoaldosteronism.
  - Addison's disease (primary adrenal insufficiency).
  - Certain drugs, e.g. angiotensin inhibitors, non-steroidal anti-inflammatory drugs, heparin and potassium-sparing diuretics (e.g. Spironolactone).

Management

In acute hyperkalaemia, the aim is to protect the myocardium and increase intracellular potassium. There is limited evidence to guide treatment, and practice varies. However, treatment generally includes:

- Intravenous calcium salt (gluconate or chloride) to temporarily protect against myocardial excitability.
- Intravenous insulin–glucose infusion to reduce serum potassium concentrations.

Any prescribed drugs exacerbating hyperkalaemia should be discontinued if possible. Chronic hyperkalaemia is usually managed by using cation-binding resins, diuretics (where appropriate) and dietary restriction of potassium. Renal replacement therapy, such as haemodialysis, peritoneal dialysis and kidney transplantation, may be necessary.

Calcium

Calcium (Ca^{2+}) is the body's most abundant divalent cation and has vital roles in regulating neuromuscular function, hormone release, myocardial contractibility and enzyme activity. The most significant effect of altered plasma calcium concentrations is related to the excitability of the nervous system. Serum calcium is under tight homeostatic control; hence, even when calcium intake is inadequate, blood calcium remains normal, but at the expense of bone loss. About half of the total serum calcium is bound to protein, and the remaining free ionised calcium is physiologically active. Therefore, before making a diagnosis of hypercalcaemia or hypocalcaemia, serum calcium levels must be corrected for albumin levels. Fibre, in general, and the binders phytate and oxalate inhibit calcium absorption, but unless consumed in excess they are not a significant contributor to calcium loss. Severe hypocalcaemia and hypercalcaemia are both potentially life threatening, requiring urgent treatment.

Hypocalcaemia

Causes of hypocalcaemia include:

- Low parathyroid hormone (PTH).
  - Hypoparathyroidism.
  - Hypomagnesaemia.
- Hungry bone syndrome (post parathyroidectomy).
- Acute pancreatitis.
- Vitamin D deficiency.
- Hyperphosphataemia.
- Large-volume blood transfusions.
- Critical illness.
- Drugs (e.g. bisphosphonates).
- Rhabdomyolysis.
- Refeeding syndrome.

Management

Acute hypocalcaemia is normally treated with intravenous calcium gluconate, but it is also essential to determine the underlying cause and commence specific treatment as early as possible. Magnesium deficiency (which reduces parathyroid hormone secretion) or alkalosis should be corrected if present. In chronic hypocalcaemia, treatment is designed to increase intestinal calcium absorption through calcium and vitamin D supplementation.

Hypercalcaemia

The most common causes of hypercalcaemia are malignancy and primary hyperparathyroidism. Other causes include:

SECTION 6

- Prolonged immobilisation.
- Drug related (e.g. lithium; calcium co-prescribed with antacid, milk-alkali syndrome, or vitamin D intoxication; thiazide diuretics; hypervitaminosis A).
- Granulomatous disease including tuberculosis and sarcoidosis.
- Adrenal insufficiency.
- Chronic kidney disease.

Management

Severe hypercalcaemia often occurs in conjunction with ECF depletion, and expansion of the ECF compartment with intravenous fluids may be effective in slowly reducing the serum calcium levels; however, it is usually not the only treatment, and it may lead to fluid overload. The use of loop diuretics is controversial, but they are sometimes used to treat hypercalcaemia once hypovolaemia has been corrected. Intravenous infusion of bisphosphonates may be required for long-term control in symptomatic or more severe hypercalcaemia. Any prescribed drugs exacerbating hypercalcaemia should be discontinued if possible.

Mild hypercalcaemia may not require immediate therapy, but drugs contributing to hypercalcaemia should be stopped or reduced if appropriate, and serum levels of calcium repeated. Treatment of chronic hypercalcaemia depends on the primary cause, and a referral should be made to the relevant specialist.

Phosphate

Phosphate (PO_4^{3-}) is the body's most abundant trivalent anion and is essential for all intracellular processes and for the structural integrity of cell membranes. It regulates the affinity of haemoglobin for oxygen and thus regulates oxygen delivery to tissues. It is also important in the renal acid–base buffer system.

Hypophosphataemia

A range of clinical conditions can result in hypophosphataemia, including:

- Redistribution
  - Respiratory alkalosis.
  - Glucose/insulin therapy.
  - Sepsis.
  - Catecholamines.
  - Rapid cell uptake (e.g. hungry bone syndrome, acute leukaemia).
  - Refeeding syndrome.
  - Recovery from DKA.
- Increased renal excretion
  - Metabolic acidosis.
  - Volume expansion.
  - Diuretics.
  - Corticosteroids.
  - Tubular disorders.
  - Hyperparathyroidism.
- Decreased intestinal absorption:
  - Malabsorption.
  - Phosphate-binding agents.
  - Vitamin D deficiency.
  - Secretory diarrhoea and steatorrhoea.
  - Vomiting.
  - Antacid abuse.

Management

Acute management is usually only necessary with moderate to severe hypophosphataemia. Intravenous administration of phosphate can lead to extraskeletal calcification, and oral supplementation is therefore often safer; however, absorption can be unpredictable.

Hyperphosphataemia

Causes of hyperphosphataemia include:

- Renal insufficiency.
- Hypoparathyroidism.
- Hypovolaemia.
- Cell breakdown (release of phosphorus into ECF), e.g. rhabdomyolysis, haemolysis, chemotherapy, tumour lysis syndrome, profound catabolic stress.
- Increased intake:
  - Phosphate enemas and laxatives.
  - Vitamin D intoxication.

Management

The treatment of acute hyperphosphataemia includes volume expansion, oral phosphate binders and dialysis; nevertheless, in normal or mild to moderate kidney disease, it is usually self-resolving, owing to the continued ability of the kidney to excrete phosphate loads. Chronic hyperphosphataemia is usually due to chronic kidney disease, and is treated with dietary phosphate restriction and oral phosphate binders.

Magnesium

Magnesium (Mg^{2+}) is the second most abundant intracellular cation. It is a co-factor in more than 300 enzyme reactions and is important for the synthesis of proteins, RNA and DNA. It is essential for muscle contractions and relaxation, heart rhythm, nerve function, vascular tone and bone formation. Circulating magnesium is under close homeostatic regulation, primarily through renal reabsorption and excretion.

Hypomagnesaemia

Serum magnesium is a poor predictor of total body magnesium content, because only 0.3% is found in serum. Only 30–50% of total dietary magnesium is absorbed, and other nutrients such as fibre, phytates, oxalates, and phosphates can bind the cation and decrease its absorption. Causes of hypomagnesaemia include:

- Reduced intake (e.g. malnutrition, alcoholism).
- Gastrointestinal losses:

    - Vomiting, diarrhoea, malabsorption (e.g. IBD/coeliac disease), short bowel syndrome, intestinal fistulae, excessive use of laxatives, long-term use of proton pump inhibitors.
- Renal losses.
- Renal tubular disorders.
- Drugs (loop and thiazide diuretics, tacrolimus, nephrotoxins e.g. cyclosporine, cisplatin, pentamidine, amphotericin and aminoglycosides).
- Endocrine.
- Diabetes mellitus/DKA.
- Hyperthyroidism.
- Hyperaldosteronism.
- Hungry bone syndrome.
- Others
    - Acute pancreatitis.
    - Refeeding syndrome.
    - ECF expansion.

Management

There are no universal guidelines for repletion of magnesium, and varying practices exist. Magnesium sulphate ($MgSO_4$) is most commonly used for intravenous administration. Intravenous repletion should be given slowly, over a period of hours. A slow rate of infusion is essential as the renal reabsorption threshold is affected by plasma magnesium concentrations; abrupt elevation above the normal range will reduce retention, and up to 50% of the infused magnesium will be excreted in the urine. The absorption of magnesium from the gastrointestinal tract is poor, and magnesium salts can cause diarrhoea, which leads to further electrolyte losses. Mild hypomagnesaemia is often treated by giving oral magnesium supplements in divided doses three to four times per day to reduce their laxative side effects. It should be noted that sufficient renal function is required prior to providing magnesium supplementation.

Hypermagnesaemia

Causes of hypermagnesaemia include:

- Kidney disease – acute or chronic.
- Administration of magnesium-containing drugs or salts (e.g. antacids, laxatives and enemas).
- Iatrogenic (e.g. high doses of magnesium supplementation given in error).
- Tissue breakdown – rhabdomyolysis, burns, DKA.

Management

Treatment is initially by removing the underlying cause and then by removing excess magnesium. If this is associated with renal disease, dialysis may be necessary. In severe hypermagnesaemia, intravenous calcium may be given to counteract the cardiac effects of magnesium.

Acknowledgement

The editor acknowledges the prior contribution of Alan Torrance.

Further reading

Adrogué HJ, Madias NE. (2000) *Hyponatremia. N. Engl. J. Med.* 342(21):1581–1589.

Adrogué HJ, Madias NE. (2000) *Hypernatremia. N. Engl. J. Med.* 342(20): 1493–1499.

Assessment of hyponatraemia. (2018) *BMJ Best Practice* [Online]. Available at http://bestpractice.bmj.com/best-practice/monograph/57/overview/aetiology.html. Accessed 12 October 2018.

Canada TW, Tajchman SK, Tucker AM, *et al.* (eds) (2015) *ASPEN. Fluids, Electrolytes, and Acid-Base Disorders Handbook.* Chicago: ASPEN.

Cooper MS, Gittoes NJ. (2008) Diagnosis and management of hypocalcaemia. *BMJ*, 336(7656): 1298–1302.

Jahnen-Dechent W, Ketteler M. (2012) Magnesium basics. *Clin. kidney J.* 5: i3–i14.

Liamis G, Milionis HJ, Elisaf M. (2010) Medication-induced hypophosphatemia: a review. *QJM* 103: 449–459.

Minisola S, Pepe J, Piemonte S, *et al.* (2015) The diagnosis and management of hypercalcaemia. *BMJ* 350: h2723.

Palmer BF. (2015) Regulation of potassium homeostasis. *Clin. J. Am. Soc. Nephrol.* 10(6): 1050–1060.

Rastergar A, Soleimani M. (2001) Hypokalaemia and hyperkalaemia. *Postgrad. Med. J.* 77(914): 759–764.

Silverthorn DU. (2016) *Human Physiology*, 7th edn. San Francisco: Pearson.

Viera AJ, Wouk N. (2015) Potassium disorders: hypokalemia and hyperkalemia. *Am. Fam. Physician.* 92(6): 488–495.

SECTION 7

Clinical dietetic practice

7.1 Respiratory disease

Peter Collins and C. Elizabeth Weekes

Key points

- Malnutrition is common in patients with chronic obstructive pulmonary disease (COPD) and tuberculosis (TB).
- Routine nutritional screening using a validated screening tool should be carried out in all patients to identify those at risk and to initiate treatment.
- Nutritional requirements in COPD and TB have yet to be fully established.
- Nutritional support is an effective treatment in the management of malnutrition in COPD, but its role in the management of TB has yet to be determined.

Many conditions affect the lungs (Table 7.1.1), which impact on breathing ability and cause mortality and morbidity (British Thoracic Society, 2006). In the UK, one person in seven is affected by chronic respiratory disease, most commonly chronic obstructive pulmonary disease (COPD) or asthma. Globally, it is estimated that about 3 million deaths were caused by COPD in 2015, and this prevalence is likely to increase due to higher smoking prevalence and aging populations (WHO, 2016). The WHO (2016) predicts that COPD will become the third leading cause of death worldwide by 2030.

A number of symptoms that result from respiratory disease can affect nutritional intake and nutritional status, e.g. dyspnoea, cough and excess sputum production. At any stage in the illness, these symptoms may be compounded by acute exacerbations and infection, and influenced by age, the social and psychological effects of chronic illness, and the presence of comorbidities. Any patient with respiratory disease may present with malnutrition; however, two respiratory conditions strongly associated with a high prevalence of malnutrition are COPD (Vermeeren *et al.*, 2006) and tuberculosis (TB) (Schwenk & Macallan, 2000). While adequate pharmacological treatment of TB often results in a cure and subsequent improvement in nutritional status (Schwenk *et al.*, 2004), the chronic nature of COPD means that it is often progressively debilitating with an increasing impact on nutritional status. All respiratory diseases affect lung function to varying degrees, but some, particularly COPD and TB, are also associated with chronic systemic inflammation that can have profound effects on skeletal muscle (sarcopenia and cachexia) and bone (osteoporosis).

Chronic obstructive pulmonary disease

The term COPD, applies to emphysema, bronchitis or a combination of both. It was recently defined as '*...a common preventable and treatable disease, characterized by persistent airflow limitation that is usually progressive and associated with an enhanced chronic inflammatory response in the airways and the lung to noxious particles or gases. Exacerbations and comorbidities contribute to the overall severity in individual patients*' (Vestbo *et al.*, 2013).

Patients usually present with a history of increasing dyspnoea over several years, chronic cough, muscle weakness and poor exercise tolerance secondary to muscle wasting; recurrent bronchial infections or weight loss may also be reported. Although COPD is incurable, early diagnosis and treatment can alleviate respiratory symptoms that compromise nutritional intake. The aetiology of malnutrition and respiratory decline in COPD is complex, and the exact causality is yet to be established. The progressive nature of the disease, leading to worsening respiratory function and nutrition impact symptoms, is one cause for worsening nutritional status. Conversely, poor nutritional status resulting in fat-free mass (FFM) losses and weakness, particularly in muscles associated with breathing, could result in an impaired ability to expectorate. This could increase the risk of recurrent pulmonary infections and hasten the progression of the

Manual of Dietetic Practice, Sixth Edition. Edited by Joan Gandy.

Companion website: www.manualofdieteticpractice.com

Table 7.1.1 Characteristics of respiratory disease

	Examples
Chronic respiratory diseases	
Obstructive	COPD
	Asthma
Restrictive	Pulmonary fibrosis
	Sarcoidosis
Vascular	Pulmonary embolism
	Pulmonary hypertension
	Cor pulmonale
Infective	TB
Environmental	Pneumoconiosis
	Asbestosis
Genetic	Cystic fibrosis
	Alpha-1-antitrypsin deficiency
Acute respiratory disease	
Multiple causes	Adult respiratory distress syndrome (ARDS)
Infective	Pneumonia

Table 7.1.2 Grading of chronic obstructive disease (COPD) obstruction severity

COPD severity classification	Lung function
GOLD I: mild	$FEV_1 \geq 80\%$ predicted
GOLD II: moderate	$FEV_1 \leq 50–80\%$ predicted
GOLD III: severe	$FEV_1 \leq 30–<50\%$ predicted
GOLD IV: very severe	$FEV_1 < 30\%$ predicted[a]

[a]Or $FEV_1 < 50\%$ predicted in the presence of chronic respiratory failure (GOLD, 2017; NICE, 2010); FEV_1, forced expiratory volume in 1 second; FVC, forced vital capacity.

disease. More recently, a small, randomised trial investigating a dietary shift to a higher consumption of antioxidant-rich foods found a preserved respiratory function in COPD patients (Keranis *et al.*, 2010); larger studies are required to confirm this effect.

Diagnostic criteria and classification

Diagnosis relies on medical history and an assessment of symptoms at presentation, together with the identification of comorbidities, and requires post bronchodilator spirometry to establish lung function (forced expiratory volume in one second (FEV_1) and forced vital capacity (FVC)) (Vestbo *et al.*, 2013). Lung function results are compared with age-specific and gender-specific standards to determine disease severity using the GOLD criteria (see Table 7.1.2).

Disease processes

While exposure to tobacco smoke (either active smoking or second-hand smoke) is the primary cause of COPD, other risk factors include exposure to indoor and outdoor air pollution and occupational dusts and fumes. (WHO, 2016). Genetic predisposition also plays a role (Lomas & Silverman, 2001). In addition to airflow limitation, pathological changes and inflammation-induced damage in the lungs can lead to excess mucus secretion, ciliary dysfunction, pulmonary hyperinflation and gas exchange abnormalities, and may result in pulmonary hypertension and cor pulmonale. Patients with COPD have an increased susceptibility to infection and often suffer acute recurrent exacerbations of the disease, the majority of which are infective by nature (IECOPD).

Burden of disease

In the UK, 1.2 million individuals have been diagnosed with COPD (British Lung Foundation, 2016); however, it is estimated 3 million have the disease (NICE, 2010). Around 30,000 people die as a result of COPD each year (British Thoracic Society, 2006). With an ageing population, increasing awareness of the disease and improved diagnostic methods, the number of individuals diagnosed with COPD in the UK has recently risen (Adeloye *et al.*, 2015). COPD is the second largest cause of emergency admissions to UK hospitals, accounting for 130,000 admissions/year (British Lung Foundation, 2007), placing a huge operational burden on hospitals by taking up 1 million bed days annually (British Thoracic Society, 2006). A recent study involving an Australian cohort of COPD patients found malnutrition to be independently associated with this increased healthcare use (Hoong *et al.*, 2017). Although a burden to hospital systems, patients with COPD are primarily managed in the community and account for 1.4 million GP consultations/year (Healthcare Commission, 2006). While the incidence of COPD has been associated with levels of deprivation, social deprivation has also been found to be a significant predictor of malnutrition in COPD (Collins *et al.*, 2018). The disease also has a profound effect on patients' quality of life, which significantly declines as disease severity increases (Rutten-van Mölken *et al.*, 2006), with the presence of malnutrition compounding this effect (Arslan *et al.*, 2016).

Nutritional impact

In epidemiological studies, a diet low in fruit and vegetables and high in meat and potatoes has been associated with an increased likelihood of developing COPD (Kaluza *et al.*, 2017; McKeever *et al.*, 2010). There is a lack of studies investigating the potential benefits of dietary interventions to prevent the development of COPD in at-risk populations. Following the study by Keranis *et al.* (2010), another small randomised controlled trial investigated the impact of increasing the intake of fruit and vegetables on outcome in patients with COPD (Baldrick *et al.*, 2012). The intervention group, patients with moderate to severe COPD, were provided with a variety of fruit and vegetables for 12 weeks. However, there was no impact on airways, systemic oxidative stress or inflammation. The effects of such interventions require longer-term, adequately powered trials in order to allow to control for significant lifestyle and behavioural confounders.

Weight loss and being underweight are associated with poor prognosis and increased mortality, independent of disease severity (Landbo *et al.*, 1999). While malnutrition has been found to be independently associated with increased healthcare use and costs (Hoong *et al.*, 2017), it was suggested, until recently, to be an inevitable part of the disease progression and, as such, unresponsive to nutritional intervention. However, it is now recognised that the weight loss observed in COPD is reversible, and that weight gain is associated with a number of functional improvements (Collins *et al.*, 2012, 2013; Ferreira *et al.*, 2012), as well as reduced mortality (Schols *et al.*, 1998).

The exact prevalence of malnutrition in COPD is unknown since an accepted definition of malnutrition does not exist. However, in a recent study of 121 hospitalised patients with COPD (Ingadottir *et al.*, 2017), 21% met the ESPEN criteria for malnutrition (Cederholm *et al.*, 2015). Reported prevalence rates vary considerably from 9 to 63%, depending on the criteria used to define malnutrition, e.g. <90% ideal body weight (Metropolitan Life Insurance Company, 1959) or >5% recent weight loss, and the population studied, e.g. inpatients or outpatients (Weekes, 2005). Compared with chronic bronchitis, patients with emphysema are more likely to have a BMI and to report unintentional weight loss (Guerra *et al.*, 2002). Little has been reported on the pattern of weight loss; however, Weekes and Bateman (2002) reported significant unintentional weight loss (>5%) in 22% of COPD outpatients. In those who unintentionally lost weight, 41% reported a recent chest infection. Although many patients describe gradual weight loss over a number of years, in a subgroup of patients, weight loss and muscle wasting follows a stepwise pattern related to acute illness (Schols & Brug, 2003). In contrast to observations in the healthy population, survival in COPD appears to be improved in those who are overweight or obese (Landbo *et al.*, 1999; Vestbo *et al.*, 2006). This *obesity paradox* extends beyond reduced mortality in COPD, with one study finding that overweight patients had lower early readmission rates (Steer *et al.*, 2010), and another that overweight and obese patients had fewer emergency hospital admissions and shorter lengths of stay (Collins *et al.*, 2011a).

Assessment of body weight alone is unlikely to be sensitive enough to detect all of those at nutritional risk, since a subgroup of COPD patients demonstrate loss of FFM despite maintaining normal weight (De Benedetto *et al.*, 2000; Schols *et al.*, 1993). Depletion of FFM may have more profound effects on functional measures than depletion of body weight *per se* (Schols *et al.*, 1993). The proportion of patients with FFM depletion increases with disease severity (Schols *et al.*, 1993; Vermeeren *et al.*, 2006). Altered body composition can be attributed to a number of factors, including the disease process itself (systemic inflammation), energy imbalance (positive or negative), medication treatment (oral corticosteroids) and lifestyle (inactivity). Loss of FFM, which often occurs with ageing, can be accelerated in the presence of chronic inflammatory disease.

Nutritional screening and nutritional assessment

As COPD patients readily pass between primary and secondary care, routine nutritional screening should be performed in all patients across both settings. Outpatients with COPD identified as at risk of malnutrition using a validated tool are at increased risk of hospitalisation, longer hospital stays and increased mortality (Steer *et al.*, 2010; Weekes *et al.*, 2007). Studies are needed to establish whether prompt identification and nutritional intervention in these patients reduce their poor clinical outcomes.

Anthropometry

Guidelines for the management of COPD recommend the anthropometric assessment of patients to determine BMI. Unfortunately, the guidelines make no recommendation for formal nutritional screening and the assessment of unintentional weight change (NICE, 2010). Anthropometric assessment in COPD is not straightforward, owing to changes in body composition and the presence of oedema, which is challenging since there are no agreed adjustment factors for oedema. In the presence of severe oedema, assessment of upper-arm anthropometry is useful. A mid-upper-arm circumference (MUAC) of <23 cm often indicates a BMI of <20 kg/m^2 (Powell-Tuck & Hennessy, 2003). Mid-arm muscle area (MAMA) of the non-dominant arm has been reported to be a better predictor of mortality in COPD than BMI (Soler-Cataluña *et al.*, 2005). Bioelectrical impedance analysis is increasingly being used in COPD to assess changes in FFM and as an illness indicator to help predict prognosis. Currently, there is no universal reference population for COPD using this technique, and research is ongoing in this area.

Biochemistry

Hospitalised patients should be assessed for hydration status, clinical condition (e.g. raised C-reactive protein, white cell count and low serum albumin levels), and nutritional markers. Patients could be at risk of refeeding syndrome (see Chapter 6.4, Enteral nutrition) if dietary intake has been poor for a prolonged period or there is a history of excessive alcohol consumption, and phosphate, potassium, calcium and magnesium levels should be reviewed prior to implementation of nutritional support in all patients with known risk factors (NICE, 2006a).

Clinical

Patients with COPD often present with several nutritionally relevant comorbidities (e.g. diabetes, gastro-oesophageal reflux, osteoporosis or depression) whose management may require a large number of different drugs (polypharmacy). Assessment of clinical condition should take account of any relevant changes in either comorbidities or pharmacological interventions. Altered swallowing physiology in COPD, particularly around the time of IECOPD, may increase aspiration risk (Teramoto *et al.*, 2002).

Dietary

Stable patients with COPD consume close to recommended daily amounts for both energy and protein (Vermeeren *et al.*, 1997; Weekes *et al.*, 2009); however, intake is compromised during IECOPD (Slinde *et al.*, 2003; Vermeeren *et al.*, 1997). Low intakes of calcium and vitamin D have been found in outpatients (Andersson *et al.*, 2007; Weekes, 2005), with a reported non-starch polysaccharide intake of <15 g/day (Weekes, 2005). This, together with a sedentary lifestyle and limited fluid intake, might predispose to constipation.

Economic and social status

Strong links exist between social deprivation and both the development of COPD and clinical outcome (Prescott *et al.*, 1999). Deprivation is a significant independent risk factor for malnutrition in outpatients with COPD, and should be a consideration in their nutritional management (Collins *et al.*, 2018). Many patients with COPD are unable to continue in employment as their disease progresses or have to decrease their working hours (Eisner *et al.*, 2002). Financial resources may therefore be limited and compromise ability to purchase food. A significant proportion of patients with COPD are housebound (Bestall *et al.*, 1999), which may be accompanied by social isolation and limited access to affordable food. Strategies for improving nutritional intake may need to include the use of meals-on-wheels-type services and socialised eating opportunities such as lunch clubs.

Clinical management

Available treatments rely almost exclusively on symptom management and should be relevant to the patient's clinical condition on presentation (Vestbo *et al.*, 2013). The recent GOLD strategy document recognises the following three conditions and makes treatment recommendations accordingly: stable COPD; acute exacerbations; and management of comorbidities such as cardiovascular disease, skeletal muscle dysfunction, osteoporosis and depression (Vestbo *et al.*, 2013). Infective exacerbations of the disease are usually treated with inhaled and/or oral corticosteroid medication and antibiotics. The increased appetite and food intake that often accompanies courses of oral steroids is usually short term, since patients are put on reducing doses as soon as possible to avoid complications of long-term therapy. Many patients take medications to counteract osteoporosis. Gastrointestinal disturbances are known complications of antibiotic therapy and may impact on nutritional intake during and immediately after IECOPD.

Recent interest has focused on the levels of vitamin D in COPD patients as the vitamin is not only involved with bone physiology but also plays an important role in muscle function and adaptive immunity (Janssens *et al.*, 2009). Vitamin D deficiency is common in COPD and correlates with disease severity (Janssens *et al.*, 2010). In COPD patients waiting for lung transplantation, 50% were found to be vitamin D deficient (Forli *et al.*, 2004). Immobility, reduced sunlight exposure, reduced capacity of ageing skin to synthesise vitamin D, and medications used to manage COPD all influence the osteoporosis risk in COPD. Vitamin D and calcium intakes should be considered in all COPD patients due to the high prevalence of both osteoporosis and vitamin D deficiency.

In patients receiving home oxygen therapy, consideration should be given to the possible effects on mobility, access to food and social life, all of which might impact adversely on nutritional intake. Prolonged periods on oxygen can cause dry mouth, and this may affect the ability to taste, chew and swallow foods. Smoking cessation is a major aim of COPD management. Current smoking status has been shown to be a significant predictor of malnutrition risk (Collins *et al.*, 2011b). An average weight gain of 3.8 kg in females and 2.8 kg in males has been observed in individuals who successfully stopped smoking for >1 year (Williamson *et al.*, 1991). Baseline weight in males did not affect the level of weight gained; however, in underweight females, the likelihood of gaining 13 kg or more was increased fourfold in those who stopped smoking.

An increasing number of patients have lung volume reduction surgery, and this has been shown to result in spontaneous weight gain (Christensen *et al.*, 1999), possibly due to a combination of reduced work of breathing, improved gas exchange and reduced post-prandial dyspnoea.

Nutritional requirements

Nutritional requirements will depend on nutritional status, clinical condition, physical activity level, nutritional goals and likely duration of nutritional support (NICE, 2006a).

Energy

The energy requirements have yet to be fully characterised, and studies of COPD have reported considerable individual variation in total energy expenditure (TEE) (Slinde *et al.*, 2006). While published prediction methods may provide adequate estimates of requirements for groups of patients, they have a poor predictive value for individuals (see Chapter 6.1, Nutritional requirements in clinical practice). Weight-stable outpatients with COPD may have requirements similar to others of their age and gender, but if their physical activity levels are compromised, energy requirements may be lower than for healthy individuals of the same age and gender (Slinde *et al.*, 2011). In stable outpatients, a modest increase in energy intake of 200–300 kcal/day has been shown to result in weight gain (Collins *et al.*, 2012; Weekes *et al.*, 2009), and therefore energy requirements are unlikely to be much above normal.

In IECOPD, resting energy expenditure (REE) may be up to 15–20% above predicted basal metabolic rate

(BMR) (Schols *et al.*, 1991; Nguyen *et al.*, 1999; Vermeeren *et al.*, 1997), but since acute illness is usually accompanied by a decrease in physical activity, TEE may be similar to, or even slightly lower than, normal. During IECOPD, some patients may be identified as at high risk of refeeding syndrome; however, this is less likely with oral nutritional support than enteral or parenteral nutrition since acute illness is usually accompanied by a loss of appetite that limits spontaneous dietary intake. Practitioners should, however, take care not to overprescribe nutritional support (NICE, 2006a) and to follow national or evidence-based local protocols for the management of refeeding in those patients identified as at high risk.

There is little evidence that disease-specific oral nutritional supplements (ONS) are more effective than standard ONS in this group of patients. There is a growing body of evidence demonstrating the effectiveness of immune modulatory enteral feeds in patients with acute respiratory distress syndrome (Gadek *et al.*, 1999) and acute lung injury (Singer *et al.*, 2006) who are ventilated. However, the efficacy of such feeds outside of intensive care in COPD patients hospitalised for IECOPD remains to be established.

Protein

While elevated protein turnover rates have been reported in COPD (Engelen *et al.*, 2000), there is currently no evidence to support prescribing protein intakes above general recommendations for chronic or acute illness (Table 7.1.3). It has been suggested that protein intakes at the upper end of those recommended by NICE (2006a), i.e. 1.5 g/kg/day, might be optimal during IECOPD (Vermeeren *et al.*, 1997). Indeed, these levels would be more in line with the recommendations of the PROT-AGE group for individuals aged 65 years and over (Bauer *et al.*, 2013).

Micronutrients

Micronutrient intake is likely to be compromised in individuals who have diets deficient in energy and protein. Prescriptions for nutritional support should provide adequate electrolytes, minerals and other micronutrients, accounting for pre-existing deficits, excessive losses or increased demands (NICE, 2006a). It may therefore be necessary to recommend the use of a multivitamin and mineral supplement if intake from diet and/or ONS is unlikely to be adequate.

Nutritional support

The reversibility of weight loss in COPD is dependent on the ability to address the underlying cause. An imbalance between energy intake and expenditure, which commonly occurs during IECOPD and is accompanied by significant worsening of nutrition impact symptoms (e.g. anorexia, early satiety, dry mouth), should be amenable to targeted nutritional support. However, during

Table 7.1.3 Nutritional management of chronic obstructive pulmonary disease (COPD)

Condition	Treatment goals	Requirements	Interventions
Stable COPD (outpatient)	Maintain nutritional status *or* improve nutritional status (e.g. post-IECOPD).	25–35 kcal/kg/day. 0.8–1.5 g protein/kg/day. 30–35 mL of fluid/kg/day (NICE, 2006a)[a]. *For patients who are not severely ill or injured, nor at risk of refeeding syndrome*. Alternatively, use PENG guidelines (Todorovic & Micklewright, 2011).	Patients identified as at risk of malnutrition or as malnourished should either be managed by referral to a dietitian or by staff using protocols drawn up by dietitians, with referral as necessary (NICE, 2006a); provision of ONS should be considered in those with a BMI of <20 kg/m² (Collins *et al.*, 2012; NICE, 2010).
Acute exacerbation (inpatient)	Minimise effects on nutritional status.	No specific recommendations can be made for energy due to the heterogeneity of the patient group and the changing clinical course during the acute phase. Intakes up to 1.5 g of protein/kg/day may be justified in exacerbating COPD patients (Vermeeren *et al.*, 1997).	Maximise oral intake within limits of patient's clinical condition using low-volume ONS between meals (Anker *et al.*, 2006). Consider supplementary tube feeding if unlikely to meet requirements for more than 5 days (NICE, 2006a).
Mechanical ventilation (ICU/HDU)	Minimise effects on nutritional status while avoiding complications of overfeeding.	No specific recommendations can be made in this setting as conditions leading to the requirement for ventilation are often highly changeable. Monitoring in this setting is vital in order to meet the nutritional needs of the patient. In patients requiring prolonged ventilation, avoid overfeeding (see PENG guidelines (Todorovic & Micklewright, 2011) for maximal energy and macronutrient profiles for ventilated patients).	Commence enteral tube feeding as soon as possible; if high risk of delayed gastric emptying and aspiration, use post-pyloric feeding (Heyland *et al.*, 2001). In acute respiratory distress disorder (ARDS) and acute lung injury (ALI), consider formulas containing n-3 fatty acids and antioxidants (Kreymann *et al.*, 2006).

IECOPD, infective exacerbations of chronic obstructive lung disease; ONS, oral nutritional supplements; ICU, intensive care unit; HDU, high dependency unit; PENG, Parenteral and Enteral Nutrition Group.

the acute phase, in the face of significant inflammation, improvements with nutritional support are hard to achieve. Studies have shown that ONS are able to overcome energy and protein deficits at this time, while not affecting oral intake (Vermeeren *et al.*, 2004), and lead to significant improvements in respiratory function and a tendency for improved general well-being (Saundy-Unterberger *et al.*, 1997).

At different periods during the course of their disease, patients may experience one or any number of symptoms that could adversely affect intake. The most frequently reported symptoms likely to affect nutritional intake in COPD are anorexia, early satiety and dyspnoea (Cochrane & Afolabi, 2004). Patients with anorexia and post-prandial dyspnoea may benefit more from low-volume, high-energy/protein ONS and/or advice on food fortification. In the presence of early satiety, small, frequent meals and snacks and/or energy-dense ONS are recommended (Anker *et al.*, 2006).

While some symptoms experienced by patients with COPD may be amenable to nutritional intervention alone, others may require a combination of nutritional intervention and other therapeutic and/or pharmacological strategies. For example, in the management of eating-related dyspnoea, liaison with the medical team or respiratory nurse could optimise oxygen therapy if appropriate, while nutritional interventions should be tailored to minimise the effects on dyspnoea of preparing and eating food.

Since most patients report experiencing several symptoms that affect dietary intake at any time, a range of dietetic strategies may be required to achieve an increase in intake. In a progressive, debilitating disease such as COPD, strategies may have to change over time to avoid taste fatigue and/or take into account changes in clinical, psychological or social status (Table 7.1.4).

Evidence base for nutritional support

Recent systematic reviews and meta-analyses suggest that nutritional support in COPD is effective in terms of increasing energy and protein intake, promoting weight gain and improving anthropometric and functional status (Collins *et al.*, 2012, 2013; Ferreira *et al.*, 2012; Schols *et al.*, 2014). Further trials are required to examine the cost-effectiveness of nutritional support in improving clinical outcomes. The current evidence for nutritional support is almost entirely based on ONS and is lacking for other forms of nutritional intervention. There is a need for trials comparing different nutritional intervention strategies, and their effects on mortality, clinical outcomes and cost-effectiveness (Schols *et al.*, 2014). Since ONS presumably produce clinical benefits through increased nutrient intake, a similar increase in nutrient intake achieved by dietary counselling and/or food fortification should result in similar benefits (NICE, 2006a). Confirmation of this should be a priority in dietetic research as it underpins many of the principles of the profession (Baldwin & Weekes, 2011). There is a particular need for robust trials around food fortification and dietary counselling, as these are often recommended as a first-line treatment for malnutrition in COPD despite a paucity of evidence.

One randomised trial showed individualised dietary counselling by a dietitian together with a 6-month supply of whole-milk powder (WMP) to be effective in improving intake and body weight in COPD (Weekes *et al.*, 2009). An important finding from this trial was that simply providing patients with dietary advice literature, without dietetic-input-tailoring advice, failed to result in any improvements. The efficacy of tailored dietary advice delivered by a dietitian and the provision of supportive literature in the absence of WMP remains unknown and urgently needs addressing. A post hoc cost analysis suggests that it might be cost-effective for a dietitian to provide dietary counselling to individuals with COPD (Weekes *et al.*, 2006), but this needs to be supported by larger, adequately powered studies.

The most effective setting for nutritional intervention in COPD is likely to be in outpatients, as these patients tend to be metabolically stable, less acutely unwell and more mobile. The nutritional enhancement of pulmonary rehabilitation (PR) is an area that is receiving increasing interest as multimodal therapy has been found to result in significant improvements not only in malnourished

Table 7.1.4 Factors influencing progression from latent to active TB (source: adapted from Bates *et al.*, 2004)

Individual	Household/community	Environmental
Age	Socioeconomic status	Availability of health services
Gender	Migrant status	Quality of healthcare
Nutritional status	Place of residence	Availability of appropriate treatment
Immune status	Access to health services	Drug resistance
Genetic predisposition	Access to treatment	Public policy
Behaviour	Informal care arrangements	Public awareness
Poverty	Access to formal care services	
Education		
Knowledge and attitudes		
Diet		
Employment status		

patients but also in adequately nourished patients with COPD, suggesting a role for nutrition beyond simply treating malnutrition (Schols *et al.*, 2014). The British Thoracic Society guidance on pulmonary rehabilitation notes that the optimal approaches for addressing malnutrition, sarcopenia or obesity in COPD are uncertain; however, the guideline group concluded that attendance at a pulmonary rehabilitation course presents an ideal opportunity to screen and educate patients on nutrition (Bolton *et al.*, 2013).

Tuberculosis

Tuberculosis (TB) is an infectious bacterial disease caused by *Mycobacterium tuberculosis* and is transmitted via droplets from the throat and lungs of people with active TB. It most commonly affects the lungs but can affect almost any part of the body, with infections of the central nervous system and abdomen being the most severe. The global prevalence of TB was 14 million in 2004, with >60% of cases in sub-Saharan Africa and Asia (WHO, 2008). Although active TB cases have declined in Europe over the past 50 years, there has been an increase in some countries since the 1990s, including in the UK (Health Protection Agency, 2010). Globally, 9.2 million new cases and 1.7 million deaths from TB occurred in 2006, and, while the number of new cases per capita is falling in some regions of the world, this is not the case in Africa and Europe (WHO, 2008).

Diagnostic criteria

TB is diagnosed by sputum smear microscopy followed by culture testing (NICE, 2006b). Patients with active TB usually present with symptoms of persistent cough, fever, night sweats, dyspnoea, haemoptysis (coughing up blood), weight loss and chest pain.

Disease processes

Following TB exposure, healthy individuals mount a cell-mediated immune response involving T cells, macrophages and cytokines, which usually controls the infection. The majority of individuals remain in this asymptomatic (latent) phase, and only about 10% go on to develop active TB, usually when their immunity is compromised. Worldwide, more than 13 million individuals are coinfected with HIV and TB, and, in many individuals infected with HIV, development of active TB is the first sign of AIDS. A number of individual factors such as genetic predisposition (Malik & Godfrey-Faussett, 2005) interact with community and environmental factors (e.g. poverty and poor housing) to influence susceptibility to infection and progression to active TB (Table 7.1.4).

Disease consequences

TB is among the top 10 causes of illness, disability and death, and is the leading cause of death from a curable infectious disease (WHO, 2008). It is currently estimated that about one-quarter of the world's population is infected. The main burden of disease in the UK is concentrated in certain urban areas, with 38% of cases in London (Health Protection Agency, 2010). The majority of cases occur in young adults and among non-UK-born black African and South Asian ethnic groups. Since most cases occur during the economically productive years of life (19–49 years), the earning capacity of patients can be severely compromised (Frieden *et al.*, 2003). With the advent of effective anti-TB therapy in recent decades, mortality rates have decreased dramatically in industrialised countries.

Clinical investigations and management

In confirmed smear positive cases, the standard treatment is short-course chemotherapy for 6–8 months. A combination of drugs and high adherence is necessary to achieve a cure, and treatment usually takes place in two phases. The initial phase lasts 2–3 months and aims to kill active and dormant bacilli, and is followed by the continuation phase, which usually lasts 4–6 months. Patients with HIV coinfection will also be prescribed a variety of antiretroviral drugs that will significantly increase the pill burden, potentially impacting negatively on adherence.

Nutritional impact

The nutritional consequences of active TB are well recognised; yet, little is understood of the complex interactions between TB treatment and nutritional status. Many patients experience severe weight loss and vitamin and mineral deficiencies. People with TB/HIV coinfection have a worse nutritional status, as TB worsens malnutrition and malnutrition weakens immunity, thereby increasing the likelihood of progressing from latent to active disease. Similar to other chronic diseases, a consistent relationship exists between TB incidence and BMI, with one review reporting that TB incidence increases exponentially as BMI decreases (Lönnroth *et al.*, 2010). Patients presenting with active TB are more likely to be wasted or to have a lower BMI than healthy controls (Paton & Ng, 2006). Nutritional status usually improves with anti-TB therapy, although recent evidence suggests that those who fail to put on weight during the early phase of treatment are more likely to suffer poorer outcomes, including death (Bernabe-Ortiz *et al.*, 2011; Khan *et al.*, 2006).

Nutritional management

The evidence surrounding best practice for nutritional management of TB is very limited, particularly in developed countries. However, the recent WHO guideline on nutritional support and care for patients with TB describes nutritional assessment as an essential prerequisite for treatment and makes recommendations for screening, nutritional counselling and management (WHO, 2013). Patients with HIV/TB coinfection face particular challenges and poorer outcomes than those with either infection alone. For more information on the nutritional management of HIV/TB coinfection, see Houtzager *et al.* (2010) and Chapter 7.11.3 (Human immunodeficiency virus). In patients with active TB, dietary intake is likely to have been poor for some time prior to diagnosis, and in those with disordered lifestyles (e.g. substance abusers) or limited access to food and drink (e.g. the shelter living homeless), nutritional intervention will need to include strategies for ensuring adequate intake throughout the treatment period. Similarly, exploration of the diet of recent immigrants and their potential access to traditional versus native foods may be necessary in order to provide appropriate advice to which patients are likely to adhere.

Nutritional requirements

Energy

There is a lack of adequately powered studies designed to determine the energy requirements of patients with TB, and it is therefore not possible to draw any firm conclusions about the energy needs of patients with TB (Raj *et al.*, 2006; WHO, 2013). Pragmatically, in the early acute phase of illness, any increase in BMR secondary to the inflammatory response is likely to be accompanied by a decrease in physical activity; thus, TEE may be similar to, or even slightly lower than, normal.

Protein

Protein loss occurs due to the catabolism induced by infection, and this loss should be made good through the provision of additional protein. The capacity to retain protein is enhanced during the recovery phase of infection, and it is essential that needs are met during this time (NICE, 2006a). There is no evidence to suggest that patients with TB require a significantly greater protein intake than patients with other acute infectious conditions, i.e. up to 1.5 g protein/day.

Micronutrients

At the time of diagnosis, patients with active TB may have low levels of several micronutrients, including vitamins C and E, retinol, zinc, iron and selenium (Papathakis, 2008). Daily micronutrient supplementation may be beneficial in those who have deficiencies, especially during the early months of therapy (Abba *et al.*, 2008), but, in the case of vitamin D, possibly only those with specific genotypes will benefit (Martineau *et al.*, 2011). In a recent Cochrane review, the authors concluded that, although blood levels of some vitamins may be low in people starting treatment for active TB, there is currently no reliable evidence that routinely supplementing micronutrients above recommended daily amounts has clinical benefits (Grobler *et al.*, 2016).

Nutritional support

Benefits in terms of weight gain and increased energy intake have been reported (Kennedy *et al.*, 1996; Paton *et al.*, 2004; Schwenk *et al.*, 2004; Sudarsanam *et al.*, 2011). However, it is difficult to distinguish whether the improvement in nutritional status was due to control of the disease or to nutritional support, since nutritional status is related to both effective TB treatment and increased dietary intake. Currently, there is a lack of good-quality evidence regarding the effects of nutritional support in patients with active TB on outcomes such as hospitalisation, quality of life or functional measures. In a recent systematic review, it was concluded that there was moderate-quality evidence that macronutrient supplementation provided during the treatment of active TB resulted in weight gain (Grobler *et al.*, 2016). However, the authors of the review emphasised that all studies were too small to reliably prove or exclude clinically important benefits on mortality, cure or treatment completion.

SECTION 7

References

Abba K, Sudarsanam TD, Grobler L, *et al.* (2008) Nutritional supplements for people being treated for active tuberculosis. *Cochrane Database Syst. Rev.* 4: CD006086.

Adeloye A, Chua S, Lee C, *et al.* (2015) Global and regional estimates of COPD prevalence: Systematic review and meta-analysis. *J. Glob. Health* 5(2):020415.

Andersson I, Grönberg A, Slinde F, *et al.* (2007) Vitamin and mineral status in elderly patients with chronic obstructive pulmonary disease. *Clin. Respir. J.* 1(1): 23–29.

Anker SD, John M, Pederson PU, *et al.* (2006) ESPEN Guidelines on Enteral Nutrition: Cardiology and Pulmonology. *Clin. Nutr.* 25: 311–318.

Arslan M, Soylu M, Kaner G, *et al.* (2016) Evaluation of malnutrition detected with the Nutritional Risk Screening 2002 (NRS-2002) and the quality of life in hospitalized patients with chronic obstructive pulmonary disease. *Hippokratia* 20(2):147–152.

Baldrick F.R., Elborn J.S., Woodside J.V. *et al.* (2012) Effect of fruit and vegetable intake on oxidative stress and inflammation in COPD: A randomized controlled trial. *Eur. Respir. J.* 39: 1377–1384.

Baldwin C, Weekes CE. (2011) Dietary advice with or without oral nutritional supplements for disease-related malnutrition in adults. *Cochrane Database Syst. Rev.* (9): CD002008.

Bates I, Fenton C, Gruber J, *et al.* (2004) Vulnerability to malaria, tuberculosis and HIV/AIDS infection and disease. Part 1: determinants operating at individual and household level. *Lancet Infect. Dis.* 4(5): 267–277.

Bauer J, Biolo G, Cederholm T, *et al.* (2013) Evidence-based recommendations for optimal dietary protein intake in older people: a position paper from the PROT-AGE Study Group. *J. Am. Med. Dir. Assoc.* 14(8): 542–559.

Bernabe-Ortiz A, Carcamo CP, Sanchez JF, *et al.* (2011) Weight variation over time and its association with tuberculosis treatment outcome: a longitudinal analysis. *PLoS ONE* 6(4): e18474.

Bestall JC, Paul EA, Garrod R, *et al.* (1999) Usefulness of the Medical Research Council (MRC) dyspnoea scale as a measure of disability in patients with chronic obstructive pulmonary disease. *Thorax.* 54: 581–586.

Bolton CE, Bevan-Smith EF, Blakey JD, *et al.* (2013) British Thoracic Society guideline on pulmonary rehabilitation in adults. *Thorax.* 68: ii1–ii30.

British Lung Foundation. (2007) *Invisible lives: Chronic Obstructive Pulmonary Disease (COPD): Finding the Missing Millions.* London: British Lung Foundation.

British Lung Foundation. (2016) *Chronic Obstructive Pulmonary Disease (COPD) statistics.* Available at https://statistics.blf.org.uk/copd. Accessed 21 February, 2019.

British Thoracic Society. (2006) *The Burden of Lung Disease*, 2nd edn. London: British Thoracic Society.

Cederholm T, Bosaeus I, Barazzoni R, *et al.* (2015) Diagnostic criteria for malnutrition: an ESPEN consensus statement. *Clin. Nutr.* 34(3): 335–340. 10.1016/j.clnu.2015.03.001.

Christensen PJ, Paine R, Curtis JL, *et al.* (1999) Weight gain after lung volume reduction surgery is not correlated with improvement in pulmonary mechanics. *Chest.* 116: 1601–1607.

Cochrane WJ, Afolabi OA. (2004) Investigation into the nutritional status, dietary intake and smoking habits of patients with chronic obstructive pulmonary disease. *J. Hum. Nutr. Diet.* 17: 3–11.

Collins PF, Stratton RJ, Kurukulaaratchy R, *et al.* (2011a) The 'obesity paradox' in chronic obstructive pulmonary disease. *Thorax* 65: 74.

Collins PF, Stratton RJ, Elia M. (2011b) The influence of smoking status on malnutrition risk and 1-year mortality in outpatients with chronic obstructive pulmonary disease. *J. Hum. Nutr. Diet.* 24(4): 382–383.

Collins PF, Stratton RJ, Elia M. (2012) Nutritional support in chronic obstructive pulmonary disease: a systematic review and meta-analysis. *Am. J. Clin. Nutr.* 95(6): 1385–1395.

Collins PF, Elia M, Stratton RJ. (2013) Nutritional support and functional capacity in chronic obstructive pulmonary disease: a systematic review and meta-analysis. *Respirology.* 18: 616–629.

Collins PF, Elia M, Kurukulaaratchy RJ, *et al.* (2018) The influence of deprivation on malnutrition risk in outpatients with chronic obstructive pulmonary disease (COPD). *Clin. Nutr.* 37: 144–148. 10.1016/j.clnu.2016.11.005

De Benedetto F, Del Ponte A, Marinari S, *et al.* (2000) In COPD patients, body weight excess can mask lean tissue depletion: a simple method of estimation. *Monaldi. Arch. Chest Dis.* 55(4): 273–278.

Eisner MD, Yelin EH, Trupin L, *et al.* (2002) The influence of chronic respiratory conditions on health status and work disability. *Am. J. Public Health* 92: 1506–1513.

Engelen MPKJ, Deutz NEP, Wouters EFM, *et al.* (2000) Enhanced levels of whole-body protein turnover in patients with chronic obstructive pulmonary disease. *Am. J. Respir. Crit. Care Med.* 162: 1488–1492.

Ferreira IM, Brooks D, Lacasse Y, *et al.* (2012) Nutritional supplementation for stable chronic obstructive pulmonary disease. *Cochrane Database Syst. Rev.* 12:CD000998.

Forli L, Halse J, Haug E, *et al.* (2004) Vitamin D deficiency, bone mineral density and weight in patients with advanced pulmonary disease. *J. Intern. Med.* 256: 56–62.

Frieden TR, Sterling TR, Munsiff SS, *et al.* (2003) Tuberculosis. *Lancet* 362: 887–899.

Gadek J, DeMichele S, Karlstad M, *et al.* (1999) Effect of enteral feeding with eicosapentaenoic acid, gamma-linolenic acid, and antioxidants in patients with acute respiratory distress syndrome. *Crit. Care Med.* 27(8): 1409–1420.

Global Initiative for Chronic Obstructive Lung Disease (GOLD). (2017) *Pocket Guide to COPD Diagnosis, Management and Prevention.* Available at http://goldcopd.org/wp-content/uploads/2016/12/wms-GOLD-2017-Pocket-Guide.pdf. Accessed September 2017.

Grobler L, Nagpal S, SudarsanamTD, *et al.* (2016) Nutritional supplements for people being treated for active tuberculosis. *Cochrane Database Syst. Rev.* (6): Art. No.: CD006086. doi: 10.1002/14651858.CD006086.pub4

Guerra S, Sherrill DL, Bobadilla A, *et al.* (2002) The relation of body mass index to asthma, chronic bronchitis and emphysema. *Chest* 122(4): 1256–1263.

Healthcare Commission. (2006) *Clearing the Air: A National Study of Chronic Obstructive Pulmonary Disease.* London: Healthcare Commission.

Health Protection Agency. (2010) *Tuberculosis in the UK: Annual Report on Tuberculosis Surveillance in the UK.* London: Health Protection Agency.

Heyland DK, Drover JW, MacDonald S, *et al.* (2001) Effect of postpyloric feeding on gastroesophageal regurgitation and pulmonary microaspiration: results of a randomized controlled trial. *Crit. Care Med.* 29(8): 1495–1501.

Hoong JM, Ferguson M, Hukins C, *et al.* (2017) Economic and operational burden associated with malnutrition in chronic obstructive pulmonary disease. *Clin. Nutr.* 36(4): 1105–1109.

Houtzager L, Barnes M, Matters K. (2010) The nutritional management of patients living with tuberculosis and HIV co-infection. In: Pibram V (ed) *Nutrition and HIV.* Oxford: Wiley Blackwell.

Ingadottir AR, Beck AM, Baldwin C, *et al.* (2018). Two components of the new ESPEN diagnostic criteria for malnutrition are independent predictors of lung function in hospitalized patients with chronic obstructive pulmonary disease (COPD). *Clin Nutr.* 37(4):1323–1331.

Janssens W, Lehouck A, Carremans C, *et al.* (2009) Vitamin D beyond bones in chronic obstructive pulmonary disease. *Am. J. Respir. Crit. Care Med.* 179: 630–636.

Janssens W, Bouillon R, Claes B, *et al.* (2010) Vitamin D deficiency is highly prevalent in COPD and correlates with variants in the vitamin D-binding gene. *Thorax* 65: 215–220.

Kaluza J, Larsson SC, Orsini N, *et al.* (2017) Fruit and vegetable consumption and risk of COPD: a prospective cohort study of men. *Thorax.* 72(6):500–509.

Kennedy N, Ramsay A, Uiso L, *et al.* (1996) Nutritional status and weight gain in patients with pulmonary tuberculosis in Tanzania. *Trans. R. Soc. Trop. Med. Hyg.* 90(2): 162–166.

Keranis E, Makris D, Rodoulou P, *et al.* (2010) Impact of dietary shift to higher-antioxidant foods in COPD: a randomized trial. *Eur. Respir. J.* 36: 774–780.

Khan A, Sterling TR, Reves R, *et al.* (2006) Lack of weight gain and relapse risk in a large tuberculosis treatment trial. *Am. J. Respir. Crit. Care Med.* 174: 344–348.

Kreymann KG, Berger MM, Deutz NEP, *et al.* (2006) ESPEN guidelines on enteral nutrition: intensive care. *Clin. Nutr.* 25: 210–223.

Landbo C, Prescott E, Lange P, *et al.* (1999) Prognostic value of nutritional status in chronic obstructive pulmonary disease. *Am. J. Respir. Crit. Care Med.* 160: 1856–1861.

Lomas DA, Silverman EK. (2001) The genetics of chronic obstructive pulmonary disease. *Respir. Res.* 2(1): 20–26.

Lönnroth K, Williams BG, Cegielski P, *et al.* (2010) A consistent log-linear relationship between tuberculosis incidence and body mass index. *Int. J. Epidemiol.* 39(1): 149–155.

Malik ANJ, Godfrey-Faussett P. (2005) Effects of genetic variability of *Mycobacterium tuberculosis* strains on the presentation of disease. *Lancet Infect. Dis.* 5: 174–183.

Martineau AR, Timms PM, Bothamley GH, *et al.* (2011) High-dose vitamin D3 during intensive-phase antimicrobial treatment of pulmonary tuberculosis: a double-blind randomised controlled trial. *Lancet* 377: 242–250.

McKeever TM, Lewis SA, Cassano PA, *et al.* (2010) Patterns of dietary intake and relation to respiratory disease, forced expiratory volume in 1 s, and decline in 5-y forced expiratory volume. *Am. J. Clin. Nutr.* 92: 408–415.

Metropolitan Life Insurance Company. (1959) New weight standards for men and women. *Statistical Bulletin – Metropolitan Life Insurance Company* 40: 1–10.4.

NICE. (2006a) Nutrition Support in Adults: Oral Nutrition Support, Enteral Tube Feeding and Parenteral Nutrition. Available at www.nice.org.uk/cg32. Accessed 2 September 2017.

NICE: National Clinical Guideline Centre for Acute Care. (2006b) *Tuberculosis: Clinical Diagnosis and Management of Tuberculosis, and Measures for its Prevention and Control.* Available at www.nice.org.uk/nicemedia/pdf/cg033niceguideline.pdf. Accessed 2 September 2017.

NICE. (2010) Chronic Obstructive Pulmonary Disease: Management of Chronic Obstructive Pulmonary Disease in Adults in Primary and Secondary Care. *Clinical Guideline* 101. Available at www.nice.org.uk/cg101. Accessed 2 September 2017.

Nguyen LT, Bedu M, Caillaud D, *et al.* (1999) Increased resting energy expenditure is related to plasma TNF-alpha concentration in stable COPD patients. *Clin. Nutr.* 18: 269–274.

Papathakis P; for the United States Agency for International Development (USAID). (2008) *Nutrition and Tuberculosis: A Review of the Literature and Considerations for TB Control Programs*. USAID.

Paton NI, Ng YM. (2006) Body composition studies in patients with wasting associated with tuberculosis. *Nutrition* 22(3): 245–251.

Paton NI, Chua YK, Earnest A, *et al.* (2004) Randomized controlled trial of nutritional supplementation in patients with newly diagnosed tuberculosis and wasting. *Am. J. Clin. Nutr.* 80(2): 460–465.

Powell-Tuck J, Hennessy EM. (2003) A comparison of mid upper arm circumference, body mass index and weight loss as indices of undernutrition in acutely hospitalised patients. *Clin. Nutr.* 22: 307–312.

Prescott E, Lange P, Vestbo J, *et al.* (1999) Socioeconomic status, lung function and admission to hospital for COPD: results from the Copenhagen City Heart Study. *Eur. Respir. J.* 13(5): 1109–1114.

Raj T, D'Souza G, Elia M, Kurpad AV. (2006) Measurement of 24 h energy expenditure in male tuberculosis patients. *In. J. Med. Res.* 124(6):665–676.

Rutten-van Mölken MP, Oostenbrink JB, Tashkin DP, *et al.* (2006) Does quality of life of COPD patients as measured by the Generic EuroQol five-dimension questionnaire differentiate between COPD severity stages? *Chest* 130: 1117–1128.

Saundy-Unterberger H, Martin JG, Gray-Donald K. (1997) Impact of nutritional support on functional status during an acute exacerbation of chronic obstructive pulmonary disease. *Am. J. Respir. Crit. Care Med.* 156: 794–799.

Schols AMWJ, Brug J. (2003) Efficacy of nutritional intervention in chronic obstructive pulmonary disease. *Eur. Respir. Monogr.* 8(24): 142–152.

Schols AMWJ, Soeters PB, Mostert R, *et al.* (1991) Energy balance in chronic obstructive pulmonary disease. *Am. Rev. Respir. Dis.* 143: 1248–1252.

Schols AM, Soeters PB, Dingemans AM, *et al.* (1993) Prevalence and characteristics of nutritional depletion in patients with stable COPD eligible for pulmonary rehabilitation. *Am. Rev. Respir. Dis.* 147: 1151–1156.

Schols AMWJ, Slangen S, Volovics L, *et al.* (1998) Weight loss is a reversible factor in the prognosis of chronic obstructive pulmonary disease. *Am. J. Respir. Crit. Care Med.* 157: 1791–1797.

Schols AM, Ferreira IM, Franssen FM, *et al.* (2014) Nutritional support and therapy in COPD: a European Respiratory Society statement. *Eur. Respir. J.* doi: 10.1183/09031936.00070914.

Schwenk A, Macallan DC. (2000) Tuberculosis, malnutrition and wasting. *Curr. Opin. Clin. Nutr. Metab. Care* 3: 285–291.

Schwenk A, Hodgson L, Wright A, *et al.* (2004) Nutrient partitioning during treatment of tuberculosis: gain in body fat mass but not in protein mass. *Am. J. Clin. Nutr.* 79: 1006–1012.

Singer P, Thiella M, Fisher H, *et al.* (2006) Benefit of an enteral diet enriched with eicosapentaenoic acid and gamma-linolenic acid in patients with acute lung injury. *Crit. Care Med.* 34(4): 1033–1038.

Slinde F, Ellegard L, Gronberg AM, *et al.* (2003) Total energy expenditure in underweight patients with severe chronic obstructive pulmonary disease living at home. *Clin. Nutr.* 22(2): 159–165.

Slinde F, Kvarnhult K, Grönberg AM, *et al.* (2006) Energy expenditure in underweight chronic obstructive pulmonary disease patients before and during a physiotherapy programme. *Eur. J. Clin. Nutr.* 60: 870–876.

Slinde F, Grönberg AM, Svantesson U, *et al.* (2011) Energy expenditure in chronic obstructive pulmonary disease – evaluation of simple measures. *Eur. J. Clin. Nutr.* 65(12): 1309–1313.

Soler-Cataluña JJ, Sánchez-Sánchez L, Martínez-García MÁ, *et al.* (2005) Mid-arm muscle area is a better predictor of mortality than body mass index in COPD. *Chest* 128: 2108–2115.

Steer J, Norman E, Gibson GJ, *et al.* (2010) Comparison of indices of nutritional status in prediction of in-hospital mortality and early readmission of patients with acute exacerbations of COPD. *Thorax* 65: A127.

Sudarsanam TD, John J, Kang G, *et al.* (2011) Pilot randomized trial of nutritional supplementation in patients with tuberculosis and HIV–tuberculosis coinfection receiving observed short-course chemotherapy for tuberculosis. *Trop. Med. Int. Health* 16(6): 699–670.

Teramoto S, Kume H, Ouchi Y. (2002) Altered swallowing physiology and aspiration in COPD. *Chest* 122(3): 1104–1105.

Todorovic V, Micklewright A. On behalf of the Parenteral and Enteral Nutrition Group of the British Dietetic Association. (2011). *A Pocket Guide to Clinical Nutrition*. Available at www.peng.org.uk/publications/pocket-guide.html. BDA Birmingham.

Vermeeren MAP, Schols AMWJ, Wouters EFM. (1997) Effects of an acute exacerbation on nutritional and metabolic profile of patients with COPD. *Eur. Respir. J.* 10: 2264–2269.

Vermeeren MA, Wouters EF, Geraerts-Keeris AJ, *et al.* (2004) Nutritional support in patients with chronic obstructive pulmonary disease during hospitalization for an acute exacerbation: a randomized controlled feasibility trial. *Clin. Nutr.* 23(5): 1184–1192.

Vermeeren MA, Creutzberg EC, Schols AM, *et al.*; on behalf of the COSMIC Study Group. (2006) Prevalence of nutritional depletion in a large out-patient population of patients with COPD. *Respir. Med.* 100(8): 1349–1355.

Vestbo J, Prescott E, Almdal T, *et al.* (2006) Body mass, fat-free body mass, and prognosis in patients with chronic obstructive pulmonary disease from a random population sample: findings from the Copenhagen City Heart Study. *Am. J. Respir. Crit. Care Med.* 173: 79–83.

Vestbo J, Hurd SS, Agusti AG, *et al.* (2013) Global strategy for the diagnosis, management, and prevention of chronic obstructive pulmonary disease: GOLD executive summary. *Am. J. Respir. Crit. Care Med.* 187(4): 347–365. doi: 10.1164/rccm.201204-0596PP

Weekes CE. (2005) Nutritional Strategies in the Management of Chronic Obstructive Pulmonary Disease; Nutrition Screening, Dietary Counselling and Food Fortification. PhD Thesis. London: King's College.

Weekes CE, Bateman NT. (2002) Weight change in chronic obstructive pulmonary disease; not just a problem of undernutrition. *Thorax* 57(III): 60.

Weekes CE, Emery PW, Elia M. (2006) Dietary counselling and food fortification in malnourished outpatients with chronic obstructive pulmonary disease: a post hoc cost analysis. ESPEN Conference, Istanbul 19–22 October 2006, p. 237 (abstract).

Weekes CE, Emery PW, Elia M. (2007) A nutrition screening tool based on the BAPEN four questions reliably predicts hospitalisation and mortality in respiratory outpatients. *Proc. Nutr. Soc.* 66: 9A.

Weekes CE, Emery PW, Elia M. (2009) Dietary counselling and food fortification in stable COPD: a randomised trial. *Thorax* 64(4): 326–331.

WHO. (2008) Global Tuberculosis Control: Surveillance, Planning, Financing. Available at http://apps.who.int/bookorders/anglais/detart1.jsp?codlan=1&codcol=15&codcch=3659.

WHO. (2013) *Guideline: Nutritional Care and Support for Patients with Tuberculosis*. Available at http://apps.who.int/iris/bitstream/10665/94836/1/9789241506410_eng.pdf. Accessed 2 September 2017.

WHO. (2016) *The Global Burden of COPD Fact Sheet 315*. Available at http://www.who.int/mediacentre/factsheets/fs315/en/. Accessed 24 October 2018.

Williamson DF, Madans J, Anda RF, *et al.* (1991) Smoking cessation and severity of weight gain in a national cohort. *N. Engl. Med.* 324: 739–745.

7.2 Dental disorders

Ursula Arens and Kathy Cowbrough

Key points

- Dental disease has a significant impact on food intake, nutritional status and general health, particularly in older people.
- Prevalence is highest in children from socioeconomically disadvantaged groups. In older adults, root caries is a significant contributor to tooth loss.
- Dietary acid (mainly from soft drinks) causes dental erosion, resulting in irreversible tooth enamel loss and tooth destruction. The tooth enamel of young children is more susceptible and easily damaged.
- The most important preventative measures for dental health include fluoride usage, reducing the frequency of consumption of sugar-containing products and acidic drinks, and good oral hygiene.

Dental disease is a major public health problem in the UK. Dental diseases can result in acute pain, disfigurement and tooth loss. It can affect food intake, nutritional status and general health, particularly in older people (Petersen & Yamamoto, 2005; Steele *et al.*, 1998), and is therefore an important aspect of dietary assessment. Dental disease is mainly preventable and should not be viewed in isolation from other aspects of health (Moynihan, 2005). Damage to or loss of teeth may result from dental caries, acid erosion and periodontal disease.

Dental caries

Between 1993 and 2003, there was a decrease in dentine decay prevalence in 15-year-old children; approximately half were caries free, compared with just over one-third in 1993 and lesser than 10% in 1983 (Lader *et al.*, 2005). There were significant improvements in 5–8-year-olds with obvious decay in the primary milk teeth between 1993 and 2003. Since 2008, 5-year-olds have shown declines in dental caries; less than 25% of the cohort suffered tooth decay, a 20% drop (PHE, 2016). However, there was significant regional and deprivation score variations. There is also concern over high levels of tooth extractions requiring hospital inpatient care in children aged 10 years and under, and this data was used in 2016 as an indicator in the NHS Outcomes Framework for the first time (HSCIC, 2016). Rates of tooth extractions due to decay were higher in 2013/2014 as compared to 2011/2012 (462 vs 446 per 100,000), and fivefold variations were reported in regional and deprivation score data.

Improvements were also seen in the Adult Dental Health Survey 1998 and 2009 as compared to previous surveys (Kelly *et al.*, 2000; NHS 2011), but mainly in younger adults (16–44 years). Decreases in the prevalence of caries have occurred largely as a result of the effects of fluoride and better oral hygiene. Dental health is particularly poor among immigrants and refugees (Davies, 1998; Gussy *et al.*, 2006; Sheiham, 2001).

Causation

Dental caries occur when carbohydrate from food and drinks reacts with dental plaque, a sticky film of bacteria that forms on all surfaces of the teeth, to produce acid. Within minutes of exposure of the bacteria to a carbohydrate, fermentation occurs, which results in acid production. At a pH of <5.5, tooth enamel begins to be demineralised and become porous. At this stage, surface damage to tooth enamel can be repaired as enamel is constantly dissolved (demineralisation) and reformed (remineralisation). The acid produced by bacterial action dissipates after about 30 minutes and, once the pH rises above 5.5, enamel is remineralised with calcium and phosphate released from saliva. However, remineralisation requires acidity to remain above pH 5.5 for a period of time. If carbohydrate is eaten frequently, there will be insufficient time for remineralisation to take place. This results in continually repeated, gradual loss of enamel and damage to the dentine. Eventually, the enamel collapses to form a cavity, and the tooth is progressively destroyed, as illustrated in a Stephan curve in Figure 7.2.1.

Manual of Dietetic Practice, Sixth Edition. Edited by Joan Gandy.

Companion website: www.manualofdieteticpractice.com

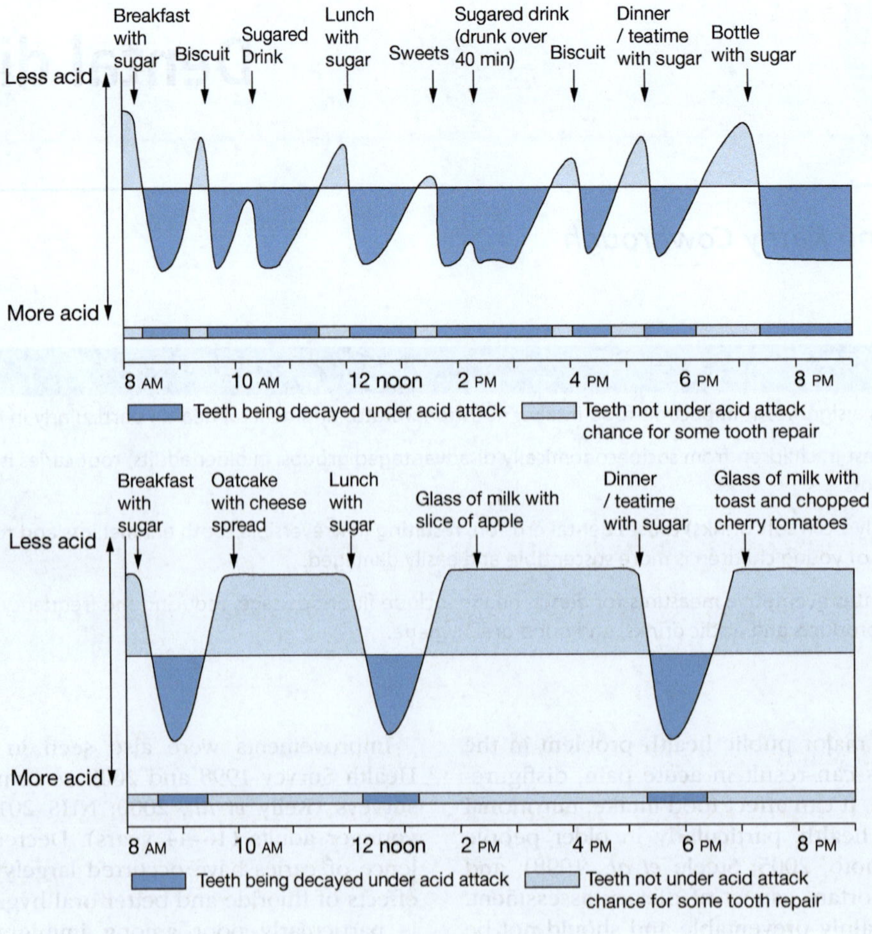

Figure 7.2.1 Stephan curve demonstrating the effect of eating frequency on mouth acidity (source: NHS Scottish Executive 2011; www.child-smile.org.uk/professionals/childsmile-manual.aspx; Appendix 5 – Stephan Curve – Example 1. Reproduced with permission from NHS Scottish Executive. Information licensed under the Open Scottish Parliament License v. 1.0)

Children's teeth are particularly vulnerable during the first 6 years of life when tooth enamel is being developed and is relatively soft. Caries can also attack the teeth roots if they become exposed due to gum recession, which is common in older adults. There is a strong relationship between the presence of root decay and the frequency of intake of sugar-rich foods (Steele *et al.*, 1998).

Factors affecting caries development

Several factors influence the formation of dental caries.

Type of carbohydrate

All carbohydrates are cariogenic, although there is considerable variation. The sugars that are potentially damaging to dental health are classified as 'free sugars', which include sugars added to foods by manufacturers, cooks or consumers, and sugars naturally present in syrups, honey and unsweetened fruit juices (SACN, 2015). Sugars naturally present in whole fruits and vegetables and in lactose in milk and dairy products are not described as 'free sugars'. There is no consensus on the risks of sugars in dried and processed fruit products. Dried fruit is included as a contributor to the 5-A-Day intake scheme, but consumption of small amounts (30 g) is scored within meals, rather than as snacks. A review of dried fruit and dental health concluded that evidence was limited and unconvincing, and so it was not possible to support firm guidelines on this (Sadler, 2016).

Starch can contribute to caries as saliva amylase breaks it down to glucose and maltose in the mouth. However, this varies with the type of starch and the way it has been processed (Grenby, 1997; WHO/FAO, 2003). Fructooligosaccharides may be as acidogenic as sucrose (Moynihan *et al.*, 2001). Sugar alcohols (e.g. xylitol, mannitol and sorbitol) are not fermentable and are hence non-cariogenic.

Frequency of exposure

Both total sugar intake and the consumption frequency are associated with caries development. However, frequency of consumption may be the more significant factor (Holt, 1991; Touger-Decker & van Loveren, 2003). Small, frequent amounts of sugars cause more damage than the same quantity consumed on a single occasion. In young children, the combination of poor oral hygiene, limited exposure to fluoride and frequent exposure to sugary snacks and drinks result in early childhood caries (ECC), particularly in infants who continually suck a bottle containing sugar-containing drinks (Ismail, 1998; Levine & Stillman-Lowe, 2009). Frequency of sugar consumption is an important aspect of dental health, but its contribution to caries development is less if there is good dental hygiene.

Food texture

Small particles of sticky foods may be left wedged between the teeth, allowing continual acid production. Therefore, foods such as dried fruit, e.g. dates and raisins, may have a much greater cariogenic potential than fresh fruit (Edgar, 1993).

Oral hygiene

Failure to clean teeth regularly results in the build-up of tooth plaque and the accumulation of food debris in teeth crevices, providing a substrate for continuous bacterial acid production. Poor oral hygiene in children has a greater impact on the levels of caries-associated microorganisms than the frequency or amount of sugar consumed (Beighton *et al.*, 1996). There is an association between caries and consumption of sugar confectionery in children whose teeth were brushed less than twice a day (Gibson & Williams, 1999). Lack of oral hygiene measures is likely to account for a significant proportion of the excessive caries prevalence in deprived groups.

Salivary flow

Saliva helps protect against dental caries by removing food particles from teeth, neutralising acids and delivering minerals to the tooth to enhance rates of remineralisation. Salivary flow can be stimulated by eating foods that require chewing or which stimulate saliva production, e.g. eating hard cheeses (Rugg-Gunn & Nunn, 1999) or chewing sugar-free gum (Murray *et al.*, 2003). Reduced saliva production may be associated with the development of root caries in older adults. Saliva flow may be reduced in poorly controlled diabetes (Chavez *et al.*, 2000).

Tooth decay resistance

There is considerable individual variability in the resistance of tooth enamel to decay due to the influence of genetic factors on tooth production. Children and the elderly (with worn enamel) are at greater risk. Fluoride markedly increases enamel resistance as it results in the formation of fluorhydroxyapatite crystals in the tooth matrix, which are more resistant to acid erosion than unfluoridated hydroxyapatite.

Dental erosion

There is a gradual loss of tooth outer substance, particularly of hard outer enamel layer, with ageing. This can be due to a triad of factors:

- Attrition – wearing away of teeth by tooth-to-tooth contact during normal chewing.
- Abrasion – wearing away of teeth as a result of external objects applied to the tooth surface, e.g. brushing teeth too vigorously or using a toothbrush with hard bristles.
- Erosion – wearing away of teeth due to acids in the mouth from foods consumed. Acids of bacterial origin do not have this effect.

The signs of dental erosion are changes to the appearance of the tooth and, at a later stage, increased sensitivity of the tooth, leading to pain when eating very hot or very cold, sweet or acidic foods. In the last two decades, there has been an increased awareness of dental erosion, particularly in children and teenagers. An increase in the observation of dental erosion in young people may be associated with recent changes in diet. The survey Children's Dental Health in the UK (O'Brien, 1994) showed that half of all 6-year-olds were found to have erosion, and, in 25%, erosion had resulted in some exposure of dentine. One-third of 14-year-old children had some erosion of their permanent teeth. A later survey of Children's Dental Health (HSCIC, 2015) reported that, in 2013, 28% of children had enamel defects (opacities), a decrease from the 35% reported in 2003. Wear of permanent teeth is a lifelong process; therefore, the extent and severity of damage can be highest in older people. However, because the most damaged teeth may have been lost or removed, occurrence figures in the remaining teeth may appear lower. Severe wear of teeth was recorded in 15% of dentate (having natural teeth)-free living participants (people aged 65 years and over) (Steele *et al.*, 1998). This figure included, but was not exclusively due to, damage from acid erosion.

Some sources of acid affecting teeth can be intrinsic. Gastric reflux increases the acidity of the mouth, and may occur occasionally during illness, or more regularly in people who are obese or alcoholic, or during pregnancy. The observation of tooth damage from acid may be a sign of bulimia. Regurgitated acids from the stomach are very erosive to teeth, and some treatments are available to inhibit reflux or neutralise the acidity of gastric juice, if this occurs regularly (O'Sullivan & Milosevic, 2008).

Extrinsic sources of acid are mainly from foods and drinks consumed in the diet. Acidic foods include many fruits, particularly citrus fruits and their juices; vinegars, salad dressings and pickles; alcoholic drinks, including wines, ciders; carbonated drinks, especially those with flavourings such as citric and phosphoric acid; fruit teas and sour-flavoured sweets. Although there is some decrease in pH in carbonated water as compared to still water, in practice carbonation does not seem to affect oral acidity.

Other factors affecting erosion

In addition to the acidity of the food, other factors may influence the risk of dental erosion to teeth.

Titratable acidity

There may be differences in pH values of foods and values obtained when adding buffering solutions to different foods (titratable acidity); the latter is thought to be a better measure of the erosive risk of the food. Buffering capacities have been shown to be high for fruit juices and fruit-based carbonated drinks, and lower for non-fruit-flavoured and sparkling waters (still water and milk have the lowest capacities) (Dugmore & Rock, 2004; Edwards *et al.*, 1999).

Frequency and timing of consumption

The frequency of exposure has a greater effect than the quantities of the risk factor. As the production of saliva is lowest during sleep, the consumption of acidic foods just before sleeping may result in greater erosive damage.

Consumption in relation to tooth brushing

If teeth are brushed after consuming acidic foods, components of the dissolved enamel will be removed, reducing subsequent remineralisation. Teeth should be brushed at least half an hour after consuming acidic foods; rinsing with water may be an alternative way to support mouth freshness after meals.

Method of consumption

Frequent sipping and swishing of acidic drinks may increase acid erosion of tooth enamel; consuming drinks through a straw may reduce tooth contact with acid liquids.

Other foods

The consumption of dairy foods may prevent the demineralisation that occurs after consuming acid foods. Eating very small amounts of cheese after consuming acid drinks supports remineralisation of the enamel; possibly due to the alkaline properties of dairy foods or promotion of salivary flow.

Periodontal disease

Gingivitis is the initial stage of periodontal disease when the gums become inflamed by plaque that accumulates next to the gum margin. In its early stages, gingivitis can be slowed by regular dental treatment to remove plaque and tartar (calcified plaque) from the gum margins. If gingivitis persists, periodontal disease develops beneath the gum surface, leading to destruction of bone and loosening of the tooth, which may eventually fall out. There is little evidence for an association between diet and periodontal disease (WHO/FAO, 2003), Periodontal disease and resultant tooth loss impairs chewing ability and can restrict food choice (Sheiham *et al.*, 1999), and, for older adults, this can have a significant impact on nutritional status. People with natural teeth are more likely to consume foods that require chewing, such as fresh fruit and vegetables, and as a result have higher intakes of some vitamins (Steele *et al.*, 1998). The prevalence of periodontal disease is increasing. In 2003, 68% of teenage boys and 56% of teenage girls had signs of dental plaque and gingivitis (Lader *et al.*, 2005). The proportion of children with plaque was highest in 8-year-olds; 71% of children were affected. The proportion of 12–15-year-olds with plaque reduced between 2003 and 2013, from 74% to 64% in 12-year-olds, and 64% to 50% in 15-year-olds (HSCIC, 2015).

Dental and oral health promotion

Dental disease is not inevitable and can be prevented by changes in behaviour. Effective and evidence-based messages to prevent dental disease should incorporate good oral hygiene practices, dietary practices and fluoride protection, as shown in Table 7.2.1.

Table 7.2.1 Practical measures to provide dental protection

Protective factors	Practical measures
Reducing the frequency of consumption of sugars	Consume sugar-containing foods and drinks with meals rather than between meals.
	Limit between-meal snacks containing sugars, particularly sticky foods such as dried fruit.
	Use sugar-free medicines wherever possible.
Reducing exposure to acid erosion	Limit consumption of acidic drinks between meals – water, tea/coffee without sugar, or plain milk are suitable.
	Avoid acidic food or drinks immediately before brushing teeth or after brushing teeth at night.
Ending a meal with foods that buffer acids	Cheese and milk assist remineralisation.
Good oral hygiene	Children's teeth should be brushed with a small, pea-sized amount of low-dose fluoride toothpaste when teeth erupt.
	Ensure correct brushing and flossing of teeth and gums to remove plaque and debris at the base of teeth.
	Avoid brushing teeth immediately after the consumption of acidic food or drinks as this may hinder remineralisation; this should not be overlooked in those unwell or those who require care.
	Essential for patients undergoing radiotherapy for head or neck cancer or chemotherapy, as they may be more susceptible to dental caries (Dreizen *et al.*, 1977; Rothwell, 1987).
Exposure to fluoride	Topical application, e.g. toothpastes, mouth rinses or tooth coating.
	Fluoridated drinking water.
	Fluoride supplements should only be prescribed by a dental practitioner on an individual basis (SIGN, 2005).
Increasing salivary flow	Consuming foods that require mastication, e.g. wholegrain foods.
	Eating foods that increase salivation, e.g. cheese, peanuts.
	Chewing sugar-free gum.
Regular dental checks	To correct early problems.
	To remove build-up of plaque and tartar.

Specific guidance for particular population subgroups

Dental health promotion is relevant to the whole population, but is particularly important for those in high-risk groups such as infants, especially at the time of weaning; children and adults living in deprived circumstances; and elderly people. Some age-specific advice for the prevention of caries has been defined in the evidence-based toolkit for prevention (PHE, 2014). Advice to all other age groups is to reduce the frequency and amounts of sugar in foods and drinks, and that sugar-containing foods and drinks should particularly be avoided at bedtime when saliva flows are reduced and buffering capacity is lower.

Infants

Dental health in infants can be improved by adhering to the following recommendations:

- Prolonged bottle-feeding should be discouraged and discontinued after 1 year.
- Infants aged >6 months should always drink from free-flowing cups, and, after the age of one, should be discouraged from drinking from a bottle.
- Infants and young children should never be given a bottle or beaker containing sugary drinks as a comforter.
- Dummies and comforters should not be dipped into honey or sugary drinks.
- Soya-based formulae can cause tooth decay as they contain sugars (SIGN, 2005).
- Sugar should not be added to weaning foods or drinks.
- Weaning practices can have a major influence on both immediate and future dental health (Holt & Moynihan, 1996); food should be low in sugars and acids.
- Milk or water are the preferred drinks; other drinks, e.g. fruit juices and concentrates, should be limited and given only at main meals. They should not be given in bottles or at bedtime.

Children

Children's dental health can be improved by:

- Limiting sugar-containing and acidic drinks, especially between meals.
- Ensuring that milk or water constitutes a major portion of drinks.
- Restricting sugary or acidic drinks at bedtime or during the night.
- Supervising teeth cleaning (ideally up to the age of 6 years) with a fluoride-containing toothpaste (SIGN, 2005).
- Regular dental check-ups.

Elderly people

Elderly people experience changes that may affect good dental health, including:

- Decreased salivary flow.
- Decreased manual dexterity.
- Impaired cognitive function.
- Polypharmacy.
- Swallowing difficulties.
- Reduced thirst and fluid intake.

Factors that should be considered include:

- Daily tooth or denture cleaning, especially in those unable to do this themselves.
- Avoiding frequent consumption of sugary foods.
- Encouraging the consumption of foods that promote salivary flow.
- Monitoring the use of over-the-counter medicines such as cough sweets, laxatives, antacids, etc.; these should be taken at mealtimes.
- Regular dental checks to identify problems and ensure that dentures fit properly.

Further reading

British Nutrition Foundation (BNF). (1999) *Oral Health. A Task Force Report*. London: BNF.

Levine RS, Stillman-Lowe CR. (2009) *The Scientific Basis of Oral Education*, 6th edn. London: British Dental Journal (BDJ) Books.

Internet resources

Scottish Intercollegiate Guidelines Network (SIGN)

Prevention and management of dental decay in the preschool child (2005) SIGN guidance 83. https://www.scottishdental.org/library/prevention-and-management-of-dental-decay-in-the-pre-school-child

Preventing dental caries in children at high caries risk. Targeted prevention of dental caries in the permanent teeth of 6–16-year-olds presenting for dental care (2000) SIGN guidance 47. https://www.scottishdental.org/library/preventing-dental-caries-in-children-at-high-caries-risk

The British Dental Health Foundation, www.dentalhealth.org.

References

Beighton D, Adamson A, Rugg-Gunn A. (1996) Associations between dietary intake, dental caries experience and salivary bacterial levels in 12-year-old English schoolchildren. *Arch. Oral Biol.* 41(3): 271–280.

Chavez EM, Taylor GW, Borrell LN, *et al.* (2000) Salivary function and glycemic control in older persons with diabetes. *Oral Surg. Oral Med. Oral Pathol. Oral Radiol. Endod.* 89(3): 305–311.

Davies GN. (1998) Early childhood caries – a synopsis. *Community Dent. Oral Epidemiol.* 26(1): 106–116.

Dreizen S, Daly TE, Drane JB, *et al.* (1977) Oral complications of cancer radiotherapy. *Postgrad. Med.* 62(2): 85–92.

Dugmore CR, Rock WP. (2004) A multifactorial analysis of factors associated with dental erosion. *Br. Dent. J.* 196: 283–286.

Edgar WM. (1993) Extrinsic and intrinsic sugars: a review of recent UK recommendations on diet and dental caries. *Caries Res.* 27(1): 64–67.

Edwards SL, Creanor RH, Hoyle W. (1999) Buffering capacities of soft drinks: the potential influence on dental erosion. *J. Oral Rehabil.* 26(12): 923–927.

Gibson S, Williams S. (1999) Dental caries in pre-school children: associations with social class, toothbrushing habit and consumption of sugars and sugar-containing foods. Further analysis of data from the National Diet and Nutrition Survey of children aged 1.5–4.5 years. *Caries Res.* 33(2): 101–113.

Grenby TH. (1997) Summary of the dental effects of starch. *Int. J. Food Sci. Nutr.* 48: 411–416.
Gussy MG, Waters EG, Walsh O, *et al.* (2006) Early childhood caries: current evidence for aetiology and prevention. *J. Paediatr. Child Health*. 42(1–2): 37–43.
Holt RD. (1991) Foods and drinks at 4 daily intervals in a group of young children. *Br. Dent. J.* 170(4): 137–143.
Holt RD, Moynihan PJ. (1996) The weaning diet and dental health. *Br. Dent. J.* 181(7): 254–259.
HSCIC. (2015) *Children's Dental Health Survey 2013*. England, Wales and Northern Ireland.
HSCIC. (2016) NHS Outcomes Framework Indicator 3.7: Tooth extraction due to decay in children admitted as inpatients to hospital aged 10 years and under. February 2016 Quarterly Publication.
Ismail AI. (1998) Prevention of early childhood caries. *Community Dent. Oral Epidemiol.* 26(1): 49–61.
Kelly M, Steele J, Nuttall N, *et al.* (2000) *Adult Dental Health Survey: Oral Health in the United Kingdom 1998*. London: The Stationery Office.
Lader D, Chadwick B, Chestnutt I, *et al.* (2005) *Children's Dental Health Survey in the United Kingdom, 2003. Summary Report.* London: Office for National Statistics.
Levine RS, Stillman-Lowe CR. (2009) *The Scientific Basis of Oral Education*, 6th edn. London: British Dental Journal Books.
Moynihan PJ. (2005) The interrelationship between diet and oral health. *Pro. Nutr. Soc.* 64: 571–580.
Moynihan PJ, McIlmoyle S, Rowshanaei R, *et al.* (2001) Acidogenic potential of fructo-oligosaccharides: incubation studies and plaque pH studies. *Caries Res.* 35: 265–316.
Murray JJ, Nunn JH, Steele JG. (2003) *Prevention of Oral Disease*, 4th edn. Oxford: Oxford University Press.
NHS (2011) *Adult Dental Health Survey 2009 – Summary report and thematic series [NS]*. Available at https://digital.nhs.uk/data-and-information/publications/statistical/adult-dental-health-survey. Accessed 25 October 2018.
O'Brien M. (1994) *Child Dental Health in the United Kingdom 1993. Office of Population Census and Surveys, Social Survey Division*. London: TSO.
O'Sullivan E, Milosevic A. (2008) UK National Clinical Guidelines in Paediatric Dentistry: diagnosis, prevention and management of dental erosion. *Int. J. Paediatr. Dent.* 18: 29–38.
Petersen PE, Yamamoto T. (2005) Improving the oral health of older people: the approach of the WHO Global Oral Health Programme. *Community Dent. Oral Epidemiol.* 33: 81–92.
PHE. (2014) Delivering better oral health: an evidence-based toolkit for prevention (3rd edn). Department of Health/NHS/The British Association for the Study of Community Dentistry. www.gov.uk.
PHE. (2016) Press release 10 May 2016: Tooth decay among 5 year olds continues significant decline. https://www.gov.uk/government/news/tooth-decay-among-5-year-olds-continues-significant-decline. Accessed 25 October 2018.
Rothwell BR. (1987) Prevention and treatment of the orofacial complications of radiotherapy. *J. Am. Dent. Assoc.* 114(3): 316–322.
Rugg-Gunn AJ, Nunn JH. (1999) *Nutrition Diet and Oral Health*. Oxford: Oxford University Press.
SACN. (2015) *Carbohydrates and Health Report*. https://www.gov.uk/government/publications/sacn-carbohydrates-and-health-report. Accessed 25 October 2018.
Sadler MJ. (2016) Dried fruit and dental health. *Int. J. Food Sci. Nutr.* 67: 944–959.
Scottish Intercollegiate Guidance Network (SIGN). (2005) *Preventing dental caries in children at high caries risk: targeted prevention of dental caries in the permanent teeth of 6–16 year olds. A national clinical guideline 138*. Available at http://www.sign.ac.uk/sign-138-dental-interventions-to-prevent-caries-in-children.html. Accessed 3 March 2018.
Sheiham A. (2001) Dietary effects of dental disease. *Public Health Nutr.* 4(2B): 569–591.
Sheiham A, Steele JG, Marcenes W, *et al.* (1999) The impact of oral health on stated ability to eat certain foods: findings from the National Diet and Nutrition Survey of older people in Great Britain. *Gerodontology*. 16(1): 11–20.
Steele JG, Sheiham A, Marcenes W, *et al.* (1998) *National Diet and Nutrition Survey: People Aged 65 Years and Over, Volume 2: Report of the oral health survey*. London: TSO.
Touger-Decker R, van Loveren C. (2003) Sugars and dental caries. *Am. J. Clin. Nutr.* 78(4): 881S–892S.
WHO/FAO. (2003) Recommendations for preventing dental diseases. In: *Joint Expert Consultation on Diet, Nutrition and Prevention of Chronic Diseases*. Geneva: World Health Organization, pp. 105–108.

7.3 Dysphagia

June Copeman

Key points

- Potential consequences of dysphagia include choking, aspiration, dehydration, malnutrition and death.
- Suitable food depends on the assessed grade of consistency required. Single-texture foods are easier to eat than foods with multiple textures. It is important that adequate nutrients and energy are consumed at all times.
- Frequent monitoring is required because the individual's condition may change.
- People with dysphagia may become dehydrated if they cannot swallow normal fluids; thickened drinks may be needed.

Swallowing is a highly complex process requiring appropriate posture of the head and neck, good lip and tongue movement, and the presence of the swallow reflex. Many factors can impair the ability to swallow, and the physical and nutritional consequences of this can be profound, even life threatening.

Dysphagia is defined as difficulty in swallowing caused by neurological or structural damage which interferes with the efficient movement of food and fluid from the mouth to the stomach. It is a common consequence of many different types of illnesses or injuries that result in mechanical or neurological impairment of the swallowing process (Table 7.3.1). Dysphagia is most likely to be encountered in patients with stroke, progressive neurological disorders (e.g. Parkinson's disease, motor neurone disease and multiple sclerosis), anoxic brain injury, and other conditions such as learning disabilities, some cancers, or injuries affecting the head and neck. The specific feeding difficulties that arise depend on the precise motor function, behaviour or cognitive deficit that has occurred. This chapter refers to dysphagic people over the age of 5 years. The normal swallow does not mature fully until this age, and details of the management of dysphagia in infants and young children should therefore be sought in paediatric textbooks.

The normal swallow

The normal swallow can be divided into four main stages, and impairment in any one of these can result in dysphagia:

- *Preparatory stage* – this stage is mainly under voluntary control, comprising the transfer of food (or liquid) into the mouth. As food or liquid approaches the mouth, the head moves forward, the tongue protrudes and the lips and jaws open in preparation. Food and drink is placed in the mouth, and the lips and jaw close to seal the mouth. The sight, smell and taste of the food will have stimulated saliva production.
- *Oral stage* – this stage, where food is prepared for passage from the mouth into the pharynx, is also mainly under voluntary control. The tongue moves the food and positions it between the teeth. Chewing (mastication) is achieved by up-and-down and rotary movements of the jaw in order to grind the food and mix it with saliva. The tongue forms a central groove to collect the food, with its tip sealed against the hard palate. The resulting bolus is propelled backwards by the posterior movement of the tongue.
- *Pharyngeal stage* – this is an involuntary stage where the food bolus passes from the mouth through the pharynx and into the oesophagus. At the same time, the airway is temporarily sealed off to prevent the entry of food or fluid into the lungs. The process is initiated when sensation of the bolus at the anterior faucal arch (towards the back of the mouth) stimulates the swallowing centre in the brain stem. The swallow reflex is then triggered:
  - The soft palate elevates to seal off the nasopharynx.
  - The larynx elevates and so forces the epiglottis down to cover the larynx.
  - The vocal cords (within the larynx) close.
  - Respiration stops momentarily.
  - Foods pass through the pharynx mainly by peristalsis (wave-like muscle contractions), i.e. the muscles of the pharynx contract and move the bolus through,

Manual of Dietetic Practice, Sixth Edition. Edited by Joan Gandy.

Companion website: www.manualofdieteticpractice.com

Table 7.3.1 Common causes of dysphagia

Mechanical	Oesophageal stricture
	Oesophageal spasm
	Cancers in the head, neck and oesophageal areas
	Cancer treatment including radiotherapy/surgery to head and neck area
	Pharyngeal pouch
	Injury or surgery to the tongue, lips, mouth or jaw
	Severe infections of the mouth or throat, e.g. oral thrush or ulcers
	Postural problems, e.g. severe kyphosis (curvature of the spine)
Neurological	Stroke
	Parkinson's disease
	Motor neurone disease
	Head injury
	Multiple sclerosis
	Cerebral palsy
	Dementia
	Huntington's disease
	Drug induced (psychotropic drugs)
Psychological	Globus hystericus
	Severe anxiety
	Severe depression

although gravity has some effect. The crico-pharyngeal sphincter relaxes and is opened by the upward pull of the larynx; the food bolus then passes into the oesophagus.

- *Oesophageal stage* – this stage is also involuntary. The food bolus passes down the oesophagus into the stomach by peristalsis and gravity, the cardiac sphincter relaxes and food enters the stomach.

Consequences of dysphagia

Dysphagia is potentially fatal; e.g. the presence of dysphagia following a stroke increases the likelihood of subsequent malnutrition (Foley *et al.*, 2009), mortality and disability at 90 days (Paciaroni *et al.*, 2004), with increased institutionalisation (Smithard *et al.*, 2007). Attempting to swallow foods or liquids without the ability to do so carries a high risk of aspiration (foods or liquids entering the lungs). This, if extensive, can cause acute asphyxiation and, in lesser degrees, is a major contributor to chest infections, lung abscesses and aspiration pneumonia (Gordon *et al.*, 1987; Ney *et al.*, 2009; Ramsey *et al.*, 2003). Aspiration may also be silent, causing no outward signs of distress but still capable of causing pulmonary complications (Marik & Kaplan, 2003; Teasell *et al.*, 1996).

An impaired ability to swallow has many nutritional implications. The physical effects of dysphagia make the process of feeding slow, difficult and tiring; and, as a result, food intake is often inadequate in terms of both quantity (sometimes further compromised by food leakages from the mouth) and variety of food consumed. Fear of choking, especially if there has been an unpleasant experience of aspiration, may cause food aversions or panic attacks at meal times. Other psychological factors such as depression or anxiety, stemming from the patient's reaction to the illness and its effects, may further depress appetite. Embarrassment, vulnerability and loss of enjoyment of eating as a social function should not be underestimated (Ekburg *et al.*, 2002; Martino *et al.*, 2009).

Physiologically, inadequate intake of food and fluid will lead to undernutrition, weight loss, compromised immune function and a high risk of dehydration. These may in turn lead to deterioration of the patient's physical or mental condition and delay recovery or hasten death. The consequences of dysphagia can be compounded by concurrent:

- General illness and frailty.
- Other comorbidities, e.g. diabetes.
- Difficulties with positioning.
- Ill-fitting or absent dentures.

The dysphagia care team

Effective treatment of dysphagia, whether in primary or secondary care (own home, community centre, care home, hospital), requires multidisciplinary care with good communication mechanisms in place. Coordinated multidisciplinary pathways for the assessment of dysphagia and feeding problems, with subsequent agreed intervention, will facilitate cost-efficient, appropriate care. Different professionals will have specific roles within the joint treatment plans, as shown in Figure 7.3.1.

Active participation of the service user and carers, whenever possible, is essential in any decision-making. Short- and long-term prognosis, ethical issues and quality of life are integral to this discussion. Joint treatment plans should enable the service user to be transferred between hospital and intermediate and community locations without compromising appropriate interventions. In the community, liaison with social workers and support personnel – such as home carers, meals-on-wheels providers or commercial ready meal home delivery services – may be essential.

Management

Dysphagia requires prompt and skilled remedial action in order to reduce the risk of aspiration and minimise nutritional deterioration, particularly if the onset has been acute (Finestone *et al.*, 1995; Odderson *et al.*, 1995). Nearly half of stroke patients admitted to hospital will have swallowing difficulties (RCP, 2016; SIGN, 2010), and considerably more among people with other neurological conditions. The primary aims of management by the team are to:

- Assess the nature of the swallowing problem.
- Determine a safe and adequate feeding route.

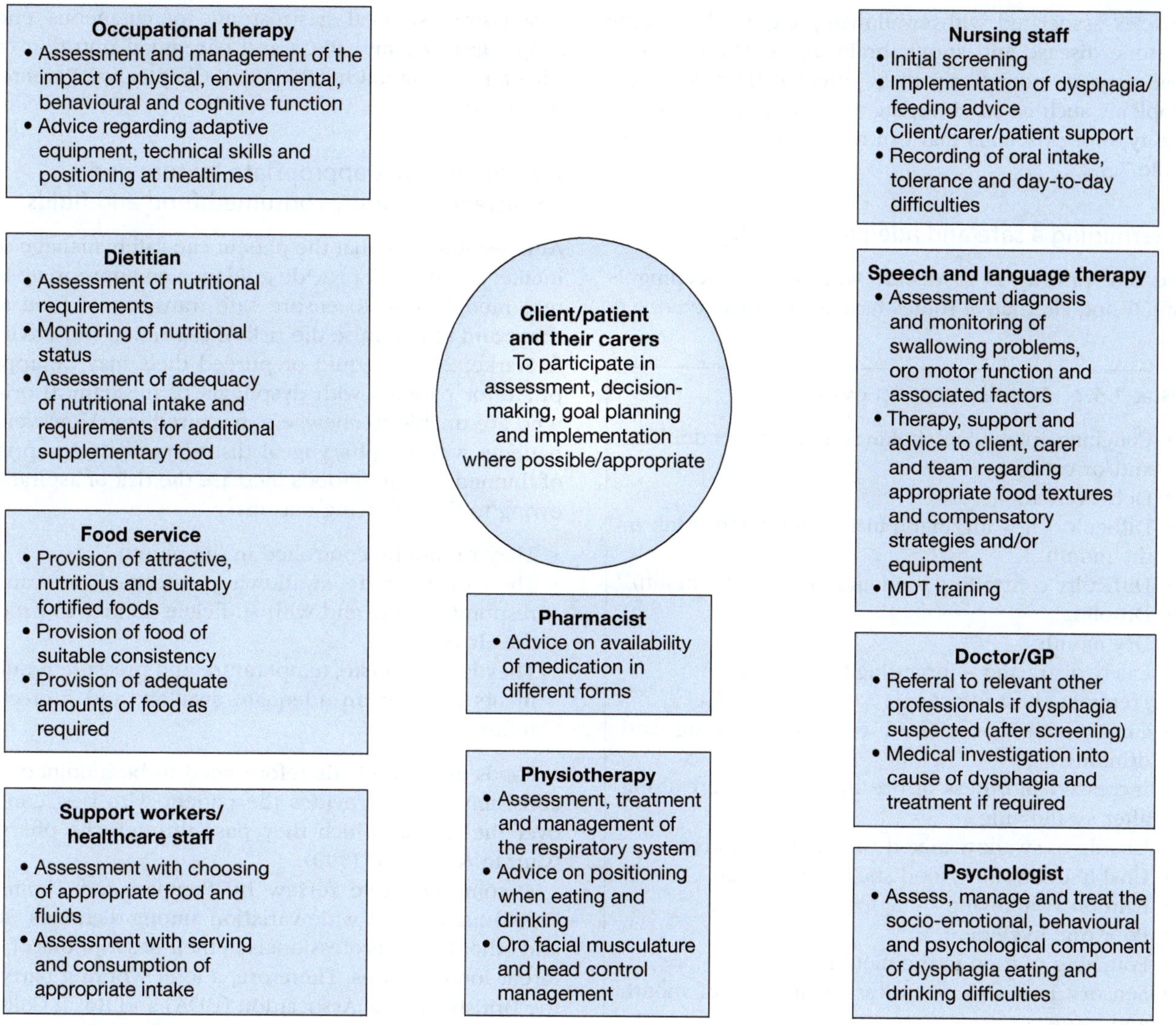

Figure 7.3.1 The role of the multidisciplinary team (MDT) in the management of swallowing and feeding disorders (modified from King's College Hospital, Multi-disciplinary Working Party, 2000)

- Determine the appropriate texture and consistency of orally consumed food and fluids.
- Ensure nutritional and fluid needs are met.
- Educate the patient, carers and other member of the care team.
- Monitor progress.
- Ensure continuity of care.

Warning signs of dysphagia

Early recognition is important to prevent unnecessary patient distress and for effective intervention. Typically, when several of the signs listed in Box 7.3.1 occur, the individual is likely to be experiencing swallowing difficulties, and an assessment is required. This is particularly important in chronic long-term conditions such as Parkinson's disease when dysphagia develops gradually.

Assessment of the swallowing problem

Suspected dysphagia should always be expertly assessed, so that it can be managed most effectively (Finestone & Greene-Finestone, 2003). Following a stroke, it is recommended that all patients be assessed using a validated tool, and local guidelines administered by designated personnel (RCP, 2016). Patients with suspected difficulties should be referred to a speech and language therapist (SLT). If the initial assessment is inconclusive (difficulties at the pharyngeal stage can be particularly difficult to ascertain), radiological examination (videofluoroscopy) may be conducted.

In primary care, a dysphagic patient identified by a GP, or a district or community nurse, should be referred to a hospital for specialist assessment if this cannot be done within the community setting. Dysphagia is a significant contributory factor to undernutrition in elderly people living in the community or care homes (Finch *et al.*, 1998; Madhavan *et al.*, 2016), but it is often regarded as being of little significance.

The first three stages of the normal swallow (preparatory, oral and pharyngeal) are most likely to be disrupted when there is neuromuscular dysfunction resulting in weakness, paralysis and/or sensory loss in the muscles associated with swallowing, e.g. stroke, motor neurone disease and anoxic brain injury. The oesophageal stage is more likely to be affected by mechanical problems such as stricture, e.g. oesophageal carcinoma. The type of problems that can result are summarised in Table 7.3.2.

Determining a safe and adequate feeding route

The first priority is to decide whether oral feeding is safe. If not, alternative routes have to be considered, e.g. nasogastric, surgical gastrostomy, percutaneous endoscopic gastrostomy (PEG) and parenteral nutrition (see Chapter 6.4, Enteral nutrition and Chapter 6.5, Parenteral nutrition).

Box 7.3.1 Warning signs of dysphagia

- Coughing/spluttering/choking during or after drinking and/or eating.
- Dehydration.
- Difficulty chewing/manipulating food and drink in the mouth.
- Difficulty controlling food and drink in the mouth.
- Drooling.
- Dry mouth.
- Easily distracted – forgetting to swallow.
- Frequent chest infections.
- Gurgly voice or altered voice after eating and drinking.
- Increased shortness of breath/change in breathing after swallowing.
- Unable to swallow mixed-consistency meals.
- Unable to swallow/food sticking in mouth.
- Pain on swallowing.
- Poor oral hygiene.
- Pouching of food in the mouth.
- Sensory loss and weakness in muscles of mouth and face.
- Spilling of food/drink from the mouth.
- Unable to clear own saliva/secretions.
- Very poor physical posture, with neck touching chest.
- Vomiting after meals.
- Weight loss.

Determining the appropriate texture and consistency of orally consumed food and fluids

After establishing that the patient can safely manage oral intake, the SLT will provide guidance on appropriate texture modification to ensure safe transport of food and drink and to minimise the risk of aspiration (Rosenvinge & Starke, 2005). Liquid or puréed diets may be appropriate for patients with dysphagia of mechanical origin who are unable to chew, e.g. fractured jaw. However, in patients with oropharyngeal disorders, diets comprised of thinned and fluid foods increase the risk of aspiration, owing to the following reasons:

- They cannot be controlled in the mouth.
- The disordered swallowing mechanism cannot respond in time and with sufficient control to protect the airway.
- They lack the taste, temperature and pressure requirements to elicit an adequate swallow and protective reflex.

Foods and liquids therefore need to be modified to a consistency that provides the patient with best control over the rate at which they pass through the pharynx (Curran & Groher, 1990).

A comprehensive review by Penman and Thomson (1998) highlighted wide variation among dietitians, SLTs and other health professionals in their descriptions of different food textures. Therefore, a joint working party of the British Dietetic Association (BDA) and Royal College of Speech and Language Therapists (RCSLT) (2002, reviewed in 2009) published national descriptors for texture modification in adults. Internationally, the need to standardise terminology to describe levels of liquid thickening or food-texture modification is recognised (Cichero *et al.*, 2013; Dietitians Association of Australia and The Speech Pathology Association of Australia Ltd,

Table 7.3.2 Disruption of the normal swallowing process

Normal swallow stages	Affected by	Consequences
Preparatory stage	Reduced range of movement of facial muscles, lips, tongue and jaw. Loss of sight, smell and/or taste.	Difficulty in getting food/liquid into the mouth. Difficulty in sealing the mouth. Reduced saliva production.
Oral stage	Reduced range of movement of facial muscles, lips, tongue and jaw, and lack of saliva. Postural problems.	Difficulty in mastication. Difficulty in forming a food bolus. Difficulty in controlling a food bolus. Difficulty in swallowing a food bolus.
Pharyngeal stage	Absence of swallow reflex.	Inability to swallow safely.
Oesophageal phase	Impaired peristalsis or obstruction.	Food fails to move into the stomach. Aspiration after the swallow.

2007); however, there is ongoing variation (Steele *et al.*, 2015). In 2015, the International Dysphagia Diet Standardisation Initiative (IDDSI) framework was released, with the subsequent quality improvement 'Kempen Pilot' to test the implementation logistics. Collective and individual staff education and communication throughout the organisation were essential for effective introduction of the texture descriptors. It is anticipated that further pilots in UK and Canada will reinforce many of the same issues (Lam *et al.*, 2017).

Poor use nationally and patient safety concerns involving recorded incidents and deaths from aspiration pneumonia resulted in a collaborative venture led by the National Patient Safety Agency (NPSA, 2011). The expert group with representatives from the BDA, RCSLT, National Nurses Nutrition Group (NNNG) and Hospital Caterers Association (HCA) developed dysphagia diet food-texture descriptors, endorsed by all organisations to be used by health professionals and food providers. The texture consistencies are described as:

B = thin purée dysphagia diet.
C = thick purée dysphagia diet.
D = premashed dysphagia diet.
E = fork-mashable dysphagia diet.

The descriptor tables are comprehensive and include the full range of textures required to manage different types of dysphagia in adults. They are intended as a resource and do not distract from an individual professional's clinical judgement and patient-informed choice. The audit checklists produced enable food items to be measured against the standards for each texture. The NPSA group recommendations for future action include the following:

- A review of descriptors should be undertaken, including the health professionals and the industry.
- All professional organisations should encourage their members to comply with the terminology and language used.
- Pictorial training aids should be developed to support texture descriptors for patients, carers and professionals.
- Industry should be encouraged to review their packaging to reflect the colour codes proposed for each texture descriptor.

Commercial thickening agents derived from food starch or xanthan gum are prescribable for dysphagia, as detailed by the Advisory Committee on Borderline Substances (ACBS), and can be added to foods or liquids to provide the desired consistency and thickness (Table 7.3.3), or prethickened ready-to-use versions can be utilised (Table 7.3.4). Xanthan gum items produce a clear product, so are often more acceptable for thickened liquids in the management of dysphagia. Thickeners based on carob seed flour such as Carobel instant powder are used to thicken infant feeds for the treatment of recurrent vomiting; but these are not suitable for the management of dysphagia.

Foods suitable or unsuitable for inclusion in an individual's diet depend on the grade of consistency required. As a general guideline, single-texture foods such as well-mashed potatoes, semolina, custards, Greek yogurt, instant desserts and sieved soups are more appropriate than combination foods such as stews or risottos. Certain foods are considered high risk (Table 7.3.5) either because of their physical structure (e.g. beans with a skin) or difficulty of manipulation within the mouth (e.g. toffees or pie crust). Foods that change consistency from solid to liquid in the mouth (e.g. ice cream and sorbet) may also be unsuitable for patients who are dysphagic to liquids.

In addition to appropriate texture modification, the SLT may suggest other measures that may assist those with oropharyngeal disorders, e.g. the use of cold or stimulating foods in those with delayed triggering of the pharyngeal swallow, or alternate mouthfuls of hot and cold foods for those with reduced oral awareness (Penman & Thomson, 1998). Other members of the care team (e.g.

Table 7.3.3 Commercial proprietary thickeners – powder (NICE, 2017)

Powder type	Product	Company
Modified maize starch – thickening of foods and liquids in dysphagia	Multi-thick	Abbott Nutrition
	Thick & Easy	Fresenius Kabi
	Thicken Aid	M & A Pharmachem
	Resource Thickened up	Nestlé Health Science
	Nutilis Powder	Nutricia Clinical
	THIXO-D Original	Sutherland Health
	Vitaquick	Vitaflo International Ltd
Xanthan gum–based food and fluid thickener	Thick & Easy Clear	Fresenius Kabi
	Resource Thickenup Clear	Nestlé Health Science
	Nutilis Clear	Nutricia Clinical
	SLO Drinks	SLO Drinks Ltd
	THIXO-D CAL-FREE	Sutherland Health

Note: The listed products are *not* normally suitable for infants and young children.

Table 7.3.4 Pre-thickened oral nutritional supplements (NICE, 2017)

Type	Product	Company
Thickened drinks	Ensure Compact Nutrition Shake	Abbott Nutrition
	Resource Thickened Drinks – syrup and custard consistencies	Nestlé Health Science
	Fresubin Thickened Stage 1	Fresenius Kabi
	Fresubin Thickened Stage 2	Fresenius Kabi
	Fresubin Juicy Drink	Fresenius Kabi
	Nutilis Complete Stage 1	Nutrica Clinical
	Nutilis Complete Stage 2	Nutrica Clinical
	SLO stage 1 Nectar	SLO Drinks Ltd
	SLO stage 2 Honey	SLO Drinks Ltd
Thickened desserts, pudding-style supplements	Ensure Original Pudding	Abbott Nutrition
	Ensure Plus Crème	Abbott Nutrition
	Fresubin YOcreme	Fresenius Kabi
	Fresubin 2kcal Creme	Fresenius Kabi
	Resource Energy Dessert	Nestlé Health Science
	Nutilis Fruit Stage 3	Nutrica Clinical
	Forticreme Complete	Nutrica Clinical
	SLO stage 3 Pudding	SLO Drinks Ltd

NB: The listed products are *not* normally suitable for infants and young children.

Table 7.3.5 High-risk foods in dysphagia[a]

Foods	Examples
Chewy foods	Chewy sweets and toffees Marshmallows Chew bars, breakfast bars Chewing gum Chewy or crispy meat, e.g. crispy duck, bacon Cooked hard cheese, e.g. cheddar
Crumbly items	Bread crusts, pie crusts Crumble Dry biscuits/cakes
Crunchy foods	Toast Flaky pastry Dry biscuits Crisps, popcorn
Floppy texture	Lettuce, cucumber, uncooked spinach leaves
Hard foods	Boiled and hard sweets, toffees Nuts and seeds Raw vegetables
Husk	Sweetcorn Granary bread, bread with grains and seeds
Mixed-consistency foods	Cereals which do not blend with milk, e.g. muesli Mince with thin gravy Soup with lumps, e.g. minestrone
Stringy, fibrous texture	Pineapple, runner beans, celery, rhubarb Steak
Vegetable and fruit skins (including bean skins)	Broad, baked, soya and black-eyed beans, peas, grapes, sweetcorn, apple with peel

[a] Modified from Joint Working Party of the British Dietetic Association and Royal College of Speech and Language Therapists, 2002, reviewed 2009, and Dietitians Association of Australia and The Speech Pathology Association of Australia Ltd, 2007.

physiotherapists or occupational therapists) may provide guidance on the best posture or sitting position for eating, or the most appropriate eating utensils and drinking vessels. Use of drinking vessels that encourage the head to tip back (e.g. feeder beakers) should be avoided. It is also important that patients and their carers be provided with specific guidance on texture-modification measures and compensatory swallowing techniques to help minimise problems such as aspiration (Elmståhl *et al.*, 1999).

Meeting nutritional needs

In addition to being of the appropriate consistency, the diet also has to be capable of meeting the individual's nutritional needs, with consideration of any other medical conditions, e.g. diabetes, as well as cultural requirements (Brody *et al.*, 2000). Where dysphagia is managed without dietetic input, these aspects are sometimes overlooked (Dietitians of Canada, 2015). Key factors to consider in improving nutritional and fluid intake for modified-texture diets are:

- Presentation and temperature of food.
- Flavour, taste and palatability.
- Texture of food.
- Nutrient dilution.
- Food fortification and/or enrichment.
- Between-meal snacks.
- Adequate fluid.
- Appropriate use of thickener.
- Posture and physical access to eating and drinking.

People with dysphagia often consume a limited variety of foods, because of constraints imposed by the need for texture modification or because patients themselves limit their intake to the few foods they know they can tolerate. Retextured food can also look unappetising. Foods such as bread, fresh fruit, meat, pulses and nuts are often absent from the diet (Table 7.3.5), and, as a result, intake of dietary fibre and micronutrients may be inadequate. In addition, dysphagia inevitably makes the process of eating difficult, requiring considerable physical effort, and the total quantity of food consumed may be insufficient to meet total energy and nutrient needs.

If intake remains inadequate, additional energy and nutrient supplementation may need to be considered (see Section 6.3). Sip feed supplements may, if necessary, be thickened to an appropriate texture with commercial thickeners (Table 7.3.3), or one of the more semi-solid fortified dessert supplements may be used (Table 7.3.4). The adequacy of these measures should be continuously reviewed along with the progress of the dysphagia itself.

Meeting fluid needs

Dehydration is a high risk, so steps need to be taken to ensure that fluid intake is adequate. Speech and language therapist guidance on the appropriate degree of thickening should be followed. It should be borne in mind that the consistency of unthickened drinks may change with time and temperature. Some liquids become thicker as they cool, e.g. gravy, homemade custard and sauces, while others become more watery, e.g. manufactured custard from cartons or cans.

Most liquids can, if necessary, be thickened with one of the commercial thickeners available (Table 7.3.3), or, alternatively, a ready-prepared thickened drink can be offered (Table 7.3.4). It is important that appropriate guidance with supporting written treatment plans, in line with a fluid texture-modification table, be given to patients, carers, and healthcare and social care professionals. Potential issues include the following:

- Thickening fluids to the correct consistency can be difficult to achieve.
- Different commercial thickeners work differently.
- Mixing techniques and timing need to be taught to achieve the best results.
- Prethickened drinks and prethickened nutritional support drinks can be a useful choice to increase fluid and nutritional intake.

Rather than focusing on thickening fluids with low palatability, it may be better to ensure sufficient fluid intake from foods of modified consistency (Vivanti *et al.*, 2009).

Educating the patient, carers and care team

Dysphagic people often need to be encouraged to eat. Factors such as anxiety or depression (often as a consequence of the underlying illness), confusion (perhaps as a result of stroke or dementia), fear (of choking), plus the physical effort of consuming food – all act as barriers to eating. There are a number of difficulties inherent in producing/providing both texture-modified food and fluids to a good standard, in addition to meeting the aesthetic, cultural and nutritional requirements of the patient. The finished puréed product is not always acceptable, owing of the following reasons:

- Some foods cannot be successfully puréed to a consistently smooth texture.
- Food served is not aesthetically acceptable owing to poor appearance, presentation, colour and flavour.
- Inconsistent preparation of puréed foods, such that the finished product is the wrong texture, can still increase the risk of aspiration.
- Food items being diluted with non-nutritional fluid, e.g. water and gravy, that also increases the volume needed to meet energy and nutrient requirements.

To improve nutritional intake, consider the following:

- Use high-energy liquids when puréeing to avoid diluting flavour and nutrient value, e.g. oil, glucose and honey.
- Provide puréed snacks, e.g. strained yoghurt, suitable dessert, fruit purées or cake, biscuits, and sandwiches prepared using a thickener soaking solution.
- Enhance flavour of puréed main meals with condiments, sauces, spices, etc.
- Employ food fortification/enhancement, e.g. oils, honey, glucose, skimmed milk powder.

- Present food attractively (purée all components separately, preferably using food moulds).
- Keep food at an appetising temperature (use plate warmers and heated dishes).
- Provide food and fluids that are hot or very cold, with or without being highly flavoured, as they can stimulate a stronger swallow.

Monitoring

In some patients, dysphagia may be regarded as stable, but in most instances this is not the case. Following stroke or acute brain injury, there is nearly always some improvement or even resolution of dysphagia. Conversely, in progressive neurological disorders or terminal illness, dysphagia may gradually (or suddenly) worsen. Management of dysphagia should therefore be regarded as a dynamic process, which is likely to change with time, rather than as a static solution to a clinical problem (Finestone & Greene-Finestone, 2003). Therefore, frequent monitoring is essential to assess whether current measures are appropriate for the level of dysphagia and to identify when they need to be modified. This monitoring process requires close collaboration between members of the care team, from carers or nursing staff who may be the first to notice feeding problems or improvements, to SLTs, dietitians and medical staff who can assess the situation and modify the care plan.

If dysphagia is resolving, patients may gradually progress towards a more normal diet in a stepwise process, utilising the audit checklist (NPSA, 2011) and local guidelines. If dysphagia is worsening, or there are signs of aspiration such as choking or recurrent chest infection, a different grade of texture modification may be required. In some cases, it may be necessary to change to an alternative feeding route such as enteral feeding, sometimes as a temporary measure until a certain amount of recovery or remission has occurred.

Continuity of care

Measures need to be in place to ensure that the dysphagic patient receives continuing assessment and support following discharge back into the community. Many areas have a liaison nurse who acts as a link between the primary and secondary care, liaising with ward staff to ascertain a patient's needs and ensuring that district nursing services are aware of and able to meet these needs.

Community dietetic provision is variable. In some areas, community dietetic services are an integral part of primary care support teams; in others, liaison with hospital-based dietetic departments will be required. When the responsibility for dietetic care is transferred from secondary to primary care, it is vital that this be accompanied by the provision of relevant information. The community dietitian will require details of the following:

- Patient, including relevant medical and contact details.
- Discharge date.
- Discharge location.
- Details of the patient's GP.
- Details of the patient's carer and home circumstances.
- Details of the initial and most recent nutritional assessment, weight, and texture requirement and prescription.
- Details of dietary measures implemented (together with their acceptability and effectiveness).
- Type of follow-up required.

The patient's GP will require:

- A summary of the dietetic management of the patient to date.
- Details of any proprietary thickeners or supplements prescribed and predicted usage.
- An indication of likely future dietetic needs.

The patient (or carer) will require:

- Name and contact details of the responsible dietitian.
- Written details of any dietary guidance.

Acknowledgement

The editor acknowledges the prior contribution of Karen Hyland.

Internet resources

British Association for Parenteral and Enteral Nutrition (BAPEN), www.bapen.org.uk
British Dietetic Association (BDA), www.bda.uk.com
British National Formulary (BNF) free online access provided by National Institute for Health and Care Excellence NICE, https://bnf.nice.org.uk/
Hospital Caterers Association, www.hospitalcaterers.org
International Dysphagia Diet Standardisation Initiative Framework (based in Canada, with developed international links), http://iddsi.org
National Patient Safety Agency (NPSA), www.npsa.nhs.uk
Royal College of Speech and Language Therapists, www.rcslt.org

Product producers

Abbott Nutrition, www.abbottnutrition.com
Fresenius Kabi Ltd, www.fresenius-kabi.co.uk
Nestlé Health Science, www.nestlehealthscience.co.uk
Nutricia Advanced Medical Nutrition UK, www.nutricia.co.uk

Texture-modified meal providers

Anglia Crown, www.angliacrown.co.uk
Apetito, www.apetito.co.uk/care-homes/apetito-food/texture-modified
Brakes Bros, www.brake.co.uk/your-business/sector-expertise/healthcare
Oakhouse Foods, www.oakhousefoods.co.uk
Tillery Valley, www.tilleryvalley.com/home/our-food/our-range-of-products.html
Wiltshire Farm Foods, www.wiltshirefarmfoods.com

References

Brody RA, Touger-Decker R, VonHagen S, *et al.* (2000) Role of registered dietitians in dysphagia screening. *J. Am. Diet. Assoc.* 100(9): 1029–1037.

Cichero J, Steele C, Duivestein J, *et al.* (2013) The need for International Terminology and definitions for texture modified foods and thickened liquids used in dysphagia management: foundations of a global initiative. *Curr. Phys. Med. Rehabil. Rep.* 1: 280–291.

Curran J, Groher ME. (1990) Development and dissemination of an aspiration risk reduction diet. *Dysphagia* 5: 6–12.

Dietitians Association of Australia and The Speech Pathology Association of Australia Ltd. (2007) Texture-modified foods and thickened fluids as used for individuals with dysphagia: Australian standardised labels and definition. *Nutr. Diet.* 64(2): S53–76.

Dietitians of Canada. (2015) Defining the role of the dietitian in dysphagia assessment and management. *Can. J. Diet. Pract. Res.* 76(2): 100. doi: 10.3148/cjdpr-2015-013

Ekburg O, Hamdy S, Woisard V, *et al.* (2002) Social and psychological burden of dysphagia: Its impact on diagnosis and treatment. *Dysphagia.* 17(2): 139–146.

Elmståhl S, Bülow M, Ekberg O, *et al.* (1999) Treatment of dysphagia improves nutritional conditions in stroke patients. *Dysphagia* 14(2): 61–66.

Finch S, Doyle W, Lowe C, *et al.* (1998) *National Diet and Nutrition Survey: People Aged 65 Years and Over. Volume 1: Report of the Diet and Nutrition Survey*. London: The Stationery Office.

Finestone HM, Greene-Finestone LS. (2003) Rehabilitation medicine: 2. Diagnosis of dysphagia and its nutritional management for stroke patients. *CMAJ.* 169(10): 1041–1044.

Finestone HM, Greene-Finestone LS, Wilson ES, *et al.* (1995) Malnutrition in stroke patients on the rehabilitation service and at follow-up: prevalence and predictors. *Arch. Phys. Med. Rehabil.* 76(4): 310–316.

Foley NC, Martin RE, Salter KL, *et al.* (2009) A review of the relationship between dysphagia and malnutrition following stroke. *J. Rehabil. Med.* 41(9): 707–713.

Gordon C, Langton Hewer R, Wade DT. (1987) Dysphagia in acute stroke. *Br. Med. J.* 295: 411–414.

Joint Working Party British Dietetic Association and Royal College of Speech and Language Therapists Working Group. (2002, reviewed 2009) *National Descriptors for Texture Modification in Adults*. Birmingham: British Dietetic Association.

King's College Hospital, Multi-disciplinary Working Party. (2000) *A Multi-disciplinary Approach to the Management of Swallowing Disorders*. London: Kings College Hospital.

Lam P, Stanschus S, Zaman R, *et al.* (2017) The International Dysphagia Diet Standardisation Initiative (IDDSI) framework: the Kempen pilot. *BJNN* 13(2): 18–26.

Madhavan A, Lagorio L, Crary M, *et al.* (2016) Prevalence of and risk factors for dysphagia in the community dwelling elderly: a systematic review. *J. Nutr. Health Aging.* 20(8): 806–815.

Marik PE, Kaplan D. (2003) Aspiration pneumonia and dysphagia in the elderly. *Chest* 124(1): 328–336.

Martino R, Beaton D, Diamant NE. (2009) Perceptions of psychological issues related to dysphagia differ in acute and chronic patients. *Dysphagia.* 25: 26–34.

National Patient Safety Agency Dysphagia Expert Reference Group (NPSA). (2011) *Dysphagia Diet Food Texture Descriptors*. NSPA.

Ney D, Weiss J, Kind A, *et al.* (2009) Senescent swallowing: impact, strategies, and interventions. *Nutr. Clin. Pract.* 24: 395–413.

NICE. (2017) *Feed Thickeners and Pre-thickened Drinks*. Available at https://bnf.nice.org.uk/borderline-substance-taxonomy/feed-thickeners-and-pre-thickened-drinks.html. Accessed 3 March 2018.

Odderson IR, Keaton JC, McKenna BS. (1995) Swallow management in patients on an acute stroke pathway: quality is cost effective. *Arch. Phys. Med. Rehabil.* 76(12): 1130–1133.

Paciaroni M, Mazzotta G, Corea F, *et al.* (2004) Dysphagia following stroke. *Eur. Neurol.* 51(3): 162–167.

Penman JP, Thomson M. (1998) A review of the textured diets developed for the management of dysphagia. *J. Hum. Nutr. Diet.* 11: 51–60.

Ramsey DJ, Smithard DG, Kalra L. (2003) Early assessments of dysphagia and aspiration risk in acute stroke patients. *Stroke* 34(5): 1252–1257.

Rosenvinge S, Starke ID. (2005) Improving care for patients with dysphagia. *Age Ageing.* 34(6): 587–593.

Royal College of Physicians (RCP) and Intercollegiate Stroke Working Party. (2016) *National Clinical Guidelines for Stroke*, 5th edn. London: RCP.

Scottish Intercollegiate Guidelines Network (SIGN). (2010) *Management of Patients with Stroke: Identification and Management of Patients with Dysphagia*. SIGN Guideline 119. SIGN.

Smithard DG, Smeeton NC, Wolfe CD. (2007) Long-term outcome after stroke: does dysphagia matter? *Age Ageing.* 36(1): 90–94.

Steele C, Alsanei W, Ayanikalath S, *et al.* (2015) The influence of food texture and liquid consistency modification on swallowing physiology and function: a systematic review. *Dysphagia.* 30(1): 2–26.

Teasell RW, McRae M, Marchuk Y, *et al.* (1996) Pneumonia associated with aspiration following stroke. *Arch. Phys. Med. Rehabil.* 77(7): 707–709.

Vivanti AP, Campbell KL, Suter MS, *et al.* (2009) Contribution of thickened drinks, food and enteral and parenteral fluids on fluid intake in hospitalised patients with dysphagia. *J. Hum. Nutr. Diet.* 22: 148–155.

7.4 Gastrointestinal disorders

7.4.1 Disorders of the upper aerodigestive tract

Poonam Gulia

Key points

- Patients with disorders of the upper aerodigestive tract are nutritionally vulnerable and pose exceptional nutritional management problems.
- Patients with oesophageal disorders may have an increased risk of developing malnutrition, and dietary advice may be required for altered food texture and to ensure nutritional adequacy.

The normal swallowing mechanism can be impaired by damage or disease that affects the oral cavity, pharynx, hypopharynx and oesophagus. This has the potential to compromise nutritional intake as it can affect the amount and types of food consumed, and impact on the time and effort experienced by the patient at each stage of the normal swallow. Even minor disorders can have a major impact on nutritional status, particularly if they are persistent and occur in people whose nutritional status is already poor. As a result, food choice and consumption can be profoundly affected in both short and long term. The upper aerodigestive tract can be affected by cancer (see Chapter 7.15.3, Cancer of the gastrointestinal tract) and several benign disorders that are described in the following text.

Benign disorders of the aerodigestive tract

Micronutrient deficiencies

The rate of epithelial cell turnover of the oral mucous membrane is faster than that of skin (3–7 days as compared to ≤28 days). As a result, the oral cavity often demonstrates early signs and symptoms of systemic diseases and nutritional deficiencies (Thomas & Giant, 2010). The presence of minor oral disorders may suggest underlying micronutrient deficiency and poor nutritional status. Both iron deficiency anaemia and pernicious anaemia (B_{12} deficiency) can result in a very red, sore and smooth tongue. Deficiencies of most of the B group vitamins affect the soft tissues of the mouth, e.g. angular stomatitis (riboflavin deficiency) and cheilosis (angular stomatitis). Although cheilosis is a classic symptom of pellagra (niacin deficiency), in the UK it is more likely to be a sign of generalised vitamin B deficiency and undernutrition. Vitamin A deficiency can cause xerostomia (dry mouth) and, in children, can result in hypoplasia of tooth enamel and dentine, increasing the susceptibility to caries.

Fractured jaw

Mandibular fractures may be treated using open (surgical) and closed (non-surgical) techniques. Fracture sites are immobilised with intermaxillary fixation (IMF) or other external or internal devices (i.e. plates and screws) to allow bone healing (Nasser *et al.*, 2013). Patients are encouraged to mobilise the jaw gently to avoid stiffness or trismus (contraction of the jaw muscles), but are advised to have a soft diet with adequate fluid replacement. The use of nutritionally complete liquid feeds is advisable to ensure that energy and nutrient needs are met, and that scrupulous oral hygiene can be maintained for the weeks following fixation. On the rare occasions of intermaxillary fixation, when the jaws remain wired for approximately 4–6 weeks, a liquid diet will be necessary. As the wires are relaxed and ultimately removed, the diet should be regraded from a liquid to a soft or semi-solid diet, with protein and energy supplements if indicated, until a normal diet can be taken.

Oesophagitis

Oesophagitis is inflammation of the mucosal lining of the oesophagus and is usually a consequence of

Manual of Dietetic Practice, Sixth Edition. Edited by Joan Gandy.

Companion website: www.manualofdieteticpractice.com

gastro-oesophageal reflux (GORD) (see Chapter 7.4.3, Disorders of the stomach and duodenum). Symptoms develop if reflux becomes frequent and the mucosa of the oesophagus becomes sensitive to the acidic reflux material. Dietary management is as for GORD, with the patient being advised to consume soft, bland and non-irritant foods and liquids while the symptoms are acute.

Achalasia

Achalasia is characterised by weak peristalsis of the oesophagus and the inability of the lower oesophageal sphincter to relax after a swallow; it is relatively uncommon. Food collects in the oesophagus, causing discomfort, and eventually may pass through the sphincter by the action of gravity and the weight of food consumed. Regurgitation of food is common but lacks the bitter taste of acid or bile that is characteristic of reflux. Aspiration of food from the oesophagus may lead to pneumonia. Repeated collection of food in the oesophagus can irritate the mucosa, resulting in secondary oesophagitis and pain. Loss of weight is uncommon unless the patient becomes fearful of eating. Relief may be obtained by advising the patient to:

- Consume small, frequent meals.
- Avoid fried foods or foods that aggravate dyspepsia.
- Avoid very hot or cold foods (these tend to increase the intake of air into the stomach).
- Avoid strong tea, coffee, large amounts of alcohol.

The patient may also find that standing up during a meal, drinking a glass of water and exhaling hard may help to force food into the stomach. If dietary measures are ineffective, surgical myotomy or mechanical dilatation may be necessary.

Oesophageal perforation

If the oesophagus perforates spontaneously, or is perforated as a result of dilatation, oesophagoscopy or caustic burns, any food or liquid consumed would enter the thoracic cavity, with potentially fatal consequences. The perforation may be allowed to heal naturally or may need surgical repair. Patients should not be fed orally; enteral tube feeding or parenteral feeding may be necessary.

Benign oesophageal stricture

Benign stricture usually results from mucosal injury, either as a consequence of chronic GORD or damage following intubation with wide-bore gastric tubes. Stricture may initially be due to muscular spasm, or it may result from physical scarring and thickening of the oesophageal wall. The first symptom is usually difficulty in swallowing solid foods or foods sticking, particularly food such as doughy bread or tough meats, which tend to remain as a bolus as they pass down the oesophagus. Dysphagia with solid foods may soon progress to dysphagia with semi-solids or liquids. Appetite is usually reduced, and severe weight loss may be reported. Patients may suffer these difficulties for some time before seeking help, and may be dehydrated and malnourished on presentation. Some patients may need intravenous rehydration and nutritional support prior to treatment, which is usually by oesophageal dilatation. If GORD has been a contributory factor, it is important that this be corrected to prevent recurrence of the stricture.

Internet resources

British Gastroenterology Society, www.bsg.org.uk
Society of Thoracic Surgeons (USA), www.sts.org

References

Nasser M, Pandis N, Fleming PS, *et al.* (2013) Interventions for the management of mandibular fractures. *Cochrane Database Syst Rev.* (7): CD006087.

Thomas DM, Giant WM. (2010) Nutrition and oral mucosal diseases. *Clin. Dermatol.* 28: 426–431.

7.4.2 Orofacial granulomatosis

Helen Campbell and Miranda Lomer

Key points

- Orofacial granulomatosis (OFG) is a rare condition defined by chronic granulomatous inflammation of the lips, oral cavity and sometimes the face.
- It is predominantly an idiopathic disease, although approximately 25% present with concurrent Crohn's disease.
- A diet cinnamon and benzoate free is the primary treatment and assumes an increased sensitivity to these compounds.

Orofacial granulomatosis (OFG) is a rare condition defined by chronic granulomatous inflammation of the lips, oral cavity and sometimes the face (Wiesenfeld *et al.*, 1985). The typical presentation involves lip swelling and erythema (Campbell *et al.*, 2011; Wiesenfeld *et al.*, 1985). Inside the mouth, the buccal mucosa (inside of the cheeks), gingivae (gums), buccal sulcus (adjoining areas between the gingivae and buccal mucosa) and floor of the mouth can be affected with swelling, erythema, nodular swelling, tags and ulcers. Lip fissures are common and can be prone to bacterial or candida infections that often exacerbate symptoms. Intraoral fissuring can also be present. The tongue, palate and throat are less commonly involved; the disease is generally painless except when ulcers are present.

OFG predominantly exists as an idiopathic disease, although approximately 25% of patients can also present with concurrent Crohn's disease (CD) (Campbell *et al.*, 2011). Consequently, OFG is often called oral CD. Other more historical nomenclature can include cheilitis granulomatosa and Miescher's cheilitis. A small proportion also present as Melkersson–Rosenthal syndrome, diagnosed when the additional features of a fissured tongue and facial palsy are present (Rogers, 1996).

Diagnosis

Expertise on this condition is rare, and patients often undergo a variety of investigations and ineffectual treatments prior to accurate diagnosis. The diagnosis is made through expert examination and exclusion of other granulomatous conditions (e.g. sarcoidosis, tuberculosis) (Grave *et al.*, 2009). Confirmation of the diagnosis is normally made from histopathological findings that identify non-caseating granulomas from biopsies of the affected sites. Patients with OFG are normally diagnosed as young adults, although it can present at any age (Campbell *et al.*, 2011).

Disease processes and consequences

The cause of OFG is unknown, but is thought to involve an allergic component. The heterogeneous nature of the condition indicates a number of different causes, and early studies identified an array of foods believed to be dietary triggers, exclusion of which often improved symptoms (Ferguson & MacFadyen, 1986; Wray *et al.*, 2000). Due to the rarity of OFG, there are no epidemiological studies. Most reports are UK based, with higher patient numbers being reported in Scotland (Gibson *et al.*, 2000) and Ireland (Fitzpatrick *et al.*, 2011). Genetic association analysis indicates that NOD2 is associated with the clinical phenotype of OFG with associated CD but not with OFG alone (Mentzer *et al.*, 2016b). Patients are most upset by the physically disfiguring and chronic nature of the disease, which is often difficult to treat and can last for months or even years.

Nutritional consequences and nutritional assessment

There are no specific nutritional consequences in patients with OFG, although, in those with severe concurrent CD, nutritional implications need to be considered (see Chapter 7.4.7, Coeliac disease). Standard nutritional and dietary assessment strategies can be used in patients.

Clinical investigation and management

Ideally, the management of OFG requires a multidisciplinary approach. Patients are referred mainly from specialists in oral medicine, gastroenterology, dermatology, allergy clinics and dentists (Campbell *et al.*, 2011). Close collaboration with colleagues in oral medicine can be helpful, particularly for expertise in objective examination and documentation of progression or regression of clinical features. In the event of gastrointestinal symptoms, patients should consult a gastroenterologist.

The treatment of OFG is challenging, and patients often suffer from episodes of relapse and recurrence that can be upsetting and frustrating. The cinnamon- and benzoate-free diet is the primary treatment of choice and assumes an increased sensitivity to these compounds (Campbell *et al.*, 2011). The mechanism remains unclear, but the diet originates from a retrospective study investigating patch test data from a series of patients with oral mucosal disorders (Wray *et al.*, 2000). Patients with OFG had increased sensitivity to cinnamon, benzoates and chocolate. A subsequent study demonstrated significant benefit from dietary elimination of cinnamon and benzoate in up to 72% of patients (White *et al.*, 2006). Other dietary measures include the use of liquid enteral feeds (taken orally), and elemental diet has proven beneficial, particularly in children (Mutalib *et al.*, 2016).

In the event of dietary failure, topical immunosuppression (e.g. beclomethasone mouthwash), topical hydrocortisone or topical tacrolimus can be used (Casson *et al.*, 2000; Leao *et al.*, 2004). Intralesional steroids can also be helpful in some cases (Fedele *et al.*, 2014). Occasionally, systemic corticosteroids may be given, although these usually only offer short-term improvement. For refractory OFG, patients may require long-term systemic immunosuppression, most commonly with a thiopurine (azathioprine or mercaptopurine). However, this is likely to be more beneficial in those with concurrent CD than in OFG alone (Mentzer *et al.*, 2016a). Anti-tumour necrosis alpha antibody infusions (infliximab and adalimumab) have been used if other treatment is unsuccessful (Elliott *et al.*, 2011; Leao *et al.*, 2004). In severe fibrotic disease, it may be necessary for patients to undergo a cheiloplasty to surgically debulk the lips (Kruse-Losler *et al.*, 2005).

Nutritional management

The cinnamon- and benzoate-free diet can be used to treat OFG and offers a non-invasive therapy which provides benefit in up to 72% of patients and can avoid the need for systemic immunosuppression in approximately 25% of patients (Campbell *et al.*, 2010; White *et al.*, 2006). For this reason, dietary treatment is commonly used first, with other therapies being employed either in refractory OFG or when diet fails to provide sufficient benefit. Dietary adherence can be difficult, although motivation is often sufficiently high, particularly in those troubled by the disfiguring nature of the disease. However, data on sources and levels of cinnamon and benzoates are scarce, and so patients are likely to be inadvertently exposed to sources. This could explain why patients often complain of recurrence despite strict adherence to the diet.

It is important to provide a structure for patients undertaking a cinnamon- and benzoate-restricted diet. Improvement in symptoms can take some time and can be frustrating, although some patients may see improvement within a few weeks. For this reason, it is important that patients are closely monitored and regularly reviewed. A diet history will identify the patient's current exposure to cinnamon and benzoates. Those regularly drinking soft drinks are most likely to be receiving the highest levels of benzoates as added preservatives. It is not uncommon for patients to be already avoiding foods that they feel contribute to their symptoms. Consequently, nutritional adequacy could be challenged with further restrictions, and this needs to be considered.

The cinnamon- and benzoate-free diet

Sources of cinnamon

Cinnamon (*Cinnamomum zeylanium* N.) is a spice commonly added to both sweet and savoury foods (Singletary, 2008). The main compound that provides the flavour and aroma is cinnamaldehyde, and it is often cited as being the component to which patients demonstrate sensitivity (Gruenwald *et al.*, 2010; Wray *et al.*, 2000). It is used in Asian cuisine and curries, but can also be added to chewing gums, sweets, chocolates, alcoholic beverages, fizzy drinks, cereals and bakery products (e.g. cakes and breads). Other products that may include cinnamon include toothpastes, mouthwashes, perfumes, perfumed creams, make-up, soaps and medicines. A food product that contains <2% of a spice is not required to be specifically labelled and can instead use the term spices or mixed spices (Food Standards Agency, 2008a, 2008b) (see Chapter 4.5, Food law and labelling). Consequently, it is necessary to avoid products labelled with these terms. In addition, products labelled as all-spice, mixed spices, curry powder and garam masala need to be avoided.

Cassia (*Cinnamomum cassia* Presl) is a close relative of cinnamon and is often used as a cheaper alternative. It has recently received some interest as it contains substantial quantities of coumarin, which is thought to be hepatotoxic and carcinogenic (Abraham *et al.*, 2010). It also contains cinnamaldehyde but in lesser quantities than cinnamon. Cassia therefore needs to be avoided on this diet.

Sources of benzoates

Rich sources of naturally occurring benzoates include a number of fruits, predominantly berries, vegetables and spices (Table 7.4.1) (Cressey & Jones, 2009; Heimhuber & Herrmann, 1990; Sieber *et al.*, 1989; Toyoda *et al.*, 1983a, 1983b). Cinnamon is also a naturally occurring source of benzoates. It is also necessary to exclude products that might contain them, e.g. soups, juices, sauces, pickles, breads and other baked goods. Vigilance with reading labels is therefore very important.

The highest contributors are benzoates used as preservatives added to foods, drinks, medicines and cosmetics. Table 7.4.2 lists the E numbers of the preservatives that should be avoided. The main foods to which these may have been added include soft drinks, pickles, jams, biscuits, cakes, pre-prepared ready meals, pickled fish, sauces, dips, yoghurts and confectionary. Therefore, all food labels need to be checked for the addition of benzoates.

A further source of benzoates and derivatives of cinnamon can include cosmetic and hygiene products. There is no current evidence that these contribute to symptoms in OFG, but absorption of benzoates through

Table 7.4.1 Natural benzoates to exclude and suitable alternative benzoate-rich foods

Benzoate-rich foods to exclude	Alternatives
Fruit	
Dried fruit, fruit sauce. Berries, e.g. blackberries, cranberries, blueberries, strawberries, raspberries. Prunes, peaches, papaya, nectarines.	All other fresh and frozen fruit, e.g. apple, orange, pear, banana, satsuma, tangerine, melon, pineapple, grapefruit, lemon, lime, grape, mango, rhubarb.
Vegetables	
Avocado, pumpkin, kidney beans, soya beans, spinach. Any juices, sauces, jams, pickles or other food products containing the preceding fruit and vegetables.	Other vegetables, e.g. broccoli, cauliflower, cabbage, carrots, green beans, runner beans, broad beans, spring greens, lettuce, cucumber, onion, peppers, bean sprouts.
Spices	
Cinnamon sticks, cinnamon powder, cassia sticks, cassia powder, cloves, nutmeg, spices, mixed spices.	Salt, pepper, all other fresh herbs, e.g. basil, parsley, mint, coriander, etc., clearly labelled single spices.
Teas	
Any tea leaves, tea bags, chai tea, green tea, rooibos tea, fruit or herbal teas with tea leaves.	Herbal infusions, coffee.
Dairy	
Blue cheeses, gorgonzola, cheese with added fruit or spices listed earlier.	All other cheeses, e.g. cheddar, feta, mozzarella, parmesan, brie, camembert, cottage cheese, etc.

Table 7.4.2 Preservatives to be avoided

E number	Benzoate
E210	Benzoic acid
E211	Sodium benzoate
E212	Potassium benzoate
E213	Calcium benzoate
E214	Ethyl 4-hydroxybenzoate or ethyl para-hydroxybenzoate
E215	Ethyl 4-hydroxybenzoate, sodium salt or sodium ethyl para-hydroxybenzoate
E216[a]	Propyl 4-hydroxybenzoate or propyl para-hydroxybenzoate
E217[a]	Propyl 4-hydroxybenzoate, sodium salt or sodium para-hydroxybenzoate
E218	Methyl 4-hydroxybenzoate or methyl para-hydroxybenzoate
E219	Methyl 4-hydroxybenzoate, sodium salt or sodium methyl-hydroxybenzoate

[a]Banned in foods produced within the European Union, but may be found in products in other countries.

the skin has been demonstrated (Nair, 2001). Anecdotally, patients often complain of sensitivity to cosmetic products. Consequently, the recommendation is currently to limit exposure to cosmetics that contain cinnamates and benzoates, particularly products that come into direct contact with the lips or face, such as lip balms, make-up, face cleansers, soaps, creams and sunscreens. Most high-street products contain cinnamates and/or benzoates. However, it is possible to find cinnamon- and benzoate-free products in specialist health food shops or on the Internet.

Other considerations

Soya

Soya is a natural source of benzoates and should be avoided in the cinnamon and benzoate free diet. Soya is increasingly used in many products, e.g. soya flour is added to bread, and soya lecithin is added as an emulsifier to many foods. The benzoate content in these foods has not been measured, but, previously, the recommendation was to avoid all products with added soya flour and lecithin (E322) that could have been sourced from soya. More recently, this recommendation has been increasingly challenged, and a recent enquiry of manufacturers suggests that the contribution of benzoates from these sources is comparatively low and perhaps negligible (Nagarajah *et al.*, 2008). Consequently, this recommendation has been changed, and baked goods with added soya flour and products with soya lecithin no longer requires avoidance.

Tomato

Patients with OFG often complain of sensitivity to tomato, particularly cooked tomato sauces. The reason for this is unclear, but tomato does contain small amounts of benzoic acid (Sieber *et al.*, 1989). It is likely that concentrated sources of tomato, such as tomato purée, could have a higher concentration of benzoic acid. Consequently, concentrated sources of tomato should be avoided. Tomato ketchup often contains benzoates as a preservative.

Chocolate

Patients often complain of sensitivity to chocolate, and patch test studies have identified chocolate hypersensitivity in OFG (Wray *et al.*, 2000). Chocolate or cocoa has not been identified as a rich source of benzoic acid or other benzoates, although certain additions such as dried fruit and cinnamon could be contributing factors. Patients should be advised to avoid chocolate for the duration of the elimination diet.

Flavourings

Flavourings do not need to be specifically named on foods labels (Food Standards Agency, 2008b), but they may be derivatives of both cinnamon and benzoates. Consequently, foods labelled as containing flavourings or natural flavourings should be excluded.

Monitoring

Objective measures are helpful as symptom change can be subtle. Photographs can prove helpful and be encouraging for many patients to demonstrate progression. A structured oral examination and documentation of disease activity and severity can be useful and should be a routine part of the multidisciplinary approach to this condition. The cinnamon- and benzoate-free diet should be tried for 12 weeks. In the event that significant benefit is demonstrated, this can be extended to maximise improvement. Prolonged or open-ended time frames on this diet are not recommended and will contribute to apathy and non-compliance. If no (or limited) improvement is demonstrated, other approaches may be considered.

Dietary reintroduction

Following a 12-week dietary restriction, foods are reintroduced one food at a time. As symptom recurrence is often reported as delayed, it is useful to undertake the challenge over 2–3 consecutive days before commencing with another food. A structured symptom diary can be useful to help identify likely triggers. The highest sources of benzoates are from soft drinks, and these are therefore often left until last (if reintroduced at all). Similarly, chocolate is often left until later. It is not uncommon to find that patients need to remain on a partially restricted diet long term, limiting exposure to overt sources of cinnamon, fizzy drinks and chocolate.

Drug–nutrient interactions

- Systemic corticosteroids can cause dyslipidaemia, affect glucose tolerance, increase the risk of osteoporosis, and cause weight gain. Grapefruit juice can affect their metabolism and should be avoided.
- Thiopurines can cause nausea, vomiting, diarrhoea and loss of appetite.

Acknowledgement

The editor acknowledges the prior contribution of Jeremy Sanderson.

Further reading

Campbell HE, Escudier MP, Patel P, *et al.* (2011) Cinnamon and benzoate free diet as a primary treatment for orofacial granulomatosis. *Aliment. Pharmacol. Ther.* 34(7): 687–701.

White A, Nunes C, Escudier M, *et al.* (2006) Improvement in orofacial granulomatosis on a cinnamon- and benzoate-free diet. *Inflamm. Bowel Dis.* 12(6): 508–514.

References

Abraham K, Wohrlin F, Lindtner O, *et al.* (2010) Toxicology and risk assessment of coumarin: focus on human data. *Mol. Nutr. Food Res.* 54(2): 228–239.

Campbell HE, Patel P, Escudier M, *et al.* (2010) The relevance of patch testing and a clinical review of the cinnamon and benzoate free diet in orofacial granulomatosis (OFG). *Oral Diseases* 16: 551–551.

Campbell H, Escudier M, Patel P, *et al.* (2011) Distinguishing orofacial granulomatosis from Crohn's disease: Two separate disease entities? *Inflamm. Bowel Dis.* 17(10): 2109–2115.

Casson DH, Eltumi M, Tomlin S, *et al.* (2000) Topical tacrolimus may be effective in the treatment of oral and perineal Crohn's disease. *Gut* 47(3): 436–440.

Cressey P, Jones S. (2009) Levels of preservatives (sulfite, sorbate and benzoate) in New Zealand foods and estimated dietary exposure. *Food Addit. Contam. Part A Chem. Anal. Control Expo. Risk Assess.* 26(5): 604–613.

Elliott E, Campbell H, Escudier M, *et al.* (2011) Experience with anti-TNF-alpha therapy for orofacial granulomatosis. *J. Oral Pathol. Med.* 40(1): 14–19.

Fedele S, Fung PP, Bamashmous N, *et al.* (2014) Long term effectiveness of intralesional triamcinolone acetonide therapy in orofacial granulomatosis: an observational cohort study. *Br. J. Dermatol.* 170(4): 794–801.

Ferguson MM, MacFadyen EE. (1986) Orofacial granulomatosis – a 10 year review. *Ann. Acad. Med. Singapore* 15(3): 370.

Fitzpatrick L, Healy CM, McCartan BE, *et al.* (2011) Patch testing for food-associated allergies in orofacial granulomatosis. *J. Oral Pathol. Med.* 40(1): 10–13.

Food Standards Agency (FSA). (2008a) *Food Labelling: Clear Food Labelling Guidance.* London: FSA.

Food Standards Agency (FSA). (2008b) *The Food Labelling Regulations 1996: Guidance Notes on Quantitative Ingredient Declarations ('QUID').* London: FSA.

Gibson J, Wray D, Bagg J. (2000) Oral staphylococcal mucositis: a new clinical entity in orofacial granulomatosis and Crohn's disease. *Oral Surg. Oral Med. Oral Pathol. Oral Radiol. Endod.* 89(2): 171–176.

Grave B, McCullough M, Wiesenfeld D. (2009) Orofacial granulomatosis – a 20-year review. *Oral Dis.* 15(1): 46–51.

Gruenwald J, Freder J, Armbruester N. (2010) Cinnamon and health. *Crit. Rev. Food Sci. Nutr.* 50(9): 822–834.

Heimhuber B, Herrmann K. (1990) Benzoe-, Phylessig-, 3-Phenylpropan- und Zimtsaure sowie benzoglucosen in einigen Obst- und Fruchtgemusearten. Deutsche Lebensmittel-Rundschau 86 jahrg. Heft 7.

Kruse-Losler B, Presser D, Metze D, *et al.* (2005) Surgical treatment of persistent macrocheilia in patients with Melkersson–Rosenthal syndrome and cheilitis granulomatosa. *Arch. Dermatol.* 141(9): 1085–11091.

Leao JC, Hodgson T, Scully C, *et al.* (2004) Review article: orofacial granulomatosis. *Aliment. Pharmacol. Ther.* 20(10): 1019–1027.

Mentzer A, Goel R, Elliott T, *et al.* (2016a) Azathioprine is effective for oral involvement in Crohn's disease but not for orofacial granulomatosis alone. *J. Oral Pathol. Med.* 45(4): 312–318.

Mentzer A, Nayee S, Omar Y, *et al.* (2016b) Genetic association analysis reveals differences in the contribution of NOD2 variants to the clinical phenotypes of orofacial granulomatosis. *Inflamm. Bowel Dis.* 22(7): 1552–1558.

Mutalib M, Bezanti K, Elawad M, *et al.* (2016) The role of exclusive enteral nutrition in the management of orofacial granulomatosis in children. *World J. Pediatr.* 12: 421–424.

Nagarajah R, Campbell H, Sanderson JD, *et al.* (2008) Dietary management of orofacial granulomatosis: quantification of benzoates in foods and cosmetics. *J. Hum. Nutr. Diet.* 21(4): 397–398.

Nair B. (2001) Final report on the safety assessment of benzyl alcohol, benzoic acid, and sodium benzoate. *Int. J. Toxicol.* 20(3): 23–50.

Rogers RS. (1996) Melkersson–Rosenthal syndrome and orofacial granulomatosis. *Dermatol. Clin.* 14(2): 371–379.

Sieber R, Butikofer U, Bosset JO, *et al.* (1989) Benzoic acid as a natural component of foods – a review. *Mitt. Geb. Lebensmittel-unters. Hyg.* 80(3): 345–362.

Singletary K. (2008) Cinnamon: overview of health benefits 160. *Nutr. Today.* 43(6): 263–266.

Toyoda M, Ito Y, Isshiki K, *et al.* (1983a) Estimation of daily intake of many kinds of food additives according to the market basket studies in Japan. *J. Jpn. Soc. Nutr. Food Sci.* 36(6): 489–497.

Toyoda M, Ito Y, Isshiki K, *et al.* (1983b) Daily intake of preservatives, benzoic acid, dehydroacetic acid, propionic acid and their salts, and esters of p-hydroxybenzoic acid in Japan. *J. Jpn. Soc. Nutr. Food Sci.* 36(6): 467–480.

White A, Nunes C, Escudier M, *et al.* (2006) Improvement in orofacial granulomatosis on a cinnamon- and benzoate-free diet. *Inflamm. Bowel Dis.* 12(6): 508–514.

Wiesenfeld D, Ferguson MM, Mitchell DN, *et al.* (1985) Oro-facial granulomatosis – a clinical and pathological analysis. *Q. J. Med.* 54(213): 101–113.

Wray D, Rees SR, Gibson J, *et al.* (2000) The role of allergy in oral mucosal diseases. *Q. J. Med.* 93(8): 507–511.

7.4.3 Disorders of the stomach and duodenum

Poonam Gulia

Key points

- Disorders of the stomach and duodenum can have a significant effect on dietary intake and nutritional status.
- Management is often a combination of medical or surgical intervention alongside dietary changes.
- Dietary advice is based on control of symptoms and ensuring nutritional adequacy.

SECTION 7

Cancers of the stomach and duodenum (see Chapter 7.15.3, Cancer of the gastrointestinal tract) and gastroparesis (see Chapter 7.4.4, Gastroparesis) are described separately. Nausea and vomiting are symptoms, rather than conditions, but are included here for completeness.

Nausea and vomiting

Nausea and vomiting can be the pathological consequences of disease or its treatment (e.g. chemotherapy), physiological (e.g. morning sickness in pregnancy), drug induced (e.g. antibiotics) or psychological (e.g. bulimia nervosa) in origin. In healthy individuals, nausea and vomiting caused by infection or food poisoning usually resolve spontaneously. Eating should be ceased until acute symptoms have eased and replaced with frequent consumption of small volumes of water, sugar-containing soft drinks or oral rehydration solutions.

Profuse or persistent nausea and vomiting may compromise intake of both food and fluids, and exacerbate an already poor nutritional status resulting from underlying disease. Dietetic management depends on the nature of the underlying problem. Measures that may help alleviate symptoms and other strategies to improve oral nutritional intake are described in Chapter 6.3 (Oral nutritional support).

Gastro-oesophageal reflux disease

Gastro-oesophageal reflux disease (GORD) is a term used to describe a range of symptoms, including acid reflux (with or without pain), heartburn and oesophagitis. Heartburn is a common accompaniment to indigestion and is characterised by a sharp, burning pain either just below the sternum or between the shoulder blades. This chest pain may be so severe that it may be mistaken for angina. It is caused by the reflux of the stomach contents (containing acid and enzymes) into the oesophagus, some of which may reach the mouth or be sensed in the back of the throat (Figure 7.4.1). This irritates the oesophageal mucosa, causing pain, and repeated attacks may cause mucosal damage and inflammation (oesophagitis). Repeated episodes of GORD can damage the lining of the oesophagus and lead to oesophageal ulceration, oesophageal stricture and Barrett's oesophagus, and possibly adenocarcinoma of the oesophagus (NICE, 2015). Reflux may occur as a result of the following conditions (Figure 7.4.2):

- Weakness of the sphincter at the junction of the oesophagus and stomach.
- High pressure within the stomach, e.g. consumption of a large quantity of food or liquid.
- High pressure from the abdominal area, e.g. obesity, pregnancy.
- Hiatus hernia resulting in impairment of the pinchcock mechanism of the diaphragm (see the section heading 'Hiatus hernia').

Although not well supported by clinical data, diet and lifestyle factors remain important instruments for the overall management of GORD (Tytgat *et al.*, 2008). The effectiveness of commonly advised measures, such as reduced intake of heavily spiced or fatty foods, alcohol intake and smoking cessation, in relieving gastro-oesophageal reflux *per se* have not been conclusively established in well-controlled trials. There is sufficient evidence that supports the fact that obesity, particularly abdominal obesity, plays a key role in determining GORD. Controlled weight loss (by diet or surgery) is effective in improving GORD symptoms and risk of

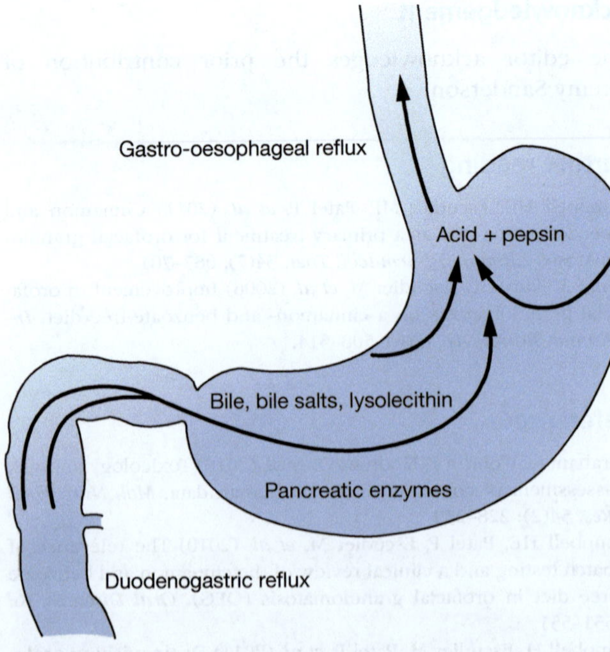

Figure 7.4.1 Constituents of gastro-oesophageal reflux

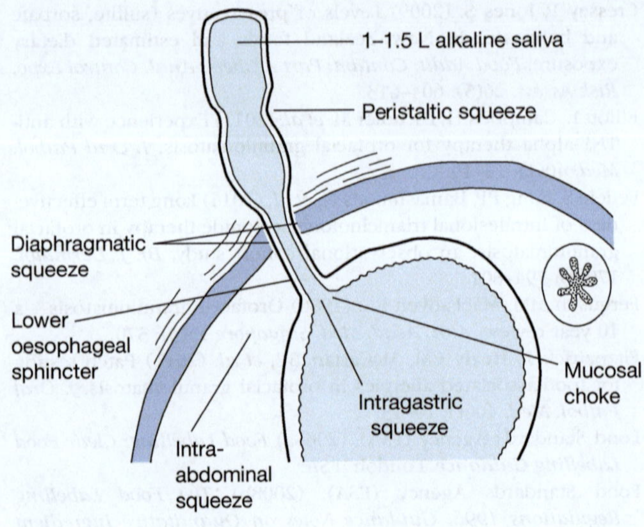

Figure 7.4.2 Factors preventing the reflux of food and regurgitation of food from the stomach

oesophageal adenocarcinoma (Festi *et al.*, 2009). Measures that are generally accepted as being helpful are:

- Eating smaller volumes at regular intervals.
- Avoiding rich or fatty foods.
- Avoiding highly spiced or irritant foods known to exacerbate symptoms.
- Avoiding excessive consumption of tea, coffee or alcohol.
- Chewing foods well.
- Avoiding eating late at night.
- Avoiding bending, lifting or lying down after meals.
- Reducing weight if obese.
- Avoiding excessive consumption of tea, coffee or alcohol.
- Smoking cessation.
- Sleeping in a semi-upright position or with the head of the bed raised a few inches to help prevent nocturnal symptoms of reflux.

Additional symptom relief is obtained by use of H2 receptor antagonists (e.g. cimetidine, ranitidine), proton pump inhibitors (e.g. lansoprazole, omeprazole), prokinetics (e.g. metoclopramide, domperidone) and alginates. The standard treatments for patients with symptomatic GORD are lifestyle modification and drug therapy. Patients who have refractory symptoms, who develop complications despite medication or who develop intolerance to medication may be considered for anti-reflux surgery (usually laparoscopic fundoplication). Several endoscopic techniques (such as endoscopic radiofrequency ablation and endoscopic injection of bulking agents) have also been used.

Dyspepsia

Dyspepsia describes a range of symptoms arising from the upper gastrointestinal tract, but it has no universally accepted definition. Dyspepsia is defined broadly to include people with recurrent epigastric pain, heartburn or acid regurgitation, with or without bloating, nausea or vomiting (NICE, 2014). It is important to establish the cause as it may be due to GORD, poor eating habits or a symptom of underlying, possibly serious, disease. Simple indigestion can nearly always be alleviated by the diet and lifestyle measures described earlier for GORD.

Hiatus hernia

The diaphragm has several openings through which the abdominal viscera can enter the thorax. The opening for the oesophagus, the hiatus, is loosely attached to the oesophagus. In middle age, this attachment weakens, and abdominal pressure may cause the hiatus to herniate (tear). This is likely to happen as a result of becoming overweight, but may also occur as a consequence of pregnancy, chronic coughing or chronic constipation due to straining. The major symptoms are pain and discomfort as a result of reflux and oesophagitis. Patients may also complain of the sensation of foods such as doughy bread or fibrous foods (e.g. salad, nuts or seeds) sticking in the gullet.

In some patients, the priority is weight loss, which will reduce abdominal pressure and may also be advisable if surgical repair is necessary. Symptom relief from GORD may be obtained by following the preventive measures listed earlier. If particular foods cause dysphagic symptoms, they should be avoided. Patients with chronic constipation should be encouraged to increase their fibre and fluid intake.

Gastritis

Gastritis, inflammation of the gastric mucosa, may be acute erosive or chronic atrophic gastritis. Alcohol, non-steroidal anti-inflammatory drugs (NSAIDs), chemical irritants and exposure to certain pathogens may trigger acute gastritis, resulting in pain, nausea and vomiting, usually of short duration. No particular dietary changes are usually required, although adequate hydration is important during any period of vomiting, and small meals should be taken at regular intervals. Chronic gastritis may follow repeated attacks of acute gastritis and is closely associated with *Helicobacter pylori* infection, which is treated by eradication (antibiotic) therapy, usually along with a proton pump inhibitor. Dietary advice should be based on the following:

- Identifying and attempting to correct dietary and lifestyle factors that are contributing to the condition, e.g. alcohol, smoking, drugs, poor eating habits.
- Encouraging a balanced diet based on healthy eating principles, together with a sensible meal pattern.
- Correcting deficiencies, e.g. iron, vitamin B_{12}, that result from repeated bleeding and reduced production of intrinsic factor.

Peptic ulcer

A peptic ulcer is erosion in the mucosal lining of the stomach or duodenum. Duodenal ulcers are more common and often occur in the duodenal cap, and duodenitis (inflammation) is invariably present in peptic ulcer. Ulceration may also occur in the pyloric antrum, and the resultant scar tissue may cause pyloric stenosis, resulting in delayed gastric emptying and the accumulation of fermenting food debris in the stomach, causing discomfort, nausea, vomiting and halitosis (bad breath). If untreated, ulcers can eventually result in perforation of the gastric or duodenal wall, a potentially fatal complication.

The principal causes of peptic ulcer are the bacterium *H. pylori* and NSAID use (Yeomans, 2011). Factors such as a stressful lifestyle, irregular meals, eating too quickly, inadequate mastication and smoking exacerbate ulcer formation and may adversely affect the healing process. Treatment of peptic ulcer has been transformed by the use of antibiotic treatment to eradicate *H. pylori*. To promote healing, this is usually accompanied by a 4–8-week course of an H2 receptor antagonist or proton pump inhibitor to reduce gastric acid production. Most patients will benefit from healthy diet and lifestyle advice to minimise the risk of recurrence.

Gastric resection and reconstruction

Gastric surgery can have a considerable impact on subsequent food intake, weight recovery and quality of life. Pouch and Roux-en-Y reconstruction following gastrectomy is associated with improved quality of life and reduced complications of gastrointestinal function post-operatively, i.e. reduced reflux symptoms and dumping effects (Zong *et al.*, 2011). Increasingly, laparoscopic techniques are being used for the removal of early gastric cancers. As a result of the combination of cachexia and chronic symptoms, such as nausea, vomiting or discomfort on eating, gastric carcinoma patients often present in a significantly malnourished state, and nutritional support measures should be instituted early, preferably perioperatively, via the enteral rather than parenteral route (see Chapter 7.15.3, Cancer of the gastrointestinal tract). Early postoperative enteral nutritional support can be established via a jejunostomy or nasojejunal tube placed intraoperatively. Jejunal feeding may also be required for certain patients receiving palliative treatment for gastric outlet obstruction (see Chapter 6.4, Enteral nutrition).

Disturbances in gastrointestinal function often occur following gastric resection and reconstruction that may affect nutritional intake and nutritional status (see Chapter 7.17.5, Surgery). Some of these problems occur soon after eating; others result from the long-term consequences of disturbed gastric function, and include the following:

- Rapid emptying of the stomach remnant or increased intestinal motility.
- Reduced secretion of intrinsic factor (check vitamin B_{12} status).
- Reduced secretion of pancreatic enzymes.
- Inadequate mixing of food with enzymes and bile.
- Reduced absorption of certain foods, especially protein and fat.
- Rapid absorption of glucose (dumping syndrome).
- Abolition of the normal pH gradient in the small intestine.

Early symptoms

Small-stomach syndrome

The majority of patients experience early satiety and may feel distended and uncomfortable during or after eating. This is particularly likely after total and partial gastrectomy, but may also occur after vagotomy and pyloroplasty. Small, frequent meals should be eaten, and fluids consumed separately from solid foods (see Chapter 6.3, Oral nutritional support).

Dumping syndrome

Early dumping occurs soon after eating and involves sweating, dizziness, faintness, hypotension, and a rapid, weak pulse as a response to the rapid and early delivery of a hyperosmolar load into the jejunum. The symptoms, which usually recede 2–3 months after surgery, may be relieved by consuming small meals, limiting the consumption of rapidly absorbed carbohydrate (low glycaemic index) and avoiding liquids with meals. Late dumping may make patients feel weak, faint, cold and sweaty about 2 hours after a meal as a result of overproduction of insulin in response to the rapid absorption of glucose. The symptoms can be managed by following the advice for early dumping along with regular consumption of starchy carbohydrates.

Diarrhoea

Diarrhoea frequently occurs following vagotomy or total gastrectomy, but may reduce with increasing time after surgery. Antidiarrhoeal agents such as codeine phosphate or loperamide may alleviate the problem.

Bile vomiting

Pancreatic and biliary secretions may accumulate in the afferent loop and, after a meal has left the stomach, can enter the gastric remnant, causing nausea and vomiting. It may be treated by prokinetics and, if refractory, may need surgical correction.

Long-term consequences of gastrectomy

Several long-term consequences of gastrectomy impact on nutrition.

Weight loss and undernutrition

Weight loss and nutritional inadequacy are common and nearly always reflect poor dietary intake. This may be precipitated by early satiety, dumping syndrome and side effects of treatments such as radiotherapy or chemotherapy. Dietary guidance should aim to improve meal frequency and nutrient density via appropriate food choice and enrichment measures; supplementation may also be indicated.

Malabsorption

Malabsorption of fat may cause steatorrhoea. Energy intake should be increased to compensate for faecal energy losses and to ensure that intake of iron, calcium and fat-soluble vitamins are not compromised. Steatorrhoea should not be treated by dietary fat restriction alone. If symptoms are particularly troublesome, a proportion of dietary fat can be isocalorically substituted by either glucose polymers or medium-chain triglycerides (MCTs). Medical management involves the use of antidiarrhoea medication, bile acid binders and, possibly, pancreatic enzyme replacements.

Anaemias

Iron deficiency anaemia can occur as a result of poor iron intake and reduced absorption; therefore, haematological status should be regularly assessed. Pernicious anaemia can be a secondary consequence of gastrectomy as a result of the loss of intrinsic factor (produced by gastric parietal cells) or reduced absorption of vitamin B_{12}, which can be supplemented by intramuscular injection. Megaloblastic anaemia may result from folate deficiency, particularly if dietary intake is poor and malabsorption is present; oral supplementation may be necessary.

Dietary guidance following gastric reconstruction should focus on the need for:

- Small, frequent, regular meals.
- Avoiding large quantities of fluids at mealtimes.
- Eating a variety of nutrient-dense, non-bulky (i.e. not high in fibre), cereal foods, and small amounts of fruit and vegetables.
- Boosting nutrient intake via food enrichment strategies if food intake is compromised.
- Nutritional supplements or micronutrient preparations as indicated.
- Suggesting remedial dietary measures for dumping syndrome or malabsorption if present.

Internet resources

Reflux Advice, www.refluxadvice.co.uk
British Society of Gastroenterology, www.bsg.org.uk

References

Festi D, Scaioli E, Baldi F, *et al.* (2009) Body weight, lifestyle, dietary habits and gastroesophageal reflux disease. *World J. Gastroenterol.* 15: 1690–1701.

NICE. (2014) *Gastro-oesophageal reflux disease and dyspepsia in adults: investigation and management*. Available at https://www.nice.org.uk/guidance/cg184. Accessed 18 February 2017.

NICE. (2015) *Dyspepsia and gastro-oesophageal reflux disease in adults – Quality Standard.* Available at https://pathways.nice.org.uk/pathways/dyspepsia-and-gastro-oesophageal-reflux-disease. Accessed 18 February 2017.

Tytgat GN, McColl K, Tack J, *et al.* (2008) New algorithm for the treatment of gastro-oesophageal reflux disease. *Aliment. Pharmacol. Ther.* 27: 249–256.

Yeomans ND. (2011) The ulcer sleuths: The search for the cause of peptic ulcers. *J. Gastroenterol. Hepatol.* 26: 35–41.

Zong L, Chen P, Chen Y, *et al.* (2011) Pouch Roux-en-Y vs no pouch Roux-en-Y following total gastrectomy: a meta-analysis based on 12 studies. *J. Biomed. Res.* 25(2): 90–99.

7.4.4 Gastroparesis

Angela Cleaver and Laura Thomas

Key points

- *Gastroparesis* is defined as delayed gastric emptying in the absence mechanical obstruction.
- Symptoms include nausea, vomiting, bloating and epigastric discomfort and may lead to serious nutritional consequences.
- Treatment is supportive and aims to improve symptoms, restore nutritional status and optimise glycaemic control in patients with diabetes.
- Dietary advice may include a reduction in the size, fat and fibre content of meals, and texture modification. Enteral or parenteral nutritional support may be indicated if oral intake is inadequate or poorly tolerated.

Gastroparesis is a chronic condition describing disordered motility of the stomach. It is defined as a delay in gastric emptying in the absence of any obstruction, with the cardinal symptoms of early satiety, postprandial fullness, nausea, vomiting, bloating and upper abdominal symptoms (Camilleri *et al.*, 2013).

Normal gastric motility

Relaxation of the fundus (proximal stomach) allows the stomach to accommodate large volumes of food. Contractions of the antrum (distal stomach) grind food and gastric juices into liquid chyme. Coordinated contractions between the stomach and duodenum pump chyme through the pylorus in tightly controlled spurts. Gastric motility is controlled by the smooth muscles lining the gut and the interstitial cells of Cajal within the smooth muscles, which act as electrical pacemakers to generate contractions (Sanders *et al.*, 2006).

The rate of gastric emptying is influenced by complex neural and hormonal signals produced in response to meal composition (Karamanolis & Tack, 2006). Receptors in the small intestine detect distension, pH and the products of digestion, such as fatty acids, peptides and amino acids. Gut mucosal cells release various hormones in response to these products of digestion, which either stimulate or inhibit gastric emptying (Camilleri, 2006). This feedback process is regulated by the autonomic and enteric nervous system, as shown in Figure 7.4.3.

Disease process

It is thought that gastroparesis is primarily caused by neuropathy or myopathy resulting in impaired fundus

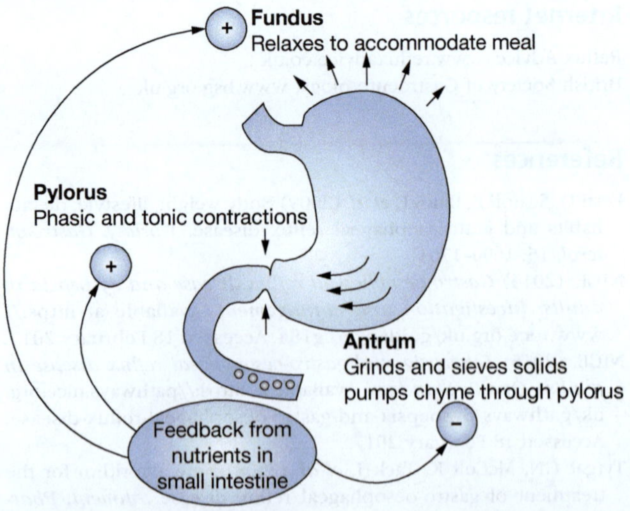

Figure 7.4.3 Motor events during normal gastric emptying (source: Rayner and Horowitz, 2005. Reproduced with permission from Macmillan Publishers Ltd)

relaxation, decreased antral contractions, spasm of the pylorus, gastric arrhythmia or a combination of these factors (Soffer *et al.*, 2009). The result is undigested food that remains in the stomach for longer than normal, leading to mild to severe gastrointestinal symptoms. Gastroparesis is more common in women than men (Keld *et al.*, 2011). Associated conditions include the following (Parkman *et al.*, 2004):

- Diabetes.
- Surgery affecting the vagus nerve.
- Critical illness.
- Gastro-oesophageal reflux disease.
- Chronic liver, renal or pancreas disease.
- Cancer, e.g. pancreatic, gastric, oesophageal.
- Connective tissue disorders, e.g. scleroderma.
- Neurological disorders, e.g. Parkinson's disease.
- Conditions affecting the nervous system, e.g. enteric neuropathy.
- Motility disorders, e.g. chronic intestinal pseudo obstruction, constipation.
- Infection, e.g. virus.
- Anorexia nervosa.
- Medication-induced conditions.

Idiopathic causes may affect up to one-third of patients with gastroparesis. Acute onset occurs in 50% of patients with idiopathic gastroparesis (Parkman et al., 2011a), and it is suspected that viral infection may be responsible for gastroparesis in this subgroup (Bityutskiy *et al.*, 1997).

Diabetic gastroparesis makes up approximately 36% of the causes of gastroparesis (Hyett *et al.*, 2007); it is more common in patients with type 1 diabetes. Chronic hyperglycaemia causes damage to the vagus nerve, which regulates gastric emptying. Loss of the interstitial cells of Cajal and neuronal nitric oxide synthase (nNOS) may also play a role in the pathogenesis (Kashyap & Farrugia, 2010). Gastroparesis may worsen glycaemic control as the stomach does not empty regularly, leading to episodes of hyperglycaemia and hypoglycaemia. Acute hyperglycaemia may itself slow the rate of gastric emptying (Bytzer *et al.*, 2002). Poor glycaemic control as a result of gastroparesis may inaccurately imply poor concordance with dietetic advice.

Post-surgical gastroparesis has been reported after gastric, oesophageal, and/or pancreatoduodenal surgery (Keld *et al.*, 2011), and is the third most common cause of gastroparesis. It is thought to result from damage to the vagus nerve during surgery.

Certain medications, dietary components and recreational drugs have also been found to delay gastric emptying (Parkman *et al.*, 2004):

- Fibre.
- Alcohol.
- Tobacco.
- Marijuana.
- Antacids.
- Opioids.
- Calcium channel blockers.
- Proton pump inhibitors.
- L-dopa.
- Lithium.
- High-dose tricyclic antidepressants.
- Anticholinergics.
- Progesterone.
- Octreotide.

Symptoms

Symptoms can range from mild to severe, and may include (Jung *et al.*, 2009):

- Nausea.
- Vomiting.
- Abdominal bloating.
- Early satiety and/or postprandial fullness.
- Abdominal pain.
- Weight loss.

Symptoms usually occur >1 hour after a meal (Karamanolis & Tack, 2006). More immediate symptoms suggest a psychosomatic or other cause (Bouras & Scolapio, 2004). The gastroparesis cardinal symptom index (GSCI) is a validated patient questionnaire that can be used to quantify the severity of symptoms (Revicki *et al.*, 2004). However, Cassilly *et al.* (2008) showed that the relationship between GSCI scores for nausea, vomiting and early satiety with gastric emptying rate is poor, suggesting that other factors, such as visceral hypersensitivity, may contribute to symptoms.

Nutritional consequences

Patients with gastroparesis are at risk of malnutrition and nutritional abnormalities due to their symptoms.

Even though 54% of individuals with gastroparesis are normal or underweight, 46% are classed as overweight or obese, and therefore signs of malnutrition may be missed (Parkman *et al.*, 2011a) without nutritional screening. Symptoms may lead to anorexia, food aversions and an unbalanced or reduced oral intake. Inadequate oral intake has been identified in this patient group (Parkman *et al.*, 2011b), possibly resulting in protein energy malnutrition, weight loss and micronutrient deficiencies.

Deficiency of vitamins A, B_6, B_{12}, C, D, K, thiamine, potassium and zinc; inadequate oral intake of calories, protein and other micronutrients; anaemia; and dehydration have been observed (Bharadwaj *et al.*, 2016; Ogorek *et al.*, 1991; Parkman *et al.*, 2011b). However, there is a need for further robust research to identify the nutritional status of patients with gastroparesis and the efficacy of different nutritional interventions.

Clinical consequences

Vomiting may result in oesophagitis, fluid and electrolyte disturbances, pulmonary aspiration and harm dentition (Bouras & Scolapio, 2004). Long-term poor glycaemic control may increase the risk of microvascular and macrovascular complications of diabetes. Delayed gastric emptying may result in impaired absorption of medications, affecting the treatment of other medical conditions. Undigested food in the stomach may form into solid masses called bezoars, which can exacerbate symptoms and cause obstruction (Tack, 2007). Gastro-oesophageal reflux disease (see Chapter 7.4.3, Disorders of the stomach and duodenum) and small intestinal bacterial overgrowth has been linked to gastroparesis (Bharadwaj *et al.*, 2016), and may further compromise nutritional intake. Many patients endure symptoms for many years before receiving an accurate diagnosis, and suffer from depression and anxiety (Hasler *et al.*, 2010; Parkman *et al.*, 2011b). Gastroparesis has been shown to affect quality of life and increase financial burden on healthcare (Lacy *et al.*, 2018). Poor oral intake, weight loss and electrolyte losses from vomiting may result in a high risk of refeeding syndrome.

Nutritional assessment

Anthropometry

- Weight, height, waist circumference (consider ascites, oedema).
- Weight history and percentage weight loss.
- Body mass index or mid-upper-arm circumference.
- Consider grip strength if oedema or ascites present.
- Calculate nutritional requirements based on the need for weight gain or loss, or if the underlying aetiology indicates additional stress, e.g. cancer, post-surgery

Biochemistry

- Urea, creatinine, sodium, potassium, magnesium, phosphate and corrected calcium to assess hydration, renal function, electrolyte depletion and risk of refeeding syndrome.
- Blood glucose levels pre- and post-meals, and HbA1c for patients with diabetes.
- Haemoglobin, ferritin, folate and B_{12} levels to detect anaemia.
- Liver function – may be affected by parenteral nutrition
- If micronutrient or trace element deficiency is suspected, check 25-hydroxycholecalciferol (vitamin D), zinc, selenium and copper

Clinical status

- Establish underlying aetiology.
- Observations, e.g. temperature, fluid balance.
- Medication.
- Bowel form, frequency and incidence of constipation or diarrhoea.
- Symptom history. Severity of symptoms can be rated using the GSCI questionnaire. A food and symptom diary may help to identify any patterns.
- If the patient has diabetes, review frequency of blood sugar monitoring, insulin injection site, incidence and treatment of hypoglycaemia.
- Intake of herbal or sports supplements, laxatives, vitamin and mineral preparations, prescription and non-prescription medication.

Dietary assessment

- Diet history – current intake versus usual intake.
- Previous dietary measures tried.
- Foods that are reported to provoke or alleviate symptoms.
- Percentage of oral intake vomited if relevant.
- Meal pattern.
- Portion sizes.
- Tolerance to different textures – solid, soft, pureed, liquid.
- Dietary balance.
- Fibre intake – soluble/insoluble sources.
- Fluid intake – alcohol, carbonated drinks, caffeine.
- Dietary sources of iron, folate, thiamine, calcium, vitamin D, vitamin C and other at-risk micronutrients.

Socioeconomic status

- Smoking (Pasricha *et al.*, 2015).
- Illicit drugs use.
- Physical activity.
- History of depression and/or stress (Pasricha *et al.*, 2015).
- Patient's understanding of digestion and nutrition.
- Cooking skills and facilities, e.g. equipment to blend food.

Service user focus

Poorly managed and severe gastroparesis is associated with multiple hospital admissions and longer lengths of stay (Kashyap & Farrugia, 2010), and therefore symptom management and maintenance of quality of life are the focus for the service user.

Clinical investigation and management

Gastroparesis is diagnosed by demonstrating delayed gastric emptying after other causes are ruled out, such as obstruction by endoscopy or barium studies, and any psychological cause, such as bulimia nervosa or rumination syndrome.

Investigations

Gastric emptying scintigraphy is considered the definitive diagnostic test for gastroparesis. The test in non-invasive and assesses solid and liquid emptying (Camilleri *et al.*, 2013). Retention of >10% of gastric contents after 4 hours of an isotope-labelled test meal or 60% after 2 hours indicates abnormal emptying (Abell *et al.*, 2008).

Other emerging measures of gastric emptying include the Smart Pill and ^{13}C-octanoic acid breath testing; however, they require further validation before they can be considered as alternative diagnostic tests (Camilleri *et al.*, 2013). Magnetic resonance imaging and ultrasonography have also been used to investigate gastroparesis; however, these tests are expensive and largely only available in the research setting.

Treatment

Treatment requires a systematic approach and aims to optimise management of the underlying cause of gastroparesis, improve glycaemic control in patients with diabetes, reduce symptoms and restore nutrition and hydration.

Medication

Prokinetics are used as first-line treatment to accelerate gastric emptying, with metocholpamide, domperidone and erythromyacin being most commonly used in practice (BMJ Best Practice, 2016). Prokinetics are used in conjunction with antiemetic and dietary advice to manage symptoms. Low-dose antidepressants may relieve symptoms of nausea, vomiting and pain (Lustman *et al.*, 2000; Sawhney *et al.*, 2007). Timing of administration of medication is imperative to ensure optimum effect. Pharmacological management of diabetes should be discussed with the multidisciplinary team as some diabetes medications have been found to delay gastric emptying (e.g. Byetta, Symlin), while others have been shown to have no effect (e.g. Sitagliptin) (Camilleri, 2010).

Botox

A systematic review (Bai *et al.*, 2010) found that botulinum toxin injected into the pylorus to reduce pylorospasm showed no benefit in symptom relief of gastroparesis.

Gastric electrical stimulation (GES)

This involves the surgical insertion of a gastric pacemaker to stimulate gastric contractions. The National Institute for Health and Care Excellence (NICE, 2014) has approved the use of GES in specialist units for patients with chronic intractable nausea and vomiting secondary to gastroparesis.

Continuous insulin pump

This may improve glycaemic control in patients with diabetes through the more precise use of short-acting insulin (see Chapter 7.12, Diabetes mellitus). Research is being undertaken into the potential benefit in patients with gastroparesis.

Surgery

A venting gastrostomy may relieve symptoms in some patients and protect dental health (Bouras & Scolapio, 2004; Kim & Nelson, 1998). This can be considered for symptom management in conjunction with other feeding routes (Maple *et al.*, 2005). Surgical options available for the treatment include pyloroplasty, pyloromyotomy, and partial or total gastric resection; however, the decision for surgical management should be made after consultation with a gastroenterologist with expertise in the management of gastroparesis (Jones & Maganti, 2003).

Psychological measures

A systematic review identified that acupuncture may be of benefit to improve post-operative gastroparesis (Cheong *et al.*, 2014), and several studies, including a small single-blinded randomised pilot study, identified that acupuncture may be of benefit in diabetic gastroparesis (Wang *et al.*, 2008). Due to the low qualities of the studies, further high-quality randomised controlled trials are needed.

Nutritional management

Dietary modification may improve tolerance to oral intake, although there is little evidence to support this. Controlled studies are scarce, and the majority of recommendations are made upon clinical experience (Karamanolis & Tack, 2006). Dietetic priority should be to ensure that nutritional status is restored or maintained through the provision of fluid, electrolytes, and macronutrients and micronutrients using the safest and best tolerated form of oral, enteral or parenteral support.

The diet currently recommended is one based on small, frequent meals that are low in fat and fibre, and texture modified (Bharadwaj *et al.*, 2016). Large, nutrient-dense meals may slow gastric emptying, owing to the time required for the stomach to grind contents down and the negative feedback from the small intestine (Camilleri, 2006). A randomised controlled trial demonstrated that a small partial-size diet improved symptoms of gastroparesis in diabetic patients (Olausson *et al.*, 2014).

A randomised controlled trial of 12 individuals with idiopathic and diabetic gastroparesis demonstrated that a high-fat solid meal increased overall symptoms of gastroparesis, whereas liquid meals were reasonably well tolerated. With regards to nausea, high- or low-fat liquid meals were better tolerated than solid meals (Homko *et al.*, 2015), indicating that the use of fat in a liquid diet maybe tolerated in individuals who require nutrition support. The effects of fibre on gastric emptying in gastroparesis has not been fully evaluated; however, foods rich in fibre take longer to empty from the stomach and have a lower energy density, which may be counterproductive in patients who require nutrition support. Water-soluble fibre delays gastric emptying (Cummings, 2001), and, in one study, the removal of fibre naturally present in food accelerated gastric emptying (Benini *et al.*, 1995). Soluble fibre may increase symptoms of bloating (Bianchi & Capurso, 2002). Insoluble fibre has been reported to induce bezoar and phytobezoar formation (non-digestible fibrous food material that can become trapped in the GI tract) (Abell *et al.*, 2006; Rayner & Horowitz, 2005), and are therefore best avoided. A variety of foods have been identified to provoke or alleviate symptoms (Wytiaz *et al.*, 2015); however, further research is needed to consolidate findings. Carbonated beverages can exacerbate gastric distention (Parkman *et al.*, 2004), and therefore may aggravate symptoms of bloating. Excess alcohol has been shown to delay gastric emptying (Bujanda, 2000).

The advice given should consider overall dietary balance, fluid and micronutrient intake, as well as glycaemic control in patients with diabetes. Adequate fluid intake should be encouraged to replace losses and prevent constipation.

Dietetic strategies

As there is a lack of evidence, the following strategies should be tried and adapted to individual patient symptoms (Camilleri *et al.*, 2013; Homko *et al.*, 2015; Olausson *et al.*, 2014):

- Small, frequent meals: 4–6 meals/day (consider volume tolerance).
- Limit fried foods.
- Fat in liquid form may be tolerated and is a useful source of energy.
- Limit intake of insoluble fibre/indigestible fibrous foods.
- Identify specific foods reported to provoke or alleviate symptoms.
- Limit alcohol and carbonated drinks.
- Modify texture.
    - Trial liquid, puréed, or soft foods that may be better tolerated than solid meals.
    - Adapt texture to symptoms, e.g. if symptoms are worse at night, encourage greater intake of liquid energy during the evening.
- Optimise glycaemic control.
    - Establish regular meal pattern.
    - Encourage frequent blood sugar monitoring before and after meals.
    - Consider short-acting insulin after meals rather than before.
    - Ensure appropriate treatment of hypoglycaemia.
- Other
    - Multivitamin supplementation if diet is inadequate.
    - Patients may benefit from sitting upright during meals.
    - Encourage patients to chew food well.
    - Reduce stress at meal times.

Nutritional support

Patients unable to maintain an adequate oral intake may require enteral or parenteral nutritional support. Oral liquid supplements are often well tolerated, including those containing fat. Patients with diabetes should be offered milk-style supplements in preference to juice-style ones as a first-line measure to minimise possible blood sugar disturbances. A trial of nasojejunal feeding is recommended for patients with vomiting and nausea who are unable to tolerate gastric feeding (Camilleri *et al.*, 2013). If successful, jejunostomy placement may maintain hydration and nutrition (Parkman *et al.*, 2004); however, it can be associated with complications (Bharadwaj *et al.*, 2016). A surgically placed needle–catheter jejunostomy may be preferable to a gastrostomy with a jejunal extension, as the extension tubes often migrate back into the stomach (Karamanolis & Tack, 2006).

There is limited evidence identifying the most appropriate administration of jejunal feeding in gastroparesis; however, continuous feeding is reported to generally be better tolerated, beginning at a low rate and typically increasing to at least 60 mL/hour (Camilleri *et al.*, 2013). There is limited research about the type of feed that should be used, and therefore selection of feed should be determined according to tolerance or any other clinical conditions (see Chapter 6.4, Enteral nutrition). Refeeding risk should be considered when initiating feeding, owing to possible poor oral intake, weight loss and/or electrolyte disturbances from vomiting.

Parenteral nutrition may be indicated during acute exacerbations of symptoms or for patients with severe intestinal dysmotility who do not tolerate jejunal feeding (Bouras & Scolapio, 2004; Staun *et al.*, 2009).

Effective recognition and management of patients with gastroparesis requires a systematic approach with close liaison between medical and surgical teams, nursing staff, dietitian, psychologist and pharmacist.

Acknowledgement

The editor acknowledges the prior contribution of Sarah Wilson.

Internet resources

Gastroparesis and Intestinal Failure Trust, www.giftuksupport.org
National Institute of Diabetes, Digestive and Kidney Disease, www.niddk.nih.gov/health-information/health-topics/digestive-diseases/gastroparesis/Pages/facts.aspx

References

Abell TL, Malinowski S, Minocha A. (2006) Nutrition aspects of gastroparesis and therapies for drug-refractory patients. *Nutr. Clin. Pract.* 21: 23–33.

Abell TL, Camilleri M, Donohoe K, *et al.* (2008) Consensus recommendations for gastric emptying scintigraphy: a joint report of the American Neurogastroenterology and Motility Society and the Society of Nuclear Medicine. *J. Nucl. Med. Technol.* 36(1): 44–54.

Bai Y, Xu MJ, Yang X, *et al.* (2010) A systematic review on intrapyloric botulinum toxic injection for gastroparesis. *Digestion.* 81(1): 27–34.

Benini M, Castellani G, Brighenti F, *et al.* (1995) Gastric emptying of a solid meal is accelerated by the removal of dietary fibre naturally present in food. *Gut.* 36(6): 825–830.

Bharadwaj S, Meka K, Tandon P, *et al.* (2016) Management of gastroparesis-associated malnutrition. *J. Dig. Dis.* 17: 285–294.

Bianchi M, Capurso L. (2002) Effects of guar gum, ispaghula and microcrystalline cellulose on abdominal symptoms, gastric emptying, orocaecal transit time and gas production in healthy volunteers. *Dig. Liver Dis.* 34(2): S129–133.

Bityutskiy LP, Soykan I, McCallum RW. (1997) Viral gastroparesis: a subgroup of idiopathic gastroparesis – clinical characteristics and long-term outcomes. *Am. J. Gastroenterol.* 92: 1501–1504.

BMJ Best Practice. (2016) *Gastroparesis.* Available at http://bestpractice.bmj.com/best-practice/monograph/642/treatment/details.html. Accessed 23 October 2016.

Bouras EP, Scolapio JS. (2004) Gastric motility disorders: management that optimizes nutritional status. *J. Clin. Gastroenterol.* 38: 549–557.

Bujanda L. (2000) The effects of alcohol consumption upon the gastrointestinal tract. *Am. J. Gastroenterol.* 95(12): 3374–3382.

Bytzer P, Talley NJ, Hammer J, *et al.* (2002) GI symptoms in diabetes mellitus are associated with both poor glycemic control and diabetic complications. *Am. J. Gastroenterol.* 97: 604–611.

Camilleri M. (2006) Integrated upper gastrointestinal response to food intake. *Gastroenterology.* 131: 640–658.

Camilleri M. (2010) Clinical practice. *Diabetic gastroparesis. N. Engl. J. Med.* 356: 820–829.

Camilleri M, Parkman H, Shafi MA, *et al.* (2013) Clinical guideline: management of gastroparesis. *Am. J. Gastroenterol.* 108: 18–38.

Cassilly DW, Wang RY, Friedenberg FK, *et al.* (2008) Symptoms of gastroparesis: use of the gastroparesis cardinal symptom index in symptomatic patients referred for gastric emptying scintigraphy. *Digestion.* 78: 144–151.

Cheong KB, Zhang JP, Huang Y. (2014) The effectiveness of acupuncture in post-operative gastroparesis syndrome – a systematic review and meta-analysis. *Complement. Ther. Med.* 4: 767–786.

Cummings JH. (2001) The effect of dietary fibre on faecal weight and composition. In Spiller G (ed) *Dietary Fibre in Human Nutrition.* Boca Raton, FL: CRC Press, pp. 183–252.

Hasler WL, Parkman HP, Wilson LA, *et al.* (2010) Psychological dysfunction is associated with symptom severity but not disease etiology or degree of gastric retention in patients with gastroparesis. *Am. J. Gastroenterol.* 105: 2357–2367.

Homko CJ, Duffy F, Friedenberg FK, *et al.* (2015) Effects of dietary fat and food consistency on gastroparesis symptoms in patients with gastroparesis. *Neurogastroenterol. Motil.* 27: 501–508.

Hyett B, Martinez FJ, Gill BM. (2007) Delayed radioneucleotide gastric emptying studies predict morbidity in diabetes with symptoms of gastroparesis in Olmstead County, Minnesota, from 1996 to 2006. *Gastroenterology.* 137: 445–452.

Jones MP, Maganti K. (2003) A systematic review of surgical therapy for gastroparesis. *Am. J. Gastroenterol.* 98: 2122–2129.

Jung HK, Choung RS, Locke GR 3rd, *et al.* (2009) The incidence, prevalence, and outcomes of patients with gastroparesis in Olmsted Count, Minnesota, from 1996 to 2006. *Gastroenterology.* 136: 1225–1233.

Karamanolis G, Tack J. (2006) Nutrition and motility disorders. *Best Pract. Res. Clin. Gastroenterol.* 20: 485–505.

Kashyap P, Farrugia G. (2010) Diabetic gastroparesis: what we have learned and had to unlearn in the past 5 years. *Gut.* 59: 1716–1726.

Keld R, Kinsey L, Athwal V, *et al.* (2011) Pathogenesis, investigation and dietary and medical management of gastroparesis. *J. Hum. Nutr. Diet.* 24(5): 421–430.

Kim CH, Nelson DK. (1998) Venting percutaneous gastrostomy in the treatment of refractory idiopathic gastroparesis. *Gastrointest. Endosc.* 47(1): 67–70.

Lacy BE, Crowell MD, Mathias C, *et al.* (2018) Gastroparesis: quality of life and healthcare utilization. *J. Clin. Gastroenterol.* 52(1): 20–24.

Lustman PJ, Griffith LS, Clouse RE, *et al.* (2000) Fluoxetine for depression in diabetes: a randomized double-blind placebo-controlled trial. *Diabetes Care.* 23: 618–623.

Maple JT, Petersen BT, Baron TH, *et al.* (2005) Direct percutaneous endoscopic jejunostomy: outcomes in 307 consecutive attempts. *Am. J. Gastroenterol.* 100: 2681–2688.

NICE. (2014) *Gastroelectrical stimulation for patients with diabetes.* Available from https://www.nice.org.uk/guidance/ipg489/resources/gastroelectrical-stimulation-for-gastroparesis-pdf-474904660165. Accessed 25 October 2018.

Ogorek CP, Davidson L, Fisher RS, *et al.* (1991) Idiopathic gastroparesis is associated with a multiplicity of severe dietary deficiencies. *Am. J. Gastroenterol.* 86: 423–428.

Olausson EA, Storsrud S, Grundin H, *et al.* (2014) A small partial size diet reduces upper gastrointestinal symptoms in patients with diabetic gastroparesis: a randomized control trial. *Am. J. Gastroenterol.* 109(3): 375–385.

Parkman HP, Hasler WL, Fisher RS. (2004) American Gastroenterological Association technical review on the diagnosis and treatment of gastroparesis. *Gastroenterology.* 127(5): 1592–1622.

Parkman HP, Yates K, Hasler WL, *et al.* (2011a) Clinical features of idiopathic gastroparesis vary with sex, body mass, symptom onset, delay in gastric emptying and gastroparesis emptying. *Gastroenterology.* 140(1): 101–115.

Parkman HP, Yates K, Hasler WL, *et al.* (2011b) National Institute of Diabetes and Digestive and Kidney Diseases Gastroparesis Clinical Research Consortium. *Dietary intake and nutritional deficiencies. Gastroenterology.* 141: 486–498.

Pasricha PJ, Yates KP, Nguyen L, *et al.* (2015) Outcomes and factors associated with reduced symptoms in patients with gastroparesis. *Gastroenterology.* 149: 1762–1774.

Rayner CK, Horowitz M. (2005) New management approaches for gastroparesis. *Nature Clinical Practice Gastroenterology & Hepatology* 2: 454–462.s

Revicki DA, Rentz AM, Dubois D, *et al.* (2004) Gastroparesis Cardinal Symptom Index (GCSI): development and validation of a patient reported assessment of severity of gastroparesis symptoms. *Qual. Life Res.* 13: 833–844.

Sanders KM, Koh SD, Ward SM. (2006) Interstitial cells of Cajal as pacemakers in the gastrointestinal tract. *Annu. Rev. Physiol.* 68: 307–343.

Sawhney MS, Prakash C, Lustman PJ, *et al.* (2007) Tricyclic antidepressants for chronic vomiting in diabetic patients. *Dig. Dis. Sci.* 52: 418–424.

Soffer E, Abell T, Lin Z, *et al.* (2009) Review article: gastric electrical stimulation for gastroparesis – physiological foundations, technical aspects and clinical implications. *Aliment. Pharmacol. Ther.* 30: 681–694.

Staun M, Pironi L, Bozzetti F, *et al.* (2009) ESPEN Guidelines on Parenteral Nutrition: home parenteral nutrition in adult patients. *Clin. Nutr.* 28:467–479.

Tack J. (2007) The difficult patient with gastroparesis. *Best Pract. Res. Clin. Gastroenterol.* 21: 379–391.

Wang CP, Kao CH, Chen WK, *et al.* (2008) A single-blinded, randomized pilot study evaluating effects of electroacupuncture in diabetic patients with symptoms suggestive of gastroparesis. *J. Altern. Compliment. Med.* 14: 833–839.

Wytiaz V, Homko C, Duffy F, *et al.* (2015) Foods provoking and alleviating symptoms in gastroparesis: patient experiences. *Dig. Dis. Sci.* 60:1052–1058.

7.4.5 Disorders of the pancreas

Mary Phillips

Key points

- Pancreatic disease presents complex multifactorial nutritional challenges.
- Enteral feeding with a peptide feed is the feeding regimen of choice in acute pancreatitis, with emphasis on achieving this early in the disease process.
- Pancreatic cancer and chronic pancreatitis are both associated with progressive malnutrition, and patients benefit from early dietetic intervention.
- Pancreatic surgery is highly complex, and preoperative and postoperative optimisation of nutritional status are required.
- Screening for long-term micronutrient deficiencies is recommended.
- Blind nasojejunal tube placement is contraindicated after pancreaticoduodenectomy or gastrojejunostomy due to the risk of tube placement in the afferent limb (blind loop).

Pancreatic disorders may be benign or malignant, and include acute and chronic pancreatitis and pancreatic cancers. The nutritional consequences of these conditions are diverse and often complicated to manage, thus presenting many dietetic challenges. The pancreas has three main functions that are essential for digestion (Neoptolemos & Bhutani, 2008a, 2008b):

- Endocrine: insulin and glucagon from islet cells mainly located in the tail of the pancreas.
- Exocrine:
  - Digestive enzymes from acinar cells found mainly in the head of the pancreas.
  - Bicarbonate secretion to neutralise gastric acid.

Pancreatic enzyme release is stimulated in three phases. Taste and smell of food stimulates an initial surge of enzymes (cephalic phase). This is followed by the second (gastric) phase, which is associated with gastric distension. The third and most significant phase (intestinal) occurs when the products of digestion are delivered into the duodenum. This final stage is responsible for the ongoing release of enzymes for 2–3 hours post-prandially (Keller & Layer, 2005).

Acute pancreatitis

Acute pancreatitis (AP) is an inflammatory condition with an overall mortality of 10–15% (Corfield *et al.*, 1985); it is most commonly associated with gallstone disease or high alcohol intakes. Other causes include trauma, surgery, hypertriglyceridaemia, endoscopic retrograde cholangiopancreatography (ERCP) and drug reactions. In some patients, the cause is unknown (Neoptolemos & Bhutani, 2008a, 2008b). AP usually presents with severe abdominal pain, caused by the auto activation of pancreatic enzymes. In the initial stages, the treatment is conservative, consisting of pain relief and organ support where necessary.

On admission, patients are scored to predict disease severity using one of a number of scoring systems. The Atlanta criteria defines the systemic inflammatory response syndrome (SIRS); the presence of this for more than 48 hours is suggestive of severe pancreatitis (Zaheer *et al.*, 2013). Other scoring methods include Apache II, RANSON criteria, modified Glasgow (or Imrie) score or CRP (UK Working Party on Acute Pancreatitis, 2005). In cases of mild pancreatitis, most patients are kept nil by mouth until the pain has resolved; however, some studies suggest that early oral diet may reduce length of stay as compared to fasting or clear fluids only (Eckerwall *et al.*, 2007; Sathiaraj *et al.*, 2008). Hospital stay is usually short; if gallstones are the cause of the pancreatitis, a laparoscopic cholecystectomy should be performed urgently to prevent recurrence.

Patients with severe acute pancreatitis (SAP) may present with, or develop, multi-organ failure. These patients require intensive care support and may need multiple interventions, with hospital admissions over many weeks or months. Comprehensive nutritional support is indicated, and enteral nutrition (EN) is considered to be the gold standard (Working Group IAP/APA Acute Pancreatitis Guidelines, 2013). However, parenteral nutrition (PN) may be needed when EN is poorly tolerated, either as a sole source of nutrition or, ideally, in addition to slow-rate EN (Neoptolemos & Bhutani, 2008a, 2008b; Sakorafas *et al.*, 2010).

Many complications of pancreatitis are septic in origin, and the use of EN to reduce bacterial translocation has been widely studied (Sakorafas *et al.*, 2010). There are many complications of SAP that can influence the delivery and tolerance of EN, including the following:

- Hyperglycaemia.
- Malabsorption.
- Significant weight and muscle mass loss.
- Delayed gastric emptying, nausea, vomiting and high nasogastric (NG) aspirates.

- Prolonged periods of nil by mouth for multiple procedures.
- Paralytic ileus secondary to electrolyte imbalance.
- Antibiotic-related diarrhoea.
- Peripheral oedema.
- Gastrointestinal oedema – diarrhoea, obstruction.
- Ascites.
- Gastric varices.
- Colonic necrosis and faecal peritonitis.
- Fluctuating inotrope requirements.
- Respiratory failure.

SAP is usually treated aggressively with multi-organ support. If necrosis develops, the necrotic tissue is removed surgically with either a minimally invasive or endoscopic necrosectomy. The degree and location of necrosis and damage arising from inflammation will help predict any long-term exocrine or endocrine insufficiency. Extensive disease in the head of the pancreas is likely to result in long-term pancreatic exocrine insufficiency (PEI), requiring pancreatic enzyme replacement therapy (PERT), whereas disease in the tail of the pancreas is likely to lead to endocrine insufficiency (type 3c diabetes mellitus).

Chronic pancreatitis

Chronic pancreatitis (CP) is a progressive inflammatory disease resulting in the destruction of the pancreas. The incidence is 20–200 per 100,000. The aetiology is excessive alcohol consumption in 70–90% of cases (Layer & Melle, 2005; Neoptolemos & Bhutani, 2008a, 2008b). In severe cases, CP causes intractable pain and severe malnutrition, leading to multiple admissions for procedures to reduce pain. These include coeliac or endoscopic plexus blocks; gastric and biliary bypass surgery; ductal drainage procedures; or pancreatic resection. A multidisciplinary team approach is crucial in managing patients with CP to prevent malnutrition, while managing PEI and optimising pain control. Alcohol and smoking cessation is a crucial part of disease management.

Pancreatic cancer

Pancreatic cancer is the fifth-most common cause of cancer death in the UK, with a median survival following diagnosis of 6 months. The high mortality is due to vague early symptoms (including nausea and vomiting, back pain and weight loss), resulting in late diagnosis, often after the tumour has metastasised. Early symptoms may include jaundice and new-onset diabetes. Unfortunately, 85% of patients with pancreatic cancer are identified as having non-resectable tumours at diagnosis (Neoptolemos & Bhutani, 2008a, 2008b).

Patients who have operable disease and are fit for surgery will have one of the following procedures:

- Whipple's procedure – removal of the duodenum, head of the pancreas, distal common bile duct, gallbladder and distal stomach.
- Pylorus-preserving pancreaticoduodenectomy (PPPD) – Whipple's procedure, without gastric resection.
- Distal pancreatectomy – removal of the pancreatic tail and usually the spleen.
- Central pancreatectomy – removal of the body of the pancreas.
- Total pancreatectomy – removal of the duodenum, the entire pancreas, distal common bile duct, gallbladder, usually the spleen, and sometimes the distal stomach.

Postoperatively, patients may experience delayed gastric emptying and/or dumping syndrome (depending on the extent of gastric resection), early satiety, endocrine and exocrine insufficiency, brittle type 3c diabetes (especially following total pancreatectomy), and, in the long term, vitamin and mineral deficiencies. There is a high risk of bacterial overgrowth and bile acid malabsorption after pancreatic head resection, and, consequently, uncontrolled symptoms should be investigated (Phillips, 2015).

Treatment options for non-resectable disease include chemotherapy, radiotherapy, palliative surgery (including gastric and biliary bypass), palliative biliary and duodenal stenting, and, eventually, palliative care (see Chapter 7.15.3, Cancer of the gastrointestinal tract). Dietetic management of postoperative complications are shown in Table 7.4.3.

Nutritional consequences of pancreatic disease

Regardless of the cause of pancreatic damage, the nutritional consequences are similar, and can be classified according to their aetiology.

Pain

Pain is a key symptom in both benign and malignant disease, and plays a significant role in the development of malnutrition. Pain may be continuous, but is often associated with eating; patients may avoid eating in an attempt to minimise pain. Some patients benefit from

Table 7.4.3 Dietetic management of postoperative complications

Complication	Dietetic intervention
Pancreatic leak/fistula	Sips of water only. Nasojejunal (NJ) or parenteral nutrition (PN) to reduce stimulation of the pancreas (Kaushik *et al.*, 2005); in combination with sandostatin analogues (Haddad *et al.*, 2009).
Chyle leak	Dietary fat restriction, low-fat, medium-chain triglyceride peptide-based EN. In severe cases, PN may be needed (Abu Hilal *et al.*, 2013).
Postoperative ileus	PN may be required.
Delayed gastric emptying	NJ feeding. If no NJ tube, PN may be required.
Pancreatic exocrine insufficiency	Routine pancreatic enzyme replacement therapy use is recommended after pancreatic head resection (Phillips, 2015).

soft or liquid-based diets, which are thought to reduce pancreatic stimulation (Jacobson *et al.*, 2007). In some cases, pancreatic rest can be used; this involves distal jejunal feeding and restriction of oral intake to small volumes of clear fluids (Lordan *et al.*, 2009). Patients are often prescribed high-dose opiates, which can cause constipation and nausea.

Endocrine insufficiency

Islet cells, which produce insulin, are predominantly located in the tail of the pancreas (Wittingen & Frey, 1974). Therefore, diabetes is more common in disease in the tail of the pancreas; this type of diabetes is classified as type 3c (pancreatogenic diabetes) (Ewald & Bretzel, 2013). Type 3c diabetes may be brittle, with patients prone to sudden episodes of hypoglycaemia due to the lack of glucagon. Insulin is often required, and care must be taken to ensure that malnourished patients do not receive inappropriate energy-restrictive advice.

Exocrine insufficiency

Malabsorption causes a variety of symptoms, including steatorrhoea (frequent, pale, loose, floating stools), abdominal bloating and flatulence, unexplained weight loss, and micronutrient deficiencies, such as anaemia and fat-soluble-vitamin deficiency. Malabsorption is managed with PERT.

Management

Low-fat diets

Historically PEI has been managed through restriction of dietary fat. It is now widely accepted that the use of low-fat diets exacerbate malnutrition, and therefore strict fat restriction is only recommended for symptom control in those who do not respond to PERT (Lankisch, 1999). If nutritional support is indicated, patients should receive high-energy, high-protein, moderate-fat advice in conjunction with PERT.

Pancreatic enzyme replacement therapy

Recommendations for the use of PERT are as follows:

- Enzymes are required for the digestion of fat, protein and carbohydrate.
- Enzymes should be prescribed with all meals, snacks and nutritional supplements.
- Enzymes are most frequently prescribed in capsule form, although tablet, granules or powered forms are also available.
- Capsules should be swallowed whole, with the first capsule at the beginning of the meal, and subsequent capsules spread out throughout the meal.
- Enzymes should be swallowed with a cold drink to prevent heat denaturation.
- Enzymes will only work on food and fluids that they mix with. They should be taken regularly with sip feeds and meals of long duration, to allow enzymes to mix properly with food.

Granular or powdered enzymes should be mixed with an acidic fruit purée, swallowed immediately without chewing, and the mouth rinsed to prevent premature activation and proteolytic damage to the oral mucosa (severe mouth ulcers).

Peptide or elemental feeds should be used for EN; these feed formulae do not normally require the use of PERT for digestion. Where PERT is required alongside EN, advice should be sought from a tertiary pancreatic centre.

Micronutrient deficiencies

Multiple micronutrient deficiencies have been associated with pancreatic insufficiency in both benign and malignant disease (Armstrong *et al.*, 2007; Dujsikova *et al.*, 2008). The most clinically significant is vitamin D deficiency, which is associated with osteopenia and osteoporosis (Dujsikova *et al.*, 2008). Routine supplementation with a calcium and vitamin D supplement (Armstrong *et al.*, 2007), regular monitoring of vitamin D and parathyroid hormone (PTH), and DXA scans are recommended routinely for patients with chronic pancreatitis (Duggan *et al.*, 2010). Case reports have highlighted incidences of deficiencies in vitamin A (Livingstone *et al.*, 2003), iron, selenium, zinc and vitamin E (Armstrong *et al.*, 2007).

Enteral feeding

Acute pancreatitis

Historically, patients with SAP were kept nil by mouth for considerable periods of time, and, if patients were fed, it was usually parenterally (Mitchell *et al.*, 2003). Over the last 20 years, however, evidence has shown that EN is safer and associated with reduced morbidity and mortality, and best practice is now to establish EN early in the evolution of disease (Petrov *et al.*, 2008). A Cochrane review concluded that EN was associated with a trend towards reduced length of stay, as well as significant reduction in the development of multiorgan failure, systemic complications, need for surgical interventions, and overall mortality when compared to patients receiving PN (Al-Omran *et al.*, 2010). Although this review included studies involving patients with pancreatitis of any severity, a subgroup analysis of patients with SAP found similar conclusions.

The European Society for Clinical Nutrition and Metabolism (ESPEN) guidelines concluded that there was strong evidence that enteral feeding in the first 5–7 days of mild pancreatitis was of no benefit, but that it was indicated in severe disease, even in the presence of complications such as fistula, pseudocyst and ascites, and that a peptide-based feed should be used (Meier *et al.*, 2006). Although EN is acknowledged to be the optimal feeding route for patients with acute pancreatitis, debate remains as to whether nasogastric (NG) or nasojejunal (NJ) feeding is more suitable, and how early enteral feeding should be initiated. Several studies have compared NG and NJ feeding, but are limited by definitions of NJ feeding, and the exclusion of those with the most severe disease (Eatock *et al.*, 2005; Kumar *et al.*, 2006; Piciucchi *et al.*, 2010; Singh *et al.*, 2012). In practice, many patients present with nausea and vomiting, in which case NJ feeding is the feeding route of choice.

Patients with SAP do not normally commence oral intake until the abdominal pain has resolved, and enteral feeding should continue until an oral intake level that is sufficient to satisfy their requirements is achieved. In practice, these patients have a significant energy deficit, and adequate oral intake is difficult to achieve; hence, patients will often require supplementary enteral feeding.

Chronic pancreatitis

Up to 10% of patients with CP have intractable pain and malnutrition that do not respond to oral nutritional support. Enteral feeding is often used in these cases, and jejunal feeding may be helpful in cases of duodenal stenosis, delayed gastric emptying or food avoidance due to pain (Meier *et al.*, 2006).

Postoperative enteral feeding

Many pancreatic centres use NJ after pancreatic surgery, although the route, feed formulation and timing of initiation of enteral feeding vary widely. A solid evidence base is needed to determine best practice (Phillips *et al.*, 2009). Enhanced recovery protocols have suggested that routine nutritional assessment may not be necessary (Lassen *et al.*, 2013), but there is conflicting evidence showing significant malnutrition, sarcopenia, and malabsorption preoperatively which is associated with increased morbidity and re-admissions (Hari & Rosenzweig, 2012; Jo *et al.*, 2006; Peng *et al.*, 2012; Tan *et al.*, 2009) (see Chapter 7.17.5, Surgery).

Some patients require long-term nutritional support postoperatively, particularly if symptoms of delayed gastric emptying are prolonged. NJ tubes inserted postoperatively must be inserted by an endoscopist or radiologist with experience of this anatomy, as there is significant risk to the patient if the tube is placed into the afferent limb. Bedside techniques are contraindicated in patients who have undergone a pancreaticoduodenectomy or gastrojejunostomy.

Novel substrates

Probiotics and immune-enhancing products

There has been conflicting data regarding the use of probiotics in acute pancreatitis (Olah *et al.*, 2002; Olah & Romics, 2010; Qin *et al.*, 2008). However, probiotics are currently not recommended in acute pancreatitis following a large, multi-centred, randomised, double-blind, placebo-controlled trial in patients with SAP where probiotic administration was associated with a significant increase in the incidence of bowel ischaemia and mortality (Bessekink *et al.*, 2008).

Antioxidants

Several studies have examined the use of antioxidants for pain control in CP. While some studies appear promising, (Bhardwaj *et al.*, 2009), a meta-analysis concluded that there was insufficient evidence to support antioxidant therapy (Mohseni Salehi Monfared *et al.*, 2009).

Eicosapentaenoic acid

Many studies have examined the use of fish oils in managing the dramatic weight loss seen in patients with advanced cancer, particularly pancreatic cancer. Some studies have shown weight gain and improved quality of life when eicosapentaenoic acid (EPA) supplements are used (Fearon *et al.*, 2003). However, a Cochrane review concluded there was insufficient data to recommend oral EPA (Dewey *et al.*, 2007). However, the incidence of exocrine insufficiency is not assessed in these trials, and there is a need for research on the use of EPA supplements alongside PERT to promote absorption.

Drug interactions

Octreotide (Sandostatin®) is used to inhibit pancreatic secretions, and therefore can worsen malabsorption. This may be used postoperatively to prevent or treat pancreatic leaks, or to treat neuroendocrine tumours (Witt & Pedersen, 1989). Lanreotide® and Sandostatin LAR® are long-acting versions of octreotide.

References

Abu Hilal M, Layfield DM, Di Fabio F, *et al.* (2013) Postoperative chyle leak after major pancreatic resections in patients who receive enteral feed: risk factors and management options. *World J. Surg.* 37: 2918–2926.

Al-Omran M, Albalawi ZH, Tashkandi MF, *et al.* (2010) Enteral versus parenteral nutrition for acute pancreatitis. *Cochrane Database Syst. Rev.* (1): CD002837.

Armstrong T, Strommer L, Ruiz-Jasbon F, *et al.* (2007) Pancreaticoduodenectomy for peri-ampullary neoplasia leads to specific micronutrient deficiencies. *Pancreatology* 7(1): 37–44.

Bessekink MGH, van Santvoort HC, Buskens E, *et al.* (2008) Probiotic prophylaxis in predicted severe acute pancreatitis: a randomised, double blind, placebo-controlled trial. *Lancet* 371: 651–659.

Bhardwaj P, Garg PK, Maulik SK, *et al.* (2009) A randomised controlled trial of antioxidant supplementation for pain relief in patients with chronic pancreatitis. *Gastroenterology.* 136(1): 149–159.

Corfield AP, Cooper MJ, Williamson RC. (1985) Acute pancreatitis: a lethal disease of increasing incidence. *Gut.* 26: 724–729.

Dewey A, Baughan C, Dean T, *et al.* (2007) Eicosapentaenoic acid (EPA, an omega 3 fatty acid from fish oils) for the treatment of cancer cachexia. *Cochrane Database Syst. Rev.* (1): CD004597.

Duggan S, O'Sullivan M, Feehan S, *et al.* (2010) Nutrition treatment of deficiency and malnutrition in chronic pancreatitis: a review. *Nutr. Clin. Pract.* 25(4): 362–370.

Dujsikova H, Dite P, Tomandl J, *et al.* (2008) Occurrence of metabolic osteopathy in patients with chronic pancreatitis. *Pancreatology.* 8(6): 583–536.

Eatock FC, Chong P, Menezes N, *et al.* (2005) A randomized study of early nasogastric versus nasojejunal feeding in severe acute pancreatitis. *Am. J. Gastroenterol.* 100: 432–439.

Eckerwall GE, Tingstedt BB, Bergenzaun PE, *et al.* (2007) Immediate oral feeding with mild acute pancreatitis is safe and may accelerate recovery – a randomised clinical study. *Clin. Nutr.* 26(6): 758–763.

Ewald N, Bretzel RG. (2013) Diabetes mellitus secondary to pancreatic diseases (type 3c) – are we neglecting an important disease? *Eur. J. Intern. Med.* 24: 203–206.

Fearon KCH, von Meyenfeldt MF, Moses AGW, *et al.* (2003) Effect of a protein and energy dense n-3 fatty acid enriched oral supplement on loss of weight and lean tissue in cancer cachexia: a randomised double blind trial. *Gut.* 52: 1479–1486.

Haddad LB, Scatton O, Randone B, *et al.* (2009) Pancreatic fistula after pancreaticoduodenectomy: the conservative treatment of choice. *HPB (Oxford)* 11: 203–209.

Hari M, Rosenzweig M. (2012) Incidence of preventable post-operative readmissions following pancreaticoduodenectomy: implications for patient education. *Oncol. Nurs. Forum.* 39: 408–412.

Jacobson BC, Vander Vliet MB, Hughes MD, *et al.* (2007) A prospective, randomized trial of clear liquids versus low-fat solid diet as the initial meal in mild acute pancreatitis. *Clin. Gastroenterol. Hepatol.* 5(8): 946–951.

Jo S, Choi SH, Heo JS, *et al.* (2006) Missing effect of glutamine supplementation on the surgical outcome after pancreaticoduodenectomy for periampullary tumors: a prospective, randomized, double-blind, controlled clinical trial. *World J. Surg.* 30: 1974–1982; discussion 1983–1984.

Kaushik N, Pietraszewski M, Holst JJ, *et al.* (2005) Enteral feeding without pancreatic stimulation. *Pancreas.* 31: 353–359.

Keller J, Layer P. (2005) Human pancreatic exocrine response to nutrients in health and disease. *Gut.* 54(VI): vi1–vi28.

Kumar A, Singh N, Prakash S, *et al.* (2006) Early enteral nutrition in severe acute pancreatitis: a prospective randomized controlled trial comparing nasojejunal and nasogastric routes. *J. Clin. Gastroenterol.* 40: 431–434.

Lankisch PG. (1999) What to do when a patient with pancreatic exocrine insufficiency does not respond to pancreatic enzyme substitution: a practical guide. *Digestion.* 60: 97–103.

Lassen K, Coolsen MM, Slim K, *et al.* (2013) Guidelines for perioperative care for pancreaticoduodenectomy: Enhanced Recovery After Surgery (ERAS®) Society recommendations. *World J. Surg.* 37: 240–258.

Layer P, Melle U. (2005) Chronic pancreatitis: definition and classification for clinical practice. In: Dominguez-Munoz JE, Malfertheiner P (eds) *Clinical Pancreatology for Practising Gastroenterologists and Surgeons*, chapter 21. Oxford: Blackwell Publishing.

Livingstone C, Davis J, Marvin V, *et al.* (2003) Vitamin A deficiency presenting as night blindness during pregnancy. *Ann. Clin. Biochem.* 40: 292–294.

Lordan JT, Phillips M, Chun JY, *et al.* (2009) A safe, effective, and cheap method of achieving pancreatic rest in patients with chronic pancreatitis with refractory symptoms and malnutrition. *Pancreas.* 38(6): 689–692.

Meier R, Ockenga J, Pertkiewicz M, *et al.* (2006) ESPEN guidelines on enteral nutrition: Pancreas. *Clin. Nutr.* 25: 275–284.

Mitchell RM, Byrne MF, Baillie J. (2003) *Pancreatitis. Lancet.* 361: 1447–1455.

Mohseni Salehi Monfared SS, Vahidi H, Abdolghaffari AH, *et al.* (2009) Antioxidant therapy in the management of acute, chronic and post-ERCP pancreatitis: a systematic review. *World J. Gastroenterol.* 15(36): 4481–4490.

Neoptolemos JP, Bhutani MS. (2008a) Acute pancreatitis. In: *Fast Facts: Diseases of the Pancreas and Biliary Tract.* Oxford: Health Press Limited, pp. 62–70.

Neoptolemos JP, Bhutani MS. (2008b) Pancreatic cancer. In: *Fast Facts: Diseases of the Pancreas and Biliary Tract.* Oxford: Health Press Limited, pp. 93–94.

Olah A, Romics L. (2010) Evidence-based use of enteral nutrition in acute pancreatitis. *Langenbecks. Arch. Surg.* 395(4): 309–316.

Olah A, Belagyi T, Issekutz A, *et al.* (2002) Randomised clinical trial of specific lactobacillus and fibre supplement to early enteral nutrition in patients with acute pancreatitis. *Br. J. Surg.* 89(9): 1103–1107.

Peng P, Hyder O, Firoozmand A, *et al.* (2012) Impact of sarcopenia on outcomes following resection of pancreatic adenocarcinoma. *J. Gastrointest. Surg.* 16: 1478–1486.

Petrov MS, Correia MI, Windsor JA. (2008) Nasogastric tube feeding in predicted severe acute pancreatitis. A systematic review of the literature to determine safety and tolerance. *JOP.* 9(4): 440–448.

Phillips ME. (2015) Pancreatic exocrine insufficiency following pancreatic resection. *Pancreatology* 15: 449–455.

Phillips M, Lordan JT, Menezes N, *et al.* (2009) Feeding patients following pancreaticoduodenectomy; A UK national survey. *Ann. R. Coll. Surg. Engl.* 91(5): 385–388.

Piciucchi M, Merola E, Marignani M, *et al.* (2010) Nasogastric or nasointestinal feeding in severe acute pancreatitis. *World J. Gastroenterol.* 16: 3692–3696.

Qin HL, Zheng JJ, Tong DN, *et al.* (2008) Effect of *Lactobacillus plantarum.* Enteral feeding on the gut permeability and septic complications in the patients with acute pancreatitis. *Eur. J. Clin. Nutr.* 62: 923–930.

Sakorafas GH, Lappas C, Mastoraki A, *et al.* (2010) Current trends in the management of infected necrotizing pancreatitis. *Infect. Disor. Drug Targets* 10(1): 9–14.

Sathiaraj E, Murthy S, Mansard MJ, *et al.* (2008) Clinical trial: oral feeding with a soft diet compared with clear liquid diet as initial meal in mild acute pancreatitis. *Aliment. Pharmacol. Ther.* 28(6): 777–781.

Singh N, Sharma B, Sharma M, *et al.* (2012) Evaluation of early enteral feeding through nasogastric and nasojejunal tube in severe acute pancreatitis: a noninferiority randomized controlled trial. *Pancreas.* 41: 153–159.

Tan BH, Birdsell LA, Martin L, *et al.* (2009) Sarcopenia in an overweight or obese patient is an adverse prognostic factor in pancreatic cancer. *Clin. Cancer Res.* 15: 6973–6979.

UK Working Party on Acute Pancreatitis. (2005) UK Guidelines for the management of acute pancreatitis. *Gut.* 54: 1–9.

Witt K, Pedersen NT. (1989) The long-acting somatostatin analogue SMS 201-995 causes malabsorption. *Scand. J. Gastroenterol.* 24(10): 1248–1252.

Wittingen J, Frey CF. (1974) Islet concentration in the head, body, tail and uncinate process of the pancreas. *Ann. Surg.* 179: 412–414.

Working Group IAP/APA Acute Pancreatitis Guidelines. (2013) IAP/APA evidence-based guidelines for the management of acute pancreatitis. *Pancreatology.* 13: e1–15.

Zaheer A, Singh VK, Qureshi RO *et al.* (2013) The revised Atlanta classification for acute pancreatitis: updates in imaging terminology and guidelines. *Abdom Imaging* 38:125–136.

7.4.6 Malabsorption

Helen Truby, Kathryn Hart and Janeane Dart

Key points

- Malabsorption may be nutrient specific, i.e. affecting one nutrient (e.g. fat or vitamin B_{12}) or more generalised.
- It may be the manifestation of a primary absorptive defect or a symptom of another underlying condition.
- Tests for malabsorption commonly measure malabsorbed compounds in urine or faeces, absorbed compounds in blood or breath, or the activity of digestive enzymes.
- Dietary treatment aims for symptom relief and achievement of nutritional adequacy.

Malabsorption has many different causes (Table 7.4.4); it may be short term (e.g. inflammation associated with an acute flare of Crohn's disease) or long term, and, in some cases, permanent. Dietary measures can be used to alleviate symptoms, and nutritional supplementation may be necessary to correct nutritional depletion or prevent further deterioration. It is, however, vital that the cause of the malabsorption be identified and, if possible, treated.

Diagnostic features of malabsorption

Some or all of the following:

- Diarrhoea or change in stool consistency.
- Abdominal distension.
- Flatulence or wind.
- Loss of weight in adults or growth failure in children.
- Hypoproteinaemia (low serum albumin/prealbumin).
- Iron deficiency anaemia or low serum ferritin.

Generalised nutrient deficiencies are likely, and the risk of specific deficiencies is heightened by disease or resection in particular sites of the gastrointestinal tract, chronic diarrhoea and/or self-imposed dietary restriction (Figure 7.4.4). The elderly, infants and young children are particularly at risk of dehydration with loss of fluid and electrolytes during acute episodes of diarrhoea.

Very loose stools, with or without urgency, is the most common presenting feature, and the nature of the stool often indicates the type or site of the malabsorption:

Table 7.4.4 Common causes of malabsorption

Reason for malabsorption	Possible causes
Reduced absorptive capacity	Intestinal resection.
	Short bowel syndrome.
	Villous atrophy, e.g. coeliac disease
	Active inflammatory bowel disease.
	Gastro- and jejuno-colic fistulae.
	Infiltration, e.g. scleroderma, lymphoma.
	Vascular insufficiency.
	Mucosal damage, e.g. drugs, irradiation, following surgery or serious gastroenteritic infection.
	Some bariatric surgery procedures: biliopancreatic diversion with duodenal switch procedure, Roux-en-Y gastric bypass.
Enzyme deficiencies	Disaccharidase deficiency, e.g. primary alactasia or secondary lactase deficiency.
	Lipase and/or proteolytic enzyme deficiency, e.g. pancreatic insufficiency.
Intraluminal factors	High pH in duodenum, e.g. achlorhydria.
	Low pH in duodenum, e.g. Zollinger–Ellison syndrome.
	Bile salt deficiency, e.g. obstructive jaundice.
Infection	Deconjugation of bile salts by bacterial colonisation of the small intestine, e.g. blind loop syndrome.
	Competition for nutrients, e.g. parasitic infections.
	Rapid intestinal transit time, e.g. gastroenteritis.
Impaired transport mechanisms	Impaired fat transport, e.g. congenital lymphangiectasia.
	Impaired monosaccharide transport, e.g. congenital primary malabsorption of glucose and galactose.

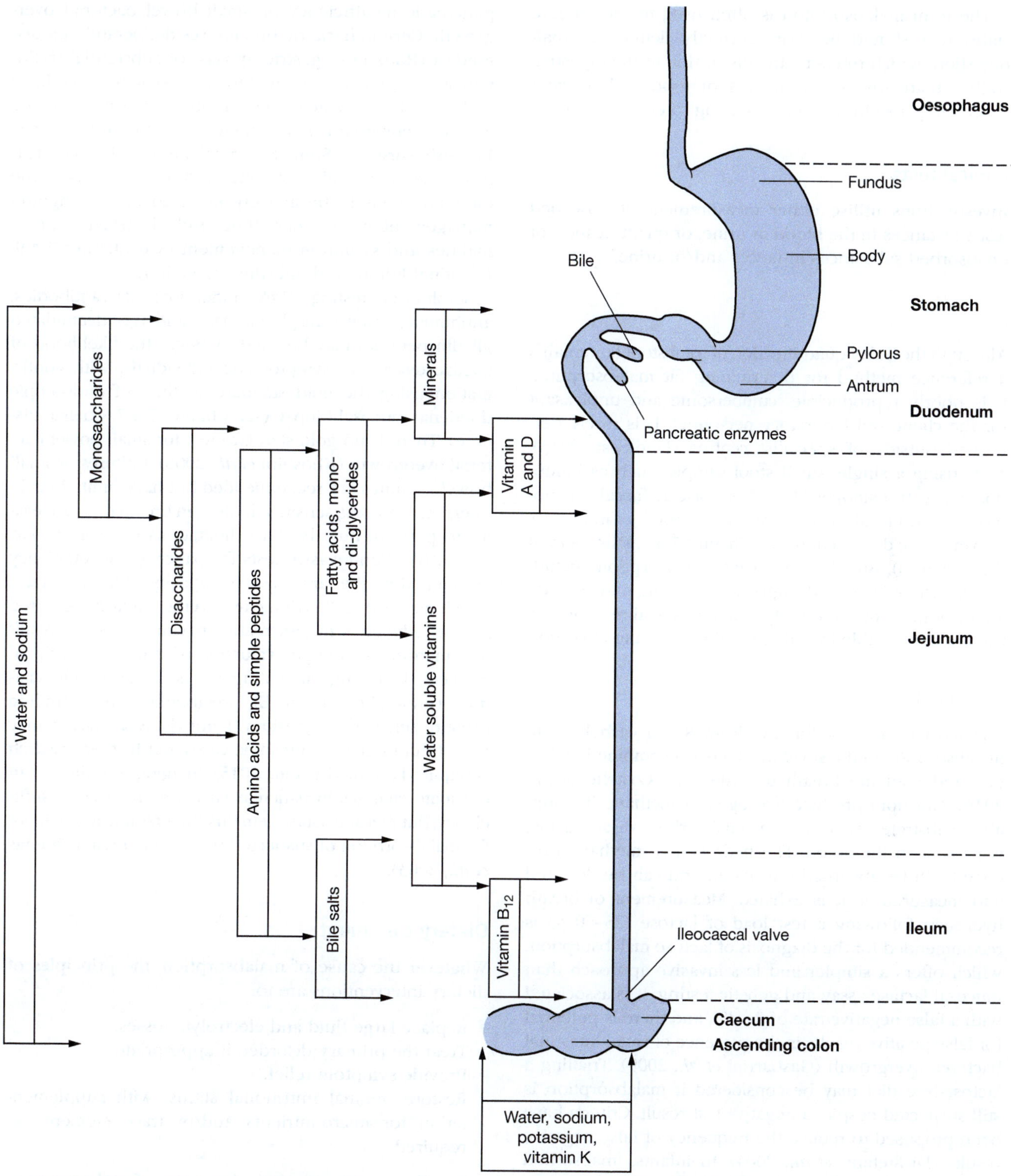

Figure 7.4.4 Principal absorption sites for nutrients

- Fat malabsorption results in steatorrhoea, pale, malodorous, greasy and unformed stools that are often difficult to flush and may leave a greasy residue in the toilet.
- Carbohydrate malabsorption typically results in watery and frothy diarrhoea due to the presence of fermented sugars.
- If more than one nutrient is malabsorbed, e.g. due to loss of absorptive surface or pancreatic insufficiency, this distinction is less clear-cut, and, for milder forms of malabsorption, no stool abnormalities may be reported, e.g. iron deficiency anaemia is a common presenting feature of adults with untreated coeliac disease.

The term malabsorption is often used to incorporate states that should be more correctly defined as maldigestion, which refers to any disruption to the digestive (rather than absorption) phases of food and nutrient processing, specifically those relating to enzyme activity.

Clinical tests

Investigations utilise either measurement of absorbed test substances in the blood or urine, or quantification of unabsorbed substances in faeces and/or urine.

Fat

Although the 3-day quantification of total stool fat remains a reference method for determining fat malabsorption, it is poorly reproducible, cumbersome and unpleasant for the client and laboratory personnel. It is rarely performed outside of specialist centres (Lindkvist, 2013). Tests using a single, small stool sample, such as immunoreactive trypsinogen, faecal elastase-1, faecal chymotrypsin and faecal microscopy, are all used as indicators of pancreatic dysfunction (see Chapter 7.4.5, Disorders of the pancreas). Breath tests for fat malabsorption, including the use of ^{13}C-mixed triglyceride fat load, may provide an assessment of both lipolysis and absorption in adults, but are not suitable for infants and very young children.

Carbohydrate

The most useful test for the diagnosis of carbohydrate malabsorption in the small intestine is a combined hydrogen and methane breath test (de Lacy Costello *et al.*, 2013). Gut flora produce hydrogen or methane if a suitable substrate, such as an unabsorbed disaccharide, is present in the colon. The hydrogen or methane produced will be absorbed into blood and can be detected and measured as it is exhaled. Measurement of breath hydrogen following a test load of lactose (25–50 g) is recommended for the diagnosis of lactose malabsorption, which offers a simpler and less invasive approach than mucosal lactase assay and genetic testing. It is associated with a false negative rate of 2–43%, and there is potential for false positive results in the presence of small intestinal bacterial overgrowth (Gasbarrini *et al.*, 2009). Trialling a lactose-free diet may be considered if malabsorption is still suspected despite a negative test result. Criteria have been proposed to reduce the frequency of false negative results (Di Stefano *et al.*, 2004). In infants, unabsorbed lactose in the stool can be clearly identified by paper chromatography or other tests for reducing substances.

The generic methods of breath testing, mucosal enzyme assays (via endoscopic biopsy) and oral tolerance tests can be applied to other disaccharides if specific malabsorption is suspected.

Tests for non-nutrient-specific malabsorption

Non-nutrient-specific malabsorptive diarrhoea may be caused by generalised loss of absorptive capacity, pancreatic insufficiency or small bowel bacterial overgrowth. Certain bariatric procedures deliberately induce modest (Roux-en-Y gastric bypass) or substantial (biliopancreatic diversion with duodenal switch procedure) malabsorption, which then require specific dietetic advice to ensure nutrient sufficiency (see Chapter 7.13.3, Bariatric surgery). Similarly, malabsorption is a key feature of short bowel syndrome, and, in these cases, the dietitian needs to be actively involved in the ongoing management of nutrient, fluid and electrolyte abnormalities and symptom management (see Chapter 7.4.9, Intestinal failure and intestinal resection).

Serological testing (IgA antiendomysial antibodies, antihuman tissue transglutaminase and IgG deamidated gliadin peptide) may be used to assess the likelihood of coeliac disease in symptomatic individuals, with confirmation using the gold standard method of endoscopic duodenal mucosal biopsy (see Chapter 7.4.7, Coeliac disease). There is no gold standard test for small bowel bacterial overgrowth (Khoshini *et al.*, 2008). Cultures of small bowel aspirates are recommended but have limitations in interpretation; less sensitive hydrogen breath tests are easier to perform but also have limitations (Gibson & Barrett, 2010). Non-invasive tests for pancreatic insufficiency are limited by the large reserve capacity of the pancreas, which means that 90% tissue involvement may be required before reductions in pancreatic enzyme secretions result in symptoms. Thorough evaluation of multiple nutritional markers, including circulating levels of fat-soluble vitamins (preferably vitamin E), prealbumin, retinol-binding protein, zinc and magnesium (Lindkvist *et al.*, 2012), may be helpful in diagnosing some cases, but further research is required (Lindkvist *et al.*, 2015). Imaging techniques can elucidate changes in pancreas structure in severe insufficiency, but faecal elastase remains the first-line assessment for malabsorption of suspected pancreatic origin (Thomas *et al.*, 2003).

Dietary treatment

Whatever the cause of malabsorption, the principles of dietary interventions are to:

- Replace large fluid and electrolyte losses.
- Treat the primary disorder, if appropriate.
- Provide symptom relief.
- Restore optimal nutritional status, with supplementation for micronutrients and/or trace elements as required.

Specific aspects of particular types of malabsorption are considered in the following text.

Fat malabsorption

The main nutritional implication of the loss of fat is the associated loss of energy and fat-soluble vitamins. Unabsorbed fatty acids may form complexes with minerals such as calcium and iron, thus inhibiting their absorption. This can increase the risk of long-term complications such as iron deficiency anaemia or osteoporosis. In those with proven chronic malabsorptive states, supplements of fat-soluble vitamins are indicated. In cases of persistent malabsorption, a micellised (water-soluble) form or injection is preferable. In children, deficiency of essential fatty acids can occur, necessitating supplementation. Zinc status can be compromised, and measurement of plasma or red blood cell zinc can guide the need for supplementation.

Steatorrhoea compromises nutritional status due to energy loss via the stool and may be exacerbated by patient selection of low-fat foods for symptom relief. Steatorrhoea due to pancreatic insufficiency can be treated with pancreatic enzymes, and clinical practice guidelines exist for cystic fibrosis (see Chapter 7.4.13, Cystic fibrosis) and pancreatitis (see Chapter 7.4.5, Disorders of the pancreas). If, despite additional drug therapy (options include the addition of a proton pump inhibitor or acid suppression with an H2 blocker), steatorrhoea continues unabated, electrolyte disturbances and/or mineral deficiencies may occur. Dietary fat intake can be reduced (30% energy), replacing energy via modular carbohydrate supplementation (see Chapter 6.3, Oral nutritional support). Alternatively, or additionally, a proportion of long-chain triglycerides can be substituted with medium-chain triglycerides (MCTs). MCTs are readily hydrolysed by pancreatic enzymes, and about one-third of ingested MCTs can directly enter the mucosal cells being hydrolysed by a mucosal lipolytic system; the medium-chain fatty acids then pass into the portal vein (Papamandjaris *et al.*,1998). Intervention studies generally use MCT-containing supplements and formulae as pure MCT oil is poorly tolerated. If used for cooking, MCT oil must not be heated above 150–160°C, or its palatability will be further impaired. MCTs can cause osmotic diarrhoea, and hence small, divided doses may improve tolerance (10 mL, qds).

In acute pancreatitis, elemental or semi-elemental feeds are effective when delivered via a tube placed past the ligament of Treitz; there is less evidence of effectiveness of this approach in mild or moderate pancreatitis, although this is accepted in practice (Pancreatitis Practice Guidance Summary, www.pennutrition.com).

Carbohydrate malabsorption

Lactose malabsorption

The enzyme lactase is required for the breakdown of the disaccharide lactose into galactose and glucose, which are absorbed. Varying degrees of deficiency of lactase can lead to lactose remaining within the intestine, causing osmotic diarrhoea. Colonic bacteria further ferment the lactose, resulting in symptoms such as abdominal distension, flatulence and explosive watery diarrhoea, which is often acidic in nature and may cause perianal dermatitis. Lactose intolerance occurs in three main forms as described in the following text.

Congenital alactasia

This is a rare autosomal recessive disorder characterised by the complete absence of lactase, and requires total and permanent lactose exclusion. The symptoms of profuse watery diarrhoea appear soon after initial feeding with lactose-containing milk. Breastfeeding is contraindicated, and the use of lactose-free infant formulae is essential. Paediatric dietetic expertise will be required to ensure that the diet remains lactose free but nutritionally adequate from weaning onwards (Shaw, 2015).

Primary lactase deficiency

A gradual reduction in lactase production (lactase non-persistence) causes symptoms of lactose maldigestion in older children and adults (Enattah *et al.*, 2002). This autosomal recessive trait is particularly common in people with their genetic origins in Asia, India, the Middle East, Africa and South America. Prevalence may exceed 50% in South America, Africa and Asia, and 100% in some Asian countries (Lomer *et al.*, 2008), as compared to Northern Europeans, North Americans and Australasians (5–17%).

Undigested lactose and the products of its bacterial fermentation can cause gastrointestinal symptoms, although not everyone with low lactase levels becomes symptomatic (Lomer *et al.*, 2008). The clinical effects are dose related and only become marked at high levels of intake, e.g. >50 g. Many people can tolerate moderate intakes of milk products, so the complete avoidance of lactose is unnecessary. Instead, symptoms should be stabilised at a low intake, and lactose-containing foods reintroduced in gradually increasing amounts. The individual level of tolerance varies, but most people with low lactase levels can consume 12 g lactose (as a single dose) with no or minor symptoms (Shaukat *et al.*, 2010). In some cases, up to 25 g/day (spread throughout the day) or sufficient dairy products to provide 1500 mg of calcium/day may be well tolerated (Suarez *et al.*, 1997, 1998). Fermented milk products may be better tolerated, perhaps due to delayed gastric emptying and increased transit time, along with the positive effects of certain probiotic strains of bacteria. Yogurts that contain some microbial beta-galactosidase can result in the beneficial proliferation of colonic flora (e.g. bifidobacteria), which can metabolise lactose, and regular lactose ingestion can improve tolerance over time (de Vrese *et al.*, 2001; Hertzler & Savaiano, 1996). Exogenous lactase via drops or tablets can be added to milk to reduce lactose load and improve tolerance, but this has mixed results (Lomer *et al.*, 2008; Suarez *et al.*, 1997). Ready-to-drink reduced lactose/lactose-free milks, yoghurts and cheeses are available.

Symptoms may be less likely to occur if lactose is consumed with food rather than in isolated liquid form between meals (Shaukat *et al.*, 2010). There is some evidence that temperature may also be related to tolerance, with warm milk being less well tolerated, but there is individual variation (Peuhkuri *et al.*, 2000).

Since the clinical effects of lactose intolerance are similar to those of irritable bowel syndrome, the possibility of primary lactase deficiency should be considered, particularly in genetically susceptible groups or in children complaining of recurrent abdominal pain, after more common organic causes have been excluded. Prevalence of lactose intolerance may be overestimated, with similar gastrointestinal symptoms resulting from a range of other physiological and psychological factors, including milk aversion (McBean & Miller, 1998; Rosado, 1997; Suarez & Levitt, 1996). In those with irritable bowel syndrome (IBS), tolerance to fermentable carbohydrates (particularly fructose and lactose) may need further investigation as they have been demonstrated to elicit IBS symptoms in some individuals (Gibson & Shepherd, 2010). Quantification of fructans and other short-chain carbohydrates in grains and cereals is available (Biesiekierski *et al.*, 2011) (see Chapter 7.4.10, Irritable bowel syndrome).

Secondary lactase deficiency

This is a common, usually temporary, consequence of damage to the intestinal brush border as a result of severe gastroenteritis, intestinal surgery, a flare of Crohn's disease, or chemotherapy. It is characterised by diarrhoea that persists after the primary disorder has been treated. Severe secondary lactose intolerance is sometimes accompanied by secondary sucrose intolerance.

Although transient, it may take weeks rather than days for lactase secretion to be adequately re-established. Most lactase production takes place in the older cells at the tips of the villi rather than in the newer basal cells. Lactase production is therefore the first of the disaccharidases to be affected by damage to the villi, and the last to be restored.

Management depends on symptom severity. In adults and children, avoidance of lactose for a few days will cause symptoms to subside, and it can then gradually be reintroduced into the diet with the use of foods such as lactose-reduced milk, fermented milk products such as yogurt and hard cheeses. As tolerance improves, the range of lactose-containing foods and their level of consumption can be increased. Because the condition is usually resolved within a relatively short timescale, the avoidance of milk and milk-based foods, even by children, is unlikely to pose a nutritional problem. However, if restriction of lactose (and consequently of certain dairy products) is required for >3–4 weeks, the question of nutritional adequacy in terms of calcium, protein and energy needs to be addressed with alternatives.

Formula-fed infants with secondary lactase deficiency may require lactose-free infant formula as a temporary substitute. Breast milk is usually tolerated, but, in severe cases, partial or total substitution by a lactose-free formula may be necessary. If the secondary lactase intolerance resulted from a cow's milk protein intolerance, alternative milk-free, lactose-free formula can be used (see Chapter 7.11.2, Food hypersensitivity).

Other disaccharides

Primary disaccharidase deficiencies

Congenital disorders such as sucrose–isomaltase deficiency occurs, but is rare. Management requires total avoidance of the disaccharide substrate.

Secondary disaccharidase deficiency

Production of sucrase and maltase is less likely to be affected by intestinal damage than lactase, but severe enteropathies or infections, particularly in children, may result in malabsorption of disaccharides, e.g. sucrose, coexisting alongside lactose malabsorption. Temporary avoidance of major sucrose sources followed by gradual reintroduction may be necessary.

Monosaccharide malabsorption

Fructose

Fructose occurs naturally in fruit, vegetables and honey, either in the monosaccharide form or as a disaccharide. In processed foods, high-fructose corn syrup (HFCS) has different properties and is derived from hydrolysed corn starch. Excess consumption of fructose, and HFCS in particular, may contribute to adiposity, dyslipidaemia, metabolic syndrome and non-alcoholic fatty liver disease (Bantle *et al.*, 2000; Elliott *et al.*, 2002; Jegatheesan & De Bandt, 2017).

Fructolysis occurs in the small intestine, with fructose being transported to the liver via the GLUT5 mechanism, which does not require insulin (Jones *et al.*, 2011). Unabsorbed fructose enters the colon, where it is a substrate for bacteria, which produce short-chain fatty acids, organic acids, hydrogen and methane. Gastrointestinal disturbances such as bloating, abdominal pain, loose stools and flatulence are symptomatic consequences of these colonic fermentation by-products (Beyer *et al.*, 2005).

In very young children, consumption of apple and pear juices that contain a large proportion of free fructose have been linked to toddler diarrhoea, which spontaneously resolves when dietary fructose is limited (see Chapter 3.8.12, Paediatric gastroenterology). The breath hydrogen test can be used alongside diet and symptom diaries to gauge individual tolerance to fructose (Jones *et al.*, 2013).

Secondary malabsorption of monosaccharides

This may occur in infants following surgery, protein energy malnutrition or gastroenteritis. An initial period of intravenous fluids is often necessary to correct water and electrolyte imbalances, followed by a carbohydrate-free formula. Careful monitoring for hypoglycaemia is necessary. The problem is thought to be monosaccharide malabsorption, since disaccharidase activity is normal. The ability to tolerate carbohydrates slowly improves, and glucose or fructose may be added to the diet in increasing increments of 1% of normal carbohydrate intake. These children are often underweight and gravely ill, and parenteral nutrition may be essential if resumption of adequate oral nutrition is delayed (Shaw, 2015) (see Chapter 3.8.11, Paediatric parenteral nutrition).

Protein malabsorption

Dietary restriction of protein is not indicated when malabsorption is due to deficiency of enzymes or proenzymes involved in protein digestion, e.g. enterokinase or trypsinogen. When increased protein losses occur due to an enteropathy or malabsorption, a high protein intake (0.5–1.5 g/kg/day) should be prescribed to allow for the decreased efficiency of absorption. If fat malabsorption is present, foods with a high protein but low fat content are advised. Modular protein supplements can be used in conjunction with glucose polymers (see Chapter 6.3, Oral nutritional support and Appendix A6, Nutritional supplements and enteral feeds).

Pancreatic enzyme replacement therapy remains a central aspect of the management of such malabsorption and maldigestion states that lead to pancreatic insufficiency (Toouli *et al.*, 2010), and more specifically in cystic fibrosis (see Chapter 7.4.13, Cystic fibrosis).

Internet resources

Pancreatitis Practice Guidance Summary, www.pennutrition.com

References

Bantle JP, Raatz SK, Thomas W, *et al.* (2000) Effects of dietary fructose on plasma lipids in healthy subjects. *Am. J. Clin. Nutr.* 72(5): 1128–1134.

Beyer PL, Caviar EM, McCallum RW. (2005) Fructose intake at current levels in the United States may cause gastrointestinal distress in normal adults. *J. Am. Diet. Assoc.* 105(10): 1559–1566.

Biesiekierski JR, Rosella O, Rose R, *et al.* (2011) Quantification of fructans, galacto-oligosacharides and other short-chain carbohydrates in processed grains and cereals. *J. Hum. Nutr. Diet.* 24(2): 154–176.

de Vrese M, Stegelmann A, Richter B, *et al.* (2001) Probiotics – compensation for lactase insufficiency. *Am. J. Clin. Nutr.* 73(2): 421S–429S.

de Lacy Costello BPJ, Ledochowski M, Ratcliffe NM. (2013) The importance of methane breath testing: a review. *J. Breath Res.* 7(2): 024001. Available at https://www.ncbi.nlm.nih.gov/pubmed/23470880.

Di Stefano M, Missanelli A, Miceli E, *et al.* (2004) Hydrogen breath test in the diagnosis of lactose malabsorption: accuracy of new versus conventional criteria. *J. Lab. Clin. Med.* 144(6): 313–318.

Elliott SS, Keim NL, Stern JS, *et al.* (2002) Fructose, weight gain, and the insulin resistance syndrome. *Am. J. Clin. Nutr.* 76(5): 911–922.

Enattah NS, Sahi T, Savilahti E, *et al.* (2002) Identification of a variant associated with adult-type hypolactasia. *Nat. Genet.* 30(2): 233–237.

Gasbarrini A, Corazza GR., Gasbarrini G, *et al.* (2009) Methodology and indications of H2-breath testing in gastrointestinal diseases: the Rome Consensus Conference. *Aliment. Pharmacol. Ther.* 29(S1): 1–49.

Gibson PR, Barrett JS. (2010) The concept of small intestinal bacterial overgrowth in relation to functional gastrointestinal disorders. *Nutrition.* 26: 1038–1043.

Gibson PJ, Shepherd SJ. (2010) Evidence-based dietary management of functional gastrointestinal symptoms: the FODMAP approach. *J. Gastroenterol. Hepatol.* 25(2): 252–258.

Hertzler SR, Savaiano DA. (1996) Colonic adaptation to daily lactose feeding in lactose maldigesters reduces lactose intolerance. *Am. J. Clin. Nutr.* 64: 232–236.

Jegatheesan P, De Bandt J-P. (2017) Fructose and NAFLD: the multifaceted aspects of fructose metabolism. *Nutrients.* 9(3): 230. doi:10.3390/nu9030230

Jones HF, Butler RN, Brooks DA. (2011) Intestinal fructose transport and malabsorption in humans. *Am. J Physiol. Gastrointest. Liver Physiol.* 300(2): G202–206. doi: 10.1152/ajpgi.00457.2010

Jones HF, Butler RN, Moore D, *et al.* (2013) Developmental changes and fructose absorption in children: effect on malabsorption testing and dietary management. *Nutr. Rev.* 71(5): 300–309.

Khoshini R, Dai S-C, Lezcano S, *et al.* (2008) A systematic review of diagnostic tests for small intestinal bacterial overgrowth. *Dig. Dis. Sci.* 53: 1443–1454.

Lindkvist B. (2013) Diagnosis and treatment of pancreatic exocrine insufficiency. *World J. Gastroenterol.* 19(42): 7258–7266.

Lindkvist B, Domínguez-Muñoz JE, Luaces-Regueira M, *et al.* (2012) Serum nutritional markers for prediction of pancreatic exocrine insufficiency in chronic pancreatitis. *Pancreatology.* 12: 305–310.

Lindkvist B, Phillips ME, Domínguez-Munoz JE. (2015) Clinical, anthropometric and laboratory nutritional markers of pancreatic exocrine insufficiency: prevalence and diagnostic use. *Pancreatology.* 15(6): 589–597.

Lomer MC, Parkes GC, Sanderson JD. (2008) Lactose intolerance in clinical practice – myths and realities. *Aliment. Pharmacol. Ther.* 27(2): 93–103.

McBean LD, Miller GD. (1998) Allaying fears and fallacies about lactose intolerance. *J. Am. Diet. Assoc.* 98: 671–676.

Papamandjaris AA, Macdougall DE, Jones PJH. (1998) Medium chain fatty acid metabolism and energy expenditure: Obesity treatment implications. *Life Sci.* 62(14): 1203–1215.

Peuhkuri K, Vapaatalo H, Nevala R, *et al.* (2000) Temperature of a test solution influenced abdominal symptoms in lactose tolerance tests. *Scand. J. Clin. Lab. Invest.* 60(1): 75–80.

Rosado JL. (1997) Lactose digestion and maldigestion: Implications for dietary habits in developing countries. *Nutr. Res. Rev.* 10: 137–149.

Shaukat A, Levitt MD, Taylor BC, *et al.* (2010) Systematic review: effective management strategies for lactose intolerance. *Ann. Intern. Med.* 152: 797–803.

Shaw V. (2015) Gastroenterology. In: *Clinical Paediatric Dietetics*, 5th edn. Chichester: John Wiley & Sons Ltd., pp. 104–142.

Suarez FL, Levitt MD. (1996) Abdominal symptoms and lactose: the discrepancy between patients' claims and the results of blinded trials. *Am. J. Clin. Nutr.* 64: 251–252.

Suarez FL, Savaiano D, Arbisi P, *et al.* (1997) Tolerance to the daily ingestion of two cups of milk by individuals claiming lactose intolerance. *Am. J. Clin. Nutr.* 65: 1502–1506.

Suarez FL, Adshead J, Furne JK, *et al.* (1998) Lactose maldigestion is not an impediment to the intake of 1500 mg calcium daily as dairy products. *Am. J. Clin. Nutr.* 68: 1118–1122.

Thomas PD, Forbes A, Green J, *et al.* (2003) Guidelines for the investigation of chronic diarrhoea. *Gut.* 52: v1–v15.

Toouli J, Biankin AV, Oliver MR, *et al.* (2010) Management of pancreatic exocrine insufficiency. *Med. J. Aust.* 193(8): 461–467.

7.4.7 Coeliac disease

Katie Kennedy

Key points

- The prevalence of coeliac disease is 1 in 100, affecting all age groups; the average age of diagnosis is 40–60 years.
- It is a multisystem disease that affects many organs, not just the gastrointestinal tract.
- Treatment is a lifelong gluten-free diet that avoids wheat, rye, barley and contaminated oats.
- Dietetic management aims to optimise absorption of nutrients and help prevent or treat complications, e.g. osteoporosis.
- The prevalence of type 1 diabetes and autoimmune thyroid disease is increased among patients with coeliac disease.

Coeliac disease is an inflammatory condition of the small intestinal mucosa that is induced by the ingestion of gluten and which improves clinically and histologically when gluten is excluded from the diet. It is alternatively termed coeliac sprue or gluten-sensitive enteropathy. Gluten is often used as a generic term to describe all of the cereal proteins that are toxic to individuals with coeliac disease. Wheat, barley and rye have all been shown to cause intestinal inflammation in coeliac patients; however, recent consensus suggests that uncontaminated oats are suitable (BSG, 2014; NICE, 2015). Coeliac disease can present at any age and has a wide range of clinical manifestations. The average age of diagnosis is 40–60 years, with a tendency towards more frequent diagnosis among females (BSG, 2014).

Traditionally, coeliac disease has been associated mainly with gastrointestinal symptoms, e.g. diarrhoea, abdominal pain and bloating, as chronic inflammation of the small intestine is a feature of the immune response to gluten. However, increasingly, non-gastrointestinal features of coeliac disease have been recognised; some people with coeliac disease have no obvious symptoms (asymptomatic presentation) (NICE, 2015). Coeliac disease is a multisystem disorder that can affect a variety of organs and can present with non-specific symptoms that may be overlooked at diagnosis or confused with other, more common conditions, including irritable bowel syndrome (IBS) (Card *et al.*, 2013).

Intolerance to gluten is permanent; the sole treatment is lifelong adherence to a gluten-free diet, which can be difficult to accept and follow. The degree of compliance to the gluten-free dietary regimen is varied and may be associated with a variety of factors. Recent research suggests that dietary compliance among certain groups of coeliac patients may be as low as 40%, with lowest compliance associated with increasing age, male gender and time since diagnosis (Comino *et al.*, 2016). Persistent problems are most often due to non-compliance, but other possible reasons are co-existing IBS, refractory coeliac disease, lactose intolerance and microscopic colitis (Leffler *et al.*, 2007a). Gluten intolerance can also manifest itself as dermatitis herpetiformis, which appears as a cutaneous rash and may be associated with gastrointestinal symptoms.

Coeliac disease is more prevalent in people with autoimmune conditions such as type 1 diabetes or autoimmune thyroid disease, and in first-degree relatives of people with coeliac disease (NICE, 2015). Primary complications of undiagnosed or untreated coeliac disease are osteoporosis and malignancy; however, recent work shows that the risk of malignancy is not as significant as previously thought (NICE, 2015).

Coeliac disease results from an immune reaction to antigenic fractions within gluten. The responsible fraction of gluten in wheat is gliadin, an alcohol-soluble prolamin that is a mixture of proteins. The different gluten peptides are involved in different ways. Some peptides cause mucosal damage by triggering an immunological pathway that has a rapid effect (innate immune response), whereas others stimulate a different immunological response (adaptive immune response) (Ciccocioppo *et al.*, 2005).

In addition to gliadin in wheat, prolamins found in other cereals, e.g. secalin in rye and hordein in barley, also trigger the immunological response leading to coeliac disease. Similar proteins (avenins) are found in oats, but these are not thought to be harmful to the majority of people with coeliac disease.

Onset and prevalence

Coeliac disease can develop and be diagnosed at any age. It was historically only associated with childhood, but now only 9% of all coeliac patients are diagnosed under 18 years of age, with highest incidence rates among individuals aged 40–70 years (West *et al.*, 2014). This is largely due to improved diagnosis among the adult population.

The actual prevalence of coeliac disease has been difficult to determine due to the wide variety of clinical presentations and asymptomatic disease. Contemporary studies estimate the overall seroprevalence of coeliac disease to be fairly static, at around 1% in most Westernised populations (BSG, 2014); however, some studies suggest that the prevalence may be increasing (Catassi *et al.*, 2010; Lohi *et al.*, 2007; White *et al.*, 2013). There is a clear gap between estimated prevalence (1 in 100) and reported incidence of coeliac disease, thus highlighting the clinical variability of the disease and the difficulties encountered by clinicians in making a correct diagnosis. While the diagnosis of coeliac disease has improved over recent years, it remains low, with only 24% of those with the condition having received a diagnosis (West *et al.*, 2014). Coeliac UK estimate that patients wait an average of 13 years before receiving an accurate diagnosis (Coeliac UK, unpublished data).

The prevalence of coeliac disease is at least 10% in first-degree relatives and approximately 2% in second-degree relatives (Hogberg *et al.*, 2003). Coeliac disease is associated with a particular human leukocyte antigen (HLA) genotype, with the HLA DQ heterodimer appearing to confer disease susceptibility. Approximately 95% of people with coeliac disease have the HLA DQ antigen, and studies looking at identical twins have found concordance levels of 75–90% (Greco *et al.*, 2002) (see Chapter 5.1, Genetics and nutritional genomics).

Clinical presentation

In children and adults, coeliac disease can present with a broad range of signs and symptoms, the most frequent being:

- Abdominal pain, bloating or distension.
- Chronic or intermittent diarrhoea.
- Faltering growth in children.
- Fatigue.
- Iron deficiency anaemia.
- Nausea or vomiting.
- Weight loss.
- Recurrent mouth ulcers.

Symptoms in children with coeliac disease depend on the age at presentation, and can develop following weaning and the introduction of foods that contain gluten at 6–24 months (Fasano, 2005). Under the age of 2 years, the clinical picture is characterised by a lethargic or irritable child, with loose, pale, offensive-smelling stools and a bloated abdomen. In infants, vomiting, anorexia and constipation may be seen. Between 2 and 16 years of age, coeliac disease presents with gastrointestinal symptoms, dental enamel defects, nutritional deficiencies, impaired growth, delayed puberty and general failure to thrive.

A retrospective case-finding study involving coeliac patients diagnosed at a specialist UK gastroenterology centre in the UK between 1990 and 2000 found that the ratio of typical to atypical symptoms was 1:2.5 (Sanders *et al.*, 2002). Moreover, Tucker *et al.* (2012) found that almost half of coeliac patients were diagnosed with a BMI of 25 or over, thus further challenging the traditional clinical picture associated with this condition.

The absence of symptoms associated with malabsorption among some patients can be explained by the fact that coeliac disease affects mainly the proximal small bowel, resulting in considerable functional reserve. In adults, anaemia may be a particularly important indicator of coeliac disease (Lebwohl *et al.*, 2014). In coeliac patients identified by serological screening (with subsequent confirmatory biopsy), over 80% did not have gastrointestinal symptoms, but over half were anaemic (Hin *et al.*, 1999). Coeliac disease should therefore be considered in any patient with anaemia or symptoms of prolonged fatigue (NICE, 2015).

The prevalence of coeliac disease among patients with an existing diagnosis of IBS is significantly higher than for the general population (Sanders *et al.*, 2002). A recent meta-analysis suggests that coeliac disease may be up to 4.5 times more common among this group of individuals (Irvine *et al.*, 2017). As a result, a diagnosis of IBS may often mask the correct identification of coeliac disease. Current NICE guidelines for the diagnosis and management of IBS recommend that all patients who meet the diagnostic criteria for IBS should undergo serological testing to rule out a possible diagnosis of coeliac disease (NICE, 2017).

Diagnosis

Biochemistry

Specific circulating antibodies are present and titres decrease when a gluten-free diet is commenced. Serological testing for coeliac disease involves the identification of immunoglobulin A tissue transglutaminase (IgA tTG) antibodies and specific endomysial antibodies (EMA). Total IgA should be determined in order to rule out IgA deficiency and reduce the risk of a false negative result. People with coeliac disease are more likely to be IgA deficient, 2.5% in coeliac disease as compared to 0.25% in the general population (Lenhardt *et al.*, 2004). In patients with known IgA deficiency, immunoglobulin G (IgG) EMA, immunoglobulin G deamidated gliadin peptide (Ig A DGP) or IgG tTG may be used in order to support the diagnosis (BSG, 2014; NICE, 2015). It is essential that patients consume a gluten-containing diet prior to and during diagnostic investigation as results may normalise on a gluten-free diet. Current guidelines recommend that gluten-containing foods be eaten in at least one meal every day for a minimum of 6 weeks prior to testing (NICE, 2015).

Small bowel histology

Patients with positive serological test results should be referred to a gastroenterologist for endoscopic intestinal biopsy to confirm or exclude coeliac disease (NICE, 2015). Duodenal biopsy carries minimal risk, and has high positive and negative predictive values. Since the small bowel damage (villous atrophy) induced by coeliac disease may be patchy, a minimum of four biopsy specimens should be obtained, including a duodenal bulb biopsy (BSG, 2014). Current guidelines also recommend that duodenal biopsy be considered in patients with negative serology but who show signs of malabsorption (e.g. anaemia, diarrhoea, severe unexplained weight loss) or a family history of coeliac disease (BSG, 2014). As with serological testing, it is essential that a gluten-containing diet be maintained before a biopsy is carried out.

Marsh classification

The stages of damage to the small bowel seen in coeliac disease are graded by the Marsh (1992) classification:

Marsh 0: normal mucosa.
March 1: increased number of intraepithelial lymphocytes.
Marsh 2: increased lymphocytes and crypt depth.
Marsh 3: partial or complete villous atrophy – classic coeliac lesion.
Marsh 4: villous atrophy without lymphocytes – rare and typically unresponsive to diet.

Biopsies in children

The European Society for Paediatric Gastroenterology, Hepatology and Nutrition (ESPGHAN) (2012) suggest that duodenal biopsies do not need to be performed in order to confirm a positive diagnosis of coeliac disease in children who have symptoms suggestive of coeliac disease; whose IgA tTG levels exceed 10 times the upper limit of normal; whose EMA antibodies are positive (on a separately taken blood sample); and who are HLA-DQ2 or HLA-DQ8 positive. These guidelines reflect the improved accuracy and reliability of modern serological tests employed to detect coeliac disease. Endoscopies are invasive and potentially distressing for children and families; furthermore, the waiting lists for such procedures risk delaying diagnosis and treatment of a vulnerable patient group. Although this approach remains controversial, the British Society of Paediatric Gastroenterology, Hepatology and Nutrition (BSPGHAN), together with Coeliac UK, have published a joint guideline supporting ESPGHAN's approach (BSPGHAN & Coeliac UK, 2013).

Malignancy

Coeliac disease is associated with a modest increase in the risk of malignant small intestinal lymphomas, mainly non-Hodgkin's lymphoma (Catassi *et al.*, 2005; West *et al.*, 2004a). It has also been suggested that the risk of lymphoma is reduced by adherence to a strict gluten-free diet; and, after approximately 5 years, the risk is likely to have been reduced to the level of the general population (Askling *et al.*, 2002; Holmes *et al.*, 1989). Coeliac disease also increases the risk of small bowel adenocarcinoma (Holmes *et al.*, 1989; Howdle *et al.*, 2003). A recent meta-analysis showed a fourfold increased risk of non-Hodgkin's lymphoma as compared to the general population, with an estimated 1:2000 coeliac patients developing lymphoma annually (Kane *et al.*, 2011). Although there is an increased risk of malignancy with undiagnosed coeliac disease, the overall risk of developing specific cancers is low (NICE, 2015).

Osteoporosis

Undiagnosed coeliac disease is related to low bone mineral density, osteoporosis and increased risk of fractures (BSG, 2014). Approximately 75% of adults with untreated coeliac disease suffer from osteopenia or osteoporosis (Corazza *et al.*, 2005). Even in people with few symptoms of coeliac disease, bone mineral density can be significantly lower than in the general population. Evidence suggests that both treated and untreated people with coeliac disease have an increased risk of osteoporosis and bone fracture. Bone fractures are almost twice as common in individuals with clinically diagnosed coeliac disease as compared to those without the disease. Moreover, coeliac disease at baseline was associated with a 30% increase in the risk of any fracture and a 69% increase in the risk of hip fracture (Heikkila *et al.*, 2015). It is well established that the villous atrophy observed in coeliac disease leads to the malabsorption of many micronutrients (e.g. calcium and vitamin D) which are essential for maintaining bone health. This increased risk of osteoporosis has been attributed to calcium malabsorption stimulating the release of parathyroid hormone, which increases bone turnover, ultimately resulting in increased bone loss (Walters, 1994). Risk factors specifically related to coeliac disease that may reduce bone mineral density and increase the risk of osteoporosis include:

- Late or delayed diagnosis of coeliac disease in adulthood.
- Chronic malabsorption of calcium prior to diagnosis.
- Reduced intake of calcium following diagnosis; bread and cereal foods contribute approximately 30% of daily calcium intake (Public Health England, 2014).
- Lapses from the glute-free diet.
- Persistent villous atrophy.
- Lactose intolerance and subsequent removal of dairy foods.
- Low BMI.

Excess risk of osteoporosis and fracture in coeliac disease may be reduced with good dietary adherence to a calcium-rich, gluten-free diet, and the subsequent reversal of villous atrophy (Bai *et al.*, 1997; Ciacci *et al.*, 1997; Valdimarsson *et al.*, 1996). A gluten-free diet is the core management strategy for the prevention of osteoporosis among coeliac patients (BSG, 2014). The prevalence of reduced bone density after 1 year of following a gluten-free diet is similar to that after 3 years. This suggests that the extent of bone mass gain in the first year of dietary treatment is indicative of overall bone mineral density improvement (Corazza *et al.*, 2005) (see Chapter 7.9.1, Osteoporosis).

Calcium requirements

Adult patients with coeliac disease should have a calcium intake of at least 1000 mg per day (BSG, 2014). Postmenopausal women, in particular, may require calcium supplementation to achieve sufficient intake. There are no guidelines recommending a higher requirement for calcium in children with coeliac disease. It is recommended that an individualised, calcium-rich, gluten-free diet be followed that uses reference nutrient intake values (DH, 1991).

Associated conditions

The association between coeliac disease and type 1 diabetes mellitus is due to a common genetic predisposition involving both HLA and non-HLA genes. In patients with type 1 diabetes, the presence of the HLA-DQ 2.5 haplotype provides the highest risk for developing both conditions (Gutierrez-Achury *et al.*, 2015). There is a 6% prevalence of coeliac disease among patients with type 1 diabetes (NICE, 2015). Consequently, patients with type 1 diabetes should be offered serological screening for coeliac disease at diagnosis (NICE, 2015).

There are no specific guidelines regarding the frequency of screening for coeliac disease among people with type 1 diabetes; however, coeliac disease should be suspected in patients with gastrointestinal symptoms, unexplained weight loss (faltering growth in children) or unexplained anaemia. Adherence to the gluten-free diet has been shown to improve growth parameters in children and long-term blood glucose control in people with type 1 diabetes (Saadah *et al.*, 2004). However, in patients with diabetes and asymptomatic coeliac disease, objective data is limited regarding the benefits of adopting a gluten-free diet on their diabetes control, bone health or quality of life. It is hoped that the Celiac Disease and Diabetes Dietary Intervention and Evaluation Trial (CD-DIET), a multicentre, randomised controlled trial aimed at evaluating the efficacy and safety of a gluten-free diet in adults and children with a dual diagnosis, will shed further light on this subject (Mahmud *et al.*, 2015).

Autoimmune thyroid disease

The link between coeliac disease and autoimmune thyroid disease is well recognised. Pooled prevalence data suggests a prevalence of 2.4% among people with coeliac disease (NICE, 2015). Graves' disease (hyperthyroidism) and Hashimoto's thyroiditis (hypothyroidism) are the most common conditions (Ch'ng *et al.*, 2005; Valentino *et al.*, 2002). Screening patients with these thyroid disorders for coeliac disease is recommended (NICE, 2015).

Down syndrome

The higher prevalence of coeliac disease in people with Down syndrome, estimated to be in the region of 3–4% (NICE, 2015), is likely to be explained by genetic factors, although the exact nature of the linkage remains to be determined (Morris *et al.*, 2000). Serological testing for coeliac disease should be considered among those with Down syndrome (NICE, 2015).

Turner syndrome

Turner syndrome is a genetic disorder that only affects females. Pooled prevalence data suggests a prevalence of coeliac disease in the region of 5–6% among people with this condition, and, as such, serological testing for coeliac disease should be considered (NICE, 2015).

Dermatitis herpetiformis

Dermatitis herpetiformis is the skin presentation of coeliac disease. It is characterised by a persistent, itchy, blistering rash that usually occurs on the knees, elbows, buttocks and back, although it can affect any area of skin. Total or subtotal villous atrophy is found in approximately 70% of patients with dermatitis herpetiformis (Fry *et al.*, 1974); however, gastrointestinal symptoms are likely to be mild or absent, with less than 10% of patients reporting gastrointestinal symptoms characteristic of coeliac disease (Caproni *et al.*, 2009). NICE guidance (2015) recommends that people with dermatitis herpetiformis be screened for coeliac disease.

Dermatitis herpetiformis is less common than coeliac disease, with a UK incidence of about 1 in 10,000; it is more common in men and usually presents at 15–40 years, being rare in children. As with coeliac disease, there is an inherited tendency to develop the disease, and there are links with autoimmune thyroid disease and type 1 diabetes (Reunala & Collin, 1997), with both patients with dermatitis herpetiformis and family members being at increased risk of developing these disorders (Hervonen *et al.*, 2004).

The condition is managed by a gluten-free diet, but as it can often take several months before the rash improves and nearly 2 years before it disappears completely, a range of medications may need to be prescribed to control the rash, including dapsone.

Patients with dermatitis herpetiformis are affected by the same long-term complications at those with coeliac disease, including lymphoma (Hervonen *et al.*, 2005). There is a high prevalence of anaemia, which may be exacerbated if dapsone is used. There is also increased risk of osteoporosis (Reunala & Collin, 1997); it is therefore important that attention be paid to the overall nutritional content of the diet, particularly regarding micronutrients, in addition to gluten avoidance.

Management

Diet therapy is essential in the management of patients with coeliac disease, and the dietitian has a key role to play in supporting patients to effectively manage this condition, both in terms of optimising nutrient intake and maintaining quality of life. Guidelines for the diagnosis and management of Coeliac disease (CD) are available for children (BSPGHAN & Coeliac UK, 2013) and adults (BSG, 2014; NICE, 2015).

Dietary management

All newly diagnosed coeliac patients should have a nutritional assessment with a dietitian to establish overall dietary adequacy and associated goals. Patients with coeliac disease also require follow-up by a dietitian and/or clinician with a specific interest or expertise in coeliac disease (BSG, 2014). The recently published quality standard for coeliac disease (NICE, 2016) states that service providers (e.g. general practices, community healthcare providers and secondary care) should ensure that processes are in place for newly diagnosed patients to discuss how to follow-up a gluten-free diet with a healthcare professional who has specialist knowledge of coeliac disease, such as a dietitian.

Dietary objectives

The dietary objectives are to ensure that people with coeliac disease:

- Exclude all dietary sources of gluten.
- Know which foods and ingredients are naturally free from gluten.
- Substitute gluten-containing foods and ingredients with gluten-free alternatives to improve dietary acceptability, nutritional adequacy and compliance.
- Consume a balanced diet which helps maintain health and prevent or manage associated diseases, particularly osteoporosis.

The dietitian needs to ensure that the diet is sufficiently energy and nutrient dense to meet increased needs and help restore losses. At diagnosis, iron deficiency is common, as well as subclinical deficiencies of other vitamins and minerals, especially folate, vitamin D and calcium. Additional vitamin and mineral supplementation, particularly of iron, may be required for a period of weeks or months in those shown to have deficiencies.

The limited period (typically 20–30 minutes) allocated to an outpatient appointment for a newly diagnosed coeliac patient rarely allows all topics to be discussed. There is great variability in the dietetic services offered to patients with coeliac disease across the UK. Increased diagnosis rates are undoubtedly applying pressure to the resources available, and, as a result, dietetic services are evolving to meet demand. Several centres in the UK have initiated successful dietetic-led group interventions (in place of one-to-one consultations) for both newly diagnosed and review patients of coeliac disease (Trott, 2016).

A new patient appointment checklist is available from Coeliac UK to assist dietitians in covering the most important issues, such as a simple explanation of the principles of a gluten-free diet, provision of written information on gluten-containing foods, obtaining gluten-free products, symptoms, cross-contamination and eating out. Individuals should be encouraged to join Coeliac UK to gain access to the annually updated food and drink directory, gluten-free prescription product list and recipe database. Coeliac UK also provides a nationwide support group network and a wide range of information leaflets and electronic apps to help support patients to adhere to a gluten-free diet.

Symptoms of coeliac disease such as bloating and diarrhoea usually improve within a few weeks of commencing a gluten-free diet. It often takes >12 months for mucosal damage to the small bowel to be completely repaired and villi to return to normal (Tuire *et al.*, 2012), so other symptoms such as anaemia may take longer to improve. A dramatic drop in antibody levels will be seen in the first month of treatment, but antibodies may still be present 12 months after commencement of the diet. For this reason, positive antibodies or a degree of villous atrophy in the first 12 months following diagnosis may be poor predictors of dietary adherence (Midhagen *et al.*, 2004). It is also of note that the presence of IBS-type symptoms in coeliac disease is common, and, while these are more common among non-adherent patients, those who are adherent to a gluten-free diet are still more likely to experience symptoms as compared to controls (Sainsbury *et al.*, 2013). As a result, detailed and skilled dietetic assessment of adherence among patients with persistent symptoms is required in order to determine the likely cause.

Dietary sources of gluten

Gluten is derived from multiple sources, and a gluten-free diet therefore necessitates the calculated avoidance of many foods. The term 'glute' is used here as a generic term to encompass all the proteins derived from wheat (gliadins), rye (secalins) and barley (hordeins). Oats contain the gluten-like protein avenin. A small number of people with coeliac disease may be sensitive to avenins (Garsed *et al.*, 2007; Haboubi *et al.*, 2006); however, current guidance recommends that gluten-free oats are acceptable to be included at any stage (NICE, 2015). Furthermore, the inclusion of oats in a gluten-free diet may help to improve variety and provide a valuable source of fibre, particularly soluble fibre. Wheat flour is a particularly ubiquitous constituent of a modern diet, being contained in bread, breakfast cereals, pasta, pizza, pastry, biscuits, cakes and sauces. The presence of gluten in such foods is easy to identify. However, gluten is also a less obvious component of many manufactured foods and can be present in almost any type of product. Under European law, food ingredient labels must now clearly highlight the presence, or possible presence, of all gluten-containing cereals (see Chapter 4.5, Food law and labelling).

Food labelling

Manufactured foods may contain gluten as a result of wheat flour being added as an ingredient, processing aid, binder, filler or a carrier for flavourings and spices. Although wheat flour may only be present in small amounts, this can still be significant in terms of gluten content. In compliance with allergen labelling law (EU, 2011), all foods that contain gluten-containing cereals as ingredients must clearly identify this on the label within the ingredients list (see Chapter 4.5, Food law and labelling). Some ingredients that are derived from gluten-containing cereals, such as glucose syrup and maltodextrin, are exempt from this labelling as the level of gluten contained in them is below the level that is toxic in coeliac disease. In 2009, the European Commission introduced new labelling standards (EC, 2009) that set maximum permitted levels of gluten for foods labelled as either 'gluten free' or 'very low gluten'. These standards were designed to help protect the long-term health of people with coeliac disease. The levels of gluten permitted are based on recognised scientific evidence, and are as follows:

- Gluten free: 20 parts per million (ppm) of gluten or less
- Very low gluten: 21–100 ppm of gluten

All foods, including specialist substitute products such as gluten-free breads and flours which may contain gluten-free wheat starch, can be labelled as 'gluten free' providing they contain no more than the maximum permitted levels of gluten outlined earlier. The 'gluten free' label may also be used for uncontaminated oat products that meet the gluten-free standard (i.e. $\leq$20 ppm). This regulation applies to all foods (both pre-packed and loose) sold in a variety of outlets, including shops and catering establishments. It is important to note that only foods containing cereal ingredients which have been specially processed to reduce the level of gluten can make a 'very low gluten' claim.

Coeliac UK licenses the Crossed Grain symbol (Figure 7.4.5) to a growing number of manufacturers who produce gluten-free foods and drinks. It is an internationally recognised symbol and a registered trademark. Many food manufacturers and supermarkets use their own symbols to identify gluten-free foods.

Contamination

Gluten may also be present due to cross-contamination during production. Contamination with wheat, rye, barley, or oats can occur during food production or storage. For example, flour particles from foods being made in one area can be suspended in the atmosphere and cross-contaminate supposedly gluten-free foods being produced in another area. Manufacturers frequently use statements such as 'May contain' to show that there could be small amounts of an allergen in a food product caused by cross-contamination during production. There are several different statements which manufacturers use on food packing labels to warn of possible allergen cross-contamination, such as 'May contain x', 'Made in a factory that also handles x', etc. These statements are simply meant to provide the consumer with information on how the risk arises as opposed to the severity of the risk. In the home, practical measures that patients can take to reduce the risk of contamination include the following:

Figure 7.4.5 The Coeliac UK Crossed Grain symbol licensed to manufacturers to indicate a gluten food product (source: Coeliac UK. Reproduced with permission from Coeliac UK, www.coeliac.org)

- Wash surfaces, chopping boards and utensils thoroughly before preparing food, or use a separate utensils.
- Use a separate toaster for gluten-free breads, or use toaster bags or foil on a clean grill to make gluten-free toast.
- Cook gluten-free food in separate pans/baking trays.
- Wash hands after handling gluten-containing food.
- Serve gluten-free food with separate utensils.
- Use separate containers for butter, jams, chutneys, etc., or ensure that a clean knife or spoon is always used to serve them.
- Store gluten-free food in sealed containers
- Use foods and ingredients naturally free from gluten.

Most foods that have not been processed, such as fresh meat, fish, eggs, cheese, milk, fruit and vegetables, can be safely included in a gluten-free diet (see Table 7.4.5).

Prescription of gluten-free products

Foods including gluten-free bread, flour mixes, crackers and pasta are prescribable according to the Advisory Committee on Borderline Substances for people medically diagnosed with coeliac disease or dermatitis herpetiformis. These products are commonly fortified with additional micronutrients of particular relevance to coeliac patients, e.g. calcium, iron and folic acid. The types of gluten-free foods available are summarised in Table 7.4.6. Further details can be found in the British National Formulary, the Monthly Index of Medical Specialities (MIMS), the Drug Tariff, or obtained directly from the manufacturers. It should be noted that the names of both the producers and products are liable to change. A full list of all currently available proprietary gluten-free foods can be obtained from Coeliac UK.

Gluten-free prescribing guidelines were produced for healthcare professionals by a collaboration of Coeliac UK, BDA, BSPGHAN and Primary Care Society for Gastroenterology (PCSG) (2011, updated 2012). These national guidelines were based on a review of data from the National Diet and Nutrition Survey (Henderson *et al.*, 2003), and provide recommendations that suggest reasonable amounts of gluten-free foods that should be prescribed as part of a balanced diet. These guidelines are based on the consumption of 50% of total energy as carbohydrate, with gluten-free prescribable foods providing 15% of total energy. Gluten-free sources of carbohydrate, such as potatoes, rice and breakfast cereals, make up the remaining 35% of total energy. Energy requirements of the different sexes and ages are taken into account, as well as variables such as a high activity level, pregnancy and breastfeeding. The guidance provides a minimum monthly requirement in unit values that are based on carbohydrate content and cost. The guidance is not mandatory, and products are prescribed at the discretion of the general practitioner (GP). Over recent years, the significant financial burdens faced by the NHS have

Table 7.4.5 Gluten content categorisation of some foods

Foods	Gluten free	May contain gluten	Gluten containing
Cereals and flours	Manufactured gluten-free products, including gluten-free oats Rice (white, brown, wild, rice flour, ground rice) Maize (corn), maize starch, cornmeal, popping corn Polenta Potato flour, potato starch Soya, soya flour Bean flours (chick pea flour, split pea flour) Sago, tapioca, cassava Arrowroot Amaranth Buckwheat Millet Quinoa Sorghum Teff Cornflour		Wheat, rye, barley Bulgar wheat, durum wheat Spelt, triticale, kamut Wheat flour (e.g. plain/self-raising/strong flour) and other flours derived from rye, barley, spelt, triticale and oats Wheat starch Wheatgerm Wheat bran Semolina, couscous Standard oats and oat products Malt and malted barley
Bread, cakes and biscuits	Manufactured gluten-free products, e.g. bread, rolls, crispbread, biscuits Pastry, cakes biscuits made with gluten-free flours or mixes Rice cakes Cakes made without flour (e.g. macaroons) Gluten-free pizza bases		Bread and bread products containing wheat, rye, barley, including croissants, brioche, naan bread, pitta bread, chapattis, parathas, ciabatta, rye bread Ordinary biscuits, crispbread, crackers, matzos, rusks Ordinary cakes and pastries, muffins and scones Pizza, pastry, croutons Batter, pancakes, Yorkshire pudding
Pasta	Manufactured gluten-free pasta Corn pasta; rice pasta	Rice noodles, buckwheat noodles	Fresh, dried or canned pasta and noodles
Breakfast cereals	Manufactured gluten-free muesli Buckwheat flakes Gluten-free porridge oats/oatmeal	Cornflakes Rice cereals	Wheat-based breakfast cereals Muesli Standard porridge oats/oatmeal
Fruit, vegetables, pulses and nuts	Fresh, frozen, canned, dried, whole or sliced fruit Fresh, frozen, canned vegetables Peas, beans, lentils Plain, roasted, salted nuts	Chips Instant mashed potato Vegetables in sauce Canned fruit pie fillings Canned baked beans Dry roasted nuts	Vegetables and potatoes coated with batter, breadcrumbs or flour Fruit pies, pasties or fruit coated with batter or flour
Milk and dairy products	Whole, semi-skimmed, skimmed milk Dried skimmed milk Evaporated and condensed milk Sterilised and ultra heat treated (UHT) milk Soya milk Rice milk Goat's milk Cream Cheese including cheese spreads and processed cheese	Yogurts and fromage frais Coffee and tea whiteners Artificial cream Ready-grated cheese	Milk with added fibre Yogurt and fromage frais containing muesli or cereals
Meat and meat products	Fresh red meat, poultry, game and offal Meat, canned or prepacked in its own juices or in jelly Smoked or cured pure meat, such as bacon or ham Gluten-free sausages Continental sausages that are 100% meat	Beef burgers Canned meat products Meat pastes, pâtés	Any type of meat coated in breadcrumbs or batter Meat pies and puddings Haggis Ordinary sausages and sausage meat Faggots and rissoles
Fish and shellfish	All fresh fish and other seafood Smoked, kippered and dried fish Fish canned in oil or brine Gluten-free fish fingers	Fish in sauce Fish pastes and pâtés	Fish/shellfish in batter or breadcrumbs Fish cakes Fish fingers Taramasalata

Table 7.4.5 (*Continued*)

Foods	Gluten free	May contain gluten	Gluten containing
Eggs	Whole eggs Egg yolk Egg white Meringue (free from flour)	Egg substitutes	Scotch eggs
Desserts and puddings	Jelly Sorbets Milk puddings made with gluten-free ingredients Custard powders	Icecream Instant dessert Mousses	Semolina and macaroni milk puddings Trifle Sponge and suet puddings
Fats and oils	Butter Lard Vegetable oils, margarines and fat spreads Reduced and low-fat spreads		Suet
Soups, sauces and seasonings	Salt, peppercorns Tomato purée Garlic, herbs and spices Wine and cider vinegars Pickled vegetables in vinegar Gluten-free stuffing mix	Canned and packet soups Packet sauces and sauce mixes 'Cook-in' sauces Bottled sauces and ketchups Stock and stock cubes Gravy browning and mixes Mustard powder Curry powder Mayonnaise, salad cream, salad dressings Pickles and chutneys Tamari (Japanese soy sauce)	Soya (Chinese soy sauce) Mixed seasonings and spices that specify flour on the label Stuffing and stuffing mixes
Savoury snack foods	Plain potato crisps Homemade popcorn Prawn crackers Poppadums	Flavoured crisps and snacks	Snack products made from wheat, rye, barley Pretzels
Preserves and spreads	Sugar, glucose, golden syrup, treacle, molasses Jam, conserves, honey, marmalade Peanut and other nut butters	Mincemeat Lemon curds and cheeses Chocolate or other sweet spreads	
Confectionery	Boiled sweets/jellies	Sweets, chocolate, toffees, etc. Iced lollies Chewing gum	
Beverages	Tea, coffee Fruit juices, fruit squash Mineral water Clear fizzy drinks Cocoa Milk Spirits, wines, liqueurs, cider, sherry, port Complan, Build-up Specialist gluten-free beers	Herbal teas Chocolate powders and drinks Milk shakes and mixes Sports and health drinks	Vending machine chocolate drinks Barley waters Cloudy fizzy drinks Malted milk drinks Beer and lager, ale and stout, home-brewed beers, low-alcohol beers and lagers.
Miscellaneous	Gelatine Bicarbonate of soda, cream of tartar Fresh and dried yeast Tofu Food colourings, essences and flavourings Cake coverings and decorations Marzipan Meat, vegetable and yeast extracts	Baking powder	Icecream cones and wafers Communion wafers Quorn

Table 7.4.6 Prescribable gluten-free foods

Type of product	Gluten-free products available	Comments
Bread and rolls	White, brown, wholemeal bread (sliced/ unsliced), rolls, baguettes High-fibre and seeded breads	Fresh or long-life options available. Some breads and rolls are vacuum packed and either fully or partially baked. Fresh products may need to be ordered/delivered in larger case sizes
Flour substitutes	Flour mixes (white, brown, high-fibre, multipurpose or specifically designed to make bread) Standard flours	Can be used for home baking
Biscuits	Digestives, tea biscuits Crackers/savoury biscuits Crispbread	Sweet biscuits only to be prescribed in exceptional circumstances (e.g. underweight/ malnourished patients) – see revised Coeliac UK prescribing guidelines
Pasta	Fusilli, lasagne, macaroni, penne, rigati, spaghetti, spirals, tagliatelle	
Convenience foods	Pizza bases	

resulted in a large number of clinical commissioning groups (CCGs) reducing or removing the provision of gluten-free foods on prescription. Furthermore, in March 2017, the Department of Health (DH) launched a national consultation regarding the future of gluten-free prescribing in England (DH, 2017). At the time of printing, the findings of this consultation have not been published. Resulting recommendations have the potential to significantly impact the current arrangements for gluten-free prescribing, including the possibility of complete removal of this provision for coeliac patients living in England. Gluten-free specialist foods have been available on prescription since the late 1960s; since this time, the range of products on prescription has increased dramatically, as has the availability of such foods in retail outlets. However, recent research suggests that the availability of gluten-free products remains variable, with smaller, budget supermarkets and local or corner shops typically stocking little or no gluten-free foods (Burden *et al.*, 2015). Specialist gluten-free food products are up to five times more expensive than their gluten-containing counterparts (Singh & Whelan, 2011). Furthermore, access to gluten-free food on prescription has been shown to negatively influence adherence (Muhammad *et al.*, 2017), however the removal of this provision may therefore reduce compliance, particularly among low-income patients and the elderly (Hall, 2013; MacColloch & Rashid, 2014; Singh & Whelan, 2011). The BDA Policy Statement (2015) regarding the provision of gluten-free food on prescription states that '*Coeliac disease is a condition that warrants the continued availability of staple GF foods on prescription*'. Methods for increasing efficiency and reducing the costs associated with the provision of gluten-free foods on prescription may offer alternatives to their removal. The Scottish Gluten-free Food Service, involving the management of gluten-free food prescriptions by community pharmacies, has demonstrated advantages in terms of reduced GP time, product usage and patient satisfaction (Scottish Government, 2015). Similar schemes in England have shown reductions in cost of approximately 20% (Carr, 2011).

A large variety of gluten-free foods, covering virtually all product categories from bakery to chilled convenience meals are available to purchase in most supermarkets. The cost of these products remains comparatively high, and availability can be variable, particularly in smaller outlets; however, their use may make the diet more appealing, inclusive and socially acceptable.

Dietetic follow-up

Review and follow-up of patients with coeliac disease allows the healthcare team to monitor dietary adherence, symptoms and the emergence of disease complications; refresh advice; and identify the need for additional support. Optimal follow-up support should feature both gastrointestinal and dietetic expertise (BSG, 2014). NICE recommends that healthcare professionals (including dietitians, consultants, and GPs) offer an annual review to people with coeliac disease, and encourage them to attend by giving them information about why they may need a review. The BSG (2014) recommends that, once the patients are stable and feel confident in managing their diet, annual follow-up appointments should be initiated, involving assessment of the full blood count, vitamin and mineral status, associated autoimmune conditions (thyroid function tests and serum glucose levels), liver function and coeliac-specific auto-antibodies (Ig A tTG or EMA/ DGP).

The following topics should be discussed at a review appointment:

- Gluten content of the diet.
- Calcium intake.
- Dietary compliance.
- Symptomatic improvement.
- Nutritional status.
- Blood test results.
- Gluten-free prescriptions.
- Membership of Coeliac UK, and use of the food and drink directory.

Ongoing dietetic support is essential both at diagnosis and follow-up to assess and review nutritional status and to review possible nutritional issues or deficiencies. It is essential for good compliance, as well as for promoting an overall healthy, balanced diet for long-term health (Haines *et al.*, 2008). Compliance to a gluten-free diet is improved by regular dietetic intervention (Pietzak, 2005; Wylie *et al.*, 2005), and patients prefer to see a dietitian for long-term follow-up, with a doctor available if needed (Bebb *et al.*, 2006). Serology markers cannot replace a trained dietitian's evaluation of adherence to the gluten-free diet (Leffler *et al.*, 2007b).

In addition, weight gain after diagnosis is common and may contribute to long-term morbidity (West *et al.*, 2004a). Patients may have additional medical conditions, such as diabetes, which also require dietetic input. It is important that dietitians work collaboratively with patients to ensure that the dietary advice meets their needs. This should be carried out on an ongoing basis, alongside the provision of patient-centred information, in order to improve healthcare outcomes and quality of life.

Diet-related problems

Poor compliance

Evaluating compliance is particularly important as the difficulties in following a gluten-free diet and the consequences of living with a long-term health condition should not be underestimated. A recent meta-analysis found that adherence to a gluten-free diet significantly improves (but does not normalise) health-related quality-of-life (HRQoL) outcomes for coeliac patients, and that better adherence results in higher HRQoL scores (Burger *et al.*, 2017). Many patients are tempted to deviate from dietary constraints in some circumstances, especially if there are no obvious penalties such as unpleasant symptoms. Compliance is particularly likely to be a problem in people found with silent coeliac disease where the benefits from gluten avoidance are even less obvious (Westman *et al.*, 1999). Studies indicate that compliance varies greatly in adults, with reported strict adherence rates ranging between 42 and 91% (Hall *et al.*, 2009).

The dietitian and other healthcare professionals should actively support the individual in developing behaviour management strategies, e.g. using behaviour change techniques (see Chapter 1.3, Changing health behaviour). Dietitians with skills in motivational interviewing can encourage behavioural change and help with dietary adherence (Stucky *et al.*, 2009).

The ubiquity of gluten in food may mean that some people inadvertently consume gluten, assuming a food to be gluten free or due to cross-contamination, e.g. eating gluten-free bread that has been sliced on the same board as gluten-containing bread, or eating foods cooked in oil previously used to cook a flour-coated product. These aspects should be explored during a dietetic consultation. Catassi *et al.* (2007) showed that changes in the height of the villous lining of the gut can occur at an intake of just 50 mg of gluten/day, thereby demonstrating the potential damage of inadvertent gluten exposure.

While dietitians should remind patients of the reasons for compliance with a gluten-free diet, it is important that they also help foster a positive dietary outlook by emphasising the many foods that can be eaten, by encouraging appropriate use of prescribable gluten-free foods (where available) and by suggesting ways in which particular difficulties can be overcome. Patients should also know where to obtain further advice on queries or problems, so that they feel they have a constant source of support.

Continuing symptoms

The most common cause of continuing symptoms or a poor response to the diet is inadvertent or deliberate gluten exposure (BSG, 2014). A troubleshooting approach in dietetic management of coeliac patients is needed when patients present with ongoing symptoms. A focused dietary history is essential for the elimination of all possible sources of gluten, including those from contamination. A further reason for poor response may be the development of a co-existing condition, including IBS, secondary lactose intolerance, pancreatic insufficiency, small bowel bacterial overgrowth, microscopic colitis or cow's milk protein sensitivity.

Refractory coeliac disease

Refractory coeliac disease is described as '*persistent or recurrent malabsorptive symptoms and signs with villous atrophy, despite a strict gluten-free diet for more than 12 months*' (Ludvigsson *et al.*, 2013). Patients with refractory coeliac disease should be referred to a specialist tertiary centre to optimise their management (BSG, 2014).

Codex wheat starch

Codex wheat starch (sometimes referred to as gluten-free wheat starch) is a highly processed specialised ingredient that improves the texture and taste of gluten-free foods, and has a trace level of gluten within the permitted Codex standard (<20 ppm). Products containing this are mainly obtained on prescription (Table 7.4.6). They are labelled as gluten free and are suitable for all people with coeliac disease. Patients with a concomitant wheat allergy or intolerance may be unable to tolerate Codex wheat starch products, and should be directed towards foods that are both gluten and wheat free.

Coexisting disorders requiring dietary intervention

The presence, or subsequent development, of other disorders, including type 1 diabetes or hyperlipidaemia, requires dietetic input. Weight-reducing or vegetarian diets also require individual dietetic consultation to ensure nutritional adequacy, especially with respect to calcium intake.

Constipation

The gluten-free diet may lead to a reduction in the intake of fibre due to reduced consumption of cereals, resulting in constipation. This may be alleviated by the following advice:

- Increasing fibre intake from fruit and vegetables, especially dried fruit, potato skins and pulses (peas, beans and lentils).

- Using higher-fibre varieties of prescribable gluten-free bread, mixes and crackers, and gluten-free muesli.
- Increasing consumption of wholegrain gluten-free cereals such as brown rice and buckwheat.
- Increasing fluid consumption.
- Increasing activity level.

Lactose intolerance
Newly diagnosed patients with coeliac disease may also suffer from secondary lactose intolerance as a result of gut inflammation, which results in a lactase deficiency. Lactase is found in the brush border of the small intestine. Symptoms of lactose intolerance are similar to some of the symptoms of coeliac disease, such as bloating, excess wind and diarrhoea. Once established on a gluten-free diet, the inflammation should subside and lactose digestion return to normal. Lactose intolerance is therefore usually temporary. However, it can take a couple of years for lactase production to return to normal. It is essential that, during this time, dietary advice be given to ensure adequate calcium intake from non-dairy sources (fortified gluten-free bread or rolls, soya milk or yoghurt).

Type 1 diabetes
Dietary management of the combined diseases requires professional guidance from a dietitian. The aim of dietary management is to improve blood glucose control as well as to support people with the gluten-free diet. Children with coeliac disease and type 1 diabetes mellitus should have their growth and development carefully monitored (see Chapter 3.8.12, Paediatric gastroenterology). Gluten-free alternatives to bread, pasta, biscuits and flour have approximately the same glycaemic index (GI) as their gluten-containing counterparts (Packer *et al.*, 2000). Hence, glycaemic control need not be compromised, and these alternative products can be incorporated into the diet in the same way as normal products. Patients should be encouraged to choose higher-fibre gluten-free foods where possible (see Chapter 7.12, Diabetes mellitus).

Dietary considerations in particular groups

For more information on weaning and celiac disease in children and teenagers, see Macdonald (2015).

Weaning

Previously, recommendations regarding the introduction of gluten encouraged the avoidance of early (<4 months) and late (7 or more months) gluten introduction, as well as the introduction of gluten while the infant was still being breastfed (Agostini *et al.*, 2008). However, more recently, two randomised controlled trials in children at genetic risk of this condition, examining the effect of age of gluten introduction on the risk of developing coeliac disease, have contradicted previous recommendations (Lionetti *et al.*, 2014; Vriezinga *et al.*, 2014). Furthermore, a systematic review evaluating evidence from prospective observational studies concluded that neither breast-feeding *per se* nor breast-feeding during time of gluten introduction reduces the risk of developing coeliac disease during childhood (Szajewska *et al.*, 2015). As a result of these new findings, ESPGHAN recently published an updated position paper concerning the introduction of gluten and the risk of coeliac disease (ESPGHAN, 2016), concluding with the following points:

- Gluten may be introduced anytime between 4 and 12 completed months of age.
- In children at high risk of coeliac disease, earlier introduction of gluten (4 *vs* 6 months or 6 *vs* 12 months) is associated with earlier development of coeliac autoimmunity (defined as positive serology) and coeliac disease, but the cumulative incidence of each in later childhood is similar.
- Based on observational data on the association between the amount of gluten intake and the risk of coeliac disease, consumption of large quantities of gluten should be avoided during the first weeks after gluten introduction and during infancy.
- The optimal amounts of gluten to be introduced at weaning are still to be identified.

It is important to remember that much of the evidence regarding the optimal time to introduce gluten in the diets of infants is derived from studies of those most at risk of developing this condition (i.e. those with a first-degree relative with the condition), rather than the general population. Exclusive breastfeeding from birth, until the introduction of solid foods, remains the optimal way to feed young infants. The BDA position paper (2013) on complementary feeding of infants recommends the introduction of solid food at around 6 months of age in accordance with DH guidance (see 3.8.2, Growth, nutritional assessment and nutritional assessment). The introduction of solid food should commence no later than 6 months (26 weeks) of age, but not before 4 months (17 weeks) (BDA, 2013). Complementary feeding is currently being reviewed by SACN.

Children

The British Society of Paediatric Gastroenterology, Hepatology and Nutrition (BSPGHAN), in collaboration with Coeliac UK, have produced guidelines regarding the diagnosis and management of children with coeliac disease (BSPGHAN & Coeliac UK, 2013). It is recommended that dietetic support be provided to children and their families within the first 1–2 weeks of diagnosis, with follow-up consultations offered at 3–6-month intervals within the first year, and annually thereafter. Factors to monitor closely include growth, symptom resolution, nutritional status and intake (particularly calcium and iron), and dietary adherence. Ongoing monitoring by an experienced paediatric dietitian and a paediatric gastroenterologist, or a paediatrician with a special interest in coeliac disease, is necessary to ensure long-term adherence.

Many families may require support to ensure that nurseries, schools and other care providers are fully informed and well equipped to help cater to the needs of their coeliac child. The provision of standard letters and simple fact sheets may be useful, in addition to ideas regarding suitable lunch-box foods and snacks to be eaten while away from home. Younger children may come in to contact with wheat flour from the use of homemade play dough commonly used in early years settings; recipes for gluten-free versions of play dough are widely available. Children's parties and play dates may be a further cause for concern, and families should be encouraged to discuss requirements with host parents in advance and offer to supply some suitable gluten-free foods for the occasion.

Teenagers

Adolescence is a period of significant emotional, social and physical development. The pressures of managing a long-term health condition, alongside those associated with a period of great change, present a significant challenge for teenagers with coeliac disease and their families. Only 50—65% teenagers with coeliac disease adhere to a gluten-free diets (Kumar *et al.*, 1988; Mayer *et al.*, 1991; Roma *et al.*, 2010). White *et al.* (2016) found that adolescents living with coeliac disease face stigmatisation and isolation in social situations. Factors associated with poor adherence in this group of patients included older age, an absence of immediate symptoms and difficulties in eating out with peers. Conversely, better emotional support and stronger organisation skills are associated with improved adherence. Teenagers should be reminded of the benefits of maintaining a gluten-free diet. Offering practical advice (e.g. a list of suitable foods/likely menu options that can be eaten outside of the home) and providing tips on how to prevent accidental or intentional gluten exposure (by carrying suitable snacks and researching suitable food outlets in advance) may also assist compliance. Parents should also consider that the appetites of teenagers, particularly boys, can be voracious, and that dietary indiscretions are more likely to occur when they are hungry; providing plenty of suitably filling gluten-free food options may help. Transition to adult services is obviously a critical period, and should be addressed in a timely and sympathetic manner to meet the needs of the young person.

Adults

The greatest difficulties usually arise when eating away from home, but can be averted to some extent by advance planning. At work, some canteens will, with notice, provide gluten-free meals, and others will be willing to microwave a preprepared meal supplied by the person with coeliac disease. Hotels and restaurants can be scoped in advance and, if necessary, sent information about the diet. Many airlines will provide gluten-free meals if sufficient notice is given. Nevertheless, carrying a supply of gluten-free rolls, crackers or similar foods is a wise precaution when travelling, on holiday or going to social functions, so that suitable foods are always available.

Pregnancy

There are no specific dietary guidelines for pregnant women with coeliac disease. Those who are diagnosed and adhering to a gluten-free diet prior to conception should follow the same advice as non-coeliac pregnant women (see Chapter 3.2, Preconception and pregnancy). A recent meta-analysis (Saccone *et al.*, 2016) concluded that women with coeliac disease (both treated and untreated) had a significantly higher risk of developing a number of pregnancy-associated complications, including pre-term birth and stillbirth, and of delivering low-birth-weight and small-for-gestational-age infants. Importantly, a 20% reduction in risk was observed among women with diagnosed and treated coeliac disease as compared with those with undiagnosed/untreated coeliac disease, thus highlighting the importance of strict dietary adherence during pregnancy.

Older people

Older patients are likely to find it particularly challenging to change long-term eating habits, but many will do so successfully if given sufficient help in making suitable dietary substitutions. Some will also welcome the feeling of improved health and energy levels while following a gluten-free diet, after perhaps years of having had undiagnosed coeliac disease. Gluten avoidance may be more difficult in those dependent on others for meals. Meals-on-wheels services may not provide gluten-free diets, although most will endeavour to provide suitable food choices (e.g. a piece of fruit instead of a starchy pudding) once they understand the nature of the diet. Since the prevalence of coeliac disease among elderly people is increasing, it is particularly important to educate residential and care homes regarding the needs of coeliac patients.

Acknowledgement

The editor acknowledges the prior contribution of Helen Fraser-Mayall.

Further reading

Coxon K. (2013) *Coeliac Disease – the Essential Guide* Need2Know: Peterborough.

Gazzola A. (2015) *Coeliac Disease. What You Need to Know (Revised)*. London: Sheldon Press.

Internet resources

British Society of Gastroenterology, www.bsg.org.uk

British Society of Paediatric Gastroenterology, Hepatology and Nutrition (BSPGHAN), www.bspghan.org.uk

Coeliac Society of Ireland, www.coeliac.ie

Coeliac UK, www.coeliac.org.uk

European Society for Paediatric Gastroenterology, Hepatology and Nutrition (ESPGHAN), www.espghan.org

Free from food manufacturers

Several of the larger specialist producers will send welcome packs or samples, as well as provide information and advice on coeliac disease and gluten-free diets, to both consumers and health professionals, including the following:

Genius Gluten Free, www.geniusglutenfree.com
Glutafin Gluten Free, www.glutafin.co.uk
Juvela, www.juvela.co.uk
Newburn Bakehouse by Warburtons, www.newburnbakehouse.com
Schär, www.schaer.com

References

Agostoni C, Decsi T, Fewtrell M, *et al.* (2008) Complementary Feeding: A Commentary by the ESPGHAN Committee on Nutrition. *J. Pedi. Gastro. Nutr.* 46(1): 99–110.

Askling J, Linet M, Gridley G, *et al.* (2002) Cancer incidence in a population-based cohort of individuals hospitalised with coeliac disease or dermatitis herpetiformis. *Gastroenterology.* 123(5): 1428–1435.

Bai J, Gonzalez D, Mautalen C, *et al.* (1997) Long-term effect of gluten restriction on bone mineral density of patients with coeliac disease. *Aliment. Pharmacol. Ther.* 11(1): 157–164.

BDA. (2013) *Complementary Feeding: Introduction of Solid Food to an Infant's Diet.* Available at www.bda.uk.com/policies/WeaningPolicyStatement.pdf. Accessed 22 November 2016.

BDA. (2015, September) *Gluten Free Food on Prescription.* Available at www.bda.uk.com/news/view?id=106. Accessed 22 November 2016.

Bebb JR, Lawson A, Knight T, *et al.* (2006) Long-term follow up of coeliac disease – what do coeliac patients want? *Aliment. Pharmacol. Ther.* 23: 827–831.

British Society of Gastroenterology (BSG). (2014) *Diagnosis and Management of Adult Coeliac Disease: Guidelines from the BSG.* Available at www.bsg.org.uk. Accessed 22 November 2016.

Burden M, Mooney P, Blanshard R, *et al.* (2015) Cost and availability of gluten-free food in the UK: in store and online. *Postgrad. Med. J.* 91(1081): 622–626.

Burger J, de Brouwer B, IntHout J, *et al.* (2017) Systematic review with meta-analysis: Dietary adherence influences normalization of health-related quality of life in coeliac disease. *Clin. Nutr.* 36: 39–406. doi: 10.1016/j.clnu.2016.04.021.

Caproni M, Antiga E, Melani L, *et al.* (2009) Guidelines for the diagnosis and treatment of dermatitis herpetiformis. *J. Eur. Acad. Dermatol. Venereol.* 23: 633–638.

Card TR, Siffledeen J, West J, *et al.* (2013) An excess of prior irritable bowel syndrome diagnoses or treatments in Celiac disease: evidence of diagnostic delay. *Scand. J. Gastroenterol.* 48(7): 801–807.

Carr L. (2011) Prescribing of gluten free specialist foods. Coeliac UK's Position. *Dietetics Today* 37: 8–9.

Catassi C, Bearzi I, Holmes G. (2005) Association of celiac disease and intestinal lymphomas and other cancers. *Gastroenterology.* 128: S79–S86.

Catassi C, Fabiani E, Iacono G, *et al.* (2007) A prospective, double blind, placebo-controlled trial to establish a safe gluten threshold for patients with coeliac disease. *Am. J. Clin. Nutr.* 85: 160–166.

Catassi C, Kryszak D, Bhatti B, *et al.* (2010) Natural history of celiac disease autoimmunity in a USA cohort followed since 1974. *Ann. Med.* 42(7): 530–538.

Ch'ng CL, Biswas M, Benton A, *et al.* (2005) Prospective screening for coeliac disease in patients with Graves' hyperthyroidism using anti-gliadin and tissue transglutaminase antibodies. *Clin. Endocrinol. (Oxf).* 62(3): 303–306.

Ciacci C, Maurelli L, Klain M, *et al.* (1997) Effects of dietary treatment on bone mineral density in adults with celiac disease: factors predicting response. *Am. J. Gastroenterol.* 92(6): 992–996.

Ciccocioppo R, Di Sabatino A, Corazza GR. (2005) The immune recognition of gluten in coeliac disease. *Clin. Exp. Immunol.* 140(3): 408–41Coeliac UK. (Unpublished data) *Unpublished Statistics Relating to Delayed Diagnosis.* Available at www.coeliac.org.uk/coeliac-disease/myths-about-coeliac-disease. Last accessed 22 November 2016.

Coeliac UK, BDA, BSPGHAN and Primary Care Society for Gastroenterology (PCSG) (2011, updated 2012) Gluten-free foods: a revised prescribing guide. https://www.coeliac.org.uk/document-library/378-gluten-free-foods-a-revised-prescribing-guide/?return=/healthcare-professionals/resources/guidance-documents/. Accessed 25 October 2018.

Comino I, Fernández-Bañares F, Esteve M, *et al.* (2016) Fecal gluten peptides reveal limitations of serological tests and food questionnaires for monitoring gluten-free diet in celiac disease patients. *Am. J. Gastroenterol.* 111(10): 1456–1465.

Corazza GR, Di Stefano M, Maurino E, *et al.* (2005) Bones in coeliac disease: diagnosis and treatment. *Best. Pract. Res. Clin. Gastroenterol.* 19(3): 453–465.

DH. (1991) *Dietary Reference Values for Food Energy and Nutrients for the United Kingdom.* London: TSO.

DH. (2017) *Consultation on the Availability of Gluten Free Foods on NHS Prescription.* Available at www.gov.uk/government/consultations/availability-of-gluten-free-foods-on-nhs-prescription. Last accessed 15 December 2017.

EC. (2009) *Regulation No. 41/2009 Concerning the Composition and Labelling of Foodstuffs Suitable for People Intolerant to Gluten.* Available at http://data.europa.eu/eli/reg/2009/41/oj. Last accessed 22 November 2016.

EU. (2011) *Regulation No. 1169/2011 on the Provision of Food Information to Consumers.* Available at http://data.europa.eu/eli/reg/2011/1169/oj. Last accessed 22 November 2016.

European Society Paediatric Gastroenterology Hepatology and Nutrition (ESPGHAN). (2012) *Guidelines for the Diagnosis of Coeliac Disease.* Available at https://www.coeliac.ie/wp-content/uploads/2015/05/European_Society_for_Pediatric_Gastroenterology_.28.pdf. Accessed 22 November 2016.

European Society Paediatric Gastroenterology Hepatology and Nutrition (ESPGHAN). (2016) *Gluten Introduction and the Risk of Coeliac Disease: A Position Paper by the European Society for Pediatric Gastroenterology, Hepatology, and Nutrition.* Available at http://espghan.org/fileadmin/user_upload/guidelines_pdf/Hep_Nutr/Gluten_Introduction_and_the_Risk_of_Coeliac.32.pdf Accessed 22 November 2016.

Fasano A. (2005) Clinical presentation of coeliac disease in the paediatric population. *Gastroenterology.* 128: S68–S73.

Fry L, Seah P, Harper P, *et al.* (1974) The small intestine in dermatitis herpetiformis. *J. Clin. Pathol.* 27(10): 817–824.

Garsed K, Scott B. (2007) Can oats be taken in a gluten-free diet? A systematic review. *Scand. J. Gastroenterol.* 42: 171–178.

Greco L, Romino R, Coto I, *et al.* (2002) The first large population based twin study of coeliac disease. *Gut.* 50: 624–628.

Gutierrez-Achury J, Romanos J, Bakker S, *et al.* (2015) Contrasting the Genetic Background of Type 1 Diabetes and Celiac Disease Autoimmunity. *Diabetes Care.* 38(2): S37–44.

Haboubi NY, Taylor S, Jones S. (2006) Coeliac disease and oats: a systematic review. *Postgrad. Med. J.* 82: 672–678.

Haines M, Anderson R, Gibson P. (2008) Systematic review: the evidence base for long-term management of coeliac disease. *Aliment. Pharmacol. Ther.* 28(9): 1042–1066.

Hall N. (2013) Intentional and inadvertent nonadherence in adult coeliac disease. *A cross-sectional survey. Appetite.* 68: 56–62.

Hall NJ, Rubin G, Charnock A. (2009) Systematic review: adherence to a gluten-free diet in adult patients with coeliac disease. *Aliment. Pharmacol. Ther.* 30: 315–330.

Heikkila K, Pearce J, Maki M, *et al.* (2015) Coeliac disease and bone fractures: a systematic review and meta-analysis. *J. Clin. Endocrinol. Metab.* 100(1): 25–34.

Henderson L, Gregory J, Swan G. (2003) *The National Diet and Nutrition Survey 2002.* TSO: London.

Hervonen K, Viljamaa M, Collin P, *et al.* (2004) The occurrence of type 1 diabetes in patients with dermatitis herpetiformis and their first-degree relatives. *Br. J. Dermatol.* 150(1): 136–138.

Hervonen K, Vornanen M, Kautiainen H, *et al.* (2005) Lymphoma in patients with dermatitis herpetiformis and their first-degree relatives. *Br. J. Dermatol.* 152(1): 82–86.

Hin H, Bird G, Fisher P, *et al.* (1999) Coeliac disease in primary care: case finding study. *BMJ.* 318: 164–167.

Hogberg L, Faith-Magnusson K, Grodzinsky E, *et al.* (2003) Familial prevalence of coeliac disease: a twenty year follow-up study. *Scand. J. Gastroenterol.* 38(1): 61–65.

Holmes GKT, Prior P, Lane MR, *et al.* (1989) Malignancy in coeliac disease – effect of a gluten free diet. *Gut.* 30: 333–338.

Howdle PD, Jalal PK, Holmes GK, *et al.* (2003) Primary small-bowel malignancy in the UK and its association with coeliac disease. *QJM.* 96: 345–353.

Irvine A, Chey W, Ford A. (2017) Screening for celiac disease in irritable bowel syndrome: an updated systematic review and meta-analysis. *Am. J. Gastroenterol.* 112(1): 65–76. doi: 10.1038/ajg.2016.466. [Epub ahead of print]

Joint BSPGHAN and Coeliac UK. (2013) *Guidelines for the Diagnosis and Management of Coeliac Disease in Children.* Available at www.bspghan.org.uk. Accessed 22 November 2016.

Kane E, Newton R, Roman E. (2011) Non-Hodgkin lymphoma and gluten-sensitive enteropathy: estimate of risk using meta-analyses. *Cancer Causes Control.* 22(10): 1435–1444.

Kumar PJ, Walker-Smith J, Milla P, *et al.* (1988) The teenage celiac: follow up study of 102 patients. *Arch. Dis. Child.* 63: 916–920.

Lebwohl B, Ludvigsson J, Green P. (2014) The unfolding story of celiac disease risk factors. *Clin. Gastroenterol. Hepatol.* 12(4): 632–635.

Leffler D, Dennis M, Hyett B, *et al.* (2007a) Etiologies and predictors of diagnosis in nonresponsive celiac disease. *Clin. Gastroenterol. Hepatol.* 5(4): 445–450.

Leffler D, Edwards George JB, Dennis M, *et al.* (2007b) A prospective comparative study of five measures of gluten-free diet adherence in adults with CD. *Aliment. Pharmacol. Ther.* 26: 1227–1235.

Lenhardt A, Plebani A, Marchetti F. (2004) Role of human-tissue transglutaminase IgG and anti-gliadin IgG antibodies in the diagnosis of coeliac disease in patients with selective immunoglobulin A deficiency. *Dig. Liver Dis.* 36(11): 730–734.

Lionetti E, Castellaneta S, Francavilla R, *et al.* (2014) Introduction of gluten, HLA status, and the risk of celiac disease in children. *N. Engl. J. Med.* 371: 1295–1303.

Lohi S, Mustalahti K, Kaukinen K, *et al.* (2007) Increasing prevalence of coeliac disease over time. *Aliment. Pharmacol. Ther.* 26(9): 1217–1225.

Ludvigsson JF, Leffler DA, Bai JC, *et al.* (2013) The Oslo definitions for coeliac disease and related terms. *Gut.* 62(1): 43–52.

MacColloch K, Rashid M. (2014) Factors affecting adherence to the gluten free diet in children with coeliac disease. *Paediatr. Child Health* 19(6): 304–305.

Macdonald S. (2015) Gastroenterology In Clinical paediatric dietetics 4th Ed Shaw V (Ed) Oxford: WIley Blackwell.

Mahmud F, De Melo E, Noordin K, *et al.* (2015) The Celiac Disease and Diabetes-Dietary Intervention and Evaluation Trial (CD-DIET) protocol: a randomised controlled study to evaluate treatment of asymptomatic coeliac disease in type 1 diabetes. *BMJ Open.* 5(5): e008097. doi: 10.1136/bmjopen-2015-008097.

Marsh MN. (1992) Gluten, major histocompatibility complex, and the small intestine. A molecular and immunobiologic approach to the spectrum of gluten sensitivity ('celiac sprue'). *Gastroenterology.* 102: 330–354.

Mayer M, Greco L, Troncone R, *et al.* (1991) Compliance of adolescents with coeliac disease on a gluten free diet. *Gut.* 32: 881–885.

Midhagen G, Aberg AK, Olcen P, *et al.* (2004) Antibody levels in adult patients with coeliac disease during gluten-free diet: a rapid initial decrease of clinical importance. *J. Intern. Med.* 256: 519–524.

Morris MA, Yiannakou JY, King AL, *et al.* (2000) Coeliac disease and Down syndrome: associations not due to genetic linkage on chromosome 21. *Scand. J. Gastroenterol.* 35(2): 177–180.

Muhammad H, Reeves S, Ishaq S, *et al.* (2017) Adherence to a gluten free diet is associated with receiving gluten free food on prescription and understanding food labelling. *Nutrients.* 9(7): E705.

NICE (2017) *Irritable Bowel Syndrome in Adults: Diagnosis and Management. Clinical Guideline (CG61).* Available at https://www.nice.org.uk/Guidance/CG61. Accessed 25 October 2018.

NICE (2015) *Coeliac Disease: Recognition, Assessment & Management of Coeliac Disease. Guideline NG20.* Available at https://www.nice.org.uk/guidance/ng20. Accessed 25 October 2018.

NICE (2016) *Coeliac Disease Quality Standard QS134.* Available at https://www.nice.org.uk/guidance/qs134. Accessed 25 October 2018.

Packer SC, Dornhurst A, Frost GS. (2000) The glycaemic index of a range of gluten-free foods. *Diabet. Med.* 17(9): 657–660.

PHE. (2014) *National Diet and Nutrition Survey: Headline Results from Years 1, 2, 3 and 4 (combined) of the Rolling Programme 2008/9–2011/12.*

Pietzak MM. (2005) Follow-up of patients with celiac disease: achieving compliance with treatment. *Gastroenterology.* 128: S135–S141.

Reunala T, Collin P. (1997) Diseases associated with dermatitis herpetiformis. *Br. J. Dermatol.* 136(3): 315–318.

Roma E, Roubani A, Kolia E, *et al.* (2010) Dietary compliance and life style of children with coeliac disease. *J. Hum. Nutr. Diet.* 23(2): 176–182.

Saadah OI, Zacharin M, O'Callaghan A, *et al.* (2004) Effect of gluten-free diet and adherence on growth and diabetic control in diabetics with coeliac disease. *Arch. Dis. Child.* 89: 871–876.

Saccone G, Berghella V, Sarno L, *et al.* (2016) Celiac disease and obstetric complications: a systematic review and meta-analysis. *Am. J. Obstet. Gynaecol.* 214(2): 225–234.

Sainsbury A, Sanders DS, Ford AC. (2013) Prevalence of irritable bowel syndrome-type symptoms in patients with celiac disease: a meta-analysis. *Clin. Gastroenterol. Hepatol.* 11(4): 359–365.

Sanders D, Hurlstone D, Stokes R, *et al.* (2002) Changing face of adult coeliac disease: experience of a single university hospital in South Yorkshire. *Postgrad. Med. J.* 78(915): 31–33.

Scottish Government. (2015) Review of the Gluten-free Food Additional Pharmaceutical Service. Available at www.gov.scot/Publications/2015/09/5884. Last accessed 22 November 2016.

Shaw V. (2015) *Clinical Paediatric Dietetics*, 4th edn. Chichester: Wiley.

Singh J, Whelan K. (2011) Limited availability and higher cost of gluten free foods. *J. Hum. Nutr. Diet.* 24: 479–486.

Stucky C, Lowdon J, Howdle P. (2009) Joint BAPEN and British Society of Gastroenterology Symposium on 'Coeliac disease: basics and controversies'. *Dietitians are better than clinicians in following up coeliac disease. Proc. Nutr. Soc.* 68: 249–251.

Szajewska H, Shamir R, Chmielewska A, *et al.* (2015) Systematic review with meta-analysis: early infant feeding and coeliac disease – update 2015. *Aliment. Pharmacol. Ther.* 41: 1038–1054.

Trott N. (2016) *Dietitian led group coeliac clinics in comparison to dietetic standard care in newly diagnosed patients.* Available at www.coeliac.org.uk/campaigns-and-research/our-research-conference/research-conference-2016/day-2-diagnosis-and-management-of-coeliac-disease-time-for/group-dietetic-clinics-vs-individual-appointments/. Accessed 21 January 2017.

Tucker E, Rostami K, Prabhakaran S, *et al.* (2012) Patients with coeliac disease are increasingly overweight or obese on presentation. *J. Gastrointestin. Liver Dis.* 21(1): 11–15.

Tuire I, Marja-Leena L, Teea S, *et al.* (2012) Persistent duodenal intraepithelial lymphocytosis despite a long-term strict gluten-free diet in celiac disease. *Am. J. Gastroenterol.* 107: 1563–1569.

Valdimarsson T, Löfman O, Toss G, *et al.* (1996) Reversal of osteopenia with diet in adult coeliac disease. *Gut.* 38(3): 322–327.

Valentino R, Savastano S, Tommaselli AP. (2002) Markers of potential coeliac disease in patients with Hashimoto's thyroiditis. *Eur. J. Endocrinol.* 146: 479–483.

Vriezinga SL, Auricchio R, Bravi E, *et al.* (2014) Randomized feeding intervention in infants at high risk for celiac disease. *N. Engl. J. Med.* 371: 1304–1315.

Walters JR. (1994) Bone mineral density in coeliac disease. *Gut.* 35(2): 150–151.

West J, Fleming K, Tata L, *et al.* (2014) Incidence and prevalence of celiac disease and dermatitis herpetiformis in the UK over two decades: population-based study. *Am. J. Gastroenterol.* 109(5): 757–768.

West J, Logan R, Smith C, *et al.* (2004a) Malignancy and mortality in people with coeliac disease: population-based cohort study. *BMJ.* 329: 716–719.

West J, Logan RFA, Card TR, *et al.* (2004b) Risk of vascular disease in adults with diagnosed coeliac disease: a population-based study. *Aliment. Pharmacol. Ther.* 20: 1–7.

Westman E, Ambler GR, Royle M, *et al.* (1999) Children with coeliac disease and insulin-dependent diabetes mellitus – growth, diabetes control and dietary intake. *J. Pediatr. Endocrinol. Metab.* 12: 433–442.

White LE, Merrick V, Bannerman E, *et al.* (2013) The rising incidence of celiac disease in Scotland. *Pediatrics.* 132(4): e924–931.

White LE, Bannerman E, Gillett PM. (2016) Coeliac disease and the gluten-free diet: a review of the burdens; factors associated with adherence and impact on health-related quality of life, with specific focus on adolescence. *J. Hum. Nutr. Diet.* 29(5): 593–606.

Wylie C, Geldart S, Winwood P. (2005) Dietitian-led coeliac clinic: a successful change in working practice in modern healthcare. *Gastroenterol. Today* 15(1): 11–12.

7.4.8 Inflammatory bowel disease

Katie Keetarut

Key points

- Malnutrition is common in inflammatory bowel disease; good nutrition is crucial for optimal clinical outcome.
- Exclusive enteral nutrition using elemental, peptide or polymeric feeds are commonly used to induce remission in children and adolescents and should be offered as a treatment option in adults.
- Limited evidence suggests a role for partial enteral nutrition in disease maintenance as adjunctive treatment to optimise medical therapies, and prevent postoperative recurrence or as nutritional support.
- Appropriate dietetic support is required to ensure patients maintain optimal nutritional status.

Crohn's disease (CD) and ulcerative colitis (UC) are the main types of inflammatory bowel diseases (IBDs), with a rarer type unclassified IBD-U accounting for approximately 10% of all cases (Silverberg *et al.*, 2005). Although these are distinct disorders with differences in presentation and management, they share several common features. IBD is a progressive disease driven by mucosal inflammation that follows a relapsing and remitting disease course, which can significantly impair quality of life (Bernklev *et al.*, 2005; Pariente *et al.*, 2011). The lifetime medical costs associated with the care of a person with IBD can be comparable to other major chronic diseases such as diabetes mellitus or cancer (IBD Standards, 2013). Nutrition therapy is pivotal in IBD, whether as a primary treatment or in a supportive role.

Both UC and CD have a peak incidence between the ages of 20 and 40 years (Marshall & Hilsden, 2003). Approximately 25% of all cases are diagnosed in childhood, and the disease is often more severe than if presenting in adulthood, with major consequences on lifelong morbidity (Van Limbergen *et al.*, 2008). In 1995, the prevalence of IBD was estimated at approximately 387 per 100,000 people (243 per 100,000 UC and 144 per 100,000 CD) (Rubin *et al.*, 2000). Differences in the rates of IBD also exist, such that the prevalence of CD is increasing faster than that of UC (Rubin *et al.*, 2000). There is a south–north gradient to the incidence of IBD in the UK, with rates being highest in Scotland. Compared with the non-Jewish Caucasian population, IBD occurs more frequently in Ashkenazi Jews and at about the same level in families originating from Africa or the Caribbean. For second-generation Indian and Pakistani families, the incidence of CD is about the same, but is higher for UC (Silverberg *et al.*, 2005).

Causation and risk factors

The cause of IBD remains unknown, yet is likely multifactorial, involving a combination of genetic and environmental triggers. Much research is focused on understanding the role of bacteria in the gut and the many different parts of the immune system's response to external triggers (Xavier & Podalsky, 2007).

Genetic factors

A genetic predisposition increases the risk of IBD about tenfold in first-degree relatives of an IBD patient. There have been over 160 genes identified that play a role in the initiation or perpetuation of IBD, which may determine the pattern and severity of the disease in any individual patient. However, only 25% of genes are thought to be

IBD risk contributors, suggesting that the rise in the incidence of CD over the last 50 years cannot be attributed to genetic factors alone (Abraham & Cho, 2009; Xavier & Podalsky, 2007).

Environmental factors

The incidence of IBD in previously low-incidence countries such as Japan has increased three to fivefold in the last decade, creating a strong interest in the transition to more Westernised eating patterns (Ahuja & Tandon, 2010; Orholm *et al.*, 1991). Fast food consumption confers a three to fourfold increased risk of CD (Persson *et al.*, 1992). Refined sugars and fats have been linked to IBD risk (Amre *et al.*, 2007). Saccharin and sucralose have also been linked to the rise of IBD, potentially due to damage to the gut barrier (Qin, 2012). Fruit, vegetables and fibre have been found to be protective against CD development in children (Reif *et al.*, 1997). Animal studies have shown that milk fat, commonly used in processed foods and confectionary, induces gut inflammation (Devkota *et al.*, 2012), and that certain emulsifiers (Polysorbate 80 and E466) increase intestinal permeability and causes increased gut bacterial translocation (Roberts *et al.*, 2013).

The European Prospective Investigation into Cancer and Nutrition study found that a high intake of n-6 linoleic acid increased the risk of developing UC by 30%, whereas a high intake of n-3 fatty acids was associated with a 77% reduced risk (Hart, 2009). Smoking is consistently documented in association with IBD. Smokers are more likely to develop CD, have a poorer prognosis and have significantly higher chances of surgical resection, with postoperative recurrence at the anastomosis site (Mahid *et al.*, 2006; Mowat *et al.*, 2011). Smoking cessation is associated with a 65% reduction in the risk of a relapse in CD (Johnson *et al.*, 2005). In contrast, smoking decreases the risk of developing UC (Mahid *et al.*, 2006).

Clinical features and symptoms

The main presenting symptoms of IBD are:

- Abdominal pain.
- Diarrhoea, sometimes with blood and mucus in the stool.
- Urgency and tenesmus (the constant sensation of needing to pass stool accompanied by cramping and straining).
- Weight loss.
- Fatigue.

Inflammation can occur in other areas of the body, including the joints, skin, liver or eyes, and are known as extra-intestinal manifestations, affecting 25–30% of IBD patients (Orchard *et al.*, 2011). CD can affect any part of the gastrointestinal tract from the mouth to the anus, but most commonly affects the terminal ileum, with the rectum often spared. It is characterised by distinct areas of inflammation, often associated with granulomas and deep fissuring ulceration, interspersed with areas of unaffected bowel tissue (Orchard *et al.*, 2011).

The disease often progresses with each flare-up and features stricturing and penetrating lesions (Pariente *et al.*, 2011). Strictures are characterised by localised, persistent narrowing of the bowel wall and can be inflammatory or fibrotic in nature, potentially leading to obstruction (Silverberg *et al.*, 2005). Penetrating lesions (fistulae) are where the disease creates holes in the bowel wall that can allow faecal content to leak out (Pariente *et al.*, 2011). UC affects the large bowel only and usually starts in the rectum and extends up the colon to varying degrees. It is characterised by an area of continuously inflamed mucosa that bleeds readily (Orchard *et al.*, 2011).

Diagnosis criteria

Diagnosis is usually confirmed by a combination of clinical, haematological, endoscopic, histological and imaging-based investigations. Laboratory investigations should include a full blood count, urea and electrolytes, liver function tests, erythrocyte sedimentation rate and C-reactive protein (Dignass *et al.*, 2010, 2012; Mowat *et al.*, 2011). The most common test used to diagnose IBD is a colonoscopy with multiple biopsies. Imaging is often used to support the diagnosis and assess disease extent. Faecal calprotectin levels are commonly used to detect colonic inflammation and to distinguish between functional and active disease (NICE, 2013).

Several disease activity indices are available to quantify disease activity and can be useful in combination with other clinical measures. The Harvey Bradshaw Index (HBI) (Harvey & Bradshaw, 1980) is a validated simplified version of the Crohn's Disease Activity Index (CDAI) (Best *et al.*, 1976). The CDAI is often used in clinical trials, but it is more complex and time consuming than the HBI, and, as the results of both tools correlate well, the HBI is more often used in clinical practice (Vermeire *et al.*, 2010). The HBI is based on scoring for five items namely general well-being, abdominal pain, number of stools per day, presence of an abdominal mass and other complications. A score of ≤3 indicates disease remission and >6 indicates active disease. The Simple Clinical Colitis Activity Index (SCCAI) is used in UC (Walmsley *et al.*, 1998) and is based on six items, including 24-hour bowel frequency, blood in the stool, general well-being and extracolonic features. A score of <2.5 defines remission, and a score of 5 or more defines relapse (Higgins *et al.*, 2005).

Management

Drug therapy in IBD is a rapidly evolving field, and, due to the complexity of the disease, each patient may follow a different treatment course (see Table 7.4.7).

Surgery

Between 50 and 70% of patients with CD will undergo surgery within 5 years of diagnosis. The lifetime surgery rates in UC are about 20–30%. In patients with chronic

Table 7.4.7 Main IBD drug and indications

Drug type	Names	Indication	Drug–nutrient interaction
Antibiotics	Metronidazole Ciprofloxacin	Control infection Reduce postoperative recurrence (Shen *et al.*, 2001). Treat abscess or bacterial overgrowth (Castiglione *et al.*, 2003).	Limited interactions but can cause diarrhoea and nausea
Immunomodulators	Thiopurines (Azathioprine/6-Mercaptopurine) Methotrexate	Maintain remission in IBD and can be used in combination with anti-TNF therapy to increase efficacy	Can suppress normal bone marrow function, causing anaemia Methotrexate can cause folic acid deficiency, leading to anaemia (Wang *et al.*, 2015).
Biological therapies (anti-TNFα agents)	(Infliximab, Adalimumab)	Induction and maintenance of remission in peri-anal CD and refractory IBD and as salvage therapy in acute severe UC. Newer biologic agents include Vedolizumab, which is used for induction and maintenance therapy in refractory IBD.	
5-Aminosalicylic acid (5-ASA)	Sulfasalazine/ Mesalamine	Used for induction and maintenance of remission in UC. The main types are Pentasa, Asacol, and Mezavant XL. These work mainly in the terminal ileum and colon.	Folic acid antagonist. Long-term use can cause megaloblastic anaemia Folate deficiency is also associated with hyper-homocysteinaemia, which increases the risk of thromboembolic disease in IBD (Chande *et al.*, 2015)
Corticosteroids	Prednisolone Budesonide	Induce remission in both UC and CD Thirty percent of patients will fail to respond to corticosteroids or are intolerant of them. These patients may then be considered for anti-TNFα therapies or surgery. Causes fewer side effects as not absorbed systemically. Its uses limited to the terminal ileum and colon.	Prolonged use may cause growth retardation in children, muscle wasting, diabetes, peptic ulcer, osteoporosis, and liver and renal damage.

relapsing UC, about 50% will need a colectomy, although rates vary between countries and regions (Oresland, 2006; Roberts *et al.*, 2007).

The most common forms of surgery for CD are removal of part of the small bowel, with or without partial or total removal of the colon and/or rectum (proctocolectomy) and formation of a stoma, which may be permanent. For people with UC, a restorative panproctocolectomy is curative and involves removal of the entire colon and rectum, combined with the fashioning of an ileo-anal pouch made from the terminal ileum and joined to the anus to form a reservoir. This replaces the rectum, thus avoiding the need for a permanent ileostomy (Orchard *et al.*, 2011; Parks & Nicholls, 1978). Corticosteroids are the biggest risk factor in postoperative complications (Dignass *et al.*, 2010).

Dietary management

The aims of dietary management in IBD are to:

- Achieve and maintain good nutritional status during active disease and remission.
- Help alleviate clinical symptoms in combination with medical and/or surgical treatment.
- Help treat clinical complications in combination with medical treatment.
- Induce remission in CD patients when enteral nutrition is used as a primary treatment.

Malnutrition is present in up to 85% of patients with IBD; and weight loss occurs in up to 80% of patients with CD and 18–62% of patients with UC (Gassull & Cabre, 2001; Geerling *et al.*, 1999). However, the rising obesity epidemic may mask current rates of malnutrition in IBD (Flores *et al.*, 2015). The cause of malnutrition is multifactorial, including: cytokine-induced anorexia in active disease, protein losses from the inflamed bowel, malabsorption of nutrients (Yakut *et al.*, 2010), drug–nutrient interactions (Hwang *et al.*, 2012) and an increased resting energy expenditure (Gassull & Cabre, 2001). Growth retardation has been reported in up to 40% of children and adolescents; up to 60% have decreased muscle and body fat stores (Lochs *et al.*, 2006). Nutritional status should be assessed at regular intervals, and the growth of children and young people closely monitored.

Patients report that access to a dietitian is vital (Prince *et al.*, 2016). The IBD standards (2013) recommend that all patients should have dietetic access, be weighed and their nutritional needs assessed. A high proportion of IBD patients attribute diet as a trigger in both disease causation and flare-up (Limdi *et al.*, 2016). Patients should be encouraged to follow as normal a diet as possible for their clinical state. During active disease, appetite can be poor, and patients may benefit from eating small, frequent meals of high energy and nutrient density. Food fortification strategies or supplements may be necessary (see Chapter 6.3, Oral nutrition support). The importance of adequate fluid intake in the presence of diarrhoea, pyrexia or fistulae should be stressed.

Nutritional considerations

Specific vitamin and mineral deficiencies are common in IBD, including iron, zinc, copper, beta-carotene, folate, and vitamins B_{12}, B_6, E, C and D. These persist in remission, do not always correlate with inadequate dietary intake, and present in healthy and overweight patients. Routine multivitamin supplementation in IBD patients is recommended (Filippi *et al.*, 2006; Vagianos *et al.*, 2007; Yakut *et al.*, 2010). In cases where diarrhoea is prolonged, bloody or severe, poor absorption of nutrients including potassium, sodium, zinc, magnesium and iron can occur, leading to anaemia, dehydration, severe weight loss and nutritional depletion. Nutritional deficiencies in energy and protein can occur due to the catabolic effects of chronic inflammation, increasing nitrogen losses, poor appetite and drug side effects. Ileal resection or small intestinal bacterial overgrowth in CD can cause B_{12} deficiency and lactase deficiency.

There is evidence that IBD patients avoid dairy products more often than necessary, and it is less likely to be associated with UC (Banos-Madrid *et al.*, 2004; Ginard *et al.*, 2003). Consideration of calcium intake may need to be addressed when dairy foods are limited (see Chapter 7.9.1, Osteoporosis). Vitamin D deficiency is common in IBD patients and is associated with worsened disease severity. Appropriate monitoring and treatment of low levels is an important part of IBD management. Whether vitamin D deficiency preceded the severe outcomes, or if poor disease control resulted in reduced physical activity, food intake (particularly of foods containing vitamin D, e.g. dairy foods) or sunlight exposure, leading to low vitamin D levels, is unclear (Kabbani *et al.*, 2016). Osteoporosis is common in IBD (Tilg *et al.*, 2007), and is likely due to a combination of inflammatory activity, leading to poor nutrient intake or malabsorption and medication use. Recent studies suggest that CD acts as a small independent risk factor for low bone mineral density, whereas UC does not (Targownik *et al.*, 2014). The daily recommendation for calcium intake in patients with IBD is 1000 mg (Lewis & Scott, 2007), and ideally should be obtained from dietary sources (Reid, 2014).

Iron deficiency is the primary cause of anaemia in IBD, resulting from dietary restrictions, intestinal bleeding loss, malabsorption due to inflammation or ulceration, and under-treatment (Filmann *et al.*, 2014). Functional bowel symptoms are reported in 33% of UC and 57% of CD patients and, in longstanding remission, are two to three times higher than in the normal population (Simren *et al.*, 2002). They have been reported to be more problematic than symptoms due to inflammation (Camilleri, 2011). Some IBD patients may need to avoid specific foods that appear to exacerbate symptoms, but unnecessary food avoidance should be discouraged. The low FODMAP diet has been shown to help alleviate functional symptoms in IBD, including abdominal pain, bloating, wind and diarrhoea (Gearry *et al.*, 2008), with up to 78% of patients reporting adequate relief of symptoms when followed for a minimum of 6 weeks (Prince *et al.*, 2016).

Specific aspects of dietary management of CD

People with CD are at particular risk of nutritional deficiencies due to:

- High prevalence in children and young adults with high energy requirements.
- Increased risk of nutrient malabsorption due to small bowel resections and inflammation.
- Repeated surgery to treat complications such as strictures or fistulae.

Restoring and maintaining good nutritional status is a treatment priority at all stages of the disease. Many patients will avoid irritant foods, including greasy or spicy foods and caffeinated drinks, in an attempt to minimise symptoms. However, the nutritional impact of any food restrictions imposed by patients needs to be carefully explored. Fat malabsorption may worsen symptoms, necessitating fat restriction to tolerance levels, but care must be taken to avoid compromising energy intake. Substitution of some long-chain triglycerides with medium-chain triglycerides, or dietary fortification with carbohydrate polymers, may be necessary. Additional fat-soluble vitamins and a daily multivitamin supplement may be required if food intake remains inadequate or malabsorption is pronounced.

In specific circumstances, parenteral nutrition (PN) is indicated, such as when the absorptive capacity of the gut is reduced in short bowel syndrome, or in the perioperative care of patients with significant (>15%) weight loss or low BMI (NICE, 2006). This may mean commencing home PN in patients with intestinal failure. Approximately 20% of home PN patients in Europe have underlying CD, which is about one case per 1.5 million population (Bakker *et al.*, 1999).

Diet therapy in active disease

Withdrawal of all food and drink except water and replacement with exclusive enteral nutrition (EEN) is recommended as primary treatment for active CD in children and adolescents. Several randomised controlled trials (RCTs) have shown remission rates of up to 80% (Griffiths *et al.*, 1995; Zachos *et al.*, 2007). If the gut is working and accessible, PN is rarely used to induce remission as it is invasive, carries risks of serious complications and leads to gut atrophy arising from complete bowel rest (Lomer, 2011). EEN can support adequate growth and development while avoiding drug-related side effects (Sandhu *et al.*, 2010). The exact mechanism of action of EEN is unclear and is hypothesised as a result of improved nutritional status, bowel rest, reduced dietary antigens and reduced gastrointestinal microbial activity (Bannerjee *et al.*, 2004; Gassull, 2004; Tsujikawa *et al.*, 2003).

In adults with CD, the evidence for EEN to induce disease remission is slightly weaker, with a response rate of 53–80% after 3–6 weeks on an intention-to-treat basis (Lee *et al.*, 2014; Zachos *et al.*, 2007). Adherence and inadequate dietetic provision may be limiting factors in adult success rates (Lomer *et al.*, 2014). It is a safe alternative to medical therapy with no associated long-term health consequences, and should therefore be offered (Mowat *et al.*, 2011).

The different types of feeds used to induce remission in CD include elemental, peptide and polymeric formulae with no difference in efficacy (Zachos *et al.*, 2007). Choice of feeds can depend on patient preference and local policy. Close support from a dedicated dietetic service is required (King *et al.*, 1997). EEN is usually prescribed for 6–8 weeks; however, the optimal length of EEN is not clearly defined and varies from 2 to 12 weeks (Ruemmele *et al.*, 2014). By day 10, there should be a clinical response, and patients can go into disease remission (Giaffer *et al.*, 1990). In order for mucosal healing to occur, EEN of 8 weeks or more may be required (Borrelli *et al.*, 2006; Fell *et al.*, 2000). Close dietetic monitoring is essential, and some of the problems that can occur and strategies for dealing with them are summarised in Table 7.4.8.

Diet therapy in remission

Partial enteral nutrition (PEN), where 35–50% of energy requirements are replaced with either an elemental or polymeric formula, has a role as adjunctive treatment to medical and surgical therapies and for nutritional support (Akobeng & Thomas, 2007; Zachos *et al.*, 2007). PEN has been shown to help prolong remission when provided for up to 12 months (Akobeng & Thomas, 2007), reduce surgical recurrence (Yamamoto *et al.*, 2013) and increase medication efficacy in adults with CD (Hirai *et al.*, 2013).

Food reintroduction diets

There are no specific guidelines on food reintroduction following EEN. Patients can be apprehensive about which foods to eat and may eliminate certain foods, fearing that they may worsen symptoms and cause a relapse, posing the risk of developing nutritional inadequacy. If food intolerance is found, patients require structured advice to ensure that a balanced diet can be resumed. Single-food elimination diets or low-fat fibre-limited exclusion (LOFFLEX) diets can be useful (Riordan *et al.*, 1993; Woolner *et al.*, 1998). High-fibre diets are not normally indicated as food reintroduction diets (Jones *et al.*, 1985). The LOFFLEX diet was developed as an easier and less time-consuming method of food reintroduction than the single-food elimination diet, with similar levels of efficacy in disease maintenance (Woolner *et al.*, 1998). It is based on eliminating foods that have been reported by >5% of CD patients as causing symptoms. Patients follow the basic diet for 2–4 weeks while weaning off EEN, and, provided the patient is still in a state of remission, further food reintroduction follows from a list of 25 specific foods, which are tested over 3–4 days. Low-fibre diets are often used in clinical practice because patients find them easier to follow, and as they are less limiting and more nutritionally adequate than exclusion or elimination diets. A study in paediatric CD patients looked at relapse rates following rapid food reintroduction (over 3 days) versus slow food reintroduction (over 5 weeks) and found that time to first relapse was similar in both groups (Faiman *et al.*, 2014).

Table 7.4.8 Problems associated with use of formula diets in patients with Crohn's disease

Problem	Cause and/or solution
Loss of weight	May be due to not meeting nutritional requirements in the first few days. If weight loss continues into the second week, increase the prescribed quantity of feed. Monitor symptoms.
Tiredness	Ensure the patient is meeting requirements for feed and fluid. Encourage rest.
Postural hypotension	Often occurs in first few days if fluid intake is inadequate.
Hunger	Seldom occurs if an adequate amount of feed is prescribed and consumed. Increase the frequency, concentration or quantity of drinks.
Headache	May be due to caffeine withdrawal or inadequate fluid intake.
Bad breath	Ensure good oral hygiene. Brushing teeth three times per day, using mouthwash and consuming water after each meal.
Green liquid stools	Infrequent, mild side effect.
Diarrhoea	May be osmotic; advise drinking the product slowly or diluting it with water. If given nasogastrically, slow administration rate.
Dislike of drink	Many people will become accustomed to the taste in time. Suggest different flavours, consuming from a covered glass with ice and a straw, or freezing/warming the drinks.

SECTION 7

Diet therapy in stricturing Crohn's disease

In stricturing disease, advice should be provided to help patients both alter and reduce their fibre intake to help prevent the risk of bowel obstruction and reduce associated symptoms (Lee *et al.*, 2014; Meier & Gassull, 2004). The degree of dietary restriction will be dependent on the nature (inflammatory and/or fibrotic) and extent (tightness and length) of the stricture (Lomer, 2011). Typically, high-fibre foods and foods that are difficult to mechanically break down (e.g. gristle, skin on meat or fish) are avoided (Lomer, 2011). EEN provided for 12 weeks has been shown to effectively treat inflammatory strictures with symptomatic and clinical remission achieved in 81.4% and 64.6% of patients, respectively, and the luminal cross-sectional area at the stricture site increased by 331% (Hu *et al.*, 2014).

Specific aspects of dietary management of ulcerative colitis

There is no indication for the use of EEN to treat active UC. At diagnosis, 35% of patients have protein energy malnutrition (Sawczenko & Sandhu, 2003), and nutrition remains of primary importance in preventing the detrimental effects of malnutrition (Burke *et al.*, 1997; Gonzalez-Huix *et al.*, 1993).

Diet therapy in ulcerative colitis

Low-fibre diets are often used for symptom relief during a disease flare-up. Patients suffering from a mild or moderate attack, or recovering from a more severe attack, will usually have lost weight and need to increase dietary intake of energy and protein, and oral nutritional supplements can be helpful. Peri- and postoperative nutrition support to maintain an adequate nutritional state is very important, and attention should be paid to micronutrient requirements. In the absence of massive bleeding, perforation, toxic megacolon or obstruction, EN rather than PN should be used. During clinical remission, patients should be encouraged to consume a varied, well-balanced diet, and unnecessary food exclusions should be discouraged.

Other aspects of nutrition in inflammatory bowel disease

There is much interest in the role of the specific carbohydrate diet (SCD) in IBD. The SCD is hypothesised to decrease intestinal inflammation by changing the faecal microbiome from a pro-inflammatory state to non-inflammatory state through exclusion of foods high in complex carbohydrates. This is achieved by excluding most starchy carbohydrates (potatoes, corn, gluten and rice), as well as food additives and preservatives, and allows certain fruits and vegetables, nuts, homemade fermented yoghurt, meats, eggs, butters and oils (Gottschall, 1994). Improved clinical and biochemical parameters have been shown in paediatric IBD patients (Chinonyelum *et al.*, 2016; Cohen *et al.*, 2014). A proportion of IBD patients following the SCD were able to discontinue immunosuppressive agents (Kakodkar *et al.*, 2015). The diet should be implemented with caution, as there are high risks of nutritional deficiencies due to its restrictive nature.

Curcumin, the active component of turmeric, may potentially be a safe alternative therapy in UC, and has been shown to suppress pro-inflammatory cytokines (Brumatti *et al.*, 2014); to be superior to placebo in the maintenance of remission (Hanai *et al.*, 2006); and, when used in combination with a 5-ASA, induced remission in mild to moderate UC (Lang *et al.*, 2015).

There is evidence for the effectiveness of probiotics in UC but not CD (Rolfe *et al.*, 2006). The probiotics most studied are *Escherichia coli Nissle 1917, VSL#3, Lactobacillus rhamnosius GC, Bifidobacterium and Saccharomyces boulardii* (Mowat *et al.*, 2011; Pham *et al.*, 2008). *VSL#3* is licensed as treatment for pouchitis (Gionchetti *et al.*, 2003; Mimura *et al.*, 2004), and may be of benefit in the maintenance and treatment of UC (Bibiloni *et al.*, 2005; Miele *et al.*, 2009). Three randomised placebo-controlled studies have shown that *E. coli Nissle 1917* (Mutaflor®), 200 mg daily, is equivalent to standard doses of mesalazine in maintaining remission in UC (Schultz, 2008). Therefore, this may be an option for patients who are unable or unwilling to take mesalazine.

Acknowledgement

The editor acknowledges the prior contribution of Derbhla O'Sullivan.

Internet resources

British Society of Gastroenterology, www.bsg.org.uk
CORE (Digestive Disorders Foundation), www.corecharity.org.uk
Crohn's and Colitis UK, www.crohnsandcolitis.org.uk
Crohn's in Childhood Research Association (CICRA), www.cicra.org
NHS Evidence, www.evidence.nhs.uk
The Crohn's and Colitis Foundation of America, www.ccfa.org

References

Abraham C, Cho JH. (2009) Inflammatory bowel disease. *N. Engl. J. Med.* 361: 2066–2078.

Ahuja V, Tandon RK. (2010) Inflammatory bowel disease in the Asia-Pacific area: a comparison with developed countries. *J. Dig. Dis.* 11: 134–147.

Akobeng AK, Thomas AG. (2007) Enteral nutrition for maintenance of remission in Crohn's disease. *Cochrane Database Syst. Rev.* (3): CD005984.

Amre DK, D'Souza S, Morgan K, *et al.* (2007) Imbalances in dietary consumption of fatty acids, vegetables and fruits are associated with risk for Crohn's disease in children. *Am. J. Gastroenterol.* 102: 2016–2025.

Bakker H, Bozzetti F, Staun M, *et al.* (1999) Home parenteral nutrition in adults: a European multicentre survey in 1997. ESPEN-Home Artificial Nutrition Working Group. *Clin. Nutr.* 18: 135–140.

Bannerjee K, Camacho-Hubner C, Babinska K, *et al.* (2004) Anti-inflammatory and growth-stimulating effects precede nutritional restitution during enteral feeding in Crohn's disease. *J. Pediatr. Gastroenterol. Nutr.* 38: 270–275.

Banos-Madrid R, Salama-Benerroch H, Moran-Sanchez S, *et al.* (2004) Lactose malabsorption in patients with inflammatory bowel disease without activity; would it be necessary to exclude lactose products in the diet of all patients? *An. Med. Interna.* 21: 212–214.

Bernklev T, Jahnsen J, Schulz T. (2005) Course of disease, drug treatment and health-related quality of life in patients with inflammatory bowel disease 5 years after initial diagnosis. *Eur. J. Gastroenterol. Hepatol.* 17(10): 1037–1045.

Best WR, Becktel WR, Singleton JW, *et al.* (1976) Development of a Crohn's disease activity index. National Cooperative Crohn's Disease Study. *Gastroenterology.* 70(3): 439–444.

Bibiloni R, Fedorak RN, Tannock GW, *et al.* (2005) *VSL#3* probiotic mixture induces remission in patients with active ulcerative colitis. *Am. J. Gastroenterol.* 100: 1539–1546.

Borrelli O, Cordischi L, Cirulli M, *et al.* (2006) Polymeric diet alone versus corticosteroids in the treatment of active pediatric Crohn's disease: a randomized controlled open-label trial. *Clin. Gastroenterol. Hepatol.* 4: 744–753.

Brumatti LV, Marcuzzi AL, Tricarico PM, *et al.* (2014) Curcumin and inflammatory bowel disease: potential and limits of innovative treatments. *Molecules.* 19: 21127–21153.

Burke A, Lichtenstein GR, Rombeau JL. (1997) Nutrition and ulcerative colitis. *Baillieres. Clin. Gastroenterol.* 11: 153–174.

Camilleri M. (2011) Managing symptoms of irritable bowel syndrome in patients with inflammatory bowel disease. *Gut.* 60: 425–428.

Castiglione F, Rispo A, Di Girolamo E, *et al.* (2003) Antibiotic treatment of small bowel bacterial overgrowth in patients with Crohn's disease. *Aliment. Pharmacol. Ther.* 18: 1107–1112.

Chande N, Patton PH, Tsoulis DJ, *et al.* (2015) Azathioprine or 6-mercaptopurine for maintenance of remission in Crohn's disease. *Cochrane Database Syst. Rev.* (1): CD000067.

Chinonyelum O, Ghassan W, Lee D, *et al.* (2016) Specific carbohydrate diet for pediatric inflammatory bowel disease in clinical practice within an academic IBD center. *Nutrition.* 32: 418–425.

Cohen SA, Gold BD, Oliva S, *et al.* (2014) Clinical and mucosal improvement with specific carbohydrate diet in pediatric Crohn disease. *J. Pediatr. Gastroenterol. Nutr.* 59: 516–521.

Devkota S, Wang Y, Musch MW, *et al.* (2012) Dietary-fat-induced taurocholic acid production promotes pathobiont and colitis in IL-10-/-mice. *Nature.* 487: 104–108.

Dignass A, Van Assche G, Lindsay JO, *et al.* (2010) The second European evidence-based consensus on the diagnosis and management of Crohn's disease: current management. *J. Crohns Colitis.* 4: 28–62.

Dignass A, Lindsay JO, Sturm A, *et al.* (2012) Second European evidence-based consensus on the diagnosis and management of ulcerative colitis part 2: current management. *J. Crohns Colitis.* 6: 991–1030.

Faiman A, Mutalibb M, Moylanb A. (2014) Standard versus rapid food reintroduction after exclusive enteral nutritional therapy in paediatric Crohn's disease. *Eur. J. Gastroenterol. Hepatol.* 26: 276–281.

Fell JM, Paintin M, Arnaud-Battandier F, *et al.* (2000) Mucosal healing and a fall in mucosal pro-inflammatory cytokine mRNA induced by a specific oral polymeric diet in paediatric Crohn's disease. *Aliment. Pharmacol. Ther.* 14: 281–289.

Filippi J, Al-Jaouni R, Wiroth JB, *et al.* (2006) Nutritional deficiencies in patients with Crohn's disease in remission. *Inflamm. Bowel Dis.* 12: 185–191.

Filmann N, Rey J, Schneeweiss S, *et al.* (2014) Prevalence of anemia in inflammatory bowel diseases in European countries: a systematic review and individual patient data meta-analysis. *Inflamm. Bowel Dis.* 20: 936–945.

Flores A, Burstein E, Cipher DJ, *et al.* (2015) Obesity in inflammatory bowel disease: a marker of less severe disease. *Dig. Dis. Sci.* 60(8): 2436–2445.

Gassull MA. (2004) Review article: the roe of nutrition in the treatment of inflammatory bowel disease. *Aliment. Pharmacol. Ther.* 20(4): 79–83.

Gassull MA, Cabre E. (2001) Nutrition in inflammatory bowel disease. *Curr. Opin. Clin. Nutr. Metab. Care* 4: 561–569.

Gearry RB, Irving PM, Barrett JS, *et al.* (2008) Reduction of dietary poorly absorbed short-chain carbohydrates (FODMAPs) improves abdominal symptoms in patients with inflammatory bowel disease – a pilot study. *J. Crohns Colitis.* 3(1): 8–14.

Geerling BJ, Stockbrugger RW, Brummer RJ. (1999) Nutrition and inflammatory bowel disease: an update. *Scand. J. Gastroenterol. Suppl.* 230: 95–105.

Giaffer MH, North G, Holdsworth CD. (1990) Controlled trial of polymeric versus elemental diet in treatment of active Crohn's disease. *Lancet* 335: 816–819.

Ginard D, Riera J, Bonet L, *et al.* (2003) Lactose malabsorption in ulcerative colitis. *A case–control study. Gastroenterol. Hepatol.* 26: 469–474.

Gionchetti P, Rizzello F, Helwig U, *et al.* (2003) Prophylaxis of pouchitis onset with probiotic therapy: a double-blind, placebo-controlled trial. *Gastroenterology.* 124: 1202–1209.

Gonzalez-Huix F, Fernandez-Banares F, Esteve-Comas M, *et al.* (1993) Enteral versus parenteral nutrition as adjunct therapy in acute ulcerative colitis. *Am. J. Gastroenterol.* 88: 227–232.

Gottschall E (ed). (1994) *Breaking the Vicious Cycle*, 2nd edn. Baltimore, ON: Kirkton Press Limited.

Griffiths AM, Ohlsson A, Sherman PM, *et al.* (1995) Meta-analysis of enteral nutrition as a primary treatment of active Crohn's disease. *Gastroenterology.* 108: 1056–1067.

Hanai H, Lida T, Takeuchi K, *et al.* (2006) Curcumin maintenance therapy for ulcerative colitis: randomized, multicenter, double-blind, placebo-controlled trial. *Clin. Gastroenterol. Hepatol.* 4(12): 1502–1506.

Hart, A and The IBD in EPIC Study Investigators (2009). Linoleic acid, a dietary n-6 polyunsaturated fatty acid, and the aetiology of ulcerative colitis: a nested case–control study within a European prospective cohort study. *The IBD in EPIC Study Investigators. Gut* 58: 1606–1611.

Harvey RF, Bradshaw MJ. (1980) Measuring Crohn's disease activity. *Lancet.* 1: 1134–1135.

Higgins PDR, Schwartz M, Mapili J, *et al.* (2005) Patient defined dichotomous end points for remission and clinical improvement in ulcerative colitis. *Gut.* 54(6): 782–788.

Hirai F, Ishihara H, Yada S, *et al.* (2013) Effectiveness of concomitant enteral nutrition therapy and infliximab for maintenance treatment of Crohn's disease in adults. *Dig. Dis. Sci.* 58(5): 1329–1334.

Hu D, Ren J, Wang G, *et al.* (2014) Exclusive enteral nutritional therapy can relieve inflammatory bowel stricture in Crohn's disease. *J. Clin. Gastroenterol.* 48(9): 790–795.

Hwang C, Ross V, Mahadevan U. (2012) Micronutrient deficiencies in inflammatory bowel disease: from A to zinc. *Inflamm. Bowel Dis.* 18: 1961–1981.

IBD Standards Update. (2013) *Standards for the healthcare of people who have inflammatory bowel disease (IBD).* Available at http://s3-eu-west-1.amazonaws.com/files.crohnsandcolitis.org.uk/Publications/PPR/ibd-standards.pdf. Accessed 26 October 2018.

Johnson GJ, Cosnes J, Mansfield JC. (2005) Smoking cessation as primary therapy to modify the course of Crohn's disease. *Aliment. Pharmacol. Ther.* 21: 921–931.

Jones VA, Dickinson RJ, Workman E. (1985) Crohn's disease: maintenance of remission by diet. *Lancet.* 2: 177–180.

Kabbani MD, Koutroubakis IE, Schoen RE, *et al.* (2016) Association of vitamin D level with clinical status in inflammatory bowel disease: a 5-year longitudinal study. *Am. J. Gastroenterol.* 111: 712–719.

Kakodkar S, Farooqui A J, Mikolaitis S L, *et al.* (2015). The Specific Carbohydrate Diet for Inflammatory Bowel Disease: A Case Series. *J. Am. Acad. Nutr. Diet.* 115(8):1226–1232.

King T.S, Woolner J T. and Hunter J O. (1997). The dietary management of Crohn's disease. *Aliment. Pharmacol. Ther.*11:17–31.

Lang A, Salomon N, Justin CY. *et al.* (2015) Curcumin in combination with mesalamine induces remission in patients with mild-to-moderate ulcerative colitis in a randomized controlled trial. *Clin. Gastroenterol. Hepatol.* 13: 1444–1449.

Limdi JK, Aggarwal D, McLaughlin JT. (2016) Dietary practices and beliefs in patients with inflammatory bowel disease. *Inflamm. Bowel Dis.* 22(1): 164–170.

Lee J, Allen R, Ashley S, *et al.* (2014) British Dietetic Association evidence-based guidelines for the dietary management of Crohn's disease in adults. *J. Hum. Nutr. Diet.* 27: 207–218.

Lewis NR, Scott BB. (2007) *Guidelines for osteoporosis in inflammatory bowel disease and coeliac disease.* British Society of Gastroenterology; London.

Lochs H, Dejong C, Hammarqvist F, *et al.* (2006) ESPEN guidelines on enteral nutrition: gastroenterology. *Clin. Nutr.* 25: 260–274.

Lomer MCE. (2011) Dietary considerations in IBD. In: Whayman K, Duncan J, O'Connor M (eds) *Inflammatory Bowel Disease Nursing.* London: Quay Books, pp. 139–159.

Lomer MCE, Gourgey R, Whelan K. (2014) Current practice in relation to nutritional assessment and dietary management of enteral nutrition in adults with Crohn's disease. *J. Hum. Nutr. Diet.* 27(2): 28–35.

Mahid SS, Minor KS, Soto RE, *et al.* (2006) Smoking and inflammatory bowel disease: a meta-analysis. *Mayo Clin. Proc.* 81: 1462–1471.

Marshall JK, Hilsden RJ. (2003) Environment and epidemiology of inflammatory bowel diseases. In: Satsangi J, Sutherland RL (eds) *Inflammatory Bowel Diseases.* London: Elsevier, pp. 17–28.

Meier R, Gassull M. (2004) Consensus recommendations on the effects and benefits of fibre in clinical practice. *Clin. Nutr.* 1(2): 73–80.

Miele E, Pascarella F, Giannetti E, *et al.* (2009) Effect of a probiotic preparation (*VSL#3*) on induction and maintenance of remission in children with ulcerative colitis. *Am. J. Gastroenterol.* 104: 437–443.

Mimura T, Rizzello F, Helwig U, *et al.* (2004) Once daily high dose probiotic therapy (*VSL#3*) for maintaining remission in recurrent or refractory pouchitis. *Gut.* 53: 108–114.

Mowat C, Cole A, Windsor A, *et al.* (2011) Guidelines for the management of inflammatory bowel disease in adults. *Gut.* 60: 571–607.

NICE. (2006) *Nutrition Support in Adults. Oral Nutrition Support, Enteral Tube Feeding and Parenteral Nutrition.* Available at https://www.nice.org.uk/guidance/cg32. Accessed 18 February 2017.

NICE. (2013) *Faecal calprotectin diagnostic tests for inflammatory diseases of the bowel.* Available at https://www.nice.org.uk/guidance/dg11. Accessed 18 February 2017.

Orchard TR, Goldin RD, Tekkis PP, *et al.* (2011) *An Atlas of investigation and Management: Inflammatory Bowel Disease.* Oxford. UK: Warner Chilcott.

Oresland T. (2006) Colon-saving medical therapy vs. colectomy in ulcerative colitis – the case for colectomy. *Aliment. Pharmacol. Ther.* 24(3): 74–79.

Orholm M, Munkholm P, Langholz E, *et al.* (1991) Familial occurrence of inflammatory bowel disease. *N. Engl. J. Med.* 324: 84–88.

Pariente B, Jacques Cosnes MD, Silvio Danese MD, *et al.* (2011) Development of the Crohn's disease digestive damage score, the Lémann score. *Inflamm. Bowel Dis.* 17(6): 1415–1422.

Parks AG, Nicholls RJ. (1978) Proctocolectomy without ileostomy for ulcerative colitis. *BMJ* 2: 85–88.

Persson PG, Ahlbom A, Hellers G. (1992) Diet and inflammatory bowel disease: a case control study. *Epidemiology.* 3: 47–52.

Pham M, Lemberg DA, Day AS. (2008) Probiotics: sorting the evidence from the myths. *Med. J. Aust.* 188: 304–308.

Prince A, Myers CE, Joyce T, *et al.* (2016) Fermentable carbohydrate restriction (low FODMAP diet) in clinical practice improves functional gastrointestinal symptoms in patients with inflammatory bowel disease. *Inflamm. Bowel Dis.* 22(5): 1129–1136.

Qin X. (2012) Etiology of inflammatory bowel disease: a unified hypothesis. *World J. Gastroenterol.* 18(15): 1708–1722.

Reid I R. (2014). Should we prescribe calcium supplements for osteoporosis prevention? *J Bone metab* 21: 21–28.

Reif S, Klein I, Lubin F. (1997) Pre-illness dietary factors in inflammatory bowel disease. *Gut.* 40: 754–760.

Riordan AM, Hunter JO, Cowan RE, *et al.* (1993) Treatment of active Crohn's disease by exclusion diet: East Anglian multicentre controlled trial. *Lancet.* 342: 1131–1134.

Roberts SE, Williams JG, Yeates D, *et al.* (2007) Mortality in patients with and without colectomy admitted to hospital for ulcerative colitis and Crohn's disease: record linkage studies. *BMJ* 335: 1033.

Roberts CL, Rushworth SL, Richman E, *et al.* (2013) Hypothesis: increased consumption of emulsifiers for the rising incidence of Crohn's Disease. *J. Crohns Colitis.* 7: 338–341.

Rolfe VE, Fortun PJ, Hawkey CJ, *et al.* (2006) Probiotics for maintenance of remission in Crohn's disease. *Cochrane Database Syst. Rev.* (4): CD004826.

Rubin GP, Hungin AP, Kelly PJ, *et al.* (2000) Inflammatory bowel disease: epidemiology and management in an English general practice population. *Aliment. Pharmacol. Ther.* 14: 1553–1559.

Ruemmele FM, Veres G, Kolho KL, *et al.* (2014) Consensus guidelines of ECCO/ESPGHAN on the medical management of paediatric Crohn's disease. *J. Crohns Colitis.* 8: 1179–1207.

Sandhu BK, Fell JM, Beattie RM, *et al.* (2010) Guidelines for the management of inflammatory bowel disease in children in the United Kingdom. *J. Pediatr. Gastroenterol. Nutr.* 50(1): S1–S13.

Sawczenko A, Sandhu BK. (2003) Presenting features of inflammatory bowel disease in Great Britain and Ireland. *Arch. Dis. Child.* 88: 995–1000.

Schultz M. (2008) Clinical use of *E. coli Nissle 1917* in inflammatory bowel disease. *Inflam. Bowel Dis.* 14: 1012–1018.

Shen B, Achkar JP, Lashner BA, *et al.* (2001) A randomized clinical trial of ciprofloxacin and metronidazole to treat acute pouchitis. *Inflamm. Bowel Dis.* 7(4): 301–305.

Silverberg MS, Satsangi J, Ahmad T, *et al.* (2005) Toward an integrated clinical, molecular and serological classification of inflammatory bowel disease: report of a Working Party of the 2005 Montreal World Congress of Gastroenterology. *Can. J. Gastroenterol.* 19(A): 5–36.

Simren M, Axelsson J, Gillberg R, *et al.* (2002) Quality of life in inflammatory bowel disease in remission: the impact of IBS-like symptoms and associated psychological factors. *Am. J. Gastroenterol.* 97: 389–396.

Targownik LE, Bernstein CN, Leslie WD. (2014) Risk factors and management of osteoporosis in inflammatory bowel disease. *Curr. Opin. Gastroenterol.* 30: 168–174.

Tilg H, Moschen AR, Kaser A, *et al.* (2007) Gut, inflammation and osteoporosis: basic and clinical concepts. *Gut.* 57: 684–694.

Tsujikawa T, Andoh A, Fujiyama Y. (2003) Enteral and parenteral nutrition therapy for Crohn's disease. *Curr. Pharma. Des.* 9: 323–332.

Van Limbergen J, Russell RK, Drummond HE, *et al.* (2008) Definition of phenotypic characteristics of childhood-onset inflammatory bowel disease. *Gastroenterology.* 135(4): 1114–1122.

Vagianos K, Bector S, McConnell J, *et al.* (2007) Nutrition assessment of patients with inflammatory bowel disease. *JPEN J. Parenter. Enteral Nutr.* 31: 311–319.

Vermeire S, Schreiber S, Sandborn WJ, *et al.* (2010) Correlation between the Crohn's disease activity and Harvey-Bradshaw indices in assessing Crohn's disease severity. *Clin. Gastroenterol. Hepatol.* 8(4): 357–363.

Walmsley RS, Ayres RCS, Pounder RE, *et al.* (1998) A simple clinical colitis activity index. *Gut.* 43: 29–32.

Wang Y, MacDonald JK, Vandermeer B, *et al.* (2015) Methotrexate for maintenance of remission in ulcerative colitis. *Cochrane Database Syst. Rev.* (8): CD007560.

Woolner JT, Parker TJ, Kirby GA, *et al.* (1998) The development and evaluation of a diet for maintaining remission in Crohn's disease. *J. Hum. Nutr. Diet.* 11: 1–11.
Xavier RJ, Podolsky DK. (2007) Unravelling the pathogenesis of inflammatory bowel disease. *Nature.* 448: 427–434.
Yakut M, Ustun Y, Kabacam G, *et al.* (2010) Serum vitamin B_{12} and folate status in patients with inflammatory bowel diseases. *Eur. J. Intern. Med.* 21: 320–323.
Yamamoto T, Shiraki M, Nakahigashi M, *et al.* (2013) Enteral nutrition to suppress postoperative Crohn's disease recurrence: a five-year prospective cohort study. *Int. J. Colorectal Dis.* 28(3): 335–340.
Zachos M, Tondeur M, Griffiths AM. (2007) Enteral nutritional therapy for induction of remission in Crohn's disease. *Cochrane Database Syst. Rev.* (1): CD000542.

7.4.9 Intestinal failure and intestinal resection

Alison Culkin

Key points

Intestinal failure

- Patients with a jejunostomy are recommended a diet high in energy, protein, fat and sodium, but restricted in fibre and fluid. Patients will require an oral rehydration solution and fluid restriction.
- Patients with a colon in continuity are recommended a diet high in energy, protein and carbohydrate, and moderate in fat, to achieve energy balance while avoiding steatorrhoea. A reduced oxalate intake is advised to prevent oxalate kidney stones.

Resection of the large intestine

- Sodium and fluid balance should be closely monitored, and an oral rehydration solution may be required.
- A well-balanced diet based on the principles of healthy eating should be encouraged without unnecessary food restrictions.

Intestinal failure

The European Society of Parenteral and Enteral Nutrition (ESPEN) has defined intestinal failure (IF) as *'the reduction of gut function below the minimum necessary for the absorption of macronutrients and/or water and electrolytes, such that intravenous supplementation is required to maintain health and/or growth'* (Pironi et al., 2016). Patients who do not require parenteral nutrition (PN) are now considered to experience intestinal insufficiency. The classification has been established by utilising functional, pathophysiological and clinical parameters.

Functional classification

On the basis of onset, metabolic and expected outcome criteria, IF is classified as:

- *Type I* – acute, short-term and usually self-limiting condition.
- *Type II* – prolonged acute condition, often in metabolically unstable patients, requiring complex multidisciplinary care and intravenous supplementation over periods of weeks or months.
- *Type III* – chronic condition, in metabolically stable patients, requiring intravenous supplementation over months or years. It may be reversible or irreversible.

Pathophysiological classification

IF can be classified into five major pathophysiological conditions, which may originate from various gastrointestinal or systemic diseases:

- Short bowel.
- Intestinal fistula.
- Intestinal dysmotility.
- Mechanical obstruction.
- Extensive small bowel mucosal disease.

Clinical classification of chronic intestinal failure

On the basis of the requirements for energy and the volume of the intravenous (IV) supplementation, chronic IF is categorised into 16 subtypes (Table 7.4.9). Types 1 and 2 are often referred to as acute IF. The worldwide prevalence of chronic IF is unknown, but, in the UK, estimates range from 10 to 15% of patients undergoing intestinal surgery (Carlson, 2003). ESPEN have published guidelines on the management of acute IF which includes information on sepsis control, fluid and electrolyte management, optimising nutritional status, wound care, surgery and rehabilitation (Klek *et al.*, 2016). The detection and management of abdominal sepsis is a priority, as this is the most common cause of death if not aggressively managed. The introduction of enhanced recovery after surgery (ERAS) protocols moderates the metabolic effects of surgery and prevents fluid and sodium overload, and may minimise the development of type 1 IF in the future (Gustafsson *et al.*, 2012). The worldwide incidence of type 3 IF remains unknown. Data collected as part of the British Artificial Nutrition Survey (BANS) estimates a prevalence of 10 per million, which is likely to be an underestimate due to the voluntary nature of reporting (Smith

Table 7.4.9 ESPEN recommendations: definition and classification of IF (source: Pironi *et al.*, 2016. Reproduced with permission from Elsevier)

IV energy supplementation[b] (kcal/kg body weight)	Volume of IV supplementation[a] (mL)			
	≤1000 (1)	1001–2000 (2)	2001–3000 (3)	>3000 (4)
0 (A)	A1	A2	A3	A4
1–10 (B)	B1	B2	B3	B4
11–20 (C)	C1	C2	C3	C4
>20 (D)	D1	D2	D3	D4

[a]calculated as daily mean of the total volume infused per week = (volume per day of infusion × number of infusions per week)/7.
[b]calculated as daily mean of the total energy infused per week = (energy per day of infusion × number of infusions per week)/7.

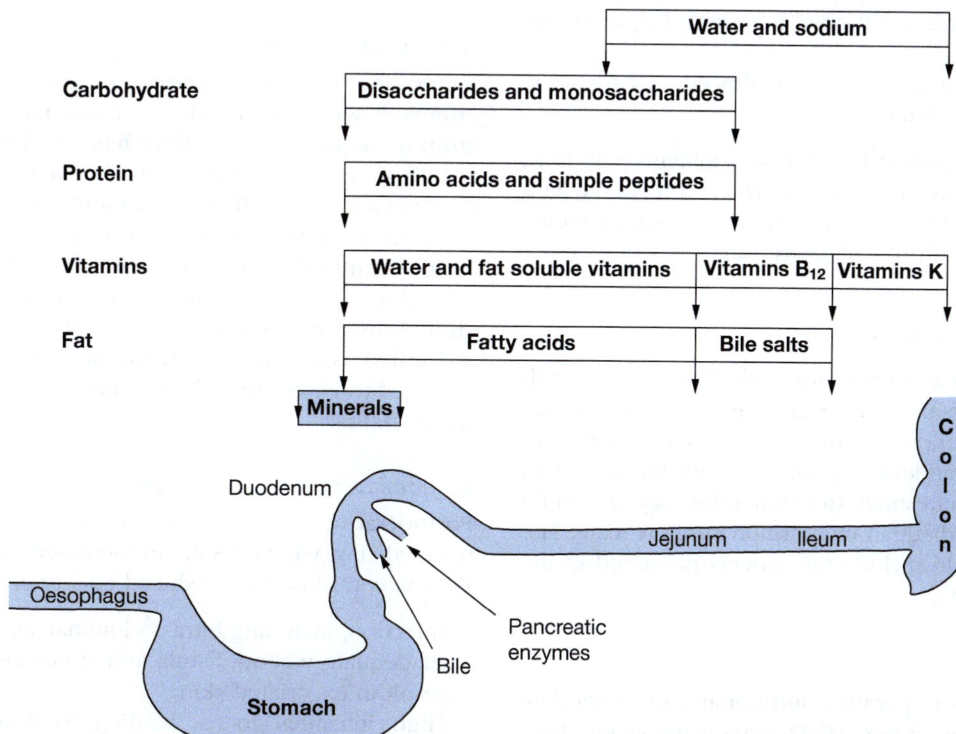

Figure 7.4.6 Sites of nutrient absorption (adapted from Thomas & Bishop, 2007, figure 4.1. Reproduced with permission from Blackwell Publishing)

et al., 2016). Patients with type 3 are those requiring long-term parenteral support, usually at home.

Disease consequences (morbidity, mortality, patient perspective)

Although IF is relatively rare, it can result in significant morbidity and mortality if not managed by experienced healthcare professionals (Pironi *et al.*, 2012). Mortality data ranges from 15 to 47%, with underlying disease or complications relating to liver disease and catheter-related sepsis often the cause of death (Schalamon *et al.*, 2003). Patients on home PN experience a quality of life similar to patients on haemodialysis, with fatigue being a major symptom. Patients also report reduced sleep quality due to nocturia induced by night-time infusions (Hofstetter *et al.*, 2013). Therefore, removing or reducing dependence on PN is a goal of therapy.

Nutritional consequences of intestinal failure and short bowel

The effect of intestinal resection is best understood by considering where nutrients are normally absorbed. Most nutrients are absorbed within the first 100–150 cm of the jejunum. Exceptions are vitamin B_{12} and bile salts, which are absorbed at specific receptor sites in the terminal ileum (Figure 7.4.6). Resection of the small bowel will therefore affect absorption, but the outcome for the patient will depend on the type, length and quality of the remaining small bowel and the presence or absence of a functioning colon. Extensive resection may result in the remaining end of the small intestine being anastomosed to the colon (jejunocolic or ileocolic anastomosis) or ending at a stoma on the abdomen (jejunostomy or ileostomy). The loss of the ileum and some of the jejunum considerably impairs digestive and absorptive function. A residual small bowel length of <200 cm can be deemed as short bowel, and can lead to nutritional, fluid and electrolyte depletion if not adequately managed. When the absorptive function of the colon is no longer available, more fluid and electrolytes will be lost. The following lengths of small bowel are inadequate to be managed on diet alone, and parenteral support is required (Nightingale *et al.*, 1992):

- <100 cm of jejunum will need long-term parenteral fluid and electrolyte replacement.
- <75 cm of jejunum will need long-term PN, fluid and electrolytes.
- <50 cm of jejunum plus colon will need long-term PN, fluid and electrolytes.

All patients with short bowel have problems with fluid and electrolyte balance, particularly in the immediate postoperative period, with nutrient requirements increased as a result of malabsorption.

Nutritional assessment

It is important that all patients with IF have a through nutritional assessment, as significant fluid shifts can result in dehydration, electrolyte depletion and malnutrition. Patients undergoing surgery who fail to regain adequate gastrointestinal function after day 5 should be referred to a dietitian or nutrition support team. The assessment should include the aspects discussed in the following sections.

Anthropometry

Determine the perioperative nutritional status including weight, body mass index (BMI), percentage weight loss, mid-arm circumference (MAC), triceps skinfold thickness (TST), mid-arm muscle circumference (MAMC) and grip strength. Inappropriate prescribing of IV fluids can lead to oedema, which can mask significant loss of lean body tissue, and is often a cause of type 1 IF (Lobo *et al.*, 2002). If oedema is present, an estimated dry weight should be used.

Biochemistry

Determine the hydration status of the patient; do they appear dehydrated or overloaded? The administration of excessive volumes of 0.9% sodium chloride is common and can exacerbate postoperative ileus (Lobo *et al.*, 2002). Routine haematology and biochemistry, including urinary sodium, should be monitored. A random urinary sodium is invaluable in assessing hydration status; a value of <20 mmol/L indicates dehydration (NICE, 2013). Consider if there are any other electrolyte deficiencies (e.g. magnesium) as requirements are high with intestinal losses? Consider the risk of micronutrient deficiencies, i.e. folate, iron, selenium, zinc, vitamin D and B_{12}. If a vitamin, mineral or trace element deficiency is demonstrated, an appropriate supplement can be prescribed. If >100 cm of terminal ileum is resected, then the patient will become depleted in vitamin B_{12} and will require replacement via an intramuscular injection every 3 months.

Clinical

Determine the underlying cause of IF. How likely is it to resolve? Is the patient septic? Ongoing sepsis will result in increased nutritional requirements and a higher risk of metabolic and infective complications. Assessment of fluid balance is crucial (NICE, 2013). Intestinal function should be assessed regularly to permit the transition from parenteral to enteral nutrition.

Dietary assessment

Determine the perioperative nutritional intake and compare with estimated requirements. Is nutritional support required? If a patient has failed or is expected to fail to establish feeding with enteral nutrition, or is expected to fail, then PN should be considered. An assessment of the adequacy of oral diet once weaned from parenteral or enteral nutrition is important to prevent deterioration in nutritional status. Patients with short bowel experience malabsorption, and therefore a detailed assessment of intake and intestinal output is required to assess the effect of malabsorption on nutritional status.

Economic and social assessment

Postoperative complications prolong the length of hospital stay, which results in increased healthcare cost. Factors contributing to reduced quality of life include:

- Infection, including intra-abdominal sepsis.
- Inadequate wound, fistula and stoma care, which can result in excoriated skin.
- High intestinal losses leading to dehydration and electrolyte disturbances.
- Poor provision of nutrition, resulting in malnutrition.
- Immobility.
- Depression.

All of the preceding factors increase the length of rehabilitation, during which the patient is unable to return to work and family life.

Clinical investigations

Radiology is invaluable to investigate the presence of intra-abdominal sepsis or the presence of an anastomotic leak as occurs in type 1 IF. The management of abdominal sepsis is the most important aspect of care and can predict mortality and morbidity. Before considering reconstructive surgery in a patient with type 2 IF, it is important that radiological assessment be completed, which will provide a detailed understanding of the postoperative anatomy and the likelihood of parenteral independence (Carlson, 2003; Klek *et al.*, 2016).

Clinical management

Fluid and sodium management of short bowel

The focus of treatment aims to reduce intestinal losses, thereby preventing dehydration and electrolyte disturbances. Restricting oral fluid intake and using an oral rehydration solution achieves this. In some patients (known as 'secretors'), intestinal losses of fluid and electrolytes exceed the amount taken orally, and parenteral replacement will be required. This is particularly likely to occur if the stoma is situated <100 cm along the jejunum (Nightingale *et al.*, 1990). Secretors may be in constant negative fluid and sodium balance. Those who can maintain sodium balance will still lose considerable amounts of sodium from their stoma or fistula, and these losses will need to be replaced. Patients with an intestinal output of <1500 mL/day can usually maintain their sodium balance by adding extra salt to food during cooking and by eating salty foods. When losses are greater than this, an oral rehydration solution (such as St Mark's solution), will be required with a sodium content of ≥90 mmol/L (containing 20 g of glucose, 35 g of sodium chloride and 2.5 g of sodium bicarbonate). The patient should be encouraged to slowly sip 1 L of an oral rehydration solution throughout the day. The solution can be unpalatable, and adding a small amount of juice or cordial, chilling it, and sipping through a straw may enhance its acceptability. Double-strength Diarolyte® can also be used, but may result in hyperkalaemia. Oral hypotonic fluids with a lower sodium concentration, such as water or tea, should be restricted to <1 L/day, as they will increase intestinal losses (Nightingale, 1994). Some patients will not be able to achieve adequate fluid and sodium balance via the oral route and will require either subcutaneous or intravenous saline, possibly with additional magnesium, which can be administered at home (Martinez-Riquelme *et al.*, 2005). Renal impairment is common in patients with type 3 IF as a result of chronic dehydration (Lauverjat *et al.*, 2006), and therefore ongoing monitoring of renal function is essential in this patient group.

Although it is common practice to encourage patients to consume foods and fluids separately, there is no evidence to support this advice. Woolf *et al.* (1987) found that restricting fluid intake around meals did not improve nutrient absorption in stable patients either with or without a colon. However, many patients with high intestinal losses anecdotally report a benefit.

Pharmaceutical management

Other factors such as increased gastric acid production and reduced intestinal transit time exacerbate dehydration and sodium depletion in patients with short bowel (Lennard-Jones, 1994). Gastric antisecretory drugs such as proton pump inhibitors have been shown to reduce intestinal losses by 1.5 kg/24 hours (Nightingale *et al.*, 1991). Patients who fail to absorb oral preparations may benefit from parenteral administration (Jeppesen *et al.*, 1998). Antidiarrhoeal agents such as loperamide and codeine phosphate benefit patients by decreasing the frequency and weight of intestinal output and prolonging the transit time (Mainguet & Fiasse, 1977). These drugs are usually needed in very high doses and should be taken 30–60 minutes before meals. Colestyramine is a bile acid sequestrant and can be helpful in patients experiencing high intestinal losses due to bile salt malabsorption. It is not recommended for patients with a colon in continuity except as a possible treatment for hyperoxaluria (Lennard-Jones, 1994). Octreotide is a somatostatin analogue that reduces gastric, pancreatic and biliary secretions (Rodrigues *et al.*, 1989). However, its use should be reserved for patients with very high intestinal losses refractory to other measures, as it is given by a subcutaneous injection, three times daily. If there is no improvement after 3 days, it should be discontinued. Octreotide is frequently used in an attempt to heal fistulae, but results are variable (Lloyd *et al.*, 2006; Rahbour *et al.*, 2012). Magnesium deficiency is common and often due to sodium depletion, which can usually be corrected using an oral rehydration solution or 0.9% saline. Hypomagnesaemia can be treated with oral magnesium salts, although this can result in increased intestinal output. If oral supplements are ineffective, then magnesium sulphate can be added to 0.9% saline and given subcutaneously or intravenously to maintain plasma concentrations (Martinez-Riquelme *et al.*, 2005). Vitamin D concentrations should be measured and replaced if found to be deficient, as vitamin D increases the intestinal and renal absorption of magnesium (Nightingale, 2001).

Nutritional management

The nutritional management of IF is a dynamic process that involves overlap or transition between diet, enteral and PN as the patient's condition changes. The judgement to instigate nutrition support in type 1 IF is often difficult. The 'wait and see' approach or the presence or absence of bowel sounds is misleading and can result in significant time without adequate nutrition in those who may benefit from PN. Despite the obvious benefits of PN in patients with type 1 and 2 IF, a recent report on the use of PN reported good standards of care in only 19% of UK hospitals. The report highlighted a lack of adequate consideration of enteral nutrition, delays in the initiation of PN, and inadequate assessment and monitoring, resulting in avoidable metabolic and infective complications (National Confidential Enquiry into Patient Outcome and Death (NCEPOD), 2010)). It is common for patients who develop enterocutaneous fistulas to be nil by mouth, and to start PN and octreotide in an attempt to heal fistulas (Lloyd *et al.*, 2006). However, in patients in whom closure is unlikely to occur spontaneously, oral diet can be introduced. Patients with intestinal fistulae who have >75 cm of normal small intestine distal to the fistula may be candidates for fistuloclysis, a technique in which EN is infused into the distal small intestine (Coetzee *et al.*, 2014).

The general principles of nutritional management are as follows:

- Postoperatively, PN will be required immediately. Close attention should be paid to fluid and electrolyte balance (especially sodium and magnesium as losses may be very high).

- Enteral intake should be introduced as soon as possible while still continuing parenteral support. Initially, the patient's oral fluid intake should not exceed 500 mL/day.
- When fluids are tolerated, small meals and snacks can be gradually introduced. Food introduction to patients with very short bowel and likely to need long-term PN should aim to find a balance between eating for quality of life and avoiding high intestinal losses. For those likely to manage on diet alone, the aim should be to maximise intake to achieve adequate absorption.
- PN can be reduced as oral intake and absorption increases. However, parenteral fluids and/or oral rehydration solutions are likely to be needed until gut adaptation occurs. Additional nutritional support in the form of polymeric supplements or overnight enteral nutrition may be required. If the patient requires enteral nutrition, sodium needs to be added to increase the sodium content to >90 mmol/L. This can be achieved by adding 10 mL of 30% sodium chloride (50 mmol) to each litre of the ready-to-hang feeds; this may allow the patient to stop taking oral rehydration solution, or it can be used for flushing the enteral tube.
- As adaptation occurs, gradual transition to a more normal diet can be made, with inadequacies in nutrition or fluid intake being compensated by nutritional support measures.
- Since restoration of intestinal lactase levels is one of the last adaptive mechanisms to occur, large lactose loads may need to be avoided initially. However, there is no evidence that stable patients, either with or without a colon, benefit from a lactose-free diet (Arrigoni *et al.*, 1994). Therefore, foods containing lactose can be included in the diet as they are a valuable source of macro- and micronutrients.

For patients with short bowel, it is imperative they adhere to an appropriate regimen to maximise the remaining intestine and reduce dependence on PN. Patients who have significant bowel resections need to consume excessive oral nutrition to overcome malabsorption and avoid malnutrition. The exact composition of the diet depends on intestinal anatomy (Nordgaard *et al.*, 1994). Balance studies have shown energy requirements exceeding 2.5 times basal (30–60 kcal (125–250 kJ)/kg/day) and nitrogen intakes of 0.2–0.25 g/kg/day are required to prevent protein energy malnutrition (Crenn *et al.*, 2004; Messing *et al.*, 1991; Woolf *et al.*, 1987); the promotion of a hyperphagic diet is now established practice. For patients who have difficulties in achieving recommended oral macronutrient intakes, oral nutritional supplements or enteral nutrition may be required. Nocturnal enteral nutrition is often utilised to maximise absorption by increasing the length of time the bowel is exposed to nutrients. McIntyre *et al.* (1986) compared elemental versus polymeric formula and found no significant differences in macronutrient absorption. Cosnes *et al.* (1992) compared semi-elemental versus polymeric formula and demonstrated no differences, except improved nitrogen absorption with semi-elemental. The contrasting results in nitrogen absorption are likely to be related to the composition of the formulae investigated. Elemental formula has a higher osmolality and requires larger volumes to meet estimated nutritional requirements in comparison to polymeric formula. Therefore, if additional nutritional support is required, then a polymeric formula is recommended. Joly *et al.* (2009) found increased absorption of energy, nitrogen and fat with no increase in intestinal output while providing continuous enteral feeding as compared to usual diet alone. The continuous method of feeding may improve intestinal absorption to an extent that patients no longer require PN and should, therefore, be a treatment option for all patients with >75 cm of small bowel.

In practice, there are two types of patients with short bowel and it has become apparent that patients differ in their response to dietary manipulation depending on the presence or absence of a colon, and this determines whether the additional energy requirements should be provided from fat or carbohydrate (Table 7.4.10).

Patients with a jejunostomy

Patients have varying lengths of jejunum, ileum and colon removed. The remaining small bowel is then brought

Table 7.4.10 Summary of evidence-based recommendations for the dietary treatment for patients with short bowel

	Jejunocolic anastomosis	Stoma (jejunostomy)
Total energy	30–60 kcal/kg/day (125–250 kJ/kg/day)	30–60 kcal/kg/day (125–250 kJ/kg/day)
Nitrogen	0.2–0.25 g/kg/day	0.2–0.25 g/kg/day
Protein	1.25–1.5 g/kg/day	1.25–1.5 g/kg/day
Fat (% of total energy)	20–30	30–40
MCT (% if total fat)	50	No proven benefit
Carbohydrate (% of total energy)	50–60	40–50
Fibre	Low to moderate	Low
Sodium chloride	Normal	Additions usually required
Enteral nutrition	Polymeric	Polymeric

MCT, medium chain triglyceride.

to the surface of the abdomen to create a stoma (jejunostomy) (Figure 7.4.7). Patients have immediate problems postoperatively due to large intestinal losses from the jejunostomy leading to fluid and electrolyte depletion. Malnutrition will occur if appropriate nutritional support is not started. In addition, the patient will also experience a rapid transit time, reducing the potential for nutrient absorption and resulting in subsequent weight loss and malnutrition. Patients with short bowel absorb, on average, 50% of their oral fat intake (Crenn *et al.*, 2004). The role of fat restriction was controversial, with conflicting results from different studies (Andersson *et al.*, 1974; Hessov *et al.*, 1983; McIntyre *et al.*, 1986; Ovesen *et al.*, 1983; Woolf *et al.*, 1983). Overall, it appears that there is no significant benefit to patients following a low-fat diet, and, since fat provides a concentrated form of energy and makes the diet palatable in addition to providing essential fatty acids, malnourished patients should be encouraged to have a high intake of fat.

Due to rapid transit through the intestine, dietary fibre should be limited. McIntyre *et al.* (1986) conducted a randomised controlled trial in four jejunostomy patients who received diets with variable amounts of fat, fibre and carbohydrate over a 2–3-day period. No significant differences were observed, and they concluded there was no benefit from manipulating fibre in the diet. No further trials have investigated this, and, despite a lack of evidence, patients anecdotally report a reduction in intestinal output on a low-fibre diet. This advice is also recommended for patients with adhesions and/or strictures.

Patients with a jejunocolic anastomosis

Patients with a jejunocolic anastomosis have had the ileum and some jejunum resected, and the remaining jejunum anastomosed to the colon (Figure 7.4.8). Postoperatively, they experience diarrhoea and/or steatorrhoea with resultant malabsorption, weight loss and malnutrition. The presence of the colon in continuity is advantageous because it enables fluid and sodium to be absorbed, and results in a slower intestinal transit, aiding nutrient absorption. A comparison of the effects of a diet either high in carbohydrate (60%) and low in fat (20%), or vice versa (20% carbohydrate and 60% fat), found that patients with a colon absorbed more energy on the high-carbohydrate, low-fat diet. This suggests that patients with a colon salvage energy as a result of the fermentation of unabsorbed carbohydrate to short-chain fatty acids, which are easily absorbed (Nordgaard *et al.*, 1994). Colonic digestion can supply up to 1000 kcal (4.19 kJ)/day (Nordgaard *et al.*, 1996); therefore, patients should be encouraged to consume a high-carbohydrate diet without causing bloating due to increased gas production. A reduction in fat intake is often helpful as this decreases magnesium and calcium losses, and reduces steatorrhoea/diarrhoea and oxalate absorption (Lennard-Jones, 1994). However, a reduced fat intake will also reduce energy intake, and so, in practice, a compromise has to be found between including fat for energy and avoiding steatorrhoea. Replacement of long-chain triglycerides (LCTs) with medium-chain triglycerides (MCTs) has been shown to increase energy and fat absorption in patients with a colon (Jeppesen &

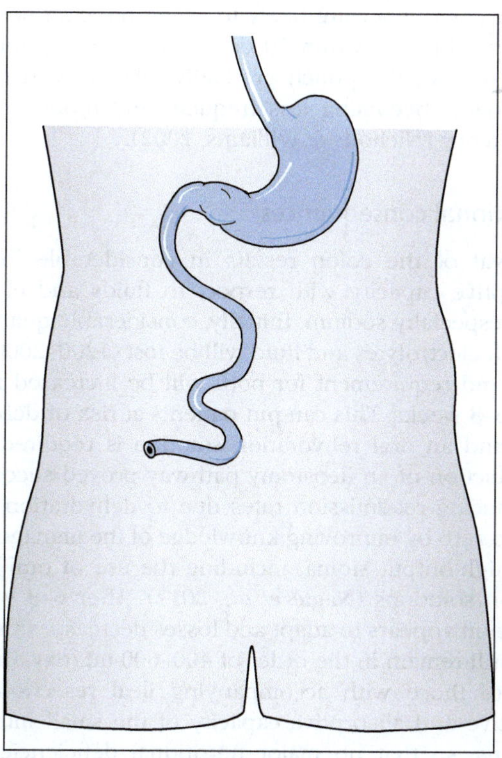

Figure 7.4.7 Jejunostomy (courtesy of Northwest London Hospital Trust, Medical Illustrations Department)

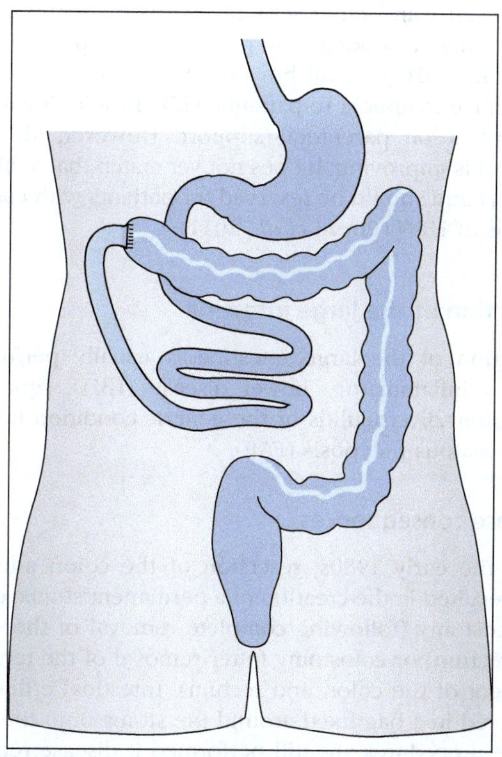

Figure 7.4.8 Jejunocolic anastomosis (courtesy of Northwest London Hospital Trust, Medical Illustrations Department)

Mortensen, 1998). A secondary consequence of steatorrhoea is the greater risk of calcium oxalate renal stones, owing to increased colonic oxalate absorption and the resultant hyperoxaluria. A low-oxalate diet is advisable that restricts intake of tea, spinach, beetroot, rhubarb, peanuts and chocolate. Avoiding chronic dehydration is also important for reducing the risk of renal stones (Nightingale *et al.*, 1992).

In conclusion, patients with short bowel need to consume more than the average estimated requirements of energy and protein to compensate for lack of absorptive capacity. Patients with a jejunostomy will benefit from a high-fat diet, whereas those with a colon should focus on increasing the carbohydrate content of the diet (see Table 7.4.10). Close dietetic supervision is vital during the early stages and until intestinal adaptation has taken place. Manipulation of the diet and changes in medication should be staged, with several days allowed for each stage to assess the impact of each change on intestinal output. Each patient is unique, and a lot of time and patience will hence be needed to find the optimum combination for each individual. Patients benefit from the support of a multidisciplinary team where there is close liaison between doctors, nurses, dietitians and pharmacists.

Future advances in treatment

Glucagon-like peptide 2 (GLP 2), a hormone secreted by the intestine, has been shown to increase the growth of normal cells in the intestine, allowing the intestine to absorb more fluid and nutrients, which may help to reduce dependency on PN. An analogue of GLP 2 (teduglutide) has demonstrated improvements in nutritional status and reductions in parenteral requirements in patients dependent on parenteral support (Jeppesen *et al.*, 2011). Small bowel transplantation offers an alternative treatment to patients with chronic IF who are dependent on parenteral support. However, although survival is improving, it does not yet match that achieved by HPN and should be reserved for patients with complications of HPN (Pironi *et al.*, 2011).

Resection of the large intestine

Resection of the large intestine is usually performed due to inflammatory bowel disease (IBD), cancer of the colon, diverticulitis or the genetic condition familial adenomatous polyposis (FAP).

Disease consequences

Until the early 1980s, resection of the colon and rectum resulted in the creation of a permanent stoma, either an ileostomy (following complete removal of the colon and rectum) or colostomy (after removal of the terminal segment of the colon and rectum). Intestinal effluent is collected in a bag fixed around the stoma onto the skin. These procedures are still performed if disease requires such extensive rectal resection that no functioning muscle tissue in the anal area remains, e.g. IBD. A major improvement has occurred with the development of the restorative proctocolectomy, a procedure that involves the creation of a pouch reservoir from a segment of ileum, which is then joined to the anus. The pouch acts as an artificial rectum, thus conserving anal continence and avoiding the need for a stoma. This technique is commonly used to treat patients with ulcerative colitis or FAP, and is much more acceptable to patients than a permanent ileostomy.

Ileal pouches derive their name from the number of limbs of ileum used in their fashioning (J pouch, S pouch and W pouch). These surgical procedures, which anastomose different pouch types to the anal canal (the ileal pouch anal anastomosis), share a common methodology. Ileal reservoirs can also be constructed without an ileal pouch by anal anastomosis, e.g. the continent ileal reservoir or Kock pouch, but these procedures are now less frequently performed (Sofo *et al.*, 2016).

Pouch creation is complex, and the operation is often done in two stages. First, colectomy (removal of the colon) and proctectomy (removal of diseased rectal mucosa) are performed, leaving the rectal muscular cuff and anal sphincter intact. A pseudo-rectum (pouch) is constructed by joining a portion of the terminal ileum to the anal canal, and a temporary ileostomy is created to divert bowel contents away from the newly formed pouch, allowing it to heal. A further operation then anastomoses the pouch to the intestine and reverses the ileostomy. The safety, feasibility and short-term outcome of performing this operation laparoscopically has demonstrated no difference in mortality and complications as compared to open surgery (Ahmed Ali *et al.*, 2009). Following surgery, problems with stool frequency and/or consistency are likely to occur, but continence is usually achieved within 10 days, and, over a period of about 1 year, the pouch gradually adapts, with bowel movements becoming less frequent and more solid in consistency (Nicholls & Williams, 2002).

Nutritional consequences

Removal of the colon results in considerable loss of absorptive capacity with respect to fluids and electrolytes, especially sodium. Initially, considerable quantities of both electrolytes and fluid will be lost (1200–2000 mL/day), and requirement for both will be increased for at least 6–8 weeks. This can put patients at risk of dehydration, and an oral rehydration solution is required. The introduction of an ileostomy pathway proved successful in reducing readmission rates due to dehydration from 15% to zero by improving knowledge of the management of a high-output stoma, including the use of oral rehydration solutions (Nagle *et al.*, 2012). After 6–8 weeks, the ileum appears to adapt and losses decrease, although they still remain in the order of 400–600 mL/day. In contrast to those with accompanying ileal resection, the digestive and absorptive capacity of the small intestine remains, so that no major nutritional deficiencies are to be expected, except for vitamin B_{12} and bile acids, which occur in about one-third of patients (Christl & Scheppach, 1997). Patients with an ileostomy may be chronically dehydrated and have depleted calcium and magnesium stores, putting them at risk of renal impairment, renal stones and bone demineralisation, supporting the use of oral rehydration solutions (Ng *et al.*, 2013).

Nutritional assessment

Anthropometry

Patients may be malnourished prior to surgery, and their nutritional risk will need to be identified and action taken in order to avoid a deterioration in nutritional status and poor surgical outcome (Fulham, 2004). Assessment of nutritional status should include weight, BMI, percentage weight loss, MAC, TST, MAMC and grip strength.

Biochemistry

Do they appear dehydrated or overloaded? The administration of excessive volumes of 0.9% sodium chloride is common and can exacerbate postoperative ileus (Lobo *et al.*, 2002). Are there any electrolyte deficiencies, i.e. potassium, magnesium, sodium? Urine sodium is a useful indicator of dehydration. Are there any micronutrient deficiencies, i.e. folate, iron, selenium, zinc, vitamin D or B_{12}. If >100 cm of terminal ileum is resected, the patient will require vitamin B_{12} injections every 3 months.

Clinical assessment

Ongoing sepsis will result in increased nutritional requirements and a higher risk of metabolic and infective complications. Assessment of fluid balance is crucial (NICE, 2013), aiming for an intestinal output of <1500 mL/day.

Dietary assessment

Determine the perioperative nutritional intake and compare with estimated requirements. Patients undergoing surgery who fail to regain adequate gastrointestinal function after day 5 should be referred to a dietitian or nutrition support team.

Economic and social assessment

Postoperative complications can cause prolonged hospital stay, resulting in increased healthcare cost. Factors contributing to reduced quality of life for patients include:

- Infection, including intra-abdominal sepsis.
- Inadequate wound and stoma care, which can result in excoriated skin.
- High intestinal losses leading to dehydration and electrolyte disturbances.
- Poor provision of nutrition, resulting in malnutrition.
- Immobility.
- Depression.

All of the preceding factors increase the length of rehabilitation, during which the patient is unable to return to work and family life.

Clinical management

Perioperative fasting in gastrointestinal surgery is no longer recommended, and early enteral feeding should be encouraged (Fearon *et al.*, 2005; Gustafsson *et al.*, 2012; Osland *et al.*, 2011). The long-term consequences in terms of faecal volume and biochemistry appear to be similar in patients after restorative proctocolectomy with a J pouch and conventional panproctocolectomy and permanent ileostomy (Okamoto *et al.*, 1995). However, due to the kidneys' attempt to conserve water and sodium, both groups of patients are at greater risk of uric acid stones as a result of producing urine that is low in volume and pH, and with a high concentration of calcium and oxalate (Christie *et al.*, 1996). In addition, J pouch patients may be at increased risk of calcium stones and abnormal bile acid metabolism. Pouchitis, inflammation within the pouch, can occur in up to 50% of patients. Symptoms include increased pouch frequency, reduced stool consistency and urgency, and patients usually respond well to antibiotics. The probiotic *VSL#3* may be beneficial in maintaining remission of pouchitis (Singh *et al.*, 2015).

Nutritional management

While the ileum is adapting and the stool or stomal effluent remains liquid, fluid losses should be replaced by 1.5–2 L/day of fluid. Additional salt, e.g. up to 1 tsp added to food during the course of a day, may be necessary in hot weather or if losses are particularly high. As stool frequency and consistency improve, losses will decrease, but it remains important to ensure adequate fluid and sodium provision. An episode of vomiting or diarrhoea can rapidly create an electrolyte imbalance, and the provision of extra potassium (via fruit juices) and sodium (via extra salt in food or salty beverages such as soup or meat extracts) is advisable (Pearson, 2008). An oral rehydration solution is recommended, and, in severe cases, parenteral saline may be necessary. High-output stomas (>2 L/d) are common, and require identification of the cause and ongoing fluid and electrolyte therapy in conjunction with nutrition support (Baker *et al.*, 2011).

Many patients will be nutritionally depleted after colorectal surgery, particularly if they suffered chronic ill health beforehand and nutritional intake was poor. If, as in the case of pouch patients, two, or even three, operations are required, this is a further strain on the nutritional status. It is therefore important that patients are encouraged to consume small, frequent, nutrient-dense meals and snacks, and that additional oral nutritional support measures are instituted when necessary. A return to normal body composition in ulcerative colitis patients undergoing J pouch has been described (Christie & Hill, 1990; Jensen *et al.*, 2002).

Dietary guidance for ileostomy and pouch patients is similar. People should be encouraged to:

- Adopt a regular meal pattern. Some may need smaller meals at more frequent intervals. Those with pouches may need to avoid eating late at night to avoid nocturnal stool production.

- Eat a varied diet based on healthy eating principles.
- Consume meals slowly, and chew foods well.
- Drink plenty of fluids (1.5–2 L/day) and more in hot weather.
- Consume extra fluid and salt if stool or stoma losses suddenly increase, or during episodes of vomiting or fever. Medical advice may be needed if losses are severe or persistent.

The range of foods consumed can be gradually increased, and patients should be encouraged to eat a healthy normal diet. No foods are specifically contraindicated for ileostomy or pouch patients, but some foods can cause unpleasant symptoms such as stool odour or flatulence. Blockage with undigested food can occur, particularly if the stoma or anastomosis is tight. Occasionally, a low-fibre diet is required if obstruction regularly occurs. However, in most people, this is unnecessary, and avoidance of the specific foods that typically cause the problem is sufficient. There is a small amount of evidence (Culkin, 2014; Pearson, 2008) on food-related problems in ileostomy/pouch patients, and commonly reported associations include the following:

- *Poorly digested foods (most likely to cause blockage)* – grapefruit, lettuce, mushrooms, sweetcorn, fruit or vegetable skins, lentils, peas, nuts, seeds, tomatoes, coconut, fibrous fruit and vegetables such as celery or pineapple, and Chinese food.
- *Increased stool odour* – onions, garlic, brassica vegetables, beans, fish and eggs.
- *Increased flatulence/bloating* – baked beans, lentils, peas, onions, garlic, brassica vegetables, fizzy drinks, beer and lager.
- *Increased stool frequency* – beer, spirits, Chinese food, whole-wheat cereals, corn, apples, wine, fried and spicy foods, strawberries, potatoes, bread, bananas, fruit, fruit juice and vegetables.
- *Decrease in stool consistency* – beer, wine, fried fish, strawberries, corn, popcorn, spirits, coleslaw, grapefruit, turnips, raspberries and fruit juice.
- *Perianal irritation* – spicy foods, citrus fruit, raw carrot, nuts and seeds.

It appears that the majority of patients with an ileal pouch report that some dietary restriction is required to help prevent unpleasant symptoms, and that this impacts on quality of life (Coffey *et al.*, 2002). However, it should be remembered that individual tolerance may vary considerably, so patients should be encouraged to discover for themselves which foods are best managed. Patients should also be warned that foods such as beetroot could change the colour of the stool to such an extent that it can be mistaken for bleeding. Continuing problems with stool frequency may be treated with loperamide. There is no evidence that supplementary fibre in the form of pectin or methylcellulose is helpful in this respect (Thirlby & Kelly, 1997). A proof-of-concept study investigated the effect of a fermentable oligo-, di- and mono-saccharides and polyols (FODMAP) diet on bowel function in patients without a colon and reported a high prevalence of carbohydrate malabsorption, which the authors hypothesised may benefit from a reduction in FODMAP intake (Croagh *et al.*, 2007). All patients should receive regular follow-up to ensure that diet-related problems are remedied, unnecessary food restrictions avoided, and adequate fluid status and nutritional status are maintained.

Drug–nutrient interactions

The following should be noted:

- ***Proton pump inhibitors*** – no interaction with food or nutrients demonstrated.
- *Loperamide* – no interaction with food or nutrients demonstrated. Aim to avoid syrup formulations, as these contain sorbitol, which can act as a laxative.
- *Octreotide* – no information available.
- *Codeine* – no information available.
- *Colestyramine* – no interaction with food or nutrients demonstrated. Other drugs should be taken at least 1 hour before or 4–6 hours after food intake to reduce possible interference with absorption.

Further reading

Birch J. (2008) *Stomacare*, 1st edn. Chichester: Wiley Blackwell, p. 210.

Culkin A. (2014) Intestinal failure and nutrition. In: Lomer M (ed) *Advanced Nutrition and Dietetics in Gastroenterology*, 1st edn. Chichester: Wiley Blackwell, p. 210.

Culkin A. (2014) Stomas and nutrition. In: Lomer M (ed) *Advanced Nutrition and Dietetics in Gastroenterology*, 1st edn. Chichester: Wiley Blackwell, p. 218.

Langnas A, Goulet O, Quigley E, Tappenden K. (2008) *Intestinal Failure*, 1st edn. New York, NY: John Wiley & Sons.

Williams J. (2002) *The Essentials of Pouch Care Nursing*, 1st edn. London: Whurr, p. 165.

Internet resources

Crohn's and Colitis UK (formerly known as NACC), www.crohnsandcolitis.org.uk

Ileostomy and Internal Pouch Support Group, www.iasupport.org.uk

Patients on Intravenous and Nasogastric Nutrition Therapy (PINNT), www.pinnt.com

References

Ahmed Ali U, Keus F, Heikens J, *et al.* (2009) Open versus laparoscopic (assisted) ileo pouch anal anastomosis for ulcerative colitis and familial adenomatous polyposis. *Cochrane Database Syst. Rev.* (1): CD006267.

Andersson H, Isaksson B, Sjögren B. (1974) Fat-reduced diet in the symptomatic treatment of small bowel disease: metabolic studies in patients with Crohn's disease and in other patients subjected to ileal resection. *Gut.* 15: 351–359.

Arrigoni E, Marteau P, Briet F, *et al.* (1994) Tolerance and absorption of lactose from milk and yogurt during short bowel syndrome in humans. *Am. J. Clin. Nutr.* 60: 926–929.

Baker M, Williams R, Nightingale J. (2011) Causes and management of a high-output stoma. *Colorectal Dis.* 13(2): 191–197.

Carlson GL. (2003) Surgical management of intestinal failure. *Proc. Nutr. Soc.* 62(3): 711–718.

Christie PM, Hill GL. (1990) Return to normal body composition after ileoanal J-pouch anastomosis for ulcerative colitis. *Dis. Colon Rectum*. 33: 584–586.

Christie PM, Knight GS, Hill GL. (1996) Comparison of relative risks of urinary stone formation after surgery for ulcerative colitis: conventional ileostomy vs. *J-pouch. A comparative study. Dis. Colon Rectum*. 39: 50–54.

Christl SU, Scheppach W. (1997) Metabolic consequences of total colectomy. *Scand. J. Gastroenterol. Suppl.* 222: 20–24.

Coetzee E, Rahim Z, Boutall A, *et al.* (2014) Refeeding enteroclysis as an alternative to parenteral nutrition for enteric fistula. *Colorectal Dis.* 16(10): 823–830.

Coffey JC, Winter DC, Neary P, *et al.* (2002) Quality of life after ileal pouch-anal anastomosis: an evaluation of diet and other factors using the Cleveland Global Quality of Life instrument. *Dis. Colon Rectum*. 45: 30–38.

Cosnes J, Evard D, Beaugerie L, *et al.* (1992*) Improvement in protein absorption with a small-peptide-based diet in patients with high jejunostomy. Nutrition*. 8: 406–411.

Crenn P, Morin MC, Joly F, *et al.* (2004) Net digestive absorption and adaptive hyperphagia in adult short bowel patients. *Gut*. 53: 1279–1286.

Croagh C, Shepherd SJ, Berryman M, *et al.* (2007) Pilot study on the effect of reducing dietary FODMAP intake on bowel function in patients without a colon. *Inflamm. Bowel Dis.* 13: 1522–1528.

Culkin A. (2014) Stomas and nutrition. In: Lomer M (ed) *Advanced Nutrition and Dietetics in Gastroenterology*, 1st edn. Chichester: Wiley Blackwell, p. 218.

Fearon KC, Ljungqvist O, Von Meyenfeldt M, *et al.* (2005) Enhanced recovery after surgery: A consensus review of clinical care for patients undergoing colonic resection. *Clin. Nutr.* 24: 466–477.

Fulham J. (2004) Improving the nutritional status of colorectal surgical and stoma patients. *Br. J. Nurs.* 13: 702–708.

Gustafsson U, Scott M, Schwenk W, *et al.* (2012) Guidelines for perioperative care in elective colonic surgery: Enhanced Recovery After Surgery (ERAS®) Society recommendations. *Clin. Nutr.* 31(6): 783–800.

Hessov I, Andersson H, Isaksson B. (1983) Effects of a low-fat diet on mineral absorption in small-bowel disease. *Scand. J. Gastroenterol.* 18: 551–554.

Hofstetter S, Stern L, Willet J. (2013) Key issues in addressing the clinical and humanistic burden of short bowel syndrome in the US. *Curr. Med. Res. Opin.* 29(5): 495–504.

Jensen MB, Houborg KB, Vestergaard P, *et al.* (2002) Improved physical performance and increased lean tissue and fat mass in patients with ulcerative colitis four to six years after ileoanal anastomosis with a J-pouch. *Dis. Colon Rectum*. 45: 1601–1607.

Jeppesen PB, Mortensen PB. (1998) The influence of a preserved colon on the absorption of medium chain fat in patients with small bowel resection. *Gut*. 43: 478–483.

Jeppesen PB, Staun M, Tjellesen L, *et al.* (1998) Effect of intravenous ranitidine and omeprazole on intestinal absorption of water, sodium, and macronutrients in patients with intestinal resection. *Gut*. 43: 763–769.

Jeppesen P, Gilroy R, Pertkiewicz M, *et al.* (2011) Randomised placebo-controlled trial of teduglutide in reducing parenteral nutrition and/or intravenous fluid requirements in patients with short bowel syndrome. *Gut*. 60(7): 902–914.

Joly F, Dray X, Corcos O, *et al.* (2009) Tube feeding improves intestinal absorption in short bowel syndrome patients. *Gastroenterology*. 136: 824–831.

Klek S, Forbes A, Gabe S, *et al.* (2016) Management of acute intestinal failure: a position paper from the European Society for Clinical Nutrition and Metabolism (ESPEN) Special Interest Group. *Clin. Nutr.* 35(6): 1209–1218.

Lauverjat M, Hadjaissa A, Vanhems P, *et al.* (2006) Chronic dehydration may impair renal function in patients with chronic intestinal failure on long-term parenteral nutrition. *Clin. Nutr.* 25(1): 75–81.

Lennard-Jones JE. (1994) Review article: practical management of the short bowel. *Aliment. Pharmacol. Ther.* 8: 563–577.

Lloyd DA, Gabe SM, Windsor AC. (2006) Nutrition and management of enterocutaneous fistula. *Br. J. Surg.* 93: 1045–1055.

Lobo DN, Bostock K, Neal KR, *et al.* (2002) Effect of salt and water balance on recovery of gastrointestinal function after elective colonic resection: a randomised controlled trial. *Lancet*. 359: 1812–1818.

Mainguet P, Fiasse R. (1977) Double-blind placebo-controlled study of loperamide (Imodium) in chronic diarrhoea caused by ileocolic disease or resection. *Gut*. 18: 575–579.

Martinez-Riquelme A, Rawlings J, Morley S, *et al.* (2005) Self-administered subcutaneous fluid infusion at home in the management of fluid depletion and hypomagnesaemia in gastro-intestinal disease. *Clin. Nutr.* 24: 158–163.

McIntyre PB, Fitchew M, Lennard-Jones JE. (1986) Patients with a high jejunostomy do not need a special diet. *Gastroenterology*. 91: 25–33.

Messing B, Pigot F, Rongier M, *et al.* (1991) Intestinal absorption of free oral hyperalimentation in the very short bowel syndrome. *Gastroenterology*. 100: 1502–1508.

Nagle D, Pare T, Keenan E, *et al.* (2012) Ileostomy pathway virtually eliminates readmissions for dehydration in new ostomates. *Dis. Colon Rectum* 55(12): 1266–1272.

National Confidential Enquiry into Patient Outcome and Death (NCEPOD). (2010) *A mixed bag: an enquiry into the care of hospital patients receiving parenteral nutrition*. Available at https://www.ncepod.org.uk/2010pn.html. Accessed 26 October 2018.

Ng D, Pither C, Wootton S, *et al.* (2013) The 'not so short-bowel syndrome': potential health problems in patients with an ileostomy. *Colorectal Dis.* 15(9): 1154–1161.

NICE. (2013) *Intravenous fluid therapy in adults in hospital: guidance and guidelines*. Available at https://www.nice.org.uk/Guidance/cg174. Accessed 26 October 2018.

Nicholls RJ, Williams J. (2002) The ileo-anal pouch. In: Williams J (ed) *The Essentials of Pouch Care Nursing*. London: Whurr Publishers Ltd, pp. 68–98.

Nightingale JMD. (1994) Clinical problems of a short bowel and their treatment. *Proc. Nutr. Soc.* 53: 373–391.

Nightingale JMD. (2001) Management of a high-output jejunostomy. In: Nightingale JMD (ed) *Intestinal Failure*. London: Greenwich Medical Media Limited, pp. 375–392.

Nightingale JMD, Lennard-Jones JE, Walker ER, *et al.* (1990) Jejunal efflux in short bowel syndrome. *Lancet*. 336: 765–768.

Nightingale JMD, Lennard-Jones JE, Gertner DJ, *et al.* (1992) Colonic preservation reduces the need for parenteral therapy, increases incidence of renal stones, but does not change the high prevalence of gall stones in patients with a short bowel. *Gut*. 33: 1493–1497.

Nightingale JMD, Walker ER, Farthing MJG, *et al.* (1991) Effect of omeprazole on intestinal output in the short bowel syndrome. *Aliment. Pharmacol. Ther.* 5: 405–412.

Nordgaard I, Hansen BS, Mortensen PB. (1994) Colon as a digestive organ in patients with short bowel. *Lancet*. 343: 373–376.

Nordgaard I, Hansen BS, Mortensen PB. (1996) Importance of colonic support for energy absorption as small bowel failure proceeds. *Am. J. Clin. Nutr.* 64: 222–231.

Okamoto T, Kusunoki M, Kusuhara K, *et al.* (1995) Water and electrolyte balance after ileal J pouch-anal anastomosis in ulcerative colitis and familial adenomatous polyposis. *Int. J. Colorectal Dis.* 10: 33–38.

Osland E, Yunus R, Khan S, *et al.* (2011) Early versus traditional postoperative feeding in patients undergoing resectional gastrointestinal surgery. *JPEN J. Parenter. Enteral Nutr.* 35(4): 473–487.

Ovesen L, Chu R, Howard L. (1983) The influence of dietary fat on jejunostomy output in patients with severe short bowel syndrome. *Am. J. Clin. Nutr.* 38: 270–277.

Pearson M. (2008) Nutrition. In: Birch J (ed) *Stoma Care*. Chichester: Wiley Blackwell, pp. 210–232.

Pironi L, Arends J, Bozzetti F, *et al.* (2016) ESPEN guidelines on chronic intestinal failure in adults. *Clin. Nutr.* 35(2): 247–307.

Pironi L, Goulet O, Buchman A, *et al.* (2012) Outcome on home parenteral nutrition for benign intestinal failure: a review of the literature and benchmarking with the European prospective survey of ESPEN. *Clin. Nutr.* 31(6): 831–845.

Pironi L, Joly F, Forbes A, *et al.* (2011) Long-term follow-up of patients on home parenteral nutrition in Europe: implications for intestinal transplantation. *Gut.* 60(1): 17–25.

Rahbour G, Siddiqui M, Ullah M, *et al.* (2012) A meta-analysis of outcomes following use of somatostatin and its analogues for the management of enterocutaneous fistulas. *Ann. Surg.* 256(6): 946–954.

Rodrigues CA, Lennard-Jones JE, Thompson DG, *et al.* (1989) The effects of octreotide, soy polysaccharide, codeine and loperamide on nutrient, fluid and electrolyte absorption in the short-bowel syndrome. *Aliment. Pharmacol. Ther.* 3: 159–169.

Schalamon J, Mayr J, Hallwarth M. (2003) Mortality and economics in short bowel syndrome. *Best Pract. Res. Clin. Gastroenterol.* 17(6): 931–942.

Singh S, Stroud A, Holubar S, *et al.* (2015) Treatment and prevention of pouchitis after ileal pouch-anal anastomosis for chronic ulcerative colitis. *Cochrane Database Syst. Rev. Cochrane Database Syst. Rev.* (11): CD001176.

Smith T, Naghibi M, *on behalf of the BANS committee* (2016) *BANS Report 2016 Artificial Nutrition Support in the UK 2005–2015 Adult Home Parenteral Nutrition & Home Intravenous Fluids.* Available at http://www.bapen.org.uk/images/pdfs/reports/bans-report-2016.pdf. Accessed 26 October 2018.

Sofo L, Caprino P, Sacchetti F, *et al.* (2016) Restorative proctocolectomy with ileal pouch-anal anastomosis for ulcerative colitis: a narrative review. *World J. Gastrointest. Surg.* 8(8): 556–563.

Thirlby RC, Kelly R. (1997) Pectin and methylcellulose do not affect intestinal function in patients after ileal pouch-anal anastomosis. *Am. J. Gastroenterol.* 92: 99–102.

Woolf GM, Miller C, Kurian R, *et al.* (1983) Diet for patients with a short bowel: high fat or high carbohydrate? *Gastroenterology.* 84: 823–828.

Woolf GM, Miller C, Kurian R, *et al.* (1987) Nutritional absorption in short bowel syndrome. Evaluation of fluid, calorie, and divalent cation requirements. *Dig. Dis. Sci.* 37: 8–15.

7.4.10 Irritable bowel syndrome

Yvonne McKenzie

Key points

- Irritable bowel syndrome is a common, chronic gastrointestinal disorder of gut–brain interaction.
- Management aims to improve symptoms and quality of life, and may require a combined lifestyle, dietary and pharmacological approach.
- Dietary management is evidence-based with first-line (healthy eating and lifestyle) and second-line (low-fermentable oligo-, di-, mono-saccharides and polyol (FODMAP) diet) approaches.
- Successful management requires advanced dietetic knowledge with an understanding of potential physiological and co-existing or differential pathophysiological mechanisms, adequate clinical time and up-to-date, accurate patient resources.
- For long-term self-management, patient empowerment should be supported.

Irritable bowel syndrome (IBS) is a common, chronic fluctuating gastrointestinal disorder characterised by recurrent abdominal pain associated with defaecation or a change in bowel habits (Lacy *et al.*, 2016). Global prevalence is 7–21% (Lovell & Ford, 2012). With functional dyspepsia, IBS accounts for 40–60% of all gastroenterology outpatient referrals (Jones *et al.*, 2000). It was first described in 1818 (Thompson, 2006). Since then, diagnostic criteria and treatment options have evolved, but the heterogeneity of IBS continues to challenge clinicians. Patients frequently alter what they eat in an attempt to alleviate symptoms (Halpert *et al.*, 2007). Dietitians have an important role in the first-line and second-line management of IBS (NICE, 2015c). Globally, the BDA were the first to publish fully comprehensive evidence-based guidelines for the dietary management of IBS in adults using a robust methodology (McKenzie *et al.*, 2016), an update to their initial ones for national clinical practice (McKenzie *et al.*, 2012).

Diagnostic criteria

There is no test to objectively diagnose IBS. NICE (2008) gives positive, cost-effective symptom-based diagnostic criteria (Box 7.4.1), reinforced by their Quality Standard for primary care clinical practice to reduce over-investigation (NICE, 2016). Red flag indicators prompt secondary care referral for investigation of more serious pathologies, such as signs and symptoms of cancer in line with the NICE (2015a) guidance NG12, or inflammatory markers for inflammatory bowel disease (NICE, 2016). In research, the more complex Rome criteria are used. The most recent are the Rome IV criteria (Drossman & Hasler, 2016), a major update over the last 25 years, with a shift away from IBS being termed a functional disorder, in which no organic, biochemical or metabolic abnormalities have been identified, to one of gut–brain interaction.

Box 7.4.1 Positive diagnostic criteria for IBS (NICE, 2008)

For at least 6 months:

Abdominal pain or discomfort
Relieved by defaecation or
Associated with altered bowel frequency or stool form

And, at least *two* of the following:

Altered stool passage (straining, urgency, incomplete evacuation)
Abdominal bloating
Symptoms made worse by eating
Passage of mucus.
Supporting diagnosis – lethargy, nausea, backache and bladder symptoms

Tests: full blood count (FBC), erythrocyte sedimentation rate (ESR), C-reactive protein (CRP), and antibody testing for coeliac disease – endomysial antibodies (EMA) or tissue transglutaminase (TTG).

Classification

The Rome IV symptom-based diagnostic criteria (Lacy *et al.*, 2016) use the Bristol Stool Scale (Heaton *et al.*, 1992) to assess stool consistency and classify four recognised subtypes of IBS (Table 7.4.11). The criteria are as follows:

- Recurrent abdominal pain, on average, at least 1 day a week in the last 3 months, agreeing with two or more of the following:
  1. Related to defecation.
  2. Associated with a change in frequency of stools.
  3. Associated with a change in form (consistency) of stools.
- Symptom onset must have started at least 6 months before diagnosis and must be present for the last 3 months.

Disease processes

Many mechanisms have been proposed to explain pathophysiology and symptom generation. These include genetic and psychological factors, visceral hypersensitivity, motility disturbance, low-grade inflammation, immune-mediated reactions and food hypersensitivity, as well as altered gastrointestinal microbiota (dysbiosis) (Farmer & Aziz, 2014).

Table 7.4.11 IBS subtypes and predominant stool forms

IBS with	Subtype	Bristol Stool Form Scale: predominant form
Diarrhoea	IBS-D	Types 6, 7
Constipation	IBS-C	Types 1, 2
Diarrhoea/ constipation – mixed	IBS-M	Types 6, 7 and 1, 2
Unspecified	IBS-U	Type 3, 4

Disease consequences

IBS depreciates quality of life and is associated with substantial healthcare costs (Agarwal & Spiegel, 2011). Symptoms vary both within and between individuals. Bloating is the second-most bothersome symptom after pain (Ringel *et al.*, 2009); distension may cause the abdominal girth to increase by >10 cm during the day. There are no long-term complications of IBS, although an insufficient dietary fibre intake is associated with diverticular disease (Painter, 1985). Comorbidity with somatic and chronic pain disorders, such as in fibromyalgia, chronic fatigue syndrome, temporomandibular joint disorder, chronic pelvic pain, non-ulcer dyspepsia, biliary dyskinesia, anxiety, depression and migraine, can exacerbate symptoms (Quigley *et al.*, 2016; Spiller *et al.*, 2007). Individuals with IBS have a normal life expectancy (Chang *et al.*, 2010).

Patient perspective

Many people with IBS suffer in silence due to lack of awareness of the condition or ineffective treatment, but they should not feel alone with the burden of their diagnosis (Brandt *et al.*, 2009). Misconceptions exist about IBS being caused by dietary habits and colitis, worsening with age, causing malnutrition or developing into cancer (Halpert *et al.*, 2007). Therefore, patient reassurance, management of patient expectations and follow-up (NICE, 2016) are important once diagnosis is established.

Gastroenterology patients view diet as having an important role in their condition, and, while a large proportion of patients are interested in receiving dietary advice, few expect to receive it in clinic (Adesokan & Neild, 2012). Individuals may self-manage symptoms by having food intolerance testing. There is international expert agreement that serum IgG4 is irrelevant in the diagnosis of food allergy or intolerance and should not be measured to account for food-related symptoms (Bock, 2010; Carr *et al.*, 2012; Stapel *et al.*, 2008).

Public health aspects

Access to clean public toilets can be a major issue for individuals with IBS. The UK's national charity for IBS, The IBS Network, supports people with IBS, and campaigns on their behalf. They offer a Radar key to help members access public toilets, and a 'Can't Wait' card scheme for the members' international use as well as within the UK.

Nutritional consequences

Studies report that 62–89% of IBS patients limited or avoided food items or food groups (e.g. dairy) to improve symptoms (Böhn *et al.*, 2013; Hayes *et al.*, 2014; Monsbakken *et al.*, 2006). However, in general, the dietary intakes of IBS patients are likely to be similar to that of the general population's intakes and recommendations, as seen from the EPIC food frequency questionnaire (Williams *et al.*, 2011) and an unvalidated Swedish questionnaire (Böhn *et al.*, 2013). The nutritional consequences of self-imposed first-line and second-line dietary management are unknown. In dietitian-led low-fermentable oligo-, di-, mono-saccharides and polyol (FODMAP) dietary intervention, specific attention to energy, carbohydrate and calcium intakes may be warranted (Staudacher, 2017). Longer-term data showed that calcium intakes met nutrient recommendations using dietitian-led delivery with expertise in FODMAP education (Martin *et al.*, 2015). Restriction of FODMAPs reduces the short-chain oligosaccharide components of dietary fibre by 4 g/day as compared to habitual diet (Staudacher *et al.*, 2012). Advice on increasing intake of low-FODMAP high-fibre foods may be warranted to meet recommendations on dietary fibre (SACN, 2015), and those on healthy eating for the general population (PHE, 2014).

Assessment

Most patients are diagnosed and managed in primary care (Thompson *et al.*, 2000). Guidelines for the diagnosis and management of IBS in primary care (NICE, 2015c addendum) highlight the importance of avoiding unnecessary investigations to confirm diagnosis and of good communication with the patient, supported by evidence-based information. Dietitians should use evidence-based IBS guidelines (McKenzie *et al.*, 2012, 2016). Assessment should follow the ABCDE format.

Anthropometry

Bodyweight, body mass index (BMI) and weight history should be assessed.

Biochemistry

The tests shown in Box 7.4.1 should be conducted to exclude other diagnoses. Check that coeliac disease screening was done when the individual was consuming gluten in more than one meal every day for at least 6 weeks (NICE, 2015b). If coeliac serology (endomysial antibodies, or tissue transglutaminase) has not been checked, it should be measured prior to changing gluten intake. Other biochemistry, e.g. haematinics, should be normal (see Chapter 7.4.7, Coeliac disease).

Clinical

Clinical history should record the presence of allergies, family history of gastrointestinal problems (e.g. coeliac disease, inflammatory bowel disease), IBS medication, and use of food/nutritional supplements. Patient-reporting of the IBS symptom profile before and after intervention is essential. There is no widely adopted, validated method for measuring IBS symptom outcomes in clinical practice. The Bristol Stool Form Scale (Heaton *et al.*, 1992) enables IBS subtyping (Lacy *et al.*, 2016). In research, the IBS Symptom Severity Score (IBS-SSS) (Francis *et al.*, 1997) and the Gastrointestinal Symptom Rating Scale (GSRS) (Svedlund *et al.*, 1988) are the most widely recognised validated tools. It is important to discuss IBS with patients to ensure they understand that it is a positive diagnosis.

Faecal calprotectin is a cost-effective sensitive marker of intestinal inflammation that is used to differentiate functional symptoms from active IBD in secondary and primary care (NICE, 2013). Hydrogen breath testing may help to identify the dietary management strategy that is the most appropriate (see Chapter 7.4.8, Inflammatory bowel disease).

Dietary assessment

Individuals may already have excluded certain foods, and their ideas on how these foods affect their IBS symptoms should be explored. Certain food avoidances may require nutritional intake assessment, e.g. energy, carbohydrate, calcium. A food and symptom diary may help identify poor dietary patterns and provide motivation to undertake dietary interventions.

Economic and social assessment

An empathic understanding of lifestyle circumstances is important and relevant to treatment options and for concordance with dietary intervention, e.g. any stressors affecting a patient's quality of life, including physical activity, work, education and family circumstances.

Management

Clinical management

Management aims to improve IBS symptoms and quality of life, and guidelines recommend general lifestyle and dietary modification and physical activity as the first-line options (NICE, 2008). Other options, either singly or in combination, include pharmacological and behavioural interventions (NICE, 2015c). These should be discussed with each individual to provide the most appropriate care pathway (NICE, 2015c), imparting education to support long-term self-management of symptoms (NICE, 2016). Self-help information covering lifestyle modification should be considered in primary care (NICE, 2015c).

Prescribed drugs to manage IBS include:

- Antispasmodics – antimuscarinics and smooth muscle relaxants are used to reduce motility, e.g. for meal-induced symptoms. Peppermint oil capsules, hyoscine butylbromide and mebeverine provide modest global symptom improvement (Enck *et al.*, 2010; Ford *et al.*, 2008).
- Osmotic, bulk-forming and stimulant laxatives (e.g. macrogols, ispaghula husk, senna); NICE (2016) discourages lactulose.
- Antidiarrhoeal agents, e.g. loperamide.
- Tricyclic analgesics (e.g. amitriptyline, nortriptyline), usually at low doses 5–30 mg nightly if first-line antispasmodics and loperamide are ineffective. Selective

serotonin reuptake inhibitors are a further option if tricyclics are ineffective.
- Linaclotide, a guanylate cyclase-C receptor agonist if first-line laxatives are ineffective and constipation has been present for 12 months (NICE, 2015c).

Behavioural interventions and psychological therapy – such as cognitive behaviour therapy, relaxation techniques, and psychodynamic interpersonal therapy – may reduce pain and other symptoms and improve quality of life (Spiller *et al.*, 2007). Reflexology and acupuncture showed no benefit and are not recommended, and evidence is lacking to recommend relaxation, computerised CBT and mindfulness therapy (NICE, 2015c). Follow-up is important, and individuals should be encouraged to make contact to arrange their appointment; this will empower them to self-manage their symptoms (NICE, 2016). Self-help organisations, such as The IBS Network, can help individuals to self-manage and come to terms with their disorder.

Dietary management

Evidence-based practice guidelines for the dietetic management of IBS in adults (McKenzie *et al.*, 2016) are available for dietitians' use in the clinical setting. They give graded evidence statements, clinical and research recommendations, and practical considerations stemming from 13 systematic reviews relating to IBS symptom improvement, as well as chosen dietary topics on healthy eating and lifestyle (alcohol, caffeine, spicy food, fat and fluid intakes, and dietary habits), milk and dairy, dietary fibre, fermentable carbohydrates, gluten, probiotics and elimination diets/food hypersensitivity. An IBS dietary algorithm (Figure 7.4.9), a logical two-tiered sequence of assessments and interventions for successful dietary management, forms the basis of these guidelines for clinical practice use. Clinical practice guidance is summarised in Box 7.4.2; for further details, see McKenzie *et al.* (2016).

Second-line dietary management relates to short-chain fermentable carbohydrates, also known as the 'low-FODMAP' (fermentable oligo-, di- and mono-saccharides, and polyols) diet. Examples of foods high in FODMAPs include wheat- and rye-based staples, e.g. bread, pasta, pizza, onion, garlic, pulses, apple, pear, stone fruit, sugar-free chewing gum, mammalian milks and yoghurts. Examples of foods low in FODMAPs are oats, potato, rice, gluten-free bread and pasta, carrot, pepper, spinach, tomato, raspberry, strawberry, citrus fruit, lactose-free cow's milk and yoghurt, and calcium-enriched almond milk. An initial consultation may last 45–60 minutes to enable education on this intervention, with explanation on the physiological mechanisms; guidance on alternative, suitable foods; eating pattern; and nutritional intake adequacy. Dietitian-led low-FODMAP education groups have been shown to be clinically and cost-wise effective as compared to one-to-one appointments (Whigham *et al.*, 2015). With patient-reported satisfactory symptom relief after 3–6 weeks, a second consultation

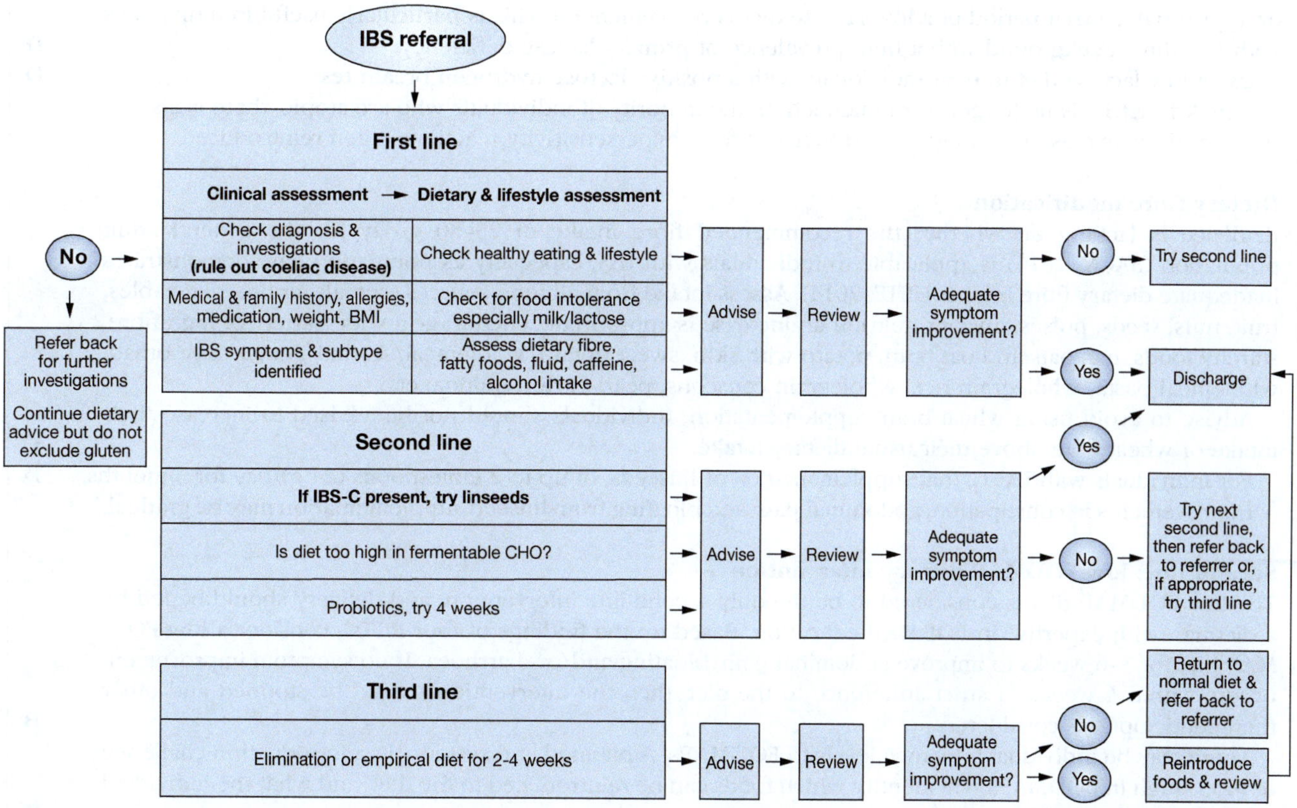

Figure 7.4.9 Algorithm for the management of IBS (source: British Dietetic Association, 2013. Reproduced with permission from the British Dietetic Association, www.bda.uk.com). CHO, carbohydrate; BMI, body mass index; IBS-C, irritable bowel syndrome-C.

Box 7.4.2 Clinical guidance for the dietary management of irritable bowel syndrome (IBS) (adapted from McKenzie *et al.*, 2016)

PEN (2015) evidence grading shown in bold after points as appropriate.

First line: Healthy eating and lifestyle management

Alcohol – alcohol can induce or worsen IBS symptoms. Assess intake and screen for binge drinking. Recommend alcohol consumption to be within safe national limits. **C**

Caffeine – can induce or worsen symptoms. There was insufficient evidence to make a recommendation. If suspected to relate to IBS symptoms, assess intake and consider reducing intake.

Dietary habits – despite insufficient evidence to make a recommendation, assess dietary habits. Advise on how to achieve a healthy, balanced diet with a regular meal pattern (breakfast, lunch and evening meal, with snacks as appropriate), in line with national healthy eating guidelines. Good eating lifestyle includes sitting down to eat, taking time over meals, chewing food thoroughly and not eating late at night.

Fat – a decrease in fat intake may relieve IBS symptoms, particularly meal-associated abdominal pain and discomfort. If related to symptoms during or after eating, assess fat intake and ensure it is in line with national healthy eating guidelines. **C**

Fluid – despite no evidence to make a recommendation, a gradual increase in fluid intake is recommended (aim for a total intake of 1.5–3.0 L per day) to improve stool frequency and decrease the need for laxatives in constipation-predominant symptoms.

Gluten – there was conflicting evidence, and no recommendation could be made for a gluten-free diet to treat IBS symptoms.

Probiotics – considered safe, although there was insufficient evidence to recommend any specific probiotic product. Individuals who choose to trial probiotics should try one product at a time for at least 4 weeks at the dose recommended by the manufacturer. **B**

Advise that substantial improvement in all IBS symptoms is unlikely, and that, if symptom benefit is gained, the long-term effects are unknown.

Spicy foods – can induce IBS symptoms. If suspected to relate to symptoms, assess intake and trial restriction. **C**

Other components of spicy meals can contribute to symptoms (e.g. FODMAPs in onion, garlic).

Removing milk and dairy products to improve IBS symptoms

In individuals in whom sensitivity to milk is suspected and a lactose hydrogen breath test is not available or appropriate, a trial period of a low-lactose diet is recommended. This is particularly useful in individuals with an ethnic background with a high prevalence of primary lactase deficiency. **D**

Use a low-lactose diet to treat individuals with a positive lactose hydrogen breath test. **D**

A milk-free trial is no longer recommended. In the minority of individuals who are atopic, there is a small risk that dairy exclusion can induce anaphylactic food hypersensitivity reactions when reintroduced.

Dietary fibre modification

Evidence is lacking on whether the recommended fibre intake of 25–30 g/day for the general adult population (SACN, 2015) is applicable to individuals with IBS, especially as population data demonstrates inadequate dietary fibre intakes (PHE, 2014). Assess intake from all food sources (cereals, grains, vegetables, fruit, nuts, seeds, pulses, mycoprotein). If an increase is appropriate, encourage a wide variety of high-fibre, starchy foods, e.g. oats and oat bran, potato with skin, sweet potato, wholemeal/seeded/granary/rye bread, wholemeal pasta, wholegrain rice, wholegrain couscous, pearl barley, quinoa, etc.

Advise to avoid using wheat bran supplementation. Individuals should not be advised to increase their intake of wheat bran above their usual dietary intake. **C**

For individuals with IBS-C, trial supplementation of linseeds, of up to 2 tablespoons (24 g)/day for 3 months. **D**

Improvements in constipation, abdominal pain and bloating from linseed supplementation may be gradual.

Second line: low-FODMAP dietary intervention

The low-FODMAP diet is considered to be the only second-line intervention, and delivery should be led by a dietitian with expertise in FODMAP education. Based on the findings of four RCTs[1], consider a low-FODMAP diet for 3–6 weeks to improve abdominal pain, bloating and/or diarrhoea. If no symptom improvement occurs within 4 weeks of strict adherence to the diet, then the intervention should be stopped and other therapeutic options considered. **B**

There may be individual tolerance levels to FODMAPs. A planned and systematic reintroduction challenge of foods high in FODMAPs will identify which foods can be reintroduced to the diet, and what the individual tolerance levels are. **D**

Evidence is lacking to support its use for IBS-C.

[1] Böhn *et al.*, 2015; Halmos *et al.*, 2014; Pedersen *et al.*, 2014; Staudacher *et al.*, 2012.

should take place, taking 30–45 minutes, to guide on planned and structured reintroduction of foods high in these carbohydrates. This is to verify effective treatment and individual tolerance to fermentable carbohydrates; increase dietary variety; and support long-term self-management. To achieve successful adherence and symptom management, provide up-to-date, detailed verbal and written information on the low-FODMAP dietary intervention and reintroduction phase. Software for mobile devises, such as FODMAP FM or Monash University's Low FODMAP Diet App, may be supportive.

A strict low-FODMAP diet alters faecal microbiota in the short term (Halmos *et al.*, 2014; Staudacher *et al.*, 2012). The long-term implications are unknown. Therefore, patients should be encouraged to include high-FODMAP foods in their diet, so that these prebiotic foods are not unnecessarily avoided. Where patient motivation or adherence is compromised or expertise in providing FODMAP education is lacking, other treatment options, such as traditional dietary advice based on NICE/BDA (NICE, 2008), should be considered. If the intervention is ineffective, then the individual should stop the intervention, return to a normal healthy diet and consider other therapeutic options.

Internet resources

The IBS Network, www.theibsnetwork.org

UK training on the low-FODMAP diet and functional gastrointestinal disorders, www.kcl.ac.uk/fodmaps

For further low-FODMAP information and recipes, www.monashfodmap.com

Patient resources

BDA IBS Food Fact Sheet, www.bda.uk.com/foodfacts/IBSfoodfacts.pdf

Nutrition and Diet Resources (NDR), www.ndr-uk.org

Smartphone applications

Australia, www.monashfodmap.com/i-have-ibs/get-the-app

UK, foodmaestro.me/fodmap-app

Healthcare professional resources

BDA Key Fact sheet on IBS, www.bda.uk.com/improvinghealth/healthprofessionals/keyfacts/ibstrustadietitian

Lomer M (ed). (2014) *Advanced Nutrition and Dietetics in Gastroenterology*. Chichester: Wiley-Blackwell, pp. 226–242.

References

Adesokan A, Neild P. (2012) Attitudes and expectations of gastroenterology outpatients about the importance of diet and possible relationship to their symptoms. *Front. Gastroenterol.* 3: 278–282.

Agarwal N, Spiegel BM. (2011) The effect of irritable bowel syndrome on health-related quality of life and health care expenditures. *Gastroenterol. Clin. North. Am.* 40(1): 11–19.

Bock SA. (2010, June) AAAAI support of the EAACI Position Paper on IgG4. *J. Allergy Clin. Immunol.* 125(6): 1410.

Böhn L, Störsrud S, Törnblom H, *et al.* (2013) Self-reported food-related gastrointestinal symptoms in IBS are common and associated with more severe symptoms and reduced quality of life. *Am. J. Gastroenterol.* 108: 634–641.

Böhn L, Störsrud S, Liljebo T, *et al.* (2015, November) Diet low in FODMAPs reduces symptoms of irritable bowel syndrome as well as traditional dietary advice: a randomized controlled trial. *Gastroenterology.* 149(6): 1399–1407.

Brandt LJ, Chey WD, Foxx-Orenstein AE, *et al.* (2009) An evidence-based systematic review on the management of irritable bowel syndrome. *Am. J. Gastroenterol.* 104: S1–S35.

Carr S, Chan E, Lavine E, *et al.* (2012) CSACI Position statement on the testing of food-specific IgG. *Allergy Asthma Clin. Immunol.* 8(1): 12.

Chang JY, Locke III GR, McNally MA, *et al.* (2010) Impact of functional gastrointestinal disorders on survival in the community. *Am. J. Gastroenterol.* 105(4): 822–832.

Drossman DA, Hasler W. (2016) Rome IV-functional GI disorders: disorders of Gut–Brain interaction. *Gastroenterology.* 150: 1257–1261.

Enck P, Junne F, Klosterhalfen S, *et al.* (2010) Therapy options in irritable bowel syndrome. *Eur. J. Gastroenterol. Hepatol.* 22(12): 1402–1411.

Farmer AD, Aziz Q. (2014) Irritable bowel syndrome pathogenesis (Chapter 3.18). In: Lomer M (ed) *Advanced Nutrition and Dietetics in Gastroenterology*. Oxford: Wiley Blackwell, pp. 226–232.

Ford AC, Talley NJ, Spiegel BM, *et al.* (2008) Effect of fibre, antispasmodics, and peppermint oil in the treatment of irritable bowel syndrome: systematic review and meta-analysis. *BMJ* 337: a2313.

Francis CY, Morris J, Whorwell PJ. (1997) The irritable bowel severity scoring system: a simple method of monitoring irritable bowel syndrome and its progress. *Aliment. Pharmacol. Ther.* 11(2): 395–402.

Halmos EP, Power VA, Shepherd SJ, *et al.* (2014) A diet low in FODMAPs reduces symptoms of irritable bowel syndrome. *Gastroenterology.* 146(1): 67–75.

Halpert A, Dalton CB, Palsson O, *et al.* (2007) What patients know about irritable bowel syndrome (IBS) and what they would like to know. National Survey on Patient Educational Needs in IBS and development and validation of the Patient Educational Needs Questionnaire (PEQ). *Am. J. Gastroenterol.* 102: 1972–1982.

Hayes P, Corish C, O'Mahoney E, *et al.* (2014) A dietary survey of patients with irritable bowel syndrome. *J. Hum. Nutr. Diet.* 27(2): 36–47.

Heaton KW, Radvan J, Cripps H, *et al.* (1992) Defecation frequency and timing, and stool form in the general population: a prospective study. *Gut.* 3: 818–824.

Jones J, Boorman J, Cann P, *et al.* (2000) British Society of Gastroenterology guidelines for the management of the irritable bowel syndrome. *Gut.* 47(2): ii1–19.

Lacy B, Mearin F, Chang L, *et al.* (2016) Bowel disorders. *Gastroenterology.* 150: 1393–1407.

Lovell RM, Ford AC. (2012) Global prevalence of and risk factors for irritable bowel syndrome: a meta-analysis. *Clin. Gastroenterol. Hepatol.* 10: 712–721.

Martin L, van Vuuren C, Seamark L, *et al.* (2015) OC-104 Long term effectiveness of short chain fermentable carbohydrate (FODMAP) restriction in patients with irritable bowel syndrome. *Gut.* 64(1): A51–A52.

McKenzie YA, Alder A, Anderson W, *et al.* on behalf of Gastroenterology Specialist Group of the British Dietetic Association. (2012) British Dietetic Association evidence-based practice guidelines for the dietary management of irritable bowel syndrome in adults. *J. Hum. Nutr. Diet.* 25: 260–274.

McKenzie Y, Bowyer R, Leach H, *et al.* (2016) British Dietetic Association systematic review and evidence-based practice guidelines for the dietary management of irritable bowel syndrome in adults (2016 update). *J. Hum. Nutr. Diet.* 29(5): 549–575.

Monsbakken KW, Vandvik PO, Farup PG. (2006) Perceived food intolerance in subjects with irritable bowel syndrome – etiology, prevalence and consequences. *Eur. J. Clin. Nutr.* 60: 667–672.

NICE. (2008) *Irritable Bowel Syndrome in Adults: Diagnosis and Management of Irritable Bowel Syndrome in Primary Care. CG61.*
NICE. (2013) *Faecal Calprotectin Diagnostic Tests for Inflammatory Diseases of the Bowel. DG11.*
NICE. (2015a) *Suspected Cancer: Recognition and Referral. NG12.*
NICE. (2015b) *Coeliac Disease: Recognition, Assessment and Management. NG20.*
NICE. (2015c) *Irritable Bowel Syndrome in Adults: Diagnosis and Management of Irritable Bowel Syndrome in Primary Care. CG61 addendum.*
NICE. (2016) *Irritable Bowel Syndrome: Quality Standard 114.*
Painter NS. (1985) The cause of diverticular disease of the colon, its symptoms and its complications. Review and hypothesis. *J. R. Coll. Surg. Edinb.* 30(2): 118–122.
Pedersen N, Andersen NN, Vegh Z, *et al.* (2014) Ehealth: low FODMAP diet vs. *Lactobacillus rhamnosus* GG in irritable bowel syndrome. *World J. Gastroenterol.* 20(43): 16215–16226.
Practice-based Evidence in Nutrition (PEN) Global. (2015) *PEN Global evidence grades.* Available from https://www.pennutrition.com/aboutpen.aspx. Accessed 20 November 2016.
Public Health England (PHE), Food Standards Agency. (2014) National Diet and Nutrition Survey: Results from Years 1, 2, 3 and 4 (combined) of the Rolling Programme (2008/2009 – 2011/2012). Available from https://assets.publishing.service.gov.uk/government/uploads/system/uploads/attachment_data/file/594361/NDNS_Y1_to_4_UK_report_full_text_revised_February_2017.pdf. Accessed 26 October 2018.
Quigley EM, Fried M, Gwee KA, *et al.* (2016) World gastroenterology organisation global guidelines irritable bowel syndrome: a global perspective update. *J. Clin. Gastroenterol.* 50(9): 704–713.
Ringel X, Williams RE, Kalilani L, *et al.* (2009) Prevalence, characteristics, and impact of bloating symptoms in patients with irritable bowel syndrome. *Clin. Gastroenterol. Hepatol.* 7(1): 68–72.
SACN. (2015) *Carbohydrate and health report.* Available at https://www.gov.uk/government/publications/sacn-carbohydrates-and-health-report. Accessed 26 October 2018.
Spiller R, Aziz Q, Creed F, *et al.* (2007) Guidelines on the irritable bowel syndrome: mechanisms and practical management. *Gut.* 56: 1770–1798.
Stapel SO, Asero R, Ballmer-Weber BK, *et al.* (2008) Testing for IgG4 against foods is not recommended as a diagnostic tool: EAACI Task Force Report. *Allergy.* 63: 793–796.
Staudacher HM. (2017) Nutritional, microbial and psychosocial implications of the low FODMAP diet. *J. Gastroenterol. Hepatol.* 32(1): 16–19.
Staudacher HM, Lomer MC, Anderson JL, *et al.* (2012) Fermentable carbohydrate restriction reduces luminal bifidobacteria and gastrointestinal symptoms in patients with irritable bowel syndrome. *J. Nutr.* 142(8): 1510–1518.
Svedlund J, Sjodin I, Dotevall G. (1988) GSRS – a clinical rating scale for gastrointestinal symptoms in patients with irritable bowel syndrome and peptic ulcer disease. *Dig. Dis. Sci.* 33: 129–134.
Thompson WG. (2006) The road to Rome. *Gastroenterology.* 130: 1552–1556.
Thompson WG, Heaton KW, Smyth GT, *et al.* (2000) Irritable bowel syndrome in general practice: prevalence, characteristics and referral. *Gut.* 46: 78–82.
Whigham L, Joyce T, Harper G, *et al.* (2015) Clinical effectiveness and economic costs of group versus one-to-one education for short-chain fermentable carbohydrate restriction (low FODMAP diet) in the management of irritable bowel syndrome. *J. Hum. Nutr. Diet.* 28(6): 687–696.
Williams E, Nai X, Corfe B. (2011) Dietary intakes in people with irritable bowel syndrome. *BMC Gastroenterol.* 11: 9.

7.4.11 Other disorders of the colon and rectum

Angela Cleaver and Laura Thomas

Key points

- Acute diarrhoea can cause severe dehydration, especially in young children and elderly people. The management of chronic diarrhoea depends on the underlying cause.
- Constipation may be a primary disorder associated with inadequate fluid, fibre or activity levels, or a secondary consequence of medication or underlying disease. Management may require a combination of dietary, behavioural and pharmacological strategies.
- Diverticular disease is a common disorder of the colon: a high-fibre diet can prevent disease progression.

The main functions of the colon are to help maintain fluid and electrolyte balance and to form stools from the waste products of digestion; this process is completed in the rectum, allowing the stool to be stored until being expelled via the anus. The colon has a small role to play in digestion and absorption of nutrients as a result of the bacterial fermentation of carbohydrates. This fermentation produces acetate, butyrate and propionate. These short-chain fatty acids can provide energy, and butyrate also helps to maintain the colonic cells themselves.

Duration of movement through the colon varies widely, usually taking 12–30 hours. Transit time in the colon depends on several factors: (i) the ability of the colonic muscle to perform co-ordinated peristaltic waves; (ii) successful digestion in the small intestine; (iii) the fibre and fluid content of the diet; (iv) the type of bacteria present; and (v) lifestyle.

Disorders of the colon commonly present with abdominal pain, altered bowel habit (diarrhoea or constipation) and bloating. It is important to establish if there is an underlying condition causing the symptoms.

Diarrhoea

Diarrhoea is described as an abnormally frequent discharge of semi-solid or fluid faecal matter from the bowel; it can be categorised as follows:

- *Acute diarrhoea* – three or more abnormally loose or watery stools in the preceding 24 hours.
- *Chronic diarrhoea* – diarrhoea which lasts ≥14 days.
- *Faecal incontinence* – inability to control bowel movements, with the involuntary passing of liquid or solid stools; this may be due to overflow around hard, constipated stools.

Diagnostic criteria

Diarrhoea is normally a symptom rather than a condition: Table 7.4.12 shows the common causes of diarrhoea. A diagnosis of functional diarrhoea is made if no underlying cause is found and the patient fulfils the following criteria, defined by the Rome III Committee (Drossman, 2006); '*loose (mushy) or watery stools without pain occurring in at least 75% of stools for the last 3 months with symptoms starting 6 months before the diagnosis*'. Stool types 5–7 on the Bristol Stool Chart (Lewis & Heaton, 1997) describe diarrhoea.

Disease processes

Acute diarrhoea is usually a symptom of a bowel infection by a virus (e.g. norovirus), a bacterial infection (e.g. food poisoning), consumption of contaminated food or water, or caused by antibiotics. *Clostridium difficile* is a common cause of hospital-acquired diarrhoea (Baldi *et al.*, 2009). Disruption of the bowel microflora by antibiotics creates an environment in which *C. difficile* can proliferate. Other causes of acute diarrhoea include anxiety, drinking excessive alcohol or caffeine-containing fluids, chemotherapy, adjusting to enteral feeding, acute radiation enteritis, intestinal ischaemia and the early presentation of a chronic cause, e.g. inflammatory bowel disease (IBD). Many drugs can cause diarrhoea, e.g. antacids containing magnesium, non-steroidal anti-inflammatory drugs (NSAIDs), statins, selective serotonin reuptake inhibitors (SSRIs), some chemotherapy agents and laxatives. Chronic diarrhoea has a broader range of possible causes than acute diarrhoea (see Table 7.4.12).

Disease consequences

Acute infectious diarrhoea is one of the commonest illnesses worldwide, particularly in developing countries, where it is the primary cause of childhood mortality. In 2012, there were 56 million deaths worldwide; 1.5 million (2.7%) were attributed to diarrhoeal diseases (World Health Organization (WHO), 2014). The prevalence of chronic diarrhoea in the general population has been reported as 3–5% (Juckett & Trivedi, 2011). Diarrhoea causes faecal incontinence in 1–10% of the UK population, and is socially stigmatising and isolating (NICE, 2007). The prognosis of chronic diarrhoea will depend on the underlying cause.

Table 7.4.12 Causes of chronic diarrhoea

Cause	Example
Chronic infection	Functional disorders such as IBS may follow infection
Small bowel	Coeliac disease
	Crohn's disease
	Bile acid malabsorption – resection, damage or disease of the terminal ileum leads to increased bile salts in the colon that can stimulate diarrhoea
	Lactase deficiency, lactose intolerance
	Fructose intolerance
	Small bowel bacterial overgrowth
	Mesenteric ischaemia
	Radiation enteritis
	Lymphoma
Colonic	Irritable bowel syndrome
	Diverticular disease
	Colon cancer
	Ulcerative colitis and Crohn's colitis
	Microscopic colitis
	Late effects of pelvic radiation
Pancreatic – associated with steatorrhoea	Chronic pancreatitis causing pancreatic insufficiency
	Pancreatic cancer
	Cystic fibrosis
Other	After gastrectomy or bariatric surgery
	Cow's milk protein or other food allergy
	Hyperthyroidism
	Diabetes – may be related to metformin or autonomic neuropathy
	Laxative use
	Medication, e.g. NSAIDs, magnesium-containing antacids

Nutritional consequences

Consequences of prolonged diarrhoea include dehydration, malnutrition, weight loss, anaemia and electrolyte imbalances.

Nutritional assessment

Consider the following:

- Anthropometry – weight, height, BMI, percentage weight loss, strength, mid-arm muscle circumference and triceps skinfold thickness.

SECTION 7

- Biochemistry – potassium and sodium due to rapid losses in acute diarrhoea, dehydration markers. Iron, folate, vitamin B_{12} and zinc status. Inflammation and/or infection markers, C-reactive protein (CRP), white cell count (WCC), erythrocyte sedimentation rate (ESR). Coeliac screen.
- Clinical assessment – bowel frequency, duration of symptoms, stool consistency and colour. Symptoms of dehydration including decreased urine output and dark urine. Medical diagnosis that could cause diarrhoea. Medications that may cause diarrhoea.
- Dietary assessment –A food and symptom diary (sent with the appointment letter if possible) can highlight trends in intake. If not available, take a diet history and evaluate fat, caffeine, alcohol and fibre intake. Assess FODMAP intake, particularly polyols from foods such as sugar-free sweets and gum. Has the patient noticed any associations? Assess the types and volumes of fluid being drunk, particularly caffeinated drinks and alcohol.
- Economic and social assessment – history of anxiety and food safety issues that may increase the risk of food poisoning.
- Service user focus – Patients are normally focused on reducing the severity and frequency of symptoms.

Clinical investigation and management

Acute diarrhoea often resolves without complications in a few days. If a bacterial infection is suspected, a stool sample is needed to confirm whether antibiotic therapy is appropriate. Initial investigations for chronic diarrhoea will include blood and stool tests; these, together with a detailed history from the patient, can help establish whether the symptoms have an organic or functional cause. Symptoms of <3 months duration, continuous or nocturnal diarrhoea and a significant weight loss are suggestive of an organic disease. Coeliac disease should be excluded. Abdominal pain with intermittent diarrhoea and constipation is suggestive of IBS once other causes have been eliminated (Longstreth *et al.*, 2006). A diagnosis of overflow diarrhoea due to faecal impaction should be excluded. Rectal examination, colonoscopy or flexible sigmoidoscopy and biopsy can be used to exclude cancer, microscopic colitis and IBD. A selenium homocholic acid taurine (SeHCAT) test or a trial of cholestyramine will help to determine if bile acid malabsorption is the cause (Wilcox *et al.*, 2014), and a glucose or lactulose hydrogen breath test can indicate small bowel bacterial overgrowth (Grace *et al.*, 2013).

Loperamide, an antidiarrhoeal medication, slows down the contractions in the bowel, decreasing gastrointestinal transit time, but is not appropriate when the diarrhoea is caused by a bacterial infection (NHS, 2018). More recently, there has been interest in faecal microbiota transplantation for the treatment of *C. difficile523* (Borody *et al.*, 2015) and as a possible treatment when standard treatment has failed (NICE, 2014; Wilcox, 2013).

Nutritional management

Acute diarrhoea

As episodes of acute diarrhoea are usually brief and self-limiting, and the focus of advice should be on the prevention of dehydration by encouraging a good fluid intake, such as water, soft drinks (preferably not fruit juices) and savoury drinks. Oral rehydration solutions increase water absorption by stimulation of sodium glucose transport in the small intestine, and should be encouraged. There is little evidence to support fasting as a treatment for acute diarrhoea (Wingate *et al.*, 2001).

There is a lot of interest in the role of probiotics in the treatment of diarrhoea. Probiotics appear to have beneficial effects in shortening the duration and reducing stool frequency in acute infectious diarrhoea (Allen *et al.*, 2010). A meta-analysis by Goldenberg *et al.* (2013) concluded that the short-term use of probiotics in patients who are not immuno-compromised or severely debilitated reduces the risk of *C. difficile*–associated diarrhoea, but there was not enough evidence to recommend a particular strain or dose of probiotic.

Chronic diarrhoea

If chronic diarrhoea is due to a functional cause, a low fermentable oligo-, di- and mono-saccharides and polyols (FODMAP) diet can be effective (Halmos *et al.*, 2014) (see Chapter 7.4.10, Irritable bowel syndrome). General advice that may be given includes:

- Maintaining a good fluid intake to help replace intestinal losses. Exclude milk if it is perceived to worsen the diarrhoea, until symptoms have settled.
- Continue to eat small, frequent meals, choosing soft, low-fibre foods such as white bread, mashed potato, plainly cooked pasta or rice, white fish, plainly cooked chicken, plain biscuits or crackers and jelly.
- Avoid high-fibre foods – such as wholegrain breads, whole-wheat cereals, nuts and seeds, fruit skins and pith, and vegetable skins and stalks – since these may increase intestinal transit time and exacerbate symptoms. If the diet is high fat, low fibre, then increasing the fibre content of the diet and avoiding fatty foods may be required.
- Foods known to aggravate symptoms should be excluded; spicy and greasy foods may stimulate diarrhoea.
- Drinking large volumes of undiluted fruit juice, caffeinated drinks and alcohol should be discouraged.

If there are concerns about nutritional adequacy, advice on food fortification and oral nutritional supplements may be needed.

Constipation

Constipation is a common gastrointestinal complaint; rates vary from 3 to 34% of populations, depending on the diagnostic criteria used and the demographics of the study population. Constipation is more prevalent with increasing age, particularly in those aged >60 years who are institutionalised or bedbound. Rates in women tend to be higher, but this may be due to an increase in reporting. Socioeconomic status, diet, obesity and immobility have also been linked (Mugie *et al.*, 2011). However, there are difficulties in establishing a diagnosis and selecting the most appropriate treatment (Garrigues *et al.*, 2004). Patients may report unsatisfactory defaecation due to fewer bowel movements than usual, difficulty passing stools, which may be hard or soft, and feelings of incomplete evacuation of stools (tenesmus). About 40% of pregnant women complain of constipation (Cullen & O'Donoghue, 2007).

The word constipation has a different meaning to different people. While some believe that they are constipated if they do not have a daily bowel movement, normal stool elimination may be three times a day or twice a week, depending on the person. Constipation is defaecation that is unsatisfactory because of infrequent stools, difficult stool passage or a feeling of incomplete evacuation; the stool type and size may vary. Constipation is a symptom, not a disease. Factors associated with an increased risk of constipation include a low fluid intake, a low-fibre diet and reduced mobility. A high fibre intake is associated with a lower prevalence of constipation (Dukas *et al.*, 2003).

Diagnostic criteria

McCallum *et al.* (2009) discuss the potential of underreporting when using the Rome criteria; however, combined with the Bristol Stool Chart (Lewis & Heaton, 1997), it is a useful tool for quantifying a patient's symptoms and measuring response to treatment. A diagnosis of chronic constipation is made when the Rome III criteria (Drossman, 2006) have been met for 3 months, with the onset of symptoms at least 6 months prior to the diagnosis. The Rome III criteria:

1. Must include two or more of the following:
    - Straining during at least 25% of defaecations.
    - Lumpy or hard stools in at least 25% of defaecations.
    - Sensation of incomplete evacuation for at least 25% of defaecations.
    - Sensation of anorectal obstruction or blockage for at least 25% of defaecations.
    - Manual manoeuvres to facilitate at least 25% of defaecations, e.g. digital evacuation, support of the pelvic floor.
    - Fewer than three defaecations per week.
2. Loose stools are rarely present without the use of laxatives.
3. Insufficient criteria for IBS.

Disease processes

Constipation is a common gastrointestinal complaint that can cause physical and psychosocial problems. The cause of constipation may be multifactorial, but it can be divided into primary/functional and secondary constipation. Primary/functional constipation is chronic constipation where there is no underlying disease but there is a psychological, psychosomatic or undiagnosed neurological cause. A drug or medical condition, as shown in Table 7.4.13, causes secondary constipation.

Primary constipation can be further classified into three categories:

- Normal-transit constipation – stool passes through the colon at a normal rate, but patients perceive difficulty in emptying their bowels; most common in young women.

Table 7.4.13 Causes of secondary constipation (NICE, 2015)

Cause	Example
Endocrine and metabolic diseases	Diabetes (autonomic myopathy)
	Hypercalcaemia
	Hypokalaemia
	Hyperparathyroidism
	Hypothyroidism
	Uraemia
Myopathic conditions	Amyloidosis
	Scleroderma
	Myotonic dystrophy
Neurological diseases	Autonomic neuropathy
	Stroke
	Guillain-Barré syndrome
	Hirschsprung's disease
	Multiple sclerosis
	Parkinson's disease
	Spinal cord injuries or tumours
Structural abnormalities	Anal fissures or strictures
	Haemorrhoids
	Colonic strictures
	Inflammatory bowel disease
	Colorectal cancer
	Rectal prolapse
	Volvulus
	Megacolon or megarectum
	Postnatal damage to the pelvic floor
Drugs	Opioid analgesics – codeine, morphine, fentanyl
	Diuretics
	Iron supplements
	Aluminium antacids
	Antispasmodics – dicycloverine, hycoscine
	Antidepressants – commonly tricyclic antidepressants
	Antiepileptics – carbamazepine, gabapentin, pregabalin, phenytoin, oxcarbazepine.
	Antipsychotics
	Calcium supplements
	Sedating antihistamines
	Calcium channel blockers – verapamil
	Antiemetics – Ondansetron
Other	Pregnancy
	Irritable bowel syndrome

SECTION 7

- Slow-transit constipation – there are infrequent bowel movements, decreased urgency or straining to have bowels open and an increased colonic transit time.
- Pelvic floor dysfunction that is characterised by dysfunction of the pelvic floor or anal sphincter and can follow childbirth (NICE, 2015).

Those diagnosed with functional constipation may be particularly affected by behavioural or psychological factors. They may regularly ignore the urge to have a bowel movement, feel uncomfortable using toilets outside the home or have limited access to toilet facilities. Constipation is common in those with a history of depression, anxiety, eating disorders, sexual abuse and physical abuse (Levy *et al.*, 2006). Changes in routine, such as travel and reduced levels of exercise or mobility, can lead to an alteration in bowel habits.

Disease consequences

Chronic constipation has a detrimental effect on quality of life due to the associated physical and psychosocial problems (Dennison *et al.*, 2005; Talley, 2004). Chronic constipation can result in faecal impaction, where faecal retention is so pronounced that the ability to expel a stool is lost. This leads to an increase in urinary tract infections, faecal incontinence, rectal bleeding and prolapse. Faecal impaction needs treating cautiously with laxatives. Chronic constipation can also lead to diverticular disease.

Nutritional consequences

Constipation often results in a poor appetite; this can have an impact on the patient's weight, macronutrient and micronutrient intake, and can also slow transit time further, increasing the constipation. Patients with a low intake of fruit and vegetables are at risk of micronutrient deficiencies, particularly vitamin C, B_{12} and folate.

Nutritional assessment

A nutritional assessment should include the following:

- *Anthropometry* – weight, height, BMI.
- Weight loss – constipation is more common in those with a history of an eating disorder or previous laxative abuse.
- *Biochemistry* – diabetes control, raised calcium, raised potassium, thyroid function, urea status, hydration status, valid coeliac screen, full blood count to eliminate anaemia.
- *Clinical assessment* – bowel frequency, stool type, medical diagnosis or medication that may increase risk of constipation, relevant psychosocial factors, reduction in mobility.
- *Dietary assessment* – food and symptom diary to evaluate dietary trends or diet history to review meal patterns and fibre and fluid intake, previous dietary management strategies.
- *Economic and social assessment* – concerns about lack of income or knowledge to achieve a well-balanced diet, relevant psychosocial factors, e.g. avoiding public toilets.
- *Service user focus* – clarify the patient's expectations of treatment.

Clinical investigation and management

The medical history and a physical examination will be used in conjunction with the Rome criteria to establish a diagnosis and investigate the possibility of an underlying cause, which may warrant further investigation such as a colonoscopy or colonic transit studies. Abdominal X ray and other more invasive tests are not required if 'red-flags' have been excluded (McCallum *et al.*, 2009). Red flags such as blood in the stool, unintentional weight loss and a family history of colon cancer warrant further investigation, especially in patients over 50 years of age.

Lifestyle

Patients should be advised to try to establish a routine for emptying their bowels, e.g. trying to go first thing in the morning, or approximately 30 mins after eating, to make the most of the gastro-colic reflex and, where possible, not to ignore the urge to go (NICE, 2015). Increased physical activity and positioning on the toilet can also help. When seated on the toilet, patients should use a small stool to raise their knees in line with or just above their hips, place their elbows on their legs and lean forwards (McCallum *et al.*, 2009). Bed bound patients may be more likely to empty their bowels when hoisted.

Medication

Faecal impaction should be dealt with first using an osmotic or stimulant laxative with care, under the direction of a doctor. The use of any constipating medication should be reviewed and, where possible, adjusted. If dietary and lifestyle measures have not helped, laxatives should be considered. First-line laxatives are bulk forming to improve transit time. Additional fluids should also be considered. If the stools remain hard, an osmotic laxative should be used as an alternative or in addition. If the stool is soft, but hard to pass, consider a stimulant laxative. If two laxatives have been tried from different groups at the highest tolerated dose for 6 months without success, NICE (2015) has approved the use of prucalopride (5HT4-receptor agonist) for women or lubiprostone (chloride channel activator) for men and women; linaclotide is licensed for use in patients with constipation-dominant irritable bowel syndrome. Only a doctor with experience in managing chronic constipation should prescribe prucalopride and linaclotide. Once the stools have become soft and easy to pass, the laxatives should be gradually withdrawn. Some medical causes of constipation or the use of constipatory medication may make this impossible. Patients suffering from chronic constipation as a result of spinal injury or neurological conditions (e.g. Guillain-Barré syndrome) may require a bulking agent or stool softener and a stimulant

Table 7.4.14 Laxatives commonly used in the management of constipation

Category of laxative	Example	Mode of action
Bulking agents	Ispaghula husk (Fybogel), methylcellulose, sterculia (Normacol), frangula	Increase fibre intake, increasing the weight and water absorbent properties of the stool. Good fluid intake needed
Stimulant laxatives	Senna, bisacodyl, sodium picosulfate (Dulcolax)	Increase intestinal motility by stimulation of colonic nerves
Faecal softeners	Liquid paraffin	Softens stool, but use is discouraged due to adverse effects, i.e. anal seepage, irritation
Osmotic laxatives	Lactulose, macrogols (Laxido or Movicol), magnesium salts (e.g. Epsom salts)	Softens stool by increasing water content Lactulose may also have a stimulant effect. Magnesium salts are not recommended due to the potential intensity of their action
Rectal laxatives	Suppositories: glycerol, bisacodyl, sodium phosphate, sodium bicarbonate	Lubricate the stool Stimulate the rectum Effervescent action
	Enemas: sodium citrate, sodium phosphate	Osmotic

laxative on alternate days, coupled with suppositories and manual evacuation, to prevent faecal impaction. See Table 7.4.14 for more information on commonly used laxatives.

Biofeedback

This is a non-invasive bowel training programme run by specialist nurses or physiotherapists, involving the retraining of muscles and nerves to coordinate and produce satisfactory effort to empty the bowel (Burch & Collins, 2010). Benefits from biofeedback therapy are limited to patients with pelvic floor dysfunction (Frattini & Norgueras, 2008).

Surgery

This is only considered in a minority of patients, because the results of total or partial removal of the colon to improve bowel function are often poor. Even if there is an improvement in bowel habits, the postoperative quality of life can be adversely affected by abdominal pain, postoperative incontinence or diarrhoea (Fitzharris *et al.*, 2003; Riss *et al.*, 2009). Kamm *et al.* (1988) recommended that those with normal transit constipation being considered for surgery have a preoperative psychosocial assessment, as it is recognised that many of these patients have psychological issues that can predispose them to a poor surgical outcome.

Nutritional management

Encourage regular meals within a balanced diet, containing wholegrains, fruit and vegetables. Adults should aim to eat 18–30g of fibre/day. Patients should be advised to increase their fibre intake gradually to help minimise bloating and flatulence (NICE, 2015). Fibre increases the bulk of the stool, which distends the colon and stimulates propulsive activity and colonic transit. The beneficial effects of a higher fibre intake may take several weeks to be evident. More specific advice about the types of dietary fibre may be of benefit to those with chronic constipation. There is evidence to support increasing the soluble fibre intake of the diet for constipation (Suares & Ford, 2011), and for decreasing insoluble fibre intake in patients with slow-transit constipation (Wald, 2007). In practice, it is easier to discuss fibre in general terms as many fibre sources contain both soluble and insoluble fibres. Increasing fibre intakes can be difficult due to financial constraints and a lack of cooking skills or facilities. While linseeds have been shown to have some benefit in constipation-dominant IBS, there is insufficient evidence to draw firm conclusions for their role in functional constipation (Staudacher & Parkes, 2014). Products such as Resource Optifibre can be useful to demonstrate the benefits of increased fibre intake, particularly in those with a poor appetite. It can then be decreased gradually as the fibre intake from food increases.

The beneficial effects of following a high-fibre diet can be enhanced by increasing fluid intake to 1.5–2.0L/day (Anti *et al.*, 1998). An increased fluid intake is needed with bulking agents and osmotic laxatives. However, elderly patients and those with decreased mobility may find the associated increase in urine output difficult to manage. The fluid requirements of patients with additional cardiac or renal problems should be established on an individual basis and monitored. There is some strain-specific evidence for the use of probiotics (improvements in transit time, faecal frequency and stool consistency); however, the evidence is too limited to allow the recommendation of any particular product (Causebrook & Speed, 2014).

Diverticular disease

Diverticular disease is a common condition that occurs when small pouches, termed diverticula, form in the wall of the colon. The terminology used can be confusing; the following definitions are most commonly used:

- Diverticulum – a single herniation of the colonic mucosal wall.
- Diverticula – several diverticulum.
- Diverticulosis – the presence of diverticula without symptoms.
- Diverticulitis – diverticulosis with evidence of inflammation.
- Complicated diverticulitis – diverticulitis with associated abscesses, fistula, obstruction or perforation.
- Diverticular disease – an overarching term for asymptomatic or symptomatic diverticula.

Diagnostic criteria

Diverticular disease can be difficult to diagnose from symptoms alone; these include left-sided abdominal pain and a change in bowel habit. A colonoscopy or barium enema may be carried out to confirm the presence of diverticula.

Disease process

The prevalence increases with age; from <10% in those under 40 years to 50% in those aged over 80 years. Men are more likely to have diverticular disease in the <40-year group and women in the older age group (Parks, 1975 cited by Williams *et al.*, 2007). The true incidence of diverticulosis is unknown, as it is asymptomatic.

Diverticular disease is more common in Western Europe, America and Japan than the rest of Asia or Africa (Delvaux, 2003). A diet low in fibre is thought to be a significant risk factor for the development of diverticular disease (Painter & Burkitt, 1971). A low dietary fibre intake is thought to slow gut transit, leading to constipation and an increased intraluminal pressure in the sigmoid colon, which causes segmentation and herniation of the mucosa through the muscle. More recent research has found that a high-meat diet may affect colonic bacterial metabolism, which may play a role in the development of diverticula (Jeyarajah, 2014).

Disease consequences

Complications of diverticulitis include the development of abscesses, fistulae, obstruction, diverticular haemorrhage and perforation of the bowel. Uncomplicated recurrence of diverticulitis is reported as 19–34%, with 5–10% of patients having complications requiring emergency surgery or stoma formation (Thomas *et al.*, 2013). Diverticular disease is predominantly a disease of the elderly and is an increasingly important health burden as a result of our ageing population.

Nutritional consequences

Dehydration is a potential consequence in acute diverticulitis. If a low-fibre diet has contributed to the development of diverticular disease and is not rectified, the patient is at risk of complicated diverticulitis, and potential micronutrient deficiencies such as vitamin C, B_{12} and folate.

Nutritional assessment

This will include the following:

- *Anthropometry* – weight, height, BMI. Diverticular disease is not normally associated with weight changes.
- *Biochemistry* – signs of dehydration, infection/inflammation markers (CRP, WCC, ESR), valid coeliac screen.
- *Clinical assessment* – history of abdominal pain or a change in bowel habit, concurrent IBS.
- *Dietary assessment* – assess fibre and fluid intake using a diet history or food and symptom diary.
- *Economic and social assessment* – concerns about lack of income, facilities or knowledge to achieve a well-balanced diet.
- *Service user focus* – patients are usually focused on reducing symptoms and preventing acute episodes.

Clinical investigation and management

Diverticulosis does not require medical management until diverticulitis develops. When there is a history of diverticular disease, a diagnosis of diverticulitis may be made by physical examination, taking a medical history and carrying out a blood test to look for signs of infection. An ultrasound scan may be performed to look for an abscess or perforation. Mild diverticulitis can be managed with paracetamol and oral antibiotics. Complicated diverticulitis will require intravenous antibiotics and fluids, and a blood transfusion if there has been significant rectal bleeding. In rare cases, surgery is required to remove the damaged area of the colon, and this may require stoma formation (see Chapter 7.4.9, Intestinal failure and intestinal resection). Possible new treatments for diverticular disease include the use of 5-aminosalicylate compounds (Di Mario *et al.*, 2006). Physical activity can help to reduce the risk of developing this condition (Vermeulen *et al.*, 2010).

Nutritional management

If a patient presents with diverticulitis, a fluid-only diet may be recommended until symptoms start to improve. Generally, after 2–3 days, advice on supplementation with nutritious fluids may be required. There is little research on diet and diverticulitis, but avoiding foods that can irritate the bowel, such as fruit and vegetable skins, seeds and nuts, and spicy foods, may be beneficial until symptoms have settled.

No treatment is routinely offered for asymptomatic diverticular disease; a high-fibre diet is unlikely to do harm, and there is some evidence to suggest that it will slow disease progression (Jeyarajah, 2014). Cereal fibres were found to be less protective than insoluble fibres from fruit and vegetables. A high-fibre diet has also been suggested as beneficial for those with complications and recurrences of diverticulitis (Hyland & Taylor, 1980).

The role of probiotics in maintaining remission of symptomatic, uncomplicated diverticular disease is still equivocal (Lamiki *et al.*, 2010).

Drug–nutrient Interaction

- Stimulant laxatives (e.g. senna and herbal preparations containing aloe or liquorice) can cause hypokalaemia.
- Bulking agents may delay the absorption of some medications.
- High-fibre diets can decrease the bioavailability of digoxin and lovastatin (Schmidt & Dalhoffi, 2002).

Acknowledgement

The editor acknowledges the prior contribution of Diane Brundrett.

Further reading

World Gastroenterology Organisation (WGO). (2012) *Acute Diarrhoea in Adults and Children; A Global Perspective*. Available at www.worldgastroenterology.org. Accessed 26 October 2016.

Internet resources

British Society of Gastroenterology, www.bsg.org.uk
Disability Rights UK, https://disabilityrightsuk.org
Guts UK https://gutscharity.org.uk
The Rome Foundation, https://theromefoundation.org

References

Allen SJ, Martinez EG, Gregorio GV, *et al.* (2010) Probiotics for treating acute infectious diarrhoea. *Cochrane Database Syst. Rev.* (11): CD003048.

Anti M, Pignataro G, Armuzzi A, *et al.* (1998) Water supplementation enhances the effect of high fibre diet on stool frequency and laxative consumption in adult patients with functional constipation. *Hepatogastroenterology.* 45(21): 727–732.

Baldi F, Bianco MA, Nardone G, *et al.* (2009) Focus on acute diarrhoeal disease. *World J. Gastroenterol.* 15(27): 3341–3348.

Bernaola Aponte G, Bada Mancilla CA, Carreazo NY, *et al.* (2013) Probiotics for treating persistent diarrhoea in children. *Cochrane Database Syst. Rev.* (8): CD007401.

Borody T, Fischer M, Mitchell S, *et al.* (2015) Fecal microbiota transplantation in gastrointestinal disease: 2015 update and the road ahead. *Expert Rev. Gastroenterol. Hepatol.* 9: 1379–1391.

Burch J, Collins B. (2010) Using biofeedback to treat constipation, faecal incontinence and other bowel disorders. *Nurs. Times* 106: 18, 20–21.

Causebrook Y, Speed C. (2014) Constipation and nutrition. In: Lomer M (ed) *Advanced Nutrition and Dietetics in Gastroenterology*. Oxford: John Wiley and Sons.

Cullen G, O'Donoghue D. (2007) Constipation and pregnancy. *Best Pract. Res. Clin. Gastroenterol.* 21(5): 807–818.

Delvaux M. (2003) Diverticular disease of the colon in Europe: epidemiology, impact on citizen health and prevention. *Aliment. Pharmacol. Ther.* 18(3): 71–74.

Dennison C, Prasad M, Lloyd A, *et al.* (2005) The health-related quality of life and economic burden of constipation. *Pharmacoeconomics.* 23(5): 461–476.

Di Mario F, Comparato G, Fanigliulo L, *et al.* (2006) Use of mesalazine in diverticular disease. *J. Clin. Gastroenterol.* 40: S155–159.

Drossman DA. (2006) The functional gastrointestinal disorders and the Rome III process. *Gastroenterology* 130: 1377–1390.

Dukas L, Willet WC, Giovannucci EL. (2003) Association between physical activity, fiber intake, and other lifestyle variables and constipation in a study of women. *Am. J. Gastroenterol.* 98: 1790–1796.

Fitzharris GP, Garcia-Aguilar J, Parker SC, *et al.* (2003) Quality of life after subtotal colectomy for slow-transit constipation: both quality and quantity count. *Dis. Colon Rectum* 46: 433–440.

Frattini JC, Norgueras JJ. (2008) Slow transit constipation: a review of a colonic functional disorder. *Clin. Colon Rectal Surg.* 21(2): 146–152.

Garrigues V, Gálvez C, Ortiz V, *et al.* (2004) Prevalence of constipation: agreement among several criteria and evaluation of the diagnostic accuracy of qualifying symptoms and self-reported definition in a population-based survey in Spain. *Am. J. Epidemiol.* 159: 520–526.

Goldenberg JZ, Ma SSY, Saxton JD, *et al.* (2013) Probiotics for the prevention of *Clostridium difficile* – associated diarrhoea in adults and children. *Cochrane Database Syst. Rev.* (5): CD006095.

Grace E, Shaw C, Whelan K, *et al.* (2013) Review article: small intestinal bacterial overgrowth – prevalence, clinical features, current and developing diagnostic tests, and treatment. *Aliment. Pharmacol. Ther.* 38: 674–688.

Halmos EP, Power VA, Shepherd SJ, *et al.* (2014) A diet low in FODMAPs reduces symptoms of irritable bowel syndrome. *Gastroenterology.* 146(1): 67–75.

Hyland JMP, Taylor I. (1980) Does a high fibre diet prevent the complications of diverticular disease? *Br. J. Surg.* 67(2): 77–79.

Jeyarajah S. (2014) Diverticular disease and nutrition. In: Lomer M (ed) *Advanced Nutrition and Dietetics in Gastroenterology.* Oxford: John Wiley and Sons Ltd.

Juckett G, Trivedi R. (2011) Evaluation of chronic diarrhea. *Am. Fam. Physician.* 84(10): 1119–1126.

Kamm MA, Hawley PR, Lennard-Jones JE. (1988) Outcome of colectomy for severe idiopathic constipation. *Gut.* 29(7): 969–973.

Lamiki P, Tsuchiya J, Pathak S, *et al.* (2010) Probiotics in diverticular disease of the colon: an open label study. *J. Gastrointestin. Liver Dis.* 19(1): 31–36.

Levy RL, Olden KW, Naliboff BD, *et al.* (2006) Psychosocial aspects of the functional gastrointestinal disorders. *Gastroenterology.* 130: 1447–1458.

Lewis SJ, Heaton KW. (1997) Stool form scale as a useful guide to intestinal transit time. *Scand. J. Gastroenterol.* 32(9): 920–924.

Longstreth GF, Thompson WG, Chey WD, *et al.* (2006) Functional bowel disorders. *Gastroenterology.* 130: 1480–1491.

McCallum IJ, Ong S, Mercer J. (2009) Chronic constipation in adults. *BMJ* 338: b831.

Mugie SM, Benninga MA, Di Lorenzo C. (2011) Epidemiology of constipation in children and adults. *Best Pract. Res. Clin. Gastroenterol.* 25(1): 3–18.

NHS. (2018) https://www.nhsinform.scot/illnesses-and-conditions/stomach-liver-and-gastrointestinal-tract/diarrhoea. Accessed 26 October 2018.

NICE. (2007) *Faecal Incontinence in Adults: Management.* Available at http//www.nice.org.uk/guidance/cg49. Accessed 24 October 2016.

NICE. (2014) *Faecal Microbiota Transplantation for Recurrent* Clostridium difficile *Infection. IPG 485.* Available at http//www.nice.org.uk. Accessed 24 October 2016.

NICE. (2015) *NHS Evidence. Clinical Knowledge Summaries. Constipation.* Available at https://cks.nice.org.uk/constipation. Accessed 26 October 2018.

Painter NS, Burkitt DP. (1971) Diverticular disease of the colon: a deficiency disease of Western civilization. *BMJ* 2: 450–454.

Riss S, Herbst F, Birsan T, *et al.* (2009) Postoperative course and long term follow up after colectomy for slow transit constipation – is surgery an appropriate approach? *Colorectal Dis.* 11(3): 302–307.

Schimdt L, Dalhoof K. (2002) Food-drug interactions. *Drugs* 62(10): 1481–1502.

Staudacher H, Parkes G. (2014) Irritable bowel syndrome dietary management. In: Lomer M (ed) *Advanced Nutrition and Dietetics in Gastroenterology.* Oxford: John Wiley and Sons.

Suares NC, Ford AC. (2011) Systematic review: the effects of fibre in the management of chronic idiopathic constipation. *Aliment. Pharmacol. Ther.* 33(8): 895–901.

Talley NJ. (2004) Definitions, epidemiology and impact of chronic constipation. *Rev. Gastroenterol. Disord.* 4(2): S3–S10.

Thomas PD, Forbes A, Green J, *et al.* (2003) *Guidelines for the Investigation of Chronic Diarrhea*, 2nd edn. *Gut* 53(Suppl V): v1–v15.

Vermeulen J, van der Harst E, Lange JF. (2010) Pathophysiology and prevention of diverticulitis and perforation. *Neth. J. Med.* 68(10): 303–309.

Wald A. (2007) Chronic constipation: advances in management. *Neurogastroenterol. Motil.* 19(1): 4–10.

WHO. (2014) *The Top 10 Causes of Death*. Available at www.who.int/mediacentre/factsheets/fs310/en/. Accessed 28 October 2016.

Wilcox C, Turner J, Green J. (2014) Systematic review: the management of chronic diarrhoea due to bile acid malabsorption. *Aliment. Pharmacol. Ther.* 39: 923–939.

Wilcox M. (2013) *Updated Guidance on the Management and Treatment of Clostridium difficile Infection*. London: Public Health England.

Williams JG, Roberts SE, Ali MF, *et al.* (2007) Gastroenterology services in the UK. The burden of disease and the organization and delivery of services for gastrointestinal and liver disease: a review of the evidence. *Gut.* 56: 1–113.

Wingate D, Phillips SF, Lewis SJ, *et al.* (2001) Guidelines for adults on self-medication for the treatment of acute diarrhoea. *Aliment. Pharmacol. Ther.* 15(6): 773–782.

7.4.12 Liver and biliary disease

Lynsey Spillman and Gillian Gatiss

Key points

- Malnutrition and sarcopenia are common in cirrhosis in both obese and non-obese individuals.
- Dietetic assessment of nutritional status in all patients is essential and should include anthropometric measurements, clinical evaluation and review of dietary intake.
- Nutritional support should be provided to meet high requirements, while considering specific nutrient deficiencies.
- Restriction of essential nutrients should be assessed in individual cases and should be avoided unless indicated.

Liver disease refers to any disorder of the liver, including steatosis, fibrosis, hepatitis, cirrhosis or cancer. Liver disease is the third-most common cause of premature death in the UK (Williams *et al.*, 2014), and mortality from liver disease has been steadily rising for over 20 years (NHS Right Care, 2013).

Anatomy and function of the liver

The liver is the largest solid organ in the body, weighing approximately 1.5 kg in adults. It lies in the right upper quadrant of the abdomen, behind the rib cage. The liver has two anatomical lobes, with a larger right lobe (Figure 7.4.10). The portal vein provides blood from the splanchnic circulation and carries 75% of the blood entering the liver, which is rich in the end products of digestion. Approximately 25% of blood inflow is from the hepatic artery, supplying the liver with oxygen. The venous outflow from the liver is via the hepatic vein into the vena cava (Hill, 2009).

Sixty percent of the liver consists of hepatocytes that are arranged in thin layers, resulting in a larger surface area for exchange of substances with blood. Bile canaliculi are very small channels between adjacent hepatocytes that allow bile, produced in the liver, to pass to the common bile duct. This travels via the cystic duct to the gall bladder for concentration and storage or into the duodenum via the common bile duct. The liver plays an essential role in the function of many processes, including the metabolism of nutrients (Table 7.4.15).

Classification of liver disease

Acute liver failure

Acute liver failure, also known as fulminant liver failure, is rare and presents as acute abnormal liver blood tests without underlying chronic liver disease. There are multiple definitions of acute liver failure, as described by the European Association for the Study of the Liver (EASL, 2017a). The most common cause of acute liver failure in the UK is paracetamol toxicity (Bernal *et al.*, 2010) (Table 7.4.16). Other causes include medication and hepatitis A, B and E, with 17% of cases being of unknown cause (Bernal *et al.*, 2010). Prognosis depends on the cause of acute liver failure but has improved since the introduction of emergency liver transplantation. Patients who survive acute liver failure usually make a full recovery (EASL, 2017a).

Chronic liver disease

Chronic liver disease has multiple aetiologies (Table 7.4.17). Hepatocellular damage may occur over several years initially via a build-up of fat in the liver (fatty liver), which develops via inflammation and scarring (fibrosis) to irreversible cirrhosis (Figure 7.4.11). In response to liver injury, e.g. alcohol, non-alcoholic fatty liver disease (NAFLD) or chronic hepatitis C infection (HCV), fatty liver progresses to fibrosis.

If the causative agent is removed (e.g. abstinence from alcohol, weight loss or antiviral treatment), normal hepatocyte structure can be restored at this stage. If the

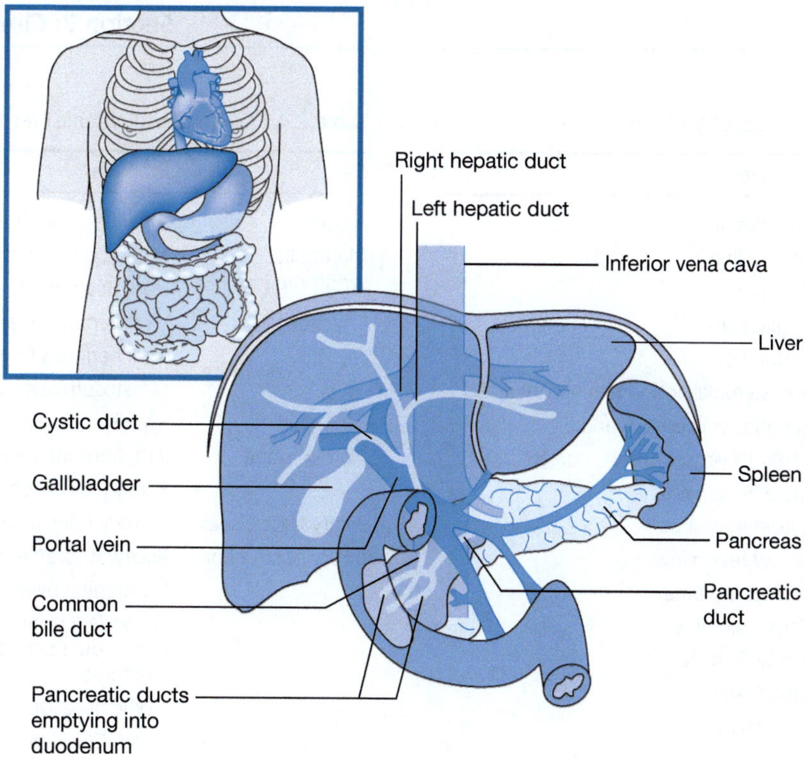

Figure 7.4.10 Anatomy of the liver (source: The British Liver Trust. Reproduced with permission from the British Liver Trust, www.britishlivertrust.org.uk)

Table 7.4.15 Major functions of the liver (Kallis & Westaby, 2014)

Function	Examples
Digestion	Bile acid production
Carbohydrate metabolism	Maintenance of glucose homeostasis
	Storage of glycogen
	Gluconeogenesis
	Mobilisation of glucose in response to hypoglycaemia
Protein metabolism	Utilisation of amino acids for protein synthesis and gluconeogenesis
	Deamination of amino acids into urea for excretion
	Regulation of amino acid supply to peripheral tissues
	Synthesis of plasma albumin, prothrombin, fibrinogen and clotting factors
Lipids and lipoproteins	Production of triglycerides and lipoprotein formation
	Synthesis of phospholipids and cholesterol
	Synthesis and degradation of non-esterified fatty acids
	Ketogenesis
Vitamins	Storage of vitamins A, B_2, B_3, B_6, B_{12}, K, folate
	Synthesis of prothrombin and factor VII, requiring vitamin K
	Conversion of tryptophan to nicotinic acid
	Hydroxylation of vitamin D
Detoxification/deactivation	Oxidation of alcohol → acetaldehyde → acetate → CO_2 + fatty acids + H_2O
	Deactivation of drugs in the cytochrome P450 system
	Conjugation of oestrogens, corticosteroids and other steroid hormones for excretion
Excretion	Excretion of porphyrins, drugs, environmental toxins and heavy metals via bile secretion
Immune function	Adaptive immune system – T and B lymphocyte production
	Innate immune system
	Cytokine and inflammatory signalling cell production
	Kupffer cell formation (mononuclear phagocyte system)
	Tumour necrosis factor alpha (TNF-α) production
Haematological function	Synthesis of haem
	Regulation of iron metabolism

Table 7.4.16 Common causes of acute liver failure

Cause	Examples
Drugs	Paracetamol
	Tetracycline
	Halothane
	Troglitazone
	Antibiotics
	Non-steroidal anti-inflammatory drugs
Viral infections	Hepatitis viruses A, B and E
	Hepatitis viruses non-A, non-B
	Epstein–Barr virus
	Cytomegalovirus
	Yellow fever virus
	Reye's syndrome
	Herpes simplex
Alcohol	Alcoholic hepatitis
Non-viral infections	Toxoplasmosis
	Leptospira
Bacterial infections	Tuberculosis
	Pyogenic liver abscess
Protozoal infections	Malaria
	Amoebiasis
Toxins	Amanita phalloides
	Aflatoxin
	Carbon tetrachloride
Other	Acute fatty liver of pregnancy
	Wilson's disease
	Herbal medicines
	Budd–Chiari
	Idiopathic
	HELLP syndrome of pregnancy

Table 7.4.17 Causes of chronic liver disease

Cause	Examples
Alcohol	Alcoholic liver disease
Metabolic syndrome	Non-alcoholic fatty liver disease (NAFLD)
	Non-alcoholic steatohepatitis (NASH)
Infections	Viral hepatitis B and C (most common)
	Viral hepatitis D, E and G
	Schistosomiasis
	Syphilis
Autoimmune	Autoimmune hepatitis
	Primary biliary cholangitis
Biliary tract disease	Primary sclerosing cholangitis
Biliary obstruction	Biliary atresia/neonatal hepatitis
	Congenital biliary cysts
	Secondary biliary cirrhosis as a result of bile duct occlusion by gallstones or strictures
	Cystic fibrosis
Vascular disorders	Budd–Chiari syndrome
	Veno-occlusive disease/portal vein
	Thrombosis
Drugs and toxins	Methotrexate
	Amiodarone
	Isoniazid
Metabolic disorders	Tyrosinaemia
	Wilson's disease
	Haemochromatosis
	Alpha-1-antitrypsin deficiency
	Porphyria
	Glycogen storage diseases
Bacterial infections	Tuberculosis
	Pyogenic liver abscess
Miscellaneous	Sarcoidosis
	Jejunoileal bypass
	Caroli's syndrome
Cryptogenic	Liver disease of unknown aetiology

injury is chronic or recurrent, fibrosis can progress to cirrhosis, which is irreversible (see Figure 7.4.11). The fibrous progression disrupts the architecture of the liver and impairs liver function. An acute episode of liver failure may also be superimposed on pre-existing chronic disease (Muir, 2015).

Cirrhosis can take many years to develop and is classified as either compensated or decompensated. In compensated cirrhosis, there are no symptoms of liver disease present, as the liver performs vital functions sufficiently, despite being cirrhotic. In decompensated cirrhosis, symptoms of liver disease are present, e.g. ascites, jaundice, varices or hepatic encephalopathy (HE). Decompensation can be part of progressive liver disease or can result from a sudden insult to an already cirrhotic liver. It is possible for the liver to shift between compensated and decompensated states (Muir, 2015).

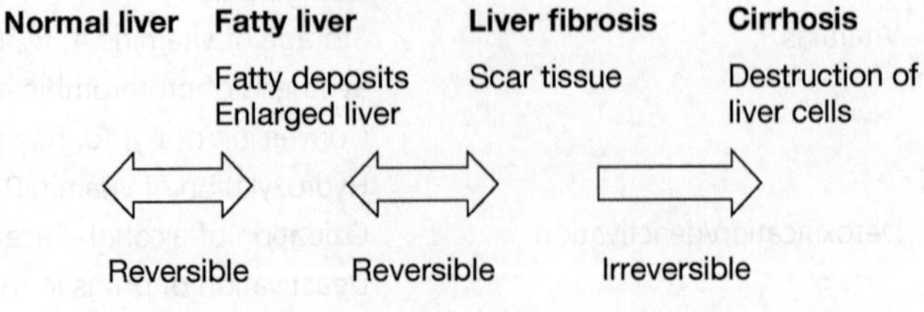

Figure 7.4.11 Stages of liver disease

Liver disease severity

Cirrhosis is often scored using the Child–Pugh score (sometimes the Child–Turcotte–Pugh score). It is used to determine prognosis as well as the required level of treatment, and is one of the scoring systems used when considering the need for referral for liver transplantation. The score employs five clinical measures of liver disease (Table 7.4.18). Each measure is scored 1–3, with 3 indicating the most severe derangement. Chronic liver disease is classified into Child–Pugh class A, B or C, using the added score from Table 7.4.19. In primary sclerosing

SECTION 7

Table 7.4.18 Severity of cirrhosis using grading scores – modified Child–Pugh classification for cirrhosis (source: Friedman & Keeffe, 2004)

Measure	1 point	2 points	3 points
Total bilirubin (μmol/L or mg/dL)	<34 (<2)	34–50 (2–3)	>50 (>3)
Serum albumin (g/L)	>35	28–35	<28
Prothrombin time (seconds increased)	1–3	4–6	>6
Ascites	None	Mild	Moderate/severe
Hepatic encephalopathy	None	Grade I–II (or suppressed with medication)	Grade III–IV (or refractory)

Table 7.4.19 Classification of Child–Pugh score (source: Pugh *et al.* (1973) Transection of the oesophagus for bleeding oesophageal varices. *British Journal of Surgery* 60: 646–649)

Points	Class
5–6	A
7–9	B
10–15	C

cholangitis (PSC) and primary biliary cholangitis (PBC), the bilirubin references are altered to reflect the fact that these diseases feature high conjugated bilirubin levels (Pugh *et al.*, 1973).

Other measures have become more common in assessing the severity of liver disease, prognosis and need for referral for liver transplantation. The 'model for end-stage liver disease' (MELD) and the 'UK end-stage liver disease' (UKELD) scoring systems are used to predict mortality among patients on the waiting list for liver transplantation (Cholongitas & Burroughs, 2012). A systematic review with meta-analysis found that MELD and Child–Pugh had similar prognostic values when compared (Peng *et al.*, 2016). The inclusion of other mortality risk factors within prognostic scores has been proposed, e.g. a measure of sarcopenia (Montano-Loza *et al.*, 2015) and HE (Montagnese *et al.*, 2015).

Disease processes

Alcoholic liver disease

In Europe, alcohol is the main cause of liver disease (Blachier *et al.*, 2013); globally, it accounts for 48% of all deaths from cirrhosis (Liangpunsakul *et al.*, 2016). The disease ranges from steatosis (fatty liver) through hepatitis to cirrhosis (EASL, 2012a). The risk of developing alcoholic liver disease increases with overall alcohol intake. However, when alcohol intake is high, and of long duration, 90–100% of consumers will have fatty liver, but only 20–35% develop alcoholic hepatitis, and 8–20% develop cirrhosis (Barve *et al.*, 2008). The risk

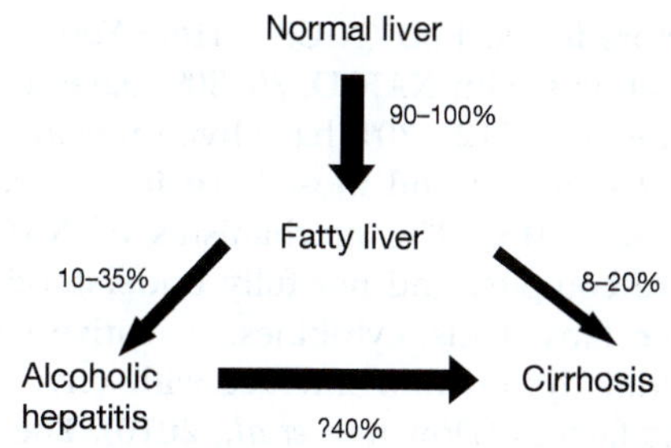

Figure 7.4.12 Progression of alcoholic liver disease in heavy drinkers (source: McCullough & O'Connor, 1998. Reproduced with permission from Wiley-Blackwell Publishing)

of developing alcoholic liver disease has been associated with female gender, obesity, metabolic syndrome, drinking outside of meals, ethnic differences, chronic infection with HCV, iron overload and genetic predisposition (EASL, 2012a). Oxidative stress, proinflammatory cytokines and reduced levels of adiponectin (which has anti-inflammatory properties) have been implicated as the pathways of injury as a result of alcohol (Tilg *et al.*, 2011).

Alcoholic hepatitis

Alcoholic hepatitis presents as an acute decompensation of liver function in a person with a history of alcohol misuse (Sougioultzis *et al.*, 2005). Typical age of presentation is 40–60 years. The female gender, elevated body mass index (BMI) and genetic predisposition have been identified as risk factors (Mitchell *et al.*, 2017; Yeluru *et al.*, 2016). Uniquely, alcoholic hepatitis does not lead to cirrhosis and is distinct from cirrhosis caused by long-term alcohol consumption. The progression of alcoholic liver disease in heavy drinkers is shown in Figure 7.4.12 (McCullough & O'Connor, 1998). Patients with alcoholic hepatitis usually present with rapid onset of jaundice, fever, hepatomegaly and anorexia. Symptoms of portal hypertension may also be involved, such as ascites, HE and variceal bleeding (Yeluru *et al.*, 2016).

Non-alcoholic fatty liver disease

The European Association for the Study of the Liver (EASL) define NAFLD *as 'the presence of liver fat accumulation exceeding 5% of hepatocytes in the absence of significant alcohol intake, viral infection, or any other specific aetiology of liver disease'* (Blachier *et al.*, 2013). NAFLD is a spectrum of fatty liver diseases in which there is a build-up of fat in liver cells. NAFLD include two different conditions with different prognoses – namely, non-alcoholic fatty liver (NAFL), also known as 'steatosis', and non-alcoholic steatohepatitis (NASH). NASH is an inflammatory fibrosing disease, which includes fibrosis, cirrhosis and hepatocellular carcinoma (HCC) (EASL–EASD–EASO, 2016). It is estimated that 20–30% of the population have NAFLD (Bellentani *et al.*, 2010). Obesity, wide waist circumference, hyperlipidaemia, type 2 diabetes and metabolic syndrome are all risk factors for NAFLD (NICE, 2016a; Younossi *et al.*, 2016). In patients with NAFLD, 20–80% have dyslipidaemia (Souza *et al.*, 2012), 70% have hypertension, 40–50% have type 2 diabetes and most have insulin resistance (Dyson *et al.*, 2015). The mechanisms of NAFLD progression are complex and not fully understood. Factors such as free fatty acids, cytokines, oxidative stress and mitochondrial dysfunction interact with environmental and genetic factors (Dowman *et al.*, 2010). The majority of patients with NAFLD are asymptomatic or have non-specific symptoms such as fatigue or abdominal pain (O'Sullivan & McAnenny, 2014).

Secondary non-alcohol fatty liver disease

It is possible for some conditions to lead to the same clinical picture as NAFLD; this is known as secondary NAFLD. Secondary NAFLD/NASH is rare in adults and is unrelated to insulin resistance or metabolic syndrome. Causes of secondary NAFLD/NASH include pregnancy-related fatty liver disease and intestinal jejunoileal bypass surgery (Adams & Angulo, 2006).

Primary biliary cholangitis

PBC (previously known as primary biliary cirrhosis) is a chronic and progressive autoimmune disease where the bile ducts become inflamed and are destroyed, resulting in reduced flow of bile into the gastrointestinal tract. It can lead to end-stage biliary cirrhosis (Hirschfield *et al.*, 2017). The estimated incidence of PBC in Europe is 1–2 per 100,000 population per year, and it predominantly affects women, with a female:male ratio reported as 10:1 (Lleo *et al.*, 2016). Onset usually occurs between 40 and 60 years of age (Hirschfield *et al.*, 2017). The aetiology is largely unknown, although genetic, immune system and environmental factors have been considered (Levy & Lindor, 2003). Symptoms include osteoporosis, pruritus (itching), fatigue and jaundice. Patients with advanced PBC and cirrhosis may develop ascites and HE. An association between PBC and coeliac disease has been found, with the incidence ranging between 0 and 11% (Rubio-Tapia & Murray, 2007).

Primary sclerosing cholangitis

PSC is a chronic progressive disorder characterised by inflammation and fibrosis of the biliary tree, leading to liver cirrhosis (Lazaridis & LaRusso, 2016). The incidence ranges from 0 to 1.3 per 100,000 population per year (Boonstra *et al.*, 2012). Approximately 60% are male, and the median age of diagnosis is 41 years (Lazaridis & LaRusso, 2016). The aetiology is still unclear, although PSC could be caused by autoimmune, genetic or inflammatory disease (Lazaridis & LaRusso, 2016). It is associated with inflammatory bowel disease in 60–80% of cases (Rossi *et al.*, 2016).

Autoimmune hepatitis

Autoimmune hepatitis is a progressive disease of unknown aetiology, where an exaggerated immune reaction towards hepatic tissue occurs in a genetically susceptible person. The incidence is reported as 0.8–3 per 100,000 population in Western Europe (van Gerven *et al.*, 2016). At least 70% of patients are female, with half younger than 40 years of age; however, onset may range from childhood to the elderly (Makol *et al.*, 2011). Clinical presentation can be from mild to severe symptoms, including abdominal and joint pain, fatigue and jaundice, or as acute liver failure (van Gerven *et al.*, 2016).

Viral hepatitis

Viral hepatitis is mainly caused by the hepatitis B virus (HBV) and HCV. Other causes include hepatitis A, D and E virus.

Hepatitis C virus

Globally, an estimated 71 million people have chronic HCV infection, with a prevalence of 1.5% in Europe (WHO, 2017a) and 0.5–1% in the UK (HSE, 2017a). It causes chronic hepatitis, leading to cirrhosis, with increased risk of hepatocellular carcinoma and intrahepatic cholangiocarcinoma (El-Serag *et al.*, 2009). Transmission is usually via infected blood, which can include drug use, blood products prior to HCV screening, tattooing or piercing.

Hepatitis B virus

It is estimated that 257 million people are living with HBV worldwide, and it is more common in developing countries. The prevalence of hepatitis B in Europe is 1.6% (WHO, 2017b) and 0.1–0.5% in the UK (HSE, 2017b). It is transmitted by the blood and body fluids of an infected person, and can be transmitted from mother to child at birth. HBV may cause an acute illness or develop into a chronic disease, which causes cirrhosis and possibly liver cancer. Most people do not experience symptoms with acute infection but some have jaundice, fatigue, nausea, vomiting and abdominal pain (WHO, 2017b).

Hepatitis E virus

Every year, there are an estimated 20 million infections with hepatitis E virus worldwide, but only 3.3 million symptomatic cases. The virus is spread via the faecal–oral route in contaminated water and via ingestion of undercooked infected animal meat. For most, the virus is self-limiting, with symptoms including fever, anorexia, nausea, vomiting, abdominal pain, itching, rash and jaundice that lasts 1–6 weeks (WHO, 2017c). In some cases, acute hepatitis E can be severe, and result in acute liver failure and death. Several reports have implicated hepatitis E virus in the deterioration of liver function in people with pre-existing compensated liver disease, with a higher mortality rate than those without underlying liver disease (Goel & Aggarwal, 2016).

Metabolic liver disease

Wilson's disease

This is an autosomal recessive genetic disorder in which copper accumulates in tissues, resulting in acute or chronic liver disease with neuropsychiatric symptoms. It is estimated that the prevalence of Wilson's disease is 1 per 30,000; however, this figure is debated (Coffey *et al.*, 2013). Wilson's disease constitutes 6–12% of acute failure referred for liver transplant, with a female:male ratio of 4:1. Fulminant Wilson's disease is usually fatal without transplantation (EASL, 2012b). Chronic Wilson's disease usually presents with hepatitis or cirrhosis and symptoms of hepatomegaly, ascites or jaundice. The progression of disease depends on the effectiveness of chelation treatment (Eapen *et al.*, 2016).

Haemochromatosis

Haemochromatosis is an autosomal genetic recessive disease characterised by the abnormal accumulation of iron in major organs, leading to accumulation in tissues and primarily the liver, causing cirrhosis (Salgia & Brown, 2015). Iron deposits can also accumulate in endocrine organs and the heart. The prevalence of haemochromatosis varies across geographical regions; those with Northern European ancestry have a higher risk of the genetic mutation responsible (Powell *et al.*, 2016). Being male and excessive alcohol consumption are risk factors for haemochromatosis, and clinical presentation of advanced disease are liver cirrhosis, diabetes, fatigue and skin pigmentation (Powell *et al.*, 2016).

Alpha-1-antitrypsin deficiency

This is an autosomal recessive genetic disorder caused by the defective production of alpha-1-antitrypsin (A1AT) protein in the liver, which affects the liver and lungs. A1AT accumulates in the liver and damages liver cells, and can lead to fibrosis, cirrhosis, liver failure and HCC (Teckman & Mangalat, 2015). There is no treatment other than symptom management and liver transplantation. A1AT accounts for 1.1% of all adult liver transplants (Lomas *et al.*, 2016).

Hepatocellular carcinoma

Liver cancer is increasing in incidence and is the third-most common cause of cancer-related deaths. It accounts for 90% of liver cancers (EASL–EORTC, 2012). The predominant risk factors for HCC are HBV in developing countries and HCV in developed countries (Park *et al.*, 2015). Cirrhosis is a risk factor for HCC, and one-third of those with cirrhosis will develop HCC. The average age in the UK at which HCC develops is 66 years; risk increases with age, and it is more prevalent in men (Ryder, 2003).

Disease consequences

Mortality

In contrast to improvements in life expectancy from chronic disorders such as stroke, heart disease and many cancers, liver disease mortality in the UK continues to rise. Standardised mortality rates have increased 400% since 1970, and by almost 500% in people younger than 65 years (Williams *et al.*, 2014). Liver disease is the third-biggest cause of premature mortality in the UK, and it has been included in the UK government's *Big Five* campaign to reduce premature avoidable mortality (DH, 2014).

Public health aspects and prevention

As the major causes of liver disease are largely avoidable (e.g. excess alcohol consumption, NAFLD-associated obesity and chronic viral hepatitis), effective prevention strategies or treatments can decrease the risk of developing cirrhosis, liver cancer and its associated mortality (Williams *et al.*, 2014). Examples of early prevention measures include early identification and treatment of HCV and HBV infection through screening and antiviral medication; identification of hazardous drinking through screening; and interventions for obesity.

Alcohol

The hazardous and harmful use of alcohol contributes to death, disease and injury at the global level, with the highest alcohol consumption occurring in the developed world, including Europe (WHO, 2011). Alcohol misuse and alcohol-related problems are a major public health concern in the UK. In 2015, there were 8 758 alcohol-related deaths in the UK (Office for National Statistics, 2015). It is estimated that alcohol-related harm costs the UK economy £17.7–£25.1 billion per year. In England, it costs the NHS up to £2.7 billion a year to treat the chronic and acute effects of drinking alcohol (DH, 2008).

Increasing-risk drinking is considered to be regularly consuming 22–50 units per week (men) or 15–35 units per week (women). Higher-risk drinking is considered to be regularly consuming over 50 alcohol units per week (men) or over 35 units per week (women) (NICE, 2010). It is estimated 3 million people in the UK drink alcohol at hazardous levels (Robinson & Bulger, 2008). The Chief Medical Officer's guideline for both men and women is reported in Box 7.4.3.

Box 7.4.3 UK government drinking guidelines (source: Chief Medical Officer, 2016)

To keep health risks from alcohol to a low level, it is safest not to drink more than 14 units a week on a regular basis.

If regularly drinking as much as 14 units per week, it is best to spread drinking evenly over 3 days or more. If having one or two heavy drinking episodes a week, there is an increased risk of death from long-term illness, and from accidents and injuries.

The risk of developing a range of health problems (including cancers of the mouth, throat and breast) increases with volume and frequency of drinking.

A good way to cut down on alcohol consumed is to have several drink-free days each week.

Prevention

Alcohol

Primary prevention strategies in the UK have focused on reducing the alcohol consumption (Williams *et al.*, 2014). Increases in alcohol duty since 2008 has resulted in a slight fall in consumption, but this policy has since been abolished (Hudson *et al.*, 2017; Williams *et al.*, 2014). Secondary prevention strategies have focused on brief alcohol interventions (early identification of hazardous drinking and brief advice), which have proved effective in reducing alcohol consumption (Bertholet *et al.*, 2005; Kaner *et al.*, 2013). More recently, NICE (2016b) have recommended that men and women drinking more than 50 and 35 units of alcohol a week, respectively, be offered transient elastography (FibroScan®) to exclude cirrhosis. However, whether this is a cost-effective strategy for the NHS is debated (Hudson *et al.*, 2017).

Obesity and non-alcoholic fatty liver disease

The Health Survey for England (Fuller *et al.*, 2016) shows that 27% of adults and 14% of children are obese, and these individuals have an increased risk of type 2 diabetes. Obesity and diabetes are associated with fatty infiltration of the liver (NICE, 2016a). The prevalence of NAFLD in the general population in Western countries is 20–30%. The prevalence of NAFLD is 80–90% in obese adults, 30–50% in patients with diabetes and up to 90% in patients with hyperlipidaemia (Bellentani *et al.*, 2010). Interventions for obesity management and UK government strategies to deal with this public health problem are discussed in Chapter 4.2 (Public health nutrition). The greatest effect on reducing NAFLD will come from reducing levels of obesity across the whole population (Williams *et al.*, 2014).

Viral hepatitis

Hepatitis C virus

The emergence of new, well-tolerated, direct-acting antiviral (DAA) drugs for chronic infection of HCV, with viral clearance in more than 90% of people, has led to the aim to eliminate HCV as a global public health threat by 2030 (Public Health England (PHE), 2017a). The cost of these newer antivirals is high, and this has restricted treatment numbers in the UK (Burstow *et al.*, 2017; Gelson & Alexander, 2017). In the UK, there are indications that DAAs may be starting to have an impact, with a 32% fall in liver transplants for HCV cirrhosis in 2015 (PHE, 2017a).

Hepatitis B virus

HBV is not considered a public health issue for liver disease in the same way as HCV. This is because, unlike HCV, an effective vaccine exists against HBV (Williams *et al.*, 2014). As the prevalence of chronic infection of HBV in the UK is less than 1%, only high-risk groups are offered vaccination, e.g. healthcare workers, injecting drug users, individuals who frequently change sexual partners, and infants born to mothers who have HBV (HSE, 2017b). From 2017, all babies born in the UK receive HBV vaccine as part of infant immunisation (PHE, 2017b).

Patient perspectives

Valery *et al.* (2015) conducted a systematic review of the perspectives, experiences and concerns of people with chronic liver disease (mainly patients with viral hepatitis). Twenty-six international studies were included, and they identified five key domains of supportive care needs, as follows:

- Informational or educational (e.g. educational material, educational sessions).
- Practical (e.g. daily living).
- Physical (e.g. controlling pruritus and fatigue).
- Patient care and support (e.g. support groups).
- Psychological (e.g. anxiety and sadness).

The authors noted a lack of literature from the population likely to have the most supportive care needs, i.e. those with cirrhosis. There are many liver-disease-related patient support groups in the UK (see the section 'Internet resources'). In 2016, the priority areas for alcohol-related liver disease research were, for the first time, agreed on jointly by patients, carers and health professionals (James Lind Alliance, 2016).

Nutritional consequences

Malnutrition as a consequence of liver disease has been recognised for decades (Dasarathy & Merli, 2016). Older studies quote a prevalence of malnutrition of up to 20% in compensated cirrhosis (Coltorti *et al.*, 1991), 75–90% in decompensated cirrhosis (Carvalho & Parise, 2006; DiCecco *et al.*, 1989) and almost 100% for those awaiting liver transplantation (Figueiredo *et al.*, 2000). These older studies have used various nutritional methods for assessing malnutrition and have not focused on skeletal muscle mass (Dasarathy, 2012).

More recently, the emergence of radiographic image analysis, e.g. computed tomography (CT) and magnetic resonance imaging (MRI), has allowed precise measurement of skeletal muscle mass and the diagnosis of sarcopenia (Dasarathy & Merli, 2016). Sarcopenia is defined as the presence of both low muscle mass and low muscle function (Cruz-Jentoft *et al.*, 2010), and it occurs in 30–70% of cirrhotic patients (Dasarathy & Merli, 2016). Sarcopenia can be found in combination with loss of fat mass (hepatic cachexia) or increased fat mass (sarcopenic obesity) (Dasarathy, 2012). Preferential loss of fat mass has been found in women as compared to muscle mass in men (Dasarathy & Merli, 2016; Morgan *et al.*, 2006). Malnutrition is associated with the following:

- Reduced survival (Durand *et al.*, 2014; Montano-Loza *et al.*, 2012; Tandon *et al.*, 2012).
- Development of other complications of cirrhosis, e.g. ascites, HE and hepatorenal syndrome (Huisman *et al.*, 2011; Merli *et al.*, 2013; Sam & Nguyen, 2009).
- Reduced quality of life (Shiraki *et al.*, 2013).

Poor post-liver-transplant outcomes (e.g. postoperative infections) lead to increased ventilator requirements and extended hospital stay (Kalafateli *et al.*, 2017).

Causes of malnutrition

Changes in metabolism

Carbohydrate and fat metabolism have been demonstrated to be altered in cirrhosis following an overnight fast (Owen *et al.*, 1983). Cirrhotic patients develop starvation-type metabolism similar to that of a 2–3-day fast in healthy people. This is due to decreased hepatic glycogen stores and reduced glycogenolysis. Fat and protein are metabolised as a short-term energy source, which creates an accelerated response to starvation (Greco *et al.*, 1998; Petersen *et al.*, 1999).

Altered glucose metabolism is common in chronic liver disease, with up to 96% exhibiting impaired glucose tolerance (Garcia-Compean *et al.*, 2016; Hickman & Macdonald, 2007), and up to 35% developing diabetes (Garcia-Compean *et al.*, 2012; Muller *et al.*, 1994). In these patients, insulin resistance has been implicated by reduced hepatic degradation and increased secretion of insulin, with elevated plasma levels of insulin alongside normal glucose tolerance (Matos *et al.*, 2002).

Metabolism of protein and amino acids may be altered in liver disease, but the mechanism is not fully understood. Studies investigating protein metabolism in liver cirrhosis have produced conflicting results, with increased, unaltered or decreased protein breakdown and decreased or unaltered protein synthesis (Dasarathy, 2012).

Branched-chain amino acids

Reduced levels of circulating branched-chain amino acids (BCAAs), leucine, isoleucine and valine, and increased levels of circulating methionine and aromatic amino acids (AAAs), phenylalanine, tryptophan and tyrosine, have been found in liver disease (Tajiri & Shimizu, 2013). BCAAs are metabolised by skeletal muscle, rather than the liver. The increase in AAAs is related to the reduced capacity of liver clearance. The proposed cause for HE is enhanced passage of AAAs through the blood–brain barrier, resulting in the creation of false neurotransmitters which cause HE symptoms. It is thought that BCAAs compete with AAAs for passage across the blood–brain barrier and facilitate ammonia detoxification through supporting glutamine synthesis (Amodio *et al.*, 2013).

Reduced nutrient intake

Reduced nutrient intake has been described by O'Brien and Williams (2008), Cheung *et al.* (2012), Johnson *et al.* (2013) and Mouzaki *et al.* (2014), and is a result of the following factors:

- Loss of appetite due to the presence of cytokines, e.g. tumour necrosis factor.
- Early satiety, commonly found when ascites results in reduced gastric capacity.
- Inability to eat due to severe encephalopathy.
- Altered sleep patterns resulting in missed meals and snacks.
- Unnecessary dietary restrictions further exacerbating the choice and volume of food.
- Nausea and vomiting due to gastroparesis, small bowel dysfunction and bacterial overgrowth.
- High alcohol intakes replacing food energy, or reduced intake due to oesophagitis, gastritis or pancreatitis.
- Altered taste sensation due to deficiency of zinc or magnesium.
- Weakness or fatigue affecting inclination to eat or prepare food.
- Repeated investigations that require prior fasting.
- Increase in leptin levels.
- Altered energy expenditure.

Studies using indirect calorimetry to measure resting energy expenditure (REE) show that 15–34% of patients with cirrhosis are hypermetabolic, i.e. REE > 120% of predicted values (Madden & Morgan, 1999; Muller *et al.*, 1999; Peng *et al.*, 2007). The cause of this increase in energy expenditure in some patients with cirrhosis is unclear. Some studies have shown an increase in energy expenditure with ascites and hepatocellular carcinoma (Cheung *et al.*, 2012), but others have found no association between hypermetabolism and these factors (Peng *et al.*, 2007). In clinical practice, predictive equations are used to estimate REE (Todorovic & Micklewright, 2011). Due to variations in body composition between patients, others would advocate the use of indirect calorimetry to measure REE (Glass *et al.*, 2012; Madden & Morgan, 1999).

Malabsorption

Malabsorption and maldigestion of gastrointestinal nutrients frequently exist in patients with liver disease. However, the extent to which they occur can vary considerably, depending on the underlying disease and the individual. Ulcerative colitis is commonly seen in people with PSC, and coeliac disease in those with PBC. Additionally, in alcoholic liver disease, pancreatic insufficiency is common. One study has showed an incidence of chronic pancreatitis of 18% in cirrhosis (Pace *et al.*, 2009). Other reasons for malabsorption can include bacterial overgrowth resulting from impaired small bowel motility or the administration of medications such a cholestyramine, lactulose and antibiotics. Malabsorption of fat-soluble vitamins is common, especially in cholestatic disease, where reduced absorption of carbohydrates, protein, water-soluble vitamins and minerals has also been demonstrated (Juakiem *et al.*, 2014).

Protein loss

Patients lose approximately 13 g protein for every litre of ascites removed in paracentesis. Normally, for every litre of ascites removed, 8 g protein is replaced with human albumin solution, giving a net loss of 5 g protein per litre (Salvioli *et al.*, 1993).

Vitamins

In chronic liver disease, deficiencies of pyridoxine, vitamin B_{12} and thiamine may result in peripheral neuropathy and neurologic disturbances (Johnson *et al.*, 2013). In particular, there is a high risk of Wernicke's encephalopathy in alcohol-related liver disease as the metabolism of alcohol increases the body's requirement for thiamine (Thomson & Marshall, 2006). There is a high incidence of fat-soluble vitamin deficiencies in liver disease, with levels related to the severity of disease (Abbott-Johnson *et al.*, 2011). Vitamin A deficiency may cause dry corneas and night blindness (Johnson *et al.*, 2013). In PBC, vitamin A deficiency is seen in 20% of cases, but is often clinically asymptomatic (Talwalkar & Lindor, 2003). In advanced PSC, up to 82% of patients will be deficient in vitamin A (Lee & Kaplan, 2002). More than 90% of those with chronic liver disease are vitamin D deficient, with severe deficiency found in 29% (Arteh *et al.*, 2010). Deficiency of vitamin E is rare, but can be seen in chronic cholestatic liver disease. Symptoms include muscle weakness, ataxia and haemolysis, and, in advanced PSC, these can be seen in 40–50% of patients (Lee & Kaplan, 2002). Vitamin K is an important clotting factor, and therefore bleeding is a common sign of deficiency (Johnson *et al.*, 2013).

Minerals

Magnesium

Serum magnesium levels are decreased in liver cirrhosis, which may be attributed to decreased intake or increased excretion (Das *et al.*, 2011). Serum magnesium was negatively associated with salt perception and overall taste score in a study by Madden *et al.* (1997).

Zinc

The liver plays an important role in zinc homeostasis. Zinc deficiency in cirrhosis is associated with impaired liver function and alteration in taste perception. Zinc deficiency may be a result of multiple factors, including decreased intestinal absorption, increased urinary losses through diuretics and reduced circulating albumin levels, which results in reduced binding of zinc to albumin. Malnutrition in cirrhotic patients is also likely to contribute to zinc deficiency (Grungreiff *et al.*, 2016). The pathogenesis of HE may be related to zinc deficiency, and oral zinc supplementation resulted in improved performance in patients with HE (Chavez-Tapia *et al.*, 2013).

Steatorrhoea

This develops if secretion of bile is significantly impaired (cholestasis) and, as a result, reduced amounts of bile salts reaching the duodenum. Bile acids also act as cofactors for digestive lipases, protecting them from the proteolytic effects of other digestive enzymes. Steatorrhoea is a frequent symptom in cholestatic diseases such as PBC and PSC. Steatorrhoea may be so severe that it compromises the nutritional status of the patient and may be a direct cause of malnutrition (Vidas, 2014).

Metabolic bone disorders

The primary metabolic bone disorder found in chronic liver disease is osteoporosis. Prevalence of osteoporosis is highest in cholestatic disease, with a prevalence of 20–45% in PBC and 15% in PSC (Guarino *et al.*, 2016). Clinically, patients present with bone pains, backache, reduced height, fractures and scoliosis (Goel & Kar, 2010). The reasons for this are multifactorial, including poor intake and absorption of calcium, altered vitamin D synthesis, malnutrition and steroid use in certain liver conditions. Other risk factors for osteoporosis include low BMI, alcohol excess and physical inactivity (see Chapter 7.9.1, Osteoporosis).

Nutritional assessment

Detailed nutritional assessment is critical in patients with liver disease in order to provide optimal nutritional support. Some markers of nutritional status used in other clinical areas are not useful in liver disease, as symptoms, dietary intake and nutritional status are prone to rapid change. Nutritional status must be monitored regularly, and alterations made to treatment plans to reflect these changes.

Screening tools

The Malnutrition Universal Screening Tool ('MUST') (Elia, 2003) was developed in order to categorise patients for risk of malnutrition. However, 'MUST' has poor sensitivity of 43% for identifying the risk of malnutrition in patients with fluid overload (Arora *et al.*, 2012a). The performance of 'MUST' improved when accurately calculated dry weights were used (Arora *et al.*, 2012a). Adequate training is essential to ensure that dry weight and dry weight loss are calculated accurately. The Royal Free Hospital Nutritional Prioritising Tool (RFH-GA; see Figure 7.14.1 and Appendix A7) has been developed and validated to identify malnutrition risk in patients with liver cirrhosis, with a sensitivity of 100% and specificity of 73% (Arora *et al.*, 2012b). This tool asks different questions depending on the presence of fluid overload.

Royal Free Hospital Global Assessment

This tool uses dry-weight BMI, MAMC and an assessment of nutritional intake to categorise patients into adequately, moderately (or suspected of being so) or severely malnourished. Morgan *et al.* (2006) validated the RFH-GA tool, which is simple, reproducible and capable of predicting outcome in patients with cirrhosis (Figure 7.4.13). The tool predicted reduced survival in those who were moderately or severely malnourished, and those with decompensated liver disease were more likely to be malnourished than those with compensated liver disease. A BMI of <20 kg/m^2 was associated with reduced survival. The subjective override can be used to change nutritional status by a single category if indicated, e.g. weight loss or severe steatorrhoea.

Further confirmation of the RFH-GA predictive power was found when it was compared with the Child–Pugh and MELD scores (Gunsar *et al.*, 2006). Dietitians use this tool as part of the patient assessment at UK liver transplant centres. Malnutrition assessed using this tool has been found to correlate with post-transplant infections, length of ventilation and length of ICU stay, but not length of hospital stay or mortality (Kalafateli *et al.*, 2017).

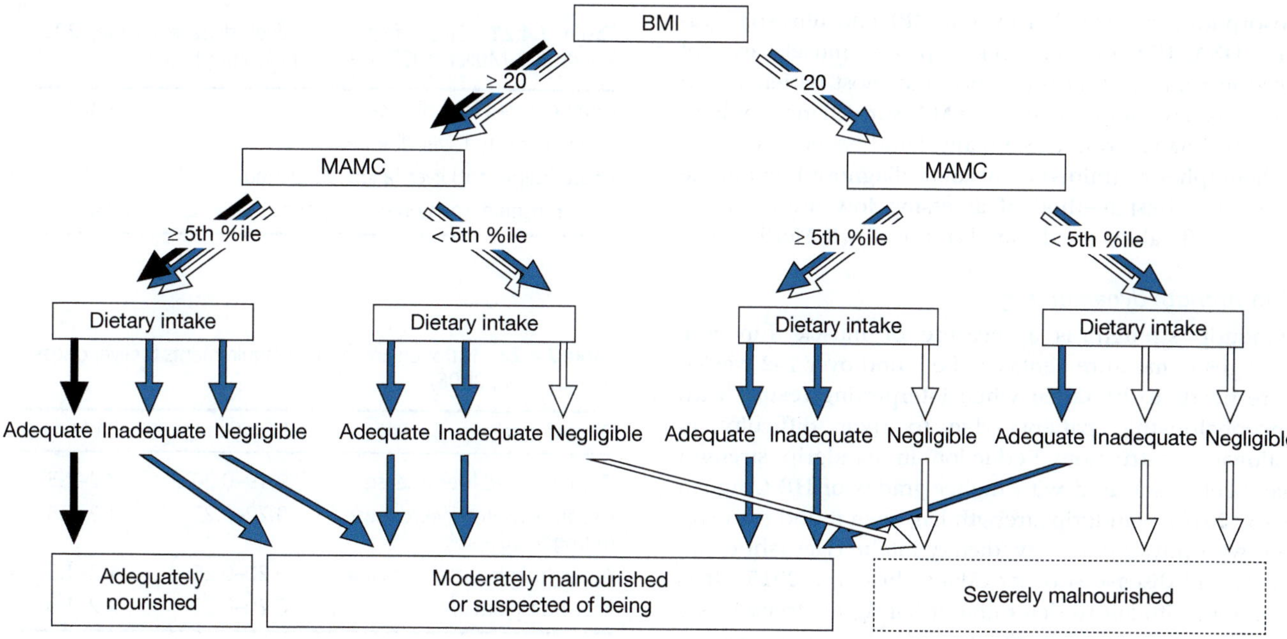

Figure 7.4.13 Royal Free Hospital Global Assessment (RFH-GA) scheme for determining nutritional status in patients with cirrhosis (source: Morgan *et al*., 2006. Reproduced with permission from Nature Publishing Group). BMI, body mass index; MAMC, mid arm muscle circumference; %ile, percentile.

Anthropometry and functional tests

Weight

The correct interpretation of the weight of fluid in patients with ascites and oedema is vital. BMI, percentage weight loss and nutritional requirements must be calculated using dry weights or estimated dry weights. Dry weight can be estimated using the following formula:

Dry weight = wet weight − estimated weight of ascites or oedema

The amount of ascites and oedema can be calculated using Mendenhall (1992) estimates (Table 7.4.20). These estimates have limitations, and patients often have more fluid than this estimate advises. Weight histories and dry weight following paracentesis can provide the best estimate of actual flesh weight, with adjustment if necessary for peripheral oedema. Patients may have up to 20–30 L of fluid retention, and therefore 20–30 kg must be taken off the wet weight.

Table 7.4.20 Estimation of fluid weight in ascites or oedema (source: Mendenhall, 1992, pp. 363–384. Reproduced with permission from Taylor & Francis)

Severity	Ascites (kg)	Peripheral oedema (kg)
Minimal	2.2	1.0
Moderate	6.0	5.0
Severe	14.0	10.0

Body mass index

BMI can be grossly misleading in interpreting the level of malnutrition in liver disease if adjustments for fluid retention are not made. Furthermore, BMI does not assess body composition; liver disease patients with normal, overweight and obese BMI have been found to have low muscle mass (Cruz *et al*., 2013).

Upper-arm anthropometry

Measurement of mid-arm circumference (MAC), triceps skinfold thickness (TSF) and mid-arm muscle circumference (MAMC) should be taken to identify fat and muscle stores (see Chapter 2.2, Assessment of nutritional status). Comparison to age- and gender-matched reference values is a useful method to diagnose malnutrition (Madden & Smith, 2014). The upper arm is usually unaffected by fluid retention (Newsome *et al*., 2012), so can be particularly useful for the assessment of patients with ascites and oedema where weight and BMI are unreliable. Guidelines recommend anthropometry and handgrip strength to identify malnutrition (Plauth *et al*., 2006). MAMC correlated with muscle mass assessed using CT imaging of abdominal muscle in patients with liver cirrhosis (Kalafateli *et al*., 2017).

Bioelectrical impedance analysis

The validity of bioelectrical impedance analysis (BIA) for patients with ascites and oedema is debated. Kyle *et al*. (2004) suggested that BIA was not adequately validated; however, Plauth *et al*. (2006) suggested that the estimation of body cell mass with BIA could be used despite limitations in patients with ascites. However, BIA is not used routinely in clinical practice.

Other methods of assessing muscle mass

A number of methods have been used in research to identify low muscle mass, including dual-energy X-ray absorptiometry (DXA), BIA, CT, MRI and ultrasonography. DXA, BIA and ultrasonography of muscle are not used in routine clinical practice, but most patients with cirrhosis have abdominal CT or MRI surveillance for liver lesions. Images from these scans could be assessed by a radiographer or trained clinician to diagnose low muscle mass. The best method of assessing low muscle mass and cut-off values are debated (Dasarathy & Merli, 2016).

Grip strength dynamometry

Handgrip strength is a measure of muscle function. Changes in measurements can be found over 1–2 weeks. Care needs to be taken when interpreting results with encephalopathic patients due to their difficulty in following instruction. Reduction in handgrip strength has been associated with higher grades of HE (Augusti *et al.*, 2016). Handgrip strength has been found to correlate with physical activity, dietary intake (Hayashi *et al.*, 2013) and disease severity (Maharshi *et al.*, 2015). It is therefore difficult to determine if handgrip strength is a measure of disease severity, functional status or malnutrition, but it is likely to be influenced by multiple factors and should be used and interpreted as one measurement in a global assessment of nutritional status.

Dietary assessment

Patterns of eating should be identified. It is important to establish when symptoms, such as fatigue, nausea, early satiety, altered sleep pattern or abdominal pain, may affect appetite and nutritional intake. Encephalopathic patients may not reliably recall their intake, and relatives may help to provide a more accurate history.

Malabsorption

A subjective diagnosis can be made on classic steatorrhoea symptoms such as loose, bulky, greasy, pale and floating stools with an offensive smell following ingestion of food containing fat. Oily droplets may appear in the toilet or on toilet tissue. The initial dietetic assessment and review of patients with jaundice, PBC and PSC should include consideration of steatorrhoea.

Estimation of energy and protein requirements

In clinical practice, either the ESPEN guidelines (Plauth *et al.*, 2006) of 35–40 kcal/kg of body weight/day or estimation of basal metabolic rate (BMR) using the Henry (2005) equations (see Chapter 6.1, Nutritional requirements in clinical practice) with added stress and activity factors (Todorovic & Micklewright, 2011) are used (Table 7.4.21). It is important for both methods to use estimated dry weight as previously described. Anecdotally, in clinical practice, the stress factor chosen is related to the symptoms present, e.g. if only ascites is present, then a 30% stress factor is appropriate, and multiple symptoms require a 40% stress factor. Nitrogen or protein requirements are shown in Table 7.4.22 (Plauth *et al.*, 2006). Based on nitrogen balance studies, Swart *et al.* (1988) established the minimum protein requirements for liver cirrhosis as 1.2 g/kg/day.

Table 7.4.21 Stress factors for liver disease (Hasse, 2001; Kondrup & Muller, 1997; Plauth *et al.*, 2009)

Compensated liver disease	0–20%
Decompensated liver disease	30–40%
Acute (fulminant) liver failure/ventilated	20–30%
Post-transplant (postoperative period)	30%

Table 7.4.22 Nitrogen and protein requirements for liver disease (Plauth *et al.*, 2006)

Disease state	Nitrogen (g)	Protein (g)
Compensated liver disease	0.19–0.20	1.2–1.3
Decompensated liver disease (nitrogen balance)	0.20–0.25	1.2–1.5
Acute (fulminant) liver failure	0.20–0.25	1.2–1.5
Post-transplant	0.20–0.25	1.2–1.5

Obesity

There is a lack of evidence regarding energy requirements in patients with liver disease who have a high BMI; however, the following may be used:

- For compensated liver disease, weight loss can be appropriate. Requirements for BMR are estimated using dry weight, omitting stress and activity factors.
- For decompensated liver disease, weight loss, even in those with a high BMI, should not be actively encouraged unless the patient can be closely monitored. Requirements for energy are calculated as described previously, adding stress and activity factors. Energy intake may be reduced only under close monitoring of muscle mass with anthropometry. It should be ensured that 0.5–1 kg/week weight loss is not exceeded (Newsome *et al.*, 2012).

Nitrogen and protein requirements should be adjusted according to BMI (Todorovic & Micklewright, 2011):

$$\text{BMI} > 30\,\text{kg/m}^2 \times 0.75$$
$$\text{BMI} > 50\,\text{kg/m}^2 \times 0.65$$

These recommendations are a guide for the estimation of energy and nitrogen requirements for maintenance of nutritional status. The key elements are the monitoring of nutritional status, i.e. weight, (if not fluid-overloaded), upper-arm anthropometry and handgrip strength. On monitoring, it may become necessary to increase requirements upwards.

Requirements for repletion

For repletion, it may be necessary to add 400–1000 kcal/day to previous totals with adequate anthropometric monitoring (Todorovic & Micklewright, 2011). Patients with liver disease require significantly higher protein intakes to maintain nitrogen balance. Most guidelines suggest an intake of 1.2–1.5g of protein/day to achieve nitrogen balance and accrual of lean body mass (Plauth *et al.*, 2006). However, Nielsen *et al.* (1995) suggested that dietary protein retention remains efficient at intakes of up to 2g/kg/day without adverse effects, including in encephalopathy. Kondrup and Muller (1997) suggested that protein intakes of 1.5–2g/kg may be required in patients with decompensated liver disease for nitrogen repletion. Where anthropometric monitoring indicates no improvement in nutritional status, these higher levels may be tried.

Biochemical monitoring for the possible adverse effects of high energy and protein provision is important.

Economic and social assessment

It is important to explore and address the economic, social and cultural factors influencing the nutritional intake of individual patients. For example, financial constraints may result in barriers to achieving the required eating pattern for liver disease (see Chapter 3.4, People in low-income groups), or there may be cultural differences in food choices (see Chapter 3.5, Working with minority ethnic groups).

Assessment in acute liver failure

The sudden onset of liver failure means this group of patients is likely to be better nourished than those with chronic liver disease; however, severity of symptoms can result in a rapid decline in nutritional status. Where possible, a full nutritional assessment should be undertaken. Patients with acute liver failure often require critical care support (see Chapter 7.17.1, Critical care).

Clinical investigation and management

Patients commonly present with elevated liver enzymes, symptoms of liver disease (Figure 7.4.14) or non-specific symptoms such as malaise, pruritis and lethargy. Many patients are asymptomatic until routine blood tests reveal abnormal liver function tests, which require further investigation.

Patient history, physical examination, blood tests, genetic testing, imaging and liver biopsies are all useful for investigating liver disease. Detailed personal, social, travel and family histories provide clues for the cause of disease. Physical examination can help to determine which symptoms of liver disease are present and provide further clues to causation. For example, scratch marks may indicate pruritus, which could be suggestive of cholestatic liver disease. To reach a diagnosis, investigations are performed that are relevant to the patient's history and presentation. Some common investigations are listed in Table 7.4.23, but this list is by no means exhaustive.

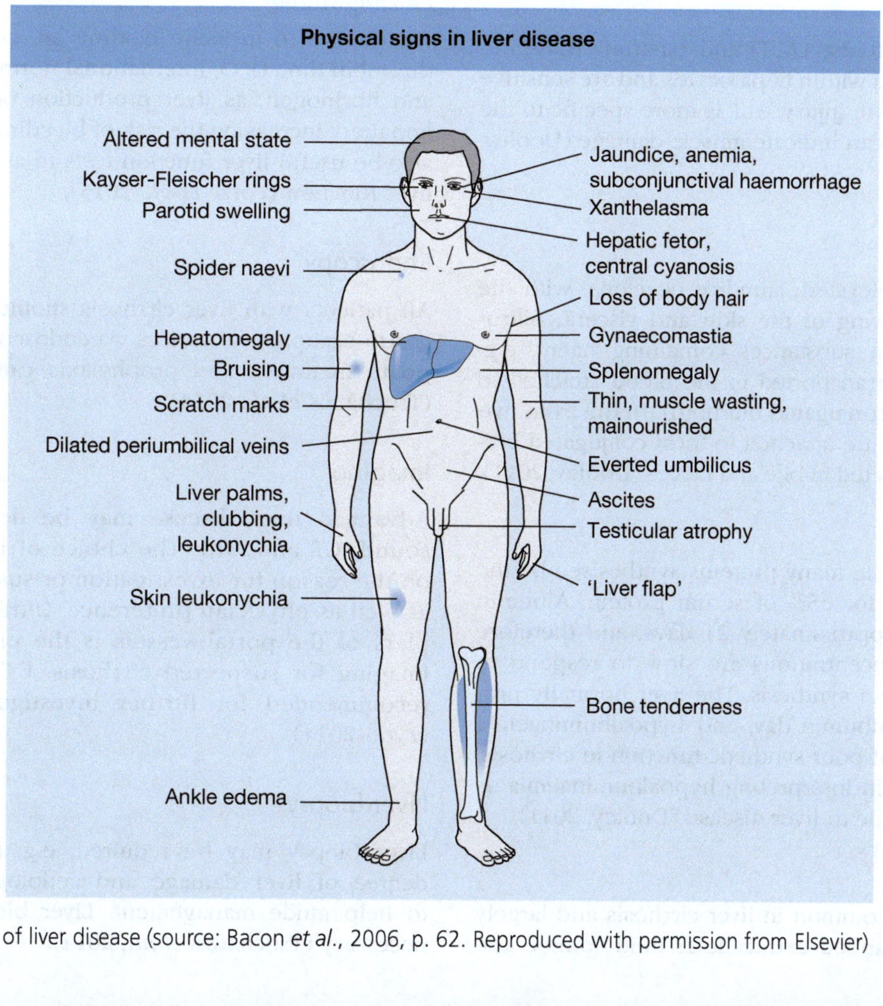

Figure 7.4.14 Signs of liver disease (source: Bacon *et al.*, 2006, p. 62. Reproduced with permission from Elsevier)

Table 7.4.23 Common investigations for liver disease aetiology, complications or comorbidities

Test	Abnormality	Interpretation
Hepatitis B surface antigen	Positive	Implies chronic infection
Hepatitis C antibody	Positive	Suggests chronic infection
Alpha-1-antitrypsin level	Low	Investigations in alpha-1-antitrypsin deficiency
Ferritin and iron binding studies	Elevated	Suggestive of haemochromatosis
Autoantibodies and immunoglobulins	ASM/ANA positive IgG	Suggestive of autoimmune hepatitis
	ANA positive	Suggestive of PBC
Full blood count	Macrocytosis	Specific for alcohol excess only if gamma-glutamyltransferase is elevated
	Thrombocytopenia	Suggestive of hypersplenism (portal hypertension)
Antiendomysial antibodies	Positive	Suggestive of Coeliac disease
Ceruloplasmin	Low	Suggestive of Wilson's disease

Biochemistry

Alkaline phosphatase

Alkaline phosphatase (ALP) is mainly found in the bile ducts of the liver. Elevated levels with high glutamyl transpeptidase (GGT) can indicate obstructive or cholestatic liver disease. Elevated ALP with normal GGT is most likely of bone origin (Dooley, 2011).

Alanine aminotransferase and aspartate transaminase

Alanine aminotransferase (ALT) and aspartate transaminase (AST) are found within hepatocytes and are sensitive markers of hepatocyte injury. ALT is more specific to the liver than AST. AST can indicate muscle damage (Dooley, 2011).

Bilirubin

When bilirubin is elevated, jaundice develops, with the characteristic yellowing of the skin and viscera. Bilirubin is formed from substances containing haem, e.g. haemoglobin. It is transported in the blood attached to serum albumin (unconjugated bilirubin). In the liver, two glucaronate groups are attached to form conjugated bilirubin, which is excreted in bile and faeces (Dooley, 2011).

Albumin

Albumin is one of the many proteins synthesised by the liver and accounts for 65% of serum protein. Albumin has a half-life of approximately 21 days, and therefore serum albumin concentrations are slow to respond to alterations in protein synthesis. The liver normally produces 12–15 g of albumin/day, and hypoalbuminaemia may be indicative of poor synthetic function in cirrhosis. Caution is needed in interpreting hypoalbuminaemia as it may not be specific to liver disease (Dooley, 2011).

Sodium

Hyponatraemia is common in liver cirrhosis and largely occurs due to expanded extracellular fluid volume and renal impairment. Patients may also experience hyponatraemia due the use of diuretics or with gastrointestinal losses (Gianotti & Cardenas, 2014).

Creatinine and glomerular filtration rate (GFR)

Liver disease is associated with renal failure, the cause of which is multifactorial. Elevated creatinine and reduced GFR indicate renal impairment and poorer outcomes (Cárdenas & Ginès, 2009).

Clotting studies

Blood tests to measure clotting are common, e.g. prothrombin time (PT), international normalised ratio (INR) and fibrinogen, as liver production of these factors is impaired, increasing the risk of bleeding. PT and INR can also be useful liver function tests to assess the extent of liver function (Potze *et al.*, 2015).

Endoscopy

All patients with liver cirrhosis should be screened for gastro-oesophageal varices via endoscopy, so that appropriate treatment and prophylaxis can be commenced (Tsochatzis *et al.*, 2014).

Imaging

Advanced liver disease may be detected by ultrasound, CT and MRI. The choice of imaging depends on the reason for investigation or suspected aetiology as well as physician preference. Ultrasound with dopplers of the portal vessels is the preferred first-line imaging for suspected cirrhosis. CT or MRI may be recommended for further investigation (Tsochatzis *et al.*, 2014).

Liver biopsy

Liver biopsy may be required, e.g. to determine the degree of liver damage and aetiology of disease, or to help guide management. Liver biopsy is often not necessary (Tsochatzis *et al.*, 2014).

Non-alcoholic fatty liver disease

Investigation

Secondary causes of liver disease and the exclusion of daily alcohol intake of ≥30 g for men and ≥20 g for women is required for the diagnosis of NAFLD (EASL–EASD–EASO, 2016). The presence of NAFLD risk factors, such as the components of metabolic syndrome, are important to assess. Often, the ratio of AST to ALT is >1, which differentiates NAFLD from alcohol-related fatty liver disease (Day, 2002). Liver biopsy remains the gold standard for NAFLD diagnosis (NICE, 2016a); however, this is invasive and expensive, so ultrasound is the preferred first-line method of assessing liver steatosis. Clinical assessment, biochemistry or imaging cannot distinguish steatosis from NASH; therefore, NASH has to be diagnosed with liver biopsy. It is important to differentiate steatosis from NASH, as NASH increases the risk of fibrosis, cirrhosis and HCC. Fibrosis can be assessed using scores that incorporate serum markers, such as enhanced liver fibrosis (ELF). It is important to assess and monitor the extent of fibrosis as fibrosis is correlated with morbidity and mortality (NICE, 2016a). Liver biopsy may still be required to investigate fibrosis (EASL–EASD–EASO, 2016).

Management

Symptoms of decompensated NASH cirrhosis should be treated or managed as with other causes of decompensated liver disease. Patients with NAFLD will require treatment of each aspect of the metabolic syndrome. There is evidence that pioglitazone and vitamin E could be beneficial for advance fibrosis with NAFLD. These medications are recommended only in the secondary or tertiary care setting with close monitoring (NICE, 2016a). It is advisable for NAFLD patients to continue taking statins unless liver enzymes double within 3 months of commencing them (NICE, 2016a).

Hepatitis C virus

HCV is often symptom-free or presents with non-specific symptoms such as fatigue. Those with risk factors are considered for testing. HCV is usually diagnosed with two blood tests. A positive anti-body test indicates exposure to the virus but does not diagnose current infection. A positive polymerase chain reaction (PCR) blood test indicates HCV infection.

Management

Until recently, HCV was treated mainly with a combination of pegylated interferon and ribavirin. Recently, interferon-free DAA medications have become available. These medications require shorter courses and have fewer side-effects as compared to interferon-based treatment. Treatments and combination therapy depend on the genotype of disease, liver function, disease stage, comorbidities, infection risk to others, HCV complications, viral load and response to treatment. Some of the HCV treatments and their side effects are summarised in Table 7.4.24 (EASL, 2017b). This is a rapidly changing field, with regular updates to treatment guidelines.

Ascites

Ascites is a common complication of cirrhosis, and approximately 60% of patients with compensated cirrhosis develop ascites within 10 years. The development of ascites in cirrhosis indicates a poor prognosis, with survival probability approximately 85% at 1 year and 56% at 5 years (Pose & Cardenas, 2017). Patients with cirrhosis and ascites are at high risk for other liver disease complications, including refractory ascites, spontaneous bacterial peritonitis (SBP), hyponatraemia or hepatorenal syndrome (HRS) (Moore & Aithal, 2006). The absence of these ascites-related complications qualifies ascites as uncomplicated.

Table 7.4.24 Hepatitis C virus treatment and potential side effects (EASL, 2017b)

Medication	Combination therapy	Side effects
Peginterferon alpha	Ribavirin	Fatigue, headache, nausea, vomiting, fever, insomnia, anorexia, dermatological symptoms, depression
Elbasvir–grazoprevir (Zepatier)	Ribavirin	Headache, fatigue, nausea
Daclatasvir (Daklinza)	Sofosbuvir, peginterferon alpha, ribavirin	Headache, fatigue, nausea
Dasabuvir (Exviera)	Ombitasvir–paritaprevir–ritonavir (Viekirax), ribavirin	Insomnia, nausea, itching, weakness, fatigue, anaemia
Ledipasvir–sofosbuvir (Harvoni)	Ribavirin	Fatigue and headache
Simeprevir (Olysio)	Peginterferon alpha, ribavirin	Rash, itching, nausea, constipation, breathlessness, photosensitivity
Sofosbuvir (Sovaldi)	Daclatasvir (Daklinza), peginterferon alpha, ribavirin	Headache, fatigue, nausea, insomnia
Ombitasvir–paritaprevir–ritonavir (Viekirax)	Dasabuvir (Exviera), ribavirin	Insomnia, nausea, itching, weakness, fatigue and anaemia
Sofosbuvir–velpatasvir (Epclusa)	Ribavirin	Headache, fatigue, nausea
Glecaprevir–pibrentasvir	Ribavirin	Headache, fatigue, nausea

Ascites only occurs when portal hypertension has developed, and is related to an inability to excrete an adequate amount of sodium into urine, leading to a positive sodium balance. Hypoalbuminaemia contributes by reducing vascular oncotic pressure, retaining fluid within the vessels and fluid leaks into the peritoneal space (Solà *et al.*, 2016). EASL (2010a) has graded ascites and given suggestions for treatment. The risk of SBP is decreased with a reduction in ascites volume, and this also reduces stress on the respiratory system and the risk of pleural effusion.

Diuretic-resistant ascites and diuretic-intractable ascites are collectively known as refractory ascites. Once refractory ascites has developed, the median survival of patients is approximately 6 months, and liver transplantation may be considered (Guevara & Ginés, 2005; Moreau *et al.*, 2004).

Investigation

Investigation of patients with ascites should include abdominal ultrasound and tests for liver disease. A diagnostic paracentesis is required to exclude other causes of ascites and test for SBP. Serum-ascites albumin gradient can differentiate the cause of ascites, and a neutrophil count should be obtained to rule out SBP (EASL, 2010a).

Management

Sodium restriction

See the following section 'Nutritional management' for detailed information.

Diuretics

Diuretics are prescribed when patients present with the first episode of grade 2 (moderate) ascites. Aldosterone antagonists, e.g. spironolactone, are prescribed initially, and, depending on response, the dose is increased to a maximum of 400 mg. If there is poor response (<2 kg/week fluid weight loss), or if patients develop hyperkalaemia, loop diuretics are added, e.g. furosemide (Angeli *et al.*, 2010).

Aldosterone antagonists are potassium-sparing and weak natrietics. If patients develop hyperkalaemia of >6 mmol/L in the absence of renal failure, this should resolve with the discontinuation of the drug, and long-term potassium restriction is unlikely to be necessary. Loop diuretics such as furosemide may be used in combination with aldosterone antagonists. These are potassium-losing and powerful natrietics. The dose is 40 mg, increasing in increments of 40 mg to 160 mg/day. If patients develop severe hypokalaemia (<3 mmol/L), loop diuretics are discontinued (Angeli *et al.*, 2010). The maximum recommended weight loss during diuretic therapy is 0.5 kg/day in patients without oedema and 1 kg/day in patients with oedema (EASL, 2010a).

Fluid restriction

Fluid intake should be restricted only in patients with dilutional hyponatraemia with a serum sodium level of 120–125 mmol/L (Moore & Aithal, 2006). Fluid restriction to 1 L/day is only effective at increasing serum sodium in a minority of patients, but may help to prevent further reduction (EASL, 2010a).

Paracentesis

Paracentesis is the therapeutic drainage of ascites from the abdomen using a catheter. The volume of ascitic fluid removed may vary from 20 mL for diagnostic purposes to over 20 L to relieve abdominal distension. Large-volume paracentesis is the first-line therapy in patients with large ascites (grade 3). It is performed together with the administration of 8 g of albumin for every litre of ascitic fluid removed (EASL, 2010a). This is required to maintain circulating blood volume, prevent rapid shifts of body fluid and subsequent hypovolaemic shock. Serial paracentesis may be the only means of treating refractory ascites.

Implanted subcutaneous drainage

Under general anaesthetic, a battery-powered drainage system is implanted. A pump removes ascitic fluid from the peritoneal cavity into the bladder, which is eliminated with urine. This method of removing ascites is currently only used in research. Early results show reduced need for paracentesis, improved quality of life, improved nutrition and reduced infections and hospital admissions (Nair *et al.*, 2015; NICE, 2014). Results of a randomised controlled trial are awaited.

Transjugular intrahepatic portosystemic shunts

A transjugular intrahepatic portosystemic shunt (TIPS) decompresses the portal system with a shunt inserted within the liver between the high-pressure portal venous area and the low-pressure hepatic venous area. This reduces portal pressure and is effective in the control of recurrent ascites. It may improve renal function and have beneficial effects on nitrogen balance and body weight (Plauth *et al.*, 2004). A major complication after TIPS insertion is the development of HE, which occurs in 30–50% of patients undergoing the procedure (Routhu *et al.*, 2017).

Hepatorenal syndrome

Hepatorenal syndrome (HRS) is defined as the occurrence of renal failure in a patient with advanced liver disease in the absence of an identifiable cause of renal failure (EASL, 2010a). The precipitating factors are often a bacterial infection of the background of vasodilatation in the splanchnic arterial bed and a cardiac output that is insufficient for the patient's needs (Baraldi *et al.*, 2015).

Investigation

Diagnosis of HRS includes the presence of cirrhosis with ascites, serum creatinine >133 µmol/L, absence of shock, absence of hypovolaemia, no recent treatment with nephrotoxic drugs and absence of parenchymal renal disease. Approximately 20% of cirrhotic patients will develop HRS. There are two types of HRS (Baraldi *et al.*, 2015). Type 1 is a rapidly progressive acute renal failure, with precipitating factors such as sepsis, SBP and acute alcoholic hepatitis. Only 10% of patients with type 1 HRS survive longer than 90 days. Type 2 occurs in patients with refractory ascites, and there is a steady, but moderate, degree of functional renal failure, often with rapid sodium retention. Following onset, the average survival rate is 6–8 months.

Management

Early identification and treatment of precipitating infection is important. Diuretics may initially be stopped. Furosemide may be restarted to maintain urine output and offload fluid, but spironolactone is contraindicated due to the risk of hyperkalaemia. Renal function can often be improved by using vasoconstrictor drugs, such as terlipressin, to increase arterial pressure. Renal replacement therapy may be necessary when the patient becomes severely fluid-overloaded or hyperkalaemic, or develops metabolic acidosis. Fluid management is important, and fluid restriction may be necessary. Liver transplantation is the best treatment for HRS, and the majority of patients will regain renal function post-transplant (EASL, 2010a).

Encephalopathy

Hepatic encephalopathy (HE) is defined as '*a brain dysfunction caused by liver insufficiency and/or portal systemic shunting; it manifests as a wide spectrum of neurological or psychiatric abnormalities ranging from subclinical alterations to coma*' (AASLD-EASL, 2014). HE can present with symptoms ranging from reduced attention and memory, disturbance to the sleep–wake cycle, personality changes, disorientation, inappropriate behaviour and loss of postural tone, through to stupor or coma (Landis *et al.*, 2016).

Investigation

Clinical examination and a clinical decision is the basis of HE diagnosis as well as exclusion for other causes of cognitive dysfunction. Various tests that measure cognitive and psychomotor functions or changes in cerebral activity are used, and the choice of test depends on the setting, availability, local norms and cost. Brain imaging and ammonia levels are not useful for HE diagnosis but may help to rule out other causes of impaired cognition or to assess the effectiveness of ammonia-lowering medication (AASLD-EASL, 2014). The severity, time course, underlying disease and precipitating factors (Box 7.4.4) should all be considered. HE is commonly graded using the West Haven criteria (Ferenci *et al.*, 2002) (Table 7.4.25). The management of encephalopathy in acute and chronic liver failure involves the treatment and prevention of its precipitants.

Encephalopathy secondary to both acute and chronic liver failure involves the treatment and prevention of its precipitants.

Management

Sepsis

Patients with chronic liver disease are more susceptible to infections including SBP. Good infection control management, full septic screen when an infection is suspected and the use of antibiotics, if appropriate, is necessary.

Box 7.4.4 Precipitating factors of acute encephalopathy

Portosystemic shunting: 30–50% incidence post shunting
Sepsis/infections (including bacterial peritonitis)
Constipation
Dehydration caused by vomiting and/or diarrhoea/ poor nutritional intake
Uraemia/azotaemia, e.g. diuretic induced
Gastrointestinal bleeding/variceal bleeding
Electrolyte disturbances
Acid–base disturbances
Drugs (sedatives, alcohol)

Table 7.4.25 West Haven criteria for grading encephalopathy (source: Ferenci *et al.*, 2002. Reproduced with permission from Wiley-Blackwell Publishing)

Grade	
1	Trivial lack of awareness; euphoria or anxiety; shortened attention span; impaired performance in addition or subtraction
2	Lethargy or apathy; minimal disorientation for time or place; subtle personality change; inappropriate behaviour
3	Somnolence to semi-stupor, but responsive to verbal stimuli; confusion; gross disorientation
4	Coma (unresponsive to verbal or noxious stimuli)

Constipation and gut microbiota

Current treatment of HE assumes that colonic bacteria produce ammonia, and constipation must be avoided in patients with HE. Patients are prescribed laxatives so that they pass two to four soft or loose stools daily. Lactulose is commonly prescribed and has a prebiotic effect, promoting the growth of beneficial microbiota, and therefore reducing ammonia production. Lactulose also has an acidifying and osmotic laxative effect, resulting in ammonia removal. There is a risk of overuse of lactulose and resulting dehydration, skin irritation or hypernatraemia, which could precipitate HE (AASLD-EASL, 2014). Rifaximin, an antibiotic, is also used to treat HE as an add-on therapy to lactulose. Rifaximin is thought to reduce gut inflammation and gut-derived toxins such as ammonia (Patidar & Bajaj, 2013).

Wernicke's encephalopathy

The Wernicke–Korsakoff syndrome develops in thiamine-deficient people, and those with a history of alcohol misuse are at risk. Thiamine is an essential cofactor in the metabolism of carbohydrate and alcohol. Symptoms include confusion, ataxia, disorientation, apathy, impaired memory, drowsiness or stupor. These clinical abnormalities may develop acutely or evolve over several days. It is reversible with thiamine administration (Donnelly, 2017). Korsakoff's psychosis is an amnesic state in which there is profound impairment of memory but relative preservation of other intellectual abilities; confabulation may be a feature. Korsakoff's psychosis generally develops after an acute episode of Wernicke's encephalopathy and is irreversible (NICE, 2010). Initially, parenteral thiamine is required, followed by oral preparations of 300 mg/day. As thiamine requirements are linked to carbohydrate intake, it is important that thiamine be administered with any form of nutrition support (e.g. intravenous dextrose, oral or enteral nutrition) (NICE, 2010).

Diabetes

It can be more challenging to diagnose diabetes in patients with liver cirrhosis as fasting serum glucose can be normal with elevated post-prandial levels. Furthermore, glycated haemoglobin (HbA1c) may not reflect glycaemic control in those with liver cirrhosis, but the reason for this is not understood. Glucose tolerance testing has therefore been recommended (Elkrief *et al.*, 2016). Maintaining tight blood glucose control and optimising insulin and/or oral hypoglycaemic therapies is important in liver disease.

Hepatocellular carcinoma

Investigation

Diagnosis of hepatocellular carcinoma (HCC) is based on imaging, including CT and MRI, or pathology. The diagnostic method depends on the size of the mass. Guidelines recommend the Barcelona Clinic Liver Cancer classification to determine the stage of HCC. This method of staging provides a way of predicting prognosis and determining the most suitable treatment (EASL–EORTC, 2012).

Management

Surgery

Surgery is the main treatment for HCC, including hepatic resection and liver transplantation, which are curative and have the best outcomes. Resection is the first-line treatment for single tumours in patients with preserved liver function. Liver transplant is the first-line treatment for single tumours less than 5 cm or three or fewer tumours that are each 3 cm or less in size. Local ablation with percutaneous ethanol injection (TEI), where alcohol is injected into the tumour site or radiofrequency ablation (RFA) using the heat, is the first-line treatment for early-stage HCC that is not suitable for surgery, and can also cure HCC. Chemoembolisation (TACE), with concentrated chemotherapy drugs delivered to the tumour, is first-line therapy for intermediate stage of HCC that is not suitable for surgery. Median survival with intermediate-stage HCC is 16 months, and TACE increases this to 19–20 months. Sorafenib offers systemic therapy for patients with advanced HCC and preserved liver function. Median survival with advanced HCC is 6 months; sorafenib may increase this to 10.7 months. There is a median survival of 3–4 months with end-stage HCC, and end-of-life care with symptom management is recommended (EASL–EORTC, 2012).

Liver transplantation

Liver transplant cures liver disease. Patients meeting transplant criteria should be offered a transplant only if it is felt they have a >50% probability of survival at 5 years after transplantation, with a quality of life that is acceptable to the patient (Neuberger *et al.*, 2008). Survival to 1 year after transplant is 93.4%, and at least 50% live for 20 years (NHS Blood and Transplant, 2016).

Nutritional management

When taking into account the incidence and consequence of malnutrition and specific micronutrient deficiencies, meeting patients' estimated requirements and monitoring nutritional status is pivotal to their management. ESPEN guidance recommends frequent small meals, high protein intake, a late-evening snack and the use of oral nutritional supplements (ONS) or tube feeding to help meet requirements (Plauth *et al.*, 2006). Although there were no clear benefits on morbidity and mortality of oral, enteral or parental nutrition support in a Cochrane review, the findings were limited by high levels of study bias (Koretz *et al.*, 2012). The studies included in the review did find improvements in nitrogen balance, reduction in postoperative complications and improvements in symptoms such as ascites and HE with nutrition support. A subgroup analysis in another meta-analysis found reduction in mortality with ONS (Ney *et al.*, 2013).

Oral nutrition

The pattern of food intake can influence energy balance in liver cirrhosis. Consuming four to six carbohydrate-rich meals or snacks per day to avoid periods of fasting greater than 2–3 hours is recommended to reduce gluconeogenesis. This eating pattern may also help patients with early satiety and disease-related anorexia to achieve adequate intake. Counselling patients to choose snacks that contain both protein and carbohydrate will help to meet this eating pattern and high protein requirements. Interestingly, Le Cornu *et al.* (2000) found that nutritional counselling may produce similar outcomes when compared with ONS, and therefore these simple changes can be very effective.

A late-evening snack, which reduces fasting periods overnight, should include 50 g of carbohydrate, and examples of suitable snacks are listed in Box 7.4.5. If patients experience altered sleep patterns and are awake during the night, encouragement should be given to consume meals, snacks and ONS when awake. In hospital, thought should be given to snack and meal times in order to allow carbohydrate snacks between meals and the provision of at least a 50 g carbohydrate snack in the evening.

Patients who are unable to meet their nutritional requirements from diet may require ONS (see Chapter 6.3, Oral nutritional support). Standard polymeric ONS can be used according to patient preference, and should be prescribed to make up the energy and protein deficit. This

Box 7.4.5 Examples of 50 g carbohydrate snacks

2 crumpets with 200 mL of milk
1–1.5 milk-based 1.5 kcal/mL ONS (dependent on composition)
1 juice-based 1.5 kcal/mL ONS (dependent on composition)
2½ thick slices of bread
Breakfast cereal (30 g) with milk
1 slice of fruit cake
Scone with jam and 300 mL of milk
5 dried dates and 200 mL of milk
Small square of flapjack and 300 mL of milk

group of patients may need to use long-term sip feeds, and therefore it is vital that time be spent establishing flavour and product preferences in order to aid compliance, with regular review of tolerance. Fluid restrictions and early satiety create increased difficulty when trying to meet requirements; the use of low-volume, high-protein ONS may be helpful, and close liaison with the MDT is vital.

Enteral nutrition

If patients are unable to tolerate an oral diet or fail to achieve adequate requirements orally, a nasogastric (NG) tube feed should be considered (see Chapter 6.4, Enteral nutrition). Clinical condition, prognosis and the risks and benefits of tube feeding for each individual patient must be taken into account, and close liaison with the MDT is essential for this. There should be a low threshold for initiation of tube feeding as patients deteriorate quickly, with the priority to meet nutritional requirements consistently. Historically, there has been a reluctance to pass NG tubes when varices are present; however, this is not supported by evidence (Borderie *et al.*, 1997; Plauth *et al.*, 2006). Cabré *et al.* (1990) demonstrated that albumin levels and Child–Pugh scores were improved with enteral nutrition in severely malnourished patients with cirrhosis. Campillo *et al.* (2005) found an improvement of liver function and an increase in dietary intake after 6 weeks of tube feeding. For those with inadequate oral intake or deteriorating anthropometric measurements, overnight feeding decreases the fasting period, may allow more activity during the day and helps meet nutritional requirements.

An energy-dense and high-protein feed should be used to achieve estimated requirements within smaller volumes for those who have delayed gastric emptying, complain of bloating or require fluid restrictions. Generally, whole-protein feeds are recommended. The rate of feed should be built up according to local enteral feeding and refeeding syndrome guidelines.

Nasojejunal feeding

There are few specific guidelines regarding the use of nasojejunal (NJ) feeding tubes in liver disease. In practice, NJ tubes may be used for patients who have poor absorption, indicated by high aspirates, nausea, vomiting or early satiety. Continuous infusion of enteral feed into the small bowel has the added benefit of avoiding fasting times, thereby optimising carbohydrate oxidation and improving nitrogen balance.

Gastrostomy and jejunostomy feeding

The placement of percutaneous endoscopic gastrostomy (PEG) tubes is associated with a higher risk of complications due to ascites, varices and altered coagulopathy, and is contraindicated according to Plauth *et al.* (2006). A case series found that the mortality of cirrhotic patients undergoing PEG placement was high, with greatest risk in those with ascites (Baltz *et al.*, 2010). Jejunostomy tubes have been used historically for post-liver-transplant patients, and they are placed during surgery. Their use has declined significantly as patients can be adequately fed with NG or NJ tubes. Elective placement of jejunostomy tubes in post-transplant patients can still be considered for prolonged feeding of patients with gastric aspirate or vomiting issues.

Parenteral nutrition

Parenteral nutrition (PN) should be reserved for patients for whom there is no enteral feeding route available (Plauth *et al.*, 2009) (see Chapter 6.5, Parenteral nutrition). Hepatic abnormalities, e.g. hepatic steatosis, intrahepatic cholestasis or elevated liver function tests, can occur in up to 75% of adults receiving PN (Guglielmi *et al.*, 2006). When there is a deterioration in liver function (LFTs), causes other than PN must be identified, e.g. sepsis. Usually, only monitoring or a small reduction in the energy content of the feed is required (Kumpf, 2006). Guidelines from the ESPEN (Plauth *et al.*, 2009) have further clarified the use of PN in liver disease.

Alcoholic hepatitis

A randomised trial by Cabré *et al.* (2000) investigated both the short- and long-term effects of steroids (prednisolone 40 g/day) or total enteral nutrition (TEN) (2000 kcal/day) in patients with alcoholic hepatitis. The trial concluded that TEN is no worse than steroid treatment in the short-term management of alcoholic hepatitis. Moreno *et al.* (2016) randomised patients with alcoholic hepatitis treated with steroids to either intensive enteral nutrition via feeding tube for 14 days or conventional nutrition, and found no difference between groups for 6-month mortality. However, a greater proportion of patients with <21 kcal/kg/day intake died than those with higher energy intake, suggesting nutritional intake is a determinant of mortality. The study also found that tube feeding was withdrawn early in 48.5% of participants, demonstrating the challenge of enteral feeding in this patient group. Patients fed after a period of reduced nutritional intake and alcohol misuse are at risk of developing refeeding syndrome (Todorovic & Micklewright, 2011). The management of refeeding syndrome is discussed further in Chapter 6.4 (Enteral nutrition).

Acute liver failure

HE symptoms may hide those of hypoglycaemia; therefore, continuous glucose infusions and monitoring is critical. EASL guidelines recommend avoiding fluid overload or under-filling, monitoring ammonia with enteral nutrition, and maintaining serum sodium within 140–150 mmol/l (EASL, 2017a). There is risk of high aspirates and aspiration pneumonia as HE progresses, and therefore monitoring aspirates and post-pyloric feeding or PN may be indicated (EASL, 2017a).

Wilson's disease

Zinc may be used alone for presymptomatic patients or in those with neurological disease (EASL, 2012b), or in combination with a chelating agent. Food and water high in copper, including chocolate, liver, nuts, mushrooms and shellfish, are best avoided, especially in the first year of treatment (EASL, 2012b).

Liver transplant nutrition

Initially following a liver transplant, patients require nutrition support with ONS or tube feeding to meet requirements and food safety advice. Long-term management involves weight maintenance and lifestyle advice. Some immunosuppression medication can cause hyperkalaemia and diabetes; this is often transient, but diabetes medication and short-term low-potassium diets may be indicated (Anastacio & Davisson Correia, 2016). If required, further advice can be obtained from specialist transplant centres.

Haemochromatosis

Haemochromatosis cannot be treated with a low-iron diet. It is managed by reducing the systemic iron overload through therapeutic phlebotomy to achieve a serum ferritin of 50–100 μg/L (EASL, 2010b). A systematic review found no studies investigating diet as treatment for haemochromatosis (Moretti *et al.*, 2013). Patients are often reluctant to eat foods rich in iron; therefore, the following advice can be given:

- Avoid vitamin and mineral supplements containing iron and vitamin C, as vitamin C aids iron absorption.
- Avoid foods fortified with iron.
- Avoid drinking fresh fruit juice with meals due to their high vitamin C content.
- Limit intake of red meat to 70 g cooked weight/day in line with healthy-eating guidelines.
- Do not avoid fruit and vegetables, including leafy green iron-rich ones, as phytates and oxalates reduce iron bioavailability.
- Alcohol can accelerate disease progression; therefore, reduced alcohol intake is recommended.
- Calcium and tannins inhibit iron absorption, so drinking dairy products and tea with meals may inhibit dietary iron absorption.

Non-alcoholic fatty liver disease

Obesity

Weight reduction improves NAFLD risk factors and can reverse progression. Guidelines recommend a target of 7–10% weight loss (EASL–EASD–EASO, 2016). Studies have found that a weight loss of ≥5% improved hepatic steatosis, and ≥7% improved NAFLD activity scores. Achieving ≥10% weight loss can induce NASH resolution or fibrosis regression (Hannah & Harrison, 2016). However, too-rapid weight loss can worsen liver function, accelerate fibrosis or result in decompensation (Farrell & Larter, 2006). Weight loss exceeding 1 kg/week should be discouraged. Monitoring liver function (LFTs) may be necessary if patients lose weight rapidly, as this may precipitate deterioration in liver function (Day, 2006). Dietary changes alone are associated with high failure rate in achieving and maintaining weight loss for multifactorial reasons. Obesity and further strategies for its management are discussed in Chapter 7.13.2 (The management of obesity and overweight in adults).

Non-cirrhotic patients

It is important to assess the stage of liver disease as the advice for a cirrhotic NASH patient differs from a patient with a fatty liver or fibrosis. At initial assessment, the stage of liver disease, weight, BMI and waist circumference should be obtained, and clear goals for weight loss discussed with the patient, with advice to avoid excessive weight loss. Exercise should be encouraged, as this improves liver fat content independently of change in weight (NICE, 2016a). Each aspect of the metabolic syndrome should be addressed individually and treated with dietary therapy as appropriate (see Chapters 7.12, Diabetes mellitus and 7.14, Cardiovascular disease). The basic principles of lifestyle intervention in NAFLD pre-cirrhosis are to:

- Aim for a BMI of <25 kg/m^2.
- Aim for a reduction of 10% from baseline weight over 6–12 months.
- Restrict energy to achieve a 0.5–1 kg (1–2 lb) per week weight loss.
- Avoid weight loss that exceeds 1 kg/week.
- Encourage exercise of at least moderate intensity for 30 minutes on 5 days per week. Advise that this can be undertaken in one 30-minute session, or in several sessions of 10 minutes or more duration. Explain that greater duration and frequency of exercise may be required.
- When a healthy BMI is achieved, encourage weight maintenance through long-term lifestyle changes.
- Give food group advice based on the Eatwell Guide (see Chapter 2.1, Dietary reference values and food-based dietary guidelines). European Guidelines recommend the Mediterranean diet (EASL–EASD–EASO, 2016); however, it is uncertain if wine should be avoided (Romero-Gomez *et al.*, 2017).

SECTION 7

- For those who choose to drink, NICE (2016a) recommends that alcohol be limited to the national guidance. Hepatology teams may recommend abstinence.

There are few trials comparing different diets for NAFLD. Both low-carbohydrate and low-fat diets have shown benefits for NAFLD and insulin resistance. It is difficult to determine if benefits have been due to weight loss or the specific diet (Hannah & Harrison, 2016). There is some evidence that probiotics may be beneficial for NAFLD (Ma *et al.*, 2013), but current guidelines do not recommend probiotics. There are concerns that high fructose intake may contribute to NAFLD, and opinions that n-3 and coffee could prevent or treat it. However, NICE (2016a) found no conclusive evidence to make recommendations about fructose, coffee or n-3. EASL–EASD–EASO (2016) recommends avoiding fructose-containing food and drink.

Cirrhotic patients

Overweight and obese patients with cirrhosis have excessive adipose tissue but may have low muscle mass or risk becoming muscle depleted (sarcopenic obesity), and could be at risk of micronutrient and energy malnutrition. There have been no studies investigating the benefits and risks of adopting an eating pattern of four to six carbohydrate-rich meals or snacks per day and a 50 g bedtime carbohydrate snack in obese patients with cirrhosis. Therefore, a full dietetic assessment and frequent monitoring is required to ensure that the recommended eating pattern for cirrhosis is not contributing to further adipose tissue gain. Weight loss should not be recommended in cirrhotic patients with decompensated end-stage liver disease due to the risk of malnutrition (Newsome *et al.*, 2012). For obese patients with stable compensated cirrhosis, it may be appropriate to try and achieve weight loss before proceeding to or while waiting for liver transplantation (Newsome *et al.*, 2012), but close monitoring with regular anthropometric measurement is essential.

Hepatitis C virus

Symptoms of decompensated liver disease should be managed as described in this chapter. However, many people have no symptoms at all. If patients are well, there is no evidence for any sort of therapeutic diet. Patients should be encouraged to eat a healthy, well-balanced diet, such as those promoted by the Eatwell Guide (see Chapter 2.1, Dietary reference values and food-based dietary guidelines), and maintain a BMI within a healthy range. There is growing evidence that obesity and insulin resistance can accelerate HCV progression and increase the risk of HCC in chronic HCV (Dyal *et al.*, 2015). Obesity can also reduce the effectiveness of interferon treatment, so patients with a BMI of >30 kg/m^2 should be advised to lose weight prior to starting interferon, as this may help the antiviral response (Iwane *et al.*, 2015). Weight loss is not recommended during anti-viral treatment due to the risk of malnutrition with medication side effects.

Alcohol

Regular alcohol consumption in HCV leads to accelerated fibrosis progression and reduced response to antiviral therapy (Gitto *et al.*, 2014), and is associated with poor adherence to medication regimens (Mathes *et al.*, 2014). Alcohol advice depends on the patients, their clinical state and previous alcohol history; medical staff should direct the decision regarding alcohol intakes.

Ascites and oedema

There is no evidence to support the prophylactic use of salt restriction in cirrhotic patients who have never had ascites, nor is bed rest advocated as a treatment of ascites (EASL, 2010a). By the time patients have developed ascites, they have advanced cirrhosis, and nutritional support is often necessary due to poor appetite and early satiety. The volume of abdominal fluid can also reduce mobility, limiting the ability to shop, cook and prepare meals. It is important that nutritional requirements are met while keeping sodium intake within the recommended levels. No-added-salt advice should be given to patients with grade 2 (moderate) ascites or above. Salt should be restricted to 4.6–6.9 g (80–120 mmol sodium) per day (EASL, 2010a). Sodium intakes vary enormously between patients, and each patient should be assessed individually. Very often, reducing a few key foods can have a profound impact on daily net sodium intake. No-added-salt advice includes the following:

- Do not add salt to meals.
- Avoid salty snacks such as crisps, salted nuts and salted crackers. Choose alternatives without salt added.
- Reduce processed foods, e.g.:
  - Bacon, ham, sausages, pâté.
  - Smoked fish and meat.
  - Fish and meat pastes.
  - Readymade soups.
  - Stock cubes, soya sauce, monosodium glutamate (or choose reduced-salt alternatives).
  - Food tinned in brine.
  - Meat and vegetable extracts.

Advise patients to look at food labels and calculate whether food is high, medium or low in salt using the following figures:

High salt: >1.5 g/100 g (0.6 g of sodium).
Medium salt: 0.3–1.5 g/100 g portion (0.6–1 g of sodium).
Low salt: 0.3 g/100 g (0.1 g of sodium).

If there is only a figure for sodium on the label, patients should be advised to multiply this by 2.5 to obtain the salt content. Patients should be advised to avoid potassium chloride–based salt substitutes due to risk of hyperkalaemia.

Nutritional support

Most milk-based ONS contain 8–10 mmol of sodium, while juice-based ONS have very small amounts. However, milk-based ONS contain more protein and may be useful to meet elevated protein requirements in patients having serial paracentesis. If tube feeding is necessary, sodium content of enteral feeds is suitable as they contain <40 mmolL sodium. High-energy and high-protein feeds are often required as they provide more energy and protein in smaller volumes. Tolerance to larger volumes due to early satiety and bloating may be difficult, and fluid restrictions need to be considered.

Hepatorenal syndrome

Serum potassium levels should be monitored on a daily basis, and diet therapy and nutritional support adjusted as necessary. Patients may be symptomatic of uraemia, and antiemetics may be required. Careful consideration of protein intake is necessary, and protein may need to be reduced to 1.2 g/kg of dry body weight if uraemia is problematic (EASL, 2010a).

Hepatic encephalopathy

Low-protein diets are not recommended (Amodio *et al.*, 2013); there is a lack of evidence that they contribute to any improvement in HE, and may cause harm due to worsening nutritional status and loss of muscle mass (Cordoba *et al.*, 2004; Plauth *et al.*, 2006). Periods of fasting should be minimised as endogenous waste from protein catabolism can precipitate encephalopathy (Merli *et al.*, 2013). Nutrition support can lead to improved nitrogen balance and HE (Koretz *et al.*, 2012).

The eating pattern of four to six carbohydrate-rich meals or snacks per day and a 50 g bedtime carbohydrate snack is recommended for minimising fasting times. Consensus guidelines advise that a diet rich in vegetable and dairy protein should be recommended for persistent HE, despite lack of evidence for this from clinical trials (Amodio *et al.*, 2013). The prebiotic effects of vegetable protein may help to reduce ammonia production, and these sources of protein are low in the amino acids implicated in the development of HE (Amodio *et al.*, 2013). It should be noted that the higher fibre and low energy content of such diets may make it difficult to meet energy requirements.

If enteral nutrition is the sole source of nutrition, 24-hour enteral feeding may be required to avoid the fasting period, and to avoid protein boluses until the encephalopathic episode resolves. Placement of NG tubes can be difficult as increasing confusion leads to tubes becoming dislodged, resulting in suboptimal nutritional intake. The MDT is essential in order to discuss the local management of these patients, which may involve increased nursing care, secure taping of the tube, or fixation devices.

Branched-chain amino acids

The BCAAs, especially leucine, appear to have an important anabolic role in protein synthesis. Studies in liver cirrhosis have shown that BCAAs reduce protein breakdown and increase muscle mass (Ruiz-Margain *et al.*, 2017; Tsien *et al.*, 2015), and may improve nutritional status and survival (Amodio *et al.*, 2013). It has been reported that supplementation with oral BCAAs improved energy metabolism in cirrhotic patients (Als-Nielsen *et al.*, 2003; Tsuchiya *et al.*, 2005).

Gluud *et al.* (2017) found that BCAAs improved HE in a Cochrane review of 16 randomised clinical trials. Subgroup analysis found a beneficial effect of oral, but not intravenous, BCAAs on overt, but not minimal, HE. Beneficial effect was found when excluding trials with lactulose or neomycin as a control group, but not in the analysis limited to these two control groups. The study found that about 1 in 10 people experienced nausea or diarrhoea with BCCAs. The authors concluded that BCAAs should be considered in the management of HE, and that there was need for further research in evaluating the effectiveness of BCAAs in combination with other treatments, such as lactulose, and for managing mild HE. Clinical guidelines recommend that BCAAs be used as an alternative or additional treatment in patients not responding to conventional management (AASLD-EASL, 2014).

There is no consensus on the recommended dose of BCAAs to date, although there is a recommendation to take them at night, as BCAAs are used as energy during the day but are used for protein synthesis at night (Fukushima *et al.*, 2003). In the UK, BCAAs have not been adopted in clinical practice, nor is a palatable product available as yet. However, this is a developing area, and specialist centres should be contacted for advice regarding any UK developments.

Probiotics

Probiotics have been studied as a treatment for HE, given the theory of altered ammonia production causing confusion. Dalal *et al.* (2017) reviewed evidence from 21 trials in a Cochrane review and found that probiotics may improve overt HE as compared to no treatment or placebo with no evidence of adverse events. However, quality of evidence was low, with high risk of bias, and it was uncertain if probiotics were better than lactulose for treating HE.

Zinc

Guidelines recommend that zinc deficiency and correction be considered when treating HE (AASLD-EASL, 2014).

Sepsis

Preserving the integrity of the gut wall to reduce the risk of bacterial translocation could help reduce sepsis, and can be achieved with small frequent meals or enteral nutrition in cognitively impaired patients (MacFie, 2004).

Diabetes

In non-cirrhotic patients with conditions such as NAFLD, poor glycaemic control is associated with disease progression, increased cardiovascular risk and increased infection rates (Hazlehurst *et al.*, 2016). Diabetes is associated with mobilisation of adipose tissue, fatty acids, and increased protein catabolism, which plays a role in the aetiology of muscle wasting (Morley *et al.*, 2014). In addition, patients with liver cirrhosis and diabetes are at increased risk of poorer survival, ascites, renal dysfunction, HE and infections (Elkrief *et al.*, 2016). Studies are needed to evaluate the effect of good glycaemic control in cirrhosis (Elkrief *et al.*, 2016).

Dietary intervention

Standard healthy-eating diabetic dietary advice should only be used in well-nourished patients who are not at risk of malnutrition. Priority should be given to meeting elevated nutritional requirements and the recommended eating pattern. In malnourished patients or those at risk of malnutrition, healthy-eating advice is inappropriate, and diabetes dietary advice includes the following:

- Reduce refined carbohydrate, e.g. sugar, sweets, sugary drinks.
- Include complex carbohydrates if appetite and levels of satiety allow.
- Small, frequent carbohydrate-containing meals and snacks, including 50 g carbohydrate evening snack.
- Include protein with meals and snacks.
- Fruit and vegetables used in moderation, as they have low energy density and can result in early satiety.
- ONS as necessary, and prioritise milk-based over juice-based ONS. Consider carbohydrate-free ONS in patients with poor glycaemic control.
- With all methods of nutrition support, close liaison is required with diabetes teams to optimise insulin and oral hypoglycaemic regimens.

Hypoglycaemia

Patients should be advised to avoid fasting and encouraged to eat small, frequent meals with adequate quantities of carbohydrate and regular snacks. It is also advisable to have a meal or snack prior to exercising.

Steatorrhoea

Fat restriction

If indicated, the aim of dietary treatment is to improve symptoms, and to prevent decline in nutritional status and fat-soluble vitamin deficiencies. Fat is an important and palatable source of energy for any patient requiring nutritional support. For patients with liver disease, a reduction in fat intake should only be used if:

- Symptoms of steatorrhoea distress the patient, reducing quality of life.
- Steatorrhoea is causing uncontrollable weight loss or muscle wasting.

The degree of fat tolerance will vary between patients and needs to be assessed on an individual basis. A detailed diet history is necessary from the patient to assess which foods cause symptoms, and advice should be to reduce the intake of these initially. If patients cannot determine which foods are causing symptoms, and the steatorrhea is severe, they should initially reduce foods that are high in fat. Steatorrhoea caused by pancreatic exocrine insufficiency can be treated with pancreatic enzyme replacement therapy (see Chapter 7.4.5, Disorders of the pancreas). Pancreatic enzyme replacement therapy is not indicated in biliary steatorrhea.

Nutritional support

Meeting the nutritional requirements for energy and protein of patients with steatorrhoea remains a priority. There is potential for energy deficit from fat restriction, and nutrition support must include appropriate replacement energy sources, as follows:

- Carbohydrates and protein should be increased. Complex carbohydrate intake can be increased in patients with a good appetite. Refined carbohydrates can be useful in patients without diabetes.
- Medium-chain triglycerides (MCTs) can be used as they do not require bile salts for emulsification, but may require gradual introduction to improve tolerance.

ONS are useful, especially juice-based ONS, which contain minimal fat and are fortified with fat-soluble vitamins. Some high-protein ONS are also low in fat and well tolerated.

If tube feeding is required, consideration should be given to the fat source:

- MCT-based feeds provide a greater percentage of fat as MCTs and should be gradually introduced to aid tolerance. Some are low in energy and protein.
- Low-fat semi-elemental feeds may be indicated, but have the disadvantage that a high volume may be needed to meet nutritional requirements.

Fat-soluble vitamins

Patients with steatorrhoea are at risk of developing deficiencies of the fat-soluble vitamins (Hirschfield *et al.*, 2017). If deficiency is suspected, levels should be checked and supplemented if necessary. Aqueous preparations of fat-soluble vitamins are recommended to improve absorption. Patients with steatorrhea without clinical signs of deficiency may benefit from a daily multivitamin supplement, including fat-soluble vitamins (Vidas, 2014). Current practice regarding fat-soluble vitamin screening and supplementation varies throughout UK liver centres. It is important that dietitians check which supplements are available and what dosage is recommended in local guidelines and with their hospital pharmacy.

Vitamin D

Vitamin D deficiency should be corrected according to local policy. In 2002, UK guidelines recommended that cirrhotic patents be routinely supplemented with 800 IU of vitamin D and 1000 mg of calcium (Collier *et al.*, 2002). However, more recent reviews have recommended individual assessment of vitamin D status, malabsorption and osteoporosis risk (Guarino *et al.*, 2016; Hirschfield *et al.*, 2017). In patients with increased cardiovascular risk, such as those with NAFLD, or renal stones, DXA scanning may be performed to confirm osteoporosis or osteopenia prior to commencing supplements (Bolland *et al.*, 2011).

Coffee

A systematic review found that patients who consumed coffee had a decreased risk of progression of liver disease to cirrhosis and HCC, and reduced mortality rate as compared to non-coffee drinkers. Coffee consumption was associated with improved response to interferon antiviral therapy in HCV, and inversely associated with steatohepatitis in NAFLD (Saab *et al.*, 2014). EASL recommend prospective studies are needed to identify the amount and type of coffee required for improved outcomes before incorporating coffee advice into guidelines (Petta and Marchesini, 2017).

Physical activity

Historically, strenuous exercise has not been recommended due to the risk of increased portal hypertension and bleeding (Berzigotti *et al.*, 2016). Recently, the importance of physical activity, with a combination of resistance and endurance exercise, has been recognised as having the potential to prevent and treat sarcopenia (Dasarathy & Merli, 2016). Although not nutritional management, dietitians should be aware of the importance of physical activity. Light–moderate activity, such as walking, should be recommended (Toshikuni *et al.*, 2014); however, more strenuous exercise should be discussed with the MDT. Studies investigating the benefits and risks of activity in cirrhosis are needed.

Drug–nutrient interactions

The following should be noted:

- *Neomycin* – malabsorption of calcium, iron and potassium.
- *Metronidazole* – avoid alcohol, consider sodium content.
- *Furosemide* – malabsorption of calcium, magnesium, potassium and zinc.
- *Spironolactone* – limit alcohol, risk of hyperkalaemia.
- *Tacrolimus and cyclosporine* – grapefruit, Seville oranges and pomegranate increase medication bioavailability, risk of hyperkalaemia.

Further reading

Dasarathy S, Merli M. (2016) Sarcopenia from mechanism to diagnosis and treatment in liver disease. *J. Hepatol.* 65: 1232–1244.

Johnson TM, Overgard EB, Cohen AE, *et al.* (2013) Nutrition assessment and management in advanced liver disease. *Nutr. Clin. Pract.* 28: 15–29.

Lomer M. (2014) *Advanced Nutrition and Dietetics in Gastroenterology*. Chichester: Wiley Blackwell.

Plauth M, Cabre E, Riggio O, *et al.* (2006) ESPEN guidelines on enteral nutrition: liver disease. *Clin. Nutr.* 25: 285–294.

Sargent S. (2009) *Liver Diseases – An Essential Guide for Nurses and Health Care Professionals*. Chichester: Wiley Blackwell.

Internet resources

UK charities and support groups

Addaction, https://www.addaction.org.uk
British Liver Trust, https://www.britishlivertrust.org.uk
Drinkaware, https://www.drinkaware.co.uk
HCV Action, http://www.hcvaction.org.uk
Hepatitis B Positive Trust, http://www.hepbpositive.org.uk
Hepatitis C Trust, http://www.hepctrust.org.uk
Liver4Life, http://www.liver4life.org.uk
PBC Foundation, https://www.pbcfoundation.org.uk
PSC Support, http://www.pscsupport.org.uk
The Haemochromatosis Society, http://haemochromatosis.org.uk
Wilson's Disease Support Group UK, http://www.wilsonsdisease.org.uk

Professional associations

American Association for the Study of Liver Diseases, https://www.aasld.org
British Association for the Study of Liver Disease, https://www.basl.org.uk
British Society of Gastroenterology, http://www.bsg.org.uk
European Association for the Study of the Liver, https://www.easl.eu
National Health Service Blood and Transplant, https://www.nhsbt.nhs.uk

Acknowledgement

The book editor acknowledges the prior contribution of Susie Hamlin and Julie Leaper.

References

Abbott-Johnson W, Kerlin P, Clague A. *et al.* (2011) Relationships between blood levels of fat soluble vitamins and disease etiology and severity in adults awaiting liver transplantation. *J. Gastroenterol. Hepatol.* 26: 1402–1410.

Adams LA, Angulo P. (2006) Treatment of non-alcoholic fatty liver disease. *Postgrad. Med. J.* 82: 315–322.

Als-Nielsen B, Koretz RL, Kjaergard LL, *et al.* (2003) Branched-chain amino acids for hepatic encephalopathy. *Cochrane Database Syst Rev.* (2): CD001939.

American Association for the Study of Liver Diseases (AASLD) and European Association for the Study of the Liver (EASL) (2014) Hepatic encephalopathy in chronic liver disease. *J. Hepatol.* 61: 642–659.

Amodio P, Bemeur C, Butterworth R, *et al.* (2013) The nutritional management of hepatic encephalopathy in patients with cirrhosis: International Society for Hepatic Encephalopathy and Nitrogen Metabolism Consensus. *Hepatology.* 58: 325–336.

Anastacio LR, Davisson Correia MI. (2016) Nutrition therapy: integral part of liver transplant care. *World J. Gastroenterol.* 22: 1513–1522.

Angeli P, Fasolato S, Mazza E. (2010) Combined versus sequential diuretic treatment of ascites in non-azotaemic patients with cirrhosis: results of an open randomised clinical trial. *Gut.* 59: 98–104.

Arora S, Mattina C, McAnenny C, *et al.* (2012a) OC-075 Assessment of nutritional status in patients with cirrhosis: must is not a must. *Gut.* 61: A32–A32.

Arora S, Mattina C, Catherine M, *et al.* (2012b) The development and validation of a nutritional prioritising tool for use in patients with chronic liver disease. *Gut.* 61: A90–A90.

Arteh J, Narra S, Nair S. (2010) Prevalence of vitamin D deficiency in chronic liver disease. *Dig. Dis. Sci.* 55: 2624–2628.

SECTION 7

Augusti L, Franzoni LC, Santos LA, *et al.* (2016) Lower values of handgrip strength and adductor pollicis muscle thickness are associated with hepatic encephalopathy manifestations in cirrhotic patients. *Metab. Brain Dis.* 31: 909–915.

Bacon BR, O'Grady JG, Di Bisceglie AM, *et al.* (2006) *Comprehensive Clinical Hepatology*. Elsevier Health Sciences.

Baltz JG, Argo CK, Al-Osaimi AM, *et al.* (2010) Mortality after percutaneous endoscopic gastrostomy in patients with cirrhosis: a case series. *Gastrointest. Endosc.* 72: 1072–1075.

Baraldi O, Valentini C, Donati G, *et al.* (2015) Hepatorenal syndrome: update on diagnosis and treatment. *World J. Nephrol.* 4: 511–520.

Barve A, Khan R, Marsano L, *et al.* (2008) Treatment of alcoholic liver disease. *Ann. Hepatol.* 7: 5–15.

Bellentani S, Scaglioni F, Marino M, *et al.* (2010) Epidemiology of non-alcoholic fatty liver disease. *Dig. Dis.* 28: 155–161.

Bernal W, Auzinger G, Dhawan A, *et al.* (2010) Acute liver failure. *Lancet.* 376: 190–201.

Bertholet N, Daeppen JB, Wietlisbach V, *et al.* (2005) Reduction of alcohol consumption by brief alcohol intervention in primary care: systematic review and meta-analysis. *Arch. Intern. Med.* 165: 986–995.

Berzigotti A, Saran U, Dufour JF. (2016) Physical activity and liver diseases. *Hepatology.* 63: 1026–1040.

Blachier M, Leleu H, Peck-Radosavljevic M, *et al.* (2013) The burden of liver disease in Europe: a review of available epidemiological data. *J. Hepatol.* 58: 593–608.

Bolland MJ, Grey A, Avenell A, *et al.* (2011) Calcium supplements with or without vitamin D and risk of cardiovascular events: reanalysis of the Women's Health Initiative limited access dataset and meta-analysis. *BMJ.* 342: d2040.

Boonstra K, Beuers U, Ponsioen CY. (2012) Epidemiology of primary sclerosing cholangitis and primary biliary cirrhosis: A systematic review. *J. Hepatol.* 56: 1181–1188.

Borderie C, Ripault MP, Silvain C, *et al.* (1997) Early feeding or enteral nutrition in patients with cirrhosis after bleeding from esophageal varices? A randomized controlled study. *Dig. Dis. Sci.* 42: 536–541.

Burstow NJ, Mohamed Z, Gomaa AI, *et al.* (2017) Hepatitis C treatment: where are we now? *Int. J. Gen. Med.* 10: 39–52.

Cabré E, Gonzalez-Huix F, Abad-Lacruz A, *et al.* (1990) Effect of total enteral nutrition on the short-term outcome of severely malnourished cirrhotics. *A randomized controlled trial. Gastroenterology.* 98: 715–720.

Cabré E, Rodriguez-Iglesias P, Caballeria J, *et al.* (2000) Short- and long-term outcome of severe alcohol-induced hepatitis treated with steroids or enteral nutrition: a multicenter randomized trial. *Hepatology.* 32: 36–42.

Campillo B, Richardet JP, Bories PN. (2005) Enteral nutrition in severely malnourished and anorectic cirrhotic patients in clinical practice. *Gastroenterol. Clin. Biol.* 29: 645–651.

Cárdenas A, Ginès P. (2009) A patient with cirrhosis and increasing creatinine level: What is it and what to do? *Clin. Gastroenterol. Hepatol.* 7: 1287–1291.

Carvalho L, Parise ER. (2006) Evaluation of nutritional status of non-hospitalized patients with liver cirrhosis. *Arq. Gastroenterol.* 43: 269–274.

Chavez-Tapia NC, Cesar-Arce A, Barrientos-Gutierrez, *et al.* (2013) A systematic review and meta-analysis of the use of oral zinc in the treatment of hepatic encephalopathy. *Nutr. J.* 12: 74.

Cheung K, Lee SS, Raman M. (2012) Prevalence and mechanisms of malnutrition in patients with advanced liver disease, and nutrition management strategies. *Clin. Gastroenterol. Hepatol.* 10: 117–125.

Chief Medical Officer. (2016) *UK Chief Medical Officers' Low Risk Drinking Guidelines.* Available at https://www.gov.uk/government/uploads/system/uploads/attachment_data/file/545937/UK_CMOs__report.pdf. Accessed 17 June 2017.

Cholongitas E, Burroughs AK. (2012) The evolution in the prioritization for liver transplantation. *Ann. Gastroenterol.* 25: 6–13.

Coffey AJ, Durkie M, Hague S, *et al.* (2013) A genetic study of Wilson's disease in the United Kingdom. *Brain.* 136: 1476–1487.

Collier JD, Ninkovic M, Compston JE. (2002) Guidelines on the management of osteoporosis associated with chronic liver disease. *Gut.* 50: i1–i9.

Coltorti M, Del Vecchio-Blanco C, Caporaso N, *et al.* (1991) Liver cirrhosis in Italy. A multicentre study on presenting modalities and the impact on health care resources. National Project on Liver Cirrhosis Group. *Ital. J. Gastroenterol.* 23: 42–48.

Cordoba J, Lopez-Hellin J, Planas M, *et al.* (2004) Normal protein diet for episodic hepatic encephalopathy: results of a randomized study. *J. Hepatol.* 41: 38–43.

Cruz RJ Jr, Dew MA, Myaskovsky L, *et al.* (2013) Objective radiologic assessment of body composition in patients with end-stage liver disease: going beyond the BMI. *Transplantation.* 95: 617–622.

Cruz-Jentoft AJ, Baeyens JP, Bauer JM, *et al.* (2010) Sarcopenia: European consensus on definition and diagnosis: Report of the European Working Group on Sarcopenia in older people. *Age Ageing.* 39: 412–423.

Dalal R, McGee RG, Riordan SM. *et al.* (2017) Probiotics for people with hepatic encephalopathy. *Cochrane Database Syst. Rev.* 2: Cd008716.

Das B, Chandra P, Thimmaraju K. (2011) Serum magnesium level in patients with liver cirrhosis. *Int. J. Biomed. J. Res.* 2: 709–711.

Dasarathy S. (2012) Consilience in sarcopenia of cirrhosis. *J. Cachexia. Sarcopenia Muscle.* 3: 225–237.

Dasarathy S, Merli M. (2016) Sarcopenia from mechanism to diagnosis and treatment in liver disease. *J. Hepatol.* 65: 1232–1244.

Day CP. (2002) Non-alcoholic steatohepatitis (NASH): where are we now and where are we going? *Gut.* 50: 585–588.

Day CP. (2006) Non-alcoholic fatty liver disease: current concepts and management strategies. *Clin. Med. (Lond).* 6: 19–25.

DH. (2008) *The cost of alcohol harm to the NHS in England: an update to the cabinet office (2003) study.* DH: TSO London.

DH. (2014) *Living well for longer. National support for local action to reduce premature avoidable mortality.* London: Department of Health. Available at https://assets.publishing.service.gov.uk/government/uploads/system/uploads/attachment_data/file/307703/LW4L.pdf Accessed 26 October 2018.

DiCecco SR, Wieners EJ, Wiesner RH, *et al.* (1989) Assessment of nutritional status of patients with end-stage liver disease undergoing liver transplantation. *Mayo Clin. Proc.* 64: 95–102.

Donnelly A. (2017) Wernicke–Korsakoff syndrome: recognition and treatment. *Nurs. Stand.* 31: 46–53.

Dooley J. (2011) *Sherlock's Diseases of the Liver and Biliary System.* Chichester: Wiley Blackwell.

Dowman JK, Tomlinson JW, Newsome PN. (2010) Pathogenesis of non-alcoholic fatty liver disease. *QJM.* 103: 71–83.

Durand F, Buyse S, Francoz C, *et al.* (2014) Prognostic value of muscle atrophy in cirrhosis using psoas muscle thickness on computed tomography. *J. Hepatol.* 60: 1151–1157.

Dyal HK, Aguilar M, Bhuket T, *et al.* (2015) Concurrent obesity, diabetes, and steatosis increase risk of advanced fibrosis among HCV patients: a systematic review. *Dig. Dis. Sci.* 60: 2813–2824.

Dyson JK, Anstee QM, Mcpherson S. (2015) Republished: non-alcoholic fatty liver disease: a practical approach to treatment. *Postgrad. Med. J.* 91: 92–101.

Eapen BA, Ammu A, Thomas JE, *et al.* (2016) Wilson's disease: a review on clinical presentation, diagnostic methods and treatment. *Int. J. Health Sci. Res.* 6: 443–450.

European Association for the Study of the Liver (EASL), European Association for the Study of Diabetes (EASD) and European Association for the Study of Obesity (EASO). (2016) EASL–EASD–EASO clinical practice guidelines for the management of non-alcoholic fatty liver disease. *Diabetologia.* 59: 1121–1140.

European Association for the Study of the Liver (EASL) and the European Organization for Research and Treatment of Cancer (EORTC). (2012) EASL–EORTC clinical practice guidelines: management of hepatocellular carcinoma. *J. Hepatol.* 56: 908–943.

European Association for the Study of Liver. (2010a) EASL clinical practice guidelines on the management of ascites, spontaneous bacterial peritonitis, and hepatorenal syndrome in cirrhosis. *J. Hepatol.* 53: 397–417.

European Association for the Study of Liver. (2010b) EASL clinical practice guidelines for HFE hemochromatosis. *J. Hepatol.* 53: 3–22.

European Association for the Study of Liver. (2012a) EASL clinical practical guidelines: management of alcoholic liver disease. *J. Hepatol.* 57: 399–420.

European Association for the Study of Liver. (2012b) EASL clinical practice guidelines: Wilson's disease. *J. Hepatol.* 56: 671–685.

European Association for the Study of Liver. (2017a) EASL clinical practical guidelines on the management of acute (fulminant) liver failure. *J. Hepatol.* 66: 1047–1081.

European Association for the Study of Liver. (2017b) EASL recommendations on treatment of hepatitis C 2016. *J. Hepatol.* 66: 153–194.

El-Serag HB, Engels EA, Landgren O, *et al.* (2009) Risk of hepatobiliary and pancreatic cancers after hepatitis C virus infection: a population-based study of U.S. veterans. *Hepatology.* 49: 116–123.

Elia M. (2003) *Screening for Malnutrition: A Multidisciplinary Responsibility. Development and use of the malnutrition universal screening tool ('MUST') for adults.* Birmingham: BAPEN.

Elkrief L, Rautou PE, Sarin S, *et al.* (2016) Diabetes mellitus in patients with cirrhosis: clinical implications and management. *Liver Int.* 36: 936–948.

Farrell GC, Larter CZ. (2006) Nonalcoholic fatty liver disease: From steatosis to cirrhosis. *Hepatology.* 43: S99–S112.

Ferenci P, Lockwood A, Mullen K, *et al.* (2002) Hepatic encephalopathy – definition, nomenclature, diagnosis, and quantification: final report of the working party at the 11th World Congresses of Gastroenterology, Vienna, 1998. *Hepatology.* 35: 716–721.

Figueiredo FA, Dickson ER, Pasha TM, *et al.* (2000) Utility of standard nutritional parameters in detecting body cell mass depletion in patients with end-stage liver disease. *Liver Transpl.* 6: 575–581.

Friedman LS, Keeffe EB. (2004) *Handbook of Liver Disease.* Edinburgh: Churchill Livingstone.

Fukushima H, Miwa Y, Ida E, *et al.* (2003) Nocturnal branched-chain amino acid administration improves protein metabolism in patients with liver cirrhosis: comparison with daytime administration. *JPEN J. Parenter. Enteral Nutr.* 27: 315–322.

Fuller E, Mindell J, Prior G. (2016) *Health Survey for England 2015.* London: NHS Digital.

Garcia-Compean D, Gonzalez-Gonzalez JA, Lavalle-Gonzalez FJ, *et al.* (2016) Current concepts in diabetes mellitus and chronic liver disease: clinical outcomes, hepatitis C virus association, and therapy. *Dig. Dis. Sci.* 61: 371–380.

Garcia-Compean D, Jaquez-Quintana JO, Lavalle-Gonzalez FJ, *et al.* (2012) The prevalence and clinical characteristics of glucose metabolism disorders in patients with liver cirrhosis. *A prospective study. Ann. Hepatol.* 11: 240–248.

Gelson W, Alexander G. (2017) Is elimination of hepatitis C from the UK by 2030 a realistic goal? *Br. Med. Bull.* 123: 59–67.

Gianotti RJ, Cardenas A. (2014) Hyponatraemia and cirrhosis. *Gastroenterol. Rep. (Oxf).* 2: 21–26.

Gitto S, Vitale G, Villa E, *et al.* (2014) Update on alcohol and viral hepatitis. *J. Clin. Transl. Hepatol.* 2: 228–233.

Glass C, Hipskind P, Cole D, *et al.* (2012) Handheld calorimeter is a valid instrument to quantify resting energy expenditure in hospitalized cirrhotic patients: A prospective study. *Nutr. Clin. Pract.* 27: 677–688.

Gluud LL, Dam G, Les I, *et al.* (2017) Branched-chain amino acids for people with hepatic encephalopathy. *Cochrane Database Syst. Rev.* 5: Cd001939.

Goel A, Aggarwal R. (2016) Advances in hepatitis E – ii: Epidemiology, clinical manifestations, treatment and prevention. *Expert Rev. Gastroenterol. Hepatol.* 10: 1065–1074.

Goel V, Kar P. (2010) Hepatic osteodystrophy. *Trop. Gastroenterol.* 31: 82–86.

Greco AV, Mingrone G, Benedetti G, *et al.* (1998) Daily energy and substrate metabolism in patients with cirrhosis. *Hepatology.* 27: 346–350.

Grungreiff K, Reinhold D, Wedemeyer H. (2016) The role of zinc in liver cirrhosis. *Ann. Hepatol.* 15: 7–16.

Guarino M, Loperto I, Camera S, *et al.* (2016) Osteoporosis across chronic liver disease. *Osteoporos. Int.* 27: 1967–1977.

Guevara M, Ginès P. (2005) Hepatorenal syndrome. *Dig. Dis.* 23: 47–55.

Guglielmi FW, Boggio-Bertinet D, Federico A, *et al.* (2006) Total parenteral nutrition–related gastroenterological complications. *Dig. Liver Dis.* 38: 623–642.

Gunsar F, Raimondo ML, Jones S, *et al.* (2006) Nutritional status and prognosis in cirrhotic patients. *Aliment. Pharmacol. Ther.* 24: 563–572.

Hannah WN Jr, Harrison SA. (2016) Lifestyle and dietary interventions in the management of nonalcoholic fatty liver disease. *Dig. Dis. Sci.* 61: 1365–1374.

Hasse JM. (2001) Nutrition assessment and support of organ transplant recipients. *JPEN J. Parenter. Enteral Nutr.* 25: 120–131.

Hayashi F, Matsumoto Y, Momoki C, *et al.* (2013) Physical inactivity and insufficient dietary intake are associated with the frequency of sarcopenia in patients with compensated viral liver cirrhosis. *Hepatol. Res.* 43: 1264–1275.

Hazlehurst JM, Woods C, Marjot T, *et al.* (2016) Non-alcoholic fatty liver disease and diabetes. *Metabolism.* 65: 1096–1108.

HE. (2017a) *Hepatitis C in the UK 2017 Report.* Available at https://assets.publishing.service.gov.uk/government/uploads/system/uploads/attachment_data/file/632465/HCV_in_the_uk_report_2017.pdf. Accessed 26 October 2018.

HE. (2017b) *Hepatitis B: The Green Book, chapter 18 (Born on or After 1 August 2017).* Available at https://www.gov.uk/government/uploads/system/uploads/attachment_data/file/628602/Greenbook_chapter__18.pdf. Accessed 18 June 2017.

Health and Safety Executive. (2017a) *Hepatitis C Virus (HCV).* Available at http://www.hse.gov.uk/biosafety/blood-borne-viruses/hepatitis-c.htm. Accessed 14 June 2017.

Health and Safety Executive. (2017b) *Hepatitis B Virus (HBV).* Available at http://www.hse.gov.uk/biosafety/blood-borne-viruses/hepatitis-b.htm. Accessed 14 June 2017.

Henry CJK. (2005) Basal metabolic rate studies in humans: Measurement and development of new equations. *Public Health Nutr.* 8(7A): 1133–1152.

Hickman IJ, Macdonald GA. (2007) Impact of diabetes on the severity of liver disease. *Am. J. Med.* 120: 829–834.

Hill H. (2009) Anatomy and physiology. In: Sargent S (ed) *Liver Diseases: An Essential Guide for Nurses and Health Care Professionals.* Chichester: Wiley Blackwell.

Hirschfield GM, Beuers U, Corpechot C, *et al.* (2017) EASL clinical practice guidelines: the diagnosis and management of patients with primary biliary cholangitis. *J. Hepatol.* 67: 145–172.

Hudson M, Sheron N, Rowe IA, *et al.* (2017) Should we screen for cirrhosis? *BMJ.* 358: j3233.

Huisman EJ, Trip EJ, Siersema PD, *et al.* (2011) Protein energy malnutrition predicts complications in liver cirrhosis. *Eur. J. Gastroenterol. Hepatol.* 23: 982–989.

Iwane S, Mizuta T, Kawaguchi Y, *et al.* (2015) Impact of body weight reduction via diet and exercise on the anti-viral effects of pegylated interferon plus ribavirin in chronic hepatitis C patients with insulin resistance: a randomized controlled pilot trial. *Intern. Med.* 54: 3113–3119.

James Lind Alliance. (2016) *Alcohol-related Liver Disease Top 10.* Available at http://www.jla.nihr.ac.uk/priority-setting-partnerships/alcohol-related-liver-disease/top-10-priorities.htm. Accessed 18 June 2017.

Johnson TM, Overgard EB, Cohen AE, *et al.* (2013) Nutrition assessment and management in advanced liver disease. *Nutr. Clin. Pract.* 28: 15–29.

Juakiem W, Torres DM, Harrison SA. (2014) Nutrition in cirrhosis and chronic liver disease. *Clin. Liver Dis.* 18: 179–190.

Kalafateli M, Mantzoukis K, Choi Yau Y, *et al.* (2017) Malnutrition and sarcopenia predict post-liver transplantation outcomes independently of the model for end-stage liver disease score. *J. Cachexia. Sarcopenia Muscle.* 8: 113–121.

Kallis YN, Westaby D. (2014) Physiology and function of the hepatobiliary tract. In: Lomer M (ed) *Advanced Nutrition and Dietetics in Gastroenterology*. Oxford: Wiley Blackwell.

Kaner E, Bland M, Cassidy P, *et al.* (2013) Effectiveness of screening and brief alcohol intervention in primary care (sips trial): pragmatic cluster randomised controlled trial. *BMJ.* 346: e8501.

Kondrup J, Muller MJ. (1997) Energy and protein requirements of patients with chronic liver disease. *J. Hepatol.* 27: 239–247.

Koretz RL, Avenell A, Lipman TO. (2012) Nutritional support for liver disease. *Cochrane Database Syst. Rev.* (5):CD008344.

Kumpf VJ. (2006) Parenteral nutrition–associated liver disease in adult and pediatric patients. *Nutr. Clin. Pract.* 21: 279–290.

Kyle UG, Bosaeus I, De Lorenzo AD, *et al.* (2004) Bioelectrical impedance analysis – part i: review of principles and methods. *Clin. Nutr.* 23: 1226–1243.

Landis CS, Ghabril M, Rustgi V, *et al.* (2016) Prospective multicenter observational study of overt hepatic encephalopathy. *Dig. Dis. Sci.* 61: 1728–1734.

Lazaridis KN, LaRusso NF. (2016) Primary sclerosing cholangitis. *N. Engl. J. Med.* 375: 2501–2502.

Le Cornu KA, McKiernan FJ, Kapadia SA, *et al.* (2000) A prospective randomized study of preoperative nutritional supplementation in patients awaiting elective orthotopic liver transplantation. *Transplantation.* 69: 1364–1369.

Lee YM, Kaplan MM. (2002) Management of primary sclerosing cholangitis. *Am. J. Gastroenterol.* 97: 528–534.

Levy C, Lindor KD. (2003) Current management of primary biliary cirrhosis and primary sclerosing cholangitis. *J. Hepatol.* 38(1): S24–S37.

Liangpunsakul S, Haber P, Mccaughan GW. (2016) Alcoholic liver disease in Asia, Europe, and North America. *Gastroenterology.* 150: 1786–1797.

Lleo A, Jepsen P, Morenghi E, *et al.* (2016) Evolving trends in female to male incidence and male mortality of primary biliary cholangitis. *Sci. Rep.* 6: 25906.

Lomas DA, Hurst JR, Gooptu B. (2016) Update on alpha-1 antitrypsin deficiency: New therapies. *J. Hepatol.* 65: 413–424.

Ma YY, Li L, Yu CH, *et al.* (2013) Effects of probiotics on nonalcoholic fatty liver disease: a meta-analysis. *World J. Gastroenterol.* 19: 6911–6918.

MacFie J. (2004) Current status of bacterial translocation as a cause of surgical sepsis. *Br. Med. Bull.* 71: 1–11.

Madden AM, Bradbury W, Morgan MY. (1997) Taste perception in cirrhosis: its relationship to circulating micronutrients and food preferences. *Hepatology.* 26: 40–48.

Madden AM, Morgan MY. (1999) Resting energy expenditure should be measured in patients with cirrhosis, not predicted. *Hepatology.* 30: 655–664.

Madden AM, Smith S. (2014) Body composition and morphological assessment of nutritional status in adults: a review of anthropometric variables. *J. Hum. Nutr. Diet.* 29: 7–25.

Maharshi S, Sharma BC, Srivastava S. (2015) Malnutrition in cirrhosis increases morbidity and mortality. *J. Gastroenterol. Hepatol.* 30: 1507–1513.

Makol A, Watt KD, Chowdhary VR. (2011) Autoimmune hepatitis: a review of current diagnosis and treatment. *Hepat. Res. Treat.* 2011: 390916.

Mathes T, Antoine SL, Pieper D. (2014) Factors influencing adherence in hepatitis C infected patients: a systematic review. *BMC Infect. Dis.* 14: 203.

Matos C, Porayko MK, Francisco-Ziller N, *et al.* (2002) Nutrition and chronic liver disease. *J. Clin. Gastroenterol.* 35: 391–397.

McCullough AJ, O'Connor JF, (1998) Alcoholic liver disease: proposed recommendations for the American College of Gastroenterology. *Am. J. Gastroenterol.* 93: 2022–2036.

Mendenhall CL. (1992) Protein-calorie malnutrition in alcoholic liver disease. In: Watson RRW (ed) *Nutrition and Alcohol*. Boca Raton: CRC Press.

Merli M, Giusto M, Lucidi C, *et al.* (2013) Muscle depletion increases the risk of overt and minimal hepatic encephalopathy: results of a prospective study. *Metab. Brain Dis.* 28: 281–284.

Mitchell MC, Friedman LS, Mcclain CJ. (2017) Medical management of severe alcoholic hepatitis: expert review from the clinical practice updates committee of the AGA institute. *Clin. Gastroenterol. Hepatol.* 15: 5–12.

Montagnese S, De Rui M, Schiff S, *et al.* (2015) Prognostic benefit of the addition of a quantitative index of hepatic encephalopathy to the MELD score: The MELD-EEG. *Liver Int.* 35: 58–64.

Montano-Loza AJ, Duarte-Rojo A, Meza-Junco J, *et al.* (2015) Inclusion of sarcopenia within MELD (MELD-Sarcopenia) and the prediction of mortality in patients with cirrhosis. *Clin. Transl. Gastroenterol.* 6: e102.

Montano-Loza AJ, Meza-Junco J, Prado CM, *et al.* (2012) Muscle wasting is associated with mortality in patients with cirrhosis. *Clin. Gastroenterol. Hepatol.* 10: 166–173.

Moore KP, Aithal GP. (2006) Guidelines on the management of ascites in cirrhosis. *Gut.* 55(6): vi1–vi12.

Moreau R, Delegue P, Pessione F, *et al.* (2004) Clinical characteristics and outcome of patients with cirrhosis and refractory ascites. *Liver Int.* 24: 457–464.

Moreno C, Deltenre P, Senterre C, *et al.* (2016) Intensive enteral nutrition is ineffective for patients with severe alcoholic hepatitis treated with corticosteroids. *Gastroenterology.* 150: 903–910.

Moretti D, Van Doorn GM, Swinkels DW, *et al.* (2013) Relevance of dietary iron intake and bioavailability in the management of HFE hemochromatosis: a systematic review. *Am. J. Clin. Nutr.* 98: 468–479.

Morgan MY, Madden AM, Soulsby CT, *et al.* (2006) Derivation and validation of a new global method for assessing nutritional status in patients with cirrhosis. *Hepatology.* 44: 823–835.

Morley JE, Malmstrom TK, Rodriguez-Manas L, *et al.* (2014) Frailty, sarcopenia and diabetes. *J. Am. Med. Dir. Assoc.* 15: 853–859.

Mouzaki M, Ng V, Kamath BM, *et al.* (2014) Enteral energy and macronutrients in end-stage liver disease. *JPEN J. Parenter. Enteral Nutr.* 38: 673–681.

Muir AJ. (2015) Understanding the complexities of cirrhosis. *Clin. Ther.* 37: 1822–1836.

Muller MJ, Bottcher J, Selberg O, *et al.* (1999) Hypermetabolism in clinically stable patients with liver cirrhosis. *Am. J. Clin. Nutr.* 69: 1194–1201.

Muller MJ, Pirlich M, Balks HJ, *et al.* (1994) Glucose intolerance in liver cirrhosis: Role of hepatic and non-hepatic influences. *Eur. J. Clin. Chem. Biochem.* 32: 749–758.

Nair S, Robinson E, Fiona S, *et al.* (2015) PWE-141 ALFA pump for the treatment of refractory ascites: A 'real world' experience from the UK. *Gut.* 64: A274–A275.

Neuberger J, Gimson A, Davies M, *et al.* (2008) Selection of patients for liver transplantation and allocation of donated livers in the UK. *Gut* 57: 252–257.

Newsome PN, Allison ME, Andrews PA, *et al.* (2012) Guidelines for liver transplantation for patients with non-alcoholic steatohepatitis. *Gut.* 61: 484–500.

Ney M, Vandermeer B, van Zanten SJ, *et al.* (2013) Meta-analysis: oral or enteral nutritional supplementation in cirrhosis. *Aliment. Pharmacol. Ther.* 37: 672–679.

NHS Right Care. (2013) *Liver disease: The NHS atlas of variation in healthcare for people with liver disease*. Available at https://fingertips.phe.org.uk/documents/Atlas_2013%20Liver%20Disease.pdf. Accessed 01 June 2017.

NHS Blood and Transplant. (2016) *Annual Report on Liver Transplantation. Report for 2015/2016. [Online].* Available at https://nhsbtdbe.blob.core.windows.net/umbraco-assets-corp/1314/organ_specific_report_liver_2016.pdf. Accessed 05 July 2017.

NICE. (2010) *Alcohol-Use Disorders.* London: NICE.

NICE. (2014) *Subcutaneous implantation of a battery-powered catheter drainage system for managing refractory and recurrent ascites.* London: NICE.

NICE. (2016a) *Non-alcoholic fatty liver disease (NAFLD): Assessment and management.* London: NICE.

NICE. (2016b) *Cirrhosis in over 16s: assessment and management.* London: NICE.

Nielsen K, Kondrup J, Martinsen L, *et al.* (1995) Long-term oral refeeding of patients with cirrhosis of the liver. *Br. J. Nutr.* 74: 557–567.

O'Brien A, Williams R. (2008) Nutrition in end-stage liver disease: principles and practice. *Gastroenterology.* 134: 1729–1740.

O'Sullivan N, McAnenny C. (2014) Non-alcoholic fatty liver disease and hereditary haemochromatosis and nutrition. In: Lomer M (ed) *Advanced Nutrition and Dietetics in Gastroenterology.* Chichester: Wiley Blackwell.

Office for National Statistics (ONS). (2015) Alcohol-related deaths in the UK: registered in 2015. Available at https://cy.ons.gov.uk/peoplepopulationandcommunity/healthandsocialcare/causesofdeath/bulletins/alcoholrelateddeathsintheunitedkingdom/registeredin2015. Accessed 16 June 2017.

Owen OE, Trapp VE, Reichard GA, *et al.* (1983) Nature and quantity of fuels consumed in patients with alcoholic cirrhosis. *J. Clin. Invest.* 72: 1821–1832.

Pace A, De Weerth A, Berna M, *et al.* (2009) Pancreas and liver injury are associated in individuals with increased alcohol consumption. *Clin. Gastroenterol. Hepatol.* 7: 1241–1246.

Park JW, Chen M, Colombo M, *et al.* (2015) Global patterns of hepatocellular carcinoma management from diagnosis to death: the BRIDGE study. *Liver Int.* 35: 2155–2166.

Patidar KR, Bajaj JS. (2013) Antibiotics for the treatment of hepatic encephalopathy. *Metab. Brain Dis.* 28: 307–312.

Patta S, Marchesini (2017) Coffee and tea breaks for liver health. *J Hepato* 67(2): 221–223.

Peng S, Plank LD, Mccall JL, *et al.* (2007) Body composition, muscle function, and energy expenditure in patients with liver cirrhosis: a comprehensive study. *Am. J. Clin. Nutr.* 85: 1257–1266.

Peng Y, Qi X, Guo X. (2016) Child–Pugh versus MELD score for the assessment of prognosis in liver cirrhosis: a systematic review and meta-analysis of observational studies. *Medicine (Baltimore).* 95: e2877.

Petersen KF, Krssak M, Navarro V, *et al.* (1999) Contributions of net hepatic glycogenolysis and gluconeogenesis to glucose production in cirrhosis. *Am. J. Physiol.* 276: e529–535.

Plauth M, Cabre E, Campillo B, *et al.* (2009) ESPEN guidelines on parenteral nutrition: hepatology. *Clin. Nutr.* 28: 436–444.

Plauth M, Cabre E, Riggio O, *et al.* (2006) ESPEN guidelines on enteral nutrition: Liver disease. *Clin. Nutr.* 25: 285–294.

Plauth M, Schutz T, Buckendahl DP, *et al.* (2004) Weight gain after transjugular intrahepatic portosystemic shunt is associated with improvement in body composition in malnourished patients with cirrhosis and hypermetabolism. *J. Hepatol.* 40: 228–233.

Pose E, Cardenas A. (2017) Translating our current understanding of ascites management into new therapies for patients with cirrhosis and fluid retention. *Dig. Dis.* 35: 402–410.

Potze W, Porte RJ, Lisman T. (2015) Management of coagulation abnormalities in liver disease. *Expert Rev. Gastroenterol. Hepatol.* 9: 103–114.

Powell LW, Seckington RC, Deugnier Y. (2016) *Haemochromatosis. Lancet.* 388: 706–716.

Pugh RN, Murray-Lyon IM, Dawson JL, *et al.* (1973) Transection of the oesophagus for bleeding oesophageal varices. *Br. J. Surg.* 60: 646–649.

Robinson S, Bulger C. (2008) *General Lifestyle Survey 2008: Smoking and Drinking Among Adults, 2008.* In: Statistics, O. F. N. (ed). Norwich: Crown.

Romero-Gomez M, Zelber-Sagi S, Trenell M. (2017) Treatment of NAFLD with diet, physical activity and exercise. *J. Hepatol.* 67(4): 829–846.

Rossi RE, Conte D, Massironi S. (2016) Primary sclerosing cholangitis associated with inflammatory bowel disease: an update. *Eur. J. Gastroenterol. Hepatol.* 28: 123–131.

Routhu M, Safka V, Routhu SK, *et al.* (2017) Observational cohort study of hepatic encephalopathy after transjugular intrahepatic portosystemic shunt (tips). *Ann. Hepatol.* 16: 140–148.

Rubio-Tapia A, Murray JA. (2007) The liver in celiac disease. *Hepatology.* 46: 1650–1658.

Ruiz-Margain A, Macias-Rodriguez RU, Rios-Torres SL, *et al.* (2017) *Effect of a high-protein, high-fiber diet plus supplementation with branched-chain amino acids on the nutritional status of patients with cirrhosis. Revista de Gastroenterologia de Mexico.* [online] Available at http://www.sciencedirect.com/science/article/pii/S0375090617300605?via%3Dihub. Accessed 17 July 2017.

Ryder S. (2003) Guidelines for the diagnosis and treatment of hepatocellular carcinoma (HCC) in adults. *Gut.* 52: iii1–iii8.

Saab S, Mallam D, Cox GA, *et al.* (2014) Impact of coffee on liver diseases: a systematic review. *Liver Int.* 34: 495–504.

Salgia RJ, Brown K. (2015) Diagnosis and management of hereditary hemochromatosis. *Clin. Liver Dis.* 19: 187–198.

Salvioli G, Tata C, Panini R, *et al.* (1993) Composition of ascitic fluid in liver cirrhosis: Bile acid and lipid content. *Eur. J. Clin. Invest.* 23: 534–539.

Sam J, Nguyen GC. (2009) Protein-calorie malnutrition as a prognostic indicator of mortality among patients hospitalized with cirrhosis and portal hypertension. *Liver Int.* 29: 1396–1402.

Shiraki M, Nishiguchi S, Saito M, *et al.* (2013) Nutritional status and quality of life in current patients with liver cirrhosis as assessed in 2007–2011. *Hepatol. Res.* 43: 106–112.

Solà E, Solé C, Ginès P. (2016) Management of uninfected and infected ascites in cirrhosis. *Liver Int.* 36: 109–115.

Sougioultzis S, Dalakas E, Hayes PC, *et al.* (2005) Alcoholic hepatitis: From pathogenesis to treatment. *Curr. Med. Res. Opin.* 21: 1337–1346.

Souza MR, Diniz Mde F, Medeiros-Filho JE, *et al.* (2012) Metabolic syndrome and risk factors for non-alcoholic fatty liver disease. *Arq. Gastroenterol.* 49: 89–96.

Swart GR, van den Berg JW, Wattimena JL, *et al.* (1988) Elevated protein requirements in cirrhosis of the liver investigated by whole body protein turnover studies. *Clin. Sci. (Lond).* 75: 101–107.

Tajiri K, Shimizu Y. (2013) Branched-chain amino acids in liver diseases. *World J. Gastroenterol.* 19: 7620–7629.

Talwalkar JA, Lindor KD. (2003) Primary biliary cirrhosis. *Lancet.* 362: 53–61.

Tandon P, Ney M, Irwin I, *et al.* (2012) Severe muscle depletion in patients on the liver transplant wait list: Its prevalence and independent prognostic value. *Liver Transpl.* 18: 1209–1216.

Teckman JH, Mangalat N. (2015) Alpha-1 antitrypsin and liver disease: mechanisms of injury and novel interventions. *Expert Rev. Gastroenterol. Hepatol.* 9: 261–268.

Thomson AD, Marshall EJ. (2006) The treatment of patients at risk of developing Wernicke's encephalopathy in the community. *Alcohol Alcohol.* 41: 159–167.

Tilg H, Moschen AR, Kaneider NC. (2011) Pathways of liver injury in alcoholic liver disease. *J. Hepatol.* 55: 1159–1161.

Todorovic ME, Micklewright A. (2011) *A Pocket Guide to Clinical Nutrition.* Birmingham: PEN Group Publications.

Toshikuni N, Arisawa T, Tsutsumi M. (2014) Nutrition and exercise in the management of liver cirrhosis. *World J. Gastroenterol.* 20: 7286–7297.

Tsien C, Davuluri G, Singh D, *et al.* (2015) Metabolic and molecular responses to leucine-enriched branched chain amino acid supplementation in the skeletal muscle of alcoholic cirrhosis. *Hepatology.* 61: 2018–2029.

Tsochatzis EA, Bosch J, Burroughs AK. (2014) Liver cirrhosis. *Lancet*. 383: 1749–1761.
Tsuchiya M, Sakaida I, Okamoto M, *et al.* (2005)The effect of a late evening snack in patients with liver cirrhosis. *Hepatol Res*. 31(2): 95–103.
Valery PC, Powell E, Moses N, *et al.* (2015) Systematic review: Unmet supportive care needs in people diagnosed with chronic liver disease. *BMJ Open*. 5: e007451.
van Gerven NM, de Boer YS, Mulder CJ, *et al.* (2016) Auto immune hepatitis. *World J. Gastroenterol*. 22: 4651–4661.
Vidas NA. (2014) Primary biliary cirrhosis and primary sclerosing cholangitis and nutrition. In: Lomer M (ed) *Advanced Nutrition and Dietetics in Gastroenterology*. Chichester: Wiley Blackwell.
WHO. (2011) *Global Status Report on Alcohol and Health*. Available at http://apps.who.int/iris/bitstream/10665/112736/1/9789240692763_eng.pdf?ua=1. Accessed 17 June 2017.
WHO. (2017a) *Hepatitis C*. Available at http://www.who.int/mediacentre/factsheets/fs164/en/. Accessed 14 June 2017.
WHO. (2017b) *Hepatitis B*. Available at http://www.who.int/mediacentre/factsheets/fs204/en/. Accessed 14 June 2017.
WHO. (2017c) *Hepatitis E*. Available at http://www.who.int/mediacentre/factsheets/fs280/en/. Accessed 14 June 2017.
Williams R, Aspinall R, Bellis M, *et al.* (2014) Addressing liver disease in the UK: a blueprint for attaining excellence in health care and reducing premature mortality from lifestyle issues of excess consumption of alcohol, obesity, and viral hepatitis. *Lancet*. 384: 1953–1997.
Yeluru A, Cuthbert JA, Casey L, *et al.* (2016) Alcoholic hepatitis: risk factors, pathogenesis, and approach to treatment. *Alcohol. Clin. Exp. Res*. 40: 246–255.
Younossi ZM, Koenig AB, Abdelatif D, *et al.* (2016) Global epidemiology of nonalcoholic fatty liver disease – meta-analytic assessment of prevalence, incidence, and outcomes. *Hepatology*. 64: 73–84.

7.4.13 Cystic fibrosis

Alison Morton

Key points

- Cystic fibrosis is a multisystem disorder mainly affecting the respiratory and gastrointestinal systems.
- Many have increased energy requirements, increased energy losses and poor oral intake: optimising nutrition is vital as there is a positive association between nutritional status, lung function and survival.
- Regular dietetic counselling aims to achieve a good nutritional status by minimising the effects of malabsorption with pancreatic enzyme replacement therapy and optimising nutritional intake.
- With increased longevity, new nutritional challenges emerge, including diabetes, disordered eating, transplantation and obesity.

The first description of cystic fibrosis (CF) was by Andersen in 1938. Dietary management of CF and optimising nutrition are integral to the improved life expectancy of patients. The replacement of the traditional low fat diet with a high-fat diet in the 1980s and the introduction of acid-resistant pancreatic enzyme replacement therapy (PERT) were milestones in management. CF is a complex multisystem disorder. Intestinal malabsorption occurs in approximately 90% of patients. Historically, malnutrition, weight loss and poor growth were inevitable consequences of disease progression, leading to impaired respiratory muscle function, immunological impairment, respiratory failure and premature death. Achieving and maintaining normal nutritional status and growth are integral parts of CF management and have contributed to improving life expectancy.

Prevalence

CF is the most common autosomal recessively inherited disease in the UK, mainly affecting Caucasians. One in 25 people in the UK are carriers of a CF gene mutation, leading to an incidence of approximately 1 in 2500 births (Dodge *et al.*, 2007). The incidence in non-Caucasians is lower, and estimated to be 1 in 100,000 in Oriental populations and 1 in 20,000 in Africans (Corey *et al.*, 1988). In the UK, approximately 10,400 people have CF, with more than half being adults (CF Trust, 2017).

Aetiology

The genetic defect is located on the long arm of chromosome 7 and results in abnormal production and function of a protein called the CF transmembrane conductance regulator (CFTR). CFTR acts as a chloride channel regulating sodium, chloride, bicarbonate and water transport across epithelial cell membranes. The lack of production or reduction of CFTR results in thick mucus secretions that can obstruct small airways, causing fibrosis and bronchiectasis. CFTR is widespread throughout the body, resulting in a multisystem condition. The two major systems affected are the respiratory system and the gastrointestinal tract. Although over 90% of the CF population in the UK share the same genetic defect (p.Phe508del mutation) (CF Trust, 2017), >2000 different mutations have been identified (CFTR2 Mutation Database, 2017). Different gene mutations and genotypes result in different disease expression and disease severity through differing mechanisms (see Chapter 5.1, Genetics and nutritional genomics). New treatments target these mechanisms.

Diagnostic criteria and classification

National newborn screening for CF was introduced in the UK in 2005 and was universal from 2007. Newborn screening involves a heel prick blood sample being taken from all babies to test for a number of diseases. The screen for CF looks at the concentration of immunoreactive trypsin (IRT), which is raised in neonates with CF. If positive, the infant is referred for a sweat test and genetic screening to confirm the diagnosis. An elevated chloride concentration in the sweat test is diagnostic of CF. CF is usually confirmed by two positive sweat tests or by the identification of two genetic mutations. The gene mutations are determined from a sample of blood or cells from the oral mucosa. Initially, only the four most common mutations are looked for (followed by a 29–32 mutation panel). Infants presenting with meconium ileus should also have a sweat test and genetic testing. Most patients are now diagnosed early by newborn screening or after presenting with meconium ileus. In people with rare mutations and those born prior to national newborn screening, the diagnosis may be made later in life. Symptoms that are suggestive of CF include the following:

- Recurrent respiratory symptoms.
- Prolonged diarrhoea and pale, greasy, offensive stools.
- Failure to thrive in children, delayed puberty or undernutrition in adults.
- Male infertility.
- Pancreatitis.
- Rectal prolapse.

Disease process

Respiratory function

People with CF may have chronic and severe respiratory infections. The presence of viscid mucus in the lungs increases the risk of colonisation by pathogens. Chronic chest infections cause inflammation, irreversible lung damage and progressive lung disease. Infection and reduction in lung function may contribute to increased energy requirements and reduced energy intake. Regular antibiotic therapy, anti-inflammatory drugs and physiotherapy are aimed at preventing lung damage and preserving lung function.

Gastrointestinal function

CFTR dysfunction at the apical surface of epithelial cells of pancreatic ducts may result in ductal plugging, obstruction, and progressive damage to the pancreas, preventing secretion of pancreatic enzymes and resulting in malabsorption. Approximately 90% of patients in Northern Europe are diagnosed with pancreatic insufficiency (PI), which results in significant fat malabsorption and steatorrhoea. Symptoms include frequent, pale, oily and offensive stools; abdominal pain; poor growth; malnutrition; and deficiencies of fat-soluble vitamins and essential fatty acids. Malabsorption is multifactorial, with contributory factors including abnormal ion transfer in the gut due to CFTR, and altered bile salt composition, motility and transit time (Littlewood *et al.*, 2006). Pancreatic enzyme replacement therapy can be inactivated by increased duodenal acidity due to pancreatic bicarbonate deficiency, which may result in bile salt precipitation. Patients with milder mutations are often pancreatic sufficient (PS).

Prognosis

CF was once a life-limiting disease of childhood. Life expectancy, although still reduced, has increased dramatically due to many factors, including specialist centre care, better nutritional support and improved treatment of respiratory infections. Recent introduction of CFTR modulators aimed at correcting the basic defect in some genotypes are encouraging. Median survival in the UK is currently 45.1 years and has been predicted to be 47 years for those born between 2012 and 2016. Over 60% of patients with CF in the UK are now 16 years or older (CF Trust, 2017).

Nutritional consequences

Impaired energy intake

Poor energy intakes are frequently reported in patients; this may be a consequence of poor appetite worsened by infection-related anorexia during pulmonary exacerbations, abdominal pain, vomiting and gastro-oesophageal reflux disease. As the disease progresses, it is difficult to maximise oral intake due to dyspnoea, early satiety or taste changes due to oxygen or drug therapy. Behavioural factors, including food refusal, psychosocial issues, depression and disordered eating, further contribute to poor food intakes and nutrient deficits.

Increased energy expenditure

Energy requirements in CF vary greatly, but are largely related to frequency and severity of respiratory infections, inflammation and the extent of lung disease. Some medications used to treat respiratory symptoms may increase resting energy expenditure (Kalnins *et al.*, 2013). With increased longevity, nutritional comorbidities including CF-related diabetes (CFRD), CF-related low bone mineral density, renal disease, obesity and transplantation are more common. However, pregnancy is still seen in fewer than 100 women with CF in the UK each year (CF Trust, 2017).

Impaired nutrient absorption

Lack of pancreatic enzymes has a devastating effect on nutritional status. Fat digestion is not clearly impaired until lipase output is <10% of normal. Pancreatic enzyme replacement therapy should be started if a patient has two CFTR mutations associated with PI. In addition, patients who present with obvious symptoms of malabsorption should commence PERT on diagnosis of CF. PI should always be confirmed by measuring faecal pancreatic elastase (FPE) (Smyth *et al.*, 2014). If clinical symptoms of malabsorption are absent, measurement of FPE to establish pancreatic status should be undertaken, and PERT should only be commenced if PI is diagnosed (CF Trust Nutrition Working Group, 2016). Some patients have difficulty controlling malabsorption despite optimal PERT, experiencing increased losses of protein, fat and fat-soluble nutrients in the stool. Undigested fat may bind other minerals and lead to increased excretion.

Fat-soluble vitamins

Biochemical evidence of deficiencies of fat-soluble vitamins (A, D, E and K) is found early in infants diagnosed by newborn screening (Neville & Ranganathan, 2009; Sokol *et al.*, 1989). Traditionally, vitamin status was considered in terms of overt deficiency resulting in the classically recognised deficiency symptoms. Subclinical deficiencies are of increasing importance (Maqbool & Stallings, 2008), and most PI patients require daily supplements. Individual assessment and advice for PS patients is required, but many require supplementation with vitamin D as a minimum.

Vitamin A

The major consequence of vitamin A deficiency is ocular, with night blindness and xerophthalmia being reported (Petersen *et al.*, 1968). Asymptomatic conjunctival xerosis with abnormal dark adaptation despite vitamin A supplementation has been reported (Huet *et al.*, 1997). Although such problems are rare, the consequence of subclinical deficiency may be significant. Subclinical vitamin A deficiency may impair the integrity of the respiratory epithelium (McCullough *et al.*, 1999). Loss of ciliated cells and increased mucus secretion make bacterial adherence and colonisation of the lung more likely (Biesalski & Nohr, 2003). Linking subclinical vitamin A deficiency and lung function is difficult. There is a correlation between low vitamin A levels, an increased number of respiratory exacerbations (Hakim *et al.*, 2007) and low lung function (Aird *et al.*, 2006). Cross-sectional data suggests that FEV_1 correlates positively with serum retinol levels in CF (Rivas-Crespo *et al.*, 2013), although this finding is not repeated in all studies (Woestenenk *et al.*, 2015a).

Beta-carotene is a precursor of vitamin A and has antioxidant properties, acting as a free-radical scavenger that may slow oxidative damage in the lung. There is currently insufficient evidence to recommend routine supplementation with beta-carotene for its antioxidant properties alone. Further studies are needed before a firm conclusion regarding optimal dose, timing and effects of antioxidant supplementation can be made (CF Trust Nutrition Working Group, 2016).

Vitamin E

Severe vitamin E deficiency is rare in modern CF care; historically, it is associated with neurological degeneration (Sitrin *et al.*, 1987), haemolytic anaemia (Wilfond *et al.*, 1994) and decreased cognitive function (Koscik *et al.*, 2005). Vitamin E is an important antioxidant, helping to protect the lungs from damage during the inflammatory response to infection. However, a recent study suggests that there is no evidence that higher serum α-tocopherol levels have a protective effect on lung function in CF (Woestenenk *et al.*, 2015b).

Vitamin D

There is increasing interest in vitamin D's role in lung disease through its action on regulating inflammation (Pincikova *et al.*, 2017), inducing antimicrobial peptides, and/or its action on muscle (Finklea *et al.*, 2011; Konstantinopoulou & Tipia, 2017). Vitamin D status has also been positively associated with improved lung function (Green *et al.*, 2008; Stephenson *et al.*, 2007) and a reduction in pulmonary exacerbations in CF (McCauley *et al.*, 2014). However, the precise relationship between vitamin D status and lung health remains unclear.

Overt vitamin D deficiency in CF is rare, but both rickets and osteomalacia have been reported (Elkin *et al.*, 2002; Scott *et al.*, 1977). Subclinical vitamin D status may be significant in the context of health outcomes (Maqbool & Stallings, 2008). There is currently no consensus on optimal vitamin D levels to maintain bone health in the CF population. A level of 20 ng/mL (50 nmol/L) has been recommended in European Guidelines (Sermet-Gaudelus *et al.*, 2011; Turck *et al.*, 2016), while the recommendation from the UK CF Trust (2007) and the North American CF Foundation (Tangpricha *et al.*, 2012) is a minimum level of 30 ng/mL (75 nmol/L). Suboptimal vitamin D levels are common in patients with CF despite routine and high-dose supplementation (Green *et al.*, 2010). Studies do not report a direct link between low vitamin D levels and low bone density, but it is likely that suboptimal vitamin D status contributes to the aetiology of low bone mineral density in CF (Sermet-Gaudelus *et al.*, 2011).

Vitamin K

Severe vitamin K deficiency prolongs bleeding time. In CF, it has been associated with coagulopathies, including haematomas, intracerebral haemorrhage and severe life-threatening bleeds (Hamid & Khan, 2007; McPhail, 2010). Subclinical vitamin K deficiency is common in PI patients and universal in patients with CF-related liver disease (Rashid *et al.*, 1999). It is reported in more than half of pre- and post-lung-transplant patients (Hubert *et al.*, 2016). This level of deficiency has been linked to reduced bone mineral density (Conway *et al.*, 2005).

Nutritional assessment

Individual assessment is essential to determine the interventions that are both appropriate and acceptable for each patient. Factors to be considered include age, clinical condition, nutritional status and history, pancreatic status, nutritional requirements, family circumstances, financial constraints, religious and cultural beliefs, and food preferences. Assessment should include the following as a minimum:

- Anthropometry
  - Accurate measurement of weight, height and body mass index (BMI) (and head circumference in young children) should be undertaken at every clinic visit and plotted on the appropriate percentile chart in children (CF Trust Nutrition Working Group, 2016) (see Chapter 3.8, Paediatric clinical dietetics and childhood nutrition).
  - Assessment of pubertal stage in peripubertal children until puberty is complete (Sermet-Gaudelus *et al.*, 2011).
  - Assessment of bone mineral density and body composition by dual-energy X ray absorptiometry should be performed from around 8–10 years of age (Turck *et al.*, 2016).
- Biochemistry
  - Annual assessment of fat-soluble vitamin status (A, D and E) (Turck *et al.*, 2016).
  - Assessment of vitamin A status in CF is difficult as both retinol and retinol-binding protein (RBP) decrease during the acute phase response to infection; RBP is depressed in plasma zinc deficiency. Vitamin A status should be measured at a time of clinical stability together with RBP, plasma zinc and a positive acute-phase protein such as C-reactive protein (Stephenson & Gildengorin, 2000).
  - Serum or plasma vitamin E levels are used to assess vitamin E status. Vitamin E circulates in the blood bound to lipoproteins, and therefore the status is more accurately assessed using the vitamin E to total lipid ratio in patients with high or low lipid levels (Turck *et al.*, 2016).
  - Plasma 25 hydroxyvitamin D is the conventional marker of status. There should be awareness of seasonal variation in levels.
  - Assessment of vitamin K deficiency is difficult as prothrombin time is not a sensitive marker of vitamin K status. Protein or prothrombin induced by vitamin K absence/antagonism (PIVKA II) and undercarboxylated osteocalcin are more sensitive markers, but are mostly used in research.
  - Urea and electrolytes, liver function, and full blood count, at least annually.
  - Annual oral glucose tolerance test.
- Dietary assessment (annual)
  - Dietary intake, including appetite.
  - Contribution of oral supplements and enteral tube feeds.
  - Knowledge and titration of PERT, including assessment of symptoms of malabsorption.
  - Fat-soluble vitamin supplementation.
  - Use of non-prescribed supplements.
  - Control of CFRD.
  - Other aspects, e.g. body image.
  - Formal assessment of dietary intake using a written diet and enzyme diary should be targeted at selected individuals only (Conway *et al.*, 2014).

Nutritional management

Nutritional status has important prognostic significance, with a positive association between body weight, height, BMI and survival (Beker *et al.*, 2001; Corey *et al.*, 1988) and between nutritional status and lung function (Panagopoulou *et al.*, 2014; Pedreira *et al.*, 2005; Vandenbranden *et al.*, 2012). A diet that achieves and maintains good nutritional status is required to ensure that growth is optimised, resistance to infection maximised, and outcomes improved. Current recommendations state that children and adolescents should achieve a BMI ≥50th percentile, adult females ≥22 kg/m² and adult males ≥23 kg/m² (Stallings *et al.*, 2008). Good nutrition education from diagnosis is needed to achieve these aims. Optimal PERT is an essential part of this education.

Pancreatic enzyme replacement therapy

The main aims of PERT are to:

- Enable eating a normal-fat to high-fat diet.
- Control signs and symptoms associated with maldigestion and malabsorption.
- Promote and maintain normal nutritional status and growth.
- Achieve optimal fat-soluble vitamin and essential fatty acid status.

Types of enzyme preparations

The enteric coated, acid-resistant microsphere and minimicrosphere preparations are significantly more effective than powder-based and enteric-coated tablet formulations in correcting fat malabsorption. The enzymes are protected from inactivation by gastric acid and are only active when the pH rises above 5.5 in the duodenum, resulting in improved fat and nitrogen absorption (Littlewood *et al.*, 2006). Currently, animal-derived enzymes represent an established standard of care; however, the growing study of plant- and microbe-derived enzymes offers great promise.

High-strength enzyme preparations

High-strength enzyme preparations became available in the mid-1980s. They were developed to improve PERT by reducing the number of capsules taken per meal. In the early 1990s, there were concerns about their safety, which were linked with the development of fibrosing colonopathy (colonic strictures), particularly in children (Smyth *et al.*, 1994). As a result, the UK Committee on the Safety of Medicines (CSM, 1995) advised that:

- The total dose of lipase should not usually exceed 10,000 units/kg body weight/day.
- Pancrease HL® and Nutrizym 22® should not be used in children under 15 years.

In the UK, the high-strength preparations Creon 25000® and Creon 40000®, which do not contain methyl acrylic copolymer, are used for adults and some children. Patients must receive detailed advice and assessment before they change their enzyme preparation.

Enzyme dosage and administration

There is no evidence on the relative dose of enzymes needed for people with different degrees of PI, optimum time to start treatment and dose variations based on the types of meals and meal sizes (Somaraju & Solis-Moya, 2016). Enzyme therapy is based on experiential learning, historical recommendations and consensus statements. Internationally, guidelines give recommendations for dosing PERT based on lipase units/kg/meal (Borowitz *et al.*, 2009; Turck *et al.*, 2016) and lipase units/g of fat consumed (Anthony *et al.*, 1999; Saxby *et al.*, 2017). Enzyme dose is most often based on the fat content of meals and snacks, and PERT should be taken with all fat-containing food and drinks. The lowest effective dose of PERT should be used. There is large individual variation in the enzyme dose required, but it should not usually exceed 10,000 units of lipase/kg/day. Patients exceeding this dose need assessment and further investigation. The recommendations are (Turck *et al.*, 2016) as follows:

- *Infants*: 2000–4000 U lipase/120 mL formula or breast-milk, and approximately 2000 U lipase/g of fat in food.
- *1–4 years*: 2000–4000 U lipase/g dietary fat titrating dose as needed, to a maximum of 10,000 U lipase/kg/day.
- *>4 years*: Consider starting at 500 U lipase/kg/meal, titrating upwards to a maximum dose of:
  - 1000–2500 U lipase/kg/meal or
  - 10,000 U lipase/kg/day
  - 2000–4000 U lipase/g of fat with all fat-containing meals, snacks and drinks.

Individual requirements for PERT depend upon a number of factors, including the following:

- Degree of residual pancreatic function.
- Pharmacological and dissolution characteristics of the preparation; some patients may respond better to one product than another.
- Timing and method of enzyme administration.
- Fat content of the diet.
- Factors affecting pH within the gastrointestinal tract.

It is important to stress to patients that dose adjustment should be dietetically or medically supervised to avoid inappropriate or excessive enzyme intake.

The method of enzyme administration is important. Microspheres should not be chewed, crushed, or sprinkled on (or mixed with) the whole meal, as exposure to hot food or food with a pH of >5.5 reduces efficacy. For infants and young children, microspheres should be mixed with a small amount of expressed breast milk, infant formula or a little semi-solid food (e.g. apple purée), and given from a teaspoon with feeds. The capsules should be swallowed whole as early as possible; most children will manage this by 4–5 years of age (CF Trust Nutrition Working Group, 2016). Enzymes are usually given in a divided dose, with half to two-third of the total dose given before the meal, and half to one-third during the meal, although this may vary between individuals, and adjustment of the timing of administration may be necessary. Guidelines on PERT are summarised in Box 7.4.6.

Monitoring effectiveness

Even with modern PERT, maldigestion and malabsorption may still occur. Factors that may contribute to this include the following:

- *Patients failing to recognise or report steatorrhoea* – patients become accustomed to their normal stool pattern and may fail to recognise symptoms of steatorrhoea, and that enzyme dosage needs adjusting.
- *Inadequate education* – knowledge of enzyme titration according to dietary fat intake and timing of administration may be inadequate.
- *Lack of regular dietetic assessment* – regular assessment is essential to achieve an appropriate balance between PERT and food intake.
- *Non-adherence with guidance given* – patients may not take their PERT or adhere to advice given with

Box 7.4.6 Guidelines for the use of pancreatic enzyme preparations

Enzymes should be taken with all fat-containing meals, snacks and drinks.

Enzymes are usually given in a divided dose, with half of the total dose before the meal and half during the meal, or two-third before the meal and one-third during the meal.

If meals last longer than 30 minutes, enzymes should be taken before, during and towards the end of the meal.

The dose should be titrated according to the fat content of the food or snack.

Enzymes should not be taken with fat-free snacks and drinks, e.g. soft drinks, fruit, boiled or jelly sweets.

Capsules containing enteric-coated tablets or microspheres should be swallowed without being chewed (to avoid losing their effectiveness). For young children, the capsules should be opened and the contents mixed with a little soft food or fruit purée and administered from a teaspoon. Granules must not be sprinkled over a meal.

Enzyme dose should not be increased if adherence is poor.

Under medical/dietetic supervision, the enzyme dose should be increased gradually if the stools are fatty, loose, offensive or frequent.

Adequate hydration is important, especially with higher-strength enzyme preparations.

Enzymes should be taken with all fat-containing enteral tube feeds; they should not be added to the feed or routinely administered via the feeding tube.

respect to timing or dosage. People with CF should be encouraged to openly discuss any adherence issues they experience.
- Other factors, including low duodenal pH, e.g. due to excessive production of gastric acid or reduced pancreatic bicarbonate, can result in inappropriate release or inactivation of enzymes. Practical considerations such as enzyme storage and stock rotation are also important.

The efficacy of PERT can be assessed by the measurement of faecal fat and calculation of the coefficient of fat absorption or stool weight, although these are used as research tools in the UK. The effectiveness of PERT is usually monitored by assessment of growth, nutritional status and abdominal symptoms.

Nutritional requirements

Energy

Dietary energy requirements vary widely between people with CF and in individuals during the course of their life, but are usually higher than those recommended for the general population. This is due to increased energy expenditure resulting from inflammation and infection, and continuing energy losses due to malabsorption. Historically, energy requirements were estimated to be approximately 120–150% of the estimated average requirement for the normal population. Energy needs are now recognised to be 110–200% of healthy individuals of the same age and gender (Stallings *et al.*, 2008; Turck *et al.*, 2016). Nutritional needs should be assessed on an individual basis, and SACN (2011) reference values should be used when estimating energy requirements.

Protein

There are no evidence-based recommendations for daily protein intake for patients with CF. Protein needs are likely to be higher to compensate for loss of nitrogen in the faeces and sputum. Optimal protein needs will depend on each individual's condition (Engelen *et al.*, 2014).

Fat

Fat restriction to reduce symptoms of steatorrhoea is not necessary with modern PERT. Restricting fat compromises energy intake, fat-soluble vitamins and essential fatty status. It is usually recommended that fat provide 35–40% of energy, although studies show that this is difficult to achieve (White *et al.*, 2004). With increasing longevity and a greater variability in health, a high fat intake should not be achieved by an overdependence on saturated fat. The consumption of mono- and polyunsaturated fats should be encouraged. Patients should be individually assessed and advised, and, if overweight, fat restriction may now be appropriate. The dietary intake of the n-3 fatty acids should be as recommended for the general population. More research is required to determine the efficacy of intervention with pharmacological doses. The use of medium-chain triglyceride oil in cooking is no longer recommended as it is unpalatable, and PERT is still required.

Dietary fibre

The need for an energy-dense diet means that fibre intake may be low. A low fibre intake with poor hydration is associated with distal intestinal obstruction syndrome (Munck *et al.*, 2016). Recommendations for fibre intake are limited, and further research is needed due to the complexity of the CF gut.

Water-soluble vitamins

Routine supplementation is unnecessary; diets should be assessed individually for dietary adequacy. Parenteral vitamin B_{12} may be required following resection of the terminal ileum for meconium ileus (Turck *et al.*, 2016). For women planning pregnancy, folic acid supplementation is required in the preconception period and throughout the first trimester of pregnancy.

Fat-soluble vitamins

Vitamins A, D, E and K should be provided from diagnosis onwards in PI patients. Vitamin requirements vary, so regimens may combine a multivitamin preparation (or A and D capsules), and a vitamin E and a vitamin K supplement. Additional vitamin D supplements may be necessary to avoid vitamin A toxicity. Specific CF vitamin supplements are available, but these may need the addition of individual vitamins. It is essential that all patients be individually assessed, and that doses be adjusted depending on plasma levels. Annual monitoring of plasma levels is recommended as a minimum for all patients, and 3–6 months after a dose change (Turck *et al.*, 2016). Vitamin D supplementation is often required in PS patients to achieve adequate levels. Hypervitaminosis A and E have been reported in patients with CF following lung transplantation (Ho *et al.*, 2011), and higher plasma levels have also been found in children and young adults as compared to the general population (Huang *et al.*, 2006; Maqbool *et al.*, 2008). Deficiency is the primary concern in patients with CF, but, with early diagnosis and improved treatments, high levels are now also a concern.

Current recommendations for fat-soluble vitamin supplementation in PI patients are based on historical data, and vary internationally. The recommended starting doses per day are (CF Trust Nutrition Working Group, 2016) as follows:

- Vitamin A
  - <1 year: 1500 IU (455 µg)
  - >1 year: 1500–10,000 IU (455–3000 µg)
- Vitamin E
  - <1 year: 40–80 mg
  - 1–3 years: 50–150 mg
  - 4–7 years: 150–300 mg
  - ≥8 years 150–500 mg
- Vitamin D – vitamin D_3 (colecalciferol) is preferable to D_2 (ergocalciferol)

  - <1 year: 400–2000 IU (10–50 μg)
  - >1 year and adults: 400–5000 IU (10–125 μg/day)
- Vitamin K – vitamin K_1 (phytomenadione) is considered the safest supplement
  - <2 years: 300 mg/kg/day, rounded to the nearest mg
  - 2–7 years: 5 mg
  - >8 years: 5–10 mg

Minerals and trace elements

Sodium

CF results in an abnormally high concentration of sodium excreted in sweat, and sodium losses are increased in conditions causing excessive sweating, e.g. hot climates. In these circumstances, salt supplements are recommended. Sodium deficiency can be a particular problem for infants, as it can lead to impaired growth.

Iron

Iron deficiency is common, and risk increases with age (von Drygalski & Biller, 2008). It is related to disease severity, malabsorption and loss of iron in the sputum rather than dietary deficiency. There should be awareness of increased iron requirements.

Calcium

Reduced bone mineral density is common in adolescents and adults with CF. Negative calcium balance may be due to malabsorption, increased endogenous faecal losses of calcium (Schulze *et al.*, 2003) and vitamin D insufficiency. Attention to calcium intake is important, and supplementation may be necessary.

Dietary intervention

All people with CF should receive preventative or anticipatory nutritional counselling regardless of their age and clinical or nutritional status. A progressive approach to intensification of nutrition interventions is recommended (Turck *et al.*, 2016). Interventions should be tried stepwise for a limited period of time until nutritional status is optimised.

First-stage intervention – improving food and energy intake

Providing practical dietary advice on matters such as increasing meal frequency, choosing energy-dense foods and food fortification are the first stage of intervention (CF Trust Nutrition Working Group, 2016; Turck *et al.*, 2016). In the USA, behavioural intervention and nutritional counselling are recommended in children aged 1–12 years to promote weight gain (Stallings *et al.*, 2008).

Second-stage intervention – oral nutritional supplements

The emphasis on the use of normal food is important, but if nutritional status remains poor despite encouraging a high-energy diet, addressing behavioural factors, ensuring optimal PERT and excluding CFRD, then oral nutritional supplements (ONS) are the next stage of intervention. Smyth and Rayner (2017) found insufficient evidence for the efficacy of ONS in CF; they concluded that nutritional supplements may be used but should not be regarded as an essential part of care (Smyth & Rayner, 2017).

A multicentre study of a high-fat, milk-based supplement demonstrated significant weight gain in individuals with CF (Skypala *et al.*, 1998). However, a small study comparing oral supplements with dietary counselling over a 3-month period found no significant change in energy intake or nutritional status in either group (Kalnins *et al.*, 2005). ONS have been shown to significantly increase energy intakes in adults as compared to diet alone (White *et al.*, 2004). A large randomised controlled trial of ONS in mild to moderately malnourished children with CF found no improvement in nutritional status or other clinical outcomes. It concluded that '*oral supplements should not be regarded as an essential part of the management of mildly malnourished children with CF*' (Poustie *et al.*, 2006). However, the study did not consider the use of supplements in adult patients, severely malnourished individuals, and those with end-stage lung disease, or short-term use in acute situations. ONS may be considered on an individual basis (Saxby *et al.*, 2017) in people with CF who have suboptimal growth and nutritional status, despite optimising oral dietary intake and PERT (Turck *et al.*, 2016). A CF-specialist dietitian should monitor the introduction, use and efficacy of supplements. The type and quantity of supplement recommended depends on the patient's age, preference and nutritional requirements, and should be taken in addition to normal food to increase total energy intake.

Third-stage intervention – enteral tube feeding

Enteral tube feeding (ETF) is considered when dietary education, behavioural intervention and ONS fail to improve nutritional status. Feeds can be provided via a fine-bore nasogastric tube, gastrostomy or, more rarely, jejunostomy. In the UK, the use of enteral tube feeding in CF is decreasing, with 5.6% of patients being gastrostomy fed and 1.0% being nasogastrically fed (CF Trust, 2017), as compared to 20% and 5%, respectively, in 2010 (CF Trust, 2011). There is no evidence to show which route is most effective; the choice depends largely on the likely duration of supplementary feeding (Schwarzenberg *et al.*, 2016). Studies of ETF are limited by methodology, sample size and duration, but weight gain or improved growth, stabilisation or slowing of the rate of decline in lung function, and improved quality of life are reported (Morton & Wolfe, 2015). A Cochrane Systematic Review reported no randomised controlled trials assessing the efficacy of long-term ETF in CF (Morton & Wolfe, 2015).

Earlier intervention with gastrostomy feeding is associated with improved outcomes (Oliver *et al.*, 2004; Truby *et al.*, 2009). Placement of percutaneous or surgical tubes should be avoided during acute illness (Schwarzenberg *et al.*, 2016). It is recommended that enteral tube feeds be administered overnight and provide 30–65% of total energy requirements (Schwarzenberg *et al.*, 2016). Some patients may receive a greater proportion of their energy needs via enteral feeding if oral intake is particularly poor or requirements are exceptionally high.

Feed formulae

Recent evidence-informed guidelines were unable to recommend for or against the use of a specific type of formula for ETF in people with CF (Schwarzenberg *et al.*, 2016). Whole-protein, polymeric feeds are the most common, and are usually well tolerated. Adults and older children are usually given energy-dense polymeric feeds (1.5–2.4 kcal/mL). Occasionally, additional fat may be added as an emulsion to increase energy density, allowing smaller volumes of feed to be administered. Young children are usually given paediatric whole-protein feeds providing 1.5 kcal/mL. Infants should be given a high-energy infant formula.

Low-fat elemental feeds are not usually required for patients with CF. It has been hypothesised that they are better absorbed, but they have a high osmolality and a lower energy density than whole-protein feeds. There remains controversy as to whether these preparations require PERT. Elemental formulae or feeds containing MCT may be beneficial if a polymeric feed is not tolerated. Optimum feed type has yet to be established and may vary with clinical situations.

Enzyme administration during enteral tube feeds

There are no clinical trials regarding the use of PERT or the most efficacious route of administration with ETF (Schwarzenberg *et al.*, 2016). In clinical practice in the UK, PERT is usually administered orally at the beginning of the feed, and sometimes during or at the end of the feed. Enzyme requirements are dependent on the rate of infusion, type and fat content of the feed. If the feed is infused continuously over a long period, lower doses of enzymes are required than would normally be administered with a meal of equivalent fat content. Increased gastric lipase production may also help fat digestion from continuously infused feeds. Recently, the US Food and Drug Administration approved an in-line enzyme delivery system for enteral tube feeds in adults with CF (Relizorb®); evaluation of its benefits should be considered before use (Schwarzenberg *et al.*, 2016).

Problems with enteral tube feeding

Complications of ETF in CF are rare: NG tube displacement may occur due to coughing, vomiting or physiotherapy. Nocturnal hyperglycaemia requiring insulin therapy may occur in patients given nocturnal feeds. Blood glucose levels should be monitored mid-feed and immediately post-feed in those with CFRD, as well as on introduction of feeds, and monthly thereafter (Moran *et al.*, 2014).

Parenteral nutrition

Parenteral nutritional support is not routinely recommended but may be useful for short-term support when enteral tube feeding is contraindicated, e.g. after major gastrointestinal surgery or in severely ill patients awaiting transplantation (Saxby *et al.*, 2017; Turck *et al.*, 2016).

Special considerations

Infants

The success of screening programmes depends on appropriate interventions for identified infants and improved outcomes. The focus is now on maintaining health by preventing nutritional and respiratory complications (Sermet-Gaudelus *et al.*, 2010). There is a lack of well-designed clinical trials to support practice. The North American CF Foundation developed recommendations for the management of infants based on a systematic review of the evidence and expert opinion (Borowitz *et al.*, 2009), while the European CF Society used a modified Delphi methodology to provide a consensus framework for the management of screened infants (Sermet-Gaudelus *et al.*, 2010). Most infants will thrive if given breast milk or standard infant formula, and breastfeeding should be encouraged. The routine use of hydrolysed formula is not recommended, but may be required for infants who have undergone surgical resection for meconium ileus or those with malabsorption unrelated to CF, e.g. cows' milk protein intolerance (Turck *et al.*, 2016). If fat malabsorption is adequately controlled, infants will usually thrive on energy intakes of 100–130 kcal/kg of body weight/day. If the infant fails to thrive despite optimising milk intake and PERT, energy intakes should be adapted to achieve normal growth. A higher-energy infant formula should be prescribed. Alternatively, breast-fed infants may be offered complimentary formula feeds.

All PI infants should be commenced on PERT at a starting dose of 2000 units of lipase/120 mL of standard formula or breastmilk. The dose should be increased if there are symptoms of malabsorption or inadequate weight gain, but the lipase intake should be kept at <10,000 units/kg of body weight/day (Sermet-Gaudelus *et al.*, 2010). Enteric-coated microspheres/mini-microspheres should be given in a teaspoon with all feeds, mixed with a small amount of the infant's milk or a small amount of fruit purée. They should not be added directly to a bottle of feed.

Gastro-oesophageal reflux is common in infants with CF (Heine *et al.*, 1998), and may compromise growth and exacerbate respiratory symptoms. Treatments include thickening feeds, using a prethickened infant formula, reducing gastric acid using H2 receptor antagonists and/or proton pump inhibitors and motility stimulants. All PI infants should be given fat-soluble vitamin supplements from diagnosis. Sodium chloride supplementation should be considered for all infants with CF, and increased during hot weather or other times of increased salt loss, e.g. diarrhoea (Sermet-Gaudelus *et al.*, 2010).

Weaning foods should be introduced between 4 and 6 months of age, and a normal weaning diet should be established by the end of the first year. The dose of PERT should be adjusted to the fat content of the weaning food.

Preconception

There is little evidence upon which to base recommendations for nutritional management of women with CF in the preconceptional period, during pregnancy and postpartum. Recommendations are based on the recommendations for the non-CF population, adapted to incorporate understandings of the nutritional requirements of CF. Detailed guidelines for the management of pregnancy in women with CF are available (Edenborough *et al.*, 2008). As nutritional status is important in the preconceptional period and throughout pregnancy, thorough preconceptional nutritional assessment and counselling should be undertaken. This should include the following:

- Assessment of weight, height and BMI.
- Dietary assessment and review of PERT, gastrointestinal symptoms and absorption.
- Assessment of glycaemic status by oral glucose tolerance test in the non-diabetic patient.
- Optimising glycaemic control in those with CFRD.
- Increasing awareness of food safety issues.
- Measurement of fasting plasma vitamins A, D and E, and review of vitamin therapy (including non-prescription items).
- Commencement of folic acid supplementation.
- Care should be taken to avoid excessive intakes of vitamin A because of the risk of teratogenicity. In practice, supplemental retinol is usually continued at a dose of <10,000 IU/day, and plasma levels are closely monitored (Edenborough *et al.*, 2008; Saxby *et al.*, 2017).

Pregnancy

Due to increased life expectancy, pregnancy is more common in CF; however, less than 100 women with CF become pregnant each year (CF Trust, 2017). Pregnancy is generally well tolerated, although there are increased risks to both mother and child. Prepregnancy lung function and nutritional status are important predictors of foetal and maternal outcome (Renton *et al.*, 2016). Poor foetal outcomes have been associated with a poor prepregnancy weight (BMI <20 kg/m^2) and a forced expiratory volume of <60% predicted values (Lau *et al.*, 2011). A high incidence of gestational diabetes has been reported (Lau *et al.*, 2011). Early participation of the MDT is essential to ensure an optimal outcome. During pregnancy, the primary nutritional aims are to:

- Achieve adequate weight gain – regular monitoring of nutritional status and weight gain is essential to optimise outcomes. ONS or ETF may be required.
- Minimise the impact of pregnancy-related problems on oral intake. Due to hormonal and mechanical changes in pregnancy, gastro-oesophageal reflux, vomiting and constipation may be more common in women with CF. Guidance on ways to alleviate these problems and improve nutrient intake are essential.

Successful breastfeeding has been achieved in mothers with CF (Gilljam *et al.*, 2000). Breastfeeding increases maternal nutritional requirements. Individual advice about infant feeding should be given according to the mother's clinical condition and circumstances. Many drugs pass into breastmilk, and therefore may be contraindicated during pregnancy and lactation, or are a contraindication to breastfeeding (Edenborough *et al.*, 2008).

Cystic fibrosis–related diabetes

CF-related diabetes (CFRD) is the most common comorbidity, and data suggest incidences of 2% in children, 19% in adolescents and 40–50% in adults (Moran *et al.*, 2014). Glycaemic abnormalities begin very early in CF (Yi *et al.*, 2016). Few people with CF have normal glucose tolerance, and CFRD is part of a spectrum of glucose tolerance abnormalities (Moran *et al.*, 2010). CF-related diabetes shares features of type 1 and type 2 diabetes, but is a distinct entity, being classified as other forms of diabetes or pancreatogenic diabetes (American Diabetes Association, 2016). Insulin deficiency is the primary defect in CFRD, in part caused by loss of insulin production. More recently, the CF gene has been shown to have a role in regulating insulin secretion, and treatment with Ivacaftor® in patients with CF carrying gating mutations has improved insulin secretion (Tsabari *et al.*, 2016). Insulin resistance also plays a role at specific times, e.g. in acute illness and in those on corticosteroids.

CF-related diabetes mainly occurs in people with the most severe CF mutations associated with exocrine PI (Lewis *et al.*, 2015). The importance of early detection, treatment and optimising control cannot be overemphasised, as CFRD is associated with deterioration in respiratory function, clinical and nutritional status, and increased mortality (Lewis *et al.*, 2015). Optimising control of CFRD is important as microvascular complications are increasingly reported. Screening plays a crucial role in the identification of these complications, and is therefore strongly recommended (Saxby *et al.*, 2017).

Patients with CFRD should be managed by a specialised multidisciplinary team with expertise in diabetes and CF. Oral diabetic agents are not recommended, as the primary problem in CFRD is insulin insufficiency; insulin is the medical treatment of choice (Moheet & Moran, 2018; Moran *et al.*, 2014). While some CF centres use oral medications to help control diabetes, the Cystic Fibrosis Foundation (USA) clinical practice guidelines support the use of insulin therapy, and this remains the most widely used treatment method. The aims of CFRD treatment are to maintain growth, optimise nutritional status, achieve good blood glucose control and avoid diabetic complications. At diagnosis, all patients should have a dietary review, and individualised advice should be given based on nutritional and clinical status. The maintenance of a diet high in energy, fat, protein and sodium to compensate for losses is important for most patients. The diet should also be healthy and well balanced, and it may be necessary to consider energy restrictions in those who are overweight. The use of carbohydrate counting to guide insulin therapy can help to optimise control. If a patient with CFRD is malnourished, overnight ETF with an adjusted insulin regimen should be given.

Cystic fibrosis–associated liver disease

CF-associated liver disease (CFLD) occurs in 27–35% of patients, and 5–10% will develop multilobular cirrhosis in the first decade of life. Portal hypertension often develops during the second decade, and liver failure usually occurs in adulthood (Debray *et al.*, 2011). Liver disease may make it increasingly difficult to meet nutritional requirements. It further exacerbates malnutrition by increasing steatorrhoea, which is often unresponsive to increasing enzyme dosage. Oral intake may be reduced as a result of nausea, early satiety resulting from an enlarged liver and/or spleen, and abdominal pain. Impaired liver function is associated with worsening pulmonary function.

Nutritional support is an essential part of the treatment of CFLD, and optimising nutritional status is the primary goal. Close monitoring is essential, especially if the disease progresses to end-stage ascites and encephalopathy. Nasogastric feeding may be required to meet energy requirements. Gastrostomy feeding is not recommended in advanced liver disease because of the risk of a gastric haemorrhage (Debray *et al.*, 2011).

Distal intestinal obstruction syndrome

Distal intestinal obstruction syndrome (DIOS) is caused by the accumulation of viscous mucus and intestinal contents that completely or partially block the intestinal lumen. Incomplete or impending DIOS is common, and patients present with a short history of abdominal pain and/or distension and a faecal mass in the ileocaecum. Complete DIOS is less common, and results in the patient having complete intestinal obstruction with vomiting of bilious material and/or fluid levels in the small intestine on abdominal X ray, in addition to the features of incomplete DIOS (Columbo *et al.*, 2011). Risk factors for DIOS include a severe genotype associated with PI (although it does occur in PS patients), a history of meconium ileus at birth, previous episodes of DIOS, poorly controlled fat absorption, high ambient temperatures, dehydration and CFRD (Munck *et al.*, 2016).

Initially, both DIOS and incomplete DIOS are managed medically. Assessment of PERT and absorption should be undertaken, including knowledge of enzyme titration, timing and adherence with therapy. Avoidance of dehydration is important, and advice on adequate fluid intake is important. The role of increasing fibre intake is unclear (van der Doef *et al.*, 2011), and this should only be done with caution.

Lung or heart–lung transplantation

Lung transplantation has become a viable option for some patients with end-stage lung disease. Some may be declined transplantation based on low weight, as poor nutritional status is linked with increased mortality and poorer outcomes. Most patients will have had intensive nutritional input throughout life, and that makes nutritional management in the pretransplant period challenging, or existing interventions more complex. Maximising oral intake can be difficult due to anorexia, dyspnoea, early satiety, nausea, or taste changes due to oxygen or drug therapy. In addition, exceptionally high energy requirements, metabolic consequences of respiratory failure, recurrent respiratory exacerbations and the need for non-invasive ventilation in some can all make ETF challenging. Some centres may use appetite stimulants at this time.

In the early postoperative period, a clean diet is usually recommended with awareness of food safety issues. Restoring and maintaining optimal nutritional status is a priority. In the long term, other nutritional problems may emerge, e.g. diabetes due to corticosteroids and immunosuppressive therapy, dyslipidaemia and high plasma levels of the fat-soluble vitamins.

Cystic fibrosis–related low bone mineral density

Reduced bone mineral density is common in adolescents and adults with CF. Bone mineral content (BMC) and bone mineral density (BMD) are usually normal in well-nourished children with good lung function, although several cross-sectional studies report low BMC/BMD in some children with CF (Sermet-Gaudelus *et al.*, 2011). The aetiology of bone disease in CF is multifactorial. Risk factors include poor nutritional status; reduced lean body mass; vitamin D, vitamin K and calcium deficiencies; delayed puberty; corticosteroid use; physical inactivity; CFTR dysfunction; and infective pulmonary exacerbations (Sermet-Gaudelus *et al.*, 2011). Bone mineral acquisition in childhood, especially during the pubertal growth spurt in adolescence, is a major determinant of adult bone health. Prevention strategies should be implemented from diagnosis to address issues relating to bone health in people with CF. Dietetic management should focus on the following:

- Optimising weight gain and growth, with particular attention to lean body mass.
- Optimising vitamin D and vitamin K status through appropriate supplementation protocols.
- Optimising skeletal accretion of calcium by attention to calcium intakes and supplementation where necessary.
- Encouraging appropriate physical activity with the support of the CF-specialist physiotherapist.

CFTR modulators

Recent advances in therapies that target correction of the underlying defective CFTR protein may be nutritionally important. These treatments are called 'CFTR modulators' and are categorised into two groups, CFTR potentiators and CFTR correctors. These drugs are targeted towards specific gene mutations, e.g. Ivacaftor® for those with the G551D mutation, and Orkambi® for people who are homozygous for the p.Phe508del mutation. Significant improvements in CFTR activity; respiratory, nutritional and quality-of-life outcomes (Barry *et al.*, 2014); and improved insulin secretion ameliorating CFRD (Tsabari *et al.*, 2016) are documented in people receiving Ivacaftor®. The response has been less significant for those receiving Orkambi® (Wainwright *et al.*, 2015). CFTR modulators may change the nutritional needs of people with CF. Close monitoring and further research are required on their nutritional implications, especially the effects on nutritional requirements, body composition, pancreatic and gastrointestinal function, and CFRD.

Drug-nutrient interactions

The following should be noted:

- *Vitamin A* – hepatotoxic drugs, retinoids, tetracycline antibiotics, warfarin.
- *Vitamin E* – anticoagulant drugs, cyclosporine, warfarin.
- *Vitamin K* – warfarin.
- *Calcium* – bisphosphonates, quinolone antibiotics, tetracycline antibiotics.
- *Orkambi and ivacaftor* – grapefruit, grapefruit juice or Seville oranges.

Acknowledgement

Sue Wolfe, Consultant Dietitian, Leeds Teaching Hospitals NHS Trust.

Internet resources

CFTR2 mutation website, www.cftr2.org
Cystic Fibrosis Foundation, www.cff.org
Cystic Fibrosis Trust, www.cftrust.org.uk
Thoracic Society of Australia and New Zealand: Nutrition Guidelines for Cystic Fibrosis in Australia and New Zealand, 2017, www.thoracic.org.au/journal-publishing/area?command=record&id=46

References

Aird, FK, Greene SA, Ogston SA *et al.* (2006) Vitamin A and lung function in CF. *J. Cystic Fibrosis* 5(2):129–131.

American Diabetes Association. (2016) Standards of Medical Care in Diabetes 2016. *Diabetes Care.* 39(1): S13–S22.

Andersen DH. (1938) Cystic fibrosis of the pancreas and its relation to celiac disease: a clinical and pathological study. *Am. J. Dis. Child.* 56: 344–399.

Anthony H, Collins CE, Davidson G, *et al.* (1999) Pancreatic enzyme replacement therapy in cystic fibrosis: Australian guidelines. *Paediatric Gastroenterological Society and the Dietitians Association of Australia. J. Paediatr. Child Health.* 35: 125–129.

Barry PJ, Plant BJ, Nair A, *et al.* (2014) Effects of ivacaftor in patients with cystic fibrosis who carry the G551D mutation and have severe lung disease. *Chest.* 146: 152–158.

Beker LT, Russek-Cohen E, Fink RJ. (2001) Stature as a prognostic factor in cystic fibrosis survival. *J. Am. Diet. Assoc.* 101: 438–442.

Biesalski HK, Nohr D. (2003) Importance of vitamin-A for lung function and development. *Mol. Aspects Med.* 24: 431–440.

Borowitz D, Robinson KA, Rosenfeld M, *et al.* (2009) Cystic Fibrosis Foundation evidence-based guidelines for management of infants with cystic fibrosis. *J. Pediatr.* 155: S73–93.

Columbo C, Ellemunter H, Houwen R, *et al.* (2011) Guidelines for the diagnosis and management of distal intestinal obstruction syndrome in cystic fibrosis patients. *J. Cyst. Fibros.* 10: S24–S28.

Committee on Safety of Medicines (CSM). (1995) *Report of the Pancreatic Enzyme Working Party.* Medicines Control Agency UK.

Conway SP, Wolfe SP, Brownlee KG, *et al.* (2005) Vitamin K status among children with cystic fibrosis and its relationship to bone mineral density and bone turnover. *Pediatrics.* 115: 1325–1331.

Conway S, Balfour-Lynn IM, De Rijcke K, *et al.* (2014) European Cystic Fibrosis Society Standards of Care: Framework for the Cystic Fibrosis Centre. *J. Cyst. Fibros.* 13(1): S3–S22.

Corey M, McLaughlin FJ, Williams M, *et al.* (1988) A comparison of survival, growth and pulmonary function in patients with cystic fibrosis in Boston and Toronto. *J. Clin. Epidemiol.* 41: 583–591.

Cystic Fibrosis Trust. (2007) *Bone Mineralisation in Cystic Fibrosis. UK Cystic Fibrosis Trust Bone Mineralisation Working Group.* Bromley: Cystic Fibrosis Trust.

Cystic Fibrosis Trust. (2011) *UK CF Registry Annual Data Report 2009.* Bromley: Cystic Fibrosis Trust.

Cystic Fibrosis Trust. (2017) *UK Cystic Fibrosis Registry Annual Data Report 2016.* London: Cystic Fibrosis Trust.

Cystic Fibrosis Trust Nutrition Working Group. (2016) *Nutritional Management of Cystic Fibrosis.* London: Cystic Fibrosis Trust.

Debray D, Kelly D, Houwen, R, *et al.* (2011) Best practice guidance for the diagnosis and management of cystic fibrosis-associated liver disease. *J. Cyst. Fibros.* 10: S29–S36.

Dodge JA, Lewis PA, Stanton M, *et al.* (2007) Cystic fibrosis mortality and survival in the UK: 1947–2003. *Eur. Respir. J.* 29: 522–526.

Edenborough FP, Borgo G, Knoop C, *et al.* (2008) Guidelines for the management of pregnancy in women with cystic fibrosis. *J. Cyst. Fibros.* 7: S2–S32.

Elkin SL, Vedi S, Bord S, *et al.* (2002) Histomorphometric analysis of bone biopsies from the iliac crest of adults with cystic fibrosis. *Am. J. Respir. Crit. Care Med.* 166: 1470–1474.

Engelen MP, Com G, Deutz NEP. (2014) Protein is an important but undervalued macronutrient in the nutritional care of patients with cystic fibrosis. *Curr. Opin. Clin. Nutr. Metab. Care.* 17: 515–520.

Finklea JD, Grossmann RE, Tangpricha V. (2011) Vitamin D and chronic lung disease: a review of molecular mechanisms and clinical studies. *Adv. Nutr.* 2: 244–253.

Gilljam M, Antoniou M, Shin J, *et al.* (2000) Pregnancy in cystic fibrosis. Fetal and maternal outcome. *Chest.* 118: 85–91.

Green D, Carson K, Leonard A, *et al.* (2008) Current treatment recommendations for correcting vitamin D deficiency in pediatric patients with cystic fibrosis are inadequate. *J. Pediatr.* 153(4): 554–559.

Green DM, Leonard AR, Paranjape SM, *et al.* (2010) Transient effectiveness of vitamin D_2 therapy in pediatric cystic fibrosis patients. *J. Cyst. Fibros.* 9: 143–149.

Hakim F, Kerem E, Rivlin J, *et al.* (2007) Vitamin A and E and pulmonary exacerbations in patients with cystic fibrosis. *J. Pediatr. Gastroenterol. Nutr.* 45: 347–353.

Hamid B, Khan A. (2007) Cerebral hemorrhage as the initial manifestation of cystic fibrosis. *J. Child Neurol.* 22: 114–115.

Heine RG, Button BM, Olinsky A, *et al.* (1998) Gastro-oesophageal reflux in infants under 6 months with cystic fibrosis. *Arch. Dis. Child.* 78: 44–48.

Ho T, Gupta S, Brotherwood M, *et al.* (2011) Increased serum vitamin A and E levels after lung transplantation. *Transplantation.* 92: 601–606.

Huang SH, Schall JI, Zemel BS, *et al.* (2006) Vitamin E status in children with cystic fibrosis and pancreatic insufficiency. *J. Pediatr.* 148: 556–559.

Hubert G, Chung TT, Prosser C, *et al.* (2016) Bone mineral density and fat-soluble vitamin status in adults with cystic fibrosis undergoing lung transplantation: a pilot study. *Can. J. Diet. Pract. Res.* 77: 199–202.

Huet F, Semama D, Maingueneau C, *et al.* (1997) Vitamin A deficiency and nocturnal vision in teenagers with cystic fibrosis. *Eur. J. Pediatr.* 156: 949–951.

Kalnins D, Corey M, Ellis L, *et al.* (2005) Failure of conventional strategies to improve nutritional status in malnourished adolescents and adults with cystic fibrosis. *J. Pediatr.* 147: 399–401.

Kalnins D, Pencharz PB, Grasemann H, *et al.* (2013) Energy expenditure and nutritional status in pediatric patients before and after lung transplantation. *J. Pediatr.* 163: 1500–1502.

Konstantinopoulou S, Tapia IE. (2017) Vitamin D and the lung. *Paediatr. Respir. Rev.* 24: 39–43.

Koscik RL, Lai HC, Laxova A, *et al.* (2005) Preventing early, prolonged vitamin E deficiency: an opportunity for better cognitive outcomes via early diagnosis through neonatal screening. *J. Pediatr.* 147: S51–S56.

Lau EMT, Barnes DJ, Moriarty C, *et al.* (2011) Pregnancy outcomes in the current era of cystic fibrosis care: A 15-year experience. *Aust. N. Z. J. Obstet. Gynaecol.* 51: 220–224.

Lewis C, Blackman SM, Nelson A, *et al.* (2015) Diabetes-related mortality in adults with cystic fibrosis. *Role of genotype and sex. Am. J. Respir. Crit. Care Med.* 191: 194–200.

Littlewood JM, Wolfe SP, Conway SP. (2006) Diagnosis and treatment of intestinal malabsorption in cystic fibrosis. *Pediatr. Pulmonol.* 41: 35–49.

Maqbool A, Stallings VA. (2008) Update on fat-soluble vitamins in cystic fibrosis. *Curr. Opin. Pulm. Med.* 14: 574–581.

Maqbool A, Graham-Marr RC, Schall J, *et al.* (2008) Vitamin A intake and elevated serum retinol levels in children and young adults with cystic fibrosis. *J. Cyst. Fibros.* 7: 137–141.

McCauley LA, Thomas W, Laguna TA, *et al.* (2014) Vitamin D deficiency is associated with pulmonary exacerbations in children with cystic fibrosis. *Ann. Am. Thorac. Soc.* 11: 198–204.

McCullough FSW, Northrop-Clewes CA, Thurnham DI. (1999) The effect of vitamin A on epithelial integrity. *Proc. Nutr. Soc.* 58: 289–293.

McPhail GL. (2010) Coagulation disorder as a presentation of cystic fibrosis. *J. Emerg. Med.* 38: 20–322.

Moheet A, Moran A. (2018) Pharmacological management of cystic fibrosis related diabetes. *Expert Rev. Clin. Pharmacol.* 11: 185–191.

Moran A, Brunzell C, Cohen RC, *et al.*; CFRD Guidelines Committee. (2010) Clinical care guidelines for cystic fibrosis-related diabetes. A position statement of the American Diabetes Association and a clinical practice guideline of the Cystic Fibrosis Foundation, endorsed by the Pediatric Endocrine Association. *Diabetes Care* 22: 2697–2708.

Moran A, Pillay K, Becker DJ, *et al.* (2014) ISPAD Clinical Practice Consensus Guidelines 2014. Management of cystic fibrosis-related diabetes in children and adolescents. *Pediatr. Diabetes.* 15(2): 65–76.

Morton A, Wolfe S. (2015) Enteral tube feeding for cystic fibrosis. *Cochrane Database Syst. Rev.* (4): CD001198.

Munck A, Alberti C, Colombo C, *et al.* (2016) International prospective study of distal intestinal obstruction syndrome in cystic fibrosis: associated factors and outcome. *J. Cyst. Fibros.* 15: 531–539.

Neville LA, Ranganathan SC. (2009) Vitamin D in infants with cystic fibrosis diagnosed by newborn screening. *J. Pediatr. Child Health.* 45: 36–41.

Oliver MR, Heine RG, Ng CH, *et al.* (2004) Factors affecting clinical outcome in gastrostomy-fed children with cystic fibrosis. *Pediatr. Pulmonol.* 37: 324–329.

Panagopoulou P, Fotoulaki M, Nikolaou A, *et al.* (2014) Prevalence of malnutrition and obesity among cystic fibrosis patients. *Pediatr. Int.* 56: 89–94.

Pedreira CC, Robert RG, Dalton V, *et al.* (2005) Association of body composition and lung function in children with cystic fibrosis. *Pediatr. Pulmonol.* 39: 276–280.

Petersen RA, Petersen VS, Robb RM. (1968) Vitamin A deficiency with xerophthalmia and night blindness in cystic fibrosis. *Am. J. Dis. Child.* 116: 662–665.

Pincikova T, Paquin-Proulx D, Sandberg JK, *et al.* (2017) Clinical impact of vitamin D treatment in cystic fibrosis: a pilot randomized, controlled trial. *Eur. J. Clin. Nutr.* 71(2): 203–205.

Poustie VJ, Russell JE, Watling RM, *et al.*: CALICO Trial Collaborative Group. (2006) Oral protein energy supplements for children with cystic fibrosis; CALICO multicentre randomised controlled trial. *BMJ.* 332: 632–636.

Rashid M, Durie P, Andrew M, *et al.* (1999) Prevalence of vitamin K deficiency in cystic fibrosis. *Am. J. Clin. Nutr.* 70: 378–382.

Renton M, Priestley L, Bennett L, *et al.* (2015) Pregnancy outcomes in cystic fibrosis: a 10-year experience from a UK centre. *Obstet. Med.* 8: 99–101.

Rivas-Crespo MF, González Jiménez D, Acuña Quirós MD, *et al.* (2013) High serum retinol and lung function in young patients with cystic fibrosis. *J. Pediatr. Gastroenterol. Nutr.* 56: 657–662.

SACN. (2011) *SACN Dietary Reference Values for Energy.* London: TSO.

Saxby N, Painter C, Kench A, *et al.* and the Australian and New Zealand Cystic Fibrosis Nutrition Guideline Authorship Group. (2017) *Nutrition Guidelines for Cystic Fibrosis in Australia and New Zealand* (Scott C. Bell, ed). Sydney: Thoracic Society of Australia and New Zealand.

Schulze KJ, O'Brien KO, Germain-Lee EL, *et al.* (2003) Endogenous fecal losses of calcium compromise calcium balance in pancreatic-insufficient girls with cystic fibrosis. *J. Pediatr.* 143: 765–771.

Schwarzenberg SJ, Hempstead SE, McDonald CM, *et al.* (2016) Enteral tube feeding for individuals with cystic fibrosis: Cystic Fibrosis Foundation evidence-informed guidelines. *J. Cyst. Fibros.* 15: 724–735.

Scott J, Elias E, Moult PJ, *et al.* (1977) Rickets in adult cystic fibrosis with myopathy, pancreatic insufficiency and proximal tubular dysfunction. *Am. J. Med.* 63: 488–492.

Sermet-Gaudelus I, Mayell SJ, Southern KW. (2010) Guidelines on the early management of infants diagnosed with cystic fibrosis following newborn screening. *J. Cyst. Fibros.* 9: 323–329.

Sermet-Gaudelus I, Bianchi ML, Garabedian M, *et al.* (2011) European cystic fibrosis bone mineralisation guidelines. *J. Cyst. Fibros.* 10: S16–S23.

Sitrin MD, Lieberman F, Jensen WE, *et al.* (1987) Vitamin E deficiency and neurologic disease in adults with cystic fibrosis. *Ann. Intern. Med.* 107: 51–54.

Skypala IJ, Ashworth FA, Hodson ME, *et al.* (1998) Oral nutritional supplements promote weight gain in cystic fibrosis patients. *J. Hum. Nutr. Diet.* 11: 95–104.

Smyth AR, Bell SC, Bojcin S, *et al.* (2014) European Cystic Fibrosis Society Standards of Care: best practice guidelines. *J. Cyst. Fibros.* 13(1): S23–42.

Smyth RL, van Velzen D, Smyth AR, *et al.* (1994) Strictures of ascending colon in cystic fibrosis and high-strength pancreatic enzymes. *Lancet.* 343: 85–86.

Smyth RL, Rayner O. (2017) Oral calorie supplements for cystic fibrosis. *Cochrane Database Syst. Rev.* (11): CD000406.

Sokol RJ, Reardon MC, Accurso FJ, *et al.* (1989) Fat-soluble vitamin status during the first year of life in infants with cystic fibrosis identified by screening of newborns. *Am. J. Clin. Nutr.* 50: 1064–1071.

Somaraju UR, Solis-Moya A. (2016) Pancreatic enzyme replacement therapy for people with cystic fibrosis. *Cochrane Database Syst. Rev.* (10): CD008227.

Stallings VA, Stark LJ, Robinson KA, *et al.* with Clinical Practice Guidelines on Growth and Nutrition Subcommittee; Ad Hoc Working Group. (2008) Evidence-based practice recommendations for nutrition-related management of children and adults with cystic fibrosis and pancreatic insufficiency: Results of a systematic review. *J. Am. Diet. Assoc.* 108: 832–839.

Stephenson CB, Gildengorin G. (2000) Serum retinol, the acute phase response, and the apparent misclassification of vitamin A status in the third National Health and Nutrition Examination Survey. *Am. J. Clin. Nutr.* 72: 1170–1178.

Stephenson A, Brotherwood M, Robert R, *et al.* (2007) Cholecalciferol significantly increases 25-hydroxyvitamin D concentrations in adults with cystic fibrosis. *Am. J. Clin. Nutr.* 85: 1307–1311.

Tangpricha V, Kelly A, Stephenson A, *et al.* (2012) An update on the screening, diagnosis, management, and treatment of vitamin D deficiency in individuals with cystic fibrosis: evidence-based recommendations from the Cystic Fibrosis Foundation. *J. Clin. Endocrinol. Metab.* 97: 1082–1093.

Tsabari R, Elyashar HI, Cymberknowh MC, *et al.* (2016) CFTR potentiator therapy ameliorates impaired insulin secretion in CF patients with a gating mutation. *J. Cyst. Fibros.* 15: e25–27.

Truby H, Cowlishaw P, O'Neil C, *et al.* (2009) The long term efficacy of gastrostomy feeding in children with cystic fibrosis on anthropometric markers of nutritional status and pulmonary function. *Open Respir. Med.* 3: 112–115.

Turck D, Braegger CP, Colombo C, *et al.* (2016) ESPEN–ESPGHAN–ECFS guidelines on nutrition care for infants, children, and adults with cystic fibrosis. *Clin. Nutr.* 35: 557–577.

van der Doef HPJ, Kokke FTM, van der Ent CK, *et al.* (2011) Intestinal obstruction syndromes in cystic fibrosis: meconium ileus, distal intestinal obstruction syndrome and constipation. *Curr. Gastroenterol. Rep.* 13: 265–270.

Vandenbranden SL, McMullen A, Schechter MS, *et al.* (2012) Lung function decline from adolescence to young adulthood in cystic fibrosis. *Pediatr. Pulmonol.* 47: 135–143.

von Drygalski A, Biller J. (2008) Anemia in cystic fibrosis: incidence, mechanisms, and association with pulmonary function and vitamin deficiency. *Nutr. Clin. Pract.* 23: 557–563.

Wainwright CE, Elborn JS, Ramsey BW. (2015) Lumacaftor–ivacaftor in patients with cystic fibrosis homozygous for Phe508del CFTR. *N. Engl. J. Med.* 373: 1783–1784.

White H, Morton AM, Peckham DG, *et al.* (2004) Dietary intakes in adult patients with cystic fibrosis – do they achieve guidelines? *J. Cyst. Fibros.* 3: 1–7.

Wilfond BS, Farrell PM, Laxova A, *et al.* (1994) Severe haemolytic anemia associated with vitamin E deficiency in infants with cystic fibrosis: implications for neonatal screening. *Clin. Pediatr.* 33: 2–7.

Woestenenk JW, Broos N, Stellato RK, *et al.* (2015a) Vitamin E intake, α-tocopherol levels and pulmonary function in children and adolescents with cystic fibrosis. *Br. J. Nutr.* 113: 1096–1101.

Woestenenk JW, Broos N, Stellato RK, *et al.* (2015b) Serum retinol levels and pulmonary function in children and adolescents with cystic fibrosis. *J. Cyst. Fibros.* 14: 392–397.

Yi Y, Norris AW, Wang K, *et al.* (2016) Abnormal glucose tolerance in infants and young children with cystic fibrosis. *Am. J. Respir. Crit. Care Med.* 194: 974–980.

7.5 Renal disorders

7.5.1 Chronic kidney disease and acute kidney injury

Sue Perry, Harriet Williams and Bruno Mafrici

Key points

- Nutrition has a central role in the management of both chronic kidney disease and acute kidney injury.
- This includes reduction of cardiovascular disease risk, monitoring of nutritional status and limiting the effects of reduced kidney function.
- Several dietary elements usually require consideration and may change over time.

Nutritional treatment has a central role in the management of both chronic kidney disease (CKD) and acute kidney injury (AKI). Dietetic interventions to reduce cardiovascular disease (CVD) risk are important in early CKD. Regular monitoring of nutritional status and limiting the effects of reduced kidney function are important considerations in AKI, progressive CKD and kidney failure. As several dietary elements usually require consideration, an appreciation of both medical and dietetic aspects of care is required in order to produce appropriate and individualised dietetic treatment plans.

Each kidney contains up to 1 million nephrons, with each nephron being a filtering unit of tiny blood vessels (glomeruli) attached to a tubule. The glomeruli normally filter approximately 100 mL of plasma/min. The rate at which this takes place is known as the glomerular filtration rate (GFR). The kidney has a number of important functions, including the excretion of waste products; electrolyte homeostasis (including sodium, potassium, calcium and phosphate); regulation of fluid, acid–base balance and metabolic processes; hormone production, including erythropoietin and renin; and activation of vitamin D.

The GFR is the best index of overall kidney function. In clinical practice, serum creatinine levels are used to monitor kidney function as levels rise with decreasing GFR. However, the kidneys have a large functional reserve, and serum creatinine levels only rise when at least 50% of kidney function is lost (GFR <60 mL/min). Creatinine is also subject to non-renal influences, which make it insufficiently sensitive to detect moderate CKD on its own. Therefore, an estimate of GFR (eGFR) is made using an equation that corrects for some of the more significant influences, such as age, gender and ethnicity. Serum creatinine also correlates with muscle mass. In those with increased muscle mass, GFR is underestimated; in those with reduced muscle mass, GFR is overestimated.

Definitions of kidney disease

Chronic kidney disease (CKD) is defined as a long-term condition that describes abnormal kidney function and/or structure (proteinuria, haematuria or anatomical abnormality), or a GFR of <60 mL/min/1.73 m^2 present on at least two occasions that are 90 days apart.

AKI is characterised by a rapid reduction in kidney function resulting in a failure to maintain fluid, electrolyte and acid–base homeostasis, and is potentially reversible (Kidney Disease; Improving Global Outcomes (KDIGO), 2012b). The term acute kidney injury, encompasses a spectrum of injury from moderate to severe deterioration of kidney function. Many people make a complete recovery from AKI, but some are left with CKD or may require renal replacement therapy (RRT).

Chronic kidney disease

Diagnostic criteria and classification

In order to quantify the degree of dysfunction, CKD is classified using a combination of categories for both

Manual of Dietetic Practice, Sixth Edition. Edited by Joan Gandy.

Companion website: www.manualofdieteticpractice.com

eGFR and albumin–creatinine ratio (ACR). Increased ACR or decreased eGFR increase the risk of adverse patient outcomes. A combination of both increased ACR and decreased eGFR multiply this risk. It was originally classified into five stages, based mainly on eGFR. These stages (stage 1, 2, 3a, 3b, 4 and 5) are still used in clinical practice and reflect the new stages (G1, GE, G3a, G3b, G4 and G5, respectively) (see Figure 7.5.1). When eGFR declines to and is sustained at stage 5 CKD, the term 'established stage 5 CKD' may be used; at this point, the disease may be deemed irreversible, and RRT will be considered.

There has been debate about the implications of having a reduced GFR, but evidence suggests that, if eGFR is <60 mL/min, there is an increased risk of mortality. As normal GFR is approximately 100 mL/min, reduced kidney function can be explained to patients as a percentage of normal function.

Aetiology

There is extensive clinical evidence that diabetes, hypertension and the presence of proteinuria are risk factors

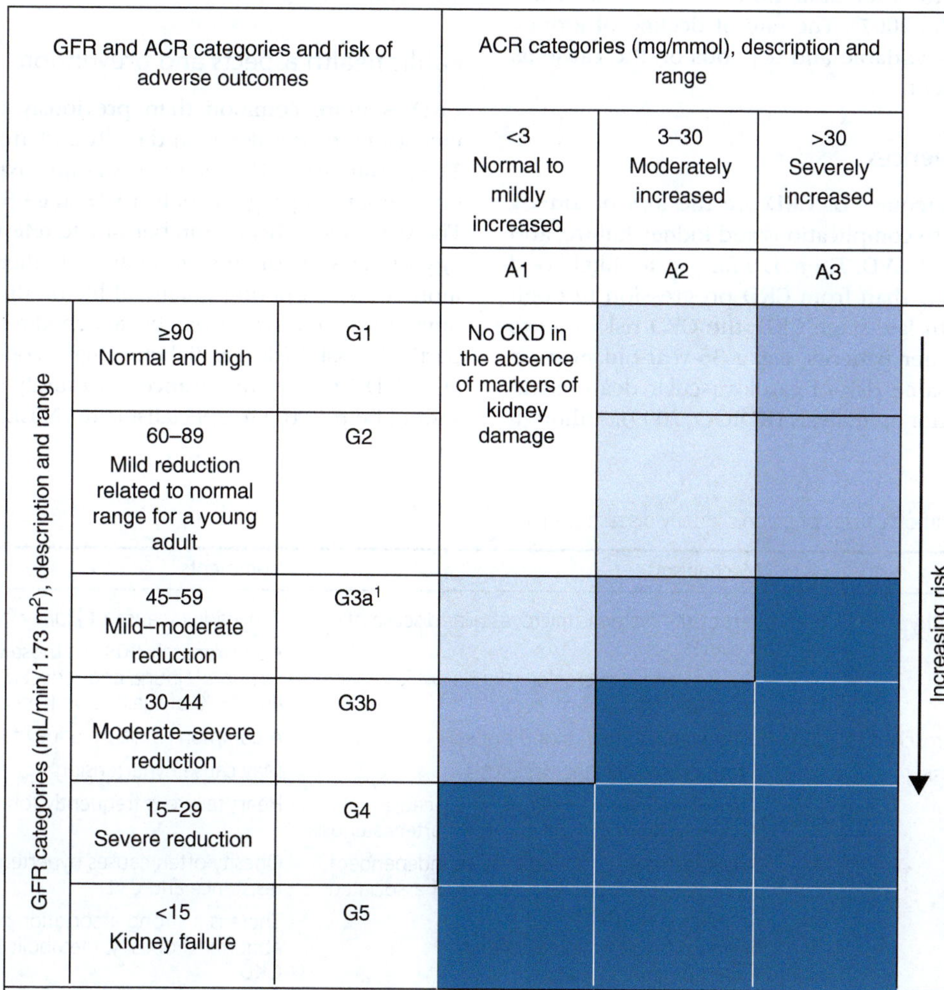

[1] Consider using eGFRcystatinC for people with CKD G3aA1 (See recommendations 1.1.14 and 1.1.15)

Abbreviations: ACR, albumin:creatinine ratio; CKD, chronic kidney disease; GFR, glomerular filtration rate

Adapted with permission from Kidney Disease; Improving Global Outcomes (KDIGO) CKD Work Group (2013) KDIGO 2012 clinical practice guideline for the evaluation and management of chronic kidney disease; Kidney International (Suppl. 3); 1–150

Figure 7.5.1 Classification of CKD stage (© NICE, 2014; Classification of CKD Stage. Available from https://www.nice.org.uk/guidance/cg182/chapter/1-recommendations#classification-of-chronic-kidney-disease-2; all rights reserved)

for the progression of CKD (NICE, 2014a). The most common causes of CKD are shown in Table 7.5.1. Despite the wide range of causes of kidney injury, once there is a significant loss of nephrons, the result is a common pathway characterised by hypertension, proteinuria and progressive decline in GFR (Metcalfe, 2007). The remaining nephrons develop glomerular hypertension, and the GFR increases for each nephron (hyperfiltration). This causes increased glomerular permeability and excessive protein filtration. In addition, hypertension and hyperlipidaemia stimulate the abnormal production of growth factors and cytokines that, together with glomerular hypertension, eventually lead to interstitial fibrosis and glomerulosclerosis (Metcalfe, 2007). The rate of decline of kidney function is highly variable and depends on the cause as well as its treatment.

Disease consequences

The two main outcomes of CKD are the loss of kidney function, leading to complications and kidney failure, and the development of CVD. There is a far greater likelihood of death from CVD than from CKD progression through to stage 5 CKD. In late-stage CKD, the CVD risk is more apparent in younger patients, e.g. a 35-year-old man on dialysis has the same risk of cardiovascular death as an 80-year-old man not on dialysis (KDIGO, 2009). Although CKD becomes more prevalent with increasing age, people aged >70 years who have a stable eGFR between 45 and 59 mL/min and no other evidence of kidney damage are unlikely to experience complications related to CKD. The greatest risks are to those who have progressive CKD.

For those who do reach stage 5 CKD and start RRT, mortality rates are very high. Five-year mortality rates in incident RRT patients are 50–73% for patients >65 years of age (Zoccali *et al.*, 2010). The main cause of death is CVD, although, in addition to hypertension and hypercholesterolaemia, the presence of CKD mineral and bone disorder (CKD–MBD), and anaemia, may complicate and accelerate vascular disease.

Public health aspects and prevention

CKD is more common than previously thought and is increasing in prevalence in the UK and around the world. The prevalence of CKD in the UK is approximately 13% but only about 2% progress onto CKD stage 5 (NICE, 2014a). There are a significant number of late referrals to nephrology services of patients who have a higher morbidity and mortality and a poorer quality of life on dialysis. NICE recommends that those at risk be screened for CKD. Those at particular risk includes diabetes, high blood pressure, AKI and CVD. Those with advanced or rapidly worsening CKD should be referred to specialist care (NICE, 2014a).

Table 7.5.1 Common causes of chronic kidney disease (CKD)

Cause	Mechanism	Comments
Diabetic nephropathy	Part of the systemic microvascular disease of diabetes The first sign is microalbuminuria, which presents when GFR is normal	The leading cause of kidney failure in the UK Approximately 50% of those with diabetes have proteinuria and reduced kidney function, and 75% of these have hypertension
Hypertensive atherosclerosis	Long-standing high blood pressure	A common cause of kidney failure
Renal artery stenosis	Often caused by atherosclerosis	May cause hypertension
Heart failure	Age, diabetes and smoking can all cause ischaemic heart disease and renal artery stenosis	Heart failure is frequently found with CKD
Obesity	A risk factor for CKD, both as an independent factor and through the presence of associated diabetes and hypertension More likely to develop glomerular hyperfiltration and albuminuria	Obesity often causes hypertension, insulin resistance and CVD There is a strong association between abdominal obesity, metabolic syndrome and CKD
Polycystic kidney disease	Multiple cysts that gradually enlarge	Inherited, often causes kidney failure in middle age
Reflux nephropathy	Reflux of urine from the bladder back up the ureters	Often inherited
Glomerular disease	Many different types of glomerulonephritis May occur in children	Usually diagnosed by renal biopsy Usually proteinuria and/or haematuria.
Nephrotic syndrome (a term used to describe the consequences of excessive urinary protein losses)	Caused by a wide range of glomerular diseases	Combination of heavy proteinuria (>3 g/24 h), hypoalbuminuria and oedema Often severe hyperlipidaemia
Microscopic vasculitis	Inflammation of the small blood vessels	For example, Wegener's granulomatosis
Myeloma	Bence Jones proteins precipitate in kidney tubules	Can cause AKI or CKD

CVD, cardiovascular disease; GFR, glomerular filtration rate.

SECTION 7

Nutritional consequences and complications

Most of the complications seen in CKD have nutritional causes or consequences. They are most often seen in stages 4 and 5, although some may start to develop during stage 3 (Table 7.5.2).

Protein energy wasting

Malnutrition is a concern in this patient group, although its onset and severity are related to GFR. By CKD stage 4, it affects between 28% (Lawson *et al.*, 2001) and 48% (Heimburger *et al.*, 2000) of individuals, which has an adverse impact on mortality rates. Individuals who are malnourished on starting dialysis are four times more likely to die within 2 years than those who are well nourished (Chung *et al.*, 2000). Malnutrition is often caused by a reduction in protein and energy intake; however, in the presence of kidney disease, other factors also play a role. These include inflammation, acidosis, inter-current infections, metabolic changes, hyperparathyroidism and nutrient losses during dialysis. This condition has been termed protein energy wasting (PEW) (Fouque *et al.*, 2008). From stage 4 CKD, serum cholesterol and serum albumin levels begin to decline. Low serum albumin is a strong predictor of adverse outcomes. However, the association between albumin and poor survival mainly reflects its associations with inflammation, comorbidity and fluid overload, as well as poor nutrition (Jones, 2001; Kaysen *et al.*, 2002).

Low protein and energy intakes become more common as GFR falls, particularly when eGFR falls <25 mL/min (Ikizler *et al.*, 1995). Uraemia is common at this stage, causing nausea, lethargy and taste changes, which adversely affect appetite. Metabolic acidosis (low plasma bicarbonate) is also common, and is associated with increased protein catabolism and reduced synthesis of serum albumin (de Brito-Ashurst *et al.*, 2009).

Initially, dialysis leads to an improvement in both appetite and nutritional status. However, a gradual but significant decline is often seen in all nutritional markers with increasing years on dialysis (Chumlea *et al.*, 2003). Both a low percentage of body fat at the start of dialysis and fat loss over time have been found to be independently associated with higher mortality. In particular, a BMI of >23 kg/m^2 is associated with reduced mortality in dialysis patients, and a BMI of <20 kg/m^2 is associated with the highest mortality rates (Leavey *et al.*, 2001).

Dyslipidaemia

Plasma triglycerides start to increase early in CKD and show the highest concentrations in nephrotic syndrome and in those receiving dialysis (NICE, 2014b). However, there is often a reduction of total, high-density (HDL) and low-density lipoprotein (LDL) cholesterol concentrations when GFR is <60 mL/min. Chronic inflammation is a common feature in dialysis patients and may cause PEW and progressive atherosclerotic CVD (Stenvinkel & Alvestrand, 2002).

Mineral and bone disorder

The kidneys play an essential role in the regulation of serum phosphate. When kidney function is normal, serum phosphate is maintained within a tight range despite wide fluctuations in dietary phosphorus intake through variations in urinary phosphorus excretion. In response to a high dietary phosphorus intake, fibroblast growth factor 23 (FGF23) is secreted by osteocytes and osteoblasts. FGF23 is a hormonal factor that promotes urinary phosphorus excretion and decreases the production of active vitamin D by the kidneys (leading to reduced phosphorus absorption from the GI tract). FGF23 concentrations increase progressively beginning in early CKD, presumably as a physiological adaptation to maintain normal serum phosphate levels (Wahl & Wolf, 2012). From CKD

Table 7.5.2 Complications seen in CKD stages 3–5

CVD	Main cause of death in patients with CKD
Hypertension	Both a cause and a complication of CKD Elevated blood pressure is associated with a faster rate of decline in GFR
Dyslipidaemia	Very prevalent in CKD and is influenced by renal function and degree of proteinuria
Increased risk of diabetic complications	Poor glycaemic control is associated with faster rate of decline in GFR Increased risk of CVD and retinopathy in patients with both diabetes and CKD
CKD mineral and bone disorder	Caused by alterations in the control mechanisms for calcium and phosphorus homeostasis
Protein energy wasting	Serum albumin, dietary protein and energy intake may fall as GFR falls
Metabolic acidosis	Kidneys become unable to remove sufficient H^+ ions, and serum bicarbonate levels fall
Hyperkalaemia	Can be life threatening, especially if K^+ is >6.5 mmol/L
Fluid (and sodium) retention	Can be a problem, e.g. in nephrotic syndrome
Anaemia	Kidneys become unable to produce sufficient erythropoietin as GFR falls
Gout	Blood urate level rises as GFR falls, leading to increased risk of gout
Depression	As with any chronic disease, CKD may be associated with depression, especially if there are physical symptoms

GFR, glomerular filtration rate; CVD, cardiovascular disease.

stage 4, hyperphosphataemia becomes more common, as the kidneys are unable to excrete all the excess dietary phosphorus. High serum phosphate levels can increase parathyroid hormone (PTH) secretion, leading to the development of secondary hyperparathyroidism. Vitamin D insufficiency is common in CKD and may also be a cause of early increases in serum PTH levels. Observational studies show an association between low vitamin D levels and adverse clinical outcomes.

Without therapeutic intervention, CKD mineral and bone disorder (CKD–MBD) will develop (Figure 7.5.2). This term defines the complex syndrome that includes both renal bone disease (renal osteodystrophy) and vascular and soft tissue calcification (KDIGO, 2017). As a result, it is associated with an increased prevalence of CVD and ultimately increased mortality. Hyperphosphataemia is one of the commonest biochemical abnormalities in CKD and poses significant challenges for management.

Hyperkalaemia

Hyperkalaemia has potentially adverse cardiac effects, causing arrhythmias and cardiac arrest. It can be life threatening, especially if potassium levels are >6.5 mmol/L. Patients may present with associated muscle weakness and feel generally unwell, or they may be completely asymptomatic. Hyperkalaemia is rarely caused by renal dysfunction alone until GFR has fallen to <30 mL/min (Bakris *et al.*, 2000). Some patients may develop hyperkalaemia as early as CKD stage 3, usually as a result of the side effects of taking medications such as angiotensin-converting enzyme (ACE) inhibitors or angiotensin receptor blockers (ARBs). If serum potassium levels are ≥6.0 mmol/L, and other drugs that promote hyperkalaemia have been discontinued, ACE inhibitors or ARBs should be stopped (NICE, 2014b). At this point, other causes of raised potassium levels, including diet, should be investigated. These include:

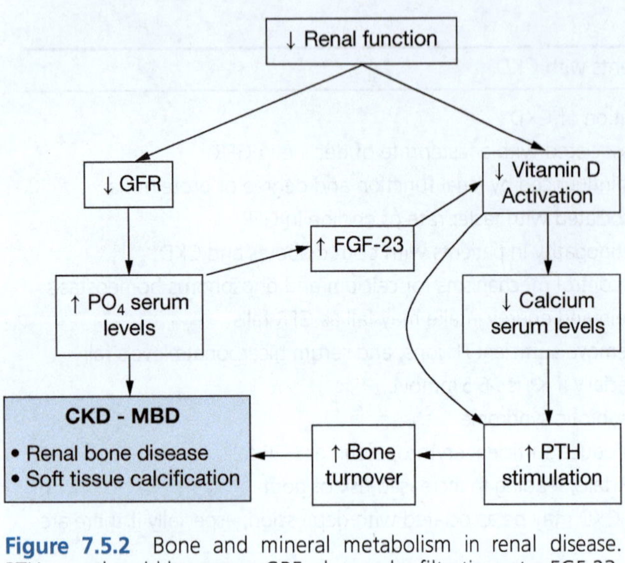

Figure 7.5.2 Bone and mineral metabolism in renal disease. PTH, parathyroid hormone; GRF, glomerular filtration rate; FGF-23, fibroblast growth factor-23; CKD–MBD, chronic kidney disease–mineral and bone disorder

- Potassium-sparing diuretics, e.g. spironolactone.
- Metabolic acidosis.
- Uncontrolled diabetes or insulin deficiency.
- Catabolism as a result of trauma or weight loss.
- Constipation.
- Dehydration.
- Sudden decline in residual renal function.
- Blood transfusion.
- Haemolysed blood sample.

Fluid and sodium retention

As kidney function deteriorates, the ability to excrete excess sodium is reduced, and sodium retention can occur. Serum sodium level is a poor indicator of sodium status, but a better indicator of hydration. Hence, hypernatraemia and hyponatraemia usually indicate dehydration and overhydration, respectively. Excess dietary sodium leads to increased thirst, which can compound problems of fluid balance. Fluid retention is unlikely in early CKD, except in nephrotic syndrome, when it is common. When urine output is reduced and fluid intake exceeds output, fluid accumulates in the body, causing hypertension and oedema. Severe fluid overload, or even mild overload in individuals with heart failure, can result in pulmonary oedema and shortness of breath. Although ankle swelling can indicate fluid overload, patients may have several excess litres of fluid without oedema. Acute changes in body weight usually represent changes in fluid balance in these patients. Clinical examination or bioelectrical impedance may be useful in determining fluid status.

Nutritional assessment

Nutritional monitoring should take place regularly in all patients from stage 4 CKD onwards, as PEW becomes more prevalent. Several criteria should be considered to diagnose PEW; these include biochemistry, body weight, weight loss, reduced total body fat, loss of muscle mass and low protein or energy intakes. Additional measures of nutrition and inflammation, e.g. C-reactive protein (CRP), are also helpful (Fouque *et al.*, 2008).

Anthropometry

As a minimum, (oedema-free) body weight, percentage weight change and BMI should be measured. Careful interpretation of weight change is important; a history of oedema or rapid weight loss or gain may be due to changes in fluid status. Attention should be paid to dry weight for those with oedema or on dialysis. For longitudinal measures, the use of skinfold callipers to assess mid-upper-arm circumference (MUAC) and triceps skinfold thickness (TST) are useful. In haemodialysis (HD) patients, high MUAC is a predictor of greater survival, particularly in those with low BMIs (Noori *et al.*, 2010).

Biochemistry

Serum cholesterol, urea, creatinine, eGFR, potassium, phosphate, serum albumin, CRP, PTH, urinary protein loss and fluid status should be measured (Renal Association, 2010).

Clinical history

This should include appetite, comorbidities and the presence of oedema.

Dietary assessment

A 24-h recall or 3-day food diary should be used to assess dietary protein and energy intake.

Functional assessment

This assesses the ability to conduct the activities of daily living. Measurement of handgrip strength has been found to correlate well with lean body mass (Heimburger *et al.*, 2000), and is likely to be a very practical measure in clinical practice. Handgrip strength shows better inter-user repeatability, requiring less skill or training than the measurement of MUAC and TST. The Dukes Activity Status or GP Physical Activity Questionnaires may be useful in monitoring trends in activity levels.

Subjective global assessment

This has been validated for use in stage 5 CKD and is linked with adverse outcomes and mortality (Enia *et al.*, 1993). In dialysis patients, the seven-point subjective global assessment may distinguish degrees of PEW associated with increasing risks of mortality (de Mutsert *et al.*, 2009). In addition, social and economic factors should be taken into account, e.g. patients living alone can be at greater nutritional risk. Ideal body weight (IBW) should be calculated from height and ideal BMI:

- 20 kg/m^2 for those with an actual BMI of <20 kg/m^2.
- 25 kg/m^2 for those with a BMI >25 kg/m^2.
- Use actual BMI if BMI 20–25 kg/m^2 (Renal Association, 2010b).

Management of CKD stages 1–3

Clinical management

The medical management of CKD consists of interventions to slow the rate of decline in renal function and limit any associated complications, e.g. CVD. In addition, specific treatments such as immunosuppressive therapy for autoimmune disorders may also be required. The medical management of all patients with CKD stages 1–3 should include reduction of all modifiable cardiovascular risk factors, including the following:

- Strict control of hypertension (blood pressure 140/90 mmHg; 130/80 mmHg in diabetes mellitus).
- Tight blood glucose control in diabetes (HbA1c 48–58 mmol/mol).
- Healthy weight (BMI 20–25 kg/m^2).
- Lipid lowering (total cholesterol <4 mmol/L; LDL <2 mmol/L).
- Smoking cessation if appropriate.
- Regular exercise.
- Limiting alcohol intake (<14 units a week).

Of these, the interventions that have been found to be particularly effective at reducing the progression of CKD are strict blood pressure control (KDIGO 2016), use of ACE inhibitors or ARBs, strict glucose control in diabetes and the use of statins (National Kidney Foundation, 2002). Uncomplicated CKD stages 1–3 can usually be managed in primary care. Serum creatinine and eGFR should be regularly monitored, as should proteinuria and albuminuria. Most people in this category will not develop stage 5 CKD, and the information provided should concentrate on cardiovascular risk reduction. However, those with rapidly declining eGFR (>5 mL/min/year) or significant proteinuria are likely to require nephrology referral.

Hypertension

There is strong evidence that lowering blood pressure reduces cardiovascular risk and the progression of CKD (NICE, 2014b). Interventions that inhibit the renin angiotensin aldosterone system activity, such as ACE inhibitors or ARBs, provide cardiovascular and renal protection (together with a reduction in proteinuria) (National Kidney Foundation, 2002). However, they can cause hyperkalaemia.

Hyperlipidaemia

Statins are safe and effective at reducing cardiovascular mortality. Statins, and particularly atorvastatin, should be considered for primary or secondary prevention of CVD in CKD stages 1–4, and in transplant patients with a >20% risk of CVD over 10 years (NICE, 2014b).

Alcohol, smoking and exercise

People should be encouraged to exercise, achieve a healthy weight and stop smoking to reduce CVD risk. Alcohol consumption should be reduced if patients drink excessively; this can reduce blood pressure and has broader health benefits (NICE, 2014b).

Dietetic management

Most of the evidence for dietetic treatment in early CKD comes from research that focused on dietetic interventions to reduce CVD. Good glycaemic control in those with diabetes, weight reduction in those with obesity and nutritional support in those with PEW improve patient outcomes. The main aims of dietetic treatment in these patients are to reduce the progression of CKD and CVD.

Protein

Protein restriction has been found to help alleviate uraemic symptoms and was thought to possibly delay the progression of renal disease (Bennett *et al.*, 1983), although evidence for this is inconclusive (Levey *et al.*, 1996; NICE, 2014a). The risk of developing PEW in patients following low-protein diets (LPDs) led to concern (Kopple *et al.*, 1997). There is insufficient evidence to recommend an optimal protein level, but it is generally considered that dietary protein intake should not be <0.8 g/kg/day (SIGN, 2008).

Energy

Energy requirements are not increased as many patients with early CKD have diabetes or hypertension, and obesity is common; weight management is an important part of the dietetic treatment. Those with, or at a high risk of, CVD should modify their fat intake and include oily fish once a week in their diet.

Obesity

Obesity is associated with CKD progression and stage 5 CKD (Hsu *et al.*, 2006; Kramer *et al.*, 2006). While the exact mechanisms remain unknown, factors including insulin resistance, dyslipidaemia and inflammation contribute to obesity-related kidney damage (MacLaughlin, 2016). Weight loss has been shown to reduce proteinuria, blood pressure and rate of renal decline (Navaneethan *et al.*, 2009). Weight reduction also has beneficial effects on associated risk factors, including insulin resistance, diabetes, dyslipidaemia and left ventricular hypertrophy (Abrass, 2004). Patients who may benefit the most from weight loss are those with BMI of ≥30 kg/m², type 2 diabetes or an increased waist circumference (Renal Association, 2010; Teta, 2010).

Modifications in lifestyle, physical activity and individualised dietary advice tailored to food preferences are the initial measures. For sustainable weight loss, a gradual decrease in energy intake by 500–600 kcal/day is recommended. This should be accompanied by close dietetic supervision to avoid exacerbation of uraemic symptoms (Teta, 2010). High-protein diets for weight loss may be unsafe for patients with CKD. Protein intake of >20% of total energy is not recommended, due to the potential detrimental effects on kidney function (Friedman, 2004). Pharmacological measures are generally unsafe, except for orlistat, which has been used with some success. Bariatric surgery may be considered in severe obesity (see Chapter 7.13.3, Bariatric surgery).

Diabetes

Strict glycaemic control has been found to delay the onset and slow the progression of microvascular complications in type 1 diabetes (Diabetes Control and Complications Trial Research Group, 1993). In type 2 diabetes, improved glycaemic control appears to provide a similar benefit.

Salt

Reducing dietary salt considerably reduces blood pressure in CKD and reduces proteinuria. Salt reduction represents a cost-effective and low-risk strategy to reduce blood pressure for people with CKD (McMahon *et al.*, 2015). Current evidence-based clinical guidelines recommend an intake target of <6 g/day salt (100 mmol; 2300 mg sodium) for people with CKD, although achieving long-term adherence to this target can be problematic. (KDIGO, 2012a; McMahon *et al.*, 2015)

The dietary approach to stop hypertension sodium (DASH) trials showed that increasing fruit and vegetable, wholegrain and fish intake, while reducing the intake of salt, fat, saturated fats, sugar and red meat, led to lower blood pressures as compared to a control group. However, this trial did not include adults with CKD. Subsequently, two small studies have found that the DASH diet appears to be safe in CKD stage 3 (Tyson *et al.*, 2016; Wells *et al.*, 2015). However, due to the potential for increased potassium and phosphate levels, this dietary approach may not be suitable for all patients with CKD stage 4; however, the principle of salt reduction is still recommended (see Chapter 7.14.4, Hypertension).

Around 75% of salt consumed is added during food manufacturing (PHE, 2014), and patients may need help in interpreting the varying information on food labels. A small amount of salt may be used in cooking, but extra salt should not be added at the table. Herbs and spices should be encouraged, but salt substitutes should be avoided due to their potassium content (SIGN, 2008). Infrequently, some patients with later stages of CKD lose excessive amounts of sodium, for instance, via the urine or ileostomies. Dietary sodium intake in these individuals should not be restricted as they may become salt and fluid depleted.

Fluid

Most patients do not need to change from the usual recommendation, and an adequate fluid intake should be encouraged to promote the excretion of waste products. Some may need a higher fluid intake, such as those with kidney stones or those with a salt-losing enteropathy. However, those with a tendency to fluid retention, such nephrotic syndrome, may need to limit both their salt and fluid intakes (see the subsection on HD in the following section, 'Management of CKD stage 5' for further information).

Potassium

Limiting dietary potassium is usually not required, unless patients are receiving medications that promote hyperkalaemia. Dietary potassium should only be limited when serum levels are raised after considering other non-dietary causes, as many foods containing potassium are required for a healthy, balanced diet. Both dietary restrictions and serum potassium levels should be regularly monitored (NICE, 2014a) (see the following section 'Management of CKD stage 4' for further information).

Phosphate

Parathyroid hormone levels may start to increase from CKD stage 3 onwards; there is no evidence to support a low-phosphate diet at this stage.

Nephrotic syndrome

Limiting salt intake is an important part of the nutritional treatment in nephrotic syndrome, as this will enhance the antiproteinuric effects of medical treatment (KDIGO, 2012a). To prevent exacerbation of urinary protein losses, high-protein diets should be avoided (Kaysen *et al.*, 1986). A protein intake of 0.8–1.0 g protein/kg IBW/day is recommended (KDIGO, 2012a; Mansy *et al.*, 1989). There is very limited evidence to recommend an LPD (<0.8 g protein/kg IBW/day) (Giordano *et al.*, 2001). Patients with oedema will benefit from a combination of salt and fluid restriction. Hyperlipidaemia usually resolves as serum albumin levels normalise; however, where this is not the case, dietary intervention is indicated (Kaysen *et al.*, 1992).

Management of CKD stage 4

Clinical management

In addition to the reduction of modifiable cardiovascular risk factors, treatments of renal anaemia, metabolic acidosis and

SECTION 7

CKD–MBD are important parts of management. Nephrology reviews usually include measurement of eGFR, haemoglobin, calcium, phosphate, potassium, bicarbonate and PTH. Ideally, these patients should be managed in a dedicated multidisciplinary team clinic (Renal Association, 2014). Patients with progressive CKD should also be offered appropriate education programmes aimed at improving their understandings of CKD and the treatment options, e.g. RRT (HD, peritoneal dialysis (PD), transplant), or conservative care (NICE, 2014a; Renal Association, 2014). It can take up to 1 year to prepare fully for RRT, but this programme should enable a planned start using an established access (such as a fistula for HD or a PD catheter), or by pre-emptive renal transplantation.

Renal anaemia

Treatment is with iron and erythropoiesis-stimulating agents (ESAs) as required, with regular monitoring of serum ferritin and haemoglobin levels.

Metabolic acidosis

Sodium bicarbonate supplementation is recommended to correct metabolic acidosis. This may also help to reduce protein catabolism and retard the progression of CKD (de Brito-Ashurst *et al.*, 2009).

Mineral and bone disorder

Management of CKD–MBD involves the correction of biochemistry by limiting dietary phosphorus intake (without compromising protein intake), together with the use of medications. It can be difficult to achieve an effective combination, and frequent monitoring of blood levels and adjustments may be required. To help achieve adequate phosphate control, phosphate binders may be required in addition to any dietary changes. These work by limiting the absorption of phosphorus from the gastrointestinal tract. Although they are used in patients with CKD stage 4, most of the evidence regarding their effectiveness comes from their use in patients on dialysis. NICE (2013) guidelines recommend calcium acetate as the first-line phosphate binder, with consideration of calcium carbonate if calcium acetate is not tolerated or if patients find it unpalatable. In comparison with non-calcium-containing binders, these are inexpensive and relatively well tolerated (Navaneethan *et al.*, 2011). However, there are concerns that their use is associated with vascular calcification (Goodman *et al.*, 2000; Guerin *et al.*, 2000; London *et al.*, 2003). Where calcium levels are raised above the upper limit of normal, or where the PTH levels are low, a switch to non-calcium-based binders such as sevelamer hydrochloride/carbonate, lanthanum carbonate and sucroferric oxyhydroxide should be considered (NICE, 2013). Poor adherence to phosphate binders is widespread and reported to range between 22 and 74% (mean 51%). High pill burden is an important contributory factor in this patient group (Carrero *et al.*, 2016).

Vitamin D levels are often measured at baseline in CKD stage 3b and above, with a view to correction as necessary. Routine supplementation of vitamin D (without checking vitamin D status) is not recommended (Renal Association, 2015). Alfacalcidol is an active vitamin D analogue that is also used in the management of CKD–MBD. It can be effective at suppressing PTH levels, but also promotes calcium and phosphorus absorption. Careful biochemical monitoring is therefore required, and its use should be balanced against other effects (Table 7.5.3). Where PTH levels remain high, tertiary hyperparathyroidism has developed. Treatment involves either a parathyroidectomy or cinacalcet therapy. Cinacalcet is a calcimimetic agent that increases the sensitivity of calcium-sensing receptors in the parathyroid gland, thereby inhibiting PTH secretion. It is expensive, and NICE (2007) currently recommends that cinacalcet be reserved for individuals in whom surgery is contraindicated.

Dietetic management

The aim is to promote a healthy, well-balanced diet, while considering the nutritional treatment of comorbidities. Other factors, particularly the monitoring of both serum electrolyte levels and nutritional status, become more important in order to provide appropriate and timely dietetic advice. By CKD stage 4, complications such as fluid and electrolyte imbalance, metabolic acidosis, anaemia and uraemia are common. Although these have an adverse effect on nutrition, well-being and blood levels, they vary greatly between individuals. Some patients experience hyperkalaemia with mild renal impairment, while others will maintain normal levels even in advanced disease. Careful review of each

Table 7.5.3 Recommended levels in CKD – mineral bone disorder (Renal Association, 2015)

	Serum phosphate (mmol/L)	Serum calcium[a] (mmol/L)	Serum parathyroid hormone (PTH)
CKD stage 3–5 patients (not on dialysis)	0.9–1.5[b]	Kept within normal reference range	Consider treatment where levels are progressively increasing and remain persistently higher than upper reference limit
Dialysis patients (stage 5D)	1.1–1.7[b]	2.1–2.5[b]	Between two and nine times upper limit of normal Marked changes in levels in either direction within range should prompt initiation or change in therapy

[a] Adjusted for albumin concentration.
[b] KDIGO now suggest lowering elevated phosphate levels towards the normal range and avoiding hypercalcaemia rather than aiming for a specific reference range (KDIGO, 2017).

patient is required. Dietary recommendations depend on biochemistry, normal dietary intake, comorbidities and nutritional status.

NICE (2014a) guidelines recognise the importance of dietary advice in the management of hyperkalaemia, hyperphosphataemia, and salt and water intake for people with advanced CKD (eGFR <20 mL/min). Dietary advice should be offered about potassium, phosphate, energy and salt intake appropriate to the severity of CKD. This should occur within the context of education, detailed dietary assessment and supervision to ensure that malnutrition is prevented.

Protein

As with earlier stages of CKD, there is debate as to the optimal level of protein intake. High-protein diets should be avoided as they increase hyperfiltration, worsen proteinuria, and hasten decline in kidney function (Burton & Harris, 1996). Advocates of dietary protein restriction claim that LPDs delay CKD progression, although this view is not supported by major randomised controlled trials (RCTs). In addition, LPDs are very demanding of both patient's and dietitian's time, and are associated with a reduction in nutritional status (Kopple *et al.*, 1997). The recommendation for CKD stage 4 or 5 is a protein intake of 0.8 g/kg IBW/day (National Kidney Federation KDIGO, 2012a). Protein provision should not exceed 1.3 g protein/kg IBW/day in patients with CKD at risk of progression of the disease (Naylor *et al.*, 2013). A high protein intake may also increase metabolic acidosis. Changes in appetite may result in a decline in protein intake, and this should be regularly monitored.

Energy

Energy expenditure is similar to that of healthy individuals (Monteen *et al.*, 1986). An intake of 35 kcal/kg/day should be adequate (Kopple *et al.*, 1986), but 30 kcal/kg may be more appropriate in those aged >60 years when energy expenditure is reduced. However, it is important to ensure adequate energy intake in order to prevent negative nitrogen balance and weight loss. Careful interpretation of weight change is important, as a history of oedema or rapid weight change may be due to changes in fluid status.

Sodium and fluid

Almost all patients will be advised to restrict salt intake to reduce fluid retention and thirst. An intake of 5–6 g is usually recommended (KDIGO, 2012a; Renal Association, 2011b); sodium bicarbonate given to correct acidosis may also contribute significantly to sodium intake. If individuals become oedematous, fluid intake will also need to be restricted. A daily limit of 500–750 mL plus the previous day's urine output is the minimum amount usually advised, although this may vary depending on local practice. Good blood glucose management is essential to achieve good adherence to fluid restriction in patients with diabetes.

Potassium

Hyperkalaemia becomes increasingly common as GFR falls. However, not all patients with stage 4 CKD will require potassium restriction. A low-potassium diet should only be used after considering other possible medical causes of hyperkalaemia. Potassium levels should be monitored closely when medications known to increase levels are started. However, it is important to ensure that the diet is not overly restrictive, as potassium levels at the lower end of normal are not advisable. The lowest mortality risk may be between 4.1 and 5.5 mmol/L (Korgaonkar *et al.*, 2010). The level of potassium restriction should be individualised according to dietary intake, blood levels and medical treatment, but, as a guide, intakes of approximately 1 mmol/kg IBW may be required. Non-essential foods high in potassium should be limited or avoided first, e.g. coffee and chocolate. Fruit, vegetables and potatoes contain significant amounts of potassium, as do meat, fish and milk. However, as these are important dietary components, limitations should be applied within the wider context of maintaining a balanced intake of essential nutrients. Cooking methods may need to be adapted, e.g. boiling potatoes and vegetables lowers their potassium content. Some people have been found to have low serum vitamin C levels on a low-potassium diet (Pollock *et al.*, 2005). Patients should be able to consume up to five 80 g portions of fruit and vegetables daily, but should also be provided with appropriate education on limiting or avoiding foods that are particularly high sources of potassium, e.g. bananas and dried fruit.

Patients with diabetes following a low-potassium diet should be advised against the use of higher-potassium choices such as pure fruit juice or milk as treatments for hypoglycaemia, and instead encouraged to use glucose tablets. Table 7.5.4 gives an example of a first-line low-potassium diet that could be used until personalised dietary advice can be provided. The task of the dietitian involves limiting those foods that are high in potassium and have the least nutritional value, while considering patient preference and nutritional adequacy.

Phosphate

Hyperphosphataemia becomes increasingly common when eGFR falls below 30 mL/min. Its treatment primarily involves limiting dietary phosphorus intake, without compromising protein intake; this is often combined with the use of phosphate binders. Current guidelines recommend that serum phosphate levels be maintained at 0.9–1.50 mmol/L for CKD stages 4 and 5 (not on dialysis) (Renal Association, 2015). Phosphate contains both phosphorus and oxygen. Phosphorus itself is highly reactive, so it is usually found in combination with other elements or molecules. Phosphorus is found in almost every food, mainly from proteins, phytates, and food additives. Two types exist, organic and inorganic, depending on the dietary source. Inorganic phosphorus is present in processed-food additives. Organic phosphorus is found in animal- and plant-derived protein-rich foods; however, the phosphorus-to-protein ratio differs markedly, depending on the food source. In animal and plant foods, phosphorus is naturally found in phosphoproteins, phospholipids, adenosine di and tri phosphates

Table 7.5.4 First-line potassium-lowering dietary advice (source: BDA, 2013. Reproduced with permission from the British Dietetic Association, www.bda.uk.com)

	Foods high in potassium – limit intake of the following	Lower-potassium alternatives
Fruit	Avocado, bananas, dried fruit, e.g. apricots, currants, dates, figs, prunes, raisins, sultanas	Fruit should be limited to a maximum of three portions/day A portion is 80 g or a handful
Vegetables	Vegetables that have not been boiled, e.g. steamed, stir fried or raw Beetroot (fresh), sundried tomatoes, tomato purée	Two to three small (80 g) portions of other vegetables Boil vegetables if possible Limit salads to one small bowl/day
Starchy foods	Jacket/baked potatoes Oven, microwave or retail chips Manufactured potato products, e.g. hash browns, frozen roast potatoes, potato waffles, potato wedges Unboiled sweet potato, cassava, plantain, taro, yam	Boiled potatoes, potatoes that have been par-boiled, then roasted or fried Boiled sweet potatoes, cassava, plantain, taro, yam Have no more than one serving of potato or starchy vegetable/day Pasta, rice, noodles, breads.
Snacks	Potato crisps/snacks, nuts, chocolate, fudge Biscuits and cakes containing lots of nuts, dried fruit or chocolate	Corn- or maize-based snacks Boiled, chewy and jelly sweets Marshmallows, mints, popcorn Biscuits and cakes not containing dried fruit, nuts or chocolate
Drinks	Coffee, malted milk drinks (e.g. Horlicks, Ovaltine), drinking chocolate, cocoa, fruit and vegetable juices, smoothies Limit milk to 400 mL (two-third pint)/day, or 200 mL (one-third pint) milk plus one yogurt/day Beer, cider, stout and wine	Tea, herbal tea, squash and cordial, mineral water, flavoured water, fizzy drinks Spirits are generally lower in potassium than other alcoholic drinks; remember to keep within safe limits for alcohol intake
Salt substitutes	Do *not* use salt substitutes, e.g. Lo-salt, SOLO, low sodium salt	Other seasonings, e.g. pepper, herbs, spices

Note: This is initial advice only, and should only be used until a registered dietitian can provide personalised dietary advice.

(ADP and ATP), and deoxyribonucleic acid and ribonucleic acid (DNA and RNA). In plant foods, a significant amount of phosphorus is bound to phytates. Humans lack phytase, required for the digestion of phytate, and hence phytate degradation is low. As a result, the phosphorus in wholegrain foods and nuts has a low absorption rate from the gastrointestinal tract, 20–50% (Kalantar-Zadeh, 2013; Williams *et al.*, 2013). In animal protein foods, a greater proportion of phosphorus, usually 40–60%, is absorbed from the gastrointestinal tract (Kalantar-Zadeh, 2013). In contrast, 90–100% of inorganic phosphorous is absorbed (Kalantar-Zadeh, 2013).

Additives can contribute an additional 600–800 mg phosphorus per day. Sodium is commonly combined with phosphorus in food additives, and an additive-rich diet may provide an additional 60% of dietary sodium and phosphorus (Carrigan *et al.*, 2014). Inorganic phosphorus is also found in some carbonated and alcoholic drinks.

In a typical Western diet, >50% of dietary phosphorus originates from animal proteins (Noori *et al.*, 2010). Dietary phosphorus is also strongly related to dietary protein intake; hence, any restriction may limit the intake of meat, fish, poultry, eggs and milk. To ensure that protein intake is not compromised by dietary phosphorus restriction, foods with a high protein to phosphorus ratio should be encouraged (Kalantar-Zadeh *et al.*, 2010; NICE, 2013). Consideration should be given to the individual's nutritional status, and care taken to ensure an adequate protein intake. Where possible, commonly eaten high-phosphorus foods should be substituted with nutritionally equivalent foods that are lower in bioavailable phosphorus (St-Jules *et al.*, 2016).

One of the difficulties in clarifying the best choices with regard to dietary phosphorus intake is that nutrient data tables are unable to distinguish between inorganic and organic phosphorus. There is some evidence that consuming a greater proportion of the diet as wholegrains or plant foods may help to control serum phosphate levels (Williams *et al.*, 2013), although there may be an increased risk of hyperkalaemia in those with CKD stage 4 (Moorthi *et al.*, 2014). NICE recommends that a specialist renal dietitian, supported by healthcare professionals with the necessary skills and competencies, give individualised information and advice on dietary phosphate management (NICE, 2013). KDIGO (2017) states that it is reasonable to consider the phosphate source (e.g. animal, vegetable, additives) in making dietary recommendations, and that efforts to restrict dietary phosphate must not compromise adequate protein intake. Points to consider when advising on a low-phosphate diet (NICE, 2013; St-Jules *et al.*, 2016) are shown in Table 7.5.5.

Management of CKD stage 5

Clinical management

Once eGFR falls below 15 mL/min, and uraemia, fluid overload or PEW are more likely to develop despite medical treatment, RRT should commence if the patient has opted to dialyse. Ideally, this should be planned so that dialysis can start with an arteriovenous fistula or PD catheter. Those patients who have opted not to dialyse should continue to have conservative management of their kidney disease. In all cases, regular monitoring of kidney function is an essential part of the continuing care of these patients.

Dietetic management

The aims will vary, depending on the mode of RRT, or if the patient is managed conservatively. In 2014, transplantation continued as the most common treatment modality (53%); HD was used in 41% and PD in 6% of RRT patients (Renal Registry, 2015). There have been more studies in patients on dialysis than in earlier stages of CKD, particularly focusing on the treatment of PEW and CKD–MBD, as these are both associated with increased morbidity and mortality. Recently, the HD population has shown a demographic shift from predominantly undernutrition to overnutrition (Kramer *et al.*, 2006), and this should be taken into account when providing dietetic advice.

Management of haemodialysis

Clinical management

HD is the main mode of dialysis in most developed countries. In 2014, HD was the established mode of dialysis for 83% of patients (Renal Registry, 2015). In HD, blood is circulated through a machine that passes it through very small tubes made from a semipermeable membrane. Surrounding these tubes is the dialysate, which consists of sterile water and electrolytes. Blood cells and proteins are too large to pass through the pores in the membranes, but small molecules such as urea, water and electrolytes pass through into the dialysate. In this way, excess water and uraemic toxins are removed, and electrolyte and acid–base balance are restored. However, amino acids, glucose, vitamins and trace elements may also be removed by dialysis. The best access to the patient's blood is via an arteriovenous fistula, although a central venous catheter (usually into the internal jugular vein) can be used when access is needed immediately.

HD usually takes place three times per week, but several forms of more frequent HD, including daily and nocturnal, have recently been evaluated and are associated with improved outcomes. Although usually hospital based, 4.3% of dialysis patients in the UK are undergoing home HD (HHD).

Dietetic management

The main aims of the dietetic management of HD are:

- Regular monitoring of nutritional status to prevent or treat PEW.
- Regular monitoring and dietetic advice to help maintain electrolytes within acceptable ranges.
- To help control fluid balance.
- To promote a healthy, well-balanced diet, taking into account the nutritional treatment of comorbidities.

Dietetic assessment should be provided on initiation of dialysis to identify those who require nutritional supplementation and/or fluid removal, and to balance this with advice on any dietary restrictions that may be required. After 6–8 weeks of commencing dialysis, many patients notice an improvement in symptoms, and dietary advice may need to change. For stable patients, nutritional changes are likely to be gradual after this. Multidisciplinary working is a vital part of ensuring appropriate

Table 7.5.5 Points to consider when advising on a low-phosphate diet (NICE, 2013; St-Jules *et al.*, 2016)

Points	Details
Where possible, choose fresh foods rather than processed foods and prepare foods at home	This is likely to reduce both phosphate and sodium intake. *Note*: This requires that patients have the time, skills/abilities and facilities to prepare foods.
Where possible, choose commercial foods and drinks prepared without phosphorus-containing food additives Check food labels and reduce your intake of foods containing the words phosphate or phosphoric acid on them, including the following: diphosphates; triphosphates; polyphosphates; calcium phosphate; mono-, di- and tri- sodium phosphates; sodium tripolyphosphate; ammonium phosphate; magnesium phosphate; phosphoric acid	Examples of foods containing these additives include ham, sausages, processed meats, breaded chicken, pizza, battered fish, instant sauces, cake mixes, frozen desserts, ice cream Dark carbonated drinks, beers, lagers, wines *Note*: Choosing additive-free foods may have cost implications
Ensure that dietary protein intake is adequate for the stage of CKD. Control the intake of foods that have a high phosphorus content per gram of protein	Where possible, commonly eaten high-phosphorus foods should be substituted with nutritionally equivalent foods that are lower in bioavailable phosphorus. *Note*: This requires dietetic expertise

treatment for these patients (Renal Association, 2010). Regular dietetic monitoring is likely to be beneficial and may lead to both a significant reduction in the proportion of patients with PEW and a significant decrease in phosphate levels (Campbell *et al.*, 2009).

Protein

In HD, protein requirements are increased, partly due to the loss of amino acids through the dialysis filter, although dialysis itself can increase protein catabolism (Fouque *et al.*, 2007). A safe level of protein intake is likely to be ≥1.1–1.2 g/kg IBW to achieve nitrogen balance (Fouque *et al.*, 2007; Naylor *et al.*, 2013; Renal Association, 2010). There is currently no evidence to support recommendations on the proportion of protein that should be of high biological value. However, high protein intakes of >1.4 g/kg may not improve survival and may be harmful (Shinaberger *et al.*, 2006).

Energy

Energy expenditure does not appear to be increased (Cuppari & Avesani, 2004). The recommended energy intake is 30–35 kcal/kg IBW/day, depending on age and physical activity (Renal Association, 2010). Energy intakes are often lower than this, and may be as low as 20–25 kcal/kg/day (Rocco *et al.*, 2002); energy intake may be insufficient, particularly on dialysis days. Even if protein intake is adequate, an inadequate energy intake is likely to result in a negative nitrogen balance. When assessing energy intake, a food diary that includes a dialysis day, a non-dialysis day and a weekend day as a minimum, or several dietary interviews, can be helpful (Fouque *et al.*, 2007).

Obesity

There is an association between higher body mass index (BMI) and improved survival in HD patients, known as the *obesity paradox*, with large observational studies suggesting that a higher BMI is protective against mortality. However, the evidence for the obesity paradox is entirely associative, and many studies are short term. The survival advantage associated with obesity is short term, due to the acute catabolic effects of dialysis and kidney failure, and the association is less robust in those who survive the early years of dialysis (MacLaughlin, 2016). However, obese patients on dialysis who are eligible for a kidney transplant will often be encouraged to lose weight, as patients with a BMI of >35 kg/m^2 may be denied transplantation in some centres (Segev *et al.*, 2008).

Diabetes

Intensive glucose control in type 2 diabetes may have less of a protective effect against cardiovascular events in these patients (Reaven *et al.*, 2009), and the aims of treatment should be balanced against the increased risk of hypoglycaemia. The HbA1c target for patients on maintenance HD should be individualised, but if the patient is on hypoglycaemia-inducing medication, it should be 58–68 mmol/mol. Dose reduction should be considered for these patients if HbA1c is <58 mmol/mol. Dietary advice should be personalised and include information on both diabetes and the renal aspects of the diet (JBDSIC, 2016).

Sodium and fluid

Most patients show a progressive reduction in urine output. Limiting sodium and fluid intake is required to control blood pressure and to prevent excessive fluid weight gains. In HD, very high fluid weight gains between dialysis sessions (intradialytic weight gain, or 'IDWG') are associated with increased mortality, particularly cardiovascular risk (Kalantar-Zadeh *et al.*, 2009). Patients with very little fluid weight gain between dialysis sessions are at highest risk of death, but this is due to the association with poor nutritional status and may reflect poor oral intake (Lopez-Gomez *et al.*, 2005).

It is very difficult to ignore thirst, since the overriding stimulus is plasma osmolality, with serum sodium being the main contributor (Tomson, 2001). Patients with poorly controlled diabetes may also be extremely thirsty. Reducing sodium intake suppresses thirst and therefore excessive IDWG. Patients on a low-sodium diet (with advice to drink only when thirsty) have been found to gain significantly less weight than those on a standard diet and fluid intake (Rigby-Matthews *et al.*, 1999). A low-sodium diet also improves blood pressure control and may result in the withdrawal of antihypertensive treatment (Krautzig *et al.*, 1998). Hence, for most patients, the focus should be on limiting salt intake rather than on fluid intake.

When fluid needs to be considered, the current guidelines for fluid intake vary from 500 to 1000 mL in addition to daily urine output in order to achieve an IDWG of 2–2.5 kg or 4–4.5% of dry body weight (Fouque *et al.*, 2007). In order to achieve this, drinks and food with a high fluid content (sauces, soup, ice cream, etc.) should be counted as part of the daily fluid allowance. The water content in other foodstuffs such as fruit and vegetables is not counted. Drinking from a full small cup is usually more helpful than using a part-filled larger cup or mug. However, any fluid allowance given should be reassessed regularly as residual renal function (urine output) is likely to change. Reducing sodium and fluid in addition to both potassium and phosphate, while ensuring that protein and energy intake is adequate, is difficult, and a stepwise approach to educate the patient is most important (Fouque *et al.*, 2007).

Potassium

Hyperkalaemia is a common indication for emergency dialysis in patients already on HD, and 3–5% of deaths in dialysis patients have been attributed to hyperkalaemia. The highest mortality rate occurs when potassium levels are >5.6–6.0 mmol/L (Kovesdy *et al.*, 2007). Serum potassium levels (measured at the start of dialysis) should be 4–6 mmol/L (Renal Association, 2009). Dietetic advice to reduce dietary potassium intake should be provided when serum potassium levels approach 6 mmol/L, but other causes for hyperkalaemia should be investigated and corrected. For these patients, a daily intake of potassium of 50–70 mmol (1950–2730 mg) or 1 mmol/kg IBW may be required (Fouque *et al.*, 2007).

Conversely, low potassium levels may lead to an increased mortality rate, especially when pre-dialysis levels are <4 mmol/L (Kovesdy *et al.*, 2007). Hypokalaemia towards the end or immediately after dialysis may be corrected by relaxing dietary potassium or by increasing the dialysate potassium concentration. Information regarding the dietary advice required for a low-potassium diet has been provided earlier in text.

Phosphate

The treatment of hyperphosphataemia and secondary hyperparathyroidism involves dietary phosphorus restriction, without compromising protein intake, combined with the use of phosphate binders. Detailed information regarding low-phosphate diets and the use of phosphate binders, vitamin D compounds and calcimimetics has been presented earlier in text. It is important to ensure an adequate dietary protein intake while on dialysis to avoid PEW and improve survival. Balancing dietary phosphorus and protein intake can be achieved by using the phosphorus-to-protein ratio to select protein sources with the least serum phosphorus cost (Kalantar-Zadeh, 2013), as well as by minimising the intake of inorganic phosphorus from food additives.

There is growing evidence that dietetic intervention is effective in lowering serum phosphate levels in patients on dialysis. Educating HD patients to avoid phosphorus-containing food additives led to modest improvements in hyperphosphatemia (Sullivan *et al.*, 2009). Dietetic education helps reduce serum phosphate levels in hyperphosphataemic patients with CKD, particularly in those on dialysis (Caldeira *et al.*, 2011), and the implementation of a systematic approach to patient care in patients on HD had led to a reduction in serum phosphate even while protein intake increased (Campbell *et al.*, 2009).

The recommended serum phosphate level is 1.1–1.7 mmol/L (measured at the start of each dialysis session) (Renal Association, 2015). Both low and high phosphate levels are associated with increased mortality in dialysis patients. Some patients may have both PEW and CKD–MBD; the association between low serum phosphate levels and increased mortality rate may be due to a decline in protein intake and worsening PEW (Shinaberger *et al.*, 2008).

Home haemodialysis

The nutritional needs of those undergoing HHD vary greatly. Patients undergoing more frequent, i.e. daily, HD sessions are less likely to require potassium restriction. Those undergoing nocturnal HHD can achieve in excess of 40 h dialysis weekly, often reversing the need for potassium and phosphorus restriction and sometimes necessitating dietary advice to increase potassium and phosphorus intake to maintain serum levels. Dialysates used in HD are typically formulated to suit the needs of traditional dialysis regimens. In nocturnal HHD, patients may require pharmaceutical addition of phosphate to dialysate to prevent hypophosphatemia. Fluid restrictions are likely to be liberal in those undergoing more frequent (daily) dialysis sessions. Individual assessment and close monitoring of electrolyte regimens while establishing HHD should guide tailored dietetic input.

Management of peritoneal dialysis

Clinical management

In PD, the dialysis fluid is introduced into the peritoneal cavity via a dialysis catheter in the patient's abdomen, where it draws waste products and excess water out of the blood using the peritoneal membrane as a filter. Most people dialyse daily either by manual exchanges performed four to five times a day (continuous ambulatory PD (CAPD)) or overnight using a machine (automated PD (APD)). The fluid must stay inside the peritoneal cavity for a period of time (a dwell) to allow the removal of waste products and fluid. Different dialysis regimens can be prescribed to maximise an individual's dialysis to ensure efficiency.

Dietetic management

The main aims of the dietetic management of PD are:

- Regular monitoring of nutritional status to prevent or treat PEW.
- Regular monitoring and dietetic advice to help maintain electrolytes within acceptable range.
- To help control fluid balance.
- To promote a healthy, well-balanced diet, taking into account the nutritional treatment of comorbidities.

Dietetic assessment should be undertaken on initiation of dialysis to give a baseline. Any symptoms of uraemia at this time usually start to recede, and appetite improves. As residual renal function is relatively preserved in this patient group, and dialysis is performed each day, some dietary and fluid restrictions may be more relaxed than in HD.

Protein

Protein requirements are increased to compensate for protein losses into the dialysis fluid. The actual amount lost in individuals is variable and is dependent on the properties of their peritoneal membrane and the dialysis regimen. Recommendations for protein requirements group have become more conservative, with increasing evidence to suggest that neutral nitrogen balance can be achieved at much lower intakes than previously recommended. Current consensus suggests aiming for a protein intake of 1.2 g protein/kg IBW (Renal Association, 2010), although intakes of a minimum of 1.0–1.2 g of protein/kg IBW may be adequate for many individuals with no adverse effect on nutritional status (Dombros *et al.*, 2005; Naylor *et al.*, 2013). Protein losses may be considerably higher during episodes of peritonitis, which in turn is likely to increase protein requirements.

Energy

Energy requirements are 30–35 kcal/kg IBW (including energy contribution from dialysis fluid), although older, less active patients may achieve neutral energy balance with lower intakes. Monitoring actual body weight will help to assess if energy intake is appropriate for an individual. Unlike other renal patient groups, energy intake is obtained by the absorption of glucose from the PD fluid as well as from diet. Glucose acts as an osmotic agent to ultrafiltrate fluid (UF) from the patient; hence, while it is in contact with the peritoneal membrane, not only does it facilitate fluid removal, but it is also absorbed, thereby contributing to the total energy intake. The amount of energy obtained from the PD fluid is dependent on the amount of glucose in the bags (increased in some bags to increase UF) and the characteristics of the individual's peritoneal membrane. In CAPD, approximately 60% of the daily dialysate glucose load is absorbed in those with a normally functioning membrane (Dombros *et al.*, 2005), which can be 300–800 kcal/day. Those using high glucose concentration bags will regularly be absorbing large amounts of energy, which may cause undesirable weight gain.

To minimise glucose absorption (and therefore non-nutritive energy), other bags are available that use alternative osmotic agents, e.g. icodextrin (a non-absorbable glucose polymer) and amino acids. Icodextrin is often used to maximise UF, particularly for longer dwells, and amino acid bags can be indicated in those with poor nutritional intake. These may be useful glucose-sparing strategies for those with obesity or diabetes. Glucose absorption from the PD fluid can make meeting other dietary requirements more difficult, as there needs to be a higher concentration of nutrients in the recommended reduced dietary energy intake.

Obesity

The energy load provided by PD treatment can lead to weight gain. Those on PD are at greater risk of development or worsening of central obesity, hyperlipidaemia and insulin resistance (Renal Association, 2010). Practically, it can also be difficult to achieve an adequate dialysis dose in these. There is no evidence to suggest a protective effect of obesity for those undergoing PD. As for HD, obesity, and particularly a BMI of >35 kg/m^2, may limit access to transplantation.

Diabetes

Glycaemic control can become more difficult to manage due to the glucose absorbed from the PD fluid. This may require an increase in insulin or oral hypoglycaemic drugs (Reaven *et al.*, 2009). Some individuals may have a set dialysis regimen against which diabetes medications can be titrated; however, patients may alter dialysis regimens to address their fluid balance on a day-to-day basis, so tight glycaemic control can become challenging. To avoid false readings, patients should be provided with blood glucose monitors that do not measure icodextrin, as these may be affected by dialysate solutions.

Sodium and fluid

The fluid requirement for those on PD depends on an individual's residual renal function (urine output) and the UF achieved by PD. While limiting fluid helps prevent fluid overload, an appropriate dialysis regimen individualised to best match the UF potential is the most important predictor of adequate fluid balance. The use of high glucose bags is associated with detrimental changes in peritoneal membrane function, which can occur over time as well as with weight gain and poor glycaemic control in diabetes (Renal Association, 2010). Limiting sodium and fluid intake helps to minimise the need for their use. Fluid intake is usually restricted to 750 mL plus the volume of the previous day's urine output.

Potassium

Most patients receiving PD are able to have a normal potassium intake. For some, the removal of potassium by dialysis can be so efficient that a high potassium intake is required to maintain normal potassium levels. High serum potassium levels may indicate ineffective dialysis. Monitoring potassium levels will inform the level of dietary potassium required.

Constipation

Constipation is associated with PD catheter malfunction and peritonitis, which can result in PD failure. Constipation needs to be dealt with in a proactive, preventative manner. Laxatives are often taken regularly; however, if changing the diet, fibre should be increased gradually, and the potassium and fluid content should also be considered to ensure that target potassium levels are achieved and fluid overload is prevented (Lee, 2011).

Phosphate

The same dietetic principles apply to patients on PD as those on HD, and the same serum phosphate levels are recommended.

Protein energy wasting

Although felt to be diminishing, PEW is still prevalent, particularly among those with other comorbidities. In PD, several factors are associated with PEW. The frequency of gastrointestinal symptoms is high, varying from diarrhoea, constipation, abdominal pain, delayed gastric emptying, and nausea and vomiting (Cano *et al.*, 2007b). Management of these symptoms may help improve appetite and food intake. For those who have fluid in their peritoneal cavity in the day, bloating and satiety may also be experienced. Inadequate dialysis has been implicated in contributing to PEW (Churchill *et al.*, 1996; Paniagua *et al.*, 2002), and the level of residual renal function is thought to be directly related to nutritional intake independent of dialysis dose (Caravaca *et al.*, 1999; Wang *et al.*, 2001). The peritoneal membrane characteristics are also associated with PEW, and fluid overload caused by poor volume management is associated with poorer nutritional status (Cheng *et al.*, 2005; Wang *et al.*, 2003). Although some of these factors are difficult to manage or cannot be altered, it is important they be considered when formulating clinical treatment plans to address PEW.

Complications

A serious but uncommon complication of PD is encapsulating peritoneal sclerosis. It is characterised by bowel obstruction and marked sclerotic thickening of the peritoneal membrane. Symptoms such as anorexia, nausea, vomiting and weight loss are common. In cases with milder gastrointestinal features, nutritional status may be maintained by ensuring adequate food intake with oral nutritional supplements and antiemetics as required.

However, more severe cases may warrant enteral tube feeding if the gastrointestinal tract allows, or parenteral feeding when it is impossible to establish adequate nutrition using the gut.

Management of kidney transplantation

Clinical management

Renal transplantation is the most common solid organ transplant procedure and is considered the gold standard for RRT; a successful transplant can lead to the restoration of renal function. Survival following renal transplantation is better than that for age-matched individuals remaining on the transplant waiting list (Wolfe *et al.*, 1999). The longer the patients receive dialysis, the greater is their risk for post-transplantation morbidity and mortality.

A transplant is considered to be the first choice for patients who are considered fit for major surgery and for chronic immunosuppression (Renal Association, 2011b). During a kidney transplant, the donor kidney is usually placed in the iliac fossa, and the existing kidneys are not removed. Almost all transplants will provoke a powerful immunological rejection response in the recipient, which will destroy renal tissue; therefore, immunosuppression is needed to avoid rejection. Acute rejection generally occurs days to weeks after surgery. Chronic rejection, however, occurs slowly over months or years and leads to progressive loss of renal function. Eventually, as transplant function declines, the patient is likely to suffer symptoms of advancing kidney failure. As with patients with CKD, dietary changes may be required at some stage. The most frequently used immunosuppressive medications are tacrolimus and ciclosporin. Other immunosuppressives used are mycophenolate mofetil, azathioprine, sirolimus and corticosteroids. Some of their adverse effects have nutritional implications, as shown in Table 7.5.6.

The medical and dietetic management of transplantation can be divided into three main periods, and the aims for medical management are:

- *Pre-transplant* – to correct or improve complications of stage 5 CKD in order to optimise outcome.
- *Immediate post-transplant phase* – to prevent acute rejection, optimise graft function and minimise infection.
- *Later post-transplant phase (3–6 months after surgery)* – to preserve good graft function and prevent the long-term consequences of immunosuppression, including premature CVD (Renal Association, 2011b).

Dietetic management

The main aims are:

- *Pre-transplant phase* – to correct or improve nutritional status and CKD–MBD, and to treat obesity.
- *Immediate post-transplant phase* – to monitor nutritional status and ensure adequate protein and energy intake, monitor electrolyte levels and treat as appropriate, and provide food safety advice.

Table 7.5.6 Drug–nutrient interactions

Medication	Nutrient interactions	Nutritional implications
ACE inhibitors/ARBs	Enhanced hypotensive effect when taken with alcohol	Can cause hyperkalaemia
Potassium-sparing diuretics, e.g. spironolactone		Can cause hyperkalaemia
Atorvastatin, simvastatin	Grapefruit juice can increase the plasma concentration of statins	
Ciclosporin, tacrolimus	Grapefruit juice can increase the plasma concentration of these medications	Hyperkalaemia Hypercholesterolaemia
Sirolimus		Hyperlipidaemia Hypokalaemia
Erythropoietin		Correct iron or folate deficiencies before starting Supplemental iron may improve response
Corticosteroids		Weight gain Glucose intolerance Lipid abnormalities Osteoporosis
Calcium-based phosphate binders, e.g. calcium acetate, Calcichew	Interacts with iron tablets. For 2 h after taking these medications, iron tablets should not be taken	May cause hypercalcaemia
Alfacalcidol, calcitriol		May cause hypercalcaemia
Cinacalcet		May cause hypocalcaemia

ACE inhibitors, angiotensin-converting enzyme inhibitors; ARB, angiotensin receptor blocker.

- *Later post-transplant phase* – to provide adequate, but not excessive, protein intake and to promote a healthy, well-balanced diet, taking into account the nutritional treatment of comorbidities to reduce CVD risk.

Obesity and transplantation

Kidney transplantation in obese patients is associated with delayed graft function, more surgical wound infections, and increased CVD morbidity, but not with overall mortality or graft survival. High BMI alone should not be a limiting factor for kidney transplantation. Individualised assessment of risks and benefits is recommended in obese patients on HD, considering factors such as age, time on dialysis, potential for kidney transplantation, malnutrition risk and coexisting cardiovascular risk factors. Further research in obesity and CKD is needed to examine the effect of weight gain or intentional weight loss on outcomes such as quality of life, kidney transplantation listing, changes in kidney function, cardiovascular events and mortality (MacLaughlin, 2016).

Pre-transplant phase

The aim of pre-transplant nutritional management is to optimise outcomes in the early and late transplant periods. Ideally, a multidisciplinary team (MDT) approach should be taken, including diet, lifestyle changes and medication to aid in the correction or improvement of PEW, dyslipidaemia, obesity, CKD–MBD and hypertension. The presence of these comorbidities is predictive of related complications in post-transplant. Poor nutritional status during the pre-transplant period is associated with higher post-transplant morbidity and mortality (Chan *et al.*, 2011).

Immediate post-transplant phase

A successful kidney transplant enables previous dietary restrictions to be relaxed. However, some patients find it difficult to relax their diet and fluid intake.

Protein and energy

In the first 4 weeks after transplantation, a diet providing 1.2–1.3 g of protein/kg of body weight may prevent negative nitrogen balance (Chan *et al.*, 2011; Teplan *et al.*, 2009). An energy intake of 30–35 kcal/kg is advised, as it helps to ensure positive nitrogen balance (Danovitch, 2005; Teplan *et al.*, 2009).

Sodium and fluid

A low-sodium diet may aid in the management of post-transplant hypertension and fluid overload (Danovitch, 2005). As kidney function improves, patients become polyuric and need encouragement to drink lots of fluid. This may be difficult for patients who have spent years on dialysis trying to reduce their fluid intake; encouragement and reassurance are essential.

Potassium

Hyperkalaemia is associated with ciclosporin and tacrolimus, especially during the immediate post-transplant period when dosages are high. This may be exaggerated by graft dysfunction. Treatment may require limitation of dietary potassium.

Phosphate

Hypophosphataemia is very common during the early weeks post-transplant due to phosphaturia (Kasiske *et al.*, 2000). Oral phosphate supplementation may be needed where profound hypophosphataemia persists despite a liberal dietary intake. Phosphate binders should be discontinued as renal function improves to avoid severe hypophosphataemia.

Food-borne infections

Immunosuppressive medications weaken the immune system's ability to fight infections, increasing the risk of all types of infection, including food-borne ones. Bacteria, viruses or parasites present in food are all potential sources of infection. It is important to recommend the use of good food hygiene when choosing, preparing and storing foods, and to avoid certain high-risk foods known to carry certain bacteria such as *Escherichia coli*, *Listeria* and *Salmonella*, and viruses such as hepatitis E virus. During the early post-transplant period, the likelihood of food-borne infection is high due to significant suppression of the immune system (Chan *et al.*, 2011). However, basic food safety principles should continue for the lifetime of the transplant as the immune system will remain suppressed, particularly if there are changes to the immunosuppressive medications (BDA RNG, 2016). These are:

- Washing hands properly and keeping them clean.
- Cooking food properly.
- Chilling food properly.
- Avoiding cross-contamination.

Transplant recipients should also be advised to avoid foods which pose a higher risk to contracting food-borne illness, including raw meat, raw poultry and raw eggs; unpasteurised milk and unpasteurised soft cheeses; raw shellfish; Slush Puppies and ice cream from ice cream vans and other soft-serve machines; ready-to-eat foods such as pâté, rotisserie chickens and cured meats; foods from salad bars and deli counters; and unwashed fruits, vegetables and salad (BDA RNG, 2016).

Long-term dietetic management

Protein

A protein intake of 0.8 g/kg/day, as well as limiting sodium intake, can stabilise long-term renal function and maintain an adequate nutritional status in the kidney transplant recipient (Bernardi *et al.*, 2003). High protein intakes should be discouraged due to the risk of protein-induced hyperfiltration. For stable patients, a normal protein intake of 0.8–1.0 g/kg IBW should be the aim.

Energy

Energy intake and expenditure should be balanced to maintain desirable body weight and prevent weight gain. For stable transplant patients who require weight reduction, a daily energy intake of 25 kcal/kg IBW is a reasonable starting point.

Nutritional consequences and complications

Long-term immunosuppression is associated with several nutrition-related problems including obesity, dyslipidaemia, glucose intolerance, hypertension and CKD–MBD.

Obesity

Weight gain and obesity are common, due to several factors, including a feeling of well-being after transplantation with increased food intake, improved quality of life (physical and psychological), freedom from dietary restrictions, a sedentary lifestyle, hyperphagia and higher body fat accumulation related to corticosteroids. Obesity is associated with CVD events and mortality (KDIGO, 2009). Diet and other behaviour modifications have been shown to aid weight loss over the short term (KDIGO, 2009).

Dyslipidaemia

CVD remains the main cause of long-term mortality in the transplant population. Management of complications of atherosclerotic CVD is the same as in the general population (KDIGO, 2009). A diet in line with the latest lipid management guidelines for the general population is likely to benefit transplant recipients with dyslipidaemia (Chan *et al.*, 2011), although statins are usually required.

New-onset diabetes mellitus

This is common and may reflect increased dietary intake, weight gain and the use of immunosuppressive agents, specifically corticosteroids, tacrolimus, sirolimus and, to a lesser extent, ciclosporin. The incidence of new-onset diabetes mellitus after transplantation is highest in the first 3 months after transplantation. It is associated with poorer outcomes, including increased graft failure, mortality and CVD (KDIGO, 2009). Diet and exercise provide the basis for the initial management (Davidson *et al.*, 2003). Oral hypoglycaemic agents or insulin may also be required.

Hypertension

Hypertension is an important risk factor for CVD as well as graft survival. Weight loss and exercise in the obese hypertensive patient may play an important role in its treatment. Hypertensive patients are likely to benefit from limiting sodium intake to 2–3 g/day (Chan *et al.*, 2011).

Chronic kidney disease–mineral and bone disorder

CKD–MBD is common in transplant recipients. Calcium, phosphate and vitamin D metabolism are influenced by several factors resulting from the earlier period of CKD. Corticosteroids may cause osteoporosis, which may further affect MBD management. Hypercalcaemia is common and is usually due to hyperparathyroidism that persists from the preceding period of CKD (KDIGO, 2009). Hypophosphataemia may persist, and dietary phosphate intake should be individualised according to blood levels. A vitamin D supplement (or analogue) may be required.

Management for those receiving conservative management

The number of people who choose not to have dialysis continues to rise, possibly as a result of an ageing population with multiple comorbidities. For these patients, regular review is important, and the focus of care is symptom management. The main aims are to provide all aspects of clinical care, with the exception of dialysis, including the management of anaemia, together with ongoing support by the MDT in liaison with community and palliative care services. Little is known about the appropriate level of nutritional intervention, and there are no documented recommendations. Realistically, an approach that promotes enjoyment of food and mealtimes combined with symptom control would appear prudent.

Nutrition support in CKD

Nutrition support advice should be individualised, based on food fortification while relaxing dietary restrictions dependent on current biochemistry. The use of sugary foods, sweet drinks and/or high-fat foods should be encouraged unless the patient has other dietary issues. As cholesterol levels are often lower in CKD stages 4 and 5, it is debatable as to whether a strict cardioprotective diet is as important at this time. Oral nutritional supplements should be added if oral intake cannot be improved following dietetic intervention (Renal Association, 2010). The choice of supplement should be based on nutritional requirements, electrolyte levels, fluid status and patient preference. Renal-specific supplements low in potassium and/or phosphate may be required if potassium and/or phosphate levels are elevated. Caution should be taken with powdered milkshake-style products, which may not be appropriate due to electrolyte content and volume (BDA RNG, 2015) (see Chapter 6.3, Oral nutritional support).

Enteral tube feeding should be considered if the nutrient intake remains suboptimal despite oral supplements, although percutaneous endoscopic gastrostomy feeding is difficult in patients on PD due to complications such as peritonitis. Another type of nutritional support that may be used is intradialytic parenteral nutrition (IDPN), a form of parenteral nutrition given via the venous return while on HD; evidence for this is limited (Bossola *et al.*, 2010; Cano *et al.*, 2007a).

It has not yet been established whether provision of nutritional support to patients prior to developing stage 5 CKD, or those on RRT, leads to reduced morbidity and mortality. There is some evidence in HD to show an improvement in nutritional parameters, such as nutritional intake, serum albumin and weight, with both oral and enteral nutrition support, small studies of PEG feeding, and IDPN (Bossola *et al.*, 2010; Holley & Kirk, 2002; Stratton *et al.*, 2005), but there is no evidence as yet to show that this leads to increased survival. Patients receiving artificial nutrition support require close monitoring and frequent review (see Chapter 6.4, Enteral nutrition).

Nutrition support in CKD for those who are metabolically stressed

Overall, there is insufficient evidence to advise on the optimal nutritional requirements in patients with CKD who are metabolically stressed and require nutritional support (e.g. an inpatient with CKD and a pressure ulcer). Energy and protein requirements will be based on the patient's underlying clinical condition (as well as kidney disease). Protein restriction (to prevent or delay the progression of kidney disease or to prevent or delay the start of dialysis) should not be promoted in patients with CKD (and not on dialysis) who are metabolically stressed in the acute setting (KDIGO, 2012a). However, strict monitoring (urea, creatinine, proteinuria) is crucial in these patients, especially if protein provision exceeds 1.0 g/kg IBW/day. Protein provision should not exceed 1.3 g protein/kg IBW/day in patients with CKD at risk of progression (KDIGO, 2012a), and not exceed 1.4 g protein/kg IBW/day in patients on dialysis (Naylor *et al.*, 2013). In clinical practice, if protein provision is increased in CKD, fluid provision should also increase, unless clinically contraindicated. Energy intake should be optimal.

An individual dietetic assessment focusing on the underlying clinical condition and a tailored approach with close monitoring (nutritional status, fluid balance and kidney function) should guide dietitians, rather than the sole use of equations.

Considerations for long-term dietetic care

Nutritional treatment can be complex as several nutrients need to be managed simultaneously, the diet needs to change over time and comorbidities may need to be considered. The complexity of a regimen has been one of the most frequently identified barriers to patient compliance (Mitch & Klahr, 1993). Although a stepwise approach to educating the patient is important, giving knowledge alone does not necessarily lead to a change in behaviour. Behavioural change techniques are appropriate for patients with CKD as they can enhance patient motivation by reducing resistance to change. People with CKD appreciate advice on what they can have to eat rather than lists of what they should avoid (DH, 2004) (see Chapter 1.3, Changing health behaviour).

Priorities may change over time, e.g. a moderate salt intake and cardioprotective diet that is important in early CKD is likely to be a lower priority if there is a greater need for nutritional support, and ensuring a high energy intake and adequate protein may mean foods that are higher in fat, sugar and salt are included in the diet. Cardiovascular death in later stages of CKD is more likely to be due to non-traditional risk factors such as phosphate control. Good glycaemic control is important in preventing or delaying the progression of early CKD in those with diabetes; however, in stage 5 CKD, opinion suggests that less strict glycaemic control may be preferable because this may reduce the risk of hypoglycaemia (JBDSIC, 2016).

Micronutrients

Individuals with CKD who are advised to follow dietary restrictions may be at increased risk of low vitamin status. However, there are no specific recommendations for the routine vitamin, mineral or trace element supplementation of this group. Patients should be assessed on an individual basis. The task of the dietitian, when advising on dietary restrictions, is to maintain adequate intakes of micronutrients from dietary sources as far as possible. CKD results in a rise in vitamin A levels, up to 20% above baseline, primarily due to an increase in retinol-binding protein; however, toxicity is rare as the vitamin is bound to protein and is therefore inactive. High-dose supplements of folic acid, pyridoxine and vitamin B_{12} in CKD have no beneficial effect on cardiovascular morbidity or mortality, and are not recommended (Jamison *et al.*, 2007; Mann *et al.*, 2008; Zoungas *et al.*, 2008). Limited evidence suggests that patients with CKD following low-potassium diets may have low serum levels of vitamin C. However, a high intake of vitamin C (>2000 mg g/day) is not recommended as it is associated with hyperoxalosis; this may result in oxalate-containing kidney stones and exacerbate CKD. A lower dose (100 mg/day) does not appear to alter serum oxalate in patients on dialysis (Gilmour *et al.*, 1998). Iron deficiency is common when erythropoietin therapy is used; oral supplementation is ineffective, and parenteral iron is often required.

Abnormal renal metabolism, inadequate intake and/or gastrointestinal absorption and dialysis losses account for vitamin deficiencies among dialysis patients (Fouque *et al.*, 2007). ESPEN recommends 1 mg folic acid, 10–20 mg pyridoxine and 30–60 mg vitamin C daily for these patients. Routine water-soluble vitamin prescription is also supported by the Renal Association (2010). This may be particularly relevant for those on HHD, where it is likely that water-soluble vitamin losses are further increased due to the greater time spent on dialysis. The provision of water-soluble vitamins is associated with significantly lower mortality rates; however, few UK units prescribe these (Fissell *et al.*, 2004). This may be due to conflicting opinion that, despite the theoretical need for vitamin supplementation, there is insufficient evidence to support routine supplementation, with the suggestion that previous studies may be limited by outdated dietary patterns and dialysis technologies. In practice, vitamin supplementation may be based on individual assessments (Bryan *et al.*, 2015).

HD does not induce significant trace element losses, and routine supplementation is not recommended; however, supplementation of zinc (15 mg/day) and selenium (50–70 mg/day) may be useful in depleted patients (Cano *et al.*, 2006; Gilmour *et al.*, 1998). There are no recommendations regarding vitamin supplementation for PD; the limited research in this area suggests that there may be deficiency of some B vitamins and vitamin C. Individual dietary assessment will help establish if supplementation is necessary. For those with a successful renal transplant, regular supplementation is not needed (Martins *et al.*, 2004). Table 7.5.7 summarises the requirements of the key nutrients to be considered in kidney disease.

Acute kidney injury

Acute kidney injury (AKI) describes the abrupt deterioration in kidney function. The definition of AKI has

Table 7.5.7 Dietary components and kidney disease

	Protein	Energy	Potassium	Phosphate	Sodium and fluid
Significance	Sufficient quantities needed to avoid PEW	Sufficient quantities required to maintain energy balance and prevent PEW	Hyperkalaemia may cause cardiac arrhythmias/arrest	Hyperphosphataemia involved with development of CKD–mineral and bone disorder	Excess intake leads to fluid overload and hypertension
AKI	0.8–1.7 g/kg BW (up to 2.5 g/kg BW in critical care setting)	20–30 kcal/kgBW/day	As required	As required	As required
CKD stages 1–3	>0.8 g/kg BW	Aim to achieve ideal weight	Unlimited unless hyperkalaemic	No limitation	5–6 g salt (rarely fluid overloaded)
Nephrotic syndrome	0.8–1.0 g/kg IBW	30–35 kcal/kg IBW	Unlimited unless hyperkalaemic	Unlimited unless hyperphosphataemic	5–6 g salt + fluid limited if overloaded
CKD stage 4	0.8–1.3 g/kg IBW	30–35 kcal/kg IBW	Unlimited unless hyperkalaemic	If phosphate or PTH levels raised: Limit intake of food additives Ensure adequate protein intake	5–6 g salt + fluid limited if overloaded
Haemodialysis	Minimum 1.1–1.2 g/kg IBW (No more than 1.4 g/kg)	30–40 kcal/kg IBW	Intake may be limited to approximately 1 mmol/kg of BW if hyperkalaemic	If phosphate or PTH levels raised: Limit intake of food additives Ensure adequate protein intake	5–6 g salt + fluid limitation usually required
Peritoneal dialysis	Minimum 1.0–1.2 g/kg IBW	30–35 kcal/kg IBW (including glucose absorbed from dialysate)	Unlimited unless hyperkalaemic	If phosphate or PTH levels raised: Limit intake of food additives Ensure adequate protein intake	5–6 g salt + fluid limitation usually required
Transplant	0.8–1 g/kg, long term	Aim to maintain desirable weight	Unlimited unless hyperkalaemic	Hypophosphataemia is common	5–6 g salt

Recommended intakes are for daily amounts. CKD, chronic kidney disease; PTH, parathyroid hormone; BW, body weight; IBW, ideal body weight.

changed in recent years, and detection is now mostly based on monitoring creatinine levels, with or without urine output. Criteria such as RIFLE (Bellomo *et al.*, 2004) and AKIN (Mehta *et al.*, 2007) have been used to diagnose AKI. KDIGO (2012b) has produced a clinical practice guideline for AKI, which includes a globally acceptable definition by merging aspects of both RIFLE and AKIN, defining its severity in three stages. This should enable the comparison of incidence, management and outcomes of AKI (Table 7.5.8).

In general terms, AKI differs from CKD, in that the decline in renal function is rapid, taking place over hours or days, and is potentially reversible. It covers a broad spectrum of conditions and clinical settings. Forms of kidney injury can be mild or severe, and the condition of individuals may vary from being mobile around the ward with a short-term episode, to being cared for in the critical care unit with multi-organ failure. RRT may or may not be required. The causes of AKI are shown in Table 7.5.9. There is an overlap between the first two groups as any prerenal cause can lead to ischemic

Table 7.5.8 Stages of acute kidney injury

Stage	Serum creatinine	Urine output
Stage 1	1.5–1.9 × baseline OR ≥0.3 mg/dl (≥26.5 μmol/L) increase	<0.5 mL/kg/h for 6–12 h
Stage 2	2.0–2.9 times baseline	<0.5 mL/kg/h for ≥12 h
Stage 3	3.0 × baseline OR Increase in serum creatinine to ≥4.0 mg/dL (≥352.6 μmol/L) OR Initiation if RRT OR In patients <18 years, decrease in eGFR to <35 mL/min per 1.73 m²	<0.3 mL/kg/h for ≥ 24 h OR Anuria for ≥12 h

SECTION 7

Table 7.5.9 Causes of acute kidney injury

Location	Cause	Example
Prerenal	Reduced intravascular volume	Blood loss, gastroenteritis, diuretics, hypoalbuminaemia, burns
	Cardiac failure	Sepsis
	Vasodilatation	Renal artery disease
	Increased resistance to renal blood flow	Renal vein thrombosis
	Hepatorenal syndrome[a]	
Renal	Glomerular disease	Primary renal disease, or as part of a multisystem disorder (includes any cause of acute glomerulonephritis)
	Intrarenal vascular disease	Vasculitis
		Atheroembolic disease
		Haemolytic uraemic syndrome
	Tubulointerstitial disease	Acute tubular necrosis: post-ischaemic (prerenal)[b]
		Toxic agents: drugs, poisons, X ray contrast
		Acute interstitial nephritis: infective, infiltration (e.g. lymphoma), drug reaction
Post-renal	Intrarenal obstruction	Crystals: uric acid, oxalate, calcium
Obstruction to the flow of urine can be at any level, from the intrarenal tubules to the urethra		Abnormal proteins, e.g. myeloma
	Ureteric obstruction (needs to be bilateral unless only one functioning kidney)	
	Bladder outflow obstruction	Prostate or bladder tumours, calculi
	Urethral obstruction	Tumours, strictures

[a]The hepatorenal syndrome is an incompletely understood syndrome in which AKI occurs in association with liver failure. Liver failure is the primary lesion, and renal function generally improves as the hepatic failure recovers.
[b]Acute tubular necrosis can result from any prerenal cause if of sufficient duration and intensity. It is most commonly seen in the context of sepsis, trauma, major surgery and cardiac failure.

damage to the kidney, causing the pathological acute tubular necrosis.

AKI is estimated to affect 13–18% of general hospital admissions (NICE, 2013) and between 20% (Hegarty *et al.*, 2005) and 57% of critically ill patients (Hoste *et al.*, 2015). In emergency hospital admissions, up to one in five are believed to be associated with AKI (Wang *et al.*, 2012). It is more likely to develop in individuals with pre-existing CKD, and is more common in older individuals. Patients may present with a reduced urine volume or with general symptoms such as nausea and vomiting. More serious presentations include pulmonary oedema, pericarditis, confusion or depressed levels of consciousness. It may also be detected incidentally following blood tests performed either routinely or to investigate other complaints.

Outcome is dependent on the cause of AKI; patients die from the severity of the underlying disease and complications rather than from AKI. Nevertheless, AKI has been associated with a more than fourfold increased likelihood of death (Wang *et al.*, 2012), and a prolonged length of hospital stay by 2 days (Liangos *et al.*, 2006) as compared to hospital patients without AKI. Low energy intake, high CRP level, the presence of oedema, negative nitrogen balance and lower resistance measured during bioelectrical impedance analysis were significantly associated with risk of death in patients with AKI (Berbel *et al.*, 2014). Hypercatabolism was most closely related to increased mortality in AKI. PEW (or malnutrition) is an important predictor of mortality in patients with AKI, independent of complications and comorbidities (Fiaccadori *et al.*, 1999). Up to 42% of patients with AKI present with signs of severe malnutrition (Cano *et al.*, 2006).

Appropriate nutritional support may improve outcomes; however, recommendations are based on expert opinion only (Fiaccadori *et al.*, 2013a; KDIGO, 2012b; Kopple *et al.*, 2013; Renal Association, 2011a). The diagnosis of PEW in patients affected by AKI is difficult. There is insufficient evidence to support the effectiveness of nutritional support in AKI, and further high-quality studies are required (Li *et al.*, 2012).

Management of acute kidney injury

The medical and nutritional management of patients with AKI are closely linked, and are dependent on the patient's clinical state. Consequently, treatment regimens will need to be tailored to the particular needs of the individual.

Medical management

Unless the patient presents with a life-threatening indication for urgent RRT (e.g. pulmonary oedema, severe hyperkalaemia or pericarditis), initial treatment will be aimed at the underlying cause of AKI. This will involve efforts to preserve kidney function, together with investigations to elucidate the cause of kidney failure. Since the kidneys are dependent on an adequate blood supply, measures to restore the circulating blood volumes and blood pressure are important. Other important general measures include aggressive treatment of sepsis and measures to improve cardiac function if impaired. Patients with an intrinsic renal cause will need further investigation, possibly including a renal biopsy, to ascertain whether any specific therapy is needed. More general management includes withdrawal of potentially nephrotoxic agents from the patient's therapy. Where the patient's urinary tract is obstructed, prompt relief of the obstruction may preserve renal function.

If the cause of AKI cannot be reversed, then it is likely that RRT will become necessary. A number of treatment options are available, and the modality chosen will reflect the clinical need, together with the facilities available locally. Intermittent HD (IHD), as discussed earlier in CKD, can be used in AKI patients who are stable. Dialysis treatment will usually be undertaken on alternate days or, in some cases, daily. If the patient is oliguric, fluid balance becomes a critical aspect of management since intermittent HD provides limited opportunity for fluid removal. For individuals with cardiovascular instability, continuous RRT (CRRT) is the most suitable mode of RRT. It provides efficient correction of blood biochemistry and the steady removal of fluid, making it suitable for treating the sickest of patients. Continuous RRT can take a number of different forms, with haemofiltration being commonly employed. This technique involves blood passing across a filter to remove waste products and electrolytes. A sterile replacement solution infusion maintains fluid balance. Running continuously over the day, CRRT enables large volumes of fluid to be removed. Sustained low-efficiency dialysis (SLED) is a recent new type of RRT in which conventional HD machines are used to provide extended duration RRT (8–12h vs 3–4h with classic intermittent HD). SLED has emerged as an alternative to CRRT in patients with hemodynamic instability (Kitchlu *et al.*, 2015).

There is very little research on nutritional losses and nutritional requirements in SLED. A small study showed that the amino acid losses are similar to those of CRRT; however, in view of the lack of evidence, no clear recommendations can be made (Umber *et al.*, 2014). Other preliminary data showed that unadjusted losses of free amino acids and 18 trace elements in IHD and sustained low-efficiency diafiltration (SLED-F) appear to be similar, despite theoretical concerns that the extended hybrid treatment might confer increased risk of micronutrient loss (Oh *et al.*, 2015).

Dietetic management

The general aim is to maintain nutritional status while limiting the complications of AKI. Early intervention is preferable since the timescale is much shorter in AKI than in CKD. Nutritional requirements are influenced by a number of factors, and can vary greatly between individuals (Table 7.5.10). Individualised assessment will enable the nutritional prescription to be matched to the patient's needs. It is recommended that a dietitian conducts this assessment (Renal Association, 2011a).

Energy requirements

AKI has no effect on an individual's energy requirements (KDIGO, 2012b; Schneeweiss *et al.*, 1990). Even in patients with AKI and multiorgan failure, measured energy requirements are only 20–30% above resting (Bouffard *et al.*, 1987; Fiaccadori *et al.*, 2013a; KDIGO, 2012b; McCarthy & Phipps, 2014). Where possible, actual energy requirements should be evaluated by indirect calorimetry (McClave *et al.*, 2016). This is often not available in clinical practice, and an individualised assessment using standard or specific formulae can be undertaken. Some authors recommend a total energy intake of 20–30kcal/kg/day in patients with any stage of AKI, highlighting the importance of avoiding overfeeding; targeting a plasma blood glucose of between 6.1 and 8.3mmol/L; promoting 20kcal/kg/day to start with; and adjusting this according to the individual patient's needs (KDIGO, 2012b; McCarthy & Phipps, 2014). Others suggest 25–30kcal/kg/day in patients with AKI in the critical care setting (McClave *et al.*, 2016).

Protein

While absolute protein requirements are not well documented, they are influenced by the patient's clinical condition, together with any RRT they receive. While the stages for AKI (Table 7.5.8) refer to the degree of AKI, from a dietetic point of view, AKI can be further classified depending on level of catabolism; however, it is important to interpret catabolism as a phase and not as present or absent. Common causes of AKI in a non-catabolic state include dehydration, nephrotoxins and urinary obstruction. In these cases, protein turnover rates are not increased, and the recommended daily intakes are 0.8–1.0g protein/kg of body weight when RRT is not required, and 1.1–1.5g/kg of body weight where RRT is required (KDIGO, 2012b; Naylor *et al.*, 2013). The recent ESPEN-endorsed recommendation for protein intake in patients aged >65years with an acute illness was 1.2–1.5g/day or higher (Deutz *et al.*, 2014). However, AKI is not mentioned in these guidelines, and, as a result, these guidelines should be interpreted with caution. Oral diet alone, or with nutritionally dense supplementary sip feeds, will frequently be sufficient to meet nutritional needs. If not, artificial nutritional support should be implemented. Wherever possible, this should be provided

Table 7.5.10 Nutritional requirements in acute kidney injury

	AKI in a non-catabolic state			AKI in a catabolic state		
	No RRT (KDIGO, 2012b)	IHD (Naylor *et al.*, 2013)	CRRT	RRT	IHD (KDIGO, 2012b)	CRRT (KDIGO, 2012b)
Protein (g/kg BW/day)	0.8–1.0	≥1.1	1.1–1.5	≥1.0	1.0–1.5 (Cano *et al.*, 2006; KDIGO, 2012b) 1.5–2.0 (Gervasio *et al.*, 2011; Patel *et al.*, 2017)	Up to 1.7 in hypercatabolism (KDIGO, 2012b) 1.5–2.5 in critically ill patients (McClave *et al.*, 2016; Patel *et al.*, 2017)
Energy	Not affected by AKI. Tailored to individual requirements, clinical state and metabolic response. Some authors suggest 20–30 kcal/kg/day (100–130% of resting energy expenditure; KDIGO, 2012b) even in the critical care setting. Others instead promote 25–30 kcal/kg/day in ICU patients with AKI (McClave *et al.*, 2016).					
Fluid	Fluid requirements need individual medical assessment. Standard fluid equations are unlikely to be helpful. Fluid balance and daily weights should be monitored closely. Fluid requirements are usually increased in stage 1 and 2, and sometimes restricted in stage 3. Post-AKI patients may enter a polyuric phase in which requirements increase significantly: daily monitoring and liaising with the medical team is key.					
Electrolytes	Monitor and adjust intake as required on an individual basis. This will vary depending on disease state and type of treatment. Solutions used in CRRT may contain electrolytes. Equally, electrolytes may drop significantly as a result of CRRT. Ongoing monitoring is required.					
Micronutrients	Requirements are not well documented. Levels of fat-soluble vitamins and anti-oxidant status may be low (although this does not necessarily translate into nutritional deficiency as other causes may contribute to this). CRRT has a negative effect on the balance of some vitamins and trace elements. Whether micronutrient supplementation improves outcomes is unknown (Oh *et al.*, 2015).					

Recommendations for kg/body weight refer to actual body weight; however, special care should be taken to avoid refeeding in obese individuals (where IBW may be used). Critical care specific equations and/or other methods may be used for patients in intensive care units to avoid the risk of overfeeding (Frankenfield *et al.*, 2004).

IHD, intermittent HD; RRT, renal replacement therapy; CRRT, continuous RRT.

via the enteral route. Nutritionally dense feeds, with or without reduced electrolyte content, are useful when the control of fluid balance and/or serum phosphate and potassium levels is an issue. Most patients with AKI in a non-catabolic state do not require RTT; however, in some situations, RRT may be required (e.g. patients admitted with drug toxicity such as lithium may not be metabolically stressed but require RRT to remove the toxins).

Fluid and electrolytes

Fluid and electrolyte intake should be individualised according to blood biochemistry and fluid status. Frequent monitoring of blood biochemistry is essential to guide provision. Indications for potassium, phosphate, sodium and fluid restriction are similar to those in CKD. However, allowing a more liberal phosphate intake may be a better management approach if it helps to promote food intake. In the short term, maintaining a good nutritional intake is more of a priority than achieving serum phosphate control. Dietary restrictions are likely to be required until renal function begins to improve; patients may become polyuric at this stage. An increased fluid intake (adequate to cover the large urine volumes and insensible losses) should then be maintained. As serum potassium and phosphate levels normalise, any dietary restrictions must be lifted. Sometimes these levels drop in the polyuric phase, and they may require supplementation.

Nutrition support in acute kidney injury for those in a catabolic state

The causes of AKI in a catabolic state include sepsis and trauma; protein turnover rates in these patients are increased, and negative nitrogen balance results. Patients will frequently have multiorgan failure and be managed in an intensive care unit. They present complex therapeutic challenges and require a broad appreciation of the management of nutrition in critical illness. Such issues are beyond the scope of any discussion, but major considerations in relation to AKI are outlined in the following text (see also Chapter 7.17.1, Critical care).

Artificial nutritional support will usually be required. Where the enteral route cannot be used, parenteral nutrition support should be considered. Energy should be provided as a balance of carbohydrate and fat, since patients will have both impaired glucose tolerance and reduced lipid clearance (Druml *et al.*, 1983; Fiaccadori *et al.*, 2010; Kopple *et al.*, 2013). Nitrogen should be sourced from a standard mixture of essential and non-essential amino acids (Brown *et al.*, 2010), as some non-essential amino acids become conditionally essential in AKI and critical illness.

During CRRT, care is needed to avoid the potential overprovision of energy from hidden sources. The metabolism of glucose, lactate and citrate contained in some of the solutions and anticoagulants used during CRRT may result in significant energy gains; 1 mmol of lactate provides 0.32 kcal (Casaer *et al.*, 2008). However, in clinical practice, it is difficult to estimate net energy gains from lactate, as this is based on an assumption that all lactate provided is entirely oxidised. In newer replacement solutions, bicarbonate has replaced lactate as a buffer, and consequently there will be no energy gain. Another potential source of CRRT-derived energy is citrate (an anti-coagulant used instead of heparin solutions); 1 mmol of citrate provides 0.59 kcal. However, the net energy gain depends on the dose infused and the amount removed by CRRT (Balik *et al.*, 2016; Oudemans-van Straten & Ostermann, 2012). This area is explored in more detail elsewhere (Hartley, 2011; McCarthy & Phipps, 2014). Continuous RRT also has a negative influence on nutrient balance with significant losses of amino acids, up to 10% of those provided (Davies *et al.*, 1991; Frankenfield *et al.*, 1993; McCarthy & Phipps, 2014). Protein intakes should be increased to compensate for these losses and the patient's catabolic rate (Brown *et al.*, 2010; Fiaccadori *et al.*, 2005). A daily protein intake up to a maximum 1.7 g/kg for hypercatabolic individuals on CRRT has been recommended (Cano *et al.*, 2009; KDIGO, 2012b; Renal Association, 2011a). However, some authors suggest that it may be safe to provide up to 2.0 g/kg/day in patients with hypercatabolism receiving RTT (Gervasio *et al.*, 2011; Patel *et al.*, 2017), and others suggest 2.5 g/kg/day in the ICU setting and CRRT (McClave *et al.*, 2016; Patel *et al.*, 2017). It is important to remember that these recommendations are based on small sample sizes of patients, the majority of who were fed via parenteral nutrition (Brown *et al.*, 2010; Patel *et al.*, 2017). Careful interpretation of these studies is required for clinical practice. In addition, such an increase in protein provision should provide sufficient energy to meet requirements; it is often difficult to meet these high protein requirements in clinical practice. Concerns have been raised regarding the safety of protein intakes of >2.5 g/kg/day, as the provided nitrogen may be used as an energy source or could even have a pro-inflammatory effect (Casaer *et al.*, 2008). To achieve high protein intakes in enterally fed patients without excessive energy, protein-rich supplements can be added to feeds to increase the nitrogen-to-energy ratio.

Continuous RRT allows feed volumes and electrolyte intake to be liberalised; clearance rates are so great that intravenous supplementation with phosphate and other electrolytes may be required. However, technical advances have led to the development of newer solutions that should result in less supplementation being required. A significant decline in serum phosphate levels during CRRT is associated with higher incidence of prolonged respiratory failure requiring tracheostomy (Bellomo *et al.*, 2004; Demirjian *et al.*, 2011; McCarthy & Phipps, 2014). Frequent monitoring is essential.

Nutrition support in acute kidney injury for those not on dialysis with increased protein requirements

Patients who present with AKI and either a pressure ulcer or a large wound, but who do not need dialysis, are likely to have higher protein requirements. However, a high protein intake may also increase endogenous ureagenesis. Absolute protein requirements are not well documented in AKI without dialysis, but will be influenced by the underlying clinical condition. It is recommended to avoid restricting protein intake with the aim of preventing or delaying the initiation of RRT. Nutritional management should aim at supplying sufficient protein to maintain metabolic balance (National Kidney Federation KDIGO, 2012b).

Nutrition and hydration play important roles in preserving skin and tissue viability and in supporting tissue repair for pressure ulcer healing (Posthauer *et al.*, 2015). Recent guidelines suggest a protein provision of 1.25–1.5 g/kg of body weight/day (NPUAP/EPUAP/PPPIA, 2014). In patients with AKI (but without the need for dialysis) who are metabolically stressed, protein provision should start with at least 1 g/kg BW/day. If a higher protein intake is provided, frequent monitoring (urea and creatinine) of these patients will be required, as renal function can change rapidly (Fiaccadori *et al.*, 2010). However, it is important to remember that protein provision is not the only factor affecting urea production. Corticosteroids, gastrointestinal bleeding, hypokalaemia, hyperglycaemia and intravascular volume depletion too can also affect urea levels (Krenitsky & Rosner, 2011). An increase in protein provision in these patients should be aligned with increased fluid provision, unless this is clinically contraindicated (Kopple *et al.*, 2013).

Micronutrients in acute kidney injury

Micronutrient requirements in AKI are not well defined. Plasma levels of vitamins A, D, E (Druml *et al.*, 1998; Lai *et al.*, 2013), together with selenium and zinc (Berger *et al.*, 2004; Story *et al.*, 1999), are lower in AKI than in normal subjects. Levels of water-soluble vitamins are usually low, with mixed results reported for vitamin C (Berger *et al.*, 2004; Renal Association, 2011a). Micronutrient losses on CRRT may be significant, but they have not been carefully quantified (McCarthy & Phipps, 2014). Documented daily ultrafiltrate losses include 100 mg vitamin C (Bellomo & Boyce, 1993), 290 µg folate (Fortin *et al.*, 1999) and 4 mg thiamine (Berger *et al.*, 2004). Since the losses of vitamin C, thiamine and selenium exceed the amounts provided by commonly used parenteral sources, and for some of these nutrients in many enteral feeds, selective micronutrient supplementation may be needed. In patients receiving CRRT, some experts (McCarthy & Phipps, 2014) recommend a supplementation of thiamine (25–100 mg/day), folate (1 mg/day) and pyridoxine (10 mg/day), although these are based on expert opinion only (Gervasio *et al.*, 2011; Renal Association, 2011). On the other hand, other experts suggest that it is not yet known whether micronutrient losses are clinically significant, or whether their replacement would improve patient outcomes (Oh *et al.*, 2015).

Megadoses of vitamin C are potentially toxic because of the danger of secondary oxalosis in kidney disease. Cases of severe oxalosis have been reported in individuals with AKI receiving daily vitamin C supplements of 500 mg intravenously (Friedman *et al.*, 1983) or 5000 mg orally (Mashour *et al.*, 2000). Therefore, it is recommended not to exceed 100 mg per day in patients not requiring CRRT; some experts allow supplementation of up to 200 mg per day for patients requiring CRRT (McCarthy & Phipps, 2014), while others suggest to not provide any vitamin C supplementation (Renal Association, 2011a).

No safe level for vitamin A supplementation has been determined due to concerns of deficient retinol degradation (McCarthy & Phipps, 2014). Very little is known about the role of vitamin D in AKI. An RCT in a general population of critically ill patients with vitamin D deficiency showed that supplementation did not reduce the length of stay or reduce mortality, with the exception of a subgroup of patients with vitamin D levels less than 30 ng/mL (Amrein *et al.*, 2014). An ongoing trial is investigating whether there is a difference in vitamin D between critically ill adult patients with and without AKI (NIHR, 2016).

Acknowledgment

The editor acknowledges the prior contribution of George Hartley, Christel Lyell and Nicki Ruddock.

Internet resources

BDA Renal Nutrition Group, www.bda.uk.com
Kidney Disease; Improving Global Outcomes, http://www.kdigo.org
Kidney Patient Guide, www.kidneypatientguide.org.uk
National Kidney Foundation (USA), http://www.kidney.org
NICE Clinical guideline 169: Prevention, detection and management of AKI up to the point of renal replacement therapy, http://www.nice.org.uk/cg169
NICE Pathways Chronic Kidney Disease Overview, http://pathways.nice.org.uk/pathways/chronic-kidney-disease/chronic-kidney-disease-overview
Renal Association, www.renal.org
UK National Kidney Federation, www.kidney.org.uk

Useful recipe books

Jackson H, Cassidy A, James G. (2006) *Eating Well with Kidney Failure*. London: Class Publishing.
Jackson H, Green C, James G. (2009) *Eating Well for Kidney Health*. London: Class Publishing.

References

Abrass CK. (2004) Overview: obesity: what does it have to do with kidney disease? *J. Am. Soc. Nephrol.* 15: 2768–2772.

Amrein K, Schnedl C, Holl A, *et al.* (2014) Effect of high dose vitamin D on hospital length of stay in critically ill patients with vitamin D deficiency. *JAMA*. 312: 1520–1530.

Bakris GL, Siomos M, Richardson D, *et al.* (2000) ACE inhibition or angiotensin receptor blockade: impact on potassium in renal failure. *Kidney Int.* 58: 2084–2092.

Balik M., Zakharchenko M. (2015) *Bioenergetic Gain of Citrate-Anticoagulated Continuous Renal Replacement Therapy*. In: Rajendram R., Preedy V.R., Patel V.B. (eds) Diet and Nutrition in Critical Care. Springer, New York, NY.

BDA Renal Nutrition Group. (2015) *Consensus statement on nutrition support and the use of oral nutritional supplements in patients with stages 4–5 chronic kidney disease*. Available at https://nutrition.abbott/uk/news/improved-nutritional-management-for-CKD-patients. Accessed 6 January 2018.

BDA Renal Nutrition Group. (2016) *Dietary Advice Post Renal Transplantation*. Available at www.bda.uk.com/regionsgroups/groups/renal/dietary_advice_post_renal_transplant_toolkit. Non-members should contact BDA directly, www.bda.co.uk. Accessed 26 October 2018.

Bellomo R, Boyce N. (1993) Acute continuous hemodiafiltration: a prospective study of 110 patients and a review of the literature. *Am. J. Kidney Dis.* 21(5): 508–518.

Bellomo R, Ronco C, Kellum JA, *et al.* (2004) Acute renal failure – definition, outcome measures, animal models, fluid therapy and information technology needs: the Second International Consensus Conference of the Acute Dialysis Quality Initiative (ADQI) Group. *Crit. Care*. 8(4): R204–R212.

Bennett SE, Russell GI, Walls J. (1983) Low-protein diets in uraemia. *Br. Med. J.* 287: 1344–1345.

Berbel MN, De Goes CA, Balbi AL, *et al.* (2014) Nutritional parameters are associated with mortality in AKI. *Clinics (Sao Paulo)*. 69: 476–482.

Berger MM, Shenkin A, Revelly JP, *et al.* (2004) Copper, selenium, zinc, and thiamine balances during continuous venovenous hemodiafiltration in critically ill patients. *Am. J. Clin. Nutr.* 80(2): 410–416.

Bernardi A, Biasia F, Pati T, *et al.* (2003) Long-term protein intake control in kidney transplant recipients: effect in kidney graft function and in nutritional status. *Am. J. Kidney Dis.* 41(3 Suppl 1): S146–152.

Bossola M, Tazza L, Giungi S, *et al.* (2010) Artificial nutritional support in chronic hemodialysis patients: a narrative review. *J. Ren. Nutr.* 20(4): 213–223.

Bouffard Y, Viale JP, Annat G, *et al.* (1987) Energy expenditure in the acute renal failure patient mechanically ventilated. *Intensive Care Med.* 13: 401–404.

Brown RO, Compher C; American Society for Parenteral and Enteral Nutrition. (2010) A.S.P.E.N. clinical guidelines: nutrition support in adult acute and chronic renal failure. *JPEN J. Parenter. Enteral Nutr.* 34(4): 366–377.

Bryan M. Tucker, DO, Sami Safadi, MD, et al. (2015) Is routine multivitamin supplementation necessary in US chronic adult hemodialysis patients? A systematic review. *J. Renal Nutr.* 25(3): 257–264.

Burton C, Harris KP. (1996) The role of proteinuria in the progression of chronic renal failure. *Am. J. Kidney Dis.* 27: 765–775.

Campbell KL, Ash S, Zabel R, *et al.* (2009) Implementation of standardised nutrition guidelines by renal dietitians is associated with improved nutrition status. *J. Ren. Nutr.* 19(2): 136–144.

Caldeira D, Amaral T, David C, *et al.* (2011) Educational strategies to reduce serum phosphorus in hyperphosphatemic patients with chronic kidney disease: systematic review with meta-analysis. *J. Ren. Nutr.* 21(4): 285–294.

Cano N, Fiaccadori E, Tesinsky P, *et al.* (2006) ESPEN guidelines on enteral nutrition: adult renal failure. *Clin. Nutr.* 25: 295–310.

Cano NJM, Fouque D, Roth H, *et al.*; and the French Study Group for Nutrition in Dialysis. (2007a) Intradialytic parenteral nutrition does not improve survival in malnourished hemodialysis patients: a 2-year multicenter, prospective, randomised study. *J. Am. Soc. Nephrol.* 18: 2583–2591.

Cano AE, Neil AK, Kang JY, *et al.* (2007b) Gastrointestinal symptoms in patients with end-stage renal disease undergoing treatment by hemodialysis or peritoneal dialysis. *Am. J. Gastroenterol.* 102: 1990–1997.

Cano NJ, Aparicio M, Brunori G, *et al.*; ESPEN. (2009) ESPEN guidelines on parenteral nutrition: adult renal failure. *Clin. Nutr.* 28(4): 401–414.

Caravaca F, Arrobas M, Dominguez C. (1999) Influence of residual renal function on dietary protein and calorie intake in patients on incremental peritoneal dialysis. *Perit. Dial. Int.* 19(4): 350–356.

Carrero J, Burrowes J, Warner C. (2016) A long road to travel: adherence to dietary recommendations and adequate dietary phosphorus control. *J. Ren. Nutr.* 26(3): 133–135.

Carrigan A, Klinger A, Choquette S, *et al.* (2014) Contribution of food additives to sodium and phosphorus content of diets rich in processed foods. *J. Ren. Nutr.* 24(1): 13–19, 19e1.

Casaer MP, Mesotten D, Schetz MR. (2008) Bench-to-bedside review: metabolism and nutrition. *Crit. Care* 12: 222–252.

Chan M, Patwardhan A, Ryan C, *et al.* (2011) Evidence based practice guidelines for the nutritional management of adult kidney transplant recipients. *J. Ren. Nutr.* 21(1): 47–51.

Cheng LT, Tang W, Wang T. (2005) Strong association between volume status and nutritional status in peritoneal dialysis patients. *Am. J. Kidney Dis.* 45(5): 891–902.

Chumlea WC, Dwyer J, Bergen C, *et al.* (2003) Nutritional status assessed from anthropometric measures in the HEMO study. *J. Ren. Nutr.* 13: 31–38.

Chung SH, Lindholm B, Lee HB. (2000) Influence of initial nutritional status on continuous ambulatory peritoneal dialysis patient survival. *Perit. Dial. Int.* 20: 19–26.

Cuppari L, Avesani C. (2004) Energy requirements in patients with chronic kidney disease. *J. Ren. Nutr.* 14(3): 121–126.

Danovitch GM. (2005) *Handbook of Kidney transplantation, 4th edn. Nutrition in the Kidney Transplant Recipient.* Philadelphia: Lippincott Williams & Wilkins.

Davidson J, Wilkinson A, Dantal J, *et al.* (2003) New-onset diabetes after transplantation: 2003 international consensus guidelines. *Transplantation.* 75(10): SS3–SS24.

Davies SP, Reaveley DA, Brown EA, *et al.* (1991) Amino acid clearances and daily losses in patients with acute renal failure treated by continuous arteriovenous hemodialysis. *Crit. Care.* 19(12): 1510–1515.

de Brito-Ashurst I, Varagunam M, Raftery MJ, *et al.* (2009) Bicarbonate supplementation slows progression of CKD and improves nutritional status. *J. Am. Soc. Nephrol.* 20: 2075–2084.

Demirjian S, Teo BW, Guzman JA, *et al.* (2011) Hypophosphatemia during continuous hemodialysis is associated with prolonged respiratory failure in patients with AKI. *Nephrol. Dial. Transplant.* 26: 3508–3514.

de Mutsert R, Grootendorst DC, Boeschoten EW, *et al.* (2009) Subjective global assessment of nutritional status is strongly associated with mortality in chronic dialysis patients. *Am. J. Clin. Nutr.* 89: 787–793.

Deutz NEP, Bauer JM, Barazzoni R, *et al.* (2014) Protein intake and exercise for optimal muscle function with aging: recommendation from ESPEN Expert Group. *Clin. Nutr.* 33: 929–936.

DH. (2004) *The National Service Framework for Renal Services.* Available at http://webarchive.nationalarchives.gov.uk/+/http://www.dh.gov.uk/en/Healthcare/Longtermconditions/Vascular/Renal/DH_4102636. Accessed 3 January 2018.

Diabetes Control and Complications Trial (DCCT) Research Group. (1993) The effect of intensive treatment of diabetes on the development and progression of long-term complications in insulin-dependent diabetes mellitus. *N. Engl. J. Med.* 329: 977–986.

Dombros N, Dratwa M, Feriani M, *et al.* (2005) European best practice guidelines for peritoneal dialysis. 8 Nutrition in peritoneal dialysis. *Nephrol. Dial. Transplant.* 20(9): ix28–ix33.

Druml W, Laggner AN, Widhalm K, *et al.* (1983) Lipid metabolism in acute renal failure. *Kidney Int. Suppl.* 16: S139–S142.

Druml W, Schwarzenhofer M, Apsner R, *et al.* (1998) Fat-soluble vitamins in patients with acute renal failure. *Miner. Electrolyte Metab.* 24: 220–226.

Enia G, Sicuso C, Alati G, *et al.* (1993) Subjective global assessment of nutrition in dialysis patients. *Nephrol. Dial. Transplant.* 8: 1094–1098.

Fiaccadori E, Lombardi M, Leonardi S, *et al.* (1999) Prevalence and clinical outcome associated with pre-existing malnutrition in acute renal failure: a prospective cohort study. *J. Am. Soc. Nephrol.* 10: 581–593.

Fiaccadori E, Maggiore U, Rotelli C, *et al.* (2005) Effects of different energy intakes on nitrogen balance in patients with acute renal failure: A pilot study. *Nephrol. Dial. Transplant.* 20: 1976–1980.

Fiaccadori E, Regolisti G, Cabassi A. (2010) Specific nutritional problems in AKI, treated with non-dialysis and dialytic modalities. *NDT. Plus* 3: 1–7.

Fiaccadori E, Regolisti G, Maggiore U. (2013a) Specialized nutritional support interventions in critically ill patients on renal replacement therapy. *Curr. Opin. Clin. Nutr. Metab. Care* 16: 217–224.

Fiaccadori E, Maggiore U, Cabassi A, *et al.* (2013b) Nutritional evaluation and management of AKI patients. *J. Ren. Nutr.* 23: 255–258.

Fissell RB, Bragg-Gresham JL, Gillespie BW, *et al.* (2004) International variation in vitamin prescribing and association with mortality in the Dialysis Outcomes and Practice Patterns Study (DOPPS). *Am. J. Kidney Dis.* 44(2): 293–299.

Fortin MC, Amyot SL, Geadah D, *et al.* (1999) Serum concentrations and clearances of folic acid and pyridoxal-5-phosphate during venovenous continuous renal replacement therapy. *Intensive Care Med.* 25(6): 594–598.

Fouque D, Vennegoor M, Wee PT, *et al.* (2007) EBPG guideline on nutrition. *Nephrol. Dial. Transplant.* 22(2): ii45–ii87.

Fouque D, Kalantar-Zadeh K, Kopple J, *et al.* (2008) A proposed nomenclature and diagnostic criteria for protein–energy wasting in acute and chronic kidney disease. *Kidney Int.* 73: 391–398.

Frankenfield DC, Badellino MM, Reynolds HN, *et al.* (1993) Amino acid loss and plasma concentration during continuous hemodiafiltration. *JPEN J. Parenter. Enteral Nutr.* 17(6): 551–561.

Frankenfield DC, Smith IS, Cooney RN. (2004) Validation of 2 approaches to predicting resting metabolic rate in critically ill patients. *JPEN J. Parenter. Enteral Nutr.* 28(4): 259–264.

Friedman A. (2004) High-protein diets: potential effects on the kidney in renal health and disease. *Am. J. Kidney Dis.* 44(6): 950–962.

Friedman AL, Chesnelof RW, Gilbert FF. (1983) Secondary oxalosis as a complication of parenteral alimentation in ARF. *A. J. Nephrol.* 3: 248–252.

Gervasio J, Garmon W, Holowatyj M. (2011) Nutrition support in AKI. *Nutr. Clin. Pract.* 26: 374–381.

Gilmour ER, Hartley GH, Goodship THJ. (1998) Trace elements and vitamins in renal disease. In: Mitch WE, Klahr S (eds) *Handbook of Nutrition and the Kidney*, 3rd edn. New York: Lippincott-Raven, pp. 105–122.

Giordano M, De Feo P, Lucidi P, *et al.* (2001) Effects of dietary protein restriction on fibrinogen and albumin metabolism in nephrotic patients. *Kidney Int.* 60(1): 235–242.

Goodman WG, Goldin J, Kuizon BD, *et al.* (2000) Coronary-artery calcification in young adults with end-stage renal disease who are undergoing dialysis. *N. Engl. J. Med.* 342(20): 1478–1483.

Guerin AP, London GM, Marchais SJ, *et al.* (2000) Arterial stiffening and vascular calcifications in end-stage renal disease. *Nephrol. Dial. Transplant.* 15(7): 1014–1021.

Hartley GH. (2011) Nutrition in kidney disease. In: Todorovic VE, Micklewright A (eds) *A Pocket Guide to Clinical Nutrition*, 4th edn. Birmingham: British Dietetic Association.

Hegarty J, Middleton RJ, Krebs M, *et al.* (2005) Severe acute renal failure in adults: place of care, incidence and outcomes. *QJM.* 98(9): 661–666.

Heimburger O, Quereshi AR, Blaner WS, *et al.* (2000) Hand-grip muscle strength, lean body mass, and plasma proteins as markers of nutritional status in patients with chronic renal failure close to start of dialysis therapy. *Am. J. Kidney Dis.* 36: 1213–1225.

Holley JL, Kirk J. (2002) Enteral tube feeding in a cohort of chronic hemodialysis patients. *J. Ren. Nutr.* 12(3): 177–182.

Hoste EAJ, Bagshaw SM, Bellomo R, *et al.* (2015) Epidemiology of AKI in critically ill patients: the multinational AKI-EPI study. *Intensive Care Med.* 41: 1411–1423.

Ikizler TA, Green JH, Wingard RL, *et al.* (1995) Spontaneous dietary protein intake during progression of chronic renal failure. *J. Am. Soc. Nephrol.* 6: 1386–1391.

Jamison RL, Hartigan P, Kaufman JS, *et al.* (2007) Effect of homocysteine lowering on mortality and vascular disease in advanced chronic kidney disease and end-stage renal disease: a randomized controlled trial. *JAMA.* 298(10): 1163–1170.

Joint British Diabetes Societies for Inpatient Care (JBDSIC). (2016) Management of adults with diabetes on the haemodialysis unit. Available at http://www.diabetologists-abcd.org.uk/JBDS/JBDS_RenalGuide_2016.pdf. Accessed 3 January 2018.

Jones CH. (2001) Serum albumin – a marker of fluid overload in dialysis patients? *J. Ren. Nutr.* 11: 59–61.

Kalantar-Zadeh K. (2013) Patient education for phosphorus management in chronic kidney disease. *Patient Prefer Adherence.* 7: 379–390.

Kalantar-Zadeh K, Regidor DL, Kovesdy CP, *et al.* (2009) Fluid retention is associated with cardiovascular mortality in patients undergoing long-term hemodialysis. *Circulation.* 119: 671–679.

Kalantar-Zadeh K, Gutekunst L, Mehrotra R, *et al.* (2010) Understanding sources of dietary phosphorus in the treatment of patients with chronic kidney disease. *Clin. J. Am. Soc. Nephrol.* 5: 519–530.

Kasiske BL, Vazquez MA, Harmon WE, *et al.* (2000) Recommendations for the outpatient surveillance of renal transplant recipients. *American Society of Transplantation. J. Am. Soc. Nephrol.* 11: S1–S86.

Kaysen GA, Dubin JA, Muller H, *et al.* (2002) Relationships among inflammation nutrition and physiologic mechanisms establishing albumin levels in hemodialysis patients. *Kidney Int.* 61: 2240–2249.

KDIGO. (2009) KDIGO clinical practice guideline for the care of kidney transplant recipients. *Am. J. Transplant.* 9(S3): S131–S155.

KDIGO. (2012a) *Clinical Practice Guideline for the Evaluation and Management of Chronic Kidney Disease.* Available at http://www.kdigo.org/clinical_practice_guidelines/pdf/CKD/KDIGO_2012_CKD_GL.pdf. Accessed 3 January 2018.

KDIGO. (2012b) Clinical practice guideline for AKI. *Kidney Int. Suppl.* 2(1): 1–138.

KDIGO. (2016) *Clinical Practice Guideline for the Management of Blood Pressure in Chronic Kidney Disease.* Available at http://www.kdigo.org/clinical_practice_guidelines/pdf/KDIGO_BP_GL.pdf. Accessed 3 January 2018.

KDIGO. (2017) Clinical practice guideline update for the diagnosis, evaluation, prevention, and treatment of Chronic Kidney Disease-Mineral and Bone Disorder (CKD–MBD). *Kidney Int. Suppl.* 7: 1–59.

Kitchlu A, Adhikari N, Burns KE, *et al.* (2015) Outcomes of sustained low efficiency dialysis versus continuous renal replacement therapy in critically ill adults with AKI: a cohort study. *BMC Nephrol.* 16: 127.

Kopple JD, Monteon FJ, Shaib JK. (1986) Effect of energy intake on nitrogen metabolism in nondialysed patients with chronic renal failure. *Kidney Int.* 29: 734–742.

Kopple JD, Levey AS, Greene T, *et al.* (1997) Effect of dietary protein restriction on nutritional status in the modification of diet in renal disease study. *Kidney Int.* 52: 778–791.

Kopple JD, Massry SG, Kalanta-Zadeh K. (2013) *Nutritional Management of Renal Disease: Nutritional Management of AKI,* chapter 36, 3rd edn. London: Academic Press; Elsevier, pp. 605–627.

Korgaonkar S, Tilea A, Gillespie BB, *et al.* (2010) Serum potassium and outcomes in CKD: insights from the RRI–CKD Cohort Study. *Clin. J. Am. Soc. Nephrol.* 5: 762–769.

Kovesdy CP, Regidor DL, Mehrotra R, *et al.* (2007) Serum and dialysate potassium concentrations and survival in haemodialysis patients. *Clin. J. Am. Soc. Nephrol.* 2: 999–1007.

Kramer HJ, Saranathan A, Luke A, *et al.* (2006) Increasing body mass index and obesity in the incident ESRD population. *J. Am. Soc. Nephrol.* 17: 1453–1459.

Kramer HJ, Saranathan A, Luke A, *et al.* (2006) Increasing body mass index and obesity in the incident ESRD population. *J. Am. Soc. Nephrol.* 17: 1453–1459.

Krenitsky J, Rosner MH. (2011) Nutritional support for patients with AKI: how much protein is enough or too much? *Pract. Gastroenterol.* 35: 28–42.

Krautzig S, Janssen U, Koch KM, *et al.* (1998) Dietary salt restriction and reduction of dialysate sodium to control hypertension in maintenance haemodialysis patients. *Nephrol. Dial. Transplant.* 13: 552–553.

Lai L, Qian J, Yang Y, *et al.* (2013) Is the serum vitamin D level at the time of hospital-acquired AKI diagnosis associated with prognosis? *PLoS One.* 8(5): e64964.

Lawson JA, Lazarus R, Kelly J. (2001) Prevalence and prognostic significance of malnutrition in chronic renal insufficiency. *J. Ren. Nutr.* 11: 16–22.

Leavey SF, McCullough K, Hecking E, *et al.* (2001) Body mass index and mortality in 'healthier' as compared to 'sicker' haemodialysis patients. Results from the dialysis outcomes and practice patterns study (DOPPS). *Nephrol. Dial. Transplant.* 16: 2386–2394.

Lee A. (2011) Constipation in patients on peritoneal dialysis: a literature review. *Ren. Soc. Aust. J.* 7(3): 122–129.

Levey AS, Adler S, Caggiula AW, *et al.* (1996) Effects of dietary protein restriction on the progression of moderate renal disease in the Modification of Diet in Renal Disease Study. *J. Am. Soc. Nephrol.* 7: 2616–2626.

Li Y, Tang X, Zhang J, *et al.* (2012) Nutritional support for AKI. *Cochrane Database Syst. Rev.* 8: CD005426.

Liangos O, Wald R, O'Bell JW, *et al.* (2006) Epidemiology and outcomes of acute renal failure in hospitalized patients: a national survey. *Clin. J. Am. Soc. Nephrol.* 1: 43–51.

London GM, Guerin AP, Marchais SJ, *et al.* (2003) Arterial media calcification in end-stage renal disease: impact on all-cause and cardiovascular mortality. *Nephrol. Dial. Transplant.* 18(9): 1731–1740.

Lopez-Gomez JM, Villaverde M, Jofre R, *et al.* (2005) Interdialytic weight gain as a marker of blood pressure, nutrition, and survival in hemodialysis patients. *Kidney Int. Suppl.* (93): S63–S68.

MacLaughlin H. (2016) Dialysis patients and obesity: do we know enough to guide practice? *J. Kidney Care.* 1: 68–71.

Mann JF, Sheridan P, McQueen MJ, *et al.*; HOPE-2 investigators. (2008) Homocysteine lowering with folic acid and B vitamins in people with chronic kidney disease – results of the renal Hope-2 study. *Nephrol. Dial. Transplant.* 23(2): 645–653.

Mansy H, Goodship THJ, Tapson JS, *et al.* (1989) Effect of a high protein diet in patients with the nephrotic syndrome. *Clin. Sci.* 77(4): 445–451.

Martins C, Pecoits-Filho R, Riella MC. (2004) Nutrition for the post renal transplant recipients. *Transplant. Proc.* 36: 1650–1654.

Mashour S, Turner JF, Merrell R. (2000) Acute renal failure, oxalosis, and vitamin C supplementation: a case report and review of the literature. *Chest* 118(2): 561–563.

McCarthy MS, Phipps SC. (2014) Special nutrition challenges: current approach to AKI. *Nutr. Clin. Pract.* 29: 56–62.

McClave SA, Taylor BE, Martindale RG, *et al.* (2016) Guidelines for the Provision and Assessment of Nutrition Support Therapy in the Adult Critically Ill Patient: Society of Critical Care Medicine (SCCM) and American Society for Parenteral and Enteral Nutrition (A.S.P.E.N.). *JPEN J. Parenter. Enteral Nutr.* 40: 159–211.

McMahon EJ, Campbell KL, Bauer JD, *et al.* (2015) Altered dietary salt intake for people with chronic kidney disease. *Cochrane Database Syst. Rev.* (2): CD010070.

Mehta RL, Kellum JA, Shah SV, *et al.* (2007) AKI Network: report of an initiative to improve outcomes in AKI. *Crit. Care* 11(2): R31.

Metcalfe W. (2007) How does early chronic kidney disease progress? *Nephrol. Dial. Transplant.* 22(9): ix26–ix30.

Mitch WE, Klahr S. (1993) *Handbook of Nutrition and the Kidney*, 3rd edn. New York: Little, Brown and Company.

Monteen FJ, Laidlaw SA, Shaib JK, *et al.* (1986) Energy expenditure in patients with chronic renal failure. *Kidney Int.* 30: 741–747.

Moorthi RN, Armstrong C, Janda K, *et al.* (2014) The effect of a diet containing 70% protein from plants on mineral metabolism and musculoskeletal health in CKD. *Am. J. Nephrol.* 40: 582–591.

National Kidney Foundation. (2002) K/DOQI Clinical practice guidelines for chronic kidney disease: evaluation, classification and stratification. *Am. J. Kidney Dis.* 39: S1–S266.

National Pressure Ulcer Advisory Panel, European Pressure Ulcer Advisory Panel and Pan Pacific Pressure Injury Alliance (NPUAP/EPUAP/PPPIA). (2014) *Prevention and Treatment of Pressure Ulcers: Quick Reference Guide*. Available at www.npuap.org. Accessed 2 January 2018.

Navaneethan SD, Yehnert H, Moustarah F, *et al.* (2009) Weight loss interventions in chronic kidney disease: a systematic review and meta-analysis. *Clin. J. Am. Soc. Nephrol.* 4(10): 1565–1574.

Navaneethan SD, Palmer SC, Vecchio M, *et al.* (2011) Phosphate binders for preventing and treating bone disease in chronic kidney disease patients. *Cochrane Database Syst. Rev.* (2): CD006023.

Naylor HL, Jackson H, Walker GH, *et al.*; Renal Nutrition Group of the British Dietetic Association, British Dietetic Association. (2013) British Dietetic Association evidence-based guidelines for the protein requirements of adults undergoing maintenance haemodialysis or peritoneal dialysis. *J. Hum. Nutr. Diet.* 26: 315–28.

NICE. (2007) *Cinacalcet for the treatment of secondary hyperparathyroidism in patients with end-stage renal disease on maintenance dialysis therapy*. Available at https://www.nice.org.uk/guidance/ta117. Accessed 3 January 2018.

NICE. (2011) *Hypertension in adults: diagnosis and management.* Available at https://www.nice.org.uk/guidance/cg127/chapter/1-guidance?unlid=93108836201611212141O. Accessed 3 January 2018.

NICE. (2013) *Chronic kidney disease (stage 4 or 5): management of hyperphosphataemia (CG157)*. Available at http://guidance.nice.org.uk/CG157. Accessed 3 January 2018.

NICE. (2014a) Chronic kidney disease in adults: assessment and management. Available at http://www.nice.org.uk/Guidance/CG182. Accessed 3 January 2018.

NICE. (2014b) Cardiovascular disease: risk assessment and reduction, including lipid modification. Available at https://www.nice.org.uk/guidance/cg181/chapter/1-Recommendations#lipid-modification-therapy-for-the-primary-and-secondary-prevention-of-cvd-2. Accessed 3 January 2018.

NICE. (2016) *Vitamin D in critically ill patients with AKI. UK Clinical Trials Gateway*. Available at https://clinicaltrials.gov/ct2/show/NCT02869919. Accessed January 2018.

Noori N, Kopple JD, Kovesdy CP, *et al.* (2010) Mid-arm muscle circumference and quality of life and survival in maintenance haemodialysis patients. *Clin. J. Am. Soc. Nephrol.* 5: 2258–2268.

Oh WC, Gardner DS, Devonald MAJ. (2015) Micronutrient and amino acid losses in acute renal replacement therapy. *Curr. Opin. Clin. Nutr. Metab. Care* 18: 593–598.

Oudemans-van Straten HM, Ostermann M. (2012) Bench-to bedside review: citrate for continuous renal replacement therapy, from science to practice. *Crit. Care* 16: 249.

Paniagua R, Amato D, Vonesh E, *et al.*; Mexican Collaborative Study Group. (2002) Effects of increased peritoneal clearances on mortality rates in peritoneal dialysis: ADEMEX, a prospective, randomised, controlled trial. *J. Am. Soc. Nephrol.* 13: 1307–1320.

Patel JJ, McClain CJ, Sarav M, *et al.* (2017) Protein requirements for critically ill patients with renal and liver failure. *Nutr. Clin. Pract.* 32 (S1): 101S–111S.

Pollock C, Voss D, Hodson E, *et al.*; Caring for Australasians with Renal Impairment (CARI). (2005) The CARI guidelines. Nutrition and growth in kidney disease. *Nephrology (Carlton)* 10(5): S177–230.

Posthauer ME, Banks M, Dorner B, *et al.* (2015) The role of nutrition for pressure ulcer management: national pressure ulcer advisory panel, European pressure ulcer advisory panel and the pan pacific pressure injury alliance white paper. *Adv. Skin Wound Care* 28: 177–188.

Public Health England. (2014) *National Diet and Nutrition Survey: Assessment of Dietary Sodium Adults (19 to 64 years) in England, 2014*. Available at http://www.gov.uk/. *Accessed 6 January 2018*.

Reaven PD, Moritz TE, Schwenke DC, *et al.* (2009) Intensive glucose lowering therapy reduces cardiovascular disease events in Veterans Affairs diabetes trial participants with lower calcified coronary atherosclerosis. *Diabetes*. 58(11): 2642–2648.

Renal Association. (2009) *Haemodialysis*. Available at http://www.renal.org/guidelines. Accessed 6 January 2018.

Renal Association. (2010) *Nutrition in CKD*. Available at www.renal.org/guidelines. Accessed 6 January 2018.

Renal Association. (2011a) *Clinical Practice Guidelines – AKI*. Available at www.renal.org/guidelines. Accessed 6 January 2018.

Renal Association. (2011b) *Assessment of the Potential Kidney Transplant Recipient*. Available at www.renal.org/Clinical/Guidelines. Accessed 6 January 2018.

Renal Association. (2014) *Planning, Initiating and Withdrawal of Renal Replacement Therapy*. Available at http://www.renal.org/guidelines. Accessed 6 January 2018.

Renal Association. (2015) *CKD Mineral and Bone Disorders*. Available at http://www.renal.org/guidelines. Accessed 6 January 2018.

Renal Registry. (2015) UK Renal Registry 18th Annual Report: Chapter 2UK Renal Replacement Therapy Prevalence in 2014: National and Centre-specific Analyses. https://www.renalreg.org/wp-content/uploads/2017/09/02-Chap-02.pdf. Accessed 6 January 2018.

Rigby-Matthews A, Scriber BH, Ahman S. (1999) Control of interdialytic weight gain does not require fluid restriction in hemodialysis patients. *J. Am. Soc. Nephrol.* 10: 267A.

Rocco MV, Paranandi L, Burrowes JD, *et al.* (2002) Nutritional status in the HEMO Study cohort at baseline. *Am. J. Kidney Dis.* 39(2): 245–256.

Schneeweiss B, Graninger W, Stockenhuber F, *et al.* (1990) Energy metabolism in acute and chronic renal failure. *Am. J. Clin. Nutr.* 52: 596–601.

Scottish Intercollegiate Guidelines Network (SIGN). (2008) *Diagnosis and management of chronic kidney disease: A national clinical guideline*. Available at http://www.sign.ac.uk. Accessed 6 January 2018.

Segev DL, Simpkins CE, Thompson RE, *et al.* (2008) Obesity Impacts Access to Kidney Transplantation. *J. Am. Soc. Nephrol.* 19(2):349–55.

Shinaberger CS, Kilpatrick RD, Regidor DL, *et al.* (2006) Longitudinal associations between dietary protein intake and survival in hemodialysis patients. *Am. J. Kidney Dis.* 48(1): 37–49.

Shinaberger CS, Greenland S, Kopple JD, *et al.* (2008) Is controlling phosphorus by decreasing dietary protein intake beneficial or harmful in persons with chronic kidney disease? *Am. J. Clin. Nutr.* 88(6): 1511–1518.

Stenvinkel P, Alvestrand A. (2002) Review articles: Inflammation in end-stage renal disease: sources, consequences, and therapy. *Semin. Dial.* 15: 329–337.

St-Jules DE, Woolf K, Pompeii M, *et al.* (2016) Re-examining the phosphorus–protein dilemma: does phosphorus restriction compromise protein status? *J. Ren. Nutr.* 26(3): 136–140.

Story DA, Ronco C, Bellomo R. (1999) Trace element and vitamin concentrations and losses in critically ill patients treated with continuous venovenous hemofiltration. *Crit. Care Med.* 27(1): 220–223.

Stratton RJ, Bircher G, Fouque D, *et al.* (2005) Multinutrient oral supplements and tube feeding in maintenance dialysis: a systematic review and meta-analysis. *Am. J. Kidney Dis.* 46: 387–405.

SECTION 7

Sullivan C, Sayre S, Leon J, *et al.* (2009) Effect of food additives on hyperphosphatemia among patients with end-stage renal disease: a randomized controlled trial. *JAMA* 301(6): 629–635.

Teplan V, Valkovsky I, Teplan V Jr, *et al.* (2009) Nutritional consequences of renal transplantation. *J. Ren. Nutr.* 19(1): 95–100.

Teta D. (2010) Weight loss in obese patients with chronic kidney disease: who and how? *J. Ren. Care* 36(1): 163–171.

Tomson CR. (2001) Advising dialysis patients to restrict fluid intake without restricting sodium intake is not based on evidence and is a waste of time. *Nephrol. Dial. Transplant.* 16: 1538–1542.

Tyson C, Lin P, Corsino L, *et al.* (2016) Short-term effects of the DASH diet in adults with moderate chronic kidney disease: a pilot feeding study. *Clin. Kidney J.* 9(4): 592–598.

Umber A, Wolley MJ, Golper TA, *et al.* (2014) Amino acid losses during sustained low efficiency dialysis in critically ill patients with AKI. *Clin. Nephrol.* 81: 93–99.

Wahl P, Wolf M. (2012) FGF23 in chronic kidney disease. *Adv. Exp. Med. Biol.* 728: 107–25.

Wang AY, Sea MM, Ip R, *et al.* (2001) Independent effects of residual renal function and dialysis adequacy on actual dietary protein, calorie and other nutrient intake in patients on continuous ambulatory peritoneal dialysis. *J. Am. Soc. Nephrol.* 12: 2450–2457.

Wang AY, Sanderson J, Sea MM, *et al.* (2003) Important factors other than dialysis adequacy associated with inadequate dietary protein and energy intakes in patients receiving maintenance peritoneal dialysis. *Am. J. Clin. Nutr.* 77(4): 834–841.

Wang HE, Muntner P, Chertow GM, *et al.* (2012) AKI and mortality in hospitalized patients. *Am. J. Nephrol.* 35: 349–355.

Wells LM, Hannah J, Jones CH. (2015) The feasibility of using the dietary approaches to stop hypertension (DASH) diet in people with chronic kidney disease (CKD) and hypertension. *Nephrol. Dial. Transplant.* 30(3): iii51–iii52.

Williams C, Ronco C, Kotanko P. (2013) Whole grains in the renal diet – is it time to re-evaluate their role? *Blood Purif.* 36: 210–214.

Wolfe RA, Ashby VB, Milford EL, *et al.* (1999) Comparison of mortality in all patients on dialysis, patients on dialysis awaiting transplantation and recipients of a first cadaveric transplant. *N. Engl. J. Med.* 341: 1725–1730.

Zoccali C, Kramer A, Jager KJ. (2010) Chronic kidney disease and end-stage renal disease—a review produced to contribute to the report 'the status of health in the European union: towards a healthier Europe'. *NDT. Plus* 3: 213–224.

Zoungas S, McGrath BP, Branley P, *et al.* (2008) Cardiovascular morbidity and mortality in the Atherosclerosis and Folic Acid Supplementation Trial (ASFAST) in chronic renal failure: a multicenter, randomized, controlled trial. *J. Am. Coll. Cardiol.* 47(6):1108–1116.

7.5.2 Kidney stones

Karen Thomsett

Key points

- Prevalence of kidney stones is increasing, likely due to dietary and lifestyle changes.
- Fluid intake is the most important factor in the dietary treatment of stones.
- Intake of calcium, protein and sodium should be considered in the management of calcium stones.
- Urolithiasis is linked with chronic kidney disease, bone loss and fractures, obesity and other non-communicable diseases.

Most urinary stones (urolithiasis) are kidney stones; bladder stones are less common. The condition is painful, ranging from a dull loin pain if the stone is in the renal pelvis to agonising colic if lodged in the ureter. Nephrocalcinosis refers to diffuse renal calcifications and is commonly present in primary hyperparathyroidism, distal renal tubular acidosis (RTA) and medullary sponge kidney disease. Nephrolithiasis refers to stones in the kidney. Approximately 80% of stones are composed of calcium salts, usually calcium oxalate and, less commonly, calcium phosphate (Worcester & Coe, 2010). The remaining 20% are composed of uric acid, struvite (magnesium ammonium phosphate) or cystine. Stones with any other composition are very rare (<1%) (Daudon *et al.*, 2004) (see Table 7.5.11). Guidelines on the diagnosis and treatment of urolithiasis have been published in Europe and the USA (Pearle *et al.*, 2014; Türk *et al.*, 2016).

Nephrolithiasis is a worldwide public health issue affecting 5–15% of the population with a recurrence rate >50% within 5–7 years (Prezioso *et al.*, 2015). In the UK, up to 5% of the population is affected (peak age 20–50 years), with a lifetime risk of passing a kidney stone of 8–10%, increasing twofold if there is a family history. Previously, males outnumbered females 2:1, but women are increasingly being affected, such that the ratio has dropped to 1.49:1 (Scales *et al.*, 2012) to 1.3:1 (Strope *et al.*, 2010). Globally, the incidence is increasing across gender, age and race; prevalence appears to have doubled over the past 30 years and is associated with socioeconomic status. The overweight and obese are at increased risk (Romero *et al.*, 2010); this association is greater in females. Kidney stones are associated with a small, but significant, increased risk of chronic and end-stage renal disease, with young women being at greater risk (Shoag *et al.*, 2014).

SECTION 7

Stone formation

Urine in normal individuals is often supersaturated with calcium oxalate, calcium phosphate and sodium urate, and is a metastable solution liable to precipitate upon small

Table 7.5.11 Main classification of kidney stones

Type of stone	Occurrence (%)	Composition
Calcium oxalate ± calcium phosphate	75	Calcium oxalate, calcium phosphate
Struvite (infection stones)	15	Magnesium ammonium phosphate (triple phosphate)
Pure calcium phosphate	5–7	Calcium phosphate
Uric acid	5–8	Uric acid

changes in surface properties (e.g. epithelial irregularity) or composition (Laube *et al.*, 2014). Inhibitors of stone formation include citrate, magnesium, phosphonates, and the organic substances glycosaminoglycans, prothrombin F1 fragment and Tamm–Horsfall glycoprotein. Promoters include calcium, sodium, oxalate, low urine volume and low urine pH (Basavaraj *et al.*, 2007). In addition, anatomical factors can influence stone formation.

There are three main phases of stone formation: crystal nucleation, growth and aggregation. Nucleation requires supersaturated urine, when dissolved substances become solid. Ionic concentration depends on urinary pH, ionic strength and solute concentration. Nucleation is followed by retention of the initial nucleus crystal, growth, aggregation and retention. Both environmental and nutritional factors affect stone formation by their effects on urinary constituents and pH (Basavaraj *et al.*, 2007).

Assessment and diagnosis

Biochemistry

Accurate 24-h urine collection is essential. Creatinine, pH, calcium, chloride, oxalate, citrate and urate should be measured while consuming the usual diet and fluid intake. Concentrations will guide treatment for stone prevention (Walker *et al.*, 2013). Serum concentrations of creatinine, calcium, phosphorous, potassium, bicarbonate, sodium, oxalate, uric acid and parathyroid hormone (PTH) should also be measured. Ideally, stones should be analysed by X ray diffraction or infrared spectroscopy.

The urinary parameters (Ferraro *et al.*, 2015; Türk *et al.*, 2016) are as follows:

- Low urine volume: <1 L/day
- Hypercalciuria calcium: >7.5 mmol/day for men/ 6.25 mmol/day for women
- Hyperoxaluria oxalate: >0.5 mmol/day
- Hyperuricosuria urate: >4.8 mmol/day for men/ 4.5 mmol/day for women
- Hypocitraturia citrate: <1.5 mmol/day
- Hypercystinuria cystine: >0.8 mmol/day

Note: Always check normal values for the laboratory where samples are analysed.

Medical history

Risk factors include family history, gout, type 2 diabetes, obesity, malabsorption conditions, RTA and hyperparathyroidism. Prolonged immobilisation leads to bone reabsorption and consequent hypercalcaemia and hypercalciuria. Intake of vitamin C, calcium and/or vitamin D supplements; protease inhibitors; and carbonic anhydrase inhibitors should be noted (Morgan & Pearle, 2016). Computerised tomography (CT) scan is the method of choice for diagnosis of kidney stones, although abdominal X ray and renal ultrasound help in identifying stones not detected by other means and in determining the number of renal calculi.

Dietary history

A dietary history will determine the past and present intake of all relevant nutrients to guide dietary intervention and to establish if hypercalciuria and/or hyperoxaluria is due to diet or hyperabsorption, e.g. hypercalciuria on a low or normal calcium diet (<700 mg/day) indicates hyperabsorption.

Social history

Past and present occupations may have caused long periods of dehydration and/or increased insensible losses, e.g. long-distance lorry drivers. People who have lived in a hot climate are at similar risk.

Calcium-based stones

Calcium oxalate is the main component of 80% of kidney stones (Parmar, 2004). Increased urinary calcium precipitates insoluble calcium salts and inactivates urinary inhibitors. Most (80%) are idiopathic; in the remaining 20%, the stone is secondary to other factors.

Idiopathic calcium stone disease

This is a syndrome of normal plasma calcium and unexplained hypercalciuria, distinguished from primary hyperparathyroidism by normal serum calcium levels. There are three subtypes (Paliouras *et al.*, 2012):

- *Absorptive hypercalciuria* – increased urinary calcium excretion due to increased intestinal absorption.
- *Renal leak hypercalciuria* – increased intestinal calcium absorption with reduced renal tubular calcium reabsorption.
- *Resorptive hypercalciuria* – due to primary hyperparathyroidism with increased bone mineral turnover and/ or increased intestinal calcium absorption.

Contributory factors include the following:

- *Gender* – men are particularly susceptible.
- *Age* – more common between 20 and 49 years of age, rising in the fourth decade.
- *Ethnicity* – risk is highest for Caucasians, followed by Asians and Hispanics, then Blacks.

- *Low urine volume* – low intake of fluid plays a pivotal role in all types of stone formation (Borghi *et al.*, 2006).
- *Social class* – the incidence is greater in social classes I and II, possibly associated with higher dietary animal protein.
- Dietary factors include high intakes of calcium, protein, sodium, sucrose and fructose, and possibly vitamin D; a poor intake of fibre, notably phytate, has been linked with stone formation. However, some of these associations remain equivocal.
- *Obesity* – stone formation is positively associated with a higher urinary oxalate and calciuria (Taylor & Curhan, 2008b), as is arterial hypertension (Borghi *et al.*, 1999).
- Insulin resistance increases intestinal absorption and excretion of calcium (Kerstetter *et al.*, 1991).
- *Increased intestinal absorption of calcium* – the cause is unknown but may result from either increased synthesis of 1,25 dihydroxycholecalciferol (calcitriol) or the presence of calcitriol intestinal receptor sites (Dretler, 1998). This raises serum calcium-reducing endogenous PTH production, leading to decreased renal tubular reabsorption of calcium and higher urinary excretion to maintain normal serum calcium.
- Impaired tubular reabsorption of calcium – secondary hyperparathyroidism stimulates calcitriol synthesis, increasing intestinal calcium (and phosphate) reabsorption (Pak, 1998).
- *Hyperoxaluria* – significantly increases stone risk.
- *Hypocitraturia* – may be due to metabolic acidosis, hypokalaemia or idiopathic. Citrate binds to calcium, inhibiting calcium oxalate and phosphate crystals forming.
- *Acidic urinary pH* – promotes the precipitation of calcium phosphate and, to a lesser extent, calcium oxalate.
- *Hyperuricosuria* – up to one-third of calcium oxalate stone formers have higher urinary uric acid excretion (Goldfarb *et al.*, 2013), which may reduce the activity of urinary inhibitors.

Pharmacological therapy of idiopathic hypercalciuria

- Thiazide diuretics promote renal calcium reabsorption, reducing urinary calcium by about 30% when sodium is also restricted (Yendt *et al.*, 1966). However, hypokalaemia, hypocitraturia and hyperuricosuria may result.
- Potassium citrate or bicarbonate, plus a thiazide, prevents hypokalaemia and increases citraturia (Pak, 1994). Potassium phosphate suppresses calcitriol synthesis, decreasing calcium absorption (Parmar, 2004).
- Orthophosphates reduce vitamin D levels and thus calcium absorption, and reduce calciuria by increasing renal tubular reabsorption, but gastrointestinal side effects may limit their use. In resistant cases of oxalate stones, the combination of orthophosphates and thiazides are highly effective.
- Bisphosphonates remove calcium from circulation by increasing bone deposition, reducing calciuria and improving bone calcium density.

Role of diet in calcium stones

Dietary recommendations for calcium-based stones include:

- Increased fluid intake aiming for urine output of >2–2.5 litres per day.
- Increased intake of citrate (e.g. lemon juice in water).
- Reduction of sodium (80–100 mmol/day).
- Moderate animal protein intake (0.8–1.0 g/kg/day).
- Moderate calcium intake.

Fluid

A fluid intake sufficient to produce a urine output of >2–2.5 L/day (3–3.5 L of fluid intake) is the most important conservative strategy in stone prevention (Borghi *et al.*, 1996). A high intake of fluid has been shown to be effective when used as the only method of stone prevention (Preminger *et al.*, 2007). In a trial in stone formers who were stone free after shock wave lithotripsy, those randomised to increased fluid intake to achieve a urine output of >2.5 L/day for 2–3 years had a stone recurrence rate of 8% as compared to 56% in those allocated to no treatment (Sarica *et al.*, 2006). The importance of extra fluids in hot weather and hot climates must be stressed. Fluid should be taken during the evening, before bedtime, and on waking at night to override the circadian rhythm for urine production (Robert *et al.*, 1994).

Citrate

Citrate is a stone inhibitor that binds calcium anions in the tubular lumen, forming a highly soluble complex. This decreases the ionic concentration of calcium and the relative saturation of urinary calcium oxalate and calcium phosphate, inhibiting oxalate and phosphate stone formation. Renal acidosis decreases, and alkalosis increases the tubular production and excretion of citrate. Diets rich in fruits and vegetables are alkaline. Lemon juice is often recommended as a source of citrate. A recent review found that evidence was conflicting for the use of lemon juice in the prevention of hypocitraturic nephrolithiasis (Wang *et al.*, 2016). Hydroxycitrate appears to be a superior inhibitor than citrate (Chung *et al.*, 2016).

Sodium

A high sodium intake increases urinary sodium and calcium excretion, and decreases urinary citrate (Parmar, 2004). Hypercalciuric patients may be more sensitive to the calciuric effect of a sodium load. High sodium intake also increases the saturation of monosodium urate, the crystals of which can act as a basis for calcium crystallisation. No randomised, prospective trials investigating the role of sodium *per se* in reducing stone formation have been carried out. A randomised controlled trial of stone formers with high salt intakes (~13 g/day) investigated the effect of a low-salt diet (approximately 4 g/day) over 3 months

(Nouvenne *et al.*, 2010). Idiopathic hypercalciuria was corrected in 30% of cases, indicating that there are populations of salt-dependent and salt-independent hypercalciuric stone formers. Sodium intake should be reduced to 80–100 mmol/day, or, if possible, to 55–80 mmol/day (Türk *et al.*, 2016).

Protein

Protein intake increases the excretion of calcium, oxalate and uric acid, and reduces citraturia. Following a protein load, there is a brief period of metabolic acidosis (due largely to sulphur-containing amino acids), and calcium phosphate and calcium oxalate are less soluble in acid conditions. Acid is produced when sulphur is oxidised to sulphate, which then forms soluble calcium sulphate, reducing calcium reabsorption, thus increasing hypercalciuria. In hypercalciuric men, dietary protein has been found to increase oxaluria and uricosuria, which are associated with urolithiasis (Borghi *et al.*, 2002). Moderate protein restriction to 0.8–1.0 g/kg/day in patients with idiopathic hypercalciuria reduces urinary excretion of urea, calcium, uric acid and oxalate, and increases urinary citrate excretion (Giannini *et al.*, 1999). Some of these effects are thought to be due to a reduction in bone resorption, an increase in renal tubular calcium reabsorption, and reduced renal loss of calcium due to the decreased exogenous acid load (Moe & Huang, 2006).

Protein restriction should focus on poultry, fish and meat, while dairy products (preferably low salt) should not be restricted. Dairy protein was associated with lower stone risk in the Nurses' Health Study II, probably due to calcium binding to oxalate in the gut (Ferraro *et al.*, 2016a).

Calcium

For many years, it was assumed that a high calcium intake increased the risk of stone formation. However, severe calcium restriction (<400 mg/day) does not reduce the frequency of new stone formation in patients with recurrent urolithiasis, and may be detrimental as negative calcium balance and secondary hyperoxaluria can occur (Parmar, 2004). The evidence for recommending high calcium intakes is conflicting. Analysis of a large, longitudinal study has shown that increased dietary calcium was associated with a 5–28% reduced risk of incident kidney stones (Sorensen *et al.*, 2012). Earlier, large epidemiological studies of younger women and previous non-stone-forming men showed similar results (Curhan *et al.*, 1993, 2004). Another large prospective study concluded that restriction of dietary calcium should not be recommended for the prevention of calcium kidney stone (Taylor *et al.*, 2013). One large prospective cohort of women at risk of stone formation found that risk was slightly increased in women who took supplemental calcium (Curhan & Curhan, 1997). This may be attributed to the timing of administration of supplements, as they were not consumed at mealtimes, so decreasing calcium's ability to chelate oxalate. However, another study of young females found that supplemental calcium was not associated with increased risk (Curhan *et al.*, 2004). The effect of dietary calcium on the rate of stone formation is likely attributable to calcium binding with oxalate in the intestinal lumen, forming an insoluble complex excreted in the faeces (Hess *et al.*, 1998). Calcium intake should be dietary rather than from supplements; and, if supplements are used, they should be taken with meals to optimise oxalate chelation.

Oxalate

Most kidney stones contain oxalate, implying that oxalate intake should be reduced. However, approximately 60% of urinary oxalate is endogenous, being produced from the metabolism of glycine, glycolate and hydroxyproline, or synthesised from glyoxylate metabolism (Holmes & Assimos, 1998). Glyoxylate is metabolised in hepatic peroxisomes to glycine and glycolate by alanine glyoxylate aminotransferase and glyoxylate reductase hydroxypyruvate reductase, respectively. The inherited defects of these enzymes lead to oxalate hyperproduction.

Total oxalate is found as two main fractions, soluble and insoluble. Soluble oxalate contains oxalic acid and the water-soluble salts of sodium and ammonia. When bound to calcium, iron and magnesium, oxalate become insoluble, and absorption is restricted. Absorption occurs in the small and large intestines and ranges from 10 to 100% (Grieff & Bushinsky, 2013). About 30% of ingested oxalate is degraded by anaerobic intestinal microflora. *Oxalobacter formigenes* supports oxalate homeostasis by using oxalate for its biosynthesis. Its absence from the intestinal lumen is associated with increased oxalate absorption and calcium oxalate nephrolithiasis (Hatch *et al.*, 2006).

Average daily oxalate intake is extremely variable, ranging between 44 and 351 mg/day, and can exceed 1000 mg/day when foods such as spinach or rhubarb are eaten (Holmes & Kennedy, 2000). The amount absorbed depends on the amount of oxalate-binding cations (e.g. calcium) in the gut lumen, oxalate bioavailability, and gastric emptying/transit time. Absorption tests have shown that absorption in healthy individuals ranges from 2.2 to 18.5%; 15% is considered hyperabsorption (von Unruh *et al.*, 2003). Urine levels peak 2–4 hours after oxalate ingestion (Holmes *et al.*, 2005).

The effectiveness of dietary restriction of oxalate alone is equivocal; restrictions should be confined to patients who normally have a high consumption of oxalate-rich foods (Table 7.5.12). Analyses of foods are limited, and much of the information is conflicting. The oxalate content of food varies between plants of the same species, possibly as a result of differences in soil quality, ripeness, climate, method of harvesting and storage, and analytical methodology. Foods containing moderate amounts of oxalate should be taken in limited quantities, i.e. gooseberries, raspberries and strawberries, okra, sweet potato and potato.

Body weight

Taylor and Curhan (2008b) showed that BMI and urinary creatinine are positively and independently associated with urinary oxalate. It appears that endogenous oxalate production increases with body weight. Rapid or extreme

Table 7.5.12 Principal dietary sources of oxalate (Harvard School of Public Health, 2007; Kasidas & Rose, 1980)

Food	Oxalic acid content (mg/100 g)
Beetroot – pickled	500
Beetroot – boiled	675
Carob powder	73
Chocolate	117
Cocoa	623
Nuts	Most nuts are high in oxalate[a]
Almonds	435
Pecans	202
Peanuts	187
Parsley (can be used in small amounts)	100
Rhubarb	600–860
Spinach	600–750
Swiss chard	645
Tea infusion (mg/100 mL) – without milk	55–78
Wheat germ	269

[a] Pistachios and chestnuts have very low levels of gastric-soluble oxalate, and are suitable in moderation (Ritter & Savage, 2007).

weight gain or loss may precipitate stone development (Stoller & Bolton, 1995); thus, gradual weight loss should be encouraged.

Vitamin C

Vitamin C is excreted in urine in its unmetabolised form and as oxalate. There remains uncertainty as to the definitive effect of vitamin C on stone formation. In one large study, there was no increased risk associated with high intakes of vitamin C (Curhan *et al.*, 1999). This contrasts with two prospective studies in America and Europe which showed that ascorbic acid supplements (1000 mg) increased the risk of incident calcium oxalate stones in men (Ferraro *et al.*, 2016b; Thomas *et al.*, 2013). In the European study, there was a dose-dependent twofold increased risk. This may not be generalisable to women, but advice to avoid supplemental vitamin C is prudent.

Other dietary factors

Caffeine

The risk of stone formation is decreased by 10% for each serving of both caffeinated and decaffeinated coffee in stone-forming men (Curhan *et al.*, 1996). Further analysis of prospective studies in previous non–stone formers showed that caffeine intake (from tea and coffee) is independently associated with 26–31% lower risk of incident (predominantly calcium oxalate) kidney stones (Ferraro *et al.*, 2014).

Cranberry juice

In healthy subjects, cranberry juice is citraturic, reducing oxalate and phosphate excretion (McHarg *et al.*, 2003). Gettman *et al.* (2005) showed that cranberry juice exerted a mixed effect on urinary stone formation; it increased the risk of calcium oxalate and uric acid stone formation, but decreased the risk of brushite stones. Current advice should be to avoid cranberry juice and tablets (Terris *et al.*, 2001) for oxalate stones.

Sucrose and fructose

A high sucrose intake increases calciuria independently of calcium intake, although the mechanism is unknown. In one large study in stone-forming men with high baseline sugar-sweetened beverage consumption, reducing these drinks lowered the risk of recurrence at 3 years as compared to the control group (Shuster *et al.*, 1992). A positive association between sucrose intake and new kidney stone formation has been shown in women but not men (Curhan *et al.*, 2004). Taylor and Curhan (2008a) concluded that fructose intake was independently associated with an increased risk of incident stones. However, in a small group of healthy subjects, increasing dietary fructose for a week had no effect on the excretion of oxalate, calcium, or uric acid (Knight *et al.*, 2010). Current evidence remains insufficient to recommend restriction of sucrose and/or fructose *per se*. However, intake should be addressed when managing the metabolic syndrome, diabetes and obesity, which are associated with stone formation.

Vitamin D

Vitamin D stimulates the small bowel's absorption of calcium and phosphate, enhances renal filtration, decreases PTH levels and reduces renal tubular calcium absorption. The role of vitamin D in stone formation is unclear, with conflicting results from studies assessing the effects of low vitamin D and vitamin D supplements (Eisner *et al.*, 2012; Yalamanchili & Gallagher, 2012; Rathod *et al.*, 2015). Calcium stone formers with normal vitamin D levels should be discouraged from self-medication of multivitamin preparations or fish liver oil capsules containing vitamin D. Repletion of low vitamin D levels is appropriate with monitoring for hypercalciuria (Dion *et al.*, 2016).

Fibre

There are conflicting epidemiological studies on the role of fibre. Phytate binds to calcium, preventing crystallisation of calcium oxalate and calcium phosphate. Observational data have shown that phytate was inversely associated with incident kidney stone formation (Curhan *et al.*, 2004). However, in a prospective study of men, phytate was not associated with stone formation (Taylor *et al.*, 2004). Until further studies are conducted, no conclusions can be made on the role of fibre in stone formation.

Secondary calcium stone disease

This may result from one of the following conditions:

- *Primary hyperparathyroidism* – treatment is parathyroidectomy. If delayed or unsuccessful, a low-calcium diet may be considered. In some cases, surgical removal of the stone may be required.

- *Medullary sponge kidney* – tiny cysts form in the medulla, giving a sponge-like appearance, and preventing urine from flowing freely through the tubules. Hypercalciuria, incomplete distal RTA and hypocitraturia are common. Increasing fluid intake is vital.
- *RTA* – this is caused by primary or secondary damage to the renal tubules in which urine cannot be acidified because of a failure of bicarbonate reabsorption; therefore, calcium phosphate stones are formed. Urine pH levels of >5.8 suggest RTA. It is treated with alkalis and/or diet to normalise serum bicarbonate and pH. A diet rich in animal protein increases urinary acidity, so reducing animal protein intake may help.
- *Primary hyperoxaluria* – three genetic forms have been recognised. Two enzyme deficiencies have been identified – namely, absence of alanine glyoxyflate aminotransferase (type 1), and of D-glycerate dehydrogenase (type 2). The majority of cases are type 1. No enzyme deficiency has yet been identified in type 3. In primary hyperoxaluria, the production and excretion of oxalic acid is significantly increased. Calcium oxalate stones readily form, leading to kidney failure. Systemic oxalate deposition in the heart, bones, joints, eyes and other tissues is common, signifying a poor prognosis.

Treatment of primary hyperoxaluria

Patients should be referred to specialist centres (Türk *et al.*, 2016); treatment options include the following:

- Increasing fluid intake, such that urinary volume is 3 L/24 hours.
- Pyridoxine supplements – although not all patients respond to pyridoxine, it remains the main treatment. Pyridoxine is a cofactor in the alanine glyoxylate pathway, reducing oxalate production by inducing enzyme activity (Parmar, 2004).
- Patients may be advised to follow a low-oxalate diet; however, there is little benefit in the long term as the overriding problem is excessive endogenous production of oxalate.
- In those with hypercalciuria, oral citrate supplements, given with thiazide diuretics, is beneficial. Oral phosphate supplements may be considered.
- *Oxalobacter formigenes* may be given orally.
- Haemodialysis can be used to remove oxalate and may need to be done daily.
- Combined liver and kidney or isolated liver transplantation (i.e. removal of the hepatic source of oxalate production) may be considered.

Secondary hyperoxaluria

There are several causes of secondary hyperoxaluria:

- *Iatrogenic* – hyperoxaluria may occur as a result of the treatment used for idiopathic hypercalciuria.
- *Enteric hyperoxaluria* – the consequence of fat malabsorption from any cause, including gastric bypass (e.g. bariatric Roux-en-Y surgery) (Lieske *et al.* 2015), chronic pancreatitis, Crohn's disease, absent/non-functioning terminal ileum (e.g. short-bowel syndrome), and use of gastrointestinal lipase inhibitors (Robijn *et al.*, 2011). Steatorrhoea may result in fatty acids binding with calcium in the gut in preference to oxalate. Consequently, more oxalate is passively absorbed, leading to oxaluria. Two additional mechanisms increase oxaluria: (1) bile acids and fatty acids, which increase intestinal mucosal permeability to oxalate, and (2) the inhibition of intestinal oxalate-degrading bacteria by bile acids (Robijn *et al.*, 2011).
- Excessive vitamin C intake (dose >1000 mg) has been implicated as a risk factor due to ascorbate being metabolised to oxalate.
- Transient hyperoxaluria after renal transplantation risks calcium oxalate accumulating within the graft (Robijn *et al.*, 2011).

Dietary treatment focuses on a high fluid intake, reducing oxalate, decreasing fats (to reduce steatorrhoea), and increasing low-fat dairy products. Medium-chain triglyceride oil has no effect on oxalate absorption, and can be used to increase energy intake. Calcium supplements bind with oxalate in the intestinal lumen and, if prescribed, should be taken with meals; cholestyramine can be used to bind fatty acids, bile acids and oxalate. Citrate supplements are beneficial.

Calcium phosphate stones

There are two main types of calcium phosphate (CaP) stones: carbonate apatite or hydroxyapatite ($Ca_{10}(PO_4)_6(OH)_2$), and brushite ($CaHPO_4 \cdot 2H_2O$). Hypercalciuria, reduced citrate excretion and alkaline pH are all present. Bacterial infections (with apatite stones) and systemic alkalosis (e.g. chronic vomiting) are associated with CaP stones (Pak *et al.*, 2003), as are RTA and hyperparathyroidism (Gambaro *et al.*, 2016). Pregnant women are twice as likely to have CaP stones as compared to age-matched non-pregnant women, and are two to three times more likely to have CaP stones than oxalate stones (Ross *et al.*, 2008). Glomerular filtration rate and calciuria are raised during pregnancy, and urine pH is higher from the second trimester, all factors predisposing to CaP stones. Stone burden is significant with brushite stones, which are often bilateral and resistant to shock wave lithotripsy. Recurrence is frequent (Moreira *et al.*, 2013). Brushite is the precursor stage of hydroxyapatite.

Treatment

Urinary tract infections, RTA and hyperparathyroidism should be treated. Minimising hypercalciuria (e.g. low-sodium diet and thiazide-type diuretics) and reducing urinary pH with L-methionine (Türk *et al.*, 2016) are the treatments of choice.

Struvite stones

Struvite stones contain magnesium ammonium phosphate and CaP (as apatite), and are more common in women than men. All struvite stone formers are at high risk of recurrence. The main causes are recurrent infection of the urinary tract with a urea-splitting bacteria, and anatomical predisposition. The bacteria break down urea, producing ammonia, resulting in alkaline urine. Magnesium ammonium phosphate and CaP are extremely insoluble in alkaline conditions; once urinary pH is >7.2, struvite precipitates spontaneously with a rapid rate of growth.

Treatment

Stones are removed by percutaneous nephrolithotomy. Other than a good fluid intake, the diet has no role in the treatment of struvite stones. Prevention is by eradicating the infection's source; after clearance of the struvite calculi, at least 3 months of oral, culture-specific, antibiotic treatment is recommended. The urease inhibitor acetohydroxamic acid inhibits the bacterial enzyme urease, preventing ammonia release. It is given with antibiotics, but is contraindicated in women of childbearing age. Up to 30% of patients cannot tolerate acetohydroxamic acid because of side effects, including deep vein thrombosis and haemolytic anaemia (Parmar, 2004; Türk *et al.*, 2016). Methionine or ammonium chloride is recommended to acidify urine (Türk *et al.*, 2016).

Uric acid stones

All uric acid stone formers are at high risk of recurrence. Uric acid is produced by the metabolism of dietary and endogenous purines. Factors leading to uric acid calculi formation include (Pak *et al.*, 2001) the following:

- *Acidic urine* – this is the primary urinary abnormality in idiopathic stone formers (pH <5.5), not elevated urinary uric acid levels (Paterson *et al.*, 2010). Causes include very high animal protein intake, diarrhoea and endogenous overproduction associated with insulin resistance (e.g. metabolic syndrome) (Türk *et al.*, 2016).
- *Hyperuricosuria* – causes include diet, increased endogenous synthesis, myeloproliferative disorders (e.g. chronic myeloid leukaemia), diuretics and tumour lysis syndrome.
- Low urine volume.

Treatment

Dietary modification

Uric acid stones are associated with obesity, the metabolic syndrome and type 2 diabetes. Patients tend to have a lower urinary pH with a decreased rate of ammonium excretion, associated with renal tubule insulin resistance (Maalouf *et al.*, 2007). Weight loss and/or a lacto-vegetarian diet is recommended to reduce protein intake, promote urine alkalinity and provide a source of calcium. A high protein intake increases the acid load, increasing the amount of less soluble urate. Patients should be advised to avoid foods rich in purines (see Chapter 7.9.3, Gout). Severe purine restriction has been superseded by the use of allopurinol.

Fluid intake

High fluid intake to maintain a urine output of 2–3 L/day is essential. Patients without a colon, with large gastrointestinal losses of fluid (e.g. high ileostomy output) and/or chronic diarrhoea, are at risk due to the loss of fluid and bicarbonate, which promotes uric acid supersaturation. In patients with an ileostomy, the amount of fluid required to maintain an adequate urine output may result in excessive stoma output; a balance may have to be achieved between the two.

Alkalinisation of urine

Potassium citrate increases urinary pH, reducing urate precipitation (Parmar, 2004). In patients with chronic diarrhoea, using potassium salts to replace alkali can cause intestinal irritation, and sodium citrate or bicarbonate may be preferred. However, the use of a sodium-based alkali is counterintuitive, owing to sodium's association with an increased risk of stone formation.

Cystine stones

Cystinuria is a rare (1:7000 births) genetic disorder affecting the renal tubular reabsorption of cystine, arginine, lysine and ornithine. Symptoms typically start between 10 and 30 years of age. In adults, 1% of stones are cystine, while in children the figure is 6–8% (Türk *et al.*, 2016). The cause is a reduction in reabsorption of filtered cystine, which is relatively insoluble (Coe *et al.*, 2005). Cystinuria is associated with high rates of surgical intervention when compared with individuals with other forms of urolithiasis (Parr *et al.*, 2015).

Treatment

Dilution of urine

A urine volume of 3–3.5 L per day is crucial. A fluid plan should be advised to ensure an adequate regular intake, including at bedtime and during the night. Hyponatraemia may result from the high fluid intake.

Pharmacological therapy

Alkalinisation therapy with potassium citrate to increase urine pH to >7.5, thus increasing cystine solubility, is recommended (Türk *et al.*, 2016). Thiol-binding agents (D-penicillamine, alpha-mercaptopropionylglycine (tiopronin) or captopril) form soluble cysteine–drug complexes. Alpha-mercaptopropionylglycine is the agent of choice (Türk *et al.*, 2016). To maximise the effectiveness of thiol drugs, alkali therapy should be used concurrently (Asplin *et al.*, 2013). However, a urine pH of >7.5 may predispose to the formation of CaP stones.

Diet

Salt restriction (80–100 mmol/day) reduces cystine excretion (Pearle *et al.*, 2014). Restricting animal protein reduces the intake of the cystine precursor methionine as well as cystine. Such a diet is restrictive and difficult to follow; animal protein from meat, fish, cheese, eggs and milk has to be strictly limited, with an increase in vegetable protein. However, in a multidisciplinary cystinuria clinic, there was overwhelming patient satisfaction with the dietetic service, illustrating that, with regular support by specialist dietitians, patients are able to follow complex, restrictive diets (Doherty *et al.*, 2012).

Melamine stones

In 2008, 294,000 infants in China were affected by melamine-contaminated infant formula, with 5000 hospitalised and six deaths. Melamine was used as a nitrogen-bulking agent to artificially increase the apparent protein content. Renal damage was thought to be the result of kidney stones formed from melamine and uric acid, or from melamine and its cocrystallising chemical derivative, cyanuric acid (Zheng *et al.*, 2013). Treatment was mainly conservative with hydration and alkalinisation; lithotripsy dissolved many stones, but some children needed dialysis.

Ketogenic diet

Nephrolithiasis has been observed in children following a ketogenic diet (e.g. for refractory epilepsy). Prevalence ranges from 3 to 10%, as compared to one in several thousand in the general population. Stone analysis shows a varied picture, with uric acid stones predominating (Furth *et al.*, 2000). Major causative factors include hypercalciuria due to increased bone demineralisation with acidosis, hypocitraturia and acidic urine (see Chapter 3.8.16, Neurology and the ketogenic diet). Urine alkalinisation with potassium citrate has been used successfully (Hallböök *et al.*, 2015).

Acknowledgement

The editor acknowledges the prior contribution of Sharon Underwood.

Further reading

Finlayson B. (1978) Physicochemical aspects of urolithiasis. *Kidney. Int.* 13: 344–360.

Lotan Y, Daudon M, Bruyère F, *et al.* (2013) Impact of fluid intake in the prevention of urinary system diseases: a brief review. *Curr. Opin. Nephrol. Hypertens.* 22: S1–10.

References

Asplin DM, Asplin JR. (2013) The interaction of thiol drugs and urine pH in the treatment of cystinuria. *J. Urol.* 189(6): 2147–2151.

Basavaraj DR, Biyani CS, Browning AJ, *et al.* (2007) The role of urinary stone inhibitors and promoters in the pathogenesis of calcium containing stones. *EAU-EBU Update Series* 5: 126–136.

Borghi L, Meschi T, Amato F, *et al.* (1996) Urinary volume, water and recurrences in idiopathic calcium nephrolithiasis: a 5-year randomized prospective study. *J. Urol.* 155: 839–843.

Borghi L, Meschi T, Guerra A, *et al.* (1999) Essential arterial hypertension and stone disease. *Kidney Int.* 55(6): 2397–2406.

Borghi L, Meschi T, Maggiore U, *et al.* (2006) Dietary therapy in idiopathic nephrolithiasis. *Nutr. Rev.* 64: 301–312.

Borghi L, Schianchi T, Meschi T, *et al.* (2002) Comparison of two diets for the prevention of recurrent stones in idiopathic hypercalciuria. *N. Engl. J. Med.* 346: 77–84.

Chung J, Granja I, Taylor MG, *et al.* (2016) Molecular modifiers reveal a mechanism of pathological crystal growth inhibition. *Nature.* 536(7617): 446–450.

Coe FL, Evans A, Worcester E. (2005) Kidney stone disease. *J. Clin. Investig.* 115(10): 2598–2608.

Curhan GC, Curhan SG. (1997) Diet and urinary stone disease. *Curr. Opin. Urol.* 7: 222–225.

Curhan GC, Willett WC, Rimm EB, *et al.* (1993) A prospective study of dietary calcium and other nutrients and the risk of symptomatic kidney stones. *N. Engl. J. Med.* 328: 833–838.

Curhan GC, Willett WC, Rimm EB, *et al.* (1996) Prospective study of beverage use and the risk of kidney stones. *Am. J. Epidemiol.*143(3): 240–247.

Curhan GC, Willett WC, Speizer FE, *et al.* (1999) Intake of vitamin B_6 and C and the risk of kidney stones in women. *J. Am. Soc. Nephrol.* 10(4): 840–845.

Curhan GC, Willett WC, Knight EL, *et al.* (2004) Dietary factors and the risk of incident kidney stones in younger women: Nurses' Health Study II. *Arch. Intern. Med.* 164(8): 885–891.

Daudon M, Bounxouei B, Santa Cruz F, *et al.* (2004) Composition of renal stones currently observed in non-industrialized countries. *Prog. Urol.* 14(6): 1151–1161.

Dion M, Ankawi G, Chew B, *et al.* (2016) CUA guideline on the evaluation and medical management of the kidney stone patient – 2016 update. *Can. Urol. Assoc. J.* 10(11–12): E348.

Doherty A, Wong K, Thomas K, *et al.* (2012) Patient satisfaction and dietary outcomes from attending a multidisciplinary cystinuria clinic. *Kidney Res. Clin. Pract.* 31(2): A29.

Dretler SP. (1998) The physiologic approach to the medical management of stone disease. *Urol. Clin. North Am.* 25(4): 613–623.

Eisner BH, Thavaseelan S, Sheth S, *et al.* (2012) Relationship between serum vitamin D and 24-hour urine calcium in patients with nephrolithiasis. *Urology.* 80(5): 1007–1010.

Ferraro PM, Taylor EN, Gambaro G, *et al.* (2014) Caffeine intake and the risk of kidney stones. *Am. J. Clin. Nutr.* 100(6): 1596–1603.

Ferraro PM, Robertson WG, Johri N, *et al.* (2015) A London experience 1995–2012: demographic, dietary and biochemical characteristics of a large adult cohort of patients with renal stone disease. *QJM.* 108: 561–568.

Ferraro PM, Mandel EI, Curhan GC, *et al.* (2016a) Dietary protein and potassium, diet–dependent net acid load, and risk of incident kidney stones. *Clin. J. Am. Soc. Nephrol.* 11(10): 1834–1844.

Ferraro PM, Curhan GC, Gambaro G, *et al.* (2016b) Total dietary and supplemental vitamin C intake and risk of incident kidney stones. *Am. J. Kidney Dis.* 7(3): 400–407.

Furth SL, Casey JC, Pyzik PL, *et al.* (2000) Risk factors for urolithiasis in children on the ketogenic diet. *Pediatr. Nephrol.* 15(1–2): 125–128.

Gambaro G, Croppi E, Coe F, *et al.* (2016) Metabolic diagnosis and medical prevention of calcium nephrolithiasis and its systemic manifestations: a consensus statement. *J. Nephrol.* 29(6): 715–734.

Gettman MT, Ogan K, Brinkley LJ, *et al.* (2005) Effect of cranberry juice consumption on urinary risk factors. *J. Urol.* 174(2): 590–594.

Giannini S, Nobile M, Sartori L, *et al.* (1999) Acute effects of moderate dietary protein restriction in patients with idiopathic hypercalciuria and calcium nephrolithiasis. *Am. J. Clin. Nutr.* 69(2): 267–271.

Goldfarb DS, et al. (2013) Kidney stones and the risk of coronary heart disease. *Am. J. Kidney Dis.* 62(6): 1039–41. doi: 10.1053/j.ajkd.2013.10.007.

Grieff M, Bushinsky DA. (2013) Nutritional prevention of kidney stones. In: Kopple JD, Massry SG, Kalantar-Zadeh K (eds) *Nutritional Management of Renal Disease*, 3rd edn. New York: Academic Press.

Hallböök T, Sjölander A, Åmark P, *et al.* (2015) Effectiveness of the ketogenic diet used to treat resistant childhood epilepsy in Scandinavia. *Eur. J. Paediatr. Neurol.* 19(1): 29–36.

Harvard School of Public Health. (2007) Oxalate content of foods Available at https://regepi.bwh.harvard.edu/health/Oxalate/files. Accessed 27 October 2018.

Hatch M, Cornelius J, Allison M, *et al.* (2006) *Oxalobacter* sp. reduces urinary oxalate excretion by promoting enteric oxalate secretion. *Kidney Int.* 69: 691–698.

Hess B, Jost C, Zipperle L, *et al.* (1998) High-calcium intake abolishes hyperoxaluria and reduces urinary crystallization during a 20-fold normal oxalate load in humans. *Nephrol. Dial. Transplant.* 13(9): 2241–2247.

Holmes RP, Assimos DG. (1998) Glyoxylate synthesis, and its modulation and influence on oxalate synthesis. *J. Urol.* 160: 1617–1624.

Holmes RP, Kennedy M. (2000) Estimation of the oxalate content of foods and daily oxalate intake. *Kidney Int.* 57(4): 1662–1667.

Holmes RP, Ambrosius WT, Assimos DG. (2005) Dietary oxalate loads and renal oxalate handling. *J. Urol.* 174(3): 943–947.

Kasidas GP, Rose GA. (1980) Oxalate content of some common foods: determination by an enzymatic method. *J. Hum. Nutr.* 34: 255–266.

Kerstetter J, Caballero B, O'Brien K, *et al.* (1991) Mineral homeostasis in obesity: effects of euglycemic hyperinsulinemia. *Metabolism.* 40: 707–713.

Knight J, Assimos DG, Easter L, *et al.* (2010) Metabolism of fructose to oxalate and glycolate. *Horm. Metab. Res.* 42: 868–873.

Laube N, Berg W, Bernsmann F, *et al.* (2014) Induced urinary crystal formation as an analytical strategy for the prediction and monitoring of urolithiasis and other metabolism-related disorders. *EPMA J.* 5(1): 13.

Lieske JC, Mehta RA, Milliner DS, *et al.* (2015) Kidney stones are common after bariatric surgery. *Kidney Int.* 87(4): 839–845.

Maalouf NM, Cameron MA, Moe OW, *et al.* (2007) Low urine pH: a novel feature of the metabolic syndrome. *Clin. J. Am. Soc. Nephrol.* 2: 883–888.

McHarg T, Rodgers A, Charlton K. (2003) Influence of cranberry juice on the urinary risk factors for calcium oxalate stone formation. *BJU Int.* 92: 765–768.

Moe OW, Huang CL. (2006) Hypercalciuria from acid load: renal mechanisms. *J. Nephrol.* 19: S53–61.

Moreira DM, Friedlander JI, Hartman C, *et al.* (2013) Differences in 24-hour urine composition between apatite and brushite stone formers. *Urology.* 82(4): 768–772.

Morgan MSC, Pearle MS. (2016) Medical management of renal stones. *BMJ.* 352: i52.

Nouvenne A, Meschi T, Prati B, *et al.* (2010) Effects of a low-salt diet on idiopathic hypercalciuria in calcium-oxalate stone formers: a 3-month randomized controlled trial. *Am. J. Clin. Nutr.* 91: 565–570.

Pak CYC. (1994) Citrate and renal calculi: an update. *Miner. Electrolyte Metab.* 20: 371–377.

Pak CYC. (1998) Kidney stones. *Lancet.* 351: 1797–1801.

Pak CYC, Sakhaee K, Peterson RD, *et al.* (2001) Biochemical profile of idiopathic uric acid nephrolithiasis. *Kidney Int.* 60: 757–761.

Pak CY, Sakhaee K, Moe O, *et al.* (2003) Biochemical profile of stone-forming patients with diabetes mellitus. *Urology* 61(3):523–527.

Paliouras C, Tsampikaki E, Alivanis P, *et al.* (2012) Pathophysiology of nephrolithiasis. *Nephron Rev.* 4: e14, 58–65.

Parmar MS. (2004) Kidney stones. *BMJ* 328: 1420–1424.

Parr JM, Desai D, Winkle D. (2015) Natural history and quality of life in patients with cystine urolithiasis: a single centre study. *BJU Int.* 116(S3): 31–35.

Paterson R, Fernandez A, Razvi H, *et al.* (2010) Evaluation and medical management of the kidney stone patient. *Can. Urol. Assoc. J.* 4(6): 375–379.

Pearle MS, Goldfarb DS, Assimos DG, *et al.* (2014) Medical management of kidney stones: AUA guideline. *J. Urol.* 192(2): 316–324.

Preminger GM, Tiselius HG, Assimos DG, *et al.* (2007) Guideline for the management of ureteral calculi. *J. Urol.* 178(6): 2418–2434.

Prezioso D, Strazzullo P, Lotti T, *et al.* (2015) Dietary treatment of urinary risk factors for renal stone formation. A review of CLU Working Group. *Arch. Ital. Urol. Androl.* 87(2): 105–120.

Rathod A, Bonny O, Guessous I, *et al.* (2015) Association of urinary calcium excretion with serum calcium and vitamin D levels. *Clin. J. Am. Soc. Nephrol.* 10(3): 452–462.

Ritter MMC, Savage GP. (2007) Soluble and insoluble oxalate content of nuts. *J. Food Compos. Anal.* 20: 169–174.

Robert M, Roux JO, Bourelly F, *et al.* (1994) Circadian variations in the risk of urinary calcium oxalate stone formation. *Br. J. Urol.* 74: 294–297.

Robijn S. Hoppe B, Vervaet BA, *et al.* (2011) Hyperoxaluria: a gut–kidney axis? *Kidney Int.* 80(11): 1146–1158.

Romero V, Akpinar H, Assimos DG. (2010) Kidney stones: A global picture of prevalence, incidence and associated risk factors. *Rev. Urol.* 12(2–3): e86–e96.

Ross AE, Handa S, Lingeman JE, *et al.* (2008) Kidney stones during pregnancy: an investigation into stone composition. *Urol. Res.* 36(2): 99–102.

Sarica K, Inal Y, Erturhan S, *et al.* (2006) The effect of calcium channel blockers on stone regrowth and recurrence after shock wave lithotripsy. *Urol. Res.* 34(3): 184–189.

Scales CD Jr, Smith AC, Hanley JM, *et al.*;. Urologic Diseases in America Project. (2012) Prevalence of kidney stones in the United States. *Eur. Urol.* 62(1): 160–165.

Shoag J, Halpern J, Goldfarb DS, *et al.* (2014) Risk of chronic and end stage kidney disease in patients with nephrolithiasis. *J. Urol.* 192(5): 1440–1445.

Shuster J, Jenkins A, Logan C, *et al.* (1992) Soft drink consumption and urinary stone recurrence: a randomized prevention trial. *J. Clin. Epidemiol.* 45(8): 911–916.

Sorensen MD, Kahn AJ, Reiner AP, *et al.* (2012) Impact of nutritional factors on incident kidney stone formation: a report from the WHI OS. *J. Urol.* 187(5): 1645–1649.

Stoller ML, Bolton DM. (1995) Urinary stone disease. In: Tanagho EA, McAninch JW (eds) *Smith's General Urology*. New Jersey: Prentice-Hall International Inc, pp. 276–304.

Strope SA, Wolf JS Jr, Hollenbeck BK. (2010) Changes in gender distribution of urinary stone disease. *Urology.* 75(3): 543–546.

Taylor EN, Curhan GC. (2008a) Fructose consumption and the risk of kidney stones. *Kidney Int.* 73: 207–212.

Taylor EN, Curhan GC. (2008b) Determinants of 24-hour urinary oxalate excretion. *Clin. J. Am. Soc. Nephrol.* 50: 1453–1460.

Taylor EN, Curhan GC. (2013) Dietary calcium from dairy and non-dairy sources, and risk of symptomatic kidney stones. *J. Urol.* 190(4): 1255–1259.

Taylor EN, Stampfer MJ, Curhan GC. (2004) Dietary factors and the risk of incident kidney stones in men: new insights after 14 years of follow-up. *J. Am. Soc. Nephrol.* 15(12): 3225–3232.

Terris MK, Issa MM, Tacker JR. (2001) Dietary supplementation with cranberry concentrate tablets may increase the risk of nephrolithiasis. *Urology.* 57: 26–29.

Thomas LDK, Elinder CG, Tiselius HG, *et al.* (2013) Ascorbic acid supplements and kidney stone incidence among men: a prospective study. *JAMA Intern. Med.* 173(5): 386–388.

Türk C, Petřík A, Sarica K, *et al.* (2016) EAU guidelines diagnosis and conservative management of urolithiasis. *Eur. Urol.* 69(3): 468–474.

von Unruh GE, Voss S, Sauerbruch T, *et al.* (2003) Reference range for gastrointestinal oxalate absorption measured with a standardized [13 C 2] oxalate absorption test. *J. Urol.* 169(2): 687–690.

Walker V, Stansbridge EM, Griffin DG. (2013) Demography and biochemistry of 2800 patients from a renal stones clinic. *Ann. Clin. Biochem.* 50(2): 127–139.

Wang CJ, Hsu CS, Chen HW, *et al.* (2016) Long-term effects of lemonade therapy on hypocitraturic nephrolithiasis and stone recurrence: a mini review. *Int. J. Nephrol. Kidney Failure* 2(1) doi http://dx.doi.org/10.16966/2380-5498.123.

Worcester EM, Coe FL. (2010) Clinical practice. Calcium kidney stones. *N. Engl. J. Med.* 363: 954–963.

Yalamanchili V, Gallagher J. (2012) Incidence of hypercalciuria and hypercalcemia during a vitamin D trial in postmenopausal women. *Endocr. Rev.* 33: OR38-1.

Yendt ER, Gagne RJ, Cohanim M. (1966) The effects of thiazides in idiopathic hypercalciuria. *Am. J. Med. Sci.* 251(4): 449–460.

Zheng X, Zhao A, Xie G, *et al.* (2013) Melamine-induced renal toxicity is mediated by the gut microbiota. *Sci. Transl. Med.* 5(172): 172ra22.

7.6 Neurological disease

7.6.1 Parkinson's disease

Karen Green

Key points

- Parkinson's disease (PD) is a progressive neurodegenerative disorder and the most common form of parkinsonism.
- Parkinson's disease can have a considerable impact on nutritional intake as a result of the effects of the disease and side effects of drug treatment.
- Nutritional inadequacies should be identified and corrected as early as possible. Dietetic intervention may be necessary to prevent undesirable weight gain or loss.
- More than 80% of people will develop swallowing difficulties that need to be addressed promptly by the dietitian and speech and language therapist to prevent weight loss and malnutrition.
- PD is associated with a changing profile of weight as the disease advances; some gain weight, while a significant proportion loses weight.

Parkinson's disease (PD) is a chronic and relentlessly progressive neurodegenerative disease; it is the primary and most common form of parkinsonism. Parkinsonism is an umbrella term used to cover a range of conditions, which share the main symptoms of slow movement, possible tremor, rigidity and problems with walking (Parkinson's UK (PUK), 2017). The European prevalence has been estimated to affect up to 160 individuals per million. It is expected that the prevalence in Europe will increase to 4.3 million by 2022. In the UK, one in every 500 individuals has PD, or approximately 127,000 individuals (PUK, 2016). It is characterised by the signs and symptoms listed in Table 7.6.1, which can be remembered by the mnemonic 'TRAP'.

Other motor symptoms include hypomimia (lack of facial expression), dysarthria (speech difficulty), dysphagia, sialorrhoea (excessive secretion of saliva) and poor manual dexterity. Non-motor symptoms include cognitive impairment, depression, dementia, sleep disorders, orthostatic hypotension, fatigue and olfactory dysfunction (loss of taste and smell functions). Gastrointestinal dysfunction is receiving increasing attention and recognition as an important clinical component (Pfeiffer, 2011). These symptoms are usually more apparent in the advanced stages of the disease.

Diagnostic criteria and classification

Onset of PD at ages over 50 years is considered to be late-onset PD; 5–10% are diagnosed before 50 years. PD is classified as juvenile onset when diagnosed under the age of 20 years, or early onset when diagnosed between 20 and 50 years (PUK, 2016).

Disease process

The disease process develops as cells are destroyed (by an unknown trigger or event) in parts of the brain stem, particularly the substantia nigra. Nerve cells in the substantia nigra send out fibres to tissue located in both sides of the brain. There, the cells release dopamine (a neurotransmitter), which helps control movement and coordination (Lang & Lozano, 1998). Loss of dopamine in the corpus stratia is the primary defect, and symptoms usually appear when at least 80% dopamine is lost. As a result, dopamine deficiency affects the nerves and

Manual of Dietetic Practice, Sixth Edition. Edited by Joan Gandy.

Companion website: www.manualofdieteticpractice.com

Table 7.6.1 Signs and symptoms of Parkinson's disease

Feature	Description	Effect
Tremor at rest	Involuntary shaking of the upper and lower limbs, e.g. hands, fingers and legs. Classical PD tremor is the pill rolling tremor.	It is most apparent when the affected part is at rest or the person is under stress. Although the tremor is rarely disabling, it is one of the symptoms that bothers patients the most.
Rigidity	Muscles remain in a constantly contracted state, causing symptoms such as muscle stiffness, weakness or aching.	Patients are less aware of impaired movement but this may be obvious to a carer, e.g. raising the patient's arm results in ratchet-like jerky movements (cogwheel rigidity).
Akinesia	Slowness of movement, which is often the most disabling feature of the disease.	Normal activities such as washing and dressing may take hours. There may also be slowness in speech and delayed reaction to conversation.
Postural instability	Impaired balance and coordination result in general unsteadiness in movement, particularly while turning, and increased risk of falls.	Patients often develop a forward lean or sometimes a stooped posture, with the head bowed and the shoulders dropped. Gait disturbance becomes more obvious; some patients may halt mid-stride, sometimes toppling over as a result; others may shuffle along with knees flexed; and, ultimately, some may be unable to walk unaided.

muscles controlling movement and coordination, and may also be responsible for associated cognitive decline.

Genetics

Known genetic causes of PD account for approximately 10% of cases, with around 15% of those with PD having a family history of the disease (Parkinson's Disease Foundation, 2016). Incidence increases with age (Hirsch *et al.*, 2016). Men were 1.5 times more likely than women to develop PD (Alves *et al.*, 2009); however, this difference was only statistically significant for males in the age range 60–79 years (Hirsch *et al.*, 2016).

Disease consequences

PD is associated with disability, morbidity, institutionalisation, high demand on healthcare input and mortality (Aarsland *et al.*, 2009; Elbaz *et al.*, 2002; Leibson *et al.*, 2006; Mutch *et al.*, 1986; Parashos *et al.*, 2002; Shulman *et al.*, 2001). Due to the progressive nature of the disease, it is generally expected that the signs and symptoms of the disease will be progressive. The natural history of PD is very variable, and it is extremely difficult to accurately predict how, or how quickly, the disease will progress. Life expectancy and age at the time of death are reduced for all onset ages, but this reduction is greatest in those with young-onset PD (Ishihara *et al.*, 2007).

Public health aspects and prevention

Although the cause of PD remains unknown, a number of factors that increase the risk of developing this disease have been identified, including early diet, genetics and environment. In patients treated with levodopa (L-dopa), plasma homocysteine levels are elevated, which exhibits multiple neurotoxic effects involved in the pathogenesis of several neurodegenerative disorders including PD (Kuhn *et al.*, 1998; Prins *et al.*, 2002; Sheshadri *et al.*, 2002).

Higher intake of vitamin B_6 lowers the risk of PD; however, there was no evidence for folate and vitamin B_{12} (Shen, 2015). Constipation and physical activity are associated with the risk of developing PD (Bellou *et al.*, 2016). There is substantial evidence that many environmental factors are associated with PD; however, more well-designed studies are needed. Knekt *et al.* (2010) found a relationship between higher serum 25-hydroxyvitamin D (25 [OH]D) and lower risk of PD; however, this was not found in a larger prospective US study by Shrestha *et al.* in 2016. Recent research is looking at the influence of selenium on the development of PD (Ellwanger *et al.*, 2016). However, there is limited research to support these claims.

Nutritional consequences

Symptoms vary from individual to individual; therefore, everyone will experience varying degrees of nutritional inadequacies because of the disease. Some of the most commonly reported nutritional consequences of the disease are discussed in the following text.

Weight loss

Weight loss is a major feature, whether it is progressive weight loss or obvious malnutrition. Approximately 30–70% of patients will experience unintentional weight loss (Vikdahl *et al.*, 2014), and about three-quarters will experience eating difficulties (Cushing *et al.*, 2002; Palhagen *et al.*, 2005). It has been reported that women are more prone to weight loss than men (Durrieu *et al.*, 1992), and that they are prone to develop dyskinesia than men (Hassain-Baer *et al.*, 2011). It has been suggested that weight loss can result from reduced energy intake;

however, Chen *et al.* (2003) reported that weight loss is not caused by reduced energy intake in early-onset patients. Barichella *et al.* (2016a) found that, although patients had a lower BMI, they reported a higher food intake than their control group. Increased energy requirements, secondary to increased rigidity and possibly due to dyskinesia, may also play a role (Markus *et al.*, 1993). Sharma and Turton (2012) found that olfactory dysfunction, and anosmia in particular, led to significant weight loss over a 5-year period. Dysphagia and gastrointestinal dysfunction contribute to weight loss due to reduced energy intake in more advanced-disease patients (Uc *et al.*, 2006). In addition, the decline in cognition can lead to lowered energy intake by affecting interest in food and eating habits. Cognitive impairment varies, depending on which part of the brain is impaired, and the timing of onset and progression of the disease (Watson & Leverenz, 2010). As the disease progresses, individuals with PD are four times more likely to lose 4.5 kg more than age-matched controls (Beyer *et al.*, 1995; Sharma & Turton, 2012).

More than 80% of people with PD will develop swallowing difficulties (Suttrup & Warnecke, 2016). This needs to be addressed promptly by a dietitian and a speech and language therapist (SLT) to prevent and/or treat weight loss and malnutrition as appropriate. The risk of aspiration is often overlooked, and, as a consequence, pneumonia is a commonly reported cause of death in this group (Miller *et al.*, 2009; Robbins *et al.*, 2008).

The on–off syndrome can occur in patients on long-term antiparkinsonian medication, which causes sudden alterations in or loss of functional ability The main feature of the off period is increased muscle tone (rigidity), and, of the on period, increased involuntary movements (dyskinesias). Off periods, also known as motor fluctuations, are unpredictable and may last for a few minutes or many hours. Drug adjustment is often titrated to overcome this problem; however, at some stage, this syndrome affects the ability of the patients to prepare meals and feed themselves, and thereby increases the risk of the patients developing malnutrition.

Autonomic failure

Autonomic failure occurs in 30–60% of patients with PD (Velseboer *et al.*, 2011), and the associated symptoms can impact on nutritional intake (see Chapter 7.6.3, Rare neurological conditions).

Bone health and osteoporosis

Hypovitaminosis D is prevalent in people living with PD (Evatt *et al.*, 2008; Sato *et al.*, 1997), and disease severity and bone density are correlated (Sato *et al.*, 1997). Patients with PD have been found to have a defect in the renal synthesis of 1,25-dihydroxyvitamin D (1,25[OH]2D (Jackson *et al.*, 2007). Some researchers have suggested that people with PD should be supplemented with alpha-hydroxyvitamin D_3 (vitamin D_3), the more active form of vitamin D, which can help increase bone density and lower fracture risk in these patients (Boonen *et al.*, 2007). Lee *et al.* (2010) has suggested that supplementation with homocysteine-lowering therapy may prevent bone loss in those taking L-dopa. It is essential for patients who are bed bound or immobile to have calcium and vitamin D status assessed early in the disease to prevent or decrease the incidence of osteoporosis.

Constipation

Constipation is common (Cassani *et al.*, 2011), with 80–90% of PD patients experiencing it (Fasano *et al.*, 2015). The possible causes of constipation include the following:

- Gastroparesis, found in >70% of PD patients (Marrinan *et al.*, 2014).
- Lack of fibre due to difficulties in chewing fibrous food or when following a texture-modified diet, e.g. puréed food.
- Lack of fluid intake as a response to problems with urgency and frequency of micturition or incontinence.
- Reduced mobility.
- Antiparkinsonian medications.

Weight gain

In contrast to the weight loss that develops as part of the disease, weight gain has been reported following deep brain stimulation (DBS) surgery (Tuite *et al.*, 2005). Sauleau *et al.* (2009) found that 38% were overweight, with a BMI of 26–29.9 kg/m^2 recorded 6 months after DBS surgery. This was attributed to the improvement in motor control, rather than any improvement in energy intake. Weight gain may also occur in individuals treated with dopaminergic agonists, sometimes as a result of impulse control difficulty with compulsive eating (Nirenberg & Waters, 2006).

Nutritional assessment

Nutritional assessment should include the following aspects.

Anthropometry

Weight, height, BMI and a validated nutritional screening score (e.g. 'MUST') are used to determine nutritional status, and baseline measurements recorded to allow progress to be monitored. Mid-upper-arm circumference (MUAC) should be considered, although severe rigidity or motor fluctuations may make these impossible.

Biochemistry

There are no specific tests that track the progress of PD; however, during periods of illness in a hospital setting (e.g. aspiration), inflammatory markers will monitor the clinical status.

Clinical assessment

Clinical observations will vary depending on the treatment. However, it is worth noting the fluid balance (dehydrated or overloaded), bowel movements (frequency and consistency), temperature, swallowing difficulties, motor function (on–off periods) and drug regimens. Consider any comorbidity when devising an individually tailored care plan.

Dietary assessment

Food charts in a hospital setting or food diaries in a community setting are important. There may be difficulties in communicating with the patient for various reasons, including on–off periods, speech difficulties or poor memory due to dementia. The appropriateness of the method of nutritional support that the individual is currently receiving and his or her tolerance to the prescribed regimen should be considered. This will help when devising and updating the care plan. Focus should be on total energy intake versus requirements, and any food avoidance or changes to dietary intake should be noted.

Economic and social assessment

To ensure streamlined, holistic care, links should be made where appropriate with carers and community teams who are involved in the patient's care at all levels. The focus should be on the living arrangements, and on the difficulties in obtaining food, meal preparation and cooking.

Management

Clinical management

Although there is no treatment available yet that is capable of slowing or stopping the progression of the disease, current treatments can effectively relieve the symptoms, especially in the early years. Many people who are adequately treated notice very little or no progression of symptoms over the first few years. However, within 5–10 years of onset, symptoms will disrupt activities of daily living. Clinical management is therefore directed at minimising symptoms and disabilities.

Drug management

Many of the available medications have significant side effects; therefore, the aim of drug therapy is to find a balance between effective symptom control and the avoidance of side effects. The following are commonly used drugs in the management of PD: L-dopa, dopamine agonists, selegiline, anticholinergics and catechol-O-methyltransferase (COMT) inhibitors. L-dopa is used to replace or mimic dopamine in the brain and, in conjunction with COMT inhibitors, to limit the conversion of L-dopa to dopamine in the peripheral tissues, thereby facilitating a greater proportion of L-dopa to cross the blood–brain barrier. Dopamine agonists, which mimic dopamine, are usually the first drugs prescribed for those diagnosed with juvenile-onset PD (Uitti *et al.*, 1999). It is also used alongside L-dopa. The efficiency of drug therapy tends to diminish with time, and the duration of benefit after each dose becomes progressively shorter; this is known as end dose failure.

Surgical procedures

DBS is used to treat the debilitating symptoms of PD, such as tremor, rigidity, stiffness, slowed movement and walking problems. Currently, the procedure is used only for patients whose symptoms cannot be adequately controlled with medications. It uses a surgically implanted neurostimulator, which is likened to a heart pacemaker and about the size of a stopwatch. It delivers electrical stimulation to targeted areas in the brain that control movement, blocking the abnormal nerve signals that cause tremor and PD symptoms. Research is ongoing to ascertain its long-term effectiveness.

Continuous intrajejunal infusion of duodopa

A new therapeutic treatment for patients with advanced PD is a cabidopa/L-dopa combination (duodopa) using continuous, modulated administration via percutaneous endoscopic transgastric jejunostomy (PEG-J). Duodopa (an aqueous gel) administered over 12–16h has been shown to significantly alleviate motor complications in PD (Abbruzzese *et al.*, 2012; Antonini *et al.*, 2014; Fernandez *et al.*, 2013). The PEG-J cannot be used for administering fluids of enteral feeds during the 12-h period, as it will dilute the duodopa, thereby reducing the effectiveness of the treatment. If clinically indicated, enteral feeding and fluids can be administered via the gastric port only at night. Close liaison with the MDT and the clinical nurse specialist is recommended.

Nutrition management

Nutrition management aims to:

- Identify nutritional inadequacies at an early stage.
- Implement measures to correct deficiencies or related problems.
- Minimise the practical difficulties associated with eating or swallowing.
- Prevent undesirable weight gain or loss.
- Lessen the impact of drug therapy side effects on dietary intake.
- Ensure regular monitoring of nutritional status throughout the progression of the disease.

It is important to establish and maintain good eating habits from diagnosis and throughout the course of the condition (Glynn, 2003). Information should be provided on how to adopt the healthy eating guidelines; this will help prevent undesirable weight gain. As the disease progresses, more specific diet therapy may be needed to help overcome problems that affect nutritional intake and status.

Weight loss and poor oral intake

Guidance on how to optimise nutrient intake with nutrient-dense foods, food fortification measures or nutritional supplements may be necessary. Other strategies to help overcome problems such as anorexia, sensory impairment and fatigue may also be helpful (see Chapter 6.3, Oral nutritional support). Due to a lack of research on energy requirements in PD, advice is based on best practice and clinical experience. Requirements are based on the Henry equation. Weight gain factors range from additional 600 to 1000 to promote weight gain, if necessary, or 25–35 kcal/kg ideal body weight (NICE, 2006b), especially in underweight patients.

Dysphagia

Dysphagia needs to be addressed promptly; significant swallowing problems require SLT assessment and guidance regarding food texture modification (see Chapter 7.3, Dysphagia). Altered-texture diets may be nutritionally inadequate and not sufficiently energy dense to meet the patient's nutritional requirements, and additional use of energy-dense nutritional supplements may be indicated. However, these may be contraindicated in patients who require thickened fluids. Available prethickened nutritional supplements include Fresubin Thickened Stage 1 & 2 (1.5 kcal/mL) (Fresenius Kabi) and Nutilis Complete Stage 1 (2.4 kcal/mL) (Nutricia), and would benefit patients with dysphagia and weight loss.

Bone health

People with PD should be routinely supplemented with 1000–1500 mg of calcium and 10–15 μg (400–600 IU) of vitamin D daily (Sato *et al.*, 2001). Recent research suggests that intake should exceed 20 μg (800 IU) of vitamin D to prevent falls and for optimal skeletal health (Bischoff-Ferrari *et al.*, 2006; Knekt *et al.*, 2010). Dietary sources of calcium and vitamin D should also be encouraged if possible.

Pressure ulcers

Risk of pressure ulcers may be increased as the disease advances, where mobility is reduced and in those who are bedbound (see Chapter 7.17.6, Wound healing, tissue viability and pressure sores). Nutritional requirements are based on the European and US National Pressure Ulcer Advisory panels guidelines (EPUAP) (2014).

Constipation

Dietary advice is aimed primarily at softening and increasing the bulk of the stool. This should be the first treatment strategy, and is usually effective. Drinking fermented milk containing probiotic strains and prebiotic fibre may improve constipation in the PD population (Barichella *et al.*, 2016b).

Fluid

Patients should drink at least six to eight glasses (1.6–2 L) of fluid per day. Fluids that can be suggested include water, cordial fruit juice, prune juice, vegetable juice, tea, coffee, smoothies and drinking yoghurt. People living with PD often have a weaker sense of thirst and, if necessary, should be helped and encouraged to drink at regular intervals throughout the day.

Fibre

Fibre-rich foods that are easy to manage, e.g. high-fibre breakfast cereals, wholemeal bread, easy-to-peel fruit, dried fruit and golden linseeds, are suitable. Golden linseeds should be introduced into the diet slowly (e.g. start with 1 teaspoon/day up to a maximum of 1 tablespoon/day over a week), and can be added to foods such as breakfast cereal, yoghurts or soups. The use of vegetables, peas, beans and lentils as meal components should be encouraged. The common practice of adding bran to foods should not be encouraged, as this is more likely to create problems than solve them. Advice on increasing fibre (30 g/day) and fluid (up to 2.5 L/day) simultaneously should be given to prevent exacerbating symptoms of constipation.

Protein manipulation

Advising advanced PD patients with motor fluctuations to manipulate protein consumption is not supported by convincing and well-designed randomised controlled trials. It was well documented that patients who followed a protein-restricted diet (PRD) experienced an increase in total energy expenditure (Barichella *et al.*, 2007; Cereda *et al.*, 2009), resulting in weight loss over time (Barichella *et al.*, 2006; Paré *et al.*, 1992). However, the long-term adequacy of protein-controlled dietary regimens has not been established. More recently, Barichella *et al.* (2016a) suggested that protein requirements should be based on 0.8 g protein/kg and a PRD to optimise L-dopa absorption; however Wolfe *et al.* (2008) suggested 0.8 g/kg of ideal body weight or using the dietary reference values. Timing of medications around meal times should be addressed to avoid protein–L-dopa interaction. Poor L-dopa absorption can also be attributed to a high-fat, high-fibre meal and constipation. It is important to stress that you may have to support a patient who decides to embark on a PRD or similar diet based on the advice of the lead neurologist responsible.

In the absence of curative treatment, the management of PD remains largely palliative, despite the huge advances that have been achieved in medical knowledge. NICE (2006a) advises, '*Palliative care should be applied throughout the course of the disease and not limited to the terminal end of life period*'. Achievement of the best possible quality of life for patients and their carers and families is the goal of palliative care. The palliative stage of the disease is defined by an inability to tolerate dopaminergic therapy, unsuitability for surgery (e.g. DBS) and the presence of advanced comorbidity (MacMahon & Thomas, 1998). Medication may be stopped due to lack of drug efficacy and increasing sensitivity to side effects such as hallucinations. Active and aggressive nutritional support may also be withdrawn if it causes discomfort or distress. Regular contact with the palliative care team is advised, and it is very important that there be good, effective and open communication within the multidisciplinary team (see Chapter 7.16, Palliative and end-of-life care).

Drug–nutrient interactions

Levodopa (L-dopa) and protein

Large, neutral amino acids in dietary proteins compete with L-dopa for intestinal absorption and transport across the blood–brain barrier. This limits L-dopa's efficacy, and results in motor fluctuations. Taking L-dopa 45 minutes before meals, with a carbohydrate source such as a cracker or a biscuit, can help alleviate this. Reducing the amount of protein to less than recommendations for general health is not advised.

Internet resources

BDA in association with Parkinson's UK Best practice guidelines for dietitians on the management of Parkinson's. (2010) Produced by, www.parkinsons.org.uk/advice/publications/professionals/dietitians_best_practice_guide.aspx

European Parkinson's Disease Association (EPDA), http://epda.eu.com

National Parkinson Foundation, www.parkinson.org

National Service Framework for Long-term (Neurological) Conditions (2005), www.dh.gov.uk/en/Publicationsandstatistics/Publications/PublicationsPolicyAndGuidance/DH_4105361

NICE Clinical guideline on the diagnosis and management of Parkinson's disease in primary and secondary care in England and Wales. (2006) CG 35. *Note*: Endorsed in Northern Ireland, www.nice.org.uk/guidance/CG35 Parkinson's UK; www.parkinsons.org.uk

The Multiple System Atrophy Trust, http://www.msatrust.org.uk

The Parkinson's Disease Foundation, http://www.pdf.org

The Professional's Guide to Parkinson's Disease (2007), www.parkinsons.org.uk/pdf/B126_Professionalsguide.pdf

The PSP Association, http://www.pspassociation.org.uk

References

Aarsland D, Marsh L, Schrag A. (2009) Neuropsychiatric symptoms in Parkinson's disease. *Mov. Disord.* 24: 2175–2186.

Abbruzzese G, Barone P, Bonuccelli U, *et al.* (2012) Continuous intestinal infusion of levodopa/carbidopa in advanced Parkinson's disease: efficacy, safety and patient selection. *Funct. Neurol.* 27: 147–154.

Alves G, Muller B, Herlofson K, *et al.* (2009) Incidence of Parkinson's disease in Norway: the Norwegian Park West study. *J. Neurol. Neurosurg. Psychiatry.* 80: 851–857.

Antonini A, Yegin A, Preda C, *et al.* (2014) Global long-term study on motor and non-motor symptoms and safety of levodopa–carbidopa intestinal gel in routine care of advanced Parkinson's disease patients: 12 interim outcomes. *Parkinsonism Relat. Disord.* 21: 231–235.

Barichella M, Marczewska A, De Notaris R, *et al.* (2006) Special low-protein foods ameliorate postprandial off in patients with advanced Parkinson's disease. *Mov. Disord.* 21: 1682–1687.

Barichella M, Savardi C, Mauri A, *et al.* (2007) Diet with LPP for renal patients increases daily energy expenditure and improves motor function in parkinsonian patients with motor fluctuations. *Nutr. Neurosci.* 10: 129–135.

Barichella M, Cereda E, Cassani E, *et al.* (2016a) Dietary habits and neurological features of Parkinson's disease patients: implications for practice. *Clin. Nutri.* 36(4): 1054–1061. 10.1016/j.clnu.2016.06.020

Barichella M, Pacchetti C, Bolliri C, *et al.* (2016b) Probiotics and prebiotic fiber for constipation associated with Parkinson disease. *Neurology.* 87: 1274–1280.

Bellou V, et al. (2016) Environmental risk factors and Parkinson's disease: an umbrella review of meta-analyses. *Parkinsonism Relat Disord.* 23:1–9.

Beyer PL, Palarino MY, Michalek D, *et al.* (1995) Weight change and body composition in patients with Parkinson's Disease. *J. Am. Diet. Assoc.* 95(9): 979–983.

Bischoff-Ferrari HA, Giovannucci E, Willett WC, *et al.* (2006) Estimation of optimal serum concentrations of 25-hydroxyvitamin D for multiple health outcomes. *Am. J. Clin. Nutr.* 84(1): 18–28.

Boonen S, Lips P, Bouillon R, *et al.* (2007) Need for additional calcium to reduce the risk of hip fracture with vitamin D supplementation: Evidence from a comparative meta-analysis of randomised controlled trials. *J. Clin. Endocrinol. Metab.* 92(4): 1415–1423.

Cassani E, Privitera G, Pezzoli G, *et al.* (2011) Use of probiotics for the treatment of constipation in Parkinson's disease patients. *Minerva Gastroenterol. Dietol.* 57(2): 117–121.

Cereda E, Pezzoli G, Barichella M. (2009) Role of an electronic armband in motor function monitoring in patients with Parkinson's disease. *Nutrition.* 26(2): 240–242.

Chen H, Zhang SM, Hernan MA, *et al.* (2003) Weight loss in Parkinson's disease. *Ann. Neurol.* 53: 676–679.

Cushing ML, Traviss KA, Calne SM. (2002) Parkinson's disease: Implications for nutritional care. *Can. J. Diet. Pract. Res.* 63(2): 81–87.

Durrieu G, Llau ME, Rascol O, *et al.* (1992) Parkinson's disease and weight loss: a study with anthropometric and nutritional assessment. *Clin. Auton. Res.* 2: 153–157.

Elbaz A, Bower JH, Maraganore DM, *et al.* (2002) Risk tables for parkinsonism and Parkinson's disease. *J. Clin. Epidemiol.* 55: 25–31.

Ellwanger JH, Franke SR, Bordin DL, *et al.* (2016) Biological functions of selenium and its potential influence on Parkinson's disease. *Ann. Brazilian Acad. Sci.* 88: 1655–1674.

EPUAP (2014) International Pressure Ulcer Guidelines. http://www.epuap.org/pu-guidelines/#2014guidelines&qrg. Accessed 29 October 2018.

Evatt ML, Delong MR, Khazai N, *et al.* (2008) Prevalence of vitamin D insufficiency in patients with Parkinson disease and Alzheimer disease. *Arch. Neurol.* 65(10): 1348–1352.

Fasano A, Visanji NP, Liu LW, et al. (2015) Gastrointestinal dysfunction in Parkinson's disease. *Lancet Neurol.* 14(6): 625–639.

Fernandez HH, Vanagunas A, Odin P, *et al.* (2013) Levodopa–carbidopa intestinal gel in advanced Parkinson's disease open-label study: interim results. *Parkinsonism Relat. Diord.* 19: 339–345.

Glynn K. (2003) Nutritional issues in Parkinson's disease. *Complete Nutr.* 3(4): 13–16.

Hassain-Baer S, Molchadski I, Cohen OS, *et al.* (2011) Gender effect on time to levodopa-induced dyskinesias. *J. Neurol.* 258: 2048–2053.

Hirsch L, Jette N, Frolkis A, et al. (2016) The Incidence of Parkinson's Disease: A Systematic Review and Meta-Analysis. *Neuroepidemiology* 46(4):292–300. doi: 10.1159/000445751. Epub 2016 Apr 23.

Ishihara L, Cheesbrough A, Brayne C, *et al.* (2007) Estimated life expectancy of Parkinson's patients compared with the UK population. *J. Neurol. Neurosurg. Psychiatry.* 78: 1304–1309.

Jackson C, Gaugris S, Sen SS, *et al.* (2007) The effect of cholecalciferol (vitamin D_3) on the risk of fall and fracture: a meta-analysis. *QJM.* 100: 185–192.

Knekt P, Kilkkinen A, Rissanen H, *et al.* (2010) Serum vitamin D and the risk of Parkinson disease. *Arch. Neurol.* 67(7): 808–811.

Kuhn W, Roebroek R, Blom H, *et al.* (1998) Hyperhomocysteinaemia in Parkinson's disease. *J. Neurol.* 245: 811–812.

Lang AE, Lozano AM. (1998) Parkinson's disease: second of two parts. *N. Engl. J. Med.* 339(16): 1130–1143.

Lee SH, Kim MJ, Kim BJ, *et al.* (2010) Hyperhomocysteinemia due to levodopa treatment as a risk factor for osteoporosis in patients with Parkinson's disease. *Calcif. Tissue Int.* 86(2): 132–141.

Leibson C, Long KH, Maraganore DM, *et al.* (2006) Direct medical costs associated with Parkinson's disease: a population-based study. *Mov. Disord.* 21: 1864–1871.

MacMahon DG, Thomas S. (1998) Practical approach to quality of life in Parkinson's disease: the nurse's role. *J. Neurol.* 245: S19–S22.

Marrinan S, Emmanuel AV, Burn DJ. (2014) Delayed gastric emptying in Parkinson's disease. *Mov. Disord.* 29: 23–32.

Markus HS, Tomkins AM, Stern GM. (1993) Increased prevalence of undernutrition in Parkinson's disease and its relationship to clinical disease parameters. *J. Neural Transm. Park. Dis. Dement. Sect.* 5: 117–125.

Miller N, Allcock L, Hildreth AJ, *et al.* (2009) Swallowing problems in Parkinson disease: frequency and clinical correlates. *J. Neurol. Neurosurg. Psychiatry.* 80(9): 1047–1049.

Mutch W, Strudwick A, Roy SK, *et al.* (1986) Parkinson's disease: disability, review, and management. *Br. Med. J. (Clin Res Ed).* 293: 675–677.

NICE. (2006a) *Parkinson's Disease: National Clinical Guideline for Diagnosis and Management in Primary and Secondary Care.* London: NICE.

NICE. (2006b) *Nutrition support in adults: oral nutrition support, enteral tube feeding and parenteral nutrition. Clinical guideline (32).* Available at www.nice.org.uk/CG032. Accessed 29 October 2018.

Nirenberg MJ, Waters C. (2006) Compulsive eating and weight gain related to dopamine agonist use. *Mov. Disord.* 21: 524–529.

Palhagen S, Lorefalt B, Carlsson M, *et al.* (2005) Does L-dopa treatment contribute to reduction in body weight in elderly patients with Parkinson's disease? *Acta Neurol. Scand.* 111(1): 12–20.

Parashos S, Maraganore DM, O'Brien PC, *et al.* (2002) Medical services utilization and prognosis in Parkinson disease: a population-based study. *Mayo Clin. Proc.* 77: 918–925.

Paré S, Barr SI, Ross SE. (1992) Effect of daytime protein restriction on nutrient intakes of free-living Parkinson's disease patients. *Am. J. Clin. Nutr.* 55: 701–707.

Parkinson's Disease Foundation (2016) https://parkinson.org/understanding-parkinsons/what-is-parkinsons. Accessed 29 October 2018.

Parkinson's UK (PUK). (2011) *National Parkinson's Audit.* Available at https://www.parkinsons.org.uk/professionals/uk-parkinsons-audit-transforming-care. Accessed 29 October 2018.

Pfeiffer RF. (2011) Gastrointestinal dysfunction in Parkinson's disease. *Parkinsonism Relat. Disord.* 17(1): 10–15.

Prins ND, Den Heijer T, Hofman A, *et al.* (2002) Homocysteine and cognitive function of the elderly: The Rotterdam Scan Study. *Neurology.* 59: 1375–1380.

Robbins J, Gensler G, Hind J, *et al.* (2008) Comparison of 2 interventions for liquid aspiration on pneumonia incidence: a randomized trial. *Ann. Intern. Med.* 148(7): 509–518.

Sato Y, Kikuyama M, Oizumi K. (1997) High prevalence of vitamin D deficiency and reduced bone mass in Parkinson's disease. *Neurology.* 49(5): 1273–1278.

Sato Y, Kaji M, Tsuru T, *et al.* (2001) Risk factors for hip fracture among elderly patients with Parkinson's disease. *J. Neurol. Sci.* 182(2): 89–93.

Sauleau P, Leray E, Rouaud T, *et al.* (2009) Comparison of weight gain and energy intake after subthalamic versus pallidal stimulation in Parkinson's disease. *Mov. Disord.* 24(14): 2149–2155.

Sharma JC, Turton J. (2012) Olfaction, dyskinesia and profile of weight change in Parkinson's disease: identifying neurodegenerative phenotypes. *Parkinsonism Relat. Disord.* 18: 964–970.

Shen L. (2015) Associations between B vitamins and Parkinson's disease. *Nutrients.* 7: 7197–7208.

Sheshadri S, Beiser A, Selhub J, *et al.* (2002) Plasma homocysteine as a risk factor for dementia and Alzheimer's disease. *N. Engl. J. Med.* 346: 476–483.

Shrestha S, Lutsey PL, Alsonso A (2016) Serum 25-hydroxyvitamin D concentrations in Mid-adulthood and Parkinson's disease risk. *Movement Disorders* 31(7):972–978.

Shulman L, Taback RL, Bean J, *et al.* (2001) Comorbidity of the nonmotor symptoms of Parkinson's disease. *Mov. Disord.* 16: 507–510.

Suttrup I, Warnecke T. (2016) Dysphagia in Parkinson's Disease. *Dysphagia.* 31(1): 24–32.

Tuite PJ, Maxwell RE, Ikramuddin S, *et al.* (2005) Weight and body mass index in Parkinson's disease patients after deep brain stimulation surgery. *Parkinsonism Relat. Disord.* 11: 247–252.

Uc EY, Struck LK, Rodnitzky RL, *et al.* (2006) Predictors of weight loss in Parkinson's disease. *Mov. Disord.* 21: 930–936.

Uitti R, Ottman R, Goldman SM, *et al.* (1999) Parkinson's disease. *Neurosci. News.* 2: 36–43.

Velseboer DC, de Haan RJ, Wieling W, *et al.* (2011) Prevalence of orthostatic hypotension in Parkinson's disease: a systematic review and meta-analysis. *Parkinsonism Relat. Dis.* 17(10): 724–729.

Watson SG, Leverenz JB. (2010) Profile of cognitive impairment in Parkinson disease. *Brain Path.* 20(3): 640–645.

Wolfe RR, Miller SL, Miller KB. (2008) Optimal protein intake in the elderly. *Clin. Nutr.* 27: 675–684.

Vikdahl M, Carlsson M, Linder J, *et al.* (2014) Weight gain and increased central obesity in early phase of Parkinson's disease. *Clin. Nutr.* 33(6):1132–1139.

7.6.2 Motor neurone disease

Elaine Cawadias and Alan Rio

Key points

- Motor neurone disease (MND) patients require coordinated care from a multidisciplinary team that includes dietetic expertise. Nutritional assessment, guidance and monitoring should commence at the earliest possible stage of the disease.
- Body weight loss of >5% from pre-diagnosis weight is related to shorter survival time, and is a clinical indicator for oral nutritional supplementation.
- Clinical indicators for gastrostomy are dysphagia, weight loss and declining respiratory function.
- Discussion regarding gastrostomy, including patient preferences, risks and benefits, should be initiated early and continue through the disease course.

Motor neurone disease (MND), also known as amyotrophic lateral sclerosis (ALS), is a group of closely related disorders characterised by degeneration of the motor neurones in the brain, brain stem and spinal cord. This degeneration leads to weakness and wasting of muscles. Early symptoms of limb-onset MND include awkwardness in fine finger movement and dexterity, wasting in the limbs, foot drop, neck weakness and stiffness in the fingers. Cramping and fasciculations (muscle twitches) in the forearm, upper arm and shoulder girdle may also appear. Early bulbar symptoms include changes in speech (such as in articulation), throat clearing and difficulty chewing or swallowing some foods.

There is wide variability in disease progression including appearance of symptoms, speed of progression and individual patient experiences; it does not affect the senses. Cognitive function usually remains intact but there is increasing evidence of a dementia component or frontotemporal dementia (FTD), which may have implications for patient decision-making and choices concerning treatment options and interventions. Criteria for the diagnosis of FTD syndromes in ALS have been proposed (Strong *et al.*, 2009).

The progression of the disease can be profound and highly distressing for patients and carers; support and forward planning are key elements of care. As the disease progresses, physical tasks, speech, swallowing and, ultimately, breathing may become affected. The course of the disease varies according to the site of onset, but prognosis is poor, with survival estimated at 2–5 years from symptom onset. In some patients, the disease progression is rapid, and survival may only be a matter of months. Death is usually due to ventilatory failure (Victor & Ropper, 2001).

MND can affect adults at any age, the highest incidence being in the 50–70-year age range, with males affected slightly more frequently than females. The incidence of MND in the UK is approximately 2 per 100,000. Current estimates suggest that approximately 5000 people in the UK have MND (MNDA, 2000).

The cause of MND is unknown in 90–95% of cases, and is classified as sporadic. Approximately 5–10% of patients have the familial form of MND (FALS). A number of genetic mutations have been identified, including SOD1, TDP43 and FUS. About 20% of FALS is caused by the SOD1 mutation, with the remaining known mutations accounting for about 65%. The most common inheritance pattern for FALS is autosomal dominant, with each offspring having a 50% chance of inheriting the gene.

Types

The physical manifestations of the disease depend on which motor neurones are affected. Neurological lesions may primarily occur in the upper motor neurones (from the brain to the spinal cord, termed bulbar onset and affecting the swallowing function), lower motor neurones (from the spinal cord to muscles, termed 'spinal onset' and affecting limbs), or both. It can be difficult to diagnose MND in the early stages as its initial symptoms may be indistinguishable from those of other neurological disorders. Diagnosis can therefore take up to 18 months due to the complexity of the investigations and the need for an accurate diagnosis. Clinical diagnostic tools include electromyography (EMG), nerve conduction studies (NCSs), physical neurological examination, magnetic resonance imaging (MRI) and cerebral spinal fluid protein (Leigh *et al.*, 2003). The El Escorial criteria are often used, with certainty of diagnosis being termed as clinically possible, probable or definitive (World Federation of Neurology Research Group on Neuromuscular Disease, 1994). MND is broadly classified into the following types, although they become less distinguishable as the disease progresses, and may overlap.

Amyotrophic lateral sclerosis

This is the most common form of the disease (about two-thirds of cases), typically occurring between 40 and 70 years. It involves both upper and lower motor neurone lesions, causing muscle weakness and wasting, spasticity (stiffness), hyperactive reflexes (jerking of limbs) and fasciculations. Bulbar onset ALS is seen in about 20% of cases. Symptoms include changes in speech (articulation, volume) and swallowing (food and/or fluids). Limb onset is more common, with symptoms including foot drop, and leg, hand or arm weakness. Most patients with limb onset will eventually develop some bulbar symptoms. Survival time from diagnosis is approximately 2–5 years, although 8–10% survive 10 years (Mitsumoto & Munsat, 2001).

Progressive muscular atrophy

This is a rarer form of MND, accounting for only about 7.5% of cases. It tends to occur at a younger age (often <50 years), and is much more common in men than women (3–4:1). It is predominantly a degeneration of lower motor neurones, causing:

- Diminished or absent tendon reflexes.
- Muscle weakness and wasting.
- Fasciculation, often starting in the small muscles of one hand.
- Weight loss.

The 5-year survival time is 72% in patients with onset under the age of 50 years and 40% in those with onset over the age of 50 years.

Progressive bulbar palsy

This accounts for about 20–25% of cases, mostly occurring in people between the ages of 50 and 70 years: it is slightly more common in women than men. Progressive bulbar palsy (PBP) affects the upper motor neurones and causes paralysis of the bulbar muscles that control speech, chewing and swallowing. Therefore, it tends to present in a different way from the other two forms of the disease discussed earlier. There is debate about whether PBP is a subtype of ALS or a separate disease; however, about 25% of patients with PBP will progress to ALS (Swash & Desai, 2000). Early symptoms are:

- Slurred or nasal-type speech.
- Tongue atrophy with or without fasciculations.
- Pharyngeal weakness.
- Emotional lability.
- Choking on certain foods.

Progression is often rapid, with the median survival time being 2–3 years; such rapid progression may have implications for nutritional support.

Primary lateral sclerosis

This is an extremely rare type of MND with an unknown prevalence. It affects the corticospinal tracts that travel from the brain and are responsible for movement (upper motor neurones). Any part of the body can be affected, and changes include brisk reflexes, increased muscle tone at rest and spasticity. Age of onset is typically in the 50s and is unrelated to the speed of progression of the disease. Unlike most forms of MND, the lifespan of the PLS patient is essentially normal. However, it may progress to MND–ALS after a significant period of time, e.g. more than 25 years after PLS diagnosis.

Management

There is no cure for MND, and management is targeted at changes in nutrition, respiration and physical functions, and includes supportive measures such as non-invasive positive pressure ventilation (NIPPV) and gastrostomy feeding. Riluzole, which acts by inhibiting the release of glutamate and protecting cells from glutamate-mediated damage, is the only NICE-approved drug for MND. It extends survival by about 3 months, primarily in the early stages of the disease. Unlike some neurodegenerative disorders, there is no remission in MND, although there may be temporary plateaus during which no further deterioration occurs.

Multidisciplinary care is crucial, with forward planning and good communication within the healthcare team being cornerstones of care (Miller *et al.*, 2011b). For dietitians working with patients with MND, a multidisciplinary team (MDT) approach will greatly assist in the assessment and planning of nutritional care and plays a key role in supporting the patient between the hospital and community (Table 7.6.2). Early dietetic referral is encouraged (Motor Neurone Disease Association (MNDA), 2000), and ensures that appropriate nutritional advice and monitoring are integrated into patient care (Rio *et al.*, 2005). The benefits of integrated patient care provided by a multidisciplinary clinic are improved prognosis and enhanced survival as compared to MND patients attending a general neurology clinic (Traynor *et al.*, 2003).

Nutritional management

MND affects each patient differently in terms of disease progression. Nutritional management will therefore depend on the nature of the individual symptoms. Patients can experience periods of rapid weight loss leading to profound reduction in mobility, a weakened physical state, respiratory muscle weakness and susceptibility to opportunistic oral infections. Nutritional support has a central role in patient management, and dietitians can influence decisions on nutritional care. The Royal College of Nursing (RCN, 2001) identified three stages of the disease process: diagnostic, palliative and terminal. Patients will not remain in these stages for any set period of time, and may progress so rapidly that they may move straight from diagnosis to the terminal stage. The dietitian needs to be empathetic and show a flexible and adaptable approach to patient care.

Nutritional assessment

Malnutrition in MND resembles marasmus with declining muscle and adipose tissue reserves. Malnutrition at

Table 7.6.2 Multidisciplinary team roles in the management of motor neurone disease

Team member	Role
Dietitian	Nutritional support, texture modification, artificial nutrition and hydration, tube feeding and aftercare, continuing support.
Speech and language therapist	Speech and swallow assessment, assisted communication aides, texture modification, postural modification for safe feeding, liaison with team regarding timing of alternative feeding methods.
Clinical nurse specialist	Educational role, symptom management control, psychological support, coordinated patient care, liaison with community team, advice on tube feeding aftercare.
Occupational therapist	Assessment of functional ability, adaptive aides including cutlery and feeding devices, advice on moving and hoisting, support with adjusting to changing lifestyle.
Physiotherapist	Exercise, mobility, head support, neck collar, assisted cough, respiratory care including chest clearance and NIPPV use.
District nurse	Continuing support, nursing care, feeding tube care, medication, liaison with palliative care and hospice teams.
Pharmacist	Medication, alternative methods of administration, i.e. oral versus tube, solid/crushed/liquid, side effects.

NIPPV, non-invasive positive pressure ventilation.

the time of diagnosis, a weight loss of 10% of usual body weight, has been associated with shorter survival (Limousin *et al.*, 2010). Risk of death is increased 7.7-fold, with nutritional status acting as an independent prognostic factor (Desport *et al.*, 1999). Twenty percent of patients with MND will develop malnutrition, even those without swallowing difficulties (Worwood & Leigh, 1998). However the incidence of malnutrition depends on the criteria used. A number of studies using a BMI of less than $18.5\,kg/m^2$ as an indicator of malnutrition found that 6–53% of patients were malnourished. Although frequently cited, this marker has a number of drawbacks, most notably lack of sensitivity in this patient group. If reduced energy intake is used, 70–100% are affected (Tandan *et al.*, 1999). It has also been suggested that initial BMI at diagnosis can be used as a predictor of rate of decline of function or disease progression (Reich-Slotky *et al.*, 2013). The slowest progression was seen in patients with a BMI of 30. For non-obese patients, a higher BMI was predictive of a slower decline; obese patients (BMI > 30) showed a somewhat faster decline.

Percentage of body weight loss is useful. More than 50% of patients experience weight loss of more than 5% (Marin *et al.*, 2011). Even a 5% weight loss was associated with a 30% increased risk of death. For each additional 5% weight loss, the risk increased by 14%. Anthropometric arm measurement, including mid-arm circumference (MAC) and %MAC, could also be useful in routine monitoring (Salvion *et al.*, 2015).

Nutritional requirements

Reliance on standard equations may lead to either under- or overfeeding (Sherman *et al.*, 2004). Resting metabolic rate (RMR) appears to change over the course of the disease, and this should be factored into calculations. Despite a paradoxically low physical activity level, people with ALS are hypermetabolic by about 10% as compared to matched controls (Tandan *et al.*, 1999), and this increases as the disease progresses (Vaisman *et al.*, 2009). Patients may also have defective energy homeostasis, whereby the hypermetabolic state may accelerate the disease (Dupuis *et al.*, 2004). However, in end-stage disease with mechanical ventilation, RMR is lower and approximates the total energy expenditure (Siirala *et al.*, 2010).

Box 7.6.1 ALS-specific equation to estimate energy requirements (Kasarskis *et al.*, 2014)

Calculate BMR using the Harris Benedict equation = X (kcal)

Adjust for ALS functional status (ALSFRS 6) total scores for the following:

1. Speech
4. Handwriting (with dominant hand prior to ALS onset)
6. Dressing and hygiene
7. Turning in bed/adjusting bed clothes
8. Walking
10. Dyspnoea

$$(55.96 \times \text{ALSFRS 6score}) - 168 = Y$$

$$\text{Daily energy requirements} = X + Y \text{ kcal}$$

A disease-specific equation to estimate energy requirements has been developed (Kasarskis *et al.*, 2014), which is based on six elements of the ALS Functional Rating Scale (ALSFRS) that relate to physical activity (Box 7.6.1). As ALSFRS scores change due to disease progression and declining function, energy requirements can be recalculated to more accurately estimated energy needs.

No disease-specific protein requirements have been established. Nitrogen requirements are calculated using percentage body weight loss and malnourished state. Suggested nitrogen requirements are as follows:

- 0.17 g/kg/day for patients in the early stages of disease.
- 0.2 g/kg/day for patients with body weight loss of 10%.

- 0.25 g/kg/day for malnourished patients and body weight loss of greater than 20%.

Fluid intake should be 30–35 mL/kg of body weight. Fibre intake should aim to meet the current recommendation of 18 g/day. Requirements for vitamins and minerals are not affected by the disease state and, although patients may become severely malnourished, overt deficiencies are rare. Requirements for other nutrients have not been well studied; however, abnormalities in iron regulation have been noted. Patients with MND have disrupted iron homeostasis with significantly higher plasma ferritin levels but normal (or lower) iron and transferrin levels (Goodall *et al.*, 2008; Mitchell *et al.*, 2010; Molfino *et al.*, 2009). It is unclear if this is a result of an increase in stored iron, ongoing muscle degradation or an inflammatory process.

There have been few studies on the effectiveness of nutritional supplements. A systematic review of studies on creatine supplements confirmed that doses of 5–10 g daily had no significant effect on survival, ALSFRS or respiratory function (Pastula *et al.*, 2012).

Metabolic changes including weight, insulin resistance and cholesterol levels have been identified in several neurodegenerative disorders (Ahmed *et al.*, 2016). There appears to be similar changes associated with MND and FTD. Further research is required to clarify the reasons and implications of these changes.

Dietary guidance

Nutritional education should commence as soon as MND is suspected or diagnosed. The basic principles of nutritional support apply, with emphasis on nutrient-dense food and drinks, a variety of foods, ease of food preparation, meal planning and adoption of a liberal and unrestricted diet. Initially, nutritional intake may be boosted by food fortification and by the consumption of frequent small meals and snacks. However, prescribable energy supplements may be necessary if dietary intake fails to meet requirements, or if 10% of body weight is lost (see Chapter 6.3, Oral nutritional support). High-calorie supplements, both high-fat and high-carbohydrate, are suitable (Dorst *et al.*, 2013).

Constipation is common, with causes including decreased physical activity, fibre intake and fluid intake due to swallowing difficulties; increased dependence for toileting; weakness in abdominal or pelvic muscles required to push; medications to control drooling or pain; and slow bowel transit time. Management of constipation focuses on the underlying causes, and may include increasing fibre intake or fibre supplements, increasing fluid intake including thickened fluids, promoting good bowel habits and establishing a bowel routine, careful use of stool softeners or laxatives and control of medications (types, dosage, timing). Unresolved constipation can lead to faecal impaction due to poor dietary intake, dehydration or muscle weakness. Symptoms of faecal impaction include bloating, abdominal distension and, on abdominal X ray, stools and gas throughout the small bowel. Faecal impaction is resolved with macrogols, inert polymers of ethylene that sequester fluid in the bowels, at dosage of 1–3 sachets/day. If this is ineffective, eight sachets in 1 L of water for a maximum of 3 days are recommended.

Dietitians should not forget that, even in the most debilitated patient, the ability to taste, smell and feel the texture of food remains intact, and eating should be made as pleasurable as possible. Patients may enquire about the use of alternative diets, vitamin supplements and plant extracts, and dietitians can help them make an informed choice based on open discussion of their likely efficacy and cost (Cameron & Rosenfeld, 2002; Rosenfeld & Ellis, 2009) (see Chapter 5.4, Alternative and complementary therapies).

Dysphagia

Approximately 70–80% of patients will develop dysphagia. A SLT can assess the severity and nature of the dysphagia and advise on safe swallowing strategies, including chin tuck, head position, texture modification and the use of food and fluid thickeners. Saliva drooling can be managed with medications including sublingual atropine, amitriptyline, glycopyrronium, dermal hyoscine patches, Botox or low-dose radiation. Patients with severe dysphagia have an increased risk of aspiration pneumonia and may be advised to be nil by mouth. However, this measure denies the pleasures associated with eating and drinking. Discussions with the patients and their carers regarding the risks of continuing oral intake is advisable. Some patients may choose to take small amounts of food or fluids of an appropriate texture or consistency for pleasure and quality of life (QoL).

Artificial nutrition and hydration

Artificial nutrition and hydration (ANH) is indicated in MND patients who have (Miller *et al.*, 2009a):

- Severe dysphagia with risk of aspiration pneumonia or recurring chest infections.
- Malnutrition with weight loss of >10% from the prediagnosis weight.
- Suboptimal energy intake.

The goals of ANH should be to (Heffernan *et al.*, 2004):

- Provide additional energy and protein.
- Stabilise body weight.
- Correct malnutrition.
- Act as a route for hydration and medications.
- Decrease the risk of aspiration (although there will still be a risk of aspirating saliva and secretions).

The most common method of providing ANH is gastrostomy, either percutaneous endoscopic gastrostomy (PEG) or percutaneous radiological gastrostomy (PRG). Respiratory status pregastrostomy will help define the suitability for PEG or PRG insertion (Leigh *et al.*, 2003). Current evidence demonstrates that PEG or PRG can be inserted any time during the disease, but that the nutritional benefits diminish as patients enter the terminal phase. Ideally, ANH should be for more than 4–6 weeks, and careful patient selection is crucial to avoid early post-procedure mortality. Pregastrostomy assessment should consider:

- *Respiratory function* – symptoms of poor respiratory function include morning headache, breathlessness, constant shallow breathing, raised PCO_2 levels and reduced forced vital capacity (FVC). Patients with respiratory failure require acclimatisation to NIPPV before gastrostomy. Single-step intervention allows patients to adapt and for their response to be fully evaluated while minimising complications.
- *Stage of the disease* – patients in the terminal phase are unlikely to benefit from gastrostomy.
- *Malnutrition* – patients presenting with severe malnutrition may benefit from NG feeding.
- *QoL* – gastrostomy may reduce QoL by increasing the burden for both patient and carer, and increasing the number of hospital visits. Alternatively, gastrostomy feeding can increase QoL, reducing the amount of time spent consuming food and the distressing symptoms associated with dysphagia.

When considering ANH, the MDT should evaluate the risk–benefit ratio of the gastrostomy procedure. Gastrostomy insertion is a relatively routine procedure and can be performed any time during the course of the disease. However, PEG insertion in MND patients with respiratory failure or respiratory muscle weakness can be life threatening (Mathus-Vliegen *et al.*, 1994), and the 30-day mortality rate following gastrostomy in MND patients is 2–25% (Forbes *et al.*, 2004). There is a median survival of 185 days post-PEG, with worse outcomes in patients with weight loss of >10% of healthy body weight and FVC <65% (Chio *et al.*, 1999). A report into patient outcomes and death in the UK showed a less positive experience for patients having PEG; 43% of patients died within 1 week, and 19% of advisers considered PEG a futile procedure (Cullinane *et al.*, 2004). However, it should be noted that the MND component in this study was quite small (7%). This wide variation in mortality represents differing selection criteria and timing, varying respiratory function and nutritional status of the population, and the expertise of the clinician involved.

The survival benefit to MND patients once associated with PEG is now unclear. Early evidence suggested improved survival (Mazzini *et al.*, 1995), although few studies confirm this increase in survival. One such study (Spataro *et al.*, 2011) showed increased survival in both limb- and bulbar-onset MND patients. Otherwise, it has been suggested that PEG be used for symptom control and improved QoL rather than for survival (Chio *et al.*, 1999). A recent study showed that PEG improves survival in dysphagic ALS patients with few side effects, and that the procedure is safe and applicable even in patients with impaired respiratory function (Spataro *et al.*, 2011). This may be a reflection of the increased experience of clinicians with this patient population. While FVC is commonly used as a guide to respiratory function, it is not a wholly reliable indicator of survival post-PEG. In a group of MND patients with FVC of less than 50% (Gregory *et al.*, 2002), survival was similar to that of a patient group with FVC above the 50% threshold. In a small group of patients with advanced MND, PEG was successfully inserted without respiratory complications (Boitano *et al.*, 2001). While a low FVC should not deprive patients of gastrostomy, thorough respiratory, nutritional and medical assessments are needed to reduce the 30-day mortality rate (Rio & Leigh, 2001).

Thorough assessment by the MDT as to fitness for the procedure can help identify those MND patients likely to benefit. Dietitians should be aware that not all patients with MND progress to requiring a gastrostomy. When PEG or PRG is indicated, it should be offered early in the course of the disease when respiratory function is good and procedural complications are fewer. Early placement also has the advantage of greater nutritional benefit (Table 7.6.3). However, patients choose gastrostomy in their own time and for different reasons. Some patients may want to delay having a gastrostomy for as long as possible. Patients may have misconceptions or misinformation regarding AHN, which delays their decision. Dietitians have a key educational role in helping patients reach this important decision by offering sensitive and timely information. An early referral allows the dietitian to get to know the patient and their family, enabling a relationship to be developed. Initiating education and discussion early allows for a non-crisis decision-making process. Knowledge of the patient's attitude to eating and its importance to them can be helpful in predicting acceptance or rejection of AHN (Johnson *et al.*, 2012). Patients who found interventions such as gastrostomy (and tracheotomy) acceptable when treatment options were first discussed (when recently diagnosed) made choices consistent with these preferences (Albert *et al.*, 1999). However, patients may change their mind, which is their prerogative. Keeping the lines of communication open for ongoing discussion is important to ensure that they are making the decision of their choosing.

Percutaneous endoscopic gastrostomy

Percutaneous endoscopic gastrostomy is the standard nutritional intervention, although insertion poses a number of clinical challenges. Risks associated with the procedure, while serious, are relatively uncommon. They include infection at the insertion site, bleeding, temporary diarrhoea, cramping, nausea and vomiting (all major or minor), oesophageal perforation, and injury to the bowel (Mitchell *et al.*, 2008). Decreased respiratory function and a high-lying stomach may be contraindications.

Percutaneous radiological gastrostomy

This technique, often called radiologically inserted gastrostomy (RIG), is suitable for patients with MND as tube placement does not require oral access. This technique is therefore suitable for patients with bulbar symptoms, although this group is required to lie supine.

Table 7.6.3 Implications of early and late gastrostomy placement

	Early placement	Late placement
Clinical condition	Disease progression at an early stage	Disease state usually advanced
Respiratory status	Good respiratory function (FVC >50%)	Respiratory function often impaired
		Patients using NIPPV due to poor respiratory function or advanced disease state
Nutritional status	Minimal weight loss	Weight loss >10%
	Meal times prolonged but dietary intake may be adequate	Dietary intake likely to be limited and the patient malnourished
Dysphagia	Swallow function mildly affected	Swallow function poor
Potential risks of gastrostomy insertion	Perceived to be fewer	Respiratory (NIPPV) support needed for procedure
	Procedure related	Increased risk of mortality
		Stoma site infection
Benefits	Additional energy and protein intake	Symptom control, including constipation management and reduced risk of aspiration
	Weight stabilisation (individual weight gain is variable)	Improved hydration
		Alleviates anxiety associated with eating and drinking (tube feeding likely to become the sole source of nutrition)
		Small weight gain/weight stabilisation
		May help stabilise respiratory function

FVC, forced ventilatory capacity; NIPPV, non-invasive positive pressure ventilation.

Preprocedural oximetry and a history of desaturation while lying supine should be obtained to prevent unnecessary distress.

Preprocedural abdominal X rays should be taken to investigate either faecal impaction or abdominal gas. The presence of one of these factors can lead to problems after PRG insertion, which include pain, discomfort and bowel perforation. Serious complications, including bowel perforation, occur in approximately 2–5%, which, importantly, are avoidable (Rio *et al.*, 2010). Faecal impaction or gas in the bowel should be resolved prior to the procedure. The standard medications for treatment of chronic constipation are suitable for this patient group and should be prescribed for a minimum of 5–7 days. A repeat abdominal X ray is advised prior to tube placement to check if constipation has resolved; some patients may require a longer duration of laxative use.

Nutritional care of patients with a gastrostomy

Nutritional care of the MND patient with a gastrostomy is similar to that of the other patient group. Some patients may receive all their nutrition via the gastrostomy, or they may choose (where appropriate) to use the gastrostomy to supplement oral intake of food or fluids. Intake should provide adequate energy and adequate, but not excessive, protein, and meet fluid requirements from the formula and additional water. Considerations in choosing a formula include energy density, protein content, fibre or non-fibre content, and special requirements (diabetes and renal disease). Studies comparing the benefits of high-fat or high-carbohydrate formulas have not been conclusive (Wills *et al.*, 2014). Feeding schedules are individualised, depending on full or supplemental feedings, lifestyle and method of administration (pump, gravity or syringe). Given that some patients may have disturbances in iron metabolism, attention to iron status and the amount of iron in the formula may be warranted (Molfino *et al.*, 2009).

Nutritional care of patients assessed unsafe for gastrostomy

Patients with advanced disease presenting with respiratory failure and malnutrition will benefit from the input of the palliative care team. Patients may consider enteral feeding as symbolic of their fight against the disease; however, gastrostomy placement at this time may not be advisable due to the limited benefit of nutritional support. Nutritional support should be carefully considered alongside anticipated goals (Ersek, 2003). Palliation of symptoms and comfort should take priority, while QoL is of paramount importance (see Chapter 7.16, Palliative and end-of-life care).

Nutritional support with nasogastric tube (NGT) feeding is advisable in this group of patients with advanced disease. Fine-bore NGTs are the primary and most frequently used route of tube feeding in the acute hospital setting. However, patients may find an NGT cosmetically unappealing and socially intrusive. Treatment with NGT has a number of advantages:

- Less invasive than PEG or PRG.
- Risk of aspiration is the same as with PEG or PRG.
- Allows immediate delivery of nutrition and hydration.

Feeding via NGT can be a temporary route where expectations of extended survival and return to normal body weight are not sought. Importantly, NGT feeding also allows the response to enteral nutrition to be fully evaluated while the benefit–risk ratio of PEG or PRG is assessed. Nutritional requirements should be calculated in the usual way (see Chapter 6.4, Enteral nutrition), but feeds should be administered gradually over several days as per patient tolerance. Risk of aspiration can be reduced by:

- Effective saliva/secretion management.
- Limiting oral intake or placing patients nil by mouth.
- Using a daytime feeding regimen.
- Ensuring patients are sat upright during feeding.

Discharge into the community with an NGT requires the support of the local team, including the GP, district nurse, home enteral nutrition team and palliative care team. Community support of patients with a NGT may vary, and information for tube replacement and tube care should be provided in advance of discharge. Dietitians have a key leadership role in the coordination and discharge of these patients.

Management of patients who refuse artificial nutrition and hydration therapy

Not all patients with MND will choose to be tube fed. Despite dysphagia, prolonged meal times, aspiration pneumonia and the presence of malnutrition, some patients will choose to maintain oral nutritional intake. Reasons why patients refuse ANH will vary and may include (Cawadias & Carroll-Thomas, 2001):

- Denial of the diagnosis.
- Reluctance to have an invasive procedure.
- Decision to let the disease take its course due to preference, age or comorbidities.
- Unwillingness to accept that a milestone has been reached.
- Misperceptions about the procedure and how the gastrostomy can be used.
- Fear of the unknown.
- Dislike of change of lifestyle.
- Belief that they will be connected to a feeding pump for lengthy periods.
- Inability to manage equipment due to decreased arm function.
- Lack of social support.

Support from the dietitian is vital for these patients, and both the acute and community teams should be involved. The MNDA regional care advisor can also offer input and act as a valuable link with the different care services. Ongoing dietetic input and good communication between team members can help these patients maintain their QoL and dignity. Some patients may initially refuse tube feeding and then suddenly decide they want to go ahead with a gastrostomy. As stated earlier, caution should be exercised, and a thorough assessment of medical fitness for the procedure and likely benefit should be conducted before a decision is made.

Multidisciplinary team in nutritional care

Working in a small team, dietitians may be challenged by the implications of MND and feel overwhelmed. Discussing QoL issues and end-of-life decisions may be unfamiliar to many dietitians. Service provision differs greatly across the UK, and this includes provision for dietetic and multidisciplinary care. Some areas may provide high standards of care, while other dietitians may find themselves working in isolation and with limited resources (Rio & Cawadias, 2007). Where services are limited, dietitians can encourage good practice by regular patient review, adoption of the MNDA nutrition guidelines, liaison with the SLT, communication with the patient's GP, consulting with a specialist MND centre dietitian and involving the patients in any decisions that affect their care. Confidence in working with this patient population comes with experience. Some patients may visit tertiary referral centres for review, clinical trials or respiratory management. Liaison with the team dietitian, centre coordinator, clinical nurse specialist or neurologist is highly recommended. Not only will this help in terms of patient care, but it also provides a source of professional support and further information.

Further reading

Motor Neurone Disease Association (MNDA). (2000) *MND Resource File: A Patient and Carer Centred Approach for Health and Social Care Professionals*. Northampton: MNDA.

Internet resources

Amyotrophic Lateral Sclerosis Association, www.alsa.org
Motor Neurone Disease (MND) Association, www.mndassociation.org
World Federation of Neurology – Research Group on Motor Neurone Disease, www.wfnals.org

References

Ahmed RM, Irish M, Piguet O, *et al.* (2016) Amyotrophic lateral sclerosis and frontotemporal dementia: distinct and overlapping changes in eating behaviour and metabolism. *Lancet Neurol.* 15(3): 332–342.

Albert SM, Murphy PL, Del Bene ML, *et al.* (1999) A prospective study of preferences and actual treatment choices in ALS. *Neurol.* 53(2): 278–283.

Boitano LJ, Jordan T, Benditt JO. (2001) Noninvasive ventilation allows gastrostomy tube placement in patients with advanced ALS. *Neurology.* 56: 413–414.

Cameron A, Rosenfeld J. (2002) Nutritional issues and supplements in amyotrophic lateral sclerosis and other neurodegenerative disorders. *Curr. Opin. Clin. Nutr. Metab. Care* 5: 631–643.

Cawadias E, Carroll-Thomas S. (2001) *Nutritional support in ALS: supporting the decision for oral feeding. Poster presentation*. Dietitians of Canada Annual Conference, Winnipeg, Canada.

Chio A, Finocchiaro E, Meineri P, *et al.* (1999) Safety and factors related to survival after percutaneous endoscopic gastrostomy in ALS. ALS Percutaneous Endoscopic Gastrostomy Study Group. *Neurology.* 53(5): 1123–1125.

Cullinane M, Gray AJG, Hargraves CMK, *et al.* (2004) *Scoping Our Practice. The National Confidential Enquiry into Patient Outcome and Death*. London: NCEPOD. Available at www.ncepod.org.uk. Accessed 28 August 2012.

Desport JC, Preux PM, Truong TC, *et al.* (1999) Nutritional status is a prognostic factor for survival in ALS patients. *Neurology.* 53(5): 1059–1063.

Dorst J, Cypionka J, Ludolph AC. (2013) High-calorie food supplements in the treatment of amyotrophic lateral sclerosis: a prospective interventional study. *Amyotroph. Lateral Scler. Frontotemporal. Degener.* 14: 533–536

Dupuis L, Oudart H, Rene F, *et al.* (2004) Evidence for defective energy homeostasis in amyotrophic lateral sclerosis: benefit of a high-energy diet in a transgenic mouse model. *Proc. Natl. Acad. Sci. USA* 101(30): 11159–11164.

Ersek M. (2003) Artificial nutrition and hydration: clinical issues. *J. Hosp. Palliat. Nurs.* 5(4): 221–230.

Forbes RB, Colville S, Swingler RJ; Scottish Motor Neurone Disease Research Group. (2004) Frequency, timing and outcome of gastrostomy tubes for amyotrophic lateral sclerosis/motor neurone disease – a record linkage study from the Scottish Motor Neurone Disease Register. *J. Neurol.* 251(7): 813–817.

Gregory S, Siderowf A, Golaszewski AL, *et al.* (2002) Gastrostomy insertion in ALS patients with low vital capacity: respiratory support and survival. *Neurology.* 58(3): 485–487.

Goodall EF, Haque MS, Morrison KE. (2008) Increased serum ferritin level in amyotrophic lateral sclerosis (ALS) patients. *J. Neurol.* 255(11): 1652–1656.

Heffernan C, Jenkinson C, Holmes T, *et al.* (2004) Nutritional management in MND/ALS patients: an evidence based review. *Amyotroph. Lateral Scler. Other Motor Neuron. Disord.* 5(2): 72–83.

Johnson J, Leigh PN, Shaw CE, *et al.* (2012) Eating derived pleasure in amyotrophic lateral sclerosis as a predictor of non-oral feeding. *Amyotroph. Lateral Scler.* 13(6): 555–559.

Kasarskis EJ, Mendiondo MS, Matthews DE, *et al.* (2014) Estimating daily energy expenditure in individuals with amyotrophic lateral sclerosis. *Am. J. Clin. Nutr.* 99(4): 792–803.

Leigh PN, Abrahams S, Al-Chalabi A, *et al.* (2003) The management of motor neurone disease. *J. Neurol. Neurosurg. Psychiatry.* 74: iv32–iv47.

Limousin N, Blasco H, Corcia P, *et al.* (2010) Malnutrition at the time of diagnosis is associated with a shorter disease duration in ALS. *J. Neurol. Sci.* 297(1–2): 36–39.

Marin B, Desport JC, Kajeu P, *et al.* (2011) Alteration of nutritional status at diagnosis is a prognostic factor for survival of amyotrophic lateral sclerosis patients. *J. Neurol. Neurosurg. Psychiatry* 82: 628–634.

Mathus-Vliegen LM, Louwerse LS, Merkus MP, *et al.* (1994) Percutaneous endoscopic gastrostomy in patients with amyotrophic lateral sclerosis and impaired pulmonary function. *Gastrointest. Endosc.* 40(4): 463–469.

Mazzini L, Corra T, Zaccala M, *et al.* (1995) Percutaneous endoscopic gastrostomy and enteral nutrition in amyotrophic lateral sclerosis. *J. Neurol.* 242(10): 695–698.

Miller RG, Jackson CE, Kasarskis EJ, *et al.* (2009a) Practice parameter update: the care of the patient with amyotrophic lateral sclerosis: drug, nutritional, and respiratory therapies. *Neurology.* 73: 1218–1226.

Miller RG, Jackson CE, Kasarskis EJ, *et al.* (2009b) Practice parameter update: the care of the patient with amyotrophic lateral sclerosis: Multidisciplinary care, symptom management, and cognitive/behavioral impairment. *Neurology.* 73: 1227–1233.

Mitchell RM, Simmons Z, Beard JL, *et al.* (2010) Plasma biomarkers associated with ALS and their relationship to iron homeostasis. *Muscle Nerve.* 42: 95–103.

Mitchell SL, Tetroe JM, O'Connor AM. (2008) *Making Choices: Long Term Feeding Tube Placement in Elderly Patients.* Ottawa: The Ottawa Health Research Institute.

Mitsumoto, H, Munsat TL (eds). (2001) *Amyotrophic Lateral Sclerosis: A Guide for Patients and Families*, 2nd edn. New York: Demos Medical Publishing.

Molfino A, Kushta I, Tommasi V, *et al.* (2009) Amyotrophic lateral sclerosis, enteral nutrition and the risk of iron overload. *J. Neuro.* 256: 1015–1016.

Motor Neurone Disease Association (MNDA). (2000) *MND Resource File: A Patient and Carer Centred Approach for Health and Social Care Professionals.* Northampton: MNDA.

Pastula DM, Moore DH, Bedlack RS. (2012) Creatine for amyotrophic lateral sclerosis/motor neuron disease. *Cochrane Database Syst. Rev.* 12: CD005225.

Reich-Slotky R, Andrews J, Cheng B, *et al.* (2013) Body mass index (BMI) as predictor of ALSFRS-R score decline in ALS patients. *Amyotroph. Lateral Scler. Frontotemporal Degeneration.* 14(3): 212–216.

Rio A, Cawadias E. (2007) Nutritional advice and treatment by dietitians to patients with amyotrophic lateral sclerosis/motor neurone disease: a survey of current practice in England, Wales, Northern Ireland and Canada. *J. Hum. Nutr. Diet.* 20(1): 3–13.

Rio A, Leigh PN. (2001) Noninvasive ventilation allows gastrostomy tube placement in patients with advanced ALS. *Neurology.* 57(7): 1351; discussion 1351–1352.

Rio A, Ampong MA, Johnson J, *et al.* (2005a) Nutritional care of patients with MND: recent advances in management. *Br. J. Neurosci. Nurs.* 1: 38–41.

Rio A, Ellis C, Shaw C, *et al.* (2010) Nutritional factors associated with survival following enteral tube feeding in patients with motor neurone disease. *J. Hum. Nutr. Diet.* 23(4): 408–415.

Rosenfeld J, Ellis A. (2009) Nutrition and dietary supplements in motor neuron disease. *Phys. Med. Rehabil. Clin. N. Am.* 19(3): 573–589.

Royal College of Nursing (RCN); MND Nurse Specialist Working Party. (2001) *Paradigm for Disease Management in Motor Neurone Disease.* London: RCN.

Salvioni CC, Stancih P, Oliveria AS, *et al.* (2015) Anthropometry of arm: nutritional risk indicator in myotrophic lateral sclerosis. *Neurol. Int.* 7(3): 48–53.

Sherman MS, Pillai A, Jackson A, *et al.* (2004) Standard equations are not accurate in assessing resting energy expenditure in patients with amyotrophic lateral sclerosis. *J. Parenter. Enteral Nutr.* 28(6): 442–446.

Siirala W, Olkkola KT, Noponen T, *et al.* (2010) Predictive equations over-estimate the resting energy expenditure in amyotrophic lateral sclerosis patients who are dependent on invasive ventilation support. *Nutr. Metab.* 7: 70.

Spataro R, Ficano L, Piccoli F, *et al.* (2011) PEG in ALS: effect on survival. *J. Neurol. Sci.* 304(1–2): 44–48.

Strong M, Grace GM, Freedman M, *et al.* (2009) Consensus criteria for the diagnosis of frontotemporal cognitive and behavioural syndromes in amyotrophic lateral sclerosis. *Amyotroph. Lateral Scler.* 10: 131–146.

Swash M, Desai J. (2000) Motor neuron disease: classification and nomenclature. *Amyotroph. Lateral Scler. Other Motor Neuron Disord.* 1: 105–112.

Tandan R, Hiser JR, Krusinski PB, *et al.* (1999) Energy requirements in amyotrophic lateral sclerosis measured by the doubly labelled water methodology. *Neurology.* 52(2): A2–A3.

Traynor BJ, Alexander M, Corr B, *et al.* (2003) Effect of a multidisciplinary amyotrophic lateral sclerosis (ALS) clinic on ALS survival: a population based study, 1996–2000. *J. Neurol. Neurosurg. Psychiatry.* 74(9): 1258–1261.

Vaisman N, Lusaus M, Nefussy B, *et al.* (2009) Do patients with amyotrophic lateral sclerosis (ALS) have increased energy needs? *J. Neurol. Sci.* 279: 26–29.

Victor M, Ropper AH (eds). (2001) *Adams & Victor's Principles of Neurology.* New York: McGraw Hill Medical Publishing Division Worldwide.

Wills AM, Hubbard J, Macklin EA, *et al.* (2014) Hypercaloric enteral nutrition in patients with amyotrophic lateral sclerosis: a randomised, double-blind, placebo-controlled phase 2 trial. *Lancet.* 383(9934): 2065–2072.

World Federation of Neurology. (1994) Criteria for the diagnosis of amyotrophic lateral sclerosis. *J. Neurol. Sci.* 124: 96–107.

Worwood AM, Leigh PN. (1998) Indicators and prevalence of malnutrition in motor neurone disease. *Eur. Neurol.* 40(3): 159–163.

7.6.3 Rare neurological conditions

Katie Johnson, Sarah J. Cameron, Emma Gaskin and Adri De Sousa

Key points

- Patients with myasthenia gravis experience varying degrees of dysphagia due to muscle weakness and fatigue; they may require enteral nutrition support as a temporary measure.
- Huntington's disease is a complex, progressive disease in which weight loss is common due to increased requirements, dysphagia and feeding difficulties.
- Patients with multiple-system atrophy experience orthostatic hypotension and, in the later stages, often dysphagia and malnutrition.
- Duchenne's muscular dystrophy is a severe, progressive, muscle-wasting disease. Patients may require nutritional intervention throughout their lifespan for malnutrition, obesity, or dysphagia.
- Patients with Guillain–Barré syndrome may require enteral tube feeding if ventilated. Nutritional intervention should concentrate on weight maintenance and meeting nutritional requirements.

This chapter covers some of the rare neurological conditions that dietitians may be involved in treating. While the nutritional problems and dietetic interventions may vary, the dietetic assessment is fundamental to all of these conditions, as shown in Table 7.6.4.

Myasthenia gravis

Disease process

Myasthenia gravis (MG) is an autoimmune disease affecting the neuromuscular junction. It is caused by antibodies linking to neurotransmitter receptors on the muscle end plate, thus disrupting the flow of neurotransmitters from the neurone to the muscle. In the majority of cases, the antibodies link specifically to acetylcholine receptors. The disruption in the pathway leads to painless muscle weakness and fatigue. Approximately 85% of patients present with ocular muscle weakness, mostly ptosis (drooping of the eyelids) and/or diplopia (double vision). Only 17% present with ocular muscle weakness without any further muscle weakness (Grob *et al.*, 2008). Bulbar weakness is also a common symptom in MG and presents as dysarthria (disordered articulation of speech), dysphagia, dysphonia (problems with voice/pitch), nasal-sounding speech and masticatory weakness (Meriggioli & Sanders, 2009).

The Association of British Neurologists' management guidelines (Sussman *et al.*, 2015) suggest that serum anti-acetylcholine receptor (ACh-R) antibody is the first-line investigation for non-urgent patients. If negative, serum anti-muscle-specific kinase (MuSK) is indicated. A neurophysical examination aids diagnosis in seronegative patients. This includes repetitive nerve stimulation initially; if negative, single fibre electromyography should be conducted. Those with negative serology and neurophysiology and symptoms compatible with MG may have structural brain disease, and therefore an MRI scan of the brain is required; a tensilon test can be used. All patients should undergo thymus imaging and thyroid function testing. The subtypes of diagnosis include: Ach-R or MuSK, and thymoma (ocular or congenital) (Sussman *et al.*, 2015).

Disease consequences

The suggested prevalence in the UK is 15 per 100,000 (Spillane *et al.*, 2012). It affects children and adults, with children accounting for 10–15% of cases. Mortality associated with MG is usually related to myasthenic crisis, where weakness affects respiratory muscles, leading to a requirement for intubation and ventilation. Alshekhlee *et al.* (2009) reported mortality rates of 4.5% in patients in myasthenic crisis.

Nutritional consequences

Dysphagia

Dysphagia occurs in 15–40% of MG patients (Llabrés *et al.*, 2005). On initial diagnosis, the risk of dysphagia must be discussed, as this can greatly impact on the self-management of oral intake during future episodes of crisis or deterioration.

Physical and cognitive fatigue

This can impact on oral intake and the ability to consume sufficient nutrition. The drug, pyridostigmine, is active within 30–60 minutes; therefore, taking this before meal preparation, eating and physical activity can maximise oral intake and minimise fatigue.

Blood glucose management

Blood glucose should be monitored with the commencement of prednisolone, and patients should be advised regarding the potential for weight gain. Daily rather than alternate-day prednisolone may improve glycaemic

Table 7.6.4 Generic dietetic assessment for rare neurological conditions

Anthropometry and functional testing	Weight, weight history, % weight loss, weight gain in sedentary patients (use wheelchair or hoist scales for non-weight-bearing patients).
	Waist circumference to assess abdominal.
	Assessment of lean body mass – with MUAC and/or grip strength.
Biochemistry	Urea and electrolytes.
	Liver function tests.
	Annual serum 25-hydroxyvitamin D (ideally late winter) – recheck level after 3 months on treatment, PTH, calcium.
	Oral glucose.
Clinical	Effects of reduced dexterity/upper limb strength/ataxia/fatigue on ability to self-feed.
	Changes in mobility and impact of tremor/dyskinesia/dystonia on energy expenditure.
	Swallow ability and whether taking appropriate texture of food, fluid and medications.
	Pressure damage/risk when mobility reduced.
	Upper gastrointestinal symptoms, including reflux, nausea and vomiting.
	Emotional adjustment and mood (depression, anxiety) and effects on appetite.
	Bowel function – especially constipation (if present).
	Enteral feed tolerance and gastrostomy stoma health.
Dietary	Energy, protein, fluid and micronutrient intake.
	Tolerance to and palatability of altered-texture food/fluids and medications.
	Ability to communicate food and feeding preferences.
	Posture and seating at mealtimes.
Economic and social	Support required and provided for feeding/accessing food and drink.
	Physical impairment and ability to access food (shopping/ cooking).

MUAC, mid upper arm circumference.

control in patients who are having treatment for elevated blood glucose.

Bone health

Prednisolone can cause bone thinning, and therefore bone protection protocol should be followed.

Nutritional assessment

In addition to the assessment shown in Table 7.6.4, the following should be considered:

- Clinical assessment
  - Bowel function should be monitored closely due to the side effects of pyridostigmine.
  - Vital capacity (VC) readings provide an indication of respiratory function; decreasing VC indicates a worsening of the disease process, with swallow function likely to be affected.

Clinical investigation and management

Cholinesterase inhibitors reduce the breakdown of acetylcholine, thereby increasing circulating levels. This has a beneficial effect on muscle weakness, as there is more acetylcholine available for binding to receptors. Pyridostigmine is a commonly used cholinesterase inhibitor. Side effects can include abdominal cramps, diarrhoea and nausea. Immunosuppressive medications such as prednisolone or azathioprine can be used in conjunction with cholinesterase inhibitors. Plasma exchange and intravenous immunoglobulin treatment are immune therapies that are used when short-term improvement is required, e.g. during myasthenic crisis (Wendell & Levine, 2011). Surgical removal of the thymus gland may be performed as it has been implicated in the production of receptor antibodies.

Nutritional management

Tailored nutritional management is essential as severity can vary from person to person. Close liaison with the speech and language therapist (SLT) and the wider multidisciplinary team (MDT) should be encouraged in order to best facilitate the patient's nutritional needs. A texture-modified diet may be required if the patient is dysphagic. The nutritional adequacy of the diet should be assessed, especially in case of progressive dysphagia (see Chapter 7.3, Dysphagia). Patients often experience increasing fatigue towards the end of the day, and it is not uncommon for the recommendation of a texture-modified diet to vary according to individual meal times, e.g. patients may successfully manage a soft/moist diet at lunchtime, but benefit from a puréed meal in the evening.

Recommendations should be made for smaller, more frequent meals, rather than full portions. Additional snacks between meals should be encouraged, including fortified drinks and desserts and/or oral sip feeds and dessert-based supplements, to enable patients to meet their nutritional requirements (see Chapter 6.3, Oral nutritional support). Nutrition support via a nasogastric tube may be required if there are concerns regarding aspiration risk, if dysphagia is severe or if respiratory function is compromised. During myasthenic crisis, patients may require intubation and ventilation, which may warrant an intensive care admission. For these patients, requirements should be calculated as for other critical care patients (see Chapter 7.17.1, Critical care). Enteral feeding as a result of dysphagia is usually a short-term measure, as the establishment of an effective medication regimen should assist in improving swallow function. As compared to other neurological conditions, gastrostomy insertion is typically considered too aggressive in MG, due to its variable course and crisis periods (Cereda *et al.*, 2009).

Huntington's disease

Disease process

Huntington's disease (HD) is a complex, inherited, neurodegenerative disorder. It is a genetic condition caused by the autosomal dominant inheritance of an expanded cytosine–adenine–guanine (CAG) nucleotide within the Huntington gene (HTT) on chromosome 4. Subsequent brain cell dysfunction results in a progressive multisystem disease characterised primarily by the following:

- *Motor symptoms* – dyskinesia (involuntary movements), dystonia, rigidity, gait disorder.
- *Cognitive symptoms* – lack of initiation, perseveration, impulsivity, perceptual problems (poor insight) and communication problems.
- *Neuropsychiatric/behavioural symptoms* – depression, obsessive–compulsive disorder, irritability, apathy, anxiety and sleep disturbances.

HD can be described in three distinct stages. In early stages, subtle dyskinesia presents alongside mild changes to co-ordination, mood, ability to plan, organise and prioritise. By mid-stage, executive functions decline, affecting, reasoned decision-making, memory and the ability to learn new information; also, dyskinesia increases. By late stages, mobility difficulties lead to immobility, and severe cognitive decline progresses to global dementia and an inability to self-care.

Disease consequences

HD commonly manifests in adulthood, at 30–50 years, limiting lifespan to 15–20 years from clinical onset (Sackley *et al.*, 2011). It affects men and women, and all ethnic groups, with a prevalence of 6–11 per million (Aziz & Roos, 2013). Juvenile forms (onset <20 years) and late-onset forms (>70 years) exist, but are less common and present a different clinical picture.

Nutritional consequences

Weight loss

Unintended and often rapid weight loss is well documented, particularly in late-stage disease. However, evidence demonstrates that, even in premanifest HD, individuals present with a lower BMI than controls (Aziz *et al.*, 2008). Several studies demonstrate that weight loss has a significant impact on disease progression and quality of life (QoL) (Aziz & Roos, 2013). The aetiology of weight loss is not easily defined due to a complex interplay of factors. Those affecting energy intake include swallowing and feeding difficulties, side effects of medications, and mood and behavioural disturbances. Factors affecting energy expenditure include increased energy expenditure due to dyskinesia, increased metabolism due to altered pathology in the hypothalamic region of the brain (Aziz & Roos, 2013) and malabsorption. Malabsorption has been shown to affect energy balance in animal models (Van der Burg *et al.*, 2011); however, this is yet to be demonstrated in human studies. These physiological changes may explain why weight loss occurs in the presence of increased appetite and energy intake.

In assessing energy requirements using the Harris–Benedict equation, Gaba *et al.* (2008) demonstrated higher TEE in HD, suggesting the use of an activity factor of 1.7 in early- and mid-stage HD as compared to 1.4 for controls. However, this, along other studies, showed significant variations in energy requirements between individuals and throughout the course of the disease (Werner & Boozer, 2005), thus making frequent weight monitoring essential.

Feeding difficulties

Dyskinesia makes self-feeding challenging, with most patients requiring support with meals. It affects chewing, lip-seal and swallowing, making eating and drinking tiring and frustrating. Dysarthria and cognitive changes affect decision-making and the ability to communicate food preferences, which can lead to inappropriate food choices, eating too much too quickly and obsessive behaviours. The resulting frustration can present as challenging behaviour. Carers therefore need to provide simple, clear choices and prompting with meals.

Dysphagia

Marked dysphagia and impaired mouth–tongue control usually occur during mid-stage HD. Aspiration and asphyxiation are significant risks caused by increased distractibility, anxiety, inadequate mastication, difficulties with bolus formation, delayed swallow initiation and reduced pharyngeal motility (Heemskerk & Roos, 2011).

Changes to appetite

Increased appetite can lead to individuals cramming food into their mouths, causing problems with choking and food spillage. Neuronal changes and the psychological impact of HD commonly contribute to depression and anxiety, which can affect appetite. Gastrointestinal problems, including vomiting, reflux and regurgitation, can also cause patients to limit intake.

Nutritional assessment

In addition to the assessment shown in Table 7.6.4, the following should be considered:

- Clinical
  - Oral health, due to the risk of chest infections from aspiration of bacteria-laden saliva.
  - Impact of atypical neuroleptics (olanzapine/risperidone/quetiapine) on mood, appetite, gastrointestinal function, triglycerides and glucose.
- Dietary
  - Impulsive food choices can limit variety in diet.
  - Recreational drug use, alcohol or smoking, and impact on diet.
- Economic and social
  - Impact of environment on intake aiming to limit distractions.

Clinical investigation and management

Genetic testing will define if someone has a strong likelihood of developing HD; CAG repeats exceeding 40 will confirm the diagnosis. Currently, there is no cure, and management focuses on managing symptoms and improving QoL. Pharmacological management is tailored to managing individual symptoms and is often based on clinical experience due to the limited evidence base for drug therapy in HD (Novak & Tabrizi, 2011). However, timely, specialist multidisciplinary care is shown to have a significant impact on symptom control and QoL (Brotherton *et al.*, 2012).

Nutritional management

As symptoms manifest differently between individuals and throughout disease course, a person-centred approach, taking disease stage into account, is required. Establishing target weight early ensures the dietitian and MDT have clear goals regarding weight management. Nutritional goals should focus on meeting increased requirements with a balanced intake of nutrients. Advice on achieving increased requirements should be practical, while taking feeding difficulties into account. Guidance may be required on energy-dense food choices, food fortification strategies and oral nutritional supplements (see Chapter 6.3, Oral nutritional support), especially when dysphagia and dyskinesia are present.

Facilitating eating and drinking

Assessment and advice from an occupational therapist (OT) can assist in positioning and feeding techniques. The use of mealtime aids such as adapted cutlery, double-handed cups and non-slip mats can be used to facilitate eating to make mealtimes more pleasant.

Minimising risks of dysphagia

Modified-texture diets may be required for many years; therefore, sensory deprivation and taste blindness should be taken into account, and presentation and food moulds considered for aiding intake. Considering the environment by reducing distractions can reduce choking and aspiration risk, particularly in late-stage disease.

Enteral feeding

As HD progresses, maintaining weight becomes more challenging with dysphagia, and gastrostomy feeding may need to be considered. Calvert *et al.* (2005) demonstrated that PEG feeding not only improved weight but also the behaviour and distress, which are in part secondary to the hunger, anxiety and fatigue caused by chronic malnutrition. Decisions regarding artificial feeding towards the end of life pose ethical dilemmas, especially when left until the late stages. It is important that patients' wishes be documented before cognitive decline and dysarthria affect their capacity and ability to consent to treatment. An advanced directive can be developed with support of the MDT to ensure patient's wishes are formally documented and adhered to.

Monitoring nutritional progress

Basic nutritional assessments are required over the duration of the disease to identify the nutritional problems at an early stage and the steps taken to rectify them. Frequent and regular monitoring of weight to maintain a healthy weight and a BMI of 23–25 kg/m^2 is recommended (Brotherton *et al.*, 2012), ensuring adequacy of nutritional intake to prevent rapid weight loss (see Section 1.84).

Multiple system atrophy

Disease process

Multiple system atrophy (MSA) is a fatal neurodegenerative condition characterised by progressive autonomic failure, parkinsonism and cerebellar ataxia (poor balance and coordination). It is considered a sporadic disease, although it has been shown that genetic factors play a role in some families (Fanciulli & Wenning, 2015). MSA commonly presents in one of two subtypes, cerebellar subtype or parkinsonian subtype, the latter being two to four times more common in most countries. Due to its varied clinical manifestation, it can be misdiagnosed as pure autonomic failure or Parkinson's disease (PD).

Disease consequence

Prevalence is approximately 3–5 per million, increasing to 8 per million over 40 years (Fanciulli & Wenning, 2015). It affects both men and women, usually in their 50s and 60s, with a mean survival from onset of 6–10 years, with some individuals surviving for 15 years or more. It is a rapidly progressing, disabling disease, with many disability milestones accumulating over a short period of time.

Nutritional consequence

Dysphagia affects approximately 64% of patients, and its presence is associated with a poor prognosis (Fernagut *et al.*, 2012). Dysphagia commonly occurs in advanced stages along with dysphonia (which significantly affects the ability to communicate preferences relating to eating and drinking) and dysarthria. As in PD, slower gastric emptying rates are seen in MSA as commonly contributing to gastrointestinal symptoms including nausea, vomiting, reflux, abdominal bloating and constipation. Progressive weight loss is also common in advanced stages of the disease.

Nutritional assessment

In addition to the assessment shown in Table 7.6.4, the following should be considered:

- Clinical
  - Blood pressure, paying attention to post-prandial changes.
- Dietary
  - Meal pattern, paying attention to the effects of large meals on blood pressure.
  - Fluid and salt intake.

Clinical investigation and management

There is no single clinical feature or investigation that confirms MSA. However, it has been agreed that recent diagnostic criteria improve the identification of early or possible MSA. The diagnostic criteria for probable MSA (Gilman *et al.*, 2008) outline a sporadic, progressive, adult (over 30 years)-onset disease characterised by the following:

- Autonomic failure involving urinary incontinence, or an orthostatic decrease (by at least 30 mmHg systolic or 15 mmHg diastolic) in blood pressure within 3 minutes of standing
- Parkinsonism with poor levodopa response
- A cerebellar syndrome (gait ataxia with cerebellar dysarthria, limb ataxia, or cerebellar oculomotor dysfunction)

There is no specific drug therapy available, and pharmacological treatment is aimed primarily at symptom relief.

Nutritional management

Dietary measures can support the symptomatic relief of orthostatic hypotension. European guidelines for orthostatic hypotension management recommend a salt intake of 8 g/day to compensate for renal losses and a fluid intake of 2–2.5 L/ day (NGC, 2011). Avoiding large meals and alcohol can contribute to the management of postprandial hypotension. Texture-modified and energy-dense diets should be considered if fatigue impacts on oral intake or if weight loss occurs. Gastrostomy feeding should be considered when signs of dysphagia present.

Duchenne muscular dystrophy (DMD)

Disease process

Duchenne muscular dystrophy is a severe, progressive, muscle-wasting disease. It is the most severe form of muscular dystrophy and the second-most common hereditary genetic disorder (Bushby *et al.*, 2010a). Milder forms exist, including intermediate muscular dystrophy and Becker muscular dystrophy (Bushby *et al.*, 2010a). DMD occurs as a result of mutations (mainly deletions) in the dystrophin gene, which lead to defects in the protein dystrophin. Muscle degeneration usually causes patients to be wheelchair bound by 13–16 years of age. Improvements in care have led to an improved life expectancy of up to 35 years or more (Bianchi *et al.*, 2011).

Disease consequences

The incidence of DMD is 1 in every 3600 live male births (Bushby *et al.*, 2010a). Diagnosis is usually made by a neuromuscular specialist, typically at around 5 years of age. Initial symptoms may include delayed milestones, e.g. walking, running, climbing stairs or frequent falls. Patients with DMD are at risk of respiratory complications due to the progressive loss of respiratory muscle strength. Progressive cardiomyopathy is currently a major source of morbidity and mortality (Bushby *et al.*, 2010b). Treatments are aimed at delaying the loss of muscle strength and function, including pharmacological interventions and physical therapy.

Bone health is an important part of lifelong DMD care. Jeronimo *et al.* (2015) highlight the monitoring of osteoporosis risk. Speech and language deficits and cognitive delays are well documented, causing difficulties in social functioning, anxiety and withdrawal (Bushby *et al.*, 2010a). There is increased risk of neurobehavioral and neurodevelopmental disorders, including autism spectrum disorders, attention-deficit hyperactivity disorder, and obsessive–compulsive disorder (Bushby *et al.*, 2010a). Good management of DMD requires a multidisciplinary approach to improve function, QoL, and survival. Cardiac transplant could be a future consideration.

Nutritional consequences

Patients may require nutritional intervention throughout their lifespan for malnutrition, obesity or dysphagia (caused by pharyngeal weakness). The overall aim is to achieve and maintain good nutritional status and treat problems associated with DMD, relevant medications and/or therapies.

Weight changes

Patients on steroid therapy in childhood are prone to slower height gain and easier weight gain, increasing the risk of becoming overweight in early years; BMI declines as patients age (Davidson *et al.*, 2014). Shimizu-Fujiwara *et al.* (2012) showed that resting energy expenditure (REE) was significantly lower at all ages, and this was strongly associated with vital capacity, and therefore disease progression. Obesity in adolescence is common due to reduced REE, reduced mobility and steroid-induced increased appetite. However, modest weight gain should not be discouraged in childhood as nutritional status will decline with disease progression (Bushby *et al.*, 2010b), and weight gain at this age can delay the onset of malnutrition in later life. Weight loss occurs due to muscle atrophy, dysphagia and/or increased energy expenditure in later years when respiratory function declines.

Dysphagia

Dysphagia symptoms can develop gradually in young adulthood, and the impact may be under-recognised and under-reported by patients (Shinonaga *et al.*, 2008). Diet modification may be appropriate, and should be implemented in conjunction with SLT. Adaptations for wheelchair users may include elevated lap trays, adaptive straws, hands-free water pouches or turntables (Bushby *et al.*, 2010b). If aspiration risk is significant, gastrostomy placement should be discussed with the patient after MDT discussion.

Gastrointestinal symptoms

Constipation is common, especially following surgery. Contributing factors include analgesia, immobility and/or dysphagia (causing poor fluid and fibre intake) (Bushby *et al.*, 2010b). Swallowing air due to ventilator use (aerophagia) can cause gastric and intestinal dilatation. Limited mobility and scoliosis/kyphoscoliosis restricts lung function and gastric capacity, therefore contributing to gastro-oesophageal reflux (GORD) and early satiety.

Nutritional assessment

In addition to the assessment shown in Table 7.6.4, the following should be considered:

- Anthropometry
  - BMI is an ineffective measure of nutritional status due to altered body composition caused by the progressive loss of LBM.
- Clinical
  - Annual DXA scan to monitor bone density.
- Dietary assessment
  - Multivitamin supplement with vitamin D and minerals.
  - Ability to eat when requiring non-invasive ventilation.

Clinical investigation and management

Translarna, the first gene-targeted drug for DMD (Haas *et al.*, 2015), treats a specific DMD genetic mutation present in 10–15% of cases. Long-term corticosteroids are recommended to reduce morbidity (Jeronimo *et al.*, 2015), but have side effects including increased hunger, growth impairments, diabetes, hypertension, osteoporosis and increased fracture risk.

Dietary advice should take into account these side effects. Nutritional goals should aim towards limiting weight loss rather than prevention due to loss of muscle mass. Early satiety should be managed by advising on small, energy-dense snacks or meals evenly spread throughout the day. Consider food fortification and low-volume nutritional supplements. To prevent/manage constipation, ensure that appropriate laxatives have been considered, and advise on dietary fibre and fluid intake.

Supplements

There is no benefit for creatine use to prevent muscle wasting in DMD (Escolar *et al.*, 2005). There is no evidence of benefit for the use of Q10, carnitine, glutamine, arginine, fish oil, vitamin E and green-tea extract in DMD (Bushby *et al.*, 2010a).

Guillain–Barré syndrome

Disease process

Guillain–Barré syndrome (GBS) is an autoimmune disease affecting the peripheral nerves. It is characterised by bilateral weakness, numbness, pain, and, in severe cases, paralysis, which progresses up the body (Pithadia & Kakadia, 2010). GBS is a heterogeneous condition; the most common type is acute inflammatory demyelinating polyradiculoneuropathy (AIDP). Other subtypes include acute motor axonal neuropathy and acute motor and sensory axonal neuropathy (Willison *et al.*, 2016). Variants of GBS include Miller Fisher syndrome (descending weakness) and acute pandysautonomia (Khan *et al.*, 2010). It is caused by the body's immune system attacking either the myelin sheath or axons of the cells of the peripheral nervous system. The inflammation and damage to the peripheral cells leads to the characteristic pain and paralysis. A preceding unrelated virus or illness such as gastroenteritis caused by *Campylobacter jejuni*, *Cytomegalovirus*, Epstein Barr virus, influenza A virus, *Mycoplasma pneumoniae*, *Haemophilus influenza*, and Zika virus, often triggers the immune response (Esposito & Longo, 2017; Willison *et al.*, 2016; Yang *et al.*, 2016).

Disease consequences

The worldwide incidence of GBS is 2.3 in 100,000. It occurs in both sexes and at any age; however, it is more common in men than women (van Doorn *et al.*, 2008). In the majority of cases, symptoms are confined to the limbs. Frequently, however, the cranial nerves may be affected, and, in 25% of cases, weakness can rapidly spread to the respiratory and bulbar muscles, leading to a requirement for artificial ventilation (Pithadia & Kakadia, 2010; van Doorn, 2013). By definition, maximal weakness is reached within 2–4 weeks (van Doorn, 2013), followed by a recovery period that can last from months to years (Willison *et al.*, 2016). Duration and severity of the disease vary, and can range from mild weakness with spontaneous recovery, to those who become quadriplegic and ventilator dependent without signs of recovery for several months (Willison *et al.*, 2016). Mortality rates in Europe and North America vary between 3 and 7%. Many patients who survive GBS have residual complaints and deficits, which can have a substantial effect on daily activities and QoL (van Doorn, 2013; Willison *et al.*, 2016).

SECTION 7

Nutritional consequences

Weight and muscle loss can occur secondary to muscle atrophy, reduced nerve conduction to the muscles, or prolonged intensive care unit (ICU) admission. Roubenoff *et al.* (1992) suggested that, due to the infective and inflammatory response, patients with GBS are hypermetabolic and hypercatabolic. However, no studies have measured energy expenditure using validated methods for a large enough sample to establish the extent of the effect on metabolic rate.

Dysphagia

Early assessment of swallowing will identify those at risk of aspiration, necessitating the placement of a nasogastric tube (Yuki & Hartung, 2012). Dysphagia can often be a cause of reduced oral intake (see Chapter 7.3, Dysphagia).

Feeding

Limb weakness, pain and fatigue can reduce the ability to self-feed and may lead to reduced intake. Ruts *et al.* (2010) showed that, even 1 year after the acute phase, 82% of GBS patients reported pain in their extremities. Fatigue is common and may affect an individual's ability to engage in feeding for the length of time required, thereby limiting the amount of food taken at a meal.

Gastric dysmotility

Two-thirds of GBS patients develop an element of autonomic dysfunction, which could include gastric dysmotility, ileus, blood pressure instability, cardiac arrhythmia and excessive sweating (Willison *et al.*, 2016). Constipation commonly occurs as a result of gastric dysmotility or the use of pain medications, and can cause a reduction in appetite.

Nutritional assessment

In addition to the assessment shown in Table 7.6.4, the following should be considered:

- Dietary assessment
  - Use of alternative diets

Clinical investigation and management

Patients should be monitored for deterioration in respiratory function. Intubation and artificial ventilation will be required if respiratory function is compromised secondary to paralysis of respiratory muscles and the diaphragm. These patients will invariably require alternative nutrition, with enteral feeding via nasogastric tube the most preferred route. Both intravenous immunoglobulin and plasma exchange have been shown to be equally effective treatments at accelerating recovery (Willison *et al.*, 2016). Medical treatment will also be required for pain management, and potentially also for the management of autonomic failure or dysfunction (see Chapter 7.17.1, Critical care).

Nutritional management

Weight and muscle loss

As weight loss is multifactorial, the individual causes should be identified for management. Muscle wasting associated with reduced muscle use is unavoidable, and it may therefore be more appropriate to aim for weight stabilisation as a dietetic goal rather than weight gain.

Hypermetabolism

Few studies have investigated the nutritional requirements of patients with GBS. During the acute phase, when patients require intensive care input, Roubenoff *et al.* (1992) suggested that patients should be fed 40–45kcal and 2g of protein/kg of body weight. These recommendations were based on a small sample, and the study did not consider the potential risks of overfeeding. Therefore, during the acute phase in an ICU, requirements should be calculated as for other critical care patients (see Chapter 7.17.1, Critical care).

During the recovery phase, weekly weights and anthropometric measurements should be monitored. Provision of nutritional supplements may be required to reduce the rate of weight loss and to encourage weight gain; however, it should be remembered that, if the patient is immobile, weight gain may occur as adipose tissue rather than LBM (see Chapter 6.3, Oral nutritional support).

Dysphagia

An SLT can recommend the appropriate texture and consistency of food and drink. Nasogastric feeding should be considered unless contraindicated in those who are nil by mouth, intubated, or as supplementary to meet nutritional and fluid requirements in dysphagia (see Chapter 7.3, Dysphagia).

Limb weakness, pain and fatigue

If upper limb weakness is present, assistance should be offered at meals. Those providing assistance should be aware of the effect of fatigue, which may prolong mealtimes and result in the food going cold. Small, regular meals may be more appropriate than three large meals a day. Pain relief should be provided for mealtimes if appropriate. Assessment from an OT can determine whether the patient may benefit from modified cutlery for feeding.

Gastric dysmotility and constipation

If patients are suffering from large aspirates, prokinetics should be employed to increase absorption and decrease aspirate volume. Constipation can occur as a result of gastric dysmotility, so the use of enteral feeds containing fibre or higher-fibre foods may be required, alongside laxatives, to maintain adequate gut function (see Chapter 7.4.11, Other disorders of the colon and rectum). An ileus may occur with autonomic dysfunction; if it persists, parenteral nutrition may be required until it resolves and the patient can tolerate enteral intake (see Chapter 6.5, Parenteral nutrition).

Balanced eating during recovery

Once oral intake resumes and a stable weight is maintained, a balanced diet should be recommended during recovery. There is no evidence to suggest that modified diets speed up recovery or improve function. Some support groups recommend the use of diets high in essential fatty acids, postulating that this may improve the integrity of the myelin sheath of nerve cells. However, there is no evidence to suggest that taking large oral doses of essential fatty acids can help regenerate damaged myelin sheaths. Similarly, avoidance of foods or food groups has not been shown to aid recovery, and may lead to an unbalanced diet, compromising nutritional status.

Acknowledgement

The editor acknowledges the prior contribution of Suzy Yates and Angeline Brookes.

Internet resources

Huntington's Disease Association Resources for Profesionals https://www.hda.org.uk/professionals/resources-for-professionals/best-practice-in-huntington-s-disease.

References

Alshekhlee A, Miles J, Katirji B, *et al.* (2009) Incidence and mortality rates of myasthenia gravis and myasthenic crisis in US hospitals. *Neurology.* 72: 1548–1544.

Aziz N, Roos R. (2013) Characteristics, pathophysiology and clinical management of weight loss in Huntington's disease. *Neurodegener. Dis. Manag.* 3(3): 253–266.

Aziz N, van der Burg J, Landwehrmeyer G, *et al.* (2008) Weight loss in Huntington disease increases with higher CAG repeat number. *Neurology.* 71(19): 1506–1513.

Bianchi M, Morandi L, Andreucci E, *et al.* (2011) Low bone density and bone metabolism alterations in Duchenne muscular dystrophy: response to calcium and vitamin D treatment. *Osteoporos. Int.* 22: 529–539.

Brotherton A, Campos L, Rowell A, *et al.* (2012) Nutritional management of individuals with Huntington's disease: nutritional guidelines. *Neurodegener. Dis. Manag.* 2(1): 33–43.

Bushby K, Finkel R, Birnkrant D, *et al.* (2010a) Diagnosis and management of Duchenne muscular dystrophy, part 1: diagnosis, and pharmacological and psychosocial management. *Lancet Neurol.* 9: 77–93.

Bushby K, Finkel R, Birnkrant D, *et al.* (2010b) Diagnosis and management of Duchenne muscular dystrophy, part 2: implementation of multidisciplinary care. *Lancet Neurol.* 9: 177–189.

Calvert D, Butterworth G, Campos L, *et al.* (2005) Benefits of enteral feeding for patients with Huntington's disease. *J. Neurol. Neurosurg. Psychiatry.* 76(IV): A28.

Cereda E, Beltramolli D, Pedrolli C, *et al.* (2009) Refractory myasthenia gravis, dysphagia and malnutrition: a case report to suggest disease-specific nutritional issues. *Nutrition.* 25: 1067–1072.

Davidson Z, Ryan M, Kornberg A, *et al.* (2014) Observations of body mass index in Duchenne muscular dystrophy: a longitudinal study. *Eur. J. Clin. Nutr.* 68: 892–897.

Escolar D, Buyse G, Henricson E, *et al.* (2005) CINRG randomized controlled trial of creatine and glutamine in Duchenne muscular dystrophy. *Ann. Neurol.* 58: 151–155.

Esposito S, Longo MR. (2017) Guillain–Barré syndrome. *Autoimmun. Rev.* 16: 96–101.

Fanciulli A, Wenning G. (2015) Multiple-system atrophy. *N. Eng. J. Med.* 372(3): 249–263.

Fernagut P, Vital A, Canron M, *et al.* (2012) Ambiguous mechanisms of dysphagia in multiple system atrophy. *Brain.* 135: 1–3.

Gaba A, Zhang K, Moskowitz C, *et al.* (2008) Harris-Benedict equation estimations of energy needs as compared to measured 24-h energy expenditure by indirect calorimetry in people with early to mid-stage Huntington's disease. *Nutr. Neurosci.* 11(5): 213–218.

Gilman S, Wenning G, Low P, *et al.* (2008) Second consensus statement on the diagnosis of multiple system atrophy. *Neurology.* 71: 670–676.

Grob D, Brunner N, Namba T, *et al.* (2008) Lifetime course of myasthenia gravis. *Muscle Nerve.* 37: 141–149.

Haas M, Vlcek V, Balabanov P, *et al.* (2015) European Medicines Agency review of ataluren for the treatment of ambulant patients aged 5 years and older with Duchenne muscular dystrophy resulting from a nonsense mutation in the dystrophin gene. *Neuromuscul. Disord.* 25: 5–13.

Heemskerk A, Roos R. (2011) Dysphagia in Huntington's disease: a review. *Dysphagia.* 26: 62–66.

Khan F, Ng L, Amatya B, *et al.* (2010) Multidisciplinary care for Guillain–Barré syndrome (review). *Cochrane Database Syst. Rev.* (10): CD008505.

Jeronimo G, Nozoe K, Polesel D, *et al.* (2015) Impact of corticotherapy, nutrition, and sleep disorder on quality of life of patients with Duchenne muscular dystrophy. *Nutrition.* 32: 391–393.

Llabrés M, Molina-Martinez F, Miralles F. (2005) Dysphagia as the sole manifestation of myasthenia gravis. *J. Neurol. Neurosurg. Psychiatry* 76: 1297–1300.

Meriggioli M, Sanders D. (2009) Autoimmune myasthenia gravis: emerging clinical and biological heterogeneity. *Lancet Neurol.* 8: 475–490.

National Guideline Clearinghouse (NGC). (2011) Guideline summary: orthostatic hypotension. In: NGC Rockville (MD), *Agency for Healthcare Research and Quality (AHRQ)*. Available at https://www.guideline.gov. Accessed 6 November 2016.

Novak M, Tabrizi S. (2011) Huntington's disease: clinical presentation and treatment. *Int. Rev. Neurobiol.* 98: 297–324.

Pithadia A, Kakadia N. (2010) Guillain–Barré syndrome. *Pharmacol. Rep.* 62: 220–232.

Roubenoff R, Borel C, Hanley D. (1992) Hypermetabolism and hypercatabolism in Guillain–Barré syndrome. *J. Parenter. Enteral Nutr.* 16: 464–472.

Ruts L, Drenthen J, Jongen J, *et al.*; on behalf of the Dutch GBS Study Group. (2010) Pain in Guillain–Barré syndrome. *Neurology.* 75: 1439–1447.

Sackley C, Hoppitt TJ, Calvert M. (2011) Huntington's disease: current epidemiological and pharmacological management in primary care. *Neuroepidemiology* 37: 216–221.

Shimizu-Fujiwara M, Komaki H, Nakagawa E, *et al.* (2008) Decreased resting energy expenditure in patients with Duchenne muscular dystrophy. *Brain Dev.* 34(3): 206–212.

Shinonaga C, Fukuda M, Suzuki Y, *et al.* (2008) Evaluation of swallowing function in Duchenne muscular dystrophy. *Dev. Med. Child Neurol.* 50: 478–480.

Spillane J, Higham E, Kullmann D M. (2012) Myasthenia gravis. *BMJ* 345: e8497.

Sussman J, Farrugia M, Maddison P, *et al.* (2015) Myasthenia gravis: Association of British Neurologists' management guidelines. *Pract. Neurol.* 15: 199–206.

van der Burg J, Winqvist A, Aziz N, *et al.* (2011) Gastrointestinal dysfunction contributes to weight loss in Huntington's disease mice. *Neurobiol. Dis.* 44(1): 1–8.

van Doorn PA. (2013) Diagnosis, treatment and prognosis of Guillain–Barré syndrome. *Presse. Med.* 42: 193–201.

van Doorn PA, Ruts L, Jacobs BC. (2008) Clinical features, pathogenesis, and treatment of Guillain–Barré syndrome. *Lancet Neurol.* 7: 939–950.

Wendell L, Levine J. (2011) Myasthenic crisis. *Neurohospitalist.* 1: 16–22.
Werner P, Boozer C. (2005) Energy balance in early stage Huntington's disease. *Am. J. Clin. Nutr.* 81: 1335–1341.
Willison H, Jacobs B, van Doorn P. (2016) Guillain–Barré syndrome. *Lancet* 388: 717–727.
Yang B, Lian L, Liu Y, *et al.* (2016) A retrospective analysis of possible triggers of Guillain–Barré syndrome. *J. Neuroimmunol.* 293: 17–21.
Yuki N, Hartung H. (2012) Guillain–Barré syndrome. *N. Engl. J. Med.* 366: 2294–2304.

7.6.4 Multiple sclerosis

Kwunita Man and Hayley Moroney

Key points

- Multiple sclerosis is a disease affecting the brain and spinal cord. Damage to the myelin and axons of nerves can lead to significant neurological disability.
- Multiple sclerosis is the most common neurological disease among young adults; onset is usually between 20 and 40 years.
- It is an incurable, long-term condition. Medications can manage symptoms, e.g. fatigue, bladder dysfunction, pain, spasticity and weakness.
- Nutritional management depends on the symptoms and their severity, and varies from a healthy, balanced diet to nutritional support, including enteral tube feeding and dysphagia management.

Multiple sclerosis (MS) is an immune-mediated progressive disease of the central nervous system (CNS). The myelin sheaths around the brain and spinal cord are damaged, affecting the ability of the nerve cells to communicate with each other. It is the most common neurological disease among young adults, with an incidence of approximately 1 in 600 and an onset usually between 20 and 40 years. Women are three times as likely to develop MS as men. It is characterised by inflammation, demyelination of the protective myelin coating and nerve axon damage throughout the CNS. Diagnosis can be confirmed using magnetic resonance imaging (MRI), alongside interpreting clinical symptoms over time (Polman *et al.*, 2011). It is a long-term condition and can have a wide range of clinical presentations that are dependent on the severity and location of CNS damage. Some people become significantly disabled in a very short time, while others can live with minimal or no disability.

Types of Multiple sclerosis (MS)

The current clinical course descriptions of MS (Lublin *et al.*, 2014) include the following:

- *Clinically isolated syndrome* – the first presentations of disease due to inflammatory demyelination, which requires further fulfilment of criteria over time to be classified as MS.
- *Relapsing–remitting* – following diagnosis, 85% of patients follow this course. It is characterised by periods of acute attacks followed by full or near-full recovery. Relapses may last days or months and vary from mild to very severe; the latter may require hospital admission. During relapses, symptoms are exacerbated, and new symptoms may develop.
- *Secondary progressive* – approximately 50–60% of individuals with relapsing–remitting MS later develop secondary progressive MS. Symptoms gradually worsen with or without occasional relapses or minor remissions. As a result, symptoms and disability become steadily worse.
- *Primary progressive* – this affects 10–15% of patients; there is continuous and gradual worsening of the symptoms, with no distinct periods of relapse or remission of symptoms.

Disease processes

Very little is known about the mechanism and causes of MS, although immunological, environmental and genetic factors have been implicated. Environmental factors that increase the risk of MS include exposure to the Epstein–Barr virus, smoking and low serum concentrations of vitamin D (McKay *et al.*, 2016). Although vitamin B_{12} plays a role in myelin formation, no definitive relationship has been identified with vitamin B_{12} (Najafi *et al.*, 2012). The effect of vitamin D on the progression of MS is not clear; however, patients with MS do commonly have vitamin D deficiencies which should be identified through screening and treated as necessary (Alharbi, 2015). Sunlight plays an important role in the synthesis of vitamin D in our bodies, and the trend of increasing incidence of MS with distance from the equator suggests an association between lack of sunlight and the incidence of MS (Mokry *et al.*, 2015). However, it is unclear whether this is a causal effect. Studies looking at supplementation have shown no association between vitamin D supplementation and risk of MS relapse (James *et al.*, 2013).

Disease consequences

Mortality rates differ; however, MS itself is not fatal; causes of death are most commonly associated with respiratory and cardiovascular diseases and infections (Manouchehrinia *et al.*, 2016; Ragonese *et al.*, 2008). However, MS is associated with considerable morbidity and many symptoms, including the following:

- Difficulties with balance and dizziness.
- Fatigue – an overwhelming sense of tiredness.
- Visual problems such as blurred or double vision.
- Numbness, tingling or a 'pins-and-needles' feeling that can be painful.
- Bladder problems.
- Bowel problems.
- Cognitive problems, including memory and thinking.
- Stiffness or spasms in muscles – sometimes called spasticity.
- Emotional and mood changes.
- Tremor.
- Sexual problems.
- Speech difficulties.
- Swallowing difficulties (dysphagia).

People with MS can present with diverse and multiple symptoms of varying severity related to the location of nervous system damage. There is also consistent evidence that health-related quality of life is compromised (Ruddick & Miller, 2008).

Nutritional assessment

The key aspects of nutritional assessment to consider in MS are discussed in the following subsections.

Anthropometry

Specialised weighing scales (wheelchair, sitting scales or hoist scales) will be required for patients who are unable to stand unsupported, or alternative measurements such as mid-upper-arm circumference and waist circumference can be used if scales are unavailable.

Biochemistry

There has been much research around vitamin D and the management of MS. Recent NICE guidance (2014) suggests that the overall benefits of vitamin D supplementation are not felt to be significant enough to outweigh the potential negative effects; however, it should be noted that research is ongoing. In view of this, the vitamin D levels should be checked before advising on vitamin D supplementation on an individual basis.

Clinical assessment

Identification of MS subtype, presenting symptoms or disability will inform likely nutritional priorities:

- If positioning in bed or chair is difficult, pressure areas may be present, and these may affect nutritional requirements (see Chapter 7.17.6, Wound healing, tissue viability and pressure sores).
- Bladder dysfunction may make people self-limit fluid intake, potentially leading to dehydration.
- Constipation is common in MS, with 50–60% of patients experiencing this in the literature, although the pathophysiology of this is unclear (Levinthal *et al.*, 2013; Preziosi *et al.*, 2013). However, reduced mobility, reduced fluid intake and other dietary changes may play a part.

Dietary assessment

The dietary assessment should consider the following:

- Dysphagia may affect food choices; certain food types and textures may need to be avoided.
- Ability to self-feed may be affected by weakness or lack of coordination of arm and/or hand muscles (ataxia); varying degrees of assistance may be needed to eat and drink.
- Fatigue can be debilitating, leaving the person without energy to shop, prepare food or even to eat a meal.
- Some patients decide to follow alternative diets, e.g. Swank, Best Bet and the Overcoming MS Programme; some of these are extremely restrictive and may result in reduced energy and/or protein intake.

There are no specific guidelines on energy and protein requirements in MS; however, energy requirements may be increased with tremor or spasticity, or decreased, with patients requiring support for weight management.

Clinical investigation and management

There is no known cure for MS, although stem cells trials are currently being conducted. Non-curative treatment with medications is common in MS. Drug therapy is aimed at the management of therapy and slowing disease progression.

Symptom management

Symptoms such as spasticity; ataxia and tremor; fatigue; pain; and bladder, bowel and sexual dysfunction can be treated with medication. For example, spasticity may be managed by medications such as baclofen, botulinum toxin or gabapentin, and rehabilitative physiotherapy. Where fatigue is impacting on daily life, modafinil and amantadine may be prescribed to increase alertness along with fatigue management programs. As with all medications, side effects may impact on nutritional intake and/or nutritional status. For example, baclofen (which acts as a skeletal muscle relaxant) can induce nausea, with possible consequent reduction in food intake. A review by Thompson *et al.* (2010) provides a comprehensive overview of drugs prescribed for symptom management in MS, their efficacy and associated side effects.

Disease-modifying therapies

Since the early 1990s, an increasing number of drugs have been licensed for the treatment of MS, including beta interferon (Avonex and Rebif), natalizumab (Tysabri), fingolimod (Gilenya), dimethyl (Tecfidera) and glatiramer acetate (Copaxone). Fingolimod and Tecfidera are taken orally, whereas the others are given via injection or intravenous infusion. All these drugs affect the immune system and are known as disease-modifying therapies (DMTs). The evidence for efficacy of DMTs in relapsing–remitting MS is far greater than for primary or secondary progressive MS. Nonetheless, there are ongoing trials to evaluate whether the course of progressive forms of MS can be influenced by DMTs, including the use of high-dose simvastatin in secondary progressive MS (Chataway *et al.*, 2014). For further information, Scolding *et al.* (2015) has revised guidelines on the prescription of DMTs in MS.

Rehabilitation

Multidisciplinary rehabilitation is also an important aspect of MS management. While there is no evidence that multidisciplinary rehabilitation programmes influence the level of functional impairment, they can improve the experience of people with MS in relation to activity and participation and help in symptom management, as described earlier (Khan *et al.*, 2007).

Nutritional management

As with any long-term condition, healthy eating should be an integral part of daily life. The Eatwell Guide should be used as a tool for empowering individuals to achieve optimum nutrition, especially at the beginning of the pathway following diagnosis (see Chapter 2.1, Dietary reference values and food based dietary guidelines). Emphasis is given to eating at least five portions of fruit and vegetables a day, adequate protein, and aiming for plant-based unsaturated fats and oily fish. Wholegrain bread and cereals are encouraged, as is enough fluids for body size and adequate dairy intake. As the disease progresses, other priorities may take precedence, e.g. weight loss or weight gain. Constipation is common in MS, and advice on its prevention by dietary means can be very helpful. Individualised high-fibre advice, including the use of golden linseeds and prune juice, can help minimise constipation.

Obesity

Obesity in MS can occur for a variety of reasons, including reduced activity as a consequence of disability, treatment with steroids, depression leading to comfort eating, and excessive intake of high-fat and/or high-sugar foods. Existing data on BMI in MS patients is inconsistent (Wens *et al.*, 2013); however, measurement of waist circumference can be a useful tool in monitoring obesity and health-related risks. Successful treatment depends on an empathetic approach, facilitating behaviour change. Appropriate follow-up, ideally in conjunction with the rest of the multidisciplinary team, can be successful. Obesity may not be successfully treated in all patients, and weight loss may not be a realistic goal for some. It may be that prevention of further weight gain is a better approach in some cases.

Alternative diets

Many people with MS follow alternative diets and complementary therapies to help control their symptoms. Surveys suggest that up to 70% of people with MS have tried one or more complementary therapies (Yadav *et al.*, 2010). In addition to relatively minor dietary modifications, people with MS may choose to follow a variety of alternative or extreme diets with a view to influencing the course of their disease. Diets that offer hope of improvement of symptoms or a cure are very attractive to many people with MS, and therefore will have followers. The Swank, Best Bet diet and the Overcoming MS programme are some of the common alternative diets for MS; some patients may also follow gluten-free or alternative diets such as Paleo. There is no substantiated evidence that following an alternative diet will affect the MS disease process. While being mindful that restrictive diets can increase the risk of certain nutritional deficiencies, the health beliefs of individuals must be respected, and support provided to ensure that their diet is nutritionally adequate and that nutritional risk is minimised.

Swank diet

Swank *et al.* (1952) demonstrated a correlation between MS and diet, and devised this diet. A low-fat diet was advised because of an apparent association between fat intake and MS. A group of 144 people on the Swank diet were followed for up to 34 years, with good results reported in long-term disability. Those who adhered strictly to the diet and who were experiencing mild symptoms had slower disability progression than those who had not adhered strictly to the diet. However, there was no control group in this study, and therefore there is a likelihood of a self-selection bias arising from the probability that only patients who perceived a benefit from the treatment would continue with it. It is therefore impossible to know whether the good results represent a genuine improvement over the entire population of MS patients. The principles of the diet are as follows:

- Saturated fat kept to 15 g or less/day.
- No red meat for the first year, then 75 g/week.
- Unsaturated fat kept to 20–50 g/day.
- No processed foods containing saturated fat.
- Dairy products must contain 1% or less fat.
- Three eggs per week, and no more than one per serving.
- Suggested daily: cod liver oil and a multivitamin and mineral supplement.

Best Bet diet

The Best Bet diet is a strict exclusion diet based on the premise that undigested food proteins with a similar structure to the protein in myelin pass across a leaky gut and cross the blood–brain barrier. This triggers an autoimmune attack on myelin, thereby causing, or worsening, MS.

A wide range of food types are restricted, including:

- Red meat.
- Dairy products.
- Legumes and grains.

In addition, over 24 dietary supplements have been recommended. Achieving a well-balanced diet will be a challenge and may also be expensive. At the time of writing, no clinical trials or results in relation to the Best Bet diet have been published in any peer-reviewed journal.

The Overcoming MS Programme

The Overcoming MS Programme is a programme developed by Jelinek (2010). It is a holistic approach focusing on:

- A plant-based diet avoiding saturated fat as far as practical.
- An n-3 fatty acid supplement or flaxseed oil daily.
- B group or vitamin B_{12} supplement if needed.
- Vitamin D_3 supplement of at least 5000 IU.
- 30 minutes of meditation daily.
- 20–30 minutes of exercise five times a week.

A large observational cohort study was started in 2011, recruiting online and using surveys to assess the association of diet on quality of life and disability. Current results indicate an improved health-related quality of life and disability rate; however the methodology is based on self-reports, which could include inaccuracies and bias (Hadgkiss *et al.*, 2015). Research is currently ongoing.

Polyunsaturated fatty acids

Previous guidelines have recommended n-3 and n-6 polyunsaturated fatty acids (PUFAs), which have anti-inflammatory properties, and may be beneficial to patients with MS. However, NICE guidelines (2014) advise not to recommend supplementation of n-3 and n-6 PUFAs due to lack of evidence to support this. A review of dietary interventions for MS by Farinotti *et al.* (2012) showed that PUFAs have no major effect on MS disease progression. However, given that n-3 and n-6 PUFAs are accepted as being beneficial to overall health, their intake should be encouraged in those with all types of MS as part of a varied and balanced diet.

A low intake of saturated fat should also be promoted, as several ecological studies have shown that MS is high in countries that have a high intake of saturated fat (Farinotti *et al.*, 2012). Naturally, this advice must be implemented using clinical judgement, as the nutritional priorities of people with MS can differ, depending on the stage of disease. Early in the disease process, when disability may be relatively mild, more attention should be paid to promoting PUFA intake, particularly where people are motivated to make positive lifestyle changes. However, this dietary advice may become more flexible once disease and disability have progressed, or where malnutrition becomes a concern.

Dysphagia

More than 30% of patients with MS experience dysphagia (Guan *et al.*, 2015). Consequences of dysphagia can be severe, such as the development of pneumonia from aspiration of food or fluid into the lungs. Dysphagia can lead to significant weight loss and dehydration as a result of the inability to meet nutritional and fluid requirements. With progressive forms of MS and where dysphagia exists, swallowing function may deteriorate over time. Where dysphagia is a feature of MS, nutritional management should ideally be undertaken with input from a speech and language therapist, who can advise on modification of food and fluid textures, positioning for eating and drinking, and swallowing strategies to reduce the risk of aspiration with oral intake. Nutritional support (oral or artificial) will be required where dysphagia is associated with a prolonged inability to meet nutritional requirements (see Chapter 7.3, Dysphagia).

Malnutrition and nutritional support

It is well recognised that unintentional weight loss and malnutrition can occur in MS (Habek *et al.*, 2010). Contributory factors include (but are not limited to):

- Dysphagia.
- Fatigue.
- Difficulties in self-feeding.
- Cognitive impairment.
- Restrictive alternative diet.

Where malnutrition or a high risk of malnutrition has been identified, nutritional support strategies should be implemented.

Oral nutritional support

Food fortification advice and a food-first approach should be recommended in the first instance, with consideration of supplementation with prescribed nutritional support products if this is inadequate to meet requirements. If thickened fluids are required to manage dysphagia, prethickened sip feeds are available.

Artificial nutritional support

Use of artificial nutritional support (such as nasogastric or gastrostomy feeding) in people with MS has not been studied extensively. It will only be relevant in a small minority of cases where advanced-stage MS has resulted in an inability to meet nutritional and fluid requirements. It is acknowledged that enteral tube feeding impacts on people's quality of life (Brotherton & Judd, 2007); therefore, quality-of-life considerations, discussions with the patients and their families, and a multi-professional team approach should always guide decision-making regarding artificial tube feeding. This may include advanced care planning and capacity assessments.

Acknowledgement

The editor acknowledges the prior contribution of Catherine Dunn and Maryanne Harrison.

Internet resources

Multiple Sclerosis Society, www.mssociety.org.uk
Multiple Sclerosis Trust, www.mstrust.org.uk

Further reading

BDA Policy Statement. (2015) *Use of Alternative Diets and Supplementation in the Management of Multiple Sclerosis*. Available at https://www.bda.uk.com/improvinghealth/healthprofessionals/ms_management. Accessed July 2015.

References

Alharbi F. (2015) Update in vitamin D and multiple sclerosis. *Neurosciences (Riyadh)* 20(4): 329–335.

Brotherton A, Judd P. (2007) Quality of life in adult enteral tube feeding patients. *J. Hum. Nutr. Diet.* 20: 513–522.

Chataway J, Schuerer N, Alsanousi A, *et al.* (2014) Effect of high dose simvastatin on brain atrophy and disability in secondary progressive multiple sclerosis (MS-STAT): a randomised, placebo-controlled, phase 2 trial. *Lancet.* 383(9936): 2213–2221.

Farinotti M, Vacchi L, Simi S, *et al.* (2012) Dietary interventions for multiple sclerosis. *Cochrane Database Syst. Rev.* 12: CD004192.

Guan XL, Wang H, Huang HS, *et al.* (2015) Prevalence of dysphagia in multiple sclerosis: a systematic review and meta-analysis. *Neurol. Sci.* 36(5): 671–681.

Habek M, Hojsak I, Brinar VV. (2010) Nutrition in multiple sclerosis. *Clin. Neurol. Neurosurg.* 112(7): 616–620.

Hadgkiss EJ, Jelinek GA, Weiland TJ, *et al.* (2015) The association of diet with quality of life, disability, and relapse rate in an international sample of people with multiple sclerosis. *Nutr. Neurosci.* 18(3): 125–136.

James E, Dobson R, Kuhle J, *et al.* (2013) The effect of vitamin D-related interventions on multiple sclerosis relapses: a meta-analysis. *Mult. Scler. J.* 19: 1571–1579.

Jelinek G. (2010) *Overcoming Multiple Sclerosis: An Evidence-Based Guide to Recovery*. Allen & Unwin: Crows Nest Australia.

Khan F, Turner-Stokes L, Ng L, *et al.* (2007) Multidisciplinary rehabilitation for adults with multiple sclerosis. *Cochrane Database Syst. Rev.* (2): CD006036.

Levinthal DJ, Rahman A, Salman N, *et al.* (2013) Adding to the burden: gastrointestinal symptoms and syndromes in multiple sclerosis. *Mult. Scler. Int.* 2013: 319201.

Lublin FD, Reingold SC, Cohen JA, *et al.* (2014) Defining the clinical course of multiple sclerosis. *Neurology.* 83(3): 278–286.

Manouchehrinia A, Tanasescu R, Tench CR, *et al.* (2016) Mortality in multiple sclerosis: meta-analysis of standardised mortality ratios. *J. Neurol. Neurosurg. Psychiatry.* 87(3): 324–331.

McKay KA, Jahanfar S, Duggan T, *et al.* (2016) Factors associated with onset, relapses or progression of multiple sclerosis: a systematic review. *Neurotoxicology.* [Online 1 April 2016] 10.1016/j.neuro.2016.03.020.

Mokry LE, Ross S, Ahmad OS, *et al.* (2015) Vitamin D and risk of multiple sclerosis: a mendelian randomization study. *PLoS Med.* 12(8): e1001866.

Najafi MR, Shaygannajad V, Mirporian M, *et al.* (2012) Vitamin B12 deficiency and multiple sclerosis; is there any association? *Int. J. Prev. Med.* 3(4): 286–289.

NICE. (2014) *Clinical Guideline CG186: Multiple Sclerosis in Adults: Management*. [Online 1 August 2016]. Available at https://www.nice.org.uk/guidance/CG186.

Polman CH, Reingold SC, Banwell B, *et al.* (2011) Diagnostic criteria for multiple sclerosis: 2010 revisions to the McDonald criteria. *Ann. Neurol.* 69(2): 292–302.

Preziosi G, Raptis DA, Raeburn A, *et al.* (2013) Gut dysfunction in patients with Multiple Sclerosis and the role of spinal cord involvement in the disease. *Eur. J. Gastroenterol. Hepatol.* 25(9): 1044–1050.

Ragonese P, Aridon P, Salemi G, *et al.* (2008) Mortality in multiple sclerosis: a review. *Eur. J. Neurol.* 15: 123–127.

Ruddick RA, Miller DM. (2008) Health-related quality of life in multiple sclerosis: current evidence, measurement and effect of disease severity and treatment. *CNS Drugs* 22(10): 827–839.

Scolding N, Barnes D, Cader S, *et al.* (2015) Guidelines for prescribing disease modifying treatments in multiple sclerosis. *Pract. Neurol.* 15(4): 273–279.

Swank RL, Lerstad O, Strøm A, *et al.* (1952) Multiple sclerosis in rural Norway. Its geographic and occupational incidence in relation to nutrition. *N. Engl. J. Med.* 246: 721–728.

Thompson AJ, Toosy AT, Ciccarelli O. (2010) Pharmacological management of symptoms in multiple sclerosis: current approaches and future directions. *Lancet Neurol.* 9(12):1182–1199.

Wens I, Dalgas U, Stenager E, *et al.* (2013) Risk factors related to CVD and the metabolic syndrome in multiple sclerosis – a systematic review. *Mult. Scler.* 19(12): 1556–1564.

Yadav V, Shinto L, Bourdette D. (2010) Complementary and alternative medicine for the treatment of multiple sclerosis. *Expert Rev. Clin. Immunol.* 6(3): 381–395.

7.6.5 Chronic fatigue syndrome/myalgic encephalomyelitis

Jennifer McIntosh

SECTION 7

Key points

- Chronic fatigue syndrome/myalgic encephalomyelitis is now classified as a neurological illness.
- It is a poorly understood, chronic disabling condition affecting both adults and children, with 60–70% reporting irritable bowel syndrome symptoms.
- Dietary advice includes recommendations for small, frequent meals as part of a balanced diet to improve the patient's energy levels.

Chronic fatigue syndrome (CFS), also known as myalgic encephalomyelitis (ME), continues to cause debate regarding its definition, aetiology, diagnosis and treatment (Mallet *et al.*, 2016). Many health professionals fail to recognise CFS/ME, despite the World Health Organization classifying it as a neurological illness. This is partly due to the unexplained aetiology, although several factors have been suggested, including the neurological, endocrine, immunological, genetic and infectious aspects (NICE, 2007).

CFS/ME is defined as persisting or recurrent debilitating fatigue that is not lifelong, not the result of ongoing exertion, not alleviated by rest, not explained by other conditions and resulting in substantial reduction in function (NICE, 2007). It is a relatively common clinical condition with a suggested prevalence of 0.76% worldwide (Johnston *et al.*, 2013). It causes prolonged illness and disability, having a substantial impact on the family and individual, including job loss, reduced financial security and relationship difficulties (Pountley, 2009). The physical symptoms are as disabling as other chronic conditions such as multiple sclerosis, rheumatoid arthritis and congestive heart failure (NICE, 2007). The symptoms vary and often fluctuate in intensity and severity between individuals but also within the individual, making it difficult for family, friends and health professionals to understand the condition.

Diagnostic criteria and classification

There is no diagnostic test for CFS/ME, and diagnosis is made on the basis of a recognisable pattern of characteristic symptoms and the exclusion of other known causes. There are several sets of diagnostic criteria; but, in the UK, NICE (2007) diagnostic criteria are used (Box 7.6.2). Diagnosis is considered if symptoms have persisted for 4 months in an adult or 3 months in a child or young person. In a child or young person, the diagnosis should be made or confirmed by a paediatrician. If the following features are present, they should be investigated before a diagnosis of CFS/ME is made:

- Localising or focal neurological signs.
- Significant weight loss.
- Sleep apnoea.
- Clinically significant lymphadenopathy.
- Signs and symptoms of inflammatory arthritis or connective tissue disease.
- Signs and symptoms of cardiorespiratory disease.

Classification of symptom severity

The severity of CFS/ME can vary enormously and is classified as mild, moderate or severe (NICE, 2007):

- *Mild* – present as mobile, able to care for themselves and perform light domestic tasks with difficulty. Most are still working or in education but, to manage the disease, have stopped all leisure and social pursuits, often taking days off work or school to recover.
- *Moderate* – present with reduced mobility and restricted in all activities of daily living, although they may have peaks and troughs in their symptom levels and ability to perform activities. They have usually stopped work, school or college, and need rest periods, often sleeping in the afternoon for 1 or 2 hours. Their sleep at night is generally of poor quality and disturbed.

Box 7.6.2 Criteria for diagnosis of CFS/ME (© NICE, 2007; Chronic fatigue syndrome/myalgic encephalomyelitis (or encephalopathy): diagnosis and management; available from https://www.nice.org.uk/guidance/cg53/resources/chronic-fatigue-syndromemyalgic-encephalomyelitis-or-encephalopathy-diagnosis-and-management-pdf-975505810885; all rights reserved)

Fatigue with all of the following features:
- New, or had a specific onset, i.e. not lifelong.
- Persistent and/or recurrent.
- Unexplained by other conditions.
- Has resulted in a substantial reduction in activity levels.
- Characterised by post-exertional malaise and/or fatigue (typically delayed, e.g. by at least 24 hours, with slow recovery over several days).

And one or more of the following symptoms
- Difficulty with sleeping, such as insomnia, hypersomnia, unrefreshing sleep, a disturbed sleep–wake cycle.
- Muscle and/or joint pain that is multi-site and without evidence of inflammation.
- Headaches.
- Painful lymph nodes without pathological enlargement.
- Sore throat.
- Cognitive dysfunction, such as difficulty thinking, inability to concentrate, impairment of short-term memory, and difficulties with word finding, planning/organising thoughts and information processing.
- Physical or mental exertion makes symptoms worse.
- General malaise or 'flu-like' symptoms.
- Dizziness and/or nausea.
- Palpitations in the absence of identified cardiac pathology.

- *Severe* – often struggle with daily activities such as having a shower, may depend on a wheelchair for mobility and are unable to leave the house, or may have severe and prolonged aftereffects if they do so. These issues can be compounded by severe cognitive difficulties. They are often bedridden, leading to associated medical risks such as postural hypotension, deep vein thrombosis and pressure sores (McDermott *et al.*, 2014).

Prevalence

CFS/ME affects people of every age, gender, ethnicity and socioeconomic group, although it is four times more common in women as men. The common age of onset for children are 11 or 15–16 years, and 40–50 years for adults. The prevalence is estimated as 0.76% worldwide (Johnston *et al.*, 2013) and 0.1–2% for children (Mackenzie & Wray, 2012).

Prognosis

Most patients will show some degree of improvement over time, especially with treatment. A substantial number of patients will pursue a fluctuating course with periods of relative remission and relapse, and a significant minority becomes severely and perhaps permanently disabled (Cairns & Hotopf, 2005; Department of Health, 2002).

Nutritional considerations

CFS/ME is a chronic condition impacting on nutritional health is varied. This can be challenging for the affected individuals, their families, and the health professionals involved. Simple tasks such as shopping, preparing and cooking can prove challenging when energy levels are impaired. Patients often report fluctuating good and bad days, depending on energy levels, and may require meals with minimal preparation and effort to eat. Those who are severely affected may require nutritional support ranging from nutritional supplements to enteral feeding.

Weight gain

It is generally recognised that many patients gain weight, averaging 12–18kg, owing to multifactorial reasons such as reduced activity levels, eating to boost energy levels and comfort eating. Weight gain can impact on fatigue and pain, increasing other health risks, such as the development of diabetes and heart disease (see Chapter 7.13.1, General aspects and prevention of obesity).

Weight loss

This tends to be more common in children and young people, and those with symptoms of nausea. Some patients can be severely underweight, which impacts on fatigue levels. For some this may lead to extreme malnourishment, resulting in emergency hospital admission (McDermott *et al.*, 2014) (see Chapter 6.2, Malnutrition). It is important to exclude possible eating disorder diagnosis in these cases (refer to Chapter 7.10.2, Eating Disorders).

Irritable bowel syndrome

Approximately 60–70% of CFS/ME patients (Rao *et al.*, 2009) report irritable bowel syndrome (IBS) symptoms, ranging from mild to severe (see Chapter 7.4.10, Irritable bowel syndrome).

Nausea

Nausea and abdominal pain are more common in children and young people, and can affect the ability to eat. There is some evidence for delayed gastric emptying (Burnet & Chatterton, 2004). Antiemetics may be useful for some patients (see Chapter 7.4.3. Disorders of the stomach and duodenum).

Food intolerances

Food intolerances are frequently self-reported, and alternative diets (e.g. anti-candida diets and stone-age/Paleo diets) are commonly adopted. Currently, there is no evidence to support their use, and their impact can lead to nutritional deficiencies further impacting on energy levels.

Osteoporosis

Osteoporosis can occur due to lack of exposure to sunlight, especially in those severely affected. Lack of weight-bearing exercise, dietary self-restriction and vitamin D deficiency can increase the likelihood of osteoporosis (see Chapter 7.9.1, Osteoporosis).

Fluid

Patients can report either over- or under-drinking, due to increased thirst as part of their symptoms or forgetting to drink due to change in lifestyle, respectively. Patients can mistakenly use caffeine to improve energy levels, but accentuate the highs and lows. For a small minority, this can result in consuming copious amounts of caffeine, which can be difficult to change. A number of patients also report intolerance to alcohol.

Reactive hypoglycaemia

Patients may report a craving for sweet foods when tired, followed by symptoms similar to reactive hypoglycaemia, although there is no evidence to support this.

Other symptoms that may lead to a restrictive diet include difficult or painful swallowing or sore throat, sensitivity to smell or taste of food, and disturbed sleep patterns.

Nutritional assessment

- Anthropometry
  - Weight, height, BMI.

- Biochemistry – the following routine blood tests are used to exclude other possible diagnosis (NICE, 2007):
  - Full blood count.
  - Creatinine, urea, and electrolytes.
  - Thyroid and liver function tests.
  - Erythrocyte sedimentation rate and C-reactive protein.
  - Random blood glucose or HbA1c.
  - Urinalysis for protein, blood and glucose.
  - Serum calcium.
  - Creatine kinase.
  - Coeliac screen.
  - Serum ferritin levels for children and young people.
- Clinical assessment
  - Detailed weight history, both prior to CFS/ME and current.
  - Depending on the reason for referral, potential food allergies and intolerance beliefs should be explored.
  - If symptoms of IBS or nausea are present, further information needs to be gathered to aid advice.
  - An awareness of concentration and short-term memory is important; having a companion present may be useful for the retention of dietary advice, in addition to providing written information.
- Dietary assessment
  - Building therapeutic relationships with patients, using a range of behavioural change techniques, is vital to understanding their relationships with food and providing motivation to change.
  - Detailed diet history, particularly noting use of nutritional supplements, alcohol and caffeine.
  - As energy levels may fluctuate, it is useful to understand if food intake is affected, e.g. patients often report good and bad days, which can impact on food provision, preparation and intake.
- Economic and social assessment
  - Patients may be unable to work, or may work only part time, which may affect their financial situation; less money for food may limit dietary choices.
  - It is important to assess their support network for shopping, food preparation and cooking, and overall emotional support.

Management

There is no single management approach that has been found universally beneficial, and currently there is no known cure for CFS/ME. Most patients are managed in primary care, but, ideally, will have access, if required, to a specialised team, which may include a specialist physiotherapist, occupational therapist, dietitian and psychologist or cognitive behaviour therapist.

Pharmacological interventions

There is no known pharmacological treatment for CFS/ME, and limited evidence on the overall benefits of pharmacological treatments. The focus is on symptom control for sleep, mood disturbance and pain management. Some patients report sensitivity to medications, and, although there is no substantial evidence for this, lower doses than normal may be given. The most common drugs include antidepressants and analgesics. Tricyclic antidepressants (amitriptyline or nortriptyline) are used at low doses and may be prescribed for poor sleep or pain. Anticonvulsants (gabapentin or pregabalin) are an alternative to tricyclic drugs; however, there is a potential for dependence and misuse. Analgesics such as non-steroidal anti-inflammatory drugs (Ibuprofen or naproxen) may be effective with muscular–skeletal symptoms with stiffness. Selective serotonin reuptake inhibitors (SSRIs – fluoxetine, citalopram) may be used for symptoms of depression or anxiety, although there is inconsistent evidence for their use (BACME, 2015). Side effects can include weight gain, constipation or diarrhoea (see Chapter 7.10.1, Nutrition and mental health). Melatonin may be considered for children and young people who have sleep difficulties, but only under specialist supervision, as it is unlicensed in the UK for those under 55 years of age. Melatonin is responsible for regulating the body's biological clock and is produced naturally in the pineal gland; deficiency can lead to insomnia.

Non-pharmacological interventions

The main interventions recognised as beneficial are cognitive behavioural therapy (CBT), graded exercise therapy (GET) and incremental pacing (NICE, 2007).

Cognitive behavioural therapy

This aims to reduce the level of symptoms, disability and distress as part of the overall management. A number of randomised controlled trials (Prins *et al.*, 2001; Sharpe *et al.*, 1996; Stulemeijer *et al.*, 2005) have reported beneficial effects with CBT on fatigue and global improvement, with the main aim to increase functional levels. However, two studies showed no significant difference (Cox, 2002; Friedberg & Krupp, 1994). It is recommended that CBT be offered to people with mild or moderate CFS/ME (NICE, 2007; White *et al.*, 2011, 2013); it is particularly effective if comorbid anxiety and depression symptoms are present (Castell *et al.*, 2011).

Graded exercise therapy

Graded exercise therapy (GET) involves gradually increasing physical activity to improve fitness and normalise the body to activity. Initially, an achievable baseline of physical activity is agreed on, followed by gradual and planned increases that are individually tailored to the patient. Several randomised controlled trials (Powell *et al.*, 2001; Moss-Morris *et al.*, 2005; Wallman *et al.*, 2004) on GET have reported significant improvements in fatigue and physical function. NICE (2007) and White *et al.* (2011, 2013) recommend GET for those with a mild or moderate CFS/ME presentation.

Incremental pacing

Incremental pacing is managed by the patient and is defined as '*energy management with the aim of maximising cognitive and physical activity, while avoiding*

SECTION 7

setbacks/relapses due to overexertion' (NICE, 2007); the evidence to date to support incremental pacing is equivocal.

Other interventions that may be beneficial include activity management, sleep management, relaxation techniques and mindfulness (Sampalli *et al.*, 2009; Surawy *et al.*, 2005). Due to the nature of CFS/ME, patients may experience setbacks or relapses, the navigation of which are built into management strategies.

Nutritional management

The evidence base for the use of nutrition in CFS/ME is small and conflicting. Current management programmes are based on available evidence and clinical experience. Patients have access to a large amount of nutritional information, often via the Internet, which can be conflicting. A healthy dietary approach is recommended (Baumer, 2005; Morris & Stare, 1993; NICE, 2007). Currently, the following is recommended:

- Eating a balanced diet according to the Eatwell Guide.
- Incorporating low-glycaemic-index foods to improve energy levels, particularly in relation to hypoglycaemic-type symptoms.
- Eating every 3–4 hours, i.e. three meals with the addition of three snacks in between to improve energy levels.
- Reducing caffeine intake if sleep is affected, or if it impacts adversely on energy levels or bowel symptoms.
- Encouraging adequate fluid intake.
- Possibly reducing or avoiding alcohol, depending on the reported impact on symptoms.
- Practical dietary advice regarding problem-solving for reduced energy levels, e.g. ready meals or Internet food shopping.

Explaining the psychological and physical benefits of dietary advice is important to aid understanding and improve compliance. It is important to recognise that this patient group's somatology is extremely diverse; and, as such, so are the nutritional problems, which may be one aspect (e.g. weight management) of a more complex presentation incorporating several nutritional problems (e.g. food intolerances, nutritional supplements and irritable bowel syndrome). Patients can also feel a sense of loss of control, which food may help combat, resulting in potential disordered eating or overuse of nutritional supplements. It is therefore important to individualise all dietary advice while remaining open-minded and compassionate.

Weight management

Initially, it is helpful to assess the reasons for weight gain, which can be multifactorial, as discussed earlier. In view of reduced activity levels, weight loss may be slower, e.g. 1–2 kg/month. Dietary advice can then be tailored to the individual situation.

Nutritional support

The reasons for weight loss can be multifactorial and linked to physical symptoms (e.g. nausea) or psychological reasons (e.g. anxiety), or both, which may impact on the rate of weight gain. Dietary advice should be tailored to the individual, e.g. food fortification, or frequent, small meals and snacks.

Nausea

Little and often should be encouraged, and standard dietary advice for nausea given. If nausea is severe, antiemetic drugs may be considered (NICE, 2007).

Food allergy and food intolerances

There is no evidence that CFS/ME patients have a greater incidence of immunoglobulin (IgE)-mediated food allergy than the general population. However, some patients believe that food allergies or food intolerances may be the cause. Explaining the difference between food allergy and food intolerance, and how they are diagnosed, can be helpful. Exclusion diets are not generally recommended for managing CFS/ME; however, they can be helpful for symptom management, especially with IBS symptoms. Exclusion diets should only be undertaken under the supervision of a dietitian (see Chapter 7.11.2, Food hypersensitivity).

Bowel symptom management

Patients often benefit from strategies employed in the management of IBS, particularly modified dietary fibre. There have also been some studies recommending the use of probiotics (Lakhan & Kirchgessner, 2010; Rao *et al.*, 2009; Sullivan *et al.*, 2009). Low-sugar and low-yeast diets are popular; however, Hobday *et al.* (2008) and Morris and Stare (1993) found no more benefit in these as compared to healthy eating (see Chapter 7.4.10, Irritable bowel syndrome).

Nutritional supplements

There is insufficient evidence for the use of nutritional supplements; however, patients report a high usage. It is important to provide advice about the potential side effects associated with high doses of vitamins and minerals e.g. vitamin B_6, and the related neurological symptoms. If the diet is inadequate or supplementation is advised, a multivitamin and mineral supplement within the recommended daily amount should be prescribed. In those with moderate to severe CFS/ME, especially those who are housebound, a vitamin D supplement (10 µg/day) may be recommended to prevent osteoporosis (Berkovitz *et al.*, 2009; NICE, 2007).

Evidence for the use of supplements is conflicting. Cox *et al.* (1991) showed an improvement in energy and pain, emotional reactions and general health with magnesium. However, all other studies have found no conclusive evidence. Nicotinamide adenine dinucleotide was shown by Forsyth *et al.* (1999) to improve the quality of life and general health, but Santaella *et al.* (2004) reported no significant difference. Werbach (2000) showed very limited evidence for vitamin B_{12} injections. Essential fatty acid supplementation studies are also conflicting. One randomised control trial reported no improvements, while another slightly larger controlled trial reported an overall beneficial effect (Behan *et al.*, 1990; Maes & Leunis, 2008; Puri *et al.*, 2004; Warren *et al.*, 1999). There is no evidence to support the use of coenzyme Q10, vitamin C and B complex supplementation.

Complementary and alternative therapies

There is insufficient evidence that complementary therapies are effective treatments (Alraek *et al.*, 2011; NICE, 2007), with a recent study reporting no clinical improvement with complementary therapies (Lewith *et al.*, 2016). However, people with CFS/ME may choose these therapies due to the frustration of there being no conventional cure for CFS/ME. More evidence is required in this area.

Further reading

Department of Health CFS/ME Working Group. (2002) *A Report to the Chief Medical Officer of an Independent Working Group*. London: DepartmentofHealth.Availableathttp://webarchive.nationalarchives.gov.uk/+/http://www.dh.gov.uk/en/Publicationsandstatistics/Publications/PublicationsPolicyAndGuidance/DH_4064840.

NICE. (2007) *Clinical guideline for the diagnosis and management of CFS/ME*. Available at www.nice.org.uk/cg53.

Internet resources

British Association for CFS/ME (BACME), https://www.bacme.info
The Chronic Fatigue Society, www.remembercfs.org.uk

References

Alraek T, Lee MS, Choi TY, *et al.* (2011) Complementary and alternative medicine for patients with chronic fatigue syndrome: a systemic review. *BMC Complement. Altern. Med.* 11: 3–87.

BACME (2015) Guide to pharmacology. https://www.meassociation.org.uk/wp-content/uploads/BACME-guide-with-pharmacology-30-06-2015-copy.pdf. Accessed 29 October 2018.

Baumer JH. (2005) Management of chronic fatigue syndrome/myalgic encephalopathy (CFS/ME). *Arch. Dis. Child. Educ. Pract. Ed.* 90: 46–50.

Behan PO, Behan WM, Horrobin D. (1990) Effect of high doses of essential fatty acids on the postviral fatigue syndrome. *Acta Neurol. Scand.* 82: 209–216.

Berkovitz S, Ambler G, Jenkins M, *et al.* (2009) Serum 25-hydroxy vitamin D levels in chronic fatigue syndrome: a retrospective survey. *Int. J. Vitam. Nutr. Res.* 79(4): 250–254.

Burnet RB, Chatterton BE. (2004) Gastric emptying is slow in chronic fatigue syndrome. *BMC Gastroenterol.* 4: 32.

Cairns R, Hotopf M. (2005) A systematic review describing the prognosis of chronic fatigue syndrome. *Occup. Med. (Lond).* 55: 20–23.

Castell BD, Kazantzis N, Moss-Morris RE. (2011) Cognitive behavioural therapy and graded exercise for chronic fatigue syndrome: a meta-analysis. *Clin. Psychol. Sci. Pract.* 18(4): 311–324.

Cox DL. (2002) Chronic fatigue syndrome: An evaluation of an occupational therapy inpatient intervention. *Br. J. Occu. Therapy* 65: 461–468.

Cox IM, Campbell MJ, Dowson D. (1991) Red blood cell magnesium and chronic fatigue syndrome. *Lancet*. 337: 757–760.

Department of Health CFS/ME Working Group. (2002) *A Report to the Chief Medical Officer of an Independent Working Group*. London: DepartmentofHealth.Availableathttp://webarchive.nationalarchives.gov.uk/+/http://www.dh.gov.uk/en/Publicationsandstatistics/Publications/PublicationsPolicyAndGuidance/DH_4064840.

Forsyth LM, Preuss HG, MacDowell AL, *et al.* (1999) Therapeutic effects of oral NADH on the symptoms of patients with chronic fatigue. *Ann Allergy, Asthma Immunol.* 82: 185–191.

Friedberg F, Krupp LB. (1994) A comparison of cognitive behavioural treatment for chronic fatigue syndrome and primary depression. *Clin. Infect Dis.* 18(1): S105–110.

Hobday RA, Thomas S, O'Donovan A, *et al.* (2008) Dietary Intervention in chronic fatigue syndrome. *J. Hum. Nutr. Diet.* 21: 141–149.

Johnston S, Brenu EW, Staines D, *et al.* (2013) The prevalence of chronic fatigue syndrome/myalgic encephalomyelitis: a meta-analysis. *Clin. Epidemiol.* 5: 105–110.

Lakhan SE, Kirchgessner A. (2010) Gut inflammation in chronic fatigue syndrome. *Nutr. Metab. (Lond).* 7: 79.

Lewith G, Stuart B, Chalder T, *et al.* (2016) Complementary and alternative healthcare use by participants in the PACE trial of treatments for chronic fatigue syndrome. *J. Pschosomc. Res.* 87: 37–42.

Mackenzie C, Wray A. (2012) Chronic fatigue syndrome in children and young people. *J. Paediatr. Child Health*. 23: 35–39.

Maes M, Leunis JC. (2008) Normalization of leaky gut in chronic fatigue syndrome (CFS) is accompanied by a clinical improvement: effects of age, duration of illness and the translocation of LPS from gram-negative bacteria. *Neuro Endocrinol. Lett.* 29(6): 901–910.

Mallet M, King E, White PD. (2016) A UK based review of recommendations regarding the management of chronic fatigue syndrome. *J. Psychosom. Res.* 88: 33–35.

McDermott C, Al Haddabi A, Akagi H, *et al.* (2014) What is the current NHS service provision for patients severely affected by chronic fatigue syndrome/myalgic encephalomyelitis? A national scoping exercise. *BMJ Open*. 4: e005083.

Morris DH, Stare FJ. (1993) Unproven diet therapies in the treatment of the chronic fatigue syndrome. *Arch. Fam. Med.* 2: 181–186.

Moss-Morris R, Sharon C, Tobin R, *et al.* (2005) A randomised controlled graded exercise trial for chronic fatigue syndrome: outcomes and mechanisms of change. *J. Health Psychol.* 10: 245–259.

NICE. (2007) *Clinical guideline for the diagnosis and management of CFS/ME*. Available at www.nice.org.uk/cg53 Accessed 29 October 2018.

Prins JB, Bleijenberg G, Bazelmans E, *et al.* (2001) Cognitive behaviour therapy for chronic fatigue syndrome: a multicentre randomised controlled trial. *Lancet*. 357: 841–847.

Pountley D. (2009) Identifying and managing chronic fatigue syndrome. *Br. J. Neurosci. Nurs.* 5(10): 460–462.

Powell P, Bentall RP, Nye FJ, *et al.* (2001) Randomised controlled trial of patient education to encourage graded exercise in chronic fatigue syndrome. *BMJ*. 322: 387–390.

Prins JB, Bleijenberg G, *et al.* (2001) Cognitive behaviour therapy for chronic fatigue syndrome: a multicentre randomised controlled trial. *Lancet*. 357: 841–847.

Puri BK, Holmes J, Hamilon G. (2004) Eicosapentaenoic acid-rich essential fatty acid supplementation in chronic fatigue associated with symptom remission and structural brain changes. *Int. J. Clin. Pract.* 58: 297–299.

Rao AV, Bested AC, Beaulne TM, *et al.* (2009) A randomized, double-blind, placebo-controlled pilot study of a probiotic in emotional symptoms of chronic fatigue syndrome. *Gut. Pathog.* 1: 1–6.

Sampalli T, Berlasso E, Fox R, *et al.* (2009) A controlled study of the effect of a mindfulness-based stress reduction technique in women with multiple chemical sensitivity, chronic fatigue syndrome and fibromyalgia. *J. Multidiscip. Healthc.* 2: 53–59.

Santaella ML, Font I, Disdier OM. (2004) Comparison of oral Nicotinamide Adenine Dinucleotide (NADH) versus conventional therapy for chronic fatigue syndrome. *P. R. Health Sci. J.* 23: 89–93.

Sharpe M, Hawton K, Simkin S, *et al.* (1996) Cognitive behaviour therapy for the chronic fatigue syndrome: a randomised controlled trial. *BMJ* 312: 22–26.
Stulemeijer M, de Jong LW, Fiselier TJ, *et al.* (2005) Cognitive behavioural therapy for adolescents with chronic fatigue syndrome: randomised controlled trail. *BMJ* 330: 14.
Sullivan A, Nord CE, Evengard B. (2009) Effect of supplement with lactic-acid producing bacteria on fatigue and physical activity in patients with chronic fatigue syndrome. *Nutr. J.* 8: 4.
Surawy C, Roberts J, Silver A. (2005) The effect of mindfulness training on mood and measures of fatigue, activity and quality of life in patients with chronic fatigue on a hospital waiting list: a series of exploratory studies. *Behav. Cogn. Psychother.* 33: 103–109.
Wallman KE, Morton AR, Goodman C, *et al.* (2004) Randomised controlled trial of graded exercise in chronic fatigue syndrome. *Med. J. Aust.* 180: 444–448.
Warren G, McKendrick M, Peet M. (1999) The role of essential fatty acids in chronic fatigue syndrome: a case-controlled study of red-cell membrane essential fatty acids (EFA) and a placebo-controlled treatment study with high dose of EFA. *Acta Neurol. Scand.* 99: 112–116.
Werbach MR. (2000) Nutritional strategies for treating chronic fatigue syndrome. *Altern. Med. Rev.* 5(2): 93–108.
White PD, Goldsmith KA, Johnson AL, *et al.* (2011) Comparison of adaptive pacing therapy, cognitive behaviour therapy, graded exercise therapy, and specialist medical care for chronic fatigue syndrome (PACE): a randomised trial. *Lancet.* 377: 823–836.
White PD, Goldsmith K, Johnson T, *et al.* (2013) Recovery from chronic fatigue syndrome after treatments given in the PACE trial. *Psychol. Med.* 43: 2227–2235.

7.6.6 Neurorehabilitation

Emma Craig, Jennie Dunwoody, Lydia Fletcher and Tanita Manton

Key points

- Neurorehabilitation requires effective collaboration, goal setting, outcome measures, and communication between members of the interdisciplinary team to enable individuals to achieve their maximum potential.
- The neurological effects of brain injury can have a significant impact on an individual's nutritional status.
- It is essential that dietitians are aware of the extent and nature of these effects to ensure effective assessment and management.

Rehabilitation is a process of assessment, treatment and management, during which the individuals, their families and carers are supported in order to achieve the maximum potential for the individuals' physical, cognitive, social and psychological functions; to enhance their participation in society; and to optimise their quality of life. Individuals requiring specialist rehabilitation are often those with complex disabilities. Such individuals typically present with a diverse mixture of medical, physical, sensory, cognitive, communicative, behavioural and social challenges. These individuals often require specialist input from a wide range of rehabilitation disciplines, as well as specialist medical input. A subgroup of individuals will have profound disability. These will require all of their care needs to be anticipated in addition to specialist interventions, e.g. spasticity management, postural support programmes and highly specialist equipment (Turner-Stokes *et al.*, 1998).

This chapter concentrates on the neurorehabilitation of individuals who have an acquired brain injury (ABI), which can be divided into traumatic (e.g. road traffic accidents, assaults and falls) and non-traumatic (e.g. stroke, hypoxic brain damage, infection and HIV) brain injury.

General principles

Phases of rehabilitation

Rehabilitation does not occur solely in a specialist centre or unit. It begins from the minute an individual is admitted to hospital and continues long after his or her return to the community, as shown in Figure 7.6.1. The key to its success is continuity across the phases, leading to seamless care. In an acute hospital, while an individual is waiting to move to a rehabilitation ward or unit, some maintenance interventions are still likely to be needed, such as managing positioning, maintaining range of movement, preventing contractures, establishing alternative methods of communication and many others. These interventions are primarily focused on preventing complications that could magnify later disability.

Guidelines

Neurorehabilitation should be undertaken in accordance with clinical guidelines and service frameworks outlined by the British Society of Rehabilitation Medicine (BSRM) and the Royal College of Physicians (RCP). These focus on the delivery of high-quality, effective and timely rehabilitation, in addition to planning for long-term care (BSRM, 2008; BSRM/RCP, 2003; RCP/BSRM, 2010). An increasing number of patients are being diagnosed with prolonged disorders of consciousness while on their rehabilitation pathway, and the RCP has published clinical guidelines for these disorders which provide guidance on acute admission through to long-term care, palliative pathways, and the withdrawal of nutrition and hydration (RCP, 2013).

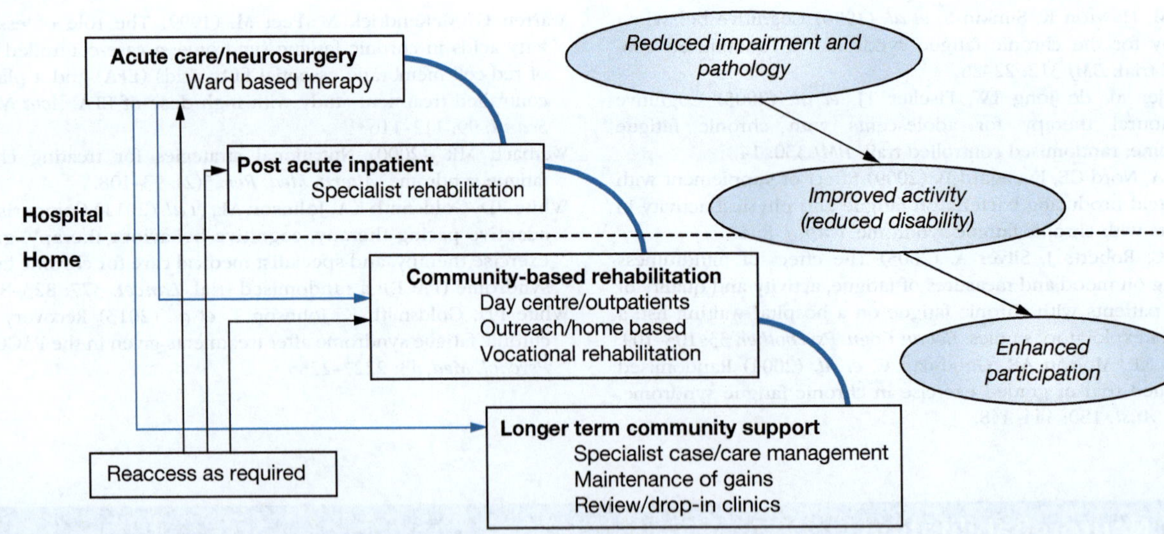

Figure 7.6.1 Phases of rehabilitation (source: National Clinical Guidelines (RCP, 2013). Reproduced with permission from the Royal College of Physicians)

The neurological rehabilitation team

Following brain injury, rehabilitation from a specialised team should be established as soon as possible. An effective team works collaboratively to provide integrated care and moves towards achieving a single set of individualised goals. The team comprises a number of healthcare professionals who work closely together in conjunction with the individual and/or carers to assess the individual's needs, devise an individual plan of care, and monitor its implementation and progress. The team may include the following members:

- Dietitian.
- Rehabilitation nurse.
- Physiotherapist.
- Consultant in rehabilitation medicine.
- Speech and language therapist (SLT).
- Occupational therapist (OT).
- Music therapist.
- Neuropsychologist.
- Social worker.
- Recreation and leisure facilitator.
- Rehabilitation assistant.

Goal planning

Neurorehabilitation should be goal driven, with regular interdisciplinary meetings to discuss, review and set specific, measureable, attainable, relevant and timely (SMART) goals. A standardised set of outcome measures (e.g. the Extended Rehabilitation Complexity Scale, Northwick Park Therapy Dependency Score, and Functional Assessment Measure) should be used as a marker of outcome within neurorehabilitation (BSRM, 2008).

Consequences of brain injury

Damage to the brain as a result of ABI can have profound effects on an individual's physical and cognitive capabilities. The effects depend on the location, nature and extent of the damage. Brain injury can be classified as mild, moderate or severe. In mild cases, patients may be able to return home and even commence paid employment. In more severe cases, however, they will be dependent on other people for many or all aspects of care for the rest of their lives.

Damage to the left hemisphere of the brain is most likely to affect:

- Language.
- Speech.
- Reading and writing ability.

Damage to the right hemisphere is most likely to affect:

- Processing of visual and spatial information.
- Recognition.
- Coordination.

Although damage to brain tissue is irreversible, since the body does not have the ability to regenerate brain cells, in certain types of brain injury, particularly stroke, the body does seem to be able to adapt to some types of damages by rerouting the way in which information is processed, hence enabling the individual in time to recover some or all of an ability, e.g. speech or swallowing. This is termed neuroplasticity.

Nutritional implications of brain injury

The neurological effects of brain injury can have significant implications in terms of nutritional status and intake. It is essential that dietitians are aware of the extent and nature of these effects to ensure accurate assessment and nutritional intervention, which will enable the individual to meet the demands of rehabilitation.

Ability to swallow

Dysphagia is a common consequence of many types of brain injury. Not only may damage to cranial nerves affect the swallowing reflex, but it may also impact on other aspects necessary for the normal swallow, including the following:

- Ability to visualise and recognise food.
- Appropriate posture of the head, neck and body.
- Effective lip and tongue movement.
- Abnormal oral reflexes, e.g. tongue thrust and bite reflex.
- Inability to concentrate.
- Fatigue and increased length of time to consume a meal.
- Fear of choking.

Any loss in swallowing ability is likely to compromise nutritional intake as a result of the following:

- Insufficient consumption of food causing energy and nutrient deficits.
- Limited choice of food leading to an imbalanced diet.
- Losses as a result of drooling and leakage of food from the mouth.

Measures that are likely to be required for brain-injured individuals with dysphagia are:

- Assessment by a specialist team and provision of appropriate assistance, e.g. techniques to trigger or strengthen the swallow reflex.
- Changes in food consistency and texture, which may necessitate either a uniform, soft consistency, e.g. purée foods, or appropriately thickened fluids, depending on the nature of the dysphagia. As altered-texture diets can lack nutritional density, individualised nutrition support may be required to meet energy, protein and micronutrient requirements.
- Maximising sensory input – foods may become more palatable and easier to swallow if they are served either hot or cold, rather than just warm or at room temperature. Chilled foods and drinks are often particularly well accepted. Main meals, initially served as hot as possible, are more likely to remain at an acceptable temperature throughout what may be a long meal duration.

The management of dysphagia is discussed in detail in Chapter 7.3 (Dysphagia).

Effects on eating behaviour

Behavioural changes

Changes in behaviours often result from frontal lobe damage and may include the following:

- Antisocial behaviour, e.g. poor table manners, spitting or throwing food.
- Aggression.
- Physical and/or verbal abuse.
- Disinhibition.
- Disinterest or apathy.
- Hyperphagia (Henson *et al*., 1993).

Mood changes

Alterations in brain function or the medications used to manage brain injury may have a direct effect on neurotransmitters and result in short- or long-term alterations in mood, e.g. depression or withdrawal, which can contribute to overeating or undereating.

Effects on appetite

Damage to the hypothalamus may result in loss of appetite control, resulting in hyperphagia (Henson *et al*., 1993) or hyperphagia for particular foods, such as a craving for sweet, carbohydrate-based foods. Drug therapy, particularly the use of mood stabilising drugs, may also affect appetite.

Effects on the physical ability to eat

Ataxia

Ataxia describes tremor or shakiness, usually as a result of damage to the cerebellum, brainstem or pyramid tracts, causing poor motor control. It can cause significant difficulties when individuals are attempting to feed themselves. This may be severe enough that the individual has to be fed by family or carers. Equipment has been devised that enables individuals with ataxia to self-feed (by creating a resistance against tremor, and therefore allowing a smooth transit from plate to mouth). However, some individuals find the equipment too large and difficult to use; others feel that it draws attention to their disability, and prefer to be discreetly fed by a carer.

Apraxia

Apraxia is the term used to describe disordered purposeful movement; it is often associated with damage to the left hemisphere and may appear in a number of forms:

- Individuals with ideomotor apraxia may be unable to perform a specific task on request despite understanding the concept and having the physical ability to do so. However, the individual may be able to carry out the task automatically.
- Individuals with ideational apraxia may be unable to select the appropriate tool to carry out a particular task, e.g. may try to use a fork as a straw.

Hemiplegia

This results in the paralysis of limbs on the side of the body that is opposite to the site of the brain injury. Other physical consequences may include muscle wasting and limb oedema on the affected side. Hemiplegia is particularly likely to compromise nutritional status, because energy requirements may be increased as a result of the reduced efficiency of movement and the presence of spasticity (Potempa *et al*., 1995). Food intake is often limited in both type and amount because of the difficulties of manipulating food with just one hand. Measures such as the use of anti-slip mats and adapted cutlery may be helpful.

Effects on the ability to communicate

Aphasia (damage to the language centre in the left hemisphere of the brain) may result in loss of or difficulties with speech (expressive aphasia). The ability to read or even interpret pictures may also be impaired (receptive aphasia). As a result of dysphasia, individuals may be unable to communicate their wishes, e.g. that they are hungry or thirsty, or express their likes and dislikes. Individuals affected by aphasia may also have difficulty in completing a hospital menu card or making sense of dietary information provided in a written or pictorial form.

Psychological effects

In addition to physical effects, the psychological consequences of having suffered ABI can affect nutritional intake.

Emotional reactions

Awareness of the nature of the injury and the prospect of permanent or progressive disability is likely to be followed by an emotional reaction similar to that of bereavement, and may include the following:

- Shock.
- Emotional lability.
- Depression.
- Realisation (which can result in further depression).
- Adjustment.

Depression may also result from, or be compounded by, chemical changes following the brain injury. Physical difficulties with eating or swallowing may be compounded by fatigue and poor concentration. This can cause frustration, irritability and feelings of resentment towards the family or healthcare professionals. It is not uncommon for these feelings to impact on an individual's engagement or participation in the rehabilitation process. The overall stress of the situation may cause the individual to become withdrawn and tearful.

Social isolation

Individuals can feel embarrassed at mealtimes due to food spillage as a result of ataxia, drooling or dribbling, or simply as a result of having to be assisted with meals. This may make individuals reluctant to eat with others or in public. Consequently, both individuals and their relatives or carers can become very isolated (Osborn & Marshall, 1993).

Nutritional management

Many individuals who have suffered ABI will commence the rehabilitation phase in a state of undernutrition as a result of the hypercatabolic effects of acute trauma and the likelihood of energy and protein deficits (see Chapter 7.17.2, Traumatic brain injury and Chapter 7.14.5, Stroke). Undernutrition is particularly likely if the injury was severe (which will result in a greater and more prolonged catabolic response) or if the individual was malnourished prior to the injury. Early nutritional intervention is indicated in individuals with ABI to minimise depletion and optimise recovery, and enteral feeding is often required immediately post-injury. Research exists on energy and protein requirements in acute ABI; however, there is little relating to the rehabilitation stage (McEvory *et al.*, 2009).

The initial nutritional priority in such individuals is thus to restore nutritional status and maximise the ability to participate in therapy sessions. As rehabilitation progresses, this objective gradually changes to helping individuals overcome, or mitigate, their neurological difficulties affecting food intake, and to ensuring that nutrient intake is adequate. With further recovery but persisting disabilities, the aim may be to prevent weight gain and overnutrition. The ultimate aim is to optimise nutritional intake in a way that maximises the individual's rehabilitation potential and quality of life. Table 7.6.5 categorises, from a nutritional perspective, the spectrum of individuals who may present on a neurorehabilitation ward.

Nutritional assessment

Many factors impact upon nutritional intake in the brain-injured individual. It is therefore essential that nutritional assessment be carried out in liaison with the interdisciplinary team (IDT), so that expert opinion on other parameters that impact on food intake can be taken into account.

The following should be considered as part of a nutritional assessment:

- The cause of the brain injury, its management and likely prognosis.
- The physical and psychological consequences of the injury on:
  - The desire to eat.
  - The ability to eat.
  - The ability to swallow.
- The ability to carry out everyday tasks, e.g. self-feeding.
- Skin integrity.
- Bowel function.
- The individual's nutritional and fluid intake, and whether this is likely to improve, worsen or remain stable.

The aim is to identify individuals who require dietetic intervention or those who need monitoring, as they may require dietetic involvement at some point in the future. Liaison with the other members of the team helps to provide a full picture of the individual's overall presenting condition and provides dietitians with the opportunity to educate other team members about the nutritional implications and management of brain-injured individuals. Dietetic interactions with other members of the IDT may include:

- Close working with the SLT to understand the individual's swallow ability and communication difficulties.
- Liaising with the OTs to understand the individuals' physical ability to get food to their own mouth, with or without specialist equipment, or to clarify if they need assistance or supervision with food and drink.
- Obtaining recommendations from the physiotherapist on posture and positioning to best enable individuals to feed themselves, if able, in addition to reducing aspiration risk.

Table 7.6.5 Feeding methods that patients may require on a neurorehabilitation ward

Feeding method	Details
Nil by mouth	All nutrition provided via nasogastric, gastrostomy or jejunal feeding tube.
Feeding tube with tastes	Assessed by a speech and language therapist as safe to commence trial of oral intake. Usually teaspoons with therapist initially, then handed over to nursing staff. Majority of nutrition, all fluid and medication via feeding tube.
Feeding tube, oral meal and some fluids	Oral intake increasing, and commence taking meals during the day. Start to reduce volume of nutrition via feeding tube, and monitor weight. May still need significant amounts of fluid via feeding tube.
Feeding tube, oral food and fluid	Managing increased oral intake of food and fluid. May start to manage medication orally. Continue to reduce nutritional provision via feeding tube. Dietitian requests oral intake record charts.
Feeding tube water only	Reached a stage where weight can be maintained by oral diet; this may be inclusive of oral nutritional supplements, but unable to drink enough to maintain hydration. It is not uncommon for individuals to be discharged from a rehabilitation setting with a feeding tube for fluids and medication only.
Full oral diet	Managing enough food and fluid orally to maintain weight and nutritional status.
Healthy eating diet for weight management	Oral intake may reach a stage where unwanted weight increases occur. Healthy-eating dietary advice will be needed; in extreme cases, individuals might become hyperphagic as a result of their brain injury.

- Advice from doctors and pharmacists on relevant drug–nutrient interactions. Individuals may be prescribed medications that reduce their level of arousal, meaning they are too tired to eat at meal times or medications may make them feel unwell.

Target weight setting

The use of target weight ranges within neurorehabilitation is a way of ensuring appropriate and timely responses to weight fluctuations. The dietitian should agree on a target weight range with an individual on admission to a rehabilitation setting. If this is not possible, the target weight should be set in the individual's best interest. Individuals in the early stages of rehabilitation, particularly if still early post-injury, may have energy requirements far greater than anticipated. This may be due to a number of reasons, including autonomic storming, high tone and spasticity, or repeated infections.

As time progresses, individuals may require far less energy as they receive appropriate postural management, and medication to manage tone and spasticity. Setting and maintaining target weights are also of great importance when considering a patient's 24-hour postural management. Large fluctuations in weight can cause issues with custom-made wheelchairs and lead to splints no longer fitting. Target weight ranges should be reviewed regularly to ensure that they remain appropriate for the individual.

Assessing the extent of nutritional depletion

Weight loss

This is usually the best way of assessing the degree of nutritional depletion in brain-injured individuals. Comparison of the individual's weight at the start of rehabilitation with the individual's usual premorbid weight provides a good indication of the extent of energy depletion. However, measurement of weight is often difficult in severely disabled ABI individuals, as appropriate scales may not be available. Hoist or weighbridge-type scales can be used, but such specialist equipment is not always available. When wheelchair or hoist scales are accessible, then a structured weighing programme can be established to ensure regular monitoring (see Chapter 7.17.3, Spinal cord injury, for details on alternative weighing scales).

Ascertaining accurate weight trends is invaluable over the period of rehabilitation. It is not uncommon for estimated energy requirements to vary considerably from actual requirements (McEvory *et al.*, 2009). In order to prevent overnutrition or undernutrition and ensure that dietary intervention is individualised, it is essential that a method of regular weight monitoring be established. The weighing programme can enable target weight ranges to be set as the dietitians can be confident they are using up-to-date information.

Adiposity measurements

These can be difficult to measure, or inappropriate, in some types of brain-injured individuals. Body mass index can only be calculated if measurements of body weight and height are available. In addition to the practicalities of measuring weight, measurement of height is particularly difficult in brain-injured individuals, because, even if standing is possible, they may not be able to stand erect or immobile for long enough. Alternative body measurements such as demispan and knee height, from which height can be derived (see Chapter 2.2,

Assessment of nutritional status), are not always appropriate alternatives, since brain-injured individuals may be unable to stretch their arms sufficiently for the former measurement or achieve the correct position for the latter. However, it is often possible to obtain an estimate of height directly from the individuals, their relatives or pre-morbid health records.

Skinfold thickness measurements, particularly triceps skinfold thickness, are fraught with problems in this population group. In those with hemiplegia, the arm on the affected side may be oedematous, have abnormal muscle wasting, and be flaccid or spastic, all of which may distort skinfold measurements. Skinfold measurements at other sites may be affected by poor posture or immobility.

Estimates of muscle mass

Measurements of, for instance, mid-arm muscle circumference, can be useful, but are inappropriate for individuals with limb paralysis (in addition to the likelihood of muscle wasting in the affected arm, there is usually a compensatory increase in muscle mass in the unaffected arm). Immobility will also result in muscle wasting.

Biochemical and haematological indices

Measurements of blood glucose, electrolytes, serum urea and urinary nitrogen are used to monitor the degree of catabolism in the acute post-injury phase. In the rehabilitation phase, the renal profile can provide useful information on the individual's hydration status (Labbe, 1986); haematological indicators may be relevant if anaemia is suspected; and biochemical markers in the rehabilitation setting are likely to be useful in an individual who is affected by autonomic storming or who has an infection.

Assessing dietary intake

It can be difficult to obtain accurate dietary information from brain-injured individuals. Many individuals will have memory and cognitive impairments, and/or dysphasia (receptive and expressive), which limit their ability to understand or communicate. Behavioural and mood changes may result in hostility or aggression towards the questioner, or withdrawal and lack of response. It is essential to understand the individual's capabilities as well as limitations, and to draw on the expertise and advice of other IDT members.

A skilled dietitian may be able to build up a useful diet history from no more than single-word responses to the display of food photographs or food models. The use of specialised computer-based packages and technology can be useful in patients with limited communication abilities, as can low-technology aids, e.g. talking mats. One of the most valuable ways of obtaining additional dietary information is by observing meal times. Not only does this give an estimate of the quantity of food and fluid consumed, but it also reveals any physical difficulties associated with eating or swallowing, together with any behavioural concerns.

Assessment tools designed to evaluate problems such as food refusal, antisocial behaviour or assistance required with feeding have been devised for individuals with dementia (VOICES, 1998; Watson, 1994a, 1994b; Watson & Deary, 1994); however, as yet, no such assessment tool has been devised for brain-injured individuals whose behaviour and care needs are very different. Food and fluid intake charts that are accurately completed can be vital when assessing dietary intake.

Managing dietary problems

Inadequate food intake is most likely to result from:

- Physical difficulties with eating or swallowing.
- Anorexia (often as a result of depression, anxiety or medication).
- Cognitive issues.
- Frustration or fatigue over the effort involved in eating.
- Level of arousal.
- Intensive therapy.
- Food refusal as a result of behavioural change or because the individual finds it embarrassing to be fed.
- Drug-induced side effects, e.g. nausea and vomiting.

Some of these problems may be remedied by quite simple measures, e.g. smaller, more frequent, energy-dense meals for those suffering from anorexia or nausea. The use of various aids to help overcome the physical difficulties of getting food into the mouth, assistance with feeding, involvement of patients in meal or menu planning groups, creating a pleasant meal atmosphere or changing the timing of the administration of drugs can help improve food intake.

Individuals with evidence of malnutrition, or at high risk of malnutrition, will require a greater level of nutritional support via:

- Food fortification (see Chapter 6.3, Oral nutritional support).
- Use of energy and protein supplements (see Chapter 6.3, Oral nutritional support).
- Enteral feeding (either overnight supplementary or total support, via the nasogastric or gastrostomy routes) (see Chapter 6.4, Enteral nutrition).

The extent, means and route of support will depend on the level of nutritional depletion, the physical and psychological effects of the injury, whether the condition is relapsing–remitting or chronically progressive, and the preferences of the individuals and carers. Specific problems that may have to be addressed are outlined in the following subsections.

Autonomic storming

Abnormal autonomic function is well recognised after brain injury. This has been variously termed autonomic dysfunction syndrome or autonomic or sympathetic storming. Features of the syndrome include increases in heart rate, respiratory rate, temperature and blood pressure, with decerebrate or decorticate posturing, increased muscle tone, and profuse sweating. Autonomic storming can greatly increase the nutritional requirements, and also lead to vastly increased fluid requirements due to increased losses from sweating.

Fluid requirements and dehydration

In order to prevent clinical dehydration and maintain biochemical markers within normal limits, patients often require significantly more than 30–35 mL/kg of fluid/day. This can be related to temperature regulation problems, autonomic storming, excess secretions due to tracheostomies, hypersalivation or diarrhoea.

Hydration status is particularly likely to be inadequate in those with poor oral or swallowing abilities. The problem often results from individuals not being encouraged to consume fluids (either in liquid or semi-solid form) at regular intervals throughout the day. This could be due to the care staff not having sufficient time, or lack of awareness of its importance. In addition, the use of medication within this patient group can be a risk factor for dehydration. The prescription of antibiotics to treat infection can cause diarrhoea. Many liquid medications that contain sorbitol can result in osmotic diarrhoea, e.g. baclofen, which is often used to manage muscle tone during neurorehabilitation.

Sodium imbalances

It is not uncommon for individuals to experience imbalances in their serum sodium levels; this is related to the role of the central nervous system in regulating sodium and water balance. Disturbances in sodium balance can have serious consequences, and working closely with the medical team to manage these disturbances is vital. Common causes of hyponatraemia in the brain-injured individual include the syndrome of inappropriate antidiuretic hormone, the cerebral salt wasting syndrome, or medications, especially some anticonvulsants (Bradshaw & Smith, 2008). Hypernatraemia can be attributed to inadequate free-water intake or excess fluid losses, central diabetes insipidus or excessive use of osmotic diuretics (Bradshaw & Smith, 2008).

Constipation

This is extremely common in individuals referred for neurorehabilitation. The following factors may contribute to constipation:

- Inadequate fluid intake.
- Low fibre intake (especially on a modified-consistency diet).
- Reduced gut motility (as a result of reduced neurological signals from the brain or muscle wasting in the gastrointestinal tract).
- Reduced mobility.
- Side effect of medication, e.g. opiates for pain relief.

Symptoms may be alleviated by increasing consumption of:

- Fluid – ideally 30–35 mL/kg/day, although some individuals may require significantly more.
- Fibre-rich foods that are compatible with the individual's eating or swallowing difficulties. Foods such as porridge, wholegrain breakfast cereals, bananas, peeled oranges or satsumas, vegetables with skins, beans, lentils and peas, and prunes and dried fruit may be suitable options. SLTs should be involved to advise on the suitability of texture-modified diets.
- Laxatives – many patients will require laxatives, suppositories, or a combination of both to achieve and maintain a regular bowel pattern.

Vestibular symptoms

The vestibular system is responsible for controlling balance, eye movement and spatial orientation. If any aspect of this system is damaged, this can result in a variety of symptoms, including dizziness, motion sickness and more generalised nausea and vomiting. A small proportion of individuals may therefore require adjustments in timings of enteral feed to allow a pause from feed prior to manual handling.

Skin integrity

Individuals undergoing neurorehabilitation are at increased risk of pressure sores due to their immobility, muscle wasting and difficulties with repositioning. Therefore, specific consideration should be given to protein intake to maintain skin integrity, minimise risk and assist with the healing of any pre-existing wounds (see Chapter 7.17.6, Wound healing, tissue viability and pressure sores).

Specific nutrients

There is ongoing research into the supplementation of specific nutrients and diets in brain injury, including, but not limited to, n-3 fatty acids, zinc, and magnesium. While these nutrients may have neuroprotective benefits, there is currently insufficient evidence to routinely include them in practice, and further research is required in this area (Vonder Haar *et al.*, 2016).

Involvement of family, friends and carers

Some families, friends or carers might be very involved in the care and management of the individual and may take an interest in the nutritional management. Regular updates on an individual's weight, progress and nutritional intake may be a key part of dietetic input. It is important to remember that family and friends may be going through a grieving process and may struggle to accept the situation. Providing day-in, day-out care for someone with serious physical or psychological difficulties is exhausting and emotionally demanding, and people who have this responsibility require considerable support if they are to maintain their own physical and mental health. The needs of family, friends and carers have been increasingly recognised in recent years, and strategies are being put in place to provide better support measures (Department of Health, 2008). Most units provide support groups or education sessions for family, friends and carers, which direct them to relevant long-term support groups, e.g. Headway. Addressing the carer's needs ensures a more holistic approach to neurorehabilitation.

Acknowledgement

The editor acknowledges the prior contribution of Emma Dresner, Katie Richards and Samantha Perry.

Internet resources

Disabled Living Foundation, www.dlf.org.uk
Headway – the brain injury association, www.headway.org.uk
Royal Association for Disability and Rehabilitation (RADAR), www.radar.org.uk
The Royal Hospital for Neuro-disability, www.rhn.org.uk
The Royal Hospital for Neuro-disability is a national medical charity, independent from the NHS. It is a hospital and a home that rebuilds the lives of adults affected by severe neurological disability, helping them to achieve the best possible quality of life.

Further reading

Braddom RL. (2004) *Handbook of Physical Medicine and Rehabilitation*. Pennsylvania: Saunders.
British Society of Rehabilitation Medicine (BSRM). (2008) *BSRM Standards for Specialist Rehabilitation Services Mapped on to the NSF for Long Term Conditions*. London: BRSM.
British Society of Rehabilitation Medicine/Job Centre Plus/Royal College of Physicians (BSRM/Job Centre Plus/RCP). (2004) *Vocational Assessment and Rehabilitation after Acquired Brain Injury – Inter-agency Guidelines*. London: RCP.
Clifton DW Jr. (2005) *Physical Rehabilitation's Role in Disability Management*. Missouri: Elsevier Saunders.
Davis S. (2006) *Rehabilitation – The Use of Theories and Models in Practice*. Oxford: Elsevier Churchill Livingstone.
DH. (2005) *The National Service Framework for Long-Term Conditions*. London: Department of Health. Available at https://www.gov.uk/government/uploads/system/uploads/attachment_data/file/198114/National_Service_Framework_for_Long_Term_Conditions.pdf.
Gronwall D, Wrightson P, Waddell P. (1998) *Head Injury – The Facts*, 2nd edn. Oxford: Oxford University Press.
Grieve J. (1993) *Neuropsychology for Occupational Therapists*. Oxford: Blackwell Science.
Kumar S. (2000) *Multidisciplinary Approach to Rehabilitation*. Massachusetts: Butterworth-Heinemann.
Laidler P. (1994) *Stroke Rehabilitation: Structure and Strategy*. London: Chapman & Hall.
Muir-Giles G, Clark-Wilson J. (1993) *Brain Injury Rehabilitation – A Neurological Approach*. London: Chapman & Hall.
NHS Confederation. (2005) *Supporting People with Long-Term Conditions. Briefing No 112*. London: NHS Confederation.
Nocan A, Baldwin S. (1998) *Trends in Rehabilitation Policy*. London: King's Fund.
Richards-Hall G. (1994) Chronic dementia – challenges in feeding an individual. *J. Gerontol. Nurs.* 20(4): 21–30.
Robinson J, Turnock S. (1998) *Investing in Rehabilitation*. London: King's Fund.
Rose FD, Johnson DA. (1996) *Brain Injury and After*. Chichester: John Wiley & Sons.
Royal College of Physicians (RCP). (2013) *Prolonged Disorders of Consciousness: National Clinical Guidelines*. London, RCP.
Sinclair A, Dickinson E. (1998) *Effective Practice in Rehabilitation*. London: King's Fund.

References

Bradshaw K, Smith M. (2008) Disorders of sodium balance after brain injury. *Continuing Education in Anaesthesia. Crit. Care Pain* 8(4): 129–133.
British Society of Rehabilitation Medicine /Royal College of Physicians (BSRM/RCP). (2003) *Rehabilitation Following Acquired Brain Injury – National Clinical Guidelines*. London: RCP. Available at https://www.headway.org.uk/media/3320/bsrm-rehabilitation-following-acquired-brain-injury.pdf. Accessed 4 February 2017.
DH. (2008) *Carers at the heart of 21st Century families and communities*. Available at https://www.gov.uk/government/uploads/system/uploads/attachment_data/file/136492/carers_at_the_heart_of_21_century_families.pdf. Accessed 24 February 2017.
Henson MB, De Castro JM, Stringer AY, *et al.* (1993) Food intake by brain-injured humans who are in the chronic phase of recovery. *Brain Inj.* 7(2): 169–178.
Labbe RF. (1986) Laboratory monitoring of nutritional support. Is more better? *Arch. Pathol Lab. Med.* 110: 775–776.
McEvory CT, Cran GW, Cooke SR, *et al.* (2009) Resting energy expenditure in non-ventilated patients recovering from serious traumatic brain injury: comparison of predictive equations with indirect calorimetry values. *Clin. Nutr.* 28(5): 526–532.
Osborn CL, Marshall MJ. (1993) Self feeding performance in nursing home residents. *J. Gerontol. Nurs.* 19(3): 7–9.
Potempa K, Lopez M, Braun LT, *et al.* (1995) Physiological outcome of aerobic exercise training in hemiparetic stroke individuals. *Stroke.* 26(1): 101–105.
Royal College of Physicians/BSRM. (2010) *Report of working party. Medical Rehabilitation in 2011 and Beyond*. London: RCP/BSRM.
Royal College of Physicians (RCP). (2013) *Prolonged Disorders of Consciousness: National Clinical Guidelines*. London: RCP.
Turner-Stokes L, Tonge P, Nyein K, *et al.* (1998) The Northwick Park Dependency Score (NPDS): a measure of nursing dependency in rehabilitation. *Clin. Rehabil.* 12(4): 304–318.
VOICES (Voluntary Organisations Involved in Caring in the Elderly Sectors). (1998) *Eating Well for Older People with Dementia*. Herts: VOICES.
Vonder Haar C, Peterson T, Martens KM, *et al.* (2016) Vitamins and nutrients as primary treatments in experimental brain injury: Clinical implications for nutraceutical therapies. *Brain Res.* 1640: 114–129.
Watson R. (1994a) Measuring feeding difficulties in individuals with dementia: developing a scale. *J. Adv. Nurs.* 19: 257–263.
Watson R. (1994b) Measuring feeding difficulties in individuals with dementia: replication and validation of the Ed Fed Scale #1. *J. Adv. Nurs.* 19: 850–855.
Watson R, Deary IJ. (1994) Measuring feeding difficulty in individuals with dementia: multivariate analysis of feeding problems, nursing intervention and indicators of feeding difficulty. *J. Adv. Nurs.* 20: 283–287.

7.7 Refsum's disease

Eleanor Baldwin

Key points

- Adult Refsum's disease is a rare autosomal recessive disorder of lipid metabolism.
- The primary management of adult Refsum's disease is dietary modification.
- Foods rich in phytanic acid must be avoided. Phytanic acid is a fatty acid found in ruminant animal products, fish and shellfish.
- Fasting and rapid weight loss must be avoided in order to prevent a rapid increase in plasma phytanic acid and deterioration in symptoms.

The Norwegian neurologist Sigvald Refsum first described adult Refsum's disease (ARD) in 1946. He documented four cases from two families, treated between 1937 and 1943. They initially presented with disturbed visual fields and subsequently developed abnormal gait, muscle wasting and paralysis (Refsum, 1946). The disorder was called heredoataxia hemeralopica polyneuritiformis', and then 'heredopathia atactica polyneuritiformis; current literature uses adult Refsum's disease.

ARD and infantile Refsum's disease (IRD) are completely different disorders, with different management strategies and prognosis. IRD is the mildest in the spectrum of a group of global disorders of the peroxisomal assembly (peroxisomal biogenesis disorders); the peroxisome is deficient in multiple enzymes responsible for different metabolic functions. It presents in infancy with severe mental and physical retardation. ARD affects one metabolic function of the peroxisome, and presentation does not usually occur until the 20s–50s with night blindness associated with retinitis pigmentosa and polyneuropathy or other signs.

Diagnostic criteria and classification

ARD is a rare autosomal recessive disorder of lipid metabolism. Straight-chain fatty acids are normally degraded by beta oxidation in the mitochondria. Fatty acids with a complicated structure, including a methyl or other functional group on carbon 3, can only be broken down by alpha or omega oxidation in the peroxisomes. Phytanic acid (3, 7, 11, 15 tetra methyl hexadecanoic acid) is a branched-chain fatty acid in the diet, derived from the microbial degradation of the phytol side chain of chlorophyll. Normally, this fatty acid is rapidly degraded by alpha oxidation, so that plasma levels are usually <10 μmol/L (normal range 0–30 μmol/L). The alternative omega oxidation pathway for phytanic acid has a much lower capacity. Patients with ARD have a mutation in an enzyme in the alpha oxidation pathway that degrades phytanic acid. As a result, patients present with plasma phytanic acid levels ranging from 100 to 6000 μmol/L.

The clinical symptoms of ARD evolve slowly. Typically, night blindness occurs in the teens, followed by a reduction in the visual fields associated with retinitis pigmentosa. On questioning, patients describe anosmia (lack of sense of smell). Some will have bony abnormalities such as short third or fourth toes or fingers. Deafness, peripheral neuropathy and cerebellar ataxia develop later. Nerve conduction studies are abnormal, with slowing of conduction velocities, and early cataracts are common. When the phytanic acid levels are very high (>1000 μmol/L), ichthyosis (rough, hard, scaly, skin), paralysis and cardiac involvement (conduction abnormalities and cardiomyopathy) can occur.

A diagnosis of retinitis pigmentosa in association with any of the symptoms described above should arouse suspicion of ARD. Suspected cases of Guillain–Barré syndrome, particularly when they present with acute demyelinating polyneuropathy that appears to be familial and recurrent, should be tested for ARD, as it can mimic Guillain–Barré syndrome (Verny *et al.*, 2006). Measurement of plasma phytanic acid and genetic testing will confirm the diagnosis of ARD.

Manual of Dietetic Practice, Sixth Edition. Edited by Joan Gandy.

Companion website: www.manualofdieteticpractice.com

Genetics

It is genetically heterogeneous; two ARD genes, phytanoyl-CoA hydroxylase (PAHX) and peroxin 7 (PEX7, the PTS2 receptor), have been identified (Jansen *et al.*, 2004). Peroxin 7 imports PAHX into the peroxisome along with a small number of other proteins. A severe deficiency in peroxin 7 function is associated with rhizomelic chondrodysplasia. Another enzyme defect in the alpha oxidation pathway involving alpha-methylacyl-CoA racemase (AMACR) can mimic ARD, although it often presents with a sensory neuropathy as opposed to night blindness, and levels of pristanic acid are more elevated than those of phytanic acid. Another Refsum-like disorder has also been identified, called polyneuropathy, hearing loss, ataxia, retinitis pigmentosa, cataract (PHARC) (Fiskerstrand *et al.*, 2010). It is caused by mutations in the alpha/beta-hydrolase domain containing 12 (ABHD12), which is involved in the metabolism of the endocannabinoid 2-arachidonyl glycerol and lysophosphatidylserine. PHARC presents with similar symptoms as ARD, but patients do not have anosmia, and plasma phytanic acid level and peroxisomal function are normal. There is no known relationship of ABHD12 to the phytanic acid degradation pathway.

Metabolism and disease processes

Clinical manifestations of ARD usually begin in adolescence with night blindness, and then progressive loss of visual field and a diagnosis of retinitis pigmentosa (Rüether *et al.*, 2010). The other clinical manifestations described earlier develop later. Phytanic acid accumulates in the plasma and all fat-containing tissues (i.e. liver, brain, adipose tissue, etc.). The mechanisms that cause these symptoms remain obscure; molecular distortion and antimetabolite hypotheses exist (Young *et al.*, 2001; Wierzbicki *et al.*, 2002); modern evidence favours a mechanism based on mitochondrial toxicity. Lifespan appears normal, provided phytanic acid levels are well controlled, and acute complications (cardiac, ichthyosis and acute neuropathy) do not develop. Retinitis pigmentosa seems to progress as people age. There can be significant differences in the clinical severity of symptoms within siblings with the condition.

Management

Treatment of people with ARD follows three approaches, discussed in the following subsections.

Dietary restriction

Dietary restriction of phytanic acid to a level (<10 mg) at which the omega oxidation pathway has the capacity to manage and gradually reduce the phytanic acid present in the plasma should be advised. Case study reports, and audits of groups of ARD patients attending ARD clinics for more than 10 years, have demonstrated that ARD patients can be successfully managed by diet, without the development of cardiomyopathy or high plasma phytanic acid levels requiring plasmapheresis (Baldwin *et al.*, 2010). Annual screening for micronutrient deficiencies is important as isolated deficiencies (vitamins A, D, E, B_{12}, selenium and copper) can occur (Baldwin *et al.*, 2016).

Supportive management of symptoms

Smoking cessation and tight management of comorbidities likely to promote visual loss or cataracts is important. Cochlear implants have successfully treated deafness in at least three Refsum's patients (personal communication). Physiotherapy can induce symptomatic improvement in physical strength and the tendency to form contractures. Emollients soothe itchy, scaly skin. Use of social services for sensory assessments and the Royal National Institute for the Blind for advice on living with visual impairment can help improve the quality of life. Psychological support, timely referral and treatment of comorbid conditions, such as depression, is important to minimise the effects they may have on the ability to eat and comply with dietary management (personal communication).

Plasmapheresis

Plasmapheresis should be offered when the plasma phytanic acid levels are very high (1000 µmol/L and above) and acute symptoms, cardiac abnormalities or acute polyneuropathy are evident, or when the clinical condition of the patient is rapidly deteriorating. More than half of phytanic acid in the plasma is localised within very-low-density (VLDL), low-density (LDL) and high-density (HDL) lipoprotein particles. Therefore, LDL- and VLDL-bound phytanic acid can be effectively eliminated from plasma with extracorporeal LDL apheresis using membrane differential filtration (Straube *et al.*, 2003).

Nutritional assessment

At diagnosis, a full dietetic assessment should be made, including:

- Anthropometry
  - Weight.
  - Height.
  - Body mass index.
  - Waist circumference or waist–hip ratio.
  - Weight history.
- Dietary assessment
  - The dietary history should assess intake of foods rich in phytanic acid (Table 7.7.1). Phytanic acid is a type of fat made by some animals (ruminants) when they digest grass. It is also found in fish as they eat algae, or eat fish that have eaten algae.
  - Fermented foods containing phytol (e.g. fermented vegetables, kimchi, preserved gherkins) should be avoided, as the phytol will be converted to phytanic acid.

SECTION 7

Table 7.7.1 Foods rich in phytanic acid, and suitable alternatives that are low in or contain virtually no phytanic acid

Foods	Foods containing phytanic acid – to be avoided	Foods low in phytanic acid
Meat, meat products and meat substitutes	Beef Beef burgers Calves' liver and kidneys Cottage pie Duck Goose Lamb Mutton Meat lasagne Rabbit Shepherd's pie	Bacon Bean curd Chicken Chicken liver Turkey Eggs Ham Pork Pork liver and kidneys Pork sausages Quorn Soya meat substitutes. Tofu
Dairy products	Cheese made from cow's, sheep's or goat's milk Milk Cream Cow's milk (full-cream or semi-skimmed) Goat's milk Sheep's milk Ice cream Yoghurt (fat-free or full-fat) Butter Ghee	Cheese made from skimmed milk and vegetable oil e.g. Locol. Cheese substitutes made from soya, or coconut oil e.g. Pure soya cheese spread, redwood soya cheeses, Bute island foods soya cheeses, Violife cheese and cheese slices Cream substitute (Alpro soya single cream, soyatoodairy free spray cream, soyatoo cooking cream and soyatoo topping cream, coconut cream substitutes) Cow's milk (skimmed only) Soya milk Swedish glace ice cream substitute Soya yoghurt-style puddings Low fat spreads made only from vegetable oil, e.g. Pure range Vegetable ghee
Other fats and oils	Suet	Vegetable suet, lard
Fish	Fish, especially oily fish such as herring, salmon and sardines Shellfish – clams, mussels, octopus, prawns, shrimps. Fish oil	Cod, coley and haddock Soya or pulse based fish substitutes such as Redwood foods fish style fingers, fish style steaks, scampi style pieces and Thai style fish cakes
Nuts	Walnuts and peanuts	Very few nuts have been analysed
Alcoholic drinks	Any drinks containing cream, e.g. cream-based liqueurs	Any alcoholic drink that does not contain cream
Bread and baked goods	Brioche, croissants, shortcrust pastry Biscuits and cakes made with butter, suet or fish oil	Puff pastry Filo pastry[a]; all bread, biscuits and cakes that do not contain butter, suet or fish oil
Breakfast cereals	Choco snaps	Breakfast cereals that do not contain milk powder (skimmed milk powder is appropriate) Small portions only of cereals containing nuts, e.g. muesli
Confectionery	Milk chocolate	Dark chocolate, carob, chocolate that does not contain milk fat or butter Fat-free sweets, e.g. boiled sweets

[a]Check ingredients label, as filo pastry is occasionally made with butter.

- Caffeine intake and recreational drug use should be assessed. Adrenergic substances theoretically increase the plasma phytanic acid levels by increasing lipolysis.

Dietary management

Advice should be given on complete avoidance of foods containing phytanic acid (Table 7.7.1), and appropriate substitutes suggested. The Westminster Diet for ARD is based on the analysis of the phytanic acid content of foods listed by Brown *et al.* (1993). The absolute level of phytanic acid in, e.g. beef and dairy products will depend on the feed that the cattle have been given (Lough, 1977) and the fat content of the carcass. Therefore, Brown's should only be taken as representative.

Foods known to contain virtually no phytanic acid include the following:

- Most breakfast cereals.
- Safflower oil, corn oil, olive oil, sunflower seed oil.
- Bread, rice, pearl barley, pasta.
- Jelly.
- Honey.
- Tea, coffee.
- Cooked green vegetables, carrots, mushrooms, onions, potatoes and swede.
- Salad vegetables.
- Fruit.

A moderate caffeine intake (200–350 mg/day for adult women, 300–450 mg/day for adult men) is advisable. A suitable n-3 fatty acid supplement should be prescribed, as increased turnover has been described in peroxisomal disorders leading to low levels (Martinez *et al.*, 2000). Oily fish is excluded in ARD (high phytanic acid); Omacor™ is the only supplement known to have a low phytanic acid content.

Anecdotal reports (Perera *et al.*, 2011) suggest that orlistat therapy may be beneficial by reducing the absorption of fat and fatty acids. However, weight loss must be monitored, and rapid weight loss avoided. It should not be used in patients with PHARC (ABHD12 deficiency).

Regular dietetic review is recommended to maximise dietary compliance. The symptoms of ARD can be controlled by diet (Baldwin *et al.*, 2010), but deterioration in vision occurs over time. This can result in practical difficulties in following the diet (cooking, shopping and reading food labels), depression and social isolation, which can also affect body weight. It is also essential to ensure rapid access to advice on nutritional support to avoid deterioration during episodes of intercurrent illness or fasting for unrelated surgery.

During weight loss or extended periods of fasting, plasma phytanic acid levels increase, doubling every 29 hours (Wierzbicki *et al.*, 2003), owing to the release of phytanic acid stored in the liver and adipose tissue. Patients often have a low BMI at diagnosis, and nutritional supplementation to promote weight gain may be required at diagnosis, during periods of intercurrent illness or pre- or post-surgery. Most nutritional supplements are suitable for use, with the exception of those containing fish oil, full-fat milk or full-fat dairy products. Weight gain can cause a reduction in plasma phytanic acid, as some of the phytanic acid will be shunted into adipose tissue deposits. Patients should be advised against weight loss unless the plasma phytanic acid levels are well controlled and their symptoms are stable. Where weight loss is advised, rates should be slow (0.25 kg or less/week), and the plasma phytanic acid levels should be closely monitored in order to detect and avoid deterioration.

Drug–nutrient interactions

The role of the peroxisome in drug metabolism is unclear, especially in patients with deficient or abnormal peroxisomal function. However, some lipid-lowering drugs (e.g. fibrates) and hypoglycaemic drugs (thiazolidinediones, also known as 'glitazones') rely on mechanisms associated with increased peroxisomal activity in animals, and should be used with caution in people with peroxisomal disorders. The only common drug known to be metabolised through the peroxisome is ibuprofen, which is metabolised through a pathway involving AMACR. Therefore, alternative non-steroidal anti-inflammatory drugs are preferred in ARD.

Adult Refsum's disease clinic

Chelsea & Westminster NHS Foundation Trust, 369 Fulham Rd, London SW10 9NH. Tel: 020 8746 8178.

Internet resources

Adult Refsum's Disease, www.refsumdisease.org: Information for patients, carers and clinicians – devised by a European Union collaborative project for research into the diagnosis, prognosis and treatment of Refsum's disease.
National Information Centre for Metabolic Diseases (CLIMB), www.climb.org.uk
Royal National Institute for the Blind, www.rnib.org.uk
The Vegan Society, www.vegansociety.com

References

Baldwin EJ, Gibberd EB, Harley C, *et al.* (2010) The effectiveness of long-term dietary therapy in the treatment of adult Refsum disease. *J. Neurol. Neurosurg. Psychiatry.* 81(9): 954–957.

Baldwin EJ, Harrington DJ, Sampson B, *et al.* (2016) Safety of long term restrictive diets for peroxisomal disorders: vitamin and trace element status of patients treated for Adult Refsum's Disease. *Int. J. Clin. Pract.* 70(3): 229–235.

Brown PJ, Mei G, Gibberd FB, *et al.* (1993) Diet and Refsum's disease. The determination of phytanic acid and phytol in certain foods and the application of this knowledge to the choice of suitable convenience foods for patients with Refsum's disease. *J. Hum. Nutr. Diet.* 6: 295–305.

Fiskerstrand T, Brahim DH, Johansson S, *et al.* (2010) Mutations in ABHD12 cause the neurodegenerative disease PHARC: an inborn error of endocannabinoid metabolism. *Am. J. Hum. Genet.* 87: 410–417.

Jansen GA, Waterham HR, Wanders RJ. (2004) Molecular basis of Refsum disease: sequence variations in phytanoyl-CoA hydroxylase (PHYH) and the PTS2 receptor (PEX7). *Hum. Mutat.* 23(3): 209–218.

Lough AK. (1977) The phytanic acid content of the lipids of bovine tissues and milk. *Lipids.* 12(1): 115–119.

Martinez M, Vázquez E, García-Silva MT, *et al.* (2000) Therapeutic effects of docosahexaenoic acid ethyl ester in patients with generalised peroxisomal disorders. *Am. J. Clin. Nutr.* 71(1): 376S–385S.

Perera NJ, Lewis B, Tran H, *et al.* (2011) Refsum's disease – use of the intestinal lipase inhibitor, Orlistat, as a novel therapeutic approach to a complex disorder. *J. Obes.* 10.1155/2011/482021.

Refsum S. (1946) Heredopathia atactica polyneuritiformis: a familial syndrome not hitherto described. A contribution to the clinical study of the hereditary disorders of the nervous system. *Acta Psychiatr. Scand.* 21: 11–303.

Rüether K, Baldwin E, Casteels M, *et al.* (2010) Adult Refsum disease: a form of tapetoretinal dystrophy accessible to therapy. *Survey Ophthalmol.* 55: 531–538.

Straube R, Gäckler D, Thiele A, *et al.* (2003) Membrane differential filtration is safe and effective for the long term treatment of Refsum syndrome – an update of treatment modalities and pathophysiological cognition. *Transfus. Apher. Sci.* 29(1): 85–91.

Verny C, Prundean A, Nicolas G, *et al.* (2006) Refsum's disease may mimic familial Guillain Barre syndrome. *Neuromuscul. Disord.* 16(11): 805–808.

Wierzbicki AS, Lloyd MD, Schofield CJ, *et al.* (2002) Refsum's disease: a peroxisomal disorder affecting phytanic acid alpha oxidation. *J. Neurochem.* 80: 727–735.

Wierzbicki AS, Mayne PD, Lloyd MD, *et al.* (2003) Metabolism of phytanic acid and 3methyladipic acid excretion in patients with adult Refsum disease. *J. Lipid Res.* 44: 1481–1488.

Young SP, Johnson AW, Muller DP. (2001) Effects of phytanic acid on the vitamin E status, lipid composition and physical properties of retinal cell membranes: implications for adult Refsum disease. *Clin. Sci. (Lond.)* 101(6): 697–705.

7.8 Inherited metabolic disorders in adults

Louise Robertson, Sarah Howe, Charlotte Ellerton, Rachel Carruthers, Heidi Chan, Sarah Ripley, Sarah Adam, Sarah Donald and Suzanne Ford

Key points

- Most inherited metabolic disorders (IMDs) require dietetic input as part of their treatment. This may include dietary modification of the amount or type of protein, fat and/or carbohydrate.
- Many IMDs need an emergency regimen as part of treatment during a metabolic decompensation.

Inherited metabolic disorders (IMDs) are a rare group of genetic diseases where a mutation in a single gene affects the production or degradation of protein, carbohydrate or fat (see Chapter 5.1, Genetics and nutritional genomics). There is often an enzyme or transport protein defect that can cause serious illness due to toxin accumulation if not treated. IMDs can develop at any time, including during adulthood; but, usually, the later they present, the less severe they are. More patients with IMDs are now surviving into adulthood, resulting in a need for adult services and a smooth transition from paediatric services. In the UK, the incidence is 1 in 800, but this varies between countries and ethnicity (Sanderson *et al.*, 2006). This chapter outlines the dietetic treatment for adults with the most common IMDs and the practical strategies to aid a successful outcome.

Phenylketonuria

Phenylketonuria (PKU) is an autosomal, recessive IMD caused by a deficiency of the enzyme phenylalanine hydroxylase (PAH), which catalyses the conversion of phenylalanine into tyrosine. High phenylalanine blood concentrations are neurotoxic during infancy and childhood, leading to irreversible brain damage if not treated from birth. The severity of PKU depends on the amount of residual activity of PAH.

Nutritional management

Dietary treatment is a restricted phenylalanine diet and involves:

- Protein substitute, which contains all the indispensable amino acids except phenylalanine: usually 60–80 g of protein equivalent, taken in three or four doses throughout the day.
- Low-protein diet and phenylalanine exchanges (one exchange = 50 mg of phenylalanine = 1 g of protein).
- Prescribed low-protein foods – bread, pasta, rice, flour, cereals and milk alternatives.
- Naturally low-protein foods – fruit, vegetables, fats and sugars.

Patients should be reviewed annually as a minimum. Blood phenylalanine concentrations in adults should be monitored monthly using dried blood spot analysis. Annual biochemical monitoring, including nutritional bloods and particularly vitamin B_{12}, is recommended (van Wegberg *et al.*, 2017). For those returning to a PKU diet, a stepwise introduction should be used. A baseline measurement of blood phenylalanine should be taken before any dietary changes are made. It is important to identify the patient's or care team's reasons for recommencing diet, as these can be later used as outcome measures to help ascertain the success of the diet.

Protein substitute should initially be given once a day, and slowly increased to the full requirement. Once the full dose is reached, high-protein foods can be safely excluded. Cow's milk should be swapped for a lower-protein alternative, and prescribed low-protein foods should be introduced to help lower phenylalanine intake, ensure sufficient energy and provide variety. If the desired phenylalanine levels are not achieved, protein exchanges should be considered. A dietary review 3–6 months after restarting the diet can ascertain the benefits of the diet, and whether it should be continued.

Manual of Dietetic Practice, Sixth Edition. Edited by Joan Gandy.

Companion website: www.manualofdieteticpractice.com

Diet for life

There is a growing body of evidence to suggest that patients with PKU should stay on diet for life: Table 7.8.1 summarises some of this evidence. The European Society for PKU (ESPKU) have recently published new guidelines to standardise care. They recommended that patients over the age of 12 years should aim for a blood phenylalanine concentration of 120–600 μmol/L (van Wegberg *et al.*, 2017).

The restrictive nature of the PKU diet can make adherence challenging, especially in adolescence. It is vital to educate patients on the benefits of adherence, but also to support their decision if they choose not to follow the diet. For women of childbearing age, the risks of conceiving off diet must be emphasised. Adult patients can be classified into four groups, each with specific problems and nutritional issues requiring different strategies for care and monitoring (see Figure 7.8.1).

Table 7.8.1 Evidence for diet for life in phenylketonuria

Study findings when off diet	Reference
Mood disturbances	Clacy *et al.* (2014)
Negative mood reported by both patient and family member	ten Hoedt *et al.* (2011)
Reduced quality of life	Bik-Multanowski *et al.* (2008)
Tremors, brisk tendon reflexes and impaired coordination	Cerone *et al.* (1999)
Lower scores on accuracy and performance speed when off diet for 5 years	Channon *et al.* (2007)
Phobias, low self-esteem, social isolation and lack of autonomy	Brumm *et al.* (2010)
Reduced reaction times	Dawson *et al.* (2011)
Neurocognitive impairment where diet relaxed in adolescence.	Weglage *et al.* (2013)

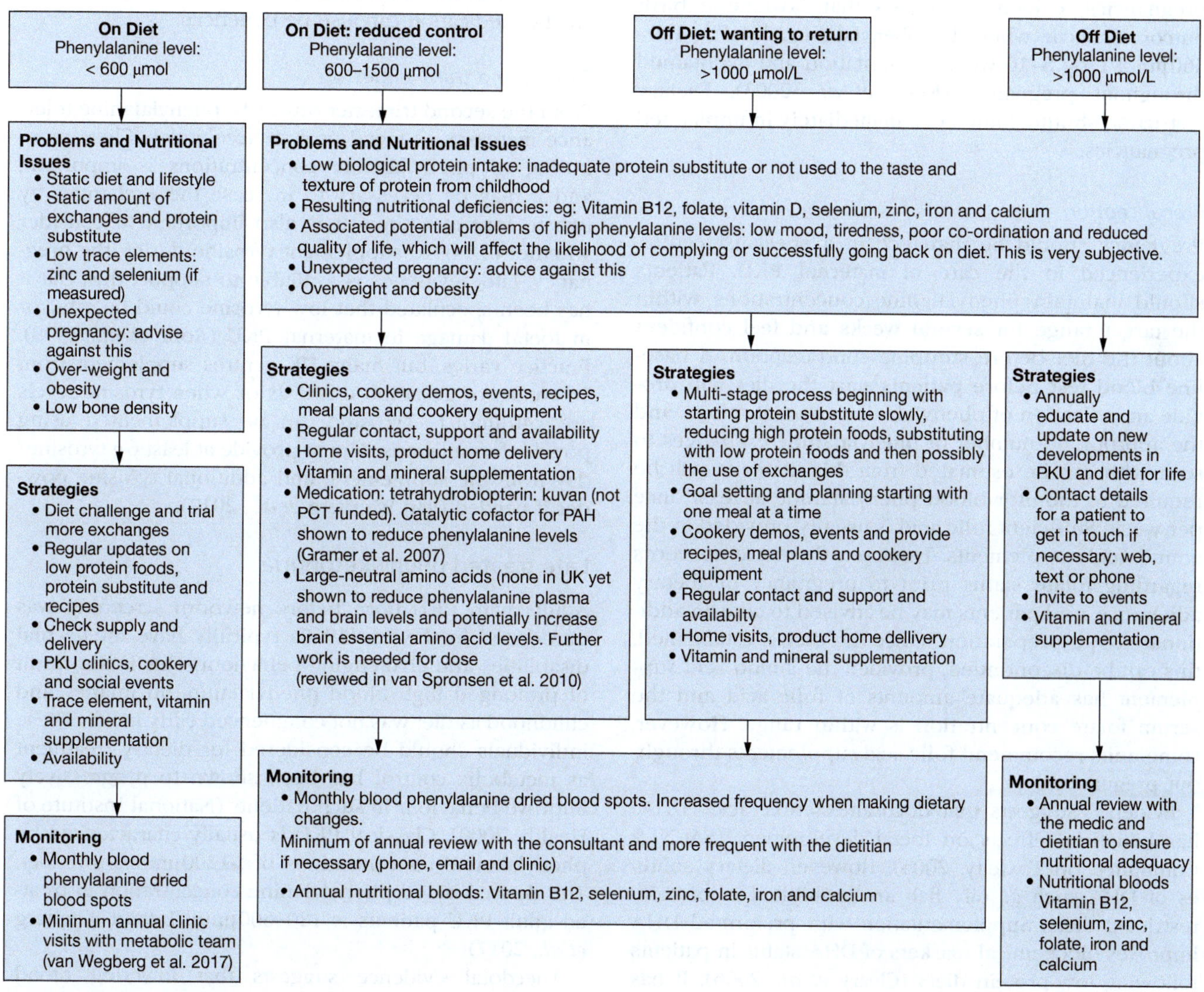

Figure 7.8.1 Challenges and strategies in adult phenylketonuria (PKU)

SECTION 7

Maternal phenylketonuria

Women with PKU must optimise metabolic control when planning a pregnancy. High phenylalanine levels are teratogenic and can cause microcephaly, mental retardation, congenital heart disease, spontaneous abortion and low birth weight (<2500 g) (Lenke & Levy, 1980). Metabolic control must be closely monitored during pregnancy, with current European guidelines recommending that maternal phenylalanine levels be maintained between 120 and 360 μmol/L (van Wegberg *et al.*, 2017). Levels of <120 μmol/L have been associated with microcephaly (Teissier *et al.*, 2012). There is also some evidence that fluctuating levels may result in suboptimal cognitive outcomes (Maillot *et al.*, 2008), and many UK centres aim for a narrower target range of 120–250 μmol/L. Strict control is necessary due to the positive amino acid gradient across the placenta, thereby exposing the foetus to higher phenylalanine concentrations than the mother (Cleary & Walter, 2001). To achieve optimal outcomes for the infant, the diet should commence before conception (Maillot *et al.*, 2008). However, for unplanned pregnancies, evidence suggests that favourable birth outcomes occur when the phenylalanine level is 120–360 μmol/L by 8–10 weeks of gestation and maintained throughout pregnancy (Koch *et al.*, 2003). Dietary restriction should commence immediately in unplanned pregnancies.

Preconception

Pregnancy should be managed in a specialist centre, experienced in the care of maternal PKU. Patients should maintain phenylalanine concentrations within the target range for several weeks and feel confident about the diet before stopping contraception. A baseline blood test before patients start the diet will provide an indication of phenylalanine concentrations, and the appropriate number of phenylalanine exchanges to start with can be estimated from this. Patients will be required to monitor blood phenylalanine at least once per week. Sufficient folic acid is usually provided in the amino acid supplements. However, there are concerns regarding folate status prior to pregnancy or dietary adherence, and patients may be advised to take an additional 400 μg preparation. Once the diet is established, this can be discontinued, provided the amino acid supplement has adequate amounts of folic acid and the serum folate concentration is within range. However, some units recommend folic acid supplements throughout pregnancy.

Evidence suggests that docosahexaenoic acid (DHA) has beneficial effects on foetal development (SACN & Committee on Toxicity, 2004). However, dietary sources of DHA such as oily fish are prohibited in protein-restricted diets. Supplementation with preformed DHA improves biochemical markers of DHA status in patients following low-protein diets (Cleary *et al.*, 2006). It has been recommended that pregnant and lactating women should have an intake of ≥200 mg DHA (FAO/WHO, 2010; Koletzko *et al.*, 2008). Some amino acid supplements contain DHA, or it can be given separately. Care should be taken to recommend DHA supplements without additional vitamins A and D.

First trimester

A frequent problem during the first trimester is pregnancy-associated nausea and vomiting. Patients may find it difficult to tolerate the amino acid supplement, and energy intake may be compromised. It may be useful to advise eating little and often, encouraging patients to have plenty of energy-dense foods and sugary, non-caffeinated drinks, and to snack on low-protein foods every 2–3 hours to prevent the phenylalanine concentrations from increasing. Reducing the volume of supplement, spreading it out over the day or changing to a tablet form may be helpful. Increasing the total dose of amino acid supplement to drive the phenylalanine concentration down is also advisable. Supplementing the diet with glucose or fat-based products will provide important extra energy (see Appendix A6). The phenylalanine concentration will increase if the mother becomes catabolic, which is detrimental to the foetus. Use of anti-emetic medication can also be beneficial.

Second and third trimesters

From the second trimester onwards, phenylalanine tolerance increases as foetal growth accelerates. Close monitoring of phenylalanine concentrations is important, and it may be necessary to increase the exchanges by two to four at a time. It is also important to consider whether or not to supplement tyrosine during the pregnancy. Little evidence is available to support this, but it has been speculated that low tyrosine could be a factor in foetal damage in maternal PKU (Rohr *et al.*, 1998). Practice varies, but many UK centres supplement from 16 weeks of gestation onwards or when tyrosine levels are <40 μmol/L. Tyrosine can be supplemented using powder formulations. Aim to provide at least 6 g tyrosine/day from the supplement, and additional tyrosine powder if needed (van Wegberg *et al.*, 2017).

Late treated phenylketonuria

Adults with PKU born before newborn screening was introduced in the late 1960s typically have intellectual disabilities and challenging behaviour. This is the result of prolonged high blood phenylalanine in infancy and childhood as diet was not commenced early in life. These individuals should be considered for dietary treatment as metabolic control has been shown to progressively improve behaviour in such patients (National Institute of Health, 2000). Classical PKU is usually characterised by phenylalanine concentrations of >1200 μmol/L pre-diet. The desired blood phenylalanine concentration in treated adult PKU patients is 120–600 μmol/L (van Wegberg *et al.*, 2017).

Anecdotal evidence suggests that lowering blood phenylalanine with a phenylalanine-restricted diet can improve communication, relationships with carers and social skills, although not all show benefit. A randomised placebo-controlled double-blind trial of a phenylalanine-restricted diet in adults with late-diagnosed PKU concluded that there are potential benefits to quality of life for the individuals and their carers (Lee *et al.*, 2009); while the overall benefit was not high, a positive effect in about three-quarters of the individuals was demonstrated. About 70% of the carers continued with the diet after the trial had ended. Another study demonstrated that giving a phenylalanine-restricted diet to adults with previously untreated PKU led to economic benefits to the UK's NHS and society in general (Brown & Guest, 1999).

Urea cycle disorders

The urea cycle metabolises the hepatic pool of nitrogen, and an enzyme defect in the pathway results in a urea cycle disorder (UCD), causing hyperammonaemia. Accumulation of ammonia in the brain may lead to damage that can result in coma and death if left untreated (Leonard, 2006). Protein aversion is common, leading to disordered eating and a poor-quality diet. Some adults may rely on artificial feeding. The UCDs are:

- Carbamoyl phosphate synthase deficiency (CPS).
- Ornithine transcarbamaylase deficiency (OTC).
- Citrullinaemia.
- Argininosuccinic aciduria (ASA).
- Arginase deficiency.
- N-acetyl glutamate synthase deficiency (NAGS).
- Ornithine amino transferase deficiency (OAT).
- Hyperornithinaemia–hyperammonaemia–homocitrullinuria (HHH) syndrome.

Clinical presentation in adults varies due to residual enzyme activity, genotype and exogenous nitrogen load (Singh, 2007). By restricting nitrogen consumption from protein, ammonia production is limited. Ammonia-scavenging drugs (sodium benzoate and/or sodium phenylbutyrate) are also used to treat pharmacologically as they provide an alternative pathway for the excretion of excess nitrogen (Häberle *et al.*, 2012).

Nutritional management

Long-term management is to restrict natural protein intake while maintaining optimal energy and nutritional status. The WHO/FAO/UNU (2007) recommends safe protein levels based on ideal body weight (>18 y 0.83 g/kg/d). If protein requirement cannot be met safely by natural protein, then an essential amino acid supplement may be indicated (Häberle *et al.*, 2012). Natural protein tolerance is greater in those with higher levels of residual enzyme and when pharmacological doses are high. Protein should be evenly distributed throughout the day along with medication, with a combination of high- and low-biological-value protein (Häberle *et al.*, 2012).

Energy provision should be sufficient to prevent fluctuations in weight. Sources include naturally low-protein foods that are high in energy, specialist low-protein prescribed foods, and high energy, non-protein nutritional supplements. Long fasts should be avoided. Patients on restricted protein diets are at risk of vitamin and mineral deficiencies, particularly iron, zinc, copper, calcium and vitamin B_{12}, and supplementation will be required (Häberle *et al.*, 2012).

Lean body mass will be broken down to produce arginine if the urea cycle does not produce sufficient quantities. Therefore, arginine becomes an essential nutrient, and oral supplementation is necessary (Singh, 2007). l-Arginine can be administered in all the UCDs except in arginase deficiency, where it does not become essential. Reports of liver transplant have been successful in adults with certain UCDs.

Treatment when unwell

Metabolic decompensation occurs when the body is in a catabolic state. This is exacerbated by infections, fever, vomiting, surgery, intense physical activity and prolonged labour. During such periods, the body requires additional non-protein energy to prevent the breakdown of lean body mass. Withdrawal of protein should be initiated immediately, and the oral emergency regimen (ER) commenced (see the section 'Emergency regimens'). The only exception to using the oral glucose emergency regime would be in citrullinaemia type 2 (citrin deficiency), where excessive glucose exacerbates hyperammonaemia. Therefore, their oral ER will consist of full-fat cow's milk to supply an alternative fuel source as fat and protein: IV dextrose is contraindicated. Ammonia scavengers need to be administered orally or intravenously, depending on the function of the gastrointestinal tract.

Organic acidaemias

Propionic acidaemia (PA) and methyl malonic acidaemia (MMA) are autosomal recessive disorders in which isoleucine, valine, methionine, threonine and odd-chain fatty acids are not metabolised fully. The deficient enzyme is propionyl-CoA carboxylase in PA, and methylmalonyl-CoA mutase, which is vitamin B_{12} dependent, in MMA (Baumgartner *et al.*, 2014). Some MMA patients respond well to vitamin B_{12} supplementation. Antibiotics are required long term to control the gut flora. Isovaleric acidaemia (IVA) affects leucine metabolism, whereas glutaric aciduria type 1 (GA1) affects lysine and tryptophan metabolism.

Nutritional management

Nutritional management for PA, MMA and IVA is similar to that of urea cycle disorders, involving a reduced natural protein diet (limiting the metabolite precursors but ensuring essential requirements) with adequate energy and micronutrient requirements and avoidance of prolonged fasting. If the WHO/FAO/UNU (2007)-recommended safe protein levels (0.83 g/kg/d) cannot be met, then precursor-free amino acids should be supplemented. Enteral feeding is often used to supplement intake due to feeding problems (Baumgartner *et al.*,

2014). Supplementation of glycine is indicated in IVA. A lysine-restricted diet is indicated in GA1 children, but there is limited evidence for this in adults. It is recommended that adults stick to a safe protein intake and continue to use their ER when unwell (Boy *et al.*, 2017). l-Carnitine supplementation counteracts urinary losses of acylcarnitine (de Baulny *et al.*, 2005). Vitamin and mineral replacement are advised to prevent deficiencies. All organic acidaemias require immediate medical and dietary treatment during illness (see the section 'Emergency regimens').

Disorders of fatty acid oxidation

Fatty acid oxidation disorders (FAODs) are autosomal recessive disorders of the mitochondrial fatty acid oxidation pathway. These conditions limit energy production from fatty acids and ketones. FAODs vary in severity. Severe mutations present in early childhood (Murphy *et al.*, 2016). Hypoglycaemia is rare in adults, and care focuses on preventing metabolic decompensations, managing pregnancy, and maintaining appropriate BMI. FAODs have three characteristic clinical presentations:

- Acute hypoketotic hypoglycaemia, with encephalopathy, hepatomegaly and liver dysfunction.
- Cardiomyopathy, arrhythmias or conduction defects.
- Myopathy with myalgia, weakness or rhabdomyolysis, which can impair renal function and require dialysis.

Nutritional management

The main emphasis in all FAODs is avoidance of fasting and the recommendation of ERs during illness (see the section 'Emergency regimens'). Further modifications are individualised per disorder and severity. Most evidence for dietary management originates from paediatric literature. Episodes of decompensation, including hypoglycaemia and encephalopathy, may result in significant neurodisability. Strong evidence to support fat restriction in newly presenting or asymptomatic adults is lacking (Murphy *et al.*, 2016).

Fatty acid oxidation consists of four stages (Stanley *et al.*, 2006), and typical dietary modifications per condition are as follows:

- Carnitine cycle defects
  - Carnitine palmitoyltransferase (CPT) I deficiency – high carbohydrate (70% energy), restriction of long-chain triglycerides (LCTs) (<20% energy), particularly during illness.
  - CPT II deficiency – normal or lower LCT, may benefit from medium-chain triglycerides (MCTs) or triheptanoin.
- Beta-oxidation defects
  - Medium-chain acyl-CoA dehydrogenase (MCAD) deficiency – regular meals, no LCT restriction, avoid MCT.
  - Long-chain 3-hydroxyacyl-CoA dehydrogenase (LCHAD) deficiency and trifunctional protein (TFP) complex – restrict LCT (<10% energy), supplement with MCT (10–20% energy), likely to require uncooked corn starch (UCCS) before bed or overnight feeding.
  - Very-long-chain acyl-CoA dehydrogenase (VLCAD) deficiency – treatment dependent on severity; asymptomatic patients advised to consume regular meals and avoid prolonged fasting; symptomatic patients will require LCT restriction (<10% energy), supplementation with MCT (10–20% energy), may require UCCS before bed or overnight feeding.
- Electron transport defects
  - Multiple acyl-CoA dehydrogenase deficiency (MADD), also known as glutaric aciduria type II, – most require low-LCT diets. Severely affected patients may require modest protein restriction; avoid MCT.
- Ketone synthesis defects
  - HMG-CoA synthase – avoid MCT.
  - HMG-CoA lyase – may require moderate protein and fat restriction: avoid MCT. Pregnancy appears to increase risk of decompensation; if nauseous, immediate hospital admission is recommended (Morris, 2016).

Supplementation

MCTs enter the mitochondria independently of carnitine, bypassing beta oxidation. To prevent exercise-induced rhabdomyolysis, supplementation with MCT, with or without carbohydrates, prior to exercise may be beneficial (Spiekerkoetter *et al.*, 2010). Triheptanoin, an ester of three C7 (odd chain) fatty acids, is thought to be more effective than MCT as its oxidation generates both propionyl-CoA and acetyl-CoA to replenish the tricarboxylic acid cycle (Roe *et al.*, 2002; Spiekerkoetter *et al.*, 2010). Side effects of MCT and triheptanoin include weight gain and gastrointestinal intolerance (Vockley *et al.*, 2016). Gradual introduction with four to five small doses, at least 3–4 hours apart, and taken with food, is recommended. Dietary counselling is necessary to prevent weight gain.

Patients consuming minimal fat risk the deficiency of essential fatty acids (EFAs) and fat-soluble vitamins, requiring supplementation. These patients should receive at least 1% total energy intake from linoleic acid and 0.2% from α-linolenic acid. Walnut oil is most commonly recommended (Dixon *et al.*, 2015a). In the absence of primary carnitine transport defect or severe carnitine deficiency, carnitine is not recommended in routine care (Spiekerkoetter *et al.*, 2010).

Alcohol

Excessive alcohol intake is hazardous (Lang, 2009): symptoms of hypoglycaemia might be mistaken as intoxication. Vomiting, loss of appetite, or lapse in judgment (such as forgetting to take UCCS or to start overnight feed) can have severe consequences. Alcohol intake should be limited and accompanied by food.

Homocystinuria

Homocystinuria (HCU) results from a deficiency of the enzyme cystathionine β synthase (CβS), which is involved in the metabolism of the amino acid methionine. CβS is dependent on a cofactor derived from pyridoxine (vitamin B_6), and the biochemical response to pyridoxine distinguishes the two phenotypes of HCU. In the pyridoxine-responsive phenotype, pharmacological doses of pyridoxine partially or completely control the biochemical abnormalities; and in the non-pyridoxine-responsive phenotype, pyridoxine has no effect. The disorder is characterised by the accumulation of homocysteine and methionine in blood. Untreated HCU can lead to developmental delay, ectopia lentis and severe myopia, skeletal abnormalities, and thromboembolism (Levy *et al.*, 2002). Newborn screening has led to early diagnosis and effective treatment, and fertility does not appear to be affected.

The biochemical aim of treatment is to control, and, if possible, normalise, the severe hyperhomocysteinaemia. The clinical aims are to prevent abnormalities in the four organ systems and optimise intelligence in patients diagnosed by newborn screening. In late-diagnosed patients, the aim is to prevent life-endangering vascular events and manage existing complications (Yap, 2003). Routine measurement of total homocysteine (tHcy) enables treatment effectiveness to be monitored. The aim is to maintain levels at 80–120 μmol/L; in the normal population, tHcy levels are 5–15 μmol/L.

Nutritional management

Treatment of non-pyridoxine-responsive HCU is through dietary methionine restriction with methionine/protein exchanges (20 mg methionine = 1 g protein) and a methionine-free amino acid preparation, e.g. HCU Lophlex LQ or HCU Cooler. Manufactured low-protein foods are available on prescription, provide variety in an otherwise very limited diet, and are a valuable energy source. The protein substitute used should contain cysteine, as this amino acid is usually formed from methionine but becomes deficient in HCU due to the metabolic block. It should be given in divided doses together with the methionine exchanges at main meals. This prevents excessive rises in plasma homocysteine, ensures a complete range of amino acids and allows protein synthesis. If vitamins and minerals are not contained in the protein substitute, these must be provided separately. Folic acid (5 mg/day) is prescribed to ensure adequate intake for use in the remethylation pathway (Walter *et al.*, 1998). The principal pathway for the metabolism of dietary methionine is through conversion of homocysteine to cysteine.

Betaine

Betaine is a methyl donor that stimulates the methylation of homocysteine and reduces homocysteine levels, but usually results in significantly increased plasma methionine levels. Oral betaine can improve biochemical control in individuals where dietary compliance is poor. However, compliance with betaine can also be an issue. The safety of betaine therapy in pregnancy has not been established, but there have been reports that suggest no adverse maternal or foetal effects (Pierre *et al.*, 2006).

Maternal homocystinuria

Newborn screening has led to early diagnosis and effective treatment. Unlike maternal PKU, no strong evidence of teratogenic effects has been found. Fertility does not appear to be affected; however, the incidence of spontaneous miscarriage is high, especially with poor control (Walter, 2000), and there is evidence of increased risk for thromboembolic complications, especially postpartum. Anticoagulant therapy during pregnancy and 6 weeks postpartum will minimise these risks (Levy *et al.*, 2002). However, there is still a high incidence of miscarriage, even with excellent metabolic control and anticoagulant therapy (personal communication).

Maple syrup urine disease

Maple syrup urine disease (MSUD) is characterised by the accumulation of the branched-chain amino acids (BCAAs), leucine, isoleucine and valine, and their metabolites, which are neurotoxic and life threatening. Leucine is thought to be one of the main toxic metabolites, and is restricted in the diet using leucine exchanges (50 mg leucine = 0.5 g protein = one exchange). Essential dietary components also include BCAA free protein substitute, vitamin and mineral supplements, and low-protein prescribed and natural foods similar to those for PKU. Dietary treatment is life long and aims to maintain plasma BCAAs within safe ranges; leucine 200–400 μmol/L, isoleucine 100–200 μmol/L and valine 100–300 μmol/L. If isoleucine and valine are low, then they will need to be supplemented. Illness is treated by an ER that should include the usual protein substitute.

Tyrosinaemia

Type 1 tyrosinaemia results in an increased plasma tyrosine and its metabolites, including succinylacetone, which damage the liver. Treatment is a combination of 2-(2-nitro 4-trifluoromethylbenzoyl)-1, 3-cyclohexanedione (NTBC) and a low-tyrosine, low-phenylalanine diet, aiming to maintain plasma tyrosine at 200–400/500 μmol/L. A tyrosine- and phenylalanine-free protein substitute is given, plus low-protein foods (as in PKU). Tyrosine is given as 1-g protein exchanges.

Galactosaemia

Galactosaemia is an autosomal recessive, rare, inherited metabolic condition in which there is an inability to metabolise galactose. It is caused primarily by the deficiency of the enzyme galactose 1 phosphate uridyl transferase (GALT). Patients present initially in the neonatal

Table 7.8.2 Dietary issues in adult galactosaemia

Dietary and monitoring issues	Evidence	References
Life-long dietary restriction of galactose	No randomised controlled trials in adults comparing patients on and off diet, therefore consensus to maintain a low-galactose diet for life. However, two case studies are available of individuals who stopped diet in childhood and developed normally.	Welling *et al.* (2016) Lee *et al.* (2003) Panis *et al.* (2006)
Alcohol	No evidence that alcohol intake should be limited.	Walter *et al.* (1999)
Bone mineral density (BMD)	Low BMD due to primary ovarian insufficiency.	Rubio-Gozalbo *et al.* (2002)
Calcium and vitamin D supplementation	Supplement calcium, vitamin D and other nutrients to ensure long-term bone health.	Welling *et al.* (2016)
Biochemical monitoring of control	Galactose-1-phosphate measurement varies in and between individuals and is better regarded as a compliance indicator. Annual monitoring suggested.	Welling *et al.* (2016)
Restriction of galactosides, free and bound galactose, galactocerebrosides	Foods containing these are allowed. There is no evidence to suggest that restriction of these foods is harmful.	Bosch (2011); Welling *et al.* (2016)

period with a life-threatening liver condition, and, after the initial crisis, are managed with a low-galactose, lactose-free diet. As a result of the enzyme deficiency, galactitol and galactonate accumulate in abnormal quantities. Increased galactitol causes cataracts, and galactonate is believed to play a role in hepatic and renal toxicity. Presentation at an adult clinic usually follows transfer from a paediatric clinic. Occasionally, patients present having been discharged from a clinic earlier in their lives, and may not be on the diet.

Ovarian dysfunction, central nervous system problems, language and speech defects, cataracts, and reduced bone mineral density have been reported (Welling *et al.*, 2016). Complications are independent of diet, and occur even if the diet is started immediately after birth (Schweizer *et al.*, 1993; Waggoner *et al.*, 1990). The cause of these problems is unknown, but may result from endogenous galactose synthesis. Endogenous production is constant in patients and is not influenced by diet. Adults have been shown to have slower rates of release of endogenous galactose than newborns. Most centres measure red blood cell galactose 1 phosphate annually, and aim for levels of <0.60 μmol/g of haemoglobin (<150 μmol/L), but the measurement varies in and between individuals and is probably most useful as a compliance monitor, for detecting severe non-compliance (Welling *et al.*, 2016).

Nutritional management

Dietary restriction of galactose is the only effective treatment for galactosaemia. There is little evidence regarding how tolerance to galactose changes with age, and therefore diet for life continues to be recommended (Welling *et al.*, 2016). Table 7.8.2 summaries the issues associated with this diet. The main source of galactose is lactose; so, all lactose is excluded from the diet. There are other non-milk sources of galactose in the diet, but there is no evidence for making the diet stricter (Welling *et al.*, 2016). The following are allowed in the diet:

- *Galactosides* – found in legumes, soya and cocoa. Although galactosides are the main subunit of these oligosaccharides, they are not hydrolysed by the intestinal mucosa.
- *Free and bound galactose* – occurs in small amounts in many fruits and vegetables, but is probably insignificant.
- *Galactose* – can also be found in offal in galactocerebrosides.

Practicalities of a lactose-free diet

Milk, all milk products and derivatives are excluded. This includes all milk (cow's, sheep's, goat's, etc.), yoghurt, most cheese, dairy desserts, butter and cream. Milk derivatives such as whey and casein must also be avoided: low-lactose milk and products are not suitable. All manufactured foods such as biscuits and cakes must be carefully checked. However, as milk is a potential allergen, all packaging should carry information on the presence of milk. The current galactosaemia guidelines (Welling *et al.*, 2016) now consider all cheese with a galactose intake of <25 mg per 100 g to be low enough to be allowed in the diet. In the UK, a number of hard, mature cheeses are now allowed, following extensive analysis. This only includes Emmental, Gruyère, Jarlsberg, French Comte, Italian Parmesan, Grana Padano, extra-mature cheddar, and vintage mature cheddar. Food additives, sodium caseinate and calcium caseinate are allowed.

Calcium requirements for teenagers are particularly high, and it is important for both adults and teenagers to have a good intake of calcium, as decreased bone mineralisation in both females and males has been reported (Batey *et al.*, 2013). A calcium-supplemented milk replacement is recommended (such as soya), and a calcium and vitamin D supplement is often necessary. Pregnancy is not common in galactosaemia due to premature ovarian insufficiency. However, spontaneous pregnancies have been reported (Briones *et al.*, 2001), and assisted conception with egg donation is possible. If pregnancy occurs, the diet should be followed, and outcome appears to be good.

Glycogen storage disorder type I

Glycogen storage disorder (GSD) type I is divided into two major subtypes, type Ia and type Ib. Type Ia is characterised by a deficiency in the enzyme glucose 6 phosphatase, and type Ib by a deficiency in glucose 6 phosphate translocase enzyme. These enzymes function together and are responsible for the breakdown of glycogen stores in order to maintain blood glucose levels (BGLs) within normal range during periods of fasting. Both phenotypically display glucose 6 phosphatase deficiency, characterised by growth retardation, hypoglycaemia, hepatomegaly and a deranged biochemical profile. Type Ib patients also suffer from chronic neutropenia and functional deficiencies of neutrophils and monocytes (Chou *et al.*, 2002).

Poor metabolic control arises as a result of frequent hypoglycaemia with subsequent secondary changes, including lactic acidaemia, hyperlipidaemia, hyperuricaemia and hypertriglyceridaemia. It has been demonstrated that metabolic control is better when the tendency toward hypoglycaemia is decreased (Weinstein & Wolfsdorf, 2002). Long-term consequences of GSD type I include hepatic adenomas, hepatocellular carcinoma, progressive renal insufficiency, short stature and hypoglycaemic brain damage (Roth, 2009). There are also reports of acute pancreatitis in some cases secondary to hypertriglyceridaemia.

Current treatment is dietary therapy to prevent and manage hypoglycaemia. These patients should avoid fasting and require ERs during periods of intercurrent illness. Biochemical markers such as lactate, cholesterol, uric acid and triglycerides should be monitored in addition to liver imaging. These patients may also require bone density and plasma micronutrient monitoring. It is essential for patients to have a facility to test BGLs.

Nutritional management

The aim of dietary treatment is to maintain normoglycaemia (blood glucose (BG) of >3.9mmol/L (Kishnani *et al.*, 2014) and ensure optimal nutritional status. Blood glucose levels of 3.5mmol/L should be treated with a source of rapid-acting carbohydrate, usually 15g, followed by a snack. The following aspects of the patient's diet need to be taken into consideration.

Percentage of total daily energy from carbohydrate

It is recommended that 65% of total energy be from carbohydrate sources, 10–15% from protein and 25% from fat (Kishnani *et al.*, 2014).

Meal and snack pattern

Most centres recommend small, frequent carbohydrate-containing meals throughout the day followed by the use of uncooked corn starch (UCCS or Glycosade®). Continuous tube feeding or uncooked corn starch is used overnight to prevent hypoglycaemia during this prolonged period of fasting, with a guideline dose of 0.2–0.25g of glucose/kg/hour (Dixon *et al.*, 2015b).

Supplementation with uncooked corn starch (Glycosade®)

UCCS is digested slowly, providing a steady release of glucose in between meal times and overnight. The amount and timing of administration depends on the patient's weight and tendency towards hypoglycaemia during fasting periods. US guidelines suggest 1.7–2.5g/kg UCCS every 4–6 hours (Kishnani *et al.*, 2014), although UK practice is often to use a smaller dose, close to 1g/kg. Some adult patients remain reliant on continuous overnight feeding with glucose polymer or enteral feed, whereas others may manage the overnight fast with a suitable weight-based dose of UUCS given at bedtime. Blood glucose testing can be used to determine the adequacy of this dosing. UCCS should not be mixed with drinks high in ascorbic or citric acid, nor should it be heated.

Weight maintenance

Importantly, a balance between energy from UCCS and normal food needs to be achieved in order to maintain weight and prevent micronutrient deficiencies. Patients should be encouraged to engage in physical activities up to individual limits, but to avoid contact sports due to the high risk of bleeding, infection and liver damage (Roth, 2009).

Fructose and galactose restriction

The degree of restriction of these foods is still debated, as restriction of two food groups renders the diet inadequate. It is not common practice in the UK.

Fasting or illness

These patients should be provided with an ER during periods of fasting or illness (see the section 'Emergency regimens').

Diabetes and glycogen storage disease

More recently, there have been some case reports of patients with GSD developing type 2 diabetes mellitus later in life. These patients may require intensive input to adjust their diet and appropriate diabetes medications to prevent hyper- and hypoglycaemia. Continuous glucose monitoring (CGM) can be useful in these patients to provide a more detailed analysis of daily glucose excursions.

Refer to Dixon *et al.* (2015b) or Hollak and Lachmann (2016) for more information on other types of glycogen storage disease.

Pregnancy in inherited metabolic disorders

An increasing number of children with IMDs are now surviving into adulthood due to expanding newborn screening, improvements in diagnostic tests and advancing therapeutic interventions. Many adults are able to lead independent lives, form relationships and have children (Lee, 2006). The main aim of managing pregnancy in IMD is to optimise maternal and foetal health through regular biochemical monitoring and nutritional status evaluation.

Preconception

It is important that all IMD patients be offered genetic counselling when planning a pregnancy. Preimplantation genetic diagnosis is widely available for X-linked IMDs such as OTC, and prenatal diagnosis is also available. Nutritional status and metabolic control should be optimised in all women on a restricted diet before conception to improve the outcome of the pregnancy (Lee, 2006), with additional considerations given to weight status and the nutrients essential for pregnancy, such as folic acid, DHA and vitamin D.

Pregnancy

Although there are clear guidelines about managing pregnancy in PKU, little has been published regarding other IMDs, apart from case reports or patient series (Langendonk *et al.*, 2012; Walter, 2000). A major risk for IMDs of energy metabolism (MSUD, UCD, FAOD, GA1 and GSD) is metabolic decompensation due to morning sickness and weight loss. This can cause reduced intake of medication or dietary supplements affecting metabolic control (Lee, 2006). It is essential that women and their obstetric teams have clear oral and intravenous emergency protocol.

The teratogenic effects of hyperphenylalaninaemia in maternal PKU have been well documented; yet, little is known about the pregnancy outcomes associated with other IMDs, although normal foetal outcome has been reported (Pierre *et al.*, 2006; Raval *et al.*, 2015; Walter, 2000). For MSUD, leucine does not appear to be a potent teratogen (Tchan *et al.*, 2013); in tyrosinaemia type II, high tyrosine (≥1000 µmol/L) may affect foetal development (Murphy, 2016). Some IMDs worsen during pregnancy, such as hypertriglyceridaemia and in lipoprotein lipase deficiency leading to pancreatitis. The risk of thromboembolic complications during pregnancy is increased in women with HCU (Pierre *et al.*, 2006). Protein requirements are increased during pregnancy and lactation (WHO/FAO/UNU, 2007). For disorders of protein metabolism, total protein intake should be carefully increased using frequent biochemical monitoring and foetal growth to guide changes; use of specialist protein supplements may be required. Increased energy needs in pregnancy may require additional overnight UCCS in GSD and/or MCT in certain FAODs.

Labour

Labour and delivery is a period of increased metabolic stress, and a clear delivery protocol must be devised beforehand. Women often require additional energy supplementation, usually as intravenous dextrose. Additional complications may include bleeding tendencies due to platelet dysfunction in GSDI or deterioration of underlying organ damage, e.g. cardiomyopathy in GSDIII (Ramachandran *et al.*, 2012).

Postpartum

The postpartum period is a time of high risk for metabolic decompensation, especially in IMDs of protein metabolism, such as MSUD, UCD and OA. This is due to the increased protein load following the involution of the uterus, and can typically last up to 6–8 weeks. Women should continue oral or intravenous ERs alongside protein restriction until metabolically stable and able to tolerate full oral intake post-delivery. Women who wish to breastfeed should be encouraged to have increased energy intake to meet demands, plus sufficient fluids and adequate calcium and vitamin D.

Emergency regimens

An ER is required in IMDs where the body has the inability to utilise one of its fuels properly (protein, carbohydrate or fat) during illness. During episodes of illness, catabolism and a fasting state secondary to poor oral intake can cause the production of metabolites that have the potential to be toxic in specific disorders. The aim of an ER is to provide an exogenous energy source to prevent catabolism, prevent or reduce production of toxic metabolites and prevent hypoglycaemia. Metabolic disorders requiring an ER during periods of illness include:

- Urea cycle disorders.
- Organic acidaemias.
- Maple syrup urine disease.
- Fatty acid oxidation disorders.
- Glycogen storage disorders.
- Fructose-1, 6-bisphosphatase deficiency.
- Disorders of ketogenesis.

The ER should be commenced immediately if the patient becomes unwell, e.g. nausea, vomiting, diarrhoea, high temperature or any illness resulting in loss of appetite and inability to take the normal diet. In adults, the ER is a 200-mL drink (25% carbohydrate solution), given every 2–3 hours, day and night. It should aim to provide adequate energy requirements over 24 h to prevent catabolism, and a total fluid volume of 2–2.4 L/24 h. For patients who are unable to take large volumes, taking smaller drinks frequently throughout the day may be easier. If the patient is tube fed, then a 24-hour feeding regimen can be devised using a 25% carbohydrate solution. Glucose polymer powders are used to make up the ER, and premeasured sachets have been shown to decrease preparation error (Gokmen-Ozel *et al.*, 2010).

Squash (cordial) can be added to improve the flavour. Alternatively, fruit juices and commercial high-sugar drinks can be used in larger amounts or extra glucose polymer added to make it up to a 25% carbohydrate solution. Fructose, sucrose and sorbitol must not be added to an ER for patients with fructose-1, 6-bisphosphatase deficiency. In disorders of protein metabolism (UCD, OA and MSUD), protein intake should be stopped initially and reintroduced gradually in 24(–48) hours to prevent catabolism from protein deficiency (Baumgartner *et al.*, 2014). In MSUD, it is important that the BCAA free protein substitute be continued, as it will help prevent muscle catabolism and stimulate endogenous protein synthesis, as well as help to protect the brain against the toxic effects of leucine.

The ER is not nutritionally complete, so should not be followed for >24–48 hours. It is advisable for patients to contact their metabolic team to inform them that the ER is in use, and for advice on diet reintroduction to prevent nutritional deficiencies.

Fat is not routinely used as part of the ER as it may not be tolerated in illness. However, in patients with a disorder of protein metabolism, if their feed includes a protein-free feed (carbohydrate, fat, vitamins and minerals), or if they frequently use the ER and are at risk of nutritional deficiency, they may benefit from using a more nutritionally complete protein-free feed for their ER if tolerated. Fat should never be added to the ER in fatty acid oxidation disorders. Dioralyte may be used to treat diarrhoea or vomiting; however, it contains very little glucose, and must be used in conjunction with glucose polymer drinks to provide adequate concentrations of carbohydrate. It may be advisable to provide a lower-concentration carbohydrate solution when the patient has diarrhoea to prevent exacerbating both the diarrhoea and the illness.

The ER should be started at home upon the first signs of illness. If the ER is not tolerated and the patient continues to vomit, they should attend an accident and emergency department immediately as they will need 10% intravenous dextrose and medical management. Over the following 24–48 hours, as the patient improves, intravenous fluids can be reduced as oral feeding is increased. If, after 48 hours, oral/enteral feeding cannot be reinstated, then parenteral nutrition should be considered to prevent further catabolism, especially in a disorder of protein metabolism (Baumgartner *et al.*, 2014).

Reintroduction of normal diet

Reintroduction of usual diet should not be delayed beyond 24–48h. For patients on low-protein diets, their normal diet should be gradually regraded over a period of 1–2 days, using their clinical condition as a guide. Patients should continue with the ER until they are eating normally, clinically improving and receiving their full energy requirements from diet.

It is important to check at clinic appointments that the patient or carer understands when the ER is needed, that the ER is up to date, that they have a supply of emergency feed at home, and that they know how to prepare the ER drinks or feed.

Acknowledgement

The editor acknowledges the prior contribution of Sarah Boocock, Avril Micciche, Charlé Maritz, Hazel Rogozinski and Pat Portnoi.

Further reading

Shaw V. (2015) *Clinical Paediatric Dietetics*, 4th edn. Oxford: Wiley Blackwell.

Internet resources

Association for Glycogen Storage Diseases, www.agsdus.org
British Inherited Metabolic Disease Group, www.bimdg.org.uk
Galactosaemia Support Group, www.galactosaemia.org
National Information Centre for Metabolic Diseases, www.climb.org.uk
National Society for Phenylketonuria, www.nspku.org

References

Batey LA, Welt CK, Rohr F, *et al.* (2013) Skeletal health in adult patients with classical galactosaemia. *Osteoporos. Int.* 24: 501–509.

Baumgartner M, Horster F, Dionisi-Vici C, *et al.* (2014) Proposed guidelines for the diagnosis and management of methylmalonic and propionic acidaemia. *Orphanet. J. Rare Dis.* 9: 130.

Bik-Multanowski M, Didycz B, Mozrzymas R, *et al.* (2008) Quality of life in non-compliant adults with Phenylketonuria after resumption of the diet. *J. Inherit. Metab. Dis.* 32(1): 126.

Bosch AM. (2011) Classic galactosemia: dietary dilemmas. *J. Inherit. Metab. Dis.* 34(2): 257–260.

Boy N, Mühlhausen C, Maier EM, *et al.* (2017) Proposed recommendations for diagnosing and managing individuals with glutaric aciduria type I: second revision. *J. Inherit. Metab. Dis.* 40(1): 75–101.

Briones P, Girós M, Martinez V. (2001) Second spontaneous pregnancy in a galactosaemic woman homozygous for the R188R mutation. *J. Inherit. Metab. Dis.* 24: 79–80.

Brown MC, Guest JF. (1999) Economic impact of feeding a phenylalanine-restricted diet to adults with previously untreated phenylketonuria. *J. Intellect. Disabil. Res.* 43: 30–37.

Brumm VL, Bilder D, Waisbren SE. (2010) Psychiatric symptoms and disorders in phenylketonuria. *Mol. Genet. Metab.* 99(1): S59–63.

Cerone R, Schiaffino MC, Di Stefano S, *et al.* (1999) Phenylketonuria: diet for life or not? *Acta Paediatr.* 88: 664–666.

Channon S, Goodman G, Zlotowitz S, *et al.* (2007) Effects of dietary management of Phenylketonuria in long-term cognitive outcome. *Arch. Dis. Child.* 92: 213–218.

Chou JY, Matern D, Mansfield BC, *et al.* (2002) Type I glycogen storage diseases: disorders of the glucose-6-phosphatase complex. *Curr. Mol. Med.* 2(2): 121–143.

Clacy A, Sharman R, McGill J. (2014) Depression, anxiety and stress in young adults with phenylketonuria: associations with biochemistry. *J. Dev. Behav. Pediatr.* 35: 388–391.

Cleary M, Walter JH. (2001) Assessment of adult phenylketonuria. *Ann. Clin. Biochem.* 38: 450–458.

Cleary MA, Feillet F, White FJ, *et al.* (2006) Randomised controlled trial of essential fatty acid supplementation in phenylketonuria. *Eur. J. Clin. Nutr.* 60(7): 915–920.

Dawson C, Murphy E, Maritz C, *et al.* (2011) Dietary treatment of phenylketonuria: the effect of phenylalanine on reaction time. *J. Inherit. Metab. Dis.* 34: 449–454.

de Baulny HO, Benoist JF, Rigal O, *et al.* (2005) Methylmalonic and propionic acidaemias: Management and outcome. *J. Inherit. Metab. Dis.* 28: 415–423.

Dixon M, Stafford J, White F, *et al.* (2015a) Disorders of mitochondrial energy metabolism, lipid metabolism and other disorders. In: Shaw V (ed) *Clinical Paediatric Dietetics*, 4th edn. Oxford: Wiley-Blackwell.

Dixon M, Staffod J, White F, *et al.* (2015b) Disorders of carbohydrate metabolism. In: Shaw V (ed) *Clinical Paediatric Dietetics*, 4th edn. Oxford: Wiley-Blackwell.

FAO/WHO. (2010) *Fats and Fatty Acids in Human Nutrition: Report of an Expert Consultation. FAO Food and Nutrition Paper 91*. Available at http://www.who.int/nutrition/publications/nutrientrequirements/fatsandfattyacids_humannutrition/en/. Accessed 2 May 2017.

Gokmen-Ozel H, Daly A, Davies P, *et al.* (2010). Errors in emergency feeds in inherited metabolic disorders: a randomized controlled trial of three preparation methods. *Arch. Dis. Child.* 95: 776–780.

Häberle J, Boddaert N, Burlina A, *et al.* (2012) Suggested guidelines for the diagnosis and management of urea cycle disorders. *Orphanet J. Rare Dis.* 7: 32.

Hollak CEM, Lachmann R. (2016) *Section 1: Disorders of Carbohydrate Metabolism. Inherited Metabolic Disease in Adults: A Clinical Guide.* Oxford Monographs on Medical Genetics.

Kishnani P, Austin SL, Abdenur JE, *et al.* (2014) Diagnosis and management of glycogen storage disease type I: a practical guideline of the American College of Medical Genetics and Genomics. *Genet. Med.* 16: E1.

Koch R, Hanley W, Levy H, *et al.* (2003) The maternal Phenylketonuria International Study: 1984–2002. *Pediatrics.* 112: 1523–1529.

Koletzko B, Lien E, Agostoni C, *et al.*; World Association of Perinatal Medicine Dietary Guidelines Working Group. (2008) The roles of long-chain polyunsaturated fatty acids in pregnancy, lactation and infancy: review of current knowledge and consensus recommendations. *J. Perinat. Med.* 36(1): 5–14.

Lang TF. (2009) Adult presentations of medium chain acyl-CoA dehydrogenase deficiency (MCADD). *J. Inherit. Metab. Dis.* 32: 675–683.

Langendonk J, Roos C, Angus L, *et al.* (2012) A series of pregnancies in women with inherited metabolic disease. *J. Inherit. Metab. Dis.* 35: 419–424.

Lee PJ. (2006) Pregnancy issues in inherited metabolic disorders. *J. Inherit. Metab. Dis.* 29: 311–316.

Lee PJ, Milburn M, Wendel U, *et al.* (2003) A woman with untreated galactosaemia. *Lancet* 362: 446.

Lee PJ, Amos A, Robertson L, *et al.* (2009) Adults with late diagnosed PKU and severe challenging behaviour: a randomised placebo controlled trial of a phenylalanine-restricted diet. *J. Neurol. Neurosurg. Psychiatry.* 80: 631–663.

Lenke RL, Levy HL. (1980) Maternal phenylketonuria and hyperphenylalaninaemia. *N. Engl. J. Med.* 303: 1202–1208.

Leonard JV. (2006) Disorders of the urea cycle and related enzymes. In: Fernandes J, Saudubray JM, van den Berghe G, *et al.* (eds) *Inborn Metabolic Diseases: Diagnosis and Treatment*, 4th edn. Berlin: Springer.

Levy HL, Vargas JE, Waisbren SE, *et al.* (2002) Reproductive fitness in maternal homocystinuria due to cystathionine β-synthase deficiency. *J. Inherit. Metab. Dis.* 25: 299–314.

Maillot F, Lilburn M, Baudin J, *et al.* (2008) Factors influencing outcomes in the offspring of mothers with phenylketonuria during pregnancy: the importance of variation in maternal blood phenylalanine. *Am. J. Clin. Nutr.* 88: 700–705.

Morris A. (2016) Disorders of ketogenesis and ketolysis. In: Hollak C, Lachmann R (eds) *Inherited Metabolic Disease in Adults: A Clinical Guide.* Oxford: Oxford University Press.

Murphy E. (2016) Tyrosinaemia type II – Chapter 14. In: Hollak CEM, Lachman RH (eds) *Inherited Metabolic Disease in Adults.* Oxford: Oxford University Press.

Murphy E, Nadjar Y, Vianey-Saban C. (2016) Fatty acid oxidation, electron transfer and riboflavin metabolism defects. In: Hollak C, Lachmann R (eds) *Inherited Metabolic Disease in Adults: A Clinical Guide.* Oxford: Oxford University Press.

National Institute of Health. (2000) Phenylketonuria: screening and management. *NIH Consens. Statement* 17(3): 1–27.

Panis B, Bakker JA, Sels JP, *et al.* (2006) Untreated classical galactosemia patient with mild phenotype. *Mol. Genet. Metab.* 89: 277–279.

Pierre G, Gissen P, Chakrapani A, *et al.* (2006) Successful treatment of pyridoxine – unresponsive homocystinuria with betaine in pregnancy. *J. Inherit. Metab. Dis.* 29: 688–689.

Ramachandran R, Wedatilake Y, Coats C, *et al.* (2012) Pregnancy and its management in women with GSD type III-a single centre experience. *J. Inherit. Metab. Dis.* 35(2): 245–251.

Raval DB, Merideth M, Sloan JL, *et al.* (2015) Methylmalonic acidemia (MMA) in pregnancy: a case series and literature review. *J. Inherit. Metab. Dis.* 38(5): 839–846.

Roe CR, Sweetman L, Roe DS, *et al.* (2002) Treatment of cardiomyopathy and rhabdomyolysis in long-chain fat oxidation disorders using an anaplerotic odd-chain triglyceride. *J. Clin. Invest.* 110: 259–269.

Rohr FJ, Lobbregt D, Levy HL. (1998) Tyrosine supplementation in the treatment of maternal phenylketonuria. *Am. J. Clin. Nutr.* 67: 473–476.

Roth K. (2009) *Genetics of glycogen-storage disease type I: treatment and medication.* Available at http://emedicine.medscape.com/article/949937-overview. Accessed 2 May 2017.

Rubio-Gozalbo ME, Hamming S, van Kroonenburgh MJ, *et al.* (2002) Bone mineral density in patients with classic galactosaemia. *Arch. Dis. Child.* 87(1): 57–60.

SACN & Committee on Toxicity. (2004) *Advice on fish consumption: benefits & risks.* Available at http://cot.food.gov.uk/cotreports/cotjointreps/sacnfishconsumption. Accessed 2 May 2017.

Sanderson S, Green A, Preece M, *et al.* (2006) The incidence of inherited metabolic disorders in the West Midlands, *UK. Arch. Dis. Child.* 91(11): 896–899.

Schweizer S, Shin Y, Jakobs C, *et al.* (1993) Long-term outcome in 134 patients with galactosaemiae. *Eur. J. Pediatr.* 152: 36–43.

Singh RH. (2007) Nutritional management of patients with urea cycle disorders. *J. Inherit. Metab. Dis.* 30: 880–887.

Spiekerkoetter U, Bastin J, Gillingham M, *et al.* (2010) Current issues regarding treatment of mitochondrial fatty acid oxidation disorders. *J. Inherit. Metab. Dis.* 33: 555–561.

Stanley CA, Bennett MJ, Mayatepek E. (2006) Disorders of mitochondrial fatty acid oxidation and related metabolic pathways. In: Fernandes J, Saudubray JM, van der Berghe G, *et al.* (eds) *Inborn Metabolic Diseases, Diagnosis and Treatment.* Berlin: Springer.

Tchan M, Westbrook M, Wilcox G, *et al.* (2013) The management of pregnancy in maple syrup urine disease: experience with two patients. *JIMD Rep.* 10: 113–117.

Teissier R, Nowak E, Assoun M, *et al.* (2012) Maternal phenylketonuria: low phenylalaninemia might increase the risk of intra uterine growth retardation. *J. Inherit. Metab. Dis.* 35: 993–999.

ten Hoedt A, de Sonnerville L, Francois B, *et al.* (2011) High phenylalanine levels directly affect mood and sustained attention in adults with phenylketonuria: a randomised double-blind, placebo controlled, crossover trail. *J. Inherit. Metab. Dis.* 34(1): 165–171.

van Wegberg MJ, MacDonald A, Ahring K, *et al.* (2017) The complete European guidelines on phenylketonuria: diagnosis and treatment. *Orphanet J. Rare Dis.* 12: 162.

Vockley J, Burton B, Berry GT, *et al.* (2016) Interim results from an open-label phase 2 study assessing the safety and clinical effects of investigational UX007 (triheptanoin) in subjects with long-chain fatty acid oxidation disorders (LC-FAOD). *J. Inherit. Metab. Dis.* 39(S1): S151.

Waggoner DD, Buist NR, Donnell GN. (1990) Long-term prognosis in galactosaemia; results of a survey of 350 cases. *J. Inherit. Metab. Dis.* 13: 802–818.

Walter JH. (2000) Inborn errors of metabolism and pregnancy. *J. Inherit. Metab. Dis.* 23: 229–236.

Walter JH, Wraith JE, White FJ, *et al.* (1998) Strategies for the treatment of cystathionine β-synthase deficiency: the experience of the Willink Biochemical Genetics Unit over the past 30 years. *Eur. J. Pediatr.* 157(S2): S71–S76.

Walter JH, Collins JE, Leonard JV. (1999) Recommendations for the management of galactosaemia: UK Galactosaemia Steering Group. *Arch. Dis. Child.* 80(1): 93–96.

Weglage J, Fromm J, van Teeffelen-Heithoff A, *et al.* (2013) Neurocognitive functioning in adults with phenylketonuria: results of a long term study. *Mol. Genet. Metab.* 110: S44–48.

Weinstein DA, Wolfsdorf JI. (2002) Effect of continuous glucose therapy with uncooked cornstarch on the long-term clinical course of type 1a glycogen storage disease. *Eur. J. Pediatr.* 161(S1): S35–S39.

Welling L, Bernstein L, Berry GT, *et al.* (2016) International clinical guideline for the management of classical galactosemia: diagnosis, treatment, and follow-up. *J. Inhert. Metab. Dis.* 40: 171–176.

WHO/FAO/UNU Expert Consultation. (2007) *Protein and Amino Acid Requirements in Human Nutrition. WHO Technical Report Series no. 935.* Singapore: United Nations University Press.

Yap S. (2003) Classical homocystinuria: vascular risk and its prevention. *J. Inhert. Metab. Dis.* 26: 259–265.

7.9 Musculoskeletal disorders

7.9.1 Osteoporosis

Jean Redmond and Inez Schoenmakers

Key points

- Osteoporosis is the most common clinical disorder of bone metabolism; it is a major and increasing public health problem.
- To maximise peak bone mass attainment and to minimise age-related bone loss, a balanced diet sufficient in calcium, good vitamin D status and regular weight-bearing physical activity are important.
- Low bone mineral density, high propensity to fall, a low body weight, and other comorbidities are risks for osteoporotic fracture.
- A high percentage of hip fracture patients are malnourished on admission to hospital, and their nutritional status may decline in the postoperative period.

Osteoporosis is the most common clinical disorder of bone metabolism, and primarily affects the elderly population (Cosman *et al.*, 2014). It is characterised by low bone mass and microarchitectural deterioration of bone tissue, with a consequent increase in bone fragility and susceptibility to fractures (WHO, 1994). Osteoporotic fractures are a significant cause of morbidity and mortality, particularly in developed countries (Johnell & Kanis, 2006). Fractures are associated with a substantial decline in functional status, a loss of independence and difficulty with normal daily activities. Fractures can cause psychosocial symptoms as patients can grapple with chronic pain, and lifestyle and cosmetic changes (Cosman *et al.*, 2014).

Most commonly, these are fractures of the hip, vertebrae, and wrist, and their incidence increases with age. Lifetime risk of any osteoporotic fracture is approximately 40–50% in women and 13–22% in men (Johnell & Kanis, 2005). Geographically, there is a greater than tenfold variation in hip fracture risk and fracture probability between countries (Kanis *et al.*, 2012). For example, in women, the lowest annual age-standardised incidences were found in Nigeria (2 per 100,000), as compared to the highest in Norway (563 per 100,000) (Kanis *et al.*, 2012). Within countries, fracture risk also differs between ethnic groups, with White Caucasians populations generally having the highest risk. For example, in the USA, American-Whites have a fourfold higher fracture risk than American-Blacks (Ballane *et al.*, 2017). The pathogenesis of osteoporosis reflects the complex interaction between genetic, metabolic and environmental factors that determine bone growth, peak bone mass (PBM) and bone loss. The increasing burden of osteoporosis means that modifiable factors such as nutrition have become of public health importance.

Functions and structure of bone, and the disease process

Bone is a specialised connective tissue, serving three major functions:

1. Metabolic – a reserve and buffer of minerals.
2. Mechanical – providing structure and muscular attachment for movement.
3. Protective – enclosing bone marrow and vital organs.

Metabolic control of calcium

The metabolic function of bone is crucial for calcium homeostasis. The plasma concentration of ionised calcium is strictly maintained for the functioning of all body cells (Ross *et al.*, 2010). When this decreases, the parathyroid hormone (PTH) concentration increases, which inhibits renal calcium excretion and stimulates the

Manual of Dietetic Practice, Sixth Edition. Edited by Joan Gandy.

Companion website: www.manualofdieteticpractice.com

liberation of calcium from bone. PTH also stimulates the renal synthesis of the active form of vitamin D, (calcitriol, 1,25(OH)2D), which, in turn, enhances intestinal calcium absorption (Ross *et al.*, 2010).

The structure of bone

Macroscopically, bone has two components: cortical (compact) bone with a dense structure for mechanical and protective functions, and a latticework of trabecular (cancellous) bone, with a metabolic function (DH, 1998). The adult human skeleton is composed of 80% cortical bone and 20% trabecular bone; different bones have different ratios of cortical to trabecular bone (Clarke, 2008). Bone consists of an extracellular mineralised matrix and a number of cell types, including osteoblasts, osteocytes and osteoclasts. The matrix consists of mineral salts (mainly hydroxyapatite ($Ca_{10}(PO_4)_6(OH)_2$) crystals) bound to proteins, largely collagen (Department of Health & Human Services, 2004). The osteoblast is the primary bone-forming cell, which creates the osteoid (pre-bone tissue) and facilitates calcification. Osteoclasts remove bone tissue and provide for the release of calcium and phosphate ions. The osteocyte has been subject to intense research in recent years. It is a multifunctional cell with an endocrine function, and also plays a role in the coordination and coupling of bone formation and resorption. Another role is to 'sense' mechanical loading. New pharmaceutical interventions targeting the osteocyte are currently in development (Dallas *et al.*, 2013).

Bone development, metabolism and the development of osteoporosis

Two processes, modelling and remodelling, mediate change in size and shape of bone during bone growth and in response to mechanical stress (Department of Health & Human Services, 2004). During childhood and adolescence, modelling allows for longitudinal and radial growth (Clarke, 2008). PBM is determined largely by genetic factors, with contributions from nutritional, endocrine and other lifestyle factors (Cosman *et al.*, 2014).

After skeletal growth is complete, bone remodelling, the continuous removing of older bone and replacing it with new bone, takes place throughout adulthood. This prevents the accumulation of micro-damage and allows for continued adaptation of the skeleton to mechanical stress (Cosman *et al.*, 2014) (see Figure 7.9.1). Net bone loss occurs with advancing age but can also occur at a younger age, associated with certain conditions and risk factors (Cosman *et al.*, 2014) (see Figure 7.9.2). The lifetime risk of developing osteoporosis is therefore determined by a combination of:

1. Attainment of maximal PBM through optimal growth in childhood, adolescence and young adulthood.
2. Maintenance of bone mass in middle age.
3. The rate of (age-related) bone loss.

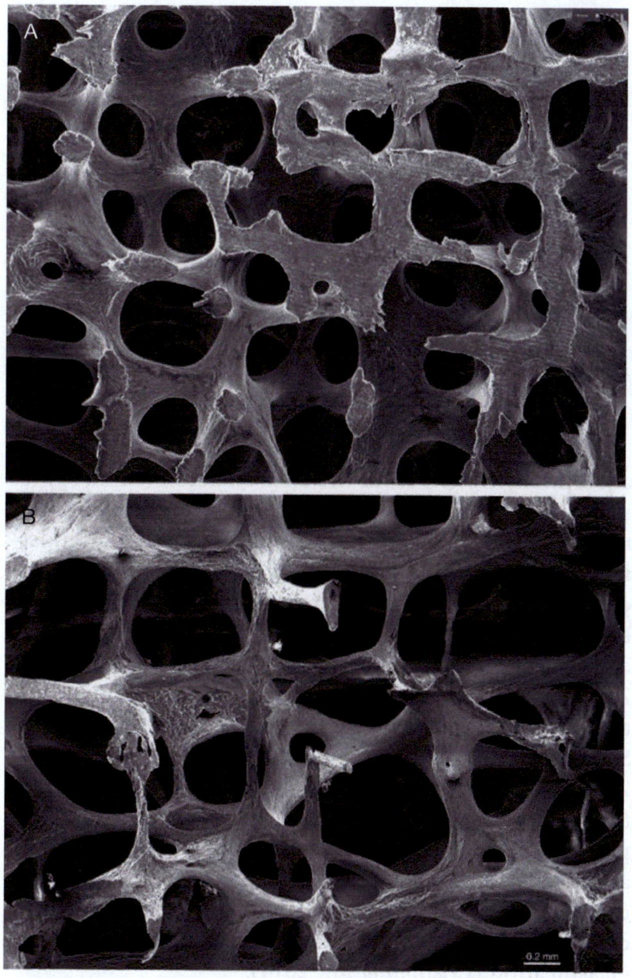

Figure 7.9.1 Comparison of (A) normal and (B) osteoporotic vertebrae, with thinning of the trabeculae (source: T. Arnett, University College London, 2013. Reproduced with permission from T. Arnett)

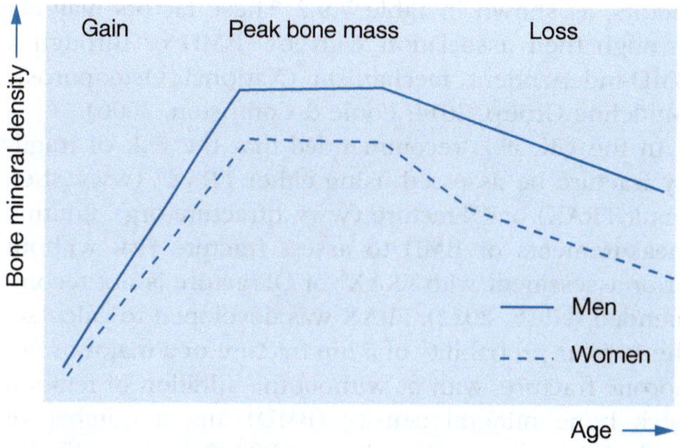

Figure 7.9.2 Age-related changes in bone mass throughout life (source: Poole & Compston, 2006; figure 5, p. 1252. Reproduced with permission from the *British Medical Journal*)

Diagnostic criteria and classification

The diagnosis of osteoporosis relies on the quantitative assessment of bone mineral density (BMD) or bone mineral content (BMC), usually by dual-energy X ray

Table 7.9.1 Classification of bone mass and osteoporosis in adults (WHO, 1994)

Normal	BMD or BMC ≤1 SD below the average value of young adults.
Low bone mass or osteopenia	BMD or BMC >1 SD below the young adult average, but ≤ −2.5 SD.
Osteoporosis	BMD or BMC >2.5 SD below the young adult average value.
Severe osteoporosis (established osteoporosis)	BMD or BMC >2.5 SD below the young adult average value, and presence of one or more fragility fractures.

Note: These cut-offs do not apply to children.

absorptiometry (DXA) of the axial skeleton (skull, spine, ribs and sternum), with the femoral neck providing the reference site (Cosman *et al.*, 2014; WHO, 1994). In postmenopausal women and men aged 50 years and older, categories of the disease are defined on the basis of bone mass, as shown in Table 7.9.1 (WHO, 1994). For other groups, it is recommended that ethnic-adjusted Z-scores be used, but that diagnosis not be made on the basis of densitometric criteria alone (International Society for Clinical Densitometry, 2013; Cosman *et al.*, 2014). In addition to DXA, a number of other imaging techniques including quantitative computed tomography (QCT), high-resolution peripheral QCT (HR-pQCT) and trabecular bone score (TBS), enable the prediction of site-specific and overall fracture risk, although these cannot yet be used according to the WHO diagnostic classification (Cosman *et al.*, 2014).

Osteoporosis is associated with an increased risk of fragility fracture, i.e. fractures caused by minimal trauma, such as a fall from a standing position. Patients are identified opportunistically on the finding of a previous fragility fracture or the presence of significant clinical risk factors, as shown in Table 7.9.2. These factors may act through their association with low BMD or through a BMD-independent mechanism (National Osteoporosis Guideline Group, 2014; Poole & Compston, 2006).

In the UK, it is recommended that the risk of fragility fracture be assessed using either FRAX® (www.shef.ac.uk/FRAX) or QFracture (www.qfracture.org). Routine measurements of BMD to assess fracture risk without prior assessment with FRAX® or QFracture is not recommended (NICE, 2012). FRAX was developed to calculate the 10-year probability of a hip fracture or a major osteoporotic fracture, with or without the addition of femoral neck bone mineral density (BMD) and a number of clinical risk factors. There is not a FRAX® tool specific for every country; in the absence of a FRAX® model, it has been suggested to use a surrogate country for which the epidemiology of osteoporosis most closely approximates the index country (Cauley *et al.*, 2011). The differential diagnosis of osteoporosis is based on the assessment of risk factors and a range of tests, depending on the severity of the disease, age at presentation, and the presence or absence of fractures (National Osteoporosis Guideline Group, 2014).

Table 7.9.2 Clinical risk factors used for the assessment of fracture probability (National Osteoporosis Guideline Group, 2014)

Risk factor
Age
Sex
Low body mass index (≤19 kg/m²)
Previous fragility fracture, particularly of the hip, wrist and spine, including morphometric vertebral fracture
Parental history of hip fracture
Current glucocorticoid treatment (any oral dose for 3 months or longer)
Current smoking
Alcohol intake ≥ 3 units/day
Propensity to fall
Specific patient groups at increased risk of osteoporosis
Rheumatoid arthritis
Inflammatory bowel disease (Crohn's disease / ulcerative colitis)
Coeliac disease
Anorexia nervosa
Athletic amenorrhea
Malabsorption syndromes
Untreated hypogonadism in men and women
Prolonged immobility
Organ transplantation
Type 1 diabetes
Hyperthyroidism and hyperparathyroidism
Chronic liver disease
Chronic obstructive pulmonary disease
Drugs that may influence bone metabolism
Corticosteroids
Thyroxine
Heparin
Loop diuretics (e.g. frusemide) increase urinary excretion of calcium (unlike thiazides, which decrease calcium loss)
Proton pump inhibitors (PPIs) interfere with calcium absorption

Nutritional aspects of bone development and osteoporosis

Bone formation requires adequate supplies of energy; amino acids; the main bone-forming minerals (calcium, phosphorus, magnesium, zinc); other ions including copper, manganese, carbonate and citrate; and the vitamins (C, D, K) that are involved in crystal and collagen formation, and cartilage and bone metabolism (Prentice *et al.*, 2006). Of these, calcium and vitamin D are the most commonly associated with bone health (EFSA, 2016; Ross *et al.*, 2010; SACN, 2016). General recommendations are to consume a calcium intake close to the reference nutrient intake (RNI), optimise vitamin D status and dietary supplementation when cutaneous sunshine exposure or synthesis is limited, be physically active, have a body weight in the healthy range, restrict salt intake, and consume plenty of fruit and vegetables (DH, 1998; EFSA, 2016; Ross *et al.*, 2010; SACN, 2016). The

National Osteoporosis Foundation (NOF) recommends that a balanced diet rich in low-fat dairy products, fruits, and vegetables provides calcium as well as numerous other nutrients needed for good health. If adequate dietary calcium cannot be obtained, dietary supplementation is indicated up to the recommended daily intake (RDA) (Cosman *et al.*, 2014).

Calcium

The evidence base of the long-term effects of dietary calcium intake on bone health through randomised controlled trials is limited, and there are knowledge gaps, particularly in children and young adults. In addition, a paradox exists between populations; while a low calcium intake is associated with an increased risk of osteoporosis in older Caucasian subjects, this may not be the case universally (Prentice, 2004). In the UK, the RNI represents a value that is likely to provide for the nutrient needs of 97.5% of the population, and is set as 700 mg for adults (>19 years) (DH, 1998) (Table 7.9.3). In the USA, the Institute of Medicine–recommended RDA for men (aged 50–70 years) is 1000 mg/day of calcium, and for women (aged >51 years) and older men (aged >71 years) is 1200 mg/day (Ross *et al.*, 2010). It has been suggested that intakes of >1200–1500 mg/day may increase the risk of developing kidney stones, cardiovascular disease, and stroke; thus, the scientific literature in this area remains highly controversial (Bolland *et al.*, 2015; Reid & Bolland, 2012).

Children

Children need to absorb 70–150 mg of calcium per day for growth and bone mineralisation, while adolescents require at least 250–300 mg per day (DH, 1998). Taking into consideration the percentage of calcium absorbed, the RNI and RDA are set between 350 and 1300 mg/day. Results from observational and intervention studies indicate that a higher intake of dietary calcium or dairy products, with and without vitamin D, significantly increases total body and lumbar spine BMC in children and reduces the risk of fractures (Goulding *et al.*, 2004; Manias *et al.*, 2006). However, data are conflicting because of the bone remodelling transient and/or the change in the rate of bone remodelling occurring when calcium intake is increased above the habitual intake (Prentice, 2004). This may result in an initial increase in BMD shortly after the onset of supplementation, with little additional effect of the intervention thereafter or after cessation of the supplementation. The current advice is to ensure a calcium intake close to the RNI or RDA, and that calcium supplementation in healthy children is unlikely to result in a decrease in fracture risk (DH, 1998; Winzenberg *et al.*, 2006).

Table 7.9.3 UK Recommendations for calcium intake (mg/day) (DH, 1998)

Age (years)	Reference nutrient intake
1–3	350
4–6	450
7–10	550
11–18 (males)	1000
11–18 (females)	800
19–50	700
50+	700

Young adults

From about the age of 35–40 years, bone mineral is lost at an average rate of 0.3–0.4 % of bone mass per year. During this time, a healthy, balanced diet should be followed, while remaining physically active and maintaining a healthy body weight.

Older age

A phase of rapid bone loss occurs in women during the first 5–10 years following menopause, after which bone loss occurs at a slower rate (see Chapter 3.1.3, Menopause). Calcium supplementation has little effect on BMD in women who are within the first 5 years after menopause (DH, 1998), although calcium may be effective in reducing bone loss during later postmenopause (>5 years) (Dawson-Hughes *et al.*, 1990). Observational studies reported that a higher lifetime and current calcium intake are associated with a reduced risk of osteoporosis (Nieves *et al.*, 2008). In contrast to this evidence, a recent meta-analysis has found that dietary calcium intake is not associated with risk of fracture, and there is no clinical trial evidence that increasing calcium intake from dietary sources prevents fractures (Bolland *et al.*, 2015). However, for the acquisition of PBM and maintenance of bone health, an adequate calcium intake throughout life is still considered necessary; if calcium intake is low, increasing dietary calcium is recommended as the first-line approach, followed by supplementation if this is not achievable (Cosman *et al.*, 2014).

Dietary sources of calcium

Calcium is present in a wide range of foods, although the bioavailability may vary appreciably. Dairy products are good sources of bioavailable calcium, and provide more calcium per calorie than any other typical food in a Western diet (Heaney, 2000). Fish with soft edible bones (e.g. whitebait, canned sardines/salmon) is a good source of calcium. In some countries, there is statutory fortification with calcium (e.g. flour in the UK), in addition to optional fortification of certain products by the food industry. For those following a vegan diet, pulses, nuts, seeds, certain dried fruit, tofu and certain green vegetables provide a source of calcium, although the bioavailability is not as high as from dairy. For those who are unable to consume foods that provide good sources of calcium, calcium supplements are advisable (see Chapter 3.6, Vegetarianism and vegan diets). The British Dietetic Association (2014) recommends a point system of calcium stars (1 star ≈ 60 mg) (British Dietetic Association, 2014) (see Appendix A2).

Vitamin D

Vitamin D status is assessed by the measurement of the plasma concentration of 25(OH)D, which serves as a reservoir for further hydroxylation to the active metabolite 1,25(OH)$_2$D. Vitamin D deficiency for the general population is defined as a plasma concentration of 25(OH)D <25 nmol/L in the UK and <40–60 nmol/L in the USA (Ross *et al.*, 2010; SACN, 2016). For specific patient groups, recommendations may also differ as related to their requirements and metabolism (Holick *et al.*, 2011). There are two forms of vitamin D: vitamin D$_3$ (cholecalciferol) and vitamin D$_2$ (ergocalciferol). These are considered to have the same anti-rachitic activity, although it is suggested that vitamin D$_3$ is more efficacious at maintaining serum 25(OH)D concentrations than vitamin D$_2$ (Tripkovich *et al.*, 2012). Vitamin D$_2$ is produced under the influence of UV irradiation in some plants, largely fungi, and is thus a suitable form of supplementation for vegetarians and vegans. Vitamin D$_3$ can be obtained from the diet and by synthesis via the UV irradiation of 7-dehydrocholesterol to pre-vitamin D$_3$ in the skin following exposure to sunlight. Egg yolks and oily fish are vitamin D$_3$–rich foods. Fortified foods and supplements may be fortified with either vitamin D$_2$ or D$_3$. Some dietary sources if vitamin D are listed in Table 7.9.4.

The proportion of vitamin D that is derived from sun exposure versus diet varies considerably worldwide, across population groups, and between individuals. If cutaneous synthesis and dietary intake are insufficient, supplements may be needed to meet the recommended intakes for vitamin D. Correction of frank vitamin D deficiency requires referral to a dietitian.

Table 7.9.4 Dietary sources of vitamin D (NOS, 2010)

Food (cooking method)	Vitamin D (µg/100 g)
Fish	
Herring (grilled)	16.1
Kipper (grilled)	9.4
Mackerel (grilled)	8.8
Mackerel (smoked)	8.0
Salmon (grilled)	7.1
Sardines (canned in tomato sauce)	8
Sardines (canned in oil)	5
Pilchards (canned in tomato sauce)	14
Cod liver oil (liquid)	210 (average 2.5 per capsule)
Fats	
Margarine	7.9
Ghee butter	1.9
Eggs	
Chicken egg (boiled)	1.8
Breakfast cereals	
Kellogg's All-Bran	1.6
Kellogg's Corn Flakes	2.6
Kellogg's Fruit 'n Fibre	2.1
Kellogg's Rice Krispies	2.1
Drinks	
Fortified milk	1.0
Horlicks powder / Ovaltine powder	4–5
Nestlé Build up! powder (shake)	4.5
Nestlé Build up! powder (soup)	4.2
Complan powder	4.4

*Adapted from NOS (2010).

Vitamin D and bone health

Classical vitamin D deficiency causes rickets in children and osteomalacia in children and adults (Munns *et al.*, 2016). In older people, it is associated with increased bone loss. Meta-analyses of vitamin D supplementation trials (most of which are with concomitant calcium supplementation) in older adults investigating the effect on BMD have concluded that vitamin D supplementation has a small beneficial effect on the femoral neck (Reid *et al.*, 2014). This analysis suggested that the effect may be limited to those who are at risk of vitamin D deficiency.

Vitamin D supplementation has also been shown to reduce the risk of falls and fractures (Murad *et al.*, 2011). Meta-analyses of vitamin D supplementation trials in older adults investigating the effect on fracture risk and falls have concluded that vitamin D supplementation with >700 IU/day (17.5 µg/day) is needed for a beneficial effect (Bischoff-Ferrari *et al.*, 2005, 2006; Francis, 2007). However, high dosages of vitamin D supplementation (≥4000 IU/day) and bolus dosages (i.e. with yearly or monthly loading administrations of 500,000 IU/year or 60,000 IU/month, given at once) have recently been shown to increase fall rates (Bischoff-Ferrari *et al.*, 2016; Gallagher, 2016; Sanders *et al.*, 2010). This indicates that the association between vitamin D and musculoskeletal health is U-shaped, and that both vitamin D deficiency and excess should be prevented. Data in infants, children and younger people are scarce (EFSA, 2016; Ross *et al.*, 2010; SACN, 2016).

Optimising bone health during development

Pregnancy

Limited data are available from randomised controlled trials of the effect of maternal vitamin D supplementation on maternal or child bone health. Observational evidence, however, shows that the risk of the development of rickets during infancy and childhood increases when a child is born to a vitamin D–deficient woman (Munns *et al.*, 2016). One recent RCT in the UK showed that supplementing women with 1000 IU/day did not result in a higher BMD and BMC in their children; however, when women who delivered in the winter were analysed separately, a significantly higher infant BMD was found in the supplementation group. This suggests a benefit if the woman is at higher risk of deficiency (Cooper *et al.*, 2016). Together, these data stress the importance for

SECTION 7

pregnant women to prevent vitamin D deficiency during pregnancy in order to prevent adverse effects on the skeletal development of their children.

Infancy and childhood

Limited data are available on the effect of vitamin D supplementation in infancy, childhood or adolescence. A number of randomised trials and observational and case studies have shown that the risk of rickets increases when plasma 25OHD falls <30 nmol/L (EFSA, 2016; Munns *et al.*, 2016; SACN, 2016). A systematic review of the effect of vitamin D supplementation in children and adolescents has shown that there is a positive effect on bone mineral content in those who had a low (25OHD <35 nmol/L) baseline vitamin D status, but not in those with a higher vitamin D status (EFSA, 2016; SACN, 2016).

In the UK and the USA, the RNI and RDA for vitamin D are based on the requirements for bone health. In the UK, the RNI is 10 μg (400 IU)/day for all people aged 4 years and over. This requirement is based on the estimation of the amount needed to maintain the plasma concentration of 25(OH)D over 25 nmol/L when UVB sunshine exposure is minimal. It includes individuals of minority ethnic groups with a darker skin. No separate recommendations are made for pregnant and lactating women, individuals confined indoors and for those in the population aged over 65 years. A recommendation could not be formulated for children younger than 4 years due to insufficient data (SACN, 2016). In contrast, the US RDA assumes a moderate contribution of cutaneous-produced vitamin D in the general public; an RDA is formulated for all age groups. For the EU, the adequate intake (AI) is 10 μg/day for children under 1 year of age, and 15 μg/day for all other age groups (EFSA, 2016).

Other nutrients and food groups

Protein

Protein intake affects bone in several ways, as it provides the organic component of the structural matrix of bone, increases the anabolic hormone insulin-like growth factor-1 (IGF-1), and influences calcium metabolism (Heaney & Layman, 2008). Amino acid precursors from dietary protein are required to build and maintain bone structure (Darling *et al.*, 2009); an inadequate anabolic drive due to insufficient dietary protein may decrease bone strength (Heaney & Layman, 2008). Elderly patients with hip fracture are often undernourished; one study has shown that those given daily oral nutrition supplements (ONS) (20 g protein, 254 kcal) showed improved clinical outcome (Delmi *et al.*, 1990).

In the general population, however, there is inconsistent evidence about the relationship between high and low protein intakes and bone health. The effect of protein may be biphasic, with potentially detrimental effects at high intakes because of its effects on calcium excretion in the urine (Prentice *et al.*, 2006). However, one recent large longitudinal cohort study of 5875 men has shown that higher protein intake (% total energy intake) was associated with a decreased risk of major osteoporotic fracture (Langsetmo *et al.*, 2017). The association between protein and fracture varied by protein source: increased dairy protein and non-dairy animal protein were associated with a decreased risk of hip fracture, whereas plant-source protein was not (Langsetmo *et al.*, 2017). Overall, this supports the advice of dietary protein intakes within recommendations, particularly for the elderly.

Phosphorus

Approximately 85% of total body phosphorus is found in the skeleton. In Western diets, phosphorous intake is usually adequate. The evidence on whether dietary phosphorus intake has any effect on bone health is inconsistent.

Potassium and sodium

Although bone does not contain appreciable amounts of potassium and sodium, these nutrients may impact on bone health through a role in maintaining calcium homeostasis. A high-potassium diet is believed to reduce urinary calcium excretion. A recent analysis of men and postmenopausal women showed an association between higher potassium intakes and higher total hip and femur neck BMD as compared to lower-potassium-intake groups (Kong *et al.*, 2017). In contrast, a high dietary sodium intake is believed to be associated with increased urinary calcium excretion in the short term, while long-term outcomes are less certain (Teucher *et al.*, 2008). A diet rich in fruit and vegetables is thought to be beneficial for bone health, owing to the high potassium and low sodium content (New, 2004).

Magnesium

Magnesium is widely distributed in soft and bony tissue; 50–60% of total body magnesium is found in bone. Results from a large observational study suggest that a lower magnesium intake is associated with lower BMD of the hip and whole body, but this result does not translate into increased risk of fractures (Orchard *et al.*, 2014). A systematic review has concluded that high intakes of magnesium were not significantly associated with risks of total hip fracture or total fractures (Farsinejad-Marj *et al.*, 2016). Overall, the exact role of magnesium in bone health remains unclear.

Vitamin K

Vitamin K is a group of fat-soluble compounds that act as a cofactor for the carboxylation of osteocalcin, a protein involved in bone formation. Levels that are sufficient to maintain blood coagulation formed the basis of the recommended dietary intake of 1 μg/kg of body weight per day, but this may be suboptimal for adult bone health (Cashman & O'Connor, 2008). Supplementation studies with vitamin K_1 in postmenopausal women showed a reduction of bone loss or improvement of BMD in some but not all sites (Bolton-Smith *et al.*, 2007; Braam *et al.*, 2003).

Other dietary factors

Vegetarian and vegan diets

Cross-sectional and longitudinal population-based studies do not suggest that there is a difference in BMD between vegetarians and omnivores, other than that which may be accounted for by differences in weight and lifestyle (New, 2004). Veganism is associated with a diet that contains a low level of bioavailable calcium (Sanders, 1999) and low protein intakes, which may be detrimental to bone. However, the evaluation of the impact of vegetarian or vegan diets on bone is complex and potentially compounded by differences in other key lifestyle factors (see Chapter 3.6, Vegetarianism and vegan diets).

Lactose intolerance

People with lactose intolerance may have a reduced calcium intake from dairy sources. The limited evidence available suggests that patients with lactose intolerance are not at an increased risk of osteoporosis, provided that their calcium requirements are met (Enattah *et al.*, 2005).

Other factors influencing bone health

Body composition

BMD is influenced by body size and weight. A meta-analysis of 12 prospective, population-based cohorts, including 60,000 adults, showed that the number of osteoporotic fractures and hip fractures were inversely related to BMI (De Laet *et al.*, 2005). Low BMI as a risk factor for fracture may be associated with muscle weakness, nutritional deficiencies (protein/vitamin D), decreased padding over the greater trochanter of the hip, or a greater liability to fall (De Laet *et al.*, 2005). Although a high BMI is associated with a lower risk of fracture in older people, recent evidence suggests a higher risk of some fractures, such as at the wrist and ankle, in obese patients. Obesity should therefore not be regarded as a protective factor for fracture risk. Rather, underweight should be regarded as a significant risk factor (De Laet *et al.*, 2005). A healthy body weight within the normal range should be encouraged.

Weight loss

Unintentional weight loss in premenopausal women is associated with fracture risk (Compston *et al.*, 2016). Weight loss, irrespective of current weight, is associated with an increased risk of fracture, and may be greater in those who suffered involuntary weight loss (Ensrud *et al.*, 1997, 2003). This may be explained by the decline in mechanical load, a decrease in nutritional intake, including calcium and protein, or be linked to alterations in levels of hormonal factors.

Sarcopenia

The presence of sarcopenia is important to consider. One longitudinal study in 1486 men aged ≥70 years suggested that the presence of sarcopenia with concurrent obesity is associated with increased fall rates and increased fracture risk over 6 years as compared to non-sarcopenic obese men (Scott *et al.*, 2017).

Subgroups of the population at particular risk

Several subgroups of the population are vulnerable to the development of osteoporosis. Anorexia nervosa is associated with a lower bone mass and an increased risk of fractures. Amenorrhea is thought to play an important role in the development of osteoporosis; other risk factors include IGF-1 deficiency, low androgen levels and hypercortisolaemia (see Chapter 7.10.2, Eating disorders).

For patients with Crohn's disease and ulcerative colitis, the relative risk of hip fractures is 1.5 and 1.4, respectively, as compared to the general population (Lewis & Scott, 2007). There is also a modest increased risk of fracture in coeliac disease (Lewis & Scott, 2007); BMD is observed to be more reduced in those with severe as compared to mild villous atrophy, and there was a significant improvement in BMD after the introduction of a gluten-free diet. Adults with IBD or coeliac disease are recommended to ensure a daily intake of calcium (from dietary sources or supplements) of 1000 mg/day (1200 mg for postmenopausal women and men aged >55 years) and to be vitamin D replete (Lewis & Scott, 2007) (see Chapter 7.4.7, Coeliac disease and Chapter 7.4.10, Irritable bowel syndrome). Chronic liver disease is associated with increased risk of osteoporosis. Therefore, the proposed guideline for these patients is to consume 1000 mg/day calcium and 800 IU/day vitamin D (Collier *et al.*, 2002).

Both type 1 and type 2 diabetes are risk factors for fragility fractures. Diabetes may negatively affect bone health through several regulatory pathways: an alteration of the balance between bone formation and resorption, an increase in inflammatory cytokines and bone marrow adiposity, and alterations in the incretin system (Napoli *et al.*, 2017). Lower BMD in rheumatoid arthritis (RA) patients relates to disease activity, severity, duration and medication use, among other factors (Coulson *et al.*, 2009). Although the majority of RA patients have one or more risk factors for osteoporosis, the minority receives preventive treatment (Coulson *et al.*, 2009). Organ transplantation is associated with an increased risk of osteoporosis and fractures, often related to the primary disease requiring transplantation or medication use. Before transplantation, it is recommended to ensure adequacy of calcium intake and vitamin D status, encourage weight-bearing exercises and treat prevalent osteoporosis (Cohen *et al.*, 2004). The most rapid rates of bone loss occur during the early post-transplantation period (6–12 months); rapid resumption of weight-bearing exercise, supplementary calcium (1000–1500 mg/day in divided doses), at least 400–800 IU/day of vitamin D, in addition to treatment with bisphosphonates or calcitriol, is recommended (Cohen *et al.*, 2004).

The presence of chronic obstructive pulmonary disease (COPD) is a risk factor for the development of osteoporosis. Patients with COPD are also at a higher risk of associated comorbidities such as a low BMI and impaired nutritional status, and are more likely to be tobacco smokers (Vrieze *et al.*, 2007). No guidelines have been established specifically for this group (Lehouck *et al.*, 2010). Osteopenia and osteoporosis are common among patients with cystic fibrosis (CF) (Conway *et al.*, 2000). A low BMD in CF patients is thought to be associated with underlying chronic inflammation, medication use, nutrient malabsorption, low physical activity and delayed puberty (Turck et *al.*, 2016). ESPEN guidelines recommend the assessment of bone health (DXA) for all patients >8 years old, every 1–5 years. In addition, for CF patients with osteopenia or osteoporosis, nutritional intervention is recommended to achieve optimal body weight, and to meet the recommended dietary calcium intake through calcium-rich foods (Turck *et al.*, 2016). Provision of supplemental calcium, vitamin D, and vitamin K may be necessary (Turck *et al.*, 2016).

Management of osteoporosis

The aim of the treatment of osteoporosis is to reduce the risk of falls and fractures. These include pharmacologic approaches, lifestyle advice and dietary interventions.

Life style advice

Exercise

Exercise, particularly weight-bearing exercise, can help to build bone and increase PBM in youth and help to maintain bone tissue in adults. It may also help to improve posture, balance and muscle power, all of which help to prevent falls. People with osteoporosis are mostly older patients who are at a higher risk of falling due to decreased muscle power and poorer balance (Cosman *et al.*, 2014). The NOF recommends regular weight-bearing and muscle-strengthening exercise to improve agility, strength, posture, and balance; maintain or improve bone strength; and reduce the risk of falls and fractures. The UK National Osteoporosis Society (NOS) recommends adults to conduct 30 minutes of moderate-intensity activity at least 5 days per week, with exercises focusing on muscle strength at least 2 days per week.

Pharmacologic treatments

These agents may act to prevent bone loss and slow the bone remodelling cycle (anti-resorptive) or stimulate bone formation and reduce bone resorption (anabolic). These drug therapies (brand name) include:

- Bisphosphonates
  - Alendronate (Fosamax)
  - Cyclical etidronate (Didronel PMO)
  - Ibandronate (Bonviva)
  - Risedronate (Actonel)
  - Zoledronic acid (Aclasta)
- Selective oestrogen receptor modulator (SERM)
  - Raloxifene (Evista)
- Human RANK-ligand antibody
  - Denosumab (Prolia)
- Other
  - Hormone replacement therapy (HRT)
  - Calcitonin
- Anabolic agents
  - Strontium ranelate (Protelos)
  - PTH treatment (Preotact, Forsteo)

In the UK, NICE guidance exists for alendronate (Fosamax), etidronate (Didronel), risedronate (Actonel), raloxifene (Evista) and strontium ranelate (Protelos) for the primary and secondary prevention of osteoporotic fragility fractures in postmenopausal women. These therapies may be used in combination or as alternating therapies (Bilezikian, 2008). Oral bisphosphonates must be taken fasted and may be associated with upper gastrointestinal side effects. Compliance to osteoporosis treatment needs to be considered in the evaluation of the patient. Pharmacological treatment strategies often include recommendations of calcium and vitamin D supplements. Patients with a poor kidney function may be prescribed calcitriol (Rocaltrol) or alfacalcidol, instead of vitamin D.

Nutritional care of the hip fracture patient

Fractures of the proximal femur (hip) are a cause of substantial morbidity and mortality in older people (Avenell & Handoll, 2010); 9 months after their hip fracture, people still have poorer quality of life than controls (Cranney *et al.*, 2005), and many fail to return to their previous state of mobility.

Nutrition status of hip fracture patients

Protein energy malnutrition is common among elderly patients hospitalised with an acute hip fracture (Delmi *et al.*, 1990; Lumbers *et al.*, 2001; Nematy *et al.*, 2006), and is associated with an increased risk of complications (Eneroth *et al.*, 2006; Houwing *et al.*, 2003). There is evidence that nutritional support, especially when overseen by a specialist dietitian and dietetic assistant, lowers the risk of postoperative complications, particularly in underweight patients (Delmi *et al.*, 1990; Duncan *et al.*, 2006; Eneroth *et al.*, 2005). ESPEN guidelines 2006 recommend ONS for this group (Volkert *et al.*, 2006), but enteral feeding may also be considered. Compliance to ONS is often low. This may have contributed to the conclusion (in a Cochrane review on ONS for hip fracture aftercare) that the evidence for the effectiveness of protein and energy feeds is weak (Avenell & Handoll, 2010). However, some evidence exists to suggest that supplementation with β-hydroxy-β-methylbutyrate (HMB) ONS is associated with improved muscle mass following a hip fracture (Malafarina *et al.*, 2017).

Assessment

Nutritional assessment of the hip fracture patient will include the following:

- Anthropometry – current weight (% weight change), current height (and height as a young adult) or demispan, and BMI. Mid-upper-arm circumference can be used as an index of malnutrition, as this correlates well with BMI in this patient group (Maffulli *et al.*, 1999).
- Biochemistry and fluid balance. Measurement of 25(OH)D for these at-risk patients is recommended.
- Clinical symptoms.
- Dietary assessment. A 24-h recall after admission and surgery is important to assess reduced voluntary oral intakes post-surgery (Nematy *et al.*, 2006; Sullivan *et al.*, 2004).

Nutritional care

Patients undergoing orthopaedic surgery have increased metabolic requirements, which are often unrecognised (Eneroth *et al.*, 2006). The total energy requirements of patients may be calculated by estimating the basal metabolic rate (BMR), adding a stress factor of 20% (to account for the increased energy requirements owing to surgical correction of the fractured femoral neck), and adding another 10–25% (based on the level of mobility) to allow for rehabilitation, physical activity and diet-induced thermogenesis (Nematy *et al.*, 2006) (see Chapter 6.1, Nutritional requirements in clinical practice and Chapter 7.17.5, Surgery).

Dietary advice should aim to achieve a high-protein, high-energy diet in small and frequent portions, potentially with the use of supplements and fortified foods. Monitoring and discharge planning are important stages in the dietetic care of a hip fracture patient.

Further reading

Nutrition

European Food Safety Authority Panel on Dietetic Products, Nutrition, and Allergies. (2016) *Scientific Opinion on Dietary Reference Values for Vitamin D*. Available at https://www.efsa.europa.eu/sites/default/files/consultation/160321.pdf.

SACN. (2016) *Vitamin D and Health*. Available at https://www.gov.uk/government/groups/scientific-advisory-committee-on-nutrition.

Exercise

Howe TE, Shea B, Dawson LJ, *et al.* (2011) *Exercise for Preventing and Treating Osteoporosis in Postmenopausal Women*. Available at https://www.cochranelibrary.com/cdsr/doi/10.1002/14651858.CD000333.pub2/epdf/full Accessed 27 February 2019.

Diagnosis and drug treatment

Cosman F, de Beur SJ, LeBoff MS, *et al.*; National Osteoporosis Foundation (NOF). (2014) Clinician's guide to prevention and treatment of osteoporosis. *Osteoporos. Int.* 25: 2359–2381.

Poole KE, Compston JE. (2006) Osteoporosis and its management. *BMJ* 333: 1251–1256.

Other

NICE. (2012) Osteoporosis: assessing the risk of fragility fracture. Available at www.nice.org.uk/guidance/cg146. Accessed 30 October 2018.

Internet resources

American Society for Bone Mineral Research, www.asbmr.org
International Osteoporosis Foundation, www.iofbonehealth.org
National Osteoporosis Society, www.nos.org.uk

References

Avenell A, Handoll HH. (2010) Nutritional supplementation for hip fracture aftercare in older people. *Cochrane Database Syst. Rev.* (11): CD001880.

Ballane G, Cauley JA, Luckey MM, *et al.* (2017) Worldwide prevalence and incidence of osteoporotic vertebral fractures. *Osteoporos. Int.* 28(5): 1531–1542.

Bilezikian JP. (2008) In: Rosen CJ (ed). *Primer on the Metabolic Diseases and Disorders of Mineral Metabolism*. Washington DC: The American Society of Bone and Mineral Research.

Bischoff-Ferrari HA, Willett WC, Wong JB, *et al.* (2005) Fracture prevention with vitamin D supplementation: a meta-analysis of randomized controlled trials. *JAMA* 293: 2257–2264.

Bischoff-Ferrari HA, Giovannucci E, Willett WC, *et al.* (2006) Estimation of optimal serum concentrations of 25-hydroxyvitamin-D for multiple health outcomes. *Am. J. Clin. Nutr.* 84: 18–28.

Bischoff-Ferrari HA, Dawson-Hughes B, Orav EJ, *et al.* (2016) Monthly high-dose vitamin D treatment for the prevention of functional decline: a randomized clinical trial. *JAMA Intern. Med.* 176(2): 175–183.

Bolland MJ, Leung W, Tai V, *et al.* (2015) Calcium intake and risk of fracture: systematic review. *BMJ* 351: h4580.

Bolton-Smith C, McMurdo ME, Paterson CR, *et al.* (2007) Two-year randomized controlled trial of vitamin K_1 (phylloquinone) and vitamin D_3 plus calcium on the bone health of older women. *J. Bone Miner. Res.* 22: 509–519.

Braam LA, Knapen MH, Geusens P, *et al.* (2003) Vitamin K_1 supplementation retards bone loss in postmenopausal women between 50 and 60 years of age. *Calcif. Tissue Int.* 73: 21–26.

British Dietetic Association. (2014) *Food Fact Sheet: Calcium*. Available at https://www.bda.uk.com/foodfacts/Calcium.pdf. Accessed 31 October 2018.

Cashman KD, O'Connor E. (2008) Does high vitamin K_1 intake protect against bone loss in later life? *Nutr. Rev.* 66: 532–538.

Cauley JA, El-Hajj Fuleihan G, Luckey MM; FRAX® Position Development Conference Members. (2011) FRAX® International Task Force of the 2010 Joint International Society for Clinical Densitometry & International Osteoporosis Foundation Position Development Conference. *J. Clin. Densitom.* 14(3): 237–239.

Clarke B. (2008) Normal bone anatomy and physiology. *Clin. J. Am. Soc. Nephrol.* 3(3): S131–139.

Cohen A, Sambrook P, Shane E. (2004) Management of bone loss after organ transplantation. *J. Bone Miner. Res.* 19: 1919–1932.

Collier JD, Ninkovic M, Compston JE. (2002) Guidelines on the management of osteoporosis associated with chronic liver disease. *Gut* 50(1): i1–9.

Cooper C, Harvey NC, Bishop NJ, *et al.*; MAVIDOS Study Group. (2016) Maternal gestational vitamin D supplementation and offspring bone health (MAVIDOS): a multicentre, double-blind, randomised placebo-controlled trial. *Lancet Diabetes Endocrinol.* 4(5): 393–402.

Compston JE, Wyman A, Fitzgerald G, *et al.* (2016) Increase in fracture risk following unintentional weight loss in postmenopausal women: the global longitudinal study of osteoporosis in women. *J. Bone Miner. Res.* 31(7): 1466–1472.

Conway SP, Morton AM, Oldroyd B, *et al.* (2000) Osteoporosis and osteopenia in adults and adolescents with cystic fibrosis: prevalence and associated factors. *Thorax.* 55(9): 798–804.

Cosman F, de Beur SJ, LeBoff MS, *et al.*; National Osteoporosis Foundation (NOF). (2014) Clinician's guide to prevention and treatment of osteoporosis. *Osteoporos. Int.* 25: 2359–2381.

Coulson KA, Reed G, Gilliam BE, *et al.* (2009) Factors influencing fracture risk, T score, and management of osteoporosis in patients with rheumatoid arthritis in the Consortium of Rheumatology Researchers of North America (CORRONA) registry. *J. Clin. Rheumatol.* 15: 155–160.

Cranney AB, Coyle D, Hopman WM, *et al.* (2005) Prospective evaluation of preferences and quality of life in women with hip fractures. *J. Rheumatol.* 32: 2393–2399.

Dallas SL, Prideaux M, Bonewald LF. (2013) The osteocyte: an endocrine cell … and more. *Endocr. Rev.* 34(5): 658–690.

Darling AL, Millward DJ, Torgerson DJ, *et al.* (2009) Dietary protein and bone health: a systematic review and meta-analysis. *Am. J. Clin. Nutr.* 90: 1674–1692.

Dawson-Hughes B, Dallal GE, Krall EA, *et al.* (1990) A controlled trial of the effect of calcium supplementation on bone density in postmenopausal women. *N. Engl. J. Med.* 323: 878–883.

De Laet C, Kanis JA, Oden A, *et al.* (2005) Body mass index as a predictor of fracture risk: a meta-analysis. *Osteoporos. Int.* 16: 1330–1338.

Delmi M, Rapin CH, Bengoa JM, *et al.* (1990) Dietary supplementation in elderly patients with fractured neck of the femur. *Lancet* 335: 1013–1016.

Department of Health & Human Services. (2004) *Bone health and osteoporosis: a report of the surgeon general.* Rockville: US Department of Health and Human Services, Office of the Surgeon General.

DH. (1998) *Nutrition and bone health with particular reference to calcium and vitamin D: Report of the Subgroup on Bone Health (Working Group on the Nutritional Status of the Population) of the Committee on Medical Aspects of Food and Nutrition Policy.* London: The Stationary Office.

Duncan DG, Beck SJ, Hood K, *et al.* (2006) Using dietetic assistants to improve the outcome of hip fracture: a randomised controlled trial of nutritional support in an acute trauma ward. *Age Ageing* 35: 148–153.

EFSA (European Food Safety Authority) Panel on Dietetic Products, Nutrition, and Allergies. (2016) Scientific Opinion on Dietary Reference Values for vitamin D. *EFSA J.* 14(10): 4547.

Enattah N, Pekkarinen T, Valimaki MJ, *et al.* (2005) Genetically defined adult-type hypolactasia and self-reported lactose intolerance as risk factors of osteoporosis in Finnish postmenopausal women. *Eur. J. Clin. Nutr.* 59: 1105–1111.

Eneroth M, Olsson UB, Thorngren KG. (2005) Insufficient fluid and energy intake in hospitalised patients with hip fracture. A prospective randomised study of 80 patients. *Clin. Nutr.* 24: 297–303.

Eneroth M, Olsson UB, Thorngren KG. (2006) Nutritional supplementation decreases hip fracture-related complications. *Clin. Orthop. Relat. Res.* 451: 212–217.

Ensrud KE, Cauley J, Lipschutz R, *et al.* (1997) Weight change and fractures in older women. Study of Osteoporotic Fractures Research Group. *Arch. Intern. Med.* 157: 857–863.

Ensrud KE, Ewing SK, Stone KL, *et al.* (2003) Intentional and unintentional weight loss increase bone loss and hip fracture risk in older women. *J. Am. Geriatr. Soc.* 51: 1740–1747.

Farsinejad-Marj M, Saneei P, Esmaillzadeh A. (2016) Dietary magnesium intake, bone mineral density and risk of fracture: a systematic review and meta-analysis. *Osteoporos. Int.* 27(4): 1389–1399.

Francis RM. (2007) The vitamin D paradox. *Rheumatology (Oxford)* 46: 1749–1750.

Gallagher JC. (2016) Vitamin D and falls – the dosage conundrum. *Nat. Rev. Endocrinol.* 12(11): 680–684

Goulding A, Rockell JE, Black RE, *et al.* (2004) Children who avoid drinking cow's milk are at increased risk for prepubertal bone fractures. *J. Am. Diet. Assoc.* 104: 250–253.

Heaney RP. (2000) Calcium, dairy products and osteoporosis. *J. Am. Coll. Nutr.* 19: 83S–99S.

Heaney RP, Layman DK. (2008) Amount and type of protein influences bone health. *Am. J. Clin. Nutr.* 87: 1567S–1570S.

Holick MF, Binkley NC, Bischoff-Ferrari HA, et al. (2011) Evaluation, treatment, and prevention of vitamin D deficiency: an Endocrine Society clinical practice guideline. *J. Clin. Endocrinol. Metab.* 96(7):1911–1930.

Houwing RH, Rozendaal M, Wouters-Wesseling W, *et al.* (2003) A randomised, double-blind assessment of the effect of nutritional supplementation on the prevention of pressure ulcers in hip-fracture patients. *Clin. Nutr.* 22: 401–405.

International Society for Clinical Densitometry. (2013) *Official Positions—Adult.* Available at http://www.iscd.org/official-positions/2013-iscd-official-positions-adult/. Accessed January 2017.

Johnell O, Kanis J. (2005) Epidemiology of osteoporotic fractures. *Osteoporos. Int.* 16(2): S3–7.

Johnell O, Kanis JA. (2006) An estimate of the worldwide prevalence and disability associated with osteoporotic fractures. *Osteoporos. Int.* 17: 1726–1733.

Kanis JA, Odén A, McCloskey EV, *et al*; IOF Working Group on Epidemiology and Quality of Life. (2012) A systematic review of hip fracture incidence and probability of fracture worldwide. *Osteoporos. Int.* 23(9): 2239–2256.

Kong SH, Kim JH, Hong AR, *et al.* (2017) Dietary potassium intake is beneficial to bone health in a low calcium intake population: the Korean National Health and Nutrition Examination Survey (KNHANES) (2008–2011). *Osteoporos. Int.* 28(5): 1577–1585.

Langsetmo L, Shikany JM, Cawthon PM, *et al.*; Osteoporotic Fractures in Men (MrOS) Research Group. (2017) The association between protein intake by source and osteoporotic fracture in older men: a prospective cohort study. *J. Bone Miner. Res.* 32(3): 592–600.

Lehouck A, van Remoortel H, Troosters T, *et al.* (2010) COPD and bone metabolism: a clinical update. *Rev. Mal. Respir.* 27: 1231–1242.

Lewis N, Scott B. (2007) Guidelines for osteoporosis in inflammatory bowel disease and coeliac disease. Available https://www.bsg.org.uk/resource/guidelines-for-osteoporosis-in-inflammatory-bowel-disease-and-coeliac-disease.html. Accessed 31 October 2018.

Lumbers M, New SA, Gibson S, *et al.* (2001) Nutritional status in elderly female hip fracture patients: comparison with an age-matched home living group attending day centres. *Br. J. Nutr.* 85: 733–740.

Maffulli N, Dougall TW, Brown MT, *et al.* (1999) Nutritional differences in patients with proximal femoral fractures. *Age Ageing* 28: 458–462.

Malafarina V, Uriz-Otano F, Malafarina C, *et al.* (2017) Effectiveness of nutritional supplementation on sarcopenia and recovery in hip fracture patients. A multi-centre randomized trial. *Maturitas.* 101: 42–50.

Manias K, McCabe D, Bishop N. (2006) Fractures and recurrent fractures in children; varying effects of environmental factors as well as bone size and mass. *Bone* 39: 652–657.

Munns CF, Shaw N, Kiely M, *et al.* (2016) Global consensus recommendations on prevention and management of nutritional rickets. *J. Clin. Endocrinol. Metab.* 101: 394–415.

Murad MH, Elamin KB, Abu Elnour NO, *et al.* (2011) Clinical review: the effect of vitamin D on falls: a systematic review and meta-analysis. *J. Clin. Endocrinol. Metab.* 96(10): 2997–3006. doi: 10.1210/jc.2011-1193

Napoli N, Chandran M, Pierroz DD, *et al.*; IOF Bone and Diabetes Working Group. (2017) Mechanisms of diabetes mellitus-induced bone fragility. *Nat. Rev. Endocrinol.* 13(4): 208–219.

National Osteoporosis Guideline Group. (2014) *Guideline for the diagnosis and management of osteoporosis in postmenopausal women and men from the age of 50 years in the UK.* Available at https://www.shef.ac.uk/NOGG/NOGG_Pocket_Guide_for_Healthcare_Professionals.pdf. Accessed 30 October 2018.

National Osteoporosis Society (2010) https://nos.org.uk/about-osteoporosis/your-bone-strength/a-balanced-diet-for-bones/vitamin-d. Accessed 31 October 2018.

Nematy M, Hickson M, Brynes AE, *et al.* (2006) Vulnerable patients with a fractured neck of femur: nutritional status and support in hospital. *J. Hum. Nutr. Diet.* 19: 209–218.

New SA. (2004) Do vegetarians have a normal bone mass? *Osteopo-ros. Int.* 15: 679–688.

NICE. (2012) *Osteoporosis: Fragility Fracture Risk.* NICE Clinical Guideline 146. National Clinical Guideline Centre.

Nieves JW, Barrett-Connor E, Siris ES, *et al.* (2008) Calcium and vitamin D intake influence bone mass, but not short-term fracture risk, in Caucasian postmenopausal women from the National Osteoporosis Risk Assessment (NORA) study. *Osteoporos. Int.* 19: 673–679.

Orchard TS, Larson JC, Alghothani N, *et al.* (2014) Magnesium intake, bone mineral density, and fractures: results from the Women's Health Initiative Observational Study. *Am. J. Clin. Nutr.* 99(4): 926–933.

Poole KE, Compston JE. (2006) Osteoporosis and its management. *BMJ* 333: 1251–1256.

Prentice A. (2004) Diet, nutrition and the prevention of osteoporosis. *Public Health Nutr.* 7: 227–243.

Prentice A, Schoenmakers I, Laskey MA, *et al.* (2006) Nutrition and bone growth and development. *Proc. Nutr. Soc.* 65: 348–360.

Reid IR, Bolland MJ. (2012) Calcium supplements: bad for the heart? *Heart.* 98(12):895–896.

Reid IR, Bolland MJ, Grey A. (2014) Effects of vitamin D supplements on bone mineral density: a systematic review and meta-analysis. *Lancet.* 383: 146–155.

Ross AC, Taylor CL, Yaktine AL, *et al.* (2010) *Dietary Reference Intakes for Calcium and Vitamin D. Committee to Review Dietary Reference Intakes for Vitamin D and Calcium.* Washington, DC, Institute of Medicine.

SACN. (2016) *Vitamin D and Health.* Available at https://www.gov.uk/government/groups/scientific-advisory-committee-on-nutrition. Accessed January 2017.

Sanders TA. (1999) The nutritional adequacy of plant-based diets. *Proc. Nutr. Soc.* 58: 265–269.

Sanders KM, Stuart AL, Williamson EJ, *et al.* (2010) Annual high-dose oral vitamin D and falls and fractures in older women: a randomized controlled trial. *JAMA.* 303(18): 1815–1822. Erratum in: *JAMA.* (2010) June 16; 303(23): 2357.

Scott D, Seibel M, Cumming R, *et al.* (2017) Sarcopenic obesity and its temporal associations with changes in bone mineral density, incident falls, and fractures in older men: the Concord Health and Ageing in Men Project. *J. Bone Miner. Res.* 32(3): 575–583.

Sullivan DH, Nelson CL, Klimberg VS, *et al.* (2004) Nightly enteral nutrition support of elderly hip fracture patients: a pilot study. *J. Am. Coll. Nutr.* 23: 683–691.

Teucher B, Dainty JR, Spinks CA, *et al.* (2008) Sodium and bone health: impact of moderately high and low salt intakes on calcium metabolism in postmenopausal women. *J. Bone Miner. Res.* 23: 1477–1485.

Tripkovic L, Lambert H, Hart K, *et al.* (2012) Comparison of vitamin D_2 and vitamin D_3 supplementation in raising serum 25-hydroxyvitamin-D status: a systematic review and meta-analysis. *Am. J. Clin. Nutr.* 95: 1357–1364.

Turck D, Braegger CP, Colombo C, *et al.* (2016) ESPEN–ESPGHAN–ECFS guidelines on nutrition care for infants, children, and adults with cystic fibrosis. *Clin. Nutr.* 35(3): 557–577.

Volkert D, Berner YN, Berry E, *et al.* (2006) ESPEN guidelines on enteral nutrition: geriatrics. *Clin. Nutr.* 25: 330–360.

Winzenberg TM, Shaw K, Fryer J, *et al.* (2006) Calcium supplementation for improving bone mineral density in children. *Cochrane Database Syst. Rev.* (2): CD005119.

WHO. (1994) Assessment of fracture risk and its application to screening for postmenopausal osteoporosis. Report of a WHO Study Group. *World Health Organization Technical Report Series.* 1994/01/01 ed. Geneva.

7.9.2 Arthritis

Martin Lau

Key points

- Weight reduction when appropriate (5–10% body weight), combined with a structured exercise programme, is effective in reducing arthritis symptoms and may halt disease progression.
- Disease activity and symptoms are intermittent; this makes it easy to misinterpret that improving symptoms is due to dietary/dietary supplement intervention.
- Fish oil supplements rich in n-3 polyunsaturated fatty acids have been found to ameliorate pain and symptoms in rheumatoid arthritis, but are inconsistent in osteoarthritis.
- There is no specific dietary regimen or food avoidance recommended for arthritis. It is therefore important to listen to patient experiences and devise a shared-decision working plan.

Musculoskeletal disorders affect the muscles, joints and bones, and is the second most common cause of disability worldwide (Vos *et al.*, 2012). Arthritis is not a single disease, and its dietary management can be complicated: the patient's own health beliefs often undermine the available scientific evidence. This chapter will discuss the dietary management of osteoarthritis (OA), rheumatoid arthritis (RA) and ankylosing spondylitis (AS).

Osteoarthritis

OA is highly prevalent, and a major cause of pain and disability in older people (Conaghan *et al.*, 2014). With the aging population and the obesity epidemic, the prevalence is set to rise. The most common risk factors include gender, age, prior joint injuries or trauma, genetics and being overweight/obese. Weakness from the supporting tendons, ligaments and muscles also contributes to the symptoms (Felson *et al.*, 2000). It is a progressive, metabolically active process, and the rate of degradation far exceeds the rate of repair.

Depending on the joints and severity, the symptoms of OA vary. The most commonly affected are the hip, knee, fingers and thumb. Pain experienced is intermittent, typically worse during and/or after weight-bearing activities. Flare-up usually associated with inflammation can happen during the course of OA. Although pain, swelling, stiffness and a reduction in physical activity are all typical outcomes of OA, structural changes in the joint may occur without accompanying symptoms. Approximately 50% of people with structural changes are asymptomatic (Hannan *et al.*, 2000). It has been suggested that OA should be subdivided into different phenotypes (post-traumatic, ageing, genetic, pain and metabolic) in order to treat effectively (Bijlsma *et al.*, 2011; Castañeda *et al.*, 2014; Felson, 2010; van der Esch *et al.*, 2015; Zhang *et al.*, 2014).

Clinical management

The current clinical management for OA aims to reduce symptoms, to prevent the progression of joint damage and to improve the quality of life. Combination of both non-pharmaceutical and pharmaceutical treatments is the most effective. Patient education along with weight reduction (if appropriate) and exercise are the cornerstones of non-pharmaceutical treatment. The use of analgesics to alleviate pain, e.g. paracetamol, and non-steroidal anti-inflammatory drugs (NSAIDs) can be useful. Injections of corticosteroids directly into the joint may be used to relieve severe local pain and inflammation. If pain becomes debilitating, joint replacement surgery may be considered (NICE, 2014).

Dietary management

Dietetic intervention has a role to play, especially in the management of risk factors such as obesity and related comorbidities. As long-term use of NSAIDs is associated with undesirable side effects, engaging in alternative health practices may offer patients hope. The use of special or elimination diets is popular among this patient group despite the lack of robust scientific evidence (Rao *et al.*, 1999). Alternative practitioners have claimed that arthritis is associated with overconsumption of acid-producing foods; hence the alkaline diet. Other foods have been considered the cause of worsening symptoms, including nightshade vegetables, e.g. tomatoes, red meat, dairy and citrus fruits. The evidence for the benefits of any particular food are limited, although Lu *et al.* (2014) found that women (not men) who consumed 400 mL/day milk had a slower rate of joint space narrowing (an indication of cartilage loss) over 4 years.

The effect of individual nutrients (e.g. dietary fat) on OA has been studied. Animal studies have shown that a high-fat diet accelerated the progression of OA (Mooney *et al.*, 2011). Human study demonstrated that a high intake of total fat and saturated fat might be associated with structural progression; this effect was not seen with polyunsaturated fat and monounsaturated fat intake (Lu *et al.*, 2017). A recent pilot study examined for 4 months the use of a Mediterranean diet on biomarkers in patients with OA. Dyer *et al.* (2016) showed a decrease in pro-inflammatory and cartilage degradation biomarkers. However, the subjects also lost 2.25 kg. Whether the reduction of the biomarkers resulted from the diet or weight loss requires further investigation.

Obesity

Obesity is a well-known risk factor for OA, especially in the knees, but also the hips and hands (Berenbaum *et al.*, 2013; Felson, 1995). Each step increases the load on the hip or knee joint by three to five times the body weight; therefore, the physical stresses imposed on the joints by excessive body weight is immense (Aspden, 2011; Messier *et al.*, 2005). This abnormal joint loading can lead to alternations in the composition, structure and metabolism of the cartilage (Guilak, 2012). Bay-Jensen *et al.* (2012) suggested that systemic factors were involved, as both weight-bearing and non-weight-bearing joints are affected in obese subjects. Weight reduction or preventing progression to obesity is an integral part of the management. Dietary intervention using low- to very-low-energy regimens has been used to promote weight loss (Bliddal *et al.*, 2011). Vincent *et al.* (2012) showed that a 5% reduction in body weight led to symptom improvement. A 10% weight loss correlated with moderate-to-large functional improvements in knee joints. It is paramount to preserve lean muscle mass during energy restriction through a structured exercise/resistance training programme. There is a dose–response relationship between percentage weight loss and symptoms improvement (Atukorala *et al.*, 2016).

Recent research into the causes of OA and its progression has focused on the biological activity of adipose tissue. It is believed that a reduction in adipose tissue, rather than body weight alone, is required for improvements in symptoms (Aspden, 2011). Toda *et al.* (1998) found that reducing fat mass gave greater symptomatic relief.

Dietary supplements

Glucosamine and chondroitin

Glucosamine is found naturally in the body; it plays an important role in the synthesis of glycosaminoglycans and glycoproteins, which are important for ligaments, tendons, cartilage and the synovial fluid of joints. It has been suggested that the way in which joint structures are built and maintained contributes to the development and the progression of OA. Studies in animals have found that glucosamine can delay degradation and repair damaged cartilage. As a supplement, glucosamine exists in two forms: glucosamine sulphate and glucosamine hydrochloride. Results from randomised controlled trials (RCTs) on the effectiveness of glucosamine alone and in combination with chondroitin are conflicting. More importantly, its specific mechanism of action in OA pain is still unknown. The current NICE guidance (2014) for OA does not recommend the use of glucosamine or chondroitin.

Herbal and other dietary supplements

Some pharmacological treatments for OA are ineffective in some patients, and some have serious side effects with long-term use. Thus, patients frequently turn to complementary/alternative medicines. While many manufacturers of dietary supplements claim that their product will reduce symptoms, there is only weak scientific evidence to support the use of nutritional supplements in the management of OA. A systematic review of herbal medicines and plant extracts in OA found only weak evidence for Devil's claw (*Harpagophytum procumbens*) and avocado/soya bean unsaponifiables, and moderate evidence for phytodor (Long *et al.*, 2001). As yet, there is no convincing evidence that fish oil supplementation confers clinical benefit in the management of OA. Hill and colleagues (2015) compared high-dose and low-dose n-3 fatty acids and found no changes in the Western Ontario and McMaster Universities Arthritis Index (WOMAC) and cartilage volume after 24 months. A review conducted in the same year found that no human trials showed consistent benefits (Boe & Vangness, 2015).

The use of rose hip or curcumin (the active component of turmeric) has gain popularity in OA due to reported anti-inflammatory effects. A meta-analysis of three RCTs (Christensen *et al.*, 2008) showed that rose hip may ameliorate the pain associated with OA. However, this conclusion must be interpreted with caution, owing to the small number of studies and participants, and potential conflicts of interest, since the studies were sponsored by a rose hip powder manufacturer (Christesen *et al.*, 2008). The latest Osteoarthritis Research Society International guidelines (2014) do not recommend the use of rose hip for non-surgical management of knee OA. Studies on the effectiveness of curcumin are difficult to interpret, owing to the different preparations of curcumin used, lack of control and/or a small sample size (Daily *et al.*, 2016).

Rheumatoid arthritis

RA is an autoimmune systemic inflammatory disease with an unknown aetiology, which affects the synovial joints as well as other tissues and organs, including the heart, lungs and eyes. It typically affects the small joints of the hands (knuckles) and feet symmetrically first. The knees, shoulders, elbows, and ankles may also be affected. Prevalence in the UK is around 400,000 (1% of the UK population), with approximately 20,000 new cases per year (Symmons *et al.*, 2002; Wiles *et al.*, 1999). It is three times more common in women and can develop at any stage of life, with a peak age of incidence of 40–60 years in the UK for both genders (NRAS, 2017). RA is associated with a high risk for cardiovascular disease (CVD), lung disease, osteoporosis and malignancy (Cronstein, 2007; Nikiphorou *et al.*, 2015).

Clinical management

The aim for patients with RA is to achieve remission by modifying the disease process. Drug treatment includes the use of paracetamol and NSAIDs (ibuprofen, naproxen, diclofenac and cyclooxygenase-2 (COX 2) inhibitors) to relieve pain and reduce joint swelling. NSAIDs can increase the risk of stomach problems (e.g. peptic ulceration), whereas COX 2 inhibitors carry a lower risk of such problems, but are associated with a greater risk of cardiovascular complications (Perry *et al.*, 2014). These drugs do not act on the disease progression of RA.

NICE (2015) guidelines for the management of RA recommend the early introduction of second-line, disease-modifying antirheumatic drugs (DMARDs); the primary immunosuppressant drugs are methotrexate (first-line medication), sulphasalazine, hydroxychloroquine and leflunomide. Corticosteroids are used to provide rapid relief of symptoms such as pain, stiffness and joint swelling. They are used on a short-term basis due to the associated side effects of weight gain, muscle weakness and loss of bone mass (NICE, 2009). In the last few decades, concerted efforts to identify the main immune modulators of RA at the cellular level, including cytokines and TNF, has resulted in the development of biological agents (biologics) to block their activity. These specifically designed immunological proteins inhibit the inflammatory pathways that cause RA, and include etanercept, infliximab, adalimumab and rituximab.

Dietary approaches

Scepticism about the dietary management of RA has been challenged (Rayman & Pattison, 2008). Dietitians, as part of the multidisciplinary rheumatology team, can guide and advise on evidence-based dietary approaches. Several studies have shown poor eating patterns and nutritionally inadequate diets in people with RA (Berube *et al.*, 2017; Goff & Basari, 1999; Morgan *et al.*, 1997; Stone *et al.*, 1997). Explanations for these findings include the following:

- Pain and fatigue associated with RA can considerably impair appetite, particularly during acute exacerbations (a characteristic of the condition).
- Joint pain and deformity have adverse effects on mobility, functional ability and manual dexterity. Shopping, food preparation, cooking and eating can become difficult, complex and tiring.
- Popular diets and alternative lifestyle regimens are very likely to compromise nutrient intake.

Pain and disability can cause challenges in the activities of day-to-day living, especially cooking. An occupational therapist can advise on adapted utensils and home modifications to improve ability in the kitchen and maintain a desirable nutritional status.

The Mediterranean diet

One of the main comorbidities for RA is CVD. Given its strong inflammatory component, and the success of dietary regimen in the management of CVD, attempts were made to evaluate whether the benefits could extend to RA. Sköldstam *et al.* (2003) found significant benefits in RA patients following a Mediterranean diet for 3 months. In a community-based project, an educational programme with an emphasis on cooking and eating a Mediterranean-type diet found that women in the intervention group reported a healthier dietary intake and showed significant improvement in patient global assessment and pain score at 6 months (McKellar *et al.*, 2007).

Vegetarian and vegan diets

Fasting followed by a vegetarian diet have long been documented to have beneficial effects (Haugen *et al.*, 1999b; Vitetta *et al.*, 2012). Fasting *per se* confers transient immunosuppression (Fraser *et al.*, 1999). Improvement in symptoms of RA, such as duration of morning stiffness, number of tender and swollen joints, and pain, were found in a small systematic review of vegetarian diet adherence (Müller *et al.*, 2001). However, the results could be confounded by the period of fasting prior to the vegetarian diet, which may have dampened inflammatory activity. Strict vegan diets comprising uncooked foods rich in lactobacilli have been reported to improve symptoms, but these studies have not been substantiated by more objective measures of disease activity (Nenonen *et al.*, 1998).

Food intolerance and exclusion diets

The withdrawal of food in patients with RA results in decreased production of the chemical mediators of inflammation; on reintroduction of food, the symptoms return (Buchanan *et al.*, 1991). Similarly, trials of elemental diets in RA patients have provided little objective evidence of benefit, with only temporary improvement in symptoms (Kavanaghi *et al.*, 1995). However, Podas *et al.* (2007) found that adhering to a liquid elemental diet (Elemental 028) for 2 weeks resulted in clinical improvements and was as effective as a course of prednisolone.

Food intolerances have been demonstrated in some RA patients. Commonly reported intolerances include milk, corn, wheat and azo dyes, but there is no evidence that prevalence is greater than in the general population (Buchanan *et al.*, 1991; van de Laar & van der Korst, 1992). Darlington and Ramsey (1993) outlined certain foods that are likely to cause intolerance in a subgroup of RA patients (Table 7.9.5). It must be recognised that this type of dietary manipulation is not universally effective and may cause nutritional deficiencies. Many patients self-impose food restrictions to gain empowerment in the

Table 7.9.5 Foods most likely to cause intolerance in patients with rheumatoid arthritis (Reproduced with permission from Darlington & Ramsey (1993), *Br. J. Rheumatol.* 32: 507–514; Table 1)

Food	Symptomatic patients affected (%)
Corn	57
Wheat	54
Bacon/pork	39
Oranges	39
Milk	37
Oats	37
Rye	34
Eggs	32
Beef	32
Coffee	32
Malt	27
Cheese	24
Grapefruit	24
Tomato	22
Peanuts	20
Sugar	20
Butter	17
Lamb	17
Lemons	17
Soya	17

management of their condition. Goff and Basari (1999) have reported that 67% of RA patients avoided a certain food or a number of foods, most commonly citrus fruit, tomatoes, vinegars, pickles, dairy products, red meat and alcohol. The same authors also highlighted that <5% of RA patients have food allergy; the same as the general population.

The effects of dietary therapy for RA remain unclear (Hagen *et al.*, 2009). Kjeldsen-Kragh (2003) highlighted that recruitment based on lifestyle change, the placebo effect, compliance to a long-term diet, high dropout rates and lack of commercial interests linked to treatment are factors contributing to inconsistent outcome. Nevertheless, in the absence of a specific intervention for RA, dietary advice should focus on achieving optimal nutritional status through a nutritionally balanced and varied eating regime.

Dietary supplements

Antioxidants

A recent systematic review of studies of antioxidants; vitamins A, C and E; and selenium supplements in RA, OA or other inflammatory conditions concluded that there is no robust evidence that antioxidant supplements confer any symptomatic benefit (Canter *et al.*, 2007).

Fatty acids

The potential benefits of changing the combination of fats in the diet of people with RA have been of interest to researchers for many years, particularly increasing the intake of marine-derived long-chain n-3 PUFAs, eicosapentaenoic acid (EPA) and docosahexaenoic acid (DHA) (Adam, 1995). There is strong evidence for the clinical efficacy of n-3 PUFAs. A meta-analysis by Fortin *et al.* (1995) concluded that dietary fish oil supplements for 3 months significantly reduce tender joint count and duration of early morning stiffness. Another meta-analysis of 17 RCTs assessed the pain-relieving effects of n-3 PUFAs in RA and in joint pain secondary to inflammatory bowel disease (Goldberg & Katz, 2007). Supplementation for 3–4 months significantly reduced patient-reported joint pain, minutes of morning stiffness, number of painful and/or tender joints and NSAID consumption. The authors concluded that n-3 PUFAs were a useful adjunctive treatment for the joint pain associated with RA.

Galarraga *et al.* (2008) undertook a randomised, double-blind, placebo-controlled study to determine whether long-chain n-3-rich cod liver oil could reduce the daily NSAID requirement. Results suggested a reduction in medication used without the worsening of disease activity. The key message from this study was that fish oil supplementation should be considered in RA patients to help reduce NSAID intake in order to attenuate the associated risk of gastrointestinal and cardiovascular adverse events. Recently, eating fish twice or more per week is has been associated with lower disease activity in patients (Tedeschi *et al.*, 2018).

Vitamin D

Vitamin D deficiency (defined as ≤53 nmol/L) has been reported in patients with RA, with 26% having severe deficiency (defined as ≤25 nmol/L) (Cecchetti *et al.*, 2016; Haroon *et al.*, 2011). In patients diagnosed with OA and inflammatory joint disease, 62% and 69%, respectively, were deficient in vitamin D. Vitamin D deficiency is associated with severe disease activity and poorer quality-of-life indices in RA patients (Lee & Bae, 2016; Raczkiewicz *et al.*, 2015). Checking vitamin D status is often now part of routine management.

Other supplements

A survey of patients with RA found that half of the respondents took some form of dietary supplement, the most common being cod liver oil. Others included evening primrose oil, iron, garlic, apple cider vinegar, vitamin C, selenium, B vitamins, calcium, general multivitamins and antioxidant supplements (Goff & Basari, 1999): these are not supported by strong evidence of clinical efficacy in symptomatic RA. A systematic review of the extract of New Zealand green lipped mussel found little evidence of efficacy in the management of RA (Cobb & Ernst, 2006). A Cochrane review of herbal interventions compared with placebo in RA found seven studies that indicated benefits of gamma-linoleic acid (GLA) supplementation from evening primrose oil, borage seed oil or blackcurrant seed oil. GLA supplementation resulted in reduced pain intensity and improved disability, but an increase in adverse events, mainly gastrointestinal (Cameron *et al.*, 2011).

SECTION 7

Comorbidities

Cardiovascular disease

Patients with RA are at an increased risk of CVD, especially ischaemic heart disease (IHD) and heart failure, and over 50% of premature deaths in RA are due to CVD (Symmons & Gabriel, 2011). It has been suggested that CVD mortality and morbidity in RA are of similar magnitude to those seen in people with type 2 diabetes mellitus (van Halm *et al.*, 2009). Some of the excess CVD risk might be explained by the adverse impact of the inflammation and immune changes of RA on blood vessel walls (Symmons & Gabriel, 2011).

Obesity

Patients with RA are generally of low body mass index, primarily due to a phenomenon known as rheumatoid cachexia. An increase in proinflammatory cytokines such as tumour necrosis factor (TNF)α and interleukin1β during the active stage of the disease contribute to the loss of lean body mass (Summers *et al.*, 2008). However, recently data from Early Rheumatoid Arthritis Study and Early Rheumatoid Arthritis Network cohorts found a threefold increase in the prevalence of obesity (Nikiphorou *et al.*, 2016). Obesity is linked to poor response to treatment and unlikely to achieve remission (Gremese *et al.*, 2014). Interestingly, the increment of fat-free mass appears to be protective against joint erosion and to decrease mortality; the so-called obesity paradox (George & Baker, 2016). However, this must not be interpreted as being obese is beneficial. Restoring muscle mass and sensible weight loss via exercise is key.

Anaemia

Anaemia is frequently observed in patients with RA; 30–60% of patients, mainly women, are anaemic, which is associated with the advanced stage of the disease (Weiss & Schett, 2013). The aetiology is multifactorial, although anaemia may independently predict joint/bone erosion (Möller *et al.*, 2013).

Osteoporosis and bone erosion

Patients with RA and other forms of inflammatory arthritis are at an elevated risk of developing osteoporosis and bone erosion. This may be due to the adverse effects on bone metabolism from the increased production of proinflammatory cytokines, synovitis or the increasing loss of bone mass caused by corticosteroid treatment. Lack of weight-bearing exercise, insufficient sunlight exposure and poor dietary intake are all detrimental to bone health (see Chapter 7.9.1, Osteoporosis).

Ankylosing spondylitis

AS belongs to a group of diseases known as axial spondyloarthropathies or axial SpA. Similar to RA, it causes systemic inflammation in the eyes, skin and gastrointestinal system. It affects three times more males than females (NHS Choices, 2016); approximately 1 in 12 patients also have inflammatory bowel disease (IBD) (NASS, 2015).

Low-starch diet

Ebringer (1977) first elucidated the molecular mimicry hypothesis in AS, postulating that *Klebsiella* carries a set of sequences resembling HLA-B27, which is a trigger for disease activities in AS. A low-starch diet was proposed to eradicate this microbe in patients, since starch is the main substrate used by *Klebsiella* (Ebringer *et al*., 2016). Advances in sequencing genetic material means new techniques are used to characterise the gut microbiota. Costello and colleagues (2015) used 16s RNA sequencing on biopsies collected from the terminal ileum of AS patients, and found no such association between *Klebsiella* and AS. This is consistent with the study by Stone *et al*. (2004), which casts doubt on the efficacy of low-starch diets.

Furthermore, a systematic review conducted on diet and AS found inconclusive evidence to warrant a dietary change (Macfarlane *et al*., 2018).

Acknowledgement

The editor acknowledges the prior contribution of Dorothy J. Pattison.

Internet resources

Arthritis Action, www.arthritisaction.org.uk
Arthritis and Musculoskeletal Alliance (ARMA), www.arma.uk.net
Versus Arthritis, www.versusarthritis.org
British Society of Rheumatology, www.rheumatology.org.uk
National Ankylosing Spondylitis Society, www.nass.co.uk
National Rheumatoid Arthritis Society, www.nras.org.uk

References

Adam O. (1995) Anti-inflammatory diet in rheumatic diseases. *E.J. Clin. Nutr.* 49: 703–717.

Arthritis Research. (2014) Arthritis in the UK – Facts and Statistics. Available at www.arthritisresearchuk.org/arthritis-information/data-and-statistics.aspx. Accessed 10 August 2016.

Aspden RM. (2011) Obesity punches above its weight in osteoarthritis. *Nat. Rev. Rheumatol.* 7: 65–68.

Atukorala I, Makovey J, Lawler L, *et al.* (2016) Is there a dose response relationship between weight loss and symptom improvement in persons with knee osteoarthritis? *Arthritis Care Res. (Hoboken)*. 68(8): 1106–1114.

Bay- Jensen A, Slagboom E, Chen-An P *et al.* (2012) Role of hormones in cartilage and joint metabolism: understanding an unhealthy phenotype in osteoarthritis. *Menopause: the Journal of the North American Menopause Society* 20(5): 578–586.

Berenbaum F, Eymard F, Houard X. (2013) Osteoarthritis, inflammation and obesity. *Curr. Opin. Rheumatol.* 25(1): 114–118.

Berube LT, Kiely M, Yazici Y *et al.* (2017) Diet quality of individuals with rheumatoid arthritis using the Healthy Eating Index (HEI)-2010. *Nutrition and Health* 23:17–24.

Bijlsma J, Berenbaum F, Lafeber F. (2011) Osteoarthritis: an update with relevance for clinical practice. *Lancet.* 377(9783): 2115–2126.

Bliddal H, Leeds A, Stigsgaard L, *et al.* (2011) Weight loss as treatment for knee osteoarthritis symptoms in obese patients: 1 year results from a randomized controlled trial. *Ann. Rheum. Dis.* 70: 1798–1803.

Boe C, Vangsness CT. (2015) Fish Oil and Osteoarthritis: Current Evidence. *Am. J. Orthop. (Belle Mead NJ)* 44(7): 302–305.

Buchanan HM, Preston PM, Brooks PM, *et al.* (1991) Is diet important in rheumatoid arthritis? *Br. J. Rheumatol.* 30: 125–134.

Cameron M, Gagnier JJ, Chrubasik S. (2011) Herbal therapy for treating rheumatoid arthritis. *Cochrane Database of Systematic Reviews* Issue 2. Art. No.: CD002948.

Canter PH, Wider B, Ernst E. (2007) The antioxidant vitamins A, C, E and selenium in the treatment of arthritis: systematic review of randomised controlled trials. *Rheumatology (Oxford)*. 46: 1223–1233.

Castañeda S, Roman-Blas J, Largo R, *et al.* (2014) Osteoarthritis: a progressive disease with changing phenotypes. *Rheumatology (Oxford)*. 53(1):1–3.

Cecchetti S, Tatar Z, Galan P, *et al.* (2016) Prevalence of vitamin D deficiency in rheumatoid arthritis and association with disease activity and cardiovascular risk factors: data from the COMEDRA study. *Clin. Exp. Rheumatol.* 34(6): 984c990.

Christensen R, Bartels EM, Altman RD *et al.* (2008) Does the hip powder of *Rosa canina* (rosehip) reduce pain in osteoarthritis patients? – A meta-analysis of randomized controlled trials. *Osteoarthritis and Cartilage* 16(9):965–972.

Cobb CS, Ernst E. (2006) Systematic review of marine nutriceutical supplement in clinical trials for arthritis: the effectiveness of the New Zealand green-lipped mussel Perna canaliculus. *Clin. Rheumatol.* 25: 275–284.

Conaghan PG, Porcheret M, Kingsbury SR *et al.* (2014) Impact and therapy of osteoarthritis: the Arthritis Care OA Nation 2012 survey. *Clin. Rheumatol.* 34(9)

Costello M-E, Ciccia F, Willner D, *et al.* (2015) Brief report: intestinal dysbiosis in ankylosing spondylitis. *Arthritis Rheumatol.* 67: 686–691.

Cronstein BN. (2007) Interleukin-6 – a key mediator of systemic and local symptoms in rheumatoid arthritis. *Bull. NYU Hosp. J. Dis.* 65(1): S11–S15.

Daily J, Yang M, Park S. (2016) Efficacy of turmeric extracts and curcumin for alleviating the symptoms of joint arthritis: a systemic review and meta-analysis of randomized clinical trials. *J. Med. Food.* 19(8): 717–729.

Darlington, LG, Ramsey, NW (1993) Review of dietary therapy for rheumatoid arthritis. *Br. J. Rheum.* 32, 507– 514.

Dyer J, Davison G, Marcora S, *et al.* (2016) Effect of a Mediterranean type diet on inflammatory and cartilage degradation biomarkers in patients with osteoarthritis. *J. Nutr. Health. Ageing.* 21: 562–566. doi:10.1007/s12603-016-0806-y

Ebringer R, Cooke D, Cawdell DR, et al. (1977) Ankylosing spondylitis: *Klebsiella* and HL-A B27. *Rheumatol. Rehabil.* 16(3):190–196.

Ebringer A, Rashid T, Wilson C. (2016) Ankylosing spondylitis, *Klebsiella* and the low starch diet in the human microbiota and chronic disease: In: Nibali L, Henderson B (eds) *Dysbiosis as a Cause of Human Pathology*. Oxford: John Wiley & Sons, pp. 317–325.

Felson D. (1995) Weight and osteoarthritis. *J. Rheumatol. Suppl.* 43: 7–9.

Felson D. (2010) Identifying different osteoarthritis phenotypes through epidemiology. *Osteoarthritis Cartilage.* 18: 601–604.

Felson D, Lawrence R, Dieppe P, *et al.* (2000) Osteoarthritis: new insights. Part 1: the disease and its risk factors. *Ann. Intern. Med.* 133: 635–646.

Fortin PR, Lew RA, Liang MH, *et al.* (1995) Validation of a meta analysis: the effects of fish oil in rheumatoid arthritis. *J. Clin. Epidemiol.* 48: 1379–1390.

Fraser DA, Thoen J, Reseland JE, *et al.* (1999) Decreased CD4+ lymphocyte activation and increased interleukin-4 production in peripheral blood of rheumatoid arthritis patients after acute starvation. *Clin. Rheumatol.* 18(5): 394–401.

Galarraga B, Ho M, Youssef HM, *et al.* (2008) Cod liver oil (n-3 fatty acids) as a non-steroidal anti-inflammatory drug sparing agent in rheumatoid arthritis. *Rheumatology (Oxford)*. 47: 665–669.

George M, Baker J. (2016) The obesity epidemic and consequences for rheumatoid arthritis care. *Curr. Rheumatol. Rep.* 18(1): 6. doi: 10.1007/s11926-015-0550-z.

Goff LM, Basari M. (1999) An assessment of the diets of people with rheumatoid arthritis. *J. Hum. Nutr. Diet.* 12: 93–101.

Goldberg RJ, Katz J. (2007) A meta-analysis of the analgesic effects of omega-3 polyunsaturated fatty acid supplementation for inflammatory joint pain. *Pain.* 129: 210–223.

Gremese E, Tolusso B, Gigante M, *et al.* (2014) Obesity as a risk and severity factor in rheumatic diseases (Autoimmune Chronic Inflammatory Diseases). *Front. Immunol.* 5(576): 1–10.

Guilak F. (2012) Biomechanical factors in osteoarthritis. *Best Pract. Res. Clin. Rheumatol.* 25(6): 815–823.

Hagen KB, Byfuglien MG, Falzon L, *et al.* (2009) The effect of diets on rheumatoid arthritis. *Cochrane Database Syst. Rev.* (1): CD006400. doi: 10.1002/14651858.CD006400.pub2.

Hannan M, Felson D, Pincus T. (2000) Analysis of discordance between radiographic changes and knee pain in osteoarthritis of the knee. *J. Rheumatol.* 27(6): 1513–1517.

Haroon M, Bond U, Quillinan N, *et al.* (2011) The prevalence of vitamin D deficiency in consecutive new patients seen over a 6-month period in general rheumatology clinics. *Clin. Rheumatol.* 30: 789–794.

Haugen M, Homme KA, Reigstad A, *et al.* (1999a) Assessment of nutritional status in patients with rheumatoid arthritis and osteoarthritis undergoing joint replacement surgery. *Arthritis Care Res.* 12: 26–32.

Haugen M, Fraser D, Førre Ø. (1999b) Diet therapy for the patient with rheumatoid arthritis. *Rheumatology. (Oxford).* 38(11): 1039–1044.

Hill C, March L, Aitken D, *et al.* (2015) Fish oil in knee osteoarthritis: a randomised clinical trial of low dose versus high dose. *Ann. Rheum. Dis.* 75: 3–9.

Kavanaghi R, Workman E, Nash P, *et al.* (1995) The effects of elemental diet and subsequent food reintroduction on rheumatoid arthritis. *Br. J. Rheumatol.* 34: 270–273.

Kjeldsen-Kragh J (2003) Mediterranean diet intervention in rheumatoid arthritis. *Ann Rheum Dis.* 62(3): 193–195.

Lee YH, Bae SC. (2016) Vitamin D level in rheumatoid arthritis and its correlation with the disease activity: a meta-analysis. *Clin. Exp. Rheumatol.* 34(5): 827–833.

Long L, Soeken K, Ernst E. (2001) Herbal medicines for the treatment of osteoarthritis: a systematic review. *Rheumatology.* 40: 779–793.

Lu B, Driban J, Duryea J, *et al.* (2014) Milk consumption and progression of medial tibiofemoral knee osteoarthritis: data from the osteoarthritis initiative. *Arthritis Care Res.* 66(6): 802–809.

Lu B, Driban J, Chang XU, et al. (2011) Dietary fat intake and radiographic progression of knee osteoarthritis initiative. *Arthritis Care Res.* 69(3): 368–375.

Macfarlane T, Abbood H, Pathan E, *et al.* (2018) Relationship between diet and ankylosing spondylitis: a systematic review. *Eur. J. Rheumatol.* 5(1): 45–52.

McKellar G, Morrison E, McEntegart A, *et al.* (2007) A pilot study of a Mediterranean-type diet intervention in female patients with rheumatoid arthritis living in areas of social deprivation in Glasgow. *Ann. Rheum. Dis.* 66: 1239–1243.

Messier SP, Gutekunst D, Davis C. (2005) Weight loss reduces knee-joint loads in overweight and obese older adults with knee osteoarthritis. *Arthritis. Rheum.* 52(7): 2062–2032.

Möller B, Scherer A, Førger F, *et al.* (2013) Anaemia may add information to standardised disease activity assessment to predict radiographic damage in rheumatoid arthritis: a prospective cohort study. *Ann. Rheum. Dis.* 73: 691–696.

Mooney RA, Sampson ER, Lerea J, *et al.* (2011) High-fat diet accelerates progression of osteoarthritis after meniscal/ligamentous injury. *Arthritis Res. Ther.* 13: R198.

Morgan SL, Anderson AM, Hood SM, *et al.* (1997) Nutrient intake patterns, body mass index and vitamin levels in patients with rheumatoid arthritis. *Arthritis Care Res.* 10: 9–17.

Müller H, de Toledo FW, Resch KL. (2001) Fasting followed by vegetarian diet in patients with rheumatoid arthritis: a systematic review. *Scand. J. Rheumatol.* 30: 1–10.

National Ankylosing Spondylitis Society (NASS). (2015) *Ankylosing Spondylitis. Guidebook: Answers and Practical Advice.* London: NASS.

Nenonen MT, Helve TA, Rauma AL, *et al.* (1998) Uncooked, lactobacilli-rich, vegan food and rheumatoid arthritis. *Br. J. Rheumatol.* 37: 274–281.

NHS Choices. (2016) Ankylosing Spondylitis. Available at www.nhs.uk/Conditions/Ankylosing-spondylitis/Pages/Introduction.aspx. Accessed on 7 November 2016.

NICE. (2009) Rheumatoid arthritis in adults: management (CG79). Available https://www.nice.org.uk/Guidance/CG79. Accessed 1 November 2018.

NICE. (2014) *Osteoarthritis: The Care and Management of Osteoarthritis in Adults. NICE Clinical Guideline 59.* Available at https://www.nice.org.uk/guidance/cg177. Accessed 2 May 2017.

NICE. (2015) *Rheumatoid Arthritis: The Management of Rheumatoid Arthritis in Adults. NICE Clinical Guideline 79.* Available at https://www.nice.org.uk/guidance/cg79. Accessed 2 May 2017.

Nikiphorou E, Demetriou C, Norton S, *et al.* (2015) The impact of comorbidities and extra-articular manifestations on 10-Year mortality risk in rheumatoid arthritis. Results from two multi-centre UK inception cohorts. *Ann. Rheum. Dis.* 74: 690–691.

Nikiphorou E, Norton S, Carpenter L, *et al.* (2016) Secular changes in clinical features at presentation of rheumatoid arthritis: Increase in comorbidity but improved inflammatory states. *Arthritis. Care. Res. (Hoboken).* 69: 21–27.

National Rheumatoid Arthritis Society (NRAS). (2017) What Is RA? Available at https://www.nras.org.uk/what-is-ra- Accessed 12 May 2017.

Perry L, Mosler C, Atkins A. (2014) Cardiovascular risk associated with NSAIDS and COX-2 inhibitors. *US Pharmacist.* 39(3): 35–38.

Podas T, Nightingale JM, Oldham R, *et al.* (2007) Is rheumatoid arthritis a disease that starts in the intestine? A pilot study comparing an elemental diet with oral prednisolone. *Postgrad. Med. J.* 83(976): 128–131.

Raczkiewicz A, Bartłomiej K, Maciej K, *et al.* (2015) Vitamin D status and its association with quality of life, physical activity, and disease activity in rheumatoid arthritis patients. *J. Clin. Rheumatol.* 21(3): 26–130.

Rao JK, Mihaliak K, Kroenke K, *et al.* (1999) Use of complementary therapies for arthritis among patients of rheumatologists. *Ann. Intern. Med.* 131: 409–416.

Rayman M, Pattison DJ. (2008) Dietary manipulation in musculoskeletal conditions. *Best Pract. Res. Clin. Rheumatol.* 22(3): 535–561.

Sköldstam L, Hagfors L, Johansson G. (2003) An experimental study of a Mediterranean diet intervention for patients with rheumatoid arthritis. *Ann. Rheum. Dis.* 62: 208–214.

Stone J, Doube A, Dudson D, *et al.* (1997) Inadequate calcium, folic acid, vitamin E, zinc and selenium intake in rheumatoid arthritis patients: results of a dietary survey. *Semin. Arthritis Rheum.* 27: 180–185.

Stone MA, Payne U, Schentag C, *et al.* (2004) Comparative immune responses to candidate arthritogenic bacteria do not confirm a dominant role for *Klebsiella* pneumonia in the pathogenesis of familial ankylosing spondylitis. *Rheumatology. (Oxford).* 43: 148–155.

Summers G, Deighton C, Rennie M, *et al.* (2008) Rheumatoid cachexia: a clinical perspective. *Rheumatology. (Oxford).* 47: 1124–1134.

Symmons DPM, Gabriel SE. (2011) Epidemiology of CVD in rheumatic disease, with a focus on RA and SLE. *Nat. Rev. Rheumatol.* 7: 399–408.

Symmons D, Turner G, Webb R, *et al.* (2002) The prevalence of rheumatoid arthritis in the United Kingdom: new estimates for a new century. *Rheumatology. (Oxford).* 41(7): 793–800.

Tedeschi S, Bathon J, Giles J, *et al.* (2018) Relationship between fish consumption and disease activity in rheumatoid arthritis. *Arthritis Care. Res. (Hoboken).* 70(3): 327–332.

Toda Y, Toda T, Takemura S, *et al.* (1998) Change in body fat, but not body weight or metabolic correlates of obesity, is related to symptomatic relief of obese patients with knee osteoarthritis after a weight control program. *J. Rheumatol.* 25: 2181–2186.

van de Laar MA, van der Korst JK. (1992) Food intolerance in rheumatoid arthritis. I. A double-blind, controlled trial of the clinical effects of the elimination of milk allergens and azo dyes. *Ann. Rheum. Dis.* 51: 298–302.

van der Esch M, Knoop J, van der Leeden M, *et al.* (2015) Clinical phenotypes in patients with knee osteoarthritis: a study in the Amsterdam osteoarthritis cohort. *Osteoarthritis Cartilage.* 23: 544–549.

van Halm VP, Peters MJ, Voskuyl AE, *et al.* (2009) Rheumatoid arthritis versus diabetes as a risk factor for cardiovascular disease: a cross-sectional study, the CARRE Investigation. *Ann. Rheum. Dis.* 68: 1395–1400.

Vincent HK, Heywood K, Connelly J, *et al.* (2012) Obesity and weight loss in the treatment and prevention of osteoarthritis. *PM R.* 4: S59–S67.

Vitetta L, Coulson S, Schloss J, *et al.* (2012) Dietary recommendations for patients with rheumatoid arthritis: a review. *Nutr. Diet. Suppl.* 4: 1–15.

Vos T, Flaxman A, Naghavi M, *et al.* (2012) Years lived with disability (YLDs) for 1160 sequelae of diseases and injuries 1990–2010: a systematic analysis for the Global Burden of Disease Study 2010. *Lancet.* 380: 2163–2196.

Weiss G, Schett G (2012) Anaemia in inflammatory rheumatic disease. *Nat. Rev. Rheumatol.* 9(4):205–215.

Wiles N, Symmons DPM, Harrison B, *et al.* (1999) Estimating the incidence of rheumatoid arthritis – trying to hit a moving target? *Arthritis Rheum.* 42(7): 1339–1346.

Zhang W, Likhodii S, Zhang Y, *et al.* (2014) Classification of osteoarthritis phenotypes by metabolomics analysis. *BMJ Open* 4(11): e006286. Available at http://bmjopen.bmj.com/content/4/11/e006286.full. Accessed on 5 October 2016.

7.9.3 Gout

Martin Lau

Key points

- Gout is a common form of inflammatory arthritis and is associated with serious comorbidities.
- Dietary or lifestyle modifications only have a small urate-lowering effect.
- Recommendations for gout management include patient education, weight management, exercise and activity, and adequate hydration.
- Dietetic advice should be tailored to manage accompanied comorbidities.

Gout is the most painful (acute) and yet common form of inflammatory arthritis, generally affecting men aged ≥40 years and women aged >65 years (Roddy & Doherty, 2010). This disease is associated with serious comorbidity such as obesity, diabetes, hypertension and cardiovascular diseases. The pathogenesis of gout is well understood; it is a true crystal deposition disease. The amount of uric acid (metabolite of purines) depends on the balance of synthesis, dietary intake and excretion (Choi, 2010). Impaired excretion of uric acid and/or overproduction will raise uric acid levels (Choi *et al.*, 2005). Chronic high levels of uric acid above the saturation threshold (380 μmol/L) result in hyperuricacidaemia. Although present in most gout patients, many with hyperuricacidaemia do not develop gout, and the urate level can be normal during an attack (Warburton, 2012). Hyperuricacidaemia, coupled with other risk factors such as physical stress, lower pH, genetics, dietary issues, and treatments of co-morbidity (e.g. diuretics), lead to the formation of monosodium urate (MSU) crystals, which precipitate in and around joints. Gout occurs when these crystals shed into the joint space causing inflammation, swelling and severe attacks of pain.

The incidence of gout in the UK is 2.68 per 1000 person years (4.42 in men and 1.32 in women) (Cea Soriano *et al.*, 2011), and the number is rising (Kuo *et al.*, 2015). Prevalence increases with age; 7% of men aged 75–84 years are affected (Mikuls *et al.*, 2005). This figure varies between countries and populations, with New Zealand Maoris having a particularly high prevalence (6.4%). This variation is probably due to genetic, environmental and dietary factors.

Diagnosis

Severe pain, swelling and erythema over a joint are strongly suggestive, but not diagnostic, of gout. A clinical diagnosis should be confirmed by demonstration of MSU crystals in the synovial fluid of the joint (Zhang *et al.*, 2006a). In chronic gout, large crystal deposits may form on joints (tophi), and joints may become eroded (Schumacher, 2008). The metatarsophalangeal joint (MTPJ), the joint between the big toe and ball of the foot, is most commonly affected. The frequency of an initial attack of MTPJ is >80% (Roddy 2011), and it is likely to reoccur during the course of the disease.

Risk factors and comorbidities

Dietary factors

An association between diet and gout has been recognised anecdotally for many years. This has now been confirmed in large, well-designed epidemiological studies. Consumption of seafood and meat are associated with relative risks (RRs) for gout of 1.51 and 1.41, respectively (Choi *et al.*, 2004a). There is no association with total protein intake or purine-rich vegetables (Lee *et al.*, 2006). Low-fat dairy products and coffee have been found to be protective (Choi *et al.*, 2007a). The RR of gout for participants drinking two or more sugar-sweetened soft drinks is 1.85; this was similar for fructose consumption, although there was no increased risk associated with the consumption of diet soft drinks (Choi & Curhan, 2008). Vitamin C may be protective, with RR being reduced to 0.55 in those who consumed >1500 mg of dietary vitamin C/day as compared to those consuming <250 mg/day (Choi *et al.*, 2009).

Alcohol

Alcohol consumption has a graded relationship, the highest risk being beer, followed by spirit (Choi *et al.*, 2004b). Women who are heavy drinkers have a threefold higher risk of developing gout than abstinent or light drinkers (Bhole *et al.*, 2010). There is also a dose-dependent relationship between an acute gout attack and the amount of alcohol consumed in the preceding 48 hours (Zhang *et al.*, 2006b).

Metabolic syndrome

There is an association between gout and the metabolic syndrome and its individual components (obesity, hypertension, type 2 diabetes and dyslipidaemia). In the NHANES, the prevalence of metabolic syndrome among patients with gout was 62.8%, as compared to 25.4% in the age- and gender-matched groups without gout (Choi *et al.*, 2007b). Primatesta *et al.* (2011) reported that 58.1% of gout patients have one or more of the comorbidities of metabolic syndrome: diabetes (15.1%), dyslipidaemia (27.0%) and hypertension (36.1%) were the most common. The presence of these comorbidities was associated with increased risk of an acute attack; women are particularly vulnerable. Gout is associated with an increased risk of myocardial infarction (Kuo *et al.*, 2013), heart failure and cardiac-associated mortality (Krishnan, 2012). Dietetic management of the components of metabolic syndrome is becoming increasingly important.

Diuretic use

There is an association between the use of diuretics and gout, although this relationship is confounded by the reason for diuretics (e.g. hypertension), which may also increase the risk of gout (Choi *et al.*, 2005; Mikuls *et al.*, 2005). There is some evidence to suggest that diuretic use may be associated with acute gout attacks (Hunter *et al.*, 2006).

Renal disease

Chronic renal disease greatly increases the risk of gout (Mikuls *et al.*, 2005), as does dialysis and transplantation.

Osteoarthritis

There is evidence to suggest enhanced deposition of MSU crystals at sites of cartilage damage in osteoarthritis (Bevis *et al.*, 2016; Roddy, 2011).

Clinical management

There are three stages of gout (Warburton, 2012):

- Asymptomatic hyperuricemia.
- Acute gout and intercritical period.
- Chronic tophaceous gout.

Acute episodes of gout are managed with non-steroidal anti-inflammatory drugs or colchicine. Once the acute phase has subsided, the condition can be controlled with urate-lowering therapy such as treatment with allopurinol.

Dietary and lifestyle management

There is a paucity of evidence from large, well-designed studies to support the use of dietary modifications and lifestyle management (Moi *et al.*, 2013). Furthermore, adhering to diet and lifestyle advice only has a small uric acid–lowering effect (1 mg/dL) (Burns & Wortman, 2012; Jordan, 2012; Holland & McGill, 2015). Overall weight loss has been found to be most effective in lowering uric acid (Richette *et al.*, 2016; Zhu *et al.*, 2010). A high-protein (30%), reduced-carbohydrate (40%) and reduced-energy regimen (1600 kcal/day) showed a weight loss of 7.7 kg and a significant reduction in monthly gout attacks (Dessein *et al.*, 2000). The use of fad or crash diets as well as ketosis and fasting is strongly discouraged, as they may worsen hyperuricemia and induce gout attacks (Fam, 2002; Lee *et al.*, 2006).

Guidelines for the management of gout, such as the American College of Rheumatology (ACR) (Khanna *et al.*, 2012), the European League Against Rheumatism (EULAR) (Richette *et al.*, 2017) and the British Society for Rheumatology (BSR) (Hui *et al.*, 2017), have attributed some importance to reducing risk factors for comorbidities by dietary and lifestyle modification, including the metabolic syndrome and its components, insulin resistance, type 2 diabetes (see Chapter 7.12, Diabetes mellitus), dyslipidaemia (see Chapter 7.14.3, Dyslipidaemia), hypertension (see Chapter 7.14.4, Hypertension) and obesity (see Chapter 7.13.2, The management of obesity and overweight in adults) (Khanna *et al.*, 2012). The recommendations of the ACR are summarised in Table 7.9.6. The dietary recommendation of the 2017 BSR guideline is very similar to the ACR. Evidence from a case-crossover trial showed that consuming cherries or drinking its juice may reduce gout flares (Zhang *et al.*, 2012).

Table 7.9.6 General health, diet and lifestyle recommendations for patients with gout (modified from Khanna *et al.*, 2012)

Weight loss for obese/overweight patients to achieve a BMI that promotes general health Healthy overall diet Exercise (achieve physical fitness) Smoking cessation Stay well hydrated		
Avoid	**Limit**	**Encourage**
Organ meats (offal) high in purines, e.g. liver, kidney, sweetbreads	Serving sizes of: Beef, lamb, pork Seafood with high purine content, e.g. sardines, shellfish, anchovies, fish roe, mackerel, sprats, whitebait	Low-fat or non-fat dairy products
High fructose corn syrup–sweetened fizzy drinks, other beverages or foods	Serving of naturally sweetened fruit juice Table sugar, sweetened beverages and desserts Table salt Sauces, gravies Meat and yeast extracts Quorn	Vegetables[a]
Alcohol >2 units/day in men and >1 unit/ day in women in all gout patients	Alcohol, particularly beer, but also wine and spirits in all gout patients	
Any alcohol during periods of frequent gout attacks or poorly controlled advanced gout		

[a] Some vegetables are moderate sources of purines, e.g. asparagus, cauliflower and spinach; however, there is no convincing evidence to recommend their avoidance.

Acknowledgement

The editor acknowledges the prior contribution of Joan Gandy.

Internet resources

Arthritis Action, www.arthritisaction.org.uk
Arthritis and Musculoskeletal Alliance (ARMA), www.arma.uk.net
Versus Arthritis, www.versusarthritis.org
British Society for Rheumatology, www.rheumatology.org.uk
UK Gout Society, www.ukgoutsociety.org

References

Bevis M, Marshall M, Rathod T, *et al.* (2016) The association between gout and radiographic hand, knee and foot osteoarthritis: a cross-sectional study. *BMC Musculoskele. Disord.* 17: 169.

Bhole V, Vera M, Rahman MM, *et al.* (2010) Epidemiology of gout in women: fifty-two-year follow up of a prospective cohort. *Arthritis Rheum.* 62: 1069–1076.

Burns C, Wortmann R. (2012) Latest evidence on gout management: what the clinician needs to know. *Ther. Adv. Chronic Dis.* 3(6): 271–286.

Cea Soriano L, Rothenbacher D, Choi HK, *et al.* (2011) Contemporary epidemiology of gout in the UK general population. *Arthritis Res. Ther.* 13: R39.

Choi H. (2010) A prescription for lifestyle change in patients with hyperuricemia and gout. *Curr. Opin. Rheumatol.* 22(2): 165–172.

Choi HK, Curhan G. (2008) Soft drinks, fructose consumption, and the risk of gout in men: prospective cohort study. *BMJ.* 336: 309–312.

Choi HK, Atkinson K, Karlson EW, *et al.* (2004a) Purine-rich foods, dairy and protein intake, and the risk of gout in men. *N. Engl. J. Med.* 350: 1093–1103.

Choi HK, Atkinson K, Karlson EW, *et al.* (2004b) Alcohol intake and risk of incident gout in men: a prospective study. *Lancet.* 363: 1277–1281.

Choi HK, Atkinson K, Karlson EW, *et al.* (2005) Obesity, weight change, hypertension, diuretic use, and risk of gout in men: the health professionals follow-up study. *Arch. Intern. Med.* 165: 742–748.

Choi HK, Willett W, Curhan G. (2007a) Coffee consumption and risk of incident gout in men: a prospective study. *Arthritis. Rheum.* 56: 2049–2055.

Choi HK, Ford ES, Li C, *et al.* (2007b) Prevalence of the metabolic syndrome in patients with gout. *Arthritis. Rheum.* 57: 109–115.

Choi HK, Gao X, Curhan G. (2009) Vitamin C intake and the risk of gout in men: a prospective study. *Arch. Intern. Med.* 169: 502–507.

Dessein P, Shipton E, Stanwix A, *et al.* (2000) Beneficial effects of weight loss associated with moderate calorie/carbohydrate restriction, and increased proportional intake of protein and unsaturated fat on serum urate and lipoprotein levels in gout: A pilot study. *Ann. Rheum. Dis.* 59: 539–543.

Fam A. (2002) Gout, diet and the insulin resistance syndrome. *J. Rheumatol.* 29(7): 1350–1355.

Holland R, McGill NW. (2015) Comprehensive dietary education in treated gout patients does not further improve serum urate. *Intern. Med. J.* 45: 189–194.

Hui M, Carr A, Cameron S, et al. (2017) The British Society for Rheumatology Guideline for the Management of Gout. *Rheumatol.* 56(7): e1–e20.

Hunter DJ, York M, Chaisson CE, *et al.* (2006) Recent diuretic use and the risk of recurrent gout attacks: the online case-crossover gout study. *J. Rheumatol.* 33(7): 1341–1345.

Jordan KM (2012) Up-to-date management of gout. *Curr. Opin. Rheumatol.* 24(2): 145–151.

Khanna D, Fitzgerald JD, Khanna PP, *et al.* (2012) American College of Rheumatology Guidelines for Management of Gout. Part 1: Systematic Nonpharmacologic and Pharmacologic Therapeutic Approaches to Hyperuricemia. *Arthritis Care Res.* 64: 1431–1446.

Krishnan E. (2012) Gout and the risk for incident heart failure and systolic dysfunction. *BMJ Open* 2: e000282.

Kuo CF, Yu KH, See LC, *et al.* (2013) Risk of myocardial infarction among patients with gout: a nationwide population-based study. *Rheumatology. (Oxford).*52(1): 111–117.

Kuo CF, Grainge MJ, Mallen C, *et al.* (2015) Rising burden of gout in the UK but continuing suboptimal management: a nationwide population study. *Ann. Rheum. Dis.* 74: 661–667.

Lee S, Terkeltaub R, Kavanaugh A. (2006) Recent developments in diet and gout. *Curr. Opin. Rheumatol.* 18(2): 193–198.

Mikuls TR, Farrar JT, Bilker WB, *et al.* (2005) Gout epidemiology: results from the UK General Practice Research Database, 1990–1999. *Ann. Rheum. Dis.* 64: 267–272.

Moi J, Sriranganathan M, Edwards C, *et al.* (2013) Lifestyle interventions for chronic gout. *Cochrane Database Syst Rev.* Available at http://onlinelibrary.wiley.com/doi/10.1002/14651858.CD010039.pub2/epdf. Accessed on 2 December 2016.

Primatesta P, Plana E, Rothenbacher D. (2011) Gout treatment and comorbidities: a retrospective cohort study in a large US managed care population. *BMC Musculoskelet. Disord.* 12: 103–109.

Richette P, Poitou C, Manivet P, *et al.* (2016) Weight loss, xanthine oxidase and serum urate levels: a prospective, longitudinal study of obese patients. *Arthritis Care Res. (Hoboken).* 68: 1036–1042.

Richette P, Doherty M, Pascual E, *et al.* (2017) 2016 updated EULAR evidence-based recommendations for the management of gout. *Annals of the Rheumatic Diseases* 76: 29–42.

Roddy E. (2011) Revisiting the pathogenesis of podagra: why does gout target the foot? *J. Foot Ankle. Res.* 4: 13. doi: 10.1186/1757-1146-4-13.

Roddy E, Doherty M. (2010) Epidemiology of gout. *Arthritis Res. Ther.* 12(6): 223.

Schumacher HR Jr. (2008) The pathogenesis of gout. *Cleve. Clin. J. Med.* 75(5): S2–4.

Warburton L. (2012) *Guidelines: Why Is Gout So Difficult to Treat?* Available at http://www.gponline.com/guidelines-why-gout-so-difficult-treat/article/1159461. Accessed 30 November 2016.

Zhang W, Doherty M, Pascual E, *et al.* (2006a) EULAR evidence-based recommendations for gout. Part I: Diagnosis. Report of a task force of the Standing Committee for International Clinical Studies Including Therapeutics (ESCISIT). *Ann. Rheum. Dis.* 65(10): 1301–1311.

Zhang Y, Woods R, Chaisson CE, *et al.* (2006b) Alcohol consumption as a trigger of recurrent gout attacks. *Am. J. Med.* 119: 800–808.

Zhang Y, Neogi T, Chen C, *et al.* (2012) Cherry consumption and decreased risk of recurrent gout attacks. *Arthritis Rheum.* 64(12): 4004–4011. doi: 10.1002/art.34677.

Zhu Y, Zhang Y, Choi HK. (2010) The serum urate-lowering impact of weight loss among men with a high cardiovascular risk profile: the Multiple Risk Factor Intervention Trial. *Rheumatology (Oxford).* 49: 2391–2399.

7.10 Mental health

7.10.1 Nutrition and mental health

Ursula Philpot

Key points

- Emerging evidence suggests that nutrition has a key role in mental health.
- The number of dietitians working in mental health is rapidly increasing.
- People with a severe mental illness are at greater risk of developing physical health problems.
- Dietitians may be managed by non-dietitians; therefore, they must articulate their key skills and be clear about their professional boundaries, duties, roles and responsibilities.

Mental health is defined by the World Health Organization (WHO, 2014) as '*a state of well-being in which every individual realizes his or her own potential, can cope with normal stresses of life, can work productively and is able to make a contribution to her or his community*'. Approximately one in four people in Britain has the diagnosis of a mental disorder or mental illness (McManus *et al.*, 2009). This is defined as a psychological or behavioural pattern associated with distress or a disability that is not a part of normal development or culture. Mental health disorders are experienced as problems with emotions, behaviours, thoughts or perceptions. The disorders can significantly affect all areas of someone's life, from problems with day-to-day functioning through to those with relationships, work and quality of life. The most common mental health disorders in the UK are depression and anxiety. Disease states such as cardiovascular disease (CVD), dyslipidaemia, high blood pressure, metabolic syndrome, type 2 diabetes and obesity are more common in people with mental illness. People with schizophrenia and bipolar disorder have 24 times the rate of CVD and five times the rate of type 2 diabetes than the general population (de Hert *et al.*, 2011).

A move towards improving the physical health of people with mental health conditions has led to growing numbers of dietetic roles within mental health settings in the UK (Kings Fund Report, 2016). Numbers vary greatly across regions, but common areas of employment include eating disorders, secure units, autism, older adults and dementia care, learning disabilities, forensic services and healthy living teams.

Causes of mental distress

There are many theories about the causes of mental distress. One view is that personality is shaped by both life experiences and genetics. This means that some people may become more vulnerable to mental health problems than others through a combination of upbringing and life events, combined with genetic factors. The following are a range of possible causes of mental distress.

Difficult family background

Growing up in an environment where feelings are not validated or spoken about, feeling uncared for or scared by a parent, or having been or are being abused in some way can affect the development of children and leave them insecure and vulnerable to mental distress. Conversely, being overprotected as a child is also a risk factor.

Hidden feelings

If children are punished for getting angry, crying or laughing too loudly, they learn that they should not feel strong emotions. This leaves them feeling bad and out of

Manual of Dietetic Practice, Sixth Edition. Edited by Joan Gandy.

Companion website: www.manualofdieteticpractice.com

control when emotions are experienced, thus leading to behaviours that try to suppress emotions, such as eating disorders, or drug or alcohol misuse.

Stressful life events

These may be traumatic events, such as the death of someone close, or longer-term struggles, such as being the victim of some form of harassment or oppression.

Biochemistry

Biochemistry can affect mood, e.g. a stressful or frightening situation will trigger the body's fight-or-flight response and drive the body to produce adrenaline. If physical activity does not use all the adrenaline, the body remains tense and the mind stays overactive.

Genetics

There is a genetic component to the risk factors for the development of disorders such as bipolar disorder, schizophrenia or eating disorders. This may be either direct or through personality traits, such as perfectionism, which may have a genetic basis.

Mental health disorders seen by dietitians

The most common mental health disorders that require dietetic input are:

- Schizophrenia.
- Depression.
- Alzheimer's disease.
- Obsessive–compulsive disorder (OCD).
- Anxiety or panic and phobias.
- Drug and alcohol problems.
- Personality disorders.
- Eating disorders (see Chapter 7.10.2, Eating disorders).
- Post-traumatic stress disorder (PTSD).
- Learning disabilities (see Chapter 3.7, People with learning disabilities).
- Bipolar disorder.

Schizophrenia

Schizophrenia is a mental illness that can severely interfere with abilities to perform everyday tasks and activities, caused by confusion and withdrawal. Symptoms can include hearing voices and seeing things that other people cannot.

Depression and anxiety

Depression and anxiety are the most common psychiatric illnesses and are increasing in prevalence worldwide (McManus *et al.*, 2009). Depression is characterised by feelings of sadness and hopelessness that interfere with normal day-to-day life. Anxiety is characterised by restlessness, with difficulty concentrating or controlling worry, and sleep problems such as problems falling or staying asleep. Both are thought to result from an imbalance of the neurotransmitters that carry messages between brain cells. This can be disturbed by many factors including stress, trauma, relationship breakdown or hormonal changes, or as a side effect of some types of medications such as steroids. Genetic influences on brain function may make some people more susceptible to depression and anxiety (Breen *et al.*, 2011).

Personality disorders

The term personality disorder refers to a diagnostic category of psychiatric disorders characterised by a chronic, inflexible and maladaptive pattern of relating to the world. This maladaptive pattern is evident in the way a person thinks, feels and behaves, which may lead to personal problems that induce extreme anxiety, distress, depression or maladaptive coping strategies like self-harm, drug and alcohol misuse, disordered eating, or overdoses. The most noticeable feature of these disorders is their negative effect on interpersonal relationships. People diagnosed with personality disorder may also be very inflexible, in that they may have a narrow range of attitudes, behaviours and coping mechanisms that they cannot change easily. They may not understand why they need to change, as they may not recognise that they have a problem, and will, instead, blame others or circumstances.

People with personality disorders may find it difficult to:

- Make or keep relationships.
- Get on with people at work.
- Get on with friends and family.
- Keep out of trouble.
- Control their feelings or behaviour.

Disordered eating

Eating disorders are considered in Chapter 7.10.2, Eating disorders. However, dietitians working in mental health settings will see a large number of service users with eating disorders not otherwise specified (EDNOS), and atypical eating disorders such as symptoms of food restriction, binge eating, vomiting and laxative misuse. This may be part of a dual diagnosis with other disorders such as depression, OCD and personality disorders. In line with NICE (2017) guidance, EDNOS should be treated along the same lines as the eating disorder it most resembles. With all disordered eating, a psychologically based multidisciplinary team (MDT) approach is the best practice. It is important to have an understanding of the psychological function of the eating behaviour in order to treat it successfully.

Assessment and diagnosis

The recognition and understanding of mental health conditions have changed over time, although there are still variations in the definition, assessment and classification of mental disorders. The ICD 10 Classification of Mental and Behavioral Disorders (WHO, 1992) and the DSM V

Classification of Mental Disorders (American Psychiatric Association, 2013) are widely accepted. Many people will suffer with a range of conditions that commonly overlap, e.g. borderline personality disorder, depression, eating disorders, and OCD are common comorbidities.

General mental health, specific conditions and their associated risk can be assessed or monitored with the help of tools and measures that look at psychosocial functioning; based on physical and mental well-being such as CORE (Clinical Outcomes in routine Evaluation) and FACE (Functional Analysis of Care Environments); or disease-specific tools such as the EDE-Q (Eating disorders Examination Questionnaire). These can act as measures of function and also as measures of treatment efficacy. Other tools such as TOMs (Therapy Outcome Measures) or GAS (Goal Attainment Scaling) may be used to measure treatment efficacy within services.

Dietitians working in mental health settings need to extend their usual assessment approaches and communication skills to include areas such as observations of mood and body language, demeanour, speech, risks to self and others, relationships, interpersonal skills, information processing, and discussing beliefs, thoughts and feelings as well as behaviours.

Treatment services in mental health

Mental health services are based in hospitals and the community. Over the past 5 years, there has been an increased focus on treating people in the community, resulting in a reduction in inpatient beds across the UK. There are a number of different mental health services spanning the age range from children and young people's mental health services (CAMHS) to adult mental health/working-age adult services and mental health services for older people (MHSOP). Specialist community treatment teams for specific mental health conditions may include early-intervention psychosis teams, eating-disorders teams, rehabilitation and recovery teams, and assertive outreach teams. Patients are usually referred to as service users within mental health services.

Forensic services

The term forensic in mental health services usually refers to secure hospitals, secure wards or secure units. These provide care and treatment to people with mental illness who are a risk to other people, and have separate wards for men and women and specific adolescent units. There are different levels of secure hospitals, and high-security hospitals treat people who need high levels of security because they could be dangerous, violent or pose a high risk to other people. They can provide different levels of secure care, as the patients there will have different needs. For example, for service users who are working towards leaving, the hospital can build up their unescorted leave. Low-security units have less physical security than medium-security units but are more secure than standard mental health wards. For example, service users may be in a low-security hospital detained under the Mental Health Act if other mental health services cannot treat them because they are a risk to other people or if their behaviour is challenging.

Most service users enter treatment voluntarily, but for some it may be involuntary. Service users may be involuntarily detained under the Mental Health Act (1983) according to specific sections; this is colloquially known as 'being sectioned'.

Healthcare professionals in mental health

Some specialist services cannot be offered in a local mental health service. These are often provided on a regional basis, are known as out-of-area placements and are with specialist tertiary services. Examples include units treating inpatient eating disorders, and high-security, forensic and alcohol detoxification units. Most services offer a multidisciplinary approach to treatment, and the following professionals are involved:

- *Psychiatrists* are medically trained doctors specialising in mental health. They are responsible for arranging admission and discharge of service users, for diagnosis, and for prescription of medication.
- *Clinical psychologists* assess and treat service users with a variety of psychological therapies. Dietitians and psychologists often work together, especially in the treatment of eating disorders. Psychologists can offer advice on the different approaches to use to support dietary change.
- *Occupational therapists* are often very experienced in working with groups and are involved in teaching life skills and activities, including shopping, cooking and budgeting. There is often close collaboration with dietitians and occupational therapists, e.g. when working on healthy lifestyle groups.
- *Psychiatric nurses* offer support to people and the families of people who have mental health problems. They assess and develop care plans, and give medication and some psychotherapy, either formally via training in techniques such as cognitive behaviour therapy (CBT), or informally.
- *Social workers* offer support for rehabilitation with regard to housing, benefits and family work. They can also assess the mental state of service users in order to determine whether sectioning under the Mental Health Act is appropriate.
- *Physiotherapists* support service users to effect physical, cognitive and behavioural change through the use of exercise, relaxation therapy, stress management, electrical modalities and manual skills.
- *Counsellors* or *psychotherapists* offer a range of talking therapies. Counsellors or psychotherapists are practitioners who work with people over the short or long term to help them bring about effective change or enhance their well-being; they are variously qualified and usually offer one form of treatment approach, e.g. CBT.

Role of dietitians in the multi disciplinary team

Allied health professionals are often the minority professions within mental health settings, although their numbers are growing. As the number of dietitians is limited, careful consideration should be given to their duty of care to ensure that they identify not only those service users most at risk, but also those most likely to benefit from dietetic input, i.e. ensuring they do the most good (or least harm) to the highest number of people within a case load population. This often involves working with carers and ward staff to ensure that the basics, such as screening tools, staff training and hospital menus, are in place, rather than seeing a high number of direct clinical cases, which can be time consuming with uncertain outcomes. They should consider prioritising areas where outcomes may be greater, e.g. early intervention psychosis. Dietitians may represent their profession alone within a service. This can be challenging and requires articulation of their key skills to the team, ensuring clarity about their professional boundaries, duties, roles and responsibilities within the team. They should also engage with regular clinical supervision from a dietitian specialising in mental health.

Community mental health teams

Most service users with a mental health problem do not need to see a psychiatrist. The general practitioner (GP) is responsible for first-line support, including assessment, medication and referrals to a counsellor or psychotherapist. However, if problems are more complicated or serious, the GP will refer the service user to a community mental health team (CMHT). This is a community-based team made up of an MDT. Usually, one member of the MDT, such as a social worker or nurse, becomes the key worker for the service user.

Key worker

This will either be a lead professional or a care coordinator for community patients, or a named nurse for an inpatient. The key worker's role is to assess the service user's specific difficulties, discuss any plans for treatment and offer counselling, information and advice. The key worker is responsible for keeping in touch with other health professionals who are involved with the service user to ensure coordinated care. All treatments are documented in the care plan, which should list the key problem, what needs to be done and who should be doing what. The service user is always involved in putting together the care plan and will usually be offered a copy of this. Dietitians should ensure that dietetic care plans follow this example, fully involving the service user in joint care planning, and, where possible, offering the service user a copy of all correspondence.

Care models

Standard care/lead professional care

Lead professional care (LPC) is appropriate for people who need secondary mental health services but have more straightforward needs, involving contact with only one professional or one agency.

Care programme approach

If service users have complex needs, or need specialist services team for a long period, they may be put on the care programme approach (CPA). Their care coordinator acts as the primary link between them and the healthcare team, organising regular meetings and updates.

The CPA is normally implemented by an MDT and aims to:

- Assess holistic health and social needs.
- Draw up a care plan in conjunction with the service user and carers.
- Monitor the quality and effectiveness of care.
- Review progress at regular intervals.

Occupational therapists, social workers and mental health nurses usually act as care coordinators or lead professionals for clients on LPC or CPA. However, because dietitians do not undertake compulsory placements in mental health settings as part of preregistration training, they require post-registration training to undertake this area of extended practice.

Legislation

Dietitians need to be familiar with two areas of mental capacity, as described in the following sections.

Mental Capacity Act

The Mental Capacity Act (MCA) (2005) applies to everyone involved in the care, treatment and support of people aged 16 years and over, living in England and Wales, who are unable to make all or some decisions for themselves. It is important to note that service users may have capacity in many areas of their lives (e.g. finances, relationships), but lack capacity in others (e.g. decisions about their health/weight).

Having mental capacity means that a person is able to make his or her own decisions. Professionals should always start from the assumption that the person has the capacity to make the decision in question, and demonstrate that they have made every effort to encourage and support the person to make the decision by himself or herself. If a person makes a decision that a healthcare professional (HCP) considers eccentric or unwise, this does not necessarily mean that the person lacks the capacity to make the decision.

Under the MCA, HCPs are required to make an assessment of capacity before carrying out any care or treatment. If capacity is lacking, it is important follow the checklist described in the code to establish the best interests of the individual concerned. The MCA says that individuals are considered as unable to make their own decision if they cannot do one or more of the following four things:

- Understand information given to them.
- Retain that information long enough to be able to make the decision.

- Weigh up the information available to make the decision.
- Communicate their decision; this could be by talking, using sign language or even simple muscle movements such as blinking an eye or squeezing a hand.

If a person has been assessed as lacking capacity, then any action taken, or any decision made for or on behalf of that person, must be made in his or her best interests. The person who has to make the decision is known as the decision-maker, and normally will be the carer responsible for the day-to-day care, or a professional such as a doctor, nurse or social worker where decisions about care need to be made. Dietitians are commonly involved in best interest meeting in areas such as learning disabilities and older adult care, where there are decisions to be made about nutritional care as an MDT rather than by the single HCP.

The Mental Health Act

The Mental Health Act (MHA, 1983) is the law that sets out when service users can be admitted, detained and treated in hospital against their wishes. It is also known as 'being sectioned'. This is used when individuals are putting their own safety or someone else's at risk, and they have a mental disorder that requires assessment and treatment. There are different sections of the Mental Health Act that have different aims. Treatment can be enforced in either a hospital or community settings for a specific time period of time, and includes Community Treatment Orders (CTOs). Dietitians maybe involved in MHA decisions for service users with conditions such as anorexia nervosa.

Standards and policies

There is a large number of policy documents, guidelines and best practice guidance that need to be considered by dietitians working within mental health settings. These change frequently and may vary locally. Some current examples include the following:

- NICE guidance for conditions including depression, schizophrenia, diabetes, eating disorders.
- Care Quality Commission (CQC), Outcome 5: Meeting Nutritional Needs.
- National Patient Safety Agency (NPSA): Ten High-Impact Nursing Standards.
- Council of Europe Resolution: Food and Nutritional Care in Hospitals.
- Essence of Care: Benchmarks for Food and Drink; Best Practice Indicators.
- Patient Environmental Action Team (PEAT) Assessment Criteria.
- Mental Health Taskforce to the NHS England (2016) The Five Year Forwards View for Mental Health.

In Scotland, the Mental Health (Care and Treatment) Scotland Act (2003); Food in Hospitals; and Food, Fluid and Nutritional Care Standards, all governed by Health Improvement Scotland (HIS) (http://www.healthcareimprovementscotland.org), formerly known as Quality Improvement Scotland (QIS), are key.

Common psychological treatments

Psychological therapies and psychiatric medication are two of the major treatment options, as are psychosocial interventions, peer support and self-help.

Psychological therapies

Psychological therapies, sometimes referred to as talking treatments, counselling or psychotherapy, are a core treatment for mental illness. Psychological therapy encompasses a broad range of treatments, including talking therapies of different models and different forms of delivery, e.g. individual, family and group. Therapy can help towards reducing distress, symptoms and risk of harm to self or others. The most appropriate treatment may vary according to the person's age, situation, diagnosis and personal preference. Therapy can either be used on its own or combined with medication. Most therapies help to identify thought, mood and behaviour patterns that have led to, or maintain, disorders. There is considerable evidence in support of the effectiveness of psychological therapies across a range of problems and settings. Common psychological therapies that are supported by good evidence include cognitive behavioural therapy, dialectical behavioural therapy, interpersonal therapy, and family-based therapies. Some therapists practice a form of integrative therapy, which draws on and blends specific types of techniques. The National Institute for Health and Care Excellence (NICE) recommends psychological therapies for mild and moderate depression and anxiety, OCD, bipolar disorder, PTSD, eating disorders and schizophrenia.

Dietitians need a broad understanding of these treatments to ensure they can work within the psychological approach taken by the team. For example, if a CBT model is used, then aligning dietetic treatment and education to use some CBT-based techniques will ensure a consistent and evidence-based approach for the service user and team. Dietitians working within specific treatment teams and modalities will need further training in these specific psychological therapies (see Chapter 1.3, Changing health behaviour).

Formulation

Case formulation is a theoretically based explanation of the information obtained from a clinical assessment. It offers a hypothesis about the development and maintenance of the problems. Formulations are used to help the service user and team to better understand the problem and provide a framework for developing the most suitable treatment approach. It is most commonly used by clinical teams.

Cognitive behavioural therapy

This therapy focuses on the here and now to identify maladaptive thinking (cognitions – ideas, mental images, beliefs and attitudes). It recognises that events in the past have shaped the way in which an individual currently thinks and behaves, with particular focus on the thought patterns and behaviours learned in childhood. However, CBT does not dwell on the past, but aims to find solutions to change current thoughts and behaviours. Cognitive behavioural therapy has a strong evidence base for phobias, anxiety, depression, OCD and bulimia nervosa, for which it is often delivered within 8–16 sessions.

Psychodynamic therapy

Psychodynamic therapy (or psychoanalytic psychotherapy) is the general name for therapeutic approaches that try to get the service user to bring to the surface their true feelings, so that they can experience them and understand them. This is often a longer-term therapy delivered over a number of years.

Systemic and family therapy

This seeks to address how people operate in a family system and not at an individual level, as is usually the focus of other forms of therapy. It looks at people in relationships, dealing with the interactions of groups, their patterns and dynamics. It includes family therapy and marriage counselling.

Didactical behavioural therapy

This is a type of CBT; its main goal is to teach the service user skills to cope with stress, regulate emotions and improve relationships with others. Didactical behaviour therapy (DBT) is designed for use by people who have the urge to harm themselves, such as those who self-harm, or who have suicidal thoughts and feelings, but has also been adapted for other conditions where the service user exhibits self-destructive behaviours, such as eating disorders and substance abuse.

Interpersonal therapy

This therapy has an evidence base for effective treatment of many psychological conditions, including depression and eating disorders. It is based on the principle that there is a relationship between the way people communicate and interact with others and their mental health.

Nutrition in mental health

Nutrition screening

All mental health service users admitted as inpatients should be screened for nutrition-related problems, and those identified as high risk should have a nutritional care plan in place that is reviewed at regular intervals by an appropriately qualified professional (CQC, Outcome 5). The Malnutrition Universal Screening Tool ('MUST') has not been validated for many mental health settings, and fails to detect selective eating, food phobias or deliberate weight loss, and disordered eating. Therefore, a number of hospitals have adapted 'MUST' or developed their own screening tool, which has then been validated for use through measurements of specificity and sensitivity locally. Other Trusts use 'MUST' to screen but have developed mental-health-specific care pathways for malnutrition and obesity, which are more appropriate to the setting.

Nutrition in mental illness

Evidence from epidemiological studies suggests that nutrition may have a key role in mental health. However, dietitians need to exercise caution when interpreting studies that involve food and mental health; criticisms of research in this area include low numbers of subjects, poor methodology, assumptions about cause and effect, and substantial heterogeneity, e.g. the trials were too different from one another to be grouped together in a meta-analysis. No single food can cure mental health conditions, but evidence for some dietary interventions is discussed in the following text; these are supported by Opie *et al.* (2016):

- Follow 'traditional'-type diets such as the Mediterranean, Norwegian, or Japanese diets. There is good evidence that traditional diets, often rich in fruit, vegetables, legumes and essential fats, are protective against conditions such as depression (Quirk *et al.*, 2013).
- In longitudinal studies, nuts, fruits, legumes and vegetables were positively weighted against depression, with moderate adherence (but not always the highest level of adherence) to diet quality scores, showing the strongest inverse association with depression Sánchez-Villegas *et al.* (2015).
- Although trial evidence of the effects of n-3 fatty acids in mental health has increased, it remains difficult to summarise the evidence because of the considerable differences between trials. However, the evidence does provide support of a benefit in individuals with diagnosed depressive illness. A meta-analysis by Li *et al.* (2016) showed that high fish consumption can reduce the risk of depression. Studies including meta-analysis by Ross *et al.* (2007) have found evidence that n-3 fatty acids can reduce symptoms of depression in clients with major depressive disorder and bipolar disorder; there are suggestions that eicosapentaenoic acid (EPA) may be better than docosahexaenoic acid (DHA) for the treatment of mood disorders. Therefore, supplementation of n-3 fatty acids, particularly EPA, should be considered if diet is deficient. A dose of around 1000 mg/day is suggested.
- Food items such as meat, meat products and sweets are found to be negatively associated with rates of depression (Sánchez-Villegas *et al.*, 2015).
- The results of a meta-analyses suggest that treatment with folate and vitamin B_{12} does not decrease the severity of depressive symptoms over a short period of time, but may be helpful in the long-term management of specific populations (Almeida *et al.*, 2015).

- Self-medication through the misuse of high-caffeine drinks and coffee is common, and contributes significant extra energy. Symptoms include headache, anxiety, agitation, chest pain and ringing in the ears, which can exacerbate conditions such as anxiety.

Physical health implications of mental illness

Diseases such as CVD, dyslipidaemia, high blood pressure, constipation, metabolic syndrome, type 2 diabetes and obesity are more common in people with mental health. The reason for this is unknown, but it is likely to be due to a combination of medication, lifestyle and the disease state itself. Numerous studies support findings that patients with schizophrenia have a poor diet, mainly characterised by a high intake of saturated fat and sugar, a low consumption of fibre and fruit, and a reliance on processed foods (Dipasquale *et al.*, 2013).

Weight gain and serious mental illness

Weight gain can result as a side effect of medication and due to the adoption of an unhealthy lifestyle, such as insufficient physical activity and unhealthy dietary preferences, with excess energy consumed through high-fat meal choices, excessive portions, snacks, carbonated drinks and takeaways. The latter may be due to boredom as a result of low occupational activity, increased thirst as a side effect of medication or the perceived positive impact on mood from the consumption of caffeine and sugar.

Dieting or weight cycling is also related to depression, with repeated diet failure and episodes of binge eating affecting mood. The use of food as a coping strategy for emotion regulation has the potential to cause overweight or obesity in those experiencing negative mood. Depression also predicts attrition from weight loss programmes, as it can prevent people from engaging in the meal planning and physical activity necessary to lose weight (Markowitw *et al.*, 2008).

Lack of knowledge or skills around meal planning and cooking can also severely limit food choice. Occupational therapy support for improving skills and confidence in the life skills required for everyday living, such as cooking, ironing, cleaning, planning and budgeting, can improve these factors. Joint work between occupational therapists and dietitians can considerably improve service users' occupational skills and healthy eating.

Weight management

Lifestyle interventions are beneficial for controlling and limiting obesity among patients with schizophrenia (Hjorth *et al.*, 2014). Many service users do not find commercial or community-based slimming groups useful due to the rapid pace of change expected, misunderstandings around the impact of the medication they are taking, and the social and interpersonal difficulties experienced in group settings. In addition, the incidence of disordered eating is high (Hudson *et al.*, 2007). Therefore, many service users will not benefit from the traditional approach where the focus is on restricting energy, and educational approaches may inadvertently reinforce beliefs about good and bad foods. Instead, the focus should be on regular meals and small changes over time.

Service users can successfully lose weight through a wide range of interventions, independent of whether they are inpatients or outpatients, and with different severity of illness. Therefore, staff and patients should select the intervention most suitable. Typically, these will be service user–led weight management groups or education groups running over 6–10 week programmes, including topics such as healthy eating principles, self-esteem, activity, meal planning and demonstrations, activity scheduling, motivation, quizzes and evaluation (Chen *et al.*, 2009; Ko *et al.*, 2010). The individual set goals and the pace of change was slow, with focus on single changes. Health strategies must be implemented within each setting as part of everyday life, as interventions must be lifelong (Hjorth *et al.*, 2014).

Additional nutritional problems for inpatient communities

Mealtimes

Hospitals have a duty of care to provide high-quality food that meets service users' preferences, satisfies nutritional health needs and offers adequate choice (CQC, Outcome 5). Weight gain caused by boredom, especially when service users have long period of residential care and are on restricted access, can be challenging to change. There may be service users who cannot access foods other than those provided by the wards, but can go as far as the vending machines or the hospital shops; this can help promote the purchasing of foods as part of a daily routine.

Service users may have disturbed sleep patterns, resulting in them staying awake at night when hospital food is not available, and sleeping through meals such as breakfast. This time might be used to snack on high-energy foods from vending machines and hospital shops, or the service users may order a takeaway. Long-stay service users report that they get bored with menus that remain the same on 3–4 week cycles and chose to order takeaways, especially if menus do not reflect service users' preferences for good-quality meat and spicy foods (Haw *et al.*, 2010).

Meals times can be a very stressful time for service users, and there are many security issues for staff to deal with. There can be difficulties in managing paranoid service users in the same communal eating space as others, sometimes necessitating a staggered approach to meals, which requires different sittings in a short space of time. Surveyed service users reported that they would prefer staff to sit and eat with them at mealtimes rather than be there just for observation, giving them an opportunity to build better relationships with staff and change the culture of mealtimes, making them a more normalised and social event (Service User Led Audit Group, 2011). The CQC makes protected mealtimes a measurable standard for all mental health trusts.

Finance

Hospital inpatients are still able to claim state benefits. If their leave is restricted, this can result in them having large amounts of cash and limited opportunities to spend this. As a result, they often purchase large quantities of high-sugar and/or high-fat drinks and snacks from vending machines and hospital cafes and/or shops. This has been further exacerbated by the recent smoking bans introduced by many mental health trusts.

Takeaways

In the 2011 Service User Led Audit in the north of England, service users gave several reasons why takeaways were important to them. Hospital food was perceived as bland; therefore, takeaways were a way by which people could have what they considered to be a 'decent meal'. Service users also viewed getting takeaways as a social experience that gives them some control over how and when they eat. It also provided an opportunity for people to eat together, often with staff and friends, in a way that normalised eating. This highlights the importance of getting the service users' inputs into food choice for the menus and dining arrangements. Takeaways in some hospitals have been successfully limited to Fridays or Saturdays, with staff placing the service users' orders. Hospitals have a duty of care to encourage healthy eating choices.

Other successful strategies include ensuring that the menus are carefully planned to give healthy choices, e.g. giving a healthy makeover to all recipes, including traditionally higher-calorie choices such as chips and curry, aiming for better taste and lower fat. Foods such as snacks may be rated, e.g. red, amber and green (RAG rated), offering service users an informed choice. Stocking non-food items such as puzzle books and magazines, rather than food, in vending machines; stocking only caffeine and sugar-free drinks; and limiting shop-sold items to small portion sizes are all ways in which hospitals have successfully started to promote healthier eating.

Service user–led groups

These are often called nutrition steering groups, and may be attended by a link from each ward. These groups can help to educate and give opportunities to expand choices and experience through activities such as 'come dine with me' groups and themed food nights. Some trusts have catering groups or service user partnership groups, where service user representatives from each ward attend meetings to provide suggestions, comments, compliments, and feedback on menus and quality of food. Service users also give suggestions for new menus; however, dietitians need to keep in mind the various policies around food in hospitals that each trust needs to adhere to.

The legal position

In the case of service users who are detained in long-stay units, the law states that the hospital is considered as the usual residence and therefore is 'home' to service users. However, because of the nature of the residence (e.g. service users cannot access any alternative environment or food provisions), it is reasonable that there may be a case for restricting or adjusting environmental factors, including food type or amount, to support the goal of treating or preventing morbidity or mortality (e.g. to control blood sugars or to prevent weight gain and coronary heart disease in service users identified as at high risk). Any restrictions that are placed on service users' food provisions must be justified and reasonable, e.g. not disproportionate to the goal of treatment. In order for this to be legal, there must be a transparent and meaningful consultation with the service users before any such restrictions are applied. All options should be explored in full, and careful consideration given to the type and severity of food restriction needed for treatment, which should be balanced against the service users' right to enjoy a normal diet. Therefore, dietitians should ensure that all these steps are followed and all actions and discussions fully documented when restricting service users' food choices or access for health reasons.

Weight loss

There is a risk of undernutrition in people with some forms of mental illness, particularly if chronic psychotic illness is associated with problems such as low income, poor housing, eating disorders or substance misuse. Malnutrition can also result as an effect of food phobia or paranoid episodes, where there is a belief that food is contaminated in some way. Some people presenting with deterioration in their mental illness may refuse to eat the food available on the ward, perhaps from fear that the food is contaminated or poisoned. Usually, food that is still packaged will be accepted, but their diet may remain limited and nutritionally unbalanced until medications have improved their condition.

Depressive illness often results in weight loss. This may be a result of taste changes leading to loss of appetite; low motivation for self-care, so that the patient does not bother to eat; a preoccupation with other problems, so that eating becomes a low-priority event; or a combination of these factors. Similarly, people suffering from anxiety are often too preoccupied to eat or may complain of food getting stuck in their throat.

Diabetes

Erratic meal patterns, binge eating, medication, excessive carbonated drink consumption and excessive sugar consumption are all common causes of unstable diabetes in mental health settings. A holistic care plan should involve the dietitian, the diabetes care team, the key worker, and the service user and carer.

Nutritional consequences of medication

A high percentage of service users with serious mental illness (SMI) use long-term medications. These types of medications are often associated with weight gain, constipation, thirst and increased appetite. In turn, increasing weight impacts on motivation and mobilisation, in addition to increasing the risk of other health problems such as metabolic syndrome and CVD. The possible effects of commonly used psychotropic drugs on nutrition are shown in Table 7.10.5.

Psychotropic medication

Psychiatric medications used to treat mental disorders are called psychotropic or psychotherapeutic medications. They cannot cure the disorder, but they make users feel better, so that they can function. Medications work differently for different people. Some people only need them for a short time, e.g. a person with depression may feel much better after taking medication for a few months, and may never need it again. People with SMI may need to take medication for much longer periods. Psychotropic medication works by affecting the brain's neurotransmitters. Neurotransmitters are chemicals that communicate information throughout the brain and the body, by relaying signals between nerve cells. There are many neurotransmitters, including:

- Gamma amino butyric acid (GABA).
- Acetylcholine (ACh).
- Bioactive amines:
  - Noradrenaline (norepinephrine).
  - Adrenaline (epinephrine).
  - Dopamine.
  - Serotonin (5HT).
  - Histamine (H1).

Monoamine neurotransmitters, which include dopamine, noradrenaline, adrenaline and serotonin, are released from neurones in both the brain and peripheral nervous system. The function of the monoamines is not clear, but they are thought to have a crucial role in arousal, emotion and cognition. Monoamines are metabolised by the enzyme monoamine oxidase (MAO) in the nerve synapses. This can result in low concentrations of the neurotransmitters, which result in disease. Most people with psychosis (schizophrenia) have unnaturally high levels of dopamine; therefore, the treatment is to lower the monoamine (dopamine) levels. Most antipsychotics (neuroleptics) involve predominately blocking or lowering the dopamine levels.

The antidepressant medication monoamine oxidase inhibitor (MAOI) inhibits the breakdown of noradrenaline and adrenaline. This leads to a build-up in the synapse, and thereby improves mood. These drugs have drug–nutrient interactions that service users must be aware of (see Table 7.10.1). Newer antidepressants, selective serotonin reuptake inhibitors (SSRIs), e.g. Prozac, increase the amount of serotonin (and, to some extent, noradrenaline) in the synaptic gap, which correlates with an improvement in mood.

Weight gain

The possible mechanisms for weight gain associated with this medication include the following:

- Blocking or lowering of ACh peripherally causes dry mouth and increased thirst. This may lead to an increase in the consumption of sugary drinks.
- Drugs that lower serotonin and histamine stimulate appetite and carbohydrate cravings. This may lead to an increase in total energy intake.
- Blocking dopamine, especially the D2 receptors, may increase appetite.
- Lithium may cause weight gain by fluid retention (due to its effect on sodium balance) and by reducing thyroxine levels (which results in a decreased metabolic rate and, therefore, a decreased energy output).

Therefore, drugs that block ACh, serotonin and histamine will have the greatest effect on body weight. Drugs that block all three of these will provoke the greatest weight gain, e.g. clozapine, olanzapine and quetiapine.

Antidepressants

The newer form of antidepressants, SSRIs (such as citalopram, paroxetine, fluoxetine and sertraline), may induce weight loss during the first few weeks and may prevent long-term weight gain. They are commonly used to treat conditions such as bulimia, panic disorder, OCD and depression.

Antipsychotic medication

Antipsychotic medications are an important treatment option for many individuals with schizophrenia. Bak *et al.* (2014), Parsons *et al.* (2009) and Norvik *et al.* (2009) reported that olanzapine and quetiapine commonly cause dramatic and long-term weight gain, with rapid gains of 30 kg over months. which continued over the 3 years of the study. Commonly, people with a healthy BMI might be more likely to increase their weight significantly, as compared to those who are already overweight when they start to take these medications.

Constipation

Constipation is a common side effect of medication and can be severe in some cases. Dehydration or an inappropriate diet can compound this.

Polydipsia and hyponatraemia

Some service users experience increased thirst sensation as a side effect of antipsychotic medication and consequently drink excessive amounts of fluid, increasing the risk of hyponatraemia. The consumption of large quantities of strong coffee or other caffeine-rich drinks may make the situation worse. Treatment may necessitate withdrawal of antidepressants, but if continued use of antidepressants is unavoidable, sodium and fluid restriction may be necessary.

Internet resources

Mental Health Taskforce to the NHS England (2016) https://www.england.nhs.uk/wp-content/uploads/2016/02/Mental-Health-Taskforce-FYFV-final.pdf.

Table 7.10.1 Possible effects of commonly used psychotropic drugs on nutrition

Drug type	Example	Licensed uses	Potential nutritional side effects
Antidepressants			
Tricyclics	Amitriptyline Imipramine Lofepramine Dosulepin Doxepin	Moderate to severe depression, particularly where sedation is required	Dry mouth, blood sugar changes, constipation or (rarely) diarrhoea, nausea and vomiting, epigastric distress, increased appetite and weight gain, syndrome of inappropriate antidiuretic hormone (SIADH) leading to hyponatraemia, anorexia (rarely)
Selective serotonin reuptake inhibitors (SSRIs)[a]	Citalopram Fluoxetine Fluvoxamine Paroxetine Sertraline Escitalopram	Moderate to severe depression Bulimia nervosa OCD Panic disorder Generalised anxiety disorder PTSD Social phobia	Anorexia, nausea and vomiting, weight loss/gain, dry mouth, dyspepsia, diarrhoea, taste disturbances, abdominal pain, SIADH
Monoamine oxidase inhibitors (MAOIs)	Isocarboxazid Phenelzine Tranylcypromine Moclobemide (reversible MAOI)	Moderate to severe depression Atypical depression Depression with phobic symptoms	Nausea and vomiting, dry mouth, constipation, increased appetite and weight gain, potentiation of action of insulin or oral hypoglycaemic with lowered blood glucose, hypertensive crisis if foods containing tyramine are ingested. *Note*: This is much less likely with the newer reversible inhibitors of monoamine oxidase A (RIMA), such as moclobemide
Presynaptic alpha 2 antagonists	Mirtazapine	Moderate to severe depression	Weight gain, increased appetite
Selective inhibitors of noradrenaline (norepinephrine) reuptake	Reboxetine	Moderate to severe depression	Dry mouth, constipation, lack of appetite, nausea, lowering of plasma potassium concentration following prolonged administration in elderly people
Serotonin and noradrenaline (norepinephrine) reuptake inhibitors (SNRIs)	Venlafaxine Duloxetine	Moderate to severe depression	Constipation, abdominal pain, nausea, vomiting, dry mouth, anorexia, weight changes, diarrhoea, dyspepsia, taste disturbances, increase in serum cholesterol during long-term treatment, SIADH
Antipsychotics			
Phenothiazines[a]	Chlorpromazine Fluphenazine Trifluoperazine	Psychoses Schizophrenia Mania Severe anxiety	Dry mouth, constipation, photosensitivity leading to sun avoidance and low vitamin D levels, appetite increase and weight gain, reduced response to hypoglycaemic agents causing elevated blood glucose
Butyrophenones	Haloperidol	Psychoses Mania Schizophrenia	Nausea, dyspepsia, loss of appetite (less effect on appetite than phenothiazines), dry mouth, constipation
Thioxanthenes	Flupentixol Zuclopenthixol	Psychoses Schizophrenia	Increased appetite and weight gain (less commonly, weight loss) May affect diabetic control
Substituted benzamides	Pimozide Sulpiride	Psychoses Schizophrenia	Nausea, dyspepsia, abdominal pain, constipation, dry mouth, changes in body weight, glycosuria
Atypical antipsychotics[a]	Clozapine Olanzapine Quetiapine Risperidone Amisulpride Aripiprazole Ziprasidone (not currently available in the UK)	Psychoses Schizophrenia Mania	Increased appetite and weight gain (likelihood of weight gain greatest with clozapine, and then in decreasing order as listed), hyperglycaemia and/or development or exacerbation of diabetes, elevated triglyceride levels, constipation, dry mouth and hypersalivation, impairment of intestinal peristalsis, dysphagia

Table 7.10.1 (*Continued*)

Drug type	Example	Licensed uses	Potential nutritional side effects
Hypnotics and anxiolytics			
Benzodiazepines	Diazepam Chlordiazepoxide Lorazepam Temazepam Nitrazepam	Short-term anxiety Alcohol withdrawal Short-term sleep disturbance	Nausea, vomiting, diarrhoea or constipation, appetite and weight changes, dry mouth, metallic taste, dysphagia. These symptoms have been reported both before and up to 6 weeks after withdrawal
Non-benzodiazepine hypnotics	Zopiclone Zolpidem Zaleplon	Short-term sleep disturbance	Metallic taste changes, nausea, vomiting, dry mouth
Mood stabilisers			
Lithium salts	Lithium carbonate Lithium citrate	Treatment of mania and hypomania Prophylactic treatment of recurrent affective disorders	Early side effects: nausea, metallic taste, increased thirst, polyuria, loose stools Later side effects: weight gain, mild oedema, polyuria, metallic taste, possible hypothyroidism, hyperglycaemia, toxic effects (can result from sodium depletion), loss of appetite, vomiting, diarrhoea
Anticonvulsants			
Benzodiazepines	Clonazepam Clobazam	All forms of epileptic seizure	As for benzodiazepines
Barbiturates	Phenobarbitone Primidone (80% of its activity is phenobarbitone)	Grand mal and focal seizures	Decreased vitamin D levels, decreased folate levels, (rarely) gastrointestinal upsets
Other antiepileptics	Carbamazepine	Temporal lobe, tonic/clonic and partial seizures. (Mood regulation as an alternative to lithium) Neuropathic pain	Mimics action of ADH on kidney, causing water retention, nausea, loss of appetite, vomiting, diarrhoea or constipation (high dose), dry mouth, lowered plasma sodium levels
	Sodium valproate	All types of seizures (mania – valproic acid)	Nausea and vomiting, anorexia, gastric irritation, increased appetite and weight gain, diarrhoea
	Phenytoin	Tonic/clonic seizures Following head injury or surgery	*Early side effects*: nausea and vomiting *Later side effects*: decreased absorption of vitamin D leading to osteomalacia, increased turnover and decreased absorption of folic acid leading to megaloblastic anaemia, gum hyperplasia and soreness, tooth decay
	Lamotrigine	Partial seizures Primary and secondary generalised tonic/clonic seizures Myoclonic seizures Lennox–Gastaut syndrome	Nausea, vomiting, diarrhoea Possibility of interference with folate metabolism during long-term therapy
	Gabapentin Pregabalin	Adjunctive treatment of partial seizures Neuropathic pain	Diarrhoea, dry mouth, dyspepsia, nausea and vomiting, weight gain, constipation, flatulence, blood glucose fluctuations in service users with diabetes
	Levetiracetam	Adjunctive treatment of partial seizures	Anorexia, diarrhoea, dyspepsia, nausea
	Topiramate	Generalised tonic/clonic seizures Partial seizures Adjunct in Lennox–Gastaut syndrome Migraine prophylaxis	Weight loss, nausea, anorexia, diarrhoea, dry mouth, taste perversion, metabolic acidosis

[a]Not all drugs licensed for all indications. OCD, obsessive compulsive disorder; PTSD, post traumatic stress disorder.

References

Almeida O, Ford A, Flicker L. (2015) Systematic review and meta-analysis of randomized placebo-controlled trials of folate and vitamin B_{12} for depression. *Int. Psychogeriatr.* 27(05): 727–737.

American Psychiatric Association. (2013) *Diagnostic and Statistical Manual of Mental Disorders*, 5th edn. Arlington, VA: American Psychiatric Publishing.

Bak M, Fransen A, Janssen J, et al. (2014) Almost all antipsychotics result in weight gain: a meta-analysis. *PLoS ONE*. 9(4): e94112.

Breen G, Webb BT, Butler AW, *et al.* (2011) A genome-wide significant linkage for severe depression on chromosome 3: the Depression Network Study. *Am. J. Psychiatry* 168: 840–847.

Chen CK, Chen YC, Huang YS. (2009) Effects of a 10-week weight control program on obese service users with schizophrenia or schizoaffective disorder: A 12-month follow up. *Psychiatry Clin. Neurosci.* 63(1): 17–22.

de Hert M, Correll CU, Bobes J, et al. (2011) Physical illness in patients with severe mental disorders. I. Prevalence, impact of medications and disparities in health care. *World Psychiatry*. 10(1): 52–77.

Dipasquale S, Pariante CM, Dazzan P, et al. (2013) The dietary pattern of patients with schizophrenia: a systematic review. *J. Psychiatr. Res.* 47(2): 197–207.

Haw C, Collyer J, Sugarman P (2010). Patients' complaints at a large psychiatric hospital: can they lead to better patient services? *International Journal of Health Care Quality Assurance*. 23:400–409.

Hjorth P, Davidsen AS, Kilian R, *et al.* (2014) A systematic review of controlled interventions to reduce overweight and obesity in people with schizophrenia. *Acta Psychiatr. Scand.* 130(4): 279–289.

Hudson J, Hiripi E, Pope HG Jr, *et al.* (2007) The prevalence and correlates of eating disorders in the National Comorbidity Survey. *Biol. Psychiatry* 61(3): 348–335.

Kings Fund Report. (2016) *Bringing together physical and mental health, A new frontier for integrated care* (Authors Chris Naylor, Preety Das, Shilpa Ross, Matthew Honeyman, James Thompson, Helen Gilburt, Available at https://www.crisiscareconcordat.org.uk/inspiration/kings-fund-bringing-together-physical-mental-health-new-frontier-integrated-care-2/. Accessed 1 November 2018.

Ko KH, Chung MS, Kim JH. (2010) The effect of a wellness program on nutritional and diet knowledge, exercise and weight control knowledge, and weight control of schizophrenia. *J. Korean Acad. Psychiatr. Ment. Health Nurs.* 19(1): 34–43.

Li F, Liu X, Zhang D. (2016) Fish consumption and risk of depression: a meta-analysis. *J. Epidemiol. Community Health*. 70(3): 299–304.

Markowitw S, Friedman MA, Arent SM. (2008) Understanding the relationship between obesity and depression; causal mechanisms and implications for treatment. *Clin. Psychol. Sci. Pract.* 15(1): 1–20.

McManus S, Meltzer H, Brugha T, *et al.* (2009) *Adult psychiatric morbidity in England, 2007. The NHS Information Centre for Health and Social Care*. Available at https://digital.nhs.uk/data-and-information/publications/statistical/adult-psychiatric-morbidity-survey/adult-psychiatric-morbidity-in-england-2007-results-of-a-household-survey. Accessed 1 November 2018.

Mental Health Act. (1983) Her Majesty's Government. The Mental Health Act (c20) Available at https://www.legislation.gov.uk/ukpga/1983/20/contents. Accessed 1 November 2018.

NICE. (2017) Eating disorders: recognition and treatment CG 69. Available at https://www.nice.org.uk/guidance/ng69. Accessed 1 November 2018.

Norvik D, Suarez D, Vieta E, Nabar D. (2009) Recovery in outservice user settings a 36 months result from The Schizophrenia Outservice Users Health Outcomes Study. *Schizophrenia Research* 108(1–3): 223–230.

Opie R, Itsiopoulos C, Parletta N, et al. (2016) Dietary recommendations for the prevention of depression. *Nutr. Neurosci.* 20(3): 161–171.

Parsons B, Allison D, Loebel A, *et al.* (2009) Weight effects associated with antipsychotics: a comprehensive database analysis. *Schizophr. Res.* 110(1–3): 103–110.

Quirk S, Williams L, O'Neil A, et al. (2013) The association between diet quality, dietary patterns and depression in adults: a systematic review. *BMC Psychiatry*. 13: 175.

Ross B, Seguin J, Sieswerda L. (2007) Omega 3 fatty acid as treatment for mental illness; which disorder and which fatty acid. *Lipids Health Dis.* 18(6): 21.

Sánchez-Villegas A, Henríquez-Sánchez P, Ruiz-Canela M, et al. (2015) A longitudinal analysis of diet quality scores and the risk of incident depression in the SUN Project. *BMC Medicine* 13: 197.

WHO. (1992) The ICD 10 Classification of Mental and Behavioral Disorders. Available at http://www.who.int/classifications/icd/en/GRNBOOK.pdf. Accessed 1 November 2018.

WHO. (2014) Mental health: a state of well-being. Available at https://www.who.int/features/factfiles/mental_health/en/ Accessed 27 February 2019.

7.10.2 Eating disorders

Kate Williams

Key points

- Dietitians in all areas of clinical practice should be alert to signs of undiagnosed disordered eating and be able to offer guidance on further investigation and support.
- Dietitians working in the field of eating disorders management should be part of a multidisciplinary team and have appropriate support and supervision.

Eating disorders are syndromes in which abnormalities of eating behaviour, driven by psychological factors, are severe and persistent enough to impair health and nutrition, interfere with social eating, and give rise to distress in sufferers and those close to them. In all areas of clinical practice, dietitians discuss eating behaviour with their patients and are often able to identify disordered eating. Although some people with eating disorders may go to great lengths to conceal them, many may welcome the opportunity to raise their concerns and begin to get help. It is important that dietitians enable patients to talk honestly about their eating, identify possible eating disorders and offer support to get the help they need. Disordered eating may severely interfere with the dietetic treatment of other conditions, so dietitians need to be alert to the possibility of disordered eating in order to achieve good outcomes of treatment.

As changing eating behaviour and improving nutrition are central to recovery from eating disorders, dietitians can make important contributions to the care and treatment of people with these conditions. There are few areas of dietetic practice that demand more skill in engaging and motivating patients, and communicating with colleagues. A warm, empathic and non-judgemental therapeutic relationship can empower a patient to discuss anxiety and distress about eating, and use help and support. For a guide to developing and using these skills, see Gable and Herrmann (2016). For detailed reviews of the contribution of the dietitian to the management of eating disorders, see Hart *et al.* (2011), Ozier *et al.* (2011), Garrett *et al.* (2005) and Herrin and Larkin (2012).

Background and historical perspective

In anorexia nervosa (AN) the central feature is deliberate and persistent restriction of food intake. It, or at least a condition with very similar features, has been described for hundreds, possibly thousands, of years (Brumberg, 1988; Grimm, 1996; Vandereycken & van Deth, 1994). AN was first named in the medical literature in the late nineteenth century by Gull (1874, 1888) and Lasègue (1873). Strikingly, these descriptions do not refer to fear of fatness as an essential feature; this seems to have emerged in Western cultures during the twentieth century, alongside increasing social valuation of thinness, especially in women (Bruch, 1973). The condition may present differently in some individuals, especially those from non-Western cultures (Nasser, 1997).

Bulimia nervosa (BN) is a condition in which there is a cycle of restriction of food intake, followed by binge eating and extreme efforts to compensate for the feared fattening effects of the binge, commonly by repeated restriction of eating, vomiting, excessive use of laxatives or over-exercising. Russell first described it in 1979 and characterised it initially as a development of AN (Russell, 1979). It quickly became clear that it might arise without any previous episodes of anorexia. The change from restricting anorexia to BN is not unusual (Fairburn & Harrison, 2003), and people with eating disorders may display different symptoms at different times. Partial syndromes are a common presentation.

In 1992, Spitzer *et al.* proposed diagnostic criteria for the binge eating disorder, in which the individual regularly binge eats, but does not compensate for the binges. The binge eating is distinguished from normal occasional overeating by its persistence and frequency, and the psychological distress associated with it. It is generally associated with obesity, which may be severe.

Diagnostic criteria and classification

Two published sets of diagnostic criteria for eating disorders are in use: the International Classification of Diseases (ICD), published by the World Health Organization (WHO), and the Diagnostic and Statistical Manual of Mental Disorders (DSM), published by the American Psychiatric Association (2013). Both set out criteria for the diagnosis of the major disorders, AN and BN, and for some partial syndromes (Table 7.10.2). DSM-5 now includes binge eating disorder and other distinct eating disorders (Box 7.10.1). These strict definitions allow the identification of the disorders for research and other purposes, but dietitians in clinical practice may encounter many people with disordered eating who do not exactly meet any of these criteria, but need help to recover.

Features and processes of eating disorders

It can be difficult to understand disorders that provoke behaviour that seems very abnormal and damaging. It may be helpful for the practitioner seeking to develop an empathic relationship with a person with an eating disorder to have some awareness of the way the disorders develop and become entrenched.

Anorexia nervosa

The central feature of AN is restriction of food intake severely enough to keep body mass index (BMI) below $17.5\,kg/m^2$ (and often much lower), with the resulting constellation of features of starvation. This is accompanied by a conviction that the restriction of food intake is appropriate for the individual, usually because they feel the need to reduce their weight.

Genetic predisposing factors (Bulik *et al.*, 2007; Gorwood *et al.*, 2003), some personality traits and thinking styles are known to increase vulnerability to developing AN. A tendency to perfectionism, rule-bound and rigid thinking, and attention to detail at the expense of a broader and more flexible approach can predispose to the disorder (Treasure *et al.*, 2010). This may underlie the association with autistic spectrum disorders (Oldershaw *et al.*, 2011). Distressing experiences in early life such as emotional or physical neglect, or physical or sexual abuse add to the risk. A very common trigger in Western cultures is dieting, which is tried by the great majority of adolescent girls and many boys. Well-publicised diets offer many detailed rules, and may seem gratifying to a person with a perfectionistic, rigid and detail-focussed approach. In vulnerable individuals, dieting may become entrenched because of anxiety about breaking self-imposed rules, and perfectionism and self-criticism driving continually increasing efforts. The pursuit of weight loss can seem rewarding and offer a distraction from persistent emotional distress, becoming increasingly extreme and fixed behaviour. Any increase in food intake may result in rapid weight gain because of repletion of glycogen stores with associated water, and so add to the belief that breaking the rules of the diet will result in uncontrollable weight increase.

From this experience develops a profound fear of fatness and weight gain, and body image distortion,

Table 7.10.2 Summarised diagnostic criteria for eating disorders

ICD-10 (WHO, 1992)	DSM-5 (American Psychiatric Association, 2013)
Anorexia nervosa	
For a definite diagnosis, all the following are required: A. Body weight is maintained at least 15% below that expected, or a BMI of ≤17.5 kg/m^2. Prepubertal patients may fail to make the expected weight gain during the period of growth. B. The weight loss is self-induced by avoidance of 'fattening foods'. One or more of the following may also be present: self-induced vomiting, self-induced purging, excessive exercise, use of appetite suppressants and/or diuretics. C. There is body image distortion, whereby a dread of fatness persists as an intrusive, overvalued idea. D. A widespread endocrine disorder involving the hypothalamic–pituitary–gonadal axis is manifest in women as amenorrhoea, and in men as loss of sexual interest and potency. There may also be elevated levels of growth hormone, raised levels of cortisol, changes in the peripheral metabolism of the thyroid gland, and abnormalities of insulin secretion. E. If onset is prepubertal, the sequence of pubertal events is delayed or even arrested. With recovery, puberty is often completed normally, but menarche is late.	A. Restriction of energy intake severe and persistent enough to result in significantly low body weight in the context of age, sex, developmental trajectory, and physical health. For children and adolescents, less than that minimally expected. B. Intense fear of gaining weight or becoming fat, or persistent behaviour that prevents weight gain. C. Disturbance in the way in which body weight or shape is experienced, undue influence of body weight or shape on self-evaluation, or persistent lack of recognition of the seriousness of the low body weight. **Restricting type:** During the last 3 months, recurrent episodes of binge eating or purging behaviour have not been present. **Binge eating/purging type:** During the last 3 months, there have been recurrent episodes of binge eating or purging behaviour. *Additional indicators of severity, including categories of BMI:* Mild, BMI ≥ 17 kg/m^2 Moderate, BMI 16–16.99 kg/m^2 Severe, BMI 15–15.99 kg/m^2 Extreme, BMI < 15 kg/m^2
Bulimia nervosa	
For a definite diagnosis, all of the following are required: A. There is persistent preoccupation with eating, and an irresistible craving for food; the patient succumbs to episodes of overeating in which large amounts of food are consumed in short periods of time. B. The patient attempts to counteract the 'fattening' effects of food by one or more of the following: self-induced vomiting; purgative abuse; periods of starvation; use of drugs such as appetite suppressants, thyroid preparations or diuretics. When bulimia occurs in diabetic patients, they may choose to neglect their insulin treatment. C. The psychopathology consists of a morbid dread of fatness. There is often, but not always, a history of an earlier episode of AN, the interval between the two disorders ranging from a few months to several years.	A. Recurrent episodes of binge eating, characterised by both of the following: 1. Eating, in a discrete period of time, an amount of food that is definitely larger than what most people would eat in similar circumstances. 2. A sense of lack of control over eating during the episode. B. Recurrent inappropriate compensatory behaviours, such as self-induced vomiting, misuse of laxatives, fasting or excessive exercise. C. The binge eating and inappropriate compensatory behaviours both occur on average at least once a week for 3 months. D. Self-evaluation is unduly influenced by body shape and weight. E. The disturbance does not occur exclusively during episodes of anorexia nervosa.

Box 7.10.1 Key diagnostic features of binge eating disorder (American Psychiatric Association, 2013)

1. Recurrent episodes of binge eating, with a sense of lack of control
2. Binge eating episodes are associated with three (or more) of the following:
   - Eating much more rapidly than normal
   - Eating until feeling uncomfortably full
   - Eating large amounts of food when not feeling physically hungry
   - Eating alone because of being embarrassed by how much one is eating
   - Feeling disgusted with oneself, depressed, or very guilty after overeating
3. Marked distress regarding binge eating
4. Binge eating happens on at least one day a week for 3 months
5. Absence of regular compensatory behaviors (such as purging).

although other anxieties may predominate in some individuals. In many individuals, the increasing hunger and food craving lead to binge eating, with anxiety-driven attempts to compensate for the binge with purging or exercise (Fairburn & Harrison, 2003). The behaviour may become very fixed because it begins at a time of rapid brain development, and the malnutrition itself may interfere with this process, in particular the maturation of emotional regulation, so that the person may find it difficult to counter the anxiety and other emotions that drive the abnormal behaviour (Harrison *et al.*, 2009; Treasure *et al.*, 2010).

Bulimia nervosa

The major feature of BN is a cycle of restriction of eating, which may be very severe, followed by food craving and uncontrolled excessive eating. This raises anxiety about the possible weight increase the binge might cause, provoking attempts to compensate, most commonly by self-induced vomiting, excessive use of laxatives or excessive exercise, and further restriction of eating. This binge–starve cycle is driven by overvaluation of thinness, and attempts to lose weight as a means to improve low self-esteem. Low mood can deprive the individual of the motivation to change (Ruhsing *et al.*, 2003). Predisposing factors include poor impulse control, and, as in AN, distressing early experience increases risk. Attempts to diet, commonly beginning in the early teenage years, may be unsuccessful in response to hunger and food craving, setting up the binge–starve cycle (Figure 7.10.1). It is possible that binge eaters have an increased drive to seek rewarding behaviour, and that the binge–starve cycle can become entrenched as food deprivation increases the reward of eating, so the drive to binge becomes increasingly powerful (Davis *et al.*, 2008; Thanos *et al.*, 2008; Wang *et al.*, 2011).

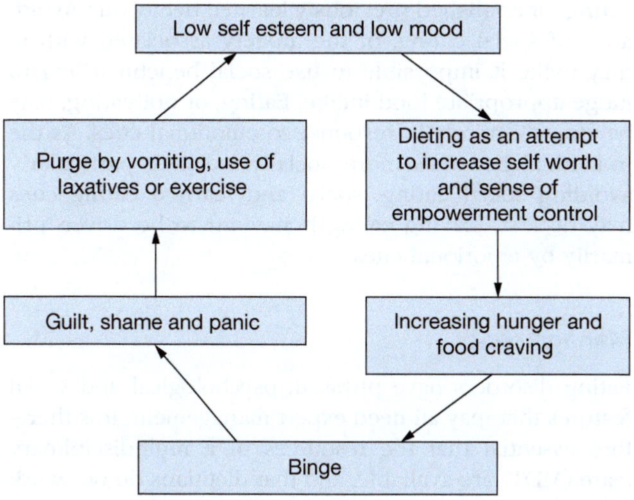

Figure 7.10.1 Binge–starve cycle in bulimia nervosa

Binge eating disorders

At present, only DSM-5 sets out diagnostic criteria for the binge eating disorder as shown in Box 7.10.1.

Partial and mixed syndromes

In any individual, the symptoms of an eating disorder may change over time, so that the person may move from one diagnostic category to another (Fairburn & Harrison, 2003). In clinical practice, the most commonly occurring eating disorders are partial syndromes that do not fully meet diagnostic criteria for AN or BN. Management strategies can be agreed on the basis of the most damaging or distressing symptoms. Binge eating disorder is characterised by repeated episodes of binge eating, without significant compensatory behaviours other than repeated attempts at dieting (Spitzer *et al.*, 1992). Levels of concern about weight and shape are similar to those in the other eating disorders, and higher than in obese people without binge eating disorder (Wilfley *et al.*, 2003). Childhood obesity, negative early experience and low self-esteem are predisposing factors (Fairburn *et al.*, 1998).

Epidemiology and public health aspects

Incidence and prevalence

Researchers considering the incidence and prevalence of eating disorders often urge caution, and suggest that published figures may be underestimates for a number of reasons, including secrecy about symptoms and reluctance to seek treatment (Hoek, 2006; Hoek & van Hoeken, 2003; Hudson *et al.*, 2007; Rooney *et al.*, 1995). For example, Keski-Rahkonen *et al.* (2007) found that, in a community sample, half of the cases of AN had not been detected by healthcare services.

Smink *et al.* (2012) reviewed the literature on incidence and prevalence, and found that they had remained relatively stable for some decades, with the highest incidence of AN in females aged 15–19 years, being 40% of cases with an incidence of 109.2 per 100,000. The incidence of BN is also highest in females, at around 40 per 100,000 person-years for females aged 10–19 years, with some evidence of decreasing age of incidence. The incidence of AN and BN is much lower in males, e.g. in data from the Netherlands and UK, incidence was found to be <1 per 100,000 person-years. Prevalence is lower in non-Western societies, but there is some evidence that it is increasing with the spread of Western cultural norms. Anorexia has long been recognised as having the highest mortality of any mental disorders (Harris & Barraclough, 1998); the review by Smink *et al.* (2012) of more recent evidence confirms this. Significant causes of death include suicide and cardiac complications, and there are concerns about the risk of death resulting from inappropriate refeeding practices (Royal College of Psychiatrists, 2014). For BN, Hoek and van Hoeken (2003) and Hoek (2006) found an incidence of about 1% among young women. For whole populations, there were incidence rates of at least 8 per 100,000 person-years for AN and 12 for BN.

Prevention

Prevention of eating disorders presents a complex challenge. It is clear that the protection of children from abuse and neglect is helpful in the prevention of eating disorders and other mental health problems. Specialist interventions targeted at the most vulnerable groups may be the most effective (Stice *et al.*, 2007). There is continuing controversy about the part played by cultural influences. In their general practice, dietitians should emphasise eating to support general health and nutrition, rather than focussing too narrowly on the control of body weight (Ozier *et al.*, 2011).

Medical and nutritional effects of eating disorders

Anorexia nervosa

Much of the information about the physical and psychological effects of starvation in otherwise healthy individuals comes from the classic work of Keys *et al.* (1950), in which healthy male volunteers ate approximately half of their energy requirement for a 12-week period (Kalm & Semba, 2005; Keys *et al.*, 1950). Starvation results in general malnutrition, affecting all tissues and organs (Mitchell & Crow, 2006). The main tissue loss is adipose tissue and muscle mass. Internal organs are not affected until the more advanced stages of malnutrition, when liver, heart and brain reduce in mass, with resulting loss of function (Casiero & Frishman, 2006; Treasure *et al.*, 2010; Winston & Stafford, 2000), and gut function is compromised (Robinson, 2000; Robinson *et al.*, 1988).

Endocrine function can be severely disturbed as an adaptation to starvation, affecting the thyroid and adrenal glands and the gonads via the hypothalamus and pituitary axis (Lawson & Klibanski, 2008; Warren, 2011). Suppression of thyroid function results in bradycardia, hypotension and hypothermia, with subjective cold sensitivity and poor sleep. The reduction in fat mass reduces leptin secretion, while cortisol secretion is increased. The tendency to central deposition of adipose tissue, which is usually a feature of hypercortisolaemia, is absent because adipose tissue is depleted; but, during recovery, a common cause of distress is the central distribution of the repleting fat mass (Lawson & Klibanski, 2008). Suppression of sex hormones results in amenorrhoea in women, and a range of other effects. These endocrine changes underlie the increased risk of osteoporosis that accompanies the nutritional deficit. The development of the illness during adolescence, when bone density should be increasing rapidly, adds further to the risk (Teng, 2011). This is a major physical complication of AN, and may not completely reverse with recovery of endocrine function, healthy body weight and good nutrition (Serpell & Treasure, 1997; Teng, 2011; Zipfel *et al.*, 2000).

The effects on the gut can make increasing food intake uncomfortable and add to its aversiveness. The direct effects of persistent vomiting may damage the teeth and the soft tissues of the mouth. Iron and riboflavin deficiency can cause glossitis and angular cheilosis, making eating uncomfortable (Frydrych *et al.*, 2005; Newton & Travess, 2000). Peristalsis is slow, causing delayed gastric emptying (Robinson *et al.*, 1988), bloating and constipation.

The volunteers in the study by Keys *et al.* also showed increases in depression, preoccupation with food to the exclusion of other interests, obsessive and bizarre eating behaviour, and social isolation (Keys *et al.*, 1950). These psychological effects are all seen in AN.

Bulimia nervosa

BN can result in erratic body weight. Vomiting and laxative use can cause disturbances in blood electrolytes, in particular low potassium (Fairburn & Harrison, 2003). Binge eating and vomiting can cause damage to the gastrointestinal tract (Mitchell & Crow, 2006; Ruhsing *et al.*, 2003), including gastro-oesophageal reflux, and acid erosion of the teeth (Frydrych *et al.*, 2005).

Binge eating disorder

This disorder is often associated with obesity, which may be extreme, and a history of weight cycling, with many attempts to reduce body weight, often including a variety of commercial diets and medication. The physical complications and excess mortality relate generally to the associated obesity (Bulik & Reichborn-Kjennerud, 2003; Wilfley *et al.*, 2003).

People with any eating disorder may find it very difficult to regulate their food intake appropriately. They may experience abnormalities of normal physiological sensations of hunger and satiety (Treasure *et al.*, 2012), and, during the development of the disorder, may have overridden them by persistent restriction or repeated binge eating, having lost the ability to respond normally. There are changes in the production of gut hormones associated with physiological appetite control, which may further serve to entrench the abnormal eating (Prince *et al.*, 2010). Erratic and distorted food choice and meal pattern may further impair physiological appetite regulation. Persistently abnormal eating may have prevented the learning needed for the development of normal eating, or abolished previously learned behaviour. Avoidance of social eating, or the anxiety associated with it, may make it impossible to use social benchmarking to judge appropriate food intake. Eating, or not eating, may be almost entirely in response to emotional cues. As the individual becomes more socially isolated, particularly avoiding social eating, social and learned eating cues may be lost, leaving eating behaviour to be driven primarily by emotional cues.

Management

Eating disorders have physical, psychological and social features that may all need expert management. It is therefore essential that the resources of a multidisciplinary team (MDT) are available, and that dietitians do not work alone (Ozier *et al.*, 2011; NICE, 2017). Good communication among the members of the MDT is therefore a high priority. There is also a particular need for good communication and effective working partnerships between specialist dietitians in eating disorders and those in acute medical or intensive care services, to which patients with AN may be admitted (Royal College of Psychiatrists, 2014). The dietitian can make a valuable contribution to the team by improving the nutritional knowledge of all team members (Cordery & Waller, 2006) and raising awareness of the risk of refeeding syndrome (Hearing, 2004).

Ambivalence about recovery and fluctuating motivation challenge everyone involved in the work towards recovery. Skills in counselling and motivation enhancement are needed for help and support to be effective (Treasure & Schmidt, 2001). Throughout the treatment process, a collaborative and motivational approach can support behaviour change and recovery (Feld *et al.*, 2001). Recovery from an eating disorder can be a difficult and complex process. This can present challenges to practitioners, so good support and governance are essential. Dietitians working in this area should seek appropriate supervision. Skilled supervision can help dietitians with the development and productive use of their skills, effective collaboration among colleagues, maintenance of professional and personal boundaries, and managing what can be a distressing experience (Ozier *et al.*, 2011; BDA, 2011).

Major elements of treatment include psychotherapy, medication to help manage depression and anxiety, and development of social skills and skills to support managing eating, such as shopping and cooking. The dietitian can contribute by managing nutritional risk, supporting nutritional rehabilitation and providing education on food and nutrition.

Identification in dietetic clinical practice

In general dietetic practice, indications of disordered eating may be apparent before a formal diagnosis is made, or at a level of severity and frequency that do not meet diagnostic criteria, but nevertheless cause distress, damage health and nutrition, and impair dietetic management. It is therefore important that dietitians are alert to signs and symptoms of disordered eating, and are able to manage them, or refer for more specialist support. It is perhaps not surprising that disordered eating arises in situations where anxiety about eating and nutrition is high, e.g. in the management of obesity (de Zwaan, 2001) and diabetes (Fairburn *et al.*, 1991).

Routine dietetic assessment may expose signs that might indicate disordered eating. Anthropometry may reveal reluctance to be weighed, underweight in the absence of known physical cause or obesity associated with a history of weight cycling. Biochemical indicators include low blood potassium, which may result from persistent vomiting or laxative abuse, or low sodium because of water loading to suppress hunger or falsify weight. Diet history may show erratic eating, restriction of amount and variety of food, rigidity and inappropriate rules about eating and food choice, binge eating or other presentations of uncontrolled overeating such as grazing or night eating, deranged eating patterns, and

Table 7.10.3 Screening questions for eating disorders

SCOFF (Morgan *et al.*, 1999)	ESP (Cotton *et al.*, 2003)
Do you make yourself sick because you feel uncomfortably full?	Are you satisfied with your eating patterns?
Do you worry that you have lost control over how much you eat?	Do you ever eat in secret?
Have you recently lost more than 1 stone in a 3-month period?	Does your weight affect the way you feel about yourself?
Do you believe yourself to be fat when others say you are too thin?	Have any members of your family suffered with an eating disorder?
Would you say that food dominates your life?	Do you currently suffer with or have you ever suffered in the past with an eating disorder?

high anxiety about eating. The SCOFF (Morgan *et al.*, 1999) and Eating disorder Screen for Primary care (ESP) tools (Cotton *et al.*, 2003) (Table 7.10.3) are very brief questionnaires designed and validated for use in primary care to help identify disordered eating. Dietitians can use them, or selected questions from them, to help confirm concerns about the presence of an eating disorder, and to encourage their patients to talk about their eating and agree to appropriate management.

If an eating disorder is suspected, patients should be promptly referred for appropriate assessment and treatment (NICE, 2017).

Dietetic assessment

Although people with eating disorders may present with a wide variety of dietetic problems, from severe underweight and malnutrition to severe obesity and weight cycling, the assessment process can be similar for all eating disorders. The aims of assessment are to begin to develop a trusting and productive therapeutic relationship that will support recovery, to develop and maintain motivation to change (Ozier *et al.*, 2011; Gable & Herrmann, 2016; Herrin & Larkin, 2012), and to gather the information needed to make a dietetic diagnosis and negotiate a treatment plan (BDA, 2009).

The structure of the process is similar to any dietetic assessment, but may require more time than average because of the ambivalence and anxiety of the patient, and the complexity of the history. It may be helpful to use more than one session to complete the process. Much information may come from previous medical assessments, e.g. diagnoses, results of blood tests and information on medication. However, the most important element is the conversation with the patient, and usually also with family members if the patient is living with them, especially if he or she is under 18 years of age. The way in which this conversation is conducted will be led to some extent by the patient, but the information needed falls into the standard dietetic assessment framework.

Anthropometry

This includes:

- Weight, height and BMI.
- For people under 18 years of age, height, weight and BMI centiles. Expected weight for height may also be useful.

Being weighed can be distressing for a person with an eating disorder. Hence, a clear explanation of the need for finding the body weight should be given, and permission sought and recorded carefully.

Biochemistry

This includes:

- *Electrolytes* – low levels of sodium, potassium and magnesium in the context of low body weight may indicate chronic low intake. Low potassium may result from the use of laxatives or self-induced vomiting. Low sodium is most likely to be due to excessive water intake to suppress hunger or falsify body weight.
- *Iron status* – haemoglobin may be low if food intake has been severely restricted for a long period, but may be protected by reduced iron loss with amenorrhoea. Much more commonly, low ferritin indicates low iron stores.
- *White cell count* – overall white cell count, or one or more elements of total white cells, may be low in chronic semi-starvation.
- *Urea* – levels will be low in chronic, severe restriction of food intake.

Low levels of urea, electrolytes and other biochemical indicators may be masked by dehydration, resulting in false normal results (Caregaro *et al.*, 2005), so care should be taken to interpret blood test results alongside indicators of hydration, such as blood pressure.

Clinical assessment

This includes:

- Eating disorder diagnosis and other diagnoses of both physical and psychological disorders.
- Endocrine function – indicators include amenorrhoea, hypotension with postural drop, bradycardia, hypothermia and subjective feeling of cold, and poor sleep.
- Low bone mineral density – a dual-energy X ray absorptiometry (DXA) scan to measure bone density is recommended for people with a history of low weight for 6 months or longer (NICE, 2017).
- Psychological effects such as low or labile mood, irritability, impaired memory or concentration.
- Medication.

Dietary assessment

This includes:

- Detailed history of weight and eating. It is helpful to take a history at least from the beginning of the eating disorder symptoms, and sometimes from infancy, to consider early feeding difficulties. The history should seek to identify periods of low or high weight; the degree of abnormality, weight cycling and instability; and any occasions when weight was normal and stable. This can help to develop a shared understanding of the way in which eating, body weight, psychological factors and life events relate to each other.
- Current diet and disordered eating symptoms:
  - Restriction in the amount and variety of foods eaten, foods avoided, foods that are acceptable.
  - Meal pattern, timing and frequency of eating, and variability of meal pattern.
  - Irrational or exaggerated rules and beliefs about eating.
  - Binge eating, grazing or other uncontrolled overeating; foods used for binge eating.
  - Purging and compensatory behaviour, such as vomiting, laxative use and excessive exercise.
  - Emotional responses to food and eating, such as anxiety or disgust.
  - Social context of eating.
  - Fluid intake, which may be restricted or excessive.
  - Alcohol intake.
  - Nutritional supplements such as vitamins.
- Impaired appetite regulation and subjective ability to control food intake.

Economic and social assessment

This includes:

- *Education or employment* – these may help to structure the day and eating pattern, or impede routine if there are changing work shifts or an erratic timetable. Education or employment may be important motivators, or worsen anxiety, distress and lower self-esteem.
- *Finance* – persistent severe binge eating may generate debt. Worries about money may add to the stress associated with buying and using food.
- *Social support* – it is useful to identify family members and friends who can support recovery.
- *Household information* – facilities for food preparation, sharing meals with other members of the household.

Feelings

Assessment of motivation and concerns is essential to begin the process of change. The assessment process can help identify the stage of change (Prochaska & DiClemente, 1983), the concerns raised by the eating disorders, and the reasons for recovery. These will inform the priorities for change in eating behaviour, identify barriers to and motivators for change, and form a basis for the treatment plan.

Dietetic treatment of eating disorders

Aims and priorities for treatment should be negotiated collaboratively by the dietitian and the sufferer, and carers when appropriate, especially when the sufferer is a child or adolescent (NICE, 2017). Modest steps towards the treatment aims can then be planned in the form

Table 7.10.4 Treatment outcomes for eating disorders

Treatment domain	Outcome
Biochemical	Normalised blood urea and electrolytes
	Normalised white cell count
	Normalised iron status (haemoglobin and ferritin)
Psychological	Reduced anxiety about eating and weight
	More stable mood
	Increased motivation to prevent relapse
Behaviour change domain	Reduced restriction of eating
	Abolition of binge eating
	Abolition of purging
	Healthier food choices
	Normal fluid intake
Physical domain	Healthy BMI
	In children and adolescents, normal growth, or catch-up growth as appropriate
	Improved bone mineral density
Symptom change domain	Reduced reflux, bloating, constipation
	Normal sleep
	Abolished faintness, giddiness
	Normal body temperature control
	Normal menstruation
Patient-focused domain	Achievement of aims for employment or education
	Avoiding hospital admission
	Independent living
	Improved personal relationships
	Improved social eating
	Appropriate physical activity

of SMART (specific, measurable, achievable, relevant and time-limited) goals. This process should proceed alongside psychological treatment to support changes in thinking and behaviour. Treatment outcomes are likely to include several domains, as shown in Table 7.10.4.

Anorexia nervosa

Evidence for the effectiveness of dietetic interventions is limited, but there is agreement in published guidance that dietetic care is an essential element of management (Hart *et al.*, 2011). Treatment may be provided in a hospital inpatient setting, day care or outpatient service. Regular weight monitoring and medical monitoring are essential at each stage of treatment, to ensure that appropriate management is in place for any problems that arise (NICE, 2017).

Treatment is in three distinct phases: medical stabilisation and management of refeeding syndrome risk; nutrition rehabilitation and increasing responsibility for normal and healthy eating; and, finally, maintenance and relapse prevention.

There is very limited evidence to guide the best approach to nutritional rehabilitation, in terms of macronutrient mix, speed of rehabilitation or method of delivery (Marzola *et al.*, 2013). In practice, the choice of type of food, use of oral nutritional supplements, or tube feeding is at least as much influenced by what is tolerable for the patient as by optimal nutritional provision, and a major part of the dietitian's contribution involves finding the best balance for the individual.

Phase 1: stabilisation

The early stage of refeeding carries risk, especially if the anorexia is severe, and it is uncomfortable and distressing. Gradual increases in food intake, with good information, clear explanations and consistent support, can help manage increased anxiety. It may be difficult to strike an optimal balance between keeping food intake low to prevent refeeding syndrome and increasing it quickly enough to reduce the risks imposed by the malnutrition (Royal College of Psychiatrists, 2014).

The evidence on the management of refeeding syndrome comes largely from critical care, where patients are acutely ill or physically traumatised (NICE, 2006a), and so are catabolic (see Chapter 7.17.1, Critical care). People with AN are generally not critically ill, but are severely starved, so rapidly become anabolic with refeeding. This difference in response to increasing food intake may affect the risk of refeeding syndrome, but evidence is lacking. However, there is a clear risk of refeeding syndrome in AN (Birmingham *et al.*, 1996; Fisher *et al.*, 2000), so caution is needed, and close monitoring is essential. This may be particularly challenging in non-specialist settings such as medical wards or intensive care units, where the guidance from the Royal College of Psychiatrists (2014) may be especially useful. The consensus is that feeding can safely be started at about 20 kcal (80 kJ)/kg of body weight/24 hours, using a tube-feeding formula or food.

To prevent Wernicke–Korsakoff syndrome, prophylactic thiamine should be given daily, following NICE guidance (NICE, 2006a) for the prevention of refeeding syndrome. There is likely to be a general deficiency of micronutrients, so multivitamins and minerals should be a part of global nutritional rehabilitation (Hadigan *et al.*, 2000; Rock & Vasantharajan, 1995; Setnick, 2010). Total fluid should be controlled, as cardiac capacity may be limited by the loss of cardiac muscle mass, and a rapid increase in blood volume may risk cardiac failure (Winston & Stafford, 2000). Weight gain may be rapid during the first 7–10 days of refeeding, owing to rehydration and, sometimes, temporary fluid retention, especially if persistent vomiting or laxative abuse are stopped. Explanation of the effect, and reassurance that it is self-limiting, may be helpful.

Tube feeding

Where tube feeding is the preferred route, bolus feeding is generally easier to manage, as it allows the patient to be mobile, and it is easier to supervise the delivery of the feed and prevent sabotage. Because the overall volume initially is low, bolus volume can be relatively low, which helps to prevent bloating and discomfort. Six boluses of 100–150 mL/day will allow the delivery of an adequate volume of feed for a person of 25–45 kg. At first, an isotonic formula is preferable, as it does not cause osmotic movement of water into the gut, which may be uncomfortable and create a pseudo-dumping syndrome, with faintness due to fall in blood pressure. As feed volume is increased, a higher-density feed may help prevent feelings of bloating (Gentile *et al.*, 2010).

Oral feeding

Initially, care should be taken to limit carbohydrate and ensure a high intake of potassium and phosphate, as blood levels can fall rapidly as part of refeeding syndrome (NICE, 2006a). This can be achieved by giving a high proportion of intake in the form of cow's milk as a source of phosphate, and fruit juice as a source of potassium. It may be more comfortable to give fruit juice diluted with water, especially if the mouth is sore. Small meals with a modest amount of food choice can help manage anxiety. Too much choice may be overwhelming.

It should be possible to accommodate vegetarian diets without difficulty. Avoidance of meat and fish is culturally common, and required by some religions, and there is no reason to challenge such a choice at this stage. If vegetarianism has developed as part of the eating disorder pathology, it may be addressed later in treatment. Vegan diets, with no animal products, present some risks, as these diets tend to have low energy density, so the patient is faced with a relatively large volume of food. The high fibre content may be uncomfortable and can possibly increase the risk of gastric dilatation or rupture (Saul *et al.*, 1981). If a vegan diet is to be used, food provision should be planned to provide adequate phosphate (most easily by using soya milk with added phosphate) and to minimise volume and fibre. Vigilant monitoring of blood and physical condition is required, and treatment adjusted according to results.

Phase 2: nutritional rehabilitation

NICE (2017) recommends recovery of healthy weight as a key goal of treatment. The aims for the rate of weight gain should be negotiated, e.g. for young people with a short duration of illness, rapid nutritional recovery supports good outcome, whereas a slower rate of weight gain may be appropriate for patients with a very long history of low weight. Setting overall aims will guide the process of agreeing on and reviewing SMART goals to progress towards recovery. The aims during this stage are to:

- Recover weight, ideally to a healthy weight that will restore normal endocrine function and reduce the risk of osteoporosis.
- Restore optimal nutritional status and normalise blood indicators of poor nutrition.
- Replete body stores of nutrients.
- Increase confidence and knowledge to support the ability to eat normally and independently, as appropriate for age and social circumstances.
- Reduce physical symptoms of malnutrition.
- Reduce anxiety about eating and preoccupation with food.
- Reduce abnormal eating behaviour.
- Abolish purging.

These goals must be aimed for alongside psychological work to reduce eating disorder psychopathology and symptoms. Strategies to achieve these aims may include the following:

- Careful calculation of energy intake to achieve weight gain at the agreed rate.
- Multivitamin and mineral supplementation (NICE, 2017).
- Negotiated meal plans to support regular eating, increasing amount and variety of food, and normalising meal pattern.
- A portion exchange system to develop flexibility.
- Planning eating to prevent anxiety associated with eating, especially when making decisions under pressure.
- Education on healthy, normal eating and body weight.
- Information about specific nutritional deficiencies such as low iron status.
- Education on natural appetite control and support to improve it.
- Practising eating, shopping and cooking with support as appropriate for the person's age, circumstances and lifestyle, to improve confidence, independence and flexibility.

Phase 3: Maintenance of improvement and relapse prevention

There is a risk of relapse of anorexia. People recovering need help to identify possible situations that may increase risk of relapse, to develop strategies to prevent relapse, and to identify relapse quickly and reverse it. Some risk situations may involve particular kinds of eating, and the dietitian can help to anticipate and plan for these. Difficulties can arise in some social situations such as celebrations or unexpected eating occasions; periods of religious fasting; and situations where the choice of food may be very limited, such as while travelling or staying with friends. Planning for these situations can help to reduce risk. Skills sin meal planning and a good knowledge of healthy, normal eating can be helpful, particularly learning and practising appropriate use of foods that may be perceived as unhealthy; usually high-fat and high-sugar foods.

Bulimia nervosa

The main element of treatment for BN is cognitive behavioural therapy (CBT) (NICE, 2017). Dietetic intervention may be helpful alongside this for patients who are finding it particularly difficult to stabilise eating, who have poor knowledge or confidence to eat healthily, or who have particular nutritional problems such as iron deficiency anaemia. As part of CBT, patients will be encouraged to self-monitor eating and purging by keeping a diary; this will also usually be used to record all food and fluid intake (Table 7.10.5). The CBT approach asks for recording of the situation, thoughts and feelings before the eating episode (antecedents); the date and time of

Table 7.10.5 Example of headings for a self-monitoring diary

Date	Time	Food and drink	Antecedents	Behaviour (meal, snack or binge)	Consequences

eating and drinking; details of the type and amount of foods and fluids consumed or avoided (behaviour); a subjective rating of whether this was a meal, snack or binge; and the thoughts, feelings and events after it (consequences). Learning this ABC (antecedents, behaviour, consequences) approach can be helpful in showing the way that dietary restriction leads to hunger and food craving, the powerful impulse to eat and the events or feelings that may then trigger binge eating.

The aims of treatment include:

- Abolition of binge eating and purging.
- Reduction of restriction of amount and variety of food.
- Establishment of regular, stable eating that is healthy and socially normal for the individual.
- Improvement in appetite regulation.
- Stabilisation of body weight in the healthy range.
- Increased confidence and reduced anxiety about eating.

There may also be a need to manage other influences on appetite, such as the use of alcohol or cannabis. Strategies to reduce hunger and the drive to binge include the following:

- Improve understanding of the ways in which restriction of food intake drives uncontrolled eating, particularly physiological hunger, which may not be recognised, and the hyper reward of eating when food-deprived.
- Ensure adequate calorie intake to maintain weight, or increase it at an agreed rate if underweight. It may be reassuring to explain how this is calculated.
- Education to improve understanding of the factors that affect body weight, particularly the effects of shifts of glycogen and fluid.
- Regular, frequent meals and snacks, normally beginning with at least six eating episodes per day. This helps to prevent excessive hunger, which may increase the drive to binge, and also helps avoid feelings of fullness, which may provoke an impulse to vomit.
- Using the foods least likely to provoke bingeing or purging. This usually means not using high-fat or high-sugar foods at first.
- Using foods most likely to reduce hunger. Low-energy-density, high-fibre and low-glycaemic-index foods may be helpful.
- Identifying times when the risk of binge eating is high, and replacing the binge with regular small snacks.
- Managing shopping and storage of food to have the planned food available, and avoid having binge food easily accessible.
- Planning meals to ensure they are available on time, and to prevent the anxiety associated with making decisions quickly.
- Encouraging the use of alternative activities to deal with emotional distress. Activities that are distracting, calming and enjoyable, such as creative activities, social contact and relaxation exercises, may be especially effective.

Strategies to reduce purging and minimise harm include the following:

- Improved understanding of body weight regulation and the factors that influence it.
- Keeping meals and snacks small initially, to prevent a feeling of fullness that may provoke vomiting or laxative use.
- Initially, encouraging the use of alternatives to specific foods that the individual finds difficult to tolerate, often high-fat, high-sugar foods. Excessively strict rules are not helpful.
- Plan activities to follow each meal and snack, as a distraction and to help reduce anxiety.
- Eating with other people may be helpful.
- Planned, appropriate exercise may help improve tolerance of regular eating.
- Stabilising fluid balance with regular fluid intake, and management of dehydrating factors such as vomiting, laxative use, alcohol and excessive caffeine intake.
- Advice on protecting teeth if vomiting does occur. Rinsing with water helps to remove acid from the mouth.
- If blood potassium is low because of vomiting or laxative use, advice on food sources of potassium, while implementing strategies to reduce purging.

As treatment progresses, the variety of foods can be increased. Difficult foods can be reintroduced in a safe context to reduce the associated anxiety. Foods such as chocolate or crisps can be taken after a meal to prevent between-meal hunger adding to the risk of uncontrolled eating. It may help to choose a single serving package, to control the amount, and to try it in a public place, where binge eating will be difficult. Individuals may be able to plan the safest situation for themselves. Success in using challenging foods in an appropriate way can help to develop confidence to tackle further goals.

Binge eating disorder

There are many similarities between binge eating disorder and BN. As with BN, CBT is recommended (NICE, 2017) to help people overcome binge eating, along with diary keeping to help link thoughts, feelings and events to binge eating, and to develop strategies to deal with them. People with binge eating disorder are generally obese and anxious to reduce their weight. Abolition of binge eating alone generally has little impact on weight. Excessive restriction of food will maintain hunger, so it may be difficult to achieve weight loss while binge eating is active, and therefore some individuals may find it easier to reduce binge eating before beginning weight reduction. It may be possible to support patients to begin weight reduction while they are reducing their binge eating behaviour by restoring regular, stable eating while maintaining a modest deficit in energy intake of about 400–500 kcal (1.7–2 MJ)/day, and ideally gradually increasing physical activity as appropriate for the individual.

As eating stabilises, binge eating reduces and confidence increases, a larger energy deficit may be tolerated, and obesity management strategies, including medication, can be applied by following NICE (2006b) guidance. In case of extreme obesity, bariatric surgery may be necessary. It is not clear whether binge eating worsens the outcome of bariatric surgery (Bocchieri-Ricciardi *et al.*, 2006; Niego *et al.*, 2007). In practice, the waiting time for bariatric surgery may be lengthy, and the time may be well spent by reducing eating pathology and body weight, and supporting the individuals to improve their knowledge and confidence to manage their eating post-surgery.

Internet resources

B-eat, www.b-eat.co.uk, the leading charity and support group for eating disorders

Eating disorders research resource, www.iop.kcl.ac.uk/sites/edu

Eating disorders resources, www.rcpsych.ac.uk/mentalhealthinfoforall/problems/eatingdisorders.aspx

Institute of Psychiatry, www.iop.kcl.ac.uk

Royal College of Psychiatrists, www.rcpsych.ac.uk

References

American Psychiatric Association. (2013) *Diagnostic and Statistical Manual of Mental Disorders, 5th edn (DSM-5)*. Washington, DC: American Psychiatric Association.

Birmingham CL, Alothman AF, Goldner EM. (1996) Anorexia nervosa: refeeding and hypophosphataemia. *Int. J. Eat. Disord.* 20(2): 211–213.

Bocchieri-Ricciardi LE, Chen EY, Munoz D, et al. (2006) Pre-surgery binge eating status: effect on eating behavior and weight outcome after gastric bypass. *Obes. Surg.* 16: 1198–1204.

British Dietetic Association (BDA). (2009) *Nutrition and Dietetic Care Process*. Birmingham: BDA.

British Dietetic Association (BDA). (2011) *Practice Supervision Guidelines*. Birmingham: BDA.

Bruch H. (1973) *Eating Disorders; Obesity, Anorexia Nervosa and the Person Within*. New York: Basic Books.

Brumberg JJ. (1988) *Fasting Girls; The History of Anorexia Nervosa*. New York: Plume.

Bulik CM, Reichborn-Kjennerud T. (2003) Medical morbidity in binge eating disorder. *Int. J. Eat. Disord.* 34(Suppl): S39–46.

Bulik CM, Slof-Op't Landt MC, van Furth EF, *et al.* (2007) The genetics of anorexia nervosa. *Ann. Rev. Nutr.* 27: 263–275.

Caregaro I, Di Pascoli L, Favaro A, *et al.* (2005) Sodium depletion and hemoconcentration – overlooked complications in patients with anorexia nervosa? *Nutrition.* 21(4): 438–445.

Casiero D, Frishman WH. (2006) Cardiovascular complications of eating disorder. *Cardiol. Rev.* 14(5): 227–231.

Cordery H, Waller G. (2006) Nutritional knowledge of healthcare professionals working in eating disorders. *Eur. Eat. Disord. Rev.* 14(6): 462–467.

Cotton M-A, Ball C, Robinson P. (2003) Four simple questions can help screen for eating disorders. *J. Gen. Intern. Med.* 18(1): 53–56.

Davis C, Levitan RD, Kaplan AS, et al. (2008) Reward sensitivity and the D2 dopamine receptor gene; a case control study of binge eating disorder. *Prog. Neuro-Psychopharmacol. Biol. Psychiatry* 32: 620–628.

de Zwaan M. (2001) Binge eating disorder and obesity. *Int. J. Obes. Relat. Metab. Disord.* 25(1): S51–55.

Fairburn CG, Harrison PJ. (2003) Eating disorders. *Lancet.* 361: 407–416.

Fairburn CG, Peveler RC, Davies B, *et al.* (1991) Eating disorders in young adults with insulin dependent diabetes mellitus: a controlled study. *BMJ* 303: 17–20.

Fairburn CG, Doll HA, Welch SL, *et al.* (1998) Risk factors for binge eating disorders: a community-based, case-control study. *Arch. Gen. Psychiatry.* 55(5): 425–432.

Feld R, Woodside DB, Kaplan AS, *et al.* (2001) Pretreatment motivational enhancement therapy for eating disorders; a pilot study. *Int. J. Eat. Disord.* 29(4): 393–400.

Fisher M, Simpser E, Schneider M. (2000) Hypophosphatemia secondary to oral refeeding in anorexia nervosa study. *Int. J. Eat. Disord.* 28(2): 181–187.

Frydrych AM, Davies GR, McDermott BM. (2005) Eating disorders and oral health: a review of the literature. *Austr. Dent. J.* 50(1): 6–15.

Gable J, Herrmann T. (2016) *Counselling Skills for Dietitians*, 3rd edn. Oxford: Blackwell.

Garrett A, Cockfield A, Philpot U, *et al.* (2005) *A Briefing Paper for Dietitians Working with Patients with Eating Disorders*. Birmingham: Mental Health Group of the British Dietetic Association.

Gentile MG, Pastorelli P, Ciceri R, *et al.* (2010) Specialised refeeding treatment fir anorexia nervosa patients suffering from extreme undernutrition. *Clin. Nutr.* 29: 627–632.

Gorwood P, Kipman A, Foulon C. (2003) The human genetics of anorexia nervosa. *Eur. J. Pharmacol.* 480: 163–170.

Grimm VE. (1996) *From Feasting to Fasting: Attitudes to Food in Late Antiquity*. London: Routledge.

Gull WW. (1874) Anorexia nervosa (apepsia hysterica, anorexia hysterica). *Trans. Clin. Soc. Lond.* 7: 22–28.

Gull WW. (1888) Clinical notes, anorexia nervosa. *Lancet* 1: 516–517.

Hadigan CM, Anderson EJ, Miller KK, et al. (2000) Assessment of macronutrient and micronutrient intake in women with anorexia nervosa. *Int. J. Eat. Disord.* 28(3): 284–292.

Harris EC, Barraclough B. (1998) Excess mortality of mental disorder. *Br. J. Psychiatry.* 173: 11–53.

Harrison A, Sullivan S, Tchanturia K, *et al.* (2009) Emotion recognition and regulation in anorexia nervosa. *Clin. Psychol. Psychother.* 16: 348–356.

Hart S, Russell J, Abraham S. (2011) Nutrition and dietetic practice in eating disorder management. *J. Hum. Nutr. Diet.* 24(2): 144–153.

Hearing SD. (2004) Refeeding syndrome. *BMJ* 328: 908–909.

Herrin M, Larkin M. (2012) *Nutrition Counselling in the Treatment of Eating Disorders*, 2nd edn. New York: Brunner-Routledge.

Hoek HW. (2006) Incidence, prevalence and mortality of anorexia nervosa and other eating disorders. *Curr. Opin. Psychiatry* 19(4): 389–394.

Hoek HW, van Hoeken D. (2003) Review of the prevalence and incidence of eating disorders. *Int. J. Eat. Disord.* 34: 383–396.

Hudson JI, Hiripi E, Pope HG, *et al.* (2007) The prevalence and correlates of eating disorders in the National Comorbidity Survey Replication. *Biol. Psychiatry.* 61(3): 348–358.

Kalm LM, Semba RD. (2005) They starved so that others be better fed: remembering Ancel Keys and the Minnesota Experiment. *J. Nutr.* 135(6): 1347–1352.

Keski-Rahkonen A, Hoek HW, Susser ES, et al. (2007) Epidemiology and course of anorexia nervosa in the community. *Am. J. Psychiatry.* 164(8): 1259–1265.

Keys A, Brozek J, Henschel A, *et al.* (1950) *The Biology of Human Starvation.* Minneapolis: University of Minneapolis Press.

Lasègue EC. (1873) De l'anorexie hystérique. *Archives Générales de Médecine* 1: 385–403.

Lawson EA, Klibanski A. (2008) Endocrine abnormalities in anorexia nervosa. *Nat. Clin. Pract. Endocrinol. Metab.* 4(7): 407–414.

Marzola E, Nasser J, Hashim S, *et al.* (2013) Nutritional rehabilitation in anorexia nervosa: review of the literature and implications for treatment. *BMC Psychiatry.* 13: 290.

Mitchell JE, Crow S. (2006) Medical complications of anorexia nervosa and bulimia nervosa. *Curr. Opin. Psychiatry.* 19(4): 438–443.

Morgan JF, Reid F, Lacey JH. (1999) The SCOFF questionnaire: assessment of a new screening tool for eating disorders. *BMJ* 319: 1467–1468.

Nasser M. (1997) *Culture and Weight Consciousness.* London: Routledge.

Newton JT, Travess HC. (2000) Oral complications. *Eur. Eat. Disord. Rev.* 8(2): 83–87.

NICE. (2006a) *Eating Disorders. National Clinical Practice Guideline No. 32.* London: NICE.

NICE. (2006b) *Obesity. National Clinical Practice Guideline No. 43.* London: NICE.

NICE. (2017) *Nutrition Support in Adults. National Clinical Practice Guideline No. 69.* London: NICE.

NICE. (2017) Nutrition support for adults: oral nutrition support, enteral tube feeding and parenteral nutrition CG32. Available at https://www.nice.org.uk/Guidance/CG32. Accessed 1 November 2018.

Niego SH, Kofman MD, Weiss JJ, *et al.* (2007) Binge eating in the bariatric surgery population: a review of the literature. *Int. J. Eat. Disord.* 40: 349–359.

Oldershaw A, Treasure J, Hambrook D, *et al.* (2011) Is anorexia nervosa a version of autism spectrum disorders? *Eur. Eat. Disord. Rev.* 19: 462–474.

Ozier AD, Henry BW. (2011) Position of the American Dietetic Association: nutrition intervention in the treatment of eating disorders. *J. Am. Diet. Assoc.* 111(8): 1236–1241.

Prince AC, Brooks SJ, Stahl D, et al. (2010) Systematic review and meta-analysis of the baseline concentrations and physiologic responses of gut hormones to food in eating disorders. *Am. J. Clin. Nutr.* 89(3):755–765.

Prochaska JO, DiClemente CC. (1983) Stages and processes of self-change of smoking: Toward an integrative model of change. *J. Consult. Clin. Psychol.* 51(3): 390–395.

Robinson PH. (2000) Review article: recognition and treatment of eating disorders in primary and secondary care. *Aliment. Pharmacol. Ther.* 14(4): 367–377.

Robinson PH, Clarke M, Barrett J. (1988) Determinants of delayed gastric emptying in anorexia nervosa and bulimia nervosa. *Gut.* 29: 458–464.

Rock CL, Vasantharajan S. (1995) Vitamin status of eating disorders patients: relationship to clinical indices and effect of treatment. *Int. J. Eat. Disord.* 18: 257–262.

Rooney B, McClelland L, Crisp AH, *et al.* (1995) The incidence and prevalence of anorexia nervosa in three suburban health districts in south west London, UK. *Int. J. Eat. Disord.* 18(4): 299–307.

Royal College of Psychiatrists (RCP). (2014) *CR189 MARSIPAN: Management of Really Sick Patients with Anorexia Nervosa*, 2nd edn. London: RCP.

Ruhsing JM, Jones LE, Carney CP. (2003) Bulimia nervosa: a primary care review. *J. Clin. Psychiatry.* 5: 217–224.

Russell GFM. (1979) Bulimia nervosa: an ominous variant of anorexia nervosa. *Psychol. Med.* 9: 429–448.

Saul SH, Dekker A, Watson CG. (1981) Acute gastric dilatation with infarction and perforation: Report of fatal outcome in patient with anorexia nervosa. *Gut.* 22: 978–983.

Serpell L, Treasure J. (1997) Osteoporosis – a serious health risk in chronic anorexia nervosa. *Eur. Eat. Disord. Rev.* 5(3): 149–157.

Setnick J. (2010) Micronutrient deficiencies and supplementation in anorexia and bulimia nervosa. *Nutr. Clin. Pract.* 25(2): 137–142.

Smink FRE, van Hoeken D, Hoek HW. (2012) Epidemiology of eating disorders: incidence, prevalence and mortality rates. *Curr. Psychiatry Rep.* 14: 406–414.

Spitzer RL, Devlin M, Walsh BT, et al. (1992) Binge eating disorder: a multisite field trial of the diagnostic criteria. *Int. J. Eat. Disord.* 11: 191–203.

Stice E, Presnell K, Gau J, Shaw H. (2007) Testing mediators of intervention effects in randomized controlled trials: An evaluation of two eating disorder prevention programs. *J. Consult. Clin. Psychol.* 75: 20–32.

Teng K. (2011) Premenopausal osteoporosis, an overlooked consequence of anorexia nervosa. *Cleve. Clin. J. Med.* 78(1): 50–58.

Thanos, PK, Michaelides M, Piyis YK, *et al.* (2008) Food restriction markedly increases dopamine D2 receptor in a rat model of obesity. *Synapse.* 62(1): 50–61.

Treasure J, Schmidt U. (2001) Ready, willing and able to change: motivational aspects of the assessment and treatment of eating disorders. *Eur. Eat. Disord. Rev.* 9(1): 4–18.

Treasure J, Claudino AM, Zucker N. (2010) Eating disorders. *Lancet.* 375: 583–593.

Treasure J, Cardi V, Kan C. (2012) Eating in eating disorders. *Eur. Eat. Disord. Rev.* 20(1): e42–49.

Vandereycken W, van Deth R. (1994) *From Fasting Saints to Anorexic Girls: The History of Self-Starvation.* London: Athlone.

Wang GJ, Geliebter A, Volkow ND, et al. (2011) Enhanced striatal dopamine release during food stimulation in binge eating disorder. *Obesity.* 19(8): 1601–1608.

Warren MP. (2011) Endocrine manifestations of eating disorders. *J. Clin. Endocrinol. Metab.* 96(2): 333–343.

WHO. (1992) *The International Classification of Diseases*, 10th edn. (ICD-10). Geneva: WHO.

Wilfley D, Schwartz MB, Spurrell EB, *et al.* (2003) Using the eating disorder examination to identify the specific psychopathology of binge eating disorder. *Int. J. Eat. Disord.* 27(3): 259–269.

Winston AP, Stafford PJ. (2000) Cardiovascular effects on anorexia nervosa. *Eur. Eat. Disord. Rev.* 8(2): 117–125.

Zipfel S, Herzog W, Beumont PJ, *et al.* (2000) *Osteoporosis. Eur. Eat. Disord. Rev.* 8: 108–116.

7.10.3 Dementias

Phil Addicott and Annette McLean

Key points

- Dementia is a syndrome associated with progressive decline in brain function; this may include memory loss and/or impaired communication, motor skills and perception, and low mood.
- Nutritional support can be essential, particularly when the individual is physically unwell or developing difficulties in preparing meals or eating independently.
- Dementia is not a natural part of ageing; however, the number of people with dementia is increasing exponentially as people are living longer.
- People with dementia can lead active and fulfilling lives if they and their families/carers are given the support they require.

Dementia is the collective term for conditions resulting from destructive pathological changes in brain tissue that cause progressive loss of intellectual function. They are defined by their cognitive and neuropsychological characteristics. Memory decline is the core feature of most disorders, many of which also have impairment of visual spatial skills, language and executive functions. Dementia can cause a wide range of symptoms, including:

- Progressive decline in the ability to remember, understand, communicate and reason.
- A loss of skills, including those needed for everyday tasks and activities.
- Changes in emotions, personality and behaviour.

Psychological symptoms in dementia can include psychosis, depression and anxiety, while behavioural changes can include wandering, restlessness, agitation, disinhibition and aggression. In time, people lose the ability to care for themselves and become totally dependent on others. In some cases, the decline may be rapid; in others, it may occur over a long period of time. Dementia is not in itself fatal, and many sufferers remain in good physical health for years. Eventually, the effects of the disease lead to increasing weakness and complications such as pneumonia and, eventually, death.

In 2014, the Alzheimer's Society, in partnership with the London School of Economics and Kings College London, produced Dementia UK Update, to provide a synthesis of best available evidence for the current cost and prevalence of dementia in the UK. It was estimated that there were 850,000 people with dementia in the UK, and this is expected to rise to 1 million by 2025. It is anticipated that the prevalence of dementia will increase as the population ages. Dementia usually occurs after the age of 40 years, and the incidence increases sharply with age, affecting 1.3% of the entire UK population but increasing to 7.1% in the population aged 65 years and over. Over the age of 80, the risk is 1 in 6. There are also currently over 40,000 people with early-onset dementia (under the age of 65 years) in the UK (Alzheimer's Society, 2014).

Nutrition in dementia progression

Nutrition plays an important role in the integrity of the brain; besides energy, the diet provides precursor amino acids for the production of neurotransmitters, thus facilitating effective synaptic communication. It is well known that severe deficiencies in several micronutrients, e.g. thiamine, folic acid and vitamin B_{12}, are accompanied by cognitive disorders. It is possible that less pronounced nutrient deficiencies might contribute to impaired cognition and aggravation of existing impairments (ESPEN, 2015). This appears supported by epidemiological evidence that suggests that, in healthy older people, specific dietary patterns may decrease the risk of dementia and cognitive decline (Lourida *et al.*, 2013). There are, however, no studies available indicating that specific dietary habits or a low intake of specific nutrients contributes to disease progression. ESPEN (2015) does not endorse the systematic use of special foods, supplementation with any specific nutrient or any other nutritional product for persons with dementia to correct cognitive impairment or prevent further cognitive decline. Nonetheless, weight loss, low body weight and malnutrition are clearly associated with a poor outcome, and contribute to disease progression, cognitive decline and, ultimately, mortality risk (ESPEN, 2015). Additionally, the relentless loss of capabilities, such as being able to shop and prepare meals, through to attention deficit and losing the ability to eat independently, invariably increases the risk of malnutrition. ESPEN (2015) recommends screening everyone with dementia for malnutrition, and positive screening should be followed by assessment and dietetic intervention, including the use of oral nutritional supplements (ONS) with the aim of improving nutritional status.

Types of dementia

Alzheimer's disease

Alois Alzheimer first identified the most common cause of dementia, Alzheimer's disease, in 1907. It results from the loss of neurones from the cortical areas of the brain, leading to reduced production of acetylcholine and other neurotransmitters, and hence impaired transmission of messages connected with thought and memory. The brain atrophies and decreases in weight, and microscopic examination reveal large numbers of neurofibrillary tangles, where nerve cells become entangled, and neuritic plaques (deposits of amyloid protein and other cellular debris) form. Age is the greatest risk factor for Alzheimer's disease; hence, it primarily affects people over the age of 65 years, and the risk continues to increase with age, with one in six people over the age of 80 years developing dementia. For reasons unknown, approximately twice as many women as men aged over 65 years develop Alzheimer's, possibly linked to a lack of oestrogen after menopause.

The cause of Alzheimer's disease is unknown, but there are genetic links. Familial Alzheimer's is a rare condition, with a relatively simple inheritance pattern due to a mutation in one specific gene. This is in contrast to the majority of Alzheimer's cases (and most other types of dementia), which follow a complex pattern of gene variants in our DNA. More than 20 gene variants have now been identified that are implicated in the risk of developing Alzheimer's disease. Apolipoprotein E (APOE) gene, found on chromosome 19, has the greatest known effect on Alzheimer's disease risk. The APOE protein plays a role in fat metabolism, including cholesterol regulation (Alzheimer's Society, 2016a). However, gene inheritance is only one aspect, and most people can significantly reduce their risk of developing dementia through healthy lifestyle choices, including smoking abstinence, engaging in regular physical exercise and eating a healthy diet.

Vascular dementia

Vascular dementia is the second most common type of dementia, affecting approximately 150,000 people in the UK (Alzheimer's Society, 2014). The term is applied to several different types of dementia caused by stroke or diseases of the blood vessels supplying brain cells with the oxygen and nutrients that they need to function.

Stroke-related dementia

This form of dementia develops when blood flow in a large vessel supplying the brain is suddenly cut off, typically when blocked by a clot, resulting in the death of a large volume of brain tissue.

Multi-infarct dementia

Multi-infarct dementia (MID) arises from two (or more) smaller or transient infarcts in the brain (often manifested as dizzy spells) that lead to increased areas of brain damage, causing symptoms of confusion, which gradually progress to dementia. In contrast to Alzheimer's disease, mental decline in MID is likely to start more abruptly, and symptoms tend to worsen in a stepwise manner following each attack. Since brain damage also tends to occur in localised areas, symptoms will vary depending on the part of the brain affected, but will often include cognitive symptoms (such as planning and concentrating) or problems with memory or language. Apathy and depression are also common, possibly as people are more aware of their difficulties.

Small vessel dementia

Small vessel dementia, also known as sub-cortical dementia, is caused by damage to tiny blood vessels that lie deep in the brain. The symptoms are less varied and develop more gradually than stroke-related dementia or MID, and are often accompanied by bladder and walking problems or problems pronouncing words.

Frontotemporal dementia

A less common type of dementia, frontotemporal dementia (FTD), is characterised by degenerative atrophy of the frontal lobes (that control behaviour, problem-solving emotions and speech) and/or the temporal lobes. The left temporal lobe typically deals with the meaning of words and names of things. The right temporal role is usually involved with recognition of faces and objects. Presentation is typically before the age of 65 years, and the rate of progression and life expectancy varies greatly. Diagnosis at a younger age is particularly difficult for families with dependent children and significant financial commitments. Symptoms of FTD are dependent on which brain lobes are damaged, but may include progressive difficulties with language and vocabulary. However, the most common variant involves early uncharacteristic behavioural changes such as disinhibition, apathy and a loss of empathy. Eating habits may also change, and individuals may overeat sweet foods and forget table etiquette (Alzheimer's Society, 2016b). Refusing to eat in protest about something is also not unusual. Personality changes such as insensitivity, rudeness or the lack of emotional warmth can be very distressing for loved ones/carers.

Dementia with Lewy bodies

Often associated with Parkinson's disease, dementia with Lewy bodies (DLB) is characterised by the presence of small spherical protein-containing structures (Lewy bodies) in brain tissue. In Parkinson's, Lewy bodies are characteristically found localised in the brain stem; however, in DLB, the Lewy bodies are more widely distributed in the cells of the cortex and subcortex. Clinical features include fluctuating cognitive function, visual hallucinations and the spontaneous motor features of Parkinsonism (Brown & Hillam, 2004).

Other causes of dementia

These include:

- *Huntington's disease* – a genetically determined progressive neurodegenerative disorder resulting in movement disturbances, depression and dementia.

- *Down's syndrome* – dementia is more common in middle-aged people with Down's syndrome than in the rest of the population (Janicki & Dalton, 2000).
- *Wernicke–Korsakoff syndrome* – caused by thiamine deficiency, usually as a result of chronic alcohol misuse leading to dementia-type symptoms.
- *Pugilistic brain injury* – repeated head blows can cause brain damage (resulting in symptoms of dementia), e.g. in boxers. The symptoms may not become apparent until 30–40 years after the end of the boxer's career. The number of fights and length of career seem to be more important than the number of knock outs (Bayer & Reban, 2004).

Diagnosis and management

Diagnosis of dementia should only be made after a comprehensive assessment. This should include a clinical cognitive assessment, which is then repeated at intervals to assess levels of decline, e.g. the Mini Mental State Examination (MMSE) test. A basic dementia screen should include biochemistry, thyroid function test, and vitamin B_{12} and folate levels (NICE, 2006). Structural imaging such as magnetic resonance imaging (MRI) should be used in the assessment to exclude other possible cerebral pathologies and to help establish the subtype diagnosis (NICE, 2006).

Early diagnosis of dementia is important because, in some cases, it may be possible to prevent disease progression. It is particularly important that people with evidence of vascular dementia receive any indicated treatment (e.g. for hypertension), which may reduce the risk of further infarction damage. Diet and lifestyle measures, such as not smoking, eating a healthy balanced diet, losing weight, exercising, and reducing salt and alcohol intake, are also important.

Medication

Medication has been developed for Alzheimer's disease that can improve symptoms, or temporarily slow down progression, in some people; however, they do not cure the condition. There are two types of drugs used to treat Alzheimer's disease:

- *Cholinesterase inhibitors* – Increased concentrations of acetylcholine lead to increased communication between the nerve cells that use acetylcholine as a chemical messenger, which may in turn temporarily improve or stabilise the symptoms, particularly in the earlier stages.
  - Aricept (donepezil hydrochloride).
  - Exelon (rivastigmine).
  - Reminyl (galantamine).
- *Glutamate blocker* – glutamate is released in excessive amounts when brain cells are damaged by Alzheimer's disease, and this causes the brain cells to be damaged further. This drug can protect brain cells by blocking the release of excess glutamate.
  - Ebixa (memantine).

NICE amended its guidance in March 2011 to recommend donepezil, galantamine and rivastigmine as options for managing mild and moderate Alzheimer's disease. Memantine is now recommended as an option for managing moderate disease in people who cannot take cholinesterase inhibitors, and as an option for managing severe disease. In terms of side effects, these drugs are typically well tolerated; however, the most frequent side effects include nausea and vomiting, diarrhoea, stomach cramps and headaches, fatigue, and loss of appetite. Such side effects are likely to have a negative effect on nutritional status.

Nutritional implications of dementia

The effects of dementia on food and fluid intake and nutritional status are considerable. The behavioural, emotional and physical changes that take place as dementia progresses can all impact on a person's eating habits and on their intake of food and drink (Alzheimer's Society, 2007).

Dementia and dietary behaviour

Depending on the type of dementia and the individual personality, each person will experience dementia in a different way. However, a typical pattern is that, in the initial stages, the individual may experience difficulty in shopping, cooking and storing food. In addition, aspects such as forgetting to eat or forgetting they have eaten, eating spoiled foods, and changes in food choices may be noted. As the dementia advances, patients may find it more difficult to open their mouth and chew; people may pool food in the mouth but not swallow; the ability to eat independently may be lost; and inedible items may be eaten. Additionally, individuals may refuse food or become aphasic and therefore unable to express pain (e.g. dental pain), or to ask for food or fluids. People may encounter chewing and swallowing difficulties or become depressed. As a result, weight loss is a common feature of progressing dementia. This is nearly always a consequence of inadequate energy intake, rather than of the disease itself (Prentice *et al.*, 1989). A systemic review (Hanson *et al.*, 2011) looking at oral feeding options for people with dementia found that high-energy supplements and other oral feeding options, such as assisted feeding and modified foods, can help people with dementia to gain weight.

Increased energy requirements

In some cases, the energy deficit may be exacerbated by increased energy requirements secondary to excessive walking or pacing. Rheaume *et al.* (1987) found that patients who wander required an additional 1600 kcal to maintain their nutritional status. Pharmacological interventions for excessive pacing can result in a poor nutritional intake due to over-sedation. Exercise and music therapy are the most acceptable non-pharmacological interventions to reduce wandering in dementia (Robinson *et al.*, 2006).

Dehydration

Inadequate oral fluid intake and subsequent dehydration are common problems, and are implicated in many of the most common ailments in people with dementia, such as constipation, urinary tract infection, electrolyte imbalance, and increased dizziness and confusion leading to falls, all of which can have a negative effect on nutritional intake. The Royal College of Nursing (2007) Hydration Best Practice Toolkit provides practical advice for healthcare staff in England and Wales on how to minimise the risk and potential harm of dehydration.

Dysphagia

Dysphagia is a common problem in dementia. Repeated chest infections, coughing at mealtimes or a prolonged oral stage (continuous chewing) can indicate dysphagia. Providing good nutrition for individuals with dementia and dysphagia can be extremely challenging, and can benefit from a multi-disciplinary approach. Some individuals require prompt assessment by a speech and language therapist who can advise on appropriate texture modifications of food and consistency of fluids with the aim of reducing risk of aspiration pneumonia (Kindell, 2002) (see Chapter 7.3, Dysphagia).

Nutritional assessment

Patients with dementia are vulnerable to developing malnutrition, and it is essential that an environment-appropriate and validated nutritional screening tool be routinely used. Patients should be weighed at regular intervals. Calculation of nutritional requirements should include factors for stress or weight gain and mobility. Food and fluid charts need to be accurately completed for patients identified as being at high risk of malnutrition. However, if food and fluid charts are not available, assessment of food intake usually depends on a combination of obtaining information from relatives or care staff and observing mealtimes. Take note of any carers' reports of weight loss; also, loose-fitting clothing may be an indicator of a problem with intake (Bayer & Reban, 2004). Features which increase the likelihood of inadequate nutritional intake are:

- Sensory impairment (e.g. smell and taste).
- Poor or missing dentition.
- Constipation or loose stools.
- Food refusal due to depression, paranoia or confusion.
- Poor mental state and challenging behaviour.
- Physical difficulties in chewing or swallowing.
- Inappropriate mealtime environment and inability to eat independently.
- Medications resulting in dry mouth and altered taste or, in particular, heavy sedation (e.g. antidepressants and antipsychotics).

It is also important to check:

- The nutritional adequacy of the offered food, requirements for texture-modified food, e.g. fork-mashable or pureed food may need fortification.
- The frequency with which food is offered and the time available for assisting people to eat. In institutions, there may be short intervals between meals; long gaps when nothing is offered; and limited time to encourage and assist patients to eat and drink.

Dietary management

Several strategies can be employed to optimise nutritional intake. These will vary according to the individual circumstances and stage of the disease, and perhaps additional clinical problems such as over-sedation, diabetes or depression. People who live alone in their own homes should be encouraged to:

- Keep a store of foods that do not require cooking and which can be opened easily, including breakfast cereals, milk, cheese, sliced ham and bananas.
- Keep a good supply of cold drinks if preparation of hot drinks is a problem.
- Make use of meal delivery services and/or meals provided in day-care or luncheon clubs.
- Remain involved in food preparation for as long as possible, and be aware of food fortification ideas.
- Sit with relatives/carers to promote the social side of eating, so that the relatives/carers can set an example or model for the confused or forgetful person.
- People with dementia, their relatives/carers and the professionals who support them need access to reliable resources, e.g. the Nutrition in the Community Settings initiative (Welsh Assembly Government, 2011).

Guidance for staff members who care for those in institutions should emphasise on the following:

- Importance of nutritional screening and the role of good nutrition in preventing weight loss, malnutrition and the prevention of pressure sores.
- Developing a high-protein and high-energy menu that includes rich sources of fibre, calcium folate and vitamins D, B_{12} and B_6.
- Importance of being able to provide, when required, appealing, nutritionally good, texture-modified meals, and of being able to accurately thicken fluids to the recommended consistency.
- Developing a finger food menu for patients who are too distracted to sit through a meal.
- Need for specialist feeding aids such as adaptive cutlery, deep-lipped plates, non-slip placemats, wide-neck and large-handled mugs, and clothing protection where necessary.
- Benefits of investing in training (e.g. how to safely assist patients to eat, or on the importance of hydration).
- Importance of adequate fluid being consumed to meet hydration needs.

- Need to recognise individual variation in terms of nutrient needs and personal likes and dislikes.
- Benefits of nutritional supplements for those with inadequate nutritional intake and weight loss.
- The importance of a robust protected mealtimes policy, and a calm and appropriate mealtime environment.

Advice to carers should focus on the need to:

- Offer small, nutritious meals and drinks at regular intervals. Not only does this help meet nutritional and fluid needs but the routine of a regular meal pattern may also provide comfort and reassurance to many people with dementia.
- Provide a variety of foods that the person likes and allow more mealtime than is usual.
- Avoid assisting people to eat when they are not fully alert or if they are lying down or anxious.
- Help maintain the person's independence by providing foods that they can manage by themselves. Deep-lipped plates, non-slip placemats, adapted utensils or finger foods may be helpful.
- Finger foods (e.g. sandwiches chips, sandwiches, biscuits) may be more appropriate for distracted or wander-some patients.
- Maximise good times of the day (typically breakfast and lunchtime) to provide foods which are good sources of nutrients and energy.
- Provide regular fluids to aid hydration.

Mealtime environment

Mealtimes should be given priority in the daily routine of people with dementia. The eating environment needs to be calm and relaxed. Patients should be advised that the mealtime is about to start after being offered the opportunity to use the toilet and reminded/assisted to wash their hands. In some cases, people with dementia can help lay the table, which can be a good source of social contact and stimulation (Kindell, 2002). People with dementia may struggle to concentrate at mealtimes if there are other distractions – therefore, televisions should be switched off, as should loud music; however, calm and soothing music can help reduce agitation (Cohen-Mansfields *et al.*, 2010).

The Social Care Institute for Excellence (2011) recommends that people with dementia be allowed to sit and eat in a place where they feel comfortable, and that carers describe the food they are offering and ensure that the food is presented colourfully and attractively. The area in which a person with dementia eats should be bright and well-lit, so they can see the food easily. Images of food can also be used for reminiscence activities; this can help stimulate discussion and interest in food and mealtimes by helping the person to reconnect with familiar foods from his or her past.

Eating assistance strategies

Relatives or carers may be able to provide advice on the level of support typically required. The following strategies may be helpful in overcoming poor dietary intake related to dementia:

- If possible, involve the person with the preparation of the meal for as long as possible (e.g. setting the table); talking about food preferences can be a useful prompt.
- Overemphasising tidy eating habits should be avoided; serving one familiar food at a time may help overcome confusion. Cutting food into smaller pieces (before the plate is taken to the patient) may be helpful (Bayer & Reban, 2004).
- If a person with dementia becomes distracted during the meal, or passively sits in front of the meal without eating, gentle verbal prompts can be useful.
- Hand-over-hand assistance can be useful for people who are having difficulty in coordinating cutlery, i.e. gently place the utensil in the person's hand and use your hand to guide them to start eating; once started, they will often be able to carry on independently.
- Take into account individual food preferences, but consider that, due to taste changes, people may prefer more sweet foods (desserts), or that foods with stronger flavour might be enjoyed.
- Food should be colourful, and presented attractively; avoid serving white foods on a white plate. Take care that foods and drinks are not too hot.
- If self-feeding is more erratic, specialist feeding aids (e.g. weighted cutlery, deep-lipped plates and non-slip placemats) may help; eventually, the person may need to be fed at least part of his or her meal.
- Some people with dementia become sensitive to foods of mixed textures (e.g. minestrone soup or cornflakes in milk) and may spit them out; if so, a softer single-texture food may be appropriate (Kindell, 2002).
- If a person walks away from an unfinished meal, be wary of assuming that the person has finished or dislikes the food. People may need some verbal prompts to come back to the table, and gesturing to the chair next to you can show the person what you mean. If the person refuses to settle, he or she may benefit from finger foods (Kindell, 2002).
- In dementia with dysphagia, position people in an upright position to reduce the risk of aspiration. Texture-modified foods may need to be fortified in order to provide adequate nutrition, and nutritional intake should be maximised when the desire to eat is higher.
- If fortifying foods and beverages proves insufficient, nutritional supplemental formulae will need to be prescribed. If a patient requires thickened fluids, consider using a pre-thickened supplement drink.

In the final stages of the illness, a multidisciplinary *best interest meeting* may need to be held in order to consider enteral feeding or intravenous hydration for a person who lacks the capacity to make this particular decision for them self. If known, the views of the patient must be considered, as well as the opinions of relatives or carers. For more information, please refer to the Mental Capacity Act (UK Government, 2005b). Each individual case must be reviewed on its individual merits.

It should be considered that dysphagia can occur earlier in the disease process, and is not always a terminal symptom as is often believed.

The needs of carers

There are estimated to be 600,000 people in the UK acting as the primary carers for people with dementia (Alzheimer's Society, 2007). Caring can be an overwhelming experience, and the financial costs of caring are significant. Many carers face financial hardship, often give up work and pay high care bills from limited incomes or private savings. The needs of those who care for dementia sufferers in the domestic setting have been increasingly recognised. Under the Carers and Disabled Children Act (UK Government, 2000), carers aged 16 years or over who provide a regular and substantial amount of care for someone aged 18 years or over have the right to an assessment of their needs as carers. Furthermore, the Carers (Equal Opportunities) Act came into force in 2005a (UK Government), and places a duty on local authorities to ensure that all carers know that they are entitled to an assessment of their needs, and to consider a carer's outside interests, i.e. work, study or leisure, when carrying out an assessment. Since 2007 (UK Government), under the Employment Act, carers have a statutory right to ask the employer for flexible working if they are caring for an adult who is a relative or lives at the same address.

NICE (2006) has produced guidelines which detail that those carrying out the assessment should seek to identify psychological distress and psychosocial impact on the carer. Care plans for carers should include tailored interventions and practical support, including access to respite and short-break services that meet the needs of both the carer and the person with dementia.

Health professionals should work closely with relatives/carers of someone with dementia for the following reasons:

- They know the persons best and are more likely to be able to identify or interpret any needs or problems.
- They may be aware of the relevant medical history, such as diabetes, gastro problems or dysphagia.
- They will be aware of the person's dietary preferences and recent body weight history.
- Carers must implement any guidance given by health professionals.

When talking to relatives/carers, bear in mind that caring for someone with dementia is extremely demanding, both physically and emotionally. Carers may feel:

- Unappreciated that they are giving a lot for little return.
- Resentful that their lives are dominated by this situation.
- Guilty that they feel like this.
- Impatient and angry, often a sign of the strain they feel.
- Depressed and bereft at the loss of the person they once knew and whose company they will be unable to enjoy again.
- Isolated, particularly if they are trying to cope alone.
- Frightened of the difficulties ahead.

Carers need to be provided with information about what dementia is and the best way of caring for a person with dementia. This can increase their confidence, decrease levels of stress and improve the care they provide for the person with dementia (Alzheimer's Society, 2007). Information such as that provided by 'Who Cares' (DH, 2007), which provides information and support for carers of people with dementia, may be useful.

Internet resources

Alzheimer's Society, www.alzheimers.org.uk

References

Alzheimer's Society. (2007) *Dementia UK*. Available at https://www.alzheimers.org.uk/info/20025/policy_and_influencing/251/dementia_uk. Accessed 25 May 2017.

Alzheimer's Society. (2014) *Dementia UK Update*. Available at https://www.alzheimers.org.uk/site/scripts/download_info.php?fileID=2323. Accessed on 13/1/2017.

Alzheimer's Society. (2016a) *Genetics of dementia Factsheet 405LP*. Available at https://www.alzheimers.org.uk/download/downloads/id/1759/factsheet_genetics_of_dementia.pdf. Accessed on 15 January 2017.

Alzheimer's Society. (2016b) *What Is Frontotemporal Dementia (FTD)? Factsheet 404LP*. Available at https://www.alzheimers.org.uk/download/downloads/id/1758/factsheet_what_is_frontotemporal_dementia.pdf. Accessed 25 May 2017.

Bayer A, Reban J. (2004) *Alzheimer's Disease and Related Conditions*. Czech Republic: MEDEA Press.

Brown J, Hillam J. (2004) *Dementia – Your Questions Answered*. London: Churchill Livingston.

Cohen-Mansfield J, Marx MS, Dakheel-Ali M, *et al.* (2010) Can agitated behavior of nursing home residents with dementia be prevented with the use of standardized stimuli? *J. Am. Geriatr. Soc.* 58(8): 1459–1464. Available at https://www.ncbi.nlm.nih.gov/pmc/articles/PMC2955178/. Accessed on 5 January 2017.

DH. (2007) Who cares? Information and support for the carers of people with dementia Available at http://webarchive.nationalarchives.gov.uk/20130105192943/http://www.dh.gov.uk/en/Publicationsandstatistics/Publications/PublicationsPolicyAndGuidance/DH_078093. Accessed 1 November 2018.

ESPEN. (2015) *Guidelines on Nutrition and Dementia*. Available at http://www.espen.info/wp/wordpress/wpcontent/uploads/2015/11/ESPEN_GL_Dementia_ClinNutr2015.pdf. Accessed on 13 December 2016.

Hanson LC, Ersek M, Gilliam R, *et al.* (2011) Oral feeding options for people with dementia: a systematic review. *J. Am. Geriatr. Soc.* 59(3): 463–472.

Janicki MP, Dalton AJ. (2000) Prevalence of dementia and impact on intellectual disability service. *Ment. Retard.* 38(3): 276–288.

Kindell J. (2002) *Feeding and Swallowing Disorders in Dementia*. Oxon: Speechmark Publishing Ltd.

Lourida I, Soni M, Thompson-Coon J, *et al.* (2013): Mediterranean Diet, Cognitive Function, and Dementia: A Systematic Review. *Epidemiology*. 24(4):479–89

NICE. (2006; amended 2011) *Dementia: Supporting people with dementia and their carers in health and social care*. Available at http://guidance.nice.org.uk/CG42. Accessed 28 July 2011.

Prentice AM, Leavesley K, Murgatroyd PR, *et al.* (1989) Is severe wasting in elderly mental patients caused by an excessive energy requirement? *Age Ageing* 18: 158–167.

Rheaume Y, Riley M, Volicer L. (1987) Meeting the nutritional needs of Alzheimer's patients who pace constantly. *J. Nutr. Elder.* 7: 43–52.

Robinson L, Hutchings D, Dickinson HO, *et al.* (2006) Effectiveness and acceptability of non-pharmacological interventions to reduce wandering in dementia: a systematic review. *Int. J. Geriatr. Psychiatry* 22(1): 9–22.

Royal College of Nursing (RCN). (2007) *Hydration Best Practice Toolkit*. Royal College of Nursing, London.

Social Care Institute for Excellence (SCIE). (2011) *Eating Well for People with Dementia*. Available at http://www.scie.org.uk/publications/dementia/eating/environment.asp. Accessed 8 August 2011.

UK Government. (2000) *Carers and Disabled Children Act*. TSO, UK. Available at http://www.legislation.gov.uk/all?title=Carers%20and%20Disabled%20Children%20Act. Accessed 23 January 2017.

UK Government. (2005a) *Carers (Equal Opportunities) Act. TSO, UK*. Available at http://www.legislation.gov.uk/all?title=Carers%20%28Equal%20Opportunities%29%20Act. Accessed 23 January 2017.

UK Government. (2005b) *The Mental Capacity Act. TSO, UK*. Available at http://www.legislation.gov.uk/all?title=Mental%20Capacity%20Act. Accessed 23 January 2017.

UK Government. (2007) *Employment Act*. The Stationary Office, UK. Available at http://www.legislation.gov.uk/all?title=Employment. Accessed 23 January 2017.

Welsh Assembly Government (WAG). (2011) *Nutrition in Community Settings – A Pathway and Resource Pack for Health and Social Care Professionals, the Third Sector, Care Home Staff, Relatives and Carers*. Cardiff: WAG.

7.11 Immunology and immune disease

7.11.1 Nutrition and immunity

Elaine Gardner

Key points

- The immune system is a complex series of processes that interact as the body's defence system.
- Nutrients play a major role in the functioning of a healthy immune system; any challenge to optimal nutritional status has an impact on the immune system.
- The immune system is linked to the pathogenesis of many everyday illnesses and diseases.
- Supplementation may be required to correct nutritional deficiencies, but caution should be exhibited. Supplementation as a treatment of illnesses and chronic diseases through their impact on the immune system requires more research.

The immune system is complex and should be viewed as a range of tissues, cells and their products. This defence mechanism guards against invasion by foreign microorganisms and molecules, protecting against illnesses and communicable diseases. A balance between destruction of foreign cells and avoidance of self-destruction is necessary, and the body's ability to distinguish and identify cells and molecules that are part of its self and those that are non-self is fundamental. There is, however, still a great deal that researchers do not understand in the field of immunology, and every year there are new discoveries, including new molecules and new theories. For example, the concept of the immune system recognising self from non-self has been challenged by a theory that suggests that the immune system is designed to recognise danger, irrespective of whether the target is self or non-self. This means that immunology is an active and rapidly changing field.

Further details of the structure and functioning of the immune system can be found in Goering *et al.* (2012). Particular attention should be given to the processes of acute and chronic inflammation.

Nutrients and the function of a healthy immune system

Adequate intakes are required for the immune system to develop and function correctly. They are required for the production of the structural components of the immune system as well as the defence responses. A deficiency can negatively influence the body's defences and impair its ability to combat infections.

Energy and protein

Infection increases energy requirements due to an increase in the basal metabolic rate. There is an increased need for protein and energy for increased production of cytokines, B and T lymphocytes, macrophages, and other leucocytes and their products, e.g. immunoglobulins. If anorexia is present, and protein and energy demands are not met, fat is mobilised. However, cytokines and other hormonal responses inhibit the efficient use of fats for energy, and the body relies on protein breakdown. If requirements are not met, especially of methionine and cysteine, wasting will occur as mobilised amino acids are prioritised for the synthesis of proteins related to the immune response.

Arginine

Nitric oxide is synthesised from arginine and is important in immune systems since the inhibition of nitric oxide production increases the body's susceptibility to infectious agents. Nitric oxide increases oxygenation and microperfusion by causing vasodilation with a subsequent increase in oxygenation. This has a positive

Manual of Dietetic Practice, Sixth Edition. Edited by Joan Gandy.

Companion website: www.manualofdieteticpractice.com

effect on the body's ability to fight infection through the recruitment of leukocytes and macrophages. Also, macrophages use L-arginine as a substrate for many of their immune functions. Nitric oxide also has inherent bactericidal activity (Bharadwaj *et al.*, 2016). Nitric oxide deficiency has been well-correlated with wound breakdown and poor wound healing. However, arginine supplementation during an inflammatory state could be detrimental due to the overwhelming production of nitric oxide (Calder, 2007).

Glutamine

Glutamine plays a crucial role in B-cell differentiation, neutrophil superoxide production, cytokine production, T-cell proliferation and phagocytosis (Bharadwaj *et al.*, 2016). Concentrations are markedly decreased in inflammatory states, which may have a suppressive effect on the immune system.

Fatty acids

Fatty acids are important in the function of the immune system because they are structural components of cell membranes. The fluidity of membranes (which is affected by the chain length and saturation of incorporated fatty acids) is important for cell surface structures such as receptors, which are crucial in immune functioning. Polyunsaturated fatty acids (PUFAs) have a direct effect on the function of immune cells as they are converted to tissue hormones (e.g. prostaglandins). n-6 and n-3 PUFAs compete in prostaglandin formation, resulting in the production of different prostaglandins. Eicosapentaenoic acid (EPA) and docosahexaenoic acid (DHA) increase the production of resolvins and protectins, which play a role in the resolution of inflammation and enhance wound healing. They also enhance immune response by improving lymphocyte function (Bharadwaj *et al.*, 2016). Diets rich in n-3 PUFAs tend to inhibit the immune response, whereas n-6 PUFA–rich diets tend to promote immune responses, which lead to inflammation (Galli & Calder, 2009). This has implications in the treatment of patients with inflammatory conditions such as rheumatoid arthritis and ulcerative colitis.

Micronutrients

Micronutrients influence the effectiveness of the immune system, and an adequate intake is required for the effective functioning of the body's defence mechanisms (Table 7.11.1). Different micronutrients have different roles, for instance: as components of enzymes required for normal immune functioning (e.g. manganese, magnesium, copper, selenium, iron); as regulatory agents (e.g. vitamin B_{12}, zinc, vitamin D, vitamin C); as components in synthesising cells (e.g. folate, retinol carotenoids, vitamin D, vitamin B_6); as stimulants of cell functions (e.g. retinol carotenoids, vitamin C); and as protectors of immune function (e.g. vitamin C, vitamin E, selenium).

It must be remembered, however, that nutrients do not work independently, but in a synergistic and interrelated manner, and focusing on single micronutrients is misleading. This is illustrated when looking at the example of HIV infection and micronutrients. The oxidative stress-induced niacin sink model (Taylor, 2010) examines the dysregulation syndrome caused by HIV infection, where several different nutrients, antioxidant vitamins, selenium, cysteine, tryptophan and niacin, interact and shift away from their normal biochemical set-points to below normal due to the actions of HIV within the body. Where deficiency states are due to metabolic dysregulation rather than inadequate intake, it appears that supplementation intended to restore them to normal levels can instead produce the symptoms of toxicity, which would normally be associated with excess consumption. It would thus seem that it is not the metabolic levels of micronutrients but their intake levels that should be the target of normalisation efforts. Thus, in people living with HIV, micronutrient intakes are not recommended above the recommended level of daily allowances for healthy non-HIV-infected persons of the same age, sex, and physical activity levels.

Table 7.11.1 Summary of nutrient requirements for the functioning of the immune system (Maggini *et al.*, 2007)

Body's defence system	Nutrients required
Skin barrier function	Vitamins A, C and E Zinc
Synergistic working to support protective activities in immune cells (cellular immunity)	Vitamins A, B_6, B_{12}, C, D and E Folic acid Iron Zinc Copper Selenium Manganese Magnesium PUFA Methionine Cysteine
Antibody production B-cell proliferation	Vitamin B_6 Selenium Copper Zinc Glutamine
Promotion of humoral immunity	Vitamins A, D and E Arginine
Indirect action on protein synthesis and/or cell growth	Vitamin B_{12} Folic acid Magnesium Manganese

Iron

Iron is essential for the growth, survival and replication of microorganisms and viruses. At the start of an infection, extracellular iron (and, to a lesser extent, zinc) shifts into the intercellular compartment; this shift is believed to make iron unavailable to some pathogens, and hence limits their potential growth (Weinberg, 2009). Supplementation with iron has the potential to increase pathogenic replication and has subsequent consequences. This has implications, especially in malaria-infected children from developing countries, who are often anaemic, and in pregnant women from these areas, who require iron-containing supplements. Guidance on iron supplementation in malaria-endemic areas can be found in the World Health Organization (2016a) guidelines for postpartum women, as well as for infants and children (2016b). There is no evidence to suggest that iron supplementation has adverse effects on infectious disease incidence or morbidity in the UK. There may, however, be possible adverse effects on individuals with HIV and children at risk of diarrhoea (SACN, 2010).

Antioxidants

The immune system is particularly at risk from oxidative stress, as many of the cells of the immune system produce reactive oxygen species during their normal functioning. Antioxidant defences have evolved to protect organisms against the damaging effects of free radicals. These defences include molecules that directly remove free radicals (e.g. vitamin E, beta-carotene, vitamin C), and antioxidant enzymes (e.g. glutathione and superoxide dismutase), which have trace metals components (e.g. manganese, copper, zinc and selenium). There is also an interaction between PUFAs and antioxidants (e.g. n-3 PUFAs and vitamin E).

The immune system and disease

Food allergy

The production of IgG or IgE antibodies in response to an allergen may be established before birth and in early childhood (through reprogramming of the immune response), and is dependent on the body's balance between types of T helper cells (Th1 or Th2 cells). Genes can increase or decrease susceptibility to allergies, and early exposure (or lack of exposure) to environmental factors, such as infectious diseases and microbial infections, may influence whether susceptible individuals become atopic (see Chapter 7.11.2, Food hypersensitivity).

Atherosclerosis

Atherosclerosis is an inflammatory disease of the arteries resulting in the deposition of plaques (Samson *et al.*, 2012). n-3 PUFAs may block the production of cytokines that promote inflammation, and so inhibit the development of atherosclerosis. Vitamin E may help prevent oxidation of low-density lipoproteins (Hansson & Hermansson, 2011) (see Chapter 7.14.1, General aspects of cardiovascular disease and Chapter 7.14.2, Coronary heart disease).

Autoimmune disease

Autoimmune disease, e.g. type 1 diabetes mellitus, multiple sclerosis, coeliac disease, Crohn's disease and rheumatoid arthritis, occurs when there is a breakdown in the self-preservation mechanism and a level of self-destruction by the immune system. A genetic predisposition; lymphocytes with receptors that can recognise the self-antigen; and environmental factors (e.g. microbial infection) that lead to the breakdown of tolerance mechanisms, which are designed to eliminate self-reactive lymphocytes; these are all necessary for autoimmune disease to occur.

Cancer

Cancer cells arise when there is malfunction of systems that promote cell growth and those that protect against excessive cell growth in a cell. A weakened immune system can increase the risk of haematological and virus-associated cancers, but there is disagreement as to whether this applies to solid tumours. Macrophages and natural killer (NK) cells are able to destroy cancer cells that occur in the tissues, but require activation. Unless there is inflammation present, activation does not occur until a tumour becomes large, and dying cancer cells activate the macrophages, which enlist help from NK cells in the blood.

Coeliac disease and gluten sensitivity

Coeliac disease derives from a mechanism that is triggered by the adaptive response of the immune system, whereas gluten sensitivity is connected to the action of the innate immune system and does not involve the function of the intestinal barrier (Sapone *et al.*, 2010, 2011) (see Chapter 7.4.7, Coeliac disease).

Critical illness and surgery

Following surgical trauma or during critical illness, an excessive inflammatory response can be induced that can be followed by an immune-suppressed state, which increases susceptibility to infection. Some nutrients, including some amino acids, antioxidant vitamins and minerals, phytochemicals, long chain n-3 fatty acids and nucleotides, may be able to influence the immune system (immunonutrition) by improving cell-mediated responses. Research is being undertaken on their use in artificial nutritional regimens (Bharadwaj *et al.*, 2016).

Gut microbiota and gut health

The gut-associated lymphoid tissue secretes antibodies to inhibit the colonisation of pathogens and to prevent the entry of harmful antigens into the blood from the digestive tract. Indigenous bacteria also contribute to the protection at the mucosal surfaces by creating a barrier effect (colonisation resistance), and are required for the development and tuning of the immune system. Commensal bacteria that normally inhabit the gut have distinct roles, which can be opposing, and a compositional balance is required to support (gut) health. When the balance of the organisms is disrupted, local immune systems may be impaired. Probiotics, prebiotics and synbiotics that rebalance gut bacteria may indirectly produce immune effects. The mechanisms involved and the impact of probiotics and prebiotics on the gut mucosal defences are reviewed in Hardy *et al.* (2013) (see Chapter 5.2, Functional foods).

Intestinal microbial inhabitants, referred to as the microbiota, are thought to facilitate the onset of and/or aggravate certain diseases, including autoimmune and allergic diseases (Milani *et al.*, 2016). Research is in its infancy to manipulate the gut microbiota through dietary intervention and to positively impact on disease, since the relationship between gut microbiota, immunity and disease is very complex. The same commensal bacteria can induce either a protective response or an inflammatory response, depending on the individual.

HIV and AIDS

The human immunodeficiency virus 1 (HIV-1) slowly overwhelms and destroys the immune system, leading to profound immune suppression. It establishes an infection that can be latent and undetectable by the killer T-cells for long periods of time, and then develops, so that the killer T-cells or antibodies no longer recognise the virus (Sompayrac, 2011). As a result, it has a high mutation rate, and is successful because it preferentially infects and disables the immune system (particularly helper T-cells, macrophages and dendritic cells) that would normally defend against it. It results in extensive immune damage and dysregulation, with the integrity of the cell-mediated immune system undermined and a chronic inflammatory state established. This is characterised by high oxidative stress, wasting and metabolic changes to fat and muscle distribution, and derangement of vitamin and mineral levels even when intakes are adequate (see Chapter 7.11.3, Human immunodeficiency virus (HIV)).

Undernutrition

In any infection, the nutritional status of the host critically determines the outcome of infection. Undernutrition compromises immunity, which increases susceptibility to infection and disease. The general effects of undernutrition on the immune system are:

- Diminished T-cell help in immune responses.
- Delayed antibody responses.
- Depressed mucosal antibody in response to mucosal infections.
- Impaired complement activation.
- Decreased lysozyme levels in leucocytes.
- Impaired activity of opsonin (a serum that attaches to bacteria to make them more attractive to phagocytes, and thus more likely to be engulfed and destroyed).
- Thymic atrophy (the primary site of T-cell development).

Infection has detrimental effects on nutritional status, which can lead to a perpetuating cycle of undernutrition

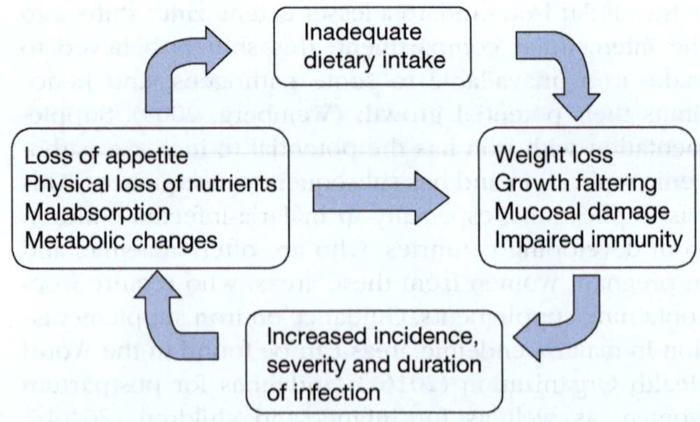

Figure 7.11.1 Cycle of undernutrition and infection [source: Tomkins & Watson, 1989. Reproduced with permission from the UN Standing Committee on Nutrition (UNSCN)]

and infection (Figure 7.11.1). In low-income countries, where low protein and/or energy intake is more common, the impact of the undernutrition and infection cycle is devastating, resulting in growth retardation in utero and in children, and increased rates of infections, parasite infestations, morbidity and mortality. A review can be found in Schaible and Kaufmann (2007). In high-income countries, undernutrition is still seen within some societal groups, such as the elderly, who are at risk from the cycle of undernutrition and infection, which results in (subclinical) nutritional deficiencies, loss of weight, poor appetite, poor wound healing, as well as increased rates of infections (see Chapter 6.2, Malnutrition).

Obesity

It has been suggested that an altered immune function contributes to the pathogenesis of obesity (de Heredia *et al.*, 2012), and that white adipose tissue inflammation may be a key factor in metabolic dysregulation (Dam *et al.*, 2016; Exley *et al.*, 2014). Research continues to fully understand the mechanisms involved. A systematic review by Dhurandhar *et al.* (2015) looked at identifying infections that potentially contribute to greater body mass index (BMI), and the differential responses of overweight and obese persons to infections. Evidence indicated that some viral infections were followed by weight gain, and that people who were overweight or obese had higher susceptibility to developing post-surgical infections, H1N1 influenza and periodontal disease. More severe infections tended to be present in people with a higher BMI, and they had a reduced response to vaccinations and antimicrobial drugs.

The immune system in infancy

Cunningham-Rundles *et al.* (2009) reviewed the development of the neonatal immune response, particularly with regard to the effects of micronutrients, concluding that nutrients moulded the developing immune system, and that, post-birth, the interactions between dietary micronutrients and microbial and environmental antigens defined the patterns of host defence in later life. Animal studies are suggestive that early-life microbial colonisation of mucosal tissues also plays a key role in the development and education of the immune system, which can facilitate tolerance to environmental exposures or contribute to the development of disease in later life. It has been postulated that these are limited to a narrow window of opportunity, and that early-life influences by the microbiota may even be evident during gestation, with microbial colonisation during pregnancy regulating the number of specific innate immune cells and their activity in the infant (Gensollen *et al.*, 2016).

The immune system in the elderly

With ageing, the immune system changes, and the ability to respond to infections and develop immunity after vaccinations progressively deteriorate (immunosenescence). As a result, there is an increased susceptibility to infections, cancers and autoimmune diseases in the elderly. Innate immunity dysfunction may be due to the increased production of proinflammatory cytokines (which may be linked to the development of diabetes, osteoporosis and atherosclerosis due to their inflammatory pathogenesis), a decline in phagocytic capacity and depressed NK cell cytotoxicity. Changes in the adaptive immune system are twofold. Humoral immunity is compromised due to the decreased production of immunoglobulin-producing B lymphocytes and the loss of immunoglobulin diversity and affinity, leading to less-well-adapted antibody responses in older people. Age-associated changes related to the thymus lead to a reduction in the functional size of the thymus, which decreases T-cell output and diversity, which may leave the elderly more susceptible to new pathogens.

Several studies have looked at the effect of vitamin B_6, vitamin E, zinc and multi-micronutrient supplementation, but the identification and levels of micronutrients necessary to slow down the immune-ageing process are still to be determined. In elderly people who are undernourished, the decrease in immune functions is highly correlated with the intensity of the nutritional deficit, and this causes a secondary immune deficiency (in addition to the primary deficiency caused by ageing per se). Refeeding may reverse secondary immune changes in the undernourished. Valiathan *et al.* (2016) and Ponnappan and Ponnappan (2011) have reviewed immune function in the elderly.

Exercise

Exercise has an impact on the immune system. Acute and chronic exercise alters the number and function of neutrophils, monocytes and NK cells of the innate immune system. Lymphocytosis is observed during and immediately after exercise, proportional to the exercise density and duration, with the number of T-cells falling below pre-exercise levels during the early stages of recovery, before returning to resting values (normally within 24 hours after the last bout of exercise). Acute bouts of moderate exercise have little impact on mucosal immunity, but there may be a link between moderate, regular exercise and a healthy immune system. However, prolonged exercise and intensive training provoke a response that has been linked to increased risk of upper tract respiratory infections during heavy training. This is linked to the elevated circulating stress hormones cortisol and adrenaline (epinephrine), which raise blood pressure and cholesterol levels and suppress the immune system. It is believed that the combined effects of small changes in the immune system may compromise resistance to minor illnesses, especially in elite athletes (Walsh *et al.*, 2011b). The protective effect of exercise against chronic inflammation–associated diseases, such as type 2 diabetes and cardiovascular disease, has been attributed to the anti-inflammatory effect of regular exercise. It has been suggested that this may be mediated via both the reduction of visceral fat mass and the establishment of an anti-inflammatory environment with each bout of exercise (Walsh *et al.*, 2011a). These authors concluded that '*nonathletes engaging in moderate physical activity programmes do not require nutritional supplements [to maintain immune function], and can obtain all needed nutrients from a healthy and balanced diet*'. The mechanisms and controversies related to exercise and immunology are reviewed by Walsh *et al.* (2011a, 2011b). Practical guidelines for athletes that can help reduce the extent of exercise-induced immunodepression and lower the risk of infection can be found in Gleeson *et al.* (2012) (see Chapter 4.3, Sports nutrition).

Further reading

Goering R, Dockrell H, Zuckerman M, *et al.* (2012) *Mims' Medical Microbiology*, 5th edn. Elsevier.

References

Bharadwaj S, Trivax B, Tandon P, *et al.* (2016) Should perioperative immunonutrition for elective surgery be the current standard of care? *Gastroenterol. Rep. (Oxf).* 4(2): 87–95.

Calder P. (2007) Immunonutrition in surgical and critically ill patients. *Br. J. Nutr.* 98(1): S133–S139.

Cunningham-Rundles S, Lin H, Ho-Lin D, *et al.* (2009) Role of nutrients in the development of neonatal immune response. *Nutr. Rev.* 67(2): S152–S163.

Dam V, Sikder T, Santosa S. (2016) From neutrophils to macrophages: differences in regional adipose tissue depots. *Obes. Rev.* 17(1): 1–17.

de Heredia FP, Gómez-Martínez S, Marcos A. (2012) Obesity, inflammation and the immune system. *Proc. Nutr. Soc.* 71(2): 332–338.

Dhurandhar NV, Bailey D, Thomas D. (2015) Interaction of obesity and infections. *Obes. Rev.* 16(12): 1017–1029.

Exley MA, Hand L, O'Shea D, *et al.* (2014) Interplay between the immune system and adipose tissue in obesity. *J. Endocrinol.* 223(2): R41–48.

Galli C, Calder PC. (2009) Effects of fat and fatty acid intake on inflammatory and immune responses: a critical review. *Ann. Nutr. Metab.* 55: 123–139.

Gensollen T, Iyer SS, Kasper DL, *et al.* (2016) How colonization by microbiota in early life shapes the immune system. *Science.* 352(6285): 539–544.

Gleeson M, Walsh NP. (2012) The BASES expert statement on exercise, immunity, and infection. *J. Sports Sci.* 30(3): 321–324.

Goering RV, Dockrell HM, Zuckerman M, *et al.* (2012) *Mims Medical Microbiology*, 5th edn. New York: Elsevier Saunders.

Hansson GK, Hermansson A. (2011) The immune system in atherosclerosis. *Nat. Immunol.* 12(3): 204–212.

Hardy H, Harris J, Lyon E, et al. (2013) Probiotics, prebiotics and immunomodulation of gut mucosal defences: homeostasis and immunopathology. *Nutrients.* 5: 1869–1912.

Maggini S, Wintergerst ES, Beveridge S, *et al.* (2007) Selected vitamins and trace elements support immune function by strengthening epithelial barriers and cellular and humoral immune responses. *Br. J. Nutr.* 98(1): S29–S35.

Milani C, Ferrario C, Turroni F, et al. (2016) The human gut microbiota and its interactive connections to diet. *J. Hum. Nutr. Diet.* 29: 539–546.

Ponnappan S, Ponnappan U. (2011) Aging and immune function: molecular mechanisms to interventions. *Antioxid. Redox Signal.* 14(8): 1551–1585.

SACN. (2010) *Iron and Health*. London: The Stationery Office.

Samson S, Mundkur L, Kakkar VV. (2012) Immune response to lipoproteins in atherosclerosis. *Cholesterol.* 2012: 571846.

Sapone A, Lammers K, Mazzarella G, *et al.* (2010) Differential mucosal IL-17 expression in two gliadin-induced disorders: gluten sensitivity and autoimmune enteropathy celiac disease. *Int. Arch. Allergy Immunol.* 152: 75–80.

Sapone A, Lammers KM, Casolaro V, *et al.* (2011) Divergence of gut permeability and mucosal gene expression in two gluten associated conditions: celiac disease and gluten sensitivity. *BMC Med.* 9: 23.

Schaible UE, Kaufmann SH. (2007) Malnutrition and infection: complex mechanisms and global impacts. *PloS Med.* 4(5): e115.

Sompayrac LM. (2011) *How the Immune System Works*, 3rd edn. Oxford: Wiley Blackwell.

Taylor EW. (2010) The oxidative stress-induced niacin sink (OSINS) model for HIV pathogenesis. *Toxicology.* 278(1): 124–130.

Tomkins AM, Watson F. (1989) *Malnutrition and infection*. A review. Geneva: Advisory Committee on Co-ordination/Subcommittee on Nutrition, World Health Organisation; 1989.

Valiathan R, Ashman M, Asthana D. (2016) Effects of ageing on the immune system: infants to elderly. *Scand. J. Immunol.* 83(4): 255–266.

Walsh NP, Gleeson M, Shephard RJ, *et al.* (2011a) Position statement. *Part one: immune function and exercise. Exerc. Immunol. Rev.* 17: 6–63.

Walsh NP, Gleeson M, Pyne DB, *et al.* (2011b) Position statement. *Part two: maintaining immune health. Exerc. Immunol. Rev.* 17: 64–103.

Weinberg ED. (2009) Iron availability and infection. *Biochim. Biophys. Acta* 1790: 600–605.

WHO. (2016a) *Guideline: Daily Iron Supplementation in Postpartum Women*. Geneva: WHO.

WHO. (2016b) *Guideline: Daily Iron Supplementation in Infants and Children*. Geneva: WHO.

7.11.2 Food hypersensitivity

Isabel Skypala and Rosan Meyer

Key points

- Food hypersensitivity is a reaction caused by food that is specific to an individual; it is divided into immune-mediated food allergy (IgE-mediated and non-IgE-mediated) and non-immune-mediated food hypersensitivity.
- The cumulative incidence of IgE-mediated food allergy in the UK in the first decade of life is 6.8%, and 3.7% in adults.
- Validated diagnostic tests exist for IgE-mediated food allergy; for other types of food hypersensitivity, diagnosis may only be achieved through strict and total exclusion and reintroduction of the suspect food.
- Food hypersensitivity can have deleterious effects on quality of life; correct diagnosis is therefore essential.
- Children with the condition must be assessed regularly for nutritional status, dietary compliance, coping strategies and potential resolution.

There has been a substantial rise in the number of patients attending hospital for food allergy events (Gupta *et al.*, 2007; Turner *et al.*, 2015), with increasing hospital admissions for severe symptoms, especially in children (Dyer *et al.*, 2015; Tejedor-Alonso *et al.*, 2015). Correct diagnosis and management is vital in order to avoid severe or even fatal reactions to food, and any nutritional consequences of unnecessary or unsupervised food avoidance, which will also affect quality of life. This chapter will cover the diagnosis and management of these adverse food reactions, usually termed food hypersensitivity (FHS) (Johansson *et al.*, 2004).

There is great disparity between perceived and actual prevalence. A UK birth cohort study found that, overall, only 15% of children with a reported reaction to food were diagnosed with a food allergy (Venter *et al.*, 2016). This pattern is repeated in adolescents and adults; only 20% of children and adults who report a food allergy are likely to have a positive food challenge (Nwaru *et al.*, 2014). In Europe, the prevalence of food-challenge-confirmed food allergy was 0.9% (Nwaru *et al.*, 2014). The cumulative incidence of challenge-proven food allergy in the UK is 6.8% in the first decade of life, with a prevalence of 3.6% (Venter *et al.*, 2016). Prevalence is higher in the very young, with up to 10% of 1-year-olds having challenge-proven food allergies (Allen & Koplin, 2012; Osborne *et al.*, 2011). The prevalence of challenge-verified food allergy in adults is 3.7% in Europe (Zuberbier *et al.*, 2004).

Diagnostic criteria and classification

Allergy has been defined as an immunologically mediated and allergen-specific hypersensitivity, and as such is a mechanism leading to disease, rather than a disease state itself (Ring 2014). A hypersensitivity reaction is an abnormally strong response to a stimulus. Adverse reactions to foods can either be due to the toxicity of the food or a hypersensitivity of the individual to that specific food (Bruijnzeel-Koomen *et al.*, 1995). The European Academy of Allergy and Clinical Immunology (EAACI) and World Allergy Organisation (WAO) (Johansson *et al.*, 2004) nomenclature classify food hypersensitivity (FHS) reactions involving immunologic mechanisms as food allergy, with all other reactions termed as non-allergic food hypersensitivity (Figure 7.11.2). The main difference between food allergy and non-allergic FHS is that, in the former, a protein interacting with the immune system causes food allergy, while there is no immune system involvement in the latter. Food-allergic reactions can be further divided into three: (1) IgE-mediated reactions, where the involvement of food-specific IgE antibodies has been demonstrated; (2) mixed IgE and non-IgE-mediated reactions; and (3) cell-mediated reactions (Muraro *et al.*, 2014c). Food-allergic symptoms may be of rapid onset (IgE-mediated, e.g. urticaria or anaphylaxis), but can also develop more slowly (non-IgE-mediated, e.g. eczema, diarrhoea, vomiting and constipation), or may be a mixture of both. Severe, generalised allergic reactions to food are classified as anaphylaxis. Reactions not involving the immune system may be due to non-immune-mediated histamine release, pharmacological effects or enzyme deficiencies. They can be acute and severe (although rarely life threatening), but are more usually chronic and diffuse, and therefore often difficult to diagnose. The terms food allergy and non-immune-mediated FHS will be used in this chapter according to the preceding EAACI definitions (Figure 7.11.3).

Reactions to food may also result from the emotional response to the thought of eating a particular food, and are termed food aversion. Food aversion is not discussed further in this chapter, but should always be considered when investigations of reported reactions to foods are being made.

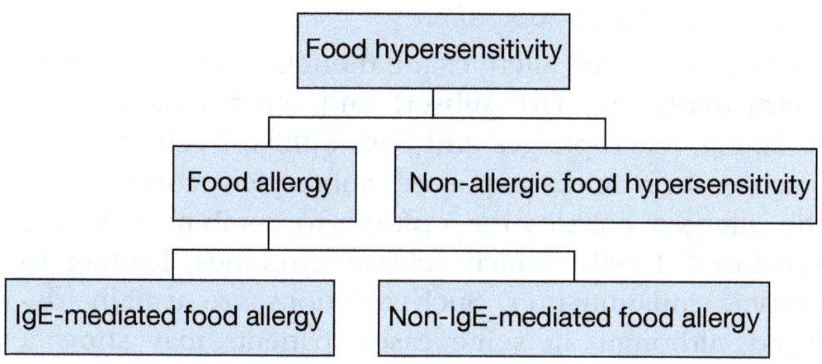

Figure 7.11.2 Proposed nomenclature for food hypersensitivity (European Academy of Allergy and Clinical Immunology Nomenclature Task Force Position Statement; Johansson et al., 2004)

Mechanisms

Immune-mediated food allergy

Food allergy results from a faulty and exaggerated response of the immune system following exposure to a foreign protein (allergen). The immune system can normally distinguish allergens that need to be destroyed, e.g. bacterial pathogens, from those that do not, e.g. food

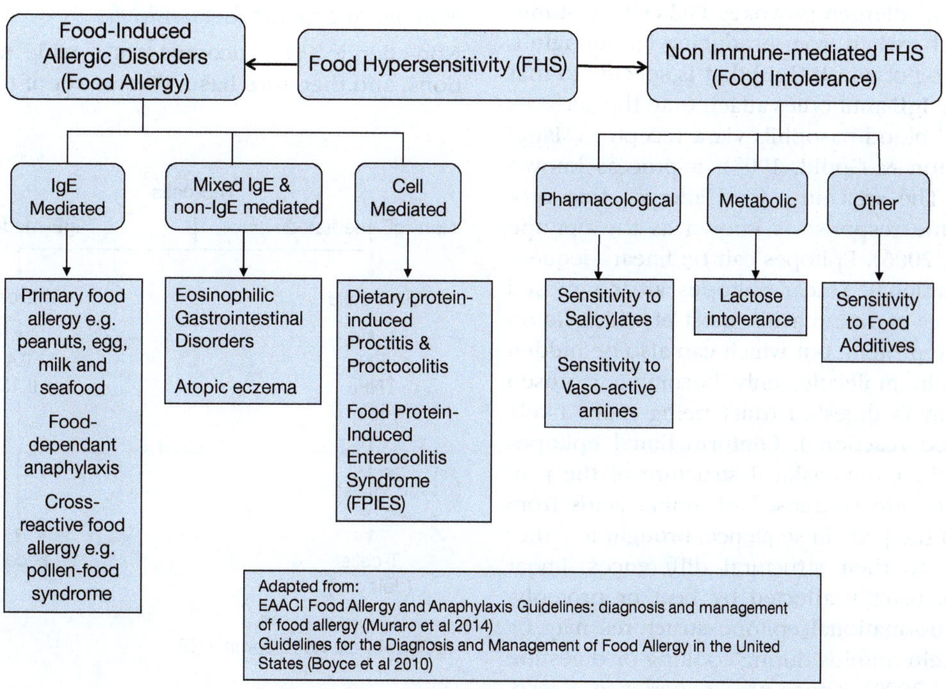

Figure 7.11.3 Nomenclature for food-allergic reactions (European Academy of Allergy and Clinical Immunology; Boyce et al., 2010; Muraro et al., 2014a)

proteins, and can mount an appropriate response to protect the body from infection and damage. In addition, the mucosal lining of the gastrointestinal tract provides a physical barrier to prevent large molecules such as proteins from entering the body.

There are two types of immunity; everyone is born with an innate immunity, but it is the cells of adaptive immunity that are involved in food allergy. The main protagonists are the T-cell lymphocytes, which recognise and destroy allergens by producing cytotoxic substances or triggering inflammatory responses. When an allergen is encountered, naive T-cells develop into either T helper 1 (Th1) or T helper 2 (Th2) cells, depending on the presence of specific mediator proteins. The other cells involved in adaptive immunity are the B-cell lymphocytes, which create antibodies (classes of immunoglobulin) to carry out further defensive reactions.

The immune system learns to do this in the early months of life, a process known as developing tolerance. If this learning process is faulty, an abnormal response to food proteins can occur, particularly to those that are encountered in early life when the immune system is still immature. Ingestion of the allergen triggers the production of inappropriately high titres of antibodies and/or altered T-cell reactivity, with consequent systemic effects.

IgE-mediated food allergy

IgE-mediated food allergy is most common in atopic individuals. Atopy is defined as a predisposition to become sensitised and produce IgE antibodies to environmental proteins (Johansson *et al.*, 2004). It is clinically defined by a positive skin prick test (SPT) and/or elevated specific IgE to one or more common environmental allergens.

Classic IgE-mediated food-allergic reactions involve the production of Th2 cells. In some individuals, exposure to a food allergen provokes Th2 cells to stimulate B-cells, which switch from producing immunoglobulin M to immunoglobulin E (IgE) that is specific to that food protein. The IgE antibodies attach onto the surfaces of mast cells and blood basophils via a receptor (Maggi *et al.*, 1992; Sutton & Gould, 1993); a process known as sensitisation. The area on a food allergen that provokes the immune response is known as the epitope (Chapman *et al.*, 2006). Epitopes can be linear (sequential) or conformational. Linear epitopes are composed of short sequences of amino acids, most of which lie on the surface of the protein, but which can also be hidden within the protein molecule, only becoming exposed when the protein is digested (thus being more likely to trigger delayed reactions). Conformational epitopes depend on the three-dimensional structure of the protein, because they are composed of amino acids from different parts of the protein sequence, brought together by folding. Due to their structural differences, linear epitopes are not usually affected by heat or proteolysis, whereas conformational epitope structures may be lost when a protein unfolds during cooking or digestion (Lin & Sampson, 2009). Those who experience a resolution of food allergy in childhood or adolescence are more likely to be sensitised to conformational epitopes (Jarvinen *et al.*, 2007; Vila *et al.*, 2001). Epitopes from different food proteins can have a degree of amino acid sequence similarity, known as homology, which enables an IgE antibody specific to one allergen to bind with another structurally similar allergen epitope. Homologous epitopes are common in food allergy, and account for the cross-reactivity between different foods and also between foods and pollens.

Many people may become sensitised to an allergen, but only a percentage will experience food-allergic symptoms on subsequent exposure to that protein. Symptoms occur when the IgE antibody recognises the allergen and the allergen epitope attaches to the binding site of the antibody. Should the allergen succeed in binding to two IgE antibodies, cross-linking them, the membrane of the mast cell perforates, and preformed mediators (e.g. histamine and leukotrienes) are released. These mediators are responsible for classic IgE-mediated food-allergic symptoms; rapid-onset sneeze, itch, red facial flush, hives and angioedema.

Non-IgE-mediated food allergy

Non-IgE-mediated allergies are thought to involve T-cells (particularly the Th1 subset) and other inflammatory cells, e.g. macrophages and eosinophils. T-cells become sensitised on initial exposure; subsequent contact with the allergen enables the epitope to combine with the sensitised T-cells, which release cytokines, leading to chronic inflammation. Such reactions are usually delayed, although, in some cases, patients may show a mixed pathology, with both IgE-mediated and cell-mediated causes. Figure 7.11.4 summarises the immune process involved in IgE-mediated and non-IgE-mediated allergic reactions.

Non-allergic food hypersensitivity

Non-allergic FHS encompasses a wide range of conditions, and therefore has a diverse set of triggers.

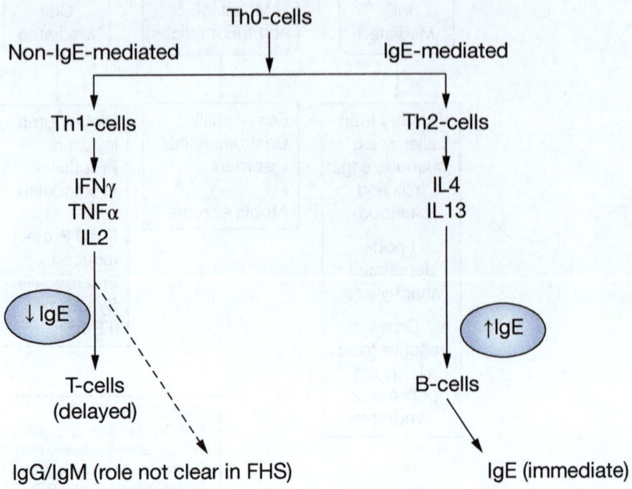

Figure 7.11.4 Food allergy – IgE-mediated and non-IgE-mediated reactions. Th, T helper; IFN, interferon, TNF, tumour necrosis factor; IL, interleukin; FHS, food hypersensitivity

Mast cell activation

Occasionally, mast cells can be directly activated by non-immunological mechanisms, after eating certain foods such as shellfish or strawberries, with the subsequent release of histamine and other mediators provoking symptoms similar to an allergic reaction. Reactions usually only occur after a significant amount of the offending food has been ingested.

Pharmacological reactions

Many foods and beverages contain substances that are pharmacologically active. Large intakes of, or undue sensitivity to, these substances can result in symptoms such as tremor, sweating, palpitations, headache or migraine, or psychological effects such as insomnia or anxiety.

Enzyme deficiencies

Partial or total deficiency of one or more enzymes in the digestive tract, e.g. lactase and disaccharidase deficiency, may result in symptoms of malabsorption when foods containing certain components are consumed.

Symptoms

The symptoms most commonly associated with FHS can broadly be divided into skin, gastrointestinal tract, respiratory system and systemic reactions (Table 7.11.2). These may occur within minutes, hours or days of ingestion.

Table 7.11.2 Symptoms experienced with food hypersensitivity

Target organ	Symptoms
Skin	Pallor
	Erythema
	Pruritus
	Urticaria
	Angio-oedema
	Eczema
	Dermatitis herpetiformis
Gastrointestinal tract	Oral allergy syndrome
	Food protein enteropathy syndrome
	Gastro-oesophageal reflux
	Allergic eosinophilic gastroenteritis/oesophagitis
	Oral itch, throat itch, lip swelling
	Diarrhoea, nausea, vomiting
	Abdominal pain
	Enteropathy
	Proctocolitis
	Enterocolitis
	Coeliac disease
	Constipation
Respiratory tract	Heiner's syndrome
	Rhinorrhoea
	Asthma
Multisystem	Hypotension
	Anaphylaxis
	Exercise-induced anaphylaxis
Controversial symptoms	Otitis media
	Hyperactivity
	Migraine/abdominal migraine
	Enuresis
Other	Irritability
	Listless with other symptoms

IgE-mediated food allergy

Clinical features

Symptoms suggestive of IgE-mediated food allergy are typically acute and may involve more than one organ. The first sign may be pruritus (itching) and mild oedema (swelling) of the oral cavity, which can precede other systemic reactions or be the sole manifestation of a condition known as oral allergy syndrome (OAS) (Amlot *et al.*, 1987). The most frequent manifestation of OAS occurs in pollen-sensitised individuals due to homologous epitopes in plant proteins that cause cross-reactivity between pollen antibodies and plant food allergens, and is usually described as pollen food allergy syndrome or pollen food syndrome (PFS), to distinguish it from other forms of OAS (Fernández-Rivas, 2015). Other clinical features of IgE-mediated food allergy include flushing, urticaria (hives), angioedema (swelling), nausea, vomiting, abdominal pain and diarrhoea; rhino-conjunctivitis and asthma may also occur, but rarely as isolated symptoms (Muraro *et al.*, 2014c). Anaphylaxis (the most severe presentation of IgE-mediated allergy) is a rapid, progressive multi-system reaction that is likely when there is acute onset of symptoms (e.g. urticaria, swelling, gastrointestinal) and either airway compromise or hypotension (Muraro *et al.*, 2014c). The onset of IgE-mediated food-allergic symptoms are usually reported soon after ingesting the offending food, typically within 30 minutes of eating. However, symptoms may be delayed up to 2 hours, especially if the reaction to the food only occurs when mediated by a cofactor such as exercise. This type of reaction is known as food-dependent, exercise-induced anaphylaxis (FDEIA), but other cofactors such as alcohol, stress, aspirin or non-steroidal anti-inflammatory drugs (NSAIDs) can also cause the same reaction (Cardona *et al.*, 2012). Those with PFS usually report more rapid onset, most often on biting or chewing the foods (Skypala *et al.*, 2011).

Non-IgE-mediated food allergy

Non-IgE-mediated food allergy mainly affects the gastrointestinal tract and the skin (Heine, 2015; Pelz *et al.*, 2016). Although symptoms tend to have a delayed onset (>2 hours), it is recognised that patients with this allergy can also have immediate IgE-mediated food/non-food triggers (Heine, 2015; Nowak-Wegrzyn *et al.*, 2015; Pelz *et al.*, 2016). Symptoms may be more diffuse and often less easy to identify (or distinguish from non-allergic FHS), and there may be differences between children and adults. For example, eosinophilic oesophagitis usually presents in children as feeding difficulties, abdominal pain, occasionally faltering growth and vomiting; however, in adolescents and adults, the most common presenting symptoms are dysphagia and food impaction (Miehlke, 2015).

Non-allergic food hypersensitivity

Non-allergic FHS can manifest with similar symptoms as both IgE-mediated or non-IgE-mediated food allergy. Reactions are usually dose dependent and, although some reactions are delayed, others can occur immediately or within 1 hour of ingestion. Anaphylactic reactions are rare, but very severe reactions can occur.

Triggers of food hypersensitivity reactions

Milk, egg and peanuts are the most prevalent allergens in children causing IgE-mediated food allergy and anaphylaxis (Grabenhenrich *et al.*, 2016). Fish, tree nuts and soy can also cause IgE-mediated reactions. For non-IgE-mediated food allergy, milk, soy, egg and wheat are the usual food culprits, but a wide range of other foods may be involved (Venter & Groetch, 2014). Milk, egg, wheat and soy allergy often remit in late childhood (Savage *et al.*, 2016), and shellfish, tree nuts, fruit and vegetables are the usual triggers of adult-onset IgE-mediated FHS (Skypala *et al.*, 2013). Non-allergic FHS reactions can be provoked by several triggers, including foods, food additives, and naturally occurring components in foods. Milk is the food most commonly reported to provoke any FHS reaction worldwide (Vierk *et al.*, 2007; Zuberbier *et al.*, 2004). More information on individual foods is available in the section Dietary management.

Links to other conditions

Rhinitis

Allergic rhinitis is directly linked to food allergy due to the close homology between plant food proteins and pollen proteins. Approximately 6% of the UK population suffers from allergic rhinitis due to tree pollen allergy, two-thirds of whom may go on to develop PFS (Bauchau & Durham, 2004; Royal College of Physicians, 2003; Skypala *et al.*, 2011). Schäfer *et al.* (2001) found that 73% of subjects reporting adverse food reactions also had allergic rhinitis. This may explain why PFS is the most prevalent food allergy in adults, affecting 2% of the UK population, mainly those with concomitant seasonal allergic rhinitis (Skypala *et al.*, 2013). Food sensitization in the first 2 years of life increased the risk of subsequent asthma and allergic rhinitis (Alduraywish *et al.*, 2016), and up to 48% of children with seasonal allergic rhinitis develop PFS (Ludman *et al.*, 2016). Climate change and increasing atmospheric carbon dioxide concentrations could also affect the severity and prevalence of allergic diseases, with exposure to diesel exhaust particles enhancing the risk of early-onset allergic rhinitis (Codispoti *et al.*, 2015; Ziska & Beggs, 2012).

Asthma

Although IgE-mediated reactions to foods can involve symptoms of both the upper and lower respiratory tracts, asthma is not commonly exacerbated by FHS, except for occupational asthma in relation to food, such as wheat flour (baker's asthma). However, there is a relationship between asthma, allergic rhinitis and food allergy in school-age children (Pénard-Morand *et al.*, 2005), and having a food allergy is independently associated with life-threatening asthma in children (Roberts *et al.*, 2003). Early food sensitisation in the first year of life can predict the onset of asthma (Caffarelli *et al.*, 2016). Asthmatic adults, who have multiple food allergies or fish allergy, may have an increased risk of hospitalisation and use of oral steroids (Berns *et al.*, 2007). Food-allergic patients with asthma are more likely to suffer from fatal or near-fatal food anaphylaxis, highlighting the need for a robust food allergy management plan (Colver *et al.*, 2005).

Eczema

Eczema is associated with food allergy, allergic rhinitis and asthma (Burks, 2003). Children with eczema have a 30% chance of having a concomitant food allergy, with those at highest risk having moderate to severe eczema unresponsive to topical treatment (NICE, 2007b; Werfel *et al.*, 2007). A recent systematic review found there was a strong and dose-dependent association between eczema, food sensitisation and food allergy, especially if the eczema is severe and chronic in nature (Tsakok *et al.*, 2016). Infants with early-onset eczema (especially within the first 1–4 months after birth) are more likely to have an increased risk of developing food allergy at 3 years of age (Shoda *et al.*, 2016). Although children and adults with eczema are often sensitised to foods, many are asymptomatic (Röckmann *et al.*, 2014; Roerdink *et al.*, 2016). Milk and egg are the two foods most often provoking IgE-mediated food allergy in children with eczema (Mavroudi *et al.*, 2017). However, early introduction of peanuts and egg into the diet of an infant who already has eczema would appear to be protective against the development of an allergy to that food (Du Toit *et al.*, 2016).

Gastrointestinal disease

Food hypersensitivity has been linked to a number of diseases of the gastrointestinal tract (see Chapters 7.4, Gastrointestinal disorders).

Migraine

A close association between migraine and allergic disease has been shown (Aamodt *et al.*, 2007), although it has been suggested that dietary restrictions are not beneficial for most migraine sufferers (Holzhammer & Wöber, 2006).

Hyperactivity and behavioural disorders

Few studies have rigorously assessed whether FHS is involved in hyperactivity disorders, and none in the last 10 years. A meta-analysis found a significant effect of artificial food colours on behaviour in hyperactive children (Schab & Trinh, 2004). A study investigating the effect of oral challenges with artificial food colourings and benzoates on hyperactivity in 3-year-old children found behaviour changes when assessed by parentally kept behaviour diaries (Bateman *et al.*, 2004). A follow-up study involving 3- and 8-year-old children taking two different additive mixes suggested that artificial colours or sodium benzoate preservative (or both) in the diet increased hyperactivity (McCann *et al.*, 2007).

Chronic disorders

People with chronic fatigue syndrome/myalgic encephalomyelitis (CFS/ME) often report experiencing FHS (NICE, 2007a). Although research evidence suggested that IgE-mediated allergy is no more common in people with CFS/ME than in the normal population, a population cohort study in China suggests that atopy is associated with CFS, particularly in patients with numerous atopic syndromes (Kowal *et al.*, 2002; Yang TY *et al.*, 2015).

Disease consequences

Food hypersensitivity can have severe consequences, with the most serious being anaphylaxis, requiring adrenaline (epinephrine). There has been a significant increase in hospital admissions for anaphylaxis (Turner *et al.*, 2015; Umasunthar *et al.*, 2015), and peanuts, tree nuts, fish or shellfish account for 33–61% of these admissions (Asai *et al.*, 2014; Jeong *et al.*, 2017; Worm *et al.*, 2014). Although mortality is low, an increasing number of severe reactions to food are suffered by a greater number of younger people, especially if asthma is present (Parlaman *et al.*, 2016). Living with a food allergy has been shown to significantly impact on quality of life for families, children and adults (Beyer *et al.*, 2016; Valentine & Knibb, 2011). Several authors have found that food allergy disrupts family/social life, and have found an increased emotional impact on parents (Primeau *et al.*, 2000; Sicherer *et al.*, 2001). Mothers seem to be affected particularly, with higher levels of stress and anxiety (King *et al.*, 2008). Parents find shopping for foods for children on restricted diets very difficult, time consuming and confusing (FSA, 2009). Results from validated health-related quality-of-life (HRQL) questionnaires found that adolescents and adults with food allergy report more pain, poorer overall health, more limitations on social activity (need to fit in with peers) and less vitality as compared to the general population (Flokstra-de Blok *et al.*, 2010; Sampson *et al.*, 2006). Those who have re-introduced foods back into their diet following a negative oral food challenge report a general improvement in their social life (Eigenmann *et al.*, 2006). The European Academy for Allergy and Clinical Immunology (EAACI) has suggested using standardised HRQL questionnaires for food allergy (Muraro *et al.*, 2014a).

Prevention

Infants born to families with a history of atopy (i.e. asthma, hay fever, eczema, food allergy) are more at risk of developing allergic diseases than those born to non-atopic families. Having a single family member with a history of allergic disease increased the risk of food allergy in the child 1.4-fold, while having two or more family members with a history of allergic disease increased the risk of food allergy 1.8-fold (Koplin *et al.*, 2015). However, many questions remain regarding the role of the maternal diet during pregnancy and breastfeeding in the development of allergic disease. Nevertheless, significant progress has been made with regards to the impact of complementary foods.

Maternal food intake in pregnancy

Maternal dietary intake has been extensively researched, particularly the effect of dietary exclusion, or the intake of dietary fats, fruit and vegetables, and fatty acids/fatty fish and fish oil supplements during pregnancy and lactation. None of these studies has led to recommendations of dietary changes during pregnancy in order to prevent allergic disease; in fact, concerns have been raised related to unwarranted elimination diets during pregnancy (Kramer & Kakuma, 2006). Current guidelines from EAACI recommend no dietary modification of the maternal diet for allergy prevention (Muraro *et al.*, 2014b).

The supplementation of probiotics during pregnancy has received a lot of attention. Many probiotic strains have been investigated, with *Lactobacillus Rhamnosus GG* yielding the most promising results (Cuello-Garcia *et al.*, 2015). Although the EAACI guidelines 2014 have found no convincing evidence to routinely suggest probiotics during pregnancy for high-risk families (Muraro *et al.*, 2014b), the more recent World Allergy Association (WAO) guidelines suggest recommending probiotics during pregnancy for the prevention of eczema; however, this is based on low-grade evidence (Fiocchi *et al.*, 2015).

Vitamin D

Vitamin D has an important immunomodulatory role (Wjst, 2012). Studies have shown an association between the rise in food allergy and vitamin D deficiency, with associations with atopic dermatitis and recurrent wheeze (Vassallo & Camargo, 2010). The proposed connection between sunshine and vitamin D includes a multiple-hit model, in which vitamin D deficiency in a developmentally critical period leads to the susceptibility of intestinal colonisation with abnormal bacterial flora, contributing to the intestinal barrier function, allowing for increased exposure to allergens. In addition, vitamin D deficiency also contributes to a pro-sensitisation immune imbalance (Vassallo & Camargo, 2010). Supplementation studies have found conflicting results about its preventative effect, with some finding no effect (Chawes *et al.*, 2016), and others finding a reduction in wheeze, such as the VDAART study (Weiss & Litonjua, 2016). A recent systematic review found no convincing evidence to support vitamin D supplementation for the prevention of allergic rhinitis, but did find an association between low vitamin D levels during pregnancy and the development of allergic rhinitis (Kim *et al.*, 2016). The WAO has published guidelines reflecting the aforementioned conflicting views, that there is currently no convincing evidence to supplement routinely with vitamin D for allergy prevention, but that this does not apply to mothers and children who require this owing to proven deficiency or being at risk of deficiency (Yepes-Nunez *et al.*, 2016). The UK Department of Health (DH) guidelines do recommend routine vitamin D supplementation for babies, children and pregnant/breastfeeding mothers (NHS Choices).

Antioxidant intake

High maternal dietary intakes of antioxidants, specifically vitamin E, during pregnancy were associated with a decreased response to allergens, which may influence the foetal immune system and affect the risk of childhood atopy (Devereux *et al.*, 2006). Some data points towards an inverse association for maternal vitamin A and E intake during pregnancy with child allergic rhinitis (Maslova *et al.*, 2014). These studies were all performed looking at current intake and not supplementation.

Vitamin C could also have a pro-oxidant effect, which may have a negative impact on allergy risk. Hoppu *et al.* (2000) found that a low maternal intake of vitamin C, coupled with a high intake of saturated fats during breastfeeding, could increase the risk of infant allergies; however, further studies have not been able to repeat these results (Hoppu *et al.*, 2000). A higher concentration of vitamin C in the breast milk of atopic mothers was associated with a reduced risk of eczema and sensitisation at 12 months; dietary intake rather than supplements determined the concentration of vitamin C in breast milk (Hoppu *et al.*, 2005). However, recent EAACI guidelines found that most studies are of low evidence quality, and therefore do not recommend routine supplementation of antioxidants during pregnancy for allergy prevention (Muraro *et al.*, 2014b).

Breastfeeding and maternal diet while breastfeeding

Gdalevich *et al.* (2001) and Mimouni *et al.* (2002) concluded that exclusive breastfeeding might have some protective effect against the development of atopic diseases, which is greater when there is a family history of atopic disease. However, some studies have found the contrary (Kramer *et al.*, 2007). Limited data exists on the preventative effect of breast milk as compared to formula milk, owing to the ethical constraints of randomisation. However, the benefits of breastfeeding in regard to the infant's immune system and later health are proven, and therefore all current allergy prevention guidelines recommend that the ideal is to breastfeed exclusively for at least 4 months, and ideally for 6 months (Fleischer *et al.*, 2013; Muraro *et al.*, 2014b). No maternal elimination diet during breastfeeding has been recommended by any of the world allergy bodies.

Use of infant formulae

Many studies have been performed using, mainly, partially hydrolysed whey formula, of which the GINI study is the most well-known (von Berg *et al.*, 2013, 2016). These studies have found that certain partially hydrolysed formulas (PHFs) and selected extensively hydrolysed formulas (EHFs) had an impact on the development of atopic disease, and have also proposed a cost benefit (Breitfelder *et al.*, 2011). However, not all studies have found a positive impact; Boyle *et al.* (2016b) found no preventative effect in the use of a PHF with prebiotics. Although Osborn and Sinn (2006) found limited evidence to suggest the use of these formulas for allergy prevention, a recent systematic review found no convincing evidence to support the use of these formulas for allergy prevention (Boyle *et al.*, 2016a). At the time of writing this chapter, guidelines have not changed to reflect this recent systematic review; however, this is expected in the updated guidelines by EAACI and the American Academy of Paediatrics (AAP), which are awaited. Current recommendations are summarised in Table 7.11.3.

Infant weaning practices

The DH recommends that complementary foods be introduced at around 6 months of age, in line with the WHO (2002) recommendations. However, EAACI, ESPGHAN and AAP all recommend that complementary foods for allergy prevention be introduced at 4–6 months of age (Agostoni *et al.*, 2008; Fleischer *et al.*, 2016). In 2015, the LEAP study on the early introduction of peanuts (from 4 months of age) in a high-risk group found compelling evidence to suggest that the early introduction of peanuts significantly reduced the development of peanut allergies. Subsequently, guidelines were adjusted to reflect the early introduction of peanuts in high-risk children (Fleischer *et al.*, 2016). Since then, the EAT study on the early introduction of all major allergens (milk, soya, egg, fish, wheat, peanuts and sesame), in a general population of infants with a background of breastfeeding, found a similar impact on the prevention, particularly, of peanut and egg allergy with early introduction (age of randomisation 13–17 weeks). When looking at the whole EAT population, in the intention-to-treat analysis, 7.1% in the standard introduction group (as DH) versus 6.6% of the early introduction group developed food allergies (Perkin *et al.*, 2016a, 2016b). See Table 7.11.3 for current guidelines.

Introduction of allergenic foods

The European Union (EU) directive (2007) lists 14 foods or food additives identified as being the source of adverse

Table 7.11.3 AAP allergy prevention advice (Fleischer *et al.*, 2013) and EAACI position statement (Muraro *et al.*, 2014b)

	AAP	EAACI
Who is at risk?	One first-degree relative (parent or sibling) with a documented allergic condition	1 or 2 parents and/or siblings with a history of allergic disease
Breastfeeding	Exclusive breastfeeding at least 4 months and up to 6 months	Exclusive breastfeeding 4–6 months
Hydrolysed formula	Hydrolysed formula: EHF may be slightly more beneficial than PHF, but data inconclusive	A documented hypoallergenic formula is recommended as formulas have varying results.
Timing of weaning	At least 4 months old, but exclusive breastfeeding is preferred until 6 months of age	After the age of 4 months
Food introductions	Do not suggest introducing one of the highly allergenic foods as one of the first complementary foods; however, once a few typical complementary foods are tolerated, highly allergenic foods may be introduced. Taken collectively, studies support the general notion that highly allergenic foods may be introduced earlier into the diet – that is, as complementary foods	No withholding or encouraging of exposure to highly allergenic foods such as cow's milk, chicken egg, and peanuts
Other	No other suggestions	No evidence to recommend prebiotics, probiotics or other dietary supplements

food reactions, namely, peanuts, tree nuts, sesame seed, mustard seed, cow's milk, eggs, fish, crustaceans, soya, wheat, celery, lupin, molluscs and sulphites. There is no need to delay the introduction of these foods beyond 6 months (Filipiak *et al.*, 2007; Zutavern *et al.*, 2008). New evidence particularly suggests the active introduction of peanuts from 4 months of age, especially if the infants are at high risk of developing peanut allergy (i.e. atopic eczema and/or egg allergy, and peanut SPT size ≤4 mm). Regarding other allergens, there is no convincing evidence to delay these beyond 6 months of age, and the results from the EAT study suggest that the early introduction of allergenic foods in sufficient amounts alongside breastfeeding may have a preventative impact (Grimshaw *et al.*, 2016). For children who have existing food allergies, no guidelines exist; however, current practice is not to delay food introductions beyond 6 months of age (if not allergic to the food).

Nutritional consequences

Children with FHS may be substantially affected by the removal of one or more food groups due to the requirements of normal growth and development Meyer *et al.* (2014b). Flammarion *et al.* (2011) report that, despite energy, protein and calcium intakes being similar, children with food allergy had weight-for-age and height-for-age z-scores lower than controls. Several studies have since confirmed the results and highlighted a low height-for-age as a particular problem (Meyer *et al.*, 2013, 2016). Vitamin and mineral deficiencies are also commonly described, and, although calcium and vitamin D has received the most focus (Slack *et al.*, 2015; Wang *et al.*, 2014), emerging evidence indicate a variety of possible deficiencies, including iodine deficiency in breastfed infants with cow's milk allergy (Meyer *et al.*, 2014a, 2015; Thomassen *et al.*, 2016).

Adults are most likely to be at nutritional risk if they are avoiding milk or wheat due to confirmed FHS, a self-imposed elimination diet, or multiple foods due to OAS/salicylates/vasoactive amines (Des Roches *et al.*, 2006). Milk avoidance is especially common in patients with asthma based on the false assumption that this causes mucus production (Wuthrich *et al.*, 2005). Such individuals may be at greater risk of poor bone density if calcium intakes are not optimal, especially in those prescribed regular corticosteroids (Kershaw, 2009). Adults newly diagnosed with coeliac disease may present with nutritional deficiencies such as anaemia, vitamin B_{12} or folate, and so should receive a nutritional assessment in order to determine any deficiency (Abenavoli *et al.*, 2015; Garcia-Manzanares & Lucendo, 2011). In eosinophilic oesophagitis, vitamin D has also been identified as being low in adults (Slack *et al.*, 2015).

Diagnosis

Allergy-focused clinical and dietary history

The diagnostic pathway starts with taking an allergy-focused diet and clinical history, followed by appropriate tests, including the gold standard of the oral food challenge (Muraro *et al.*, 2014c). Failure to diagnose FHS, due to negative test results, could risk further potentially severe reactions or ongoing chronic disease. Alternatively, a diagnosis achieved on the basis of positive tests can result in unnecessary restrictions on lifestyle and possible disease from nutrient restriction. A robust diagnostic process is key, given the disparity between reported and diagnosed food allergy. Diagnosis in children is covered by NICE (2011) guidance, and quality standards for the diagnosis of food allergy in children and young people have also been published (NICE, 2016a). The dietitian plays a key role in taking a thorough dietary history to ensure the correct trigger foods are identified, so that an elimination diet or supervised oral food challenge can be utilised to confirm or refute a diagnosis. The algorithm of FHS diagnosis is shown in Figure 7.11.5.

Standardised diet and clinical history tools have been published to ensure that sufficient relevant information is collected and correctly interpreted (Skypala *et al.*, 2015). The following information needs to be elicited, depending on the age of the patient:

- Current daily dietary intake and pattern, including foods currently being eaten or avoided.
- Detailed history of any known food reactions, including what was eaten and length of time between consumption and symptoms.
- Symptom type, speed of onset and whether local or systemic reactions are reported.
- Suspected food triggers and the quantity thought to have elicited a reaction.
- Other known allergies.
- Family history of allergy.
- Likely involvement of cofactors such as exercise, aspirin/NSAIDs, alcohol, etc.
- Regular medications.

This information should then be systematically linked to enable the formation of a working diagnosis, and inform decisions on diagnostic testing, food elimination or food challenge, should this be required (Skypala *et al.*, 2015). Cross-reactions, inaccurate recollection of events, the involvement of multiple foods or the presence of cofactors can confound the clinical history. Diet and symptom diaries may help to identify problem foods, but their efficacy has not been formally assessed. Validated diagnostic questionnaires have shown that the history can be wholly diagnostic for some types of FHS, such as PFS (Skypala *et al.*, 2011).

Diagnostic tests

Skin prick tests

SPTs measure specific IgE antibodies attached to mast cells in the skin and provide an easy method to screen patients of all ages with suspected IgE-mediated food allergy. The skin is pricked through a drop of food extract reagent, and any resultant wheal measured against the results of a positive (histamine) and negative (saline or diluent) control. The positive control indicates skin reactivity, and the negative control identifies patients with

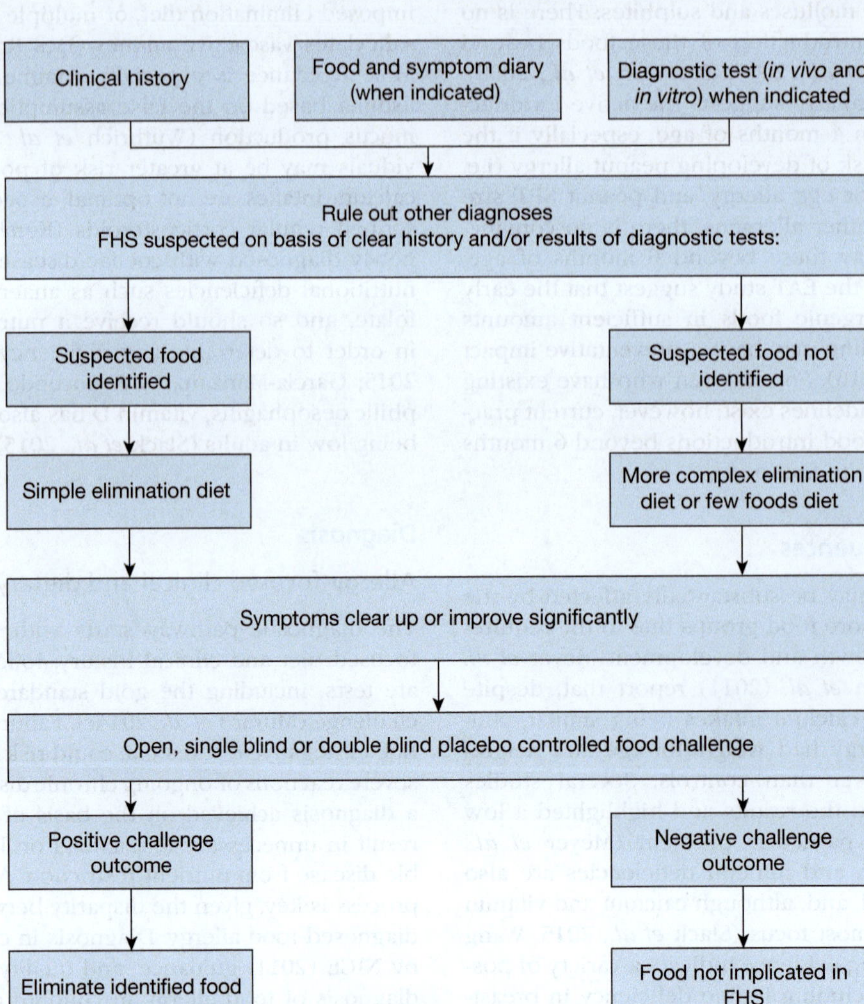

Figure 7.11.5 Algorithm for the diagnosis of food hypersensitivity (FHS) (adapted from Muraro *et al.*, 2004)

dermatographism (skin reactions to any contact, including the prick with a lancet and not necessarily the allergen applied). Allergens eliciting a wheal of ≥3 mm than the negative control are considered positive (Muraro *et al.*, 2014c). However, some recommend the use of a cut-off of 2 mm in children, especially those younger than 6 months. Studies suggest that the average diameter method of measuring SPT wheal diameter gives the best result in clinical practice (van der Valk *et al.*, 2016). SPTs have a negative predictive value of 95% or more (Sampson, 2004), so are useful in ruling out IgE-mediated food allergy. However, negative results should be verified by other tests, especially if severe symptoms have been reported. The predictive value of a positive test is low; only 50–60% of those with positive tests will have a positive oral food challenge (Bock *et al.*, 1988). Thus, a positive test needs to be of a convincing wheal size and linked to a positive clinical history before it can be considered diagnostic.

Most SPTs are undertaken using purified allergen extracts; however, the allergen content can be variable, and thus the sensitivity of SPT for some foods is low (van Kampen *et al.*, 2013; Werfel *et al.*, 2015). Fresh foods can be used in place of reagents, a procedure known as prick-to-prick testing (PPT), and may give a more accurate result (Rancé *et al.*, 1997), even though they lack standardisation.

Specific IgE tests

Specific IgE tests quantify the level of circulating IgE antibodies specific to a particular food. As with SPTs, the presence of specific IgE in the blood indicates sensitisation, but not necessarily clinical allergy. Specific IgE tests are often referred to as radioallergosorbant tests (RASTs), although the technology used now measures fluorescent enzyme-labelled IgE (CAP RAST FEIA), and is usually called an immunoassay. Specific IgE is measured as kilounits of allergen per litre (kUA/L; a test is classed as 'positive' if the result is >0.34 kUA/L. Some laboratories still grade results on a 0–6 scale, where 0 is <0.34 kUA/L. The negative predictive value of immunoassays is similar to those for SPTs, but negative tests need to be interpreted with the history, as undetectable serum food-specific IgE levels might occur in 10–25% of clinical reactions, depending on the food involved (Ives & Hourihane, 2002). In individuals with a very high level of total IgE antibody, measuring the ratio of specific IgE to total IgE may be useful; if the ratio is high, a positive test is more likely to indicate food allergy (Gupta *et al.*, 2014). As with SPT, underrepresentation of minor allergens in the test reagents can lead to false negative reactions (Muraro *et al.*, 2014c).

Both SPT and specific IgE can be used to good effect with clinical history; they have a sensitivity of 70–100%, although the specificity is poor, usually 40–70% (Soares-Weiser *et al.*, 2014), However, there may be a poor correlation between SPT and specific IgE results for the same food in children (Schoos *et al.*, 2015), but closer concordance in adults (Ling *et al.*, 2016). The SPT is often a first-line test due to ease of use, low cost and immediate results. Specific IgE blood tests may be more accessible, especially in primary care, and are useful for patients with severe eczema, dermatographism or who cannot discontinue antihistamines.

Several studies have examined the predictive value of SPT wheal diameters and specific IgE levels, but there is some variance in the results, which appears to suggest that they may be specific to particular populations (Peters *et al.*, 2012). However, it is possible to utilise such predictive values when calculating pre-test probability and likelihood rations to help interpret the results of SPT or specific IgE tests (Roberts *et al.*, 2016).

While SPTs and specific IgE tests are good first-line tests for the diagnosis of IgE-mediated food allergy, they are not useful in the diagnosis of delayed type/non-IgE-mediated food allergy or non-allergic FHS. In addition, many adults have specific IgE antibodies against foods which are tolerated (Burney *et al.*, 2014). Thus, detection of sensitisation alone is insufficient proof of clinical relevance without a supporting clinical history, so it is important not to undertake multiple tests on foods which are currently tolerated by the patient (Werfel *et al.*, 2015).

Diagnosis using individual allergens – component-resolved diagnostics

A major advance in the diagnosis of food allergy has been the sequencing of allergens and allergen epitopes. Food allergens are graded as either class 1 or class 2 allergens. Class 1 allergens are stable to heat, acids and proteases and include casein (milk), vicilins (legumes and nuts), ovomucoid (eggs) and non-specific lipid transfer proteins (plant foods). Class 2 allergens are usually sensitive to heat and enzymatic degradation, which means they cannot sensitise upon ingestion. Many allergens have been sequenced and classified according to the standard nomenclature of the WHO and International Union of Immunological Societies. Some allergens are available as single allergen component tests or as part of a large number of different allergens on a microarray Immuno-Solid-Phase Allergy Chip (ISAC). This technology can determine whether reactions are due to a class 1 or class 2 allergen and ascertain the likelihood of resolution (Matricardi *et al.*, 2016). The seed storage proteins in peanuts (Ara h 2) and hazelnuts (Cor a 14) are markers of primary allergy, whereas mono-sensitisation to the PR10 allergens Ara h 8 and Cor a 1 is indicative of PFS in symptomatic individuals (Asarnoj *et al.*, 2012; Beyer *et al.*, 2015). The wheat allergen omega-5 gliadin is useful for differentiating between wheat allergy and sensitisation to wheat due to cross-reactions to grass pollen (Nilsson *et al.*, 2015; Venter *et al.*, 2016). Milk- and egg-allergic children sensitised to casein in milk (Bos d 8) and ovomucoid in egg (Gal d 1) are less likely to have a resolving allergy, whereas mono-sensitisation to the heat-labile whey (Bos d 4 and Bos d 5) or ovomucin (Gal d 2) allergens seems to indicate tolerance to baked milk and egg and likelihood of resolving disease (Benhamou Senouf *et al.*, 2015; Caubet *et al.*, 2013). Not all studies have found component-resolved diagnostics (CRD) to be superior to standard tests, and CRD cannot replace oral food challenges in most cases (van Veen *et al.*, 2016). Also, studies using microarray technology demonstrate that sensitisation to individual allergens is widespread in populations and can still be positive in asymptomatic individuals, and those who pass oral food challenges make positive test results difficult to interpret (Lopes de Oliveira *et al.*, 2013; Scala *et al.*, 2010). There is insufficient evidence to recommend the routine adoption of microarray testing, but it may be effective for those with difficult-to-diagnose allergies (NICE, 2016a; Westwood *et al.*, 2016).

Atopy patch tests

Atopy patch testing involves food allergens being applied to a healthy area of the patient's skin, and the effects evaluated 48–72 hours later. Patch tests are usually used to determine the cause of delayed allergic reactions such as contact dermatitis, e.g. nickel. Due to the lack of standardised test substances and the lack of studies that demonstrate the advantages of atopy patch test (APT) over SPT or serum IgE, APTs are not recommended for routine diagnosis of food allergy (Turjanmaa *et al.*, 2006).

Other tests

Principal among the commercial tests are those measuring IgG antibodies. This test is not recognised as having any clinical utility in the diagnosis of either food allergy or non-immune-mediated FHS (Boyce *et al.*, 2010; Muraro *et al.*, 2014c). Similarly, other tests, including the leucocyte cytotoxic test, hair analysis, bioresonance diagnostics, auto-homologous immune therapy, kinesiology, iridology, sublingual provocative food testing, homeopathic remedies and electro-dermal testing (including electro-acupuncture and Vega testing), are not valid diagnostic tests for any type of FHS (Muraro *et al.*, 2014c).

Diagnostic exclusion diets

In some patients, the diagnosis is very straightforward, but often the history and standard tests do not give a clear diagnosis; hence, for many patients, diagnosis can only be made by means of diagnostic exclusion diets (Skypala *et al.*, 2015). A successful exclusion diet will improve the symptoms, but they should be for no longer than 2–4 weeks for IgE-mediated symptoms and 6–8 weeks for non-IgE-mediated conditions (Chebar *et al.*, 2015; Muraro *et al.*, 2014c).

Single-food exclusion diet

This excludes all sources of a single food, e.g. milk, as identified from the patient's dietary history.

Multiple-food exclusion diet

This diet excludes a number of foods at the same time, most commonly milk and egg for eczema; milk and soya for non-IgE-mediated gastrointestinal allergies (Hill & Hosking, 2004; Meyer *et al.*, 2013b); or milk, egg, soya and wheat (nuts and fish) for eosinophilic diseases (Kagalwalla *et al.*, 2011). The number and combination of foods avoided will depend on the symptoms and the likelihood of reactions based on available evidence, but can often reflect clinical practices rather than research (Berry *et al.*, 2015; McWilliam *et al.*, 2016). Parents of children and adults with FHS may report reactions to a variety of foods outside of the common food allergens. These need to eliminated based on an allergy-focused history; and, most importantly, reintroduction should occur to confirm any reactions and to avoid unnecessary elimination diets.

Elemental/amino acid and protein hydrolysate formula diets

Elemental or amino acid feeds are, in essence, the same, as both contain pure amino acids as a source of protein. However, the term amino acid formula is most commonly used in the context of infants and young children; elemental feeds are used in older children and adults. The most common reasons for using amino acid feeds in paediatrics are for eosinophilic oesophagitis and for severe multiple-food allergies that do not resolve on a standard elimination diet. However, due to their palatability, many children require a nasogastric tube which may lead to the development of feeding difficulties (Henderson *et al.*, 2012; Mukkada *et al.*, 2011). In adults, these diets are often used in the diagnosis of severe allergic symptoms, or in those suffering from a range of reported food intolerances to establish if food consumption does play a role in their symptoms (Venter *et al.*, 2009).

Oral provocation tests

If symptoms improve, dietary exclusion needs to be followed by the reintroduction of the food either during a supervised oral food challenge or a home reintroduction. Patients with a history of immediate symptoms or a positive SPT/specific IgE test should be challenged in a hospital setting (Sampson *et al.*, 2012). All other patients can undergo food reintroduction at home, but only if there is no risk of immediate severe symptoms (Venter *et al.*, 2009). For non-IgE-mediated cow's milk allergy, the milk ladder approach has gained popularity for home reintroductions (Venter *et al.*, 2013), and the British Society for Allergy and Clinical Immunology (BSACI) has guidelines with home reintroduction protocols for IgE-mediated cow's milk protein allergy (CMPA) (Luyt *et al.*, 2014). The latter should only occur with guidance from a specialist centre and using the exact published protocol.

Careful consideration should be given to deciding which patients should be challenged. This decision should be made based on their allergy test, the impact of the food elimination on their quality of life, the available services, and also the likelihood of the family reintroducing the challenge foods following the hospital challenge (DunnGalvin *et al.*, 2011). What is known is that food challenges, irrespective of positive or negative outcome, has a positive impact on HRQL (van der Velde *et al.*, 2012).

There are three types of food challenges, as discussed in the following subsections.

Open food challenges

There are three types of food challenges, as discussed in the following subsections. Examples of milk challenges for both double-blind and open challenges are shown in Box 7.11.1.

Single-blind placebo-controlled food challenges

The challenge is administered without the patient knowing which dose is active and which is placebo, i.e. the patient is blind but the healthcare professional is not. This type of food challenge is particularly useful when dealing with highly anxious children or adults who have major concerns about ingesting the particular food (Skypala & Venter, 2009).

Double-blind placebo-controlled food challenges

During this challenge, neither the patient nor the investigator knows when the active or placebo challenge is performed. This rules out measurement and reporting bias from the observer and any psychological effect from the patient.

The open food challenge is the challenge of choice in most cases when dealing with adults or children suffering from objective symptoms, e.g. urticaria, angioedema, etc. (Venter *et al.*, 2007). Blinded challenges are preferable when dealing with adults or children reporting subjective symptoms (abdominal pain, nausea, headache) or symptoms that are difficult to assess due to the nature of the disease, e.g. eczema. For research purposes, a double-blind placebo-controlled food challenge (DBPCFC) is still the preferred method of choice (Sampson *et al.*, 2012), as it is considered the gold standard for diagnosing FHS.

Step-wise approach in the planning of a food challenge

History

This should consider the following factors:

- Age and age of onset, which can help determine how difficult it may be to perform the food challenge, and also the possible food causing the symptoms.
- Food type (e.g. raw or cooked egg) and quantity causing symptoms (helps prevent false negative food challenges).
- Symptoms – speed of onset, type, duration and reproducibility of reactions.
- A thorough description of the most recent reaction – helps when designing challenges.
- Cofactors – whether a combination of foods, or the trigger food taken with exercise, alcohol or drugs, is necessary to reproduce the reaction.
- List of tolerated foods – these could be used as a placebo or vehicle to mask the challenge food.
- Factors to consider when planning a challenge.
- In any challenge, the food used should mimic the history as closely as possible.
- Dose and time intervals for immediate symptoms.

The total amount of food given in a challenge is generally based on the normal daily portion of food that is likely to be consumed by the patient, and divided into 5–10 doses of increasing size. Some clinicians prefer to start the challenge with a labial rub of the lip (Rancé & Dutau, 1999); however this is not common practice and not part of the PRACTALL guidelines (Sampson *et al.*, 2012). There is no recommended starting dose, but it should be small enough to minimise the risk of severe reactions (Bindslev-Jensen *et al.*, 2004). The dose may be doubled every 15–20 minutes or increased logarithmically, as guided by the patient's history and as outlined in the PRACTALL guidelines (Sampson *et al.*, 2012). Recent published guidelines on DBPCFC recommend a top blinded dose of 2 g of food protein, although, for some foods such as fish, this may need to be higher (Sampson *et al.*, 2012).

Dose and time intervals for delayed symptoms

Due to the time taken for symptoms to develop, patients with delayed onset of FHS are often advised to undergo a home reintroduction. Limited data exists on home reintroductions, and some studies have used gradually increasing dosages over a reintroduction period of 1–4 weeks until the full daily dose or one that triggers symptoms

Box 7.11.1 Examples of milk challenges for both double-blind and open challenges

PRACTALL – using pasteurised cow's milk (15–20-min intervals) – double blind	BSACI open-challenge protocol using fresh milk or infant formula (15–20-min intervals)	Skypala & Venter, 2009
0.1 mL	1. One drop of cow's milk placed on lower oral mucosa	For adults and children: 100–200 mL of cow's milk to be drunk or 100–200 mL of yoghurt (2 hour observation)
0.3 mL	2. 0.1 mL	
0.9 mL	3. 0.25 mL	
3 mL	4. 0.5 mL	
9.1 mL	5. 1.0 mL	
30.3 mL	6. 2.5 mL	
90.9 mL	7. 5.0 mL	
	8. 10 mL	
	9. 20 mL	
	10. 50 mL	
	11. 100 mL	

PRACTALL, PRACTical ALLergy; BSACI, British Society for Allergy and Clinical Immunology.

has been reached (Majamaa *et al.*, 1999a, 1999b). Dosages have not been standardised, and it is thought that the final dose for a home introduction should reflect the normal intake of that food. This may be 2–3 portions of milk/milk products on one day as per local guidance. Normal daily consumption can be calculated by referring to national diet and nutrition surveys. More detailed information on this is available in Venter *et al.* (2009).

Blinding/masking

When performing a DBPCFC, the challenge food should be sufficiently blinded, so that the active and placebo challenges are identical regarding taste, appearance, smell, viscosity, texture, structure and volume (Bindslev-Jensen *et al.*, 2004; Sampson *et al.*, 2012; Vlieg-Boerstra *et al.*, 2004). For validated recipes suitable for DBPCFC, see Vlieg-Boerstra *et al.* (2004), Palmer *et al.* (2005) and Vassilopoulou *et al.* (2010).

Patient information prior to the food challenge

Patients should be well informed prior to the challenge/reintroduction at home regarding food avoidance, challenge procedure and which medications should not be used. Detailed information regarding this aspect of the food challenge can found in Venter *et al.* (2009) and Ball (2005).

Interpreting food challenge and food reintroduction outcome

During supervised food challenges, the patient should be constantly monitored, and all signs, symptoms and clinical observations should be recorded on a clinical observation chart. During home challenges or food reintroduction at home, patients or their carers should keep a strict food and symptoms diary. Open food challenge/food reintroduction is considered negative in the absence of any subjective or objective clinical reaction. It is recommended that a challenge should be stopped and considered positive if a clear, clinical reaction is shown (Table 7.11.4). In the case of a questionable (subjective) reaction, a repeat dose can be given after waiting an additional 10–20 minutes to see if it elicits a more definitive allergic reaction (Niggemann, 2010).

It is recommended that a challenge be considered positive if severe, reproducible or persisting symptoms are experienced (Niggemann, 2010). In children, a mood change (e.g. becoming very quiet), ear picking, tongue rubbing (e.g. scratching food out of the mouth), or neck scratching are often the precursors of a positive challenge (Table 7.11.5). The results of a food challenge/reintroduction could be falsely negative when diseases such as eczema, chronic urticaria or functional bowel disorders are in remission, or falsely positive when they are active. Allergic reactions to inhalant allergens can also affect the challenge outcome.

For DBPCFCs, the challenge is considered negative if no symptoms are experienced during the active food challenge, or if symptoms are experienced during the placebo phase of the DBPCFC. When symptoms are experienced during both the active and placebo phases of a

Table 7.11.4 Subjective and objective symptoms during food challenge (Niggemann, 2010)

	Possible problems with interpretation
Subjective symptoms	
Nausea	All difficult to interpret due to the subjective nature of the symptoms
Sting/burning of tongue or mouth	
Itching	
Heart palpitations	
Sleeplessness	
Irritability	
Excitement	
General change of behaviour/sense of impending doom	Highly predictive of a positive challenge
Diarrhoea	Could be caused by stress
Abdominal pain and cramps	Could be caused by stress, but also a sign of impending anaphylaxis
Objective symptoms	
Flushing	Difficult to interpret if it subsides very quickly
Urticaria	Could be contact urticaria if only around the mouth; generalised urticaria (in the absence of chronic urticaria) is almost always a sign of a positive challenge
Slight worsening of eczema	Difficult to interpret/could be contact related; however, a scored index increase of >15 points is very indicative of positive reactions – may need to wait 48 hours for assessment
Vomiting	Could be caused by food aversion – may need to ensure that vomiting occurs more than once and is severe in nature for a positive result
Cardiovascular symptoms – especially a drop in blood pressure	Almost always a sign of a positive challenge
Respiratory symptoms	Could be aero-allergen-related/generally uncontrolled symptoms; however, stridor, wheeze, watery rhinitis, redness of eyes and nose, tears are almost always signs of a positive reaction
Dyspnoea/difficulty breathing	Could be aero-allergen related, but is often a sign of a positive challenge

Table 7.11.5 Major and minor criteria for outcome of challenge

Major criteria	Minor criteria
≥3 hives ≥1 site of angio-oedema Wheezing Dyspnoea Stridor Dysphonia Aphonia Severe persistent abdominal symptoms for ≥30 minutes, e.g. abdominal pain/stillness, vomiting, nausea or diarrhoea Hypotension for age	Eczematous pruritic rash (worsening to ≥10 SCORAD points)[a] 1–2 hives ≥1 of sneezing, congestion or rhinorrhoea Conjunctivitis ≥1 of nausea, vomiting or diarrhoea for <20 minutes A change in behaviour, e.g. irritability, drowsiness, decreased activity, anxiety, distress

Positive food challenge: presence of ≥1 major criteria or ≥2 minor criteria; *negative food challenge*: absence of a major or minor criteria; [a]worsening of eczema alone is not a stopping criterion during the challenge – however, if a worsening of eczema to >10 SCORAD points is observed at the end of the active arm of the DBPCFC with no worsening of eczema with the placebo challenge, the diagnosis of cow's milk allergy will be given; SCORAD: SCORing Atopic Dermatitis.

DBPCFC, the challenge needs to be repeated. Symptoms developing only during the active phase of the challenges indicates a positive food challenge (Ahrens *et al.*, 2014; Niggemann, 2010). The PRACTALL guidelines have got a useful scoring system to assess challenge outcomes, which may be useful in dietetic practice (Sampson *et al.*, 2012).

Management strategies

Once the challenge and reintroduction of food is completed, sufficient aftercare should be provided for the patient or their carers to ensure the following:

- After a positive challenge: the allergenic food is avoided (dietetic advice important), emergency medication is prescribed if needed, and appropriate training is given to administer the medication.
- After a negative challenge: the challenge food is reintroduced into the diet and regularly consumed in order to prevent any nutritional deficiencies or resensitisation.

In some cases, i.e. some primary care settings, these tests may not be available, or it may take a long time to obtain results. However, the history could give a good indication of the type and time of onset of symptoms, which should assist healthcare professionals to decide if symptoms are IgE- or non-IgE-mediated reactions, taking into account that eczema could initially present with delayed symptoms (Flinterman *et al.*, 2006; Skypala *et al.*, 2015), and then may turn into a presentation of immediate, more severe symptoms.

Dietary management

At present, the only means of treatment is avoidance of the problem food, although a number of studies have examined the efficacy of food-specific immunotherapy. This technique promotes tolerance to a food through the administration of daily oral doses of the food in increasing amounts until a maintenance dose is reached. It has been successfully used to treat some common food allergies, but cannot yet be recommended in routine practice (Fisher *et al.*, 2011).

Dietary avoidance issues

The dietary management of food hypersensitivity can be complex; unexpected ingredients are often present in a wide range of manufactured foods, and there may be poor comprehension of the dietary requirement and adherence issues. The restriction of food choices can increase the risk of overall dietary imbalance, especially if the problem food is a major contributor to nutrient intake. Dietetic support is required to advice on dietary adequacy, food shopping, eating at school/workplace, socialising and eating out, and holidays (Venter & Meyer, 2010). All children and adults with moderate to severe food allergy should also have an action plan for dietary management and drug prophylaxis (Clark & Ewan, 2008).

The patient's tolerance level or degree of avoidance required will mainly be determined by the type of FHS the patient is suffering from. Most people with IgE-mediated food allergy need to completely avoid a trigger food, even in trace amounts. However, there is evidence in both IgE-mediated milk and egg allergy that a cohort of children will tolerate baked milk/egg, and that the introduction of these foods assist in tolerance induction (Kim *et al.*, 2011; Leonard *et al.*, 2015). People with non-IgE-mediated allergy or non-immune-mediated FHS may be able to include small amounts of the food in their diet with no adverse effects. It is currently unknown whether allowing patients to eat small amounts of the trigger food (if tolerated) on a regular basis has an adverse effect on the development of tolerance, or conversely induces further tolerance. Some patients will already be aware of their own tolerance levels. The non-IgE-mediated milk ladder, now commonly used in the UK, is based on the principle that heating and processing reduce allergenicity, and finding the level of tolerance of patients with this delayed allergy (Venter *et al.*, 2013).

From a nutritional perspective, avoidance of a single food (e.g. fruit) will be of little significance if nutritionally similar foods (e.g. other fruit and vegetables) can be eaten instead. However, if food avoidance necessitates excluding a major food group (i.e. milk), the nutritional impact will be considerable. Even if the food being excluded is not in itself nutritionally significant, it may be widely present in manufactured foods, resulting in a subsequent effect on the overall dietary balance. Patients who exclude other foods because of, e.g. cultural reasons (e.g. excluding nuts and milk in a vegetarian), or because they are fussy eaters, will also need special consideration if their usual staple foods are being excluded.

Some types of FHS resolve over time; both milk and egg allergies commonly remit in most people by the teenage years (Santos *et al.*, 2010). Some forms of non-allergic FHS in adults may be transient, such as secondary lactose intolerance. The necessity for dietary exclusion should be reviewed at intervals, so that dietary restrictions are not imposed for longer than necessary, since they have a major impact on diet and lifestyle.

Food labelling

European food labelling law

Labelling of food allergens is controlled by European Directives 2003/89/EC and 2006/142/EC (European Commission Directives, 2003, 2006), which require all packaged foods to contain comprehensive ingredient listing information. The law requires 14 foods to be labelled if present in the product. Following the implementation of the EU Food Information for Consumers Regulation (EU FIC) No. 1169/2011 in 2014, allergen information must also be provided for non-packed foods, including those sold in food outlets and restaurants (EU, 2011) (see Chapter 4.5, Food law and labelling).

If the product contains one of 14 allergens on the list, it must be emphasised on the label. For example, if the product contains some form of milk, the ingredients list on packaged foods must state 'milk' in bold, even if the actual ingredient is a milk derivative such as casein or whey. Product labels are no longer allowed to have allergen warning labels; the allergen must be present in the ingredients list. Vendors of foods sold in restaurants and other food outlets have to comply with the new regulation by providing consumers with information about whether any of the 14 allergens are present in their foods. The most usual method is to provide an allergy menu that lists the ingredients of each meal and the allergen content. The 14 allergens and the products thereof required by law to be listed on all prepacked and non-packaged foods are:

1. Cereals containing gluten, i.e. wheat, rye, barley, oats, spelt, kamut or their hybridised strains, and products thereof.
2. Crustaceans.
3. Molluscs.
4. Eggs.
5. Fish.
6. Peanuts.
7. Soya beans.
8. Lupin.
9. Milk, including lactose.
10. Nuts, i.e. almond (*Amygdalus communis L.*), hazelnut (*Corylus avellana*), walnut (*Juglans regia*), cashew (*Anacardium occidentale*), pecan (*Carya illinoinensis (Wangenh.) K. Koch*), Brazil nut (*Bertholletia excelsa*), pistachio (*Pistacia vera*), macadamia nut (Queensland nut) (*Macadamia ternifolia*).
11. Celery.
12. Mustard.
13. Sesame seeds.
14. Sulphur dioxide and sulphites at concentrations of >10 mg/kg or 10 mg/L, expressed as SO_2.

The European Food Safety Authority publishes detailed information on food allergen labelling. In the UK, the full directives are available from the Food Standards Agency.

May contain labelling

If an added ingredient in a product is purposeful, even if it is in a trace amount, it has to be listed in the ingredients list. However, there is no legal requirement to state on the label that a food might contain accidental traces of a food from the production process. However, many manufacturers choose to label their products with 'may contain' warnings, to warn consumers about the possibility of accidental traces of another food in a manufactured product. The change in legislation in 2014 still permitted the use of may contain statements on labels, although the value of such information is questionable, and research has shown that allergen levels in products with label warnings are very variable (Remington *et al.*, 2015; Robertson *et al.*, 2013). Where labels carry a 'may contain' warning, patients should be advised to still check the full ingredients listing.

Major food triggers

Milk

Cows' milk is a leading cause of food allergy, especially in infants and children. The recent EuroPrevall data showed that the prevalence of cow's milk allergy Europe-wide was <1% (Schoemaker *et al.*, 2015). From this cohort, the UK had one of the highest incidence rates at 1.28%. However, several researchers have highlighted concerns that the study design may not have adequately identified non-IgE-mediated CMPA (Katz *et al.*, 2015; Koletzko *et al.*, 2015). A UK birth cohort study has shown that 2–3% of 1–3-year-olds can be confirmed as having a CMPA, but this still does not adequately reflect the prevalence of non-IgE-mediated CMPA. The prognosis of cow's milk allergy is good; although the age of tolerance seems to shift to later childhood, about 90% of children will grow out of milk allergy by adulthood (Bishop *et al.*, 1990; Santos *et al.*, 2010; Skripak *et al.*, 2007). IgE-mediated milk allergy in adults is rare, and most adults who report symptoms to milk will not usually have specific IgE antibodies to milk (Zuberbier *et al.*, 2004).

IgE-mediated CMPA

IgE-mediated CMPA is characterised by acute-onset and rapid-onset symptoms, as described in Table 7.11.2. These reactions are commonly associated with a family history of atopy, and usually develop early in infancy soon after exposure to cow's milk in the form of infant formula (Fiocchi *et al.*, 2010; Host & Halken, 1990), or during early weaning with dairy foods. Symptoms can occasionally present in an exclusively breastfed infant because the mother is consuming cow's milk (or derivatives) in her diet and the protein fractions pass through the breast milk, causing symptoms in the infant. To determine whether this is the case, a maternal elimination diet for 2–4 weeks is suggested. If the symptoms resolve, then this diet should be adhered to for the duration of breastfeeding, and the dietitian needs to ensure dietary adequacy of the mother's diet (i.e. calcium and vitamin D). There are several formulae available for infants who cannot tolerate whole cow's milk protein or lactose, and a dietitian should advise on the most suitable choice, as shown in Table 7.11.6.

Non-IgE-mediated CMPA

Non-IgE-mediated cow's milk allergy is characterised by a delayed reaction following cow's milk protein ingestion. Symptoms typically occur within a few hours, and sometimes after 2–3 days, and often include eczema, reflux, abdominal pains, constipation, diarrhoea, and flatus (Heine, 2015).

Non-immune-mediated cow's milk hypersensitivity

The most common form of non-immune reactions to cow's milk is to the milk sugar lactose. Lactose intolerance results from an impaired ability to either absorb lactose or its component monosaccharides, resulting in symptoms of malabsorption. If lactose needs to be excluded, food avoidance measures are similar to those for exclusion of cow's milk protein (Ingram *et al.*, 2009), but low-lactose cow's milk products can often be included, which is not the case for CMPA. Some foods are naturally very low in lactose, whereas others are manufactured specifically for this purpose. The presentation of non-IgE-mediated gastrointestinal allergies often overlaps with symptoms of lactose intolerance. It is therefore important to establish the diagnosis correctly (De Koker *et al.*, 2014), since, in a small cohort of children with gut inflammation related to cow's milk, a secondary lactose intolerance may be present as a result of brush border damage. The management of lactose intolerance is discussed in more detail in Chapter 7.4.6 (Malabsorption).

Congenital disorders of monosaccharide metabolism

Details of these disorders can be found in Chapter 3.8.6 (Autism) and Chapter 7.8 (Inherited metabolic disorders in adults).

Guidance when choosing a formula milk

The choice of formula milk will depend on the presenting symptoms (IgE versus non-IgE and severity), tolerance of breast milk (as ß-lactoglobulin in breast milk is similar to that of EHF), infant's requirements, taste preference, clinician experience and many other clinical and non-clinical factors (Chebar *et al.*, 2015; Host & Halken, 2004). In the last 10 years, 11 guidelines have been published worldwide in the English language on the diagnosis and management of CMPA (Caffarelli *et al.*, 2010; De Greef *et al.*, 2012; Fiocchi *et al.*, 2010; Kemp *et al.*, 2008; Vandenplas *et al.*, 2007). The UK guidelines are the milk allergy guidelines for primary care (iMAP) (Venter *et al.*, 2017), the BSACI guidelines for secondary and tertiary care (Luyt *et al.*, 2014), and the NICE (2014) guidelines. All guidelines agree that a hypoallergenic formula should have <1% immunoreactive protein on in vitro testing, and should be tolerated by 90% of children with a CMPA (with a 95% confidence interval) (Host *et al.*, 1999). In principle, the guidelines indicate that, for the majority of children with mild to moderate IgE-mediated/non-IgE-mediated CMPA, an EHF is appropriate; however, if they have anaphylaxis, eosinophilic oesophagitis, faltering growth (particularly with multiple foods eliminated), and severe symptoms, an amino acid formula (AAF) is indicated (Meyer *et al.*, 2017). In addition, if an EHF does not lead to symptom improvement, the trial of an AAF

Table 7.11.6 Nutritionally complete milk substitutes for use in cow's milk hypersensitivity

Type of milk hypersensitivity	Product type[a]	Product name (manufacturer)
Used for IgE-mediated and non-IgE-mediated cow's milk allergy	Soya based[b] Do not use before 6 months unless no other choice, e.g. vegan or refusal of all other suitable formula	Infasoy (Cow & Gate) Wysoy (SMA)
	Casein-based hydrolysed cow's milk	Nutramigen Lipil 1 and 2 (MJN) Pregestimil (with MCT oils) (MJN)
	Whey-based hydrolysed cow's milk	Pepti Junior (Cow & Gate) Pepti 1 and 2 (Aptamil)
	Amino acid	Neocate LCP (SHS) Neocate Advance and Neocate Active if over 12 months (SHS) Nutramigen AA (MJN)
Lactose intolerance only (*Note*: Some of these products may also be suitable for lactose intolerance; check prescribing indications.)	Usually contain whole cow's milk protein	Enfamil Lactofree (MJN) SMA LF (SMA)

MCT, medium-chain triglyceride.

[a]The choice of product depends on the age of the child, the level of sensitivity to milk and the presence of coexisting allergies. Check compositional details and prescribing indications for suitability. Choice may also be dictated by the infant's palate.

[b]Infants under the age of 6 months should not use a soya formula as the first choice due to their phyto-oestrogen content and the risk of becoming sensitised to soya. It can be used if other formulae are either not suitable, not acceptable or not tolerated by the infant, or if the mother is vegan. See www.bda.uk.com for the BDA Paediatric Group Position Statement on the use of soya protein for infants. Further details of products currently available and their prescribing indications can be found in the *British National Formulary* (BNF) or the *Monthly Index of Medical Specialities* (MIMS), or obtained directly from the manufacturers. Further information for dietitians is also available in the *Special Foods for Children* booklet compiled by the Dietetic Department, Children's Hospital, Birmingham, UK.

is warranted (Luyt *et al.*, 2014; Venter *et al.*, 2013). All current guidelines recommend continuing with hypoallergenic formulas until 2 years of age, unless they have a nutritional review after 1 year of age, and their diet is deemed nutritionally adequate.

Milk from goats, sheep and other mammals should not be used as an alternative to cow's milk, owing to the high degree of cross-reactivity resulting in poor tolerance (Fiocchi *et al.*, 2010). Over-the-counter milk alternatives made from soya, rice, hemp, potato nut, coconut, pea or oat are not recommended for infants under 1 year of age; even after 1 year of age, the introduction of these alternatives requires a nutritional review, as they are generally much lower in energy and protein.

Due to inorganic arsenic being a natural component of rice milks, they are not recommended for children younger than 4.5 years (FSA, 2009; Meharg *et al.*, 2008a, 2008b). When they are used, daily intake should not exceed 200 mL; these plant-based milks should be enriched with calcium, and attention should also be given to iodine content, both of which are generally low in these plant-based milks (Bath *et al.*, 2017). Products based on soya can be used after 6 months of age; these include soya yogurts, deserts, cream cheeses, hard cheeses and cream. Once solid food is introduced, care must be taken that intake remains free of cow's milk protein, not only from obvious sources such as dairy products but also from its less obvious presence in many manufactured foods. The BDA Food Allergy Specialist Group produces diet sheets with infant formulas and foods to avoid.

If a child passes a milk challenge but then refuses milk and dairy foods due to anxiety or dislike, parents will need guidance on ways to incorporate hidden milk into the diet, such as in rice pudding, white sauce, scones, creamy soups, risotto, etc. In the rare cases where milk allergy persists into adulthood, a permanent exclusion of cow's milk is necessary.

Peanuts and tree nuts

Peanuts and tree nuts are a common cause of severe IgE-mediated reactions. Between 1999 and 2006, 18 of the 44 deaths from food allergy were caused by tree nuts or peanuts (Pumphrey & Gowland, 2007). A review of emergency room visits by food-allergic individuals found that 50% had a peanut or tree nut allergy, and these foods were more frequently associated with adrenaline treatment and hospitalisation than other foods (Johnson *et al.*, 2014). Peanuts and tree nuts, along with egg, fruit/vegetables and milk, were the main cause of severe reactions and even fatalities (Versluis *et al.*, 2015). Peanut and tree nut allergies most often start in childhood, with the average age for peanut allergies being 18 months, although both can also present in later childhood or in adults, either as a primary allergy or as PFS (Savage *et al.*, 2007; Skypala *et al.*, 2011; Vereda *et al.*, 2011). Peanut and tree nut allergy are less likely to resolve; early studies reported that over 90% of tree-nut-allergic and 80% of peanut-allergic children remained sensitised and symptomatic into their adult years (Fleischer *et al.*, 2005; Skolnick *et al.*, 2001). More recent studies found that up to 39% of children had resolving peanut or tree nut allergy, usually acquiring tolerance by the age of 8 years, with symptom severity and higher specific IgE levels associated with persisting allergy (Bégin *et al.*, 2013; Neuman-Sunshine *et al.*, 2012; Peters *et al.*, 2015; Wainstein & Saad, 2015). The worldwide prevalence ranges from 1.4 to 5%, but, in UK children, the cumulative prevalence of peanut allergy is 0.7–1.4%, with no significant differences in the level of peanut allergy between 1989 and 2001 (Grimshaw *et al.*, 2016; Savage *et al.*, 2016; Venter *et al.*, 2016). In US adults, the doctor-diagnosed prevalence of peanut allergy was 0.3%, whereas 1.5% of adults reported reactions to peanuts in the UK, 0.2% of which was due to PFS (Skypala *et al.*, 2013; Vierk *et al.*, 2007).

The way peanuts are prepared can affect their allergenicity; roasting may increase the IgE reactivity of peanuts, while boiling results in loss of proteins; particularly the main sensitising allergens Ara h 2 and 6 (Beyer *et al.*, 2001; Turner *et al.*, 2014). Peanuts have similar allergen epitopes as tree nuts, especially hazelnut, Brazil nut, almond, as well as some seeds (de Leon *et al.*, 2003). Peanut-allergic individuals have a 25–40% risk of developing a co-allergy to tree nuts (Bock *et al.*, 2007; Sicherer *et al.*, 2000). A systematic review reported that challenge-confirmed IgE-mediated tree nut allergy prevalence was less than 2%, whereas probable tree nut allergy prevalence ranged from 0.05 to 4.9%; if PFS reactions to nuts were included, this rose again to 8–11.4%. (McWilliam *et al.*, 2015). Hazelnut is the dominant tree nut allergy in Europe, with Brazil nut, almond and walnut more prevalent in the UK (Ewan, 1996; McWilliam *et al.*, 2015). Walnut and cashew are the main allergenic nuts in the USA, and cashew nut allergy also predominates in Australia (Hill *et al.*, 1997; Sicherer *et al.*, 2010). Cashew nut allergy can cause severe reactions (Davoren & Peake, 2005); children with a cashew nut allergy were more likely to experience anaphylaxis than case-matched children with a peanut allergy (Clark *et al.*, 2007). As with peanuts, roasting changes the allergenicity of hazelnuts due to its effects on Cor a 1, and the same may be true for almonds (Masthoff *et al.*, 2013). This may enable those with PFS to tolerate roasted tree nuts, whereas those with a tree nut allergy cannot tolerate raw or roasted nuts.

Peanuts and tree nuts are the most frequent cause of systemic reactions on SPT, and so individuals with reported severe reactions should have serum-specific IgE testing (Sellaturay *et al.*, 2015). It is known that many with peanut allergy will be co-sensitised to tree nuts and vice versa, but only one-third of peanut-allergic individuals will be allergic to one or more tree nuts (Pumphrey *et al.*, 1999; Sampson *et al.*, 2014). Previously, peanut- and tree-nut-allergic individuals were usually advised to avoid all nuts, not only due to co-sensitisation but also because of the risk of contamination and difficulties in identifying individual nuts (Ferdman & Church, 2006). However, it is now recommended that, for peanut-allergic individuals, age, risk of cross-contamination, and implications of dietary restrictions should be considered when advising whether avoidance of tree nuts is also necessary (Lomas & Järvinen, 2015). Best practice should be to give patients advice on avoidance based on oral food challenges (Eigenmann *et al.*, 2017). It is also important to make individual risk assessments; severe reactions are significantly more frequent in teenagers and adults, asthmatic patients and those who react to inhalation (Deschildre *et al.*, 2016). If PFS is suspected, then component testing is useful, since those with PFS to one nut often tolerate other nuts and do not need to avoid those foods that state 'may contain nuts' (Skypala *et al.*, 2011).

Avoidance can be problematic, with many manufactured food products containing peanuts, nuts or derivatives (see the earlier section 'European food labelling law'). Although the labelling laws now make it clear whether the ingredients contain nuts, advisory labelling is difficult to interpret, especially as there are a variety of terminologies used (Noimark *et al.*, 2009; Pieretti *et al.*, 2009). The BDA Food Allergy Specialist Group produces diet sheets on nut allergy. Nut-allergic individuals often rely on their previous experience of food consumption and the knowledge they have developed of the brand, the provider and the country of origin (Barnett *et al.*, 2013). Anxiety in peanut-allergic individuals is associated with strict avoidance; however, one study found that both labelled and unlabelled products contained significant amounts of unintended allergen contamination, whereas another reported that many food products bearing advisory nut statements were free of peanut contamination (Deschildre *et al.*, 2016; Remington *et al.*, 2015; Robertson *et al.*, 2013).

Peanuts can sensitise via inhalation and the skin, as well as orally. It has been demonstrated that exposure to peanut antigen in household dust through an impaired skin barrier, such as in eczema, could lead to peanut sensitisation and peanut allergy (Brough *et al.*, 2013, 2015). Peanut allergens persist on hands and in saliva for several hours after consumption, and cannot easily be removed from household surfaces, even after detergent cleaning (Brough *et al.*, 2013). It has been estimated that 5–12% of accidental exposures causing reactions are due to kissing, possibly due to the longevity of some of the allergens involved (Eriksson *et al.*, 2003). In one study, the annual rate of reactions to peanuts after diagnosis was 4.7%, of which 1.6% were severe, although the severity of the reactions did not increase or decrease with repeated exposure (Neuman-Sunshine *et al.*, 2012). These data demonstrate why adrenaline (epinephrine) is often prescribed for nut-allergic individuals, and thus a good management plan giving information on how and when to use it is of paramount importance (Anagnostou & Clark, 2016). Peanut allergy sufferers have a greater risk of accidental exposure; 54% of recorded anaphylaxis fatalities between 1999 and 2006 occurred when eating restaurant or takeaway food (Pumphrey & Gowland, 2007). Thai, Indonesian, Asian and Chinese cuisines use peanuts and other nuts regularly in dishes. Chefs may add or change ingredients on an ad hoc basis, although the change in labelling law now requires all food establishments to state whether peanuts or tree nuts have been added to a dish deliberately.

Refined peanut oil is not considered to be allergenic (Hourihane *et al.*, 1997), but other nut oils (e.g. walnut, hazelnut, almond, and unrefined or cold-pressed peanut oil) may contain traces of allergens and should be avoided. Unrefined peanut oil is most likely to be used in Thai, Chinese, Indonesian or Indian cuisine; other nut oils may be used in salad dressings or garnishes.

Travelling can be problematic with a peanut or tree nut allergy. Many airlines have stopped serving peanuts due to concerns about airborne peanut particles, but this is not universal. Few studies on peanut exposure on flights are available, but one found that 9% of adults with a severe nut or seed allergy experienced an allergic reaction to food while on board an airplane (Comstock *et al.*, 2008). Another study concluded that there was a need for airline policy regarding allergy to be declared, and that it is also important to quantify the true risks of airborne allergens in the cabin (Barnett *et al.*, 2012). Translation sheets for restaurants abroad, which give details of the problem, are useful as a list of food ingredients to look out for when travelling. Some brands of products that are nut free in the UK may not be nut free when produced and purchased in other countries (even if they have the same brand name), e.g. some infant formulae or vitamin D preparations may contain peanuts. Measures such as learning the word for 'peanuts' or 'nuts' in the relevant language, wearing medic alert identification and always carrying rescue medication are strongly recommended. Support groups, such as the Anaphylaxis Campaign and Allergy UK, can provide useful advice on all of these issues.

Soya and other legumes

A recent systematic review identified 40 suitable studies on soya allergy prevalence. From these studies, a prevalence of 0–0.5% (0.27) was found for the general population, 0.4–3.1% (1.9) for patients referred for this allergy, and 0–12.9% (2.7) for allergic children (Katz *et al.*, 2014). Soya allergy is usually a transient allergy of infancy and childhood (Sicherer *et al.*, 2000). Savage *et al.* (2010) reported that 50% of the studied population had a resolution of their soya allergy by the age of 7 years (Savage *et al.*, 2010). The prevalence of concomitant soy allergy in infants with cow's milk allergy differs significantly between IgE-mediated and non-IgE-mediated allergy. Klemola *et al.* (2005) and Zeiger *et al.* (1999) found that 10% and 14% of infants with IgE-mediated CMPA, respectively, have concomitant soy allergy, whereas associated soy allergy in non-IgE-mediated CMPA is much higher (up to 60%), especially in enterocolitis/enteropathy syndromes.

Soya allergy most commonly manifests in older children and adults due to cross-reactions between homologous epitopes in soya beans and birch pollen provoking reactions, which may be severe (Kleine-Tebbe *et al.*, 2002; Mittag *et al.*, 2004). It is possible that up to

30% of adults with a peanut allergy have cross-reactivity to other legumes (Ballmer-Weber *et al.*, 2007), although this sensitisation may not be clinically relevant. Although old data indicated an association between peanut and soya allergy in children (Lack *et al.*, 2003), newer data has not found a strong association between soya and peanut allergy (Tewari *et al.*, 2006).

Soya beans are ubiquitous, especially in processed foods, and are commonly used as a binding agent, meat extender or replacement for meat in vegetarian dishes. Refined soya bean oil and soya lecithin (E322) are safe for soya-allergic patients to consume, although case reports suggest that some individuals may still react to soya lecithin (Awazuhara *et al.*, 1998; Taylor & Baumert, 2017; Gu *et al.*, 2001). The allergen associated with PFS reactions, Gly m 4, is unlikely to be present in products derived from roasted soya beans or highly fermented products such as miso or soya sauce, but is found in soya milk and dietary powders such as body building powders (Mittag *et al.*, 2004). Soya sauce is a highly fermented product containing high levels of histamine and can provoke oral symptoms in some people (Sugiura & Sugiura, 2010). The BDA Food Allergy Specialist Group produces diet sheets on soya allergy.

Allergy to other legumes, such as chickpeas and lentils, has not been extensively studied in the UK, although they are a significant issue in India and Spain (Kumar *et al.*, 2010; Martinez *et al.*, 2008). Lupin is another legume not permitted for use in the UK, but it can be found in gluten-free products and also in products containing wheat flour from other continental countries. Allergy to lupin has been reported (Peeters *et al.*, 2007, 2009), but the prevalence is low. Among those patients referred to specialist allergy services, the estimated prevalence of actual lupin allergy was only 0.3–0.8% (de Jong *et al.*, 2010).

Seeds

Sesame is the most prevalent seed allergy worldwide, being an important cause of anaphylaxis in Israel and Saudi Arabia (Patel & Bhana, 2016). Sesame allergy usually presents in the first 2 years of life and only remits in about 20% of cases (Cohen *et al.*, 2007). Diagnosis can be difficult; negative SPT and specific IgE can occur, possibly due to the removal of the allergenic lipid fraction (oleosins) during processing (Barbarroja-Escudero *et al.*, 2015). A study from the Netherlands identified oleosin as the major sesame allergen in those who had experienced anaphylaxis to sesame, but it was not a relevant allergen in milder oropharyngeal reactions (Teodorowicz *et al.*, 2016). Thus, a PPT with sesame seed paste (tahini) or sesame oil may be useful in those with a strong history but negative tests, especially as they could develop severe symptoms on oral challenge with sesame (Della-Torre *et al.*, 2013).

The sesame allergen Ses i 3 has an 80% homology with the peanut allergen Ara h 1, and also cross-reacts with tree nuts, poppy seeds, kiwi and rye (Gangur *et al.*, 2005; Vocks *et al.*, 1993). Sensitisation to sesame has been linked to a high prevalence of sensitisation to tree nuts; children reacting to both peanuts and tree nuts are more likely to be clinically allergic to sesame (Stutius *et al.*, 2010). However, sensitisation to the sesame oleosins does not appear to involve clinical cross-reactivity to peanuts and tree nuts (Teodorowicz *et al.*, 2016). There is no need for sesame-allergic individuals to avoid cross-reacting foods unless clinically indicated. Sesame and its derivatives can often be present under a variety of different names, as shown in Table 7.11.7. Sesame is a common ingredient in vegetarian dishes, and also in Thai, Indonesian, Japanese, Chinese, Middle Eastern, Greek and Turkish food. Sesame-allergic patients also need to avoid sesame oil, which has been reported to cause anaphylaxis in very small amounts (Alonzi *et al.*, 2011). The refined sesame oil found in pharmaceutical products and cosmetics (*Sesamum indicum*) is generally non-allergic, although delayed reactions to sesame oil in medications have been observed (Kelso, 2014; Phy *et al.*, 2003).

Table 7.11.7 Sesame products

Alternative names	Foods containing sesame		Dishes containing sesame
Ajonjoli	Falafel	Halva	Baba ghanoush
Benne/benne seed	Burger buns	Hummus	Banh ran
Gomasio	Bread sticks	Tahini	Dim sum
Gingelly	Pastries	Salad dressing	Gevrek
Sesamum indicum	Pretzels	Soups	Giuggiuleni
Sim sim	Bagels	Sauces	Goma-dofu
Oleum	Biscuits	Noodles	Gomashio
Teel	Rice cakes	Samosa	Khao phan
Till	Crackers	Dips	Milagi podi
	Sandwiches	Aqua Libra	Til pitha
	Crackers	Muesli bars	Tilor laru

Allergy to other seeds is less common; only a few cases of allergy to sunflower and pumpkin seeds have been reported (Patel & Bhana, 2016). The only other significant seed allergy involves mustard seed, reported to be a common allergen affecting French children (Mailhol *et al.*, 2014). Mustard can cross-react with mugwort pollen and so can cause PFS, but it can also cause anaphylaxis (Patel & Bhana, 2016). Mustard is a common ingredient in many preprepared foods and should be considered if there are multiple reactions to unrelated foods (Añíbarro *et al.*, 2007).

Fish and shellfish

Seafood is a common cause of emergency hospital visits and is linked to fatal anaphylaxis (Pumphrey, 2000). The prevalence of seafood allergy in Europe has been estimated to be 0.1–0.3% for fish and 0.1–0.9% for shellfish

(Moonesinghe *et al.*, 2016; Nwaru *et al.*, 2014). Fish allergy is more prevalent in children, whereas allergy to shellfish is more common in adults (Worm *et al.*, 2016). Reactions usually involve IgE-mediated mechanisms, but fish is also a known trigger of food protein–induced enterocolitis syndrome (FPIES), and shellfish is thought to cause a similar type of delayed non-IgE-mediated food allergy in adults (González-Delgardo *et al.*, 2016; Tan & Smith, 2014). Seafood allergy is thought to be lifelong (Daul *et al.*, 1990), although there have been no large studies on resolution.

Seafood contains highly cross-reactive allergens that cause sensitisation or symptoms through consumption, but also through inhalation due to aerosolisation during cooking (James & Crespo, 2007). Beta parvalbumin is the dominant allergen in finned fish (Hansen *et al.*, 1997). Cod is an allergenic fish because it contains a high level of β parvalbumin, whereas large migratory fish such as tuna and swordfish contain very low levels, so are less likely to provoke allergic symptoms (Kobayashi *et al.*, 2016). In one study, reactions were most frequently reported to cod and herring, whereas hake and swordfish were the least likely to cause reactions (Schulkes *et al.*, 2014). Allergy to tropical fish may involve other allergens such as enolases and aldolases when sensitisation to parvalbumin is absent (Kuehn *et al.*, 2013). Crustaceans (shrimp/prawn, lobster, crab, crayfish) and molluscs (mussels, clams, oysters, scallops, octopus, squid) also share a common allergenic protein called invertebrate tropomyosin, additionally found in cockroach, snails, house dust mite and the fish parasite *Anisakis* (Ayuso *et al.*, 2002; Reese *et al.*, 1999). Despite this, cross-reactivity between crustaceans and molluscs is low, and reported reactions to shellfish are most often to crustaceans rather than molluscs (Khan *et al.*, 2011; Lopata & Lehrer, 2009). Other shellfish allergens include arginine kinase, myosin light chain and sarcoplasmic binding protein, and these may be linked to clinical reactivity in subjects with a positive oral food challenge (Giuffrida *et al.*, 2014). The presence of pan allergens means reactions may occur to more than one type of fish or shellfish, but cross-reactivity between shellfish and vertebrate fish does not occur, although some people do report reactions to both types of seafood (Chapman *et al.*, 2006). For diagnosis, SPTs and specific IgE blood tests have good sensitivity and specificity, but if negative despite a well-taken history, then prick testing and oral food challenge with the suspected seafood is indicated (Schulkes *et al.*, 2014; Thalayasingam *et al.*, 2014). Fish allergens may be denatured sufficiently in canned fish, but most fish-allergic individuals will not tolerate fish cooked under normal conditions (Bernhisel-Broadbent *et al.*, 1992). In contrast, allergens from shellfish, which include crustaceans and molluscs, remain potent allergens after cooking. Lehrer *et al.* (2007) demonstrated shrimp allergenic activity in oil used to cook shrimp.

Most seafood is an obvious component of a meal; less obvious sources can include fish stock, Worcestershire sauce, caviar, aspic, buffet food, Asian cuisine, fish oil supplements and other health foods such as green-lipped mussels. Fish allergy has a number of differential diagnoses. In Europe, anisakiasis is caused by the consumption of raw or lightly cooked fish contaminated with *L3 Anisakis spp.* Larvae, and is prevalent where consumption of raw/marinated fish is high (Garcia-Perez *et al.*, 2015). Seafood can also provoke adverse food reactions due to the presence of the ciguatera toxin, which is present in live fish and causes vomiting and diarrhoea, but it is scombroid poisoning that most often causes the symptoms of flushing, sweating, urticaria, gastrointestinal symptoms, palpitations and bronchospasm within an hour of consumption, which may be confused with anaphylaxis (Attaran & Probst, 2000). These symptoms are due to the heat-stable toxins produced in the flesh of caught fish by marine bacteria decarboxylating fish histidine into histamine. Scombroid (tuna, mackerel, skipjack and bonito) and non-scombroid (herring, sardines, marlin and anchovies) fish can all provoke this condition (Fritz & Baldwin, 2003). The fish may not look spoiled, but a histamine concentration >50 ppm suggests decomposition, and it is known that 75 mg of liquid histamine can provoke symptoms in healthy volunteers (Wöhrl *et al.*, 2004).

Egg

Approximately 1.6–3.2% of children are reported to have egg allergy (Wright & Meyer, 2009), which usually resolves in childhood (Heine *et al.*, 2006). About half of the egg-allergic children will be tolerant by the age of 3 years, and 66% by 5 years of age (Boyano-Martinez *et al.*, 2002). Newly diagnosed egg allergy can occur in adults due to bird egg syndrome, which involves hypersensitivity to bird allergens precipitating a cross-reaction to the egg yolk allergen alpha livetin (Szepfalusi *et al.*, 1994). Asthma is a comorbidity associated with egg allergy (Tariq *et al.*, 2000).

Baking reduces the allergenicity of eggs by 70% (Wright & Meyer, 2009), and the majority of egg-allergic children are likely to be able to tolerate baked egg (Kemp, 2007). Persistent egg allergy is associated with sensitisation to the linear epitopes of the egg allergen Gal d 1 (ovomucoid), which is not degraded by heat, unlike the other main egg allergen Gal d 2 (ovalbumin) (Jarvinen *et al.*, 2007). There may be a wide variation in the type of egg-containing foods that those with egg allergy can tolerate (Table 7.11.8).

Table 7.11.8 shows the type of foods that can be classified as containing well-cooked egg, loosely cooked egg and raw egg. Egg can be a less obvious ingredient of foods such as pasta, biscuits, ice cream, egg glazes, sweets and desserts, so labels should always be carefully scrutinised for its presence. The BDA Food Allergy Specialist Group produces a diet sheet on egg, and members can download this for free.

Fruit and vegetables

The most widespread group of foods provoking food-allergic reactions in adolescents and adults is fruit, and,

Table 7.11.8 Classification of egg-containing foods

Well-cooked egg	Lightly cooked egg	Raw egg
Cakes	Scrambled egg	Fresh mayonnaise
Biscuits	Boiled egg	Fresh mousse and shop-bought mousse that contain egg
Dried egg pasta	Fried egg	Fresh ice cream
Pancakes and Yorkshire pudding	Omelette	Sorbet
Egg in sausages, both vegetarian and meat varieties, and also in other processed meats such as burgers	Egg fried rice	Royal icing (both fresh and powdered icing sugar)
Prepared meat dishes	Meringues	Homemade marzipan
Well-cooked fresh egg pasta	Some marshmallows	Raw egg in cake mix and other dishes awaiting cooking (children of all ages love to taste or lick the spoon!)
Quorn	Lemon curd	Egg glaze on pastry
Sponges and sponge fingers	Quiche	Horseradish sauce
Chocolate bars that contain nougat or dried egg, e.g. Milky Way, Mars bar or Cadbury Creme Egg	Poached egg	Tartar sauce
Some soft-centred chocolates	Pancakes	Cheese that contains egg white in the form of lysozyme
Soft fruit chews	Egg in batter	Mayonnaise
Egg in some gravy granules	Egg in breadcrumbs, e.g. on fish fingers and chicken nuggets	Salad cream
Dried egg noodles	Hollandaise sauce	
Waffles	Quiche and flans (fruity and savoury)	
Commercial marzipan	Egg custard and egg custard tarts	
	Crème caramel	
	Crème brûlée	
	Real (egg) custard	
	Tempura batter	
	Yorkshire pudding – some patients who can eat well-cooked eggs can tolerate this, but it depends on how well cooked they are and if they contain any uncooked batter inside	

to a lesser extent, vegetables (Fernández-Rivas, 2015). These reactions are usually due to pollen–food syndrome (PFS), the prevalence of which varies according to the pollens present in a particular geographical region. Up to two-thirds of those sensitised to birch tree pollen are likely to develop PFS (Skypala *et al.*, 2011). The reported prevalence of PFS in the UK is 2% (Skypala *et al.*, 2013). It used to be considered that PFS does not affect children, but studies show that PFS can occur even in young children who are sensitised to aeroallergens (Ludman *et al.*, 2016). The main trigger foods for PFS vary, depending on the pollen involved; however, in the UK, tree nuts, apples and stone fruit (such as peaches and cherries) are most regularly included (Table 7.11.9) (Skypala *et al.*, 2013).

Symptoms of PFS are usually mild and rapid in onset, occurring either on contact with the food, or 5–15 minutes after eating the food (Skypala *et al.*, 2011). More severe symptoms can occur in the pollen season, or if a large quantity of protein is consumed. For example, there is a high risk of severe reactions to fresh fruit and vegetable juices and smoothies, as well as to soy milk, owing to the high levels of the Gly m 4 allergen (De Swert *et al.*, 2012). Generally, only raw foods provoke symptoms, owing to the labile nature of the class 2 allergens involved, the pathogenesis-related (PR) 10 proteins, and profilins. The PR-10 proteins are highly homologous to the main birch pollen allergen Bet v 1, the dominant sensitizing allergen in 90% of birch-pollen-allergic subjects

Table 7.11.9 Cross-reacting plant food allergens

Birch pollen	Apple, pear, cherry, peach, nectarine, apricot, plum, kiwi, hazelnut, other nuts, almond, celery, carrot, potato
Birch/mugwort	Celery, carrot, spices, sunflower seed, honey
Grass	Melon, watermelon, orange, tomato, potato, peanut, Swiss chard
Ragweed	Watermelon and other melons, banana, courgette, cucumber
Plane tree	Hazelnut, peach, apple, melon, kiwi, peanut, maize, chickpea, lettuce, green beans
Latex	Avocado pear, chestnut, banana, passion fruit, kiwi fruit, papaya, mango, tomato, pepper, potato, celery

(García & Lizaso, 2011). In addition to birch pollen, PFS can also manifest in individuals sensitised to mugwort and grass, owing to the cross-reactivity between profilins (Fernández-Rivas, 2015).

Diagnosis of PFS can be made on history alone, with immediate oropharyngeal reactions to raw fruits and vegetables being diagnostic, although a positive SPT to birch pollen supports the diagnosis (Skypala *et al.*, 2011). Sensitisation to fruits and nuts is very common in adults (Burney *et al.*, 2014), so skin prick or specific IgE testing should only be carried out to foods reported to cause reactions. Due to the high homology between hazelnuts and birch, and peanuts and grass, positive tests to nuts in a pollen-sensitised individual should be interpreted with caution. Component test results for the PR-10 allergens in hazelnuts (Cor a 1) and peanuts (Ara h 8) can be compared to those obtained for the primary allergens in these foods (Cor a 9 and 14, Ara h 1, 2, 6) to determine whether the symptoms to nuts are due to a primary allergy or PFS (Werfel *et al.*, 2015). Getting the correct diagnosis ensures that only those foods causing symptoms will need to be avoided. The main dietary intervention for PFS involves the avoidance of raw fruits, vegetables or nuts reported to provoke symptoms, but other forms of the food may be tolerated, e.g. cooked fruits/vegetables, roasted nuts, marzipan, soy flour, and nuts in chocolate. Those who have PFS should be encouraged to try different varieties of fruit, as some may be less allergenic than others (Nybom *et al.*, 2013).

Another less prevalent manifestation of cross-reactivity is caused by antibodies to natural rubber latex (NRL) (*Hevea brasilienisis*) cross-reacting with various fruit and vegetables; 30–50% of those allergic to NRL will have associated hypersensitivity reactions to plant foods (Wagner & Breiteneder, 2002). An individual who is clinically allergic to NRL can have severe cross-reactions to foods due to the similarity between major latex allergens and those in bananas, avocado, kiwi and chestnuts. However, people sensitised but asymptomatic to NRL can also have reactions to foods, usually due to profilin sensitisation, and the resulting reactions are often mild.

Another more severe plant food allergy involves allergens known as lipid transfer proteins (LTPs). Unlike the allergens involved in PFS, LTP allergens are resistant to proteolysis, pH change and thermal treatments, enabling them to be primary sensitisers (Fernández-Rivas *et al.*, 2006). Allergy to LTP is most prevalent in the Mediterranean region, although limited data suggests it could also affect Northern Europeans (Azofra *et al.*, 2016; Salcedo *et al.*, 2004). It manifests as a primary allergy to a food, typically peaches, due to sensitisation to the peach LTP allergen Pru p 3, with some individuals experiencing symptoms to other plant foods due to cross-reactivity between Pru p 3 and other LTP allergens (Pascal *et al.*, 2012). The primary food may not always be peaches; other foods have been reported including tomatoes and lettuce (López-Matas *et al.*, 2015; Muñoz-García *et al.*, 2017). However, it is also possible that a pollen such as mugwort could be the primary sensitising agent (Gao *et al.*, 2013). LTP symptoms occur up to 30 minutes after eating and are often severe, systemic and include anaphylaxis (Fernández-Rivas, 2015). Unlike PFS, both cooked and raw versions of the trigger food need to be avoided, especially foods containing high levels of peel and seeds, such as tomato puree, sundried tomatoes, candied peel, dried fruits, etc.

Wheat

Wheat allergy is usually a transient, but important, allergy of childhood. In a recent study by the Isle of Wight, 0.48% (4/827; 95% CI 0–1%) of children had wheat allergy based on oral food challenges. From this cohort, 16.3% (96/588) were sensitised to grass pollen, 13.4% (79/588) to wheat pollen, and 78% (75/96) to both (Venter *et al.*, 2016). Almost all children with wheat allergy achieved tolerance by adolescence (Keet *et al.*, 2009), but, despite this, 0.5–0.9% of adults report reactions to wheat (Schäfer *et al.*, 2001; Vierk *et al.*, 2007; Young *et al.*, 1994). In adults, the most common manifestation is as a trigger of FDEIA (Roe *et al.*, 2016; Scherf *et al.*, 2016). Those affected by this condition can tolerate wheat, except when it is consumed within 2 hours of exercising. Anaphylaxis can be induced by exercise alone, but it is possible that, in 80% of all cases, food could be a cofactor (Yang *et al.*, 2008). Shellfish, tomatoes, celery, peanuts, maize, soya, strawberries and cheese have also been implicated as triggers of FDEIA (Shadick *et al.*, 1999). Presenting symptoms to wheat are often cutaneous, such as atopic dermatitis and urticaria, but laryngeal oedema and anaphylaxis may occur as the first manifestation (Pourpak *et al.*, 2004, 2007).

Non-IgE-mediated wheat allergy in children may present with chronic, diffuse gastrointestinal symptoms (Meyer *et al.*, 2013b). In adults, wheat is most often reported to provoke gastrointestinal symptoms, most notably in those with irritable bowel disease, although the mechanism is unknown (Monsbakken *et al.*, 2006). Rice, maize, barley and oats can all provoke allergic reactions, but are not common triggers of FHS in the UK, although they should not be ruled out, especially as corn or barley may be minor ingredients in many foods. Although it is not a cereal, buckwheat is often used to replace flour. Buckwheat noodles are a common cause of reactions in Korea (Yang *et al.*, 2008); also, buckwheat in the form of galettes (pancakes) is becoming a common allergen in France, and should be considered in cases of unexplained reactions.

Wheat allergy (IgE-mediated and non-IgE-mediated), in most cases, will require total wheat exclusion. Partial exclusion may be sufficient in non-allergic food hypersensitivity forms of wheat hypersensitivity. The threshold of sensitivity varies, and some people can obtain symptom relief by significant reduction of wheat intake. In the UK, wheat is a major component of most cereal foods and a common ingredient in many manufactured foods, ranging from sausages to ice cream. Wheat exclusion therefore has considerable impact on food choice and nutrient intake. In children, wheat may be an additional allergen excluded alongside milk and/or egg, which increases nutritional risks for calcium deficiency and makes the diet very limited, unless a good range of substitutes are introduced.

An excellent range of commercially produced wheat-free (and gluten-free) products, including bread, biscuits, pastries, pasta and ready meals, are available. Some gluten-free and wheat products are available on prescription; however, this may vary between primary healthcare community trusts. These are not prescribable for wheat FHS, but usually only for people with coeliac disease who can tolerate wheat starch, as it is present in many proprietary gluten-free foods. Gluten-free products are not suitable for people with wheat allergy unless they are specifically labelled as 'wheat free'.

Other triggers

Food additives

Approximately 4.9% of the UK population cite food additives as a trigger of food allergy (Young *et al.*, 1994), although the true prevalence ranges from 0.1 to 0.4% (Osterballe *et al.*, 2005; Young *et al.*, 1987). Studies suggest that artificial colours and the benzoate preservatives can increase hyperactivity in children (McCann *et al.*, 2007), although evidence for the efficacy of diets free from individual additives or high levels of natural food chemicals in children is sparse, and no recent studies have been undertaken (Skypala *et al.*, 2015). Synthetic azo dyes, particularly tartrazine (E102) and sunset yellow (E110), are often thought to be implicated in adverse food reactions, but the evidence is sparse. However, mistrust by the public has led to an increase in the use of natural colourings, precipitating a number of case reports of IgE-mediated food allergy, especially to carmine/cochineal, which is derived from insects (Voltolini *et al.*, 2014). Benzoates have been linked to chronic idiopathic urticaria, but the evidence is not conclusive (Di Lorenzo *et al.*, 2005). However, a cinnamon- and benzoate-free diet has been shown to provide benefit in up to three-quarters of those who have orofacial granulomatosis, a rare inflammatory disease of the lips, face and mouth (Campbell *et al.*, 2011) (see Chapter 7.4.2, Orofacial granulomatosis).

Monosodium glutamate (MSG), or E621, a common additive in savoury foods, has been linked with a number of conditions, especially headache; however, a recent systematic review concluded that there was insufficient evidence to determine a causal relationship between MSG ingestion and headache (Obayashi & Nagamura, 2016).

Reactions to sulphites have been the best characterised, and sulphites are the only food additives required by law to be declared on food labels (see Chapter 4.5, Food law and labelling). Sulphites inhibit the enzymatic and non-enzymatic reactions that control browning (Taylor *et al.*, 2003), and are primarily added to wine, cider, vinegar, pectin, clear or light-coloured fruit juices, lime and lemon juice, and dried foods such as dried fruit and dried onions (E220–E228) (Skypala *et al.*, 2015). The use of sulphites in foods was widespread. However, in the 1980s, following reports of reactions, including six deaths, the use of sulphites was regulated, and foods containing >10 ppm (10 mg/kg) of sulphites have to be labelled (Yang & Purchase, 1985). Sulphites are more likely to affect asthmatic patients, with up to 10% experiencing symptoms on exposure, especially those with steroid-dependent asthma (Bush *et al.*, 1986). Sulphites can also cause urticaria and angio-oedema, both through topical application of sulphite-containing cosmetics or skin reactions following the oral ingestion of sulphite (Ban *et al.*, 2014). Other reactions are less common but include anaphylaxis and rhinitis (Vally & Misso, 2012). Symptoms of sulphite intolerance include the development of flushing, nasal and sinus symptoms, bronchospasm and occasional gastrointestinal upset, and these symptoms surface within 45 minutes of consumption. As with many other types of FHS, sulphite intolerance is dose dependent; while a small number of people are sensitive to small amounts, most report symptoms after consuming a dose of >20 mg. Sulphite intolerance usually manifests in adults, and it is unknown whether this condition also affects children and teenagers (Skypala *et al.*, 2015).

Pharmacological food reactions

Biogenic or vasoactive amines are produced by bacteria during fermentation, storage or decay, with histamine and tyramine being most associated with food-related symptoms. Although some dispute any relationship between the oral ingestion of biogenic amines and FHS reactions, others contend that histamine intolerance is probably underestimated, especially as it is known that an increase in plasma histamine levels causes increased gastric acid secretion, flushing, headache, urticaria, pruritus and tachycardia (Jansen *et al.*, 2003; Maintz & Novak, 2007). It has been suggested that 1% of the population might be affected by histamine sensitivity, the majority of whom will be middle-aged (Maintz & Novak, 2007). Histamine responses are usually dose dependent; most people will react to a dose of 75 mg, but very sensitive individuals may respond to levels as low as 2.5 mg (Morrow *et al.*, 1991; Wöhrl *et al.*, 2004). Dietary histamine is degraded by the enzyme diamine oxidase, and it is proposed that low diamine oxidase levels are a good indicator of the need for a low-histamine diet (Rosell-Camps *et al.*, 2013). Foods rich in histamine and tyramine include strong cheeses, red wine, spinach, aubergines, yeast extract and scombroid fish such as tuna and mackerel (Skypala *et al.*, 2015).

Salicylate intolerance has been defined as '*a nonspecific antigen-induced pseudo-allergic hypersensitivity reaction to salicylic acid, its derivatives or other related organic or inorganic acids of similar chemical structure*' (Raithel *et al.*, 2005). Salicylates are signalling molecules which are widely distributed in plant foods in the form of salicylic acid. It is unknown whether naturally occurring salicylic acid in foods can provoke a response in individuals with a hypersensitivity to acetyl salicylate (aspirin) or NSAIDs. It has been suggested that 2.5% of Europeans may have salicylate sensitivity, and that salicylate intolerance could be relevant in people with a pre-existing intolerance to NSAIDs who also have lower-gastrointestinal-tract disease (Baenkler, 2008; Raithel *et al.*, 2005). A position paper also proposes that a low-salicylate diet could be effective in a percentage of those with aspirin-sensitive urticaria or angio-oedmea (Zuberbier *et al.*, 2014). However, the efficacy of the avoidance of dietary salicylate has been refuted, and few controlled studies of salicylate avoidance have been published (Dahlén *et al.*, 1994; Skypala *et al.*,

2015). The amount of salicylate in foods can vary owing to varietal differences and growing conditions, and there are large discrepancies in the amounts of salicylate attributed to specific foods by different studies (Baxter *et al.*, 2001; Mitchell & Skypala, 2013). However, curry spices are universally agreed as being high in natural salicylate, and so could be a more important dietary factor than other high-salicylate foods (Paterson *et al.*, 2006). The benefits of salicylate avoidance need to be weighed against the fact that salicylates may be beneficial for the prevention of cancer and heart disease.

Other pharmacological reactions include those reported to dietary methylxanthines, such as caffeine in coffee, cola and chocolate, and theobromine in chocolate. These substances can provoke symptoms such as anxiety and disordered sleep in sensitive individuals (Mathew & Wilson, 1990; Pollak & Bright, 2003), although both coffee and cola drinks have also been reported to trigger urticaria and anaphylaxis (Fernandez-Nieto *et al.*, 2002; Infante *et al.*, 2003). Despite chocolate being the most commonly reported food to provoke symptoms in the prevalence study by Young *et al.* (1994), allergy to chocolate bars is unlikely, owing to the extensive processing of the cocoa beans (Zak & Keeney, 1976), although it has been proposed that the availability of chocolate containing pieces of roasted or raw cacao nut could lead to an increase in reported reactions (Chapman *et al.*, 2006).

Reactions to alcohol are most commonly due to a deficiency of the enzyme alcohol dehydrogenise, which predominantly affects people of Asian ethnicity (Agarwal *et al.*, 1981). However, alcoholic drinks can provoke FHS reactions or act as a cofactor in precipitating or exacerbating these reactions. The alcoholic drink most commonly reported to cause symptoms is red wine (Linneberg *et al.*, 2008). Rarely, but occasionally, these reactions are due to the pure alcohol itself (Ehlers *et al.*, 2002), but more common precipitants are the biogenic amines or added sodium metabisulphite (Skypala *et al.*, 2015; Vally & Misso, 2012). The LTP allergens in barley, wheat and grapes have also been reported to trigger severe IgE-mediated allergic responses to beer and wine (Asero *et al.*, 2001; Herzinger *et al.*, 2004; Kalogeromitros *et al.*, 2005).

Acknowledgement

The book editor acknowledges the prior contribution of Carina Venter and Tanya Wright.

Further reading

Arshad SH. (2002) *Allergy: An Illustrated Colour Text*. London: Churchill Livingstone.

NICE. (2011) *Diagnosis of Food Allergies under 19s: Assessment and Diagnosis*. Available at https://www.nice.org.uk/guidance/cg116. Accessed 2 November 2018.

NICE. (2016a) *Anaphylaxis Quality Standards*. Available at https://www.nice.org.uk/guidance/qs119. Accessed 2 November 2018.

NICE. (2016b) *Food Allergy Quality Standards*. Available at https://www.nice.org.uk/guidance/qs118. Accessed 2 November 2018.

Skypala IJ, Venter C. (2009) *Food Hypersensitivity*. Oxford: Wiley Blackwell.

Internet resources

Allergy UK, www.allergyuk.org

Anaphylaxis Campaign, www.anaphylaxis.org.uk

Asthma UK, www.asthma.org.uk

British Dietetic Association, www.bda.uk.com

British Society for Allergy and Clinical Immunology (BSACI), www.bsaci.org

Medic Alert Foundation (medical alert bracelets), www.medicalert.org.uk

Migraine Trust, www.migrainetrust.org

National Eczema Society, www.eczema.org

References

Aamodt AH, Stovner LJ, Langhammer L, *et al.* (2007) Is headache related to Asthma, hay fever and chronic bronchitis? The Head-HUNT Study. *Headache* 47: 204–221.

Abenavoli L, Delibasic M, Peta V, *et al.* (2015) Nutritional profile of adult patients with celiac disease. *Eur. Rev. Med. Pharmacol. Sci.* 19(22): 4285–4292.

Agarwal DP, Harada S, Goedde HW. (1981) Racial differences in biological sensitivity to ethanol: the role of alcohol dehydrogenase and aldehyde dehydrogenase isozymes. *Alcohol. Clin. Exp. Res.* 5: 12–16.

Agostoni C, Decsi T, Fewtrell M, *et al.* (2008) Complementary feeding: a commentary by the ESPGHAN Committee on Nutrition. *J. Pediatr. Gastroenterol. Nutr.* 46(1): 99–110.

Ahrens B, Niggemann B, Wahn U, *et al.* (2014) Positive reactions to placebo in children undergoing double-blind, placebo-controlled food challenge. *Clin. Exp. Allergy* 44(4): 572–578.

Alduraywish SA, Lodge CJ, Vicendese D, *et al.* (2016) Sensitization to milk, egg and peanut from birth to 18 years: a longitudinal study of a cohort at risk of allergic disease. *Pediatr. Allergy Immunol.* 27: 83–91.

Allen KJ, Koplin JJ. (2012) The epidemiology of IgE-mediated food allergy and anaphylaxis. *Immunol. Allergy Clin. North Am.* 32: 35–50.

Alonzi C, Campi P, Gaeta F, *et al.* (2011) Diagnosing IgE-mediated hypersensitivity to sesame by an immediate-reading "contact test" with sesame oil. *J. Allergy Clin. Immunol.* 127: 1627–1629.

Amlot PL, Kemeny DM, Zachary C, *et al.* (1987) Oral allergy syndrome (OAS): symptoms of IgE-mediated hypersensitivity to foods. *Clin. Allergy* 17: 33–42.

Anagnostou K, Clark A. (2016) Oral immunotherapy for peanut allergy. *Annu. Rev. Med.* 67: 375–385.

Añíbarro B, Seoane FJ, Múgica MV. (2007) Involvement of hidden allergens in food allergic reactions. *J. Investig. Allergol. Clin. Immunol.* 17: 168–172.

Asai Y, Yanishevsky Y, Clarke A, *et al.* (2014) Rate, triggers, severity and management of anaphylaxis in adults treated in a Canadian emergency department. *Int. Arch. Allergy Immunol.* 164(3): 246–252.

Asarnoj A, Nilsson C, Lidholm J, *et al.* (2012) Peanut component Ara h 8 sensitization and tolerance to peanut. *J. Allergy Clin. Immunol.* 130: 468–472.

Asero R, Mistrello G, Roncarolo D, *et al.* (2001) A case of allergy to beer showing cross-reactivity between lipid transfer proteins. *Ann Allergy Asthma Immunol.* 87: 65–67.

Attaran RR, Probst F. (2000) Histamine fish poisoning: a common but frequently misdiagnosed condition. *Emerg. Med J.* 19: 474–475.

Awazuhara H, Kawai H, Baba M, *et al.* (1998) Antigenicity of the proteins in soy lecithin and soy oil in soybean allergy. *Clin. Exp. Allergy.* 28(12): 1559–1564.

Ayuso R, Reese G, Leong-Kee S, *et al.* (2002) Molecular basis of arthropod cross-reactivity: IgE-binding cross-reactive epitopes of shrimp, house dust mite and cockroach tropomyosins. *Int. Arch. Allergy Immunol.* 129: 38–48.

Azofra J, Berroa F, Gastaminza G, *et al.* (2016) Lipid transfer protein syndrome in a non-Mediterranean area. *Int. Arch. Allergy Immunol.* 169: 181–188.

Baenkler HW. (2008) Salicylate intolerance: pathophysiology, clinical spectrum, diagnosis and treatment. *Dtsch. Arztebl. Int.* 105: 137–142.

Ball HB. (2005) *Food Challenges for Children: A Practical Guide.* Enderby: Leicestershire Nutrition and Dietetic Service.

Ballmer-Weber BK, Holzhauser T, Scibilia J, *et al.* (2007) Clinical characteristics of soybean allergy in Europe: a double-blind, placebo-controlled food challenge study. *J. Allergy Clin. Immunol.* 119(6): 1489–1496.

Ban GY, Kim MA, Yoo HS, *et al.* (2014) Letter to the editor. Two major phenotypes of sulfite hypersensitivity: asthma and urticaria. *Yonsei Med. J.* 55: 542–544.

Barbarroja-Escudero J, Sanchez-Gonzalez M-J, Antolin-Amerigo D, et al. (2015) Diagnosis of IgE-mediated hypersensitivity to sesame seeds supplemented with lipid body proteins. *Allergol Int.* 64(4): 396–398.

Barnett J, Botting N, Gowland MH, Lucas JS. (2012) The strategies that peanut and nut-allergic consumers employ to remain safe when travelling abroad. *Clin. Transl. Allergy.* 2: 12.

Barnett J, Vasileiou K, Gowland MH, *et al.* (2013) Beyond labelling: what strategies do nut allergic individuals employ to make food choices? A qualitative study. *PLoS One.* 8: e55293.

Bateman B, Warner JO, Hutchinson E, *et al.* (2004) The effects of a double blind, placebo controlled, artificial food colourings and benzoate preservative challenge on hyperactivity in a general population sample of preschool children. *Arch. Dis. Child.* 89: 506–511.

Bath SC, Hill S, Infante HG, et al. (2017) Iodine concentration of milk-alternative drinks available in the UK in comparison with cows' milk. *Br. J. Nutr.* 118: 525–532.

Bauchau V, Durham SR. (2004) Prevalence and rate of diagnosis of allergic rhinitis in Europe. *Eur. Respir. J.* 24: 758–764.

Baxter GJ, Graham AB, Lawrence JR, *et al.* (2001) Salicylic acid in soups prepared from organically and nonorganically grown vegetables. *Eur. J. Nutr.* 40: 289–292.

Bégin P, Paradis L, Paradis J, *et al.* (2013) Natural resolution of peanut allergy: a 12-year longitudinal follow-up study. *J. Allergy. Clin. Immunol. Pract.* 1: 528–530.

Benhamou Senouf AH, Borres MP, Eigenmann PA. (2015) Native and denatured egg white protein IgE tests discriminate hen's egg allergic from egg-tolerant children. *Pediatr. Allergy Immunol.* 26: 12–17.

Bernhisel-Broadbent J, Scanlon SM, Sampson HA. (1992) Fish hypersensitivity. I. In vitro and oral challenge results in fish-allergic patients. *J. Allergy. Clin. Immunol.* 89: 730–737.

Berns SH, Halm EA, Sampson HA, *et al.* (2007) Food allergy as a risk factor for asthma morbidity in adults. *J. Asthma.* 44: 377–381.

Berry MJ, Adams J, Voutilainen H, *et al.* (2015) Impact of elimination diets on growth and nutritional status in children with multiple food allergies. *Pediatr. Allergy Immunol.* 26(2): 133–138.

Beyer K, Grabenhenrich L, Härtl M, *et al.* (2015) Predictive values of component-specific IgE for the outcome of peanut and hazelnut food challenges in children. *Allergy.* 70: 90–98.

Beyer K, Morrow E, Li XM, *et al.* (2001) Effects of cooking methods on peanut allergenicity. *J. Allergy Clin. Immunol.* 107: 1077–1081.

Beyer S, Franke A, Simon JC, *et al.* (2016) Measurement of health-related quality of life in adult patients with birch pollen-associated food allergy. *J. Dtsch. Dermatol. Ges.* 14(4): 397–404.

Bindslev-Jensen C, Ballmer-Weber BK, Bengtsson U, *et al.* (2004) Standardization of food challenges in patients with immediate reactions to foods – position paper from the European Academy of Allergology and Clinical Immunology. *Allergy.* 59(7): 690–697.

Bishop JM, Hill DJ, Hosking CS. (1990) Natural history of cow milk allergy: clinical outcome. *J. Pediatr.* 116(6): 862–867.

Bock SA, Muñoz-Furlong A, Sampson HA. (2007) Further fatalities caused by anaphylactic reactions to food, 2001–2006. *J. Allergy. Clin. Immunol.* 119: 1016–1018.

Bock SA, Sampson HA, Atkins FM, *et al.* (1988) Double-blind, placebo-controlled food challenge (DBPCFC) as an office procedure: a manual. *J. Allergy. Clin. Immunol.* 82(6): 986–997.

Boyano-Martinez T, Garcia-Ara C, Díaz-Pena JM, *et al.* (2002) Prediction of tolerance on the basis of quantification of egg white-specific IgE antibodies in children with egg allergy. *J. Allergy Clin. Immunol.* 110(2): 304–309.

Boyce JA, Assa'ad A, Burks AW, *et al.* (2010) Guidelines for the diagnosis and management of food allergy in the United States: report of the NIAID-sponsored expert panel. *J. Allergy Clin. Immunol.* 126(6): S1–58.

Boyle RJ, Ierodiakonou D, Khan T, *et al.* (2016a) Hydrolysed formula and risk of allergic or autoimmune disease: systematic review and meta-analysis. *BMJ* 352: i974.

Boyle RJ, Tang ML, Chiang WC, *et al.* (2016b) Prebiotic-supplemented partially hydrolysed cow's milk formula for the prevention of eczema in high-risk infants: a randomised controlled trial. *Allergy.* 71(5): 701–710.

Breitfelder A, Wenig CM, Wolfenstetter SB, *et al.* (2011) Relative weight-related costs of healthcare use by children – results from the two German birth cohorts, GINI-plus and LISA-plus. *Econ. Hum. Biol.* 9(3): 302–315.

Brough HA, Liu AH, Sicherer S, *et al.* (2015) Atopic dermatitis increases the effect of exposure to peanut antigen in dust on peanut sensitization and likely peanut allergy. *J. Allergy Clin. Immunol.* 135: 164–170.

Brough HA, Santos AF, Makinson K, *et al.* (2013) Peanut protein in household dust is related to household peanut consumption and is biologically active. *J. Allergy Clin. Immunol.* 132: 630–638.

Bruijnzeel-Koomen C, Ortolani C, Aas K, *et al.* (1995) Adverse reactions to foods. *Allergy.* 50: 623–635.

Burks W. (2003) Skin manifestations of food allergy. *Pediatrics.* 111: 1617–1624.

Burney PG, Potts J, Kummeling I, *et al.* (2014) The prevalence and distribution of food sensitization in European adults. *Allergy.* 69: 365–371.

Bush RK, Taylor SL, Holden K, *et al.* (1986) Prevalence of sensitivity to sulfiting agents in asthmatics. *Am. J. Med.* 81: 816–820.

Caffarelli C, Garrubba M, Greco C, *et al.* (2016) Asthma and food allergy in children: is there a connection or interaction? *Front Pediatr.* 4: 34.

Caffarelli C, Baldi F, Bendandi B, *et al.* (2010) Cow's milk allergy in children: a practical guide. *J. Pediatr.* 36: 5.

Campbell HE, Escudier MP, Patel P, *et al.* (2011) Review article: cinnamon- and benzoate-free diet as a primary treatment for orofacial granulomatosis. *Aliment. Pharmacol. Ther.* 34: 687–701.

Cardona V, Luengo O, Garriga T, *et al.* (2012) Co-factor-enhanced food allergy. *Allergy.* 67: 1316–1318.

Caubet JC, Nowak-Węgrzyn A, Moshier E, *et al.* (2013) Utility of casein-specific IgE levels in predicting reactivity to baked milk. *J. Allergy Clin. Immunol.* 131: 222–224.

Chapman JA, Bernstein IL, Lee RE, *et al.* (2006) Food allergy: a practice parameter. *Ann. Allergy. Asthma. Immunol.* 96: S1–S68.

Chawes BL, Bønnelykke K, Stokholm J, *et al.* (2016) Effect of vitamin D_3 supplementation during pregnancy on risk of persistent wheeze in the offspring: a randomised clinical trial. *JAMA* 315(4): 353–361.

Chebar LA, Meyer R, De Koker C, *et al.* (2015) Time to symptom improvement using elimination diets in non-IgE-mediated gastrointestinal food allergies. *Pediatr. Allergy Immunol.* 26(5): 403–408.

Clark AT, Ewan PW. (2008) Good prognosis, clinical features, and circumstances of peanut and tree nut reactions in children treated by a specialist allergy center. *J. Allergy Clin. Immunol.* 122(2): 286–289.

Clark AT, Anagnostou K, Ewan PW. (2007) Cashew nut causes more severe reactions than peanut: case matched comparison in 141 children. *Allergy.* 62: 913–916.

Codispoti CD, LeMasters GK, Levin L, *et al.* (2015) Traffic pollution is associated with early childhood aeroallergen sensitization. *Ann. Allergy Asthma. Immunol.* 114: 126–133.

SECTION 7

Cohen A, Goldberg M, Levy B, *et al.* (2007) Sesame food allergy and sensitization in children: the natural history and long-term follow-up. *Pediatr. Allergy. Immunol.* 18: 217–223.

Colver AF, Nevantaus H, Macdougall CF, *et al.* (2005) Severe food-allergic reactions in children across the UK and Ireland 1998–2000. *Acta Paediatr.* 94: 689–695.

Comstock GW, Meyer MB, Helsing KJ, *et al.* (2008) Respiratory effects of household exposures to tobacco smoke and gas cooking. *Am. J. Epidemiol.* 168: 810–815.

Cuello-Garcia CA, Brozek JL, Fiocchi A, *et al.* (2015) Probiotics for the prevention of allergy: A systematic review and meta-analysis of randomised controlled trials. *J. Allergy Clin. Immunol.* 136(4): 952–961.

Dahlén B, Boréus LO, Anderson P, *et al.* (1994) Plasma acetylsalicylic acid and salicylic acid levels during aspirin provocation in aspirin-sensitive subjects. *Allergy.* 49: 43–49.

Daul CB, Morgan JE, Lehrer SB. (1990) The natural history of shrimp-specific immunity. *J. Allergy. Clin. Immunol.* 86: 88–93.

Davoren M, Peake J. (2005) Cashew nut allergy is associated with a high risk of anaphylaxis. *Arch. Dis. Child.* 90: 1084–1085.

De Greef E, Hauser B, Devreker T, *et al.* (2012) Diagnosis and management of cow's milk protein allergy in infants. *World J. Pediatr.* 8(1): 19–24.

de Jong NW, van Maaren MS, Vlieg-Boersta BJ, *et al.* (2010) Sensitization to lupine flour: is it clinically relevant? *Clin. Exp. Allergy* 40(10): 1571–1577.

De Koker CE, Shah N, Meyer R. (2014) The differences between lactose intolerance and cow's milk protein allergy. *J. Fam. Health Care* 24(1): 14–8, 20.

de Leon MP, Glaspole IN, Drew AC, *et al.* (2003) Immunological analysis of allergenic cross-reactivity between peanut and tree nuts. *Clin. Exp. Allergy.* 33: 1273–1280.

De Swert LF, Gadisseur R, Sjölander S, et al. (2012) Secondary soy allergy in children with birch pollen allergy may cause both chronic and acute symptoms. *Pediatr. Allergy Immunol.* 23: 117–123.

Della-Torre E, Pignatti P, Yacoub MR, *et al.* (2013) In vivo tests with "Tahini" sauce: new allergenic source to evaluate IgE-mediated hypersensitivity to sesame. *Ann. Allergy Asthma Immunol.* 110: 209–210.

Des Roches A, Paradis L, Paradis J, *et al.* (2006) Food allergy as a new risk factor for scurvy. *Allergy.* 61(12): 1487–1488.

Deschildre A, Elegbédé CF, Just J, *et al.* (2016) Peanut-allergic patients in the MIRABEL survey: characteristics, allergists' dietary advice and lessons from real life. *Clin. Exp. Allergy.* 46: 610–620.

Devereux G, Turner SW, Craig LC, *et al.* (2006) Low maternal vitamin E intake during pregnancy is associated with asthma in 5-year-old children. *Am. J. Respir. Crit. Care Med.* 174(5): 499–507.

Di Lorenzo G, Pacor ML, Mansueto P, *et al.* (2005) Food additive-induced urticaria: a survey of 838 patients with recurrent chronic idiopathic urticaria. *Int. Arch. Allergy. Immunol.* 138: 235–242.

Du Toit G, Foong RM, Lack G. (2016a) Prevention of food allergy – early dietary interventions. *Allergol. Int.* 65(4): 370–377.

DunnGalvin A, Daly D, Cullinane C, *et al.* (2011) Highly accurate prediction of food challenge outcome using routinely available clinical data. *J. Allergy Clin. Immunol.* 127(3): 633–639.

Dyer AA, Lau CH, Smith TL, *et al.* (2015) Pediatric emergency department visits and hospitalizations due to food-induced anaphylaxis in Illinois. *Ann. Allergy Asthma Immunol.* 115: 56–62.

Ehlers I, Hipler UC, Zuberbier T, *et al.* (2002) Ethanol as a cause of hypersensitivity reactions to alcoholic beverages. *Clin. Exp. Allergy.* 32: 1231–1235.

Eigenmann PA, Caubet JC, Zamora SA. (2006) Continuing food-avoidance diets after negative food challenges. *Pediatr. Allergy Immunol.* 17(8): 601–605.

Eigenmann PA, Lack G, Mazon A, *et al.* (2017) Managing nut allergy: a remaining clinical challenge. *J. Allergy. Clin. Immunol. Pract.* 5(2): 296–300.

Eriksson NE, Möller C, Werner S, *et al.* (2003) The hazards of kissing when you are food allergic. *J. Investig. Allergol. Clin. Immunol.* 13: 149–154.

European Commission Directive. (2003) Directive 2003/89/EC of the European Parliament and of the Council of 10 November 2003 amending Directive 2000/13/EC as regards indication of the ingredients present in foodstuffs. *OJL* 308: 15–18.

European Commission Directive. (2006) 2006/142/EC of 22 December 2006 amending Annex IIIa of Directive 2000/13/EC of the European Parliament and of the Council listing the ingredients which must under all circumstances appear on the labelling of foodstuffs. *OJL* 368: 110–111.

European Union. (2007) Directive 2007/68/EC of the European Parliament amendment of Directive 2000/13/EC. *OJL* 310: 11.

European Union. (2011) Regulation (EU) No 1169/2011 of the European Parliament and of the Council of 25 October 2011 on the provision of food information to consumers, amending Regulations (EC) No 1924/2006 and (EC) No 1925/2006 of the European Parliament and of the Council, and repealing Commission Directive 87/250/EEC, Council Directive 90/496/EEC, Commission Directive 1999/10/EC, Directive 2000/13/EC of the European Parliament and of the Council, Commission Directives 2002/67/EC and 2008/5/EC and Commission Regulation (EC) No 608/2004 Text with EEA relevance. *OJL* 304: 18–63. 22.11.2011.

Ewan PW. (1996) Clinical study of peanut and nut allergy in 62 consecutive patients: new features and associations. *BMJ* 312: 1074–1078.

Ferdman RM, Church JA. (2006) Mixed-up nuts: identification of peanuts and tree nuts by children. *Ann. Allergy. Asthma. Immunol.* 97: 73–77.

Fernandez-Nieto M, Sastre J, Quirce S. (2002) Urticaria caused by cola drink. *Allergy.* 57: 967.

Fernández-Rivas M, Bolhaar S, González-Mancebo E, *et al.* (2006) Apple allergy across Europe: How allergen sensitization profiles determine the clinical expression of allergies to plant foods. *J. Allergy. Clin. Immunol.* 118: 481–488.

Fernández-Rivas M. (2015) Fruit and vegetable allergy. *Chem. Immunol. Allergy.* 101: 162–170.

Filipiak B, Zutavern A, Koletzko S, *et al.* (2007) Solid food introduction in relation to eczema: results from a four-year prospective birth cohort study. *J. Pediatr.* 151: 352–358.

Fiocchi A, Brozek J, Schünemann H, *et al.* (2010) World Allergy Organization (WAO) Diagnosis and Rationale for Action against Cow's Milk Allergy (DRACMA) Guidelines. *Pediatr. Allergy Immunol.* 21(21): 1–125.

Fiocchi A, Pawankar R, Cuello-Garcia C, *et al.* (2015) World Allergy Organization-McMaster University Guidelines for Allergic Disease Prevention (GLAD-P): Probiotics. *World Allergy Organ. J.* 8(1): 4.

Fisher HR, Du Toit G, Lack G. (2011) Specific oral tolerance induction in food allergic children: is oral desensitisation more effective than allergen avoidance? A meta-analysis of published RCTs. *Arch. Dis. Child.* 96(3): 259–264.

Flammarion S, Santos C, Guimber D, et al. (2011) Diet and nutritional status of children with food allergies. *Pediatr. Allergy Immunol.* 22(2): 161–165.

Fleischer D, Conover-Walker M, Matsui E, *et al.* (2005) The natural history of tree nut allergy. *J. Allergy Clin. Immunol.* 116: 1087–1093.

Fleischer DM, Spergel JM, Assa'ad AH, *et al.* (2013) Primary prevention of allergic disease through nutritional interventions. *J. Allergy Clin. Immunol. Pract.* 1(1): 29–36.

Flinterman AE, Knulst AC, Meijer Y, *et al.* (2006) Acute allergic reactions in children with AEDS after prolonged cow's milk elimination diets. *Allergy.* 61(3): 370–374.

Flokstra-de Blok BM, Dubois AE, Vlieg-Boerstra BJ, *et al.* (2010) Health-related quality of life of food allergic patients: comparison with the general population and other diseases. *Allergy.* 65(2): 238–244.

Food Allergy Research and Research Program. (2006) *Soy bean and soy lecithin.* Taylor SL. 31-1-2006. 27-11-2012.

Food Standards Agency (FSA). (2009) *Survey of total and inorganic arsenic in rice drinks.* Available at www.food.gov.uk (C01049). 21-5-2009. 9-11-2013.

Fritz SB, Baldwin JL. (2003) Pharmacologic food reactions. In: Metcalfe DD, Sampson HJ, Simon RA, eds. *Food Allergy: Adverse Reactions to Foods and Food Additives*. Oxford: Blackwell Publishing Ltd, pp. 324–341.

Gangur V, Kelly C, Navuluri L. (2005) Sesame allergy: a growing food allergy of global proportions? *Ann. Allergy. Asthma. Immunol.* 95: 4–11.

Gao ZS, Yang ZW, Wu SD, *et al.* (2013) Peach allergy in China: a dominant role for mugwort pollen lipid transfer protein as a primary sensitiser. *J. Allergy Clin. Immunol.* 131: 224–246.

García BE, Lizaso MT. (2011) Cross-reactivity syndromes in food allergy. *J. Investig. Allergol. Clin. Immunol.* 21: 162–170.

Garcia-Manzanares A, Lucendo AJ. (2011) Nutritional and dietary aspects of celiac disease. *Nutr. Clin. Pract.* 26(2): 163–173.

Garcia-Perez JC, Rodríguez-Perez R, Ballestero A, *et al.* (2015) Previous exposure to the fish parasite *Anisakis* as a potential risk factor for gastric or colon adenocarcinoma. *Medicine (Baltimore)*. 94: e1699.

Gdalevich M, Mimouni D, David M, *et al.* (2001) Breastfeeding and the onset of atopic dermatitis in childhood: a systematic review and meta-analysis of prospective studies. *J. Am. Acad. Dermatol.* 45(4): 520–527.

Giuffrida MG, Villalta D, Mistrello G, *et al.* (2014) Shrimp allergy beyond Tropomyosin in Italy: clinical relevance of Arginine Kinase, *Sarcoplasmic calcium binding protein and Hemocyanin*. *Eur. Ann. Allergy Clin. Immunol.* 46: 172–177.

González-Delgado P, Caparrós E, Moreno MV, *et al.* (2016) Clinical and immunological characteristics of a pediatric population with food protein-induced enterocolitis syndrome (FPIES) to fish. *Pediatr. Allergy Immunol.* 27: 269–275.

Grabenhenrich LB, Dölle S, Moneret-Vautrin A, *et al.* (2016) Anaphylaxis in children and adolescents: The European Anaphylaxis Registry. *J. Allergy Clin. Immunol.* 137: 1128–1137.

Grimshaw KE, Bryant T, Oliver EM, *et al.* (2016) Incidence and risk factors for food hypersensitivity in UK infants: results from a birth cohort study. *Clin. Transl. Allergy.* 6:1.

Grimshaw K, Logan K, O'Donovan S, *et al.* (2017) Modifying the infant's diet to prevent food allergy. *Arch. Dis. Child.* 102(2): 179–186.

Gu X, Beardslee T, Zeece M, *et al.* (2001) Identification of IgE-binding proteins in soy lecithin. *Int. Arch. Allergy Immunol.* 126(3): 218–225.

Gupta R, Sheikh A, Strachan DP, *et al.* (2007) Time trends in allergic disorders in the UK. *Thorax.* 62: 91–96.

Gupta RS, Lau CH, Hamilton RG, *et al.* (2014) Predicting outcomes of oral food challenges by using the allergen-specific IgE-total IgE ratio. *J. Allergy Clin. Immunol. Pract.* 2: 300–305.

Hansen TK, Bindslev-Jensen C, Skov PS, *et al.* (1997) Codfish allergy in adults: IgE cross-reactivity among fish species. *Ann. Allergy. Asthma. Immunol.* 78: 187–194.

Heine RG. (2015) Gastrointestinal food allergies. *Chem. Immunol. Allergy.* 101: 171–180.

Heine RG, Laske N, Hill DJ. (2006) The diagnosis and management of egg allergy. *Curr. Allergy. Asthma. Rep.* 6(2): 145–152.

Henderson CJ, Abonia JP, King EC, *et al.* (2012) Comparative dietary therapy effectiveness in remission of pediatric eosinophilic esophagitis. *J. Allergy Clin. Immunol.* 129(6): 1570–1578.

Herzinger T, Kick G, Ludolph-Hauser D, *et al.* (2004) Anaphylaxis to wheat beer. *Ann. Allergy. Asthma. Immunol.* 92: 673–675.

Hill DJ, Hosking CS. (2004) Food allergy and atopic dermatitis in infancy: an epidemiologic study. *Pediatr. Allergy Immunol.* 15(5): 421–427.

Hill DJ, Hosking CS, Yu Zhie C, *et al.* (1997) The frequency of food allergy in Australia and Asia. *Environ. Toxicol. Pharmacol.* 4: 101–110.

Holzhammer J, Wöber C. (2006) Alimentary trigger factors that provoke migraine and tension-type headache. *Schmerz.* 20: 151–159.

Hoppu U, Kalliomaki M, Isolauri E. (2000) Maternal diet rich in saturated fat during breastfeeding is associated with atopic sensitization of the infant. *Eur. J. Clin. Nutr.* 54(9): 702–705.

Hoppu U, Rinne M, Salo-Vaananen P, *et al.* (2005) Vitamin C in breast milk may reduce the risk of atopy in the infant. *Eur. J. Clin. Nutr.* 59(1): 123–128.

Host A, Halken S. (1990) A prospective study of cow milk allergy in Danish infants during the first 3 years of life. Clinical course in relation to clinical and immunological type of hypersensitivity reaction. *Allergy.* 45(8): 587–596.

Host A, Halken S. (2004) Hypoallergenic formulas – when, to whom and how long: after more than 15 years we know the right indication! *Allergy.* 59(78): 45–52.

Host A, Koletzko B, Dreborg S, *et al.* (1999) Dietary products used in infants for treatment and prevention of food allergy. Joint Statement of the European Society for Paediatric Allergology and Clinical Immunology (ESPACI) Committee on Hypoallergenic Formulas and the European Society for Paediatric Gastroenterology, Hepatology and Nutrition (ESPGHAN) Committee on Nutrition. *Arch. Dis. Child.* 81(1): 80–84.

Hourihane JO, Bedwani SJ, Dean TP, *et al.* (1997) Randomised, double blind, crossover challenge study of allergenicity of peanut oils in subjects allergic to peanuts. *BMJ* 314: 1084–1088.

Infante S, Baeza ML, Calvo M, *et al.* (2003) Anaphylaxis due to caffeine. *Allergy.* 58: 681–682.

Ingram CJ, Mulcare CA, Itan Y, *et al.* (2009) Lactose digestion and the evolutionary genetics of lactase persistence. *Hum. Genet.* 124(6): 579–591.

Ives AJ, Hourihane JO'B. (2002) Evidence-based diagnosis of food allergy. *Paediatr. Child Health.* 12: 357–364.

James JM, Crespo JF. (2007) Allergic reactions to foods by inhalation. *Curr. Allergy. Asthma. Rep.* 7: 167–174.

Jansen SC, van-Dusseldorp M, Bottema KC, *et al.* (2003) Intolerance to dietary biogenic amines: a review. *Ann. Allergy. Asthma. Immunol.* 91: 233–240.

Jarvinen KM, Beyer K, Vila L, *et al.* (2007) Specificity of IgE antibodies to sequential epitopes of hen's egg ovomucoid as a marker for persistence of egg allergy. *Allergy.* 62(7): 758–765.

Jeong K, Lee SY, Ahn K, *et al.* (2017) A multi-center study on anaphylaxis caused by peanut, tree nuts and seeds in children and adolescents. *Allergy.* 72(3): 507–510.

Johansson SG, Bieber T, Dahl R, *et al.* (2004) Revised nomenclature for allergy for global use: report of the Nomenclature Review Committee of the World Allergy Organization, October 2003. *J. Allergy Clin. Immunol.* 113(5): 832–836.

Johnson J, Malinovschi A, Alving K, *et al.* (2014) Ten-year review reveals changing trends and severity of allergic reactions to nuts and other foods. *Acta Paediatr.* 103(8): 862–7.

Kalogeromitros DC, Makris MP, Gregoriou SG, *et al.* (2005) Grape anaphylaxis: a study of 11 adult onset cases. *Allergy. Asthma. Proc.* 26: 53–58.

Kagalwalla AF, Shah A, Li BU, *et al.* (2011) Identification of specific foods responsible for inflammation in children with eosinophilic esophagitis successfully treated with empiric elimination diet. *J. Pediatr. Gastroenterol. Nutr.* 53(2): 145–149.

Katz Y, Gutierrez-Castrellon P, Gonzalez MG, *et al.* (2014) A comprehensive review of sensitization and allergy to soy-based products. *Clin. Rev. Allergy Immunol.* 46(3): 272–281.

Katz Y, Nowak-Wegrzyn A, Grimshaw KE, *et al.* (2015) Is it the true incidence of IgE-cow's milk allergy (CMA) or CMA or IgE-CMA in some countries and CMA in others. *Allergy.* 70(11): 1509–1510.

Keet CA, Matsui EC, Dhillon G, *et al.* (2009) The natural history of wheat allergy. *Ann. Allergy. Asthma. Immunol.* 102(5): 410–415.

Kelso JM. (2014) Potential food allergens in medications. *J. Allergy Clin. Immunol.* 133: 1509–1518.

Kemp AS. (2007) Egg allergy. *Pediatr. Allergy Immunol.* 18(8): 696–702.

Kemp AS, Hill DJ, Allen KJ, *et al.* (2008) Guidelines for the use of infant formulas to treat cows milk protein allergy: an Australian consensus panel opinion. *Med. J. Aust.* 188(2): 109–112.

Kershaw R. (2009) Nutritional consequences of avoidance and practical approaches to nutritional management. In: Skypala I, Venter C (eds) *Food Hypersensitivity*, 1st edn. Oxford: Wiley-Blackwell, pp. 243–265.
Khan F, Orson F, Ogawa Y, *et al.* (2011) Adult seafood allergy in the Texas Medical Center: a 13-year experience. *Allergy Rhinol. (Providence)*. 2: e71–77.
Kim JS, Nowak-Wegrzyn A, Sicherer SH, *et al.* (2011) Dietary baked milk accelerates the resolution of cow's milk allergy in children. *J. Allergy Clin. Immunol.* 128(1): 125–131.
Kim YH, Kim KW, Kim MJ, *et al.* (2016) Vitamin D levels in allergic rhinitis: a systematic review and meta-analysis. *Pediatr. Allergy Immunol.* 27(6): 580–590.
King RM, Knibb RC, Hourihane JO. (2008) Impact of peanut allergy on quality of life, stress and anxiety in the family. *Allergy.* 64(3): 461–468.
Kleine-Tebbe J, Vogel L, Crowell DN, *et al.* (2002) Severe oral allergy syndrome and anaphylactic reactions caused by a Bet v 1- related PR-10 protein in soybean, SAM22. *J. Allergy Clin. Immunol.* 110(5): 797–804.
Klemola T, Kalimo K, Poussa T, *et al.* (2005) Feeding a soy formula to children with cow's milk allergy: the development of immunoglobulin E-mediated allergy to soy and peanuts. *Pediatr. Allergy Immunol.* 16(8): 641–646.
Kobayashi Y, Yang T, Yu CT, *et al.* (2016) Quantification of major allergen parvalbumin in 22 species of fish by SDS-PAGE. *Food Chem.* 194: 345–353.
Koletzko S, Heine RG, Grimshaw KE, *et al.* (2015) Non-IgE-mediated cow's milk allergy in EuroPrevall. *Allergy.* 70(12): 1679–1680.
Koplin JJ, Wake M, Dharmage SC, *et al.* (2015) Cohort profile: The HealthNuts Study: Population prevalence and environmental/genetic predictors of food allergy. *Int. J. Epidemiol.* 44(4): 1161–1171.
Kowal K, Schacterele RS, Schur PH, *et al.* (2002) Prevalence of allergen specific IgE among patients with chronic fatigue syndrome. *Allergy Asthma Proc.* 23: 35–39.
Kramer MS, Kakuma R. (2006) Maternal dietary antigen avoidance during pregnancy or lactation, or both, for preventing or treating atopic disease in the child. *Cochrane. Database. Syst. Rev.* 3: CD000133.
Kramer MS, Matush L, Vanilovich I, *et al.* (2007) Effect of prolonged and exclusive breast feeding on risk of allergy and asthma: cluster randomised trial. *BMJ* 335(7624): 815.
Kuehn A, Hilger C, Lehners-Weber C, *et al.* (2013) Identification of enolases and aldolases as important fish allergens in cod, salmon and tuna: component resolved diagnosis using parvalbumin and the new allergens. *Clin. Exp. Allergy.* 43(7): 811–822.
Kumar R, Kumari D, Srivastava P, *et al.* (2010) Identification of IgE-mediated food allergy and allergens in older children and adults with asthma and allergic rhinitis. *Indian J. Chest Dis. Allied Sci.* 52(4): 217–224.
Lack G, Fox D, Northstone K, *et al.* (2003) Factors associated with the development of peanut allergy in childhood. *N. Engl. J. Med.* 348(11): 977–985.
Lehrer SB, Kim L, Rice T, *et al.* (2007) Transfer of shrimp allergens to other foods through cooking oil. *J. Allergy Clin. Immunol.* 119: S112.
Leonard SA, Caubet JC, Kim JS, *et al.* (2015) Baked milk- and egg-containing diet in the management of milk and egg allergy. *J. Allergy Clin. Immunol. Pract.* 3(1): 13–23.
Lin J, Sampson HA. (2009) The role of immunoglobulin E-binding epitopes in the characterization of food allergy. *Curr. Opin. Allergy. Clin. Immunol.* 9: 357–363.
Ling L, Ospina MB, Sideri K, *et al.* (2016) Retrospective analysis on the agreement between skin prick test and serum food specific IgE antibody results in adults with suspected food allergy. *Allergy Asthma Clin. Immunol.* 12: 30.
Linneberg A, Berg ND, Gonzalez-Quintela A, *et al.* (2008) Prevalence of self-reported hypersensitivity symptoms following intake of alcoholic drinks. *Clin. Exp. Allergy.* 38: 145–151.
Lomas JM, Järvinen KM. (2015) Managing nut-induced anaphylaxis: challenges and solutions. *J. Asthma Allergy.* 8: 115–123.
Lopata AL, Lehrer SB. (2009) New insights into seafood allergy. *Curr. Opin. Allergy Clin. Immunol.* 9(3): 270–277.
Lopes de Oliveira LC, Aderhold M, Brill M, *et al.* (2013) The value of specific IgE to peanut and its component Ara h 2 in the diagnosis of peanut allergy. *J. Allergy Clin. Immunol. Pract.* 1(4): 394–398.
López-Matas MA, Larramendi CH, Huertas AJ, *et al.* (2015) Tomato nsLTP as an "in vivo" diagnostic tool: sensitization in a Mediterranean population. *J. Investig. Allergol. Clin. Immunol.* 25: 196–204.
Ludman S, Jafari-Mamaghani M, Ebling R, *et al.* (2016) Pollen food syndrome amongst children with seasonal allergic rhinitis attending allergy clinic. *Pediatr. Allergy Immunol.* 27: 134–140.
Luyt D, Ball H, Makwana N, *et al.* (2014) BSACI guideline for the diagnosis and management of cow's milk allergy. *Clin. Exp. Allergy.* 44(5): 642–672.
Maggi I, Parronchi P, Manetti R, *et al.* (1992) Reciprocal regulatory effects of IFNγ and IL-4 on the in vitro development of human Th1 and Th2 clones. *J. Immunol.* 148: 2142–2147.
Mailhol C, Giordano-Labadie F, Lauwers-Cances V, *et al.* (2014) Point prevalence and risk factors for food allergy in a cohort of 386 children with atopic dermatitis attending a multidisciplinary dermatology/paediatric allergy clinic. *Eur. J. Dermatol.* 24(1): 63–69.
Maintz L, Novak N. (2007) Histamine and histamine intolerance. *Am. J. Clin. Nutr.* 85: 1185–1196.
Majamaa H, Moisio P, Holm K, *et al.* (1999a) Cow's milk allergy: diagnostic accuracy of skin prick and patch tests and specific IgE. *Allergy.* 54(4): 346–351.
Majamaa H, Moisio P, Holm K, *et al.* (1999b) Wheat allergy: diagnostic accuracy of skin prick and patch tests and specific IgE. *Allergy.* 54(8): 851–856.
Martinez SIM, Ibanez MD, Sanchez JJ, *et al.* (2008) Clinical features of legume allergy in children from a Mediterranean area. *Ann. Allergy Asthma Immunol.* 101(2): 179–184.
Maslova E, Hansen S, Strom M, *et al.* (2014) Maternal intake of vitamins A, E and K in pregnancy and child allergic disease: a longitudinal study from the Danish National Birth Cohort. *Br. J. Nutr.* 111(6): 1096–1108.
Masthoff LJ, Hoff R, Verhoeckx KC, *et al.* (2013) A systematic review of the effect of thermal processing on the allergenicity of tree nuts. *Allergy.* 68: 983–993.
Mathew RJ, Wilson WH. (1990) Behavioral and cerebrovascular effects of caffeine in patients with anxiety disorders. *Acta Psychiatr. Scand.* 82: 17–22.
Matricardi PM, Kleine-Tebbe J, Hoffmann HJ, *et al.* (2016) EAACI molecular allergology user's guide. *Pediatr. Allergy Immunol.* 27(23): 1–250.
Mavroudi A, Karagiannidou A, Xinias I, *et al.* (2017) Assessment of IgE-mediated food allergies in children with atopic dermatitis. *Allergol. Immunopathol. (Madr).* 45(1): 77–81.
McCann D, Barrett A, Cooper A, *et al.* (2007) Food additives and hyperactive behaviour in 3-year-old and 8/9-year-old children in the community: a randomised, double-blinded, placebo-controlled trial. *Lancet.* 370: 1560–1567.
McWilliam V, Koplin J, Lodge C, *et al.* (2015) The prevalence of tree nut allergy: a systematic review. *Curr. Allergy Asthma Rep.* 15(9): 54.
McWilliam V, Heine R, Tang ML, *et al.* (2016) Multiple food protein intolerance of infancy or severe spectrum of non-IgE-mediated cow's milk allergy? – A case series. *J. Allergy Clin. Immunol. Pract.* 4(2): 324–326.
Meharg AA, Deacon C, Campbell RC, *et al.* (2008a) Inorganic arsenic levels in rice milk exceed EU and US drinking water standards. *J. Environ. Monit.* 10(4): 428–431.
Meharg AA, Lombi E, Williams PN, *et al.* (2008b) Speciation and localization of arsenic in white and brown rice grains. *Environ. Sci. Technol.* 42(4): 1051–1057.
Meyer R, De Koker C, Dziubak R, *et al.* (2014a) Dietary elimination of children with food protein induced gastrointestinal allergy – micronutrient adequacy with and without a hypoallergenic formula? *Clin. Transl. Allergy.* 4(1): 31.

Meyer R, De Koker C, Dziubak R, *et al.* (2014b) Malnutrition in children with food allergies in the UK. *J. Hum. Nutr. Diet.* 27(3): 227–235.

Meyer R, De Koker C, Dziubak R, *et al.* (2015) A practical approach to vitamin and mineral supplementation in food allergic children. *Clin. Transl. Allergy.* 5: 11.

Meyer R, De Koker C, Dzubiak R, *et al.* (2016) The impact of the elimination diet on Growth and nutrient intake in children with food protein induced gastrointestinal allergies. *Clin. Transl. Allergy.* 6: 25.

Meyer R, Fleming C, Dominguez-Ortega G, *et al.* (2013b) Manifestations of food protein induced gastrointestinal allergies presenting to a single tertiary paediatric gastroenterology unit. *World Allergy Organ J.* 6(1): 13.

Meyer R, Groetch M, Venter C. (2017) When should infants with cow's milk protein allergy use an amino acid formula? A practical guide. *J. Allergy Clin. Immunol. Pract.* 6(2): 383–399.

Miehlke S. (2015) Clinical features of Eosinophilic esophagitis in children and adults. *Best. Pract. Res. Clin. Gastroenterol.* 29(5): 739–748.

Mimouni BA, Mimouni D, Mimouni M, Gdalevich M. (2002) Does breastfeeding protect against allergic rhinitis during childhood? A meta-analysis of prospective studies. *Acta Paediatrica* 91: 275–279.

Mitchell JE, Skypala I. (2013) Aspirin and salicylate in respiratory disease. *Rhinology.* 51: 195–205.

Mittag D, Akkerdaas J, Ballmer-Weber BK, *et al.* (2004) Ara h 8, a Bet v 1-homologous allergen from peanut, is a major allergen in patients with combined birch pollen and peanut allergy. *J. Allergy Clin. Immunol.* 114(6): 1410–1417. Available from: PM:15577846.

Monsbakken KW, Vandvik PO, Farup PG. (2006) Perceived food intolerance in subjects with irritable bowel syndrome – etiology, prevalence and consequences. *Eur. J. Clin. Nutr.* 60(5): 667–672.

Moonesinghe H, Mackenzie H, Venter C, *et al.* (2016) Prevalence of fish and shellfish allergy: A systematic review. *Ann. Allergy Asthma Immunol.* 117: 264–272.

Morrow JD, Margolies GR, Rowland J, *et al.* (1991) Evidence that histamine is the causative toxin of scombroid-fish poisoning. *N. Engl. J. Med.* 324: 716–720.

Mukkada VA, Haas A, Maune NC, *et al.* (2011) Feeding dysfunction in children with eosinophilic gastrointestinal diseases. *Pediatrics.* 126: e672–e677.

Muñoz-García E, Luengo-Sánchez O, Moreno-Pérez N, *et al.* (2017) Lettuce allergy is a lipid transfer syndrome-related food allergy with high risk of severe reactions. *J. Investig. Allergol. Clin. Immunol.* 27(2): 98–103.

Muraro A, Dubois AE, DunnGalvin A, *et al.* (2014a) EAACI food allergy and anaphylaxis guidelines. Food allergy health-related quality of life measures. *Allergy.* 69(7): 845–853.

Muraro A, Halken S, Arshad SH, *et al.* (2014b) EAACI food allergy and anaphylaxis guidelines. Primary prevention of food allergy. *Allergy.* 69(5): 590–601.

Muraro A, Werfel T, Hoffmann-Sommergruber K, *et al.* (2014c) EAACI food allergy and anaphylaxis guidelines: diagnosis and management of food allergy. *Allergy.* 69(8): 1008–1025.

Neuman-Sunshine DL, Eckman JA, Keet CA, *et al.* (2012) The natural history of persistent peanut allergy. *Ann. Allergy Asthma Immunol.* 108: 326–331.

NHS Choices. (2016) *Vitamins and Minerals: Vitamin D.* Available at https://www.nhs.uk/conditions/vitamins-and-minerals/vitamin-d/. Accessed 16 January 2018.

NICE. (2007a) *Clinical Guideline 53: Chronic fatigue syndrome/myalgic encephalomyelitis (or encephalopathy). Diagnosis and management of CFS/ME in adults and children.* Available at http://guidance.nice.org.uk/CG116. Accessed 2 November 2018.

NICE. (2007b) *Clinical Guideline 57: Atopic eczema in under 12s: diagnosis and management.* Available at https://www.nice.org.uk/guidance/cg57. Accessed 2 November 2018.

NICE. (2011) *Clinical Guideline 116: Food allergy in under 19s: assessment and diagnosis.* Available at https://www.nice.org.uk/guidance/CG116. Accessed 2 November 2018.

NICE. (2014) *Cow's milk protein allergy in children.* Available at https://cks.nice.org.uk/cows-milk-protein-allergy-in-children Accessed 28 February 2019.

NICE. (2016a) *Diagnostics Guidance DG24: ImmunoCAP ISAC 112 and Microtest for multiplex allergen testing.* Available at https://www.nice.org.uk/guidance/dg24. Accessed 2 November 2018.

NICE. (2016b) *Quality Standard 118: Food Allergy.* Available at https://www.nice.org.uk/guidance/qs118. Accessed 2 November 2018.

Niggemann B. (2010) When is an oral food challenge positive? *Allergy.* 65(1): 2–6.

Nilsson N, Sjölander S, Baar A. (2015) Wheat allergy in children evaluated with challenge and IgE antibodies to wheat components. *Pediatr. Allergy Immunol.* 26: 119–125.

Noimark L, Gardner J, Warner JO. (2009) Parents' attitudes when purchasing products for children with nut allergy: a UK perspective. *Pediatr. Allergy Immunol.* 20: 500–504.

Nowak-Wegrzyn A, Katz Y, Mehr SS, *et al.* (2015) Non-IgE-mediated gastrointestinal food allergy. *J. Allergy Clin. Immunol.* 135(5): 1114–1124.

Nwaru BI, Hickstein L, Panesar SS, *et al.* (2014) Prevalence of common food allergies in Europe: a systematic review and meta-analysis. *Allergy.* 69: 992–1007.

Nybom H, Cervin-Hoberg C, Andersson M. (2013) Oral challenges with four apple cultivars result in significant differences in oral allergy symptoms. *Int Arch. Allergy Immunol.* 161: 258–264.

Obayashi Y, Nagamura Y. (2016) Does monosodium glutamate really cause headache?: a systematic review of human studies. *J. Headache Pain.* 17: 54.

Osborn DA, Sinn J. (2006) Formulas containing hydrolysed protein for prevention of allergy and food intolerance in infants. *Cochrane Database Syst. Rev.* (4): CD003664.

Osborne NJ, Koplin JJ, Martin PE, et al; HealthNuts Investigators. (2011) Prevalence of challenge-proven IgE-mediated food allergy using population-based sampling and predetermined challenge criteria in infants. *J. Allergy Clin. Immunol.* 127: 668–676.

Osterballe M, Hansen TK, Mortz CG, *et al.* (2005) The prevalence of food hypersensitivity in an unselected population of children and adults. *Pediatr Allergy Immunol.* 16(7): 567–573.

Palmer DJ, Gold MS, Makrides M. (2005) Effect of cooked and raw egg consumption on ovalbumin content of human milk: a randomised, double-blind, cross-over trial. *Clin. Exp. Allergy* 35(2): 173–178.

Parlaman JP, Oron AP, Uspal NG, *et al.* (2016) Emergency and hospital care for food-related anaphylaxis in children. *Hosp. Pediatr.* 6(5): 269–274.

Pascal M, Muñoz-Cano R, Reina Z, *et al.* (2012) Lipid transfer protein syndrome: clinical pattern, cofactor effect and profile of molecular sensitization to plant-foods and pollens. *Clin. Exp. Allergy.* 42(10): 1529–1539.

Patel A, Bahna SL. (2016) Hypersensitivities to sesame and other common edible seeds. *Allergy.* 71: 1405–1413.

Paterson JR, Srivastava R, Baxter GJ, *et al.* (2006) Salicylic acid content of spices and its implications. *J. Agric. Food Chem.* 54: 2891–2896.

Peeters KA, Koppelman SJ, Penninks AH, *et al.* (2009) Clinical relevance of sensitization to lupine in peanut-sensitised adults. *Allergy.* 64(4): 549–555.

Peeters KA, Nordlee JA, Penninks AH, *et al.* (2007) Lupine allergy: not simply cross-reactivity with peanut or soy. *J. Allergy Clin. Immunol.* 120(3): 647–653.

Pelz BJ, Wechsler JB, Amsden K, *et al.* (2016) IgE-associated food allergy alters the presentation of paediatric eosinophilic esophagitis. *Clin. Exp. Allergy* 46(11): 1431–1440.

Pénard-Morand C, Raherison C, Kopferschmitt C, *et al.* (2005) Prevalence of food allergy and its relationship to asthma and allergic rhinitis in schoolchildren. *Allergy.* 60: 1165–1171.

Perkin MR, Logan K, Marrs T, *et al.* (2016a) Enquiring About Tolerance (EAT) study: Feasibility of an early allergenic food introduction regimen. *J. Allergy Clin. Immunol.* 137(5): 1477–1486.

Perkin MR, Logan K, Tseng A, *et al.* (2016b) Randomised trial of introduction of allergenic foods in breastfed infants. *N. Engl. J. Med.* 374(18): 1733–1743.

Peters RL, Allen KJ, Dharmage SC, *et al.* (2015) Natural history of peanut allergy and predictors of resolution in the first 4 years of life: a population-based assessment. *J. Allergy Clin. Immunol.* 135: 1257–1266.e1–2.

Peters RL, Gurrin LC, Allen KJ. (2012) The predictive value of skin prick testing for challenge-proven food allergy: a systematic review. *Pediatr. Allergy Immunol.* 23: 347–352.

Phy JL, Weiss WT, Weiler CR, *et al.* (2003) Hypersensitivity to progesterone-in-oil after in vitro fertilization and embryo transfer. *Fertil. Steril.* 80(5): 1272–1275.

Pieretti MM, Chung D, Pacenza R, *et al.* (2009) Audit of manufactured products: use of allergen advisory labels and identification of labelling ambiguities. *J. Allergy Clin. Immunol.* 124: 337–341.

Pollak CP, Bright D. (2003) Caffeine consumption and weekly sleep patterns in US seventh-, eighth-, and ninth-graders. *Pediatrics.* 111: 42–46.

Pourpak Z, Ghojezadeh L, Mansouri M, *et al.* (2007) Wheat anaphylaxis in children. *Immunol. Invest.* 36(2): 175–182.

Pourpak Z, Mansouri M, Mesdaghi M, *et al.* (2004) Wheat allergy: clinical and laboratory findings. *Int. Arch. Allergy Immunol.* 133(2): 168–173.

Primeau MN, Kagan R, Joseph L, *et al.* (2000) The psychological burden of peanut allergy as perceived by adults with peanut allergy and the parents of peanut-allergic children. *Clin. Exp. Allergy* 30(8): 1135–1143.

Pumphrey RS. (2000) Lessons for management of anaphylaxis from a study of fatal reactions. *Clin. Exp. Allergy.* 30: 1144–1150.

Pumphrey RS, Gowland MH. (2007) Further fatal allergic reactions to food in the United Kingdom, 1999–2006. *J. Allergy. Clin. Immunol.* 119: 1018–1019.

Pumphrey RS, Wilson PB, Faragher EB, *et al.* (1999) Specific immunoglobulin E to peanut, hazelnut and Brazil nut in 731 patients: similar patterns found at all ages. *Clin. Exp. Allergy.* 29: 1256–1259.

Raithel M, Baenkler HW, Naegel A, *et al.* (2005) Significance of salicylate intolerance in diseases of the lower gastrointestinal tract. *J. Physiol. Pharmacol.* 56: 89–102.

Rancé F, Dutau G. (1999) Peanut hypersensitivity in children. *Pediatr. Pulmonol. Suppl.* 18: 165–167.

Rancé F, Juchet A, Brémont F, *et al.* (1997) Correlations between skin prick tests using commercial extracts and fresh foods, specific IgE, and food challenges. *Allergy.* 32: 1031–1035.

Reese G, Ayuso R, Lehrer SB. (1999) Tropomyosin: an invertebrate pan-allergen. *Int. Arch. Allergy Immunol.* 119: 247–258.

Remington BC, Baumert JL, Blom WM, *et al.* (2015) Unintended allergens in precautionary labelled and unlabelled products pose significant risks to UK allergic consumers. *Allergy.* 70: 813–819.

Ring J (2014) Chapter 2, What is Allergy in The Global Atlas of Allergy. (Eds.) Akdis CA & Agache I. Global Atlas of Allergy. European Academy of Allergy and Clinical Immunology. Available at http://www.eaaci.org/GlobalAtlas/GlobalAtlasAllergy.pdf. Accessed 19 November 2018.

Roberts G, Ollert M, Aalberse R, *et al.* (2016) A new framework for the interpretation of IgE sensitization tests. *Allergy.* 71: 1540–1551.

Roberts G, Patel N, Levi-Schaffer F, *et al.* (2003) Food allergy as a risk factor for life-threatening asthma in childhood: a case-controlled study. *J. Allergy. Clin. Immunol.* 112: 168–174.

Robertson ON, Hourihane JO, Remington BC, *et al.* (2013) Survey of peanut levels in selected Irish food products bearing peanut allergen advisory labels. *Food Addit. Contam. Part A Chem. Anal. Control Expo. Risk Assess.* 30(9): 1467–1472.

Röckmann H, van Geel MJ, Knulst AC, *et al.* (2014) Food allergen sensitization pattern in adults in relation to severity of atopic dermatitis. *Clin. Transl. Allergy* 4: 9.

Roe C, Anderson N, Frew A, *et al.* (2016) Recognizing and managing food-dependent exercise-induced anaphylaxis. *Br. J. Hosp. Med. (Lond)* 77(3): 190–191.

Roerdink EM, Flokstra-de Blok BM, Blok JL, *et al.* (2016) Association of food allergy and atopic dermatitis exacerbations. *Ann. Allergy Asthma Immunol.* 116: 334–338.

Rosell-Camps A, Zibetti S, Pérez-Esteban G, *et al.* (2013) Histamine intolerance as a cause of chronic digestive complaints in pediatric patients. *Rev. Esp. Enferm. Dig.* 105: 201–206.

Royal College of Physicians. (2003) *Allergy: The Unmet Needs. Report of a Working Party.* London: RCP.

Salcedo G, Sanchez-Monge R, Diaz-Perales A, *et al.* (2004) Plant non-specific lipid transfer proteins as food and pollen allergens. *Clin. Exp. Allergy.* 34: 1336–1341.

Sampson HA. (2004) Update on food allergy. *J. Allergy. Clin. Immunol.* 113: 805–819.

Sampson HA, Aceves S, Bock SA, *et al.* (2014) Food allergy: a practice parameter update-2014. *J. Allergy Clin. Immunol.* 134: 1016–1025.

Sampson HA, Gerth van WR, Bindslev-Jensen C, *et al.* (2012) Standardizing double-blind, placebo-controlled oral food challenges: American Academy of Allergy, Asthma & Immunology-European Academy of Allergy and Clinical Immunology PRACTALL consensus report. *J. Allergy Clin. Immunol.* 130(6): 1260–1274.

Sampson MA, Munoz-Furlong A, Sicherer SH. (2006) Risk-taking and coping strategies of adolescents and young adults with food allergy. *J. Allergy Clin. Immunol.* 117(6): 1440–1445.

Santos A, Dias A, Pinheiro JA. (2010) Predictive factors for the persistence of cow's milk allergy. *Pediatr. Allergy Immunol.* 21(8): 1127–1134.

Savage JH, Limb SL, Brereton NH, *et al.* (2007) The natural history of peanut allergy: Extending our knowledge beyond childhood. *J. Allergy Clin. Immunol.* 120: 717–719.

Savage JH, Kaeding AJ, Matsui EC, *et al.* (2010) The natural history of soy allergy. *J. Allergy Clin. Immunol.* 125(3): 683–686.

Savage JH, Sicherer S, Wood R. (2016) The natural history of food allergy. *J. Allergy Clin. Immunol. Pract.* 4: 196–203.

Scala E, Alessandri C, Bernardi ML, *et al.* (2010) Cross-sectional survey on immunoglobulin E reactivity in 23077 subjects using an allergenic molecule-based microarray detection system. *Clin. Exp. Allergy.* 40: 911–921.

Schab DW, Trinh NT. (2004) Do artificial food colours promote hyperactivity in children with hyperactive syndromes? A meta-analysis of double-blind placebo-controlled trials. *J. Dev. Behav. Pediatr.* 25: 423–434.

Schäfer T, Bohler E, Ruhdorfer S, *et al.* (2001) Epidemiology of food allergy/food intolerance in adults: associations with other manifestations of atopy. *Allergy.* 56(12): 1172–1179.

Scherf KA, Brockow K, Biedermann T, *et al.* (2016) Wheat-dependent exercise-induced anaphylaxis. *Clin. Exp. Allergy* 46(1): 10–20.

Schoemaker AA, Sprikkelman AB, Grimshaw KE, *et al.* (2015) Incidence and natural history of challenge-proven cow's milk allergy in European children – EuroPrevall birth cohort. *Allergy.* 70(8): 963–972. Available from PM:25864712.

Schoos AM, Chawes BL, Følsgaard NV, *et al.* (2015) Disagreement between skin prick test and specific IgE in young children. *Allergy.* 70: 41–48.

Schulkes KJ, Klemans RJ, Knigge L, *et al.* (2014) Specific IgE to fish extracts does not predict allergy to specific species within an adult fish allergic population. *Clin. Transl. Allergy.* 4: 27.

Sellaturay P, Nasser S, Ewan P. (2015) The incidence and features of systemic reactions to skin prick tests. *Ann. Allergy Asthma Immunol.* 115: 229–233.

Shadick NA, Liang MH, Partridge AJ, *et al.* (1999) The natural history of exercise-induced anaphylaxis: survey results from a 10-year follow-up study. *J. Allergy Clin. Immunol.* 104(1): 123–127.

Shoda T, Futamura M, Yang L, *et al.* (2016) Timing of eczema onset and risk of food allergy at 3 years of age: a hospital-based prospective birth cohort study. *J. Dermatol. Sci.* 84: 144–148.

Sicherer SH, Muñoz-Furlong A, Godbold JH, *et al.* (2010) US prevalence of self-reported peanut, tree nut, and sesame allergy: 11-year follow-up. *J. Allergy Clin. Immunol.* 125: 1322–1326.

Sicherer SH, Noone SA, Muñoz-Furlong A. (2001) The impact of childhood food allergy on quality of life. *Ann. Allergy Asthma Immunol.* 87(6): 461–464.

Sicherer SH, Sampson HA, Burks AW. (2000) Peanut and soy allergy: a clinical and therapeutic dilemma. *Allergy.* 55(6): 515–521.

Skolnick HS, Conover-Walker MK, Koerner CB, *et al.* (2001) The natural history of peanut allergy. *J. Allergy Clin. Immunol.* 107: 367–374.

Skripak JM, Matsui EC, Mudd K, *et al.* (2007) The natural history of IgE-mediated cow's milk allergy. *J. Allergy Clin. Immunol.* 120(5): 1172–1177.

Skypala IJ, Venter C. (2009) *Food Hypersensitivity.* Oxford: Wiley-Blackwell Publishing.

Skypala IJ, Bull S, Deegan K, *et al.* (2013) The prevalence of PFS and prevalence and characteristics of reported food allergy; a survey of UK adults aged 18–75 incorporating a validated PFS diagnostic questionnaire. *Clin. Exp. Allergy.* 43: 928–940.

Skypala IJ, Calderon MA, Leeds AR, *et al.* (2011) Development and validation of a structured questionnaire for the diagnosis of oral allergy syndrome in subjects with seasonal allergic rhinitis during the UK birch pollen season. *Clin. Exp. Allergy* 41(7): 1001–1011.

Skypala IJ, Venter C, Meyer R, *et al.* (2015) The development of a standardised diet history tool to support the diagnosis of food allergy. *Clin. Transl. Allergy* 5: 7.

Slack MA, Ogbogu PU, Phillips G, *et al.* (2015) Serum vitamin D levels in a cohort of adult and pediatric patients with eosinophilic esophagitis. *Ann. Allergy Asthma Immunol.* 115(1): 45–50.

Soares-Weiser K, Takwoingi Y, Panesar SS, *et al.* (2014) The diagnosis of food allergy: a systematic review and meta-analysis. *Allergy.* 69(1): 76–86.

Stutius LM, Sheehan WJ, Rangsithienchai P, *et al.* (2010) Characterizing the relationship between sesame, coconut, and nut allergy in children. *Pediatr. Allergy. Immunol.* 21: 1114–1118.

Sugiura K, Sugiura M. (2010) Soy sauce allergy. *J. Eur. Acad. Dermatol. Venereol.* 24(7): 852–855.

Sutton BJ, Gould HJ. (1993) The human IgE network. *Nature.* 366: 421–428.

Szepfalusi Z, Ebner C, Pandjaitan R, *et al.* (1994) Egg yolk alpha-livetin (chicken serum albumin) is a cross-reactive allergen in the bird-egg syndrome. *J. Allergy Clin. Immunol.* 93(5): 932–942.

Tan JA, Smith WB. (2014) Non-IgE-mediated gastrointestinal food hypersensitivity syndrome in adults. *J. Allergy Clin. Immunol. Pract.* 2: 355–357.

Tariq SM, Matthews SM, Hakim EA, *et al.* (2000) Egg allergy in infancy predicts respiratory allergic disease by 4 years of age. *Pediatr. Allergy Immunol.* 11(3): 162–167.

Taylor SL, Bush RK, Nordlee JA. (2003) Sulfites. In: Metcalfe DD, Sampson HJ, Simon RA (eds) *Food Allergy: Adverse Reactions to Foods and Food Additives.* Oxford: Blackwell Publishing Ltd, pp. 324–341.

Taylor SL, Baumert JL. (2017) Allergenicity of Soybean Lecithin. Institute of Agriculture and Natural Resources: Food Allergy Research and Resource Program. Available at https://farrp.unl.edu/soy-lecithin. Accessed 19 November 2018.

Tejedor-Alonso MA, Moro-Moro M, Mosquera González M, *et al.* (2015) Increased incidence of admissions for anaphylaxis in Spain 1998–2011. *Allergy.* 70: 880–883.

Teodorowicz M, Terlouw RJ, Jansen A, *et al.* (2016) Immunological characterization of Dutch sesame seed-allergic patients. *Int. Arch. Allergy Immunol.* 169: 13–22.

Tewari A, Meyer R, Fisher H, *et al.* (2006) Soy milk and allergy: indications and contraindications. *Curr. Allergy Clin. Immunol.* 19(3): 126–128.

Thalayasingam M, Gerez IF, Yap GC, et al. (2015). Clinical and immunochemical profiles of food challenge proven or anaphylactic shrimp allergy in tropical Singapore. *Clin Exp Allergy.* 45(3):687–697.

Thomassen RA, Kvammen JA, Eskerud MB, *et al.* (2016) Iodine status and growth in 0-2-year-old infants with cow's milk protein allergy. *J. Pediatr. Gastroenterol. Nutr.* 64(5): 806–811.

Tsakok T, Marrs T, Mohsin M, *et al.* (2016) Does atopic dermatitis cause food allergy? A systematic review. *J. Allergy Clin. Immunol.* 137: 1071–1078.

Turjanmaa K, Darsow U, Niggemann B, *et al.* (2006) EAACI/GA-2LEN position paper: present status of the atopy patch test. *Allergy.* 61: 1377–1384.

Turner PJ, Mehr S, Sayers R, *et al.* (2014) Loss of allergenic proteins during boiling explains tolerance to boiled peanut in peanut allergy. *J. Allergy Clin. Immunol.* 134: 751–753.

Turner PJ, Gowland MH, Sharma V, *et al.* (2015) Increase in anaphylaxis-related hospitalizations but no increase in fatalities: an analysis of United Kingdom national anaphylaxis data, 1992–2012. *J. Allergy Clin. Immunol.* 135(4): 956–963.

Umasunthar T, Leonardi-Bee J, Turner PJ, *et al.* (2015) Incidence of food anaphylaxis in people with food allergy: a systematic review and meta-analysis. *Clin. Exp. Allergy* 45(11): 1621–1636.

Valentine AZ, Knibb RC. (2011) Exploring quality of life in families of children living with and without a severe food allergy. *Appetite.* 57(2): 467–474.

Vally H, Misso NL. (2012) Adverse reactions to the sulphite additives. *Gastroenterol. Hepatol. Bed. Bench.* 5: 16–23.

van der Valk JP, Gerth van Wijk R, Hoorn E, *et al.* (2016) Measurement and interpretation of skin prick test results. *Clin. Transl. Allergy.* 6: 8.

van der Velde JL, Flokstra-de Blok BM, de Groot H, *et al.* (2012) Food allergy-related quality of life after double-blind, placebo-controlled food challenges in adults, adolescents, and children. *J. Allergy Clin. Immunol.* 130(5): 1136–1143.

van Kampen V, de Blay F, Folletti I, *et al.* (2013) EAACI position paper: skin prick testing in the diagnosis of occupational type I allergies. *Allergy.* 68: 580–584.

van Veen LN, Heron M, Batstra M, *et al.* (2016) The diagnostic value of component-resolved diagnostics in peanut allergy in children attending a Regional Paediatric Allergology Clinic. *BMC Pediatr.* 16: 74.

Vandenplas Y, Koletzko S, Isolauri E, *et al.* (2007) Guidelines for the diagnosis and management of cow's milk protein allergy in infants. *Arch. Dis. Child* 92(10): 902–908.

Vassallo MF, Camargo CA Jr. (2010) Potential mechanisms for the hypothesised link between sunshine, vitamin D, and food allergy in children. *J. Allergy Clin. Immunol.* 126(2): 217–222.

Vassilopoulou E, Douladiris N, Sakellariou A, *et al.* (2010) Evaluation and standardisation of different matrices used for double-blind placebo-controlled food challenges to fish. *J. Hum. Nutr. Diet.* 23(5): 544–549.

Venter C, Groetch M. (2014) Nutritional management of food protein-induced enterocolitis syndrome. *Curr. Opin. Allergy Clin. Immunol.* 14: 255–262.

Venter C, Meyer R. (2010) Allergic disease: the challenges of managing food hypersensitivity. *Proc. Nutr. Soc.* 69(1): 11–24.

Venter C, Brown T, Meyer R, *et al.* (2017) Better recognition, diagnosis and management of non-IgE-mediated cow's milk allergy in infancy: iMAP-an international interpretation of the MAP (Milk Allergy in Primary Care) guideline. *Clin. Transl. Allergy* 7: 26.

Venter C, Brown T, Shah N, *et al.* (2013) Diagnosis and management of non-IgE-mediated cow's milk allergy in infancy – a UK primary care practical guide. *Clin. Transl. Allergy.* 3(1): 23.

Venter C, Maslin K, Arshad SH, *et al.* (2016) Very low prevalence of IgE-mediated wheat allergy and high levels of cross-sensitisation between grass and wheat in a UK birth cohort. *Clin. Transl. Allergy* 6: 22.

Venter C, Pereira B, Voigt K, *et al.* (2007) Comparison of open and double-blind placebo-controlled food challenges in diagnosis of food hypersensitivity amongst children. *J. Hum. Nutr. Diet.* 20(6): 565–579.

Venter C, Vlieg-Boerstra BJ, Carling A. (2009) The diagnosis of food hypersensitivity. In: Skypala I, Venter C (eds) *Food Hypersensitivity*, 1st edn. Oxford: Blackwell Publishing, pp. 85–103.
Vereda A, van Hage M, Ahlstedt S, *et al.* (2011) Peanut allergy: clinical and immunologic differences among patients from 3 different geographic regions. *J. Allergy Clin. Immunol.* 127: 603–607.
Versluis A, Knulst AC, Kruizinga AG, *et al.* (2015) Frequency, severity and causes of unexpected allergic reactions to food: a systematic literature review. *Clin. Exp. Allergy.* 45: 347–367.
Vierk KA, Koehler KM, Fein SB, *et al.* (2007) Prevalence of self-reported food allergy in American adults and use of food labels. *J. Allergy Clin. Immunol.* 119(6): 1504–1510.
Vila L, Beyer K, Järvinen KM, *et al.* (2001) Role of conformational and linear epitopes in the achievement of tolerance in cow's milk allergy. *Clin. Exp. Allergy.* 31(10): 1599–1606.
Vlieg-Boerstra BJ, Bijleveld CM, van der Heide S, *et al.* (2004) Development and validation of challenge materials for double-blind, placebo-controlled food challenges in children. *J. Allergy Clin. Immunol.* 113(2): 341–346.
Vocks E, Borga A, Szliska C, *et al.* (1993) Common allergenic structures in hazelnut, rye grain, sesame seeds, kiwi, and poppy seeds. *Allergy.* 48: 168–172.
Voltolini S, Pellegrini S, Contatore M, *et al.* (2014) New risks from ancient food dyes: cochineal red allergy. *Eur. Ann. Allergy Clin. Immunol.* 46: 232–233.
von Berg A, Filipiak-Pittroff B, Kramer U, *et al.* (2013) Allergies in high-risk schoolchildren after early intervention with cow's milk protein hydrolysates: 10-year results from the German Infant Nutritional Intervention (GINI) study. *J. Allergy Clin. Immunol.* 131(6): 1565–1573.
von Berg A, Filipiak-Pittroff B, Schulz H, *et al.* (2016) Allergic manifestation 15 years after early intervention with hydrolyzed formulas – the GINI Study. *Allergy.* 71(2): 210–219.
Wagner S, Breiteneder H. (2002) The latex-fruit syndrome. *Biochem. Soc. Trans.* 30: 935–940.
Wainstein BK, Saad RA. (2015) Repeat oral food challenges in peanut and tree nut allergic children with a history of mild/moderate reactions. *Asia Pac. Allergy.* 5: 170–176.
Wang SS, Hon KL, Kong AP, *et al.* (2014) Vitamin D deficiency is associated with diagnosis and severity of childhood atopic dermatitis. *Pediatr. Allergy Immunol.* 25(1): 30–35.
Weiss ST, Litonjua AA. (2016) Can we prevent childhood asthma before birth? Summary of the VDAART results so far. *Expert. Rev. Respir. Med.* 10(10): 1039–1040.
Werfel T, Asero R, Ballmer-Weber BK, *et al.* (2015) Position paper of the EAACI: food allergy due to immunological cross-reactions with common inhalant allergens. *Allergy.* 70: 1079–1090.
Werfel T, Ballmer-Weber B, Eigenmann PA, *et al.* (2007) Eczematous reactions to food in atopic eczema: position paper of the EAACI and GA2LEN. *Allergy.* 62: 723–728.
Westwood M, Ramaekers B, Lang S, *et al.* (2016) ImmunoCAP® ISAC and Microtest for multiplex allergen testing in people with difficult to manage allergic disease: a systematic review and cost analysis. *Health Technol. Assess.* 20: 1–178.
WHO. (2002) *Guiding principles for complementary feeding of the breastfed child.* Available at http://www.who.int/maternal_child_adolescent/documents/a85622/en/. Accessed 5 January 2018.
Wjst M. (2012) Is vitamin D supplementation responsible for the allergy pandemic? *Curr. Opin. Allergy Clin. Immunol.* 12(3): 257–262.
Wöhrl S, Hemmer W, Focke M, *et al.* (2004) Histamine intolerance-like symptoms in healthy volunteers after oral provocation with liquid histamine. *Allergy Asthma Proc.* 25: 305–311.
Worm M, Grünhagen J, Dölle S. (2016) (Food-induced anaphylaxis – data from the anaphylaxis registry). *Bundesgesundheitsblatt Gesundheitsforschung Gesundheitsschutz.* 59(7): 836–840.
Worm M, Eckermann O, Dolle S, *et al.* (2014) Triggers and treatment of anaphylaxis: an analysis of 4,000 cases from Germany, Austria and Switzerland. *Dtsch. Arztebl. Int.* 111(21): 367–375.
Wright, T. Meyer, R. (2009) Dietary management: milk and eggs. In: Skypala I, Venter C (eds) *Food Hypersensitivity*. Oxford: Blackwell Publishing Ltd, pp. 117–128.
Wuthrich B, Schmid A, Walther B, *et al.* (2005) Milk consumption does not lead to mucus production or occurrence of asthma. *J. Am. Coll. Nutr.* 24(6): 547S–555S.
Yang TY, Kuo HT, Chen HJ, *et al.* (2015) Increased risk of chronic fatigue syndrome following atopy: a population-based study. *Medicine (Baltimore).* 94: e1211.
Yang WH, Purchase EC. (1985) Adverse reactions to sulfites. *CMAJ.* 133: 865–867.
Yang MS, Lee SH, Kim TW, *et al.* (2008) Epidemiologic and clinical features of anaphylaxis in Korea. *Ann. Allergy Asthma Immunol.* 100(1): 31–36.
Yepes-Nunez JJ, Fiocchi A, Pawankar R, *et al.* (2016) World Allergy Organization – McMaster University Guidelines for Allergic Disease Prevention (GLAD-P): Vitamin D. *World Allergy Organ J.* 9: 17.
Young E, Patel S, Stoneham M, *et al.* (1987) The prevalence of reaction to food additives in a survey population. *J. R. Coll. Physicians. Lond.* 21: 241–247.
Young E, Stoneham MD, Petruckevitch A, *et al.* (1994) A population study of food intolerance. *Lancet* 343(8906): 1127–1130.
Zak DL, Keeney PG. (1976) Changes in cocoa proteins during ripening of fruit, fermentation and further processing of cocoa beans. *J. Agric. Food. Chem.* 24: 483–486.
Zeiger RS, Sampson HA, Bock SA, *et al.* (1999) Soy allergy in infants and children with IgE-associated cow's milk allergy. *J. Pediatr.* 134(5): 614–622.
Ziska LH, Beggs PJ. (2012) Anthropogenic climate change and allergen exposure: The role of plant biology. *J. Allergy Clin. Immunol.* 129: 27–32.
Zuberbier T, Aberer W, Asero R, *et al.* (2014) The EAACI/GA(2) LEN/EDF/WAO guideline for the definition, classification, diagnosis, and management of urticaria: the 2013 revision and update. *Allergy.* 69(7): 868–887.
Zuberbier T, Edenharter G, Worm M, *et al.* (2004) Prevalence of adverse reactions to food in Germany – a population study. *Allergy.* 59(3): 338–345.
Zutavern A, Brockow I, Schaaf B, *et al.* (2008) Timing of solid food introduction in relation to eczema, asthma, allergic rhinitis, and food and inhalant sensitization at the age of 6 years: results from the prospective birth cohort study LISA. *Pediatrics* 121: e44–e52.

7.11.3 Human immunodeficiency virus (HIV)

Karen Klassen

Key points

- Good nutritional status is important for a healthy immune system.
- Human immunodeficiency virus (HIV) disease can present with a variety of nutritional problems.
- Nutritional interventions for people with HIV can include management of weight loss, micronutrient deficiencies, gastrointestinal complaints and metabolic conditions, such as dyslipidaemia, insulin resistance and osteoporosis.

The nutritional status of people with human immunodeficiency virus (HIV) remains an important part of the medical management of HIV care worldwide. Both overnutrition and undernutrition can have important consequences for the health and well-being of patients. Although weight loss is much less common since the availability of effective antiretroviral therapy (ART), it can still occur, particularly in those who are food insecure. Even small amounts of unintentional weight loss may increase the risk of morbidity and mortality. In juxtaposition to this is the rapidly increasing occurrence of obesity and metabolic complications. The combination of HIV infection, ART and lifestyle factors are contributing to the increased risk of cardiovascular disease (CVD) and events, diabetes and osteoporosis. Good nutrition is important for the prevention and management of all these problems, and is therefore crucial in the HIV setting. The aims of dietetic intervention and nutritional care of people with HIV (PWHIV) include:

- Maintaining or achieving a healthy weight.
- Promoting a well-balanced diet to optimise macronutrient and micronutrient status.
- Preventing or managing malnutrition and opportunistic infections.
- Preventing foodborne illness.
- Improving and supporting quality of life.
- Increasing nutrition self-management skills for PWHIV and/or their carers.

The outcomes of achieving these aims can be:

- Decreasing hospitalisations, emergency room visits, morbidity and mortality, and cost of care.
- Decreasing or delaying invasive or expensive treatments by providing early, appropriate nutrition interventions.
- Improving tolerance and adherence to medications.
- Preventing or managing metabolic and morphological comorbidities.

The HIV virus was isolated and identified as responsible for acquired immune deficiency syndrome (AIDS) in 1983. HIV infection does not immediately cause AIDS; however, it grows in CD4 T-cells, a subset of lymphocytes, and causes them to decrease in most instances, although the rate of decline will vary among individuals. The first antiretroviral medicine for HIV was zidovudine (also known as AZT), which became available in 1987. Since then, the development and availability of other ART has been rapidly evolving.

In 2015, it was estimated that 36.7 million people were living with HIV infection worldwide. Just over half of all adults are women; also, 1.8 million children live with HIV, and a further 16.6 million have been orphaned due to AIDS. The rate of new HIV infections has continued to decrease, and the number of people on ART has increased from 2010 to 2015 (UNAIDS, 2016). In the UK, as a direct result of reduced mortality and improved life expectancy (May *et al.*, 2011), the number of people living with HIV is increasing. New diagnoses of HIV in the UK remain relatively stable at around 6000 people per year, and new diagnoses among men who have sex with men (MSM) remains high (54% of new diagnoses). A small proportion of individuals were infected through injecting drugs (2%), with only one individual acquiring HIV through mother-to-child transmission in the UK. In 2015, the average age of people accessing HIV care in the UK was 45 (compared with 39 in 2006) (Kirwan *et al.*, 2016). For current data, and to understand the demographic characteristics, see PHE (2017).

Diagnosis and disease classification

Diagnosis of HIV is based on detecting anti-HIV antibodies in the serum. The enzyme-linked immunosorbent antibody (ELISA) test, also known as enzyme immunoassay (EIA), was the first HIV test to be widely used; other HIV tests are now available. Most people will develop detectable levels of antibodies within 3 months of acquiring HIV. If an HIV test is positive, the most common secondary tests are CD4 T-cell count and HIV RNA (viral load). The CD4 T-cell count is a reliable indicator of the risk of acquiring opportunistic infections, and is monitored over time. Viral load is the amount of virus in the peripheral blood and is used as a surrogate marker of viral replication rate. These are also used as markers to evaluate the effectiveness of ART. These markers are strongly associated with clinical response; however, they should be interpreted along with an individual's clinical condition (Gazzard *et al.*, 2008).

Table 7.11.10 CDC classification system for HIV-infected adults and adolescents

CD4 cell category	Clinical category		
	A Asymptomatic, acute HIV or PGL	B Symptomatic conditions, not A or C	C AIDS indicator conditions
≥500 cells/μL	A1	B1	C1
200–499 cells/μL	A2	B2	C2
<200 cells/μL	A3	B3	C3

Patients in shaded categories are considered to have AIDS.
PGL, persistent generalised lymphadenopathy.

HIV disease staging and classification systems have been developed by the Centers for Disease Control (CDC) in the USA (Castro *et al.*, 1993) and the World Health Organization (WHO, 2007). These staging systems are used to track and monitor the HIV epidemic, as well as to provide clinicians and patients with information about HIV disease stage and clinical management. The WHO system can be used in resource-constrained settings, where access to CD4 cell counts or other laboratory parameters is not available. The CDC disease staging system was developed in 1986 and most recently revised in 1993, and it assesses the severity of HIV disease by CD4 cell count and the presence of specific HIV-related conditions (Table 7.11.10).

Category B symptomatic conditions

These are symptomatic conditions occurring in an HIV-infected adolescent or adult that meet at least one of the following criteria including, but not limited to, the following:

- Bacillary angiomatosis.
- Oropharyngeal candidiasis (thrush).
- Vulvovaginal candidiasis, persistent or resistant.
- Pelvic inflammatory disease (PID).
- Cervical dysplasia (moderate or severe) or cervical carcinoma in situ.
- Hairy leucoplakia, oral.
- Herpes zoster (shingles), involving two or more episodes or at least one dermatome.
- Idiopathic thrombocytopenic purpura.
- Constitutional symptoms, such as fever (>38.5 °C) or diarrhoea lasting >1 month.
- Peripheral neuropathy.

Category C AIDS indicator conditions

These include:

- Bacterial pneumonia, recurrent (two or more episodes in 12 months).
- Candidiasis of the bronchi, trachea or lungs.
- Candidiasis, oesophageal.
- Cervical carcinoma, invasive, confirmed by biopsy.
- Coccidioidomycosis, disseminated or extrapulmonary.
- Cryptococcosis, extrapulmonary.
- Cryptosporidiosis, chronic intestinal (>1 month in duration).
- Cytomegalovirus disease (other than the liver, spleen or nodes).
- Encephalopathy, HIV related.
- Herpes simplex: chronic ulcers (>1 month in duration), or bronchitis, pneumonitis or oesophagitis.
- Histoplasmosis, disseminated or extrapulmonary.
- Isosporiasis, chronic intestinal (>1 month duration).
- Kaposi sarcoma.
- Lymphoma, Burkitt's, immunoblastic or primary central nervous system.
- *Mycobacterium avium* complex (MAC) or *Mycobacterium kansasii*, disseminated or extrapulmonary.
- *Mycobacterium tuberculosis*, pulmonary or extrapulmonary.
- *Mycobacterium*, other species or unidentified species, disseminated or extrapulmonary.
- *Pneumocystis jiroveci* (formerly *P. carinii*) pneumonia (PCP).
- Progressive multifocal leukoencephalopathy (PML).
- *Salmonella* septicaemia, recurrent (non-typhoid).
- Toxoplasmosis of brain.
- Wasting syndrome caused by HIV (involuntary weight loss of >10% of baseline body weight) associated with either chronic diarrhoea (two or more loose stools/day for ≥1 month) or chronic weakness and documented fever for 1 month or longer.

Clinical investigation and management

There is no cure for HIV as such, but treatment is available to manage the condition. Life expectancy in people treated for HIV infection has increased following the availability and widespread use of ART; however, it still appears to be shorter than that of the general population (May *et al.*, 2011). If treatment is started early and as prescribed, overall health and life expectancy are greatly improved. However, in the UK in 2015, 39% of adults were diagnosed with HIV at a late stage of infection (CD4 counts <350 cells/mm^3 within 3 months of diagnosis). Treatment options have improved greatly over recent years; complex regimens with many side effects are being replaced with just one or two pills once or twice a day. Someone who is diagnosed now will have a different experience from someone who has been living with HIV for some time and gone through many different treatment options. Some people suffer side effects with ART, including nausea, diarrhoea, fatigue and headaches, especially in the first few weeks after starting treatment. Other side effects can include metabolic diseases (see the following section 'Metabolic complications with nutritional consequences and/or causes'), peripheral neuropathy, lactic acidosis, pancreatitis, mitochondrial toxicity and hepatotoxicity. In some cases, treatment may cause changes in body shape, depression and mental health issues. Other people find that they are able to lead a very healthy life with HIV and may not suffer the same side effects. In addition to managing medications and its side effects, social care, peer support and counselling are all important forms of support for PWHIV.

The British HIV Association recommends that PWHIV be given the opportunity to be involved in making decisions about their treatment, and that all PWHIV be offered ART (Waters *et al.*, 2016). The guidelines provide the rationale for treatment with antiretroviral drugs as follows:

- Preservation of specific anti-HIV immune responses that would otherwise be lost, and which are associated with long-term non-progression in untreated individuals.
- Reduction in morbidity associated with high viraemia and CD4 depletion during acute infection.
- Reduction in the risk of onward transmission of HIV.

There are many different classes of antiretroviral drugs, each targeting the virus at different stages of its life cycle (Figure 7.11.6). Each country has a slightly different list of currently available ART, which is constantly changing. To keep up to date with ART, periodically check your country's ART list by the following means:

- National HIV association's websites (such as BHIVA.org in the UK; also, the BHIVA app is available).
- Talking to a pharmacist.
- Following reputable HIV organisations on Twitter (such as aidmsmap.com in the UK).

For further reading on the pharmacology and use of ART, see Chen *et al.* (2007).

Public health aspects and prevention

Transmission

The HIV virus is found in the blood and other body fluids, such as semen, vaginal fluid and breast milk; the virus does not survive for long outside the body. The most common form of transmission is through sexual contact, but it can also be transmitted through sharing needles, and from mother to child via breastfeeding or during delivery. Occupational HIV transmission is extremely rare, but if you have had a needlestick injury or have in some way exchanged bodily fluids with your patient, talk to your clinic's nurses and follow the local procedures. By avoiding shaking hands with PWHIV, or completing anthropometric assessments on them because you are concerned about HIV transmission, you are unfairly discriminating against your patients and have no evidence to support this discrimination (see the following section, Stigma).

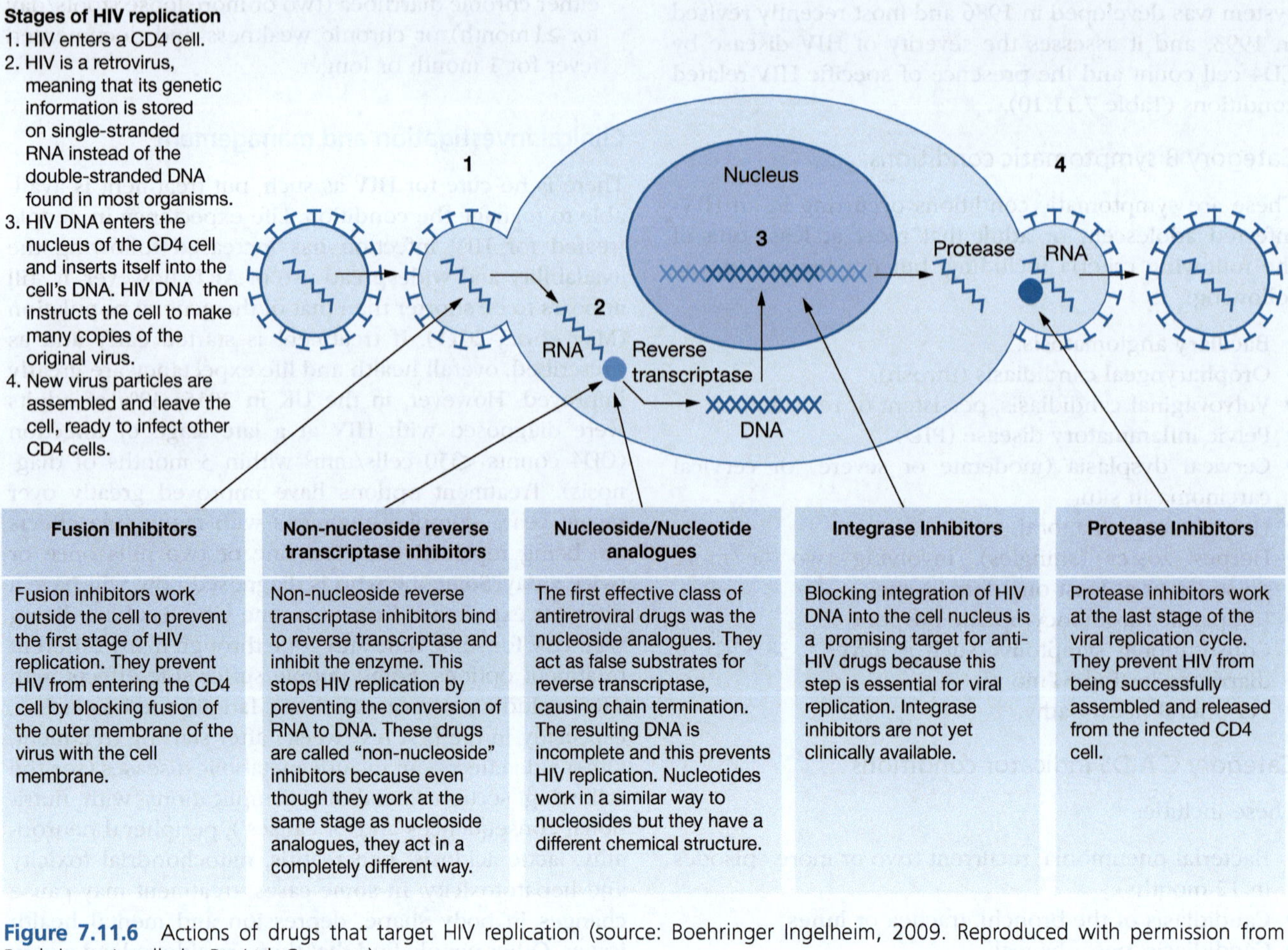

Figure 7.11.6 Actions of drugs that target HIV replication (source: Boehringer Ingelheim, 2009. Reproduced with permission from Boehringer Ingelheim Pty Ltd, Germany)

Stigma

AIDS-related stigma and discrimination refer to prejudice, negative attitudes, abuse and maltreatment directed at people living with HIV/AIDS (AVERT). Examples of this include being shunned by family, peers and the wider community; poor treatment in healthcare and education settings; an erosion of rights; and psychological damage. These can negatively affect the success of HIV testing and treatment. Although the awareness and understanding of HIV have improved in the UK over the past decade, stigma and discrimination still exist and can come from family, friends and healthcare workers. It is estimated that one-quarter of people infected with HIV in the UK are unaware of their diagnosis (Health Protection Agency, 2010). As a healthcare professional, it is essential to understand how HIV is transmitted, to use universal precautions with all patients, and to demonstrate non-judgemental attitudes towards all patients.

Nutritional assessment

Nutritional assessment of PWHIV may vary depending on the reason for referral and the individual's clinical condition. This section will highlight aspects of nutritional assessment that are specific to working with patients with HIV.

Anthropometry and related tests

Taking anthropometric measurements requires training and practice, but is a valuable skill. Several HIV guidance documents recommend anthropometry when starting ART, and annually thereafter (Asboe *et al.*, 2011; Lundgren *et al.*, 2008). Using a variety of anthropometric measurements (Table 7.11.11) is helpful in order to more accurately assess fat distribution changes and muscle mass changes. Fat-free mass (FFM) and fat mass can be lower in PWHIV, particularly in those not on ART (Fields-Gardner *et al.*, 2010). Studies evaluating anthropometry with gold standard measurements have found that anthropometry measurements correlated well with magnetic resonance imaging (MRI) (Scherzer *et al.*, 2008). Furthermore, simple anthropometric measurements, such as mid-arm muscle circumference and mid-thigh muscle circumference, were associated with health risk indicators almost as strongly as MRI-based measures.

In addition to anthropometric measurements, physical examination can provide additional evidence of nutritional status. Physical signs of malnutrition can include:

- Easily plucked or falling out hair.
- Poor skin pallor or turgor; or dry, flaky, scaly skin.
- Scooped or cracking nails.

Table 7.11.11 Anthropometric and related assessments of individuals with HIV infection

Measurements	Assessment
Anthropometry	
Weight	Overall nutritional status; however, must be interpreted in individuals with caution, and with a view to evaluating other aspects of body composition.
BMI	Good marker of nutritional status in populations; can determine if overweight, obese or underweight; interpret with caution in individuals.
Waist circumference	A good correlate of visceral fat and an indicator of metabolic syndrome. Can also be used to measure fluid changes due to ascites.
Mid-upper arm circumference	Reflection of muscle and subcutaneous fat stores; can compare with reference values and evaluate changes over time.
Triceps skinfold	Subcutaneous fat stores; can compare with reference values and serial changes in an individual.
Mid-arm muscle circumference	A good marker of lean body mass; useful in assessing changes in individuals, particularly for inpatients who cannot be weighed.
Hip circumference	On its own, can reflect buttock muscle and fat stores and can be monitored serially in individuals.
Waist-to-hip ratio	Use with reference values, but interpret in light of potential fat loss from lipoatrophy.
Other skinfold measurements	Can be used to assess overall subcutaneous fat and estimate total body fat percentage.
Other measurements	
Bioelectrical impedance analysis	Low phase angles have been shown to be of prognostic relevance in HIV-infected patients (Kyle *et al.*, 2004); however, they are not able to detect changes in body shape, nor should they be used to evaluate fat atrophy (Schwenk *et al.*, 2001). Can measure body cell mass, which is a component of some definitions of HIV-related wasting (see Table 7.11.13).
Handgrip strength	A measure of muscle strength and function; correlates well with nutritional status; however, interpret with caution as reference values are limited, and consider factors such as mood, mobility and peripheral neuropathy.

- Muscle wasting and weakness (can be visually determined by looking at the following muscles: temporalis, deltoids, biceps, quadriceps).
- Oedema.
- Loss of fat stores can be easily seen by looking at the fat pads under the eyes and by pinching (lightly) the skin behind the triceps.

Biochemical and haematological tests

Biochemistry and haematology assessment will depend on the patient's clinical condition and varies widely as patients with HIV present with a variety of clinical needs (Table 7.11.12).

Table 7.11.12 Laboratory markers used in PWHIV

Markers	Used to assess
Plasma/serum markers	
Urea	Hydration status, renal function (usually measured in an inpatient setting).
Creatinine	Renal function (also useful to calculate estimated glomerular filtration rate) (Labarga *et al.*, 2010).
Potassium	Can be low in poor nutritional states and high in chronic renal disease.
Phosphate	Measure of phosphate intake; however, hypophosphataemia is very common in PWHIV infection (Assadi, 2010), and needs to be interpreted in view of dietary intake, malabsorption, vitamin D deficiency and, importantly, tubular renal losses, most commonly due to ART and hyperparathyroidism. A fractional excretion of phosphate will help determine the cause of hypophosphataemia.
Liver function tests (LFTs)	Increased LFTs can be an indicator of liver function, especially considering the high prevalence of coinfection with hepatitis B and C; however, if only alkaline phosphatase is raised, it may be due to increased bone turnover and/or vitamin D deficiency.
CD4 T-cell count	See the section 'Diagnosis and disease classification'.
Viral load	See the section 'Diagnosis and disease classification'.
Albumin	Indicator of visceral protein status and related to inflammatory states, e.g. difficult to assess in cases of liver disease and acute infection. It is also an indicator of disease state and mortality. Can be low in malabsorption and states of protein loss.
Vitamin B_{12}, folate	Low in macrocytic anaemia, can be related to low dietary intakes or other causes.
Ferritin transferrin saturation, total iron binding capacity, etc.	Low in microcytic anaemia, can be related to low dietary intakes or other causes.
Zinc, selenium	Need to be interpreted with caution in inflammatory states (see the section 'Micronutrient deficiencies' in the following text).
Calcium	Plasma levels are bound to plasma proteins (such as albumin) and are tightly regulated, so are not a good reflector of dietary calcium intake.
Vitamin D (25-hydroxyvitamin D), parathyroid hormone (PTH)	Vitamin D deficiency can be diagnosed by measuring 25(OH)D and is common in HIV as it is in many other individuals. Vitamin D deficiency or dietary calcium deficiency can result in secondary hyperparathyroidism.
Other fat-soluble vitamins	Can be useful to measure in patients with fat malabsorption.
Hormones: testosterone, oestradiol, thyroid	Measured to rule out secondary causes of wasting and low bone mineral density.
Fasting lipids (total cholesterol, HDL, LDL, triglycerides)	Use local reference values and national guidelines for target levels.
Fasting glucose	Increased fasting or random glucose should warrant an oral glucose tolerance test to rule out diabetes, impaired glucose tolerance or impaired fasting glucose. It has been suggested that fasting insulin and glucose should be routinely measured, and HOMA-IR calculated, particularly in those at highest risk, such as those with metabolic syndrome, obesity, lipodystrophy or a longer exposure to antiretrovirals (Gianotti *et al.*, 2011).
Urine markers	
Protein: creatinine	Reflects renal protein loss and is more sensitive than a dipstick test. Should be measured annually in all patients on ART.
Fractional excretion of phosphate (FePi)	FePi = (urine phosphate × serum creatinine × 100)/(serum phosphate × urine creatinine). This should be done fasting and can be used to determine whether hypophosphataemia is a result of renal losses or inadequate dietary intake/reduced gastrointestinal absorption.
Faecal markers	
1-alpha antitrypsin	A protein synthesised in the liver that is neither actively secreted nor absorbed. Use with serum levels to determine clearance in order to help diagnose protein-losing enteropathy if indicated (Umar & DiBaise, 2010).
Pancreatic elastase	Used to determine exocrine pancreatic function that may result in fat malabsorption and diarrhoea.

Clinical assessment

Clinical assessment will include:

- Current medications (including side effects) and medication history.
- Use of supplements, vitamins, herbs and over-the-counter medicines.
- Current medical status (opportunistic infections and comorbid conditions) and medical history.
- Blood pressure.
- Appetite, nausea, vomiting, early satiety, chewing and swallowing difficulties (note dentition).
- Bowel history (including frequency and consistency) and other changes in gastrointestinal function. Gastrointestinal complaints are common in PWHIV and can sometimes be overlooked, especially in people who are reluctant to talk about their bowels or who do not look inside the toilet before flushing.
- Use risk calculators to calculate 10-year risk of CVD (e.g. www.patient.co.uk/doctor/Primary-Cardiovascular-Risk-Calculator.htm) or 10-year risk of fracture (www.shef.ac.uk/FRAX/) when indicated.

Dietary assessment

Dietary assessment can include:

- A record of dietary intake and food patterns:
    - Depending on the reason for referral, a variety of dietary history tools may be employed, e.g. 24-hour recall, food frequency questionnaire and usual intake pattern.
    - A recall of usual intake in 24 hours is also a good way to check medication adherence.
- Food allergies and intolerances.
- Other lifestyle factors should be included as a part of the dietary assessment:
    - Alcohol intake (Williams *et al.*, 2016).
    - Smoking (history and frequency).
    - Substance abuse (history and frequency).
    - Eating out.
    - Erratic meal patterns.
- Nutritional knowledge.
- Behaviour change assessment (intentions, attitudes, subjective norms, etc.).

Economic and social assessment

People living with HIV come from varied socioeconomic and ethnic backgrounds, and individual assessment is crucial. Bear in mind when you are assessing these factors that you may encounter information that is outside your scope as a dietitian. Get to know the local services, so that you can practice within your competencies and refer your patients, which will ensure that they receive the best care possible. Factors to consider include the following:

- Psychosocial factors – depression, substance abuse, dementia and other psychiatric problems that may impede appetite or the ability to prepare meals.
- Educational factors – consider basic understanding of bodily functions and key nutritional principles (i.e. food literacy).
- Living environment – homelessness, bed and breakfast rooms, access to a stove or refrigerator. Asking patients about their living environment and available cooking and food storage equipment is important for providing the appropriate nutritional advice.
- Financial factors – poverty is a common problem, and can be cyclical. Major drivers of poverty among PWHIV include:
    - Immigration system.
    - Insufficient benefits.
    - Poor physical or mental health.
    - Unemployment.
    - Inadequate housing.
    - Responsibility for children.
- Food insecurity is associated with lower CD4 cell counts and could be a potential barrier to optimal immune recovery in PWHIV (Aibibula *et al.*, 2016). In the UK, the Terence Higgins Trust and National AIDS Trust provide support to many PWHIV living in poverty.
- Functional status – the ability to shop and prepare food. Other comorbidities and/or side effects, such as peripheral neuropathy and severe weight loss, will affect energy levels and the ability to prepare food and carry shopping bags. In addition to social services, some HIV charities can provide assistance and support to patients with these conditions.
- Physical activity.
- Cultural factors – dietary restrictions and habits. Becoming acquainted with food habits common in various cultures and religions will assist in providing appropriate nutritional advice. For example, some Somalian, Ethiopian and Eritrean patients may be Orthodox Christian and may restrict meat during the Lenten season. For some, this will decrease ferritin stores, and they may require iron supplementation during this time period. In addition to religious restrictions, recent immigrants to the UK may find it difficult to access foods that they are familiar with. Knowledge of foods commonly consumed will enable the practitioner to advise on appropriate substitutes, as well as recipe modifications when necessary (see Chapter 3.5, Working with minority ethnic groups).

Energy and protein requirements

For asymptomatic PWHIV taking ART, energy requirements can increase by 10% to maintain body weight and physical activity. However, in PWHIV taking ART, energy requirements may not be different from that of the general population. During symptomatic HIV, and subsequently during AIDS, energy requirements increase by approximately 20–30% to maintain adult body weight (World Health Organization, 2003). Although studies of energy expenditure have not shown an increase in overall total energy expenditure (TEE) in patients with HIV-related wasting, this may have been the result of individuals compensating by reducing activity-related energy expenditure (AEE). Therefore, weight loss may have resulted from reduced dietary intake (Macallan *et al.*, 1995). Reviews of energy expenditure in HIV have concluded that it appears that resting energy expenditure (REE) is higher (but not always TEE) in PWHIV not on ART (Chang *et al.*, 2007; Fields-Gardner *et al.*, 2010), and a meta-analysis confirmed this (Batterham, 2005). Fewer studies have explored this in the post-ART era. Factors associated with altered REE appear to be viral load, CD4, use of ART, body composition, hormones and proinflammatory cytokines, as well as other opportunistic infections.

Protein requirements have not been specifically addressed in studies of HIV adults. They may have higher requirements to maintain lean body mass, and general recommendations are 1.2–1.5 g/kg of body weight/day (Ockenga *et al.*, 2006). Protein requirements should take into consideration the stage of HIV disease and the presence of other infections or comorbidities.

Nutritional problems and their management

It is well known that nutritional deficiencies are commonly associated with an impaired immune response (see Chapter 7.11.1, Nutrition and immunity); therefore, malnutrition in PWHIV has serious consequences. Adults living with HIV can present with a variety of nutritional problems throughout the course of HIV infection. Furthermore, patients requiring dietetic intervention may be critically unwell, have multiple medical diagnoses and mental health issues, as well as issues surrounding confidentiality, stigma and ART adherence that require a specialist team approach. The complexity of these patients requires input from a specialist dietitian trained in the area of HIV, who plays an active role in the multidisciplinary team (MDT).

The different stages of HIV infection as well as opportunistic infections, comorbidities and metabolic side effects of ART can all lead to various nutritional problems. Ideally, all patients with HIV infection should have access to a registered dietitian for nutritional advice. Table 7.11.13 shows which patients with HIV in the inpatient and outpatient settings require referral to an HIV-specialist dietitian, and a summary of the possible outcomes from the referral.

Medication side effects

Side effects are most commonly seen in people who have recently started ART; however, they can also occur due to the HIV infection itself, other opportunistic and comorbid conditions, or other medications. The most common side effects are:

- Nausea.
- Vomiting.
- Diarrhoea.
- Taste changes.
- Dry mouth.
- Flatulence.

The details of dietetic interventions for these side effects can be found in other chapters.

Wasting and weight loss

Weight loss can still be a problem for many PWHIV infections, even those on ART. In a longitudinal cohort, the prevalence of wasting and weight loss was 38% (Tang *et al.*, 2005). Several studies have shown that weight or muscle mass loss, even a 5% loss of usual weight, increases the risk of mortality (Scherzer *et al.*, 2011; Tang *et al.*, 2005). Furthermore, HIV wasting disease is defined as an AIDS-defining illness (Centers for Disease Control, 1987) that is common in states of severe immunodeficiency (Mangili *et al.*, 2006; Polsky *et al.*, 2001). Many clinicians and researchers in the area felt that this definition of an AIDS-defining illness did not fully capture all patients with HIV wasting; therefore, other definitions have been proposed (Table 7.11.14). In cases of weight loss despite adequate combination ART (cART), special consideration has to be given to other factors such as depression, gastrointestinal disease, anorexia, self-neglect (e.g. drug users), or the dry mouth/lack of saliva caused by medication (Grinspoon *et al.*, 2003).

Aetiology

Weight loss can be due to one or a combination of several factors, depending on the patient's immune function and clinical condition (Figure 7.11.7):

- *Reduced food intake* – this can be due to poor appetite, dysphagia (or oesophageal pain due to oesophageal candidiasis) or nausea.
- *Malabsorption* – can arise from other opportunistic infections, such as *Mycobacterium* spp., *Cryptosporidium*, pancreatic dysfunction or HIV enteropathy (Knox *et al.*, 2000).
- *Hypermetabolism* – REE is increased in patients not on ART and is positively correlated with viral load and C-reactive protein level (Chang *et al.*, 2007). Opportunistic infections can also increase energy requirements.
- *Endocrine abnormalities* – altered regulation of anabolic and adipocyte hormones has also been implicated in causing increased REE. Altered regulation of other hormonal axes involved in energy homeostasis could potentially result from chronic immune activation.
- *Cytokine dysregulation* – increased REE is associated with catabolic cytokines interleukin (IL) 1b and tumour necrosis factor alpha (TNFα) abnormalities.

Dietetic management of weight loss

The primary approach for weight loss and HIV-related wasting is treatment of the underlying condition that is leading to the weight loss. However, this is not always apparent and may take some time to diagnose. Therefore, to prevent further weight loss, to restore nutritional status and achieve a healthy weight in conjunction with medical/other treatment, dietetic therapy is of paramount importance. Evaluating current dietary intake

Table 7.11.13 Dietetic interventions and outcomes for treating nutritional problems in patients with HIV infection

Patients requiring a dietetic referral	Dietetic interventions and outcomes of referral
All PWHIV	Healthy eating principles that ensure adequate nutrition and promote a healthy immune system to reduce infections and prevent the development of metabolic comorbidities.
Immunocompromised (e.g. CD4+ cell count <200 cells/mL)	Food and water safety counselling to reduce the risk of developing foodborne and waterborne illnesses.
Pregnant women	Antenatal and postnatal nutrition and breastfeeding education (see Chapter 3.8.2, Growth, nutritional assessment and nutritional requirements). Improving micronutrient deficiency (including iron) and constipation.
Poor dietary intake due to disease or side effects of treatment	Nutrition strategies for symptom management, e.g. anorexia, early satiety, swallowing problems, thrush, nausea and vomiting, diarrhoea, food intolerances. Outcomes may be improved diarrhoea, and prevention of weight loss and loss of lean body mass, which is known to increase mortality.
Patients taking antiretrovirals or other medications related to opportunistic infections or comorbidities	Identifying food–medication interactions and strategies to ensure optimal medication efficacy and provide adherence support.
Loss of >5% of usual weight	Short-term alternative feeding methods, e.g. oral supplementation, tube feeding and parenteral nutrition. Outcomes may be reduced risk of infections, mortality, hospital admissions (if an outpatient) and length of stay (if inpatient), and improved patient experience (quality of life and energy levels).
Dyslipidaemia and/or lipodystrophy and/ or obesity and/or diabetes and/or insulin resistance	Strategies for treatment of body fat changes and altered metabolism (in collaboration with the clinician) include exercise, lipid-lowering medications and dietary modifications. Outcomes may be improved glycaemic control and hormonal normalisation, resulting in the prevention of CVD events, reduced hospital admissions and improved quality of life (obesity related).
Bone disease (osteoporosis, osteopaenia, osteomalacia)	Assessment of dietary and lifestyle factors influencing bone mineral density (dietary protein, calcium, phosphorus and vitamin D; exercise; risk of falls; smoking; alcohol), and advice on altering these as needed. Advising on vitamin D ± calcium supplementation. Outcomes may include prevention of falls, fractures and hospital admissions.
Allergies/intolerances or patients following special diets/taking excess supplementation	Evaluation of nutrition information; special diets; vitamin, mineral or other dietary supplementation; and other nutrition practices. Prevention of toxic effects of hypervitaminosis, improved patient experience/well-being, ensuring nutritional adequacy, prevention of interactions with ART or other medications.
Patients requiring weight loss or gain of lean body tissue	Additional activities and therapies that support good nutrition, e.g. physical exercise, medications for symptom management, chronic disease management, etc., including referral to appropriate exercise facilities. See outcomes for dyslipidaemia.
Alteration in bowel habit	Assessment of impact on quality of life and diet, dietary advice to improve symptoms (constipation/diarrhoea), discussion with patient about lifestyle factors, liaising with specialist gastroenterology team/dietitian, communication with GP if supplements or medicines are required. Outcomes may be improved quality of life, prevention of nutritional deficiencies and enhanced medication absorption.

ART, antiretroviral therapy; PWHIV, people with HIV; CVD, cardiovascular disease.

and calculating energy deficits is the first step in the nutritional management of someone who presents with weight loss. As hypermetabolism is one of the potential causes of weight loss, using indirect methods of measuring energy expenditure may help determine metabolic stress, which may be arising from opportunistic infections and other underlying conditions in addition to the HIV disease itself. In the absence of objective measurements, anthropometric measurements should be closely monitored to determine the effectiveness of nutritional intervention (see Chapter 6.1, Nutritional requirements in clinical practice).

Several studies have shown that dietary counselling with oral nutritional supplements (providing 40–50 kcal/kg; 1.6 g of protein/kg) achieved increases in dietary intake and lean body mass. When resistance exercise training was added, an even greater increase in physical functioning was achieved (Rabeneck *et al.*, 1998; Shevitz

Table 7.11.14 Definitions of HIV-related wasting

CDC (Centers for Disease Control, 1987)	Consensus panel (Wanke *et al.*, 2004)	Nutrition for Healthy Living (Wanke *et al.*, 2000)
Involuntary weight loss of >10% of baseline body weight + either chronic diarrhoea or chronic weakness and documented fever in the absence of concurrent illness or condition.	10% unintentional weight loss over 12 months. Or 7.5% unintentional weight loss over 6 months. Or 5% unintentional weight loss over 3 months. Or, in men: BCM <35% of total BW, with BMI <27 kg/m^2. Or, in women: BCM <23% of total BW, with BMI <27 kg/m^2. In either men or women, regardless of BCM: BMI <20 kg/m^2.	Unintentional loss of >10% of body weight. Or BMI <20 kg/m^2. Or unintentional loss of >5% of body weight in 6 months and persisting for at least 1 year.

BW, body weight; BMI, body mass index; BCM, body cell mass.

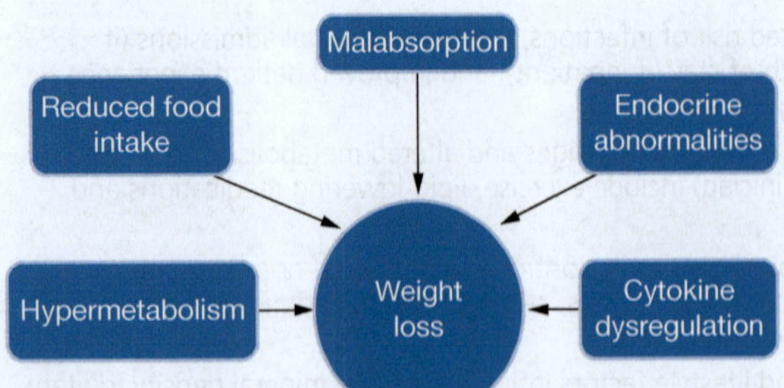

Figure 7.11.7 Potential causes of weight loss in HIV-infected individuals

et al., 2005). Another study evaluated resistance training and intramuscular testosterone injections in eugonadal men with AIDS wasting, and these combined interventions increased muscle attenuation (Fairfield *et al.*, 2001). Other randomised controlled trials (RCTs) of nutritional supplements demonstrated an improvement in both energy and protein intake for patients given macronutrient supplements, as compared to patients given placebos or no supplements, but no uniform improvements in weight, fat mass or fat-free mass were found (Grobler *et al.*, 2013). Most studies investigating the role of nutritional supplementation have not included HIV outcomes or mortality, although one trial found an increase in the CD4+ cell counts associated with nutritional supplementation (Fields-Gardner *et al.*, 2010).

There is limited evidence regarding the mode of artificial nutritional support. Enteral nutritional support is often used as supplementary intake in patients with HIV. For long-term artificial nutritional support, gastrostomy feeding is feasible in HIV patients and should be considered as an option. Parenteral nutrition should be used only in patients who are unable to feed enterally (Ockenga *et al.*, 2006).

Diarrhoea and malabsorption are common causes of weight loss and poor nutritional status in patients with HIV. Furthermore, malabsorption in the absence of clinical symptoms has been found to be common in adults with HIV (Knox *et al.*, 2000). Medium-chain triglycerides (MCTs) have been used in several studies in patients with HIV and diarrhoea. Use of MCTs results in fewer stools, decreased stool fat and weight, and increased weight gain and fat absorption (Wanke *et al.*, 1996). Several other nutritional interventions for diarrhoea in patients with HIV have been evaluated; however, these were all very small studies, and conclusions could not be drawn from them. One study looking at vitamin A and beta-carotene supplements found that they decreased gut permeability and reduced the risk of severe watery diarrhoea. Other studies have looked at elemental diets, probiotics, pancreatic enzymes, calcium carbonate, glutamine and the bananas, rice, applesauce and toast (BRAT) diet (Academy of Nutrition & Dietetics, 2008). Other dietary strategies will depend on the cause and severity of diarrhoea.

Pharmacological agents used to treat HIV wasting have included megestrol acetate, oxandrolone and dronabinol (Grinspoon *et al.*, 2003).

Metabolic complications with nutritional consequences and/or causes

Metabolic complications in PWHIV can arise from uncontrolled HIV replication, coinfections or as a side effect of some ART medicines. Metabolic complications are a common reason for referrals in dietetic services. These complications include dyslipidaemias, altered glucose metabolism, bone problems, altered body fat metabolism characterised by changes in body composition, and lactic acidaemia. The majority of antiretroviral medicines interfere with viral genetic material. Many human metabolic processes are operationally similar to those of HIV viral replication, so it is not surprising that the side effects of ART include metabolic complications. As the population living with HIV ages, the prevalence of metabolic diseases will continue to increase. Managing ageing in HIV itself is a topic of much interest to both researchers and clinicians. A multidisciplinary review of ageing with HIV found that combining the least toxic drugs and promotion of healthy lifestyle behaviours, such as a healthy diet, might be the best practice to help PWHIV age (Calcagno *et al.*, 2015). Helpful guidelines for the management of HIV-related comorbidities are produced by the European AIDS Clinical Society.

Heart disease and dyslipidaemia

Cardiovascular disease (CVD) is a concern for PWHIV. HIV infection and ART, along with traditional lifestyle factors, all seem to play a role in increasing CVD risk (Freiberg *et al.*, 2013). Cardiovascular risk can be assessed using a variety of different tools, including the HIV-specific tools found on the Centre of Excellence for Health, Immunity and Infections website (www.chip.dk/Tools) or the UK-specific QRISK tool (www.qrisk.org). Consistency in the use of tools is important. All CVD risk tools include the major predictors of heart disease: dyslipidaemia and hypertension. HIV infection or ART can also contribute to dyslipidaemia, together with lifestyle factors. The following may occur in isolation or in combination, leading to an increased risk of CVD:

- Hypertriglyceridaemia.
- Raised total or low-density lipoprotein (LDL) cholesterol.
- Decreased high-density lipoprotein (HDL) cholesterol.

Observational studies have reported that people living with HIV infection generally consume diets higher in total fat, saturated fat and dietary cholesterol, which has been related to dyslipidaemia (Hadigan *et al.*, 2001; Shah *et al.*, 2005).

Dietetic treatment

As there are several possible causes for dyslipidaemia in HIV-infected individuals, evaluating the effect of dietary interventions is a complex task. Some studies have evaluated those with isolated dyslipidaemia, and others those with dyslipidaemia in the presence of lipodystrophy. Dietary advice has also varied between studies. Low-fat dietary interventions have been investigated with varying results (Leyes *et al.*, 2008). In adults with HIV and dyslipidaemia, a retrospective review of dietary counselling found that total cholesterol decreased significantly by 13% (Batterham *et al.*, 2003; Woods *et al.*, 2009). Compliance with the dietary advice given was assessed in one trial; only 36% and 45% patients reported a good compliance with the prescribed diet at 3 and 6 months, respectively, and those with good compliance had a significant reduction in total cholesterol and triglyceride levels, as well as weight loss (Barrios *et al.*, 2002). n-3 fatty acid supplements have been shown in several trials to reduce triglycerides (De Truchis *et al.*, 2007), and, when combined with dietary advice to reduce saturated fat, had an even greater effect and lowered the risk of lipohypertrophy (Woods *et al.*, 2009). Interim results have shown that the Mediterranean Portfolio diet can lead to lower systolic blood pressure as compared to a standard low-saturated-fat diet (Stradling *et al.*, 2016). Overall, there appears to be some evidence that a combination of exercise and a healthy Mediterranean-style diet (e.g. low saturated fat, high fibre and low–moderate alcohol consumption) may improve CVD risk factors.

Altered glucose metabolism

Insulin resistance is the initial detectable step in the development of type 2 diabetes mellitus; in PWHIV, it may be accompanied by lipodystrophy. Traditional risk factors such as genetic predisposition, increased body mass index (BMI), smoking and increasing age, as well as HIV-related factors such as mitochondrial dysfunction and elevated pro-inflammatory cytokines, all play a role in the development of type 2 diabetes (Paik & Kotler, 2011). Furthermore, patients on ART are more likely to develop glucose intolerance and type 2 diabetes mellitus than controls.

Care should be taken when using HbA1C as a surrogate measure for glycaemic control in HIV patients, since ART use may result in this measure underestimating glycaemia by up to 20%, particularly in patients using nucleoside reverse transcriptase inhibitors (NRTIs) such as abacavir (Kim *et al.*, 2009). The goals of treatment are the same as in uninfected individuals (see Chapter 7.12, Diabetes mellitus). The European AIDS Clinical Society and Paik and Kotler (2011) provide further information on management considerations.

Lipodystrophy (fat redistribution)

Lipodystrophy syndrome (LDS), also referred to as fat redistribution syndrome, describes body shape changes and metabolic disorders seen in some patients with HIV infection. Although the aetiology is likely multifactorial, most believe it occurs as a result of certain ART (more commonly prescribed a decade ago and used less frequently now). Individual and viral factors such as duration of HIV disease, duration of ART, age, BMI, gender and ethnicity all seem to play a role in its development (Wohl & Brown, 2008). Limited evidence supports a relationship between low fibre or high glycaemic index (GI) and increased risk of fat deposition (Hendricks *et al.*, 2003).

Fat redistribution can occur in an individual in several ways:

- *Lipoatrophy* – the loss of subcutaneous fat tissue, most commonly in the legs, arms, buttocks and/or face.
- *Fat accumulation (sometimes called lipohypertrophy)* – the accumulation of adipose tissue in the intraabdominal space (Figure 7.11.8), the dorsocervical regions (known commonly as the buffalo hump) and the breasts.

Dietetic management

There have been few RCTs studying lifestyle interventions in the treatment of lipodystrophy; therefore, much of the advice given in clinical practice is based on observational data and case series reports. There is no effective treatment for lipoatrophy using nutrition or lifestyle interventions. However, resistance exercises may improve the appearance of limbs by bulking up muscles to compensate for the loss of fat. Lipoatrophy is managed by switching ART regimens, and several other interventional treatments have been evaluated, but with limited effectiveness to date (Wohl & Brown, 2008). For facial fat tissue loss, polylactic acid has been reported to produce lasting changes in dermal thickness of the cheeks, and is available for patients receiving care in the NHS in the UK (NICE, 2013).

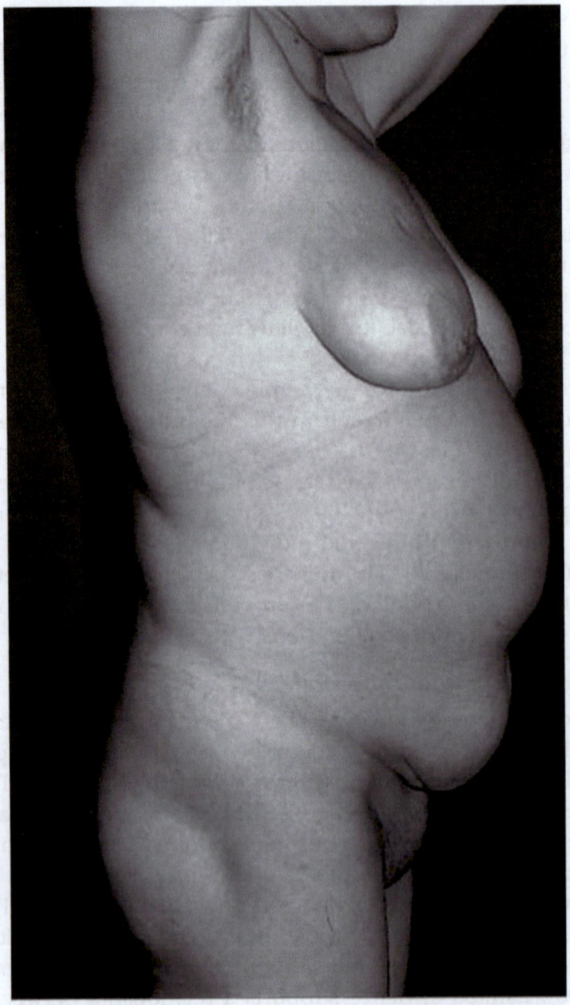

Figure 7.11.8 HIV-infected woman with lipodystrophy (source: AIDS Images Library. Reproduced with permission from AIDS Image Library, www.aids-images.ch)

Limited evidence from observational studies shows that a low-fibre diet leads to an increased risk of developing lipohypertrophy (Hendricks *et al.*, 2003). A combination of diet and exercise in interventional trials has shown small improvements in abdominal girth and blood pressure, but limited effect on lipids (Driscoll *et al.*, 2004; Engelson *et al.*, 2006). Furthermore, a combination of both aerobic and resistance training appears be the most beneficial exercise intervention in patients with HIV-associated lipodystrophy (Yarasheski & Roubenoff, 2001).

Bone problems

Three main bone diseases have been described in the HIV setting:

- Osteopenia and osteoporosis (decreased bone mineral density).
- Osteomalacia (softening of the bones or demineralisation from severe vitamin D or phosphate deficiency).
- Avascular necrosis.

The most commonly found and studied of these is reduced bone mineral density (BMD), which is associated with an increased risk of fracture. Factors associated with low BMD in PWHIV are both traditional (i.e. well known in all populations to influence BMD) and HIV related:

- Low weight, BMI.
- Duration of HIV infection.
- Older age.
- Smoking.
- Non-black/white ethnicity.
- Corticosteroid exposure.
- Postmenopausal women.
- Viral load levels.
- ART exposure (most commonly, tenofovir disoproxil fumarate and protease inhibitors).

Other risk factors also commonly found in patients with HIV include hypogonadism, vitamin D deficiency and secondary hyperparathyroidism, opiate use, and various other medical conditions (McComsey *et al.*, 2010). Lifestyle factors influencing BMD include dietary calcium intake and exercise (North American Menopause Society, 2010). These have not been well explored in PWHIV. The advice provided in Chapter 7.9.1 (Osteoporosis) is applicable for preventing and managing low BMD in PWHIV. Fracture risk can be assessed using the 10-year FRAX tool (https://www.shef.ac.uk/FRAX).

Micronutrient deficiencies

Micronutrient deficiencies are common in patients with HIV not on ART (Lanzillotti & Tang, 2005). They are also common in countries with poor overall nutritional status, mostly in the developing world. The micronutrients most commonly studied in patients with HIV are shown in Table 7.11.15.

There have been many observational studies investigating the prevalence of micronutrient deficiencies, whether they have HIV-related causes, and if they are associated with adverse outcomes. As you can see from Tables 7.11.15 and 7.11.16, the findings have been mixed. Trials of micronutrient supplements, especially individual supplements, in patients with HIV have not demonstrated consistent benefits. Micronutrient supplementation in clinical practice should be based on the individual's micronutrient levels in conjunction with available evidence from both the general and HIV-specific population (Table 7.11.16).

Obesity

Obesity in PWHIV is now similar in prevalence to obesity in the general population. A longitudinal cohort study found that participants were often overweight at the time of diagnosis and continued to gain weight after they were diagnosed with HIV (Crum-Cianflone *et al.*, 2010a). Obesity management tends to be similar in PWHIV; however, there is some evidence that, in people with untreated HIV (i.e. not on ART), a higher BMI can be protective against disease progression (Crum-Cianflone *et al.*, 2010b; Martinez *et al.*, 2016). Exercise and dietary interventions have been investigated in HIV-positive patients presenting with general obesity or metabolic syndrome. A randomised study of intensive lifestyle intervention, comprised of weekly one-on-one counselling sessions focusing on

Table 7.11.15 Observational studies of micronutrient deficiencies in relation to HIV disease

Micronutrient	Observational findings in HIV
Vitamin A	Low vitamin A levels have been associated with quicker progression of HIV disease and mortality in adults (Semba *et al.*, 1995; Tang *et al.*, 1993).
Vitamin D	Low vitamin D has been associated with HIV disease progression or CD4 cell count decline (Klassen *et al.*, 2015; Mehta *et al.*, 2010; Viard *et al.*, 2011). Different classes of ART seem to influence vitamin D metabolism at various points in the metabolism pathway (Klassen *et al.*, 2016). It can be challenging to interpret 25(OH) D levels, especially without measuring the corresponding biologically active metabolites; therefore, the best practice is to follow guidelines for the general population. In the general population, vitamin D deficiency has been associated with CVD, diabetes, immune functioning and mortality (Melamed *et al.*, 2008).
Zinc	Serum zinc levels have been linked to HIV disease progression, decreased CD4+ cell counts and increased mortality (Baum *et al.*, 1997, 2003). An association was seen between people who took over-the-counter zinc supplements and a more rapid progression to AIDS and mortality (Tang *et al.*, 1993, 1996). This may be because adults with more advanced or symptomatic HIV disease are more likely to take more supplements (Bormann *et al.*, 2009).
Selenium	Low levels have been linked with progression of HIV disease (Baum *et al.*, 1997).
Calcium	Several studies have found that a high percentage of HIV-infected individuals have inadequate dietary calcium intake (Arpadi *et al.*, 2009; Bonjoch *et al.*, 2010; Jacobson *et al.*, 2008). An increased dietary calcium intake has been associated with greater bone mineral density in HIV (McComsey *et al.*, 2007).
Iron	Iron deficiency is common, especially in women and in developing countries, and dietary iron appears to be a contributing factor (Castro & Goldani, 2009; Shet *et al.*, 2012).
Phosphate	Hypophosphataemia is commonly seen in patients with HIV regardless of ART use (Day *et al.*, 2005). It is thought that the use of tenofovir disoproxil fumarate contributes to renal tubular losses of phosphate; however, vitamin D deficiency, malabsorption and use of antacids can also be contributing factors (Assadi, 2010).

ART, antiretroviral therapy.

Table 7.11.16 Interventional studies of micronutrients in people living with HIV/AIDS

Micronutrient	Findings from RCTs
Vitamin A	No trials reviewed (Irlam *et al.*, 2010) showed a reduction in disease progression in adults with vitamin A supplementation. In children, vitamin A supplementation showed a reduction in mortality, and moderate evidence for morbidity and growth benefits.
Vitamin D	7000 IU VD3/day in 56 patients aged 9–25 years; improved neuromuscular motor skills (Brown *et al.*, 2015). One trial found that vitamin D_3 supplementation decreased the risk of developing diabetes (Guaraldi *et al.*, 2011). No risks of supplementation have been seen to date (Arpadi *et al.*, 2009; Wejse *et al.*, 2009).
Zinc	No benefit of zinc supplements has been seen in pregnant women; furthermore, zinc inhibits iron absorption, thereby mitigating increases in haemoglobin levels, which are often low in pregnancy. In drug users in Florida, those who took the dietary reference intake (DRI) of zinc as a supplement had a decrease in immunological failure (defined as CD4+ <200 cells/mm^3) and less diarrhoea, as compared to those taking placebo (Baum *et al.*, 2010). In children, supplementation reduced the risk and progression of diarrhoea in several studies (in Africa), but not prophylactically (Irlam *et al.*, 2010).
Selenium	Reduced diarrhoeal morbidity in pregnant women in Tanzania, and reduced viral load in two separate small trials in American adults (with high dropout rates) (Irlam *et al.*, 2010).
Calcium	Calcium with vitamin D supplements have been given in the control arm of several trials investigating the role of bisphosphonates in treating osteoporosis. These studies found that there was a trend for bone mineral density increases, albeit non-significantly, in those receiving calcium supplements only; however, this was significantly less than in those on bisphosphonates (McComsey *et al.*, 2007; Mondy *et al.*, 2005).
Iron and phosphate	To date, no RCTs have evaluated the influence of diet on iron or phosphate stores in patients with HIV infection. Iron supplements have been given in conjunction with multivitamins to women with hepatitis C (Semba *et al.*, 2007), and this improved their iron stores and anaemia. The results from this trial cannot be generalised to the HIV-infected population as a whole, owing to the narrow inclusion criteria and short duration.
Other	Multi-micronutrient formulations have shown a reduction in mortality in patients with a CD4 of <100 cells/mm^3 in Thailand (Jiamton *et al.*, 2003), an increase in CD4 in the USA (Kaiser *et al.*, 2006), and an improvement in benefits to mothers and offspring in Tanzania (Fawzi *et al.*, 2004).

reducing saturated fats, increasing fibre and walking, evaluated 34 HIV-positive subjects with metabolic syndrome. At 6 months, subjects assigned to the lifestyle intervention group showed a 2.6 cm decrease in waist circumference, as well as significant improvements in systolic blood pressure and HbA1C, but not lipid levels, fasting glucose or insulin resistance (Engelson *et al.*, 2006; Fitch *et al.*, 2006). Dietary advice for the obese should be based on standard dietetic practice and tailored to the individual with HIV (see Chapter 7.13.2, The management of obesity and overweight in adults).

Food and water safety

General food safety advice may benefit all individuals with HIV; however, those who are severely immunocompromised, e.g. with a CD4+ cell count of <200 cells/mm^3, may benefit from more targeted advice. Salmonellosis has been estimated to be nearly 20 times more common, and often five times more bacteraemic, in AIDS patients (Hayes *et al.*, 2003). Other microorganisms such as *Giardia lamblia*, *Entamoeba histolytica*, *Cryptosporidium*, *Salmonella*, *Shigella*, *Listeria*, *Yersinia* and *Campylobacter* spp. have been identified as the cause of enteric infections in HIV-infected patients, and have also been recognised as causing foodborne and waterborne diseases. Preventative measures should include food and water safety advice. Water safety advice is important as *Cryptosporidium* has been isolated from tap water on rare occasions. Cryptosporidiosis can be prevented by boiling tap water, using an appropriate filter or using sterile water. Bottled water or domestic water filters are not necessarily free from *Cryptosporidium* cysts, and therefore should not be recommended in place of boiled water or appropriate filters (Hunter & Nichols, 2002).

Drug–nutrient interactions

Some of the older antiretroviral drugs came with strict food requirements; however, many of the newer formulations have fewer food and timing requirements. With the exception of didanosine, all NRTIs/nucleotide reverse transcriptase inhibitors (NtRTIs) may be taken either with food or on an empty stomach. Many people find that taking NRTIs/NtRTIs with food helps reduce side effects such as nausea. It is advised to take efavirenz (a nonnucleoside reverse transcriptase) on an empty stomach to reduce side effects. Most protease inhibitors work better when taken with food; however, the new formulation of lopinavir/ritonavir and fosamprenavir have no food restrictions. Current information on antiretrovirals and food restrictions is available at www.aidsmap.com.

SECTION 7

Further reading

Hendricks KM, Dong KR, Gerrior JL (eds). (2009) *Nutrition Management of HIV and AIDS*. Chicago: American Dietetic Association.

Pribram V (ed). (2010) *Nutrition and HIV*. Oxford: Wiley Blackwell.

Internet resources

Academy of Nutrition & Dietetics HIV/AIDS Nutrition Evidence Analysis Project, www.andeal.org

Antiretroviral Drugs Chart, www.aidsmap.com/resources/Antiretroviral-drugs-chart/page/1412453

AVERTing HIV & AIDS, www.avert.org

British HIV Association, www.bhiva.org

European AIDS Clinical Society, www.eacsociety.org

HIV Care Dietitians Special Interest group of the BDA, www.dhiva.org.uk

National AIDS Manual (nam – aidsmap), www.aidsmap.com

National AIDS Trust, www.nat.org.uk

References

Aibibula W, Cox J, Hamelin A-M, *et al.* (2016) Food insecurity and low CD4 count among HIV-infected people: a systematic review and meta-analysis. *AIDS Care* 28: 1577–1585.

Academy of Nutrition & Dietetics. (2010) *HIV/AIDS Treatment of Diarrhea/Malabsorption*. Available at https://www.andeal.org/template.cfm?key=2816. Accessed 7 July 2017.

Arpadi S, McMahon D, Abrams E, *et al.* (2009) Effect of bimonthly supplementation with oral cholecalciferol on serum 25-hydroxyvitamin D concentrations in HIV-infected children and adolescents. *Pediatrics* 123: e121–126.

Asboe D, Aitken C, Boffito M, *et al.* (2011) *Routine Investigation and Monitoring of Adult HIV-1-Infected Individuals*. London: British HIV Association.

Assadi F. (2010) Hypophosphatemia: An evidence-based problem-solving approach to clinical cases. *Iran J. Kidney Dis.* 4: 195–201.

Barrios A, Blanco F, García-Benayas T, *et al.* (2002) Effect of dietary intervention on highly active antiretroviral therapy–related dyslipemia. *AIDS*. 16: 2079–2081.

Batterham MJ. (2005) Investigating heterogeneity in studies of resting energy expenditure in persons with HIV/AIDS: a meta-analysis. *Am. J. Clin. Nutr.* 81: 702–713.

Batterham MJ, Brown D, Workman C. (2003) Modifying dietary fat intake can reduce serum cholesterol in HIV-associated hypercholesterolemia. *AIDS*. 17: 1414–1416.

Baum MK, Shor-Posner G, Lai S, *et al.* (1997) High risk of HIV-related mortality is associated with selenium deficiency. *J. Acquir. Immune Defic. Syndr. Hum. Retrovirol.* 15(5): 370–374.

Baum MK, Campa A, Lai S, *et al.* (2003) Zinc status in human immunodeficiency virus type 1 infection and illicit drug use. *Clin. Infect. Dis.* 37(S2): S117–123.

Baum MK, Lai S, Sales S, *et al.* (2010) Randomized, controlled clinical trial of zinc supplementation to prevent immunological failure in HIV-infected adults. *Clin. Infect. Dis.* 50: 1653–1660.

Bonjoch A, Figueras M, Estany C, *et al.* (2010) High prevalence of and progression to low bone mineral density in HIV-infected patients: a longitudinal cohort study. *AIDS*. 24: 2827–2833.

Bormann JE, Uphold CR, Maynard C. (2009) Predictors of complementary/alternative medicine use and intensity of use among men with HIV infection from two geographic areas in the United States. *J. Assoc. Nurses AIDS Care*. 20: 468–480.

Brown TT, Hoy J, Borderi M, *et al.* (2015) Recommendations for evaluation and management of bone disease in HIV. *Clin. Infect. Dis.* 60(8):1242–1251.

Calcagno A, Nozza S, Muss C, *et al.* (2015) Ageing with HIV: a multidisciplinary review. *Infection*. 43: 509–522.

Castro L, Goldani LZ. (2009) Iron, folate and vitamin B_{12} parameters in HIV-1 infected patients with anaemia in southern Brazil. *Trop. Doct.* 39: 83–85.

Castro KG, Ward JW, Slutsker L, *et al.* (1993) *1993 Revised Classification System for HIV Infection and Expanded Surveillance Case Definition for AIDS Among Adolescents and Adults*. Morbidity and Mortality Weekly Reports: Recommendations and

Reports 41(RR-17). Available at www.cdc.gov/mmwr/preview/mmwrhtml/00018871.htm. Accessed 12 April 2018.

Centers for Disease Control (CDC). (1987) Revision of the CDC surveillance case definition for acquired immunodeficiency syndrome. Council of State and Territorial Epidemiologists; AIDS Program, Center for Infectious Diseases. *MMWR Suppl.* 36(1): 1S–15S.

Chang E, Sekhar R, Patel S, *et al.* (2007) Dysregulated energy expenditure in HIV-infected patients: a mechanistic review. *Clin. Infect. Dis.* 44: 1509–1517.

Chen LF, Hoy J, Lewin SR. (2007) Ten years of highly active antiretroviral therapy for HIV infection. *Med. J. Aust.* 186: 146–151.

Crum-Cianflone N, Roediger MP, Eberly L, *et al.* (2010a) Increasing rates of obesity among HIV-infected persons during the HIV epidemic. *PLoS One.* 5(4): e10106.

Crum-Cianflone NF, Roediger M, Eberly LE, *et al.* (2010b) Obesity among HIV-infected persons: impact of weight on CD4 cell count. *AIDS.* 24: 1069–1072.

Day SL, Leake Date HA, Bannister A, *et al.* (2005) Serum hypophosphatemia in tenofovir disoproxil fumarate recipients is multifactorial in origin, questioning the utility of its monitoring in clinical practice. *J. Acquir. Immune Defic. Syndr.* 38: 301–304.

De Truchis P, Kirstetter M, Perier A. *et al.* (2007) Reduction in triglyceride level with N-3 polyunsaturated fatty acids in HIV-infected patients taking potent antiretroviral therapy: a randomized prospective study. *J. Acquir. Immune Defic. Synd.* 44: 278–285.

Driscoll SD, Meininger GE, Lareau MT, *et al.* (2004) Effects of exercise training and metformin on body composition and cardiovascular indices in HIV-infected patients. *AIDS.* 18: 465–473.

Engelson ES, Agin D, Kenya S, *et al.* (2006) Body composition and metabolic effects of a diet and exercise weight loss regimen on obese, HIV-infected women. *Metabolism.* 55: 1327–1336.

Fairfield WP, Treat M, Rosenthal DI, *et al.* (2001) Effects of testosterone and exercise on muscle leanness in eugonadal men with AIDS wasting. *J. Appl. Physiol.* 90: 2166–2171.

Fawzi WW, Msamanga GI, Spiegelman D, *et al.* (2004) A randomized trial of multivitamin supplements and HIV disease progression and mortality. *N. Engl. J. Med.* 351: 23–32.

Fields-Gardner C, Campa A, American Dietetics Association. (2010) Position of the American Dietetic Association: nutrition intervention and human immunodeficiency virus infection. *J. Am. Diet. Assoc.* 110: 1105–1119.

Fitch KV, Anderson EJ, Hubbard JL, *et al.* (2006) Effects of a lifestyle modification program in HIV-infected patients with the metabolic syndrome. *AIDS.* 20: 1843–1850.

Freiberg MS, Chang CC, Kuller LH, *et al.* (2013) HIV infection and the risk of acute myocardial infarction. *JAMA Intern. Med.* 173: 614–622.

Gazzard BG, Anderson J, Babiker A, *et al.* (2008) British HIV Association Guidelines for the treatment of HIV-1-infected adults with antiretroviral therapy 2008. *HIV Med.* 9: 563–608.

Gianotti N, Visco F, Galli L, *et al.* (2011) Detecting impaired glucose tolerance or type 2 diabetes mellitus by means of an oral glucose tolerance test in HIV-infected patients. *HIV Med.* 12: 109–117.

Grinspoon S, Mulligan K, Department of Health and Human Services Working Group on the Prevention and Treatment of Wasting and Weight Loss. (2003) Weight loss and wasting in patients infected with human immunodeficiency virus. *Clin. Infect. Dis.* 36: S69–78.

Grobler L, Siegfried N, Visser ME, *et al.* (2013) Nutritional interventions for reducing morbidity and mortality in people with HIV. *Cochrane Database Syst. Rev.* (2): CD004536.

Guaraldi G, Orlando G, Carli F. (2011) Vitamin D3 supplementation decreases the risk of diabetes mellitus among patients with HIV infection. 18th Conference on Retroviruses and Opportunistic Infections, 2011, Boston. Poster 827.

Hadigan C, Jeste S, Anderson EJ, *et al.* (2001) Modifiable dietary habits and their relation to metabolic abnormalities in men and women with human immunodeficiency virus infection and fat redistribution. *Clin. Infect. Dis.* 33: 710–717.

Hayes C, Elliot E, Krales E, *et al.* (2003) Food and water safety for persons infected with human immunodeficiency virus. *Clin. Infect. Dis.* 36: S106–109.

Health Protection Agency (2010) HIV in the United Kingdom: 2010 Report. Available at http://webarchive.nationalarchives.gov.uk/20140714113046/http://www.hpa.org.uk/webc/HPAwebFile/HPAweb_C/1287145367237. Accessed 2 November 2018.

Hendricks KM, Dong KR, Tang AM, *et al.* (2003) High-fiber diet in HIV-positive men is associated with lower risk of developing fat deposition. *Am. J. Clin. Nutr.* 78: 790–795.

Hunter PR, Nichols G. (2002) Epidemiology and clinical features of Cryptosporidium infection in immunocompromised patients. *Clin. Microbiol. Rev.* 15: 145–154.

Irlam JH, Visser MM, Rollins NN, *et al.* (2010) Micronutrient supplementation in children and adults with HIV infection. *Cochrane Database Syst. Rev.* (12): CD003650.

Jacobson DL, Spiegelman D, Knox TK, *et al.* (2008) Evolution and predictors of change in total bone mineral density over time in HIV-infected men and women in the nutrition for healthy living study. *J. Acquir. Immune Defic. Syndr.* 49: 298–308.

Jiamton S, Pepin J, Suttent R, *et al.* (2003) A randomized trial of the impact of multiple micronutrient supplementation on mortality among HIV-infected individuals living in Bangkok. *AIDS.* 17: 2461–2469.

Joint United Nations Programme on HIV/AIDS (UNAIDS). (2010) *Global Report: UNAIDS report on the global AIDS epidemic: 2010.* Available at www.unaids.org/en/media/unaids/contentassets/dataimport/pub/report/2009/jc1700_epi_update_2009_en.pdf. Accessed 7 June 2017.

Kaiser JD, Campa AM, Ondercin JP, *et al.* (2006) Micronutrient supplementation increases CD4 count in HIV-infected individuals on highly active antiretroviral therapy: a prospective, double-blinded, placebo-controlled trial. *J. Acquir. Immune Defic. Synd.* 42: 523–528.

Kim PS, Woods C, Georgoff P, *et al.* (2009) A1C underestimates glycemia in HIV infection. *Diabetes Care.* 32: 1591–1593.

Kirwan PD, Chau C, Brown AE, *et al.* (2016) HIV in the United Kingdom – 2016 report. Available at https://www.gov.uk/government/uploads/system/uploads/attachment_data/file/574667/HIV_in_the_UK_2016.pdf. Accessed 7 June 2017.

Klassen KM, Fairley CK, Chen M, *et al.* (2015) Vitamin D deficiency may be associated with a more rapid decline in CD4 cell count to <350 cells/microL in untreated HIV-infected adults. *Curr. HIV Res.* 13: 517–523.

Klassen KM, Kimlin MG, Fairley CK, *et al.* (2016) Associations between vitamin D metabolites, antiretroviral therapy and bone mineral density in people with HIV. *Osteoporos. Int.* 27: 1737–1745.

Knox TA, Spiegelman D, Skinner SC, *et al.* (2000) Diarrhea and abnormalities of gastrointestinal function in a cohort of men and women with HIV infection. *Am. J. Gastroenterol.* 95: 3482–3489.

Kyle UG, Bosaeus I, De Lorenzo AD, *et al.*; ESPEN. (2004) Bioelectrical impedance analysis-part II: utilization in clinical practice. *Clin. Nutr.* 23: 1430–1453.

Labarga P, Albalate M, Barreiro P. (2010) Glomerular filtration (GF) determined by creatinine clearance (CCR) in 24 hours urine and cockcroft & gault (cg) and modification of diet in renal disease (MDRD) equations in a large cohort of HIV plus patients. *Retrovirology.* 7: 39.

Lanzillotti JS, Tang AM. (2005) Micronutrients and HIV disease: a review pre- and post-HAART. *Nutr. Clin. Care* 8: 16–23.

Leyes P, Martínez E, Forga Mde T. (2008) Use of diet, nutritional supplements and exercise in HIV-infected patients receiving combination antiretroviral therapies: a systematic review. *Antivir. Ther.* 13: 149–159.

Lundgren JD, Battegay M, Behrens G, *et al.* (2008) European AIDS Clinical Society (EACS) guidelines on the prevention and management of metabolic diseases in HIV. *HIV Med.* 9: 72–81.

Macallan DC, Noble C, Baldwin C, *et al.* (1995) Energy expenditure and wasting in human immunodeficiency virus infection. *N. Engl. J. Med.* 333: 83–88.

Mangili A, Murman DH, Zampini AM, *et al.* (2006) Nutrition and HIV infection: review of weight loss and wasting in the era of highly active antiretroviral therapy from the nutrition for healthy living cohort. *Clin. Infect. Dis.* 42: 836–842.

Martinez S, Campa A, Huffman F *et al.* (2016) The endotoxin-lipoprotein hypothesis, obesity and HIV. Available at http://programme.aids2016.org/Abstract/Abstract/9185. Accessed 3 November 2018.

May M, Gompels M, Delpech V, *et al.* (2011) Impact of late diagnosis and treatment on life expectancy in people with HIV-1: UK Collaborative HIV Cohort (UK CHIC) Study. *BMJ.* 343: d6016.

McComsey GA, Kendall MA, Tebas P, *et al.* (2007) Alendronate with calcium and vitamin D supplementation is safe and effective for the treatment of decreased bone mineral density in HIV. *AIDS.* 21: 2473–2482.

McComsey G, Tebas P, Shane E. (2010) Bone disease in HIV infection: a practical review and recommendations for HIV care providers. *Clin. Infect. Dis.* 51: 937–946.

Mehta S, Giovannucci E, Mugusi FM, *et al.* (2010) Vitamin D status of HIV-infected women and its association with HIV disease progression, anemia, and mortality. *PLoS One.* 5(1): e8770.

Melamed M, Michos E, Post W, *et al.* (2008) 25-hydroxyvitamin D levels and the risk of mortality in the general population. *Arch. Intern. Med.* 168: 1629–1637.

Mondy K, Powderly WG, Claxton SA, *et al.* (2005) Alendronate, vitamin D, and calcium for the treatment of osteopenia/osteoporosis associated with HIV infection. *J. Acquir. Immune Defic. Synd.* 38: 426–431.

NICE. (2013) *Deep dermal injection of non-absorbable gel polymer for HIV-related lipoatrophy.* Available at https://www.nice.org.uk/guidance/ipg439. Accessed 7 June 2017.

North American Menopause Society. (2010) Management of osteoporosis in postmenopausal women: 2010 position statement of The North American Menopause Society. *Menopause.* 17: 25–54.

Ockenga J, Grimble R, Jonkers-Schuitema C, *et al.* (2006) ESPEN Guidelines on Enteral Nutrition: Wasting in HIV and other chronic infectious diseases. *Clin. Nutr.* 25: 319–329.

Paik IJ, Kotler DP. (2011) The prevalence and pathogenesis of diabetes mellitus in treated HIV-infection. *Best Pract. Res. Clin. Endocrinol. Metab.* 25: 469–478.

Polsky B, Kotler D, Steinhart C. (2001) HIV-associated wasting in the HAART era: guidelines for assessment, diagnosis, and treatment. *AIDS Patient Care STDS.* 15: 411–423.

Public Health England (PHE). (2017) *HIV: Surveillance, Data and Management.* Available at https://www.gov.uk/government/collections/hiv-surveillance-data-and-management. Accessed 7 June 2017.

Rabeneck L, Palmer A, Knowles JB, *et al.* (1998) A randomized controlled trial evaluating nutrition counseling with or without oral supplementation in malnourished HIV-infected patients. *J. Am. Diet. Assoc.* 98: 434–438.

Scherzer R, Shen W, Bacchetti P, *et al.* (2008) Simple anthropometric measures correlate with metabolic risk indicators as strongly as magnetic resonance imaging-measured adipose tissue depots in both HIV-infected and control subjects. *Am. J. Clin. Nutr.* 87: 1809–1817.

Scherzer R, Heymsfield SB, Lee D, *et al.* (2011) Decreased limb muscle and increased central adiposity are associated with 5-year all-cause mortality in HIV infection. *AIDS.* 25: 1405–1414.

Schwenk A, Breuer P, Kremer G, *et al.* (2001) Clinical assessment of HIV-associated lipodystrophy syndrome: bioelectrical impedance analysis, anthropometry and clinical scores. *Clin. Nutr.* 20: 243–249.

Semba RD, Caiaffa WT, Graham NM, *et al.* (1995) Vitamin A deficiency and wasting as predictors of mortality in human immunodeficiency virus-infected injection drug users. *J. Infect. Dis.* 171(5): 1196–1202.

Semba RD, Kumwenda J, Zijlstra E, *et al.* (2007) Micronutrient supplements and mortality of HIV-infected adults with pulmonary TB: a controlled clinical trial. *Int. J. Tuberc. Lung. Dis.* 11: 854–859.

Shah M, Tierney K, Adams-Huet B, *et al.* (2005) The role of diet, exercise and smoking in dyslipidaemia in HIV-infected patients with lipodystrophy. *HIV Med.* 6: 291–298.

Shet A, Arumugam K, Rajagopalan N, *et al.* (2012) The prevalence and etiology of anemia among HIV-infected children in India. *Eur. J. Pediatr.* 171(3): 531–540.

Shevitz AH, Wilson IB, McDermott AY, *et al.* (2005) A comparison of the clinical and cost-effectiveness of 3 intervention strategies for AIDS wasting. *J. Acquir. Immune Defic. Synd.* 38: 399–406.

Stradling C, Thomas N, Taylor S, *et al.* (2016) 'Best foods for your heart': a pilot randomised controlled trial of dietary intervention to reduce cardiovascular risk in HIV dyslipidaemia. *Atherosclerosis.* 255: 5.

Tang AM, Graham NM, Kirby AJ, *et al.* (1993) Dietary micronutrient intake and risk of progression to acquired immunodeficiency syndrome (AIDS) in human deficiency virus type 1 (HIV-1)-infected homosexual men. *Am. J. Epidemiol.* 138: 937–951.

Tang AM, Graham NMH, Saah AJ. (1996) Effects of micronutrient intake on survival in human immunodeficiency virus type 1 infection. *Am. J. Epidemiol.* 143: 1244–1256.

Tang AM, Jacobson DL, Spiegelman D, *et al.* (2005) Increasing risk of 5% or greater unintentional weight loss in a cohort of HIV-infected patients, 1995 to 2003. *J. Acquir. Immune Defic. Synd.* 40: 70–76.

Umar SB, DiBaise JK. (2010) Protein-losing enteropathy: case illustrations and clinical review. *Am. J. Gastroenterol.* 105: 43–49; quiz 50.

Viard JP, Souberbielle JC, Kirk O, *et al.* (2011) Vitamin D and clinical disease progression in HIV infection: results from the EuroSIDA study. *AIDS.* 25: 1305–1315.

Wanke C, Kotler D, HIV Wasting Collaborative Consensus Committee. (2004) Collaborative recommendations: the approach to diagnosis and treatment of HIV wasting. *J. Acquir. Immune Defic. Synd.* 37(5): S284–288.

Wanke CA, Pleskow D, Degirolami PC, *et al.* (1996) A medium chain triglyceride-based diet in patients with HIV and chronic diarrhea reduces diarrhea and malabsorption: a prospective, controlled trial. *Nutrition.* 12: 766–771.

Wanke CA, Silva M, Knox TA, *et al.* (2000) Weight loss and wasting remain common complications in individuals infected with human immunodeficiency virus in the era of highly active antiretroviral therapy. *Clin. Infect. Dis.* 31: 803–805.

Waters L, Ahmed N, Angus B, *et al.* (2016) British HIV Association guidelines for the treatment of HIV-1-positive adults with antiretroviral therapy 2015 (2016 interim update). Available at https://www.bhiva.org/HIV-1-treatment-guidelines. Accessed 3 November 2018.

Wejse C, Gomes V, Rabna P, *et al.* (2009) Vitamin D as supplementary treatment for tuberculosis: a double-blind, randomized, placebo-controlled trial. *Am. J. Respir. Crit. Care Med.* 179: 843–850.

WHO. (2003) *Nutrient requirements for people living with HIV/AIDS: report of a technical consultation.* Available at www.who.int/nutrition/publications/Content_nutrient_requirements.pdf. Accessed 12 April 2018.

WHO. (2007) *WHO case definitions of HIV for surveillance and revised clinical staging and immunological classification of HIV-related disease in adults and children.* Available at www.who.int/hiv/pub/guidelines/HIVstaging150307.pdf. Accessed 12 April 2018.

Williams EC, Hahn JA, Saitz R, *et al.* (2016) Alcohol use and Human Immunodeficiency Virus (HIV) infection: current knowledge, implications, and future directions. *Alcohol. Clin. Exp. Res.* 40: 2056–2072.

Wohl DA, Brown TT. (2008) Management of morphologic changes associated with antiretroviral use in HIV-infected patients. *J. Acquir. Immune Defic. Synd.* 49(2): S93–S100.

Woods MN, Wanke CA, Ling PR, *et al.* (2009) Effect of a dietary intervention and n-3 fatty acid supplementation on measures of serum lipid and insulin sensitivity in persons with HIV. *Am. J. Clin. Nutr.* 90: 1566–1578.

Yarasheski KE, Roubenoff R. (2001) Exercise treatment for HIV associated metabolic and anthropomorphic complications. *Exerc. Sport Sci. Rev.* 29: 170–174.

7.12 Diabetes mellitus

Pamela Dyson

Key points

- Diabetes is one of the most common non-communicable diseases, has high rates of both morbidity and mortality, and affects over 285 million people globally.
- There are two main types of diabetes, type 1 and type 2.
- Lifestyle interventions, including diet and physical activity, are fundamental to diabetes management, and evidence is accumulating for the most effective strategies.
- The key to successful management is to tailor lifestyle advice to the individual.

Diabetes mellitus (DM) is a metabolic disorder characterised by chronic hyperglycaemia resulting from defects in insulin secretion, insulin action or both (WHO, 2006). It is one of the most common non-communicable diseases (NCD) worldwide, and is a leading cause of morbidity and premature death. The global prevalence of diabetes in adults has been estimated as 415 million in 2015 (9% of the adult population), and is projected to increase to 642 million (10% of the population) by 2040 (International Diabetes Federation (IDF), 2015). Over 75% of those with diabetes live in lower- and middle income-countries. Diabetes UK, the leading charity for people with diabetes in the UK, estimated that 3.4 million people in the UK (6.2%) were living with diabetes in 2015 (Diabetes UK, 2015); these statistics are supported by data from the NHS Quality and Outcomes Framework (Holman *et al.*, 2015).

Diabetes is a disease with high rates of morbidity and mortality (Zimmet *et al.*, 2001), and it has been estimated that diabetes caused 1.5 million deaths in 2012 (WHO Organisation, 2016). Diabetes is associated with macrovascular complications (cardiovascular disease, stroke, peripheral vascular disease) leading to heart attacks, haemiplegia and amputations, and with microvascular complications (neuropathy, retinopathy, nephropathy) causing foot ulcers, blindness and kidney failure (EURODIAB IDDM Complications Study Group, 1994; Turner *et al.*, 1995). Apart from the effects of diabetes in terms of health and quality of life, it imposes a financial burden on societies. In the UK in 2012, treatment of diabetes and its associated complications accounted for 10% of the total NHS budget, approximately £10 billion (Hex *et al.*, 2012).

Diagnostic criteria

The diagnostic criteria for diabetes have been developed and revised by the World Health Organization (WHO, 2006) and use the occurrence of diabetes-specific complications to derive diagnostic cut-points for diabetes. A diagnosis of diabetes can be made under any of the following circumstances:

- Fasting plasma glucose >7.0 mmol/L (126 mg/dL).
- 2-hour glucose >11.1 mmol/L (200 mg/dL) after ingestion of a 75-g oral glucose load (oral glucose tolerance test (OGTT)).
- Glycated haemoglobin (HbA1c) >48 mmol/mol (6.5%).

Glycaemia can be assessed by a simple blood test measuring levels of glycated haemoglobin (HbA1c), and the WHO now recommends that this test may be used in the diagnosis of diabetes, provided that stringent quality assurance tests are in place and that assays are standardised to international reference values (WHO, 2011). However, the diagnosis of diabetes in an asymptomatic person should not be made on the basis of a single HbA1c test, and an additional plasma glucose or HbA1c test is required to confirm the diagnosis.

In addition, both impaired glucose tolerance (IGT) and increased fasting glucose (IFG) have been identified as risk factors for developing diabetes, and IGT as a risk factor for cardiovascular disease (WHO, 2006). The diagnostic criteria for IGT and IFG are:

- IGT: Fasting plasma glucose <7.0 mmol/L (126 mg/dL), and 2-hour plasma glucose >7.8 and <11.1 mmol/L (140 and 200 mg/dL) after OGTT

Manual of Dietetic Practice, Sixth Edition. Edited by Joan Gandy.

Companion website: www.manualofdieteticpractice.com

- IFG: Fasting plasma glucose 6.1–6.9 mmol/L (110–125 mg/dL), and (if measured) 2-hour glucose <7.8 mmol/L (142 mg/dL)

Classification

There are two broad types of diabetes: type 1 and type 2.

Type 1 diabetes

Type 1 diabetes is an autoimmune disease characterised by destruction of the insulin-producing cells of the pancreas. Its cause is unknown, although genetic factors and certain viruses may play a part. Type 1 diabetes usually presents in children and young adults, although it can be diagnosed at any age. It accounts for approximately 10–20% of diabetes, and is treated by a combination of insulin replacement (by injection or pump therapy) and lifestyle modification.

Type 2 diabetes

Type 2 diabetes is caused by a combination of impaired insulin secretion and resistance to the action of insulin. Type 2 diabetes has a strong genetic propensity, but is also associated with lifestyle factors, and is more common in societies with low levels of physical activity and high levels of obesity. Currently, 90% of adults in England with type 2 diabetes are overweight or obese (Public Health England (PHE), 2014). Although traditionally diagnosed in people over the age of 40, it is now increasingly being diagnosed in obese children and adolescents, and as many as 1 400 children may have type 2 diabetes in the UK (Lobstein & Leach, 2004). Globally, it has been estimated that 4 million children aged 4–17 years will have type 2 diabetes by 2015 (Lobstein & Jackson-Leach, 2016). Type 2 diabetes affects approximately 80–90% of those diagnosed with diabetes and is treated by a combination of diet, physical activity, oral medications and, increasingly, injectable therapies, including insulin.

Other types of diabetes

Other types of diabetes are those that are neither type 1 nor type 2, and they are summarised in the following text:

- Maturity-onset diabetes of the young (MODY) is a hereditary form of diabetes caused by mutations in the genes, which affect insulin production.
- Latent autoimmune diabetes in adults (LADA) is a slow-progressing form of autoimmune diabetes, sometimes referred to as type 1.5. LADA is usually managed by diet and physical activity, and eventually insulin.
- Gestational diabetes mellitus (GDM) is caused by increased insulin demand during pregnancy. It may resolve after birth, but increases the risk of developing type 2 diabetes in later life.
- Secondary diabetes occurs after surgical removal of the pancreas, as a result of pancreatitis or can be induced by drugs, usually high doses of steroids.

Disease processes

Physiology of diabetes

DM is a condition in which the body is unable to utilise the glucose in the blood for energy due to complete or relative lack of insulin, insulin resistance (a condition where the body does not respond adequately to insulin) or a combination of both. Insulin is produced and secreted in the β-cells of islets of Langerhans in the pancreas, and type 1 diabetes is characterised by complete β-cell failure, leading to absolute insulin deficiency. Type 2 diabetes is characterised by progressive β-cell failure and is usually associated with peripheral insulin resistance. Complete or relative lack of insulin results in raised blood glucose levels and the diagnosis of diabetes.

Glucose is the body's primary energy source, and is provided by foods containing carbohydrate. Carbohydrate is found in starchy foods such as bread; potatoes; rice and pasta; and sugary foods such as sweets, chocolate and cakes, and occurs as natural sugars in milk and fruit. After eating, excess glucose is first stored in the liver and muscle as glycogen, to be released into the bloodstream as blood glucose levels fall. Once glycogen stores are filled, excess glucose is converted to fat and stored as adipose tissue.

Insulin is automatically released as blood glucose levels rise following carbohydrate intake or glycogenolysis. Insulin facilitates entry of glucose into the muscle and adipose tissue cells to be utilised as energy. Lack of insulin leads directly to increased blood glucose levels and the symptoms of diabetes, i.e. polyuria, polydipsia, fatigue, weight loss and increased susceptibility to infections.

Symptoms of diabetes

Blood glucose levels >12 mmol/L exceed the renal threshold, therefore glucose will appear in the urine. Glucose can be excreted by the kidneys only when accompanied by fluid, and this extra fluid causes excessive urine production (polyuria), leading to excessive thirst (polydipsia). Lack of insulin means that the body's cells are unable to utilise glucose for energy, and, despite high circulating glucose levels, the body has to rely on its stores of fat for energy. Lack of available glucose causes fatigue and weight loss. In the absence of any insulin, people with type 1 diabetes rely entirely on fat and its by-products, ketones, for energy. Small amounts of ketones can be used for energy, but large amounts cause acidity and, in combination with high blood glucose levels, this results in diabetic ketoacidosis (DKA), a life-threatening condition.

Disease consequences

It is challenging to assess mortality and morbidity rates for people with diabetes as many countries do not have diabetes registers or a system of death certification. Where death certificates do exist, diabetes is often not noted as a cause of death, and, as a result, available statistics frequently underestimate mortality.

Mortality

The IDF estimated that, in 2015, 5 million deaths in the 20–79 age group were caused by diabetes (IDF, 2015). Diabetes is associated with premature mortality from a variety of causes, including vascular disease, cancer, infectious diseases, intentional self-harm, external causes and degenerative disorders (The Emerging Risk Factors Collaboration, 2011). It doubles the risk of vascular disease, which is the cause of death in nearly 60% of people with diabetes (The Emerging Risk Factors Collaboration, 2010), and people with diabetes are 25% more likely to die of cancer. Hyperglycaemia is directly associated with risk of death, with levels of >5.6 mmol/L linked with increased risk. On average, a 50-year-old adult with diabetes and without vascular disease will die 6 years earlier than a counterpart without diabetes.

Morbidity

One of the most important features of diabetes is the association of sustained hyperglycaemia with long-term tissue damage; as a result, morbidity rates are high. There is strong evidence that intensive glycaemic control and management of cardiovascular risk factors can reduce both the morbidity and mortality associated with diabetes (DCCT Research Group, 1993; UKPDS Group, 1998). There is also evidence that improvements in care have reduced the risk of complications for people with type 1 diabetes over the past 30 years. However, even those receiving intensive treatment still show relatively high levels of complications, with over 20% developing proliferative retinopathy and 9% developing nephropathy and cardiovascular disease (Nathan *et al.*, 2009).

Macrovascular disease

Macrovascular or cardiovascular disease (CVD) affects the large blood vessels, and is the most common complication associated with diabetes. It is associated with premature mortality and poses a disproportionate risk for premenopausal women (Koerbel & Korytkowski, 2003) and ethnic minority groups with diabetes (Oldroyd *et al.*, 2005). Risk factors for CVD in people with diabetes include hyperglycaemia, hypertension, dyslipidaemia, overweight and obesity, tobacco use, high-fat diet and physical inactivity. Management of CVD risk for people with diabetes is multi-factorial, and data from long-term studies have shown significant benefits of risk factor control for both type 1 and type 2 diabetes (DCCT/EDIC Study Group, 2016; Holman *et al.*, 2008). There has been much discussion about the role of intensive glycaemic control in people with type 2 diabetes, and a review of studies that have failed to show a significant reduction in CVD events concluded that individual targets for glycaemia may be appropriate, and that management of blood pressure and lipids, smoking cessation and healthy lifestyles are a priority for CVD risk-management (Skyler *et al.*, 2009).

Microvascular disease

Microvascular disease affects the small blood vessels, especially in the eye, kidney and nerves. Diabetes is the most common cause of blindness in people of working age in the UK, and is also the most common cause of lower limb amputations and end-stage renal disease (ESRD) (Diabetes UK, 2015).

Diabetic retinopathy

This describes the narrowing or blockage of blood vessels at the back of the eye, caused by high blood glucose levels, high blood pressure, or a combination of these. It can be divided into early, reversible (background) retinopathy, and the more developed stages that require treatment and may result in blindness. It affects 10–65% of people with diabetes globally (IDF, 2015), and the prevalence is related to the duration of diabetes. In the UK, it is estimated that 25% of people with diabetes will develop retinopathy after 5 years (NHS Choices, 2011).

Diabetic nephropathy

Nephropathy affects the blood vessels in the kidney, and the first sign is the presence of small amounts of protein in the urine (microalbuminuria). Microalbuminuria may be present for many years without progression, but can lead to increased protein loss and, eventually, ESRD, requiring dialysis or transplant. Globally, 5–30% develop nephropathy, and figures for the UK suggest that 30% of people with type 2 diabetes will develop kidney disease (Stratton *et al.*, 2000).

Diabetic neuropathy

Nerve damage associated with high blood glucose levels can affect sensory nerves (resulting in loss of sensation or increased pain sensation), autonomic nerves (leading to warmer, swollen feet, or dry, cracked skin) and motor nerves (leading to muscle atrophy and deformities in the shape of the foot). Nerve damage is often associated with peripheral circulatory damage and can lead to foot ulcers, progressing to gangrene and requiring amputation. Peripheral neuropathy is estimated to affect 15–55% of people with diabetes worldwide (IDF, 2015).

Diabetic gastroparesis

Diabetic gastroparesis (DGP) is characterised by delayed gastric emptying in the absence of mechanical obstruction of the stomach, and is associated with central neuropathy affecting the vagal nerve. It leads to erratic blood glucose control and postprandial hypoglycaemia in those treated with insulin (see Chapter 7.4.4, Gastroparesis).

Sexual dysfunction

Erectile dysfunction (ED) and female sexual dysfunction (FSD) are more common in people with diabetes. ED affects 35–90% of men with diabetes and is associated with increasing age, duration of diabetes, hyperglycaemia, hypertension, hyperlipidaemia, sedentary lifestyle and smoking (Malavige & Levy, 2009). FSD has been reported in 33% of women with diabetes, but it does not appear to be associated with diabetes-related factors (Nowosielski & Skrzypulec-Plinta, 2011).

Depression

People with diabetes appear to have a twofold increased risk of depression (Anderson *et al.*, 2011), and this is true for both type 1 (Barnard *et al.*, 2006) and type 2 diabetes (Ali *et al.*, 2006). The presence of depression is associated with a reduced quality of life in people with diabetes (Schram *et al.*, 2009).

Public health aspects and prevention

There is no evidence for the prevention of type 1 diabetes as the aetiology remains unclear, but there is strong evidence from studies in different ethnic groups showing that type 2 diabetes can be prevented in high-risk individuals by lifestyle and pharmacological interventions (Paulweber *et al.*, 2010; Stevens *et al.*, 2015). Lifestyle interventions show the greatest effect, with reductions in risk of 28–59% following implementation (Walker *et al.*, 2010), and with a legacy effect of lower incidence of diabetes at 7–20 years after intervention (Knowler *et al.*, 2009; Li *et al.*, 2008; Lindstrom *et al.*, 2006). Evidence-based European guidelines for diabetes prevention and Diabetes UK lifestyle-specific guidelines have been published, and are summarised in the following text (Dyson *et al.*, 2011; Paulweber *et al.*, 2010). Diabetes prevention programs have been applied to real-world settings in a variety of countries, and, although surrogate end-points (weight loss) rather than progression to type 2 diabetes are commonly reported, there is evidence of efficacy (Aziz *et al.*, 2015; Dunkley *et al.*, 2014; Johnson *et al.*, 2013).

Components of lifestyle interventions for type 2 diabetes prevention

Weight reduction

Weight reduction in overweight or obese individuals is the most dominant factor for diabetes prevention, with weight losses of 5–7% significantly lowering risk, with a 16% reduction in risk associated with every kilogram lost (Hamman *et al.*, 2006). Although the majority of studies have promoted reduced-fat, high-fibre diets with a moderate reduction in energy intake, there is emerging evidence that alternative dietary strategies, including the Mediterranean diet and low-carbohydrate diets, are effective for weight loss and diabetes risk reduction (Walker *et al.*, 2010).

Physical activity

Increased physical activity reduces the risk of diabetes, and at least 30 minutes per day of moderate activity is recommended on at least 5 days during the week.

Diet

Studies have shown that diets high in fibre (>15 g/1000 kcal) and reduced in total fat (<35% total energy) and saturated and trans fat (<10% total energy) can induce weight loss and reduce risk. There are no head-to-head trials of different dietary strategies showing the most effective diet for type 2 diabetes prevention.

Nutritional assessment

Anthropometry

Body weight and BMI should be monitored regularly in people with diabetes, especially in those with type 2 diabetes, as they are prone to weight gain. Obesity increases the risk of diabetes-related complications, especially cardiovascular disease. Waist circumference predicts both type 2 diabetes and cardiovascular disease (Yusuf *et al.*, 2004). Waist circumference cut-off points differ by ethnicity and gender (see Chapter 2.2, Assessment of nutritional status).

Biochemistry

HbA1c measures long-term glycaemic control (over 10–12 weeks) by assessing levels of glycated haemoglobin, and should be measured 6-monthly, and more frequently if there have been changes in medication or lifestyle. In the UK, HbA1c is now expressed in mmol/mol. Lipid profiles (serum total cholesterol, high density lipoprotein (HDL) and low density lipoprotein cholesterol, and triglycerides levels) are measured to assess cardiovascular risk. Microalbumin is an indicator of early-stage kidney disease; it should be measured annually. In addition, blood creatinine measurements can be used to calculate eGFR, which provides an assessment of overall excretory kidney function.

Clinical

Blood pressure assesses cardiovascular risk, and should be measured at least once a year. Retinal screening involves dilation of the eyes and a retinal photograph, and is designed to measure diabetic eye disease. In the UK, all people with diabetes are called to have an annual retinal screening. Foot examination assesses skin, blood and nerve supply to the legs and feet, and should be part of the annual review. Injection sites should be examined in people using injection therapy to check for hyperlipotrophy, hard lumps under the skin caused by repeated injections into the same site, which affects insulin absorption.

Dietary assessment

There is some discussion about the usefulness of diet histories (including 24-hour recall) in managing chronic diseases such as diabetes. Many dietitians feel that it is impossible to give someone advice about a healthy diet unless they have some idea of the individual's usual diet, but there is no evidence that taking a diet history improves diabetes control. On the other hand, strong evidence exists that up to 67% of people under-report intake, especially snack foods. BMI is a strong determinant of under-reporting (Poslusna *et al.*, 2009). Dietary assessment can be used to evaluate an individual's wishes and willingness to change in the following areas:

- Meal patterns and usual lifestyle, and gives additional information about work and physical activity.

- Likes and dislikes, including usual food choices, and attitudes and beliefs about different foods.
- Perceptions and beliefs about food, related specifically to health.

Economic and social factors

Factors such as socioeconomic circumstances, ethnic group and occupation will influence people's willingness and ability to manage their diabetes.

Clinical management

The aims of management of diabetes are to maintain blood glucose as near to normal as possible in order to minimise both the short-term (hypoglycaemia and diabetic ketoacidosis) and long-term (macrovascular and microvascular) complications.

Targets for glycaemic control

Internationally, it is generally agreed that, for most people, the target for HbA1c level is <53 mmol/mol (7.0%). In the UK, targets for people with type 1 diabetes are set at <48 mmol/mol (6.5%) (NICE, 2015a, 2015b), and individualised targets of 48–59 mmol/mol (6.5–7.5%) are recommended for those with type 2 diabetes (NICE, 2015c). Self-blood glucose monitoring (SBGM) at least four times daily is encouraged in those with type 1 diabetes, and more monitoring may be required when exercising, driving, during sickness, in pregnancy and in those experiencing hypoglycaemia. Finger-prick testing is routinely used for SBGM, although continuous glucose monitoring is also available. Targets for self-monitored blood glucose (SMBG) levels in the UK are:

- Children with type 1 diabetes (NICE, 2015a)
  - On waking (fasting plasma glucose) 4–7 mmol/L
  - Before meals 4–7 mmol/L
  - After meals 5–9 mmol/L
- Adults with type 1 diabetes (NICE, 2015b)
  - On waking (fasting plasma glucose) 5–7 mmol/L
  - Before meals 4–7 mmol/L
  - >90 minutes postprandial 5–9 mmol/L
- Pregnancy (NICE, 2015d)
  - Fasting <5.3 mmol/L
  - 1 hour post-meal <7.8 mmol/L
  - 2 hours post-meal <6.4 mmol/L

It is now recommended that self-monitoring of blood glucose not be offered routinely to adults with type 2 diabetes, unless they inject insulin, have evidence of hypoglycaemia, are driving or operating machinery and take oral medication that increases hypoglycaemia risk, or if a woman is pregnant or planning pregnancy (NICE, 2015c).

Targets for risk-reduction of comorbidities

Targets for risk factor reduction in the UK are:

- Adults with type 1 diabetes
  - Blood pressure <135/80 mm/Hg (or <130/80 mm/Hg for those with abnormal albumin excretion or more than two features of the metabolic syndrome) (NICE, 2015b).
  - No specific targets for lipid concentrations. Therapy should be offered to those aged >40 years, with established nephropathy, or with >10% risk of CVD assessed by QRISK2 tool.
- Individuals with type 2 diabetes (NICE, 2015c)
  - Blood pressure <140/80 mm/Hg (or <130/80 mm/Hg in those with evidence of complications)
  - No specific targets for lipid concentrations (aim should be the lowest possible). Therapy should be offered to those with >10% risk of CVD assessed by QRISK2 tool
- Diabetes UK recommend the following lipid concentrations in people with diabetes:
  - Total cholesterol <4.0 mmol/L
  - LDL cholesterol <2.0 mmol/L
  - HDL cholesterol >1.0 mmol/L in men and >1.2 mmol/L in women
  - Triglycerides <1.7 mmol/L (Diabetes UK/BDA, 2015).

Pharmaceutical management of diabetes

Type 1 diabetes

Type 1 diabetes is managed by insulin replacement; there are many different insulin preparations available, and the type, dose and regimen depends on the lifestyle of the individual. Until the 1980s, insulin was only available by extraction and purification from the pancreas of cattle and pigs. This animal insulin is still in use, but has been largely replaced by human insulin that is genetically engineered. Newer analogue insulin types have been introduced in an attempt to replicate the action of naturally produced insulin in the body. Insulin can be divided into the following types:

- Rapid-acting analogue insulin with an onset of action within 5–10 minutes, peaking at 90 minutes and lasting for 4 hours. It is commonly taken with meals and can be injected at the time of, or after, eating.
- Short-acting insulin begins working within 30 minutes, peaks at 2 hours and lasts for 4–8 hours. Like rapid-acting insulin, it is usually taken with meals, but is injected 20–30 minutes before eating.
- Medium- and long-acting insulins are usually taken once or twice a day and provide background insulin over 24 hours. They have an onset of action within 90 minutes, peak between 4 and 12 hours and last 12–24 hours.
- Long-acting analogue insulin is promoted as having a flat profile, with no peak action and lasts 18–42 hours. It is usually taken once or twice a day.
- Mixed insulin consists of premixed short-acting insulin with medium- or long-acting insulin, and is usually taken twice a day, usually before breakfast and before the evening meal. It has an onset of action within 30 minutes, peaks at 2–8 hours and lasts 16–20 hours.
- Mixed analogue insulin is a mixture of rapid-acting and long-acting analogue insulin with an onset of action within 5–10 minutes, peaking at 90 minutes and lasting 6–10 hours.

New initiatives in insulin treatment include the development of longer-acting basal, faster-acting rapid, and higher-strength insulins, and combinations of fixed doses of long-acting basal insulin and incretin mimetics.

The majority of people with type 1 diabetes are encouraged to use multiple daily injection (MDI) regimens, also known as basal bolus, typically consisting of one injection of long-acting insulin and three (or more) injections of rapid-acting insulin with meals. This intensive insulin regimen has been shown to be associated with improved glycaemic control and allows for dietary flexibility (DAFNE Study Group, 2002). The traditional regimen of mixed insulin injected twice daily, usually before breakfast and before the evening meal, is less common, and is associated with increased hypoglycaemia in those who do not have regular meals.

Insulin is administered using syringe and needles, pen injection devices, or pumps (continuous subcutaneous insulin infusion (CSII). Pump therapy consists of a portable pump that delivers rapid-acting insulin through a cannula, providing background insulin and a bolus of insulin when food is eaten. Pump therapy is becoming more common; in the UK, in 2013, approximately 6% of adults and 19% of children with type 1 diabetes were using pump therapy, although this did not compare favourably with other European countries such as Germany and Norway, where 15% used pump therapy, and the USA, where 40% of people with type 1 diabetes used pump therapy (Diabetes UK, 2013). In the UK, NICE has issued guidance stating that pumps are suitable for those with disabling hypoglycaemia, or those who have failed to reach HbA1c <69 mmol/mol despite MDI therapy and structured education (NICE, 2008).

Type 2 diabetes

Type 2 diabetes is managed clinically with a combination of various oral and injectable therapies, including insulin. Various algorithms have been produced recommending a treatment cascade for those with type 2 diabetes, and all emphasise lifestyle interventions, including structured education (Inzucchi *et al.*, 2015; NICE, 2015c).

- Metformin is recommended as a first-line therapy; it belongs to the biguanide class of drugs, and its main action is to increase insulin sensitivity and reduce hepatic gluconeogenesis. It does not cause weight gain or hypoglycaemia and may be associated with a reduced risk of cardiovascular disease. Around 10% of patients do not respond to metformin, and approximately 5–10% of patients a year on metformin will need an additional agent. If maximum tolerated doses of metformin fail to achieve target glucose levels, a second agent is commonly added in.
- Sulphonylureas act directly on the pancreas to stimulate insulin production. They are associated with weight gain of approximately 3 kg, and can cause hypoglycaemia.
- Glinides are short-acting agents that are used to control postprandial rises in glucose. They are taken before main meals and stimulate insulin production for that meal. Essentially, they may be viewed as a short-acting sulphonylurea and have similar side effects, although they are generally regarded as weight neutral.
- Thiazolidinediones (also known as glitazones) are taken once daily, starting with a low dose, and are taken up to 3 months to achieve maximum effect. Their action is to reduce insulin resistance; they produce a lowering of blood glucose levels comparable to metformin or sulphonylurea. Side effects include weight gain and fluid retention. Glitazones tend to be given as second- or third-line therapy, partly because of the 10–12 weeks that it takes for them to have effect.
- Acarbose is an alpha-glucosidase inhibitor that reduces the rate of carbohydrate digestion, thus controlling postprandial blood glucose rises. This agent has unpleasant side effects such as flatulence, abdominal pain, bloating and diarrhoea. Since its effect is moderate as compared to the other agents available, it is rarely prescribed in the UK, although it is widely used in countries with higher carbohydrate intakes e.g. China.
- Incretin agonists are injectable therapies which mimic the action of naturally produced gut hormones and act by stimulating glucose-dependant insulin secretion from the pancreas, reducing glucagon secretion and inhibiting gastric emptying, thus promoting satiety and reducing weight. The most common side effects are nausea and vomiting.
- Gliptins (DPP-4 inhibitors) prevent the rapid degradation of the enzyme dipeptidyl peptidase 4 (DPP-4), and thereby increase concentrations of endogenous, naturally occurring incretin hormones. They are weight-neutral, and the most frequent side effect is that of nausea.
- Sodiumglucose linked transporter 2 (SGLT2) inhibitors are novel therapies that act by preventing reabsorption of 30–50% of glucose in the proximal tubule of the kidney. This promotes glucose excretion in the urine and lowers blood glucose concentrations. They offer a realistic chance of weight loss and do not cause hypoglycaemia, and the most common side effect is urinary tract infections.

In addition to blood glucose management, people with diabetes frequently take antihypertensives and statins, and may need further agents to treat any diabetes-related complication.

Surgical treatment of diabetes

Bariatric surgery is increasingly used as a treatment for obesity in people with type 2 diabetes, with a recent IDF statement calling for surgery to be an accepted treatment option for people with type 2 diabetes and BMI >35 (Dixon *et al.*, 2011). Surgery can induce diabetes remission, with rates of 65% reported in one meta-analysis (Yu *et al.*, 2015). Other surgical procedures to treat type 1 diabetes include islet transplantation and pancreatic transplants. Both these procedures can restore endogenous insulin secretion, but are only available to a few people because of a shortage of donors and because immunosuppressive drugs have side effects that may outweigh the benefits.

Lifestyle management

Lifestyle therapy, including diet and physical activity, is an integral part of the effective management of diabetes. It has a vital role in helping people with diabetes achieve and maintain optimal glycaemic control and reduce the risk of long-term tissue damage (Evert *et al.*, 2014). There is evidence that intensive treatment of type 1 diabetes, especially involving the diet, improves outcomes (Franz *et al.*, 2010), and that dietary change, weight loss and increased physical activity are of benefit to people with type 2 diabetes (Look AHEAD Research Group & Wing, 2010), although there are few well-designed studies investigating the most effective approach (Nield *et al.*, 2007).

Physical activity and diabetes management

The benefits of increased physical activity in people with type 2 diabetes are clear and include improved glycaemic control and reductions in cardiovascular risk, including positive effects on lipids and blood pressure. Long-term studies have shown that these benefits are translated to a reduction in cardiovascular events and improvements in mortality and quality of life (Colberg *et al.*, 2010). Physical activity does not appear to have a direct effect on BMI in people with type 2 diabetes, although there is evidence of reduction in visceral adipose tissue (Boulé *et al.*, 2001). The benefits of physical activity in people with type 1 diabetes are less clear-cut. Although physical activity improves cardiovascular risk and well-being, there is no evidence of improvement in glycaemic control in people with type 1 diabetes (Chimen *et al.*, 2012).

It is recommended that people with diabetes take at least 150 minutes of moderate activity each week. Physical activity guidelines are usually made in terms of daily activity, the most common recommendation being that moderate activity be taken on at least 5 days each week for 30 minutes. Moderate activity is defined as any activity that raises the heart rate, increases breathing rate but does not induce breathlessness, causes a feeling of warmth or promotes light sweating. For many people, brisk walking is sufficient.

Physical activity generally lowers blood glucose in people with diabetes and may increase the risk of hypoglycaemia in those taking insulin or sulphonylureas. For many people with type 2 diabetes not treated by insulin, the effects of physical activity are beneficial and do not require any adjustment to the medication or dietary intake. People with type 1 require more active management to prevent hypoglycaemia. Management of activity can be facilitated by SBGM and may require adjustment of medication and/or increased carbohydrate intake.

Before undertaking activity, people treated with sulphonylureas or insulin are advised to test their blood glucose levels, aiming for the range 6–13 mmol/L. If levels are <6 mmol/L, an additional 15–30 g of high-glycaemic-index (GI) carbohydrate should be taken, depending on the duration and intensity of exercise. Examples of high-GI carbohydrates include isotonic sports drinks, made-up squash, bananas, jelly beans and fruit pastilles. Alternatively, a reduction in meal-time insulin can be made if exercise takes place within 2 hours of the last meal. People with type 1 diabetes showing levels of >13 mmol/L should delay activity and test for the presence of ketones, as they may be at increased risk of ketoacidosis.

During activity, additional high-GI carbohydrate may be necessary, depending on the duration and intensity of exercise. As a rough guide, for any exercise session that lasts more than 60 minutes, 30–60 g/hour of high-GI carbohydrate may be needed. After prolonged or strenuous activity, the effect of exercise can be assessed by testing blood glucose levels. Consuming high-GI carbohydrates within an hour of activity will replenish liver and muscle glycogen stores, and those with type 1 diabetes may need to reduce the post-activity insulin doses.

Alcohol and diabetes

Epidemiological studies have shown that moderate alcohol intake (1–3 units/day) in people with diabetes is associated with improved glycaemic control, and reduced cardiovascular disease and all-cause mortality (Koppes *et al.*, 2006). The guidelines for alcohol intake for people with diabetes do not differ from those for the general population, but there are additional factors for consideration.

Hypoglycaemia is a well-documented side effect of alcohol in people with type 1 diabetes and can occur at relatively low levels of intake, and up to 12 hours after ingestion. There is no evidence for the most effective treatment to prevent hypoglycaemia, but pragmatic advice includes recommending insulin dose adjustment, additional carbohydrate or a combination of the two according to individual need.

The amount of carbohydrate in alcoholic drinks can vary greatly, with some (dry wines, spirits) containing little or no carbohydrates, and some (sweet liqueurs, alcopops) containing significant amounts. Consumption of alcoholic drinks containing carbohydrate raises blood glucose levels and can cause hyperglycaemia. People treated by insulin may take extra to cover the carbohydrate in drinks, but this may exacerbate hypoglycaemia.

Nutritional management of diabetes

Aims of dietary treatment

Dietetic therapy is an integral part of diabetes self-management and treatment. The aims of dietary treatment of diabetes are complementary to those of medical management and have been summarised by Diabetes UK as (Dyson *et al.*, 2011) follows:

- Supporting self-management to reduce the risk of type 2 diabetes and the comorbidities associated with diabetes.
- Promoting healthy lifestyles and quality of life.
- Providing flexibility and meeting the needs of all individuals, including those with comorbidities such as coeliac disease and cystic fibrosis.

Many countries have published nutritional recommendations for diabetes (Canadian Diabetes Association, 2008; Dyson *et al.*, 2011; Evert *et al.*, 2014; Mann *et al.*, 2004). Recent recommendations have been made in terms of topic areas rather than nutrients, stressing on the importance of tailoring nutritional advice for each individual, taking into account personal and cultural preferences, beliefs, lifestyle, and willingness and ability to change.

Nutrition management and education models

In the UK, for people with diabetes, structured education is now recommended for all individuals at the time of diagnosis, with regular (at least annual) review (NICE, 2011). Nutritional management should be included as an integrated component of structured education, and there is strong evidence of clinical effectiveness, cost-effectiveness and improved quality of life for both type 1 and type 2 diabetes. Structured education can be delivered in groups or to individuals. The four key components of structured education are:

- A structured, written curriculum, including philosophy and theoretical principles.
- Trained educators.
- Quality assurance.
- Audit and evaluation of both biomedical and quality-of-life outcomes.

More detailed criteria for education programmes include the recommendations that all programmes should:

- Be patient-centred and incorporate individual assessment.
- Be reliable, valid, relevant and comprehensive.
- Be theory-driven and evidence-based.
- Be flexible and able to cope with diversity.
- Be able to utilise different teaching techniques.
- Be resource-effective with supporting materials, written down (including philosophy, aims and objectives, timetables and detailed content).
- Be subject to robust audit and evaluation.

Although these criteria apply more to structured education in groups, the principles can be applied to all education.

Education delivery

The traditional model of delivering education is that of one-to-one interviews between the healthcare professional and the person with diabetes, and is often based on dietary histories and prescriptive advice. These didactic-based approaches have been shown to produce modest improvements in outcomes, but patient education has been shown to be more effective if it has a behavioural element rather than being didactic. Innovative approaches may be needed to deliver education to people with diabetes. Patients with chronic disease, including diabetes, state that they would like information in as many formats as possible, and as early as possible after diagnosis, and a variety of techniques, including picture charts, video techniques, computer packages, text messaging, e-mail and phone applications, can be used (Corben & Rosen, 2005). There is evidence that these strategies are acceptable to people with diabetes, and that they support self-management, but the efficacy of new technologies still awaits confirmation (Or & Tao, 2014).

Nutrition and glycaemic control

Carbohydrate has most effect on blood glucose levels after eating, and is a major nutritional consideration for people with diabetes. All carbohydrate foods are digested to glucose and appear in the blood between 10 minutes and 2 hours or more after eating, and both the amount and type will affect postprandial levels. There is no evidence for an optimal amount of carbohydrate for achieving and maintaining glycaemic control in people with diabetes, and, in people with type 1 diabetes, the emphasis is on matching insulin to carbohydrate on a meal-by-meal basis. This process is commonly called carbohydrate counting and insulin adjustment. It requires calculation of the amount of carbohydrate in each meal and snack and injection of a matching amount of insulin. There is no evidence supporting the use of carbohydrate counting for people with type 2 diabetes. People with type 1 diabetes are treated with fixed doses of insulin, and those with type 2 diabetes are advised to monitor carbohydrate intake by a variety of means, including exchanges, portions or experience-based estimation. Carbohydrate restriction, by means of low-carbohydrate diets, has recently been promoted for the treatment of type 2 diabetes (Feinman *et al.*, 2015). Low-carbohydrate diets are effective in improving glycaemic control and reducing body weight, but there is no evidence of superiority over other, higher-carbohydrate diets (van Wyk *et al.*, 2016).

Carbohydrates

Carbohydrate awareness is the process of identifying carbohydrate-containing foods, and is the first step in the process of carbohydrate estimation. Carbohydrate awareness can be facilitated with a variety of teaching aids, including food lists, picture charts, food photographs and food models. Carbohydrate budgets or portions can be facilitated by a variety of strategies. Traditionally, carbohydrate was restricted in people with diabetes by the use of the exchange system (one exchange containing 10 g carbohydrate, e.g. two-thirds slice bread, one-third pint milk, two plain biscuits), where diets were prescribed with a limited allowance of exchanges at each meal or snack. The modern use of budgets or portions encourages consistent amounts of carbohydrate at each specific meal from day to day, but does not necessarily prescribe a limited amount of carbohydrate. Teaching aids for promoting consistent portion sizes include using household measurements (spoonfuls, cupfuls and units), visual estimation with reference to food photographs, comparing portion size to hand size (e.g. fist-sized potion of starchy food such as rice, potato or pasta) and exchanges lists.

Carbohydrate counting, used by people with type 1 diabetes, is the most accurate method of carbohydrate assessment. The amount of carbohydrate in individual meals and snacks is usually calculated to the nearest 5–10 g, or expressed as carbohydrate portions (CP), each containing 10 g carbohydrate. Strategies include the use of household measures, exchange or portion lists, and visual estimation using food photographs or phone applications. Nutritional labels on packaged foods can provide useful information. It can be helpful to weigh, at least initially, individual foods such as breakfast cereals, rice and pasta where there is no recognised portion size, and food tables are then necessary for carbohydrate calculation.

Type of carbohydrate

The most significant predictor of postprandial blood glucose levels is the amount of carbohydrate eaten, but the type of carbohydrate has an effect. Relevant concepts are those of glycaemic index, sugar and dietary fibre. The GI has been widely promoted for dietary management of diabetes, but recent reviews have suggested that the evidence is mixed, and that the positive effect of low-GI diets may be due to increased intakes of dietary fibre (Yu *et al.*, 2015). The ADA and Diabetes UK no longer recommend low-GI diets as a primary strategy for the dietary management of diabetes, although they acknowledge that substituting low-GI foods for high-GI food may modestly improve glycaemic control (Dyson *et al.*, 2011; Evert *et al.*, 2014). Sugar has been traditionally restricted in people with diabetes as it is commonly assumed that the sugar content of food relates directly to blood sugar (glucose) levels. In terms of glycaemic control, sucrose has no more effect on blood glucose levels than isocaloric amounts of starchy carbohydrate, but the effects of sugar on general health have been evaluated. Both WHO and SACN now recommend that <5% of total energy intake be derived from free sugars (SACN, 2015; WHO, 2015).

Dietary fibre is promoted for its cardioprotective effects, but there is little evidence for its effect on glycaemic control in people with diabetes. Some studies report improved glycaemic control, but these use large amounts of fibre (40–50 g/day), with little evidence supporting smaller amounts. The recommendation for the general population for fibre intake should be applied to people with diabetes (SACN, 2015).

Nutrition and diabetes complications

Cardiovascular disease

As people with diabetes are at high risk, nutrition recommendations are similar to those for people with established heart disease. The aims of nutritional guidelines for cardiovascular disease are to reduce risk by improving blood lipid profiles and reducing blood pressure by addressing dietary factors including fat, salt, dietary fibre and alcohol intake.

Fat

High fat intakes, especially saturated fat, are associated with increased lipid levels and risk of heart disease, and current recommendations from both the ADA and Diabetes UK recommend that people with diabetes reduce saturated fat and replace this with unsaturated fat, and particularly monounsaturated fat. The promotion of low-carbohydrate, high-fat diets for the treatment of type 2 diabetes was evaluated by Diabetes UK in 2015, and a policy statement was issued that there is currently no evidence to support the use of high-fat diets (Diabetes UK/BDA, 2015). In addition, there is no strong evidence to support a specific amount of total fat in the diet; current guidelines reflect this, and have not formulated recommendations for exact proportions of energy derived from fat, but do recommend individual flexibility. There is little evidence about trans fat intake in people with diabetes, and the guidelines for the general population should be adopted.

High intakes of oily fish are associated with reduced rates of cardiovascular disease, and oily fish should hence be consumed at least twice weekly. There remains controversy about the use of fish oil supplements for people with diabetes, with some evidence of reduction in triglyceride levels in those with hypertriglyceridaemia. Diabetes UK indicates that fish oil supplementation may have therapeutic benefits for this sub-group.

Plant stanols and sterols

Plant sterols and stanols included in manufactured foods such as margarine, yogurt and yogurt drinks can significantly lower cholesterol levels, by up to 10%. In the UK, NICE do not recommend plant stanols and sterols as a cost-effective intervention for people with diabetes (NICE, 2014).

Salt

Salt intakes are significantly associated with blood pressure, and studies show that salt reduction lowers blood pressure. The daily average intake of salt in the UK is 8.6 g/day, and most guidelines recommend reductions to 5–6 g/day, effectively reducing consumption by one-third. Reductions in salt intake can be achieved by avoiding or reducing the salt used in cooking or added at the table, and by avoiding obviously salty foods such as savoury snacks. However, the majority of salt (75%) in the Western diet comes from processed foods, and effective salt reduction will require intervention from the food industry.

Dietary fibre

Although there is contradictory evidence for the role of dietary fibre in glycaemic control, high intakes of fibre, and especially soluble fibre, are associated with reductions in cholesterol and LDL cholesterol levels. Guidelines for people with diabetes recommend adopting the dietary reference values for the general population.

Physical activity, alcohol and weight management are all key factors for cardiovascular risk reduction, and are discussed in Chapter 7.14.1 (General aspects of cardiovascular disease). Dietary strategies to reduce cardiovascular disease combine some of the individual elements associated with risk reduction, and include the Mediterranean and dietary approaches to stop hypertension (DASH) diets. These diets recommend reducing saturated fat and substituting fish and olive oil for red meat and butter, and increasing vegetable, fruit, pulses and legumes, and wholegrain intake. The combined effects of these diets have a greater effect on blood pressure than those achieved by individual components, and significantly reduce cardiovascular risk.

Microvascular disease

The most important predictor of both development and progression of microvascular disease is glycaemic control. All nutritional strategies to maintain or improve blood glucose levels in people with diabetes can be applied to those with microvascular disease. There is very little good-quality evidence for specific nutritional management of diabetes-related microvascular disease apart from that of glycaemic control.

Hypoglycaemia

People with diabetes treated by insulin, sulphonylureas or glinides are at risk of hypoglycaemia, and this risk increases with the duration of diabetes. In people with diabetes, hypoglycaemia is defined as a blood glucose level of <4 mmol/L. Those with diabetes can be advised to 'make 4 the floor', meaning they should treat any level <4 mmol/L as soon as possible. People without diabetes are unlikely to experience hypoglycaemia due to a homeostatic response as blood glucose levels fall and the glucose stored in the liver is released into the bloodstream by the action of the counter-regulatory hormones glucagon, adrenaline and cortisol. Although this process does occur in people with diabetes, it may be overridden by the presence of excess insulin, and there is evidence of attenuated hormonal response related to the duration of diabetes. The causes of hypoglycaemia include:

- Missing or delaying a meal or snack.
- Eating less carbohydrate than normal.
- Increased physical activity or exercise.
- Drinking alcohol.
- Taking excessive amounts of insulin or tablets.

The first symptoms of hypoglycaemia are caused by adrenaline release and include sweating, shaking, increased heart rate, hunger or nausea, anxiety, irritability, tiredness and headache. As hypoglycaemia progresses, lack of glucose to the brain can cause confusion, lack of coordination, slurred speech, drowsiness and aggression, and eventually convulsions and coma. Hypoglycaemia is rarely fatal, although deaths have been reported following excessive alcohol consumption. Severe hypoglycaemia in those already at high CVD risk appears to increase this risk.

Treatment of hypoglycaemia aims to raise blood glucose levels to the normal range as quickly as possible, avoiding over-treating and associated hyperglycaemia and preventing re-occurrence of hypoglycaemia. Glucose is the preferred treatment for hypoglycaemia, and advice for treatment follows the 'rule of 15':

- 15–20 g glucose taken as soon as possible.
- If glucose levels do not rise above 4 mmol/L after 15 minutes, repeat treatment.
- A follow-up snack containing 15–20 g carbohydrate may be necessary to reduce the risk of further hypoglycaemia.

Isolated incidences of hypoglycaemia should follow the preceding guidelines, but repeated hypoglycaemic episodes need further investigation. Advice for prevention involves identifying the cause and taking steps to prevent re-occurrence by adjusting insulin dose or carbohydrate intake. General advice includes instructions to avoid missing meals, always carry glucose, monitor blood glucose levels before driving, and avoid drinking alcohol on an empty stomach.

Hypoglycaemia unawareness is a condition in which people no longer recognise the symptoms of hypoglycaemia. It is more prevalent in people with type 1 diabetes and is associated with duration of diabetes and intensive management. Symptoms can be restored after a period of maintaining glucose at higher levels, and this should be done under medical supervision.

Other nutritional considerations

Protein

There is insufficient evidence to support protein restriction to prevent the development of diabetic nephropathy, and a systematic review has concluded that there is little evidence to support protein restriction as a management strategy for established diabetic kidney disease (Robertson *et al.*, 2007). Current guidelines recommend that protein intakes for the general population be adopted for people with diabetes.

Fat

Fat has a negligible impact on blood glucose levels following ingestion, but high-fat meals may delay digestion, leading to increased postprandial glucose concentrations up to 8 hours after a meal. There is some evidence that high-fat diets are associated with increased insulin resistance.

Micronutrients

Recent research has investigated the role of vitamin D in diabetes and cardiovascular disease prevention and the association of vitamin B_1 with a reduction in the risk of kidney and heart disease in people with diabetes. There is, as yet, no firm evidence to support the use of vitamin supplements in people with diabetes. Chromium, magnesium and zinc are all utilised in carbohydrate metabolism and have been the focus of diabetes studies. Studies report conflicting results regarding the benefits of supplementation in terms of glycaemic control, and the current advice from Diabetes UK is that there is insufficient evidence to recommend any vitamin or mineral supplement for people with diabetes.

Functional foods

Food such as chilli and karela (bitter gourd) and spices (cinnamon and fenugreek) have been shown to lower blood glucose levels, and are frequently used in traditional medicine. Although they have hypoglycaemic effects, these are unpredictable, and they are not currently recommended.

Weight management

Weight loss can improve glycaemic control, and reduce cardiovascular risk and all-cause mortality in people with type 2 diabetes (Aucott *et al.*, 2004), and recent research reported that significant weight loss (10 kg) at diagnosis induced diabetes remission at 1-year follow-up in 46% of the sample (Lean *et al.*, 2018). There is little evidence for weight loss in people with type 1 diabetes. Strategies used to promote weight reduction in people with diabetes include dietary, physical activity, behavioural, pharmacological and surgical interventions.

Dietary interventions for weight loss

Studies using dietary interventions for weight loss in people with type 2 diabetes have been widely researched and reported, but many have methodological flaws and take place over the short term, so it is difficult to draw firm conclusions for clinical practice. Different dietary strategies have been used, including low-fat diets, low-calorie diets, low-carbohydrate diets, very-low-calorie liquid diets, meal replacements and commercial slimming clubs. Regardless of the diet used, dietary interventions for obesity have positive effects on body weight and improve glycaemic control, although weight loss of >5% appears to be necessary for significant benefit (Franz *et al.*, 2015). However, there is no evidence for the most effective diet for inducing weight loss in people with diabetes, and the advice from Diabetes UK is that any strategy that is recommended for people without diabetes can be adopted by those with diabetes (see Chapter 7.13.2, The management of obesity and overweight in adults).

Physical activity and weight loss

Physical activity is not an effective strategy for weight loss in people with diabetes when used in isolation (Boule *et al.*, 2001); a combination of diet and physical activity is more effective than either strategy alone (Shaw *et al.*, 2006). There are very few studies investigating the effects of different types and intensities of physical activity in weight loss, and guidelines cannot be formulated for the relative benefits of aerobic or resistance training.

Behavioural therapy and weight loss

Many different psychological techniques have been used to promote weight loss, including behavioural and cognitive therapy, group therapy, psycho-dynamic therapy and humanistic therapy. All behavioural interventions have been shown to promote significant weight loss, and adding dietary or physical activity interventions increases weight loss (Dyson, 2010). Although the majority of studies do not include people with diabetes, evidence suggests that behavioural therapy as an adjunct would improve weight loss in people with diabetes.

Pharmacological and surgical interventions

There is evidence of significant weight loss with both pharmacological and surgical interventions for people with diabetes, although, in the UK, only one pharmaceutical agent is available (Bray *et al.*, 2016). Dietary advice is part of the educational package that should be offered to those who adopt these interventions for weight loss.

Considerations for particular groups

Children and adolescents

The aims of dietary treatment of diabetes in children and adolescents are similar to those for adults, with an additional emphasis on providing sufficient energy and nutrients for optimal growth. The International Society for Pediatric and Adolescent Diabetes (ISPAD) has published clinical practice consensus guidelines, and the broad approach is that of child-centred, individualised care, based on healthy eating recommendations suitable for the whole family (Smart *et al.*, 2014). A multi-disciplinary team approach is recommended, including a specialist paediatric dietitian, providing education and support to the child, the family, the school and other carers. A summary of nutritional recommendations is shown in Table 7.12.1.

Energy balance

Childhood and adolescence are times of rapid growth, and it can be challenging to meet increased energy demands for optimal growth while maintaining target blood glucose levels. Children with diabetes have similar rates of overweight and obesity as the general population, and prevention is a key strategy of care. Energy intake can vary greatly from day to day, especially in young children, and dietary advice should be flexible, adaptable and reviewed regularly.

Carbohydrates should not be restricted in children as this may affect growth. Sugar may provide up to 10% of energy, although excessive consumption in the form of sugar-sweetened beverages has been linked to weight gain in children. Matching insulin dose to carbohydrate intake is recommended, and there are several methods

Table 7.12.1 Nutritional recommendations for children and adolescents with diabetes (ISPAD, 2014)

Nutrient	Recommendation
Carbohydrate	50–55% of total energy intake
Sucrose	Up to 10% of total energy intake
Dietary fibre	2.8–3.4 g/MJ
Total fat	25–35% of total energy intake
Saturated fat + trans fatty acids	<10% of total energy intake
Polyunsaturated fat	<10% of total energy intake
Monounsaturated fat	>10% of total energy intake
Protein	15–20% of total energy intake

that can be used, with no strong evidence for one particular strategy. Recommendations for other nutrients are no different from those for the general population, and are in line with guidelines for promoting health.

Education models for the delivery of dietary education for children have been developed, and these include food pyramids and plate models that are designed to promote optimal glycaemic control and reduce the risk of cardiovascular disease. As there are no studies showing that one method is better that another, and there is no international consensus for the most effective tool, it is recommended that appropriate education models be adapted to the needs of the individual child and family.

Physical activity should be promoted for children and adolescents, but it is the commonest cause of hypoglycaemia and needs careful planning on an individual basis. For most children, extra carbohydrate is needed for activity, and this is especially true of unplanned activity. Children taking part in regular training sessions or competitive sport will need specialist advice from a paediatric dietitian.

Teenagers often have poor glycaemic control, and although this may be partly due to lifestyle factors, the adolescent growth spurt is accompanied by increased insulin resistance, and this contributes to higher glucose levels. Body weight changes rapidly during adolescence, and both excessive weight gain or weight loss may occur. Inappropriate weight gain requires review and advice about dietary intake, insulin dose and physical activity. Weight loss may be associated with insulin omission in order to control weight and/or an eating disorder. Erratic lifestyles, rebellion and peer pressure can all affect diabetes control, and may need specialist psychological input.

Type 2 diabetes was formerly unknown in children, but its prevalence is increasing as obesity rates rise. Most children and adolescents with diabetes are obese and will require lifestyle management. There is little evidence for the most effective strategies for management, but recommendations for adults can be adapted for children and should include guidelines for weight reduction, increased physical activity, and avoiding energy-dense foods and sugar-sweetened beverages (Copeland *et al.*, 2013).

Pregnancy and lactation

Women with diabetes who become pregnant are at greater risk of miscarriage, congenital malformation, stillbirth and neonatal death. They should be offered preconception care and advice, and this should be continued during pregnancy (American Diabetes Association, 2016; NICE, 2015d). Dietary advice should be offered as part of a structured education package for women with diabetes and those who develop GDM (NICE, 2015d). Preconception care includes advice about establishing optimum glycaemic control and body weight before conception. Women planning pregnancy should aim for a HbA1c concentrations of 48 mmol/mol (6.5%) (NICE, 2015d).

Antenatal advice should include standard education about food safety and healthy eating for pregnancy, and education should be provided by a multi-disciplinary team, including a specialist dietitian. Glycaemic control is of paramount importance during pregnancy, and guidelines recommend that blood glucose levels as near to the normal ranges as possible be maintained. Hypoglycaemia is more common during the first trimester in those treated with insulin, but insulin resistance increases throughout pregnancy, and women should be advised to titrate insulin doses in order to control glucose levels. Body weight monitoring during pregnancy is not recommended by NICE in the UK, although other authorities have issued guidelines and recommend weight gains predicted by prepregnancy weight (Canadian Diabetes Association Clinical Practice Guidelines Expert Committee, 2013; Institute of Medicine, 2009).

Postnatal care includes support and advice about breastfeeding, which should be encouraged in all women. Insulin requirements are reduced following delivery, and breastfeeding may induce hypoglycaemia. Women with diabetes can manage blood glucose levels during breastfeeding by frequent blood glucose tests and a combination of insulin reductions and increased carbohydrate intake. Women with GDM are at greater risk of type 2 diabetes in the future and may benefit from dietary advice to reduce future risk, especially if they are overweight.

Gestational diabetes mellitus

GDM is one of the most common complications of pregnancy, and its prevalence has increased by 30% over the past decade (Zhu & Zhang, 2016), with one in seven births globally now affected by GDM (Guariguata *et al.*, 2014). Obesity is a strong risk factor for GDM, and women who are obese at conception are up to six times more likely to develop GDM than those of normal weight (Stang & Huffman, 2016). The evidence for effective strategies for the dietary management of GDM is limited, and three meta-analyses have suggested that total energy restriction, low-GI diets and carbohydrate management may be helpful strategies to prevent excess weight gain and manage blood glucose levels in women with GDM (Han *et al.*, 2013; Viana *et al.*, 2014; Wei *et al.*, 2016).

Older adults

Older people with diabetes show reduced physical function, health status and impaired cognitive function as compared to those without diabetes (Formiga *et al.*, 2014). There is some evidence of poorer nutritional status both in hospital and the general community. In older people, the guidelines for the management of glycaemia and cardiovascular risk are the same as in other adults; nevertheless, in older people with comorbidities, functional dependence or limited life expectancy, the targets should be relaxed, with emphasis on avoiding both symptomatic hyperglycaemia and hypoglycaemia (IDF, 2013). Nutritional assessment and support should be made available for older people with diabetes who are malnourished.

Related comorbidities

Coeliac disease, as type 1 diabetes, is an autoimmune condition, and the two are often associated. Approximately

2% of adults and 10% of children with type 1 diabetes have diagnosed coeliac disease, and many more may remain undiagnosed. Coeliac UK has produced guidelines for the dietary management of diabetes and coeliac disease in the UK, and recommend individualised advice from a specialist dietitian.

Cystic fibrosis–related diabetes (CFRD) is a unique type of diabetes with features of both type 1 and type 2 diabetes, and it occurs in 40–50% of adults with cystic fibrosis (CF). Insulin is used to treat CFRD, and the aim of treatment is to maintain both body weight and blood glucose levels as near to the normal range as possible. Most people with CF are advised to eat an energy-dense diet to maintain a healthy body weight, and this continues to apply for those with CFRD, where the emphasis is on dose adjustment of insulin to match foods eaten rather than dietary restriction.

Disorders of the pancreas, including acute and chronic pancreatitis and cancer of the pancreas, can affect insulin production and may be associated with diabetes. All these conditions are also associated with malabsorption and malnutrition, and the support of a specialist dietitian is essential.

HIV and AIDS are associated with insulin resistance and increases the risk of developing type 2 diabetes fourfold. Diabetes pharmaceutical agents are of limited use in HIV owing to interactions with antiretroviral medications, and the main options for treatment are diet and physical activity.

Eating disorders such as anorexia nervosa and bulimia are >2.4 times more common in adolescent girls with type 1 diabetes. The deliberate omission of insulin to aid weight loss, termed diabulimia by the media, has serious health consequences in terms of the development of DKA and diabetes-associated complications. Eating disorders in people with type 1 diabetes affect physical and emotional health and cause impaired metabolic control. All members of the diabetes team should be alert to the possibility of eating disorders, and insulin dose manipulation and urgent referral to eating disorder units may be necessary.

Nutrition support

There is very little evidence available for the role of nutrition support in people with diabetes, but the general recommendation is to follow local protocols and guidelines for those without diabetes. Many feeds and supplements are glucose based and will exacerbate hyperglycaemia, and this should be managed by adequate diabetes medication rather than dietary restriction. Diabetes-specific formulae (providing energy derived from monounsaturated fat and fructose) have been shown to help glycaemic control, but these are expensive, and not available in the UK.

End-of-life care

In common with guidelines for people without diabetes, end-of-life care for people with diabetes should ensure non-intrusive dietary and management regimens tailored to individual needs. The main emphasis is to avoid symptoms of hyperglycaemia and hypoglycaemia as the risk of long-term cardiovascular and microvascular complications is not relevant. In line with changes in dietary intake, adjustment of medication may be required.

Residents in external agencies

People in hospitals, prisons, care homes and boarding schools are not in charge of their own nutrition and often have restricted choice in the food they eat. It is recommended that people with diabetes, their carers and associated staff have sufficient education and/or training to enable healthy food choices where possible. All food provided should include snacks and meals that allow food choices that are in line with the dietary recommendations for diabetes. In addition, all residents with diabetes should have access to a registered dietitian, and a nutritional care plan for each individual should be developed.

Fasting

Fasting is a significant part of many religions, and, although people with diabetes are often exempt, many will choose to respect fasts. The IDF has published guidelines for the management of diabetes during Ramadan, and state that consideration should be given to timings and doses of medication, and to the carbohydrate and energy density of foods taken when the fast is broken (IDF, 2016). The main aims of nutritional therapy are to avoid hypoglycaemia during the fast period, to distribute carbohydrate intake equally among meals to minimise postprandial hyperglycaemia, and to manage comorbidities such as hypertension and dyslipidaemia.

Internet resources

American Diabetes Association (ADA), www.diabetes.org
Carbs & cals (Carbohydrate counting), www.carbsandcals.com
Diabetes UK, www.diabetes.org.uk
European Association for the Study of Diabetes (EASD), www.easd.org
Glycaemic index, www.glycemicindex.com
International Diabetes Federation (IDF), www.idf.org
Run sweet (Managing diabetes and sport), www.runsweet.com

Structured education for diabetes

Diabetes Education and Self-Management for Ongoing and Newly Diagnosed Diabetes (DESMOND), www.desmond-project.org.uk
Dose Adjustment for Normal Eating (DAFNE), www.dafne.uk.com
The X-PERT programme, www.xperthealth.org.uk
UK Diabetes Education Network, www.diabetes-education.net

Further reading

American Diabetes Association, Bantle JP, Wylie-Rosett J, *et al.* (2008) Nutrition recommendations and interventions for diabetes: a position statement of the American Diabetes Association. *Diabetes Care.* 31(1): S61–78.Diabetes UK evidence-based nutrition guidelines for the prevention and management of diabetes. Available at www.diabetes.org.uk/Documents/Reports/Nutritional_guidelines.31.05.11.pdf.

Goff L, Dyson P (ed). (2016) *Advanced Nutrition and Dietetic in Diabetes*. Oxford: Wiley Blackwell.

International Diabetes Federation (IDF). (2015) *Diabetes Atlas*, 7th edn. Brussels: IDF.

References

Ali S, Stone MA, Peters JL, *et al.* (2006) The prevalence of co-morbid depression in adults with type 2 diabetes: a systematic review and meta-analysis. *Diabet Med.* 23(11): 1165–1173.

American Diabetes Association. (2016) Standards of medical care in diabetes – 2016. *Diabetes Care.* 39(1): S1–112.

Anderson RJ, Freedland KE, Clouse RE, *et al.* (2011) The prevalence of co-morbid depression in adults with diabetes: a meta-analysis. *Diabetes Care.* 24(6): 1069–1078.

Aucott L, Poobalan A, Smith WC, *et al.* (2004) Weight loss in obese diabetic and non-diabetic individuals and long-term diabetes outcomes – a systematic review. *Diabetes Obes Metab.* 6(2): 85–94.

Aziz Z, Absetz P, Oldroyd J, *et al.* (2015) A systematic review of real-world diabetes prevention programs: learnings from the last 15 years. *Implement. Sci.*10: 172.

Barnard KD, Skinner TC, Peveler R. (2006) The prevalence of co-morbid depression in adults with type 1 diabetes: a systematic literature review. *Diabet. Med.* 23(4): 445–448.

Boulé NG, Haddad E, Kenny GP, *et al.* (2001) Effects of exercise on glycemic control and body mass in type 2 diabetes mellitus: a meta-analysis of controlled clinical trials. *JAMA.* 286(10): 1218–1227.

Bray GA, Frühbeck G, Ryan DH, *et al.* (2016) Management of obesity. *Lancet.* 387(10031): 1947–1956.

Canadian Diabetes Association. (2008) Canadian Diabetes Association 2008 clinical practice guidelines for the prevention and management of diabetes in Canada. *Can. J. Diabet.* 32(1): S1–201.

Canadian Diabetes Association Clinical Practice Guidelines Expert Committee. (2013) Clinical practice guidelines: diabetes and pregnancy. *Can. J. Diabetes.* 37: S168–183.

Chimen M, Kennedy A, Nirantharakumar K, *et al.* (2012) What are the health benefits of physical activity in type 1 diabetes mellitus? A literature review. *Diabetologia.* 55(3): 542–551.

Colberg SR, Sigal RJ, Fernhall B, *et al.*; American College of Sports Medicine, American Diabetes Association. (2010) Exercise and type 2 diabetes: the American College of Sports Medicine and the American Diabetes Association: joint position statement. *Diabetes Care.* 33(12): 147–167.

Copeland KC, Silverstein J, Moore KR, *et al.*; American Academy of Pediatrics. (2013) Management of newly diagnosed type 2 Diabetes Mellitus (T2DM) in children and adolescents. *Pediatrics.* 131(2): 364–382.

Corben S, Rosen R. (2005) *Self-Management for Long-Term Conditions*. London: King's Fund.

DAFNE Study Group. (2002) Training in flexible, intensive insulin management to enable dietary freedom in people with type 1 diabetes: dose adjustment for normal eating (DAFNE) randomised controlled trial. *BMJ.* 325(7367): 746.

DCCT Research Group. (1993) The effect of intensive treatment of diabetes on the development and progression of long-term complications in insulin-dependent diabetes mellitus. *N. Engl. J. Med.* 329: 977–986.

DCCT/EDIC Study Group. (2016) Intensive diabetes treatment and cardiovascular outcomes. The Diabetes Control and Complications Trial/Epidemiology and Complications Study 30-year follow-up. *Diabetes Care.* 39(5): 686–693.

Diabetes UK. *Diabetes and Checking Your Blood Sugars.* Available at https://www.diabetes.org.uk/Guide-to-diabetes/Monitoring/Testing/.

Diabetes UK. (2013) *The United Kingdom Insulin Pump Audit: Service Level Data.* London: Diabetes UK.

Diabetes UK. (2015) *Facts and Stats.* London: Diabetes UK.

Diabetes UK/BDA. *Policy Statement: Dietary Fat Consumption in the Management of Type 2 Diabetes.* Available at https://www.bda.uk.com/improvinghealth/healthprofessionals/policy_statements/policy_statement_diabetes. Accessed 12 November 2018.

Dixon JD, Zimmet P, Alberti KG, *et al.*; IDF Taskforce on Epidemiology and Prevention. (2011) Bariatric surgery: an IDF statement for obese type 2 diabetes. *Diabet. Med.* 28(6): 628–642.

Dunkley AJ, Bodicoat DH, Greaves CJ, *et al.* (2014) Diabetes prevention in the real world: effectiveness of pragmatic lifestyle interventions for the prevention of type 2 diabetes and of the impact of adherence to guideline recommendations: a systematic review and meta-analysis. *Diabetes Care.* 37(4): 922–933.

Dyson PA. (2010) The therapeutics of lifestyle management on obesity. *Diabetes Obes Metab.* 12: 941–946.

Dyson PA, Kelly T, Deakin T, *et al.*; Diabetes UK Nutrition Working Group. (2011) Diabetes UK evidence-based nutrition guidelines for the prevention and management of diabetes. *Diabet. Med.* 28(11): 1282–1288.

EURODIAB IDDM Complications Study Group. (1994) Microvascular and acute complications in IDDM patients: the EURODIAB IDDM complications study. *Diabetologia.* 37(3): 278–285.

Evert AB, Boucher JL, Cypress M, *et al.* (2014) Nutrition therapy recommendations for the management of adults with diabetes. *Diabetes Care.* 37(1): S120–143.

Feinman RD, Pogozelski WK, Astrup A, *et al.* (2015) Dietary carbohydrate restriction as the first approach in diabetes management: critical review and evidence base. *Nutrition.* 31: 1–13.

Formiga F, Ferrer A, Padrós G, *et al.* (2014) Diabetes mellitus as a risk factor for functional and cognitive decline in very old people: the Octabaix study. *J. Am. Med. Dir. Assoc.* 15(12): 924–928.

Franz MJ, Boucher JL, Rutten-Ramos S, *et al.* (2015) Lifestyle weight-loss intervention outcomes in overweight and obese adults with type 2 diabetes: a systematic review and meta-analysis of randomized clinical trials. *J. Acad. Nutr. Diet.* 115(9): 1447–1463.

Franz MJ, Powers MA, Leontos C, *et al.* (2010) The evidence for medical nutrition therapy for type 1 and type 2 diabetes in adults. *J. Am. Diet. Assoc.* 110(12): 1852–1889.

Guariguata L, Linnenkamp U, Beagley J, *et al.* (2014) Global estimates of the prevalence of hyperglycaemia in pregnancy. *Diabetes Res. Clin. Prac.* 103(2): 176–185.

Hamman RF, Wing RR, Edelstein SL, *et al.* (2006) Effect of weight loss with lifestyle intervention on risk of diabetes. *Diabetes Care.* 29(9): 2102–2107.

Han S, Crowther CA, Middleton P, *et al.* (2013) Different types of dietary advice for women with gestational diabetes mellitus. *Cochrane Database Syst. Rev.* (3): CD009275.

Hex N, Bartlett C, Wright D, *et al.* (2012) Estimating the current and future costs of type 1 and type 2 diabetes in the United Kingdom, including direct health costs and indirect societal and productivity costs. *Diabet. Med.* 29(7): 855–862.

Holman N, Young B, Gadsby R. (2015) Current prevalence of type 1 and type 2 diabetes in adults and children in the UK. *Diabet. Med.* 32(9): 1119–1120.

Holman RR, Paul SK, Bethel MA, *et al.* (2008) 10-year follow-up of intensive glucose control in type 2 diabetes. *N. Engl. J. Med.* 359(15): 1577–1589.

Institute of Medicine. (2009) *Weight Gain During Pregnancy: Reexamining the Guidelines.* Washington DC: The National Academies Press.

International Diabetes Federation (IDF). (2013) *Managing Older People with Type 2 Diabetes.* Brussels: IDF.

International Diabetes Federation (IDF). (2015) *Diabetes Atlas*, 7th edn. Brussels: IDF.

International Diabetes Federation (IDF). (2016) *Diabetes and Ramadan: Practical Guidelines.* Brussels: IDF.

Inzucchi SE, Bergenstal RM, Buse JB, *et al.* (2015) Management of hyperglycaemia in type 2 diabetes, 2015: a patient-centred approach: update to a position statement of the American Diabetes Association and the European Association for the Study of Diabetes. *Diabetologia.* 58(3): 429–442.

Johnson M, Jones R, Freeman C, *et al.* (2013) Can diabetes prevention programmes be translated effectively into real-world settings and still deliver improved outcomes? A synthesis of evidence. *Diabet. Med.* 30(1): 3–15.

Knowler WC, Fowler SE, Hamman RF, *et al.* (2009) 10-year follow-up of diabetes incidence and weight loss in the Diabetes Prevention Program Outcomes Study. *Lancet.* 374(9702): 1677–1686.

Koerbel G, Korytkowski M. (2003) Coronary heart disease in women with diabetes. *Diabetes Spectr.* 16(3): 148–153.

Koppes LL, Dekker JM, Hendriks HF, *et al.* (2006) Meta-analysis of the relationship between alcohol consumption and coronary heart disease and mortality in type 2 diabetic patients. *Diabetologia.* 49(4): 648–652.

Lean ME, Leslie WS, Barnes AC, *et al.* (2018) Primary care-led weight management for remission of type 2 diabetes (DiRECT): an open-label, cluster-randomised trial. *Lancet.* 391(10120): 541–551.

Li G, Zhang P, Wang J, *et al.* (2008) The long-term effect of lifestyle interventions to prevent diabetes in the China Da Qing Diabetes Prevention Study: a 20-year follow-up study. *Lancet.* 371(9626): 1783–1789.

Lindstrom J, Ilanne-Parikka P, Peltonen M, *et al.* (2006) Sustained reduction in the incidence of type 2 diabetes by lifestyle intervention: follow-up of the Finnish Diabetes Prevention Study. *Lancet.* 368(9548): 1673–1679.

Lobstein T, Jackson-Leach R. (2016) Planning for the worst: estimates of obesity and co-morbidities in school-age children in 2015. *Pediatr. Obes.* 11(5): 321–325.

Lobstein T, Leach R. (2004) Diabetes may be undetected in many children in the UK. *BMJ.* 328(7450): 1261–1262.

Look AHEAD Research Group. (2010) Long-term effects of a lifestyle intervention on weight and cardiovascular risk factors in individuals with type 2 diabetes mellitus: four-year results of the Look AHEAD trial. *Arch. Intern. Med.* 170(17): 1566–1575.

Malavige LS, Levy JC. (2009) Erectile dysfunction in diabetes mellitus. *J. Sex Med.* 6(5): 1232–1247.

Mann JI, De Leeuw I, Hermansen K, *et al.*; Diabetes and Nutrition Study Group (DNSG) of the European Association. (2004) Evidence-based nutritional approaches to the treatment and prevention of diabetes mellitus. *Nutr. Metab. Cardiovasc. Dis.* 14(6): 373–394.

Nathan DM, Zinman B, Cleary PA, *et al.* (2009) Modern-day clinical course of type 1 diabetes mellitus after 30 years' duration: the diabetes control and complications trial/epidemiology of diabetes interventions and complications and Pittsburgh epidemiology of diabetes complications experience (1983–2005). *Arch. Intern. Med.* 169(14): 1307–1316.

NHS Choices. (2011) *Diabetic Retinopathy.* London: National Health Service.

NICE. (2008) *Continuous subcutaneous insulin infusion for the treatment of diabetes.* London: NICE.

NICE. (2011) *Diabetes in adults: quality standards.* London: NICE.

NICE. (2014) *Cardiovascular disease: risk assessment and reduction including lipid modification.* London: NICE (CG181).

NICE. (2015a) *Diabetes (type 1 and type 2) in children and young people: diagnosis and management.* London: NICE.

NICE. (2015b) *Type 1 diabetes in adults: diagnosis and management (NG17).* London: NICE.

NICE. (2015c) *Diabetes in pregnancy: management from the preconception to the postnatal period.* London: NICE (NG3).

NICE. (2015d) *Type 2 diabetes in adults: management (NG28).* London: NICE.

Nield L, Moore HJ, Hooper L, *et al.* (2007) Dietary advice for treatment of type 2 diabetes mellitus in adults. *Cochrane Database Syst. Rev.* (3): CD004097.

Nowosielski K, Skrzypulec-Plinta V. (2011) Mediators of sexual function in women with diabetes. *J. Sex Med.* 8(9): 2532–2545.

Oldroyd J, Banerjee M, Heald A, *et al.* (2005) Diabetes and ethnic minorities. *Postgrad. Med. J.* 81(958): 486–490.

Or CK, Tao D. (2014) Does the use of consumer health information technology improve outcomes in the patient self-management of diabetes? A meta-analysis and narrative review of randomized controlled trials. *Int. J. Med. Inform.* 83(5): 320–329.

Paulweber B, Valensi P, Lindstrom J, *et al.* (2010) A European evidence-based guideline for the prevention of type 2 diabetes. *Horm. Metab. Res.* 41(1): S3–36.

PHE. (2014) *Adult Obesity and Type 2 Diabetes.* London: PHE.

Poslusna K, Ruprich J, de Vries J, *et al.* (2009) Misreporting of energy and micronutrient intake estimated by food records and 24 hour recalls, control and adjustment methods in practice. *Br. J. Nutr.* 101(2): S73–85.

Rao KS, Kaptoge S, Thompson A *et al.* (2011) Diabetes mellitus: fasting glucose and risk of cause-specific death. *N. Engl. J. Med.* 364(9): 829–841.

Robertson LM, Waugh N, Robertson A. (2007) Protein restriction for diabetic renal disease. *Cochrane Database Syst. Rev.* (4): CD002181.

SACN. (2015) *Carbohydrates and Health.* London TSO: SACNE.

Sarwar N, Gao P, *et al.* (2010) Diabetes mellitus, fasting blood glucose concentrations and risk of vascular disease: a collaborative meta-analysis of 102 prospective studies. *Lancet* 375: 2215–2222.

Schram MT, Baan CA, Pouwer F. (2009) Depression and quality of life in patients with diabetes: a systematic review from the European depression in diabetes (EDID) research consortium. *Curr. Diabetes Rev.* 5(2): 112–119.

Shaw K, Gennat H, O'Rourke P, *et al.* (2006) Exercise for overweight or obesity. *Cochrane Database Syst. Rev.* (4): CD003817.

Skyler JS, Bergenstal R, Bonow RO, *et al.* (2009) Intensive glycemic control and the prevention of cardiovascular events: implications of the ACCORD, ADVANCE and VA diabetes trials: a position statement of the American Diabetes Association and a scientific statement of the American College of Cardiology Foundation and the American Heart Association. *Diabetes Care.* 32(1): 187–192.

Smart CE, Annan F, Bruno LPC, *et al.* (2014) Nutritional management in children and adolescents with diabetes. *Pediatr. Diabetes* 15(20): 135–153.

Stang J, Huffman LG. (2016) Position of the Academy of Nutrition and Dietetics: obesity, reproduction, and pregnancy outcomes. *J. Acad. Nutr. Diet.* 116(4): 677–691.

Stevens JW, Khunti K, Harvey R, *et al.* (2015) Preventing the progression to type 2 diabetes mellitus in adults at high risk: a systematic review and network meta-analysis of lifestyle, pharmacological and surgical interventions. *Diabetes Res. Clin. Pract.* 107(3): 320–331.

Stratton IM, Adler AI, Neil HA, *et al.* (2000) Association of glycaemic with macrovascular and microvascular complications of type 2 diabetes (UKPDS 35): prospective observational study. *BMJ* 321(7258): 405–412.

Turner RC, Holman RR. (1995) Lessons from UK prospective diabetes study. *Diabetes Res. Clin. Pract.* 28(1): S151–157.

UKPDS Group. (1998) Intensive blood-glucose control with sulphonylureas or insulin compared with conventional treatment and risk of complications in patients with type 2 diabetes (UKPDS 33). *Lancet* 352: 837–853.

van Wyk HJ, Davis RE, Davies JS. (2016) A critical review of low-carbohydrate diets in people with type 2 diabetes. *Diabet. Med.* 33(2): 148–157.

Viana LV, Gross JL, Azevedo MJ. (2014) Dietary intervention in patients with gestational diabetes mellitus: a systematic review and meta-analysis of randomized clinical trials on maternal and newborn outcomes. *Diabetes Care.* 37(12): 3345–3355.

Walker KZ, O'Dea K, Gomez M, *et al.* (2010) Diet and exercise in the prevention of diabetes. *J. Hum. Nutr. Diet.* 23(4): 344–352.

Wei J, Heng W, Gao J. (2016) Effects of low glycemic index diets on gestational diabetes mellitus: a meta-analysis of randomized controlled clinical trials. *Medicine (Baltimore).* 95(22): e3792.

WHO. (2006) *Definition and Diagnosis of Diabetes Mellitus and Intermediate Hyperglycaemia.* WHO: Geneva.

WHO. (2011) *Use of Glycated Haemoglobin (HbA1c) in the Diagnosis of Diabetes Mellitus*. World Health Organisation: Geneva.

WHO. (2015) *Sugars Intake for Adults and Children*. WHO: Geneva.

WHO. (2016) *Global Report on Diabetes*. WHO: Geneva.

Yu J, Zhou X, Li L, *et al.* (2015) The long-term effects of bariatric surgery for type 2 diabetes: systematic review and meta-analysis of randomized and non-randomized evidence. *Obes. Surg.* 25(1): 143–158.

Yusuf S, Hawken S, Ounpuu S, *et al.*; INTERHEART Study Investigators. (2004) Effect of potentially modifiable risk factors associated with myocardial infarction in 52 countries (the INTERHEART study): case control study. *Lancet*. 364(9438): 937–952.

Zhu Y, Zhang C. (2016) Prevalence of gestational diabetes and risk of progression to type 2 diabetes: a global perspective. *Curr. Diab. Rep.* 16(1): 7.

Zimmet P, Alberti KG, Shaw J. (2001) Global and societal implications of the diabetes epidemic. *Nature*. 414(6865): 782–787.

7.13 Obesity

7.13.1 General aspects and prevention of obesity

Linda Hindle, Jamie Blackshaw and Charlene Mulhern

Key points

- Obesity prevalence in the UK has trebled in 20 years. It poses a serious health risk, reducing life expectancy and quality of life, and is associated with health inequalities. The causes are multifactorial, characterised by a combination of poor dietary habits, lack of physical activity, and sedentary lifestyles, which are compounded by a latent genetic programming to weight gain.
- Preventing obesity requires action at all levels, from supporting individuals and families to lead healthier lifestyles, through local initiatives and provision of services in communities, schools and workplaces, to government policies and approaches to support and facilitate healthier lifestyle choices.
- Dietitians have a role in obesity management and prevention as a part of their posts, but also as advocates for health in their communities.

Definition and classification of obesity

Obesity and overweight are defined by the World Health Organisation (WHO, 2016a) as '*abnormal or excessive fat accumulation that may impair health*'. Obesity is classified using the international classification for body mass index (BMI) (NICE, 2014a), as shown in Table 7.13.1. BMI is calculated as weight (kg)/height (m)^2 (measured in indoor clothing and without shoes).

Health professionals routinely use BMI as a means to identify whether an individual is underweight, overweight or obese, as it is a practical, quick and hands-off approach. This does not mean it is without its limitations, as it does not measure body composition and cannot discriminate between lean and fat tissue (Prentice & Jebb, 2001).

BMI, adjusted for age and sex, is recommended as a practical estimate of overweight in children and young people. Centiles on the UK childhood and puberty close monitoring (CPCM) BMI growth charts, 2–20 years for boys and girls, are used to express the degree to which children are overweight as they develop (see Chapter 3.8.2, Growth, nutritional assessment and nutritional requirements). A BMI above the 91st centile suggests overweight. A child above the 98th centile is very overweight (clinically obese), while a BMI above the 99.6th centile is severely obese. It should not be used for children under 2 years of age. Dietitians assessing and monitoring obese children will use the BMI charts in conjunction with Royal College of Paediatrics and Child Health Growth Charts, 2–18 years for boys and girls (RCPCH, 2017). An electronic BMI assessment tool for children and adults is available on NHS Choices (NHS Choices, 2017).

Since 2004, there has been considerable interest in the relative risks associated with obesity across diverse ethnic population groups. NICE recommends the use of lower BMI thresholds (23 kg/m^2 to indicate increased risk and 27.5 kg/m^2 to indicate high risk) to trigger action to reduce the risk of conditions such as type 2 diabetes in black African, African-Caribbean and Asian (South Asian and Chinese) groups.

Health professionals should consider using waist circumference in addition to BMI in adults with a BMI <35 kg/m^2 (NICE, 2014c). An indicative guide to waist circumference in the adult male and female population is given in the following:

- Men: waist circumference <94 cm is low, 94–102 cm is high and >102 cm is very high.
- Women: waist circumference <80 cm is low, 80–88 cm is high and >88 cm is very high.

Manual of Dietetic Practice, Sixth Edition. Edited by Joan Gandy.

Companion website: www.manualofdieteticpractice.com

Table 7.13.1 Classification of body mass index (BMI) and risk of comorbidities in adults (NICE, 2014b)

Classification	White European population, BMI (kg/m^2)	Asian population, BMI (kg/m^2)	Risk of comorbidities
Underweight	<18.5	<18.5	Underweight
Healthy weight	18.5–24.9	18.5–23	Average
Overweight	25–29.9	23–27.5	Increased risk
Obese	≥30	≥27.5	High risk

Waist circumference is not recommended as a routine measurement for children, but it may be used to give additional information on the risk of developing other long-term health problems (NICE, 2014c). While there are other alternative techniques and some emerging evidence for analysing body composition, such approaches are not recommended as substitutes to BMI (NICE, 2014c).

Prevalence

Obesity is the most common nutrition-related disorder in the world. Globally, there are more than 1.9 billion overweight adults, and at least 600 million of these are obese (WHOa, 2016). A systematic review of the economic burden of obesity worldwide concluded that obesity accounted for 0.7–2.8% of a country's total healthcare costs, and that obese individuals had medical costs 30% higher than those of normal weight (Withrow & Alter, 2011). In the UK, it is estimated that the healthcare cost of treating obesity-related conditions is now at least £6.1 billion per annum (Scarborough *et al.*, 2011). This does not account for the cost to social care, which is currently estimated as at least £352 million per annum (PHE, 2017c).

The proportion of adults categorised as obese increased from 15% in 1993 to 26% in 2014. The prevalence of morbid obesity (BMI >40 kg/m^2) increased threefold since 1993, with 2% of men and 4% of women being classified as morbidly obese (HSCIC, 2016a). By 2050, obesity is predicted to affect 60% of adult men, 50% of adult women and 25% of children (Foresight, 2007). The prevalence of obesity and overweight increases with age, peaking for women at 55–64 years and for men 65–74 years. While obesity is an issue across the social class gradient, there does appear to be a disproportionate impact for women, with obesity levels increasing with level of deprivation, from 22% in the least deprived areas to 33% in the most deprived areas (HSCIC, 2016b).

There are particular concerns about the rate of increase in overweight and obesity among children and young people, which has approximately trebled in the last 20 years. In the UK, data from the National Child Measurement Programme (NCMP) indicated that 10% of boys and 9.2% of girls (all children: 9.3%) aged 4–5 years, and 21.8% of boys and 18.1% of girls (all children: 19.8%) aged 10–11 years were classified as obese according to the British 1990 population monitoring definition of obesity (≥95th centile) (NHS Digital, 2017). Children are more likely to become obese if they have obese parents. Obese children are more likely to become obese adults than their peers, and the degree of obesity tends to increase with age. This suggests that the burden of obesity will increase markedly in the future, unless there is effective action to tackle excess weight gain (Wang *et al.*, 2011).

Impact of obesity on health

Obesity is an independent risk factor for premature death, but it is also strongly associated, probably causally, with a number of other serious medical conditions (Table 7.13.2). Overall, obese people are two to three times more likely to die prematurely than their lean counterparts, and, on average, obesity reduces life expectancy by about 3 years (Calle *et al.*, 1999), while morbid obesity reduces life expectancy by 8–10 years (NOO, 2010). The morbidity associated with obesity can be broadly divided into metabolic, mechanical and psychosocial disorders (Lee, 2009). Insulin resistance, hyperlipidaemia and hypertension are strongly associated with excess weight, especially in the abdominal region, and characterised by an increased waist circumference. The clustering of these risk factors is described as the metabolic syndrome, and it strongly predicts an increased risk of cardiovascular disease (CVD) and diabetes. The increase in the risk of developing type 2 diabetes as a result of excess weight is particularly striking (Temneanu *et al.*, 2016). It is also important to recognise that, regardless of baseline weight, further weight gain increases risk.

In recent years, the links between obesity and cancer have been recognised, and, after smoking, excess weight is considered as the most important modifiable risk factor to reduce the risk of cancer (Murray *et al.*, 2013). Obesity is particularly associated with postmenopausal breast cancer, colon cancer and cancers of the reproductive system (De Pergola & Silvestris, 2013). Other conditions such as stroke, non-alcoholic fatty liver disease, gallstones and reproductive problems, including polycystic ovarian syndrome and infertility, are all increased in obese subjects. Social research, however, suggests that there remain gaps in how individuals perceive the threat

Table 7.13.2 Health risks of obesity – relative risks[a] of developing disease by gender (adapted from NAO, 2006)

Disease	Men	Women
Type 2 diabetes	5.2	12.7
Myocardial infarction	1.5	3.2
Hypertension	2.6	4.2
Angina	1.8	1.8
Stroke	1.3	1.3
Cancer – colon	3.0	2.7
Cancer – ovary	–	1.7
Osteoarthritis	1.9	1.4

[a] All relative risk estimates are approximate.

SECTION 7

of obesity in relation to cancer, with recent research indicating that only 42% of people knew that some types of cancer are caused by obesity (PHE, 2015a).

Musculoskeletal and respiratory problems, including osteoarthritis, chronic low back pain and breathlessness, contribute to decreased mobility, reduced work productivity and impaired quality of life. Sleep apnoea is a problem for many obese patients. The health risks of obesity in young adults are particularly marked, and there is a tendency for the relative risk to increase with age.

Studies are beginning to show that the early origins of many of these conditions, especially metabolic diseases, can be seen among obese children. There is an increasing prevalence of type 2 diabetes in paediatric practice. Evidence that overweight in childhood is a risk factor independent of adult weight is limited. However, since there is tracking of weight throughout childhood (PHE, 2017c), and from childhood weight into adulthood, the health concerns for obese children are substantial (Simmonds *et al.*, 2015).

There is also an association between obesity and decreased psychological well-being, but this is not a simple relationship. Obesity does not cause psychological problems, but the social stigma attached to excess weight can leave many obese people, especially children or those with morbid obesity, susceptible to significant psychological morbidity, including depression, low self-esteem and reduced quality of life (Griffiths *et al.*, 2010). In some cases, this may contribute to a downward spiral of increasing weight and declining psychosocial functioning. Dietitians are not isolated from prevailing cultural attitudes towards obese people, and establishing an empathic, non-judgmental relationship with an obese patient makes an important contribution towards effective therapy.

Obesity is a serious health risk. There is good evidence that losing even small amounts of weight can decrease the occurrence or severity of risk factors for disease (e.g. insulin resistance and dyslipidaemia), but there is only limited evidence so far from long-term prospective studies on overall impact, such as incidence of diabetes or reduced mortality. Nonetheless, the decrease in obesity-related morbidity with weight loss of even 5–10% among obese people (15–20% in those with a BMI >35 kg/m^2) brings significant benefits to the individual, including reductions in medication for other diseases and improvements in physical functioning and quality of life (NICE, 2014a).

Aetiology

Obesity occurs as a consequence of long-term excess energy consumption relative to an individual's energy use, leading to an accumulation of excess fat. The causes of this imbalance can be traced to a number of factors, including specific genetic traits, which may convey a metabolic predisposition, behavioural factors and environmental circumstances (Sahoo *et al.*, 2015). The Foresight report (2007) referred to a complex web of societal and biological factors that have, in recent decades, exposed inherent human vulnerability to weight gain; in a complex, full-system obesity

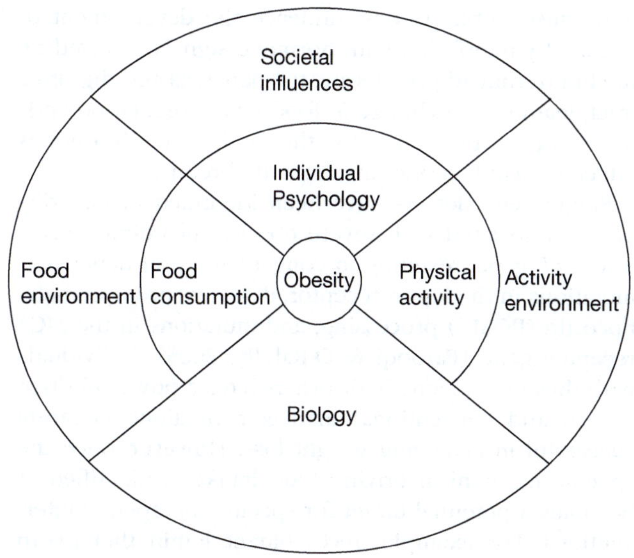

Figure 7.13.1 Factors affecting obesity – a simplified Foresight systems map (from Foresight, 2007)

map, over 100 variables directly or indirectly influence energy balance. A simplified model divided the Foresight map into seven interrelated themes, as shown in Figure 7.13.1. The themes were:

- *Biology* – the influence of genetics and ill health.
- *Activity environment* – the influence of the environment on an individual's activity behaviour.
- *Physical activity* – the type, frequency and intensity of activities an individual carries out.
- *Societal influences* – the impact of society, e.g. the influence of the media, education, peer pressure or culture.
- *Individual psychology.*
- *Food environment* – the influence of the food environment on an individual's food choices.
- *Food consumption* – the quality, quantity (portion sizes) and frequency (snacking patterns) of an individual's diet.
- *Genetics and metabolism.*

There are some diseases in which obesity is a major feature; the most significant of these are the Prader–Willi and Bardet–Biedl syndromes. A further group of patients may develop obesity because of an endocrine disorder, e.g. hypothyroidism or Cushing's syndrome. These patients represent a very small proportion of all cases of obesity and usually present with additional symptoms that can be readily identified and usually successfully treated. In children, short stature for age and weight is an indication for further medical tests (PHE, 2014a).

There has been growing interest in the impact of genetics on the development of obesity (Choquet & Meyre, 2011). The rapid rise in obesity has occurred too quickly to be due to genetic changes alone, and the obesogenic environment is considered to be the major cause of the recent epidemic. However, not everyone subject to an obesogenic environment becomes obese, and genetic studies have investigated why some people appear to be more susceptible. Genes influence the development of obesity by interfering with hormone signals received by the brain from adipose tissue, the pancreas and digestive tract, leading to a change in food intake regulation and/or energy expenditure by the brain. The hormones affected include leptin, insulin and ghrelin.

Single gene defects have been identified in rare disorders associated with severe obesity, including defects in the *ob* gene, resulting in congenital leptin deficiency, mutations in the leptin receptor, defective pro-opiomelanocortin (POMC) processing, and mutations in the MC4 receptor gene (Farooqi & O'Rahilly, 2005). Individuals with these monogenetic disorders have a powerful drive to eat, and conventional management alone is rarely successful in achieving weight loss. However, once the specific mechanism driving food intake is identified, it becomes a potential target for specific therapeutic interventions. For example, recombinant leptin therapy in children with mutations in the leptin gene has resulted in substantial weight loss (Farooqi *et al.*, 1999).

A much greater proportion of the population is likely to exhibit polymorphisms in other genes that have a significant but less dramatic effect on body weight, e.g. mutations in uncoupling proteins, the β_3 adrenergic receptor, or peroxisome proliferator–activated receptor gamma (PPARγ) (Hainer *et al.*, 2008). These genes may influence a wide range of metabolic and behavioural characteristics that together determine an individual's susceptibility to obesity. More than 50 genes have been found to be associated with obesity; however, most have small effects. Most obesity is multifactorial, a result of the complex interactions between environmental and genetic factors.

There has been extensive research into alleged metabolic differences between individuals that may account for differences in susceptibility to obesity. Previous suggestions that obese persons have a markedly lower metabolic rate than lean individuals have been categorically refuted, since increases in weight are associated with increased energy needs (Prentice & Poppitt, 1996). However, this does not preclude differences between individuals in the pre-obese period. Some studies of post-obese subjects have shown minor differences in energy expenditure as compared to age- and weight-matched never-obese controls (Astrup *et al.*, 1999). However, these studies are thwarted by difficulties in accounting for subtle differences in body composition. Defects in diet-induced thermogenesis and impairments in fat oxidation have also been suggested as metabolic defects that may increase the risk of obesity, but the net effects of these on energy expenditure are extremely small (Astrup *et al.*, 1996).

Recent research is exploring epigenetics, where environmental exposure at critical periods of human development, such as during infancy or in utero, can cause permanent changes to genetic activity, even though the gene sequence is unchanged. It is only in recent years that it has been acknowledged that behavioural traits may have a genetic basis. However, voluntary behaviour has the potential to override a genetic and metabolic susceptibility to obesity, e.g. by increasing energy expenditure through voluntary exercise (Li *et al.*, 2010).

Activity

An active lifestyle, in addition to being physically active, is considered important in maintaining a healthier weight, and thus is protective against the development of obesity. Around 50% of women and 33% of men in England are considered to be damaging their health through the lack of physical activity (HSCIC, 2013). In prospective studies, individuals who maintain a high level of activity experience smaller concurrent gains in weight than inactive people (Golubic *et al.*, 2013). There appears to be a strong association between sedentary behaviours (or physical inactivity) and obesity (DH, 2010). Television viewing, in particular, has been linked to the development of obesity because of the combination of sedentary behaviour and snacking on energy-dense foods (Avery *et al.*, 2017; Gubbels *et al.*, 2013).

Exercise alone as a weight loss programme is less effective than when combined with behaviour weight management programmes (Johns *et al.*, 2014). Interventions that deal with both diet and exercise have shown small but significant benefits on weight loss maintenance (Dombrowski *et al.*, 2014). Together, these data suggest that physical activity may help to attenuate the rate of weight gain rather than accelerating weight loss. Current UK recommendations for physical activity across the life course include (PHE, 2017a) the following:

- Children aged under 5 years who are able to walk should be physically active for 180 minutes spread throughout the day.
- Children and young people aged 5–18 years should engage in a minimum of 60 minutes of moderate–vigorous-intensity physical activity a day.
- Adults, including older adults, should aim for a minimum of 150 minutes of moderate-intensity physical activity spread over a week, with the addition of two activities focused on muscle strengthening.

A wealth of evidence shows that regular physical activity can reduce the risk of developing type 2 diabetes by 30–40% (Public Health England, 2014), as well as reduce the need for medication and the risk of complications in those who are diagnosed with the condition (Qiu *et al.*, 2012). Increases in physical activity are essential for physical and mental health and well-being. The health benefits associated with regular physical activity include reducing the risk of hypertension, depression, vascular dementia, as well as the risk of premature death from CVD and some cancers (Owen *et al.*, 2011). After reviewing the existing evidence, NICE provided advice to practitioners to encourage obese individuals to undertake physical activity; to avoid low energy expenditure; and to integrate such activities into daily life, routines and habits. Suggestions include the following:

- Increase regular walking or cycling as a form of active travel.

- Increase activities during leisure time and breaks at work or school.
- Increase activity as part of daily routine, e.g. taking the stairs instead of the lift.
- Reduce television viewing and other screen time.

In addition, NICE recognises that role modelling and broader behavioural changes can help children maintain a healthy weight; that communicating the benefits of achieving a healthier weight along with eating a healthier diet and increasing activity levels can help motivate individuals to change; and that self-monitoring is useful in helping individuals to reinforce positive behaviour.

Diet

Poor diet ranks at the top of the risk factors, along with tobacco smoking and BMI, for morbidity and mortality in England, and is arguably the most significant driver in the energy balance equation (Newton *et al.*, 2015). National surveys show that the population, across the life course, is not meeting dietary recommendations for saturated fat, non-milk extrinsic sugars and salt (PHE, 2017c). Most of the adult and child population consume more than twice the recommended (≤5% of food energy) amount of free sugars (PHE, 2015b), which demonstrates the magnitude of change that is required. Children aged 11–18 years consume more than three times the recommended amount (PHE, 2015c). Further compounding the state of the nation's diet is that population-average intakes of fruit and vegetables remain below the recommendations of at least five portions every day. For adults, the average daily intake was four portions, and, for children aged 11–18 years, the average daily intake was approximately three portions (PHE, 2017b).

These dietary patterns influence an individual's daily energy balance. While there are daily variations, it is estimated that men and women in the UK tend to consume approximately 300 and 200 calories a day, respectively, more than what is needed to maintain a healthy body weight (PHE, 2014b). For some individuals, this modest energy imbalance, linked to increased availability of energy-dense food choices, has led to a persistent consumption of excess calories, which over time has contributed to weight gain and led to the current generation's obesity problem. Sugar-sweetened beverages have been directly linked to increased energy intake, development of obesity, and risk of type 2 diabetes in children (SACN, 2015).

In recent years, action to tackle obesity, particularly in children, has become focused on how to reduce sugar intake (PHE, 2014b). While the WHO and the science and academic community have distilled the evidence to inform new dietary recommendations, what has helped drive this forward is the societal call for action. This has witnessed debate and the involvement of the government, public, dietitians and other health professionals, food industry, and popular culture icons (House of Commons, Health Committee, 2015).

Using the Scientific Advisory Committee on Nutrition's (SACN) risk assessment of the impact of carbohydrates on health as the case for change, Public Health England (PHE) investigated the evidence on how to reduce sugar intakes. It concluded that there was a series of drivers that influenced consumption, and that inclusive action across the breadth of identified approaches was needed to effect change. These approaches included changes to (PHE, 2015c) the following:

- Marketing, promotion and advertisement of high-sugar food and drinks to children.
- Reduction of sugar in, and the reformulation of, the food and drinks which contribute the most to children's intake.
- Fiscal measures such as the use of taxation.
- Controls on pack and portion sizes, both of which have increased in recent decades and are associated with greater consumption (Hollands *et al.*, 2015).
- Promotion of a balanced diet.
- Development of consistent approaches to nutrition in training and support for practitioners working with children and families.

The latest evidence on sugar complements the generally accepted position that there are several dietary factors that may protect against or, conversely, promote the risk of obesity (WHO, 2016b). A nutrient- and energy-balanced diet will help prevent obesity. This needs to take into account all macronutrients and micronutrients important for maintaining good health and energy balance. The model of a balanced diet has been updated following SACN's advice, and the Eatwell Guide (see Chapter 2.1, Dietary reference values and food-based dietary guidelines) provides a renewed focus to eat healthily. While action on dietary factors contributing to excess energy intakes is necessary to improve health outcomes, an equal focus is required to support behaviour change, so that individuals habitually consume more fruit and vegetables, which tend to be low in energy and offer other nutritional benefits. Shifting behaviour towards the Eatwell Guide has the potential to confer health benefits, and, compared with earlier models, should not lead to a significant change in the cost of diet (Scarborough *et al.*, 2016). It is a dietary model that could also confer potential benefits for the environment (The Carbon Trust, 2016).

Maintaining information on the population's food-purchasing and dietary habits is important in helping to provide a dynamic understanding about the population-level and individual-level risks of developing obesity. This is particularly so when it comes to children, who are less likely to have full control of their food and activity choices.

Environmental factors

At a global level, the marked increase in obesity that accompanies urbanisation and economic development provides strong evidence that environmental factors *per se* play a strong part in the aetiology of obesity, or unleash a latent genetic predisposition to obesity (Swinburn *et al.*, 2015). It is generally accepted that the environment (food, physical, and built) that people live, work and play in has an impact on the risk of obesity (Foresight, 2007). Over the last 50 years, technology and advances in healthcare have altered the way in which people live in developed countries; labour-saving devices, cars and Internet shopping have reduced levels of activity. In parallel, the food environment and the default choice has become subsumed by relatively inexpensive, ready-to-eat, high-energy foods, offered with incentives such as multi-item meal deals or supersize offers. Described as the obesogenic environment, this term implicates the total sum of influences in the environment that has driven obesities in individuals and populations. This has evolved over recent decades as a result of a complex web of global and local drivers, including food and agriculture policies, consumer demand, production and supply, and societal and cultural behaviours (Roberto *et al.*, 2015; Swinburn *et al.*, 2015).

Weight gain is a natural response in humans, who are designed to withstand famine rather than feast. Therefore, logically, within the context of such an environment, obesity is a potential inevitability (Prentice, 1997; Rutter, 2011). Although these drivers of obesities have an affect across the UK population, in reality, there is variability of distribution, with a disproportionate impact and burden of obesity in the most deprived children and families of society (NOO, 2012). Such phenomena are highlighted by analysing the available of data on the geographical location of food outlets and obesity prevalence. This shows that poorer neighbourhoods have a greater density of fast food outlets and higher levels of child obesity as compared to more affluent neighbourhoods (PHE, 2016). This focusses attention on the social and cultural determinants of health inequalities.

Prevention and treatment

Prevention of obesity is the long-term public health goal, including the maintenance of a healthy weight and primary prevention of weight gain. However, considering the extent to which overweight and obesity are affecting the population, there is a need for secondary prevention approaches to stop further weight gain and to help those who are overweight or obese achieve a healthier weight (NICE, 2013, 2014c). For the morbidly obese and obese individuals with comorbidities, clinical treatment and care, including pharmaceutical and elective surgery, are approaches about which NICE has provided guidance to practitioners (NICE, 2014c) (see Chapter 7.13.2, The management of obesity and overweight in adults).

Secondary prevention and treatment approaches are part of the holistic public health solution to tackling obesity. They are inextricably linked with preventative dietary and physical activity approaches by the need to ensure that environmental cues and defaults help focus strategies to avoid weight regain following successful weight loss. There is the greatest population-level gain from preventing the development of obesity, rather than treating obesity once it has occurred, although all of these are needed. The long-term, large-scale and societal commitment needed to successfully tackle the obesity epidemic is now recognised, and, encouragingly, contemporary policies and approaches tend to be commensurate with such an approach. This is a dynamic landscape with evolving key decision-making, influencers and evidence (Blackshaw, 2016).

It is accepted that there is not one single solution to preventing or tackling obesity. Such a complex issue suitably requires a sophisticated and complex response, which takes account of a life course approach and puts in place a framework of population-level and individual-centred approaches. There is sufficient evidence about the approaches that can help reduce the prevalence of obesity. Where evidence does not exist, policymakers and practitioners need to consider the ethical and moral implications to act or not to act, and how this accords with the precautionary principle and responsibility of the state to protect its population from the risk of harm.

This implies an imperative for policymakers, practitioners and research communities to take joint responsibility to provide approaches and the wherewithal to ensure that the necessary evidence framework is put into action to inform effective future decision-making. This framework needs to utilise and equip practitioners with the tools for innovation; keep abreast with digital behavioural approaches and the population's use of such technology; and, importantly, have due consideration for the population's attitudes to obesity, and how it perceives and is open, or not open, to approaches for tackling obesity and its causes. Policymakers need to weigh the relative benefit of effective interventions reaching a modest number of people against the less effective interventions reaching wider populations (Gortmaker *et al.*, 2011).

It has been argued that obesity prevention interventions should be universal across entire societies, including people of every age and regardless of risk factors, given that there is a paucity of data on effective ways to identify and manage an individual's obesity risks to justify a population strategy that would devote resources to sorting people by risk or readiness (Linde & Jeffrey, 2010). However, there are specific times in the life course that have the greatest potential to impact on obesity (NICE, 2015), including pregnancy, when there is the opportunity to affect the future health risk of the child and the mother (NICE, 2014d), and early childhood, when there is a high level of parental control and over eating, and activity patterns and preferences are being established. There are also evidenced opportunities to influence healthier choices through planning a health-promoting local environment (LGA, 2016; TCPA, 2014); by taking community approaches (NICE, 2012); and through place-based approaches, including encouraging a whole-school approach to regulate and make healthier food and activity the default choice, and to influence the family through the school (Food Standards Agency, 2010).

Dietitians have many roles to play in the prevention and management of obesity including the following:

- Using a making-every-contact-count approach with patients and families, and remaining vigilant to the potential opportunities for health promotion in everyday work.

- Anticipating the potential for excess weight gain, e.g. linked to medications, treatment and while providing mitigating support.
- Managing obesity as part of clinical practice – dietitians should be aware of commercial and community support programmes as an adjunct.
- Acting as an advocate for healthy eating and physical activity outside direct clinical practice, e.g. workplace well-being initiatives.
- Engaging in obesity prevention programmes, including inter-sectoral initiatives and broader environmental policies.

Further reading

Foresight Report. (2007) *Tackling Obesity: Future Choices*. Available at www.bis.gov.uk.

HM Government. (2016) *Childhood Obesity: A Plan for Action London*. Available at https://www.gov.uk/government/publications/childhood-obesity-a-plan-for-action/.

Internet resources

Age-specific UK Physical Activity Guidelines, www.gov.uk/government/publications/uk-physical-activity-guidelines

All Our Health Framework: evidence and guidance to support public health interventions including prevention of obesity, www.gov.uk/government/collections/all-our-health-personalised-care-and-population-health

Association for the Study of Obesity, www.aso.org.uk

Government Obesity and Healthy Eating web pages, https://www.gov.uk/government/policies/obesity-and-healthy-eating

Let's talk about weight guide: A step-by-step guide to brief interventions with adults, https://www.gov.uk/government/publications/adult-weight-management-a-guide-to-brief-interventions

Let's talk about weight guide: A step-by-step guide to brief interventions with children and families, https://www.gov.uk/government/publications/child-weight-management-short-conversations-with-patients

National Obesity Forum, www.nationalobesityforum.org.uk

National Obesity Observatory briefing papers archive, http://webarchive.nationalarchives.gov.uk/20170110170114/http://www.noo.org.uk/NOO_pub/briefing_papers

Obesity Health Alliance, www.obesityhealthalliance.org.uk

Obesity Learning Centre, www.obesitylearningcentre-nhf.org.uk

WHO, www.who.int/topics/obesity/en

World Obesity, https://www.worldobesity.org

References

Astrup A, Buemann B, Toubro S, *et al.* (1996) Defects in substrate oxidation involved in the predisposition to obesity. *Proc. Nutr. Soc.* 55: 817–828.

Astrup A, Gotzsche PC, van-de-Werken K, *et al.* (1999) Meta-analysis of resting metabolic rate in formerly obese subjects. *Am. J. Clin. Nutr.* 69: 1117–1122.

Avery A, Anderson C, McCullough F. (2017) Associations between children's diet quality and watching television during meal or snack consumption: a systematic review. *Matern. Child Nutr.* 13(4). doi: 10.1111/mcn.12428

Blackshaw J. (2016) Public health nutrition in the civil service (England): approaches to tackling obesity. *Proc. Nutr. Soc.* 75(3): 356–366.

Calle EE, Thun MJ, Petrelli JM, *et al.* (1999) Body mass index and mortality in a prospective cohort of U.S. adults. *N. Engl. J. Med.* 341: 1097–1105.

Choquet H, Meyre D. (2011) Genetics of obesity: what have we learned? *Curr. Genomics.* 12(3): 169–179

De Pergola G, Silvestris F. (2013) Obesity as a major risk factor for cancer. *J. Obes.* 2013: 291546.

DH. (2010) *Sedentary Behaviour and Obesity: Review of the Current Scientific Evidence*. London: DH.

Dombrowski SU, Knittle K, Avenell A, *et al.* (2014) Long term maintenance of weight loss with non-surgical interventions in obese adults: systematic review and meta-analyses of randomised controlled trials. *BMJ.* 348: g2646.

Farooqi IS, O'Rahilly S. (2005) Monogenic obesity in humans. *Annu. Rev. Med.* 56: 443–458.

Farooqi IS, Jebb SA, Langmack G, *et al.* (1999) Effects of recombinant leptin therapy in a child with congenital leptin deficiency. *N. Engl. J. Med.* 341: 879–884.

Food Standards Agency (FSA). (2010) *Understanding the Effectiveness of Dietary and Food Choice Interventions: A Review of Reviews*. Available from UK Government Archive. http://webarchive.nationalarchives.gov.uk/20141103171112/http://www.foodbase.org.uk/results.php?f_report_id=622. Accessed 13 November 2018.

Foresight. (2007) *Foresight trends and drivers of obesity. A literature review for the foresight project on obesity*. Available at https://www.gov.uk/government/publications/reducing-obesity-drivers-and-trends-literature-review. Accessed 12 November 2018.

Golubic R, Ekelund U, Wijndaele K, *et al.* (2013) Rate of weight gain predicts change in physical activity levels: a longitudinal analysis of the EPIC-Norfolk cohort. *Int. J. Obes. (Lond.)* 37(3): 404–409.

Gortmaker SL, Swinburn BA, Levy D, *et al.* (2011) Changing the future of obesity: science, policy, and action. *Lancet* 378: 838–847.

Griffiths LJ, Parsons TJ, Hill AJ. (2010) Self-esteem and quality of life in obese children and adolescents: a systematic review. *Int. J. Pediatr. Obes.* 5(4): 282–304.

Gubbels, JS, van Assema P, Kremers SP. (2013) Physical activity, sedentary behavior, and dietary patterns among children. *Curr. Nutr. Rep.* 2(2): 105–112.

Hainer V, Zamrazilova H, Spaloval J, *et al.* (2008) Role of hereditary factors in weight loss and its maintenance. *Physiol. Res.* 57(1): S1–S15.

Health and Social Care Information Centre. (2013) *Health Survey for England 2012. Volume 1: Chapter 2 – Physical Activity in Adults*. Leeds: Health and Social Care Information Centre. Available at http://content.digital.nhs.uk/catalogue/PUB13218/HSE2012-Ch2-Phys-act-adults.pdf. Accessed 13 November 2018.

Health and Social Care Information Centre. (2016a) *Health Survey for England 2015: Adult Overweight and Obesity*. Surrey. Health and Social Care Information Centre. Available at https://www.gov.uk/government/statistics/health-survey-for-england-health-survey-for-england-2015. Accessed 11 November 2018.

Health and Social Care Information Centre. (2016b) *Statistics on Obesity, Physical Activity and Diet – England*. Health and Social Care Information Centre. Available at http://webarchive.nationalarchives.gov.uk/20180328133204/http://digital.nhs.uk/catalogue/PUB20562. Accessed 11 November 2018.

House of Commons, Health Committee. (2015) *Childhood Obesity – Brave and Bold Action. First Report of Session 2015–2016*. London: The Stationery Office Limited. Available at https://www.publications.parliament.uk/pa/cm201516/cmselect/cmhealth/465/46502.htm. Accessed 3 June 2017.

Hollands GJ, Shemilt I, Marteau TM, *et al.* (2015) Portion, package or tableware size for changing selection and consumption of food, alcohol and tobacco. *Cochrane Database Syst. Rev.* (9): CD011045.

Johns DJ, Hartmann-Boyce J, Jebb SA, *et al.* (2014) Diet or Exercise Interventions vs Combined Behavioral Weight Management Programs: A Systematic Review and Meta-Analysis of Direct Comparisons. *J. Acad. Nutr. Diet.* 114(10): 1557–1568.

Lee YS. (2009) Consequences of childhood obesity. *Ann. Acad. Med. Singapore*. 38(1): 75–77.

Local Government Association (LGA). (2016) *Building the Foundations: Tackling Obesity Through Planning and Development*. London: LGA.

Li S, Zhao JH, Luan J, *et al*. (2010) Physical activity attenuates the genetic predisposition to obesity in 20,000 men and women from EPIC-Norfolk prospective population study. *PLoS Med*. 7(8).

Linde JA, Jeffrey RW. (2010) Population approaches to obesity prevention. In: Crawford D, Jeffrey RW, Ball K, *et al*. (eds) *Obesity Epidemiology*, pp. 208–221. Oxford: Oxford University Press.

Murray CJ, Richards MA, Newton JN, *et al*. (2013) UK health performance: findings of the Global Burden of Disease Study 2010. *Lancet*. 381(9871): 997–1020.

National Audit Office (NAO). (2006) *Tackling Child Obesity – First Steps*. Available at http://www.nao.org.uk/report/tackling-child-obesity-first-steps/. Accessed 3 June 2017.

National Obesity Observatory. (2010) *Briefing Note: Obesity and Life Expectancy*. Available at http://webarchive.nationalarchives.gov.uk/20100810035356/http://www.noo.org.uk/uploads/doc/vid_7199_Obesity_and_life_expectancy.pdf. Accessed 12 November 2018.

National Obesity Observatory. (2012) *Child Obesity and Socioeconomic Status*. Available at http://webarchive.nationalarchives.gov.uk/20170110173508/http://www.noo.org.uk/uploads/doc/vid_16967_ChildSocioeconSep2012.pdf. Accessed 14 January 2018.

Newton JN, Briggs AD, Murray CJ *et al*. (2015) Changes in health in England, with analysis by English regions and areas of deprivation, 1990–2013: a systematic analysis for the Global Burden of Disease Study 2013. *Lancet*. 365: 2257–2274.

NHS Choices. (2017) *BMI Healthy Weight Calculator – Healthy Tools*. Available at http://www.nhs.uk/Tools/Pages/Healthyweightcalculator.aspx. Accessed 12 November 2018.

NHS Digital. (2017) National Child Measurement Programme (2016–2017): England 2016 /2017 schoolyear. Available at https://digital.nhs.uk/catalogue/PUB30113. Accessed 14 January 2018.

NICE. (2012) *Obesity: Working with Local Communities [PH42]*. Available at https://www.nice.org.uk/guidance/ph42/chapter/1-recommendations. Accessed 3 June 2017.

NICE. (2013) *Managing overweight and obesity among children and young people: lifestyle weight management services*. Available at http://www.nice.org.uk/guidance/ph47. Accessed 4 June 2017.

NICE. (2014a) *Managing overweight and obesity in adults – lifestyle weight management services*. Available at https://www.nice.org.uk/guidance/ph53. Accessed 6 June 2017.

NICE. (2014b) *BMI preventing ill health and premature death in back, Asian and other minority ethnic groups [PH46]*. Available at https://www.nice.org.uk/guidance/ph46. Accessed 6 June 2017.

NICE. (2014c) *Obesity: identification, assessment and management. CG189*. Available at https://www.nice.org.uk/guidance/cg189. Accessed 6 June 2017.

NICE. (2014d) *Maternal and Child Nutrition [PH11]*. Available at https://www.nice.org.uk/guidance/ph11. Accessed 6 June 2017.

NICE. (2015) *Maintaining a healthy weight and preventing excess weight gain among adults and children*. Available at http://pathways.nice.org.uk/pathways/obesity/obesity-maintaining-a-healthy-weight-and-preventing-excess-weight-gain. Accessed 6 June 2017.

Owen N, Sugiyama T, Eakin E. *et al*. (2011) Adults' sedentary behavior: determinants and interventions. *Am. J. Prev. Med*. 41(2): 189–196.

PHE. (2014) Everybody Active Every Day: An evidence based approach to physical activity https://assets.publishing.service.gov.uk/government/uploads/system/uploads/attachment_data/file/374914/Framework_13.pdf.

PHE. (2014a) *Obesity and disability – children and young people briefing paper*. Available at https://www.gov.uk/government/news/obesity-and-disability-children-and-young-people. Accessed 12 November 2018.

PHE. (2014b) *Sugar reduction: responding to the challenge*. Available at https://www.gov.uk/government/publications/sugar-reduction-responding-to-the-challenge. Accessed 6 June 2017.

PHE. (2015a) *British social attitudes: findings from the 2015 British Social Attitudes survey*. NatCen Research. Available at http://www.bsa.natcen.ac.uk/media/39132/attitudes-to-obesity.pdf.

PHE. (2015b) *Why 5%? An explanation of the Scientific Advisory Committee on Nutrition's recommendations about sugars and health, in the context of current intakes of free sugars, other dietary recommendations and the changes in dietary habits needed to reduce consumption of free sugars to 5% of dietary energy*. Available at https://www.gov.uk/government/publications/sacns-sugars-and-health-recommendations-why-5. Accessed 12 November 2018.

PHE. (2015c) *Sugar reduction: the evidence for action*. Available at https://www.gov.uk/government/publications/sugar-reduction-from-evidence-into-action. Accessed 12 November 2018.

PHE. (2016) *Obesity and the Environment: Density of Fast Food Outlets*. London: Public Health England. Available at https://www.gov.uk/government/publications/obesity-and-the-environment-briefing-regulating-the-growth-of-fast-food-outlets. Accessed 12 November 2018.

PHE. (2017a) *Everybody Active, Every Day: Two Years On. An Update on the National Physical Activity Framework*. London: Public Health England; 2017. Available at https://www.gov.uk/government/uploads/system/uploads/attachment_data/file/601298/Everybody_active_every_day_2_years_on.pdf. Accessed 12 November 2018.

PHE. (2017b) *National Diet and Nutrition Survey: Results from Years 1, 2, 3 and 4 (combined) of the Rolling Programme (2008/2009–2011/2012) Executive summary*. Available at https://www.gov.uk/government/statistics/national-diet-and-nutrition-survey-results-from-years-1-to-4-combined-of-the-rolling-programme-for-2008-and-2009-to-2011-and-2012. Accessed 12 November 2018.

PHE. (2017c) *Economic impact: obesity, knowledge and intelligence team*. Available at http://webarchive.nationalarchives.gov.uk/20170110171204/https://www.noo.org.uk/LA/impact/economic. Accessed 12 November 2018.

Prentice AM. (1997) Obesity – the inevitable penalty of civilisation? *Br. Med. Bull*. 53: 229–237.

Prentice AM, Jebb SA. (2001) Beyond body mass index. *Obes. Rev*. 2(3): 141–147.

Prentice AM, Poppitt SD. (1996) Importance of energy density and macronutrients in the regulation of energy intake. *Int. J. Obes. Relat. Metab. Disord*. 20(2): S18–S23.

Qiu S, Sun Z, Cai X, *et al*. (2012) Improving patients' adherence to physical activity in diabetes mellitus: a review. *Diabetes Metab. J*. 36(1): 1–5.

Roberto CA, Swinburn B, Hawkes C, *et al*. (2015) Patchy progress on obesity prevention: emerging examples, entrenched barriers, and new thinking. *Lancet*. 385(9985): 2400–2409.

Royal College of Paediatrics and Child Health (RCPCH). (2017) School age charts and resources. Available from http://www.rcpch.ac.uk/child-health/research-projects/uk-who-growth-charts/uk-growth-chart-resources-2-18-years/school-age. Accessed 12 November 2018.

Rutter H. (2011) Where next for obesity? *Lancet*. 378(9793): 746–747.

SACN. (2015) *Carbohydrates and Health*. Available at https://www.gov.uk/government/publications/sacn-carbohydrates-and-health-report. Accessed 12 November 2018.

Sahoo K, Sahoo B, Choudhury AK, *et al*. (2015) Childhood obesity: causes and consequences. *J. Family Med. Prim. Care*. 4(2): 187–192.

Scarborough P, Bhatnagar P, Wickramasinghe KK, *et al*. (2011) The economic burden of ill health due to diet, physical inactivity, smoking, alcohol and obesity in the UK: an update to 2006–07 NHS costs. *J. Pub. Health*, 33(4): 527–535.

Scarborough P, Kaur A, Cobiac L, *et al.* (2016) Eatwell guide: modelling the dietary and cost implications of incorporating new sugar and fibre guidelines. *BMJ Open.* 6: e013182. doi:10.1136/bmjopen-2016-013182.
Simmonds M, Burch J, Llewellyn A, *et al.* (2015) The use of measures of obesity in childhood for predicting obesity and the development of obesity-related diseases in adulthood: a systematic review and meta-analysis. *Health Technol. Assess.* 19(43): 1–336.
Swinburn B, Kraak V, Rutter H. (2015) Strengthening of accountability systems to create healthy food environments and reduce global obesity. *Lancet.* 385: 2534–2545.
Temneanu OR, Trandafir LM, Purcarea MR. (2016) Type 2 diabetes mellitus in children and adolescents: a relatively new clinical problem within pediatric practice. *J. Med. Life.* 9(3): 235–239.
The Carbon Trust. (2016) *The Eatwell Guide: A More Sustainable Diet.* Available at https://www.carbontrust.com/resources/reports/advice/sustainable-diets/. Accessed 12 November 2018.
Town and Country Planning Association. (2014) *Planning Healthy – Weight Environments – A TCPA Reuniting Health with Planning Project.* Available at https://www.tcpa.org.uk/Handlers/Download.ashx?IDMF=7166d749-288a-4306-bb74-10b6c4ffd460. Accessed 12 November 2018.
Wang YC, McPherson K, Marsh T, *et al.* (2011) Health and economic burden of the projected obesity trends in the USA and the UK. *Lancet.* 378: 815–825.
Withrow D, Alter DA. (2011) The economic burden of obesity worldwide: a systematic review of the direct costs of obesity. *Obes. Rev.* 12: 131–141.
WHO. (2016a) *Obesity and Overweight. Fact Sheet No: 311.* Available at http://www.who.int/mediacentre/factsheets/fs311/en. Accessed 5 January 2017.
WHO. (2016b) *Consideration of the Evidence on Childhood Obesity for the Commission on Ending Childhood Obesity.* Available at http://apps.who.int/iris/bitstream/10665/206549/1/9789241565332_eng.pdf. Accessed 23 March 2017.

7.13.2 The management of obesity and overweight in adults

Catherine R. Hankey

Key points

- Moderate weight loss, usually 5–10% of body weight, is a realistic target for weight management programmes; a target ≥15% is justified when BMI ≥35 kg/m^2.
- Clinical obesity guidelines advocate structured approaches to weight loss and weight maintenance. Medication and surgical approaches are justified for some patients.
- The effectiveness of any dietary approach is dependent on the generation of an energy deficit; long-term behaviour change is required to sustain this approach.
- Weight loss usually slows after 12 weeks; after this, weight maintenance is required. More than one cycle of weight loss and maintenance are often required to achieve and maintain clinically important weight change.

The prevalence of adult overweight and obesity worldwide remains at epidemic proportions. In 2014, >1.9 billion adults were overweight, of which >600 million were obese (WHO, 2016). This is illustrated by the data for England, which estimated that 27% of adults were obese, and that 41% of men and 31% of women were overweight, but not obese. Less than one-third of adults were of a healthy BMI. Increased mean BMI is reflected in the increased prevalence of obesity and overweight across all ages (with older adults increasingly affected), as well as the numbers of individuals with a BMI of ≥35 kg/m^2. The latter, known as severe and complicated obesity (SCO), offers particular management challenges. The velocity of increase in this group is increasing internationally (WHO, 2016). In Scotland, the Scottish Health Survey (SHS, 2016) showed that SCO prevalence in adults (BMI >40 kg/m^2) had more than trebled since 1995 to 3%, increasing faster than the lower-BMI groups; yet, this is likely to be an underestimate. The incidence of severe and complicated obesity appears consistent between the Scottish data (SHS, 2016) and that collected in the comparable survey of England (Health Survey for England, 2016), at around 3%, and 2% in adults aged 16–4 years. Women are more affected, with all men at 1.8% and women at 3.6% (Health Survey for England, 2016).

These increases have direct effects on particular areas of healthcare, with one pertinent example being the increased obesity incidence among women of childbearing age. Pregnancies are frequently associated with excessive weight gain and postnatal weight retention, often in those at a social disadvantage (Heslehurst *et al.*, 2010). This presents particular management challenges, and effective approaches to manage weight in this group have proved elusive to date. Overweight and obesity are both positively associated with age. A majority of the population was overweight or obese in the 25–34 age group, with levels rising to 78% in those aged 55–74 years. Around a third of adults aged 45–74 years were obese (Scottish Government, 2016).

Obesity incurs considerable additional healthcare and other costs, which is illustrated by the example of medical prescribing in primary care for the obese. The number of prescriptions in the majority of drug categories almost doubled among the obese as compared to those for healthy-BMI individuals (Counterweight Project Team, 2005), and continues to increase. Health economic evaluations have estimated the current costs of obesity and estimated costs conservatively. This warns of the enormous financial costs that will result from continued inaction to challenge the relentless rise in obesity (National Obesity Observatory, 2011).

Approaches to challenge increasing overweight and obesity include prevention, which, while an attractive option (NIH, 2016) (see Chapter 7.13.1, General aspects and prevention of obesity), does not meet the needs of over three-quarters of adults who are already obese. Effective and clinically important weight management has been defined as weight loss of either 5–10% of body weight or, for those with raised BMI, 15–20% both maintained for a period of at least 1 year (SIGN, 2010). The SIGN (2010) guidelines suggested that a weight loss of >15% would be required to show health benefits. Adults whose BMI is >35 kg/m^2, or who have comorbidities (e.g. type 2 diabetes with a lower BMI of 30 kg/m^2), require greater weight loss to improve health. The health benefits of moderate weight loss are wide ranging and include improved physical capacity; improvements in biochemical indices (e.g. lipid profiles); as well as reductions in blood pressure, plasma insulin and glucose. Other benefits include decreases in degenerative joint pain and improved gynaecological health.

Effective weight management needs to be a structured process with clear assessment and management approaches. Weight loss is often thought of as the only element of weight management, but a weight maintenance phase, arguably of equal importance, is required to consolidate weight loss. It is in this context, rather than the target of achieving a BMI in the healthy reference range, that the different strategies for weight management in adults will be discussed. Surgical approaches for weight management, while important, are specific and fundamentally different from others (see Chapter 7.13.3, Bariatric surgery).

Assessment of overweight and obesity

The most widely used assessment method for overweight and obesity, and the associated health risks, involves the BMI. BMI cut-offs differ according to ethnicity, and South Asian and Oriental adults have lower BMI cut-offs than the Caucasian population (see Appendix A3). Waist circumference and waist–hip ratio are often used in addition to BMI, as BMI does not reflect the distribution of adipose tissue, and therefore body shape. Abdominal obesity is strongly associated with negative health effects; therefore, waist circumference or waist–hip ratio provide additional risk assessment (see Chapter 7.13.1, General aspects and prevention of obesity). Cut-offs for BMI and waist circumference are shown in Appendix A3. Descriptions of how to take anthropometry measurements are given in Chapter 2.2 (Assessment of nutritional status).

Dietetic approaches to weight loss

The accepted target for success, reflecting adequate to good compliance, with weight loss regimens is 5–20% weight reduction. The target of achieving a BMI within the healthy reference range is considered untenable for most adults. These targets should be considered in the context of populations living in obesogenic settings, such as the UK, which favour body weight increases steadily across adulthood. The rate of this weight increase has been estimated as 0.5–1 kg annually, using data from the EPIC cohort studies, which reported an increase of around 400 g/year (Romaguera *et al.*, 2010). Unintentional weight gain occurs frequently, and can reach up to 10 kg after a year of treatment in those on long-term medication, usually as treatment for a chronic disease (Leslie *et al.*, 2007). Simply arresting or slowing the almost inevitable weight gain in adulthood can therefore be considered a therapeutic success. However, health benefits from clinically important weight loss can be considerable, either in early adulthood through to older people (Han *et al.*, 2011). The effectiveness of a reduced-energy regimen in self-directed slimming is almost impossible to gauge. However, it has been estimated that a 10% decrease in overweight is achieved by only 10% of the population attempting to lose weight (Perri *et al.*, 1992). It is against such estimates that the success of weight loss programmes are currently judged. Most conventional professional dietetic approaches use one-to-one interviews, inherently expensive in terms of staff time, while group-based approaches are mainly, but not entirely, used by commercial organisations.

Evaluation of studies examining different approaches for achieving intentional weight loss is conducted in a variety of ways. This includes using data only from those who completed the study (completers analysis), data from all those who entered the study (intention-to-treat analysis (ITT)), or data from the last observation recorded for participants (last observation carried forward (LOCF)). Arguably, data ought to be analysed using at least two of the above approaches to determine the best-case scenario (completers analysis), but also to provide an insight into the initial treatment intent, and not the treatment eventually administered. An ITT analysis should minimise the risks of misleading effectiveness that can arise in any intervention research, and provide insight into how generalisable the intervention can be in usual care.

It is recognised that ITT can be useful in counteracting the effects of high attrition rates usually observed in weight management studies, some predictors of which are raised BMI, low aerobic fitness and low socioeconomic status (Roumen *et al.*, 2011); however a consistent set of predictors has not been identified (Moroshko *et al.*, 2011). An LOCF approach, which assumes that a patient's condition had stabilised before the last observation, and remained unchanged, is often implausible if patients dropout some time before the end of the trial. In theory, such patients could have received another intervention, in which case their measured weight could be quite different had if they have not made changes in their eating and activity patterns. The baseline observation carried forward (BOCF) approach, rather than LOCF, is the accepted approach (European Medicines Agency, 2010).

All approaches designed to achieve intentional weight loss are dependent on the maintenance of an energy deficit between energy intake and expenditure for success, and to allow the process of weight maintenance to commence. The most commonly used approaches to achieve such energy imbalance include dietary changes to reduce energy intake and increased physical activity to increase expenditure.

The individualised energy-deficit approach

For many years, the dietary restriction was the 1000 kcal (4.2 MJ) diet, irrespective of initial BMI; compliance, measured by body weight changes, was recognised to be poor. Frost *et al.* (1991) confirmed that a greater energy restriction did not lead to a greater weight loss in free-living subjects who were either overweight or obese, largely due to compliance issues and thus, endorsing the value of moving away from severe energy restriction. Patients were allocated to a 1200 kcal regimen or an individualised prescription based on the Lean and James formula (1986), together with a daily energy deficit close to 600 kcal below estimated energy expenditure. The prescriptions recognised, for the first time, that a person's energy requirements increase as the person becomes heavier. In addition to body weight, age and gender also influence an individuals' energy requirements. A mean prescription of 1700 kcal/day over 3 months produced a 5 kg weight loss, as compared to a 3 kg loss achieved with a standard 1100 kcal/day approach. A formal evaluation of the energy-deficit approach for 12 weeks weight loss versus a generalised low-energy (1500 kcal/day) approach using a randomised controlled design has been carried out (Leslie *et al.*, 2002). Weight loss did not differ between treatments (4.3 kg energy deficit vs. 4.9 kg generalised low-energy diet). Target weight losses, calculated using estimated energy requirements, and assuming total compliance with each approach, were 7 kg and 13 kg, respectively. The weight losses achieved using the energy-deficit approach were closer to those predicted than the generalised low-calorie approach, confirming the findings of Frost *et al.* that a greater energy deficit is not related to a greater weight loss. This moderate-energy-deficit approach was used as part of a national study of weight management in primary care, and the findings are encouraging (Counterweight Project Team, 2004b). The energy-deficit approach to weight management is advocated by current UK national weight management programmes (NICE, 2017; SIGN, 2010).

Differing macronutrient composition

Increased-protein/low-carbohydrate diets

There are consistent findings from metabolic studies and epidemiological observations that high-carbohydrate/low-fat diets assist in weight loss and help prevent regain. Increased-protein/low-carbohydrate diets, while opposing current public health advice, achieve weight loss by harnessing the positive effects of protein on controlling appetite (Weigle *et al.*, 2005). High-protein/low-carbohydrate dietary advice is not new; the Atkins diet has generated huge international interest since the publication of *Dr. Atkins' Diet Revolution* in 1972; the book has been reprinted at least once (Atkins, 1998). The dietary principles aim to achieve weight loss, weight maintenance and good health by limiting carbohydrate intake to 20–30 g per day, while consuming unprocessed foods rich in protein and fat in unlimited quantities. Foods to be eaten freely include red meat, fish, poultry, eggs and fats. Foods severely restricted are most fruits, some vegetables, rice, pasta and other grain products. Currently, there is no universal definition as to what constitutes a low-carbohydrate diet. One widely used example (Feinman *et al.*, 2015) suggests that a low-carbohydrate diet should comprise <26% of total energy, or <130 g/day.

Initial weight loss with a high-protein/low-carbohydrate diet is mostly due to glycogen losses (Eisenstein *et al.*, 2002). The satiating effects of protein also encourage weight loss, as shown by the findings of a 26-week randomised controlled trial (RCT) of overweight and obese subjects (Foster *et al.*, 2003), where the dietary advice was to consume either a high-carbohydrate or a high-protein/low-carbohydrate diet *ad libitum*. A significantly greater weight loss (−8.9 vs. −5.1 kg) was achieved with the high-protein/low-carbohydrate approach. The efficacy and safety of low-carbohydrate diets were considered in a systematic review (Bravata *et al.*, 2003), which concluded that there was insufficient evidence to make recommendations. Two 1-year studies compared low- and high-carbohydrate diets (Brinkworth *et al.*, 2004; Eisenstein *et al.*, 2002), while a 2-year study (Foster *et al.*, 2010) provided more definitive results. These longer studies reported no differences in weight loss according to dietary treatment (−4.1% vs. −2.9% and −4.4% vs. −2.5%), and, at 2 years, weight loss for all participants was 7 kg (7%). Two further systematic reviews compared low-carbohydrate (<30 g per day) and low-fat diets (<30% energy per day), confirming that both are equally effective at 12 months, achieving modest weight loss (Hession *et al.*, 2009; Nordmann *et al.*, 2006). Mean weight losses were mostly clinically important at 6 months, with a 4.1 kg difference in favour of the raised protein approach. However, at 1 year, this difference had decreased to <2 kg, indicating small and probably unimportant differences between groups. The attrition rate, usually around 30% in studies of weight management, was 36% in the studies included in this review; this was significantly lower in low-carbohydrate groups. A large worksite weight management study (Shai *et al.*, 2008) confirmed that the mean weight loss in adults who completed three different interventions were 3.3 kg for the low-fat diet, 4.6 kg for the Mediterranean diet, and 4.7 kg for the low-carbohydrate group. There was a statistically (but not clinically) important difference between weight changes for these two approaches versus the low-fat approach.

A systematic review (Noto *et al.*, 2013) reported that low-carbohydrate diets were associated with a significantly higher risk of all-cause mortality. However, these findings should be treated with caution as they rely on data from observational studies. Although no studies have reported any actual negative health effects in terms of cardiovascular risk factors, questions remain as to the long-term health effects. To determine the complex interactions between low-carbohydrate diets and cardiovascular health, long-term intervention studies are required. However, since there appears to be no advantage, at present, of following a low-carbohydrate diets in terms of weight loss at 2 years, such research may not be justified.

Low glycaemic index

Glycaemic index (GI) is defined as the incremental positive area under the blood glucose curve of 50 g of carbohydrate from a test food divided by the incremental area of 50 g of a reference food (white bread vs. glucose) (Jenkins *et al.*, 1981). Some examples of low-GI foods are lentils, pasta and apples, and of high-GI foods are cornflakes, rice and white bread. It has been proposed that a low-GI diet could have beneficial effects on appetite, reduce energy intake and induce an energy-deficit weight loss. However, there was no difference in weight loss between a low- or high-GI diet (−1.5 vs. −1.6 kg); effects on satiety did not differ (Raben, 2002). A more recent systematic review (Schwingshackl *et al.*, 2015) showed that, in obese and overweight adults and adolescents, none of the anthropometric measures (BMI, waist circumference, waist–hip ratio) were affected significantly by a low-GI/low-glycaemic-load dietary approach.

Very-low-calorie diet regimens

Very-low-calorie diets (VLCDs) and very-low-energy diets (VLEDs) provide pre-prepared meals, usually in liquid form, but occasionally a daily meal based on solid food is permitted. The term VLCD is used when the energy provision from the entire regimen is less than 800 kcal per day, as defined by the National Task Force on Prevention and Treatment of Obesity, National Institutes of Health (NTFPTO, 1993). This task force concluded that supervision by a physician and the selection of patients with a BMI of >30 kg/m^2 should provide appropriate and adequate safeguards for VLCD use. The recommended VLCD composition includes 1 g protein per kg of ideal body weight per day to minimise muscle breakdown.

Low-calorie liquid diets (LCLDs) are liquid diets based on similar ingredients as VLCDs, and provide 800–1200 kcal daily. These approaches are becoming more popular, since, unlike VLCDs, there is no requirement for provision of medical supervision. The products are mostly available in packets, and are consumed in the form of drinks. Details on the current evidence for approaches to LCLD have recently been summarised (Leeds, 2017). The recently completed DiRECT Study (Leslie *et al.*, 2016; Lean *et al.*, 2018) has shown that it is possible to put their type 2 diabetes into remission using a low-energy, liquid-diet-based weight management programme. Almost half (45.6%) of those who took part in the programme were in remission after a year. Type 2 diabetes remission and total weight loss were linked, with 86% of people who lost more than 15 kg on the programme in remission after a year, as were 57% of people who lost 10–15 kg, and 34% who lost 5–10 kg. In the comparison group, where people had the best diabetes care currently available, but did not try the new weight management approach, only 4% went into remission.

Cholelithiasis (gall stones) has been shown as the most frequent clinical complication associated with the use of VLCD, with a reported 10% incidence of clinically recognisable symptoms after 16 weeks of VLCD or LCLD therapy (Yang *et al.*, 1992). Potential dangers with VLCD are increased if there is underlying heart disease, and prolonged use. A 12–20-week period is acceptable (NTFPTO, 1993). A systematic review and meta-analysis (Tsai & Wadden, 2005) that included studies comparing VLCDs with low-calorie diets (LCDs), comprised of conventional food over both the long and short term, was performed using participants with BMI of 35–40 kg/m^2, with and without type 2 diabetes. Short-term weight loss (13 weeks) was 16% in VLCD *vs.* 10% for LCD participants. However, over the longer term, these statistically and clinically important differences were not maintained. After nearly 2 years, weight losses were 6.3 and 5%, respectively; interestingly, attrition was similar for both treatments, at 23%. In practice, VLCD compliance is rarely complete, with patients tending to revert to their usual diet and life style, using VLCDs only sporadically. However, the use of VLCD regimens can be justified in certain situations where weight loss is required quickly, such as pre-surgery or, more importantly, diabetes remission, or even routine weight management. Furthermore, it may be that a VLCD approach could be used in those who are obese with a chronic condition such as type 2 diabetes. Short-term use could be of value, illustrating to participants that they are able to lose weight. Then, other food-based weight management programmes can be discussed, suitable for longer-term use. The options are also suitable for application in the LCLD approach. Use of food replacement products may have a role in the long-term management of weight-related chronic disease, both metabolic, such as diabetes, and other chronic conditions, such as osteoarthritis-related disability.

Intermittent fasting

Intermittent fasting (IF) is a currently popular, but incorrectly described, dietary approach. The idea of the approach is that changing what you eat on a couple or more days per week to low levels of energy intake, often 600–800 kcal, would be sufficient to achieve weight loss that can be maintained over the longer term. The actual definition of IF is flexible, and no particular approach is described by the term. For example, alternate-day fasting comprises at least 3 low-energy days, whereas other intermittent interventions include VLCD approaches, or other lowered-energy approaches, which have been applied for periods of perhaps 2 weeks, and then a 2-week break.

The idea of a regular routine eating plan is attractive, and many men anecdotally indicate this to be their preference. There are a number of studies on this topic, although most are short term, with insufficient sample size; also, the majority do not include a weight maintenance period. Recent systematic reviews have considered the questions of whether short- or longer-term intermittent interventions are any more effective than a continuous daily energy restriction (CER) (Harris *et al.*, 2018a). Harris *et al.* (2018b) reported that existing data suggest IF approaches are as effective as CER approaches, but that there was no additional benefit. There was certainly insufficient data to confirm any metabolic advantage that IF may offer in terms of maintaining fat-free mass or preventing falls in resting energy expenditure. Similar conclusions (Harris *et al.*, 2017a) were evident from systematic review data of studies where the IF period was beyond 1 week. This area is one that is popular, and it may be that such an intermittent approach has value for certain adults.

Physical activity strategies in the treatment of obesity

The established health benefits of physical activity include reduced blood pressure, improved lipids (especially HDL cholesterol and triglyceride concentrations), and increased insulin sensitivity. The potential mechanisms linking exercise with weight loss include enhanced resting metabolic rate, preservation of lean tissue, increased total daily energy expenditure and post-exercise oxygen consumption (Hill *et al.*, 1994). The influences of physical activity on hunger and satiety are conflicting, with both increases and decreases being reported. A J-shaped relationship with appetite, involving a paradoxical increase in appetite with complete inactivity, has been suggested.

When physical activity or exercise alone is used in the treatment of obesity, weight losses are modest, averaging 2–3 kg (King *et al.*, 2011). When compared with no intervention, in this case, waiting list controls, physical activity achieved greater weight loss, but much less than dietary interventions (NICE, 2006). However, evidence does exist that exercise alone can produce larger reductions in weight when exercise is of sufficient frequency, intensity and duration, and there appears to be a dose–response relationship between the level of exercise and the degree of weight loss. Given the limited ability and desire of overweight and obese adults to exercise, it seems that energy restriction, rather than physical activity, should remain the focus of the weight loss element of weight management.

A combination of diet and exercise generally produces greater weight loss than diet alone (Skender *et al.*, 1996). One study randomised dieters to an exercise or no-exercise group, and found that the exercise group lost an average of 10.9 kg during the 12-week intervention period, as compared to the diet-only (no-exercise) group, which lost an average of 6.6 kg (Svendsen *et al.*, 1994). Subjects in the exercise group had improved plasma lipids, although weight loss was not different. NICE (2015) reviewed the evidence for recommending physical activity, 45 minutes, three times per week, combined with a 600-kcal energy-deficit diet versus recommending the energy-deficit diet alone. A meta-analysis examined the same issue, this time considering the long-term (2-year) effectiveness of diet plus exercise interventions vs. diet alone (Wu *et al.*, 2009). The same issues applied for any examination of this topic, with dose and durations of physical activity differing between interventions. At 2 years, there was a 1.1 kg or 0.5 kg/m^2 change in BMI, in favour of interventions that used activity and diet. Interestingly, the authors indicated that partial weight regain was evident for both types of studies.

Physical activity may be of most value in the treatment of obesity by encouraging weight maintenance. Fogelholm *et al.* (2000) randomly allocated those who had successfully lost weight to either a moderate- or higher-intensity walk programme or control. The moderate-intensity programme was as effective as the higher-intensity one in preventing weight regain, and in avoiding the 2.6 kg regain in the inactive control subjects.

A systematic review has considered the use of behavioural treatment strategies to improve adherence to lifestyle intervention programmes in adults with obesity. Findings support the use goal setting and self-monitoring as encouraging increased physical activity (17–105 minutes weekly). Such a level of activity, were it to be sustained, would be an asset, particularly to those in the weight maintenance phase (Burgess *et al.*, 2017).

Behavioural modifications in weight management

Behaviour modification has been described as a process that identifies unproductive habits, which are then replaced with adaptive behaviour patterns. Behaviour therapy in weight management addresses two main aims: first, a reduction in the food energy consumed, and second, an increase in physical activity to induce an energy deficit to facilitate weight loss. The most widely used approaches for behaviour modification are summarised by Avenell *et al.* (2006). These comprise reflective approaches that encourage the individual to reflect on their own actions, self-monitoring their food intake, identifying eating behaviour cues before introducing control methods, including stimulus control, changing eating patterns, and revising weight loss expectations in line with realistic and clinically important targets. In order to provide clarity on what elements of behavioural treatment are incorporated into any intervention study, the CALO-RE taxonomy (Michie *et al.*, 2011) was devised. This is useful to identify effective components and allow their incorporation into other interventions.

Together with education in nutrition and strategies to manage lapses, self-monitoring has been considered vital to the success of these approaches, as subjects then contribute to and define a programme of care with which they feel most comfortable. Cognitive approaches are often used in parallel with behavioural methods, to combat barriers to weight loss that exist within the patients' framework of beliefs. The administration of behaviour therapy can be through either group teaching or individual counselling. Wadden *et al.* (2005) reviewed the results of treatments that included behavioural therapy for weight reduction. Forty-two weight reduction studies were published over this period, and the rates of weight loss were 0.4–0.5 kg/week across all treatments. SIGN (2010) reviewed the effectiveness of such approaches, reporting that no studies had shown behavioural approaches alone to be effective in inducing weight loss. They reported three small studies whose focus was on behaviour, but did include a dietary element and reported an average weight loss of 3.8 kg, as compared to 0.5 kg for a passive intervention (self-help). In clinical practice, behavioural skills are important to improve communication between professionals and patients, and to encourage maximum patient participation. It is likely that some elements of behavioural approaches are already in use in dietetic practice, and that, together with dietary advice, they contribute towards effective weight management.

Conclusive studies

The concept that any study could be able to draw firm and final conclusions in any research area is unlikely, if not unknown. However, there are two US-based studies that follow randomised designs and answer questions in relation to dietary composition and long-term follow-up. Sacks and colleagues (2009) recognised the possible advantages of different dietary composition in weight loss diets. Using a factorial model, adults were randomised to one of four diets, varying in macronutrient composition, but all regimens incorporated an energy deficit of 750 kcal/day. Weight loss was 6 kg at 6 months, and then participants were followed up at 2 years. Attrition was low (20%), and, despite weight regain, losses still remained useful at 4 kg, with about 15% of participants having achieved a weight loss of >10%. The authors concluded that the reduced-energy diet, irrespective of macronutrient focus, could lead to clinically meaningful weight loss. Another 2-year study was set within primary care and illustrated how behavioural weight loss counselling could best be delivered, using lifestyle coaches (Wadden *et al.*, 2011). All participants were prescribed identical goals for diet and physical activity, but were provided with different levels of support to achieve them. Dietary advice was 1200–1500 kcal if weight was less than 113.4 kg, and up to 1800 kcal if weight was greater. All were advised to exercise for up to 180 minutes per week and given a pedometer to become aware of their activity. Usual care comprised quarterly visits of approximately 5–7 minutes duration, to review any weight change. Brief lifestyle counselling included an additional 15 minutes per month with an auxiliary healthcare provider, while an enhanced counselling option offered the option of further tools. This allowed participants to choose obesogenic medications such as orlistat, or sibutramine (no longer licensed for use in many countries) after 6 months, or some meal-replacement products. Enhanced care attempted to mimic practice in primary care, providing participants with the opportunity to influence their care, guided by practice staff, by choosing one or more of these tools. At 2 years, usual care achieved losses of 1.7 kg, lifestyle counselling 2.9 kg and the enhanced option 4.6 kg. Initial weight loss of at least 5% was seen in 21%, 26% and 34% of the participants of the three groups, respectively. The enhanced option was significantly more effective than the other group in achieving clinically important weight loss. These two studies effectively capture the short- and long-term effectiveness of weight management approaches.

Weight management in different settings

Group versus individual therapy

Group therapy offers obvious and important benefits for decreasing cost and improving professional resource management (Bitzen *et al.*, 1988; Chenoweth, 1990). While the group environment is undoubtedly unsuitable for some shy or reluctant socialisers, for those agreeable to this approach, it allows additional harnessing of structure and peer support, which is not available to a subject undergoing individual one-to-one dietary counselling. Commercial organisations utilise group setting for their sessions. The effectiveness of these has been considered earlier in the text. However, other programmes such as Counterweight also offer group-based treatments, when these are possible within the primary care setting.

The Australian *Gutbuster waist loss* programme was a group programme designed for men who were recruited to a 6-week course, and then followed for a year. It involved advice on exercise, dietary fat and alcohol intake. Average waist losses of 4% were achieved, and lifestyle advice led to lowered fat and alcohol intakes. A more advanced programme, which included six additional fortnightly sessions, saw falls in waist circumference of 10% (Egger *et al.*, 1996). In contrast to the majority of group-based interventions, this approach showed the value of group programmes for weight management in men.

There may be cost benefits from using group approaches to weight management, but this is not entirely clear, as the class size may, in some cases, be small. A systematic review (Paul-Ebhohimhen & Avenell, 2009) included RCTs, but not those examining commercial weight treatments. At 12 months, a weight difference of 1.4 kg was seen between group *vs.* individual approaches. Subanalyses indicated that financial incentives within group treatments increased weight loss. Subsequent examination of the role of financial incentives in studies designed to achieve intentional weight loss, carried out by the same authors, indicated that financial incentives themselves were not a useful tool to maximise weight loss.

The Counterweight programme: an example of weight management in primary care

Primary care has been advocated by clinical guidelines as a suitable but underutilised setting for weight management. Counterweight is a unique nationwide programme, originally set only in primary care, and harnessing the best evidence-based approaches for weight management (Counterweight Project Team, 2008). The overall aim is for patients to develop skills to manage weight in the long term. Dietary change is based either on the 600-kcal energy-deficit approach or on individualised goal setting. As with any weight management approach, the intensity of the intervention can affect the main outcome, weight change, and the cost and utility of the programme. Counterweight participants receive six appointments over 3 months, delivered on a group or one-to-one basis, and then follow-up sessions every 3 months for a year, and then annually (Counterweight Project Team, 2004b). This level of intensity probably reflects realistic implementation resource availability within the National Health Service (NHS). As the evidence underpinning the project involves harnessing current evidence, there is no requirement to prove effectiveness once again by making biochemical measures and/or using an experimental design such as an RCT. A continuous improvement model to develop the model was employed (Petticrew *et al.*, 2012), and the 5-year outcome data were the starting point for this (Counterweight Project Team, 2008). These data indicated that the mean weight loss was 3 kg at 12 months (95% CI −3.5 to −2.3 kg). At 24 months, the mean weight loss was 2.3 kg (95% CI −3.2 to −1.4). Clinically beneficial weight loss of >5% was achieved in 30.7% of the attending population at 12 months, and in 31.9% at 24 months. Counterweight achieves and maintains clinically important weight loss. New elements have been added to the regimen for severely obese patients, combining low energy, liquid diet and food reintroduction (Lean *et al.*, 2013).

Multidisciplinary weight management service in a secondary care specialist centre

The management of obesity by healthcare professionals (dietitians, doctors, nurses, physiotherapists and psychologists) is generally fragmented, and has developed largely independently of each other. Dietitians offer both inpatient and outpatient services in most general hospitals and in the community. There is little evidence that input to dietetic weight management from specialist health professionals occurs regularly. Practice nurses offer weight management advice to many overweight clients, although this appears to be on an ad hoc basis (Hoppe & Ogden, 1997). Physician-led obesity clinics are found in only a few UK NHS centres. A specialist weight management service using a multidisciplinary team-based approach, bringing together dietitians, psychologists, physiotherapists, physicians and surgeons, was advocated by SIGN (2010). This innovative service has been delivered by Greater Glasgow and Clyde Health Board. Data for follow-up at around 19 months are now published (Logue *et al.*, 2014). This phase of evaluation indicated that 34% of 5637 adult referrals participated in the programme. Of these, 1838 completed the programme after around 19 months; 238 achieved ≥5% or greater weight loss. These data indicate how challenging it is to achieve weight loss in adults referred into a service by medical practitioners (mostly from the general practitioner). Further longer-term data are eagerly awaited from this unique service, although involvement with commercial weight management services for a 3-month period is a proposed modification.

Although multidisciplinary working is widely advocated, there still appears to be a reluctance among many health professionals. A survey of general practitioners, practice nurses and dietitians found that all felt under-skilled to effectively manage both obesity and overweight (Hankey *et al.*, 2004). Similar findings were reported in a survey of secondary care consultants (Leslie *et al.*, 2005). In both studies, dietitians were identified as the professional group most likely to manage weight management, but were considered too scarce to assume a major role. It is unlikely that the views of these health professionals have altered since these studies were completed; and, in fact, it is likely that resources are scarcer, given the current financial climate.

Community pharmacy: a possible setting for community-based weight management

The sheer number of adults who are overweight or obese justifies the use of as wide a range as possible of opportunities to deliver weight management. Community pharmacists occupy a position of trust, and are easily accessible to many. Evidence evaluating the effectiveness of the community pharmacist in terms of weight management has been systematically reviewed (Gordon *et al.*, 2011). The review indicated that only scant research data exist, and that there is a dearth of robust studies of up to 12 months duration. While RCTs would appear inappropriate in this setting, further investigation into the clinical value and cost-effectiveness of weight management using pharmacies is justified. More recently, a review examining the effect of interventions in pharmacies, among others locations, found that weight loss was more encouraging and comparable to that achieved in primary care, although the cost was estimated as higher than in commercial slimming groups (Brown *et al.*, 2016).

Commercial slimming organisations

A number of commercial slimming organisations operate and offer a regular service to those seeking assistance with weight management. Slimming groups are accessible, convenient and relatively inexpensive, and currently their role in the UK is expanding, with partnership with the NHS becoming established (Jolly *et al.*, 2011). The 12-week treatment data appear promising, with a 4 kg weight loss and 1.5 kg/m^2 BMI reduction, but further data concerning both attrition rates and longer-term weight change (of at least 1 year) are required to fully assess the value of this programme.

Dansinger *et al.* (2005) compared commercial organisations with other dietary approaches and showed that, in 1-year weight loss (3 kg), the commercial organisation *Weight Watchers* was similar to the other approaches tested. Another comparison between a commercial slimming organisation and a self-help group found a 4kg weight loss at 1 year with the commercial programme and a 1kg weight loss with self-help (Heshka *et al.*, 2003). A review (Tsai & Wadden, 2005) examined evidence from commercial and self-help groups and concurred with these findings. The best result was a 3.2% weight loss at 2 years for the commercial slimming group *Weight Watchers*. The effectiveness of a primary care referral to a commercial provider for weight loss treatment was evaluated. Participants were randomly allocated to usual care, or to receive the commercial programme for 12 months. The attrition rates were similar for both groups: 39% in commercial programme vs. 46% in usual care. However, the weight loss after 12 months in the commercial setting was more than double that of usual care (5.06kg *vs.* 2.25kg). This finding is encouraging, and in excess of that achieved in any other study. The increased intensity of the commercial intervention, with either two or three appointments per month, may have strongly influenced the weight loss, favouring its greater success. The cost-effectiveness of such an intervention remains uncertain, and also whether the level of intensity applied in this study could be justified and replicated in usual care. An audit of the same commercial programme indicated that the provision of 12 sessions in an NHS referral scheme (with a median duration of attendance) was 12 weeks, resulted in a median weight change for all referrals of −2.8kg/3.1%, with an attrition rate of 46% (Jebb *et al.*, 2011).

The Internet as a setting for weight management

The Internet appears to offer promise as a tool to facilitate weight management, and, in theory, this could be cost-effective. There are relatively few studies to date; but, in general, these show moderate weight loss and some positive effects on weight maintenance. The setting itself is restricted to those who are computer literate and have Internet access. These interventions can be either commercial or delivered through healthcare routes. McConnon *et al.* (2007) examined the effect of a combination of dietary and physical activity advice, along with behaviour therapy, in an NHS setting. Patients were randomised to receive usual care or the Internet-delivered intervention. Weight loss did not differ between both treatments (<2kg). In contrast, two other Internet-based approaches were compared in a 12-month study, with weight losses of 8.3±7.9kg in those receiving usual care and 4.3±6.2kg in those also receiving behaviour therapy The higher weight loss was seen with the structured behavioural intervention, compared with a self-help approach (Gold *et al.*, 2007). Internet-based delivery appears promising, alongside challenges, such as determining the outcome of a remotely delivered intervention, and further evaluation is justified. More recently, Leahey *et al.* (2016) showed that, for those who have already lost a clinically important amount of weight (≥5%), an Internet-delivered programme can be more effective than conventional face-to-face weight management interventions. Two programmes which included some financial rewards for self-monitoring and either peer or expert coaching were compared. After 10 months, as compared to standard care, both online interventions achieved additional weight loss of 1.8±7kg and 0.5±6.4kg, respectively, while the control group gained 3.5±5.7kg. Online approaches certainly hold promise, and a web- and text-based intervention named 'Helpmedoit!' is currently being developed and evaluated (Simpson *et al.*, 2016).

Multicomponent weight loss interventions

The UK clinical guidelines for weight management advocate the use of multicomponent weight loss programmes, comprising diet, exercise/physical activity and behaviour therapy. This approach has undergone thorough investigation recently (Loveman *et al.*, 2011). A systematic review assessed the clinical effectiveness and cost-effectiveness of multicomponent weight management programmes in overweight and obese adults. The included studies, largely non-UK based, were diverse in nature, and hence meta-analysis was precluded. Weight loss was moderate across all studies, although, in general, weight change appeared to be greater in the intervention groups than the comparator groups. Some studies incorporated longer-term follow-up, in which a majority of subjects were observed to regain weight. The differences in study design precluded the drawing of firm conclusions concerning the effectiveness of multicomponent weight management. The assessment of cost-effectiveness, increasingly relevant to justify the implementation of all interventions, was also problematic. A preliminary cost-effectiveness assessment was carried out with two studies, despite each having limitations, namely, a duration of only 36 months, use of prescription anti-obesity drugs in some participants, and follow-up of less than 18 months. Each study used a particular approach, a lifetime chronic disease model, to evaluate the effect of changes in an individual's weight. The models included the costs and benefits from avoiding chronic illnesses such as coronary heart disease and type 2 diabetes. Some other models have been broader, and included a wider range of chronic diseases. However, both studies concluded that the long-term multicomponent interventions were cost-effective, with estimates varying between £473 and £7200 (US$12,640). As per cost-effectiveness studies, this was expressed per quality-adjusted life-year gained. The authors cautiously suggested that long-term multicomponent weight management interventions, in general, promoted weight loss in overweight or obese adults, but emphasised that small weight changes and regain was common. Some evidence suggested that they may be cost-effective, but this finding was by no means conclusive. As there were no UK-based RCTs included in the review, a research need was expressed to evaluate the effects of long-term multicomponent weight management interventions in a UK setting. Adults with intellectual disabilities are more prone to obesity than other sections of society, although they have fewer opportunities to receive treatment. A recent study, WELLDO (Harris *et al.*, 2017b), confirmed that this type of intervention was useful in a group of largely mild–moderate learning-disabled adults, with close to 50% of participants achieving a 5% weight loss.

Anti-obesity medication

There remains only one anti-obesity medication available for prescription by physicians for the management of obesity and comorbid conditions in the UK (tetrahydrolipstatin or orlistat), although a number of others are under development. Other medications under development for weight management operate through appetite suppression (or satiety promotion), or by thermogenesis to increase energy expenditure. Importantly, orlistat should be taken in combination with a programme of diet, exercise and behaviour therapy.

Malabsorption

Lipase inhibition induces partial malabsorption of dietary fat by the inhibition of triglyceride hydrolysis. The chemically synthesised hydrogenated derivative of lipostatin (tetrahydrolipstatin or orlistat) is a potent inhibitor of gastric, pancreatic and carboxyl ester lipase. There are possible risks, possibly correctable, of depletion of fat-soluble vitamins A, D, E and K. Predictable side effects from malabsorption, altered bowel habits, and bacterial overgrowth in the small bowel have led to a patient withdrawal of around 37% from therapy (Sjostrom *et al.*, 1998). A low-fat, low-energy diet reduces symptoms and maximises weight loss, which at 1 year was 10.2% control vs. 6.1% intervention. At 2 years, the difference in weight loss due to orlistat was 3.6 kg. About 20% of patients who took part in studies of orlistat lost at least 10% body weight, which was twice the number on placebo. This medication is now available in the UK with medical prescription or as an over-the-counter product. The success of this initiative is unknown; however, orlistat is sold over the counter at a dosage, approximately half its prescription dosage, and is expensive.

Hypoglycaemic agent for diabetes and obesity

Although not classified as an anti-obesity medication, and only appropriate for use in the management of type 2 diabetes, the glucagon-like peptide-1 (GLP-1) receptor agonist does reduce body weight close to clinically important levels. Liraglutide has been licenced for use since 2009, and shows a beneficial effect on both body weight, −3 kg at 26 weeks (Buse *et al.*, 2009), and diabetic control, with a reduction of 1.5% in HbA1C. The medication is administered subcutaneously once daily, and its mode of actions are to improve blood glucose control (mediated by increased insulin secretion), delay gastric emptying, and suppress postprandial glucagon secretion.

Medication under consideration for weight management

Lorcaserin is licensed for use in the USA for use in obesity, but is not licensed for use in the UK and Europe at present. It is a selective serotonin 2C (5HT2c) receptor agonist, administered orally twice daily. Data from a study in patients with obesity, but not diabetes, showed a weight change of 3.2 kg more than placebo. Almost double the number of patients on lorcaserin lost 5% or more weight (47 vs. 20%) (Smith *et al.*, 2010).

Maintenance of weight loss

The European-wide multicentre Diogenes study (Larsen *et al.*, 2010) examined dietary composition in the context of preventing weight regain, post-weight loss. Adults from eight European countries were randomly assigned to one of five ad libitum diets to prevent weight regain over a 26-week period. The diets were a low-protein and low-GI diet, a low-protein and high-GI diet, a high-protein and low-GI diet, a high-protein and high-GI diet, and a control diet. A mean weight loss of 11 kg was seen using a VLCD, and only the low-protein and high-GI diet was associated with clinically important weight regain (+1.7 kg). A common failing in almost all conventional approaches for weight loss has been to leave weight maintenance to chance, so that regain is usual and most often almost complete. Many researchers have found that weight loss is relatively easy to achieve, but that weight maintenance is more challenging. There are a number of follow-up studies that have examined long-term weight loss after treatment, but they are not technically addressing weight maintenance. A meta-analysis in overweight and obese adults examined long-term weight loss after diet and exercise. The findings showed that the inclusion of physical activity and diet together led to a 20% greater sustained weight loss, of 6.7 vs. 4.5 kg (diet alone), after 1 year (Curioni & Lourenco, 2005). However, in both groups, almost half the initial weight loss was regained after 1 year. Douketis *et al.* (2005) confirmed the conclusions of the present review that all dietary approaches achieve moderate weight loss, with the exception of surgery, after 2–4-year follow-up. In a bid to challenge the perception that almost no one succeeds in long-term weight maintenance, Wing and Hill (2001) identified the characteristics of successful weight losers and maintainers within the National Weight Control Registry (Wing & Hill, 2001). These individuals were defined as 10% weight losers who sustain this loss for a least 1 year, and for whom, at 5 years, the mean weight loss was 30 kg. The common characteristics of maintainers in the registry were the consumption of a low-fat diet, a high level of physical activity, and regularly weighing themselves and taking responsibility for monitoring their own weight. Although successful weight maintenance strategies have yet to be defined, there are many reflective articles that consider the reasons behind the prevention of weight gain (Swinburn & Egger, 2002). A recent editorial suggested that weight maintenance remains a key area of weight management where effective long-term approaches are urgently required (Lean & Hankey, 2018).

Conclusions

There are a range of approaches available for the achievement of weight loss. The outcome in the majority of these interventions is moderate weight loss, which has been acknowledged to confer some health benefits. Long-term weight maintenance, dependent on effective weight maintenance strategies, is increasingly recognised as a key element. The moderate-energy-deficit approach has been shown to lead to a weight loss of approximately 5 kg over 12 weeks, and has been used in longer-term studies and the Counterweight programme. The value of this approach may lie in the emphasis on eating conventional foods, and the introduction of regular meal patterns. The effect of diet composition on weight loss is minimal, although the consumption of a high-carbohydrate diet in the longer term should be advocated to reduce the risk of long-term chronic disease. Physical activity in addition to dietary intervention can offer opportunities for improved maintenance of weight loss, although physical activity programmes alone result in minimal weight losses. VLCD or LCLD approaches are valuable in inducing short-term weight loss of up to 10–15 kg, either pre-surgery or in a setting where subsequent dietary management is proposed. Medical supervision is required, together with a minimum BMI of 30 kg/m², as well as long-term management in these cases. Promising results support the case for LCLD approaches being introduced into routine care; in addition, they have been shown to result in diabetes remission.

A wide range of treatments for overweight have been tested, and the majority achieve a modest (5–10%) weight loss, sufficient to improve clinical outcomes for type 2 diabetes, plasma lipids, hypertension and other risk factors for ischaemic heart disease. This weight loss is mostly achieved over 12 weeks, after which it is difficult for many to achieve further loss. Greater weight loss is usually possible for patients with surgery.

Particular weight management challenges are offered by emerging sectors of the overweight and obese populations. These include the severe and complicated groups such as those who are obese and pregnant, and likely to retain the weight gained in pregnancy; those with intellectual disabilities; and older people for whom physical activity may be particularly challenging. There are likely to be others.

The ability to maintain weight losses is crucial if the health benefits of weight loss are to be sustainable. Weight maintenance is required to support the clinically important weight losses seen with any approaches described for weight management. However, effective approaches for weight maintenance are yet to be defined and tested. Many health professionals can contribute to effective weight management programmes; however, given the scale of the problem, the role of the dietitian is perhaps more important in terms of training others to enable them to challenge the epidemic of overweight and obesity, rather than directly dealing with the problem.

SECTION 7

Further reading

Hankey C, Whelan K (ed). (2018) *Advanced Nutrition and Dietetics in Obesity*. Advanced Nutrition and Dietetics, BDA. Chichester: Wiley-Blackwell.

Sattar N, Lean M (eds). (2009) *ABC of Obesity*. Oxford: Blackwell Publishing.

Resources

Association for the Study of Obesity, www.aso.org.uk

BDA Obesity Specialist Group, www.bda.uk.com/regionsgroups/groups/obesity/home

PHE Data and analysis tools, https://www.gov.uk/guidance/phe-data-and-analysis-tools#obesity-diet-and-physical-activity

Public Health England Obesity Updates, www.noo.org.uk/NOO_pub/KU

World Obesity, www.worldobesity.org

References

Atkins RC. (1998) *Dr Atkins's New Diet Revolution*. New York: Simon and Schuster.

Avenell A, Sattar N, Lean MEJ. (2006) ABC of obesity. Management: part I – behaviour change, diet and activity. *BMJ*. 333: 740–743.

Bitzen PO, Melander A, Schersten B, *et al.* (1988) Efficacy of dietary regulation in primary health care patients with hyperglycaemia detected by screening. *Diabet. Med.* 5: 640–647.

Bravata DM, Sanders L, Huang J, *et al.* (2003) Efficacy and safety of low-carbohydrate diets: a systematic review. *JAMA*. 289(14): 1837–1850.

Brinkworth GD, Noakes M, Keogh JB, *et al.* (2004) Long-term effects of a high-protein, low-carbohydrate diet on weight control and cardiovascular risk markers in obese hyperinsulinemic subjects. *Int. J. Obes.* 28(5): 661–670.

Brown TJ, Todd A, O'Malley C, *et al.* (2016) Community pharmacy-delivered interventions for public health priorities: a systematic review of interventions for alcohol reduction, smoking cessation and weight management, including meta-analysis for smoking cessation. *BMJ Open*. 6(2): e009828.

Burgess E, Hassmén P, Welvaert M, *et al.* (2017) Behavioural treatment strategies improve adherence to lifestyle intervention programmes in adults with obesity: a systematic review and meta-analysis. *Clin. Obes.* 7: 105–114.

Buse JB, Rosenstock J, Sesti G, *et al.* (2009) Liraglutide once a day versus exenatide twice a day for type 2 diabetes: a 26-week randomised, parallel-group, multinational, open-label trial (LEAD-6). *Lancet*. 374: 39–47.

Chenoweth DA. (1990) Health promotion programs examined through cost effectiveness analysis. *Occup. Heal. Saf.* 59: 40–41.

Counterweight Project Team. (2004a) Current approaches to obesity management in UK Primary Care: the Counterweight Programme. *J. Hum. Nutr. Diet.* 17: 183–190.

Counterweight Project Team. (2004b) A new evidence based model for weight-management in primary care: the Counterweight Programme. *J. Hum. Nutr. Diet.* 17: 191–208.

Counterweight Project Team. (2005) The impact of obesity on drug prescribing in primary care. *Br. J. Gen. Pract.* 55: 743–749.

Counterweight Project Team. (2008) Evaluation of the Counterweight Programme for obesity management in primary care: a starting point for continuous improvement. *Br. J. Gen. Pract.* 58: 548–554.

Curioni CC, Lourenco PM. (2005) Long-term weight loss after diet and exercise: a systemic review. *Int. J. Obes.* 29(10): 168–174.

Dansinger ML, Gleason JA, Griffith JL, *et al.* (2005) Comparison of the Atkins, Ornish, Weight Watchers, and Zone diets for weight loss and heart disease risk reduction: a randomized trial. *J. Am. Med. Ass.* 293(1): 43–53.

Douketis JD, Macie C, Thabane L, *et al.* (2005) Systematic review of long-term weight loss studies in obese adults: clinical significance and applicability to clinical practice. *Int. J. Obes. (Lond).* 29(10): 1153–1167.

Egger G, Bolton A, O'Neill M, *et al.* (1996) Effectiveness of an abdominal obesity reduction programme in men: the GutBuster 'waist loss' programme. *Int. J. Obes. Relat. Metab. Disord.* 20(3): 227–231.

Eisenstein J, Roberts SB, Dallal G, *et al.* (2002) High-protein weight-loss diets: are they safe and do they work? A review of the experimental and epidemiologic data. *Nutr. Rev.* 60: 189–200.

European Medicines Agency. (2010) *Guideline on Missing Data in Confirmatory Clinical Trials.* Available at http://www.ema.europa.eu/docs/en_GB/document_library/Scientific_guideline/2010/09/WC500096793.pdf. Accessed 24 January 2017.

Feinman RD, Pogozelski WK, Astrup A *et al.*, (2015) Dietary carbohydrate restriction as the first approach in diabetes management: critical review and evidence base. *Nutrition* 31(1):1–13.

Fogelholm M, Kukkonen-Harjula K, Nenonen A, *et al.* (2000) Effects of walking training on weight maintenance after a very-low-energy diet in premenopausal obese women: a randomized controlled trial. *Arch. Intern. Med.* 160(14): 2177–2184.

Foster GD, Wyatt HR, Hill JO, *et al.* (2003) A randomized trial of a low-carbohydrate diet for obesity. *N. Engl. J. Med.* 348(21): 2082–2090.

Foster GD, Wyatt HR, Hill JO, *et al.* (2010) Weight and metabolic outcomes after 2 years on a low carbohydrate versus low fat diet: a randomised trial. *Ann. Intern. Med.* 153: 147–157.

Frost G, Masters K, Kin C, *et al.* (1991) A new method of energy prescription to improve weight loss. *J. Hum. Nutr. Diet.* 4: 369–373.

Gold BC, Burke S, Pintauro S, *et al.* (2007) Weight loss on the web: a pilot study comparing a structured behavioural intervention to a commercial program. *Obesity (Silver Spring).* 15(1): 155–164.

Gordon J, Watson M, Avenell A. (2011) Lightening the load? A systematic review of community pharmacy-based weight management interventions. *Obes. Rev.* 12(11): 897–911.

Han TS, Tajar A, Lean MEJ. (2011) Obesity and weight management in the elderly. *Br. Med. Bull.* 97: 169–196.

Hankey CR, Eley S, Leslie WS, *et al.* (2004) Eating habits, beliefs, attitudes and knowledge among health professionals regarding the links between obesity, nutrition and health. *Public Health Nutr.* 7(2): 337–343.

Harris L, Hankey C, Jones N, et al. (2017a) A cluster randomised control trial of a multi-component weight management programme for adults with intellectual disabilities and obesity. *Br. J. Nutr.* 118(3): 229–240.

Harris L, Hankey C, Murray H et al. (2017b) The effects of physical activity interventions on preventing weight gain and the effects on body composition in young adults with intellectual disabilities: systematic review and meta-analysis of randomized controlled trials. *Clin. Obesity* 5(4): 198–210.

Harris L, McGarty A, Hutchinson L, *et al.* (2018a) Short-term intermittent energy restriction for weight management: a systematic review and meta-analysis. *Obes. Rev.* 19: 1–13.

Harris L, Hamiliton S, Azevedo L, *et al.* (2018b) Intermittent fasting for the treatment of overweight and obesity in adults aged 18 years and over; a systematic review and meta-analysis. *JBI Database System. Rev. Implement. Rep.* 16(2): 507–547.

Health Survey for England. (2016) Available at https://digital.nhs.uk/data-and-information/publications/statistical/health-survey-for-england/health-survey-for-england-2016. Accessed 13 November 2018.

Heshka S, Anderson JW, Atkinson RL, *et al.* (2003) Weight loss with self-help compared with a structured commercial program: a randomized trial. *JAMA.* 289(14): 1792–1798.

Heslehurst N, Rankin J, Wilkinson JR, *et al.* (2010) A nationally representative study of maternal obesity in England, UK: trends in incidence and demographic inequalities in 619 323 births, 1989–2007. *Int. J. Obes. (Lond).* 34: 420–428.

Hession M, Rolland C, Kulkarni U, *et al.* (2009) Systematic review of randomised controlled trials of low-carbohydrate vs. low-fat/low calorie diets in the management of obesity and its comorbidities. *Obes. Rev.* 10: 36–50.

Hill JO, Drougas HJ, Peters JC. (1994) Physical activity, fitness and moderate obesity. In: Bouchard C, Shephard RJ, Stephens T (eds) *Physical Activity, Fitness and Health: International Proceedings and Consensus Statement 1992.* Champaign: Human Kinetics Publishers, pp. 684–691.

Hoppe R, Ogden J. (1997) Practice nurses' beliefs about obesity and weight related interventions in primary care. *Int. J. Obes. Relat. Metab. Disord.* 21: 141–146.

Jebb SA, Ahern AL, Olson AD, *et al.* (2011) Primary care referral to a commercial provider for weight loss treatment versus standard care: a randomised controlled trial. *Lancet.* 378(9801): 1485–1492.

Jenkins DJ, Wolever TM, Taylor RH, *et al.* (1981) Glycemic index of foods: a physiological basis for carbohydrate exchange. *Am. J. Clin. Nutr.* 34(3): 362–366.

Jolly K, Lewis A, Beach J, *et al.* (2011) Comparison of range of commercial or primary care led weight reduction programmes with minimal intervention control for weight loss in obesity: lighten Up randomised controlled trial. *BMJ.* 343: d6500.

King L, Gill T, Allender S, *et al.* (2011) Best practice principles for community-based obesity prevention : development, content and application. *Obes. Rev.* 12(5): 329–338.

Larsen TM, Dalskov SM, van Baak M, *et al.* (2010) Diets with high or low protein content and glycemic index for weight-loss maintenance. *N. Engl. J. Med.* 363(22): 2102–2113.

Leahey TM, Fava JL, Seiden A, *et al.* (2016) A randomized controlled trial testing an Internet delivered cost–benefit approach to weight loss maintenance. *Prev. Med.* 92: 51–57.

Lean M, Hankey C. (2018) Keeping it off: the challenge of weight-loss maintenance. *Lancet Diabetes Endocrinol.* 6(9): 681–683. doi:10.1016/S2213-8587(17)30405-9.

Lean ME, James WP. (1986) Prescription of diabetic diets in the 1980s. *Lancet.* 1: 723–725.

Lean M, Brosnahan N, McLoone P, *et al.* (2013) Feasibility and indicative results from a 12-month low-energy liquid diet treatment and maintenance programme for severe obesity. *Br. J. Gen. Pract.* 63: e115–e124.

Lean ME, Leslie WS, Barnes AC, *et al.* (2018) Primary care-led weight management for remission of type 2 diabetes (DiRECT): an open-label, cluster-randomised trial. *Lancet.* 391(10120): 541–551.

Leeds AR. (2017) Formula diets for weight loss in obesity. In: Hankey C (ed) *Advanced Textbook of Obesity and Weight Management.* Chichester: Wiley Publishing.

Leslie WS, Hankey, CR, Lean ME. (2007) Weight gain as an adverse effect of some commonly prescribed drugs: a systematic review. *QJM.* 100: 395–404.

Leslie WS, Ford I, Sattar N, *et al.* (2016) The Diabetes Remission Clinical Trial (DiRECT): protocol for a cluster randomised Trial. *BMC Fam. Pract.* 17: 20. doi: 10.1186/s12875-016-0406-2. Accessed 7 June 2017.

Leslie WS, Hankey CR, McCombie L, *et al.* (2005) Weight management: a survey of current practice in secondary care NHS settings in 2004. *J. Eval. Clin. Pract.* 11(5): 462–467.

Leslie WS, Lean MEJ, Baillie HM, *et al.* (2002) Weight management: a comparison of existing dietary approaches in a work-site setting. *Int. J. Obes. Relat. Metab. Disord.* 26: 1469–1475.

Logue J, Allardice G, Gillies M, *et al.* (2014) Outcomes of a specialist weight management programme in the UK National Health Service: prospective study of 1838 patients. *BMJ Open*. 4(1): e003747.

Loveman E, Frampton GK, Shepherd J, *et al.* (2011) The clinical effectiveness and cost-effectiveness of long-term weight management schemes for adults: a systematic review. *Health Technol. Assess.* 15(2): 1–182.

McConnon A, Kirk SF, Cockroft JE, *et al.* (2007) The Internet for weight control in an obese sample: results of a randomised controlled trial. *BMC Health Serv. Res.* 7: 206.

Michie S, Ashford S, Sniehotta FF, *et al.* (2011) A refined taxonomy of behaviour change techniques to help people change their physical activity and healthy eating behaviours: the CALO-RE taxonomy. *Psychol. Health.* 26(11): 1479–1498.

Moroshko L, Brennan L, O'Brien P. (2011) Predictors of dropout in weight loss interventions: a systematic review of the literature. *Obes. Rev.* 12: 912–934.

National Institutes for Health. (2016) *How can obesity and overweight be prevented?* Available at https://www.nhlbi.nih.gov/health/health-topics/topics/obe/prevention. Accessed 24 January 2017.

National Obesity Observatory. (2011) *Economics of obesity*. Available at http://webarchive.nationalarchives.gov.uk/20160805122056/https://www.noo.org.uk/NOO_about_obesity/economics. Accessed 13 November 2018.

National Task Force on the Prevention and Treatment of Obesity, National Institutes of Health. (1993) Very low calorie diets. *JAMA*. 270: 967–974.

NICE. (2006) *Obesity – guidance on the prevention, identification, assessment and management of overweight and obesity in adults and children. Clinical Guideline 43*. Available at https://www.nice.org.uk/guidance/CG43/chapter/5-Other-versions-of-this-guideline. Accessed 24 January 2017.

NICE. (2017) Clinical Knowledge Obesity Summary. Available at https://cks.nice.org.uk/obesity#!topicsummary. Accessed 13 November 2018.

Nordmann AJ, Nordmann A, Briel M, *et al.* (2006) Effects of low-carbohydrate vs low-fat diets on weight loss and cardiovascular risk factors, a meta-analysis of randomised controlled trials. *Arch. Intern. Med.* 166: 285–293.

Noto H, Goto A, Tsujimoto T, *et al.* (2013) Low-carbohydrate diets and all-cause mortality: a systematic review and meta-analysis of observational studies. *PLoS One*. 8(1): e55030. doi: 10.1371/journal.pone.0055030.

Paul-Ebhohimhen V, Avenell A. (2009) A systematic review of the effectiveness of group versus individual treatments for adult obesity. *Obes. Facts* 2(1): 17–24.

Perri MG, Nezu AM. Viegner BJ. (1992) *Improving the Long Term Management of Obesity*. New York: Willey Bioscience.

Petticrew M, Chalabi Z, Jones DR. (2012) To RCT or not to RCT: deciding when 'more evidence is needed' for public health policy and practice. *J. Epidemiol. Community Health*. 66: 391–396.

Raben A. (2002) Should obese patients be counselled to follow a low-glycaemic index diet? *No. Obes. Rev.* 3(4): 245–256.

Romaguera D, Norat T, Vergnaud AC. (2010) Mediterranean dietary patterns and prospective weight change in participants of the EPIC-PANACEA project. *Am. J. Clin. Nutr.* 92(4): 912–921.

Roumen C, Feskens EJ, Corpeleijn E, *et al.* (2011) Predictors of lifestyle intervention outcome and dropout: the SLIM study. *Eur. J. Clin. Nutr.* 65: 1141–1147.

Sacks FM, Bray GA, Carey VJ, *et al.* (2009) Comparison of weight loss diets with different compositions of fat, protein and carbohydrates. *N. Engl. J. Med.* 360(9): 859–873.

Scottish Government Data. (2016) *On Adult Obesity*. Available at http://www.gov.scot/Publications/2015/09/6648/318800. Accessed 24 January 17.

Scottish Intercollegiate Guidelines Network (SIGN). (2010) *Management of obesity – a national clinical guideline No 115*. Edinburgh: Scottish Intercollegiate Guidelines Network.

Scottish Government (2016) Scottish Health Survey 2016 Available at https://www.gov.scot/publications/scottish-health-survey-2016-summary-key-findings/. Accessed 12 November 2018.

Schwingshackl L, Hobl LP, Hoffmann G. (2015) Effects of low glycaemic index/low glycaemic load vs. high glycaemic index/ high glycaemic load diets on overweight/obesity and associated risk factors in children and adolescents: a systematic review and meta-analysis. *Nutr. J.* 14: 87–97.

Shai I, Schwarzfuchs, D, Henkin Y, *et al.*; Dietary Intervention Randomized Controlled Trial (DIRECT) Group. (2008) Weight loss with a low-carbohydrate, Mediterranean, or low-fat diet. *N. Engl. J. Med.* 359: 229–241.

SIGN. (2010) *Management of obesity*. Available at https://www.sign.ac.uk/sign-115-management-of-obesity.html. Accessed 13 November 2018.

Simpson S, Coulman E, Hughes K et al. (2016) 'Help Me Do It!' a web, app and text based intervention to facilitate social support to achieve and maintain health related change in physical activity and dietary behaviour. Available at https://www.journalslibrary.nihr.ac.uk/programmes/phr/1218020/#/. Accessed 13 November 2018.

Sjostrom L, Rissanen A, Andersen T, *et al.* (1998) Randomised placebo-controlled trial of orlistat for weight loss and prevention of weight regain in obese patients. European Multicentre Orlistat Study Group. *Lancet.* 352(9123): 167–172.

Skender ML, Goodrick GK, Del Junco DJ, *et al.* (1996) Comparison of 2-year weight loss trends in behavioural treatments for obesity: diet, exercise and combination interventions. *J. Am. Diet. Assoc.* 96(4): 342–346.

Smith SR, Weissman NJ, Anderson CM, *et al.* (2010) Multicenter, placebo-controlled trial of lorcaserin for weight management. *N. Engl. J. Med.* 363(3): 245–256.

Svendsen OL, Hassager C, Christiansen C. (1994) Six months' follow-up on exercise added to a short-term diet in overweight postmenopausal women – effects on body composition, resting metabolic rate, cardiovascular risk factors and bone. *Int. J. Obes. Relat. Metab. Disord.* 18(10): 692–698.

Swinburn W, Egger G. (2002) Preventive strategies against weight gain and obesity. *Obes. Rev.* 3(4): 289–301.

Tsai AG, Wadden TA. (2005) Systematic review: an evaluation of major commercial weight loss programs in the United States. *Ann. Intern. Med.* 142(1): 56–66.

Wadden T, Berkowitz RI, Womble LG, et al. (2005) Randomized trial of lifestyle modification and pharmacotherapy for obesity. *N. Engl. J. Med.* 353(20): 2111–2120.

Wadden TA, Volger S, Sarwer D, *et al.* (2011) A two-year randomized trial of obesity treatment in primary care practice. *N. Engl. J. Med.* 365: 1969–1979.

Weigle DS, Breen PA, Matthys CC, *et al.* (2005) A high-protein diet induces sustained reductions in appetite, ad libitum caloric intake, and body weight despite compensatory changes in diurnal plasma leptin and ghrelin concentrations. *Am. J. Clin. Nutr.* 82: 41–48.

WHO. (2016) *Obesity and Overweight Facts*. Available at http://www.who.int/mediacentre/factsheets/fs311/en/. Accessed January 2017.

Wing RR, Hill, JO. (2001) Successful weight loss maintenance. *Annu. Rev. Nutr.* 21: 323–341.

Wu T, Gao X, Chem M, *et al.* (2009) Long-term effectiveness of diet-plus-exercise interventions vs. diet-only interventions for weight loss: a meta-analysis. *Obes. Rev.* 10: 313–323.

Yang H, Petersen GM, Roth MP, *et al.* (1992) Risk factors for gallstone formation during rapid loss of weight. *Dig. Dis. Sci.* 37: 912–918.

7.13.3 Bariatric surgery

Gail Pinnock and Mary O'Kane

Key points

- Bariatric surgery is an effective long-term treatment of obesity.
- Comorbidities significantly improve after surgery.
- There is a risk of micronutrient deficiencies following surgery.
- Long-term dietetic support is essential.

Surgery should be considered if weight loss associated with diet, medication and lifestyle change is insufficient to improve health, especially in those with severe and complex obesity (NICE, 2014). Bariatric surgery is the most effective long-term treatment of severe obesity (Picot *et al.*, 2009). The weight loss following bariatric surgery varies depending on the procedure; however, there have been few well-designed trials comparing procedures (Picot *et al.*, 2009; Rogers *et al.*, 2014). The benefits of surgery are well established, with resolution of comorbidities in a significant number (Karlsson *et al.*, 2007; Mechanick *et al.*, 2013). Recent data compiled from the National Bariatric Surgery Registry ((Welbourn *et al.*, 2014) showed that 61% of patients with sleep apnoea were able to stop treatment 1 year after surgery, and 65.1% with type 2 diabetes were able to stop diabetic medications 2 years after surgery.

In 2015/2016, there were over 6 438 bariatric surgery procedures undertaken within the NHS (Health and Social Care Information Centre, 2016). There are no reliable data on procedures carried out in the private sector.

Clinical guidelines

In the UK, NICE (2014) guidance recommends surgery as a treatment option if all the following criteria are met:

- BMI >40 kg/m².
- BMI >35 kg/m² with significant disease (e.g. type 2 diabetes, high blood pressure, obstructive sleep apnoea) that could be improved with weight loss.
- Appropriate non-surgical measures have been tried, but failed to achieve or maintain adequate, clinically beneficial weight loss.
- Has been receiving or will receive intensive management in a specialist obesity tier 3 service.
- Generally fit for anaesthesia and surgery, commits to the need for long-term follow-up.

For those with recent-onset type 2 diabetes, NICE (2014) recommends:

- An expedited assessment for bariatric surgery if BMI ≥35 kg/m², receiving or will receive assessment in a tier 3 service (or equivalent).
- An assessment should be considered for BMI 30–34.9 kg/m², receiving or will receive assessment in a tier 3 service (or equivalent).
- Consider an assessment for bariatric surgery if of Asian descent at BMI <29.9 kg/m² (see recommendation 1.2.8), receiving or will receive assessment in a tier 3 service (or equivalent).

Treatment centres are required to have a multidisciplinary team (MDT) that can effectively select and manage these complex patients (NICE, 2014). A comprehensive assessment in which the benefits of surgery can be balanced against the risks is essential to enable the patient to make an informed choice in consultation with the MDT. For some, the risks may be too great, and surgery declined.

Surgical procedures

Bariatric surgery works by impacting on satiety, malabsorption or a combination of both; most surgery is performed laparoscopically to shorten recovery. The choice of surgical procedure depends on several factors, including the MDT's decision, patient's comorbidities and patient preference (see Figures 7.13.2–7.13.6; Table 7.13.3).

Roux-en-Y gastric bypass (RYGB) was the most frequently performed procedure from 2011 to 2013, followed by sleeve and adjustable gastric band (AGB) (Welbourn *et al.*, 2014). Duodenal switch is rarely used because of a greater risk of malnutrition. It may be done as a two-stage procedure, and only in patients with considerable weight to lose. The intragastric balloon is placed endoscopically into the stomach and then inflated with saline. It is a short-term measure, viable for 6 months, and therefore outside NICE guidance.

It is not known which procedure gives the best long-term clinical outcomes, although the SurgiCal Obesity Treatment (SCOTS) Study (Logue *et al.*, 2015) and the By-Band-Sleeve Study (Rogers *et al.*, 2014) are being conducted in the UK. SCOTS is a 10-year longitudinal study. Novel, less invasive techniques are being developed, although they are not yet in common use in the UK.

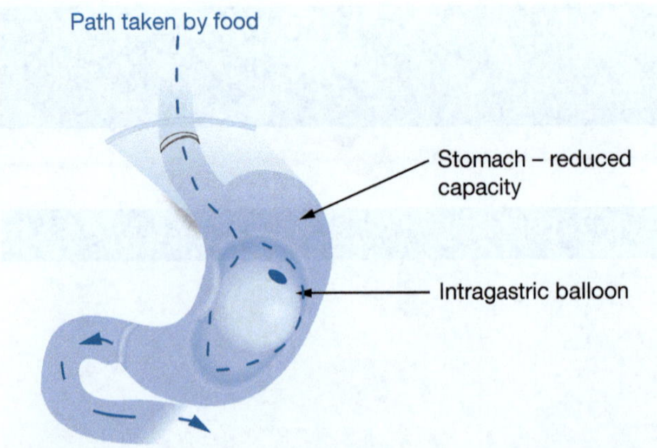

Figure 7.13.2 Intragastric balloon (source: The National Bariatric Surgery Registry: First Registry Report, 2011. Reproduced with permission from Dentrite Clinical Systems Ltd.)

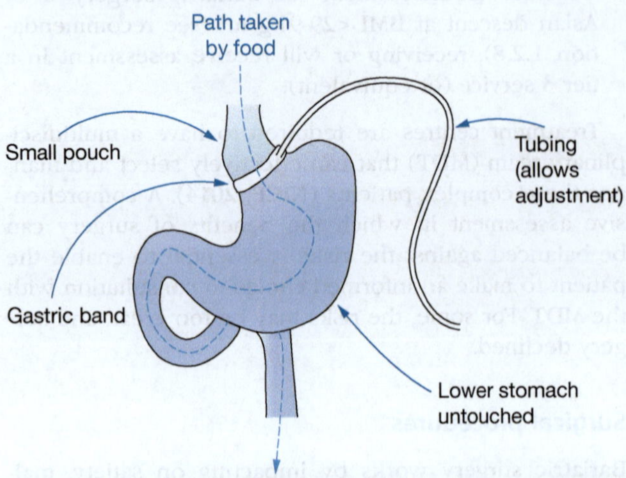

Figure 7.13.3 Adjustable gastric band (source: The National Bariatric Surgery Registry: First Registry Report, 2011. Reproduced with permission from Dentrite Clinical Systems Ltd.)

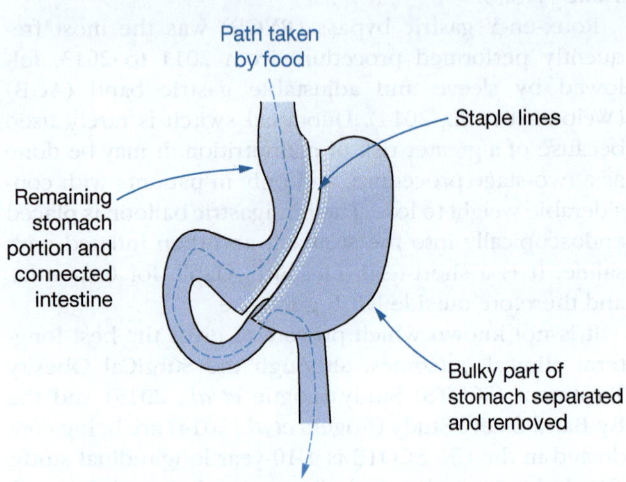

Figure 7.13.4 Sleeve gastrectomy (source: The National Bariatric Surgery Registry: First Registry Report, 2011. Reproduced with permission from Dentrite Clinical Systems Ltd.)

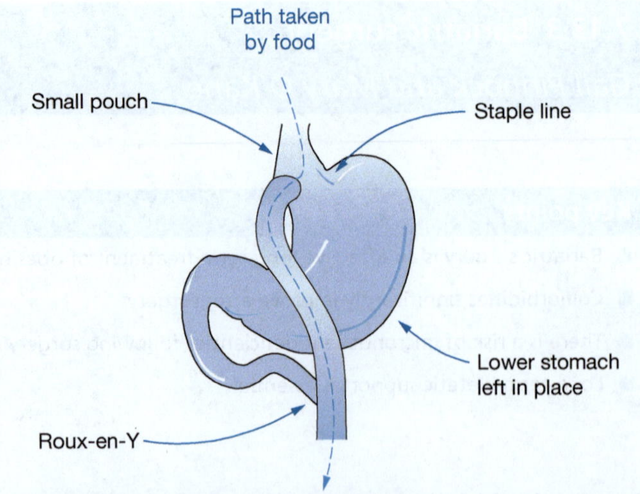

Figure 7.13.5 Roux-en-Y gastric bypass (source: The National Bariatric Surgery Registry: First Registry Report, 2011. Reproduced with permission from Dentrite Clinical Systems Ltd.)

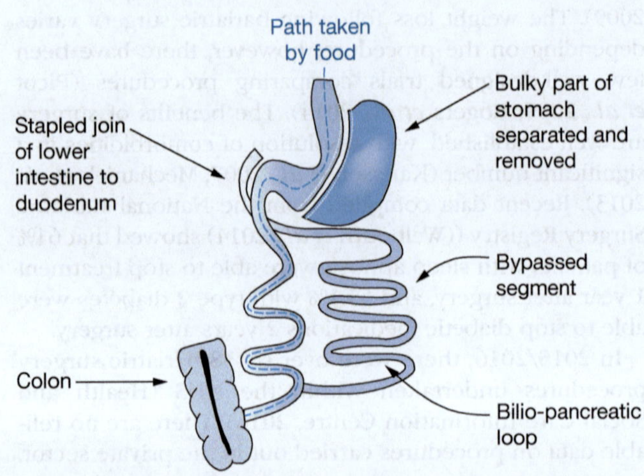

Figure 7.13.6 Duodenal switch (source: The National Bariatric Surgery Registry: First Registry Report, 2011. Reproduced with permission from Dentrite Clinical Systems Ltd.)

Gut hormones

The gastric bypass, sleeve gastrectomy, long-limb bypass and duodenal switch affect some gut hormones, including ghrelin, glucagon-like peptide-1 and peptide YY, involved in glucose regulation and appetite control. This results in improvements in glycaemic control and reduced appetite; however, appetite eventually returns. Recent evidence suggests that the beneficial effects of surgery involve changes in the gut hormones, bile acid metabolism, gut microbiota and vagal sensory neurons (Meek *et al.*, 2016; Williams *et al.*, 2016). The exact mechanism has not yet been fully elucidated.

Weight loss following surgery

The gastric bypass, sleeve gastrectomy and duodenal switch result in an initial fast weight loss, which plateaus over time; the gastric band results in a more

Table 7.13.3 Bariatric surgery procedures

Procedure	Mechanism of action	Impact on nutrition	Supplementation recommended[a]
Intragastric balloon	Increased satiety	Reduced intake	Multivitamin and mineral
Adjustable gastric band	Increased satiety	Reduced intake	Multivitamin and mineral
Sleeve gastrectomy	Increased satiety	Reduced intake	Protein (60–80 g/day)
		Calcium, iron, vitamin D and vitamin B_{12} absorption affected	Multivitamin, mineral, calcium, iron and vitamin D
Roux-en-Y gastric bypass		May experience dumping syndrome or postprandial hypoglycaemia following the gastric bypass	Vitamin B_{12} injections
Long-limb gastric bypass	Increased satiety	Reduced intake	Protein (80–100 g/day), low fat
	May experience steatorrhoea affecting absorption	Macronutrient (protein and fat) malabsorption possible	Multivitamin, mineral, calcium, iron, vitamin D and vitamin B_{12}
		Calcium, iron, vitamin D and vitamin B_{12} absorption affected	
		May experience dumping syndrome or postprandial hypoglycaemia	
Duodenal switch (biliopancreatic diversion)	Increased satiety	Reduced intake	High-protein (80–100 g/day), low-fat diet
	Malabsorptive, steatorrhoea affecting absorption	Macronutrient (protein and fat) malabsorption	Multivitamin, mineral, high doses of fat-soluble vitamins, calcium, iron and vitamin B_{12}
		Calcium, iron, vitamin B_{12}, and fat-soluble vitamin absorption affected	

[a] See O'Kane *et al.* (2014) for full recommendations.

gradual weight loss. Maximum loss is usually achieved in 18–24 months. Unless permanent lifestyle and dietary changes are made, there may be unsatisfactory weight loss or weight regain (Karlsson *et al.*, 2007).

Surgical complications

Mortality rates vary depending on the procedure, but are lower when performed by experienced surgeons in specialist high-volume centres (Welbourn *et al.*, 2014). Complications include anastomotic leaks, bleeding, infection, strictures, obstructions or incisional hernias (Mechanick *et al.*, 2008); nutritional support may be required. Careful consideration must be given to the risks and benefits of surgery before proceeding.

Long-term complications

The benefits of surgery in improving glycaemic control, hypertension, sleep apnoea and hyperlipidaemia are well established (Karlsson *et al.*, 2007; Mechanick *et al.*, 2013; Welbourn *et al.*, 2014). However, long-term problems have been reported, including nutritional deficiencies (Homan *et al.*, 2015; Mechanick *et al.*, 2013), metabolic bone disease (Muschitz *et al.*, 2015), renal stones, anastomotic ulcers, strictures and obstructions (Mechanick *et al.*, 2008).

Role of the dietitian

The dietitian is an essential and respected member of the MDT (NICE, 2014), who is involved in the presurgical assessment and preparation, through to postsurgical and long-term nutritional support and follow-up.

Presurgical assessment

The presurgical dietetic assessment covers the following (Aills *et al.*, 2008):

- Weight and dieting history.
- Dietary assessment, including eating behaviours and recognised eating disorders.
- Psychological issues – beliefs, behaviours, motivation, support mechanisms.
- Alcohol and smoking.
- Assessment of the patient's understanding of the impact of surgery on diet and lifestyle.
- Physical activity.
- Current medical history, including comorbidities.
- Past medical history, including past surgery.
- Medication.

Nutritional biochemistry should be performed as part of the tier 3 assessment, and nutritional deficiencies must be addressed before surgery (O'Kane *et al.*, 2014).

Preparation

The dietitian helps patients develop coping strategies to manage the changes needed after surgery. Patients are encouraged to follow a liver shrinkage diet for 7–14 days before surgery (Baldry *et al.*, 2014). This may be liquid or food based and low in energy and carbohydrate, which reduces liver size, making surgery easier.

Table 7.13.4 Nutritional monitoring before and annually after surgery[a]

Blood tests	Before surgery	Surgical procedure			
		Gastric band	Gastric bypass	Sleeve gastrectomy	Duodenal switch
Liver function tests	Yes	Yes	Yes	Yes	Yes
Full blood count, folate, vitamin B_{12}	Yes	Full blood count, folate	Yes	Yes	Yes
Calcium, vitamin D	Yes	Yes	Yes	Yes	Yes
Vitamin A	No	No	Possibly[b]	No	Yes
Zinc, copper	No	No	Yes	Possibly[b]	Yes
Selenium	No	No	No[b]	No[b]	No[b]

[a] See O'Kane *et al.* (2014) for full recommendations.
[b] Yes, if there is cause for concern.

Post-surgery

All bariatric procedures affect nutritional intake. The dietitian supports the patient to reintroduce different textures and foods into the diet. Typical issues include regurgitation, vomiting, food intolerances, vitamin and mineral supplementation, and changes in bowel habit. The dietitian is usually the first point of contact for patients, but they must also have access to good surgical support. If persistent vomiting occurs, thiamine deficiency may develop extremely quickly, and urgent supplementation and surgical review is essential (O'Kane *et al.*, 2014). There is an increased incidence of calcium, vitamin D, iron and vitamin B_{12} deficiency following gastric bypass, sleeve gastrectomy and duodenal switch (Mechanick *et al.*, 2013). In addition, zinc and fat-soluble vitamin deficiencies are seen following long-limb bypasses and duodenal switch (Homan *et al.*, 2015). Compliance with vitamin and mineral supplements and nutritional monitoring are essential (O'Kane *et al.*, 2014). The recommended blood tests are outlined in Table 7.13.4 (O'Kane *et al.*, 2014).

Short-term management

As the patient progresses from liquids to puréed foods and onto normal-textured foods, the dietitian must ensure that nutritional and fluid requirements are met. It is crucial that patients establish new eating behaviours, such as eating slowly, stopping before feeling full and chewing food well. They must avoid eating and drinking at the same time initially, because the small stomach makes it difficult, and subsequently because fluid pushes food through quickly, enabling them to eat more. Patients often struggle with textures such as that of bread, roast or grilled meat, and fibrous vegetables. To compensate, patients may resort to a poor-quality diet; foods such as chocolate and crisps tend to be well tolerated.

Long-term management

The patient must be encouraged to have a balanced, low-fat, low-sugar diet. Reduced stomach capacity can result in grazing throughout the day, and a regular meal pattern is necessary (Mitchell *et al.*, 2016). To minimise the risk of nutritional deficiencies, patients are advised to take multivitamin and mineral supplements long term (O'Kane *et al.*, 2014). Regular blood tests should be carried out, and supplementation adjusted as needed. Protein malnutrition may occur because of food intolerances (especially meat), and alternative sources of protein should be suggested. Following a restrictive and malabsorptive procedure, patients should be encouraged to consume 60–100 g of protein/day. Patients who experience dumping syndrome and related symptoms of postprandial hypoglycaemia will need additional support (O'Kane *et al.*, 2016). Patients need continued dietetic support throughout the weight loss phase to encourage permanent dietary and lifestyle changes, and during long-term weight maintenance.

Women of childbearing age are discouraged from becoming pregnant within 18 months of surgery (Mechanick *et al.*, 2013). Vitamin supplements should not contain vitamin A in the retinol form; however, those who have had a duodenal switch may need to continue to take high doses of fat-soluble vitamins throughout pregnancy. Pregnant women require more frequent follow-up, with nutritional monitoring being increased with every trimester (O'Kane *et al.*, 2014, 2016).

Generally, NHS bariatric surgery centres are commissioned to provide 2 years of follow-up. Following discharge from the bariatric service, NICE (2014) recommends that '*there should be at least annual monitoring of nutritional status and appropriate supplementation according to need following bariatric surgery, as part of a shared care model of chronic disease management*'. Long-term follow-up guidelines have been developed (O'Kane *et al.*, 2016), emphasising the importance of annual review and referral back to bariatric centres for those patients with complications.

Internet resources

British Obesity and Metabolic Surgery Society, www.bomss.org.uk
British Obesity Surgery Patient Association (BOSPA), www.bospa.org
NICE quality standard (QS127). (2016) Obesity: clinical assessment and management. Available at https://www.nice.org.uk/guidance/qs127.

References

Aills L, Blankenship J, Buffington C, *et al.* (2008) ASMBS Allied Health nutritional guidelines for the surgical weight loss patient. *Surg. Obes. Relat. Dis.* 4: S73–S108.

Baldry EL, Leeder PC, Idris IR. (2014) Pre-operative dietary restriction for patients undergoing bariatric surgery in the UK: observational study of current practice and dietary effects. *Obes. Surg.* 24: 416–421.

Health and Social Care Information Centre. (2016) *Statistics on obesity, physical activity and diet: England 2016*. Available at www.ic.nhs.uk. Accessed 9 July 2016.

Homan J, Betzel B, Aarts EO, *et al.* (2015) Vitamin and mineral deficiencies after biliopancreatic diversion and biliopancreatic diversion with duodenal switch – the rule rather than the exception. *Obes. Surg.* 25(9): 1626–1632.

Karlsson J, Taft C, Rydén A, *et al.* (2007) Ten-year trends in health-related quality of life after surgical and conventional treatment for severe obesity: the SOS intervention study. *Int. J. Obes. (Lond).* 31: 1248–1261.

Logue J, Stewart S, Munro J, *et al.* (2015) SurgiCal Obesity Treatment Study (SCOTS): protocol for a national prospective cohort study of patients undergoing bariatric surgery in Scotland. *BMJ Open.* 5: e008106. doi:10.1136/bmjopen-2015-008106.

Mechanick JI, Kushner RF, Sugerman HJ, *et al.* (2008) AACE, TOS and ASMBS; medical guidelines for clinical practice for the perioperative nutritional metabolic and non-surgical support of the bariatric patient. *Endocr. Pract.* 14(S1):1–83.

Mechanick JI, Youdim A, Jones DB, *et al.* (2013) Clinical practice guidelines for the perioperative nutritional, metabolic, and nonsurgical support of the bariatric surgery patient – 2013 update. *Obesity* 21(S1): S1–S7.

Meek CL, Lewis HB, Reimann F, *et al.* (2016) The effect of bariatric surgery on gastrointestinal and pancreatic hormones. *Peptides.* 77: 28–37

Mitchell JE, Christian NJ, Flum DR, *et al.* (2016) Postoperative behavioral variables and weight change 3 years after bariatric surgery. *JAMA Surg.* 151: 752–757.

Muschitz C, Kocijan R, Haschka J, *et al.* (2015) The impact of vitamin D, calcium, protein supplementation, and physical exercise on bone metabolism after bariatric surgery: the BABS study. *J. Bone Miner. Res.* 31: 672–682.

NICE. (2014) *Clinical Guideline 189. Obesity: identification, assessment and management of overweight and obesity in children, young people and adults.* Available at http://www.nice.org.uk/guidance/cg189. Accessed 11 May 2016.

O'Kane M, Parretti HM, Hughes CA, *et al.* (2016) Guidelines for the follow-up of patients undergoing bariatric surgery. *Clin. Obes.* 6: 210–224.

O'Kane M, Pinkney J, Aasheim ET, *et al.* (2014) *BOMSS guidelines on perioperative and postoperative biochemical monitoring and micronutrient replacement for patients undergoing bariatric surgery adults.* Available at http://www.bomss.org.uk/wp-content/uploads/2014/09/BOMSS-guidelines-Final-version1Oct14.pdf. Accessed August 2016.

Picot J, Jones J, Colquitt JL, *et al.* (2009) The clinical effectiveness and cost-effectiveness of bariatric (weight loss) surgery for obesity: a systematic review and economic evaluation. economic evaluation. *Health Technol. Assess.* 13(41): 1–190, 215–357.

Rogers CA, Welbourn R, Byrne J, *et al.* (2014) The By-Band study: gastric bypass or adjustable gastric band surgery to treat morbid obesity: study protocol for a multi-centre randomised controlled trial with an internal pilot phase. *Trials.* 15: 53. Available at http://www.trialsjournal.com/content/15/1/53. Accessed 11 May 2016.

Welbourn R, Small P, Finlay I, *et al.* (2014) *National Bariatric Surgery Registry: Second Registry Report 2014.* ISBN 978-0-9568154-8-4. Oxfordshire: Dendrite Clinical Systems Ltd.

Williams EK, Chang RB, Strochlic DE, et al. (2016) Sensory neurons that detect stretch and nutrients in the digestive system. *Cell* 166(1): 209–221.

7.13.4 Childhood obesity

Laura Stewart and Jenny Gillespie

Key points

- Obesity is the most common childhood nutritional disorder worldwide, and is an important area for dietitians.
- Managing childhood obesity is challenging due to the need to engage the child or young person, parents and the whole family.
- The consequences of childhood obesity are seen in childhood, adolescence and adulthood.
- Interventions should be family based, with at least one of the parents involved. Changes in diet, physical activity and screen time should be targeted equally.
- It is important to ensure that normal growth occurs when dietary intake is restricted.

Obesity is the most common childhood nutritional disorder worldwide (Lobstein *et al.*, 2004), and therefore is an important area for dietitians. Managing childhood obesity is challenging due to the need to engage not only with the child or young person but also with his or her parents and the entire family. Dietitians may see overweight and obese children individually in a clinical setting or as a group, e.g. in the community (Edwards *et al.*, 2006; Sacher *et al.*, 2010; Stewart *et al.*, 2005). This chapter explores the knowledge and skills that a dietitian requires to deliver a childhood weight management programme (Sahota *et al.*, 2010). Dietitians working in childhood obesity need to have an appreciation not only of the complex behavioural issues that need to be explored, but also of the causes and consequences of childhood obesity.

The prevalence of childhood obesity in the UK dramatically increased during the early 1990s (Chinn &

Rona, 2001; Reilly & Dorosty, 1999). Due to the complex manner in which data on child weight are collected, it is difficult to give prevalence figures across the UK. Public Health England (https://www.gov.uk/guidance/phe-data-and-analysis-tools#obesity-diet-and-physical-activity) gives up-to-date information on prevalence figures for the four UK home countries.

Aetiology

Since excess weight gain occurs in a state of positive energy balance, the aetiology of obesity is multifactorial, involving an interaction of the modern obesogenic environment and family lifestyle choices. Increased intakes of energy-dense foods (particularly fast foods and snacks), and more time spent watching television and playing computer games, with a consequential decrease in the amount of physical activity, have all been advocated as the causes of the childhood obesity epidemic (House of Commons Health Committee, 2004; Mulvihill & Quigley, 2003).

Non-lifestyle-related causes

A child or adolescent who is obese but also short for stature should be referred to a paediatric endocrinologist for further investigation to exclude possible underlying endocrine causes of their obesity, such as hypothyroidism, growth hormone deficiency, Cushing's syndrome and pseudohypoparathyroidism. Young children, particularly those under 2 years, who have had rapid weight gain, are severely obese and appear to be hyperphagic, may have a rare genetic cause to their obesity, and referral to a paediatrician for further investigations would be advisable (Han *et al.*, 2010; SIGN, 2010). There are also a number of syndromes that are associated with obesity, such as Prader–Willi, Down, and Fragile X syndromes.

Definition

Body mass index (BMI) is generally recognised as the most appropriate measure for diagnosing childhood obesity and overweight (Lobstein *et al.*, 2004; NICE, 2014; SIGN, 2010). It is calculated as for adults, as weight (kg)/height (m)^2; however, it is only meaningful when it is plotted correctly on age- and sex-specific centile charts (UK 1990 data for those aged ≥4 years; WHO data charts for those aged <4 years). UK BMI centile charts incorporating both the WHO and UK 1990 data have been developed by the Royal College of Paediatrics and Child Health (RCPCH), and are available from RCPCH (https://www.rcpch.ac.uk/resources/growth-charts). All dietitians working with obese children should use these charts for diagnosis and monitoring of management (NICE, 2014; SIGN, 2010) (see Chapter 3.8.2, Growth, nutritional assessment and nutritional requirements). There is debate about the most appropriate centile cut-off points for defining childhood overweight and obesity. However, in the UK, both NICE (2014) and SIGN (2010) recommend the use of the 98th centile on BMI charts to define obesity, and the 91st centile to define overweight for clinical use. For epidemiological studies, the 95th and 85th centiles should be used to define obesity and overweight, respectively (see Chapter 3.8.2, Growth, nutritional assessment and nutritional requirements).

Consequences

The consequences of childhood obesity have been reported in childhood, adolescence and later in adult life. Clustering of cardiovascular risk factors have been reported (such as high blood pressure, dyslipidaemia, abnormalities in left ventricular mass and/or function, abnormalities in endothelial function, and hyperinsulinaemia and/or insulin resistance). There is evidence that these cardiovascular risk factors are seen in adults who were obese in childhood or adolescence (Han *et al.*, 2010; Reilly *et al.*, 2003). Type 2 diabetes, a disease previously only seen in adults, is now reported in adolescents (Drake *et al.*, 2002; Han *et al.*, 2010; Sinha *et al.*, 2002). In girls, psychological issues in relation to low self-esteem and behavioural problems, as well as longer-term social and economic consequences of achieving a lower income, have been reported (Drake *et al.*, 2002; Sinha *et al.*, 2002).

There is good evidence to suggest that obesity in childhood and adolescence persists into adulthood, often referred to as tracking. The risk of tracking into adulthood can be compounded by parental obesity, the level of obesity and obesity in adolescence (Reilly *et al.*, 2003; Whitaker *et al.*, 2010). Therefore, it is important to treat childhood obesity as early as possible, and involving the parents/carers is considered to be important.

Assessment

At the first session with the child, the dietitian needs to obtain baseline measurements of weight and height, and to plot these on centile charts. BMI should be calculated and then plotted at the correct age on the appropriate centile chart for sex. Although measuring waist circumference can be difficult in obese children, it is a useful tool in monitoring progress in the clinic; however, there are no agreed cut-off points for defining health risk (Reilly *et al.*, 2010).

The typical day model or a lifestyle diary is useful to elicit information on the family diet and eating pattern. These are seen as more client-centred and child-friendly information collection methods, and are more effective for ascertaining information on the levels of physical activity that the child normally undertakes, as well as screen time. The number of takeaway meals the child and family has, the amount and types of snacks the child eats, and the amount of pocket money that the child spends must be considered. Other details such as age of onset of obesity, eating patterns and family dynamics are most helpful.

Management

Management should encompass the following points:

- It should only be commenced when the parents are ready and willing to make lifestyle changes.
- It should be family based, with at least one of the parents involved.
- Lifestyle changes in diet, physical activity and screen time, i.e. television watching, computer use and playing video games, should be targeted equally.
- Weight maintenance is an acceptable goal of treatment, with height increasing and the BMI decreasing over time (NICE, 2013, 2014; SIGN, 2010).

Qualitative studies have identified barriers in the initial access to, and subsequent continuation of, child weight management programmes, particularly those linked to stigma and the difficulty in recognising the child's overweight status by parents and, even in some cases, by healthcare professionals (Parry *et al.*, 2008; Reid, 2009). It is important for dietitians to be aware of this challenge and of the need to undertake appropriate training of gate keepers in both recognising overweight in children and discussing unhealthy weight in a non-judgemental manner with parents or carers (Gillespie *et al.*, 2015; Stewart, 2008).

Rapport

Childhood weight management clinics have previously reported a high dropout rate (Denzer *et al.*, 2004; Stewart *et al.*, 2004), and dietitians need to carefully consider their manner and approach with the child and family. Successful treatment of obesity demands a sustained commitment and effort from the whole family, and the dietitian must endeavour to maintain a positive attitude and help motivate the child and family towards weight control. The role of the dietitian, whether seeing children and their families individually, in community groups or as part of a multidisciplinary team (MDT), is to educate them on the necessary lifestyle changes and to help facilitate behavioural change. It is important that this be done in a positive, enthusiastic, non-judgemental and sensitive manner. Indeed, the development of rapport between the dietitian, child and family has emerged as an important element for families in considering an intervention to be successful (Sahota *et al.*, 2010; Stewart *et al.*, 2008). The whole family should be encouraged to attend sessions and to make the necessary lifestyle changes. The dietitian needs to work with the parents/carers to ensure that they are engaged.

Where group sessions are used, it is not uncommon to hold some separate sessions for the children and parents. Indeed, most parents appreciate the opportunity to discuss problems they have encountered with other parents, and with the dietitian without the child present. Dietitians working with individual children and their families should also consider seeing the parents separately from the child, as this can lead to important information being revealed that parents would not wish to discuss in front of the child (Stewart *et al.*, 2005).

Consideration needs to be given to the most appropriate model of seeing and interacting with different age groups. Although not based on evidence, there are suggestions that, for preschool and lower primary school–aged children, the intervention should be targeted directly at the parent or carer; for upper primary–aged children, jointly at the child and parent or carer; and, for teenagers, directly at the adolescent, with the parent in a supporting role.

Behavioural modification

Both NICE (2013, 2014) and SIGN (2010) guidelines suggest that the use of behavioural change tools in the management of childhood obesity is essential (NICE, 2013, 2014; SIGN, 2010). Most of these techniques are employed within lifestyle change programmes to assist clients in raising their awareness of lifestyle, focusing on the aspects of their lifestyles that require change, and developing strategies to implement and monitor those changes. In childhood obesity, using a package of tools is more effective than any one particular tool (Sahota *et al.*, 2010). Table 7.13.5 summarises the tools that a dietitian would be expected to deploy, along with supporting parents to role model and to give concrete praise to their children. Tools for problem solving, goal setting, modelling and self-monitoring should all be used to help increase self-efficacy and positive reinforcement for change (Elder *et al.*, 1999; Newman *et al.*, 2004). Behavioural change is a process, and the dietitian's role is to facilitate change by helping the child and parent or carer make small steps using SMART (specific, measurable, achievable, realistic, timed) goals (Rollnick *et al.*, 1999).

Diet

The main drive of dietary change is to reduce the total energy intake in the diet. Calorie counting is not normally used, and dietitians need to ensure that they can convey the necessary information about dietary energy reduction effectively to the child and family. Gow *et al.* (2014) showed that no one type of dietary manipulation was more effective than another in childhood obesity. Children and their families should be encouraged to reduce the total amount of energy consumed by decreasing foods high in sugar and fat, and replacing them with lower-energy foods such as fruit and vegetables. It is also important to ensure that portion sizes of all foods are appropriate for age; the most commonly used models are the UK Eatwell Guide (see Chapter 2.1, Dietary reference values and food-based dietary guidelines) and the traffic light scheme (Ho *et al.*, 2012).

It is important to ensure that normal growth occurs when dietary intake is restricted. Plotting weight and height on UK/WHO growth charts as well as tracking BMI are useful steps to ensure appropriate growth monitoring, as well as regular nutritional assessment

Table 7.13.5 Brief description of behavioural change techniques (source: Stewart *et al.*, 2008, table 2, p. 466. Reproduced with permission from Wiley-Blackwell Publishing)

Behavioural change techniques	Description
Goal setting	Goals for necessary changes in diet, physical activity levels and screen time are agreed between child, parent and dietitian. Goals should be SMART – specific/small, measurable, achievable, recorded and timed.
Contracting	The signing of a contract between the child, parent and dietitian establishes a commitment to achieving the goals in the allotted time period.
Rewards for reaching goals	The parent agrees to give a reward to the child for achieving the agreed lifestyle change goals. This is a positive reinforcement for the setting and attainment of goals. The reward should be small, inexpensive and non-food or screen time based. The parent should also be encouraged to use praise.
Self-monitoring	Recording targeted lifestyles, i.e. diet, physical activity and screen time. This enhances motivation by increasing self-awareness of lifestyle behaviours, and allows the child and parent to monitor progress towards set goals.
Environmental/ stimulus control	Encouraging changes in the environment to help: • Reduce the cues that encourage the behaviours requiring change, such as the parent not buying certain foods or the child not walking past a certain shop on the way home from school. • Promote new healthier behaviours or routines.
Problem solving	Helping the child and family to identify possible 'high-risk' situations that may make it difficult to stick to their goals (e.g. holidays, parties and wet weather), as well as identifying barriers to change and developing possible solutions to these barriers. This could be done as a paper exercise, or as simulation and role play.
Preventing relapse	Near the end of the programme, it is important to discuss and offer strategies to help avoid relapse into old behaviours. These include planning ahead for difficult situations, and continuing with or returning to goal setting and self-monitoring.

and comparison with age- and sex-appropriate nutrient requirements. Adequate, but not excessive, quantities of protein, vitamins and minerals for age need to be consumed. Occasionally, a child who dislikes certain foods and does not consume a nutritionally adequate diet may need a supplement of vitamins or minerals (particularly iron and calcium). Written information, including a list of unrestricted foods and foods to be controlled, should be given to the parents and child. Many parents find food labelling confusing, and appreciate advice and help with understanding what to look for in food packets, and how to read the labels on them.

The problem with eating outside of the home and beyond the parents' influence should be explored. Suggesting, particularly to indulgent grandparents, that money previously spent on sweets, chocolate, etc., may be used for other items of the child's choice (e.g. games, books and clothing) is sometimes useful.

Physical activity

Children should be encouraged to increase their overall activity levels to 60 minutes of moderate–vigorous activity each day (NICE, 2014; SIGN, 2010). For preschool children who are able to walk, the recommendation is 3 hours of activity during the day (DH, 2011). Many overweight and obese children dislike team sports and physical education at school, and it is important to help such children and families find local activities that they may enjoy and are not embarrassed to take part in. Research has shown that increasing lifestyle activities, such as walking and taking the stairs rather than lift, can be particularly effective in controlling weight on a long-term basis (Epstein *et al.*, 1985). Working together with local community groups and leisure partners can be helpful in supporting children and their families to increase their levels of activity and make it enjoyable.

Screen time

Current recommendations are that the amount of time children spend watching television, playing video games and using computers should be no more than 2 hours/day, or an average of 14 hours/week (Epstein *et al.*, 2000; Gortmaker *et al.*, 1996; SIGN, 2010). For children aged under 2 years, a number of countries have recommended no screen time (Okely & Janssen, 2015). Some children and parents do find this particularly difficult, and the dietitian needs to help with setting SMART goals to reduce screen time gradually.

Outcomes

Weight maintenance in combination with increasing height growth is an acceptable goal of treatment, as this will lead to BMI decreasing over time. For older adolescents, particularly those in the very severe BMI range, weight loss may be required, and a weight loss of 0.5–1 kg/month could be advised (SIGN, 2010), dependent on age and stage of growth (NICE, 2014). There is emerging evidence to suggest that a range of decrease in BMI standard deviation scores of between –0.25 (Ford *et al.*, 2010) and –0.5 (Reinehr & Andler, 2004) may lead to improvements in insulin resistance, dyslipidaemia and cardiovascular risk factors.

Radical therapies

In general, slimming foods, drinks as a replacement for meals, and extremely restrictive diets that exclude food groups are not considered appropriate for this age group. Both NICE (2014) and SIGN (2010) recommend that anti-obesity drug therapy could be considered for obese adolescents who are attending specialist weight management clinics. Currently, orlistat is the only anti-obesity drug available for use in the UK. Adolescents should only be started on drug treatment if they have physical and/or psychological comorbidities and are regularly reviewed by a specialist paediatric MDT throughout the period of use, with careful monitoring for side effects (NICE, 2014).

Although bariatric surgery in children and adolescents is uncommon in the UK, it could be considered for weight loss in post-pubertal adolescents with very severe obesity and comorbidities; importantly, surgery should only be undertaken in a centre of excellence in adult bariatric surgery (NICE, 2014; SIGN, 2010). Since long-term side effects of bariatric surgery in adolescents are unknown, it is highly desirable that follow-up should be for life.

Prevention

It has been recognised that prevention strategies that target all children, including those who fall into the healthy weight range, must be considered. There are strong arguments towards prevention as a useful approach, as it is considered to be cheaper to prevent rather that treat obesity (Barlow & Expert Committee, 2007). There is evidence to suggest that children involved in prevention interventions can change their behaviour, although the effectiveness of such interventions is still poorly understood (Summerbell *et al.*, 2009). Dietitians, particularly those working in public health, have a key role to play in prevention strategies, including the planning, development, delivery and evaluation of interventions that take place in a range of settings and at all ages, from pre-birth through to adolescence. Prevention programmes that take place in schools and also target parents would appear to be an effective route (Gortmaker *et al.*, 1999).

Government policies, such as England's Healthy Weight, Healthy Lives (DH, 2008) or Scotland's Preventing Overweight and Obesity – A Route Map Towards Healthy Weight (The Scottish Government, 2010), drive most health promotion activity related to childhood obesity prevention. Initiatives tend to be educational or health promoting in nature, and encourage healthy weight through promotion of healthier food choices and/or increased physical activity. Several countries now have examples of such programmes, including national guidance on the nutritional content of school meals, school walking buses and family-based community physical activity programmes.

Social marketing is an emerging approach to obesity prevention. Governments, businesses, health and educational organisations, and others come together in a society-wide movement with the aim of empowering whole communities, families and individuals to make positive behavioural changes linked to healthy lifestyles. French *et al.* (2010) describe social marketing as the systematic application of marketing, alongside other concepts and techniques, to achieve specific behavioural goals for a social good. Current examples of UK social marketing campaigns relevant to childhood obesity include Change4Life in England and Wales; Take life on, one step at a time in Scotland; and Get a life, get active in Northern Ireland (see Chapter 4.2, Public health nutrition).

Schools

School-based interventions tend to focus either on physical activity or diet, or a combination of the two, with the latter thought to be most useful (Brown & Summerbell, 2009). More recently, school-based obesity prevention programmes found physical activity and/or diet to be mildly effective in reducing BMI in children (Sobel-Goldberg *et al.*, 2013). Of particular interest is the fact that the studies in this review were of longer duration, combining nutrition and physical activity elements together with changes in attitudes, behavioural monitoring, modification of environment and parental support.

In the last 5 years, there has been increasing focus on intervention and prevention in early years, and thus settings such as nurseries and kindergartens are seen as places where energy-balance-related behaviours can be influenced. Early results from one such large-scale, pan-European study called 'ToyBox-study' are promising (Manios, 2012; Manios *et al.*, 2014). Small reductions in overweight and obesity prevalence overall, significant improvements in both dietary and physical activity behaviour, greater consumption of water, reduced consumption of confectionery and greater numbers of children achieving at least 10,000 steps per day were observed (The World Obesity Federation, 2014).

Summerbell *et al.* (2012) have produced a range of recommendations for preschool prevention programmes that may help policymakers by outlining best-practice approaches and easy-to-understand messages for this age group for healthy eating, physical activity and sedentary behaviours.

Internet resources

PHE Data and analysis tools, https://www.gov.uk/guidance/phe-data-and-analysis-tools#obesity-diet-and-physical-activity

World Obesity Federation. (2014) Obesity prevention in children in pre-school years: Policies and evidence. Available at http://www.toybox-study.eu/?q=en/system/files/Obesity_Prevention_in_Preschool_Children_0.pdf

References

Barlow SE, Expert Committee. (2007) Expert Committee recommendations regarding the prevention, assessment and treatment of child and adolescent overweight and obesity: summary report. *Pediatrics*. 120: S164–S192.

Brown T, Summerbell C. (2009) Systematic review of school-based interventions that focus on changing dietary intake and physical activity levels to prevent childhood obesity. *Obes. Rev.* 10: 110–141.

Chinn S, Rona RJ. (2001) Prevalence and trends in overweight and obesity in three cross sectional studies of British children, 1974–1994. *BMJ*. 322: 24–26.

Denzer C, Reithofer E, Wabitsch M, *et al.* (2004) The outcome of childhood obesity management depends highly upon patient compliance. *Eur. J. Pediatr.* 163: 99–104.

DH. (2008) *Healthy Weight, Healthy Lives: A Cross-Government Strategy for England*. Available at http://webarchive.nationalarchives.gov.uk/20100407220245/http:/www.dh.gov.uk/prod_consum_dh/groups/dh_digitalassets/documents/digitalasset/dh_084024.pdf. Accessed 13 February 2017.

DH. (2011) *UK Physical Activity Guidelines*. Available at www.gov.uk/government/publications/uk-physical-activity-guidelines. Accessed 12 November 2016.

Drake AJ, Smith A, Betts PR, *et al.* (2002) Type 2 diabetes in obese white children. *Arch. Dis. Child.* 86(3): 207–208.

Edwards C, Nicholls D, Croker H, *et al.* (2006) Family-based behavioural treatment of obesity: acceptability and effectiveness in the UK. *Euro. J. Clin. Nutr.* 60: 587–592.

Elder JP, Ayala GX, Harris S. (1999) Theories and intervention approaches to health-behavior change in primary care. *Am. J. Prev. Med.* 17(4): 275–284.

Epstein LH, Wing RR, Valoski AM. (1985) Childhood obesity. *Pediatr. Clin. North Am.* 32(2): 363–379.

Epstein LH, Paluch RA, Gordy CC, *et al.* (2000) Decreasing sedentary behaviors in treating pediatric obesity. *Arch. Pediatr. Adolesc. Med.* 154: 220–226.

Ford AL, Hunt LP, Cooper A, *et al.* (2010) What reduction in BMI SDS is required in obese adolescents to improve body composition and cardiometabolic health? *Arch. Dis. Child.* 95: 256–261.

French F, Blair-Stevens C, McVey D, *et al.* (2010) *Social Marketing and Public Health Theory and Practice*. Oxford: Oxford University Press.

Gillespie J, Midmore C, Hoeflich J, *et al.* (2015) Parents as the start of the solution – a social marketing approach to understanding triggers and barriers to entering a childhood weight management service. *J. Hum. Nutr. Diet.* 28(1): 83–92.

Gortmaker SL, Peterson K, Wiecha J, *et al.* (1999) Reducing obesity via a school based interdisciplinary intervention among youth: Planet Health. *Arch. Pediatr. Adolesc. Med.* 151: 409–418.

Gortmaker SL, Must A, Sobol AM, *et al.* (1996) Television viewing as a cause of increasing obesity among children in the United States, 1986–1990. *Arch. Pediatr. Adolesc. Med.* 150(4): 356–362.

Gow ML, Ho M, Burrows T, *et al.* (2014) Impact of dietary macronutrient distribution on BMI and cardiometabolic outcomes in overweight and obese children and adolescents: a systematic review. *Nutr. Rev.* 72(7): 453–470.

Han JC, Lawlor DA, Kimm SYS. (2010) Childhood obesity. *Lancet*. 375: 1737–1748.

House of Commons Health Committee. (2004) *Obesity: Third Report of Session 2003–04, Volume 1*. London: TSO.

Ho M, Garnett SP, Baur L, *et al.* (2012) Effectiveness of lifestyle interventions in child obesity: systematic review with meta-analysis. *Pediatrics*. 130(6): e1647–e1671.

Lobstein T, Baur L, Uauy R; IASO International Obesity Task Force. (2004) Obesity in children and young people: a crisis in public health. *Obes. Rev.* 5(1): 4–104.

Manios Y. (2012) The 'ToyBox-study' obesity prevention programme in early childhood: an introduction. *Obes. Rev.* 13(1): 1–2.

Manios Y, Androutsos O, Katsarou C, *et al.* (2014) Designing and implementing a kindergarten-based, family-involved intervention to prevent obesity in early childhood: the ToyBox-study. *Obes. Rev.* 15(3): 5–13.

Mulvihill C, Quigley R. (2003) *The Management of Obesity and Overweight: An Analysis of Reviews of Diet, Physical Activity and Behavioural Approaches. Evidence Briefing*. NHS Health Development Agency.

NICE. (2013) *Weight management: lifestyle services for overweight or obese children and young people. Public health guideline [PH47].*

NICE. (2014) *Obesity: identification, assessment and management. Clinical guideline [CG189].*

Newman S, Steed L, Mulligan K. (2004) Self-management interventions for chronic illness. *Lancet*. 364: 1523–1537.

Okely AD, Janssen X. (2015) Early physical activity and sedentary behaviours. In: Stewart L, Thompson J (eds) *Early Years Nutrition and Healthy Weight*. Chichester: Wiley Blackwell.

Parry L, Netuveli G, Parry J, *et al.* (2008) A systematic review of parental perception of overweight status in children. *J. Ambul. Care Manage.* 31(3): 253–268.

Reid M. (2009) *Debrief of a study to identify and explore parental, young people's and health professionals' attitudes, awareness and knowledge of child healthy weight. 2008/2009 RE036*. Edinburgh: NHS Health Scotland.

Reilly JJ, Dorosty AR. (1999) Epidemic of obesity in UK children. *Lancet*. 354: 1874–1875.

Reilly JJ, Kelly J, Wilson DC. (2010) Accuracy of simple clinical and epidemiological definitions of childhood obesity: systematic review and evidence appraisal. *Obes. Rev.* 11(9): 645–655.

Reilly JJ, Methven E, McDowell ZC, *et al.* (2003) Health consequences of obesity. *Arch. Dis. Child.* 88: 748–752.

Reinehr T, Andler W. (2004) Changes in the atherogenic risk factor profile according to degree of weight loss. *Arch. Dis. Child.* 89: 419–422.

Rollnick S, Mason P, Butler C. (1999) *Health Behavior Change. A Guide for Practitioners*. Edinburgh: Churchill Livingstone.

Royal College of Paediatrics and Child Health. (2017) *Growth Charts*. Available at www.rcpch.ac.uk/improving-child-health/public-health/uk-who-growth-charts/uk-who-growth-charts-0-18-years. Accessed 29 October 2016.

Sacher PM, Kalotourou M, Chadwick P, *et al.* (2010) Randomised controlled trial of the MEND program: a family community intervention for childhood obesity. *Obesity. (Silver Spring)*. 18(2): S62–68.

Sahota P, Wordley J, Woodward J. (2010) *Health Behaviour Change Models and Approaches for Families and Young People to Support HEAT 3: Child Healthy Weight Programmes*. Edinburgh: NHS Health Scotland.

Scottish Intercollegiate Guideline Network (SIGN). (2010) *Management of Obesity: A National Clinical Guideline. 115*. Edinburgh: SIGN.

Sinha R, Fisch G, Teague B, *et al.* (2002) Prevalence of impaired glucose tolerance among children and adolescents with marked obesity. *N. Eng. J. Med.* 346(11): 802–810.

Sobol-Goldberg S, Rabinowitz J, Gross R. (2013) School-based obesity prevention programs: A meta-analysis of randomized controlled trials. *Obesity* 21(12):2422–2428.

Stewart L. (2008) Recognizing childhood obesity: the role of the school nurse. *Br. J. School Nurs.* 3(7): 323–326.

Stewart L, Chapple J, Hughes AR, *et al.* (2008) The use of behavioural change techniques in the treatment of paediatric obesity: qualitative evaluation of parental perspectives on treatment. *J. Hum. Nutr. Diet.* 21(5): 464–473.

Stewart L, Deane M, Wilson DC. (2004) Failure of routine management of obese children: an audit of dietetic intervention. *Arch. Dis. Child.* 89(1): A13–16.

Stewart L, Houghton J, Hughes AR, *et al.* (2005) Dietetic management of pediatric overweight: development of a practical and evidence-based behavioral approach. *J. Am. Diet. Assoc.* 105: 1810–1815.

Summerbell CD, Moore HJ, Vögele C, *et al.* (2012) Evidence-based recommendations for the development of obesity prevention programs targeted at preschool children. *Obes. Rev.* 13(1): 129–132.

Summerbell CD, Waters E, Edmunds L, *et al.* (2009) Interventions for preventing obesity in children. *Cochrane Database Syst. Rev.* 3: CD001871.

The Scottish Government. (2010) *Preventing Overweight and Obesity in Scotland: A Route Map Towards Healthy Weight*. Edinburgh: The Scottish Government.

Whitaker KL, Jarvis MJ, Beeken RJ, *et al.* (2010) Comparing maternal and paternal intergenerational transmission of obesity risk in a large population-based sample. *Am. J. Clin. Nutr.* 91: 1560–1567.

SECTION 7

7.14 Cardiovascular disease

7.14.1 General aspects of cardiovascular disease

Katherine Paterson

Key points

- Cardiovascular disease (CVD) includes coronary heart disease, stroke and peripheral vascular disease.
- A cardioprotective diet is the first line of dietary support for those with, or at risk of, CVD.
- Additional dietary interventions may be needed to treat risk factors such as dyslipidaemia, obesity and diabetes.

Aetiology

Cardiovascular disease (CVD) includes coronary heart disease, stroke and peripheral vascular disease (PVD). CVD is caused by atherosclerosis, developing slowly over many years, and/or thrombosis (blood clots), developing suddenly and causing an acute episode, such as a myocardial infarction or stroke. Chronic kidney disease and vascular dementia also come under the umbrella term of CVD. The incidence of CVD is related to modifiable risk factors, such as dyslipidaemia and hypertension, which in turn can be linked to lifestyle factors, e.g. high saturated fat intake, smoking, lack of physical activity, diabetes mellitus and obesity. Therefore, improving lifestyle factors can lead to a reduction in cardiovascular events (ESC, 2016). The aetiology of atherosclerosis and thrombosis are discussed further in Chapter 7.14.2 (Coronary heart disease).

Prevalence and costs

Despite the improvements in outcomes for CVD over the last 20 years, CVD remains a major cause of morbidity and mortality in the UK. More patients survive their first CVD event, but remain at high further CVD risk. As levels of certain risk factors such as obesity and diabetes are increasing, more focus on prevention is required (DH, 2013). CVD is the second-most frequent cause of death in the UK, and a major cause of premature death (BHF, 2015). In 2014, approximately 150,000 people in the UK died of CVD, 27% of all deaths. It accounted for 25% and 17% of premature mortality in men and women aged under 75 years, respectively. Age-standardised death rates are highest in Scotland and the North of England, and lowest in the South of England. It is thought that this may be partly attributable to the socioeconomic differences in the populations in these areas. South Asian people living in the UK, who include immigrants from India, Pakistan, Bangladesh and Sri Lanka, have a 50% greater risk of premature death from CHD and stroke (BHF, 2015). Data from England and Wales show that African-Caribbean people have a lower-than-average risk of CHD, but a threefold higher risk of stroke. Death rates in the UK continue to remain relatively high in comparison with some other Western European Countries, despite death rates from CVD falling in the UK at one of the fastest rates in Europe (BHF, 2015). The National Service Framework launched in 2000 aimed to reduce CVD by 40% by 2010; this target was met 5 years early (DH, 2000). This is in line with the overall reduction in risk since the 1970s owing to the introduction of statins (for reducing blood cholesterol levels), improved screening, prevention and post-cardiac-event treatments, and increases in smoking cessation (BHF, 2015).

Coronary heart disease (CHD) is a major cause of mortality in patients presenting with stroke, diabetes and renal disease. Patients receiving renal replacement therapy are 16–19 times more likely to develop CHD than matched controls, with the rate for people with diabetic nephropathy being even greater (Holt & Goldsmith,

Manual of Dietetic Practice, Sixth Edition. Edited by Joan Gandy.

Companion website: www.manualofdieteticpractice.com

2010; Wheeler, 1997). New onset of type 2 diabetes *per se* is not considered a CHD risk–equivalent condition (JBS3, 2014). Longer duration of diabetes (Wannamethee *et al.*, 2011) and/or proteinuria (Preiss *et al.*, 2011), however, increase CVD risk considerably.

In addition, CVD is an economic burden for the UK. In 2012–2013, the cost of treating heart disease and stroke was estimated to be £6.8 billion (Bhatnagar *et al.*, 2015).

Cardiovascular risk

The third Joint British Societies' (JBS3) consensus recommendations (2014) for CVD prevention advocate using the JBS3 risk calculator to estimate both absolute risk of CVD over 10 years and lifetime risk (JBS3, 2014). This tool, which includes the concept of HEART AGE, in addition to indicating CVD risk in the short term, can be used to estimate risk in younger individuals whose lifetime risk is high, although 10-year risk is relatively low. Individuals with existing CVD are already at high risk of developing further events, and should be treated as such. The required information includes gender, age, systolic blood pressure, ethnicity, total cholesterol/total cholesterol to high-density lipoprotein (HDL) ratio, family history, height, weight, diabetes status, Townsend deprivation index and smoking behaviour.

JBS3 (2014) recommends:

- Intensive risk factor modification with diet, lifestyle intervention and pharmacological therapy in patients with existing CVD, without the need for estimation of CVD risk.
- Intensive risk factor modification with diet, lifestyle intervention and pharmacological therapy in individuals at particularly high risk of developing CVD, i.e. diabetics patients, those aged >40 years, patients with chronic kidney disease (CKD) stages 3–5, or those with familial hypercholesterolemia (FH) – without the need for estimation of CVD risk.
- Diet, lifestyle intervention and pharmacological therapy in people at high short-term risk. Thresholds for treatment with statins based on 10-year CVD risk (10-year CVD risk of >10% should be considered as high risk) will be informed by NICE guidelines (NICE, 2014a).
- Diet, lifestyle interventions and, for some people, pharmacological therapy, in those with increased modifiable lifetime risk as informed by JBS3 calculator metrics.

Alternative risk equations in practice include the following:

- *ASSIGN* – developed using a Scottish cohort (Woodward *et al.*, 2007).
- *QRISK 2* – recommended by Hippisley-Cox *et al.*, 2008 and NICE, 2014a.
- *SCORE* – high-risk Systemic Coronary Risk Estimation risk equation and relative risk chart (Conroy *et al.*, 2003), recommended by the European Society of Cardiology (ESC, 2016).

It should be remembered that equations can only provide an estimate of risk, and clinical judgement should always be applied to improve the accuracy of the assessment.

Both JBS3 (2014) and NICE (2014a) recommend the use non-HDL cholesterol as the treatment target for lipid-lowering therapy in preference to LDL cholesterol. Non-HDL cholesterol levels can be calculated from non-fasting blood samples of total cholesterol minus HDL cholesterol.

Prevention

It has been estimated that more than half of deaths and disability from heart disease and stroke could be prevented by modifications to lifestyle, such as diet, activity and smoking (Iqbal *et al.*, 2008). All current guidelines agree that, when treating people with elevated risk of CVD, the lifestyle factor priorities are as follows(in no particular order of priority):

- Smoking cessation.
- Increased physical activity.
- Management of blood pressure.
- Management of lipids.
- Management of diabetes.
- Healthy food choices.
- Weight management and limiting central obesity.

Further details for CHD can be found in Chapter 7.14.2 (Coronary heart disease); for dyslipidaemia in Chapter 7.14.3 (Dyslipidaemia); for hypertension in Chapter 7.14.4 (Hypertension); for stroke in Chapter 7.14.5 (Stroke); for diabetes in Chapter 7.12 (Diabetes mellitus); for management of obesity and overweight in adults in Chapter 7.13.2 (The management of obesity and overweight in adults); and for renal disease in Chapter 7.5.1 (Chronic kidney disease and acute kidney injury).

Despite a reduction in morbidity and mortality from CVD in the UK, the latest European-wide EUROASPIRE IV survey showed that the majority of surveyed patients with CHD were still not achieving the Joint European Societies' standards for secondary prevention lifestyle, blood pressure and lipid targets, despite an increase in medications and screening (Kotseva *et al.*, 2016).

The cardiovascular outcomes strategy (DH, 2013) recommends continuation of the NHS health checks introduced in 2009 to identify individuals at risk of developing heart disease, stroke, vascular dementia (for those aged 65 years and over), kidney disease or diabetes, with the focus on preventing these diseases (NHS, 2009). Health checks are offered to those aged 40–85 years who have not been diagnosed with hypertension, atrial fibrillation, transient ischaemic attacks, hypercholesterolaemia, heart failure, CVD, peripheral arterial disease or dementia. Eligible people are invited to attend every 5 years.

In an evaluation of the first 4 years of the health checks, Robson *et al.* (2016) concluded that a considerable number of comorbidities had been identified, and that the prescription of statin in 20% of those at high

10-year CVD risk would most certainly have contributed to a reduction in CVD events in the population. The national UK CVD prevention priorities are (DH, 2013; NHS, 2014) as follows:

- Diabetes prevention programme and obesity strategy.
- Early detection, which includes NHS Health Checks.
- Blood pressure awareness and atrial fibrillation.
- Integration of (CVD) services (new models of care).
- Better management in, and support for, primary care.
- Inherited cardiac conditions.
- Improved survival from out-of-hospital cardiac arrest.
- Seven-day working.
- Addressing Inequalities.
- Information provision.
- Research and innovation.

The cardioprotective diet

The cardioprotective diet is the first line of dietary advice in protection against CVD. It can be used in primary or secondary prevention, and in conjunction with specific dietary advice given on individually relevant risk factors, including diabetes, renal disease, dyslipidaemia, hypertension, overweight and obesity. NICE (2010) has produced guidance on the prevention of CVD to improve risk factors at the population level. These guidelines target food and drink providers, marketing, media, the family support sector, national non-governmental organisations (e.g. charities), and farming associations. The recommended cardioprotective diet for people with, or at high risk of, CVD includes (NICE, 2014a) the following:

- Dietary fat
  - Total fat intake ≤30% of total energy intake.
  - Saturated fats ≤7% of total energy intake.
  - Dietary cholesterol <300 mg/day.
  - Replace saturates with monounsaturates (MUFA) and polyunsaturates (PUFA).
- Overall advice
  - Reduce saturates.
  - Increase MUFA with olive oil, rapeseed oil or spreads based on these oils, and use them in food preparation.
  - Choose wholegrain varieties of starchy food.
  - Reduce intake of sugar and food products containing refined sugars, including fructose.
  - Eat at least five portions of fruit and vegetables per day.
  - Eat at least two portions of fish per week, including a portion of oily fish.
  - Eat at least four to five portions of unsalted nuts, seeds and legumes per week.
  - Do not drink >14 units of alcohol a week, it is best to spread this out over 3 or more days. Avoid binge drinking.

Unlike JBS3 (2014) and ESC (2016), NICE (2014a) recommends restricting dietary cholesterol. In addition, debate remains as to whether saturates should be replaced with PUFA or MUFA (Hooper *et al.*, 2015). While JBS3 (2014) and ESC (2016) recommend replacing saturates with PUFA, NICE (2014a) recommends either PUFA or MUFA, while emphasising the use of olive oil/rapeseed oil or spreads to replace the MUFA lost when reducing fat from animal sources.

Effectiveness

The cardioprotective diet is based on the Mediterranean diet. The value of eating a Mediterranean-style diet came into focus in the late 1950s when men living in Crete, parts of Greece and southern Italy were shown to have the least likelihood of developing CHD (Willett *et al.*, 1995). The premature death rate from heart attack for Greek men was 90% lower than that of American men, with Greek men enjoying the longest life expectancy in the world. However, this is no longer true today, as the traditional Greek diet has become increasingly Westernised. Therefore, focus has been on the benefits of the traditional Mediterranean diet prior to the 1960s. Several elements of this diet have been proposed as being especially protective, and there is now some experimental evidence from randomised controlled trials to support its protective role in high-risk populations.

Influence on cardiovascular disease

The cardioprotective diet exerts its effects on CVD by altering a wide range of risk factors in a positive way. These may include effects on the following:

- Blood pressure, lipid oxidation and inflammation (reducing injury to coronary arteries).
- Lipid profile, homocysteine levels and insulin resistance (reducing fibrous plaque formation).
- Platelet aggregation, clotting factors and arrhythmias (reducing the occurrence of thrombosis, which leads to heart attack and stroke).

The effects of the diet on the cardiovascular system and its benefits alongside statins are summarised in Chapter 7.14.2 (Coronary heart disease). Chapter 7.14.3 (Dyslipidaemia) discusses the effects of diet on blood lipids.

The Mediterranean diet is rich in plant foods (fruit, vegetables, cereals, beans, nuts and seeds) and fish; it advocates olive oil as the principal source of dietary lipids, a low consumption of red meat, and a low–moderate consumption of dairy products and wine (usually with meals). The Primary Prevention of Cardiovascular Disease with a Mediterranean Diet (PREDIMED) study showed that the risk of CVD was reduced in individuals at high risk of developing CVD when using extra virgin olive oil or 30 g mixed nuts per day (Estruch *et al.*, 2013). In addition, meta-analyses have shown a protective effect of the Mediterranean diet on cardiovascular morbidity, mortality and total mortality (Martinez-Gonzalez *et al.*, 2014; Grosso *et al.*, 2015; Rees *et al.*, 2013). Tong *et al.* (2016) showed an inverse association between greater Mediterranean dietary adherence versus CVD incidence and mortality in a prospective cohort study that assessed adherence to the Mediterranean diet in a UK cohort.

Table 7.14.1 Main sources of saturated, trans and unsaturated fats in the diet

Saturated fat	Trans fats	Unsaturated fats	
		PUFA	MUFA
Butter, lard, ghee, dripping	Baked products	Oils – sunflower, soya, linseed, sesame seed, fish	Olive oil, rapeseed oil, peanut oil (ground nut)
Fatty meats – beef, lamb, corned beef, sausages, beef burgers, streaky bacon	Cakes, biscuits, pastries		
	Convenience foods, e.g. takeaways, ready meals	Margarines	Almonds, walnuts, peanuts, avocados
Dairy products – full-fat milk, cream, full-fat yoghurt, cheese		Soya beans	
Pies, cakes, biscuits, chocolate and pastry products			
Coconut			

Fats

The main sources of saturated, unsaturated and trans fats in the diet are shown in Table 7.14.1.

Saturated fats

A systematic review of studies that replaced saturated fatty acids (SFAs) with unsaturated fats (mainly PUFA) for at least 2 years concluded that this reduced the risk of cardiovascular events (Hooper *et al.*, 2015). Replacing SFAs with carbohydrate foods did not confer any clear health effects. Practical tips for reducing saturated fat and replacing them with unsaturated fats include the following:

- Remove fat from meats and avoid processed meats.
- Remove skin from poultry.
- Avoid deep-fried snacks and dishes.
- Replace butter, ghee and lard with a vegetable oil such as olive or rapeseed oil; replace full-fat dairy products with low-fat alternatives or soya products.
- Replace high-fat snacks (such as crisps, chocolates and biscuits) with fruit and nuts.
- Read food labels; aim for <1.5 g of saturates/100 g.

Trans fatty acids

There is a lack of controlled trials concerning trans fatty acids (TFAs) and CVD (Hooper *et al.*, 2015). NICE (2014a) makes no recommendation for TFA intake; however, JBS3 recommends reducing foods that are high in TFAs, such as processed meats or commercially produced foods. ESC (2016) recommends that TFAs contribute <1% of dietary energy. TFAs are produced in the hydrogenation of vegetable oils that are used in the production of margarine and shortening, by subjecting PUFAs to high temperatures (220°C). TFAs raise low-density lipoprotein (LDL) cholesterol while lowering HDL (Ascherio & Willett, 1997). If possible, SFAs and TFAs should be replaced with unsaturated fatty acids (MUFAs and PUFAs). In the UK, TFA intake has reduced. However, there may be segments of the population eating more than the ideal amount. These include individuals consuming fast food very often, and some low-income groups (Mouratidou *et al.*, 2014).

Omega-3 fatty acids

Omega-3 fatty acids are the long-chain PUFAs, eicosapentaenoic acid (EPA) and docosahexaenoic acid (DHA). They do not have a cholesterol-lowering effect; however, they are thought to be protective by improving endothelial function, and have anti-inflammatory and antithrombotic effects. NICE (2014a) recommends that n-3 fatty acid supplements not be offered for the prevention of CVD in those being treated for primary prevention, secondary prevention, CKD, type 1 diabetes, and type 2 diabetes. Furthermore, it recommends that people be told that there is no evidence that these compounds help in preventing CVD. However, fish intake is recommended, and it is advisable to include at least two portions per week, including one portion of oily fish (ESC, 2016; NICE, 2014a). A portion is defined as 140 g, which has been calculated to provide approximately 0.45 g/day of long-chain n-3 PUFAs. Based on epidemiological evidence, JBS3 encourages oily fish consumption over white fish.

Vegetarian sources of the essential precursor fatty acid alpha-linolenic acid (ALA) include nuts, seeds, dark green vegetables, rapeseed oil, wholegrain cereals and soya products; however, conversion from ALA to the active EPA and DHA by humans appears poor, especially in men (2–10%). Despite this, NICE (2014a) recommends inclusion of nuts and seeds as part of the cardioprotective diet.

Safety of oily fish and fish oils

Concern has been expressed over the relatively high levels of dioxins and polychlorinated biphenyls (PCBs) present in fish and fish oils (MAFF, 1999). SACN and COT issued a joint report in 2004 addressing these issues, and suggesting healthy and maximal fish intakes for various population groups (SACN/COT, 2004), as shown in Table 7.14.2.

Dietary cholesterol

NICE (2014a) recommends <300 mg dietary cholesterol per day, although other guidelines do not make specific recommendations. (ESC, 2016; JBS3, 2014) However, the ESC/EAS guidelines recommend this restriction for those with high levels of cholesterol, such as those with inherited (FH – see Chapter 7.14.3, Dyslipidaemia) high cholesterol (ESC/EAS, 2016). It is known that dietary cholesterol can increase blood cholesterol levels; however, it is thought that, in the UK, dietary cholesterol is unlikely to have any significant impact on blood cholesterol levels (Leeds & Gray, 2001). Shell fish, eggs and

Table 7.14.2 Suggested population intakes of oily fish (SACN/COT, 2004)

Population group	Suggested lower limit	Suggested higher limit
Women of reproductive age and girls	One portion of oily fish/week	Two portions of oily fish/week
Pregnant and lactating women	One portion of oily fish/week (but avoid marlin, swordfish, shark and tuna)	Two portions of oily fish/week (but avoid marlin, swordfish, shark and tuna)
Women past reproductive age, boys and men	One portion of oily fish/week	Four portions of oily fish/week

offal are rich in cholesterol but are not high in saturated fat, and so can be used as healthy alternatives to fatty meats in the diet.

Stanols and sterols

Stanols and sterols are known to lower LDL cholesterol by interfering with biliary and dietary cholesterol absorption from the gut. Sterols and stanols occur naturally in the diet; however, 1.5–3 g stanol/sterol esters/day (20–30 g of margarine/spread or one yoghurt drink) is seen as an optimal intake. They have been shown to lower cholesterol by at least 10% (Thompson & Grundy, 2005). They have been granted a health claims title by the European Food Safety Authority (2010), with no known long-term adverse effects (see Chapter 4.5, Food law and labelling, and Chapter 5.2, Functional foods). To obtain beneficial effects, supplemented foods should be used for at least 2–3 weeks. Currently, stanols and sterols are not recommended for primary or secondary prevention due to the lack of studies with clinical end points (NICE, 2014a).

Salt

Prevention guidelines recommend that the adult population should decrease their salt intake to ≤6 g/day (2.4 g of sodium/day); the equivalent of one level teaspoon (JBS3, 2014; NICE, 2014a; SACN, 2003). The current intake in the UK is estimated to be 8 g/day (PHE, 2016). Public health initiatives are currently aiming to reduce salt consumption to 3 g/day by 2025 (NICE, 2010). However, in a systematic review, Adler *et al.* (2014) concluded that there was insufficient evidence to confirm clinically useful effects of dietary advice and salt substitution on clinical CVD events in normotensives or hypertensives. The authors do not support dietary advice alone as a means to reducing salt intake, suggesting a parallel population strategy. Further randomised controlled trials are needed (Adler *et al.*, 2014; ESC, 2016). Adler and colleagues estimate that the benefits of salt restriction are '*consistent with the predicted small effects on clinical events attributable to the small blood pressure reduction achieved*'. Examples of some common sources of salt in the diet include the following:

- Ready meals.
- Tinned and packet soups.
- Breads and breakfast cereals.
- Dehydrated meals.
- Processed meats such as bacon and sausages.
- Cooking and pasta sauces.
- Cheese.
- Stock cubes.
- Savoury snacks.

Practical advice to lower salt intake includes the following:

- Discourage adding salt when cooking or at the table.
- Discourage consumption of food with high salt content.
- Encourage the use of alternatives such as herbs and spices.
- Look for food containing <0.3 g of salt/100 g.

Fruit and vegetables

At least five portions of fruit and vegetables a day (80 g portion of fresh fruit or vegetables; 30 g dried fruit or 150 mL fresh unsweetened fruit/vegetable juice) (ESC, 2016; JBS3, 2014; NICE, 2014a) are recommended. All fruit and vegetables should be encouraged including tinned, fresh, frozen or juiced. Fruit and vegetables contribute to soluble fibre and antioxidants, giving them a protective effect; they are also rich in folic acid. Fruit and vegetables have relatively low energy, and therefore aid weight management.

Nuts

Nuts are recommended as part of a cardioprotective diet (ESC, 2016; JBS3, 2014; NICE, 2014a), with almonds and walnuts having been studied the most in intervention trials. A reduction of about 30% CVD risk is associated with 30 g/day consumption of nuts (Luo *et al.*, 2014). Nut consumption is associated with lowering total cholesterol and LDL cholesterol. (Mukuddem-Peterson, 2005). A Mediterranean diet supplemented with nuts was associated with reduced stroke and cardiovascular morbidity/mortality in individuals at high risk of developing CVD in one randomised controlled trial (Estruch *et al.*, 2013).

Soluble fibre

The dietary reference value for the intake of dietary fibre in adults is 30 g/day (SACN, 2015). The high viscosity of soluble fibre reduces cholesterol levels by interfering with cholesterol absorption in the gut. Soluble fibre can be found in oats and other wholegrains, beans, pulses, fruit and vegetables, with a recommended intake of 15–20 g/day (Brown *et al.*, 1999). Wholegrain foods, which can include wholemeal breads, wholegrain breakfast cereals, wholegrain pasta and brown rice, should be encouraged, to prevent constipation and help with weight control. Observational evidence has suggested that high intakes of whole grains have a protective effect on CHD risk, reducing the risk of both CVD and diabetes by up to 30%. Large intervention trials with sufficient power would be required to determine a causal link. Diets with 7–13 g soluble fibre and 25–40 g fibre through increase in wholegrains, vegetables, legumes, fruit and nuts are thought to be well tolerated (ESC/EAS, 2016).

Carbohydrates

SACN (2015) recommends that the dietary reference value for total carbohydrate should remain at a population average of 50% dietary energy. They found no evidence from prospective cohort studies that the intake of refined grains or starch were associated with cardiovascular endpoints. There is no evidence from prospective cohort studies to suggest an association between glycaemic index and CVD or CHD. Glycaemic load is associated with a greater risk of CVD, but the evidence is limited due to the small number of studies. However, low-GI diets may be beneficial in those with diabetes or metabolic syndrome, and in those with high triglycerides (see Chapter 7.12, Diabetes mellitus).

Sugar-sweetened beverages

Excessive amounts of sugar-sweetened beverages has been associated with CVD risk, type 2 diabetes onset and obesity (Malik *et al.*, 2010). Reducing intake is associated with reduced obesity in adults and children (Malik *et al.*, 2013).

Folic acid and antioxidant vitamins

Elevated levels of homocysteine have been linked with CVD (Bazzano *et al.*, 2006); in particular, high levels are thought to be a predictor for CVD. Intakes of folic acid and B vitamins (especially B_{12} and B_6) have been shown to lower homocysteine levels, but there is no evidence that B vitamin supplements should be used alone or in combination to prevent cardiovascular events (Martí-Carvajal *et al.*, 2015). Vitamins A, C, E and beta carotene supplements have not been found to improve CVD morbidity or mortality (Myung *et al.*, 2013). Some may even increase mortality, such as vitamin E, beta carotene and higher doses of vitamin A.

Garlic

Although garlic may have an effect on reducing blood pressure in hypertensive people, there is a lack of evidence for it preventing CVD events (Stabler *et al.*, 2012).

Practical aspects

Practical dietary details are given in Table 7.14.3. A low-fat diet will allow weight loss (similar to the cardioprotective diet), but will not provide protective effects. The low-fat diet contains no fruit and vegetables, is lacking in fibre and n-3 fatty acids, and is higher in salt. Cardioprotective dietary advice should always be set in the context of healthy eating guidance, such as the Eatwell Guide (see Chapter 2.1, Dietary reference values and food-based dietary guidelines), to ensure the overall diet is balanced. Excessive focus on any one nutrient (such as saturated fat reduction) can risk compromising the intake of others (such as iron and calcium) if dietary advice is not comprehensive. Other dietary therapeutic objectives, e.g. maintenance of glycaemic control in the management of diabetes, may also be relevant. For frail or elderly people, who are at risk of being nutritionally compromised, especially if appetite and food intake are poor, fruit and vegetables can be encouraged, but dietary fat content and composition should only be altered if this can be achieved with no loss of enjoyment or reduction in dietary energy density (see Chapter 3.3, Older adults).

Table 7.14.3 Comparison of traditional high-fat, low-fat and cardioprotective diets

	High-fat diet	Low-fat/low-calorie diet	Cardioprotective diet
Meal plan	Refined cereal (such as cornflakes) with whole milk. Coffee with full-cream milk.	Refined cereal (cornflakes). Skimmed milk. Black coffee.	Porridge oats made with skimmed milk/soya milk and a chopped banana. Glass of fruit juice. Coffee.
	Two slices of white bread with butter, processed ham and mayonnaise, full-fat yoghurt and a packet of crisps.	Two slices of white bread, low-fat spread, processed ham and low-fat mayonnaise. Packet of 'lite' crisps and a low-fat yoghurt. Three salted rice cakes.	Two slices of wholemeal bread with olive-based spread, turkey and salad, apple and a low-fat yoghurt. Handful of almonds.
	Two chocolate-coated biscuits. Fried fish and chips with a sprinkling of salt. Fruit pie and ice cream.	Breaded cod and oven chips, peas, with a sprinkle of salt. Low-fat ice cream.	Salmon fillet with new potatoes (flavoured with mint), carrots and peas. Stewed fruit and low-fat yoghurt.
Energy (kcals)	2310	1434	1470
Total fat (g)	135	46.1	45.5
Saturated fat (g)	48	10.9	7.4

Specific considerations

Alcohol

The American Heart Association (AHA, 2015) cautions against initiating alcohol consumption in previous abstainers. Alcohol intake should be moderate, and the risks and benefits of alcohol consumption should be discussed with a physician. It stresses the dangers associated with alcohol consumption such as high blood pressure, obesity and alcoholism. The role of alcohol in the cardioprotective diet remains unclear because of the lack of intervention studies, but there is clear evidence of the hazards of excessive intakes. Low intakes of alcohol (1–2 units/day) are associated with reduced CVD morbidity as compared to no alcohol (Ronksley *et al.*, 2011). A randomised study using individualised participant data has questioned any CVD benefit associated with moderate drinking, suggesting that CVD morbidity was lowest in abstainers, and that even very low alcohol intakes were associated with increased blood pressure and BMI (Holmes *et al.*, 2014).

Gout

Some people at high cardiovascular risk will also have gout, and may need to avoid high intakes of purines (see Chapter 7.9.3, Gout). As oily fish is rich in purines, increasing consumption may be contraindicated.

Lifestyle

The cardioprotective diet should always be discussed in the context of a healthy lifestyle, and reference should be made to activity and exercise levels, smoking cessation and the continued use of prescribed medication. Dietetic participation in CVD prevention and rehabilitation programmes helps to ensure consistency in the delivery of health messages. It also allows dietitians to reinforce the lifestyle messages, and ensures that other healthcare professionals remain well informed on dietary issues. NICE (2014a) recommends the following for people with CVD, or at high risk, to include each week:

- 150 minutes of moderate-intensity aerobic activity, or 75 minutes of vigorous-intensity aerobic activity, or a mix of moderate and vigorous aerobic activity.
- Muscle-strengthening activities on 2 or more days a week that work all major muscle groups.
- For those unable to perform these activities, exercise at the individual's maximum safe capacity is recommended.

Acceptability

Patients are often apprehensive about the perceived restrictions of a cardioprotective diet, and may be visibly relieved when the positive changes are described and encouraged. The approach to the patient should be determined by the stages of change model (see Chapter 1.3, Changing health behaviour). Those who have never contemplated change will need a different approach from those who have already started to make changes, or have previously made changes but slipped back. While many people enjoy the cardioprotective diet, there are also some who find particular elements of it very difficult. Many people struggle to increase their fruit, vegetables and oily fish intakes, while reducing and/or modifying their fat intake. Practical advice should be offered to promote dietary change, and giving examples of advocated foods will likely improve adherence, e.g. providing examples of oily fish recipes. Dietary advice should always be tailored to an individual's likes and dislikes. To help people maintain their healthier habits, regular review is advisable. This may involve dietetic review in a central location or the community, including delegation to other community staff (who must be trained, updated and provided with appropriate support materials).

Motivation can be boosted by involving the whole family (Wood *et al.*, 2008). This reduces the sense of isolation, and the whole family group (who may also be at increased genetic or lifestyle risk of CHD) should reinforce the benefits of risk reduction (Cousins *et al.*, 1992). NICE (2014a) now recommends that, when giving dietary advice, healthcare professionals should consider individual circumstances, including comorbidities, drug therapy and other lifestyle changes, and that behaviour change principles should be used (NICE, 2007).

Evaluation

Weight and waist circumference

Patients should aim for a healthy weight (BMI 18.5–25 kg/m^2) and waist circumference (<102 cm in European men, <90 cm in Asian men, <88 cm in European women and <80 cm in Asian women). See the chapter on obesity (Chapter 7.13, Obesity) for information about the therapeutic benefits of 5–10% weight loss. NICE (2014b) recommends using BMI as a first-line measure of adiposity, and advises to use clinical judgment to determine whether waist circumference measurement is indicated in BMI of <35 kg/m^2 (see Appendix A3). Different thresholds for waist circumference and BMI have been proposed to ascertain CVD and diabetes risk in different populations (NICE, 2013).

Monitoring and outcomes

Appropriate factors to consider for monitoring and evaluating CVD are shown in Table 7.14.4. The National Obesity Observatory has reviewed several dietary assessment tools for monitoring healthy eating interventions (Roberts & Flaherty, 2010). In addition, it is important to remember that the benefits from dietary change depend on the extent to which other lifestyle changes have been achieved. Both aspects therefore need to be considered in conjunction in order to assess the effectiveness of risk reduction measures. Connolly *et al.* (2017) demonstrated the outcomes of an integrated, community-based, nurse-led CVD prevention programme based on the EUROACTION model (Wood *et al.*, 2008). They reported improvements in participants' Mediterranean diet score,

Table 7.14.4 Possible factors to consider for monitoring and evaluation purposes in cardiovascular disease

Domain	Factors
Diet	Portions of fish/seafood per week (white/oily fish)
	Portions of nuts, seeds and pulses per week
	Portions of fruit and vegetables/day
	Appropriate fat spread
	Appropriate milk
	Appropriate fats in cooking
	Units of alcohol taken/day or week
	Level of fat intake
	Level of salt intake
Emotional	Acceptability of diet
	Barriers to change
	Stages of change
Lifestyle	Smoking
	Exercise levels
	Lipid reduction medication
	Hypertension medication
Risk levels	Waist circumference
	Body mass index
	Weight change
	Total cholesterol
	Triglycerides
	HDL cholesterol
	LDL cholesterol
	Non-HDL cholesterol
	Cholesterol–HDL ratio
	Blood pressure (systolic, diastolic)
	Factors relevant to diabetic or renal control
Outcomes	Myocardial infarction
	Angina frequency
	Stroke
	Coronary artery bypass graft
	Angioplasty
	Hospital admissions
	Death

HDL, high-density lipoprotein; LDL, low-density lipoprotein.

administered by dietitians, at baseline, end of programme, and at 1 year, along with improvements in risk factors, medicine adherence and quality-of-life indices.

Drug – nutrient interactions

- Potassium-containing salt substitutes are cautioned against, or not recommended, for patients at risk of hyperkalaemia, and include individuals on medications such as ACE inhibitors and angiotensin receptor blockers. Salt substitutes (≈60 mEq/tsp of potassium chloride) have been associated with hyperkalaemia when taken in combination with ACE inhibitors (Sica, 2004). Risks of potassium-based sodium replacers added to manufactured foods are currently being reviewed (SACN/COT Potassium-based Sodium Replacers Working Group, 2016).
- Grapefruit juice inhibits cytochrome P450 3A4.
- Grapefruit is contraindicated if taking simvastatin, as the blood level of simvastatin increases significantly, and thus increasing the risk of side effects. An occasional glass of grapefruit juice is thought to be safe with atorvastatin, and no restriction is given for other statins.
- Grapefruit juice increases levels of some calcium channel blockers in the blood.

Patients should be directed to read the medicines' patient information leaflets and seek advice from a pharmacist or prescriber if they wish to include grapefruit juice in their diet (NHS Choices, 2015) or consider potassium-based salt substitutes. It is also advisable to check the special product characteristics leaflets for individual medicines, which are aimed at health professionals (www.medicines.org.uk).

Acknowledgement

The editor acknowledges the prior contribution of Catherine Hames.

References

Adler AJ, Taylor F, Martin N, *et al.* (2014) Reduced dietary salt for the prevention of cardiovascular disease. *Cochrane Database Syst. Rev.* (12): CD009217. doi: 10.1002/14651858.CD009217.pub3.

American Heart Association. (2015) *Alcohol and Health*. Available at http://www.heart.org/HEARTORG/HealthyLiving/HealthyEating/Nutrition/Alcohol-and-Heart-Health_UCM_305173_Article.jsp. Accessed 14 May 2017.

Ascherio A, Willett WC. (1997) Health effects of trans fatty acids. *Am. J. Clin. Nutr.* 66: 1006S–1010S.

Bazzano LA, Reynolds K, Holder KN, *et al.* (2006) Effect of folic acid supplementation on risk of cardiovascular diseases: a meta-analysis of randomized controlled trials. *JAMA.* 296: 2720–2726.

Bhatnagar P, Wickramasinghe K, Williams J, *et al.* (2015) The epidemiology of cardiovascular disease in the UK. *Heart.* 101: 1182–1189.

British Heart Foundation (BHF). (2015) *Cardiovascular Statistics.* London: British Heart Foundation.

Brown L, Rosner B, Willett W, *et al.* (1999) Cholesterol-lowering effects of dietary fibre: a meta-analysis. *Am. J. Clin. Nutr.* 69: 30–42.

Connolly SB, Kotseva K, Jennings C, *et al.* (2017) Outcomes of an integrated community-based nurse-led cardiovascular disease prevention programme. *Heart.* 103: 840–847. doi: 10.1136/heartjnl-2016-310477

Conroy RM, Pyörälä K, Fitzgerald AP, *et al.* (2003) Estimation of ten-year risk of fatal cardiovascular disease in Europe: the SCORE project. *Eur. Heart J.* 24: 987–1003.

Cousins JH, Rubovits DS, Dunn JK, *et al.* (1992) Family versus individually oriented intervention for weight loss in Mexican American women. *Public Health Rep.* 107: 549–555.

DH. (2000) *Coronary Heart Disease: National SERVICE framework for Coronary Heart Disease Modern Standards and Service Models.* London: Department of Health.

DH. (2008) *Putting Prevention First – Vascular Checks: Risk Assessment and Management.* London: Department of Health.

DH. (2013) *Cardiovascular Disease Outcomes Strategy: Improving Outcomes for People with or at Risk of Cardiovascular Disease.* London: Department of Health.

Estruch R, Ros E, Salas-Salvadó J, *et al.* (2013) Primary prevention of cardiovascular disease with a Mediterranean diet. *N. Engl. J. Med.* 368: 1279–1290.

ESC/EAS. (2016) 2016 ESC/EAS guidelines for the management of dyslipidaemias. *Eur. Heart J.* 37: 2999–3058.

European Food Safety Authority. (2010) *Health Claims*. Brussels: European Commission.

European Society of Cardiology (ESC). (2016) European guidelines on cardiovascular disease prevention in clinical practice. *Eur. Heart J.* 37: 2315–2381.

Grosso G, Marventano S, Yang J, *et al.* (2015) A comprehensive meta-analysis on evidence of Mediterranean diet and cardiovascular disease: are individual components equal? *Crit. Rev. Food Sci. Nutr.* 57(15): 3218–3232.

Hippisley-Cox J, Coupland C, Robson J, *et al.* (2008) Predicting cardiovascular risk in England and Wales: prospective derivation and validation of QRISK2. *BMJ.* 336: 1475–1482.

Holmes MV, Dale CE, Zuccolo L, *et al.* (2014) Association between alcohol and cardiovascular disease: Mendelian randomisation analysis based on individual participant data. *BMJ.* 349: g4164.

Holt S, Goldsmith D. (2010) *Clinical Practice Guidelines: Cardiovascular Disease in CKD, 2008–2010*, 5th edn. Final Draft (26.5.10) incorporating feedback on the module from RA Members. UK Renal Association.

Hooper L, Martin N, Abdelhamid A, *et al.* (2015) Reduction in saturated fat intake for cardiovascular disease. *Cochrane Database Syst. Rev.* (6): CD011737. doi: 10.1002/14651858.CD011737.

Iqbal R, Anand S, Ounpuu S, *et al.*; INTERHEART Study Investigators. (2008) Dietary patterns and the risk of acute myocardial infarction in 52 countries: results of the INTERHEART study. *Circulation.* 118: 1929–1937.

JBS3. (2014) Joint British Societies' consensus recommendations for the prevention of cardiovascular disease (JBS3). *Heart.* 100(2): ii1–ii67.

Kotseva K, Wood D, De Bacquer D, *et al.* (2016) EUROASPIRE IV: A European Society of Cardiology survey on the lifestyle, risk factor and therapeutic management of coronary patients from 24 European countries. *Eur. J. Prev. Cardiol.* 23: 636–648. doi: 10.1177/2047487315569401.

Leeds AR, Gray J. (2001) *Dietary Cholesterol as a Cardiac Risk Factor: Myth or Reality?* Huntingdon: Smith-Gordon & Co Ltd.

Luo C, Zhang Y, Ding Y, *et al.* (2014) Nut consumption and risk of type 2 diabetes, cardiovascular disease, and all-cause mortality: a systematic review and meta-analysis. *Am. J. Clin. Nutr.* 100: 256–269.

MAFF. (1999) *Dioxins and PCBs in UK and Imported Marine Fish*. Food Surveillance Information Sheet no 184.

Malik VS, Popkin BM, Bray GA, *et al.* (2010) Sugar-sweetened beverages, obesity, type 2 diabetes mellitus, and cardiovascular disease risk. *Circulation.* 121: 1356–1364.

Malik VS, Pan A, Willett WC, *et al.* (2013) Sugar-sweetened beverages and weight gain in children and adults: a systematic review and meta-analysis. *Am. J. Clin. Nutr.* 98: 1084–1102.

Martí-Carvajal AJ, Solà I, Lathyris D, *et al.* (2015) Homocysteine-lowering interventions for preventing cardiovascular events. *Cochrane Database Syst. Rev.* (1): CD006612. doi: 10.1002/14651858.CD006612.pub4.

Martinez-Gonzalez MA, Bes-Rastrollo M. (2014) Dietary patterns, Mediterranean diet, and cardiovascular disease. *Curr. Opin. Lipidol.* 25: 20–26.

Mouratidou T, Livaniou A, Saborido CM, *et al.* (2014) Trans fatty acids in Europe: where do we stand? *JRC Science and Policy Reports*. doi: 10.2788/1070.

Mukuddem-Petersen J, Oosthuizen W, Jerling JC. (2005) A systematic review of the effects of nuts on blood lipid profiles in humans. *J Nutr.* 135(9):2082–2089.

Myung SK, Ju W, Cho B, *et al.* (2013) Efficacy of vitamin and antioxidant supplements in prevention of cardiovascular disease: systematic review and meta-analysis of randomised controlled trials. *BMJ.* 346: f10. doi: 10.1136/bmj.f10.

NHS. (2009) *NHS Health Checks*. Available at www.healthcheck.nhs.uk. Accessed 13 May 2017.

NHS. (2014) *Five Year Forward View*. London: NHS. Available at www.england.nhs.uk. Accessed 13 May 2017.

NHS Choices. (2015) *Does Grapefruit Affect My Medicine?* Available at http://www.nhs.uk/chq/Pages/2474.aspx?CategoryID=73. Accessed 14 May 2017.

NICE. (2007) *Behaviour Change: General Approaches*. Available at www.nice.org.uk/guidance/ph6. Accessed 13 May 2017.

NICE. (2010) *Cardiovascular Disease Prevention PH 25*. Available at www.nice.org.uk. Accessed 13 May 2017.

NICE. (2013) *BMI: preventing ill health and premature death in black, Asian and other minority ethnic groups. Public health guideline (PH46)*. Available at www.nice.org.uk. Accessed 13 May 2017.

NICE. (2014a) *Lipid modification: Cardiovascular risk assessment and the modification of blood lipids for the primary and secondary prevention of cardiovascular disease. CG181*. Available at www.nice.org.uk. Accessed 13 May 2017.

NICE. (2014b) *Obesity: Identification, Assessment and Management. CG189*. Available at www.nice.org.uk. Accessed 13 May 2017.

Preiss D, Sattar N, McMurray JJ. (2011) A systematic review of event rates in clinical trials in diabetes mellitus: the importance of quantifying baseline cardiovascular disease history and proteinuria and implications for clinical trial design. *Am. Heart J.* 161: 210–219.

Public Health England. (2016) *National Diet and Nutrition Survey: Assessment of Dietary Sodium Adults (19 to 64 years) in England, 2014*. London: Department of Health.

Rees K, Hartley L, Flowers N, *et al.* (2013) 'Mediterranean' dietary pattern for the primary prevention of cardiovascular disease. *Cochrane Database Syst. Rev.* 8: CD009825.

Roberts K, Flaherty SJ. (2010) *Review of Dietary Assessment Methods in PUBLIC health*. Oxford: National Obesity Observatory.

Robson J, Dostal I, Sheikh A. (2016) The NHS Health Check in England: an evaluation of the first 4 years. *BMJ Open.* 6(1): e008840. Available at 10.1136/bmjopen-2015-008840. Accessed 16 April 2017.

Ronksley PE, Brien SE, Turner BJ, *et al.* (2011) Association of alcohol consumption with selected cardiovascular disease outcomes: a systematic review and meta-analysis. *BMJ.* 342: d671.

SACN. (2003) *Salt and Health*. London: HMSO.

SACN (2015) Carbohydrates and Health. Available at https://www.gov.uk/govergnment/publications/sacn-carbohydrates-and-health-report. Accessed 13 November 2018.

SACN/COT. (2004) *Advice on Fish Consumption: Benefits and Risks*. London: HMSO.

SACN/COT Potassium-based Sodium Replacers Working Group. (2016) *Terms of Reference*. Available at https://cot.food.gov.uk/committee/committee-on-toxicity/cotwg/joint-sacn/cot-potassium-based-sodium-replacers-working-group. Accessed 14 May 2017.

Sica DA. (2004) Angiotensin-converting enzyme inhibitors side effects–physiologic and non-physiologic considerations. *J. Clin. Hypertens. (Greenwich)*. 6: 410–416. Available at http://onlinelibrary.wiley.com/doi/10.1111/j.1524-6175.2004.02866.x/full. Accessed 14 May 2017.

Stabler SN, Tejani AM, Huynh F, *et al.* (2012) Garlic for the prevention of cardiovascular morbidity and mortality in hypertensive patients. *Cochrane Database Syst. Rev.* (8): CD007653. doi: 10.1002/14651858.CD007653.pub2.

Thompson GR, Grundy SM. (2005) History and development of plant sterol and stanol esters for cholesterol-lowering purposes. *Am. J. Cardiol.* 96(1A): 3D–9D.

Tong TYN, Wareham NJ, Khaw KT, *et al.* (2016) Prospective association of the Mediterranean diet with cardiovascular disease incidence and mortality and its population impact in a non-Mediterranean population: the EPIC-Norfolk study. *BMC Med.* 14: 135. doi: 10.1186/s12916-016-0677-4.

Wannamethee SG, Shaper AG, Whincup PH, *et al.* (2011) Impact of diabetes on cardiovascular disease risk and all-cause mortality in older men: influence of age at onset, diabetes duration, and established and novel risk factors. *Arch. Intern. Med.* 171: 404–410.

Wheeler DC. (1997) Cardiovascular risk factors in patients with chronic renal failure. *J. Ren. Nutr.* 7: 182–186.

Willett WC, Sacks F, Trichopoulou A, *et al.* (1995) Mediterranean diet pyramid: a cultural model for healthy eating. *Am. J. Clin. Nutr.* 61: 1402S–1406S.

Woodward M, Brindle P, Tunstall-Pedoe H; SIGN group on risk estimation. (2007) Adding social deprivation and family history to cardiovascular risk assessment: the ASSIGN score from the Scottish Heart Health Extended Cohort (SHHEC). *Heart.* 93(2): 172–176.

Wood DA, Kotseva K, Connolly S, *et al.* (2008) Nurse-coordinated multidisciplinary, family-based cardiovascular disease prevention programme (EUROACTION) for patients with coronary heart disease and asymptomatic individuals at high risk of cardiovascular disease: a paired, cluster-randomised controlled trial. *Lancet.* 371: 1999–2012.

7.14.2 Coronary heart disease

Julie Hinchliffe and Jane Green

Key points

- Dietitians have a multi-agency role in advising on public health policy and strategy.
- Dietitians actively contribute to multi-disciplinary cardiac rehabilitation programmes for groups and individuals.
- Dietitians provide advice and training for healthcare professionals, delivering a consistent evidence-based message on nutrition.
- Dietitians provide nutrition support advice to heart failure or cardiac cachexia patients.

Coronary heart disease (CHD) is the most common form of cardiovascular disease (CVD). This chapter focuses on the aetiology and management of CHD, and the role of the dietitian in its prevention. Chronic heart failure (CHF) is the most common cause of CHD. CHD can present clinically in several different ways, which may include the following:

- Stable angina – chest pain that is controlled, except on exertion.
- Acute coronary syndrome (ACS) – myocardial infarction (MI) (heart attack) and unstable angina.
- Sudden death, with or without a history of angina, or infarction due to inherited cardiomyopathies or arrhythmias.
- Heart failure because of CHD, where cachexia is a sign of end-stage disease.

ACS is the umbrella term that encompasses the following:

- ST-elevated MI (STEMI) – the lumen of one of the main arteries is blocked by a thrombus, resulting in acute ST elevation (an abnormality in the electrocardiogram, or 'ECG'), i.e. traditional heart attack where oxygen supply is cut off, causing death to an area of the heart muscle (Table 7.14.5).
- Non-ST-elevated MI (NSTEMI) – the lumen of one of the main coronary arteries is partially occluded, or one of the minor coronary arteries is completely occluded. This results in a shortage of blood supply to the heart muscle that is less severe than in STEMI, or intermittent. There is often some damage to the heart muscle, as evidenced by a rise in the cardiac-specific serum biomarkers such as troponin.
- Unstable angina – new-onset chest pain or discomfort, or abrupt deterioration in previously stable angina, with chest pain or discomfort occurring frequently and with little or no exertion, and often with prolonged episodes. This often presents in a comparable way to acute MI, but without biomarker evidence of myocardial necrosis (NICE, 2013b).

Diagnosis will be based on a combination of presenting symptoms (e.g. chest discomfort) and investigations such as cardiac markers (e.g. troponins) and electrocardiograph changes (e.g. ST segment elevation). There will also be consideration of the patient's individual risk factors for CHD (Table 7.14.6).

CHD is the most common cause of death in the UK, being responsible for nearly 70,000 deaths a year; the most common trigger of death is a heart attack (BHF, 2015). Approximately one in seven men and one in 11 women in the UK die from CHD (BHF, 2016a). In the 1960s, more than seven out of 10 heart attacks in the UK were fatal. An estimated 915,000 people alive in the UK today have survived a heart attack. Deaths from CHD also vary across the UK (BHF, 2015), as follows:

- Highest in Scotland and Northern England, and lowest in Southern England.
- Highest in the lowest socioeconomic group, and lowest in the highest socioeconomic group.
- Higher in the South Asian community (BHF, 2010).

Dietary factors may contribute to these regional, socioeconomic and ethnic differences (e.g. variation of fruit and vegetable consumption), but they primarily reflect health inequalities see Chapter 4.2 (Public health nutrition), Chapter 3.4 (People in low-income groups) and

Table 7.14.5 Investigative procedures for coronary heart disease

Investigation	Description
Electrocardiogram (ECG)	Monitors the progressive electrical stimulation of the heart muscle. Provides a graph of the heartbeat. Used to detect arrhythmias and can help to diagnose a heart attack. Portions of the graph are labelled 'PQRST' (e.g. ST elevation describes a rise in a particular portion of this graph, which indicates ischaemia).
Exercise stress testing	ECG recorded while exercising or having been given a drug to simulate the effect. It can assess whether pain on exertion is due to heart disease.
24-hour ECG recording or Holter monitoring	Monitoring during everyday activity, including that which produces symptoms over 24–48 hours. Can help to diagnose intermittent symptoms such as palpitations.
Echocardiography	Ultrasound is used to provide a picture of the heart. Can also be used to measure the speed of blood flow.
Electrophysiological studies	Study electrical activity in detail. Can diagnose arrhythmias and identify the areas of the heart that are affected.
Angiogram (also known as coronary angiogram or cardiac catheterisation)	Radio-opaque fluid is infused into major blood vessels of the heart. It reveals the outline of the lumen of the coronary arteries and the extent of atheromatous disease. Used in the process of decision-making about coronary artery bypass grafting and angioplasty.
Magnetic resonance imaging scan	Provide a clear picture of the heart's structure and blood supply.

Table 7.14.6 Risk factors for coronary heart disease (CHD)

Type	Risk factor	Comments
Unmodifiable	Age	Risk increases with age.
	Gender	Due to the protective effects of oestrogen, premenopausal women have a lower prevalence of CHD than same-age men, although this difference can disappear in some circumstances, e.g. coexistence of diabetes.
	Genotype	Family history of CHD is strongly associated with increased risk, probably due in part to genetic differences in lipid metabolism or somatotype, e.g. propensity to central or peripheral fat distribution.
	Ethnicity	Risk is higher in the South Asians, i.e. people of Indian, Pakistani, Bangladeshi and Sri Lankan origin.
	Socioeconomic status	Risk is higher in the lowest socioeconomic groups. In all socioeconomic groups, CVD has improved substantially over the past two decades, but the gap between poorer and more affluent sections of society has widened as the rate of improvement has been fastest in the more affluent groups.
Modifiable	Smoking	Increases oxidative stress damages the inner lining of blood vessels and increases the rate of atherosclerosis.
	Diet	See the section 'Role of diet in the development of CHD'.
	Physical activity	Physical activity positively influences adiposity, insulin resistance, lipid profile (increases HDL cholesterol) and reduces hypertension.
	Hypertension	Increases risk of stroke, induces endothelial dysfunction, contributes to the instability of atherosclerotic plaque and increases the workload of the heart.
	Lipid profile	Uptake of cholesterol by macrophages causes endothelial damage, and is the core of the atherosclerotic plaque; higher LDL – carry cholesterol to be deposited in artery walls; lower HDL – carry excess cholesterol to liver for excretion; higher triglyceride level is inversely related to HDL and is also an independent risk factor. Lipids also influence thrombogenesis.
	Obesity	Effect is due to hypertension, diabetes and dyslipidaemia. The distribution of body fat is also important. A high waist circumference is a risk factor for the metabolic syndrome (IDF, 2005).
	Insulin resistance	Risk marker for CVD. Insulin resistance and abdominal obesity are important causative factors in metabolic syndrome.
	Psychosocial stress	Depression and social isolation or lack of quality support (SIGN, 2007). The way in which a person deals with stress can encourage less healthy behaviours, e.g. smoking, drinking too much alcohol and overeating.

HDL, high-density lipoprotein; LDL, low-density lipoprotein.

SECTION 7

Chapter 3.5 (Working with minority ethnic groups). While mortality rates are reducing, morbidity rates are not falling, as more people survive cardiac events. This may be a reflection of advances in treatment, such as medications and revascularisation, and reductions in major risk factors such as smoking (BHF, 2015). The current prevalence of CHD in the UK is estimated to be 2.3 million, of which 60% are male (BHF, 2015).

Pathogenesis

The pathogenesis of CHD is a complex interaction of several processes. Both atherosclerosis and thrombosis are fundamental to the development of the disease, and each is affected by diet. These two processes are described separately for ease of understanding, but, in reality, they are interlinked.

Atherosclerosis

The first step in the development of atherosclerosis is injury to the arterial endothelium (the metabolically active lining of the artery). In areas of damage, macrophages ingest low-density lipoprotein (LDL) and other atherogenic particles to form foam cells. When the macrophages die, the lipid remains in the arterial wall, accumulating over time to form a lipid core or pool (Figure 7.14.1). The formation of this fatty streak is the first stage in plaque development.

Subsequent proliferation of smooth muscle cells and the development of collagen strands, minor thrombi and calcification in this area of lipid accumulation then result in the formation of atherosclerotic plaque. As the plaque grows, it protrudes into the lumen of the artery. The plaques are covered by a fibrous cap, which can rupture. If this happens, it triggers platelet aggregation and the formation of a blood clot. The narrowing of the lumen of the coronary arteries as a result of plaque development can lead to an inadequate oxygen supply to the myocardium (heart muscle) at times of increased workload to the heart such as physical exertion. This is the cause of stable angina. Severe narrowing of the blood vessel leads to unstable angina or NSTEMI. Complete occlusion of the blood vessel by a thrombus (clot) will cut off the supply of oxygen to a section of the myocardium (heart muscle), resulting in a STEMI.

A description of lipoprotein metabolism and its influence on atherogenesis is given in Chapter 7.14.3 (Dyslipidaemia). More detailed discussion of this subject can be found in British Nutrition Foundation (BNF, 2005).

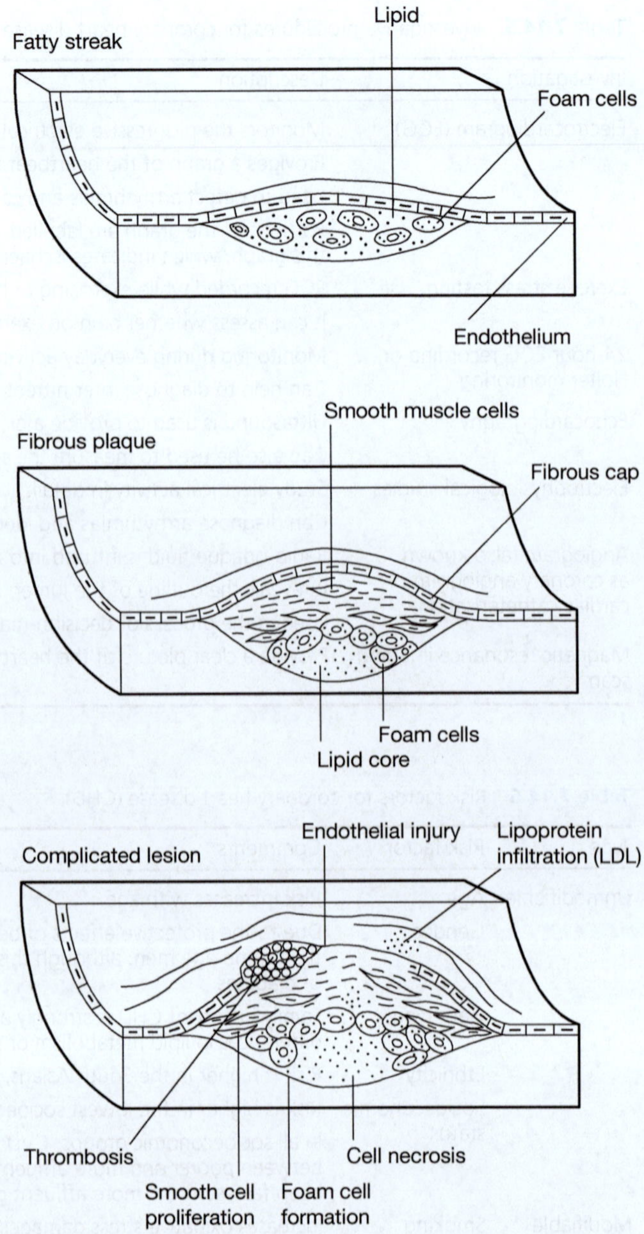

Figure 7.14.1 Stages of atherosclerosis (source: Farringdon J, Thomas B (2001) Coronary heart disease. In Manual of Dietetic Practice 3rd Edition Thomas B (Ed) Oxford: Blackwell Science Figure 4.7 page 515. Reproduced with permission from Jo Farringdon)

Thrombosis

Damage to the endothelium at the micro level, or to the cap of a plaque at the macro level, can trigger platelet activation and coagulation. In addition to being a cause of acute coronary events, thrombosis is an integral part of plaque development, as thrombi can become incorporated into the structure. The repair system is complex, because the clot needs to be assembled at the site of damage and then removed when the repair is complete. Over 50 different chemicals are involved in the process, all of which are present in plasma all the time. A shift in the balance of their activation determines whether the anticoagulants or procoagulants dominate. A brief summary of the coagulation process (Simmons, 1997) is as follows:

- *Stage 1 – vasoconstriction.* In smaller vessels, this is caused by the release of thromboxane A2 and serotonin from platelets. Thromboxane also activates other platelets.
- *Stage 2 – platelet plug formation.* Platelets become sticky when activated and form plugs that can cause

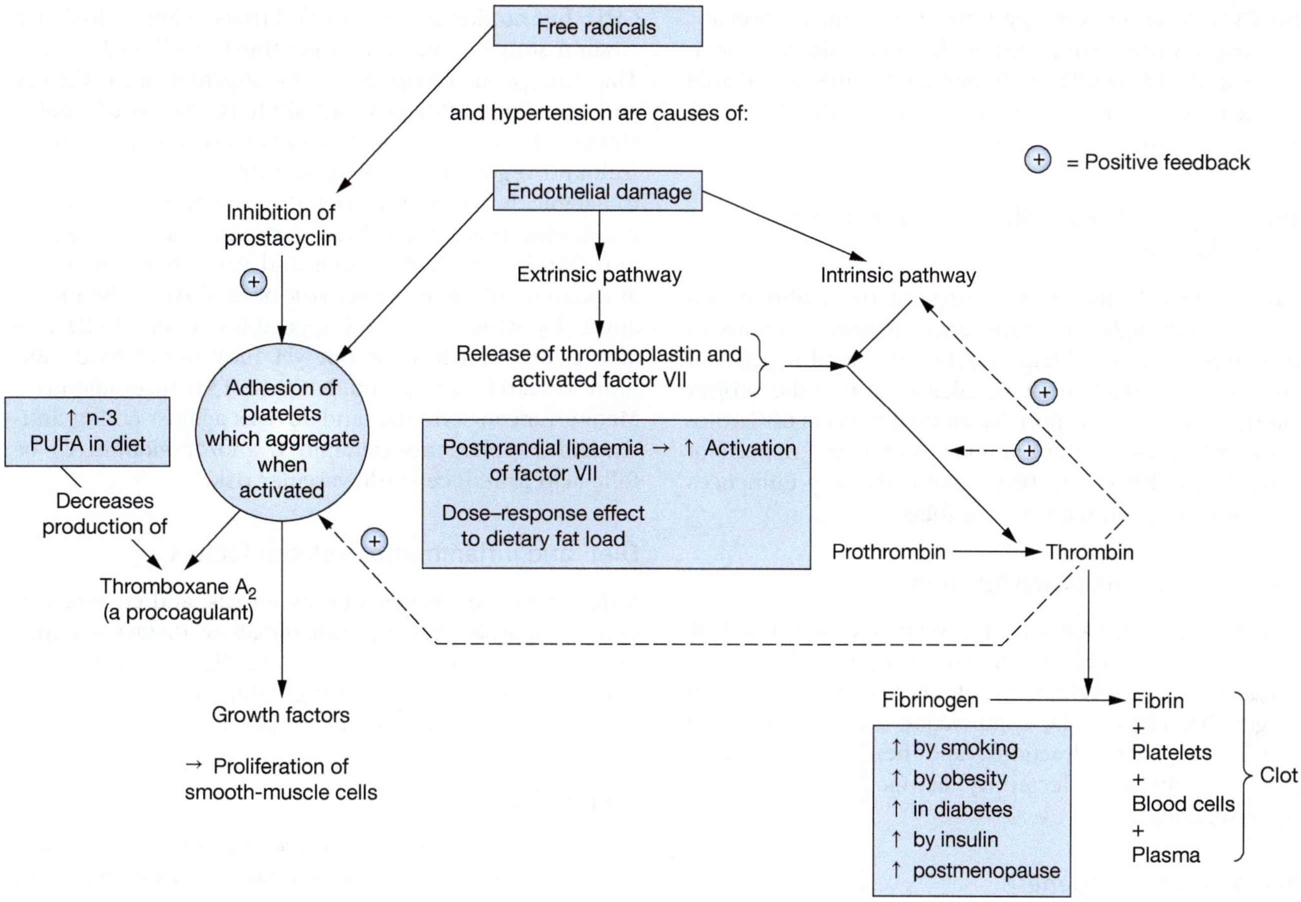

Figure 7.14.2 Diet and haemostasis (source: Thomas & Bishop, 2007, figure 4.20.2, p. 606. Reproduced with permission from Blackwell Science)

minute ruptures in small blood vessels. They also release active compounds such as growth factors, which promote smooth muscle cell proliferation, a stage in the process of atherosclerosis.

- *Stage 3 – clot formation.* Platelet aggregation combines with the extrinsic and intrinsic pathways to produce a clot (Figure 7.14.2). Prothrombin activator catalyses the split of prothrombin to form thrombin. This in turn causes the polymerisation of fibrinogen to form fibrin threads. These form a mesh, which entrap platelets, plasma and blood cells to form the blood clot; this retracts, expressing the serum.
- *Stage 4 – fibrinolysis.* Plasminogen is activated to produce plasmin, a proteolytic enzyme that digests the fibrin threads. Raised levels of plasminogen activator inhibitor-1 (PAI-1), which binds with the plasmin and so inhibits the process of clot breakdown, is a known risk factor for CHD.

Blood coagulation is a complex autocatalytic process; more detailed discussions can be found in BNF (2005).

Risk factors

There is no single cause of CHD, and many factors can contribute to its development. The major risk factors for CHD include physical and biochemical parameters, as well as features of lifestyle and behaviour. Some risk factors (such as genotype) are unmodifiable, but many are potentially modifiable and hence are the focus of disease prevention. Table 7.14.6 summarises the conventional risk factors detailed by the Scottish Intercollegiate Guidelines Network (SIGN, 2016a) and Joint British Societies (JBS3, 2014).

Reducing CHD risk requires multifactorial risk assessment and management. Correcting one risk factor alone may have little impact on CHD risk if other risk factors are ignored, e.g. correcting raised cholesterol will be less beneficial if that person continues to smoke and remains hypertensive. The benefits of diet and lifestyle change must also be considered in this context, and it is vital that dietitians take a broad perspective of CHD risk that encompasses all contributory factors. The JBS3 risk calculator supports the identification of these patients, who are at low short-term risk but high lifetime risk. The calculator is designed to communicate long-term consequences of an individual's lifestyle and the associated risk factors, as well as the substantial lowering of CVD risk which can be obtained by early lifestyle changes, and, where appropriate, by use of evidence-based drug therapies. This tool is used in the NHS Health Check programme in England (DH, 2008), which invites adults aged 40–74 years for a CVD risk assessment with their general practitioner (GP). The JBS3 risk calculator supports the CVD outcome strategy (DH, 2013). Internationally, similar prevention strategies are based on similar principles; the INTERHEART Study highlighted that modifiable risk factors (e.g. diet) account for >90% of the risk of MI worldwide (Yusuf *et al.*, 2004).

Role of diet in the development of coronary heart disease

Many dietary factors may impact on the pathogenesis of CHD, although the significance of some remains to be determined (see Chapter 7.14.1, General aspects of cardiovascular disease). A detailed review of the subject can be found in the report 'Nutritional Aspects of Cardiovascular Disease' (DH, Committee on Medical Aspects of Food Policy, 1994) and BNF (2005). The key influences are summarised in the text that follows.

Diet and endothelial dysfunction

A high intake of saturated fat increases total and LDL cholesterol, causing endothelial damage, which is the first step in the development of atherosclerosis, and can trigger thrombosis. The composition and concentration of the lipoprotein fractions, and hence their atherogenic capacity, are affected by diet (see Chapter 7.14.3, Dyslipidaemia).

Diet and thrombogenesis

Many dietary factors influence haemostasis, including the following:

- Dietary fat (quantity and type) (see Figure 7.14.2) – an increase in the total intake of fat causes postprandial activation of factor VII (FVII) and suppresses fibrinolysis (clot breakdown). Saturated fats increase platelet activity, whereas polyunsaturates have the opposite effect. n-3 Fatty acids attenuate thromboxane A2 synthesis, and thereby suppresses platelet activation. The anticoagulant effect of aspirin is also achieved by the inhibition of thromboxane A2 production.
- Energy balance – non-rapid weight loss improves fibrinolytic activity.
- Alcohol consumption – regular alcohol consumption reduces fibrinogen and FVII concentrations, but heavy drinking reduces fibrinolytic activity.

Diet and oxidative stress

Free radicals are implicated in the processes of both atherosclerosis and thrombosis via:

- Damage to the endothelium.
- Inhibition of prostacyclin, and hence increase in platelet activation and aggregation.
- Oxidation of LDL and other atherogenic lipoproteins, leading to their preferential uptake by macrophages to form foam cells.

Epidemiological data suggest that the consumption of fruit and vegetables has a protective effect against CHD, but randomised controlled trials using antioxidant vitamin supplements contradict this (Mead *et al.*, 2006). The European Prospective Investigation into Cancer and Nutrition (EPIC) – Heart study (Crowe *et al.*, 2011) showed that the consumption of at least eight portions of fruit and vegetables a day gave a 22% lower risk of fatal ischaemic heart disease (IHD), as compared to those consuming lesser than three portions a day. A one-portion (80 g) increment in fruit and vegetable intake was associated with a 4% lower risk of fatal IHD. The mechanism by which fruit and vegetables reduce CHD risk at a population level is not yet fully understood, and more research is required. NICE (2013a) recommends a Mediterranean-style diet and advises against taking antioxidant supplements (vitamin E and/or vitamin C) or folic acid to reduce cardiovascular risk.

Diet- and inflammation-related factors

Inflammation underlies atherosclerosis, and current evidence suggests that anti-inflammatory dietary components, such as n-3 fatty acids, and dietary antioxidants may have a role in reducing injury to the coronary arteries, but more research is required.

Diet and homocysteine

Hyperhomocysteinaemia has been suggested to increase the risk of fibrous plaque formation, thrombosis and arterial injury. Despite epidemiological evidence of an association between these factors, it is not yet clear whether the reduction of homocysteine levels by folic acid and other B vitamin supplementation reduces CHD events (Mead *et al.*, 2006).

Indirect dietary influences

Indirect dietary influences on CHD development include obesity and its consequences, such as hypertension, hypertriglyceridaemia and type 2 diabetes.

Management

CHD management has been shaped by the National Service Framework (NSF) (DH, 2000), the cardiac rehabilitation commissioning pack (DH, 2010a), and, more recently, the NICE cardiac rehabilitation services commissioning guide (NICE, 2013c). Alongside this, numerous guidelines have been produced to influence clinical care and the types of investigative procedures used (Table 7.14.7). Other national guidelines explicitly state the need for professional dietetic advice (British Association for Cardiac Prevention and Rehabilitation (BACPR), 2012; Joint British Societies, 2014; NICE, 2013a). Providing evidence-based dietary information to all people with CHD will save more lives than concentrating dietary advice on just those in need of weight management or lipid reduction. The practice of prioritising dietetic time in secondary prevention to those with raised lipids is out of date since the advent of statin

Table 7.14.7 Summary of coronary heart disease guidance

Society/institute	Guidance
Joint British Societies (JBS)	JBS3 consensus recommendations for the prevention of cardiovascular disease (JBS3, 2014).
British Association for Cardiac Prevention and Rehabilitation (BACPR)	The BACPR standards and core components for cardiovascular disease prevention and rehabilitation (BACPR, 2012).
Scottish Intercollegiate Guidelines Network (SIGN)	Heart disease guidelines (SIGN, 2007, 2016a, 2016b).
National Institute for Health and Care Excellence (NICE)	MI: cardiac rehabilitation and prevention of further cardiovascular disease (NICE, 2013a).
	Cardiovascular disease: risk assessment and reduction, including lipid modification (NICE, 2016b).
	Unstable angina and NSTEMI: the early management of unstable angina and NSTEMI. CG 94 (NICE, 2013b).
	Stable angina CG126 (NICE, 2016).
	Chronic heart failure: management of chronic heart failure in adults in primary and secondary care (NICE, 2018).
European Society of Cardiology (ESC)	Guidelines for the diagnosis and treatment of acute and chronic heart failure (Ponikowski *et al.*, 2016).
	Guidelines for the management of acute coronary syndromes in patients presenting without persistent ST segment elevation (Roffi *et al.*, 2016).

STEMI, ST elevation MI; NSTEMI, non-ST elevation MI.

therapy (NICE, 2013a, 2016a). The BACPR is currently developing guideline documents for the seven core components of cardiac rehab; to date, documents have been produced on the physical activity and exercise, and the health behaviour change and education components. A review is currently underway to produce the BACPR dietetic core competencies document. The BACPR–NACR national certification programme for cardiovascular rehabilitation was launched in 2015, and this enables cardiac rehabilitation programmes to voluntarily apply for assessment against the minimum BACPR standards (Furze *et al.*, 2016).

Overall, the dietary management of CHD depends on the extent to which the disease has progressed and the way in which it is being clinically treated. In the early stages, the main priority will be to change to a Mediterranean-style diet (increasing fruit and vegetables, fish and nuts, and replacing butter and cheese with products based on plant oils) (see Chapter 7.14.1, General aspects of cardiovascular disease), in conjunction with other lifestyle-related risk-reduction measures, e.g. increased physical activity. The Mediterranean diet score (MDS) tool (Schroder *et al.*, 2011) can be used to assess current eating habits and identify areas for improvement, and it is now included on the National Audit for Cardiac Rehabilitation (NACR); hence, it can be used as an outcome measure of dietetic intervention. The BACPR are currently reviewing evidence to improve the validity of MDS for the UK population. Following a major coronary event, this objective remains the same, but will need to be achieved as part of the stepwise process of cardiac rehabilitation. Invasive surgical procedures may temporarily alter dietetic priorities in favour of nutritional repletion. The development of heart failure or cachexia may necessitate permanent change in these priorities. Understanding the medical and surgical management of CHD in terms of their physical and psychological consequences (e.g. on nutritional status or patient motivation) can help determine what these priorities should be.

Medical management

The medical treatment of CHD depends largely on its manifestation, as discussed in the following subsections.

Myocardial infarction – STEMI (Roffi et al., 2016)

Medical treatment includes:

- Consideration of immediate primary percutaneous coronary intervention (PPCI) and revascularisation of the culprit lesion (see the following text).
- Initiation of appropriate pharmacological therapies for secondary prevention (see the following text).
- Assessment of left ventricular function.
- Management of cardiovascular risk factors.
- Referral to cardiac rehabilitation services.

Myocardial infarction – NSTEMI and unstable angina (NICE, 2013a)

Medical treatment includes:

- Consideration for elective coronary angioplasty.
- Assessment of left ventricular function – recommended for all MI patients, and to be considered in the management of unstable angina patients.
- Management of cardiovascular risk factors.
- Initiation of appropriate pharmacological therapies for secondary prevention (see the following text), and to improve angina symptom control as appropriate.
- Referral to cardiac rehabilitation services as appropriate.

National guidelines, e.g. Roffi *et al.* (2016), NICE (2013a) and SIGN (2016a) have identified four main prophylactic drug groups for the secondary prevention of CHD:

- *Antiplatelet drugs* – aspirin blocks the production of thromboxane, which is involved in platelet aggregation. The benefits of the long-term use of low-dose aspirin in secondary prevention are well documented. For patients with a hypersensitivity to aspirin, clopidogrel monotherapy should be considered. More potent antiplatelet agents (e.g. prasugrel or ticagrelor) are recommended as dual anti-platelet therapy in combination with aspirin in patients with ACS. Dual antiplatelet therapy is recommended for up to 12 months post-MI, with a minimum of 1 month for patients also receiving a bare-metal stent, and 6 months for patients also receiving a drug-eluting stent.

- *Statins* – intensive statin therapy is recommended for all patients following MI in the absence of contraindication/intolerance, irrespective of initial cholesterol values (see Chapter 7.14.3, Dyslipidaemia).
- *Beta-blockers* – they block the stimulating action of noradrenaline and adrenaline, thus reducing the force and speed of myocardial contraction. The increase in diastolic interval allows for better coronary perfusion during exercise and a reduction in myocardial oxygen demand. They are used in the treatment of MI, angina, heart failure, arrhythmias and hypertension. If patients post-MI have no evidence of left ventricular systolic dysfunction and none of the other conditions that indicate the use of a beta blocker, then the beta blocker may be discontinued after 12 months (NICE, 2013a).
- *Angiotensin-converting enzyme (ACE) inhibitors* – they have a vasodilatory action through the decreased formation of angiotensin II and the increase in protective bradykinin. The main indications for ACE inhibitor therapy include prophylaxis of cardiovascular events, hypertension and all grades of heart failure. Angiotensin II receptor antagonists (also referred to as angiotensin receptor blockers (ARBs)) are used when patients are intolerant to ACE inhibitors. Other vasodilators are nitrates (e.g. glyceryl trinitrate (GTN) spray for symptomatic relief of angina) and calcium channel blockers. Both work by inhibiting smooth muscle contraction in the vessel walls.

NICE (2013a) no longer routinely recommends eating oily fish or the use of n-3 capsules or supplemented foods for secondary prevention post-MI in excess of the recommendations for the general population. This is based on randomised control trials (Galan *et al.*, 2011; Kromhout *et al.*, 2010; Matsuzaki *et al.*, 2009; Rauch *et al.*, 2010). NICE also recommends that, if oily fish is consumed, there is no evidence of harm, and that fish forms part of the cardioprotective Mediterranean-style diet. SACN (2004) recommends a maximum intake of four portions of oily fish per week due to the relatively high levels of dioxins and polychlorinated biphenyls (PCBs). Hence, dietitians should recommend at least one portion of white fish (e.g. cod/haddock/hake) and one portion of oily fish per week (e.g. salmon/mackerel/trout), as per general population advice, and no more than four portions per week of oily fish in the diet. NICE makes lifestyle recommendations about physical activity, smoking cessation and alcohol consumption. NICE (2016a) also states that there is no evidence that vitamins or fish oil help stable angina.

Surgical management

Following an angiogram, patients may be referred for an angioplasty and/or coronary artery bypass graft (CABG).

Angioplasty – percutaneous coronary Intervention

A balloon is introduced at the site where blood flow through the arterial lumen has been significantly reduced as a result of atherosclerotic plaque. Once in position, the balloon is inflated to increase the size of the arterial lumen. In some cases, a small stent (a mesh tube that can be expanded to hold the artery open) is inserted. The PPCI procedure, also known as primary angioplasty, is used for the prompt restoration of flow in STEMI.

Coronary artery bypass graft

In this surgical procedure, one or more diseased coronary arteries are bypassed. Blood vessels (usually taken from the leg) are grafted onto the existing coronary arteries to bypass the occluded section. Access to the heart is gained via the sternum, which is broken in the process. CABG is a major surgical procedure, with all the metabolic and nutritional consequences that this implies. It should also be borne in mind that, if patients are advised by the surgical team to lose weight prior to the procedure, some will undergo surgery in a nutritionally depleted state as a result of inappropriate crash dieting. If weight is still an issue, post-CABG patients should be told not to lose weight until the sternum has healed, which usually takes 6 weeks. For planned CABG prehabilitation, a combination of nurse counselling and a brief cognitive behavioural intervention has been found to reduce depression and cardiac misconceptions, and improve physical functioning before CABG surgery (Furze *et al.*, 2009).

Cardiac rehabilitation

The DH (2010a) cardiac rehabilitation commissioning pack and NICE cardiac rehabilitation commissioning guide (2013c) set explicit standards for the provision of effective cardiac rehabilitation for high-priority patients. These include NSTEMI, STEMI and unstable angina patients, including all those undergoing reperfusion (e.g. CABG, PCI or PPCI), as well as newly diagnosed CHF patients or those with a step change in clinical presentation. Furthermore, the pack recommends the extension of services once high-priority patient cardiac rehabilitation services have been successfully implemented to include heart transplant patients, as well as patients who have undergone surgery to implant a cardioverter defibrillator or heart valve replacement for reasons other than ACS or heart failure. The pack recommends a seamless pathway involving six stages (Table 7.14.8), with the dietitian influencing the management of each stage. There is currently no evidence that cardiac rehabilitation is clinically or cost-wise effective for managing stable angina, and more research is needed in this area (NICE, 2016a).

Stage 1

Initial advice on lifestyle, including diet, is usually given by the ward staff (training of other healthcare professionals is an important role of the cardiac rehabilitation dietitian), but the ability of both patients and

Table 7.14.8 Role of the dietitian in cardiac rehabilitation (CR)

Stage	Service delivered by	Description (DH, 2010a)	Timescale	Role of the dietitian (Fox *et al.*, 2004; Mead *et al.*, 2006)
1	Acute services	Acute event in hospital	2–5 days as inpatient	Training CR staff or practice nurse to deliver consistent key cardioprotective dietary messages
2 and 3	Acute services and primary care	Complete initial assessment via telephone/home visit, and introduce CR core components Devise individual care plan based on patient risk factors and motivation	5–10 working days from receipt of referral/ discharge from hospital	Ensuring dietary resources are up to date Referral criteria to dietitian is not based on lipid levels, but identifies patients struggling with the cardioprotective diet
4	Acute services and primary care	Hospital rehabilitation service – high-risk patients Community-based rehabilitation service – low-risk patients Multidisciplinary approach	8–12 weeks	Deliver group sessions and/or individual consultations to achieve and sustain effective secondary prevention within multidisciplinary care
5 and 6	Primary care	Nurse-led CHD clinics by practice nurses Community exercise classes	Week 12 and beyond	

their families to assimilate information will be severely impaired by anxiety and stress in coming to terms with the diagnosis. In particular, patients receiving immediate PPCI have very short hospital stay and should receive stopgap information to ensure that they are aware of their local cardiac rehabilitation programme. Following major cardiac surgery, the immediate dietary objectives (to restore recent energy and nutrient losses) may be different from longer-term aims (e.g. to alter fat intake). Some patients may require oral nutritional support measures; therefore, healthy heart food choices from the hospital menu may not be appropriate at this stage. Good communication between dietetic, nursing and medical staff is essential to ensure that the nutritional objectives are understood and that patients are given food that is appropriate for their nutritional needs.

Stage 2

Following an initial assessment, the cardiac rehabilitation specialist nurse introduces the core components of cardiac rehabilitation:

- *Lifestyle* – diet, exercise and, if appropriate, weight management and smoking cessation.
- *Risk factor management* – cholesterol, blood pressure and, if diabetic, glucose management.
- *Cardioprotective drug therapy* – rate, rhythm, thrombotic risk management and fluid status, they can be modified by prescribing cardiac specialist nurses.
- *Psychosocial well-being* – an anxiety and depression screening tool will be used to identify high-risk clients to be referred to psychological specialists.

Stage 3

A care plan is devised, realistic goals are set from the initial assessment and the patient is enrolled into a cardiac rehabilitation programme that meets their needs. This may include home-based cardiac rehabilitation programmes, e.g. the Heart Manual (Lewin *et al.*, 1992), or a formal cardiac rehabilitation exercise programme. There is usually very little direct dietetic contact during this phase.

Stage 4

A formal cardiac rehabilitation outpatient programme typically lasts 6 weeks, with twice-weekly supervised exercise sessions followed by group education. Community-based programmes are becoming more common to improve access and increase the participation of women and ethnic minority groups. Dietetic input depends on the capacity of the service, but a dietitian will usually see the patient in group sessions and/or individually depending on the availability of local resources (BHF, 2016b). The patient's partner or carer should also be involved, as he or she has an important role in helping implement and maintain the diet and lifestyle measures necessary for secondary prevention.

Dietitians, as part of a multidisciplinary team (MDT), can support patients to achieve and sustain effective secondary prevention (Fox *et al.*, 2004). However, the EUROASPIRE II survey (Kotseva *et al.*, 2004) found that only one-third of patients attended the cardiac rehabilitation programmes, and that those who attended still did not achieve lifestyle and risk factor targets. The EUROACTION trial demonstrated that a multidisciplinary, family-based programme improved lifestyle and reduced cardiovascular risk. Patients in the intervention group reduced the consumption of saturated fat; three-quarters of patients and their partners achieved the recommended fruit and vegetable intake (as compared to just over one-third of usual-care patients), and twice as many in the former group met the recommended weekly intake

Table 7.14.9 New York Heart Association functional classification of heart failure (Ponikowski *et al.*, 2016)

Classification	Symptoms	Comments
Class I	Impaired left ventricular failure, but no symptoms, e.g. fatigue or breathlessness.	No limitations to activities of daily living.
Class II	Comfortable at rest, but ordinary physical activity results in fatigue, palpitation or dyspnoea.	Mild – slight limitations.
Class III	Comfortable at rest, but less than ordinary activity results in fatigue, palpitations or dyspnoea.	Moderate – marked limitations.
Class IV	Symptoms at rest. If any physical activity is undertaken, discomfort is increased.	Severe – inability to carry out any activities of daily living without discomfort.

of oily fish (Wood *et al.*, 2008). Nationally, cardiac rehabilitation uptake is 50% (BHF, 2016b).

Stages 5 and 6

At the patients' final discharge assessment from the cardiac rehabilitation programme, they are signposted to lifestyle maintenance programmes to encourage them to continue to exercise, e.g. local heart care support group or community exercise classes. The patient is referred back to the care of their GP. The NSF for CHD (DH, 2000) advocates the use of disease registers in primary care to provide long-term follow-up for CHD patients. For CHD, this is realised in the Quality Outcome Framework (BMA/NHS Employers, 2016/2017), with annual reviews being conducted by practice nurses. There is opportunity during this phase for referral to a dietitian to review and enhance dietary understanding and compliance.

Chronic heart failure

CHF is a complex syndrome caused by a reduction in the heart's ability to pump blood around the body. While the most common cause is CHD, other causes include hypertension, valvular heart disease, cardiomyopathy, atrial fibrillation and alcohol abuse. Prevalence of CHF increases sharply with age to about 7% in men and women over 75 years (NHS IC, 2010). Patients with CHF often have a poor quality of life, with high mortality rates (10–50%, depending on severity). They have a worse prognosis than patients with breast and prostate cancer (NHS IC, 2010). CHF has become one of the most common causes of hospital admissions. Due to the ageing population and improved survival in patients who develop CVD (such as MI), hospital admissions and the number of people diagnosed with CHF are expected to rise. To address these issues, the NSF for CHD, Standard 11 (DH, 2000), has set out a service delivery agenda, and NICE (2018) has produced clinical guidelines to improve management. Specialist CHF services are currently being developed to reduce hospital admissions/mortality rates and improve symptoms (NHS IC, 2010). The physical effects of CHF include the following:

- Inadequate cardiac output.
- Fluid imbalance.
- Pulmonary and other oedema.
- Dyspnoea.
- Fatigue.

Echocardiogram is now the gold standard for diagnosis in those patients with a medical history of MI. For patients with no previous history of MI, an echocardiogram is only needed if the B-type natriuretic peptide (BNP) test is positive (NICE, 2016a). Heart failure is a progressive condition, and is classified into four stages according to the severity of symptoms (Table 7.14.9).

Medical management

In CHF, the main treatment objectives are to:

- Prevent progressive damage to the myocardium.
- Prevent or reverse further enlargement of the heart.
- Improve quality of life through symptom management.
- Prolong life (Opie & Gersh, 2009).

The main cause of CHF is left ventricular systolic dysfunction (LVSD), for which the recommendations for pharmacological management can include the following (NICE, 2018; Ponikowski *et al.*, 2016):

- ACE inhibitors are recommended as first-line treatment. These can prolong life expectancy, delay progression and improve symptoms. ARBs may be used if ACE inhibitors are not tolerated.
- Beta-blockers are used in controlled heart failure alongside ACE inhibitors, and have been proven to reduce mortality in low doses.
- Diuretics are used routinely for the relief of congestive symptoms and fluid retention (peripheral and pulmonary oedema); the removal of fluid and reduction in blood volume reduces the workload of the heart. This can result in rapid improvement in dyspnoea and improve exercise tolerance.

In addition, other agents such as aldosterone antagonists and digoxin may be considered. Anticoagulation may be indicated in the absence of contraindication, to reduce the risk of thromboembolic complications (e.g. stroke) in CHF and atrial fibrillation. Warfarin is recommended in patients with CHF and in atrial fibrillation with a structurally abnormal heart. Where atrial fibrillation is present persistently or paroxysmally, with a structurally normal heart, novel oral anticoagulants (NOACs) may be used in the absence of CHD (e.g. dabigatran, apixaban, rivaroxaban).

Surgical management

Although medical management is the mainstay of treatment, some patients will benefit from invasive procedures (NICE, 2016a; Ponikowski *et al.*, 2016) such as:

- Mechanical support cardiac resynchronisation therapy with pacemaker function – recommended to reduce morbidity in patients in New York Heart Association (NYHA) classes III–IV who are symptomatic despite optimal medical therapy.
- Heart transplantation – however, shortage of donor organs means that many are unable to benefit from this.

Dietetic management

Many guidelines for CHF management (NICE, 2010; Ponikowski *et al.*, 2016; SIGN, 2016b) highlight the benefits of lifestyle changes, including dietary manipulation. However, there are no specific evidence-based nutritional guidelines, and more research is required. The therapeutic aims of dietary management are to:

- Maintain adequate energy intake to prevent obesity, malnutrition and cachexia.
- Reduce the workload for the heart by weight management, and sodium and fluid restriction.
- Provide a nutritionally adequate diet.
- Protect against further heart disease.

Dietetic management in CHF will therefore address the following:

- Obesity – should be avoided as it increases cardiac workload. Planned weight loss should be gradual as rapid weight loss can result in undesirable muscle loss and also increase the risk of inadequate or poor nutritional intake. Weight reduction should not be routinely recommended in moderate to severe CHF (Ponikowski *et al.*, 2016).
- Malnutrition – the combination of reduced nutritional intake and increased requirements increase the risk of malnutrition (Gibbs *et al.*, 2000). Energy intake needs to be sufficient to meet nutritional needs and prevent deterioration in nutritional status. Gains in adiposity should be distinguished from the short-term fluctuations in body weight caused by changes in fluid balance.
- Cachexia – see the following subsection.
- Sodium restriction – sodium and water retention, leading to expansion of extracellular fluid volume, are important components of CHF syndrome. Therefore, it is of little or no benefit to restrict fluid intake if patients continue to use unlimited amounts of salt. Restricting salt is more relevant in advanced CHF: severe salt restriction (<2 g/day) is rarely necessary. Where salt restriction needs to be considered, it should be at a no added salt level (see Chapter 6.6, Fluids and electrolytes). Salt substitutes should be avoided, as these are rich in potassium and may lead to hyperkalaemia, especially if patients are on ACE inhibitors and/or spironolactone. Salt restriction can affect food palatability and possibly compromise intake of energy and essential nutrients.
- Fluid restriction – excessive fluid intake should be avoided as it negates the positive effects of diuretics and induces hyponatraemia. Patients with advanced CHF, with or without hyponatraemia, may need to restrict their fluid intake. There is no evidence-based calculation for the level of fluid restriction as in the case of patients with renal failure. In practice, a restriction of 1.5–2 L/day is often advised. Daily weighing is advised for CHF patients to detect sudden or unexpected weight gains (>2 kg in 3 days), which would indicate the need for adjustment of diuretic dose.
- Maintaining nutritional adequacy – particular attention should be paid to micronutrient intake since the use of diuretics and other drugs may result in significant urinary losses of potassium and water -soluble vitamins. Since appetite is often poor, the diet may need to be relatively nutrient dense, and meal frequency may need to be increased. Social factors such as support for food purchasing and preparation, particularly if the patient lives alone, should not be overlooked. Alcohol should only be consumed in moderation, and completely avoided if CHF has been caused by alcohol abuse.
- Protect against further heart disease – the key cardioprotective dietary messages should be incorporated (see Chapter 7.14.1, General aspects of cardiovascular disease). Supplementation with 1 g/day of n-3 fatty acid may be beneficial, but further studies are needed prior to routine recommendation (GISSI, 2008).

Cardiac cachexia

CHF can lead to cardiac cachexia, a complex condition that affects many body systems (Anker & Coats, 1999). There is a loss of skeletal and heart muscle, fat and bone tissue, neurohormonal and immunological changes, and impaired functioning. Many of the common symptoms, e.g. anorexia and fatigue, are similar to the cachexia of cancer and chronic infection (see Chapter 7.15.9, Cancer cachexia). Cardiac cachexia has a poor prognosis (50% mortality rate within 18 months), with the amount of weight lost being a strong predictor of mortality. The incidence of cachexia with CHF may be about 9%, and up to 68% for hospitalised patients.

Dietary management

Nutritional support is required to address anorexia that is exacerbated by:

- Dyspnoea – this increases fatigue during eating, and swallowing exacerbates the symptoms of dyspnoea.
- Oedema.
- Palatability of food, e.g. salt restriction, ACE inhibitors impairing taste.
- Drug reactions, e.g. aspirin, digoxin and ACE inhibitors all cause anorexia.

Table 7.14.10 Key UK public health documents that influence primary CHD prevention

Key documents	Comments
Saving Lives: Our Healthier Nation (DH, 1999).	National policy on public health, e.g. reducing death rate from CHD, stroke and related disease in people <75years of age by at least 40% by 2010.
Coronary heart disease: National Service Framework (NSF) for CHD – modern standards and service models (DH, 2000).	Strategy to modernise CHD services. Standard 1 highlights that the NHS needs to work with partner agencies to address CHD prevention in the population.
Coronary Heart Disease: Guidance for Implementing the Preventative Aspects of the NSF (HDA, 2001).	Guidance on best practices to support healthier lifestyles: • Reduce smoking. • Promote healthy eating. • Promote physical activity. • Reduce overweight and obesity.
Tackling Health Inequalities. A Programme for Action (DH, 2003).	Need to address access issues, especially as low-income and minority ethnic groups are disproportionately affected by CHD.
Securing Good Health for the Whole Population (Wanless, 2004).	Describes required resources to provide high-quality health services for the future.
Coronary Heart Disease Ten Years On – Improving Heart Care (DH, 2007).	Report of progress in CHD outcomes and prevention.
Tackling Health Inequalities: 10 Years on. (DH, 2009).	Update from publication of the Acheson Report (1998), leading to strategic review of health inequalities in 2008.
Healthy Lives, Healthy People (DH, 2010b).	Updated public health strategy to promote health and aim to create a wellness service.
Our Health and Well-being Today (DH, 2010c).	Summary of evidence setting out the nation's health in 2010.
Prevention of Cardiovascular Disease at Population Level (NICE, 2010).	DH commissioned NICE to produce public health guidance for the prevention of CVD at the population level. CVD includes stroke and peripheral arterial disease.
England	
Choosing Health – Making Healthier Choices Easier (DH, 2004).	Considers wider determinants and barriers to choosing a healthy lifestyle and inequalities, etc.
Choosing a Better Diet: A Food and Health Action Plan (DH, 2005).	Government plans to improve nutrition and health.
Five Year Forward View (NHS England, 2014).	NHS 5-year plan.
Action on Cardiovascular Disease: Getting Serious about Prevention (PHE, 2016).	Aimed at clinical commissioning groups and public health workers to highlight the impact of CVD, and an overview of Public Health England's work and leadership to support the NHS.
Scotland	
Eating for Health – Meeting the Challenge: Co-ordinated Action, Improved Communication and Leadership for Scottish Food and Health Policy (Scottish Executive, 2004).	A strategic framework for food and health.
Healthy Eating, Active Living (HEAL) (Scottish Government, 2008).	An action plan to improve diet, increase physical activity and tackle obesity.
Preventing Overweight and Obesity in Scotland. A Route Map Towards Healthy Weight (Scottish Government, 2010).	Target areas – energy consumption, energy expenditure, early years, working lives.
Heart Disease Improvement Plan (Scottish Government, 2014).	Six priority areas for improvement – to improve clinical outcomes for heart disease patients.
Wales	
Food and Well-being: Reducing Inequalities through a Nutrition Strategy for Wales (Wales Assembly Government, 2003).	Addresses the widening gap in health between the most- and least-deprived communities.
Together for Health. A Heart Disease Delivery Plan (WG18538; Wales Assembly Government, 2011).	A delivery plan up to 2016 for NHS Wales and partners.
Together for Health. A Heart Disease Delivery Plan – Annual Report (WG25424; Wales Assembly Government, 2015).	Identifies progress in the last year, and five national priorities set for further improvement.
Northern Ireland	
Investing for Health (DH, Social Services and Public Safety, 2003).	Plans to improve the health of all people and reduce health inequalities.
Developing New Public Health Strategy for Northern Ireland (DH, Social Services and Public Safety, updated September 2011), www.dhsspsni.gov.uk.	An updated review of 'Investing in Health'.
Service Framework for Cardiovascular Health and Well-being (DH, Social Services and Public Safety, 2014–2017), www.dhsspsni.gov.uk.	42 standards relating to a number of specific conditions to be achieved over 3 years.

- Metabolic disturbances, e.g. hyponatraemia or renal failure.
- Depression.

The levels of sodium, fluid restriction and micronutrient needs should be discussed with the referring clinician. Overall, an MDT approach is key to ensure that weight loss is minimised as part of the need to address quality-of-life issues during palliative care. Gold standards framework is a model that makes available good practices to all people nearing the end of their lives with a life-limiting condition, including heart failure. It is now recommended that patients with two or more of the following prognostic indicators be listed on a gold standards framework register to enable a multidisciplinary approach to end-of-life care (RCGP, 2008):

- CHF NYHA III–IV – shortness of breath at rest or on minimal exertion.
- Patients thought to be in their last year of life.
- Repeated hospital admissions with symptoms of heart failure.
- Difficult physical or psychological symptoms despite optimal medical treatment.

A discussion with the patient and carer about palliative end-of-life care is essential to ensure that an appropriate care plan and support are implemented (RCGP, 2008). Dietitians are gradually becoming more involved in the management of cardiac cachexia, and at an earlier stage, but this is variable across the country. Since the number of hospital admissions for this condition is increasing, it is likely that its management will adopt a rising profile in the clinical dietetic caseload. Current research is investigating the use of anabolics, anti-inflammatory drugs, appetite stimulants and nutritional supplements, which will strengthen the evidence base for dietetic practice in this area.

Public health prevention strategies

The multifactorial nature of CHD is reflected in public health strategy. Addressing health inequalities is an important issue as poor-quality diet can result in inequalities in people's health. Poor diet can account for 30% of life years lost in early death/disability from diet-related diseases such as CHD (National Heart Forum, 2004). The key documents that have shaped primary CHD prevention to date within the public health arena are outlined in Table 7.14.10 (see Chapter 4.2, Public health nutrition). The evidence base for the dietary aspects of primary CHD prevention is well known (DH, Committee on Medical Aspects of Food Policy, 1994) and implemented in practice via the Eatwell Guide (see Chapter 2.1, Dietary reference values and food-based dietary guidelines). New evidence from the EPIC Norfolk study supports adherence to a Mediterranean diet for the prevention of CHD in the UK population (Tong *et al.*, 2016).

Drug–nutrient interactions (SIGN, 2016b)

- Cranberries and cranberry juice may increase warfarin's potency.
- Warfarin interacts with foods containing vitamin K, e.g. spinach, kale, Brussel sprouts and broccoli. Patients are advised to keep the intake of these foods consistent in the diet.
- Any herbal medicines could affect the way in which prescribed treatments work, so these should be discussed with the GP first, e.g. St John's wort should be avoided in CHF patients, as it can interact with warfarin, digoxin, eplerenone and selective serotonin reuptake inhibitors.
- Grapefruit and grapefruit juices should be avoided in patients prescribed simvastatin. Patients prescribed atorvastatin should not drink >1–2 L/day.

Internet resources

American Heart Association, www.heart.org
British Association for Cardiovascular Prevention and Rehabilitation, www.bacpr.com
British Heart Foundation, www.bhf.org.uk
EUROACTION, https://www.escardio.org/The-ESC/What-we-do/Initiatives/EuroAction
European Society of Cardiology, https://www.escardio.org
Foundation for Circulatory Health, www.ffch.org
Heart Improvement Programme, NHS, http://www.bcs.com/documents/DEA_PwSI_Cardiology_Framework.PDF
Sustain, www.sustainweb.org
The Heart Manual, www.theheartmanual.com

References

Anker SD, Coats AJS. (1999) Cardiac cachexia: A syndrome with impaired survival and immune and neuroendocrine activation. *Chest.* 115: 836–847.

British Association for Cardiac Prevention and Rehabilitation (BACPR). (2012) *Standards and Core Components for Cardiac Rehabilitation*. Available at http://www.bacpr.com/resources/46C_BACPR_Standards_and_Core_Components_2012.pdf. Accessed 13 November 2018.

British Heart Foundation (BHF). (2010) *Statistics Database. Ethnic Differences in Cardiovascular Disease*. Available at https://www.bhf.org.uk/informationsupport/publications/statistics/ethnic-differences-in-cardiovascular-disease-2010. Accessed 13 November 2018.

British Heart Foundation (BHF). (2015) *Statistics Database. Cardiovascular Disease Statistics*. https://www.bhf.org.uk/informationsupport/publications/statistics/cvd-stats-2015. Accessed 13 November 2018.

British Heart Foundation (BHF). (2016a) *Cardiovascular Disease Statistics BHF UK Factsheet*. Available from www.bhf.org/uk/research/heart-statistics. Accessed 31 May 2017.

British Heart Foundation (BHF). (2016b) *The National Audit of Cardiac Rehabilitation (NACR) Annual Statistics Report 2016*. Available at https://www.bhf.org.uk/informationsupport/publications/statistics/national-audit-of-cardiac-rehabilitation-annual-statistical-report-2016. Accessed 13 November 2018.

British Medical Association (BMA)/NHS Employers. (2016) *Quality & Outcomes Framework Guidance for General Medical Services (GMS) Contract 2016/2017*. Available at http://www.nhsemployers.org/your-workforce/primary-care-contacts/general-medical-services/quality-and-outcomes-framework Accessed 13 November 2018.

British Nutrition Foundation (BNF). (2005) *Cardiovascular Disease: Diet, Nutrition and Emerging Risk Factors*. Oxford: Blackwell Science.

SECTION 7

Crowe FL, Roddam AW, Key TJ, *et al.*; European Prospective Investigation into Cancer and Nutrition (EPIC) – Heart Study Collaborators. (2011) Fruit and vegetable intake and mortality from ischaemic heart disease: results from the European Prospective Investigation into Cancer and Nutrition (EPIC) – Heart study. *Eur. Heart J.* 32(10): 1182–1183.

DH. (1999) *Saving Lives: Our Healthier Nation*. London: The Stationery Office.

DH. (2000) *National Service Framework for Coronary Heart Disease – modern standards and service models*. Available at http://webarchive.nationalarchives.gov.uk/20130123204144/http://www.dh.gov.uk/en/Publicationsandstatistics/Publications/PublicationsPolicyAndGuidance/DH_4094275. Accessed 13 November 2018.

DH. (2003) *Tackling Health Inequalities. A Programme for Action*. Available at http://webarchive.nationalarchives.gov.uk/20031221042257/http://www.doh.gov.uk/healthinequalities/programmeforaction/. Accessed 13 November 2018.

DH. (2004) *Choosing Health – Making Healthier Choices Easier*. Available at http://webarchive.nationalarchives.gov.uk/+/http://www.dh.gov.uk/en/Publicationsandstatistics/Publications/PublicationsPolicyAndGuidance/DH_4094550. Accessed 13 November 2018.

DH. (2005) *Choosing a Better Diet: A Food and Health Action Plan*. Available at http://webarchive.nationalarchives.gov.uk/20130105040029/http://www.dh.gov.uk/prod_consum_dh/groups/dh_digitalassets/@dh/@en/documents/digitalasset/dh_4105709.pdf. Accessed 13 November 2018.

DH. (2007) *Coronary Heart Disease Ten Years On – Improving Heart Care*. London: DH.

DH. (2008) *Putting Prevention First: NHS Health Check: Vascular Risk Assessment and Management. Best Practice Guidance*. Available at http://webarchive.nationalarchives.gov.uk/+/http://www.dh.gov.uk/en/Publicationsandstatistics/Publications/PublicationsPolicyAndGuidance/DH_083822. Accessed 13 November 2018.

DH. (2009) *Tackling Health Inequalities: 10 Years on (Report 2009)*. Available at http://webarchive.nationalarchives.gov.uk/20130123195944/http://www.dh.gov.uk/en/Publicationsandstatistics/Publications/PublicationsPolicyAndGuidance/DH_098936. Accessed 13 November 2013.

DH. (2010a) *Strategic Commissioning Development Unit (SCDU) CHD & the Need for Cardiac Rehab*. London: DH.

DH HM Government. (2010b) *Healthy Lives, Healthy People*. Available at https://assets.publishing.service.gov.uk/government/uploads/system/uploads/attachment_data/file/216096/dh_127424.pdf. Accessed 13 November 2018.

DH HM Government. (2010c) *Our Health and Well-being Today*. Available at https://assets.publishing.service.gov.uk/government/uploads/system/uploads/attachment_data/file/215911/dh_122238.pdf. Accessed 13 November 2018.

DH. (2013) *Cardiovascular Disease Outcomes Strategy*. Available at https://assets.publishing.service.gov.uk/government/uploads/system/uploads/attachment_data/file/214895/9387-2900853-CVD-Outcomes_web1.pdf. Accessed 13 November 2018.

DH, Committee on Medical Aspects of Food Policy. (1994) *Nutritional Aspects of Cardiovascular Disease. Reports on Health and Social Subjects 46*. London: HMSO.

DH, Social Services and Public Safety. (2003) *Investing for Health*. Northern Ireland: DH, Social Services and Public Safety.

DH, Social Services and Public Safety. (2011 update) *Investing for Health*. Northern Ireland: DH, Social Services and Public Safety.

DH, Social Services and Public Safety. (2014–2017) *Service Framework for Cardiovascular Health and Well-being*. Northern Ireland: DH, Social Services and Public Safety.

Farringdon J, Thomas B. (2001) *Coronary heart disease*. In Manual of Dietetic Practice 3rd Edition. Oxford: Blackwell Science. Figure 4.7 page 515.

Fox K, Barber K, Muir L, *et al.* (2004) Development, implementation and audit of a cardiac prevention and rehabilitation programme for patients with coronary artery disease. *Eur. Heart. J. Suppl.* 6(SJ): J53–58.

Furze G, Dumville JC, Miles JN, *et al.* (2009) 'Prehabilitation' prior to CABG surgery improves physical functioning and depression. *Int. J. Cardiol.* 132(1): 51–58.

Furze G, Doherty P, Grant-Pearce C. (2016) Development of a UK National Certification Programme for Cardiac Rehabilitation (NCP_CR). *Br. J. Cardiol.* 23(2): 102–105.

Galan P, Kesse-Guyot E, Czernichow S, *et al.* (2011) Effects of B vitamins and omega-3 fatty acids on cardiovascular diseases: a randomized placebo-controlled trial. *BMJ.* 341:c6273.

Gibbs CR, Jackson G, Lip GYH. (2000) ABC of heart failure: Non-drug management. *BMJ.* 320: 366–369.

GISSI – HF Investigators. (2008) Effect of omega-3 polyunsaturated fatty acids in patients with chronic heart failure (the GISSI-HF trial): a randomised, double-blind, placebo-controlled trial. *Lancet.* 372: 1223–1230.

Health Development Agency (HDA). (2001) *Coronary Heart Disease: Guidance for Implementing the Preventative Aspects of the NSF*. London: HDA.

International Diabetes Federation (IDF). (2005) *The International Diabetes Federation consensus worldwide definition of the metabolic syndrome*. Available at www.idf.org.

Joint British Societies. (2014) JBS3: Joint British Societies' consensus recommendations for the prevention of cardiovascular disease. *Heart.* 100: ii1–ii67.

Kotseva K, Wood DA, De Bacquer D, *et al.* (2004) Cardiac rehabilitation for coronary patients: lifestyle, risk factor and therapeutic management. Results from the EUROASPIRE II Survey. *Eur. Heart J. Suppl.* 6(J): J17–J26.

Kromhout D, Gitlay EJ, Geleijnse JM; Alpha Omega Trial Group. (2010) n-3 fatty acids and cardiovascular disease events after myocardial infarction. *N. Engl. J. Med.* 363(21): 2015–2026.

Lewin B, Robertson IH, Cay EL, *et al.* (1992) Effects of self-help post myocardial infarction rehabilitation on psychological adjustment and use of health services. *Lancet.* 339: 1036–1040.

Matsuzaki M, Yokoyama M, Saito Y, *et al.* (2009) Incremental effects of eicosapentaenoic acid on cardiovascular events in statin treated patients with coronary heart disease. *Circ. J.* 73(7): 1283–1290.

Mead A, Atkinson G, Albin D, *et al.* (2006) Dietetic guidelines on food and nutrition in the secondary prevention of cardiovascular disease – evidence from systematic reviews of randomized controlled trials (second update). *J. Hum. Nutr. Diet.* 19: 401–419.

National Heart Forum (NHF). (2004) *Nutrition and Food Poverty: A tool kit for those involved in developing or implementing a local Nutrition strategy*. London: NHF

NHS England. (2014) *Five Year Forward View*. Available at https://www.england.nhs.uk/five-year-forward-view/. Accessed 13 November 2018.

NHS IC (The NHS Information Centre for Health & Social Care). (2010) *National Heart Failure Audit*. Available at https://www.ucl.ac.uk/nicor/audits/heartfailure/documents/annualreports/hfannual09-10.pdf Accessed 13 November 2018.

NICE. (2010) *Prevention of Cardiovascular Disease at Population Level*. NICE Public Health Guidance 25. London: NICE.

NICE. (2013a) Myocardial infarction: cardiac rehabilitation and prevention of further cardiovascular disease. Clinical guideline [CG172] Still 2013 Available at https://www.nice.org.uk/guidance/cg172. Accessed 13 November 2018.

NICE. (2013b) *Unstable Angina & NSTEMI: The Early Management of Unstable Angina & NSTEMI. CG94*. London: NICE. Available at https://www.nice.org.uk/guidance/cg94. Accessed 13 November 2018.

NICE. (2013c) *Cardiac Rehabilitation Services Commissioning Guide*. London: NICE.

NICE. (2016a) *Stable Angina. Clinical Guideline 126*. Available at https://www.nice.org.uk/Guidance/CG126. Accessed 13 November 2018.

SECTION 7

NICE. (2016b) Cardiovascular disease: risk assessment and reduction, including lipid modification. Available at https://www.nice.org.uk/guidance/CG181. Accessed 13 November 2018.

NICE. (2018) *Chronic Heart Failure: Management of Chronic Heart Failure in Adults Diagnosis and management* CG 106. Available at https://www.nice.org.uk/guidance/ng106. Accessed 13 November 2018.

Opie LH, Gersh BJ. (2009) *Drugs for the Heart*, 7th edn. Philadelphia: Saunders Elsevier.

PHE. (2016) *Action on Cardiovascular Disease: Getting Serious about Prevention*. Available at https://www.gov.uk/government/publications/cardiovascular-disease-getting-serious-about-prevention. Accessed 13 November 2018.

Ponikowski P, Voors AA, Anker SD, *et al.*; ESC Committee for Practice Guidelines (CPG). (2016) *ESC Guidelines for the diagnosis and treatment of acute and chronic heart failure 2016. Eur. Heart J.* 37: 2129–2200.

Rauch B, Schiele R, Schneider S, *et al.* (2010) OMEGA, a randomized placebo-controlled trial to test the effect of highly purified omega-3 fatty acids on top of modern guideline adjusted therapy after myocardial infarction. *Circulation.* 122(21): 2152–2159.

Roffi M, Patrono C, Collet J, P *et al.*; ESC Committee for Practice Guidelines. (2016) ESC Guidelines for the management of acute coronary syndromes in patients presenting without persistent ST-segment elevation. *Eur. Heart J.* 37: 267–315.

Royal College of General Practitioners (RCGP). (2008) *Prognostic Indicator Guidance Paper. National Gold Standards Framework Centre England.* London: RCGP.

SACN. (2004) *Advice of fish consumption- benefits and risks.* Available at https://www.gov.uk/government/uploads/system/uploads/attachment_data/file/338801/SACN_Advice_on_Fish_Consumption.pdf. Accessed 31 May 2017.

Scottish Executive. (2004) *Eating for Health Meeting the Challenge: Co-ordinated Action, Improved Communication and Leadership for Scottish Food and Health Policy*. Edinburgh: Scottish Executive.

Scottish Government. (2008) *Healthy Eating Active Living (HEAL)*. Edinburgh: Scottish Government

Scottish Government. (2010) *Preventing Overweight and Obesity in Scotland. A Route Map Towards Healthy Weight*. Edinburgh: Scottish Government.

Scottish Government. (2014) *Heart Disease Improvement Plan*. Edinburgh: Scottish Government.

Scottish Intercollegiate Guidelines Network (SIGN). (2007) *Risk Estimation and the Prevention of Cardiovascular Disease. A National Clinical Guideline. Publication No 97*. Edinburgh: SIGN.

Scottish Intercollegiate Guidelines Network (SIGN). (2016a) *Acute Coronary Syndromes. A National Clinical Guideline. Publication No 148*. Edinburgh: SIGN.

Scottish Intercollegiate Guidelines Network (SIGN). (2016b) *Management of Chronic Heart failure. A National Clinical Guideline. Publication No 147*. Edinburgh: SIGN.

Schroder H, Fito M, Estruch R, *et al.* (2011) A short screener is valid for assessing Mediterranean diet adherence among older men and women. *J. Nutr.* 141: 1140–1145.

Simmons A. (1997) *Hematology – A Combined Theoretical and Technical Approach*, 2nd edn. London: Butterworth-Heineman.

Tong YN, Wareham NJ, Khaw K. *et al.* (2016) Prospective association of the Mediterranean diet with cardiovascular disease and mortality and its population impact on a non-Mediterranean population: the EPIC – Norfolk study. *BMC Med.*14: 135.

Wales Assembly Government. (2003) *Food and Well Being: Reducing Inequalities Through a Nutrition Strategy for Wales*. Cardiff: Welsh Assembly Government.

Wales Assembly Government. (2011) *Together for Health. A Heart Disease Delivery Plan*. Cardiff: Welsh Assembly Government.

Wales Assembly Government. (2015) *Together for Health. A Heart Disease Delivery plan. Annual Report 2015*. Cardiff: Welsh Assembly Government.

Wanless D. (2004) *Securing Good Health for the Whole Population*. London: HMSO.

Wood DA, Kotseva K, Connolly S, *et al.*; EUROACTION Study Group. (2008) Nurse-co-ordinated multidisciplinary, family-based cardiovascular disease prevention programme (EUROACTION) for patients with coronary heart disease and asymptomatic individuals at high risk of cardiovascular disease: a paired, cluster-randomised controlled trial. *Lancet.* 371: 1999–2012.

Yusuf S, Hawken S, Ounpuu S, *et al.*; INTERHEART Study Investigators. (2004) Effect of potentially modifiable risk factors associated with myocardial infarction in 52 countries (the INTERHEART study): case-control study. *Lancet.* 364: 937–952.

7.14.3 Dyslipidaemia

Linda Main

Key points

- Dyslipidaemia should not be treated in isolation but in conjunction with the assessment of cardiovascular disease risk.
- Dietary treatment and advice is still relevant despite drug therapy.
- While the role of high-density lipoprotein needs further research, treatment is focused on the reduction of all atherogenic lipoproteins (by lifestyle and dietary means).
- Statins are generally safe and well tolerated, and remain the first line of therapy. Combination treatments are used to aggressively achieve individual lipid targets.

Dyslipidaemia refers to the presence of high levels of lipids (cholesterol, triglycerides and/or fat phospholipids) in the blood, or lipoproteins, the compounds in which lipids are transported. The clinical significance of dyslipidaemia depends on other risk factors that contribute to total risk. Dyslipidaemia is associated with atherosclerosis, the process by which arteries become occluded, leading to chronic conditions such as coronary heart disease (CHD), stroke and peripheral vascular disease.

Lipid metabolism

Cholesterol

Cholesterol is an essential part of all cell membranes, and a precursor of bile acids (needed for fat digestion and absorption), steroid hormones and vitamin D. Excess cholesterol can accumulate in blood vessels walls (atheroma), ultimately causing a restriction or interruption in the circulation; this process is called *atherosclerosis*. Depending on where the restriction in blood flow occurs, it can result in angina, heart attack, stroke or claudication (pain on walking), and can contribute to other conditions such as erectile dysfunction and Alzheimer's disease. Populations with low levels of blood cholesterol have low levels of CHD, and those with high levels of cholesterol have high levels of CHD (DH, 1994) (see Chapter 7.14.2, Coronary heart disease). Approximately 20% of cholesterol is derived from the diet, and the remainder is synthesised in the body. Cholesterol is produced in a multistage process mainly in the liver, although most tissues are able to make cholesterol.

Triglycerides

Triglycerides are the major storage form of fats and a major source of dietary energy. Many tissues have the ability to synthesise triglycerides, including the gut, liver, muscle and adipose tissues.

Lipoproteins

All lipids (cholesterol, phospholipids, triglycerides) are insoluble in water (hydrophobic), and therefore have to be transported in the blood as lipoproteins. Lipoproteins are classified according to their size and density. The metabolism of lipoproteins is complex. The principal features are as follows:

- Lipoproteins are globular complexes of lipids and proteins.
- The definitions of low-density lipoprotein (LDL), very-low-density lipoprotein (VLDL) and high-density lipoprotein (HDL) are artificial cut-off points.
- Each lipoprotein has several components that are metabolically active and constantly in flux, both in the circulation and within tissue fluids. They exchange components with each other.
- Lipoproteins interact with receptors and enzymes located on the surface of cells.

Chylomicrons (from exogenous production)

The composition of chylomicrons is 80–95% triglycerides, 3–7% cholesterol, and 1–2% protein. They are the largest lipoproteins, and they enter the circulation via the lymphatic system, taking triglycerides and cholesterol from digestion and newly synthesised cholesterol from the gut into the body. Lipoprotein lipase, present on the vascular endothelium of tissues, releases triglycerides from the core of the chylomicron. Triglycerides are converted into fatty acids and monoglycerides, which are taken up by the tissues. Chylomicrons quickly become depleted of triglycerides and are removed from the circulation by the liver.

Very-low-density lipoproteins (from endogenous production)

These lipoproteins consist of 60% triglycerides, 10–15% cholesterol and 15% phospholipids. They are smaller and denser than chylomicrons and account for 10–15% of total serum cholesterol. VLDLs are produced by the liver to supply tissues with triglyceride. Similar to chylomicrons, VLDLs become depleted of triglyceride over time under the influence of lipoprotein lipase.

Low-density lipoproteins (from endogenous production)

LDLs consist of 10% triglycerides, 37% cholesterol, 22% phospholipids and 20–22% protein. Raised LDL cholesterol (LDL-C) is an established risk factor for CHD. Remnant VLDLs are known as LDLs. Being smaller, they are able to cross the vascular endothelium and enter the tissues, where they are the major supplier of cholesterol for membrane repair and growth, and in the specialised tissues for hormone and vitamin D synthesis. LDL-C accounts for 60–70% of total serum cholesterol. The size of LDL particles varies, and this is significant as smaller, denser LDL particles are more atherogenic than larger ones.

High-density lipoproteins (from endogenous production)

HDLs are the smallest lipoproteins and account for 20–30% of circulating cholesterol. They consist of 20% cholesterol, 48% protein, 3% triglycerides and 27% phospholipids. HDL cholesterol (HDL-C) is inversely associated with the risk of CHD (Rader & Hovingh, 2014). It collects excess cholesterol from the tissues and returns it to the liver, where it is converted to cholesterol-rich bile acids that are excreted into the gut. This process is essential to prevent the build-up of surplus cholesterol in the tissues. Drugs which raise HDL have failed to provide clinical benefit, creating scepticism around the HDL hypothesis. However, HDL-C remains an important predictor of cardiovascular disease (CVD) risk, hence its continued role in CVD risk calculations (Rader & Hovingh, 2014). Recent evidence suggests that both low and very high HDL-C levels are highly correlated with a higher risk of both CVD and non-CVD mortality, although not a specific cardiovascular risk factor itself (Ko *et al.*, 2016).

Intermediate-density lipoproteins

Intermediate-density lipoproteins (IDLs) are short-lived intermediaries between VLDLs and LDLs.

Apolipoproteins

Apolipoproteins bind to lipids within the lipoproteins and are classified as A, B, C, etc., with further subclassifications (AI, AII, etc.). They are sometimes referred to as Apo A, Apo B, etc. The principal apolipoprotein of HDL is apolipoprotein A; and, for chylomicrons, VLDL and LDL, it is apolipoprotein B.

High levels (>50 mg/dL or 125 nmol/L) of lipoprotein (Lp(a)), a large sticky lipoprotein which is genetically determined, have been linked to early CVD, especially in people with familial hypercholesterolaemia (FH) (Banach, 2016). High levels have been shown to affect one in five people, and are more common in Asian and African populations (Kronenberg & Utermann, 2012).

Cardiovascular risk

Cholesterol

Raised LDL cholesterol is a major risk factor for CVD, which claimed 17.5 million lives worldwide in 2012 – 6 million under the age of 70 years; 7.4 million due to CHD; and 6.7 million owing to stroke (WHO, 2016). On a population basis, a 1 mmol/L reduction in LDL-C is associated with a 12% reduction in all-cause mortality, a 19% reduction in coronary mortality and a 21% reduction in vascular events (myocardial infarction (MI), coronary revascularisation and stroke) over 5 years (Cholesterol Treatment Trialists' Collaboration, 2005). The longer they remain, the benefits of cholesterol reduction seem to increase (Law *et al.*, 2003).

Blood cholesterol concentrations (including LDL-C and HDL-C) are only one of many risk factors that influence the development of CHD, and cannot by itself predict individual CHD risk. A raised level poses a greater threat to an individual at high CHD risk than to someone at low risk. Similarly, the benefits from cholesterol reduction in a particular individual will be affected by other risk factors, e.g. smoking, hypertension, overweight and physical inactivity. It is now recognised that effective prevention of CVD requires multifactorial risk assessment and intervention (see Chapter 7.14.1, General aspects of cardiovascular disease). For this reason, blood lipid measurements must always be considered in the context of other risk factors. Emphasis is placed on the reduction in non-HDL cholesterol (non-HDL-C), as this is considered the sum of all the atherogenic particles, and is easy to measure (NICE CG181, 2015). HDL-C is considered anti-inflammatory, reflects cholesterol removal, and levels 1–1.5 mmol/L are associated with lower risk (Rader & Hovingh, 2014). Very high levels of HDL-C have been reported to be atherogenic, but the mechanism is not clear (Rader & Hovingh, 2014).

Triglycerides

Circulating triglycerides are present mainly in VLDL, which is made in the liver (endogenous production), and chylomicrons, which are produced by the gut following digestion (exogenous production). Modest levels of hypertriglyceridaemia (2–10 mmol/L) are associated with increased risk of CVD, and higher levels with acute pancreatitis. Raised triglycerides are strongly associated with low HDL-C, and, until recently, it was believed that the observed associations between blood triglyceride concentration and CHD risk might simply reflect the more powerful predictive value of low HDL-C levels. However, as the HDL hypothesis comes under increasing scrutiny, there is renewed interest in the role of triglycerides. Epidemiological and genetic evidence supports the role of triglycerides in CVD; furthermore, studies using fibrates showed that a 1 mmol/L reduction in triglycerides reduced coronary events by 54% overall, and by 43% in those with high triglycerides (Nordestgaard & Varbo, 2014). Raised triglycerides are also associated with insulin resistance, highly atherogenic small LDL particles, low HDL-C and the metabolic syndrome. At present, there is no clear evidence to demonstrate that lowering triglyceride levels (independent of other risk factors) reduces major CVD events. However, REDUCE IT and STRENGTH, two large-scale trials using n-3 fatty acids, and PROMINENT, a fibrate trial in high-risk diabetics, are due to report soon (Davidson & Benes, 2016). Other novel therapies that target triglycerides are in development.

Genetic predisposition

Plasma concentrations of total cholesterol, LDL-C, HDL-C and triglycerides are inheritable risk factors for CVD (see Chapter 5.1, Genetics and nutritional genomics). Many genes are involved in lipid metabolism, and, together, these explain 25–30% of the genetic variance for each lipoprotein. Genetic diagnosis is available for FH in some parts of the UK. Genome-wide testing may, in the future, offer a valuable method of identifying those at high CVD risk who would benefit from early treatment.

Diet and lifestyle

Many aspects of diet and lifestyle affect blood lipids and can contribute to dyslipidaemia. Body mass index (BMI), alcohol, smoking and saturated fat intake are strong predictors of blood lipid levels (Constanza *et al.*, 2004; FAO, 2010). Diet is central to the treatment of dyslipidaemia, either as a first-line treatment or alongside drug therapy. Metabolic studies have demonstrated a cholesterol-lowering effect from diet in the range of 5–35%, dependent on the baseline diet and the extent of dietary changes made (Jenkins *et al.*, 2002, 2003b, 2011). For most people, 5–20% cholesterol reduction is realistic (Jenkins *et al.*, 2006, 2011).

Fat

Following a fat-containing meal, blood triglyceride levels rise, triglyceride-rich chylomicrons enter the bloodstream, and triglyceride production by the liver temporarily ceases. Individual saturated fatty acids (SFAs) have different effects on blood cholesterol levels. Lauric (C12.0), myristic (C14.0) and palmitic (C16.0) acids all increase LDL-C (Mensink, 2016); stearic acid (C18.0) has also been recently implicated (Zong *et al.*, 2016). There is also evidence that the impact of SFAs may be different, dependent on the food matrix they originate from (Praagman *et al.*, 2016).

Dietary guidelines recommend 7–10% of energy from SFAs. While restriction of SFA intake is crucial, reduction in total dietary fat may not be necessary. Sustained reduction in SFAs can reduce LDL-C and total cholesterol, provided care is taken with how this energy is replaced. Evidence currently suggests that replacement with polyunsaturated fatty acids (PUFAs) may have a greater impact on reducing LDL-C than monounsaturated fatty acids (MUFAs) or carbohydrate (Astrup *et al.*, 2011; Mensink, 2016; Zong *et al.*, 2016). Replacing 1% of energy from SFAs (C12-18) with PUFAs can reduce CHD risk by 6–8% (Zong *et al.*, 2016) and CHD incidence by 2–3% (Astrup *et al.*, 2011).

Several studies have failed to demonstrate a reduction in cholesterol and cardiovascular end points with reduction of SFAs (Chowdhury *et al.*, 2014; de Souza *et al.*, 2015; Siri-Tarino *et al.*, 2010). This can in part be explained by the lack of control over what SFA is replaced with, the predominant source of the saturated fat, and inclusion of studies where foods on the test diet were high in trans fats (de Souza *et al.*, 2015; Praagman *et al.*, 2016; Zong *et al.*, 2016).

Trans fatty acids (TFAs)

TFAs are industrially produced by partial hydrogenation of vegetable and marine oils to produce hardened fats (such as margarines) and cooking fats. They have been shown to increase total and LDL-C levels, but, unlike SFAs, they also lower HDL-C (Mensink, 2016; SACN, 2007). A 1% energy decrease in TFAs is estimated to reduce the risk of CHD by 12.5% (Oomen *et al.*, 2001). In the UK, the food and catering industries have made significant efforts to remove industrially produced TFAs from the food chain. TFAs currently provide 0.5–0.6% of food energy (Bates *et al.*, 2016), although some groups may have a higher intake. TFAs from ruminant sources are low in most diets, and evidence suggests that they are not associated with CHD risk (Bendsen *et al.*, 2011; de Souza *et al.*, 2015).

Omega-3 fatty acids

The n-3 fatty acids eicosapentaenoic acid (EPA) and docosahexaenoic acid (DHA) at doses of 2–4 g/day (in purified supplemental form) have been shown to reduce fasting and postprandial blood triglyceride levels (Castro *et al.*, 2005; Roche & Gibney, 2000). Fish or vegetable oils n-3 fatty acids do not have a significant effect on blood cholesterol levels (Hooper *et al.*, 2004).

Dietary cholesterol

Approximately 30–60% of dietary cholesterol is absorbed (Durrington, 2007), and this contributes approximately 20% of the total circulating cholesterol. Most dietary cholesterol comes from foods that are also rich in SFAs, such as full-fat dairy foods and fatty meats, and reducing SFA intake will therefore reduce dietary cholesterol. However, some foods rich in cholesterol are low in SFAs, including egg yolk, liver and shellfish (prawns, crabs, lobster, squid, octopus and cuttlefish).

UK dietary guidelines for CVD prevention and lipid modification recommend restricting cholesterol intake to <300 mg/day (NICE, 2015). Mean daily intakes of cholesterol in the UK are at 304 mg (men) and 213 mg (women) (Henderson *et al.*, 2003). Restriction of dietary cholesterol over and above that found in foods high in SFAs is unlikely to have a significant influence on blood cholesterol for most people. However, some individuals with FH may benefit from restriction.

Carbohydrate

Carbohydrate intake has not been shown to directly affect blood cholesterol levels (SACN, 2015); however, carbohydrate energy content is inversely proportional to the energy derived from fat. In practice, restricting SFA intake often results in an increase in the percentage of energy derived from carbohydrate. Increasing refined dietary carbohydrate, particularly if energy intake is excessive, can elevate endogenous production of triglyceride by the liver as VLDLs (Durrington, 2007). Patients with raised triglycerides should be encouraged to choose whole grains and carbohydrates with a low glycaemic index.

Soluble fibre

Water-soluble fibre (psyllium, guar, oat bran and pectin) reduces total and LDL-C (Anderson & Hanna, 1999; Brown *et al.*, 1999; Castro *et al.*, 2005; Truswell, 2002), whereas insoluble fibre has no effect. An increase in soluble fibre intake of 5–10 g/day can reduce LDL-C by 5%. Cereals are the most practical source of soluble fibre (especially oats and barley), followed by nuts and legumes. Some fruit and vegetables (okra, aubergine, citrus fruit, apples, bananas, cabbage, carrots, avocado and dried fruit) are good sources.

Obesity

Overweight and obesity are associated with elevated LDL-C, hypertriglyceridaemia and decreased HDL-C (Hecker *et al.*, 1999). Central obesity exaggerates lipid changes as a consequence of insulin resistance (Carmena *et al.*, 2001; Chan *et al.*, 2004). For every 1% above desirable BMI, the risk of CHD increases by 3.3% for women and 3.6% for men (Anderson & Konz, 2001). Reviews of weight loss studies predict a drop in cholesterol of 0.23 mmol/L for every sustained 10 kg weight loss in obese and severely obese individuals (Poobalan *et al.*, 2004). Reductions in total cholesterol, LDL-C and triglycerides of 1–1.3%, 0.7% and 1.6–1.9%, respectively, per kilogram of weight lost have also been reported (Anderson & Konz, 2001; Aucott *et al.*, 2011). A modest, sustained weight loss of 5–10% of body weight can therefore confer significant benefit (Aronne & Isoldi, 2007). Weight loss that is achieved through exercise is more effective at raising HDL-C levels than energy intake restriction (Rashid & Genest, 2007) (see Chapter 7.13.2, Management of obesity and overweight in adults).

Alcohol

Alcohol is a common cause of hypertriglyceridaemia and can also exacerbate existing hypertriglyceridaemia (Durrington, 2007). Complete alcohol avoidance for a month should bring about a significant reduction in triglyceride levels, but lifelong abstinence may be necessary. Moderate alcohol consumption produces a small increase in serum HDL-C (0.03–0.05 mmol/L), regardless of its source, and epidemiological studies have demonstrated a reduction in CHD incidence (Durrington, 2007). The effect is insufficient to justify alcohol intake in those who currently abstain.

Plant sterols and stanols

Plant sterols are chemically similar to cholesterol and perform similar functions in plants (see Chapter 5.2, Functional foods). They are found naturally in vegetable oils, nuts, seeds and grains, with a typical diet containing 146–405 mg, although vegetarian intakes are significantly higher (Cassidy & Dalais, 2003). By displacing cholesterol within micelles, both plant sterols and their hydrogenated form (stanols) decrease dietary cholesterol absorption and biliary cholesterol by about 50%. The unabsorbed cholesterol is eliminated in the faeces along with virtually all the plant sterols and stanols. This inhibition of cholesterol absorption results in a compensatory increase in cholesterol synthesis; however, the overall effect is a reduction in circulating LDL-C of up to 10% within a 2–3-week period.

The effect is dose responsive, with an optimal intake of 2–2.5 g/day. Few studies have been conducted with plant sterols over 4 g/day, but two studies with plant stanols at 8.8 g and 9 g per day showed a cholesterol lowering of 17% without significant increases in serum stanol concentrations or reductions in beta carotene (Gylling *et al.*, 2010; Mensink *et al.*, 2010). Such doses are unlikely to be cost-effective for most people, and a ceiling of 3 g/day is normally recommended. The health claim '*plant sterols and plant stanol esters have been shown to lower/reduce blood cholesterol. High cholesterol is a risk factor in the development of coronary heart disease*' has been approved for fortified foods (fat spreads, yoghurts, milks, cheese) (EFSA, 2010). Since plant sterols and stanols work by mixing with food in the gut, fortified foods should always be taken at meal times.

Plant sterols/stanols have been shown to reduce the absorption of beta carotene; however, this can easily be compensated for by a diet rich in fruit and vegetables. Foods fortified with sterols/stanols are not recommended in individuals without hypercholesterolaemia or in pregnant and breastfeeding women, unless medically advised. Plant sterols (but not plant stanols) are contraindicated in homozygous sitosterolaemia, a very rare metabolic lipid condition estimated to affect only 80–100 people worldwide. Modest increases in plasma plant sterols/stanols have not been shown to be associated with increased CVD risk in other groups (Ramprasath *et al.*, 2014).

Soya protein

The soya bean is low in SFAs and cholesterol; is a good source of high-quality vegetable protein, dietary fibre, vitamins, minerals and phytonutrients; and has a low glycaemic index. A number of systematic reviews have demonstrated that soya protein can reduce LDL-C (Anderson *et al.*, 1995; Harland & Haffner, 2008; Reynolds *et al.*, 2006; Zhan & Ho, 2005) via two separate mechanisms. First, soya protein is thought to interfere with LDL-C synthesis; second, the inclusion of soya protein alternatives in the diet can result in the displacement of both SFAs and cholesterol from animal proteins. Together, these effects have been estimated to lower LDL-C by up to 10.3% (4.3% intrinsic and 6% displacement) (Jenkins *et al.*, 2010). A systematic review and meta-analysis showed that even modest intakes of soya proteins (15–25 g) can result in significant reductions in cholesterol, of approximately 6% (Harland & Haffner, 2008).

Nuts

Tree nuts (almond, Brazil nut, beechnut, cashew nut, hazelnut, macadamia nut, pecan nut, pistachio nut and walnut) and peanuts (a legume) are rich in energy, with approximately 75% of the energy coming from fat (predominately MUFAs). The SFA content of nuts is relatively low (approximately 10% of energy) and should not discourage consumption. Epidemiological studies have associated the frequency of nut consumption with a reduced risk of CVD, with a dose–response effect of 35% risk reduction for CHD in those eating the most nuts (Kris-Etherton *et al.*, 2008). Studies of almonds, peanuts, pecan nuts and walnuts have shown an LDL-C lowering effect of 2–19% (Mukuddem-Petersen *et al.*, 2005). The ability of nuts to lower cholesterol may only partly be explained by their favourable lipid profile (Mukuddem-Petersen *et al.*, 2005; Nash & Nash, 2008; Ros *et al.*, 2010). Concerns over the potential of nuts to cause weight gain could be misplaced, as several studies have failed to identify weight gain as a consequence of regular consumption (Higgs, 2005; St-Onge, 2005).

Physical activity

Regular physical activity has beneficial effects on lipid metabolism in overweight and obese individuals, and these are independent of weight loss (Shaw *et al.*, 2006). Increasing aerobic activity has been shown to improve lipid profiles in overweight children and teenagers (Kelley & Kelley, 2007a), adults (Durstine *et al.*, 2001) and older adults (Kelley *et al.*, 2005). Beneficial effects have been shown in both primary (Karmisholt *et al.*, 2005) and secondary (Kelley *et al.*, 2006) prevention, and in people with diabetes (Kelley & Kelley, 2007b).

Smoking

Smoking suppresses levels of HDL-C and increases LDL-C oxidation.

Diagnosis

Biochemistry

A full lipid profile, using venous blood serum, is necessary to aid diagnosis and management of lipid disorders (see Table 7.14.11). This should include the following serum measurements:

- Total cholesterol (mmol/L).
- HDL-C (mmol/L).

Table 7.14.11 Cholesterol targets

	NICE (2015, 2017)	Joint British Societies (2014)
Primary and secondary prevention	40% reduction of non-HDL-C from baseline	Non-HDL-C <2.5 mmol/L LDL-C <1.8 mmol/L
FH	50% reduction of LDL-C from baseline	

- LDL-C (mmol/L) (by Friedwall calculation) or non-HDL-C (by subtraction).
- Total cholesterol to HDL-C ratio (by calculation).
- Triglycerides – levels are raised following a meal, so measurements may need to be made in a fasting state.
- Apolipoproteins – depending on the clinical circumstances.

Monitoring

Small variations in cholesterol and triglyceride levels, resulting from changes in diet, can be difficult to demonstrate due to the variability in many factors, including the following:

- Normal variation in testing of approximately 7% (i.e. a mean total cholesterol of 6.5 mmol/L can fluctuate by ±0.5 mmol/L).
- Menstrual cycle (cholesterol and triglycerides peak mid-cycle).
- Seasonal variations (highest in winter and lowest in summer, perhaps reflecting changes in diet and body weight).
- Inter-laboratory variations.
- Illness or trauma (can reduce cholesterol and raise triglycerides).

Clinical features

Dyslipidaemia is usually symptomless and can therefore go undiagnosed; angina or a heart attack may be the first symptom. Specific signs and symptoms usually only occur if the increase in lipid level is severe over a prolonged period. Exposure to very high cholesterol levels over time may result in:

- Xanthoma – small soft deposits of cholesterol, sometimes seen as a uniform thickening of the Achilles tendon or as nodules in the tendons of the fingers (tendon xanthoma). Palmar xanthoma may be seen as yellow lines in the creases in the palm of the hand. Tuberose xanthoma occur in the form of masses around the elbows or knees.
- Corneal arcus – a white ring visible around the iris of the eye.
- Xanthelasma – small, soft, yellow deposits of cholesterol and other fatty substances found on the skin, often on the eyelids.

Very high triglyceride levels may result in:

- Small, yellow papules with a faint red halo – often found on the skin of the buttocks, thighs and elbows.
- Lipaemia retinalis – plasma lipids visible in the retinal veins and arteries.
- Acute pancreatitis – sudden onset inflammation of the pancreas.
- Hepatosplenomegaly – enlargement of the liver and spleen.

Classification

Classification of primary (familial) dyslipidaemia

The classification and definitions of dyslipidaemia vary. Historically, primary disorders of lipid metabolism were categorised based on the type of lipoprotein that was raised (Frederickson classification), as shown in Table 7.14.12. While this is still of value, a method of classification based on aetiology (genetic cause and the type of lipid raised) is recommended (Table 7.14.13).

Elevated cholesterol

Familial hypercholesterolaemia

Prevalence is estimated at 1 in 500, but may be as high as 1 in 200–300 (Wald *et al.*, 2016), and is caused by an autosomal dominant gene. It dramatically increases the risk of premature CHD before the age of 50 years (possibly much earlier), accounting for 5–10% of early CHD deaths (Holmes *et al.*, 2011). People with FH are eight times more likely to die from CHD, but, if diagnosed and treated early, may have a normal lifespan (Holmes *et al.*, 2011). LDL-C levels are raised from birth, often two to three times higher than normal. People with FH have fewer functional LDL receptors. Most people with FH have the heterozygous form, but 1 in 1 million will have a more severe form (homozygous or compound heterozygous FH), with plasma cholesterol levels as high as 20–30 mmol/L.

It is often accompanied by tendon xanthoma and corneal arcus in undiagnosed older individuals. Diagnosis relies on the Simon Broome criteria and/or genetic testing (NICE, 2008). Children from affected parents should be tested early, ideally at 2–9 years of age. Drug treatment can be started in childhood.

Polygenic hypercholesterolaemia

Polygenic hypercholesterolaemia is common, and is characterised by raised total cholesterol and LDL-C levels (with normal HDL-C and triglyceride levels). Clinical signs such as xanthoma are rare, and LDL-C is elevated to a lesser extent than in FH. Polygenic hypercholesterolaemia results from several genetic factors and their interaction with environmental, largely nutritional, factors (see Chapter 5.1, Genetics and nutritional genomics). Treatment is based on overall cardiovascular risk.

Elevated triglycerides (Chylomicronaemias)

Familial lipoprotein lipase deficiency (LPLD)

LPLD has a prevalence of 1 in 1,000,000, results from a congenital deficiency (autosomal recessive) of the

Table 7.14.12 Fredrickson classification of dyslipidaemia

Phenotype: Fredrickson type	I	IIa	IIb	III	IV	V
Increased lipid fraction	Chylomicrons	LDL	LDL and VLDL	IDL	Triglycerides	VLDL and chylomicrons

LDL, low-density lipoprotein; VLDL, very-low-density lipoprotein; IDL, intermediate-density lipoprotein.

Table 7.14.13 Aetiological classifications of dyslipidaemia

Elevated cholesterol	Familial hypercholesterolaemia – single gene alteration. Polygenic hypercholesterolaemia – influenced by several genes.
Elevated triglycerides	Familial lipoprotein lipase deficiency (familial hypertriglyceridaemia) – single gene. Polygenic hypertriglyceridaemia – influenced by several genes.
Elevated cholesterol and triglycerides	Familial combined hyperlipidaemia (FCH). Familial dyslipoproteinaemia (broad beta disease) is an additional but rare type.

lipoprotein lipase gene, and is characterised by the presence of chylomicrons in fasting plasma. Levels of triglycerides are severely raised from childhood, but the condition may not be diagnosed until adulthood. Symptoms include recurrent abdominal pain, eruptive xanthomata and attacks of acute pancreatitis. Medication has limited benefit. The main treatment is a low-fat diet (20–40 g/day), but restrictions to 10 g or less may occasionally be required. Medium-chain triglycerides (MCTs) should be consumed with caution, as they can exacerbate triglyceride levels (Durrington, 2007). At very low fat intakes, supplements of essential fatty acids and fat-soluble vitamins are required. LPLD patients are at risk of developing type 1 diabetes.

Polygenic hypertriglyceridaemia

This is a group of disorders in which a genetic disposition interacts with environmental factors such as diet; the prevalence is 1 in 100. Plasma triglycerides are elevated, with a normal to slightly elevated cholesterol. Reductions in body weight, refined carbohydrates and alcohol are key elements of management; fish oils may also be prescribed.

Severe polygenic hypertriglyceridaemia (chylomicronaemia syndrome)

This is characterised by the gross accumulation of triglyceride-rich VLDL and chylomicrons, and has a prevalence of 1 in 50,000–100,000; cholesterol is moderately elevated. Uncontrolled diabetes mellitus is often the precipitating factor in those who already have the genetic predisposition.

Elevated cholesterol and triglycerides

Familial combined hyperlipidaemia (FCH)

This is a common disorder (prevalence 1 in 100) characterised by raised levels of VLDL triglyceride and LDL-C, and low HDL-C. The condition is associated with an increased risk of CHD, and is usually diagnosed in adulthood. Environmental factors play a significant role in its expression as people with FCH are often hypertensive and overweight, may be insulin resistant, and have diabetes or gout.

Familial dysbetalipoproteinaemia (broad beta disease, remnant removal disease, floating beta disease, Fredrickson type III)

This is a rare polygenic disorder (prevalence is <1 in 5000) in which abnormal IDL accumulates. This results in the accumulation of broad beta-lipoprotein that carries roughly equal amounts of cholesterol and triglyceride. Intermittent claudication and CHD are equally common symptoms (Durrington & Sniderman, 2005).

Secondary (acquired) dyslipidaemias

Secondary dyslipidaemias can mimic primary dyslipidaemias and have similar consequences, resulting in increased risk of premature CVD or, in the case of high levels of triglycerides, pancreatitis (Table 7.14.14). Treatment of the underlying condition or discontinuation of the offending drugs usually leads to an improvement in the dyslipidaemia. Specific lipid-lowering therapy may be prescribed in individuals at moderate and high risk.

Diabetes and metabolic syndrome

Patients with metabolic syndrome and diabetes are at increased CHD risk, with insulin resistance resulting in increased lipid levels. Dyslipidaemia in diabetes and metabolic syndrome is characterised by raised triglycerides, low HDL-C and increased small, dense LDL particles. Dyslipidaemia is often present in type I diabetes, but HDL-C levels may be increased or normal (Durrington & Sniderman, 2005).

Management

Drug treatment

Lipid-lowering drugs are being increasingly used in the treatment of dyslipidaemia, in patients with established CHD or those at significant risk of developing CHD. They include statins, fibrates, cholesterol absorption inhibitors and PCSK9 inhibitors.

Statins (3-hydroxy-3-methylglutaryl-coenzyme A reductase inhibitors)

Statins are now routinely prescribed for the management of dyslipidaemia, and have been shown to significantly

Table 7.14.14 Conditions and drugs commonly associated with changes in lipid levels (Durrington & Sniderman, 2005)

Condition	Raised cholesterol	Raised triglycerides	Reduced HDL-C
Obesity	X	X	
Excess alcohol intake		X	
Diabetes, metabolic syndrome		X	X
Hypothyroid	X	X	
Anorexia nervosa	X		
Pituitary disease		X	
Cushing's syndrome	X		
Pregnancy	X	X	
Renal disease – nephrotic syndrome	X		
Renal disease – renal failure		X	
Cholestasis	X		
Cholelithiasis, hepatocellular disease		X	
Pancreatitis		X	
Immune disorders – myeloma, macroglobulinaemia, lupus	X	X	
Hyperuricaemia, gout		X	
Drugs			
Beta-blockers		X	
Thiazide diuretics	X	X	
Microsomal enzyme-inducing agents (phenytoin, phenobarbitone, griseofulvin)	X		
Retinoic acid derivatives		X	
HIV antiretroviral therapy	X	X	
Oestrogen		X	
Progesterone	X		
Anabolic steroids	X		X
Amiodarone (antiarrhythmic agent)	X		
Antipsychotic drugs, e.g. olanzapine, clozapine	X		

HDL, high-density lipoprotein.

reduce the risk of vascular events in those at moderate and high risk. Statin therapy is considered cost-effective once the absolute risk of CVD exceeds 10% over a 10-year period (NICE, 2014). Statins reduce LDL-C levels by up to 60% by blocking the enzyme 3-hydroxy-3-methylglutaryl-coenzyme A reductase in the cholesterol production pathway in the liver. Reduced endogenous cholesterol production causes the liver to take up more cholesterol from the blood by activating the LDL receptor genes. This increases the number of effective LDL receptors on the surface of liver cells, which in turn increases uptake and consequently lowers LDL-C levels. Statins also help to stabilise atheroma; improve endothelial function; and have anti-inflammatory, antioxidant and antithrombotic effects. They can increase HDL-C by about 5% and moderately lower triglycerides.

Statins are generally well tolerated and relatively free of side effects. Occasionally, side effects such as muscle-related pain (myopathy) have been reported at higher statin doses. This is usually related to an increase in the muscle enzyme creatinine kinase (CK); elevations of CK (over 10 times normal) should be investigated. In the UK, atorvastatin, simvastatin, pravastatin, fluvastatin and rosuvastatin are available. Those taking simvastatin or atorvastatin need to avoid or restrict their intake of grapefruit juice, respectively, as it reduces statin metabolism, and therefore potentiates their effects. Exaggerated claims in the media about side effect rates have been identified as a cause of underuse and poor compliance in those at increased cardiovascular risk (Collins *et al.*, 2016).

Fibrates

These drugs (e.g. bezafibrate and gemfibrozil) are generally used for mixed dyslipidaemias, and are often used in conjunction with statins in diabetic patients in whom serum triglycerides are significantly raised. They are effective in reducing triglycerides (by reducing VLDL), improving LDL quality and increasing HDL-C.

Cholesterol absorption inhibitors

Cholesterol absorption inhibitors (e.g. ezetimibe) act at the brush border of the small intestine and prevent the absorption of cholesterol; their cholesterol-lowering ability is approximately 18% (Reckless & Morrell, 2005). They are often prescribed when statins are not tolerated, or alongside a lower statin dose.

Pro-protein convertase subtilisin/kexin type 9 inhibitors

In 2016, a new class of potent cholesterol-lowering drugs (pro-protein convertase subtilisin/kexin 9 inhibitors) became available for high-risk patients who are unable to reach lipid-lowering targets on maximum-tolerated traditional therapy. They target the PCSK9 protein, making it less effective at breaking down the LDL receptors that sit on the surface of healthy liver cells and are responsible for taking LDL cholesterol out of the circulation. They are delivered by injection every 2–4 weeks.

Other drug treatments

Other classes of lipid-lowering drugs available include the following:

- Resins or bile acid sequestrants (cholestyramine, colestipol) were used widely to treat hypercholesterolaemia before statins were available, but were poorly tolerated. A non-absorbed lipid-lowering polymer (colesevelam) is better tolerated.
- Omacor (EPA and DHA) has beneficial effects on serum triglyceride levels, lowering them by 25% at 2 g and 31% at 4 g. They may also have anti-thrombotic, anti-inflammatory and anti-arrhythmic effects that are

independent of triglyceride lowering (Davidson & Benes, 2016).

- LDL apheresis involves the complete blood of the patient undergoing a filtration procedure via an external machine (similar to renal dialysis), on a regular basis, so that LDL-C is extracted. It may be used where cholesterol levels remain high or are resistant to drug therapy; however, this technique is not widely available in the UK.

Drug–nutrient interactions

Grapefruit juice reduces the metabolism of simvastatin and atorvastatin, and therefore potentiates their effects.

Dietary treatment and regimens

Mediterranean diet

The Mediterranean diet describes a pattern of eating that is high in MUFAs (from olives and olive oil), being rich in fruit, vegetables, wholegrain cereals, low-fat dairy products, fish, poultry, nuts and pulses, with moderate red wine consumption and relatively little red meat. This dietary pattern was first described in the Seven Countries Study when differences in mean age, blood pressure, serum cholesterol and smoking habits were shown to explain 80% of variance of death from CHD in a 15-year observational study of over 11,000 middle-aged men (Keys *et al.*, 1986). Adherence to a Mediterranean-style diet is consistent with a reduced prevalence and progression of metabolic syndrome, and favourable improvements in components of metabolic syndrome, e.g. HDL-C, triglycerides, blood pressure, blood glucose and waist circumference (Kastorini *et al.*, 2010; Tong *et al.*, 2016).

Portfolio diet

Several individual dietary components have been shown to have an additive cholesterol-lowering effect. The portfolio diet combines specific daily quantities of these: 14–23g of almonds, 1g of plant sterols, 22.5g of soya protein and 10g of soluble fibre per 1000kcal (4.2MJ); together with a low-saturated-fat diet (<7% energy); low dietary cholesterol (<200mg); and 5–10 portions of fruit, vegetables and pulses (Jenkins *et al.*, 2006). Reductions in cholesterol of up to 35% have been demonstrated in metabolic studies (Jenkins *et al.*, 2003a). In free-living populations, average LDL-C reductions of 12–14% were observed. The percentage of cholesterol reduction was linked to the degree of adherence to the diet (Jenkins *et al.*, 2006, 2011), with one-third achieving a >20% reduction in LDL-C at 1 year (Jenkins *et al.*, 2006).

Ultimate cholesterol-lowering plan

The ultimate cholesterol lowering plan (UCLP) combines a step-by-step approach to cholesterol lowering with motivational interviewing techniques. It is a modified portfolio diet that encourages patient compliance through discussion, patient choice and commitment to a range of small dietary changes. The baseline diet (<10% of energy from saturated fat; five portions of fruit and vegetables, one of pulses and two of fish, one of which is oily) can be enhanced by including one or more of the four cholesterol-lowering food types (15–25g of soya protein, 1.5–2.4g of plant sterols/stanols, 30g of nuts and 15–20g of soluble fibre).

A summary of dietary advice for the management of dyslipidaemias is shown in Table 7.14.15, while Table 7.14.16 summarises the evidence for the use of dietary interventions.

Table 7.14.15 Summary of dietary advice for the management of dyslipidaemia

Raised total and LDL-C cholesterol (with normal HDL-C and triglyceride levels)	Moderately raised triglyceride levels (with normal total, LDL-C and HDL-C levels)	Raised total and LDL-C, and raised triglyceride levels	Low HDL-C
Reduce SFA intake. Partial substitution of SFAs with PUFAs and MUFAs, to a level of energy intake appropriate for body weight. Encourage the consumption of foods that actively lower cholesterol. Moderate intake of dietary cholesterol only if excessive, and in FH if failing to achieve target levels.	If obese, weight loss is the overriding treatment priority. Energy reduction should come from a reduction in SFAs and total fat, and refined carbohydrate, and activity should be increased. Remaining carbohydrates should be from more complex sources, especially those with a low glycaemic index. Encourage oily fish. Reduce or avoid alcohol intake.	If obese, weight loss is the overriding treatment priority. Reduce SFA and total fat intake. Partial substitution with PUFAs and MUFAs to a level of energy intake appropriate for body weight. Encourage the consumption of foods that actively lower cholesterol. Replace high intakes of refined carbohydrates with more complex sources of carbohydrate, especially those with a low glycaemic index. Reduce or avoid alcohol. Moderate intake of dietary cholesterol if excessive.	Modest alcohol intake (1–2 units/day) is acceptable. Ensure that total fat intake is not reduced too low. Replace some SFAs with PUFAs and MUFAs. Stop smoking (this depresses HDL-C). Encourage physical activity.

LDL-C, low density lipoprotein-cholesterol; HDL-C, high density lipoprotein-cholesterol; SAF, saturated fatty acids; MUFA, monounsaturated fatty acids; PUFA, polyunsaturated fatty acids; FH, familial hypercholesterolaemia.

Table 7.14.16 Evidence to support dietary recommendations for total fat and fatty acid intake in adults (Brouwer, 2016; FAO/WHO, 2008; Mensink, 2016)

	Convincing	Probable	Possible
Total fat		No relation with CHD events or fatal CHD.	
SFAs	Increases LDL-C and TC:HDL-C ratio when compared to PUFAs and MUFAs.		
MUFAs	Decreases LDL-C and TC:HDL-C ratio when substituted for SFAs.		Reduces risk of metabolic syndrome.
Total PUFAs	Decreases LDL-C and TC:HDL-C ratio when substituted for SFAs. Reduces risk of CHD events.		Reduces risk of metabolic syndrome. Increases lipid oxidation with high consumption, especially if vitamin E intake is low.
n-6 PUFAs	Decreases LDL-C and TC:HDL-C ratio when substituted for SFAs. Reduces risk of CHD events.	Reduces risk of metabolic syndrome.	
n-3 PUFAs	Reduces risk of CHD events (DHA and EPA).		Decreases risk of total CHD events and stroke.
TFAs	Lowers HDL-C and increases TC:HDL-C ratio in comparison to SFAs, MUFAs and PUFAs. Increases risk of CHD events.	Increases risk of metabolic syndrome. Increases risk of fatal CHD and sudden cardiac death.	

CHD, coronary heart disease; TC, total cholesterol; LDL-C, low-density lipoprotein cholesterol; HDL-C, high-density lipoprotein cholesterol; DHA, docosahexaenoic acid; EPA, eicosapentaenoic acid.

Internet resources

British Heart Foundation, www.bhf.org.uk
HEART UK – The Cholesterol Charity, www.heartuk.org.uk

References

Anderson J, Hanna T. (1999) Impact of non-digestible carbohydrates on serum lipoproteins and risk for cardiovascular disease. *J. Nutr.* 129: 1457S–1466S.

Anderson J, Konz E. (2001) Obesity and disease management: effects of weight loss on comorbid conditions. *Obes. Res.* 9: 326S–334S.

Anderson J, Johnstone B, Cook-Newell M. (1995) Meta-analysis of the effects of soy protein intake on serum lipids. *N. Engl. J. Med.* 333: 276–282.

Aronne L, Isoldi K. (2007) Overweight and obesity: key components of cardiometabolic risk. *Clin. Cornerstone.* 8: 29–37.

Astrup A, Dyerberg J, Elwood P, *et al.* (2011) The role of reducing intakes of saturated fat in the prevention of cardiovascular disease: where does the evidence stand in 2010. *Am. J. Clin. Nutr.* 93: 684–688.

Aucott L, Gray D, Rothnie H, *et al.* (2011) Effects of lifestyle interventions and long-term weight loss on lipid outcomes – a systematic review. *Obes. Rev.* 12(5): e412–425.

Banach M. (2016) Lipoprotein (a) We know so much yet have much to learn. *J. Am. Heart Assoc.* 5: e003597

Bates B, Cox L, Nicholson S, *et al.* (2016) *National Diet and Nutrition Survey: Results from Year 5 and 6 (combined) of the Rolling Programme (2012/2013).* London: PHE and FSA.

Bendsen NT, Christensen R, Bartels EM, *et al.* (2011) Consumption of industrially and ruminant trans fatty acids and risk of coronary heart disease: a systematic review and meta-analysis of cohort studies. *Eur. J. Clin. Nutr.* 65: 773–783.

Brouwer IA (2016) *Effects of trans- fatty acid intake on blood lipids and lipoproteins: a systematic review and meta-regression analysis.* Available at http://apps.who.int/iris/bitstream/handle/10665/246109/9789241510608-eng.pdf;jsessionid=DF1D672A983704B0501EB36BE2191B46?sequence=1. Accessed 14 November 2018.

Brown L, Rosner B, Willett W, *et al.* (1999) Cholesterol lowering effects of dietary fibre: a meta-analysis. *Am. J. Clin. Nutr.* 69: 30–42.

Carmena R, Ascaso J, Real J. (2001) Impact of obesity in primary hyperlipidemias. *Nutr. Metab. Cardiovasc. Dis.* 11: 354–359.

Cassidy A, Dalais F. (2003) *Nutrition and Metabolism – Phytochemicals.* Oxford: Blackwell Science.

Castro IA, Barroso LP, Sinnecker P. (2005) Functional foods for coronary heart disease risk reduction: a meta-analysis using a multivariate approach. *Am. J. Clin. Nutr.* 82(1): 32–40.

Chan D, Barrett H, Watts G. (2004) Dyslipidemia in visceral obesity: mechanisms, implications, and therapy. *Am. J. Cardiovasc. Drugs* 4: 227–246.

Cholesterol Treatment Trialists' Collaboration (CTTC). (2005) Efficacy and safety of cholesterol-lowering treatment: prospective meta-analysis of data from 90,056 participants in 14 randomised trials of statins. *Lancet.* 366: 1267–1278.

Chowdhury R, Warnakula S, Kunutsor S, *et al.* (2014) Association of dietary, circulating and supplement fatty acids with coronary risk. *Ann. Intern. Med.* 160(6): 398–406.

Collins R, Reith C, Emberson J, *et al.* (2016) Interpretation of the evidence for the efficacy and safety of statin therapy. *Lancet.* Online September 8.

Constanza MC, Cayanis E, Ross BM, *et al.* (2004) Relative contributions of genes, environment and interactions to blood lipid concentrations in a general adult population. *Am. J. Epidemiol.* 161(8): 714–724.

Davidson MH, Benes LB. (2016) The future of n3 polyunsaturated fatty acid therapy. *Curr. Opin. Lipidol.* 27: 570–578.

de Souza RJ, Mente A, Maroleanu A, *et al.* (2015) Intake of saturated and trans unsaturated fatty acids and risk of all cause mortality, cardiovascular disease, and type 2 diabetes: systematic review and meta-analysis of observational studies. *BMJ.* 351: h3978.

DH (COMA). (1994) *Nutritional Aspects of Cardiovascular Disease.* London: HMSO.

Durrington PN. (2007) *Hyperlipidaemia: Diagnosis and Management*, 3rd edn. London: Hodder Arnold.

Durrington P, Sniderman A. (2005) *Hyperlipidaemia*. Oxford: Health Press Limited.
Durstine J, Grandjean P, Davis P, *et al.* (2001) Blood lipid and lipoprotein adaptations to exercise: a quantitative analysis. *Sports Med.* 31: 1033–1062.
EFSA. (2010) *Commission Regulation (EU) No 384/2010*. Official Journal of the European Union 53.
FAO. (2010) *Fats and fatty acids in human nutrition – report of an expert consultation*. Rome: FAO.
Gylling H, Hallikainen M, Nissinen MJ, *et al.* (2010) Very high plant stanol intake and serum plant stanols and non-cholesterol sterols. *Eur. J. Nutr.* 49: 111–117.
Harland J, Haffner T. (2008) Systematic review, meta-analysis and regression of randomised controlled trials reporting an association between an intake ~25 g soy protein per day and blood cholesterol. *Atherosclerosis*. 200: 13–27.
Hecker K, Kris-Etherton PM, Zhao G, *et al.* (1999) Impact of body weight and weight loss on cardiovascular risk factors. *Curr. Atheroscler. Rep.* 1: 236–242.
Henderson L, Gregory J, Irving K, *et al.* (2003) *The National Diet and Nutrition Survey: adults aged 19–64 years: Energy, protein, carbohydrate, fat and alcohol intake. FSA, DoH, OfNS, MRC Human Nutrition Research*. London: TSO.
Higgs J. (2005) The potential role of peanuts in the prevention of obesity. *Nutr. Food Sci.* 35: 353–358.
Holmes MV, Harrison S, Talmud PJ, *et al.* (2011) Utility of genetic determinants of lipids and cardiovascular events in assessing risk. *Nat. Rev. Cardiol.* 8: 207–221.
Hooper L, Thompson RL, Harrison RA, *et al.* (2004) Omega 3 fats for the treatment and prevention of cardiovascular disease. *Cochrane Database Syst. Rev.* 4: CD003177.
Jenkins D, Kendall C, Marchie A, *et al.* (2002) Dose response of almonds on coronary heart disease risk factors: Blood lipids, low density lipoproteins, lipoprotein(a), homocysteine and pulmonary nitric oxide: a randomised, controlled, crossover trial. *Circulation*. 106: 1327–1332.
Jenkins D, Kendall C, Marchie A, *et al.* (2003a) The effect of combining plant sterols, soy protein, viscous fibers, and almonds in treating hypercholesterolemia. *Metabolism*. 52: 1478–1483.
Jenkins D, Kendall C, Marchie A, *et al.* (2003b) Effects of dietary portfolio of cholesterol-lowering foods vs lovastatin on serum lipids and C-reactive protein. *JAMA*. 290: 502–510.
Jenkins D, Kendall C, Faulkner D, *et al.* (2006) Assessment of the longer-term effects of a dietary portfolio of cholesterol-lowering foods in hypercholesterolaemia. *Am. J. Clin. Nutr.* 83: 582–591.
Jenkins D, Mirrahimi A, Srichaikul K, *et al.* (2010) Soy protein reduces serum cholesterol by both intrinsic and food displacement mechanisms. *J. Nutr.* 140(12): 2302S–2311S.
Jenkins DJA, Jones PJ, Lamarche B, *et al.* (2011) Effect of a dietary portfolio of cholesterol lowering foods given at 2 levels of intensity of dietary advice on serum lipids in hyperlipidaemia. *JAMA*. 306: 831–839.
Joint British Societies. (2014) JBS3 consensus recommendations for the prevention of cardiovascular disease. *Heart*. 100: ii1–ii67.
Karmisholt K, Gyntelberg F, Gøtzche P. (2005) Physical activity for primary prevention of disease. Systematic reviews of randomised clinical trials. *Dan. Med. Bull.* 52(2): 86–89.
Kastorini CM, Milionis HK, Esposito K, *et al.* (2010) The effect of Mediterranean diet on metabolic syndrome and its components: a meta-analysis of 50 studies and 534,906 individuals. *J. Am. Coll. Cardiol.* 57: 1299–1313.
Kelley G, Kelley K. (2007a) Aerobic exercise and lipids and lipoproteins in children and adolescents: a meta-analysis of randomized controlled trials. *Atherosclerosis* 191: 447–453.
Kelley G, Kelley K. (2007b) Effects of aerobic exercise on lipids and lipoproteins in adults with type 2 diabetes: a meta-analysis of randomized-controlled trials. *Public Health* 121: 643–655.
Kelley G, Kelley K, Tran Z. (2005) Exercise, lipids, and lipoproteins in older adults: a meta-analysis. *Prev. Cardiol.* 8: 206–214.
Kelley G, Kelley K, Franklin B. (2006) Aerobic exercise and lipids and lipoproteins in patients with cardiovascular disease: a meta-analysis of randomized controlled trials. *J. Cardiopulm. Rehabil.* 26: 131–144.
Keys A, Menotti A, Karvonen M, *et al.* (1986) The diet and 15-year death rate in the seven countries study. *Am. J. Epidemiol.* 124: 903–915.
Ko DT, Alter DA, Guo H, *et al.* (2016) High density lipoprotein cholesterol and cause specific mortality in individuals without previous cardiovascular conditions. *JACC* 68(19): 2073–2083.
Kris-Etherton P, Hu F, Ros E, *et al.* (2008) The role of tree nuts and peanuts in the prevention of coronary heart disease: multiple potential mechanisms. *J. Nutr.* 138: 1746S.
Kronenberg F, Utermann G. (2012) Lipoprotein(a): resurrected by genetics. *J. Intern. Med.* 273: 6–30.
Law MR, Wald NJ, Rudnicka AR. (2003) Quantifying effect of statins on low density lipoprotein cholesterol, ischaemic heart disease, and stroke: systematic review and meta-analysis. *BMJ*. 326: 1407–1408.
Mensink RP. (2016) *Effects of saturated fatty acids on serum lipids and lipoproteins: a systematic review and regression analysis*. WHO.
Mensink RP, de Jong A, Lutjohann D, *et al.* (2010) Plant stanols dose-dependently decrease LDL-cholesterol concentrations but not cholesterol-standardized fat-soluble antioxidant concentrations at intakes up to 9 g/d. *Am J. Clin. Nutr.* 92: 24–33.
Mukuddem-Petersen J, Oosthuizen W, Jerling J. (2005) A systematic review of the effects of nuts on lipid profiles in humans. *J. Nutr.* 135: 2082–2089.
Nash S, Nash D. (2008) Nuts as part of a healthy cardiovascular diet. *Curr. Atheroscler. Rep.* 10: 529–535.
NICE. (2017) *Familial hypercholesterolaemia CG71*. Available at https://www.nice.org.uk/Guidance/CG71. Accessed 14 November 2018.
NICE. (2014) Cardiovascular disease: risk assessment and reduction, including lipid modification. Available at https://www.nice.org.uk/guidance/CG181. Accessed 13 November 018.
NICE. (2015) *CG181: Cardiovascular disease: risk assessment and reduction, including lipid modification*. Available at https://www.nice.org.uk/guidance/CG181. Accessed 14 November 2018.
Nordestgaard B, Varbo A. (2014) Lipids and cardiovascular disease 3: triglycerides and cardiovascular disease. *Lancet*. 384: 626–635.
Oomen C, Ocke M, Feskens E, *et al.* (2001) Association between trans fatty acid intake and 10 year risk of coronary heart disease in Zutphen Elderly Study: A prospective population based study. *Lancet*. 357: 746–751.
Poobalan A, Aucott L, Smith W, *et al.* (2004) Effects of weight loss in overweight/obese individuals and long-term lipid outcomes–a systematic review. *Obes. Rev.* 5: 43–50.
Praagman J, Beulens JWJ, Alssema M, *et al.* (2016) The association between dietary saturated fatty acids and ischaemic heart disease depends on the type and source of fatty acids in the EPIC and nutrition – Netherlands cohort. *Am. J. Clin. Nutr.* 103(2): 356–365. doi: 10.3945/ajcn115.122671
Rader D, Hovingh G. (2014) Lipids and cardiovascular disease 2: HDL and cardiovascular disease. *Lancet*. 384: 618–625.
Ramprasath VR, Jenkins DJA, Lamarche B, *et al.* (2014) Consumption of a dietary portfolio of cholesterol lowering foods improves blood lipids without affecting concentrations of fat soluble compounds. *Nutr. J.* 13: 101–113.
Rashid S, Genest J. (2007) Effect of obesity on high-density lipoprotein metabolism. *Obesity (Silver Spring)*. 15: 2875–2888.
Reckless J, Morrell J. (2005) *Lipid Disorders – Your Questions Answered*. London: Churchill Livingstone.
Reynolds K, Chin A, Lees K, *et al.* (2006) A meta-analysis of the effect of soy protein supplementation on serum lipids. *Am. J. Cardiol.* 98: 633–640.
Roche HM, Gibney MJ. (2000) Effect of long-chain n-3 polyunsaturated fatty acids on fasting and postprandial triacylglycerol metabolism. *Am. J. Clin. Nutr.* 71(S1): 232S–237S.

Ros E, Tapsell L, Sabate J. (2010) Nuts and berries for heart health. *Curr. Atheroscler. Rep.* 12: 397–406.

SACN. (2007) *Update on Trans Fatty Acids and Health: Position Statement*. Available at https://www.gov.uk/government/uploads/system/uploads/attachment_data/file/339359/SACN_Update_on_Trans_Fatty_Acids_2007.pdf. Accessed 16 October 2017.

SACN. (2015) *Carbohydrates and Health*. Available at https://www.gov.uk/government/uploads/system/uploads/attachment_data/file/445503/SACN_Carbohydrates_and_Health.pdf. Accessed 16 February 2017.

Shaw K, Gennat H, O'Rourke P, *et al.* (2006) Exercise for overweight or obesity. *Cochrane Database Syst. Rev.* (3): CD003817.

Siri-Tarino PW, Sun Q, Hu FB, *et al.* (2010) Meta-analysis of prospective cohort studies evaluating the association of saturated fat with cardiovascular disease. *Am. J. Clin. Nutr.* 91(3): 535–546.

St-Onge M. (2005) Dietary fats, teas, dairy, and nuts: potential functional foods for weight control? *Am. J. Clin. Nutr.* 81: 7–15.

Tong TYN, Wareham NJ, Khaw KT, *et al.* (2016) Prospective association of the Mediterranean diet with cardiovascular disease incidence and mortality and its population impact in a non-Mediterranean population: the EPIC Norfolk study. *BMC Med.* 14: 135.

Truswell AS. (2002) Cereal grains and coronary heart disease. *Eur. J. Clin. Nutr.* 56(1): 1–14.

Wald DS, Bestwick JP, Morris JK, *et al.* (2016) Child-parent familial hypercholesterolaemia screening in primary care. *N. Engl. J. Med.* 375: 1628–1637.

WHO. (2008) *The Global Burden of Disease: 2004 Update*. Geneva: WHO.

WHO. (2016) *World Health Statistics: Monitoring the Health for the SDGs*. Available at who.int/gho/publications/world_health_statistics/en. Accessed 16 April 2018.

Zhan S, Ho S. (2005) Meta-analysis of the effects of soy protein containing isoflavones on lipid profile. *Am. J. Clin. Nutr.* 81: 397–408.

Zong G, Yanping L, Wanders AJ, *et al.* (2016) Intake of individual saturated fatty acids and risk of coronary heart disease in US men and women: two prospective longitudinal cohort studies. *BMJ.* 355: i5796.

7.14.4 Hypertension

Mary Ward and Martina Rooney

Key points

- Hypertension is the strongest modifiable risk factor for cardiovascular disease worldwide.
- Obesity, physical inactivity, high salt intake and excessive alcohol consumption are major contributory factors to the development of hypertension.
- Diet and lifestyle modification is an integral part of management of all hypertensive patients, whether on drug therapy or not.
- A reduction in blood pressure leads to significant benefits in terms of cardiovascular risk; however, despite the availability of very effective BP-lowering drugs, >40% of adults with hypertension do not achieve target BP.

Hypertension (high blood pressure) is a major risk factor for stroke, myocardial infarction (MI), heart failure, chronic kidney disease, cognitive decline and premature death (NICE, 2016). Globally, about 51% of strokes and 45% of cases of coronary heart disease (CHD) are estimated to be attributable to high systolic blood pressure (BP) (WHO, 2013). In people with diabetes, hypertension significantly increases the risk of both cardiovascular and microvascular complications, particularly diabetic nephropathy. Hypertension is responsible for 13% of global mortality (WHO, 2017), and is one of the most important preventable causes of premature morbidity and mortality (NICE, 2016).

BP is the measurement of the force exerted by the blood circulating in the arteries. The force with which the heart pumps blood, the diameter of the blood vessels and the volume of circulating blood influence BP. When taking a BP reading, two figures are recorded:

- *Systolic pressure (SBP)* – the force during contraction of the heart ventricles.
- *Diastolic pressure (DBP)* – the BP during relaxation of the heart ventricles.

BP is measured in millimetres of mercury (mmHg), and is expressed as systolic/diastolic. The most common method of measuring BP in the clinical setting is using a standard sphygmomanometer. However, it is now recognised that a one-off clinic BP reading is not the most reliable measure of an individual's true BP, and that it is subject to considerable variability (Clement *et al.*, 2003). Twenty-four-hour ambulatory BP monitoring (ABPM) is increasingly being used to confirm the diagnosis of hypertension. Current UK guidelines recommend that if clinic BP is recorded as ≥140/90 mmHg, ABPM should be used to confirm a diagnosis of hypertension, with at least two measurements per waking hour. Home BP monitoring (HBPM) may also be used, ideally to include two diurnal readings for 7 days (NICE, 2016). Using either of these methods, BP readings of ≥135/85 mmHg indicates hypertension (NICE, 2016). Used in conjunction with clinic measurements, ABPM and HBPM are now recognised as superior predictors of future cardiovascular disease (CVD) as compared to clinic BP measurements alone (Myers, 2005).

Definitions of normal and abnormal BP are summarised in the British Hypertension Society Guidelines

Table 7.14.17 Blood pressure (BP) classification (NICE, 2016; Williams *et al.*, 2004)

Category	SBP (mmHg)	DBP (mmHg)
Optimal BP	<120	<80
Normal BP	<130	<85
High normal BP	130–139	85–89
Stage 1 hypertension	140–159	90–99
Stage 2 hypertension	160–179	100–109
Severe hypertension	≥180	≥110

Note: Ambulatory blood pressure measurement (ABPM) daytime average of >135/85 mmHg is diagnostic of hypertension. SBP, systolic blood pressure; DBP, diastolic blood pressure.

(Williams *et al.*, 2004), and updated in the NICE (2016) guidelines on the clinical management of primary hypertension in adults, as shown in Table 7.14.17. Similar guidance has been reported by European and WHO expert committees (Mancia *et al.*, 2013). In healthy adults, optimal SBP is considered to be <120 mmHg, and DBP <80 mmHg (120/80). In 2017, the American Heart Association updated clinical practice guidelines for the management of BP to redefine hypertension as 130/80 mmHg, removing the pre-hypertensive cut-off. This recommendation was largely driven by results from the SPRINT trial, which demonstrated that achieving an SBP of >120 mmHg, compared to <140 mmHg, led to lower rates of fatal and nonfatal major cardiovascular events. Hypertension is usually symptomless and often only discovered as a result of routine health screening, or when overt signs of CVD develop.

Prevalence

It is estimated that 13.4 million people in England have either GP-recorded or undiagnosed hypertension, which represents approximately 24% of the population. Undiagnosed hypertension prevalence ranges from 9.4% to 14%. (PHE, 2017). Prevalence rises steeply with age, so that, by the age of 75 years, 66% of men and 78% of women are estimated to be hypertensive. Prevalence is higher among men as compared to women at all ages. The prevalence of hypertension in childhood is increasing (Din-Dzietham *et al.*, 2007). Raised BP levels in childhood are associated with higher levels in adulthood (Chen & Wang, 2008; Flynn, 2013).

A role of genetics in BP is well established. In recent years, a large number of genome-wide association studies have contributed to the understanding of how specific genetic factors contribute to changes in BP. The genetics of hypertension is complicated, with single genes not thought to play a major role; instead, multiple genes each contribute smaller effects, which in turn are influenced by different environmental factors. One recent example of a gene–nutrient interaction that has been shown to have a role in modulating BP is the association between the B-vitamin riboflavin and a common polymorphism (C677T) in the folate-metabolising enzyme methylenetetrahydrofolate reductase (MTHFR). In a series of randomised controlled trials, riboflavin, supplemented at the dietary level of 1.6 mg/day, was shown to lower BP by 5–13 mmHg in genetically at-risk adults (McNulty *et al.*, 2017). These findings have important implications for BP treatment and management in adults who carry this polymorphism, i.e. approximately 10% of UK adults, but as many as 30% in some populations.

Genetic influences on BP may be particularly marked in some minority ethnic groups. The recent SABRE study by Park *et al.* (2016) found hypertension to be significantly more prevalent in those of South Asian or African-Caribbean descent (as compared to Europeans), findings that are consistent with early studies focused on these populations (Cappuccio *et al.*, 1997).

Prognostic significance

Hypertension, smoking and raised blood cholesterol are the three main modifiable risk factors for CHD, and hypertension is the single largest risk factor for stroke. People with hypertension are three times more likely to die from heart disease and four times more likely to die from stroke as compared to people with normal BP (Centre for Disease Control and Prevention; CDC, 2014). The increased risk of cardiovascular events is associated with both SBP and DBP. The risk increases progressively in a linear relationship, starting at about 115/75 mm/Hg (Chobanian *et al.*, 2003; Lewington *et al.*, 2002). Meta-analysis of prospective data from 1 million adults has shown that each 20 mmHg increase in usual SBP, or 10 mmHg increase in DBP, doubles the risk of death from CVD (Lewington *et al.*, 2002).

Reducing BP, particularly SBP, significantly reduces the risk of CHD and stroke (Falashetti *et al.*, 2014; Mozaffarian *et al.*, 2016). Reducing BP by 10 mmHg can reduce stroke by 41% and CHD events by 22% (Law *et al.*, 2009). A recent meta-analysis showed that a decrease of 10 mmHg in SBP can reduce the risk of a major cardiovascular event by 20%, stroke by 27% and coronary heart disease by 17%, with a reduction of 13% in all-cause mortality (Ettehad *et al.*, 2016). In people with diabetes, treatment of hypertension also reduces the risk of diabetic microvascular complications, as well as CVD (UKPDS, 1998). The American Heart Association has recommended an emphasis on approaches to targeting lifestyle and treatment at the individual level (Mozaffarian *et al.*, 2016).

Risk factors

Hypertension occurs when the vessels through which the blood flows become too narrow, or the volume of circulating blood too high. Raised BP increases the workload on the heart and can damage the endothelial lining of blood vessels. It also increases the infiltration of blood components such as lipids into the arterial wall, exacerbating endothelial damage, enhancing atherosclerotic deposition and, ultimately, increasing cardiovascular risk. Primary hypertension accounts for approximately 90% of cases. The remaining 10% of cases are secondary to a specific cause such as renal or liver disease, cardiac failure and pregnancy. The pathogenesis of primary hypertension remains unknown and probably results from the interaction of a number of factors, including the effects of the ageing process on renal function and peripheral resistance, genetic susceptibility, and environmental influences, such as smoking, stress, diet and lifestyle. The most significant diet and lifestyle influences are overweight and obesity, and excess intakes of salt and/or alcohol (Williams *et al.*, 2004).

Obesity

Obesity is long established as a risk factor for hypertension, with early evidence from the Framingham study reporting that hypertension was twice as likely in obese subjects (Hubert *et al.*, 1983). The Nurses' Health Study found that the incidence of hypertension was up to six times higher in those with a BMI of >29 kg/m², as compared to those with a BMI of <22 kg/m² (Manson *et al.*, 1995); over half of those diagnosed with hypertension were obese (Ford *et al.*, 2008). It is well recognised that BP increases with increasing body mass index (BMI; Higgins *et al.*, 1988). Weight gain with age is recognised to significantly contribute to the rise in hypertension with age (Burt *et al.*, 1995; Yang *et al.*, 2007). Furthermore, and importantly, it is estimated that a weight loss of 5–10% of body weight can reduce both SBP and DBP by 5 mmHg, with further benefits observed with greater weight loss (Wing *et al.*, 2011). A sustained weight loss of 10 kg is associated with a reduction in SBP of up to 20 mmHg (Chobanian *et al.*, 2003). Raised BP is particularly linked to central adiposity, and this association is more marked in men than women (Benetou *et al.*, 2004; Canoy *et al.*, 2004; Strazzullo, 2002). Indeed, obesity may cause hemodynamic alterations in cardiac morphology and ventricular function (Alpert *et al.*, 2014).

Salt intake

Sodium, taken as dietary salt, is a major contributor to raised BP and the age-related rise. Evidence comes from a variety of sources, including epidemiological, migration, intervention, treatment, animal and genetic studies (He & MacGregor, 2010; Sacks *et al.*, 2001). The relationship between salt and BP is direct and dose related (Denton *et al.*, 1995; Ezzati *et al.*, 2002; Sacks *et al.*, 2001). Evidence from meta-analysis concluded that high dietary salt intake is associated with an increase in stoke and cardiovascular events; a 5-g higher daily salt intake is associated with a 23% increased risk of stroke, and a 17% increased risk of total CVD (Strazzullo *et al.*, 2009). An investigation into childhood BP found BMI and sodium intake to be independently associated with elevated BP (Rosner *et al.*, 2013).

Alcohol

Many epidemiological studies have shown a direct and linear association between alcohol consumption and increased BP, particularly with regular heavy consumption of alcohol or binge drinking (Klatsky *et al.*, 1977; Puddey *et al.*, 1999; Xin *et al.*, 2001). High levels of alcohol consumption are associated with a high risk of stroke, particularly in those who engage in binge drinking (Wannamethee & Shaper, 1996). Genetic polymorphisms may also have a role to play, as several single-nucleotide polymorphisms have been shown to be expressed differently in drinkers as compared to non-drinkers, with significant effects on SBP, DBP and pulse pressure (Yin *et al.*, 2015).

Management

Antihypertensive therapy can result in reductions in stroke, MI and heart failure by 20–50% (Neal *et al.*, 2000). The management of hypertension has changed in recent years, and BP levels alone no longer determine treatment. Risk models should be used to predict the likelihood of developing CHD or stroke over 10 years, taking into account gender, age, family history, diabetic status, smoking status, total cholesterol, high-density lipoprotein (HDL) cholesterol and BP (NICE, 2010). Current recommendations according to NICE guidelines (2016) are as follows:

- Pharmacological treatment should be initiated when SBP ≥160 mmHg or DBP ≥100 mmHg, and a daytime average ABPM >150/95 (stage 2 hypertension).
- When SBP is 140–159 mmHg and/or DBP is 90–99 mmHg, pharmacological treatment (stage 1 hypertension) should be decided on the basis of established CVD, diabetes, target organ damage (e.g. kidney), or an estimated CVD risk of >20% over 10 years.
- People with high normal BP (130–139/85–89 mmHg) should be given diet and lifestyle advice and reassessed annually.

For most patients, optimal goals for BP treatment are ≤140 mmHg SBP and ≤85 mmHg DBP. For patients with diabetes, renal impairment or established CVD, a lower target of ≤130/80 mmHg is recommended.

Drug treatment

Classes of drugs that may be used include the following:

- *Angiotensin-converting enzyme (ACE) inhibitors* – reduce production of the vasoconstrictor angiotensin II.
- *Angiotensin II receptor antagonists* – an alternative for people who cannot tolerate ACE inhibitors.
- *Alpha-blockers* – block alpha-adrenoceptors and have vasodilatory effects.
- *Beta-blockers* – reduce the stimulating action of noradrenaline by blocking beta-adrenoceptors in the heart and peripheral vasculature. Beta-blockers lower BP primarily by reducing the force and rate of cardiac output.
- *Calcium channel blockers* – inhibit smooth muscle contraction in blood vessel walls.
- *Thiazide diuretics* – inhibit sodium reabsorption from the distal tubules of the kidney, thereby increasing fluid loss and reducing blood volume.

Many of the drugs used to treat hypertension are also used in the management of CVD; therefore, the choice of drug will be influenced by the nature of any clinical symptoms, as well as other factors such as age and renal function. Most people require more than one drug in order to achieve an optimal level of control.

Diet and lifestyle

Guidelines on the management of hypertension emphasise the importance of diet and lifestyle changes (NICE, 2016). All people with BP above the normal range should be given diet and lifestyle advice. If implemented, such measures have been shown to avert the need for drug treatment, or to reduce the dosage of antihypertensive drugs required (Appel *et al.*, 1997; Whelton *et al.*, 1998). Diet and lifestyle measures may be the only form of treatment needed in people with stage 1 hypertension who have no other evidence of CVD. The effectiveness of lifestyle measures alone should be evaluated for up to 6 months.

People with borderline or high normal BP should also be encouraged to adopt protective diet and lifestyle measures. These can reduce the age-associated rise in BP, and hence delay or prevent the need for antihypertensive drugs in the future. Dietary advice should be given in the context of general cardioprotection, and tailored to individual risk factors and nutritional priorities. Diet and lifestyle measures that should be strongly recommended to people with hypertension are given in Table 7.14.18.

Weight management

Weight loss, whether by dietary means or physical activity, can result in clinically significant reductions in BP. A meta-analysis (Neter *et al.*, 2003) concluded that a reduction in weight by energy restriction and/or increased physical activity of 1 kg would result in a fall in both SBP and DBP of 1 mmHg. The BP-lowering effect of weight loss persists over longer periods, particularly if it is maintained (Harsha & Bray, 2008). A meta-analysis by Zomer *et al.* (2016) found that weight loss interventions significantly reduces both SBP and DBP by 2.68 mmHg and 1.34 mmHg, respectively. Weight loss of 10 kg has been shown to reduce SBP by up to 20 mmHg (Chobanian *et al.*, 2003).

Table 7.14.18 Lifestyle modifications to prevent and manage hypertension

Lifestyle modification	Approximate SBP lowering (mmHg) (Aronow *et al.*, 2011)
Lose weight if overweight or obese.	5–20 mmHg/10 kg weight loss
Reduce sodium intake to <6 g of salt/day.	2–8
Limit alcohol consumption to <3 units/day for men and <2 units/day for women. Less advisable if overweight. Binge drinking must be avoided.	2–4
Take regular aerobic physical exercise, ideally for >30 minutes/day, on at least 5 days/week.	4–9
Consume at least five portions/day of fruit and vegetables. Dietary Approaches to Stop Hypertension (DASH) diet.	8–14

SBP, systolic blood pressure.

Dietary salt reduction

The BP-lowering effect of salt restriction is widely reported. A meta-analysis (He & MacGregor, 2002) of trials of >1-month duration concluded that a 6-g reduction in dietary salt lowered BP by 7/4 mmHg in hypertensive individuals, and by 4/2 mmHg in those who were normotensive; the effects observed were in a dose-responsive manner. More recently, the same authors reported that a 4.4-g reduction in salt intake resulted in a lowering of 5.39 mmHg in SBP and 2.82 mmHg in DBP in those with hypertension, double the benefit observed in normotensives of 2.42 mmHg and 1 mmHg, respectively (He *et al.*, 2013). Taylor *et al.* (2011) reported that a decrease in salt intake of 2.3 g/day in hypertensives reduced SBP by 4.14 mmHg, while a reduction of 2 g/day was found to decrease both SBP and DBP in normotensives by 1.1 and 0.8 mmHg, respectively. Reducing salt intake to under 2 g/day was found to reduce SBP by 3.47 mmHg and DBP by 1.81 mmHg (Aburto *et al.*, 2013).

The reduction in BP in response to sodium restriction has been shown to be even more striking in patients with resistant hypertension (i.e. those who do not respond to anti-hypertensive medication; Pimenta *et al.*, 2009). Dose–response trials have clearly demonstrated that the lower the salt intake, the lower the BP (MacGregor *et al.*, 1989; Sacks *et al.*, 2001). Furthermore, salt reduction appears to influence the age-related rise observed in BP (Sacks *et al.*, 2001). The fall in BP with salt restriction is greatest in those of African origin, older people and those with hypertension (Vollmer *et al.*, 2001). This may partly be due to the diminished responsiveness of the renin angiotensin system in these individuals (He *et al.*, 1998).

Salt reduction can enhance the action of antihypertensive medication and positively influence the requirements for drug therapy (MacGregor *et al.*, 1987; Whelton *et al.*, 1998). It is also additive to other dietary treatments, such as the Dietary Approaches to Stop Hypertension (DASH) diet (Sacks *et al.*, 2001) and weight reduction (The Trials of Hypertension Prevention Collaborative Research Group, 1997; Whelton *et al.*, 1998). Evidence of the long-term benefits of salt restriction on cardiovascular outcomes comes from the 10–15-year Trial of Hypertension Prevention. This study demonstrated that those who reduced their salt intake by 25–30% (from an average of 10 g/day) had a 25% lower incidence of cardiovascular events (Cook *et al.*, 2007). A reduction of dietary salt from 10 to 5 g/day would be expected to decrease stroke rate by 23%, and CVD by 17% (Karppanen & Mervaala, 2006; Strazzullo *et al.*, 2009).

The WHO (2016) encourages population sodium reduction strategies, and has set a worldwide target for salt intake of ≤5 g/day. Several countries, including the UK, have introduced salt reduction programmes. In 1994, COMA recommended a daily maximum salt intake of 6 g (DH, 1994). A comprehensive review by SACN (2003) concluded that evidence for an adverse association between salt and BP had strengthened, and endorsed the COMA recommendation. The National Diet and Nutrition Survey (NDNS) 2000/2001 (Hoare *et al.*, 2004) estimated the UK average daily salt consumption to be 9.5 g, with 80% contributed by processed foods and food eaten outside the home. The initial target was to encourage manufacturers to reduce salt content of processed foods on a voluntary basis. The Food Standards Agency (FSA) and Consensus Action on Salt and Health (a group of scientific experts aiming to reduce the UK salt intake) supported this by conducting salt awareness campaigns and front-of-pack food labelling promotion activities to provide clear indications of salt content. These very successful strategies have resulted in a 40–50% reduction in the salt content of many processed foods (FSA). New, revised UK-wide salt reduction targets for 2017 have been published by the FSA for 76 categories of foods. These set even more challenging and wide-ranging targets than the previous 2012 targets.

The NDNS reported that the mean estimated salt intake decreased by 1.5 g per day to 8 g per day by 2014 (a decrease of 11% since 2005–2006) in response to government-led salt-reducing initiatives. The NICE guidance (2010) on the prevention of CVD at the population level set a daily salt consumption target of <6 g/day for adults by 2015, with a further reduction to <3 g/day by 2025. Children younger than 11 years are recommended to consume substantially less than adults.

Potassium

High levels of potassium in the diet are associated with lower BPs (Cappuccio & Mac-Gregor, 1991; Geleijnse *et al.*, 2003; Intersalt Cooperative Research Group, 1988). The BP-lowering effect of potassium is greater in those of African origin, in the presence of a high salt intake and in individuals with hypertension. Meta-analyses do not support the use of potassium supplements (Dickinson *et al.*, 2006a). Increasing dietary potassium is recommended as treatment for high BP, especially when a reduction in salt intake is not achieved (European Hypertension Society, 2003; Whitworth *et al.*, 2003; Williams *et al.*, 2004). At least five portions of fruit and vegetable should be eaten per day. Most healthy individuals can tolerate an increase in dietary potassium, but care should be taken in those with certain conditions (e.g. chronic kidney disease).

The Prospective Urban and Rural Epidemiological (PURE) study (Mente *et al.*, 2014) found an inverse relationship between potassium excretion and BP, where an increase of 1 g/day of excreted potassium reduced SBP significantly ($P<0.001$), by 0.75 mmHg. The European Food Safety Authority recently updated the dietary reference value (DRV) for potassium to 3 500 mg, based on its beneficial effect on BP (Aburto *et al.*, 2013; Binia *et al.*, 2015), and reported that lower intakes have been linked with increased risk of stroke (Aburto *et al.*, 2013; D'Elia *et al.*, 2014).

Calcium and magnesium

Dietary calcium intake may have a small inverse effect on BP, but studies are inconsistent (Cappuccio *et al.*, 1995); there is insufficient evidence to advocate calcium supplementation (Dickinson *et al.*, 2006b). A meta-analysis showed that there is an inverse association between risk of elevated BP and intake of low-fat dairy foods, as well as with milk and yoghurt (Ralston *et al.*, 2012). The evidence linking dietary magnesium with a positive effect on BP is also inconsistent (Burgess *et al.*, 1999; Ma *et al.*, 1995; Mizushima *et al.*, 1998), and dietary supplementation is currently not advised (Dickinson *et al.*, 2006c). Supplementation of 450 mg of magnesium reduced SBP by 20.4 mmHg and DBP by 8.7 mmHg in type 2 diabetics (Guerrero-Romero & Rodriguez-Moran, 2009). However, in a study of young diabetic men, no association was observed (Cosaro *et al.*, 2014). In the Nurses' Health Study, high magnesium intake was associated with a 13% reduced stroke risk, whereas no association with calcium was reported (Adebamowo *et al.*, 2015). Intake of low-fat dairy products may also reduce the risk of hypertension and its associated complications (McGrane *et al.*, 2011; Ralston *et al.*, 2012; Sabita Soedamah-Muthu *et al.*, 2012), and may be of more benefit to those already at risk of CVD (Maki *et al.*, 2013).

Alcohol

In a meta-analysis, Xin *et al.* (2001) found that reducing alcohol intake reduced SBP and DBP by an average of 3.3 and 2 mmHg, respectively. The effect was dose related, with the largest reductions in alcohol intake producing the greatest reductions in BP. The effects of intervention were also greater in those with higher baseline BP. Alcohol, in small amounts, has been shown to have cardioprotective properties, and should be allowed in moderation (Power *et al.*, 1998). The UK Chief Medical Officer currently recommends limiting alcohol to no more than 14 units per week, and avoiding binge drinking. Alcohol should be taken with food, as this seems to lessen the BP-raising effects (Stranges *et al.*, 2004). A meta-analysis found a J-shaped relationship between alcohol consumption and elevated BP in women; however, in men, low and moderate alcohol intake trended towards raised BP as compared to non-drinkers (Briasoulis *et al.*, 2012). The phenolic content of beer and wine, especially red wine, appear to offer some cardioprotective effect (Chiva-Blanch *et al.*, 2013).

Other dietary components

Several other dietary components have been implicated in lowering BP, although the evidence is not strong enough for these to be incorporated into management guidelines. These include cocoa (Desch *et al.*, 2010), dietary fibre (Whelton *et al.*, 2005), fish oil (Appel *et al.*,

1993), protein (Altorf-van der Kuil *et al.*, 2010) and vitamin D (Geleijnse, 2011). There may be a U-shaped relationship between coffee and BP levels. Coffee has been reported to lower BP in both abstainers and in those with high coffee intake, and to slightly raise BP (2/1 mmHg) in those with medium (five cups/day) intake (Geleijnse, 2008). Liquorice consumption may raise BP even at levels as low as 50 g/day for 2 weeks (Sigurjonsdottir *et al.*, 2001).

Studies regarding coffee consumption and stroke risk report a U-shaped curve (Larsson & Orsini, 2011; Nordestgaard *et al.*, 2016). Drinking three or more cups of coffee per day has been linked with a significant reduction in silent brain infarction (Nakaguchi *et al.*, 2016). Cocoa intake has been shown to decrease SBP by 4.8 mmHg and DBP by 3.03 mmHg in a small cohort of healthy volunteers (Grassi *et al.*, 2015a). Flavonoids in black tea have demonstrated a reduction of 3.2 mmHg in SBP and 2.6 mmHg in DBP in hypertensives (Grassi *et al.*, 2015b). Optimal vitamin D status has been shown to decrease CVD risk in middle-aged and elderly adults (Parker *et al.*, 2010). Increased BP has been reported among those with lower vitamin D status (Muldowney *et al.*, 2011); however, recent trials have illustrated little or no benefit of vitamin D supplementation on BP lowering (Pilz *et al.*, 2015; Scragg *et al.*, 2014; Vimaleswaran *et al.*, 2014). A meta-analysis of prospective studies indicated increased circulating levels of long-chain n-3 polyunsaturated fatty acids to be inversely associated with elevated BP (Yang *et al.*, 2016).

Physical activity

In addition to the benefits of physical activity in terms of energy balance and obesity, aerobic exercise may have direct hypotensive effects. A meta-analysis found that aerobic exercise reduced SBP by an average of 3.8 mmHg, and DBP by 2.6 mmHg (Whelton *et al.*, 2002). These effects occurred in both normotensive and hypertensive individuals, and also in overweight and normal-weight individuals. Physical activity has been found to have a beneficial effect on cardiovascular health (Li & Siegrist, 2012), while leisure activity, such as walking, was shown to reduce stroke risk in women (Sattelmair *et al.*, 2010).

Multiple lifestyle interventions

BP-lowering advice generally incorporates a number dietary and lifestyle factors, such as reducing salt intake, increasing intake of fruit and vegetables, limiting alcohol consumption, increasing physical activity and promoting weight loss. A number of trials have incorporated multiple lifestyle interventions; the most widely studied and promoted are the DASH trials. The original DASH diet was high in fruit and vegetables, low-fat dairy foods, wholegrain cereals, nuts and seeds, with foods rich in saturated fat and refined sugar being restricted. Thus, the DASH dietary pattern increases intakes of potassium, calcium, magnesium, fibre and protein, while lowering saturated fat. When compared with a typical US diet, the DASH diet significantly lowered SBP and DBP in hypertensive and normotensive individuals by 11.4 and 5.5 mmHg and 3.5 and 2.1 mmHg, respectively (Appel *et al.*, 1997). This reduction was achieved within 2 weeks, and was maintained for the remaining 6 weeks of the study. These dramatic effects were repeated in the DASH sodium trial (Sacks *et al.*, 2001), which demonstrated that restriction of dietary sodium had an additive effect on lowering BP. The PREMIER trial demonstrated that the DASH diet was effective in lowering BP over a longer period, and when subjects self-select their food (Aronow *et al.*, 2011). More recently, the ENCORE study showed that the addition of exercise and weight loss advice to the DASH diet for 4 months resulted in even greater BP reductions (Blumenthal *et al.*, 2010); there was a 16.1/9.9 mmHg reduction in BP with DASH and weight management, and a 11.2/7.5 mmHg reduction with the DASH diet alone. DASH diet has been observed to reduce estimated 10-year CHD risk by 18% (Chen *et al.*, 2010). In addition to reducing BP, the DASH diet may also substantially reduce the risk of CHD. DASH diet appears to have a more beneficial effect in those with higher CVD risk (Saneei *et al.*, 2014; Siervo *et al.*, 2015). A report by Mozaffarian *et al.* (2011) found increased intake of fruit, vegetables, whole grains, dairy products and fish to be cardioprotective. In US (Chobanian *et al.*, 2003) and Canadian (Hackam *et al.*, 2010) national guidelines, the DASH diet is recommended for the treatment of hypertension. Harnden *et al.* (2010) have reported BP benefits following adherence to the DASH diet in a UK population.

Summary

Strong evidence exists to support the significant health and economic benefits of early detection, adequate treatment and good control of hypertension at the population level. In the UK, strategies, including those aimed at reducing the prevalence of obesity and decreasing habitual salt intake, as well as adhering to specific dietary patterns, have been proven to result in significant cardiovascular benefit, although challenging to implement. Recent scientific advances have also enabled the identification and study of genetic and environmental factors that interact to influence BP. Prevention and control is complex, and requires a multi-stakeholder collaboration, including government agencies, health professionals, the food industry, academia and the public, working together to design and support public health strategies to bring about sustained lifestyle modifications to help prevent hypertension.

Acknowledgement

The editor acknowledges the prior contribution of Karin Harnden.

Further reading

Appel LJ, Giles TD, Black HR, *et al.* (2010) ASH position paper: dietary approaches to lower blood pressure. *J. Am. Soc. Hypertens.* 4: 79–89.

NICE. (2016) Hypertension in adults: diagnosis and management *CG127*. Available at https://www.nice.org.uk/Guidance/CG127.

PHE. (2017) *Health Matters: Combating High Blood Pressure*. Available at www.gov.uk/government/publications/health-matters-combating-high-blood-pressure.

SACN. (2003) *Salt and Health*. Available at www.sacn.gov.uk/pdfs/sacn_salt_final.pdf.

Internet resources

Blood Pressure Association, www.bpassoc.org.uk

British Hypertension Society, www.bhsoc.org

Consensus Action on Salt and Health (CASH), www.actiononsalt.org.uk

World Action on Salt and Health (WASH), www.worldactiononsalt.com

References

Aburto NJ, Ziolkovska A, Hooper L, *et al.* (2013) Effect of lower sodium intake on health: systematic review and meta-analyses. *BMJ*. 346: f1326.

ACC/AHA/AAPA/ABC/ACPM/AGS/APhA/ASH/ASPC/NMA/PCNA. (2017) Guideline for the Prevention, Detection, Evaluation, and Management of High Blood Pressure in Adults: A Report of the American College of Cardiology/American Heart Association Task Force on Clinical Practice Guidelines. *J. Am. Coll. Cardiol.* doi.org/10.1161/HYP.0000000000000065

Adebamowo SN, Spiegelman D, Willet W, *et al.* (2015) Association between intakes of magnesium, potassium, and calcium and risk of stroke: 2 cohorts of US women and updated meta-analyses. *Am. J. Clin. Nutr.* 101: 1269–1277.

Alpert MA, Omran J, Mehra A, *et al.* (2014) Impact of obesity and weight loss on cardiac performance and morphology in adults. *Prog. Cardiovasc. Dis.* 56: 391–400.

Altorf-van der Kuil W, Engberink MF, van Rooij FJ, *et al.* (2010) Dietary protein and risk of hypertension in a Dutch older population: the Rotterdam study. *J. Hypertens.* 28: 2394–2400.

Appel LJ, Miller ER, Seidler AJ, *et al.* (1993) Does supplementation of diet with 'fish oil' reduce blood pressure? A meta-analysis of controlled clinical trials. *Arch. Intern. Med.* 153: 1429–1438.

Appel LJ, Moore TJ, Obarzanek E, *et al.* (1997) A clinical trial of the effects of dietary patterns on blood pressure. DASH Collaborative Research Group. *N. Engl. J. Med.* 336: 1117–1124.

Aronow WS, Fleg JL, Pepine CJ, *et al.* (2011) ACCF/AHA 2011 Expert Consensus Document on Hypertension in the Elderly A Report of the American College of Cardiology Foundation Task Force on Clinical Expert Consensus Documents Developed in Collaboration With the American Academy of Neurology, American Geriatrics Society, American Society for Preventive Cardiology, American Society of Hypertension, American Society of Nephrology, Association of Black Cardiologists, and European Society of Hypertension. *J. Am. Coll. Cardiol.* 57: 2037–2114.

Benetou V, Bamia C, Trichopoulos D, *et al.* (2004) The association of body mass index and waist circumference with blood pressure depends on age and gender: a study of 10 928 non-smoking adults in the Greek EPIC cohort. *Eur. J. Epidemiol.* 19: 803–809.

Binia A, Jaeger J, Hu Y, *et al.* (2015) Daily potassium intake and sodium-to-potassium ratio in the reduction of blood pressure: a meta-analysis of randomized controlled trials. *J. Hypertens.* 33: 1509–1520.

Blumenthal JA, Babyak MA, Hinderliter A, *et al.* (2010) Effects of the DASH diet alone and in combination with exercise and weight loss on blood pressure and cardiovascular biomarkers in men and women with high blood pressure: the ENCORE study. *Arch. Intern. Med.* 170: 126–135.

Briasoulis A, Agarwal V, Messerli FH. (2012) Alcohol consumption and the risk of hypertension in men and women: a systematic review and meta-analysis. *J. Clin. Hypertens. (Greenwich)*. 14: 792–798.

Burgess E, Lewanczuk R, Bolli P, *et al.* (1999) Lifestyle modifications to prevent and control hypertension. 6. Recommendations on potassium, magnesium and calcium. *CMAJ* 160: S35–45.

Burt VL, Whelton P, Roccella EJ, *et al.* (1995) Prevalence of hypertension in the US adult population. Results from the Third National Health and Nutrition Examination Survey, 1988–1991. *Hypertension*. 25: 305–313.

Canoy D, Luben R, Welch A, *et al.* (2004) Fat distribution, body mass index and blood pressure in 22 090 men and women in the Norfolk cohort of the European Prospective Investigation into Cancer and Nutrition (EPIC-Norfolk) study. *J. Hypertens.* 22: 2067–2074.

Cappuccio FP, MacGregor GA. (1991) Does potassium supplementation lower blood pressure? A meta-analysis of published trials. *J. Hypertens.* 9: 465–473.

Cappuccio FP, Elliott P, Allender PS, *et al.* (1995) Epidemiologic association between dietary calcium intake and blood pressure: a meta-analysis of published data. *Am. J. Epidemiol.* 142: 935–945.

Cappuccio FP, Cook DG, Atkinson RW, *et al.* (1997) Prevalence, detection, and management of cardiovascular risk factors in different ethnic groups in south London. *Heart* 78(6): 555–563.

Centre for Disease Control and Prevention; CDC (2014) High blood pressure Facts. Available at https://www.cdc.gov/bloodpressure/facts.htm. Accessed 14 November 2018.

Chen X, Wang Y. (2008) Tracking of blood pressure from childhood to adulthood: a systematic review and meta-regression analysis. *Circulation*. 117: 3171–3180.

Chen ST, Maruthur NM, Appel LJ. (2010) The effect of dietary patterns on estimated coronary heart disease risk. *Circ. Cardiovasc. Qual. Outcomes*. 3(5): 484–489.

Chiva-Blanch G, Arranz S, Lamuela-Raventos RM, *et al.* (2013) Effects of wine, alcohol and polyphenols on cardiovascular disease risk factors: evidences from human studies. *Alcohol Alcohol.* 48: 270–277.

Chobanian AV, Bakris GL, Black HR, *et al.* (2003) The Seventh Report of the Joint National Committee on Prevention, Detection, Evaluation, and Treatment of High Blood Pressure: the JNC 7 report. *JAMA*. 289: 2560–2572.

Clement DL, De Buyzere ML, De Bacquer DA, *et al.* (2003) Prognostic value of ambulatory blood pressure recordings in patients with treated hypertension. *N. Engl. J. Med.* 348: 2407–2415.

Cook NR, Cutler JA, Obarzanek E, *et al.* (2007) Long term effects of dietary sodium reduction on cardiovascular disease outcomes: observational follow-up of the trials of hypertension prevention (TOHP). *BMJ*. 334: 885–888.

Cosaro E, Bonafini S, Montagnana M, *et al.* (2014) Effects of magnesium supplements on blood pressure, endothelial function and metabolic parameters in healthy young men with a family history of metabolic syndrome. *Nutr. Metab. Cardiovasc. Dis.* 24: 1213–1220.

D'Elia L, Iannotta C, Sabino P, *et al.* (2014) Potassium-rich diet and risk of stroke: updated meta-analysis. *Nutr. Metab. Cardiovasc. Dis.* 24: 585–587.

Denton D, Weisinger R, Mundy N, *et al.* (1995) The effect of increased salt intake on blood pressure of chimpanzees. *Nat. Med.* 1: 1009–1016.

Desch S, Schmidt J, Kobler D, *et al.* (2010) Effect of cocoa products on blood pressure: systematic review and meta-analysis. *Am. J. Hypertens.* 23: 97–103.

DH. (1994) *Nutritional Aspects of Cardiovascular Disease*. London: HMSO.

Dickinson HO, Nicolson D, Campbell F, *et al.* (2006a) Potassium supplementation for the management of primary hypertension in adults. *Cochrane Database Syst. Rev.* (3): CD004641.

Dickinson HO, Nicolson D, Cook JV, *et al.* (2006b) Calcium supplementation for the management of primary hypertension in adults. *Cochrane Database Syst. Rev.* (2): CD004639.

Dickinson HO, Nicolson D, Campbell F, *et al.* (2006c) Magnesium supplementation for the management of primary hypertension in adults. *Cochrane Database Syst. Rev.* (3): CD004640.

Din-Dzietham R, Liu Y, Bielo MV, *et al.* (2007) High blood pressure trends in children and adolescents in national surveys, 1963 to 2002. *Circulation.* 116: 1488–1496.

Ettehad D, Emdin CA, Kiran A, *et al.* (2016) Blood pressure lowering for prevention of cardiovascular disease and death: a systematic review and meta-analysis. *Lancet.* 387: 957–967.

Ezzati M, Lopez AD, Rodgers A, *et al.* (2002) Selected major risk factors and global and regional burden of disease. *Lancet.* 360: 1347–1360.

European Hypertension Society. (2003) Guidelines for the management of arterial hypertension. *J. Hypertens.* 21: 1011–1053.

Falashetti *et al.* (2014) Hypertension management in England: a serial cross-sectional study from 1994 to 2011. *Lancet* 383(9932): 1912–1918.

Flynn J. (2013) The changing face of pediatric hypertension in the era of the childhood obesity epidemic. *Pediatr. Nephrol.* 28: 1059–1066.

Ford ES, Zhao G, Li C, *et al.* (2008) Trends in obesity and abdominal obesity among hypertensive and nonhypertensive adults in the United States. *Am. J. Hypertens.* 21: 1124–1128.

Geleijnse JM. (2008) Habitual coffee consumption and blood pressure: an epidemiological perspective. *Vasc. Health Risk Manag.* 4: 963–970.

Geleijnse JM. (2011) Vitamin D and the prevention of hypertension and cardiovascular diseases: a review of the current evidence. *Am. J. Hypertens.* 24: 253–262.

Geleijnse JM, Kok FJ, Grobbee DE. (2003) Blood pressure response to changes in sodium and potassium intake: a metaregression analysis of randomised trials. *J. Hum. Hypertens.* 17: 471–480.

Grassi D, Desideri G, Necozione S, *et al.* (2015a) Cocoa consumption dose-dependently improves flow-mediated dilation and arterial stiffness decreasing blood pressure in healthy individuals. *J. Hypertens.* 33: 294–303.

Grassi D, Draijer R, Desideri G, *et al.* (2015b) Black tea lowers blood pressure and wave reflections in fasted and postprandial conditions in hypertensive patients: a randomised study. *Nutrients* 7: 1037–1051.

Guerrero-Romero F, Rodriguez-Moran M. (2009) The effect of lowering blood pressure by magnesium supplementation in diabetic hypertensive adults with low serum magnesium levels: a randomized, double-blind, placebo-controlled clinical trial. *J. Hum. Hypertens.* 23: 245–251.

Hackam DG, Khan NA, Hemmelgarn BR, *et al.* (2010) The 2010 Canadian Hypertension Education Program recommendations for the management of hypertension: part 2 therapy. *Can. J. Cardiol.* 26: 249–258.

Harnden KE, Frayn KN, Hodson L. (2010) Dietary Approaches to Stop Hypertension (DASH) diet: applicability and acceptability to a UK population. *J. Hum. Nutr. Diet.* 23: 3–10.

Harsha DW, Bray GA. (2008) Weight loss and blood pressure control (Pro). *Hypertension.* 51: 1420–1425.

He FJ, MacGregor GA. (2002) Effect of modest salt reduction on blood pressure: a meta-analysis of randomized trials. Implications for public health. *J. Hum. Hypertens.* 16: 761–770.

He FJ, MacGregor GA. (2010) Reducing population salt intake worldwide: from evidence to implementation. *Prog. Cardiovasc. Dis.* 52: 363–382.

He FJ, Li J, MacGregor GA. (2013) Effect of longer term modest salt reduction on blood pressure. Cochrane systematic review and meta-analysis of randomised trials. *BMJ.* 346: f1325.

He FJ, Markandu ND, Sagnella GA, *et al.* (1998) Importance of the renin system in determining blood pressure fall with salt restriction in black and white hypertensives. *Hypertension.* 32: 820–824.

Higgins M, Kannel W, Garrison R, *et al.* (1988) Hazards of obesity – the Framingham experience. *Acta Med. Scand. Suppl.* 723: 23–36.

Hoare J, Henderson L, Bates CJ, *et al.* (2004) *National Diet and Nutrition Survey*. London: TSO.

Hubert HB, Feinleib M, McNamara PM, *et al.* (1983) Obesity as an independent risk factor for cardiovascular disease: a 26-year follow-up of participants in the Framingham Heart Study. *Circulation.* 67: 968–977.

Intersalt Cooperative Research Group. (1988) Intersalt: an international study of electrolyte excretion and blood pressure. Results for 24 hour urinary sodium and potassium excretion. *BMJ.* 297: 319–328.

Karppanen H, Mervaala E. (2006) Sodium intake and hypertension. *Prog. Cardiovasc. Dis.* 49: 59–75.

Klatsky AL, Friedman GD, Siegelaub AB, *et al.* (1977) Alcohol consumption and blood pressure Kaiser-Permanente Multiphasic Health Examination data. *N. Engl. J. Med.* 296: 1194–1200.

Larsson SC, Orsini N. (2011) Coffee consumption and risk of stroke: a dose-response meta-analysis of prospective studies. *Am. J. Epidemiol.*, 174(9): 993–1001.

Law M, Morris JK, Wald NJ. (2009) Use of blood pressure lowering drugs in the prevention of cardiovascular disease: meta-analysis of 147 randomised trials in the context of expectations from prospective epidemiological studies. *BMJ.* 338: b1665.

Lewington S, Clarke R, Qizilbash N, *et al.* (2002) Age specific relevance of usual blood pressure to vascular mortality: a meta-analysis of individual data for one million adults in 61 prospective studies. *Lancet.* 360: 1903–1913.

Li J, Siegrist J. (2012) Physical activity and risk of cardiovascular disease – a meta-analysis of prospective cohort studies. *Int. J. Environ. Res. Public Health* 9(2):391–407.

Ma J, Folsom AR, Melnick SL, *et al.* (1995) Associations of serum and dietary magnesium with cardiovascular disease, hypertension, diabetes, insulin, and carotid arterial wall thickness: the ARIC study. Atherosclerosis Risk in Communities Study. *J. Clin. Epidemiol.* 48: 927–940.

MacGregor GA, Markandu ND, Singer DR, *et al.* (1987) Moderate sodium restriction with angiotensin converting enzyme inhibitor in essential hypertension: a double blind study. *BMJ. (Clin Res Ed).* 294: 531–534.

MacGregor GA, Markandu ND, Sagnella GA, *et al.* (1989) Double-blind study of three sodium intakes and long-term effects of sodium restriction in essential hypertension. *Lancet.* 2: 1244–1247.

Maki KC, Rains TM, Schild AL, *et al.* (2013) Effects of low-fat dairy intake on blood pressure, endothelial function, and lipoprotein lipids in subjects with prehypertension or stage 1 hypertension. *Vasc. Health Risk Manag.* 9: 369–379.

Mancia G, Fagard R, Narkiewicze K, *et al.* (2013) 2013 ESH/ESC guidelines for the management of arterial hypertension: the Task Force for the Management of Arterial Hypertension of the European Society of Hypertension (ESH) and of the European Society of Cardiology (ESC). *Blood Press.* 22: 193–278.

Manson JE, Willett WC, Stampfer MJ, *et al.* (1995) Body weight and mortality among women. *N. Engl. J. Med.* 333: 677–685.

McGrane MM, Essery E, Obbagy J, *et al.* (2011) Dairy consumption, blood pressure, and risk of hypertension: an evidence-based review of recent literature. *Curr. Cardiovasc. Risk Rep.* 5: 287–298.

McNulty H, Strain JJ, Hughes CF, *et al.* (2017) Riboflavin, MTHFR genotype and blood pressure: A personalized approach to prevention and treatment of hypertension. *Mol. Aspects Med.* 53: 2–9

Mente A, O'Donnell MJ, Rangarajan S, *et al.* (2014) Association of urinary sodium and potassium excretion with blood pressure. *N. Engl. J. Med.* 371: 601–611.

Mizushima S, Cappuccio FP, Nichols R, *et al.* (1998) Dietary magnesium intake and blood pressure: a qualitative overview of the observational studies. *J. Hum. Hypertens.* 12: 447–453.

Mozaffarian D, Appel LJ, Van Horn L. (2011) Components of a cardioprotective diet. *Circulation.* 123(24): 2870–2891.

Mozaffarian D, Benjamin EJ, Go AS, *et al.* (2016) Executive summary: Heart Disease and Stroke Statistics – 2016 Update: A Report from the American Heart Association. *Circulation.* 133: 447–454.

Muldowney S, Lucey A, Paschos G, *et al.* (2011) Relationships between vitamin D status and cardio-metabolic risk factors in young European adults. *Ann. Nutr. Metab.* 58: 85–93.

Myers MG. (2005) Ambulatory blood pressure monitoring for routine clinical practice. *Hypertension* 45(4): 483–484.

Nakaguchi H, Matsuno A, Okubo T, *et al.* (2016) Relationship between silent brain infarction and amount of daily coffee consumption in middle age. *J. Stroke Cerebrovasc. Dis.* 25: 1678–1682.

Neal B, MacMahon S, Chapman N. (2000) Effects of ACE inhibitors, calcium antagonists, and other blood-pressure-lowering drugs: results of prospectively designed overviews of randomised trials. Blood Pressure Lowering Treatment Trialists' Collaboration. *Lancet* 356: 1955–1964.

Neter JE, Stam BE, Kok FJ, *et al.* (2003) Influence of weight reduction on blood pressure: a meta-analysis of randomized controlled trials. *Hypertension.* 42: 878–884.

NICE. (2010) *Guidance on the prevention of cardiovascular disease at the population level.* Available at http://guidance.nice.org.uk/PH25. Accessed 14 November 2018.

NICE. (2016) *Hypertension – the clinical management of primary hypertension in adults in primary care.* CG127. Available at www.nice.org.uk. Accessed 14 November 2018.

Nordestgaard AT, Thomsen M, Nordestgaard BG. (2015) Coffee intake and risk of obesity, metabolic syndrome and type 2 diabetes: a Mendelian randomization study. *Int. J. Epidemiol.* 44: 551–565.

Park CM, Tillin T, March K, *et al.* (2016) Adverse effect of diabetes and hyperglycemia on arterial stiffness in Europeans, South Asians and African Caribbeans in the SABRE study. *J. Hypertens.* 34: 282.

Parker J, Hashmi O, Dutton D, *et al.* (2010) Levels of vitamin D and cardiometabolic disorders: systematic review and meta-analysis. *Maturitas.* 65: 225–236.

PHE. (2017) Health Matters: Combatting High Blood Pressure. Available at https://www.gov.uk/government/publications/health-matters-combating-high-blood-pressure/health-matters-combating-high-blood-pressure.

Pilz S, Gaksch M, Kienreich K, *et al.* (2015) Effects of vitamin D on blood pressure and cardiovascular risk factors. *Hypertension.* 71: 666–672.

Pimenta E, Gaddam KK, Oparil S, *et al.* (2009) Effects of dietary sodium reduction on blood pressure in subjects with resistant hypertension: results from a randomized trial. *Hypertension.* 54: 475–481.

Power C, Rodgers B, Hope S. (1998) U-shaped relation for alcohol consumption and health in early adulthood and implications for mortality. *Lancet.* 352: 877.

Puddey IB, Rakic V, Dimmitt SB, *et al.* (1999) Influence of pattern of drinking on cardiovascular disease and cardiovascular risk factors – a review. *Addiction.* 94: 649–663.

Ralston RA, Lee JH, Truby H, *et al.* (2012) A systematic review and meta-analysis of elevated blood pressure and consumption of dairy foods. *J. Hum. Hypertens.* 26(1): 3–13.

Rosner B, Cook NR, Daniels S, *et al.* (2013) Childhood blood pressure trends and risk factors for high blood pressure. *Hypertension* 62: 247–254.

Sacks FM, Svetkey LP, Vollmer WM, *et al.* (2001) Effects on blood pressure of reduced dietary sodium and the Dietary Approaches to Stop Hypertension (DASH) diet. DASH-Sodium Collaborative Research Group. *N. Engl. J. Med.* 344: 3–10.

SACN. (2003) *Salt and Health.* Available at www.sacn.gov.uk/pdfs/sacn_salt_final.pdf. Accessed 18 November 2017.

Saneei P, Salehi-Abargouei A, Esmaillzadeh A, *et al.* (2014) Influence of Dietary Approaches to Stop Hypertension (DASH) diet on blood pressure: a systematic review and meta-analysis on randomized controlled trials. *Nutr. Metab. Cardiovasc. Dis.* 24(12): 1253–1261.

Sattelmair JR, Kurth T, Buring JE, *et al.* (2010) Physical activity and risk of stroke in women. *Stroke.* 41: 1243–1250.

Scragg R, Slow S, Stewart AW, *et al.* (2014) Long-term high-dose vitamin D3 supplementation and blood pressure in healthy adults: a randomized controlled trial. *Hypertension* 64: 725–730.

Siervo M, Lara J, Chowdhury S, *et al.* (2015) Effects of the Dietary Approach to Stop Hypertension (DASH) diet on cardiovascular risk factors: a systematic review and meta-analysis. *Br. J. Nutr.* 113(1): 1–15.

Sigurjonsdottir HA, Franzson L, Manhem K, *et al.* (2001) Liquorice-induced rise in blood pressure: a linear dose-response relationship. *J. Hum. Hypertens.* 15: 549–552.

Soedamah-Muthu SS, Verberne LD, Ding EL, *et al.* (2012) Dairy consumption and incidence of hypertension: a dose-response meta-analysis of prospective cohort studies. *Hypertension* 60(5):1131–1137.

Stranges S, Wu T, Dorn JM, *et al.* (2004) Relationship of alcohol drinking pattern to risk of hypertension: a population-based study. *Hypertension.* 44: 813–819.

Strazzullo P. (2002) Salt-sensitivity, hypertension and cardiovascular ageing: broadening our view without missing the point. *J. Hypertens.* 20: 561–563.

Strazzullo P, D'Elia L, Kandala NB, *et al.* (2009) Salt intake, stroke, and cardiovascular disease: meta-analysis of prospective studies. *BMJ.* 339: b4567.

Taylor RS, Ashton KE, Moxham T, *et al.* (2011) Reduced dietary salt for the prevention of cardiovascular disease: a meta-analysis of randomized controlled trials (Cochrane review). *Am. J. Hypertens.* 24: 843–853.

The Trials of Hypertension Prevention Collaborative Research Group. (1997) Effects of weight loss and sodium reduction intervention on blood pressure and hypertension incidence in overweight people with high-normal blood pressure. The Trials of Hypertension Prevention, phase II. *Arch. Intern. Med.* 157: 657–667.

UK Prospective Diabetes Study Group (UKPDS). (1998) Tight blood pressure control and risk of macrovascular and microvascular complications in type 2 diabetes: UKPDS 38. *BMJ.* 317: 703–713.

Vimaleswaran KS, Cavadino A, Berry DJ, *et al.* (2014) Association of vitamin D status with arterial blood pressure and hypertension risk: a Mendelian randomisation study. *Lancet Diabetes Endocrinol.* 2: 719–729.

Vollmer WM, Sacks FM, Ard J, *et al.* (2001) Effects of diet and sodium intake on blood pressure: subgroup analysis of the DASH-sodium trial. *Ann. Intern. Med.* 135: 1019–1028.

Wannamethee SG, Shaper AG. (1996) Patterns of alcohol intake and risk of stroke in middle-aged British men. *Stroke* 27: 1033–1039.

Whelton PK, Apel LJ, Esperland MA, *et al.* (1998) Sodium reduction and weight loss in the treatment of hypertension in older persons: a randomized controlled trial of nonpharmacologic interventions in the elderly (TONE). TONE Collaborative Research Group. *JAMA.* 279: 839–846.

Whelton SP, Chin A, Xin X, *et al.* (2002) Effect of aerobic exercise on blood pressure: a meta-analysis of randomized, controlled trials. *Ann. Intern. Med.* 136: 493–503.

Whelton SP, Hyre AD, Pedersen B, *et al.* (2005) Effect of dietary fiber intake on blood pressure: a meta-analysis of randomized, controlled clinical trials. *J. Hypertens.* 23: 475–481.

Whitworth JA; World Health Organization, International Society of Hypertension Writing Group. (2003) World Health Organization (WHO)/International Society of Hypertension (ISH) statement on management of hypertension. *J. Hypertens.* 21: 1983–1992.

WHO. (2013) *A global brief on hypertension.* Available at http://www.who.int/cardiovascular_diseases/publications/global_brief_hypertension/en/. Accessed 14 November 2018.

WHO. (2016) *SHAKE the salt habit: The SHAKE technical package for salt reduction.* Available at http://apps.who.int/iris/bitstream/handle/10665/250135/9789241511346-eng.pdf?sequence=1. Accessed 14 November 2018.

WHO. (2017) *Global Health Observatory (GHO) data*. Available at http://www.who.int/gho/ncd/risk_factors/blood_pressure_prevalence_text/en/. Accessed 18 November 2017.

Williams B, Poulter NR, Brown MJ, *et al.* (2004) Guidelines for management of hypertension: report of the fourth working party of the British Hypertension Society, 2004–BHS IV. *J. Hum. Hypertens.* 18: 139–185.

Wing RR, Lang W, Wadden TA, *et al.* (2011) Benefits of modest weight loss in improving cardiovascular risk factors in overweight and obese individuals with type 2 diabetes. *Diabetes care* 34: 1481–1486.

Xin X, He J, Frontini MG, *et al.* (2001) Effects of alcohol reduction on blood pressure: a meta-analysis of randomized controlled trials. *Hypertension.* 38: 1112–1117.

Yang B, Shi MQ, Li ZH, *et al.* (2016) Fish, long-chain n-3 PUFA and incidence of elevated blood pressure: a meta-analysis of prospective cohort studies. *Nutrients.* 8: 58.

Yang G, Xiang YB, Zheng W, *et al.* (2007) Body weight and weight change in relation to blood pressure in normotensive men. *J. Hum. Hypertens.* 21: 45–52.

Yin RX, Aung LHH, Long XJ, *et al.* (2015) Interactions of several genetic polymorphisms and alcohol consumption on blood pressure levels. *Biofactors.* 41: 339–351.

Zomer E, Gurusamy K, Leach R, *et al.* (2016) Interventions that cause weight loss and the impact on cardiovascular risk factors: a systematic review and meta-analysis. *Obes. Rev.* 17(10): 1001–1011.

7.14.5 Stroke

Pauline Douglas and Alison McGlone

Key points

- Stroke is a major cause of morbidity and mortality in the UK.
- Malnutrition in stroke patients is associated with poor long-term outcomes.
- Multidisciplinary management of stroke in designated units has been shown to improve long-term survival and functional state.
- The neurological impairments of stroke can significantly impact on nutritional status, and malnutrition can have a negative knock-on effect in terms of slowed recovery and capacity for rehabilitation.

Stroke is the fourth-most common cause of death in the UK, and the third-most common in Scotland (National Records of Scotland, 2016; Office for National Statistics, 2016). Each year, in the UK, over 100,000 people have a stroke (Royal College of Physicians (RCP), 2015). More than 1.2 million people in the UK are survivors of stroke, with two-thirds leaving hospital with a disability, making it a leading cause of disability (Department of Health (DH), 2016; ISD Scotland, 2016a; NHS Digital, 2016; Welsh Government, 2016). Stroke incidence rates fell 19% from 1990 to 2010 in the UK (Feigin *et al.*, 2013). Most strokes occur in people older than 65 years, but they can occur at any age. In England, Wales and Northern Ireland, the average age for stroke in men is 74 years, and for women 80 years (RCP, 2016a). In Scotland, the ages are 71 and 76 years, respectively (ISD Scotland, 2016b). There are over 400 childhood strokes a year in the UK (Stroke Association, 2017). In 2017, the Royal College of Paediatrics and Child Health published evidence-based clinical guidelines for healthcare professionals working with children and young adults (RCPCH, 2017). There are ethnic differences, with black people twice as likely to have a stroke, and also at a younger age than white people (Wang *et al.*, 2013). Social deprivation also increases the risk of stroke (Marshall *et al.*, 2015). Research has estimated that stroke costs the UK around £9 billion/year (Saka *et al.*, 2009).

Stroke quality markers were developed as part of the National Stroke Strategy for England (DH, 2007) as a means of raising the quality of stroke prevention, treatment, care and support, and to provide guidelines to measure the quality of stroke services. However, the National Stroke Strategy ended in 2017, with no current plans to renew. Scottish Intercollegiate Guidelines Network (SIGN) guidelines for stroke are currently being updated for Scotland. The Royal College of Physicians' National Clinical Guideline for Stroke, 5th edition (RCP, 2016b), represent the current recommendations for stroke care within the UK, and this aligns with the quality standard updates in adults from NICE, 2017a.

The recommended staffing levels for dietitians per five beds are 0.15 WTE for both hyperacute and acute stroke units (RCP, 2016b). This is based on weekday working, and will need to be adjusted for 7-day working. The additional use of a therapy assistant under the supervision of a registered practitioner should also be considered in the skill mix of the team (RCP, 2016b).

Diagnostic criteria and classification

A stroke or cerebrovascular accident occurs when the blood supply to a part of the brain is disrupted. As this, in turn, affects the supply of nutrients and oxygen to that part of the brain, brain cells then become damaged or die. Various signs and symptoms then develop, depending on the area of the brain affected. These usually develop rapidly and include the following:

- Numbness or weakness of the face, arm or leg, usually on one side of the body.

- Difficulty in speaking or understanding speech.
- Blurred vision or loss of sight in one or both eyes.
- Problems with co-ordination.
- Difficulty walking.
- Dizziness or loss of balance.
- Difficulty swallowing.
- Confusion.
- Severe headache.

A transient ischaemic attack (TIA) occurs when there is a temporary disruption of blood supply to part of the brain. It can cause sudden symptoms similar to that of stroke; however, they resolve within 24 hours of onset. Following a TIA, there is increased risk of having a stroke. This can be 5% within 24 hours, 8% within a week, 12% within a month and 17% within 3 months; 1 in 12 people will have a stroke within a week of a TIA.

Classification of stroke

Strokes can be classified by their main causes. There are two main types of stroke: ischaemic stroke and haemorrhagic stroke, and they affect the brain in different ways and have different causes. Ischaemic stroke accounts for 85% of all strokes in the UK, with haemorrhagic stroke accounting for 15% (10% being intracerebral haemorrhage, and 5% being subarachnoid haemorrhage).

Ischaemic stroke

An ischaemic stroke occurs when a blood vessel in the brain becomes obstructed. There are two types of obstructions that can cause an ischaemic stroke: a thrombus, and an embolism. A cerebral thrombus refers to the obstruction being caused by a blood clot (thrombus) in the brain, and a cerebral embolus refers to the obstruction being caused by a blood clot, or other matter such as an air bubble or fatty debris (emboli), which has moved through the bloodstream from another part of the body to the brain. There are many reasons why obstructions can form and cause an ischaemic stroke, including the following:

- *Atherosclerosis* – fatty deposits (plaques) build up inside the walls of arteries, making them harder and narrower and more susceptible to blockage.
- *Arterial fibrillation* – a heart condition which is characterised by an irregular heart beat and can cause blood clots in the heart, which can travel in the bloodstream to the brain.
- *Carotid or vertebral arterial dissection* – this occurs when a small tear forms in the lining of the arterial wall, allowing blood to enter and form a clot. This can lead to thickening of the arterial wall, and subsequently impede blood flow. Alternatively, part or all of the clot can break off and cause an obstruction elsewhere in the blood vessel. This type of stroke occurs more in younger people.

Some stroke wards will further classify ischaemic stokes based on the area of circulation affected, such as a total anterior circulation (TAC), a partial anterior circulation (PAC), a posterior circulation (POC) or a lacuna (LAC) stroke.

Haemorrhagic stroke

A haemorrhagic stroke results from bleeding within the brain caused by a ruptured blood vessel. There are two main types of haemorrhagic stroke:

- An intracerebral haemorrhage results from bleeding from a blood vessel within the brain; mainly caused by hypertension.
- A subarachnoid haemorrhage (SAH) results from bleeding on the surface of the brain; 85% are caused by an aneurysm, and can be familial. Other causes include arteriovenous malformation (AVM) and cerebral amyloid angiopathy.

Morbidity and mortality

One in eight people will die within the first 30 days post-stroke (Bray *et al.*, 2016). Those who have suffered a haemorrhagic stroke have a greater risk of dying within 3 months than those who have suffered an ischaemic stroke (Mohan *et al.*, 2011). Haemorrhagic stroke occurs less often than an ischaemic stroke; however, it accounts for 40% of deaths from stroke in the UK, as the damage can be greater than that from an ischaemic stroke. Following SAH, about 70% of all people, or 85% who are admitted to a neurosurgical unit, will survive.

Effects of stroke

The effects of stroke depend on the location of the tissue damage within the brain. The right side of the brain controls functions on the left side of the body, and vice versa. Table 7.14.19 outlines the potential impairments from stroke in different areas of the brain.

The effects of a cerebellar stroke can also be related to the lobes of the brain involved: the frontal lobe, the parietal lobe, the temporal lobe or the occipital lobe.

Diagnosis and treatment

Brain imaging within 1 hour of admission to hospital is recommended to determine whether an ischaemic or haemorrhagic stroke has occurred, as this will help to determine the treatment.

Treatment of ischaemic stroke

Revascularisation treatments for acute ischaemic stroke aim to re-establish blood flow to the affected area of the brain, minimising brain tissue damage. The first line of treatment for an acute ischaemic stroke is thrombolysis. This involves the intravenous delivery of recombinant plasminogen activator (alteplase), within 4.5 hours of the onset of stroke symptoms, to dissolve the blood clot and restore blood flow to the brain. Thrombolysis with alteplase is now used with one in nine patients

SECTION 7

Table 7.14.19 The effects of stroke in different parts of the brain

Right-sided cerebral stroke	Left-sided cerebral stroke	Cerebellum stroke	Brain stem stroke
Left-sided weakness	Right-sided weakness	Inability to walk	Breathing
Sensory impairment	Speech and language problems such as in talking, reading, writing or understanding	Problems with co-ordination and balance	Heart function
Visual problems	Memory – difficulty retaining new information	Dizziness	Balance and coordination
Spatial awareness	Cautious behaviour	Headache	Paralysis
Memory problems		Nausea and vomiting	Speech
Behavioural changes, e.g. being impulsive or inappropriate			Swallowing
Reduced safety awareness			Vision
Perceptual problems			Hearing
Problem processing visual and verbal information			Locked-in syndrome

with stroke in the UK (RCP, 2016b). Thrombolysis helps to reduce the degree of long-term disability and improve clinical outcomes post–acute ischaemic stroke. Mechanical clot retrieval (thrombectomy) is becoming more commonly used for large cerebral artery occlusions. The most common type of clot retrieval device is a stent retriever. Following a cerebral angiogram to show the exact location of the arterial occlusion, a delivery catheter is inserted, usually through the femoral artery in the groin. The stent retriever, a metal mesh tube, is introduced through the delivery catheter to the occlusion under X ray guidance. The clot is captured in its mesh, and then withdrawn through the catheter, thereby removing the clot and re-establishing blood flow to the affected area of the brain. Many patients undergoing thrombectomy will have had thrombolysis initially. Treatment with thrombectomy has shown significant improvement in functional outcomes up to 90 days post-stroke (Goyal *et al.*, 2016). Neurosurgical intervention may be indicated in some patients following an ischaemic stroke in the middle cerebral artery (MCA). A decompressive hemicraniectomy may be considered. Endovascular treatments for acute ischaemic stroke should only be administered within well-organised stroke services.

Treatment of haemorrhagic stroke

Most patients with intracerebral haemorrhage do not require surgical intervention. Patients with a spontaneous SAH should be transferred to a neurosciences centre. Those diagnosed with SAH secondary to an aneurysm should be treated within 48 hours. This usually involves endovascular embolisation using metal coils or surgical clipping of the aneurysm if appropriate.

The phrase 'time is brain' emphasises the time urgency of stroke care. On average, a patient loses 1.9 million neurons each minute a stroke is left untreated. As treatments for stroke need to be administered in a timely manner, it is important to promote the rapid recognition of stroke symptoms to enable admission of patients to a stroke unit and commencement onto the stroke care pathway. This will ensure that patients are able to access multidisciplinary stroke specialist management, which has been shown to improve long-term survival and functional state. Patients with stroke who receive organised inpatient care in a stroke unit are more likely to be alive, independent and living at home 1 year after a stroke (Stroke Unit Trialists' Collaboration, 2013). The FAST (face, arm, speech, time) awareness campaign, launched by the Department of Health in 2009, has helped to improve the recognition of stroke and TIA symptoms.

In some areas, this timely access to stroke specialist assessment and imaging has been achieved via several different systems, including telemedicine, partnership on call rota systems across several organisations, and the hub and spoke system. In the latter, one hospital across a locality provides 24/7 hyperacute care, including thrombolysis and thrombectomy, and the patient is then transferred to local hospitals or services for acute care and rehabilitation.

Stroke units should participate in the National Stroke Audit to enable comparison of the clinical and organisational quality of their service with national data, and use the findings to plan and deliver service improvement. The Sentinel Stroke National Audit Programme (SSNAP) collects data from all acute stroke units in England, Wales and Northern Ireland (RCP, 2016c). Their performance is summarised against 10 key aspects of stroke care, one of which includes *'proportion of applicable patients screened for nutrition and seen by a dietitian by discharge'*. The most recent data, from April to July 2017, showed that this occurred in 82.5% of cases. In Scotland, all hospitals managing acute stroke use the Scottish Stroke Care Audit, which measures data collected against the Scottish Care Standards for Stroke.

Nutritional consequences

Dysphagia is a frequent and potentially serious complication of stroke (Smithard *et al.*, 1997), and, in some cases, may be the sole or overriding symptom (Celifarco *et al.*, 1990). Dysphagia is present in 40–78% of patients following acute stroke; poor patient outcomes are linked with dysphagia, including chest infection, disability and death (Martino *et al.*, 2005) (see Chapter 7.3, Dysphagia). It is important to screen and assess dysphagia early to prevent pneumonia (Bray *et al.*, 2016), undernutrition and dehydration (Kidd *et al.*, 1995; Smithard *et al.*, 1997; Whelan, 2001). Up to 29% of patients recover their swallow and resume full oral nutrition, although this process may take up to 31 months (ESPEN, 2006). During this period, it is important to utilise the skills of the dietitian and the speech and language therapist (SLT) to support the recovery and ensure that adequate intake of nutrition and fluids is maintained, taking into consideration the roles of enteral nutrition and texture modification. Raising awareness of nutritional risk with all multidisciplinary team (MDT members will support the recognition of malnutrition in a timely way that will enable its effective management.

Patients with acute stroke often exhibit a poor nutritional status, with 15% of cases being admitted to hospital with malnutrition. This negatively impacts on outcome and costs: length of hospital stay is extended; rehabilitation is delayed; and survival reduced (Age Concern, 2006; Axelsson *et al.*, 1988; ESPEN, 2006; King's Fund, 1992). This increases to 30% over the first week following a stroke (RCP, 2016b). Gariballa *et al.* (1998) identified that malnutrition is common and worsens within the first 2 weeks after stroke, and this affects outcome. Malnutrition will impact on the patient's ability to participate in rehabilitation, owing to its impact on fatigue, strength and concentration, thus affecting recovery and long-term outcomes.

Dietitians oversee the implementation and monitoring of nutritional screening processes and the actions arising from screening, incorporating a multidisciplinary approach to the management of dysphagia. Dietitians can then undertake a more comprehensive nutritional assessment and put a nutritional care package into place (Logemann, 1994). The nutritional status of all stroke patients should be screened, and access to dietetic services provided as necessary (Gomes *et al.*, 2016). If tube feeding is required, it needs to be considered within 24 hours of admission (RCP, 2016b). Dietitians advise patients on achieving nutritional requirements via tube feeding, food fortification or supplementation; monitor patients and adapt advice as required; and advise staff, patients and carers on how to meet nutritional requirements on a texture-modified diet. Table 7.14.20 shows the potential complications or consequences following a stroke, the impact these may have on nutritional intake, and how the dietitian can work with the patient and the other members of the MDT to reduce the impact. Vascular dementia can occur post-stroke, which can further affect nutritional status; see Chapter 7.10.3 (Dementias) for additional considerations.

To ensure nutritional outcomes are maximised, multidisciplinary working is essential. This should ideally include relevant members of the medical team, nurses, physiotherapists, occupational therapists, dietitians, SLTs, therapy assistants (including dietetic assistants), social workers, care managers, healthcare assistants, pharmacists, psychologists/neuropsychologists, orthoptists, catering staff/assistants, and orthotists.

Patient-centred goals, treatment and therapy plans should be agreed on with the patient whenever possible, and developed in partnership with the MDT to facilitate the rehabilitation of the patients post-stroke. The MAGIC (making good decisions in collaboration) improvement programme (Health Foundation, 2013) and 'Choosing Wisely' are examples of programmes to help practitioners engage more with patients in sharing decision-making.

Over one-third of patients post-stroke in England, Wales and Northern Ireland will be discharged to an Early Supported Discharge (ESD) team or community stroke rehabilitation team (RCP, 2016b), where rehabilitation is provided in the patients' own homes. There should be easy access to dietetics for these community-based teams (RCP, 2016b).

Nutritional assessment

Dietitians should assess the nutritional status of stroke patients using the model and process for nutrition and dietetic practice (see Chapter 1.1, Professional practice). The key points for consideration by the dietitian include the following:

- Type of stroke.
- Ethics of artificial nutrition.
- If swallow is unsafe, consider enteral feeding within 24 hours post-stroke, unless the patient has had thrombolysis. If so, then insertion of the nasogastric tube (NGT) should be performed 24 hours after the completion of thrombolysis.
- Patients post-SAH secondary to aneurysm normally require 3L fluid daily for an extended period. Liaise with medical staff as to how best to meet this requirement.
- For patients post-SAH secondary to aneurysm, nimodipine may be administered to prevent vasospasm by relaxing blood vessels, so that blood can flow more easily. The drug is normally prescribed for a 21-day period.
- Assess risk of refeeding syndrome and treat according to policy.
- Consider the use of nasal bridles if NGT needs frequent replacement (Beavan *et al.*, 2010).
- Consider the use of bolus, continuous or overnight feeding to best meet patients' nutritional requirements, alongside other therapy/medical interventions.
- Monitor and reassess as patients' needs change, recognising the impact of therapy on nutritional requirements, timing of therapy, increased energy expenditure and the possible fatigue due to the therapy and the stroke.
- Assess for gastrostomy insertion if:
  - Unable to tolerate NGT with nasal bridle.
  - Unable to meet nutritional needs orally by 4 weeks post-stroke.
  - High long-term risk of malnutrition.

Table 7.14.20 Impairments post-stroke, nutritional consequences and their management

Potential impairments	Nutritional consequences	Dietetic and MDT management
Activities of daily living Personal and extended activities Driving Work and leisure activities	Difficulty shopping and cooking Access to food	Provide adaptations and appropriate equipment Appropriate seating/positioning
Arm function	Limited ability to self-feed Loss of function leading to problems with eating and drinking	Provide assistance/support at meal times, which includes physical help and verbal encouragement Use of adapted cutlery, plate and/or guards
Mobility Weakness and ataxia Balance Falls and fear of falling Walking	Increased risk of falls Loss of independence	Use of appropriate moving and handling techniques Support physical activity as much as possible
Spasticity and contractures	Effects on activities of daily living, arm function and mobility, as listed in the preceding text	Take into account the use of splints and casts when weighing patients
Pain Neuropathic pain Musculoskeletal pain Shoulder pain and subluxation	Affects ability to eat and drink Can lead to decreased mood	Optimum pain control Appropriate therapy to affected area
Sensation	Sensory losses that can, in turn, affect oral intake	Sensory retraining
Vision	Only seeing food on one side of the plate/tray	Consider the position of the plate
Cognition Cognitive impairments: Apraxia Attention and concentration Executive function Memory Perception Spatial awareness	Poor engagement in dietetic consultations Reduced speed of processing information given Easily distracted when eating Poor dietary recall Forget to eat and drink Impaired object recognition, e.g. knowing how to use cutlery Difficulty analysing the position of the plate	Reduce background distractions Shorter treatment sessions Behaviour modification techniques
Communication Aphasia Dysarthria Apraxia of speech	Difficulty communicating needs such as hunger and thirst Difficulty expressing food preferences Difficulties filling out a menu or ordering food	Use of food record charts Use of a food diary – written or pictorial Ensure written information provided is aphasia-friendly where possible Include family/carers in advice giving Use of communication aids Use of interpreters when required
Mental capacity	Poor retention of information	Liaise with family/carers regarding preferences
Mood and well-being Anxiety, depression and psychological distress Emotionalism	Social isolation Decreased oral intake	Increase social interaction
Mouth care	Sore mouth, mouth ulcers and cracked lips as a result of poor oral hygiene	Maintain good oral hygiene

(*Continued*)

Table 7.14.20 (*Continued*)

Potential impairments	Nutritional consequences	Dietetic and MDT management
Fatigue	Lack of energy Reduced engagement	Help identify triggers and re-energisers
Swallowing	Need for texture modification and/or thickened drinks can reduce nutritional and fluid intake Increased risk of aspiration pneumonia Difficulties in taking prescribed medication	Swallow screening and assessment Adherence to the nationally agreed descriptors for modified-consistency food and fluids Provide written guidance for all staff/carers to use when feeding or providing fluids to patients with dysphagia Ensure medication is prescribed in an appropriate form Consider nasogastric (NG) feeding within 24 hrs of admission in patients who are unable to meet nutritional and fluid needs orally (NG tube should not be passed until 24 hours post-thrombolysis)
Hydration and nutrition	Reduced appetite Risk of malnutrition Risk of dehydration Continual dislodgement of enteral feeding tubes	Screening for the risk of malnutrition on admission, and weekly thereafter Regular monitoring of dietary intake and nutritional status Provide nutritional support for those identified as malnourished or at risk of malnutrition Monitor fluid intake Dietetic assessment, treatment and advice for patients requiring tube feeding, dietary modification or texture-modified diets Consider percutaneous endoscopic gastrostomy insertion if patients are unable to take adequate food and fluids orally 4 weeks post-stroke, or are at high long-term risk of malnutrition Consider calcium and vitamin D supplementation for those who are at high risk of, or with symptoms of, vitamin D deficiency Hold discussions regarding removing food or fluid restrictions for those receiving end-of-life care
Continence	Constipation Increased risk of skin breakdown and pressure ulcers	Management of urinary and faecal incontinence Management of constipation, which includes advice on diet, fluid intake and exercise

MDT, multidisciplinary team.

- If discharging on enteral nutrition, refer to Chapter 6.4 (Enteral nutrition) and the NICE clinical guidelines for nutrition support (NICE, 2017b).
- For patients requiring dietary modification or texture-modified diets, see Chapter 6.3 (Oral nutritional support), the NICE clinical guidelines for nutrition support (NICE, 2017b), and Chapter 7.3 (Dysphagia) for additional guidance on providing individualised specialised dietary advice.
- Consider discharge planning to ensure seamless transfer of care.

Stroke prevention

Primary prevention

Through promoting healthy living, dietitians can help manage the risk of stroke, by being able to assess and give information about smoking, diet, weight, alcohol and family history (see Chapter 7.14.1, General aspects of cardiovascular disease). Dietitians working in public health projects and programmes across the community help promote a healthier lifestyle and, in the longer term, reduce stroke (see Chapter 4.2, Public health nutrition). It is important to address the risk factors for cardiovascular disease (see Chapter 7.14.1, General aspects of cardiovascular disease).

Secondary prevention

There is an increased risk of stroke patients having a further stroke; 26% within 5 years, and 39% by 10 years post–first stroke (Mohan *et al.*, 2011). Dietitians have a key role in reducing the risk of further strokes and improving the management of conditions such as hyperlipidaemia, diabetes and hypertension, as recommended in the RCP guidelines, British Hypertension

Society Guidelines, and Diabetes UK – see Chapters 7.12 (Diabetes mellitus), 7.14.3 (Dyslipidaemia), and 7.14.4 (Hypertension). This can be delivered one to one, in group sessions, or by training other healthcare professionals to disseminate the information. To reduce the risk of further stroke, it is important to moderate the risk factors where possible, including the following:

- Smoking.
- Hypertension.
- Obesity.
- High lipid levels.
- Diabetes or insulin resistance.
- Atrial fibrillation.
- Obstructive sleep apnoea.
- Physical inactivity.
- Excessive alcohol.
- Carotid artery stenosis.
- Oral contraception.
- Hormone replacement therapy.

Dietitians have a role in reducing many of these risk factors.

Drug–nutrient interactions

A number of drugs are used to prevent a stroke. Their main actions include reducing blood pressure, reducing the risk of developing blood clots and reducing lipid levels. These, including statins and warfarin, have known interactions with some foods:

- Grapefruit – grapefruit and grapefruit juice can slow the breakdown of some medications. This causes an increase in the amount of the drug in the blood stream, which increases its effect. It is not clear how long this effect lasts. This reaction is not associated with other juices.
  - Statins – grapefruit juice should be avoided when taking simvastatin. It can be consumed in small amounts when taking other statins, e.g. atorvastin.
  - Nimodipine – grapefruit and grapefruit juice should be avoided.
- Warfarin
  - Cranberry juice can increase the effect of warfarin, so should be avoided to reduce the risk of bleeding.
  - Foods high in vitamin K (e.g. Brussels sprouts, broccoli and liver) can stop warfarin from functioning. It is advised that these foods not necessarily be avoided, but that large quantities should only be eaten infrequently. This will have a more consistent impact on warfarin levels.
- Novel (non–vitamin K antagonist) oral anticoagulants (NOACs) – rivaroxaban is first choice for stroke prevention, and has no known food interactions.

Acknowledgement

The editor acknowledges the prior contribution of Fiona Jenkins.

Internet resources

Blood Pressure Association, www.bpassoc.org.uk
British Heart Foundation, www.bhf.org.uk
British Hypertension Society, www.bhsoc.org
Diabetes UK, www.diabetes.org.uk
Foundation for Circulatory Health, www.ffch.org
NHS Improvement, www.improvement.nhs.uk
NHS – The Fast Campaign, www.nhs.uk/actfast
NICE, www.nice.org.uk
CG68 – Stroke and transient ischaemic attack in over 16s: diagnosis and initial management.
Public Health Guidance – e.g. PH42 Obesity: working with local communities; PH47: Weight management: lifestyle services for overweight and obese children and young people; PH53: Weight management: lifestyle services for overweight and obese adults.
Royal College of Physicians, www.rcplondon.ac.uk
National Clinical Guideline for Stroke, 5th edn (2016)
Profession Specific Audit (2006)
Sentinel Stroke National Audit, www.strokeaudit.org
Stroke Association, www.stroke.org.uk

References

Age Concern. (2006) *Hungry to be Heard*. Available at www.ageuk.org.uk/documents/en-gb/hungry_to_be_heard_inf.pdf?dtrk=true. Accessed August 2017.

Axelsson K, Asplund K, Norberg A, *et al.* (1988) Nutritional status in patients with acute stroke. *Acta Med. Scand.* 224(3): 217–224.

Beavan J, Conroy SP, Harwood R, *et al.* (2010) Does looped nasogastric tube feeding improve nutritional delivery for patients with dysphagia after acute stroke? A randomised controlled trial. *Age Ageing*. 39: 624–630.

Bray BD, Cloud GC, James MA, *et al.* (2016) Weekly variation in health-care quality by day and time of admission: a nationwide, registry-based, prospective cohort study of acute stroke care. *Lancet*. 388: 170–177.

Celifarco A, Gerard G, Faegenburg D, *et al.* (1990) Dysphagia as the sole manifestation of bilateral strokes. *Am. J. Gastroenterol.* 85(5): 610–613.

DH. (2007) *National Stroke Strategy HD/Vascular Programme/Stroke*. Available at http://webarchive.nationalarchives.gov.uk/20130105121530/http://www.dh.gov.uk/en/Publicationsandstatistics/Publications/PublicationsPolicyandguidance/dh_081062. Accessed August 2017.

DH. (2016) *Quality and Outcomes Framework (QOF) Achievement Data 2015/2016*. Available at http://bit.ly/2hQNsMB. Accessed August 2017.

ESPEN. (2006) ESPEN guidelines on enteral nutrition: cardiology and pulmonology. *Clin. Nutr.* 25(2): 311–318.

Feigin VL, Forouzanfar MH, Krishnamurthi R, *et al.* (2013) Global and regional burden of stroke during 1990–2010: findings from the Global Burden of Disease Study 2010. *Lancet*. 383: 245–255.

Gariballa SE, Parker SG, Taub N, *et al.* (1998) Influence of nutritional status on clinical outcome after acute stroke. *Am. J. Clin. Nutr.* 68(2): 275–281.

Gomes F, Emery PW, Weekes CE. (2016) Risk of malnutrition is an independent predictor or mortality, length of hospital stay, and hospitalization costs in stroke patients. *J. Stroke Cerebrovasc. Dis.* 25: 799–806.

Goyal M, Menon BK, van Zwam WH, *et al.* (2016) Endovascular thrombectomy after large-vessel ischaemic stroke: a meta-analysis of individual patient data from five randomised trials. *Lancet*. 387: 1723–1731.

Health Foundation. (2013) *MAGIC Programme (Making Good Decisions in Collaboration) Improvement Programme*. Available at http://www.health.org.uk/publication/magic-programme-evaluation. Accessed August 2017.

Information Services Division (ISD) Scotland. (2016a) *Quality and Outcomes Framework 2015–2016*. Available at http://bit.ly/2hPEpZv. Accessed 20 December 2016.

Information Services Division (ISD) Scotland. (2016b) *Scottish Stroke Care Audit, Scottish Stroke Improvement Programme Report – 2016*. Available at http://bit.ly/29uWaYZ. Accessed October 2016.

Kidd D, Lawson J, Nesbitt R, *et al.* (1995) The natural history and clinical consequences of aspiration in acute stroke. *QJM*. 88: 409–413.

King's Fund. (1992) *A Positive Approach to Nutrition as Treatment*. Available at www.bapen.org.uk/pdfs/bapen_pubs/pub_kings_fund.pdf. Accessed August 2017.

Logemann JA. (1994) Multidisciplinary management of dysphagia. *Acta Otorhinolaryngol. Belg.* 48(2): 235–238.

Marshall IJ, Wang Y, Crichton S, *et al.* (2015) The effects of socio-economic status on stroke risk and outcomes. *Lancet Neurol.* 14: 1206–1218.

Martino R, Foley N, Bhogal S, *et al.* (2005) Dysphagia after stroke: incidence, diagnosis, and pulmonary complications. *Stroke*. 36(12): 2756–2763.

Mohan KM, Wolfe CD, Rudd AG, *et al.* (2011) Risk and cumulative risk of stroke recurrence: a systematic review and meta-analysis. *Stroke*. 42: 1489–1494.

National Records of Scotland. (2016) *Deaths by Sex, Age and Cause, Scotland, 2015*. Available at http://bit.ly/2h671Pu. Accessed 20 December 2016.

NHS. (2016) *Quality Outcomes Framework (QOF) – 2015–2016*. Available at http://bit.ly/2gC6LWb. Accessed August 2017.

NICE. (2017a) *Clinical Guideline CG68 Stroke and transient ischaemic attack in over 16s: diagnosis and initial management*. Available at www.nice.org.uk/guidance/cg68. Accessed August 2017.

NICE. (2017b) *Clinical Guideline CG32: Nutrition support in adults: oral nutrition support, enteral tube feeding and parenteral nutrition*. Available at https://www.nice.org.uk/guidance/cg32. Accessed August 2017.

Office for National Statistics. (2016) *Deaths Registered in England and Wales: 2015*. Available at http://bit.ly/2h7Om7P. Accessed 20 December 2016.

Royal College of Paediatrics and Child Health. (2017) *Stroke in Childhood; Clinical Guideline for Diagnosis, Management and Rehabilitation*. Available at www.rcpch.ac.uk/stroke-guideline#fullclinicalguideline. Accessed August 2017.

Royal College of Physicians Sentinel Stroke National Audit Programme (SSNAP). (2015) *Is Stroke Care Improving? Second SSNAP Annual Report Prepared on Behalf of the Intercollegiate Stroke Working Party November 2015*. London: RCP. Available at https://www.rcplondon.ac.uk/projects/outputs/sentinel-stroke-national-audit-programme-ssnap. Accessed August 2017.

Royal College of Physicians Sentinel Stroke National Audit Programme (SSNAP). (2016a) *National Clinical Audit Annual Results Portfolio March 2015–April 2016*. Available at http://bit.ly/1M5R3Op. Accessed August 2017.

Royal College of Physicians Sentinel Stroke National Audit Programme. (2016b) *National Clinical Guideline for Stroke*, 5th edn. London: RCP. Available at https://www.rcplondon.ac.uk/guidelines-policy/stroke-guidelines. Accessed August 2017.

Royal College of Physicians Sentinel Stroke National Audit Programme. (2016c) *Annual Results portfolio prepared on behalf of the Intercollegiate Stroke Working Party*. London: RCP. Available a https://www.strokeaudit.org/Documents/National/AcuteOrg/2016/2016-AOANationalReport.aspx. Accessed August 2017.

Saka O, McGuire A, Wolfe C. (2009) Cost of stroke in the United Kingdom. *Age Ageing*. 38: 27–32.

Smithard DG, O'Neill PA, England RE, *et al.* (1997) The natural history of dysphagia following a stroke. *Dysphagia*. 12(4): 188–193.

Stroke Association. (2017) *State of the Nation, Stroke Statistics*. Available at https://www.stroke.org.uk/resources/state-nation-stroke-statistics. Accessed August 2017.

Stroke Unit Trialists' Collaboration. (2013) Organised inpatient (stroke unit) care for stroke. *Cochrane Database Syst. Rev.* (9): CD000197.

Wang Y, Rudd AG, Wolfe CD. (2013) Age and ethnic disparities in incidence of stroke over time: the South London Stroke Register. *Stroke*. 44: 3298–3304.

Welsh Government. (2016) *General Medical Services Quality and Outcomes Framework Statistics for Wales 2015–2016*. Available at http://bit.ly/2hQzI46. Accessed 20 December 2016.

Whelan K. (2001) Inadequate fluid intake in dysphagic acute stroke. *Clin. Nutr.* 20(5): 423–428.

7.15 Cancer

7.15.1 General aspects of cancer

Clare Shaw

Key points

- Diet is both a causative and protective environmental factor that may influence cancer development.
- Development of cancer may increase an individual's risk of becoming malnourished, owing to disease or treatment effects.
- Weight loss may increase the morbidity and mortality associated with cancer treatment.
- Appropriate nutritional advice and/or artificial nutritional support should be an integral part of the treatment plan.

It is estimated that about one-third of the UK population will be diagnosed with cancer during their lifetime; however, as treatments have developed, survival rates have increased significantly. The term cancer describes a wide range of malignant tumours that affect virtually every organ and tissue in the body. Cancer is a major cause of mortality and morbidity throughout the world. In the UK, approximately 352,197 new cases occur every year (Cancer Research UK (CRUK), 2013a).

In the UK, the most common cancer sites are the breast, lung, large bowel and prostate, which together account for over 50% of all cancer diagnoses (CRUK, 2013b). Cancer is generally a disease of increasing age, with 50% of cancers occurring in those aged over 70 years. Worldwide survival rates vary greatly; this is largely dependent on access to diagnostic and treatment services. Although the incidence rates of some of the less common cancers are increasing, overall mortality rates from cancer in middle-aged people are falling, due to improvements in treatment (CRUK, 2012). Many cancers are also treatable if detected at an early stage, and people are increasingly living with cancer; it is now recognised as a chronic disease. In the UK, there are approximately 2.5 million people living with cancer (Macmillan, 2016). The number of people surviving has doubled in the last 40 years, and the combined 10-year survival for all cancers is 50% (CRUK, 2013c).

Definition of *cancer*

Cancer is a consequence of genetic mutations which result in the production and proliferation of abnormal cells. This can occur when healthy cells are damaged and undergo replication that is outside the usual control. Some of these genetic mutations are inherited, but most occur and accumulate over time as the result of lifestyle and environmental factors. The development of cancer is a complex, multistage process that can be summarised as follows:

1. *Initiation* – exposure to substances or influences (mutagens) that are capable of initiating genetic mutations. DNA damage may or may not lead to cancer.
2. *Promotion* – under the influence of promoters, damaged DNA begins to be expressed, resulting in cellular changes. Promoters thus enhance tumour development following exposure to mutagens.
3. *Progression* – a complex process leading to the development of malignant cells that have the capacity to invade other tissues.

The term carcinogen indicates a substance that may influence one or more of these stages. Only a few carcinogens can affect all three.

Cancers spread by invading the surrounding tissue until they reach a blood or lymph vessel. Small groups of

Manual of Dietetic Practice, Sixth Edition. Edited by Joan Gandy.

Companion website: www.manualofdieteticpractice.com

cells may then break off and be carried to other parts of the body, where they may settle and grow. New cancers that develop are called secondary cancers or metastases. Cancer is therefore not a single disease but a group of diseases; there are over 200 different types of cancers arising from different cells of the body.

Development of cancer

Much remains to be learned about the complex interplay of factors that lead to cancer development, particularly hereditary influences. About 5% of cancers are thought to result from inherited genetic mutations (e.g. the *BRCA1* and *BRCA2* genes in breast cancer), but even the aetiology of this form of cancer is complex; not everyone with a cancer-predisposing genotype develops the disease (see Chapter 5.1, Genetics and nutritional genomics). Ninety-five per cent of cancers are defined as sporadic, i.e. the unpredictable consequence of a combination of genetics, environment and chance. Since little can be done to alter the influence of genetics and chance, efforts to prevent cancer must focus on identifying and minimising the risk from factors that are modifiable, i.e. environmental influences. The main environmental factors implicated in the causation of cancer are as follows:

- *Tobacco* – more than a quarter of all cancer deaths in the UK are thought to be tobacco related. Cigarette smoking causes 90% of lung cancers and increases the risk of many other cancers, particularly those in tissues most exposed to tobacco carcinogens, i.e. head and neck, oesophagus, stomach, kidney and bladder.
- *Body weight* – increased adiposity increases the risk of some cancer through effects on hormones and growth factors. Many types are more common in overweight or obese people, including breast, bowel, oesophageal and uterine cancer.
- *Diet* – can have either harmful or protective influences on cancer development, depending on its composition in terms of foods, nutrients and contaminants.
- *Infection* – certain viruses can cause genetic mutations that may result in cancer development, e.g. the Epstein–Barr virus is associated with some types of lymphatic cancer, and human papilloma virus is linked with cervical cancer. *Helicobacter pylori* infection is thought to be a major factor in the development of gastric cancer.
- *Industrial pollutants* – exposure to toxic substances (e.g. asbestos or vinyl chloride) can rapidly lead to cancer. This is more of a problem in less-developed countries where environmental safety controls are often poor.
- *Ionising radiation* – overexposure to X rays, nuclear emissions or some other sources of radioactivity increases the risk of leukaemia.
- *Sunlight* – most skin cancers are caused by the action of radiation from sunlight on the skin.
- *Physical inactivity* – has been implicated in the aetiology of some types of cancer, including breast, bowel and kidney cancer, via its influence on hormone levels in the body.

Diet and causation of cancer

Although there is a common underlying aetiology, different factors influence the development of each type of cancer. For this reason, relationships between diet and cancer are complex and variable; dietary factors may be involved in the initiation of tumour growth (carcinogens), the promotion of growth, or be protective against the development of cancer. It is thought that about half of all cancer-related deaths are preventable, many of them by diet and lifestyle measures.

Many components of the diet have carcinogenic potential. Some result from food contamination, e.g. aflatoxin, a potent carcinogen causing liver cancer that is produced by a mould that can grow on grain stored under inappropriate conditions. Other carcinogens (e.g. alkaloids, benzene derivatives or N-nitroso compounds) occur naturally in foods, or are created during the cooking or preservation processes. Alcohol may act as a carcinogen when in contact with tissues of the head, neck or oesophagus.

Diet may have a role to play in the promotion of tumour growth by encouraging cell replication. This may be caused by dietary components such as alcohol or a high-energy diet. Diet and body weight may also influence the growth of cancer cells through the promotion of hormones, e.g. oestrogens in the promotion of breast cancer.

The human body has many defences to protect it from potentially harmful dietary and non-dietary agents, and to a large extent can withstand continuous onslaught. However, the body's ability to do so depends on several factors, including immune competence, the integrity of mucosal barriers and the levels of detoxifying enzymes, all of which are affected by diet. It is therefore not unreasonable to expect that diet is likely to be one of the factors enhancing or diminishing the risk of cancer.

In 1981, Doll and Peto suggested that about one-third of cancers in Westernised countries may be attributable to dietary factors, and that as much as 70% of cancers in sites such as the large bowel, breast and prostate may be preventable by dietary modification. A major report from the World Cancer Research Fund (WCRF), in conjunction with the American Institute for Cancer Research (AICR) (WCRF/AICR, 2007), confirmed that there are many links between diet and cancer, both causal and protective. The relationships are complex and, given the quality of available evidence, difficult to ascertain. The effect on reducing cancer risk if dietary recommendations (Table 7.15.1) are followed is unclear, although a study of 36,626 women showed that following 6–9 of the WCRF recommendations over a 17-year period resulted in a 22% reduction in cancer risk, as compared to women who did not follow any recommendations. This relationship existed in women with both modifiable and non-modifiable risk factors such as height and family history of breast cancer (Nomura *et al.*, 2016).

Table 7.15.1 Dietary recommendations for cancer prevention – based on the World Cancer Research Fund–American Institute for Cancer Research report (WCRF/AICR, 2007)

Recommendation	Public health goals	Justification
Maintain a healthy weight.	Median adult body mass index (BMI) of 21–23 kg/m^2, depending on population normal range. Maintain overweight/obesity levels, preferably lower, in 10 years.	Maintenance of a healthy weight throughout life may be one of the most important ways to protect against cancer.
Be physically active as part of everyday life.	Half the proportion of the population that is sedentary every 10 years. Average physical activity levels (PALs) >1.6.	Most populations have habitual levels of activity below which humans are adapted.
Limit consumption of energy-dense foods. Avoid sugary drinks.	Average diet energy density to be lowered towards 125 kcal/100 g. Halve average consumption of sugary drinks every 10 years.	Consumption of energy-dense foods and sugary drinks increasing, and is probably contributing to the global increase in obesity.
Eat mostly foods of plant origin.	Population average consumption of non-starchy vegetables and fruit of ≥600 g/day. Relatively unprocessed cereals and/or pulses, and other natural dietary fibre sources, to contribute to a population average of ≥25 g/day of non-starch polysaccharides (NSPs).	Evidence shows that most protective diets consist mainly of foods of plant origin.
Limit intake of red meat and avoid processed meat.	Population average consumption of ≤300 g/week, very little (if any) processed.	Evidence shows that many foods of animal origin are nourishing and healthy if consumed in modest amounts.
Limit alcoholic drinks.	Proportion of the population drinking no more than the recommended limits to be reduced by one-third every 10 years.	Evidence on cancer justifies a recommendation not to consume alcoholic drinks. Other evidence shows that a modest amount of alcoholic drinks is likely to reduce the risk of coronary heart disease.
Limit consumption of salt. Avoid mouldy cereals (grains) or pulses (legumes).	Population average consumption of salt from all sources to be <5 g (2 g sodium/day). Proportion of the population consuming >6 g salt (2.4 g of sodium)/day to be halved every 10 years. Minimise exposure to aflatoxins from mouldy cereals or (legumes).	Evidence shows that salt and salt-preserved foods are probably a cause of stomach cancer, and that foods contaminated with aflatoxins are a cause of liver cancer.
Aim to meet nutritional needs through diet alone.	Maximise the proportion of the population achieving nutritional adequacy without dietary supplements.	Evidence shows that high-dose nutrient supplements can be protective or cause cancer. The studies that demonstrate such effects do not relate to widespread use among the general population, in whom the balance of the risks and benefits cannot confidently be predicted. A general recommendation to consume supplements for cancer prevention may have unexpected adverse effects. Increasing the consumption of the relevant nutrients through usual diet is preferred.
Mothers to breastfeed: children to be breastfed.	The majority of mothers to breastfeed exclusively for 6 months.	Evidence shows that sustained, exclusive breastfeeding is protective for the mother as well as the child.
Cancer survivors: follow the recommendations for cancer prevention.	All cancer survivors to receive nutritional care from an appropriately trained professional. If unable to do so, and unless otherwise advised, aim to follow the recommendations for diet, healthy weight, and physical activity.	Subject to the qualifications made in the WCRF report.

Nature of the evidence for relationships between diet and cancer

Most of the suggested associations between diet and cancer are based on data from epidemiological studies, which include the following types of study (see Chapter 1.1, Professional practice).

- *Cross-sectional studies* can provide valuable pointers but are not in themselves evidence of cause and effect, as many other relevant factors (e.g. socioeconomic, demographic, genetic, cultural and environmental factors) will also differ.
- *Case control studies* have the advantage of creating more homogeneous study populations. However, at

the same time, such homogeneity in terms of age, social class, occupation, etc., also means that dietary differences between the two groups are likely to be small, or not readily detectable, given the limitations of dietary assessment methodology. Alternatively, if dietary differences are observed, it is difficult to know whether they existed in the early stages of cancer development (perhaps before many years), or whether they are a consequence of the disease.

- *Prospective (cohort) studies* follow people until cancer develops, thus enabling dietary comparison between those who develop the disease and those who do not, and are particularly informative. The European Prospective Intervention into Cancer and Nutrition (EPIC) is a cohort study that investigates the effects of diet, lifestyle, and genetic and environmental factors on the incidence of different forms of cancer.
- *Intervention trials* evaluate the effects of dietary change in a randomised, controlled prospective trial, and can provide the clearest evidence of dietary benefit or risk. However, for reasons of cost, they are unlikely to be carried out on a sufficiently large scale, or for long enough, to evaluate the effect of major dietary manipulations on cancer (e.g. encouraging a high consumption of fruit and vegetables).

Animal studies are a valuable supplement to human studies to help explain the mechanisms of carcinogenesis and provide pointers to dietary influences on those mechanisms. However, animal studies cannot ultimately predict dietary risk in free-living human populations where many other factors will operate.

Complexity of the relationship between diet and cancer

The interrelationship between diet and the development of cancer is complex and multifactorial. The relationships between diet and cancer are hard to unravel because of the great variability of both the disease and the dietary influences on it. Different cancers are influenced by diet to a different extent. Although all cancers stem from DNA damage, the causes and effects of that damage are very variable. Some cancers, e.g. colorectal and breast, may be strongly linked with diet and body composition; others, e.g. leukaemia, have no relationships with diet at all.

Some dietary factors, e.g. NSP, may be protective against one type of cancer but have no influence on another. Also, observed dietary relationships do not always operate in the same direction; energy intake is positively associated with the development of some cancers, e.g. breast and endometrial, but negatively with others, e.g. stomach and oesophageal. A dietary influence may be heightened or diminished by non-dietary factors, e.g. a dietary component may only become a risk factor in certain circumstances, such as a person smoking. The risk or benefit from one dietary component may be affected by the presence or absence of other dietary components, e.g. the level of risk from meat may depend on the level of consumption of protective fruit and vegetables. Therefore, attempts to assess whether one particular dietary component is beneficial, harmful or neutral in effect are fraught with difficulty and open to misinterpretation. Few dietary risk factors operate in isolation, and it seems increasingly likely that it is the combination of harmful and protective influences from both dietary and non-dietary sources that determines the level of cancer risk. The relationships between diet and cancer are therefore based on judgement as to what the research evidence means, as reviewed by the WCRF/AICR (2007).

Diet and cancer care

Nutrition is an important aspect of the care of the person with cancer from diagnosis onwards. Many aspects of cancer can affect nutritional status, and impaired nutritional status can in turn affect the response to treatment, the amount of treatment required and the quality of life (Henry, 2011; NICE, 2004). Dietitians working in oncology have a vital role in ensuring that the nutritional aspects of patient management are an integral component of multidisciplinary care, and that all cancer patients receive necessary dietetic support. The National Institute for Health and Care Excellence (NICE, 2004) recommends that dietitians working in oncology have knowledge of the impact of the disease and treatment, and their complex needs, to be able to provide the high level of care. This criterion is subject to peer review in the NHS (NCAT, 2011). Dietitians need to work in close collaboration with other team members to meet patient needs. The value of dietitians and other allied health professionals and the impact they can have on improving clinical outcomes is increasingly recognised in cancer care, particularly as most people will require rehabilitation (NHS networks, 2012).

Nutritional implications of cancer

People with cancer are at high risk of nutritional depletion, owing to the physical and psychological effects of both the disease and its treatment, such as the following:

- A prolonged catabolic response to the presence of a tumour may occur, resulting in muscle wasting and weight loss (Fearon *et al.*, 2011; Laviano *et al.*, 2011). This is described as the cancer cachexia syndrome, and is a result of both nutritional and metabolic changes.
- Physical symptoms (e.g. pain, dysphagia, vomiting and diarrhoea) may impair food intake or nutrient absorption, or increase nutrient losses.
- The psychological effects of a cancer diagnosis can result in anxiety and/or depression, and may impair appetite.
- Cancer treatments often result in pronounced and debilitating side effects. Gastrointestinal consequences such as anorexia, nausea, vomiting, diarrhoea, bloating, pain or cramping inevitably have an adverse effect

on nutritional intake, and additional problems such as taste changes, dysphagia, infections and fistulae may further compromise nutritional status.

The risk of weight loss and undernutrition is therefore high. About 40% of cancer patients have been found to have significant protein energy malnutrition (Bozzetti & SCRINIO Working Group, 2009). Also, in some high-risk groups, such as those hospitalised for cancer treatment and head and neck cancer patients, up to 70–80% may have some degree of malnutrition (Shaw *et al.*, 2015). The adverse consequences of this in terms of postoperative recovery time, prevalence of complications and prognosis are well documented (see Chapter 6.2, Malnutrition). In cancer patients, undernutrition may also have implications for cancer treatment, since chemotherapy dosages use body weight to calculate body surface area, and underweight patients may not be given optimum dosages (Andreyev *et al.*, 1998). A patient with muscle wasting is also less likely to be able to withstand any side effects and will develop more toxicity (Jung *et al.*, 2015; Prado *et al.*, 2009).

Preventing and correcting nutritional depletion in order to maintain physical strength and quality of life for as long as possible are therefore important objectives in the care of the cancer patient. The ways in which this is achieved will vary according to the individual clinical circumstances, but primarily comprise the following:

- Ensuring that nutritional and hydration needs are met in an acceptable and appropriate way for each individual throughout the course of the disease.
- Restoring any nutritional inadequacies that occur.
- Minimising the nutritional consequences of the symptoms and side effects of treatment.
- Instituting additional nutritional support measures if dietary intake is inadequate.
- Reviewing the effectiveness of nutritional interventions and adjusting them as necessary.

Close interaction with other members of the multidisciplinary team is essential if these objectives are to be achieved effectively (Fearon, 2008; NICE, 2004; Shaw & Eldridge, 2015).

General aspects of the dietary care of cancer patients

Dietary care may range from offering healthy eating guidance for people who have successfully recovered from treatment, to the provision of total artificial nutritional support in those who are critically ill or unable to manage their full nutritional requirements. In practice, most people will require varying degrees of nutritional intervention throughout the treatment and disease progression. It is important to consider the whole treatment, as this may involve many weeks or months of a range of different treatments.

Nutritional assessment of individual needs and problems should be the cornerstone of dietary management.

Nutritional assessment

Anthropometry

Nutritional assessment should be undertaken as for any patient who is considered to be at risk of malnutrition (see Chapter 6.2, Malnutrition). The degree of any nutritional depletion, to some extent compounded by the cancer process itself, the extent and rapidity of recent weight loss is an important indicator of nutritional depletion (see Chapter 2.2, Assessment of nutritional status). Important considerations include the presence of ascites or oedema, which may influence body weight. The gold standard in cancer care is the patient-generated subjective global assessment (PG-SGA), which assesses weight change over 2 weeks, 1 month and 6 months, in addition to symptoms, functional status, clinical considerations and a physical examination to assess fat and protein stores (Ottery, 1996).

Biochemistry

Low plasma albumin and raised CRP are common, and reflect the disease process, the likelihood of treatment-related infection and the catabolic response to some cancer treatment. Specific biochemical abnormalities may be related to particular clinical conditions, e.g. intestinal failure (see Chapter 7.4.9, Intestinal failure and intestinal resection) and neutropenia (see Chapter 7.11.1, Other disorders of the colon and rectum).

Clinical

The diagnosis and planned treatment will have implications for the likelihood of further (or future) nutritional depletion; surgery will incur significant metabolic costs as a result of preoperative and perioperative starvation and postoperative trauma. Radiotherapy and chemotherapy often result in general disinclination to eat, in addition to causing specific problems with eating or swallowing, or exacerbating pre-existing problems. The risk of nutritional depletion is particularly high in those who are already malnourished. There are nutritional implications for specific cancers (e.g. malabsorption resulting from pancreatic cancer), consequences of surgical procedures (e.g. dumping syndrome following gastric resection), and consequences of treatment (e.g. diarrhoea or steatorrhoea following pelvic radiotherapy). These are discussed in more detail in other chapters.

Dietary assessment

Dietary intake should be assessed using standard methods (see Chapter 2.3, Dietary assessment). The dietitian should be sensitive to considerations which may affect the ability to recall dietary intake, e.g. nausea and fatigue as a result of treatment, or cognitive decline associated with admission to critical care or as a result of chemotherapy. Dietary considerations include the following:

- *Current nutritional intake* – whether this is sufficient to meet estimated nutritional needs.

- *Current nutritional problems* – the extent to which food and fluid intake is impaired by the physical or psychological effects of the disease or its treatment.

Economic and social factors

A diagnosis of cancer can have major economic and social implications, which may also impact on dietary intake. These may include temporary loss of paid employment, fatigue, social isolation and the impact of cancer treatment on lifestyle by factors such as travelling to the cancer centre (e.g. chemotherapy or radiotherapy).

Nutritional management

The importance of good nutrition should be stressed for everyone with a cancer diagnosis. People should be encouraged to continue to meet their needs via a healthy, well-balanced diet whenever possible. If nutritional intake is inadequate, the dietetic objectives are to:

- Increase energy and nutrient intake to meet nutritional requirements in ways that are acceptable to the patient.
- Tackle general and specific problems inhibiting food and fluid intake.
- Identify when further nutritional support is necessary in the context of current and future planned anticancer treatment.

Individualised dietary counselling has been demonstrated to improve nutrient and fluid intake (Baldwin *et al.*, 2012; Bourdel-Marchasson *et al.*, 2014). This may be achieved by relatively simple dietary measures which increase the frequency and energy/nutrient density of the foods and beverages consumed (see Chapter 6.3, Oral nutritional support). Food-enrichment measures (e.g. the addition of milk powder to milk, and adding cheese, butter, olive or vegetable oil or cream to foods) can be an effective. The use of additional high-energy snacks between meals has been shown to be an effective method for increasing dietary intake in addition to the avoidance of meal patterns that rely primarily on fluids (Hutton *et al.*, 2006). Remedial measures to help alleviate treatment side effects affecting food intake (e.g. mucositis, taste changes, nausea, vomiting or diarrhoea) should be suggested (see Chapter 6.3, Oral nutritional support, and other cancer chapters). Adequate symptom control is also paramount.

If oral intake remains inadequate, additional supplementation in the form of sip feeds or other supplements may be considered (Baldwin *et al.*, 2012). Artificial nutritional support (enteral/parenteral nutrition) may be necessary following some types of surgery or cancer treatment, or in those with severe or worsening malnutrition (see Chapter 6.4, Enteral nutrition, and Chapter 6.5, Parenteral nutrition). If the cancer progresses, palliative measures may become the primary consideration (see Chapter 7.16, Palliative and end-of-life care).

Some oral nutritional supplements are specifically aimed at patients with cancer cachexia as they contain n-3 fatty acids which have anti-inflammatory properties. They aim to reduce the metabolic element of cancer cachexia while providing additional energy and protein. Although the principles supporting a reduction in the inflammatory reaction in cancer cachexia are attractive in the management of cachexia, several studies have failed to confirm their efficacy (Fearon *et al.*, 2003; Murphy *et al.*, 2011; Ries *et al.*, 2012). There is interest in the use of n-3 fatty acids to help preserve body composition, although the evidence is weak (Arends *et al.*, 2016).

The dietitian has a crucial role at all stages in identifying when additional support is appropriate and what form this should take to optimise nutritional status without impairing quality of life. Social factors must also be considered in assessing nutritional needs. Those who live alone are particularly vulnerable to malnutrition when they are unwell, in pain, and find it an effort to shop, cook and eat. People should be encouraged to make use of any help offered by friends and neighbours, or other support services available in their community.

It is essential to provide written guidance to patients and carers, together with the contact details of the dietitian, or another member of the healthcare team. Patients who feel unwell may find it difficult to remember the advice given, or to later remember questions they wanted to ask. Providing appropriate dietetic support and guidance not only helps patients feel physically better, but often also psychologically better equipped to cope with what is inevitably a traumatic time.

Maintaining nutritional status may improve tolerance to treatment in terms of less medication to control symptoms, a shorter period of chemotherapy-induced nausea and vomiting, better tolerance of chemotherapy and fewer treatment delays (Ravasco *et al.*, 2012). All patients should therefore be encouraged to regard eating well as an important component of medical care, and a positive step in helping to maintain their health. Some patients may be at increased risk of gaining weight with treatment, e.g. breast cancer patients, and therefore may require advice on weight maintenance during and after treatment, as weight gain may adversely influence prognosis (WCRF, 2010).

Specific aspects of dietary management during cancer treatment

Treatment for cancer usually involves surgery, radiotherapy or chemotherapy (including hormonal treatment), and sometimes a combination of all three. Newer treatments such as immunotherapy or targeted drugs may be used in combination with standard treatments, or as part of clinical trials.

Surgery

A high proportion of patients undergoing curative treatment will have surgery at some point. Surgical removal of a tumour has several nutritional implications:

- Preparation for surgery involves a period of fasting.
- Surgery incurs a significant metabolic cost as a result of the response to trauma.

- In all cases, there will be some delay before normal feeding is resumed. If the surgery is major, or involves any part of the gastrointestinal tract, there may be considerable delay before feeding is possible via the enteral route. Surgery to the mouth, throat or digestive tract may result in prolonged problems with oral feeding (see Chapter 7.15.2, Head and neck cancer).
- Surgery may result in temporary or permanent side effects that affect food intake, digestion or absorption (e.g. dumping syndrome, intestinal failure, ileostomy).

In addition, some cancer patients will undergo surgery in an already malnourished state and be particularly at risk of severe nutritional depletion. All the preceding factors need to be taken into account when nutritional care is being planned, and may influence the following:

- Whether preoperative nutritional support is indicated, its feasibility, and, if feasible, its form. This may include the consideration of immunonutrition, which has been demonstrated to reduce postoperative infection in upper gastrointestinal cancers (Arends *et al.*, 2006, 2016).
- Whether perisurgical and postsurgical nutritional support is likely to be needed, either at an early stage or if there are delays in resumption of oral feeding or complications.
- Whether support should be total or partial.
- The extent to which the oral route will be accessible.
- Whether support is likely to be for short or long term.

As recovery progresses, every effort should be made to restore and maintain good nutritional status if necessary, by means of oral support to optimise nutritional intake. The use of enhanced recovery after surgery (ERAS) programmes can improve outcomes in terms of morbidity and length of hospital stay. Some patients will require specific guidance to alleviate the postsurgical consequences of gastric or intestinal resection. Arrangements should be made to ensure that, after discharge from hospital, the progress of any nutritionally vulnerable patient, particularly in terms of body weight and dietary intake, is monitored.

Radiotherapy

This involves the use of ionising radiation within a treatment field to destroy cancer cells. Radiotherapy damages tissue because energy dissipated from ionising radiation generates a series of biochemical events inside the cell. Free radicals are formed which disrupt DNA, preventing replication, transcription and protein synthesis. When given in combination with chemotherapy, the risk to healthy tissues may be enhanced. Individual radiation treatments, known as fractions, are usually given once daily, sometimes more often (known as hyperfractionated) or less often (hypofractionated); the radiation dose is measured in Gray (Gy). The length of treatment can vary from a single fraction to a 7-week course of five fractions/week. Radical treatment is given with curative intent, while palliative treatment is usually given for symptom control, e.g. pain or shortness of breath. Common general side effects of radiotherapy include the following:

- Anorexia.
- Nausea.
- Fatigue.
- Reduced mood, often related to physical symptoms.

Combinations of these, together with travelling for treatment each day, can have a devastating effect on food intake. Some people find that fatigue makes shopping, food preparation and eating particularly difficult. The site at which the radiotherapy is targeted will determine the severity of side effects. Techniques such as intensity-modulated radiotherapy (IMRT) aim to reduce the effect of radiotherapy on tissues and adjacent organs by targeting as closely to the tumour as possible. Side effects of radiotherapy can further impair food intake. Radiation to the head and neck often affects the ability to eat or swallow; radiation to the pelvic area often results in abdominal cramps and diarrhoea. If steps are not taken to alleviate them, the nutritional consequences can be severe. The side effects of radiotherapy may also change during the course of treatment, e.g. patients initially experiencing dry mouth may develop a sore mouth at a later stage. Regular dietetic assessment is therefore essential to ensure that appropriate and timely advice is given, as patients may experience progressive dysphagia. As patients proceed with radiotherapy treatment, there is a high risk of worsening morbidity and quality of life. Patients undergoing radiotherapy should have regular nutrition screening, and any difficulties with eating should be identified at an early stage in order for these to be addressed.

Chemotherapy

Chemotherapy has a systemic effect; the aim is to destroy cancer cells, but normal tissue will also be affected. The consequences, and side effects, are worst in rapidly dividing tissues such as the lining of the mouth and gastrointestinal tract. Chemotherapy may be given with other targeted therapies, e.g. drugs that affect the growth of cancer cells by different actions. These include monoclonal antibodies that target vascular epidermal growth factor, thereby preventing it from stimulating the growth of new blood vessels. Chemotherapy can be administered as oral tablets, a bolus, continuous infusion or combinations of these.

The number of cytotoxic drugs used to treat cancer is continually increasing, and each drug has different side effects. When drugs are used in combination, the aim is to increase toxicity to the cancer cells while minimising the side effects. Nevertheless, side effects are common, and those that may affect appetite and food intake include the following:

- Nausea and vomiting.
- Taste changes.
- Stomatitis.
- Mucositis (resulting in sore or painful mouth).

- Oesophagitis.
- Diarrhoea.
- Constipation.
- Neutropenia.

In addition to the impact on nutritional status, cytotoxic drugs may also influence certain nutrients as a result of drug–nutrient interactions. For example, methotrexate is a folate antagonist, so its use may need to be accompanied by folinic acid to speed recovery from methotrexate-induced mucositis or myelosuppression. Pyridoxine is used to treat palmar plantar erythrodysesthesia (a painful condition affecting the hands and feet) caused by capecitabine or 5-flurouracil chemotherapy.

Good symptom management is essential to minimise the impact on nutritional intake and nutritional status. Dietary measures that may help alleviate the effects of chemotherapy, such as nausea, taste changes or sore mouth, are described in Chapter 6.3 (Oral nutritional support), and these should be available to patients undergoing treatment to ensure that their dietary intake and quality of life are maximised.

Endocrine therapies

Hormonal manipulation is used in the treatment of hormone-sensitive cancers, e.g. breast and prostate. Cells may vary in their sensitivity to hormones such as oestrogens and progesterones, and sensitivity can be determined by the presence of cellular receptors (oestrogen receptor and progesterone receptor). Treatment interventions may include surgery (e.g. oophorectomy), or, more commonly, medication that blocks hormone action. For example, some endocrine therapies block at the receptor level (receptor antagonist), or block part of the process of hormone manufacture, e.g. aromatise inhibitors or luteinising hormone–releasing hormone agonists. Endocrine therapies can influence mood and cause a decrease in appetite; however, in some patients, weight gain may occur after diagnosis (Parry, 2011).

Monitoring progress of cancer patients

Nutritional assessment should be an integral part of patient monitoring following cancer treatment. Some patients with complex nutritional problems will need ongoing specialist dietetic follow-up. It is essential that all members of the healthcare team be aware of the need to look for and identify emerging nutritional problems, so that they can be rectified at an early stage. Appropriate guidance should be given to identify problems, and referrals provided for dietetic assessment and advice.

Enteral feeding may be indicated for patients with severe anorexia, dysphagia or mucositis, or in who have become nutritionally debilitated. In the short term, this is usually achieved by nasogastric or nasojejunal tube, sometimes on an overnight basis. In the long term (for 4 weeks or more), it is more likely to be via gastrostomy or jejunostomy. Parenteral nutrition should only be used when use of the gastrointestinal route is contraindicated (e.g. bowel obstruction, uncontrollable vomiting or severe malabsorption).

Post-recovery dietary guidance

Cancer patients are usually anxious to consume a diet that minimises the chance of disease progression or recurrence. Some may be tempted to follow complementary or alternative dietary regimens (see Chapter 5.4, Alternative and complementary therapies). People should be assured that current evidence suggests that a diet based on the principles of healthy eating, i.e. a well-balanced diet relatively high in starch and fibre and low in fat, will offer the most protection. Particular emphasis should be placed on the importance of plentiful consumption of fruit and vegetables and wholegrain cereal foods. However, this advice does not apply to patients who have eating difficulties or are losing weight.

Some patients may take vitamin and mineral supplements to reduce cancer growth or risk of recurrence. However, some studies have indicated that such high-dose supplements may increase risk (e.g. beta-carotene in lung cancer) or decrease risk (e.g. calcium in colorectal cancer) of disease or recurrence. At present, there is insufficient evidence to recommend the use of vitamin or mineral supplements as an adjunct to conventional therapy, apart from their use to ensure an adequate dietary intake or to correct a detected deficiency. High doses of vitamins are to be avoided as they may interact with medication, including chemotherapy.

Late effects of cancer treatment may occur, e.g. altered bowel habits following intestinal surgery or pelvic radiotherapy. It is important that persistent symptoms be investigated fully. Peer-reviewed published algorithms are available to support clinicians to investigate and manage gastrointestinal symptoms (Macmillan, 2014). Management may include dietary intervention, e.g. the use of low-fat diets for bile acid malabsorption (Watson *et al.*, 2015).

Palliative care

Sometimes cancer cannot be cured, and treatment becomes palliative, i.e. focusing on the relief of symptoms rather than treating their cause. As the disease progresses, eating and swallowing difficulties become increasingly likely. The patient's food intake is often a great concern to relatives and carers, and can even be a source of conflict. Patients become increasingly cachectic (see Chapter 7.15.9, Cancer cachexia), and the extent to which nutritional and hydration support should be used to sustain life may eventually need to be discussed. The nutritional care of people who are terminally ill is discussed in Chapter 7.16 (Palliative and end-of-life care). Some of the ethical issues involved are discussed in Chapter 1.1 (Professional practice).

Alternative diets

Many people with cancer try unconventional remedies, including alternative and complementary diets, in the hope of cure or remission (Garland *et al.*, 2013). Alternative diets claim to treat or cure cancer, and they are followed instead of conventional cancer treatment. Complementary diets constitute any unusual or unorthodox change to a normal diet and claim to benefit people with cancer; they are followed in association with accepted cancer treatments.

The rationale for trying these diets is understandable, given that the patients are faced with the prospect of a life-threatening condition. Patients may also use complementary and alternative therapies to address the emotional and spiritual aspects of the disease and to boost their immune system (Parker *et al.*, 2010). No randomised controlled trials have been conducted to evaluate the benefit of such diets, and healthcare professionals remain sceptical about their value (Cassileth *et al.*, 1991; Huebner *et al.*, 2014). In addition, cancer patients may not be aware of the potential risks of using complementary and alternative medicines, or may not always inform their doctor of their use (Werneke *et al.*, 2004). Healthcare professionals often do not ask if such therapies are being used. Alternatively, patients may choose to make lifestyle changes with the aim of managing the negative impact that cancer treatment can have on health-related quality of life (Ashing-Giwa *et al.*, 2010). These lifestyle changes include eating a healthier diet, increasing exercise, use of complementary or alternative medicine, and stress reduction. However, many alternative and complementary diets (see Table 7.15.2) are more likely to worsen nutritional status than improve it. Common features of such diets include the following:

- Being vegetarian or vegan.
- Large amounts of raw food.
- The use of organic foods.
- Low fat.
- Low sugar or sugar free.
- Low salt.
- Restricting or avoiding dairy products.
- Ketogenic diets
- Avoiding processed foods and beverages containing caffeine.
- Encouraging the use of vitamin and mineral supplements.

As a result, these diets often have low energy density (due to their high bulky fibrous food content) and low content of fat and carbohydrate (Arends *et al.*, 2016).

Table 7.15.2 Examples of alternative and complementary dietary regimens

Dietary regimen	Philosophy	Main dietary principles
Low sugar or sugar free (complementary). Diet may restrict carbohydrate intake sufficient to induce ketogenesis.	Cancer cells use glucose as the main form of substrate via aerobic glycolysis. A reduction in intake of sugar restricts the availability of glucose. This does not consider the availability of glucose to the cells due to maintenance of blood glucose levels by hormonal mechanisms.	Restrict sugar (sucrose) intake in the diet. Avoidance of all foods containing sugar, particularly processed foods. Some diets restrict total carbohydrate intake to 20–70 g per day to create a moderate-protein, high-fat ketogenic diet.
Macrobiotics (complementary).	Foods are classified as Yin foods, representing feminine, dark and negative principles, and Yang foods, representing masculine, light and positive principles. The aim is to balance these for each individual in order to obtain a healthy mind and body.	Mainly cereal grains. Vegetables, sea vegetables and fruit. Bean and bean products. Nuts and seeds. Fish. Soup made with vegetables, beans and grains. Sea vegetables seasoned with sea salt, soy sauce or miso.
Dairy-free diets (complementary).	Milk and dairy foods promote cancer growth, particularly breast and prostate cancer.	Soya foods can be substituted for dairy foods. Increase fruit and vegetable consumption (preferably organic). Avoid processed foods, including meats, oils, refined starchy foods, alcohol and fizzy drinks.
Gerson therapy (alternative).	Aim is to stimulate the body's own defence system to overcome cancer. Both the nutritional and detoxification parts of the therapy are required.	Vegan. Fresh fruit and vegetables. Freshly made fruit and vegetable juices. Supplements of digestive enzymes, niacin, liver capsules, iodine, thyroid extract, potassium compound and vitamin B_{12} injections. Coffee enemas.

Therefore, it may be difficult to eat enough to meet their needs, particularly if they have eating or swallowing problems associated with the disease or its treatment. Restrictions on food choice may cause dietary imbalances. Use of mega doses of vitamins and minerals can create other nutritional distortions and may even be hazardous.

Such regimens may also be expensive, unpalatable and time consuming to prepare. Patients accept this because they have high expectations of their success, but may then suffer feelings of anger and frustration if these are subsequently not met. They may also feel guilty if they have to abandon the diet. While there is no evidence that these regimens offer any benefit over conventional therapies, and make matters worse in some instances, some patients do claim to feel better on these regimens (Cassileth & Deng, 2004; McLay *et al.*, 2012; Werneke *et al.*, 2004). The reason for this is unclear, but may be associated with *doing something positive* to take control of the disease and treatment, and also because of the often-excellent psychological support offered along with dietary advice as part of holistic therapy.

It is important that dietitians be aware that patients may try, or are already following, alternative or complementary diets. The role of the dietitian is to explore whether patients want to discuss their dietary intake and change any aspect of their diet:

- If patients ask whether they should try a particular alternative diet, encourage them to find out all they can about the regimen and openly discuss the potential benefits and hazards.
- If patients want to try one of these diets, encourage them to follow it for a short period of time (e.g. 1 month), and to then return for further assessment and discussion.
- If an alternative diet is already being followed, discuss obvious dietary shortcomings and suggest positive measures that the patient can take to improve nutritional intake. Some patients may be prepared to compromise and will incorporate some aspects of their alternative regimen into a better balanced nutritional programme.
- If alternative or complementary medicines are being taken, refer to the pharmacy to check the supplement, dosage and any possible interaction with conventional medicines that are being prescribed (McLay *et al.*, 2012; Werneke *et al.*, 2004).

Ultimately, the patient is responsible for making the decision to follow a complementary or alternative dietary regimen. However, it is the responsibility of the dietitian to ensure that the patient has been given sufficient balanced information and advice on which to base that decision. In order to do this, it is important that dietitians keep up to date with the types of diets being suggested for cancer and their nutritional implications. The progress and dietary intake of patients following alternative diets should be monitored in order to try and ensure that good nutritional status is maintained.

Drug–nutrient interactions

Drug–nutrient interactions may occur with chemotherapeutic agents, drugs used to manage symptoms and additional medication that is being taken to manage comorbidities. These interactions can potentially occur with food, nutritional supplements and herbal preparations. Patients should be encouraged to discuss all additional over-the-counter supplements with a pharmacist before consuming them to check for any potential adverse reactions.

Further reading

Alpha-Tocopherol, Beta-Carotene Cancer Prevention Study Group (ATBC). (1994) The effect of vitamin E and beta-carotene on the incidence of lung cancer and other cancers in male smokers. *N. Engl. J. Med.* 330: 1029–1035.

Brown JK, Byers T, Doyle C, *et al.*; American Cancer Society. (2003) Nutrition and physical activity during and after cancer treatment: an American Cancer Society guide for informed choices. *CA Cancer J. Clin.* 53: 268–291.

Cassileth BR, Yeung, KS, Gubill, J. (2010) *Herb-Drug Interactions in Oncology*, 2nd edn. Hamilton, Canada: BC Decker.

Cerhan JR, Potter JD, Gilmore JME, *et al.* (2004) Adherence to the AICR cancer prevention recommendations and subsequent morbidity and mortality in the Iowa Women's Health Study Cohort. *Cancer Epidemiol. Biomarkers Prev.* 13(7): 1114–1120.

DH. (1998) *Report of the Working Group on Diet and Cancer of the Committee on Medical Aspects of Food and Nutrition Policy. Nutritional Aspects of the Development of Cancer. Report on Health and Social Subjects 48*. London: Stationery Office.

DH. (2000) *The NHS Cancer Plan: A Plan for Investment, a Plan for Reform*. London: Department of Health.

Shaw C (ed). (2011) *Nutrition and Cancer*. Oxford: Wiley Blackwell.

Internet resources

Cancer Research UK, www.cancerresearchuk.org
Macmillan Cancer Support, www.macmillan.org.uk
NHS Choices, www.nhs.uk/livewell/healthy-eating
World Cancer Research Fund, www.wcrf-uk.org

References

Andreyev HJ, Norman AR, Oates J, *et al.* (1998) Why do patients with weight loss have a worse outcome when undergoing chemotherapy for gastrointestinal malignancies? *Eur. J. Cancer.* 34(4): 503–509.

Arends J, Bachmann P. Baracos V, *et al.* (2016) ESPEN guidelines on nutrition in cancer patients. *Clin. Nutr. (Epub)* 10.1016/j.clnu.2016.07.015

Arends J, Bodoky G, Bozzetti F, *et al.* (2006) ESPEN guidelines on enteral nutrition: non-surgical oncology. *Clin. Nutr.* 25(2): 245–259.

Ashing-Giwa KT, Lim J-W, Gonzalez P. (2010) Exploring the relationship between physical well-being and healthy lifestyle change among European- and Latina-American breast and cervical cancer survivors. *Psychooncology.* 19: 1161–1170.

Baldwin C, Spiro A, Ahern R, *et al.* (2012) Oral nutritional interventions in malnourished patients with cancer: A systematic review and meta-analysis. *J. Natl. Cancer Inst.* 104: 371–385.

Bourdel-Marchasson I, Blanc-Bisson C, Doussau A, *et al.* (2014) Nutritional advice in older patients at risk of malnutrition during treatment for chemotherapy: a two-year randomized controlled trial. *PLoS One.* 9(9): e108687.

Bozzetti F; SCRINIO Working Group. (2009) Screening the nutritional status in oncology: a preliminary report on 1000 patients. *Support Care Cancer.* 17: 279–284.

Cancer Research UK. (2012) *Cancer Mortality Statistics.* Available at www.cancerresearchuk.org/cancer-info/cancerstats/mortality/. Accessed 2 December 2013.

Cancer Research UK. (2013a) *Incidence of all Cancers.* Available at http://www.cancerresearchuk.org/health-professional/cancer-statistics. Accessed 11 July 2016.

Cancer Research UK. (2013b) *Common Cancers.* Available at http://www.cancerresearchuk.org/health-professional/cancer-statistics/incidence. Accessed 11 July 2016.

Cancer Research UK. (2013c) *Cancer Survival Statistics.* Available at http://www.cancerresearchuk.org/health-professional/cancer-statistics/survival#heading-Five. Accessed 11 July 2016.

Cassileth BR, Deng G. (2004) Complementary and alternative therapies for cancer. *Oncologist* 9(1): 80–89.

Cassileth BR, Lusk EJ, Guerry D, *et al.* (1991) Survival and quality of life among patients receiving unproven as compared with conventional cancer therapy. *N. Engl. J. Med.* 324: 1180–1185.

CRUK (2018) Cancer mortality statistics. Available at https://www.cancerresearchuk.org/health-professional/cancer-statistics/mortality/all-cancers-combined#heading-One. Accessed 15 November 2018.

Doll R, Peto R. (1981) The causes of cancer; quantitative estimates of avoidable risks of cancer in the United States today. *J. Natl. Cancer Inst.* 66: 1192–1308.

Fearon KCH. (2008) Cancer cachexia: developing multimodal therapy for a multidimensional problem. *Eur. J. Cancer* 44(8): 1124–1132.

Fearon KCH, von Meyenfeldt MR, Moses AGW, *et al.* (2003) Effect of a protein and energy dense n-3 fatty acid enriched oral supplement on loss of weight and lean tissue in cancer cachexia: a randomised double blind trial. *Gut* 52: 1479–1486.

Fearon K, Strasser F, Anker SD, *et al.* (2011) Definition and classification of cancer cachexia: an international consensus. *Lancet Oncol.* 12(5): 489–495.

Garland SN, Valentine D, Desai K, *et al.* (2013) Complementary and alternative medicine use and benefit finding among cancer patients. *J. Altern. Complement Med.* 19(11): 876–881.

Henry L. (2011) Effect of malnutrition on cancer patients. In: Shaw C (ed) *Nutrition and Cancer.* Oxford: Wiley Blackwell.

Huebner J, Marienfeld S, Abbenhardt C, *et al.* (2014) Counseling patients on cancer diets: a review of the literature and recommendations for clinical practice. *Anticancer Res.* 34: 39–48.

Hutton JL, Martin L, Field CJ, *et al.* (2006) Dietary patterns in patients with advanced cancer: Implications for anorexia-cachexia therapy. *Am. J. Clin. Nutr.* 84(5): 1163–1170.

Jung HW, Kim JW, Kim JY, *et al.* (2015) Effect of muscle mass on toxicity and survival in patients with colon cancer undergoing adjuvant chemotherapy. *Support Care Cancer.* 23(3): 687–694.

Laviano A, Preziosa I, Fanelli FR. (2011) Cancer and nutritional status. In: Shaw C (ed) *Nutrition and Cancer.* Oxford: Wiley Blackwell.

Macmillan. (2014) *Guidance: The Practical Management of Gastrointestinal Symptoms of Pelvic Radiation Disease.* Available at http://www.macmillan.org.uk/documents/aboutus/health_professionals/p215trmgibooklet_aw.pdf. Accessed 11 July 2016.

Macmillan. (2016) *Statistics Fact Sheet.* Available at http://www.macmillan.org.uk/documents/aboutus/research/keystats/statisticsfactsheet.pdf. Accessed 11 July 2016.

McLay JS, Stewart D, George J, *et al.* (2012) Complementary and alternative medicines use by Scottish women with breast cancer. What, why and the potential for drug interactions? *Eur. J. Clin. Pharmacol.* 68(5): 811–819.

Murphy RA, Mourtzakis M, Chu QSC, *et al.* (2011) Nutritional intervention with fish oil provides a benefit over standard of care for patients with weight and skeletal muscle mass in patients with non-small cell lung cancer receiving chemotherapy. *Cancer.* 117: 1775–1782.

National Cancer Action Team (NCAT). (2008) *Manual for Cancer Services 2008: Rehabilitation Measures.* Available at http://cancerni.net/files/file/Revised%20Rehabilitation%20Measures%20April%202011.pdf. Accessed 19 November 2018.

NHS networks. (2012) *AHP Cancer Toolkit.* Available at https://www.networks.nhs.uk/nhs-networks/ahp-networks/ahp-qipp-toolkits. Accessed 11 July 2016.

NICE. (2004) *Improving Supportive and Palliative Care for Adults with Cancer: The Manual.* London: NICE.

Nomura SJ, Inoue-Choi M, Lazovich D, *et al.* (2016) WCRF/AICR recommendation adherence and breast cancer incidence among postmenopausal women with and without non-modifiable risk factors. *Int. J. Cancer.* 138(11): 2602–2615.

Ottery FD. (1996) Definition of standardized nutritional assessment and interventional pathways in oncology. *Nutrition.* 12(1): S15–19.

Parker PA, Cohen L, Bekele BN, *et al.* (2010) Complementary and alternative medicine (CAM) use among cancer patients in community oncology settings. *J. Clin. Oncol.* 28(15): 0732–183X.

Parry B. (2011) Nutrition and breast cancer. In: Shaw C (ed) *Nutrition and Cancer.* Oxford: Wiley Blackwell, pp. 334–362.

Prado CMM, Baracos VE, McCargar LJ, *et al.* (2009) Sarcopenia as a determinant of chemotherapy toxicity and time to tumor progression in metastatic breast cancer patients receiving capecitabine treatment. *Clin. Cancer Res.* 15(8): 2920–2926.

Ravasco P, Monteiro-Grillo I, Camilo M. (2012) Individualized nutrition intervention is of major benefit to colorectal cancer patients: long-term follow-up of a randomized controlled trial of nutritional therapy. *Am. J. Clin. Nutr.* 96(6): 1346–1353.

Ries A, Trottenberg P, Elsner F, *et al.* (2012) A systematic review on the role of fish oil for the treatment of cachexia in advanced cancer: an EPCRC cachexia guidelines project. *Palliat. Med.* 26(4): 294–304.

Shaw C, Eldridge L. (2015) Nutritional considerations for the palliative care patient. *Int. J. Palliat. Nurs.* 21(1): 7–8, 10, 12–15.

Shaw C, Fleuret C, Pickard JM, *et al.* (2015) Comparison of a novel, simple nutrition screening tool for adult oncology inpatients and the Malnutrition Screening Tool (MST) against the Patient-Generated Subjective Global Assessment (PG-SGA). *Support Care Cancer.* 23(1): 47–54.

Watson L, Lalji A, Bodla S, *et al.* (2015) Management of bile acid malabsorption using low-fat dietary interventions: a useful strategy applicable to some patients with diarrhoea-predominant irritable bowel syndrome? *Clin. Med. (Lond.)* 15(6): 536–540.

Werneke U, Earl J, Seydel C, *et al.* (2004) Potential health risks of complementary alternative medicines in cancer patients. *Br. J. Cancer* 90: 408–413.

World Cancer Research Fund/American Institute for Cancer Research (WCRF/AICR). (2007) *Food, Nutrition, Physical Activity and the Prevention of Cancer: A Global Perspective.* Washington, DC.

World Cancer Research Fund. (2010) *Breast Cancer 2010 Report Food, Nutrition, Physical Activity, and the Prevention of Breast Cancer.* London: World Cancer Research Fund. Available at http://www.wcrf.org/sites/default/files/Breast-Cancer-2010-Report.pdf. Accessed 11 July 2016.

7.15.2 Head and neck cancer

Bella Talwar

Key points

- The dietitian is a core member of the head and neck cancer care team, providing nutritional assessment, advice and support from diagnosis onwards.
- Early referral is crucial to provide timely nutritional support tailored to the patient's needs, from diagnosis to end-of-life care.
- Prophylactic tube placement is recommended if oral intake is inadequate, not possible or likely to be restricted during treatment and rehabilitation over a prolonged period. Appropriate decision-making around prophylactic tube feeding should be discussed at diagnosis as part of the treatment management plan.

Cancers of the head and neck are the sixth most common cancers worldwide, and constitute 3% of malignancies in the UK; they represent the fourth-most common diagnosis in men, and 12th-most common cancer in woman (Cancer Research UK, 2016). The majority of these cancers arise from the surface layers of the upper aerodigestive tract and include a variety of histological types, of which squamous cell carcinomas make up 95% of cancers (Argiris *et al.*, 2008). Cancers of the mouth, lip and tongue (oral cavity), the upper part of the throat and respiratory system (pharynx), and the voice box (larynx) represent 90% of head and neck malignant tumours. Cancers of the salivary glands, nose, sinuses, middle ear and those that originate in the nerve and bone of the head and neck are relatively rare (NICE, 2016).

The newly diagnosed patients are most frequently in the fifth to seventh decade of life, but it is increasing in the middle-aged adult population, and the 3:1 ratio for the prevalence in men and women is decreasing (Cancer Research UK).

Tobacco exposure and high alcohol consumption are the two strongest aetiological factors, both independently and synergistically, in the development of primary and secondary head and neck cancers (Marron *et al.*, 2010). Certain tumour sites are associated with specific risk factors. The chewing of tobacco is linked to cancers of the oral cavity (Proia *et al.*, 2006). The Epstein–Barr virus is associated with nasopharyngeal cancers in individuals of oriental origin. Human papilloma virus (HPV 16) is an increasingly recognised causative factor in oropharyngeal and oral cancer, particularly in individuals who are non-smokers or non-drinkers, and in people aged 30–50 years (BAO-HNS, 2016).

The aims of treatment are to eliminate the disease and achieve long-term survival. However, the 5-year mortality rate from head and neck cancer has not improved significantly over the last 40 years, despite advances in diagnostic tools and treatment modalities. Therefore, locoregional control (disease recurrence at the primary site or the neck), quality of life, and organ function are critical outcome considerations in describing and evaluating treatment (BAO-HNS, 2016; List & Bilir, 2004).

Nutritional status has been recognised as a fundamental long-term prognostic factor (Brookes, 1985), with the incidence of weight loss before and during treatment identified as an indicator for disease-specific survival (Langius *et al.*, 2013). Subsequently, nutrition has become an increasingly important quality-of-life issue surrounding the psychosocial and rehabilitation needs of head and neck cancer patients (BAO-HNS, 2016).

Nutritional implications

Head and neck cancer patients present a significant nutritional challenge due to the risk of malnutrition associated with lifestyle choices, cancer site, the disease process and treatment. Studies over the past 20 years have estimated that approximately 50–75% of diagnosed patients experience moderate to severe malnutrition (Hammerlid *et al.*, 1998; van Bokhorst-de van der Scheuren *et al.*, 1997), and that 80% will lose weight during multimodality treatment (BAO-HNS, 2016). Regardless of the population changes with presenting BMI, unintended weight loss of 10% in the preceding 6 months in this patient group will have significant malnutrition-associated morbidity and mortality (Findlay *et al.*, 2011) (see Chapter 6.2, Malnutrition). However, the causes and consequences of malnutrition in head and neck cancer patients at presentation are multifactorial (see Table 7.15.3). It is evident that nutrition influences patients' functional, oncological and quality-of-life outcomes, which have an impact on health economics.

Nutritional effects of treatment

Treatment options for head and neck cancers involve single- or multi-modality regimens with surgery, radiotherapy, chemotherapy and biological targeted treatment (BAO-HNS, 2016). The International Union Against Cancer (2016) TNM classification of head and neck tumours describes the anatomical extent of disease based on the size of the primary tumour (T1 4), the absence or presence and extent of regional lymph node metastasis (N1 3), and the absence or presence of distant metastasis

Table 7.15.3 Factors contributing to malnutrition in head and neck cancer (source: Talwar, 2010. Reproduced with permission from Wiley-Blackwell Publishing)

Contributory factors	Cause
Poor dietary habits	Consumption of unbalanced meals can lead to energy, protein and micronutrient deficiency.
Excessive alcohol intake	Associated with appetite suppression, inadequate nutrient intake and micronutrient deficiency.
Depression and anxiety	These can result in aversion to food and/or loss of appetite with reduced quality of life.
Difficulty with chewing	Lack of teeth, ill-fitting dentures and physical problems with jaw movement can markedly affect food choice in favour of a limited range of soft or liquid foods.
Difficulty with swallowing	Presence of the tumour mass, pain on eating, ulcerated mouth and fear of choking can compromise the safety of swallowing, and result in the consumption of a diet restricted in variety, texture and nutritional content.
Cachexia	Altered nutritional and metabolic response due to the presence of the tumour can result in symptoms such as anorexia, loss of appetite, early satiety and marked weight loss associated with muscle wasting and increased production of acute-phase protein.
Changes in body composition	Disturbance in energy balance with changes in resting energy expenditure, glucose uptake, mobilisation of fat and protein stores, and muscle protein release.
Halitosis	Anaerobic respiration with the production of lactic acid and subsequent build-up of ammonia released via the mouth.
High risk of refeeding syndrome	Combined effect of the causes and consequences of malnutrition in this patient group, leading to risk of starvation for longer than 7–10 days and unintentional significant weight loss.
Limited support network	Patients who live alone or have no family can be less motivated and often find it more challenging to maintain adequate nutrition.
Impaired wound healing	Increased risk of infection due to decreased muscle, respiratory, gut and immune functions.
Higher risk of hospital admission	Nutritional deterioration requiring feeding management with greater length and cost of hospital stay.
Poor functional status and quality of life	Increased lethargy and decreased ability to mobilise, work and socialise.
Increased morbidity and mortality	Poor nutritional status at presentation combined with malnutrition and its associated consequences, limiting the options and choice of cancer therapy due to tolerance, and therefore contributing towards poorer tumour control and survival.

(M site). The main anatomical sites in the head and neck region are shown in Figure 7.15.1.

Curative treatment options differ according to the staging and primary tumour site, with stage I or II disease managed with single-modality treatment using surgery or radiotherapy and/or chemotherapy, and stage III and IV disease requiring multimodality therapy with surgery, radiotherapy and chemotherapy. The different combination treatments have led to several competing management strategies, each with different advantages and disadvantages, and initial treatment can vary significantly between institutions (BAO-HNS, 2016).

Over the past decade, there have been significant advances in treatments. Surgical resection and reconstruction techniques have evolved, and now include minimally invasive approaches such as transoral laser and robotic approaches. Radiotherapy fractionation schedules have been modified to promote organ preservation with induction and/or concurrent chemotherapy, sparing healthy tissue by targeted coverage (BAO-HNS, 2016). Chemoradiotherapy results in an absolute survival improvement of 8% at 5 years, and is currently recognised as the gold standard treatment for advanced cancers requiring combined modality treatment. These chemotherapeutic agents are platinum based, with the dose, delivery method and timing varying between institutions, but the benefits are largely confined to delivery during (concurrent) radiotherapy rather than before (neoadjuvant) or after (adjuvant) (Blanchard *et al.*, 2011; Pignon *et al.*, 2009). Cancer treatments delivered as single-modality or multimodality therapy to the head and neck region have a permanent effect on the organs essential for normal human activities such as breathing, speaking, eating and drinking (NICE, 2016). This creates further nutritional problems and increases the risk of nutritional depletion, requiring appropriate and timely intervention (Talwar, 2010).

Surgery

Surgical resection can severely restrict or even eliminate the patient's ability to consume oral nutrition. van Bokhorst-de van der Schuer *et al.* (1997) assessed a variety of malnutrition parameters in patients undergoing major surgery for advanced cancer, and identified weight loss as the most significant. Patients with a weight loss of >10% during the 6 months presurgery had a greater risk of postoperative complications, with an incidence of between 20% and 50% (Bertrand *et al.*, 2002). A follow-on study to evaluate nutritional status

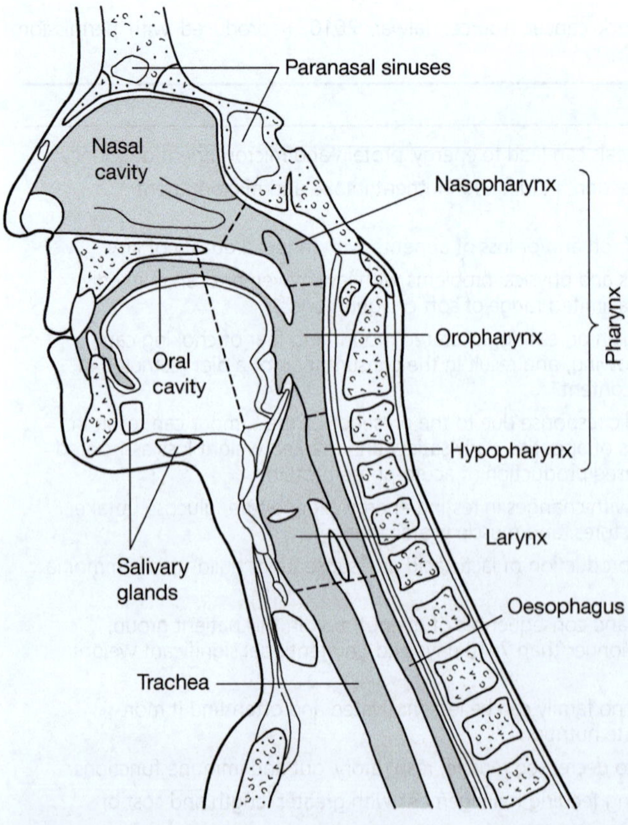

Figure 7.15.1 Main sites of head and neck cancers (adapted from Talwar, 2010. Reproduced with permission from Wiley-Blackwell Publishing)

as a prognostic value found no influence of any of the investigated nutritional parameters for the whole group. However, preoperative weight loss and the occurrence of major postoperative complications showed a marked negative influence on the survival of male patients with head and neck cancers (van Bokhorst-de van der Schuer *et al.*, 1999).

Based on these findings, the same researchers conducted a randomised controlled trial to study the effect of perioperative nutritional support on nutritional status, immune status, postoperative outcome and survival in severely malnourished patients undergoing major surgery. Although the trial concluded that 7–10 days preoperative feeding did not improve nutritional status, it did find that preoperative enteral nutrition in patients with head and neck cancer improved their functional and emotional status in the preoperative period, although this was not evident at 6 months (van Bokhorst-de van der Schuer *et al.*, 2000). This raised the question of whether preoperative enteral feeding should commence at clinical presentation when there is a strong suspicion that the diagnosis is likely to be a malignancy, to evaluate if there is a beneficial effect on nutritional status (Bradley & Donaldson, 2000).

Immunonutrition is supported by limited evidence, and therefore is not routinely recommended in this patient group; however, some benefit is observed if it is administered in the pre- or postoperative period to

Box 7.15.1 High-risk selection criteria for preoperative feeding of head and neck cancer patients (Weimann *et al.*, 2017)

Weight loss >10–15% in 6 months.
Body mass index <18.5 kg/m^2.
Subjective global assessment grade C or NRS >5.
Preoperative serum albumin <30 g/L (with no evidence of hepatic or renal dysfunction).
Unable to maintain intake above 60% of recommended intake for >10 days.

reduce fistulae rates and length of stay, and to improve 10-year survival (Findlay *et al.*, 2011); further research is required in this area. However, there is consensus guidance at the international level for best practice, recommending preoperative nutrition in patients at severe nutritional risk (BAO-HNS, 2016; Findlay *et al.*, 2011), as identified in Box 7.15.1.

There are several centres across the UK that have developed and implemented enhanced recovery programmes with the use of carbohydrate loading drinks. Evidence is currently limited, but nutritional interventions should be considered at all stages of the pathway from diagnosis to survivorship and well-being (BAO-HNS, 2016; Weimann *et al.*, 2017). The consequences of surgery are outlined in Table 7.15.4.

Radiotherapy

The side effects of radiotherapy are due to the direct effect of radiation on the tumour, or because of the involvement of healthy tissue within the field of treatment in the head and neck region (Figure 7.15.1). The severity of the reaction depends on the radiation schedule, volume and cumulative dose given to the anatomical structures in the treatment field. This treatment can be given as a single or cumulative dose, and a radical course involves the patient attending daily treatments for up to 6–7 weeks and receiving a total dose of 60–70 Gray (BAO-HNS, 2016). Radiotherapy side effects impact on the patient from the second week of treatment, peaking during the fourth–fifth week, and continuing for on average 3 weeks after completing the course (Polisena, 2010). Radiotherapy can further compromise the patient's nutritional status and make the management particularly challenging. The treatment side effects can occur in the acute stage with permanent changes, or as a late reaction during the patient's follow-up and rehabilitation (Brown *et al.*, 2015). These side effects are summarised in Table 7.15.5. Prior to starting radiotherapy, it is estimated that 44% of patients present with common symptoms associated with eating, including difficulty with mastication and/or swallowing (odynophagia), loss of appetite, and nausea; and, by the third week of treatment, patients report three or more eating problems (Larsson *et al.*, 2005).

In a small study (Larsson *et al.*, 2003), using qualitative measures to examine patient experiences during

SECTION 7

Table 7.15.4 Effects of surgery and nutritional consequences (source: Talwar, 2010. Reproduced with permission from Wiley-Blackwell Publishing)

Effects of surgery	Nutritional consequences
Loss of taste	Surgery to the tongue, salivary glands or olfactory nerve negatively influence taste acuity, leading to reduced appetite and gustation.
Loss of smell	Loss of nasal airflow via the olfactory receptors in the nasal cavity leading to reduced enjoyment of mealtimes and social interaction.
Difficulty chewing	Partial or total inability to masticate due to loss of bony supporting structure (mandible); exacerbated by dental extraction, misalignment of the jaw and trismus; leading to the requirement for texture modification, increased effort and reduced enjoyment of food, and social isolation.
Drooling and pocketing of food and fluid	Reduced pressure to move the bolus into the pharynx occurs due to surgery or nerve damage, and can be embarrassing and isolating, causing anxiety and depression.
Reduced peristalsis	Prolonged mealtimes with risk of avoiding food and fluid, leading to inadequate diet, dehydration, constipation and weight loss.
Oral regurgitation	Due to reconstruction or gastric transposition (pharyngolaryngooesophagectomy), requiring small frequent meals, remaining upright for 1 hour post-meal, and lying down with the head elevated.
Nasal regurgitation	Functional impairment of the soft palate or motor activity of the graft can be embarrassing and distressing, and require to be maintained while eating and drinking.
Dumping syndrome (pharyngolaryngooesophagectomy)	Causes nausea, bloating, abdominal cramps and explosive diarrhoea; fear of food and eating is common, and changes in eating habits are required due to prolonged mealtimes and early satiety.
Poor wound healing	Examples include flap failure, dehiscence at anastomosis, necrosis and infection. Contributing factors include previous radiotherapy, malnutrition and increased nutritional requirements, necessitating assessment for vitamin and mineral supplementation.
Fistulae	Occur in the oral cavity, pharynx or larynx, caused by previous radiotherapy, and affect tissue healing and swallowing, requiring alternative feeding.
Risk of wound infection	At wound site or chest with extensive or revision surgery and lengthy operations when entering into or resecting part of the upper aerodigestive tract, increasing nutritional requirements.
Nerve injury	Damage to the trigeminal, facial, glossopharyngeal, vagus, accessory, hyoglossal and recurrent laryngeal nerves affect swallowing coordination, chewing and taste, increasing the risk of aspiration and fatigue during meals, as well as facial disfigurement.
Aspiration	Can be a silent or reactive cough with food or fluid entering the lungs, requiring the patient to be nil by mouth and needing alternative feeding.
Chylous fistula	Tumour invasion or surgical trauma of the thoracic duct with <500 mL/day lymphatic drainage, requiring conservative management, or >600 mL/day over a prolonged period and suggesting surgical repair.
Strictures and stenosis	Complete or partial obstruction of the food bolus, requiring dilatation with texture modification, and smaller-size food bolus with plenty of fluid and multiple swallows.
Patient comorbidity factors	Diabetes, renal impairment, malnutrition, previous surgery or radiotherapy, anaesthetics for procedure and duration of the surgery.

radiotherapy, the following symptoms were reported to affect quality of life:

- Ability to chew and swallow.
- Will and desire to eat.
- Changes in saliva quantity and consistency.
- Narrowing in the throat and pain.
- Nausea.
- Taste changes.

Patients felt their way of life was disturbed as a result of having to cope with the effects of their symptoms at mealtimes, leading to loss of togetherness with family and friends. Additionally, they experienced extreme fatigue and loss of self-confidence (Larsson *et al.*, 2003). Up to 57% of head and neck cancer patients experience weight loss before starting radiotherapy, 95% of whom report this as being unintentional weight loss. Radiotherapy treatment may result in a further loss of approximately 10% of body weight (Nugent *et al.*, 2010b).

Chemoradiation

Chemotherapy is particularly likely to affect the rapidly dividing cells of the buccal and gastrointestinal mucosa, causing damage to the mucosal lining of the mouth (Van Cutsem & Arends, 2005). Chemotherapy alone is not used widely, but is administered as a neoadjuvant (before radiotherapy) and/or concurrently with radiotherapy; although it has been shown to improve survival, this is at the cost of increased toxicity (Blanchard *et al.*, 2011;

Table 7.15.5 Side effects of radiotherapy and nutritional consequences (source: Talwar, 2010. Reproduced with permission from Wiley-Blackwell Publishing)

Side effects	Nutritional consequences
Taste changes	Diminished, distorted, abnormal and/or loss of taste (described as cardboard, metallic or sandpaper), leading to food aversion and reduced intake.
Mucositis	Oral mucosal reaction that can result in pain, infection or retching.
Xerostomia	Requires good oral hygiene, artificial saliva and food texture modification.
Dysphagia	Pre-existing or post-treatment, with tissue damage impairing wound healing.
Swallowing impairment of oral phase	Reduced range of lingual motion and strength; impaired bolus formation and transport through the oral cavity; prolonged transit time; and increased residue occur in the floor of mouth resections, causing chewing difficulty, taste changes and fatigue during meals.
Swallowing impairment of pharyngeal phase	Impaired tongue base movement, delayed trigger of the swallow, reduced pharyngeal contraction, reduced laryngeal function, reduced opening of the oesophageal sphincter, resulting in impaired bolus clearance and aspiration.
Aspiration	Silent or reactive coughing on food and fluid associated with fear of eating; can be due to lethargy, weakness and reduced alertness secondary to malnutrition.
Trismus	Restricted ability to open the mouth, which can be radiation induced, or due to pre-existing tumour obstruction or reduced mastication over a prolonged period.
Osteoradionecrosis	Mandible incapable of healing itself or fighting infection due to poor blood supply, resulting in reduced ability to masticate and limited mouth opening.
Impaired wound healing	Permanent tissue damage increasing risk of poor wound healing.
Fatigue	Apathy and severe tiredness limiting physical function, as well as motivation with swallowing due to increasing time and effort at meals, with an overall reduced nutrient intake.
Dental caries	Due to poor oral hygiene, or exacerbated in the presence of xerostomia; as food and fluid stick to the teeth, there is no flushing effect from saliva, and the teeth rapidly decay.
Dehydration	Decreased salivary flow resulting in altered colonisation of the oropharynx, impaired bolus preparation due to lack of saliva and increased thickness of sputum.

Pignon *et al.*, 2009). Chemoradiation results in more severe and acute adverse effects than radiotherapy alone, and the long-term effects of radiation are also increased and can profoundly affect nutritional intake and swallowing physiology, causing significant morbidity and diminished quality of life (Patterson *et al.*, 2015). In head and neck cancer, the chemotherapeutic agents most commonly used are platinum based, and where patient comorbidities present a risk for administering systemic agents, an alternative monoclonal epidermal growth factor receptor (EGFR) inhibitor is used (cetuxmab) (BAO-HNS, 2016).

Intensity-modulated radiotherapy is the established form of radiation therapy for 70–80% of advanced-stage head and neck tumours, where sparing of the salivary gland is required with an expectation of reduced morbidity (BAO-HNS, 2016). Nutrition-related toxicity has not reduced with this approach, and therefore patients should be managed in the same way as in conventional radiotherapy (Brown *et al.*, 2015).

Chemoradiation is known to exacerbate weight loss during treatment by >5% of pretreatment weight (Nugent *et al.*, 2010b). Odynophagia (pain on swallowing food and fluids) caused by severe mucositis and nausea can markedly impair the intake and enjoyment of food, and are thought to be significant factors associated with weight loss and the difficulties experienced with eating (Kelly, 2007). Poor symptom control during radiotherapy and/or chemotherapy will result in dehydration, lethargy and severe weight loss if nutrition support is inadequate, and contribute to inadequate treatment delivery and efficacy for local regional control and survival. International nutrition guidelines recommend that patients be seen weekly by a specialist dietitian (Findlay *et al.*, 2011), although twice-weekly follow-up is provided in some UK centres (BAO-HNS, 2016). The side effects of chemotherapy on nutritional consequences are listed in Table 7.15.6.

Current treatments for head and neck cancer have adverse effects on many nutritional aspects. A prospective cross-sectional study, taking account of the stage of disease and therapeutic intervention, evaluated quality of life, nutritional status and dietary intake, and found that reduced energy and protein intakes, together with weight loss, were independent determinants of quality of life (Ravasco *et al.*, 2004). Patients at risk of severe weight loss at diagnosis and during treatment can be identified with health-related quality-of-life questionnaires (Karin *et al.*, 2005), although there is no nutrition-specific module to assess the relationship between malnutrition, nutritional status, dietary counselling and nutrition support in this patient group (Talwar, 2010).

New treatments for head and neck cancer currently being examined include robotic surgery, photodynamic therapy, and ongoing interest with biological targeted

Table 7.15.6 Side effects of chemotherapy and nutritional consequences (source: Talwar, 2010. Reproduced with permission from Wiley-Blackwell Publishing)

Side effects	Nutritional consequences
Severe mucositis	Although radiation induced, this can be exacerbated by the systemic effects of the drug and can impair wound healing.
Nausea and vomiting	Systemic or anticipatory; triggered by taste, smell and anxiety.
Anorexia	Reduced appetite accompanied by reduced intake.
Taste and smell alterations	Diminished, distorted, abnormal and/or loss of taste (described as 'cardboard', 'metallic' or 'sandpaper'), leading to food aversion and reduced intake.
Diarrhoea	Risk of dehydration and distressing to the patient.
Stomatitis	Sore mouth significantly affecting food intake.
Nephrotoxicity/ ototoxicity	Renal impairment can lead to nausea and loss of appetite.
Metabolic abnormalities	Can lead to increased energy expenditure and micronutrient deficiency.

therapy focussing on tumour suppression genes and EGFRs using cetuximab (BAO-HNS, 2016). The nutritional consequences have yet to be evaluated.

Principles of nutritional management

The organisation and structure of nutrition and dietetic services should aim to provide a quality-centred, seamless service at all stages of the patient pathway, with access to dedicated, site-specific dietitians throughout the patient journey as a core member of the multidisciplinary head and neck cancer team for optimal service delivery (BAO-HNS, 2016; Findlay *et al.*, 2011). The publication of evidence-based practice guidelines based on a systematic review of literature across the entire nutritional care pathway sets the benchmark for quality-rated nutritional interventions and outcomes (Findlay *et al.*, 2011). Best-practice nutritional care should incorporate implementation of appropriate validated tools for routine malnutrition screening, early referral to the dietitian, and regular comprehensive nutritional assessment and monitoring to optimise nutritional status (Talwar & Findlay, 2012). The patient pathway and dietetic clinical model of care is shown in in Box 7.15.2.

Nutritional screening

It is crucial that all head and neck cancer patients undergo nutritional screening to identify those who have, or are at risk of developing, malnutrition at any stage of the patient pathway. It should be an integral part of multidisciplinary clinical practice for all inpatients on admission, repeated weekly until hospital discharge, and recorded at each outpatient appointment with clear dietetic referral criteria (Findlay *et al.*, 2011; BAO-HNS, 2016). Nutritional screening tools should be validated in oncology patients, and, where used for head and neck cancer patients, should be able to identify the following groups who may benefit from full nutritional assessment (Findlay *et al.*, 2011; BAO-HNS, 2016):

- Patients who are not nutritionally compromised at diagnosis, but who are at risk of malnutrition during treatment. These patients would benefit from dietetic assessment during the planning of their cancer treatment in order to recommend an appropriate nutritional management plan.
- Patients who are disease free post-treatment, but who present with late side effects from surgery, radiotherapy, and chemoradiotherapy that may impact on their oral intake, increasing the risk of developing malnutrition.

Assessment

Effective nutritional management is dependent on appropriate nutritional assessment. Useful factors to consider include clinical observation, dietary history, calculation of requirements, proposed treatment, anthropometry, biochemistry and social information. The specific parameters for this patient group are summarised in national clinical guidance (BAO-HNS, 2016), with key reflective questions that should be considered as part of the assessment. These should include the factors discussed in the following text.

Nutritional aspects

These include:

- What is the nutritional status of the patient? Consider the percentage energy intake from alcohol, percentage body weight loss in the previous 6 months, and body mass index (BMI).
- Is the patient at risk of refeeding syndrome?
- How many cups of fluid is the patient drinking during the day?
- How long is it taking the patient to consume a meal?
- Is the patient feeling hungry or thirsty after a meal?
- Which types of food is the patient finding easy/difficult to manage?

Box 7.15.2 Patient pathway and dietetic clinical model of care (Talwar, 2010)

Diagnosis

Intervention

Assess risk factors for patient compliance.
Negotiate feeding options with team and patient.
Assess need for artificial feeding, including screening for suitability and method of insertion.
Screening of nutritional status.

Outcome

Improve or maintain nutritional status.
Identify need and determine timing and type of prophylactic tube placement.

Pretreatment

Intervention

Discuss outcomes of intensive nutritional counselling with dietary intake, and oral and enteral nutrition support
Assess presenting symptoms from previous treatment.
Discuss effects of treatment and possible impact on ability to eat and drink in the short and long term.
Discuss method of feeding options and types of feeding tubes using visual aids, psychosocial aspects relating to body image, feeding in public, physical activity.

Outcome

Assess need for pretreatment reconditioning.
Provide realistic expectations of eating and feeding issues.
Establish rapport to promote patient motivation and compliance.
Support consent process for placement and use of feeding tubes, timelines for oral and enteral nutrition and rehabilitation programme to ensure timely and appropriate tube removal.

Treatment: surgery

Intervention

Discuss effects of surgery on ability to eat and drink.
Advise patient on how to overcome dietary problems and use the feeding tube.
Tailor feeding regimen to meet patient's individual requirements.
Adjust feeding regimen accordingly following introduction of oral diet, so that optimum intake is maintained.
Prepare patient for discharge on enteral feeding, including necessary training of patient and carers, practical feeding tube management.
Liaise with all relevant community staff and feed company to ensure that discharge home on enteral feed is safe and efficient.

Outcome

Improve or maintain nutritional status to reduce risk of developing postoperative complications.
Prepare patient for safe and effective discharge, allaying any anxieties.
Adequate preparation for discharge reduces likelihood of readmission for feeding-tube-related problems.

Treatment: radiotherapy and/or chemoradiation

Intervention

Discuss any presenting or ongoing problems with eating and drinking, and the potential impact of further treatment.
Advise patient on overcoming problems associated with chemoradiation.
Monitor dietary adequacy and tolerance to treatment.

Outcome

Optimise nutritional status to minimise risk of treatment interruptions (and subsequent admission).
Provide support and advice to enhance motivation and compliance with oral nutrition support and on the appropriate use of enteral feeding to prevent tube reliance.

Post-treatment

Intervention

Assess/monitor post-treatment effect on ability to eat and drink.
Adjust dietary feeding regimen suitably with oral diet to maintain adequate nutritional intake.
Provide advice on modifying texture of diet and symptom control for side effects.
Negotiate feeding tube removal as appropriate.

Outcome

Maintain adequate nutritional status.
Maximise patient motivation and compliance.
Assist patient to re-establish eating and drinking, thus improving quality of life.

Long-term care/survivorship

Intervention

Provide ongoing nutritional care with dietary advice for oral nutrition support and enteral nutrition.
Provide psychosocial support for enteral feeding.

Outcome

Establish goals for weight management and for maintaining adequate nutrition support.
Support the patient and carers living with the effects of treatment.

- Is the patient chewing food for longer before swallowing?
- Consider the effort and time taken to eat or drink, and how this is impacting on the patient's quality of life.
- Does drinking sips of liquids between bites of food make it easier to swallow?
- Has the patient adapted his or her eating habits to make it easier to swallow? If so, how?
- Is it taking more time and effort to eat and drink throughout the day?
- Are there any problems with the patient's dentition?

Clinical aspects

These include:

- What is the size of the tumour?
- What part(s) of the anatomy does the tumour involve?
- What are the aims of treatment – cure, symptom control, palliation?
- Does the treatment plan involve combined modality treatment?
- Has the patient had previous oncological treatment?
- What is the extent of any surgical resection, and is reconstruction planned?
- What are the risk factors for postoperative complications?
- What is the radiotherapy dose and treatment field?
- What is the patient's performance status?
- Does the patient have comorbidities or contraindications if considering alternative feeding?
- What is the patient's social support network?
- What are the patient's lifestyle choices for smoking, drinking and recreational drugs?
- How motivated is the patient to assess compliance with nutritional recommendations?

Dietetic management

Dietetic input throughout the patient pathway is needed to assess and correct nutritional deficiencies, evaluate how different treatment modalities will impact on a patient's nutritional status, and recommend the most appropriate short- and long-term nutritional interventions to meet the nutritional needs of the patient and/or achieve outcomes (BAO-HNS, 2016; Findlay *et al.*, 2011). The key questions that need to be asked in order to determine the nutritional management include the following:

- Is it safe for the patient to consume oral nutrition, and/or does the patient need to be referred to a speech and language therapist (SLT)?
- Is the patient meeting his or her energy and nutrient requirement by >50% of caloric requirement over the past 7 days?
- Is the patient maintaining his or her nutritional status with oral intake alone, or is an alternative system of feeding required?
- Does the patient's symptoms and/or treatment plan indicate the need for alternative feeding in the short or long term?
- If the patient requires enteral feeding, what is the type of tube and safest technique for placement to meet his or her nutritional needs?

Table 7.15.7 Consequences of malnutrition and dehydration in head and neck cancer patients

	Consequences
Malnutrition	Swallowing impairment and increased risk of aspiration due to lethargy, weakness and reduced alertness.
	Reduced strength of the cough and mechanical clearance in the lungs.
	Impaired wound healing and increased risk of infection due to decreased muscle, respiratory, gut and immune functions.
	Higher risk of admission to hospital and greater length and cost of hospital stay.
	Poor functional status and quality of life due to lethargy and decreased ability to mobilise, work and socialise.
	Increased morbidity and mortality.
Dehydration	Decreased salivary flow resulting in altered colonisation of the oropharynx
	Impaired bolus preparation due to lack of saliva and increased thickness of sputum.
	Increased risk of aspiration due to lethargy and mental confusion.

- If the patient requires tube feeding, is there continuity with dietetic support and management until it is appropriate to remove the feeding?

Dysphagia can lead to an inadequate energy, nutrient and fluid intake, and can have a severe adverse effect on the patient's health, nutritional status and quality of life unless the cause is identified and appropriately managed. If unrecognised over a prolonged period of time, dysphagia can place the patient at risk of malnutrition or dehydration and the associated complications (Table 7.15.7).

The SLT will assess the degree of dysphagia, including the risk of aspiration, and recommend management that may include alternative texture modification and the use of swallowing techniques or postures where appropriate (RCSLT, 2002) (see Chapter 7.3, Dysphagia). The dietitian should be part of the dysphagia team, providing nutrition information to support the diagnosis of swallowing problems and subsequent management (BAO-HNS, 2016; Findlay *et al.*, 2011; Lundy *et al.*, 2009).

Nutritional support

The choice of cancer treatment will influence the need for preoperative nutrition, and may also increase the nutritional requirements for postoperative recovery – hence the need for nutritional support during radiotherapy or chemoradiation. Recently, there have been several systematic reviews to evaluate the outcomes of dietary counselling and methods of nutritional support in patients receiving treatment for head and neck cancer (Findlay *et al.*, 2011; Garg *et al.*, 2010; Nugent *et al.*, 2010a). The first-line nutritional support intervention is often food fortification, but it is imperative to evaluate the appropriateness of this, given the intensity of treatment regimens and the consequences on the patient's ability to consume and sustain adequate oral nutrition. Patients should receive individualised nutritional support that is tailored to their diagnosis and treatment plan, including early oral nutritional support and enteral nutrition (BAO-HNS, 2016).

Oral nutritional support

It is challenging for patients to remain motivated and committed to sustaining adequate nutrition while experiencing the side effects of treatment (Cady, 2007; Mayre-Chilton *et al.*, 2011). It is important that patients maintain an intake as close as possible to a normal diet in order to maintain muscle function for swallowing and to minimise feelings of loss of control with oral nutrition during their cancer care (BAO-HNS, 2016). However, a patient's ability to sustain an adequate oral intake over an extended period is often underestimated (Talwar, 2010). Randomised controlled trials evaluating the impact of dietary counselling have demonstrated improvements in patients' nutritional status, dietary compliance and quality of life (Isenring *et al.*, 2004; Ravasco *et al.*, 2005) (see Chapter 6.3, Oral nutritional support).

Enteral nutritional support

If oral nutrition is inadequate or not possible, enteral feeding should be considered without delay, as the patient's nutritional status will otherwise be compromised, leading to poor patient-centred, clinical and financial outcomes (Findlay *et al.*, 2011). Assessing the need for early instigation of partial or total artificial support should be included when treatment options are being considered for head and neck cancer patients (BAO-HNS, 2016; NICE, 2016). Details of the principles and practice of artificial nutritional support are available in Chapter 6.4 (Enteral nutrition). The benefits of increased energy and protein intake, and reduced weight loss in patients receiving enteral nutrition as compared to oral nutrition, has been known for decades from randomised controlled trials (Daly *et al.*, 1984; Hearne *et al.*, 1985). Early referral to the dietitian within a nutritional support programme and dietary counselling have also been shown to improve outcomes for enteral nutrition, with less weight loss, as well as fewer treatment interruptions and unplanned hospital admissions (Mangar *et al.*, 2006; Paccagnella *et al.*, 2010; Wood, 2005; Zhang *et al.*, 2016).

Early studies have shown gastrostomy feeding to be more advantageous than nasogastric tube feeding, with patients experiencing increased mobility, reduced anxiety with altered body image, higher energy intakes, and improved quality-of-life scores with the former (Lees, 1997; Mekhail *et al.*, 2001; Piquet *et al.*, 2002). Patients and their carers need to be supported to establish a feeding pattern and to improve their confidence with tube care before having to cope with the debilitating effects of the treatment (Mayre-Chilton *et al.*, 2011). The relative advantages of gastrostomy placement have been challenged in the last decade, with much debate regarding the optimal timing and route of enteral tube feeding (Talwar & Findlay, 2012). The TUBE trial, a feasibility study incorporating a pilot randomised controlled trial comparing nasogastric and gastrostomy tubes in patients treated with chemoradiotherapy, is currently being conducted (Paleri *et al.*, 2016).

Prophylactic placement is gastrostomy insertion before treatment and differs from interventional gastrostomy, which refers to placement as required during treatment. In a non-prospective randomised controlled trial, nasogastric tubes were compared with non-prophylactic gastrostomy placement (Corry *et al.*, 2009). The gastrostomy group used tubes for longer and had better weight outcomes as compared to the nasogastric group, who experienced greater tube dislodgement and increasing patient and carer dissatisfaction as the study progressed. These findings have been supported in a large retrospective review which showed that weight loss was less with prophylactic gastrostomy placement as compared to placement as an intervention during treatment (Nugent *et al.*, 2010a). In a randomised controlled trial, improved quality-of-life scores at 6 months have also been reported with prophylactic gastrostomy placement as compared to interventional gastrostomy placement (Salas *et al.*, 2008). A Cochrane review concluded that the method of enteral feeding remains unclear in patients receiving radiotherapy or chemoradiotherapy, but this review only included one study, and this study had a high degree of bias (Nugent *et al.*, 2010b). However, another systematic review that included 10 randomised controlled trials concluded that both dietary counselling and prophylactic gastrostomy maintained or improved nutritional status (Garg *et al.*, 2010). All of these studies used weight as a nutrition outcome, but a more recent prospective longitudinal case series evaluated other anthropometrical measures and found improvements with prophylactic tube placement before, during and after treatment (Silander *et al.*, 2010).

Zhang *et al.* (2016) compared the outcomes of nasogastric tubes and either prophylactic or reactive gastrostomy tubes in a meta-analysis. Findings included evidence that prophylactic tube feeding resulted in reduced treatment interruptions and nutrition-related hospital admissions (Zhang *et al.*, 2016). There are no consensus guidelines, and decision-making for tube type, timing of insertion and method of placement is based on the clinical expertise and experience of the institution (BAO-HNS, 2016; NICE, 2016; Talwar, 2010). Outcomes of nutritional status with different feeding tubes remain inconclusive (Zhang *et al.*, 2016), and are thought to be associated with the fact that initiation of nutrition support is reactive and usually commences when clinically indicated during treatment despite prophylactic tube placement (Brown *et al.*, 2017). A recent randomised controlled trial of early prophylactic feeding versus standardised care which identified patients using a validated multidisciplinary protocol evaluated the impact of early feeding (Brown *et al.*, 2017). Earlier work by Brown *et al.* (2016) identified a target group of well-nourished patients with minimal dysphagia to have high rates of weight loss, thus requiring further research. Findings from the randomised control trial found no impact on weight loss outcomes at 3 months post-treatment, with both groups losing 10% of their body weight, and concluded that poor adherence to the intervention impacted on the power of the study and may have affected the limitations of statistical significance between the groups (Brown *et al.*, 2017). This study supports dietetic clinical practice of patient adherence to nutritional recommendations as a complex multifactorial issue for patients who are tube fed before, during and after treatment. The concept of gastrostomy dependency exists in clinical practice and is associated with long-term swallowing impairment. Many of these clinical studies have used gastrostomy tubes as a proxy measure for poor swallowing in the absence of reviewing nutritional intervention and outcome data, swallowing rehabilitation and co-ordination of these services before, during and after treatment (BAO-HNS, 2016). The use of reactive nasogastric tube placement in this patient group has subsequently increased, and emerging reviews are highlighting regional differences with community support and safe hospital discharge. Additionally, it has been suggested that complications with tube displacement and management, admission costs during radiotherapy treatment, and emergency department attendance following discharge may vary (Cook, 2017; Coomes *et al.*, 2017).

The most recent NICE (2016) guidance for cancer of the upper aerodigestive tract assessment and management in people aged ≥16 years, addressed the specific question: '*What specific clinical and non-clinical factors allow risk stratification when selecting which people would benefit from short- or long-term enteral nutrition?*' The optimal timing for decision-making is at diagnosis, and all factors impacting on nutrition should be considered, including patient demographics, tumour site and staging, treatment modalities, nutritional status, type and placement technique of feeding tube, and associated morbidity (NICE, 2016; Talwar & Findlay, 2012).

Careful consideration needs to be given to the timing and method of gastrostomy placement, with appropriate screening and selection for endoscopic, radiological or surgical placement based on comorbidities and contraindications. Organisational needs include a coordinated approach across the head and neck, gastroenterology, and radiology services for appropriate screening and selection of placement method. Close monitoring to minimise the risk of morbidity or mortality from postoperative complications and accountable services for the insertion and removal of the feeding tube are essential (BAO-HNS, 2016; Findlay *et al.*, 2011; Talwar & Findlay, 2012).

Practical and psychosocial aspects of gastrostomy feeding

The emotional, psychological and physical stresses associated with the diagnosis and treatment of head and neck cancer can be substantial for patients and their partners (Vickery *et al.*, 2003). Patients and carers reported that gastrostomy improved nutritional status, and provided relief from the pressure of coping with the side effects of treatment during periods of extreme fatigue; they would confidently make the same decision regarding gastrostomy placement (Mayre-Chilton *et al.*, 2011). However, a gastrostomy is not without a burden in day-to-day living, and negative experiences have also been reported (Brotherton & Judd, 2007; Jordan *et al.*, 2006; Mayre-Chilton *et al.*, 2011; Silver *et al.*, 2004). These studies found the following key elements to influence the patient's and/or carers' daily activities, lifestyle choices, relationship dynamics and quality of life (Talwar, 2010):

- *Practical limitations* – physical restrictions on going out or staying at home during the day, as well as disturbed sleep at night.
- *Lifestyle restrictions* – restricted choice in clothing and for going on holiday.
- Social adjustments – difficulties in finding a place to feed, effect on eating patterns and interference with family life.
- *Psychological issues* – avoiding or missing mealtimes with others, dealing with the negative attitudes of others towards feeding, changes in body image, effects of setting up the feeds, confidence with feeding in front of others, inability to act affectionately, understanding why the tube is necessary.
- *Impact on carers* – interaction at mealtimes, burden of care, with an estimated 15–30 hours/week dedicated to feeding issues.
- *Feeding tube management* – limited knowledge of (and support for) technical difficulties, leading to complications and hospital readmission.

The preceding findings have been confirmed in a quality-of-life study that also identified the importance of effective gastrostomy counselling in the pretreatment phase, with the use of appropriate literature and visual aids, and ongoing support until the tube is removed (Rogers *et al.*, 2007). A specialist dietitian should undertake this role from the point of deciding on tube placement until tube removal (Talwar, 2010).

Nutritional monitoring

Continuous feeding can markedly restrict a patient's independence, but may be necessary to meet nutritional requirements when experiencing treatment-related side effects. Patients established on a feeding regimen should be encouraged to bolus feed during the day with or without overnight pump feeding. This will prevent nutritional inadequacy (e.g. when attending daily radiotherapy), encourage a normal eating pattern, help the transition to oral feeding, and, most importantly, release patients from being attached to a pump and thus improve their sense of being in control over feeding issues (Talwar, 2010).

Nutritional intervention post-treatment improves and maintains nutritional status and quality of life (Findlay *et al.*, 2011). The majority of patients continue to experience eating difficulties after treatment (Pauloski *et al.*, 2006), placing them at risk of ongoing weight loss; therefore, dietary manipulation and optimisation of nutritional support should continue as a priority (Schattner *et al.*, 2005). Weight loss and functional status are important predictors of quality of life in head and neck cancer patients (Karin *et al.*, 2005). Patient weight should be monitored on admission, weekly during treatment, and at each outpatient appointment (BAO-HNS, 2016). It should be routine practice to use anthropometric tools that measure functional muscle status in this patient group, especially in those on long-term nutritional support (see Chapter 2.2, Assessment of nutritional status). The specialist dietitian and SLT should set collaborative goals to optimise nutrition and swallowing outcomes – dispelling the misinterpreted concept of gastrostomy dependency and optimising safe transition with swallowing from enteral to oral nutrition, without compromising the patient's quality of life in the presence of side effects from treatment (Talwar & Findlay, 2012).

Palliative care issues

The incidence of distant metastasis at initial diagnosis is 10%, with the lung, mediastinal lymph nodes, liver and bone being the most common sites of presentation (Argiris *et al.*, 2008). The incidence of developing a second primary is 3–5% on a yearly basis (Khuri *et al.*, 2006), and the 5-year survival for all stages combined is 60% (Ries *et al.*, 2006). Mortality is usually associated with recurrent disease from the primary site. The patient's oral intake ability can be severely restricted or eliminated due to the progressive nature of the disease causing swallowing difficulties. This can lead to malnutrition and its associated consequences, and is further exacerbated by cachexia, for which the incidence in this patient group is not known (Talwar, 2010). The treatment options at this stage are the same as for curative intent, with the aim of symptom control and the goal of improving quality and extending life (BAO-HNS, 2016).

Oral and/or artificial supportive nutrition should be offered as part of palliative care for symptom control (Arends *et al.*, 2017). The specialist dietitian should discuss nutritional support with other members of the head and neck cancer care team, and facilitate the decision-making process for appropriate nutritional management (BAO-HNS, 2016; Findlay *et al.*, 2011; NICE, 2004) (see Chapter 7.16, Palliative and end-of-life care).

Further reading

British Association of Otorhinolaryngologists – Head and Neck Surgeons (BAO-HNS). (2016) *Effective Head and Neck Cancer Multidisciplinary Management, 4th Consensus Document*. London: BAO-HNS.

Findlay M, Bauer J, Brown T, *et al.* (2011) *Evidence based practice guidelines for the nutritional management of adult patients with head and neck cancer*. Sydney, Australia: Clinical Oncological Society of Australia. Available at http://wiki.cancer.org.au/australia/COSA:Head_and_neck_cancer_nutrition_guidelines. Accessed 27 October 2012.

NICE. (2004) *Improving Outcomes in Head and Neck Cancers – The Manual*. London: NICE.

NICE. (2016) *Cancer of the Upper Aerodigestive Tract: Assessment and Management in People Aged 16 and Over*. Available at https://www.nice.org.uk/guidance/ng36. Accessed 27 January 2017.

Talwar B. (2010) Head & neck cancer. In: Shaw C (ed) *Nutrition and Cancer*. Oxford: Blackwell Wiley, pp. 188–220.

Internet resources

British Association of Head & Neck Oncology Nurses (BAHNON), www.bahnon.org.uk

Head & Neck Sub Group, Oncology Group of the British Dietetic Association, www.bda.uk.com

National Association of Laryngectomee Clubs, www.laryngectomy.org.uk

References

Arends J, Bachmann P, Baracos V, *et al.* (2017) ESPEN guidelines on nutrition in cancer. *Clin. Nutr.* 36: 11–38.

Argiris A, Karamouzis M, Raben D, *et al.* (2008) Head and neck cancer. *Lancet.* 371: 1695–1709.

Bertrand P, Piquet M, Bordier I, *et al.* (2002) Preoperative nutritional support at home in head and neck cancer patients: from nutritional benefits to the prevention of the alcohol withdrawal syndrome. *Curr. Opin. Clin. Nutr. Metab. Care.* 5(4): 435–440.

Blanchard P, Baujat B, Holostenco V, *et al.* (2011) Meta-analysis of chemotherapy in head and neck cancer (MACH-NC): a comprehensive analysis by tumour site. *Radiother. Oncol.* 100: 33–40.

Bradley P, Donaldson M. (2000) Current management of the nutritional needs of the head and neck cancer patient. *Curr. Opin. Otolaryngol. Head Neck Surg.* 8(2): 107–112.

British Association of Otorhinolaryngologists – Head and Neck Surgeons (BAO-HNS). (2016) *Head & Neck Cancer: United Kingdom Multidisciplinary Guidelines (Online)*. Available at http://bahno.org.uk/wp-content/uploads/2014/03/UK-Head-and-Cancer-Guidelines-2016.pdf. Accessed 27 January 2017.

Brookes G. (1985) Nutritional status – a prognostic indicator in head and neck cancer. *Otolaryngol. Head Neck Surg.* 93: 69–74.

Brotherton AM, Judd PA. (2007) Quality of life in adult enteral tube feeding patients. *J. Hum. Nutr. Diet.* 20(6): 513–522.

Brown T, Banks M, Hughes B, *et al.* (2015) New radiotherapy techniques do not reduce the need for nutrition intervention in patients with head and neck cancer. *Eur. J. Clin. Nutr.* 69(10): 1119–1124.

Brown TE, Getliffe V, Banks MD, *et al.* (2016) Validation of an updated evidence-based protocol for proactive gastrostomy tube insertion in patients with head and neck cancer. *Eur. J. Clin. Nutr.* 70: 574–581.

Brown TE, Banks MD, Hughes BG, *et al.* (2017) Randomised controlled trial of early prophylactic feeding vs standard care in patients with head and neck cancer. *Br. J. Cancer* 117: 15–24.

Cady J. (2007) Nutritional support during radiotherapy for head and neck cancer: The role of prophylactic feeding tube placement. *Clin. J. Oncol. Nurs.* 11(6): 875–880.

Cancer Research UK. (2016) *Head & Neck Cancer Incidence (Online)*. Available at www.cancerresearchuk.org/health-professional/cancer-statistics/statistics-by-cancer-type/oral-cancer/incidence#heading-Zero. Accessed 27 January 2017.

Cook F. (2017) A prospective review from a UK tertiary cancer centre of head and neck patients discharged with naso-gastric (NG) tubes over 2 years (2015–2016). *British Association of Head and Neck Oncologists Annual Scientific Meeting* (Oral Presentation and in Preparation for Publication).

Coomes A, Mir N, McBride R, *et al.* (2017) Nasal Tube Complications in Head and Neck Cancer Patients at a London Tertiary Cancer Centre. *British Association of Head and Neck Oncologists Annual Scientific Meeting.*

Corry J, Poon W, McPhee N, *et al.* (2009) Prospective study of percutaneous endoscopic gastrostomy tubes versus nasogastric tubes for enteral feeding in patients with head and neck cancer undergoing (chemo)radiation. *Head Neck.* 31(7): 944–948.

Daly JM, Hearne B, Dunaj J, *et al.* (1984) Nutritional rehabilitation in patients with advanced head and neck cancer receiving radiation therapy. *Am. J. Surg.* 148: 514–520.

Findlay M, Bauer J, Brown T, *et al.* (2011) *Evidence based practice guidelines for the nutritional management of adult patients with head and neck cancer.* Sydney, Australia: Clinical Oncological Society of Australia. Available at http://wiki.cancer.org.au/australia/COSA:Head_and_neck_cancer_nutrition_guidelines. Accessed 27 October 2012.

Garg S, Yoo J, Winquist E. (2010) Nutritional support for head and neck cancer patients receiving radiotherapy: a systematic review. *Support Care Cancer.* 18(6): 667–677.

Hammerlid E, Wirblad B, Sandin C, *et al.* (1998) Malnutrition and food intake in relation to quality of life in head and neck cancer patients. *Head Neck.* 20(6): 540–548.

Hearne BE, Dunaj JM, Daly JM, *et al.* (1985) Enteral nutrition support in head and neck cancer: tube vs. oral feeding during radiation therapy. *J. Am. Diet. Assoc.* 85: 669–674.

International Union Against Cancer. (2016) *TNM Classification.* Available at www.uicc.org/resources/tnm. Accessed 27 January 2017.

Isenring I, Capra S, Bauer J. (2004) Nutrition intervention is beneficial in oncology outpatients receiving radiotherapy to the gastrointestinal or head and neck area. *Br. J. Cancer.* 91(3): 447–452.

Jordan S, Philpin S, Warring J, *et al.* (2006) Percutaneous endoscopic gastrostomies: the burden of treatment from a patient perspective. *J. Adv. Nur.* 56(3): 270–281.

Karin P, Ewa S, Hammerlid E. (2005) Quality of life as predictor of weight loss in patients with head and neck cancer. *Head Neck.* 27(4): 302–310.

Kelly LE. (2007) Radiation and chemotherapy. In: Ward E, van As-Brooks CJ (eds) *Head & Neck Cancer: Treatment, Rehabilitation and Outcomes.* San Diego: Plural Publishing Inc, pp. 57–86.

Khuri FR, Lee JJ, Lippman SM, *et al.* (2006) Randomised phase III trial of low-dose isotretinoin for prevention of second primary tumours in stage I and II head and neck cancer patients. *J. Nat. Cancer Inst.* 98(7): 441–450.

Langius JA, Bakker S, Rietveld DH, *et al.* (2013) Critical weight loss is a major prognostic indicator for disease-specific survival in patients with head and neck cancer receiving radiotherapy. *Br. J. Cancer* 109: 1093–1099.

Larsson M, Hedelin B, Athlin E. (2003) Lived experiences of eating problems for patients with head and neck cancer during radiotherapy. *J. Clin. Nutr.* 12(4): 562–570.

Larsson M, Hedelin B, Johansson I, *et al.* (2005) Eating problems and weight loss for patients with head and neck cancer. *Cancer Nurs.* 28(6): 425–435.

Lees J. (1997) Nasogastric and percutaneous endoscopic gastrostomy feeding in head and neck cancer patients receiving radiotherapy treatment at a regional oncology unit: a two year study. *Eur. J. Cancer Care (Engl).* 6(1): 45–49.

List M, Bilir P. (2004) Evaluations of quality of life and organ function. *Semin. Oncol.* 31: 827–835.

Lundy D, Sullivan P, Bernstein MG. (2009) Rehabilitation of swallowing and speech following treatment of head & neck malignancies. In: Petruzzelli GP (ed) *Practical Head and Neck Oncology.* San Diego: Plural Publishing Inc, pp. 591–611.

Mangar S, Slevin N, Mais K, *et al.* (2006) Evaluating predictive factors for determining enteral nutrition in patients receiving radical radiotherapy for head and neck cancer: a retrospective review. *Radiother. Oncol.* 78: 152–158.

Marron M, Boffetta P, Zhang Z, *et al.* (2010) Cessation of alcohol drinking, tobacco smoking and the reversal of head and neck cancer risk. *Int. J. Epidemiol.* 39(1): 182–196.

Mayre-Chilton K, Talwar B, Goff L. (2011) Different experiences and perspectives between head and neck cancer patients and their care-givers on their daily impact of a gastrostomy tube. *J. Hum. Nutr. Diet.* 24: 449–459.

Mekhail TM, Adelstein D, Rybicki L, *et al.* (2001) Enteral nutrition during the treatment of head and neck carcinoma. *Cancer.* 91: 1785–1790.

NICE. (2004) *Improving Outcomes in Head and Neck Cancers – The Manual.* London: NICE.

NICE. (2016) *Cancer of the Upper Aerodigestive Tract: Assessment and Management in People Aged 16 and Over.* Available at https://www.nice.org.uk/guidance/ng36. Accessed 27 January 2017.

Nugent B, Parker MJ, McIntyre IA. (2010a) Nasogastric tube feeding and percutaneous endoscopic gastrostomy tube feeding in patients with head and neck cancer. *J. Hum. Nutr. Diet.* 23: 277–284.

Nugent B, Lewis S, O'Sullivan JM. (2010b) Enteral feeding methods for nutritional management in patients with head and neck cancers being treated with radiotherapy and/or chemotherapy. *Cochrane Database Syst. Rev.* (3): CD007904.

Paccagnella A, Morello M, Da Mosto MC, *et al.* (2010) Early nutritional intervention improves treatment tolerance and outcomes in head and neck cancer patients undergoing concurrent chemoradiotherapy. *Support Care Cancer.* 18: 837–845.

Paleri V, Wood J, Patterson, *et al.* (2016) A feasibility study incorporating a pilot randomised controlled trial of oral feeding plus pretreatment gastrostomy tube versus oral feeding plus as-needed nasogastric tube feeding in patients undergoing chemoradiation for head and neck cancer (TIBE trial): study protocol. *Pilot & Feasibility Studies.* doi 10.1186/s40814-016-0069-8.

Patterson J, McColl E, Wilson J, *et al.* (2015) Head & neck cancer patients' perceptions of swallowing following chemoradiotherapy. *Support Care Cancer.* 23(12): 3531–3538.

Pauloski BR, Rademaker AW, Logemann JA, *et al.* (2006) Relationship between swallow motility disorders on videofluorography and oral intake in patients treated for head and neck cancer with radiotherapy with or without chemotherapy. *Head Neck.* 28(12): 1069–1076.

Pignon J, le Maître A, Maillard E, *et al.*; MACH-NC Collaborative Group. (2009) Meta-analysis of chemotherapy in head and neck cancer (MACH-NC): an update on 93 randomised trials and 17,346 patients. *Radiother. Oncol.* 92(1): 4–14.

Piquet M-A, Ozsahin M, Larpin I, *et al.* (2002) Early nutritional intervention in oropharyngeal cancer patients undergoing radiotherapy. *Support Care Cancer.* 10: 502–504.

Polisena CG. (2010) Nutrition concerns with the radiation therapy patient. In: McCallum PD, Polisena CG (eds) *The Clinical Guide to Oncology Nutrition.* Chicago: The American Dietetic Association.

Proia N, Paszkiewicz G, Nasca M, *et al.* (2006) Smoking and smokeless tobacco-associated human buccal cell mutations and their association with oral cancer – a review. *Cancer Epidemiology, Biomarkers & Prevention* 15: 1061–1077.

Ravasco P, Monterio-Grillo I, Marques P, *et al.* (2004) Cancer: Disease and nutrition are key determinants of patients' quality of life. *Support. Care Cancer* 12(4): 246–252.

Ravasco P, Monterio-Grillo I, Marques P, *et al.* (2005) Impact of nutrition on outcome: a prospective randomised controlled trial in patients with head and neck cancer undergoing radiotherapy. *Head Neck.* 27(8): 659–668.

Ries LG, Melbert D, Krapcho M, *et al.* (2006) *SEER Cancer Statistics Review, 1975–2004.* Bethesda, MD: National Cancer Institute.

Rogers SN, Thomson R, O'Toole P, *et al.* (2007) Patients experience with long-term percutaneous endoscopic gastrostomy feeding following primary surgery for oral and oropharyngeal cancer. *Oral Oncol.* 43(5): 499–507.

Royal College of Speech and Language Therapists (RCSLT). (2002) *Communicating quality 2 professional standards for Speech and Language Therapists.* London: RCSLT.

Salas S, Deville J-L, Giorgi R, *et al.* (2008) Nutritional factors as predictors of response to radio-chemotherapy and survival in unresectable squamous head and neck carcinoma. *Radiother. Oncol.* 87: 195–200.

Schattner M, Willis H, Raykher A, *et al.* (2005) Long-term enteral nutrition facilitates optimization of body weight. *JPEN J. Parenter. Enteral Nutr.* 29(3): 198–203.

Silander E, Nyman J, Bove M, *et al.* (2010) The use of prophylactic percutaneous endoscopic gastrostomy and early enteral feeding in patients with advanced head and neck cancer – a prospective longitudinal study. *Eur. e-J. Clin. Nutr. Metab.* doi:10.1016.

Silver HJ, Wellman NS, Arnold DJ, *et al.* (2004) Older adults receiving home enteral nutrition: enteral regimen, provider involvement, and health care outcomes. *JPEN J. Parenter. Enteral Nutr.* 28(2): 92–98.

Talwar B. (2010) Head & neck cancer. In: Shaw C (ed) *Nutrition and Cancer*, Vol. 1. Oxford: Blackwell Wiley, pp. 188–220.

Talwar B, Findlay M. (2012) When is the optimal time for placing a gastrostomy in patients undergoing treatment for head and neck cancer? *Curr. Opin. Support. Palliat. Care* 6: 41–53.

van Bokhorst-de van der Schuer M, van Leeuwen P, Sauerwein HP, *et al.* (1997) Assessment of malnutrition parameters in head and neck cancer and their relation to postoperative complications. *Head Neck.* 19(5): 419–425.

van Bokhorst-de van der Schuer M, van Leeuwen P, Kuik D, *et al.* (1999) The impact of nutritional status on the prognosis of patients with advanced head and neck cancer. *Cancer* 86(3): 519–527.

van Bokhorst-de van der Schuer M, Langendoen S, Vondeling H, *et al.* (2000) Perioperative enteral nutrition and quality of life of severely malnourished head and neck cancer patients: a randomised clinical trial. *Clin. Nutr.* 19(6): 437–444.

Van Cutsem E, Arends J. (2005) The causes and consequences of cancer-associated malnutrition. *Eur. J. Oncol. Nurs.* 9 (2): S51–63.

Vickery L, Latchford G, Hewison J, *et al.* (2003) The impact of head and neck cancer and facial disfigurement on the quality of life of patients and their partners. *Head Neck.* 25(4): 289–296.

Weimann A, Braga M, Carli F, *et al.* (2017) ESPEN guideline: clinical nutrition in surgery. *Clin. Nutr.* (36) 623–650.

Wood K. (2005) Audit of nutritional guidelines for head and neck cancer patients undergoing radiotherapy. *J. Hum. Nutr. Diet.* 18(5): 343–351.

Zhang Z, Shu Y, Ling Y, *et al.* (2016) Comparative effects of different enteral feeding methods in head and neck cancer patients receiving radiotherapy or chemoradiotherapy: a network meta-analysis. *Onco Targets Ther.* 9: 2897–2909.

7.15.3 Cancer of the gastrointestinal tract

Eva Glass, Mary Phillips and Lindsey Allan

Key points

- Cancers of the gastrointestinal tract (GIT) are associated with nutritional risk factors, including obesity.
- A range of symptoms, which greatly affect food intake and utilisation, accompany GIT cancer.
- Nutritional problems can be further exacerbated by treatment interventions such as major surgery, radiotherapy or chemotherapy.
- Nutritional intervention may involve dietary counselling and nutritional support at all stages of cancer treatment, including palliation.

This chapter discusses cancer of the gastrointestinal tract apart from hepatocellular carcinoma (liver cancer), which is discussed in Chapter 7.4.12 (Liver & Biliary Disease).

Carcinoma of the oesophagus

Eva Glass

Oesophageal cancer is the 13th most common cancer in the UK, accounting for around 8800 new diagnoses per year (ISD, 2014; NICR, 2014; ONS, 2014; WCISU, 2016). The incidence is much higher in males, with a 2:1 male to female ratio. Bosman *et al.* (2010) describes more than 20 histological subtypes of oesophageal carcinoma, although adenocarcinoma (arising from the glandular epithelium) and squamous cell carcinoma (arising from the epithelial cells) represent the majority of the diagnoses. In the Western world, adenocarcinoma incidence is seen to be increasing, whereas the incidence of squamous cell carcinoma is stable, or even decreasing (Melhado *et al.*, 2010).

There is strong evidence that being overweight or obese, and consuming tobacco, alcohol and mate (a herbal tea), increases the risk of oesophageal cancer (WCRF/AICR, 2016b). Consuming fruit and vegetables, and being physically active, decreases the risk, while consuming processed meat increases the risk of oesophageal cancer (WCRF/AICR, 2016b). Furthermore, the risk of oesophageal cancer is increased in the presence of other diseases, such as gastro-oesophageal reflux disease, oesophageal achalasia, Barrett's oesophagus, and the human papilloma virus (WCRF/AICR, 2016b).

Patients may present with weight loss, dysphagia and retrosternal pain on eating. The extent of weight loss tends to be related to the degree and duration of the dysphagia. Cancer of the oesophagus is diagnosed, and subsequently staged by endoscopy, endoscopic ultrasound, computed tomography (CT) and positron emission tomography (PET). Biopsy is required to confirm the histological diagnosis. By the time patients present with symptoms, the disease may be advanced, and deterioration may occur rapidly. Treatment may involve chemotherapy, radiotherapy, and surgery, depending on patient choice, fitness, location and stage of disease, and whether there is spread to adjacent lymph nodes or distant sites in the body. Endoscopic techniques such as dilatation, or the insertion of a stent, may also be required, depending on the progression of disease or symptoms. If the cancer is advanced, palliative chemotherapy and/or supportive care may be appropriate.

Upper gastrointestinal (UGI) cancer patients present many dietetic challenges (see Chapter 7.15.2, Head and neck cancer). The reported incidence of malnutrition in UGI patients ranges from 60% to 90% (Hebuterne *et al.*, 2014; Silvers *et al.*, 2014), with an average weight loss of approximately 16% (Bozzetti on behalf of the SCRINIO Working Group, 2009). This reported variance is due to the differences in the definition of malnutrition, and in the subjects included in studies; the highest incidences of malnutrition are normally found in those with advanced disease.

Management

Oesophageal resection

Endoscopic mucosal resection is mainly used in severe dysplasia, but its use in treating very early carcinomas is increasing. Surgical treatment of carcinoma of the oesophagus may be oesophagectomy or oesophagogastrectomy, depending on the site and extent of the cancer. Patients who are severely nutritionally depleted will require nutritional support prior to surgery. Patients who are able to swallow will require dietary advice, often with nutritional supplements. Those undergoing preoperative chemotherapy may experience an improvement in dysphagia during this time, which enables an improved dietary intake prior to surgery. The enhanced recovery programme is mainly used in other surgical areas, e.g. orthopaedics, yet there is increasing usage in the UK with oesophagectomies and gastrectomies. The programme has been shown to have positive benefits, including a lower lean body mass loss, decreased complications, and decreased length of hospital stay (Findlay *et al.*, 2014) (see Chapter 7.17.5, Surgery).

Early post-operative nutritional support is essential; enteral feeding by a route that bypasses the oesophagus and stomach is usually appropriate, e.g. jejunostomy feeding. Once the integrity of the anastomosis has been confirmed, oral feeding can resume, starting with oral fluids, followed by the gradual phasing in of solid foods (see Chapter 7.3, Dysphagia), as enteral nutrition is phased out. Ongoing dietetic supervision is essential, both during hospitalisation and following discharge. Persistent postoperative nutritional problems can include the following:

- Poor appetite.
- Early satiety.
- Fear of eating, particularly foods which were difficult to eat preoperatively.
- Difficulty in regaining or maintaining body weight.
- Nausea.
- Reflux.
- Dysphagia (due to anastomotic stricture or recurrence of disease).

Dietary management should aim to prevent further nutritional deterioration and weight loss, and attempt to restore good nutritional status, which may have been severely compromised prior to surgery. Practical guidance should focus on the following:

- Eating small, frequent meals.
- Taking time at mealtimes and chewing foods well.
- Drinking fluids separately from meals.
- Good choices of nutrient- and energy-dense foods, and useful food-enrichment strategies (see Chapter 6.3, Oral nutritional support).
- Good choices of nutrient-rich beverages.
- Avoiding foods that cause discomfort or gastrointestinal symptoms.
- Adopting strategies that reduce the likelihood of reflux, e.g. not eating late at night; not lying down soon after eating; avoiding strong tea, coffee, and alcohol.

Additional support measures, such as oral sip feed supplementation, may be indicated if nutritional needs cannot be met by these measures alone.

Radiotherapy

Radiotherapy, external beam radiation therapy (EBRT) or, occasionally, intraluminal radiation (brachytherapy) may be used to treat oesophageal carcinoma. This may be the sole treatment, or used in combination with chemotherapy or surgery. During a course of radiotherapy, the tissues will become oedematous, inflamed, and swollen, and it is therefore likely that dysphagia will worsen. These effects are usually temporary; however, these patients are often already severely malnourished and have suffered marked weight loss. It may therefore be important for the dietitian to raise the issue with the medical team, whether enteral feeding is indicated prior to, or during, treatment. The need for enteral feeding is even more imperative in those patients presenting with an already high degree of dysphagia due to the anticipated side effects experienced with radiotherapy. Nutritional support at this stage via nasogastric tube, gastrostomy, or jejunostomy may prevent further deterioration of an already poor nutritional status. If such support is implemented, it is important to explain to the patient why such intervention is advisable at this stage, i.e. to avert possible problems, and not as a sign that their condition has worsened.

During radiotherapy treatment, patients may experience sore throat and/or an increase in dysphagia. Therefore, they may find that bland foods (avoiding strong flavours, artificial or natural acidity, and spices) are best tolerated. Foods may need to have a smooth consistency (e.g. liquidised meals, strained thickened soups, custard, milk puddings), or a crumbly texture (e.g. crackers, crisp bread, or savoury cheese snacks). It is helpful to liaise with the medical team to ensure the appropriate use of medications to help with the radiotherapy symptoms, e.g. adequate analgesia.

Reintroduction of a normal diet should be gradual. Meals will need to be well moistened, and accompanied by frequent sips of drinks to assist the passage of food past the inflamed area. Sip feed supplements may be necessary to maintain adequate energy and nutrient intake. Most patients will continue with a soft diet for some time, as some difficulties with swallowing often persist. Some will also be afraid to try foods with which they associate problems, particularly meat and bread. The dietitian is key to encouraging patients to gradually increase back to normal textures in their diet. Patients may find that such foods can be well tolerated if consumed with plenty of sauce or gravy.

Chemotherapy

Side effects commonly associated with this form of therapy, such as nausea, vomiting, and taste changes, may have an additional impact on oral intake. Some general remedial measures to help alleviate these effects are discussed in Chapters 6.3 (Oral nutritional support) and 7.15.1 (General aspects of cancer).

Other treatment strategies

When radical treatment is contraindicated (e.g. due to medical history, size of disease, metastatic spread, or fitness), endoscopic techniques such as dilatation, laser therapy or the insertion of a stent can be used as palliative procedures to relieve dysphagia. An oesophageal stent is normally a permanent self-expanding metal stent that is placed under sedation. These procedures have high rates of complications such as perforation or haemorrhage, and there is an increased risk of mortality (Martinez *et al.*, 2011). However, an immediate improvement in dysphagia is usually seen, and, with appropriate guidance, many patients are able to resume a fairly normal diet. The main complication is that of stent migration, or overgrowth of tumour, which leads to a recurrence of dysphagia. If this occurs, laser therapy or placement of a further stent is required. A temporary (around 3 months) biodegradable stent is sometimes the preferred option to a permanent stent or enteral feeding. This is a measure for those who are dysphagic, but who will be receiving treatment that may ultimately improve their swallow without the need for a permanent stent.

Guidelines for the dietary management of patients who have an oesophageal stent in place vary according to the type of device inserted and local policy. There is little evidence in the literature of the best advice for such patients; nevertheless, the BDA's Oncology Group has constructed a consensus statement based on the available literature and current practice – however, this is currently being updated. Guidance for patients with oesophageal stents on texture modification may be helpful in some cases (see Chapter 7.3, Dysphagia). However, tolerance to different foods does vary between patients, and may even vary on a day-to-day basis in the same patient. It is therefore difficult to give precise guidance as to which foods will or will not cause problems, but the dietitian should give advice on ensuring small mouthfuls, positioning, and chewing food well. Many patients establish a diet of suitable texture by a process of trial and error.

Nutritional support

Whether the treatment plan is for surgery, chemotherapy, radiotherapy or supportive care, many patients will be nutritionally compromised. A common complaint is reduced appetite and cancer cachexia, often accompanied by dysphagia and other issues already outlined (Bozzetti, 2010). Consumption of a nutrient-dense diet via appropriate food choice, food enrichment strategies and, if necessary, use of proprietary supplements should be encouraged (see Chapter 6.3, Oral nutritional support). However, patients may present with cancer cachexia that cannot be fully reversed with an improvement in energy intake alone (Fearon *et al.*, 2011) (see Chapter 7.15.9, Cancer cachexia).

The use of enteral nutrition in oesophageal cancer varies, depending on the treatment planned and its expected outcome, i.e. radical or palliative treatment. As already discussed, patients with total dysphagia will often have enteral nutrition, particularly if they are to receive radical treatment of chemotherapy and surgery, or chemotherapy and radiotherapy. Those receiving palliative chemotherapy may also receive enteral nutrition if a stent is not in place. There is much debate on the use of enteral nutrition in the palliative care setting for oesophageal cancer patients who are unable to meet their nutritional requirements for reasons other than dysphagia. The multidisciplinary team may decide that it is in the patient's best interest to have a stent placed in order to improve their swallow, therefore allowing the patient to eat and improve their quality of life.

Parenteral nutrition is not routinely used in these patients, because nutritional support via the oral or enteral route is normally viable. However, it should be considered if patients are malnourished, or at risk of malnutrition, and are unable to meet their nutritional requirements orally or enterally as per NICE guidelines (2006).

Gastric carcinoma

Eva Glass

The incidence of gastric cancer is declining, due to the decrease in *Helicobacter pylori*; although survival is rapidly improving, the 5-year survival rate is 19% (ISD, 2014; Cancer Registry, 2014; WCISU, 2016). There is strong evidence that consuming three or more alcoholic drinks per day, eating salt-preserved foods and processed meat, and being overweight or obese increases the risk (WCRF/AICR, 2016a). Evidence suggests that consuming grilled or barbecued meat and fish, and having a low fruit intake, also increases the risk (WCRF/AICR, 2016a). In contrast, there is evidence suggesting that consuming citrus fruit decreases the risk of gastric cancer (WCRF/AICR, 2016a). Non-dietary risk factors for gastric cancer include *Helicobacter pylori* infection, the Epstein-Barr virus, smoking and industrial chemical exposure (WCRF/AICR, 2016a).

Gastric carcinoma is often diagnosed late because its early symptoms may be dismissed as indigestion or heartburn. By the time patients present with anorexia, nausea, vomiting, pain on eating and severe weight loss, the disease may be well advanced, possibly with metastatic spread. If the condition is operable, the preferred treatment is perioperative chemotherapy (chemotherapy before and after surgery), followed by partial or total gastrectomy as appropriate; early tumours can be endoscopically or surgically treated without chemotherapy (Smyth *et al.*, 2016). If a gastrectomy is contraindicated in patients with pyloric obstruction, a gastroenterostomy may be performed or the pylorus stented, to allow eating. If a stent is placed, then patients often tolerate a normal diet, but if not, a soft diet or a low-fibre diet, similar to that recommended with an oesophageal stent, is often advised. The additional use of supplements or other support measures is usually necessary.

However, if pyloric obstruction occurs in patients with a poor prognosis, medical management is normally conservative, involving medications such as prokinetics and palliative care. Jejunal feeding may be used for a small number of patients receiving palliative treatment for gastric outlet obstruction if their prognosis is not so poor and a stent is not placed. Parenteral nutrition may also be considered; however, this is normally used temporarily until oral or enteral nutrition can be established.

Gastric resection and reconstruction

Gastric surgery can have a considerable negative impact on subsequent food intake, weight recovery and quality of life. Gastric replacement with various enteric reservoirs has been used to improve the postprandial symptoms and nutrition of patients after total gastrectomy. To improve quality of life postoperatively, pouch and Roux-en-Y reconstructions have been shown to be most useful (Zong *et al.*, 2011). Increasingly, laparoscopic techniques are being used for the removal of early gastric cancers (Smyth *et al.*, 2016).

As a result of the combination of cancer-related cachexia and chronic symptoms such as nausea, vomiting or discomfort on eating, patients with gastric carcinoma often present significantly malnourished. Therefore, nutritional support measures should be instigated as early as possible, preferably before surgery or as soon as possible afterwards. The enteral rather than parenteral route should be used if possible.

Early postoperative enteral nutritional support (within 24 hours) can be safely established via a jejunostomy or nasojejunal tube placed intraoperatively. However, some hospitals do not provide this routinely, keeping patients nil by mouth postoperatively with or without the provision of parenteral nutrition until oral diet can be commenced (Baker *et al.*, 2011). Standard feeds are commonly given, although the use of immunonutrition is increasing; there is increasing evidence for the benefit of this following gastric resection; however the evidence is equivocal (Mabvuure *et al.*, 2013).

Disturbances in gastrointestinal function following gastric resection and reconstruction are common, and may affect nutritional intake and, subsequently, nutritional status. Gastrointestinal consequences of gastric resection and reconstruction include the following:

- Rapid emptying of the stomach remnant.
- Reduced secretion of intrinsic factor.
- Reduced secretion of pancreatic enzymes.
- Inadequate mixing of food with enzymes and bile.
- Reduced absorption of certain food substances, especially protein and fat.
- Rapid absorption of glucose.
- Abolition of the normal pH gradient in the small intestine.
- Increased intestinal motility.

Some of these problems occur soon after eating; others result from the long-term consequences of disturbed gastric function. These consequences of surgery can manifest as discussed in the following sections.

Small stomach syndrome

The majority of patients experience early satiety and may feel distended or uncomfortable during or after eating. This is particularly common after total or partial gastrectomy, but may also occur after vagotomy and pyloroplasty. Small, frequent meals should be eaten, and fluids should be consumed separately from solid food (see Chapter 6.3, Oral nutritional support).

Dumping syndrome

Early dumping

This occurs soon after eating and causes symptoms such as sweating, dizziness, faintness, rapid weak pulse, and hypotension as a response to the rapid and early delivery of a hyperosmolar meal into the jejunum. The symptoms usually recede 2–3 months after surgery. In the meantime, symptoms can be relieved by consuming small meals, limiting the consumption of refined carbohydrates and avoiding the consumption of liquids with meals.

Late dumping

Some patients may also experience symptoms similar to hypoglycaemia approximately 2 hours after a meal as a result of overproduction of insulin in response to the rapid absorption of glucose. Patients typically experience weakness, light-headedness, and feelings of cold and sweating, and these symptoms can be minimised by following the advice for early dumping, with emphasis on the regular consumption of starchy carbohydrate foods.

Diarrhoea

Diarrhoea frequently occurs following vagotomy or total gastrectomy, but may reduce with increasing time after surgery. Antidiarrhoeal agents such as codeine phosphate or loperamide may alleviate the problem.

Vomiting bile

Pancreatic and biliary secretions may accumulate in the afferent loop and, after food has left the stomach, can enter the gastric remnant, causing nausea and vomiting. Prokinetics (e.g. metoclopramide, domperidone, or erythromycin) may be useful, although surgical correction may be needed if vomiting is refractory to medical management.

Long-term consequences

Weight loss and malnutrition

Weight loss and nutritional inadequacy are common after gastric surgery, and nearly always reflect poor intake. Problems such as early satiety or dumping syndrome tend to make people reluctant to eat. In addition, treatment side effects may further affect appetite and intake. Dietary guidance should focus on improving meal frequency and nutrient density via appropriate food choice and enrichment (see Chapter 6.3, Oral nutritional support). Additional oral nutritional supplementation may be indicated. Patients should be monitored regularly, so that progress can be assessed and nutritional support measures adjusted as necessary.

Malabsorption

Malabsorption, particularly of fat, may result due to a number of alterations in gastrointestinal function following gastrectomy. It is important to ensure that energy intake is increased to compensate for faecal energy losses and ensure that micronutrient intake, particularly calcium, iron and fat-soluble vitamins, is not compromised. Treatment of steatorrhoea by dietary fat restriction alone is normally not recommended, as the resultant dietary energy content will be too low to meet needs. The cause of the steatorrhoea should be identified and appropriate management accordingly provided. This may include the use of bile acid binders, treatment of small bacterial overgrowth, pancreatic enzyme replacement therapy (PERT), or antidiarrhoea medication.

Anaemias

Iron deficiency anaemia is a common and particular risk following gastrectomy, due to poor iron intake and absorption. Haematological status should be regularly assessed and treated if necessary. Pernicious anaemia can be a secondary consequence of gastrectomy as a result of the loss of intrinsic factor (produced by gastric parietal cells) and local conditions necessary for the absorption of vitamin B_{12}. Vitamin B_{12} should be given by injection to those considered to be at risk. Megaloblastic anaemia may result from folate deficiency, particularly if dietary intake is poor and malabsorption is present; oral folate supplementation may be necessary.

Dietetic management

Dietary guidance following gastric reconstruction should focus on the following:

- Small, frequent, regular meals.
- Avoiding large quantities of fluid.
- Consuming fluids between meals rather than with them.
- Eating a variety of nutrient-dense foods (e.g. milk, dairy products, lean meat and eggs). Non-bulky (i.e. not high in fibre) cereal foods and small amounts of fruit and vegetables should also be included in the daily diet.
- Boosting nutrient intake via food-enrichment strategies if food intake is, or has been, particularly poor.
- Taking recommended nutritional supplements (either energy/nutrient supplements or vitamin/mineral preparations) if indicated.
- Advising remedial dietary measures for dumping syndrome or malabsorption if present.
- Oral nutritional support is normally the preferred method of nutritional support, but enteral nutrition may be considered if this is not sufficient.

Cancer of the pancreas

Mary Phillips

Pancreatic cancer is the tenth-most common cancer in the UK, but the fifth-most common cause of cancer-related death. The prognosis is very poor, with more than 80% of pancreatic tumours unresectable at diagnosis, and a 5-year survival of 3% (Cancer Research UK (CRUK), 2014). It is often diagnosed late, and many patients only receive palliative therapy. Pancreatic cancer causes a range of symptoms that impact on nutritional status, including pain, nausea, anorexia, jaundice, new-onset diabetes, early satiety and pancreatic exocrine insufficiency (PEI) (Davidson *et al.*, 2004). Both endocrine and exocrine functions of the pancreas may be affected. Most patients with pancreatic cancer experience worsening PEI over time, which requires aggressive treatment and frequent monitoring. PERT may be required.

Curative resection

Curative resection, when possible, consists of resection of the site of disease and surrounding tissue. Tumour infiltration of the surrounding blood vessels or metastatic disease renders pancreatic cancer inoperable. This surgery carries a considerable morbidity, and patients need to be fit. The tumour itself may sometimes be operable, but, due to comorbidities or general frailty, the patient may not be fit enough for surgery. Curative surgery is detailed in Chapter 7.4.5 (Disorders of the pancreas).

Neoadjuvant treatment

Some patients present with borderline operable cancer, and may be offered chemotherapy as first-line treatment. These patients require intensive nutritional support, as they may undergo major surgery following their chemotherapy.

Palliative treatment

The aim of management in palliative care is to improve quality of life. Symptom control is predominantly pain control, but also includes treating malabsorption, which is frequently mistaken for chemotherapy-related diarrhoea (see Chapter 7.16, Palliative and end-of-life care).

Jaundice

Patients often present with painless jaundice, indicative of obstruction of the biliary tree, and disease in the head of the pancreas or distal common bile duct (cholangiocarcinoma). PEI is likely, as the pancreatic duct is usually obstructed, and the patients usually require intensive nutritional support.

Duodenal stents

Following duodenal stenting, patients should be encouraged to commence oral fluids, slowly working up to puree/soft diets. Foods that are likely to block the stent (bread, seeds, pips and skins) should be avoided. Some patients may tolerate normal foods after duodenal stenting; others may only tolerate liquids and very moist diets. Gastric outflow obstruction may take many weeks to resolve, even with a patent stent. In those with localised disease or who are potentially operable, NJ feeding tubes can be inserted through the duodenal stent, and can prevent nutritional deterioration and dehydration.

Palliative bypass procedures

Patients who are inoperable, or for whom stenting has failed, may undergo a gastric and biliary bypass. This palliative procedure is carried out to treat jaundice and allow tolerance of oral diet. This does not always provide a quick resolution of oral intake, and NJ or jejunostomy feeding tubes may be considered, especially in patients fit to undergo chemotherapy.

Type 3c diabetes

New-onset diabetes or progressive hyperglycaemia is common. Blood glucose levels should be monitored regularly, and hyperglycaemia treated to minimise the impact on quality of life and nutritional status.

Pancreatic enzyme replacement therapy

Most patients with pancreatic cancer experience worsening pancreatic exocrine insufficiency over time, requiring aggressive treatment and frequent monitoring: PERT may be required.

Oral nutritional support

Nutritional support should be sufficient to prevent unnecessary nutritional debilitation while not being over-invasive in patients with widespread disease. The use of PERT alongside nutrition support is advised. There is emerging evidence that more aggressive nutritional support in patients with locally advanced disease may result in significant nutritional and quality-of-life benefits, with current trials examining the benefits of jejunal and parenteral nutrition in patients undergoing chemotherapy (Pelzer *et al.*, 2010; Vashi *et al.*, 2014).

Fish oils

A Cochrane review concluded that there was insufficient evidence to support the use of supplement drinks containing eicosapentaenoic acid (EPA) (Dewey *et al.*, 2007), but the lack of PERT use in the earlier studies needs addressing in future research (see Chapter 7.15.9, Cancer cachexia).

Colorectal cancer

Lindsey Allan

Colorectal cancers include those that affect the colon, rectum (including the anus) and appendix. These are the fourth-most common cancers in the UK, after breast, prostate and lung cancer, with approximately 40,000 new diagnoses/year (ISD, 2016; NICR, 2016; ONS, 2016a; WCISU, 2016). Incidence has increased by 14% since the 1970s, and diagnosis is strongly related to age, with 58% of cases found in those over 70 years (CRUK, 2016). The introduction of the NHS Bowel Screening Programme in 2006 has led to earlier diagnosis, and is predicted to reduce mortality rates by 16% (NHS Bowel Screening Programme, 2011).

Aetiology

A number of risk factors have been implicated in the development and progression of colorectal cancer, including genetic predisposition, inflammatory bowel disease, smoking, excess alcohol, lack of physical activity, obesity and diet (WCRF/AICR, 2011). Most (95%) cases are adenocarcinomas that develop from adenomatous polyps; many of these can be detected prior to molecular changes that can result in malignancies (Manne *et al.*, 2010). Obesity has been associated with increased risk (Ben *et al.*, 2012), and there is conclusive evidence to show that increased levels of physical activity lower risk (Boyle *et al.*, 2012). A positive association has been established between the intake of red and processed meat and colorectal cancer (Xu *et al.*, 2013), and there is evidence to show that dietary fibre can have a protective effect (Murphy *et al.*, 2012), particularly wholegrain intake (Kyrø *et al.*, 2013). The effect of lifestyle factors has become more convincing over the past few years, and, in theory, some cancers could be theoretically avoidable if these factors are addressed (WCRF/AICR, 2007).

Diagnosis

Colorectal cancer usually presents with symptoms such as a persistent change in bowel habit (including unresolved diarrhoea for several weeks), rectal bleeding, abdominal pain, a lump in the abdomen, unexplained tiredness, anorexia and loss of weight. If the disease is detected at an early stage, it can be cured by surgery. One-year survival rates have significantly improved over the past 40 years from 39% to 77.6% in men and 40% to 75.8% in women (Coleman *et al.*, 1999; ONS, 2016b).

Management

The prognosis and treatment modality depend on the type and grade of tumour and its degree of spread. This is determined by the Dukes clinicopathological classification and the Royal College of Pathologists' TNM5 staging (see Chapter 7.15.1, General aspects of cancer). Surgical resection is the principal first-line treatment for the majority of patients. It is undertaken either as a curative treatment or as a palliative measure to improve quality of life in those with bowel obstruction. Carbohydrate loading as part of 'enhanced recovery programmes' is now common (see Chapter 7.17.5, Surgery). Surgery will involve end-to-end anastomoses or stoma formation (ileostomy or colostomy), depending on the degree of tumour infiltration. Papillon radiotherapy (low-energy contact X ray brachytherapy) is now being used to treat low rectal tumours in patients who are not fit to undergo surgery.

Chemotherapy and/or radiotherapy can be used neoadjuvantly to reduce the tumour burden prior to surgery, and chemotherapy is used adjuvantly postoperatively to prevent the risk of recurrence. In the case of advanced metastatic disease, palliative chemotherapy is routinely offered. New surgical techniques and treatment modalities, including targeted therapies (e.g. cetuximab and bevacizumab), are being developed, and it is now recognised that optimum outcomes for patients with colorectal cancer require specialised multidisciplinary care (NICE, 2014).

Dietary management

People with colorectal cancer may present in a nutritionally depleted state as a result of chronic symptoms, side effects from treatment, and the cancer process itself. In such patients, appropriate nutritional support should be instituted as soon as possible to help manage the effects of treatment. An appropriate nutritional screening tool and dietetic referral system should be in place to identify those who are malnourished at an early stage (Arends *et al.*, 2016).

Nutritional support should aim to prevent weight loss during treatment, as undernutrition and cachexia are indicators of poor prognosis (Lin *et al.*, 2016) and can increase the risk of treatment-related toxicity (Andreyev *et al.*, 1998). The side effects experienced by colorectal cancer patients undergoing chemotherapy can include diarrhoea, constipation, nausea, taste changes and anorexia. In the first instance, it is essential to ensure that such symptoms are controlled with medication. Diet should then be manipulated accordingly to ensure that patients maximise their intake (see Chapter 7.15.1, General aspects of cancer). Dietary counselling during chemotherapy has been shown to improve nutritional status (Dobrila-Dintinjana *et al.*, 2012), and the use of oral nutritional supplements may be necessary if intake remains suboptimal and weight loss is ongoing. Supplements can result in increased energy intake and improved quality of life (Ravasco *et al.*, 2005).

Pelvic radiotherapy-related symptoms include diarrhoea, faecal incontinence, increased urgency and pain. Approximately 70% of patients experience acute small intestinal changes that can lead to gastrointestinal symptoms both during and after treatment (Andreyev *et al.*, 1998). Nutritional support is essential to prevent weight loss and manage these effects. Various approaches have been investigated, including elemental diets, probiotic supplementation, low-fat diets and reducing insoluble fibre in the form of raw vegetables, but more research is recommended (McGough *et al.*, 2004). A high-fibre diet has, however, been shown to reduce radiation-induced toxicity in pelvic radiotherapy patients as compared to a low-fibre diet (Wedlake *et al.*, 2017). Late onset of symptoms is not always initially linked to previous cancer treatment, and dietetic input may be required for several months after radiotherapy finishes. If a definitive cause cannot be established and symptoms persist, referral to a gastroenterologist for further investigation is advisable.

In case of tumour or peritoneal metastases causing a partial obstruction, the trial of a soft, low-fibre diet may be effective in reducing symptoms in the short term, but no research is available to support this approach. Patients undertaking such dietary restrictions should be advised, monitored and reviewed regularly by a dietitian. The aim is to maintain nutritional status while the obstruction is treated or palliated. This may involve the placement of a colonic stent, or the insertion of a stoma if the patient is well enough to undergo surgery.

Patients who are undergoing colorectal surgery do not routinely require artificial nutritional support postoperatively. Oral fluids and diet should be initiated at an early stage (see Chapter 7.17.5, Surgery). Nevertheless, as with all patients, nutritional status during the recovery period should be monitored, particularly if patients were malnourished preoperatively or experience postsurgical complications, or if resumption of oral food intake is slow. In such cases, appropriate nutritional support should be instigated – see Chapters 6.3 (Oral nutritional support), 6.4 (Enteral nutrition) and 6.5 (Parenteral nutrition). Symptom control, including adequate pain relief, is important as part of the overall management plan, because continuous pain, discomfort or nausea can markedly suppress appetite. Patients taking opiates to control pain are likely to develop constipation, so regular laxatives would be recommended. Specific dietary measures may be required during the initial phase of adjustment to the effects of intestinal resection and the possible creation or reversal of a stoma (see Chapter 7.4.9, Intestinal failure and intestinal resection).

In the palliative care setting, if nutrition is highlighted as an issue for either the patient or family and carers, this should be addressed as for advanced cancer of any site (see Chapter 7.16, Palliative and end-of-life care). Dietary advice for colorectal cancer survivors should be to increase dietary fibre, limit red and processed meat, maintain a healthy body weight and be regularly physical active (WCRF/AICR, 2011).

Acknowledgement

The book editor acknowledges the prior contribution of Linda Murray.

References

Andreyev HJN, Norman AR, Oates J, *et al.* (1998) Why do patients with weight loss have a worse outcome when undergoing chemotherapy for gastrointestinal malignancies? *Eur. J. Cancer* 34(4): 503–509.

Arends J, Bachmann P, Baracos V, *et al.* (2016) ESPEN guidelines on nutrition in cancer patients. *Clin. Nutr.* pii: S0261-5614(16)30181-9. doi: 10.1016/j.clnu.2016.07.015. [Epub ahead of print] Accessed on 16 November 2016.

Baker A, Wooten L-A, Malloy M. (2011) Nutritional considerations after gastrectomy and esophagectomy for malignancy. *Curr. Treat. Options Oncol.* 12(1): 85–95.

Ben Q, An W, Jiang Y, *et al.* (2012) Body mass index increases risk for colorectal adenomas based on meta-analysis. *Gastroenterology.* 142(4): 762–772.

Bosman FT, Carneiro F, Hruban RH, *et al.* (2010) *WHO Classification of Tumours of the Digestive System*, 4th edn, Vol. 3. Lyon: WHO/IARC.

Boyle T, Keegel T, Bull F, *et al.* (2012) Physical activity and risks of proximal and distal colon cancers: a systematic review and meta-analysis. *J. Natl. Cancer Inst.* 104(20): 1548–1561.

Bozzetti F. (2010) Nutritional support in patients with oesophageal cancer. *Support. Care Cancer* 18(2): 41–50.

Bozzetti F, on behalf of the SCRINIO Working Group. (2009) Screening the nutritional status in oncology: a preliminary report on 1,000 outpatients. *Support. Care Cancer.* 17(3): 279–284.

Cancer Registry. (2014) NI Cancer registry Available at http://www.qub.ac.uk/research-centres/nicr/CancerInformation/official-statistics/BySite/StomachGastric/. Accessed 2018.

Cancer Research UK (CRUK). (2014) *Pancreatic Cancer Key Stats.* Available at http://www.cancerresearchuk.org/health-professional/cancer-statistics/statistics-by-cancer-type/pancreatic-cancer. Accessed 29 December 2016.

Cancer Research UK (CRUK). (2016) *Bowel Cancer: 1979–2013.* Available at http://www.cancerresearchuk.org/health-professional/cancer-statistics/statistics-by-cancer-type/bowel-cancer/incidence#heading-Two. Accessed 16 November 2016.

Coleman MP, Babb P, Damiecki P, *et al.* (1999) *Cancer Survival Trends in England and Wales, 1971–1995: Deprivation and NHS Region. Series SMPS No. 61.* London: Stationery Office.

Davidson W, Ash S, Capra S, *et al.* (2004) Weight stabilisation is associated with improved survival duration and quality of life in unresectable pancreatic cancer. *Clin. Nutr.* 23: 239–247.

Dewey A, Baughan C, Dean T, *et al.* (2007) Eicosapentaenoic acid (EPA, an omega-3 fatty acid from fish oils) for the treatment of cancer cachexia. *Cochrane Database Syst. Rev.* (1): CD004597.

Dobrila-Dintinjana R, Trivanovic D, Zelic M, *et al.* (2012) Nutritional support in patients with colorectal cancer during chemotherapy: does it work? *Hepatogastroenterology.* 60(123): 475–480. [Epub ahead of print].

Fearon K, Strasser F, Anker SD, *et al.* (2011) Definition and classification of cancer cachexia: an international consensus. *Lancet Oncol.* 12(5): 489–495.

Findlay JM, Gillies RS, Millo J, *et al.* (2014) Enhanced recovery for esophagectomy: a systematic review and evidence-based guidelines. *Ann. Surg.* 259(3): 413–431.

Hebuterne X, Lemarie E, Michallet M, *et al.* (2014) Prevalence of malnutrition and current use of nutrition support in patients with cancer. *JPEN J. Parenter. Enteral. Nutr.* 38(2): 196–204.

Information Services Division (ISD). (2014) *Cancer Incidence in Scotland.* Available at http://www.isdscotland.org/Health-Topics/Cancer/Publications/2016-05-17/2016-05-17-Cancer-Incidence-Report.pdf. Accessed 16 October 2016.

Information Services Division (ISD). (2016) *Cancer Statistics: Colorectal Cancer.* Available at http://www.isdscotland.org/Health-Topics/Cancer/Cancer-Statistics/Colorectal/index.asp?Co=Y. Accessed 16 November 2016.

Kyrø C, Skeie G, Loft S, *et al.* (2013) Intake of whole grains from different cereal and food sources and incidence of colorectal cancer in the Scandinavian HELGA cohort. *Cancer Causes Control.* 24(7): 1363–1374.

Lin J, Peng J, Qdaisat A, *et al.* (2016) Severe weight loss during preoperative chemoradiotherapy compromises survival outcome for patients with locally advanced rectal cancer. *J. Cancer Res. Clin. Oncol.* 142(12): 2551–2560.

Mabvuure NT, Roman I, Khan OA. (2013) Enteral immunonutrition versus standard enteral nutrition for patients undergoing oesophagogastric resection for cancer. *Int. J. Surg.* 11(2): 122–127.

Manne U, Shanmugam C, Katkoori VR, *et al.* (2010) Development and progression of colorectal neoplasia. *Cancer Biomark.* 9(1–6): 235–265.

Martinez JC, Puc MM, Quiros RM. (2011) Esophageal stenting in the setting of malignancy. *Gastroenterol.* doi.org/10.5402/2011/719575.

McGough C, Baldwin C, Frost G, *et al.* (2004) Role of nutritional intervention in patients treated with radiotherapy for pelvic malignancy. *Br. J. Cancer.* 90(12): 2278–2287.

Melhado RE, Alderson D, Tucker O. (2010) The changing face of esophageal cancer. *Cancers (Basel).* 2: 1379–1404.

Murphy N, Norat T, Ferrari P, *et al.* (2012) Dietary fibre intake and risks of cancers of the colon and rectum in the European prospective investigation into cancer and nutrition (EPIC). *Public Libr. Sci.* 7(6): e39361.

NHS Bowel Screening Programme. (2011) *Press Release Issued on 8.12.2011.* Available at www.cancerscreening.nhs.uk/bowel/news/010.html. Accessed 21 December 2012.

NICE. (2006) *Nutrition support for adults: oral nutrition support, enteral tube feeding and parenteral nutrition. Clinical guideline (CG32).* Available at https://www.nice.org.uk/guidance/cg32. Accessed 25 May 2017.

NICE. (2014) *Colorectal Cancer: Diagnosis and Management.* London: NICE. Available at www.nice.org.uk. Accessed 16 November 2016.

Northern Ireland Cancer Registry (NICR). (2014) *Incidence, Prevalence and Survival Statistics: 1993–2014.* Available at http://www.qub.ac.uk/research-centres/nicr/CancerInformation/official-statistics/BySite/Oesophagus/. Accessed 15 November 2018.

Northern Ireland Cancer Registry (NICR). (2016) *Colorectal Cancer Incidence, Prevalence and Survival.* Available at http://www.qub.ac.uk/research-centres/nicr/CancerInformation/official-statistics/BySite/Colorectal/. Accessed 15 November 2018.

Office for National Statistics (ONS). (2014) *Statistical Bulletin: Cancer Registration Statistics, England.* Available at http://www.ons.gov.uk/peoplepopulationandcommunity/healthandsocialcare/conditionsanddiseases/bulletins/cancerregistrationstatisticsengland/2014. Accessed 9 October 2016.

Office for National Statistics (ONS). (2016a) *Cancer Registration Statistics England, 2014.* Available at http://www.ons.gov.uk/peoplepopulationandcommunity/healthandsocialcare/conditionsanddiseases/bulletins/cancerregistrationstatisticsengland/2014#the-most-common-cancers-registered-were-breast-prostate-lung-and-colorectal-cancers. Accessed 16 November 2016.

Office for National Statistics (ONS). (2016b) *Cancer survival in England: Patients diagnosed between 2010–2014 and followed up to 2015. Released 16 September 2016.* Available at https://www.ons.gov.uk/peoplepopulationandcommunity/healthandsocialcare/conditionsanddiseases/bulletins/cancersurvivalinenglandadultsdiagnosed/2010and2014andfollowedupto2015#1-year-survival. Accessed 16 November 2016.

Pelzer U, Arnold D, Govercin M, *et al.* (2010) Parenteral nutrition support for patients with pancreatic cancer. Results of a phase II study. *BMC Cancer.* 10: 86.

Ravasco P, Monteiro-Grillo I, Vidal PM, *et al.* (2005) Dietary counseling improves patient outcomes: a prospective, randomized, controlled trial in colorectal cancer patients undergoing radiotherapy. *J. Clin. Oncol.* 23(7): 1431–1438.

Silvers MA, Savva J, Huggins CE, *et al.* (2014) Potential benefits of early nutritional intervention in adults with upper gastrointestinal cancer: a pilot randomised trial. *Support. Care Cancer.* 22(11): 3035–3044.

Smyth EC, Verheij M, Allum W, *et al.*; ESMO Guidelines Committee. (2016) Gastric cancer: ESMO clinical practice guidelines. *Ann. Oncol.* 27(5): 38–49.

Vashi PG, Dahlk S, Popiel B, *et al.* (2014) A longitudinal study investigating quality of life and nutritional outcomes in advanced cancer patients receiving home parenteral nutrition. *BMC Cancer.* 14: 593.

Wedlake L, Shaw C, McNair H, *et al.* (2017) Randomized controlled trial of dietary fiber for the prevention of radiation-induced gastrointestinal toxicity during pelvic radiotherapy. *Am. J. Clin. Nutr.* 106: 849–857.

Welsh Cancer Intelligence and Surveillance Unit (WCISU). (2016) *Cancer in Wales 2014. Welsh Cancer Intelligence and Surveillance Unit.* Available at http://www.wcisu.wales.nhs.uk/sitesplus/documents/1111/WCISU%20Statistical%20report%20%28bilinguall%29%20rotated.pdf. Accessed 16 November 2016.

World Cancer Research Fund /American Institute for Cancer Research (WCRF/AICR). (2007) *Food, Nutrition, Physical Activity, and the Prevention of Cancer: A Global Perspective.* Washington DC: AICR. Available at www.wcrf.org. Accessed 16 November 2016.

World Cancer Research Fund/American Institute for Cancer Research (WCRF/AICR). (2011) *Continuous Update Project Report Summary. Food, Nutrition, Physical Activity, and the Prevention of Colorectal Cancer.* Available at www.wcrf.org. Accessed 16 November 2016.

World Cancer Research Fund International /American Institute for Cancer Research (WCRF/AICR). (2016a) *Diet, Nutrition, Physical Activity and Stomach Cancer.* Available at: wcrf.org/stomach-cancer-2016. Accessed 16 October 2016.

World Cancer Research Fund International/American Institute for Cancer Research (WCRF/AICR). (2016b) *Diet, Nutrition, Physical Activity and Oesophageal Cancer.* Available at wcrf.org/oesophageal-cancer-2016. Accessed 9 October 2016.

Xu X, Yu E, Gao X, *et al.* (2013) Red and processed meat intake and risk of colorectal adenomas: a meta-analysis of observational studies. *Int. J. Cancer.* 132(2): 437–448.

Zong L, Chen P, Chen Y, *et al.* (2011) Pouch Roux-en-Y vs no pouch Roux-en-Y following total gastrectomy: a meta-analysis based on 12 studies. *J. Biomed. Res.* 25(2): 90–99.

7.15.4 Breast cancer

Michelle Harvie

Key points

- Breast cancer is the most common malignancy among women.
- Increasing rates of breast cancer are linked to trends in overweight and obesity, sedentary lifestyle and increased alcohol intakes.
- Weight control and exercise are recommended to improve survival after a diagnosis of breast cancer.

Breast cancer accounts for one-third of cancer cases in women in the UK. In 2014, 54,800 women and 390 men were diagnosed, and 11,400 died from the disease. Earlier detection and improved adjuvant treatment has reduced breast cancer mortality by 40% in the past 20 years. The most recent, and undoubtedly conservative, estimates indicate that there are approximately 550,000 women living with a history of breast cancer in the UK. This equates to almost 2% of the female population, and nearly 10% of the female population aged 65 years and older. The long-term health and well-being of breast cancer patients is therefore an increasingly important consideration for researchers and healthcare professionals (Cancer Research UK (CRUK), 2016).

Risk factors and prevention

Estimated lifetime risk of breast cancer in the UK is 1 in 8 for women and 1 in 870 for men. Female UK breast cancer rates have almost doubled between 1979 and 2013 (98–170 per 100,000), with similar increases globally, particularly within Asian and developing countries that traditionally had low rates (Torre *et al.*, 2015). These increases have been linked to adverse trends in several lifestyle-related, hormonal and reproductive risk factors.

Hormonal and reproductive risk factors

The majority of breast cancers in the UK (81%) occur in postmenopausal women. Both earlier age of menarche (20% risk reduction for 5-year delay) and later age of menopause (3% for each year older at menopause) increase risk. The average age of menarche in developed countries has fallen – from 16–17 years in the mid-nineteenth century to 12–13 years today. Risk of breast cancer reduces by 7% with each full-term pregnancy, and by 4% for every 12 months of breastfeeding. Women currently taking hormone replacement therapy (HRT), particularly combined oestrogen–progestogen therapy, have a twofold increased risk as compared to non-users. Once HRT use ceases, risk returns to that of a never-user within 5 years (Prevent Breast Cancer, 2016).

Lifestyle risk factors

Observational data consistently link overweight and obesity, adult weight gain, sedentary lifestyle and alcohol intake to increased risk among women; excess weight is linked to post-menopausal, but not pre-menopausal, breast cancer. A weight gain of 20 kg during adulthood doubles the risk of postmenopausal breast cancer (Vrieling *et al.*, 2010). Alcohol and sedentary behaviour increase the risk of both pre- and post-menopausal breast cancer. An additional 10 g (1 unit)/day alcohol increases risk by 2–12% (Scoccianti *et al.*, 2014), while each additional 3 hours of moderate exercise (65–80% maximum heart rate) per week can reduce risk by 3% (Wu *et al.*, 2013). Observational studies and recent bariatric data suggest cancer risk reduction with weight loss and energy restriction, even with modest weight loss (5–10%) (Eliassen *et al.*, 2006; Harvie *et al.*, 2005a; Tee *et al.*, 2013). Energy restriction appears to be more important for prevention of breast cancer as compared to modification of dietary composition (Brennan *et al.*, 2010). Obesity is the only identified lifestyle risk factor among men, where a body mass index (BMI) of >30 kg/m^2 doubles risk (Johansen Taber *et al.*, 2010).

The proportion of breast cancer cases estimated to be preventable with weight control, exercise and limiting alcohol is contentious, but has recently been suggested to be 18–38% (Parkin *et al.*, 2011; WCRF, 2010).

Genetic factors

Of all breast cancer cases, 15% occur in women with a family history of the disease, and 2% in women with mutations in the breast cancer susceptibility genes *BRCA1* and *BRCA2*. These mutation carriers have a 45–65% chance of developing breast cancer. As with the general population, excess weight, lack of exercise, and alcohol consumption increase the risk of developing breast cancer among women with a family history. Specific evidence of links between lifestyle factors and breast cancer among known *BRCA* mutation carriers is equivocal (Harvie *et al.*, 2015).

Treatment

In countries with breast screening, approximately 76% of cancers are localised to the breast at the time of diagnosis (stages 1 and 2), 8% have local lymph involvement (stage 3) and 5% are metastatic (stage 4); stage was not reported for 11% (CRUK, 2014). Patients with stage 1–3 breast cancer generally have some form of breast and axillary lymph node surgery, followed by 15 or 19 daily sessions of radiotherapy for women who have had conservation surgery, and for some women who have had a mastectomy. Three-quarters of breast cancers in the UK are oestrogen receptor positive (ER+), and these patients receive adjuvant endocrine therapy. Standard treatment is a 10-year course of adjuvant endocrine therapy, with the selective oestrogen receptor modulator (SERM) tamoxifen for premenopausal women, or an aromatase inhibitor (anastrozole, exemestane or letrozole) for post-menopausal women (Burstein *et al.*, 2014).

Approximately 25% of breast cancer patients receive adjuvant chemotherapy (after breast surgery), and 3% receive neoadjuvant chemotherapy (before breast surgery). The 20% of patients with cancers that express the human epidermal growth factor receptor 2 (HER2) receive a targeted monoclonal antibody therapy (e.g. trastuzumab or lapatinib). Women diagnosed with advanced metastatic disease can receive endocrine therapy, chemotherapy, radiotherapy or targeted monoclonal antibody therapy.

Most men diagnosed with breast cancer undergo mastectomy with axillary lymph node clearance or sentinel node biopsy, where fewer than five lymph nodes are generally removed. Indications for radiotherapy are similar to those for female breast cancer. The majority of male breast tumours are ER+ and are treated with either tamoxifen or aromatase inhibitors, while one-third receive chemotherapy. Men with metastatic disease typically receive endocrine treatment.

Body weight

An estimated 50–65% of breast cancer patients are overweight or obese at diagnosis, while 30–50% gain significant amounts (>5%) in the first year after diagnosis, including those with a previous healthy weight (Renehan *et al.*, 2016). Gains in fat mass are usually accompanied by a loss of fat-free mass (sarcopenic obesity) (Makari-Judson *et al.*, 2014). Gains in body fat are greater during adjuvant chemotherapy as compared to endocrine therapy (2–3 kg versus 1.5 to 2–3 kg, respectively, in the first year after diagnosis) (Chaudhary *et al.*, 2014; Sestak *et al.*, 2012). Gains occur during and after chemotherapy due to increased energy intake and decreased energy expenditure linked to treatment (chemotherapy and steroids), hormonal (chemotherapy-induced menopause), psychosocial, and anxiety-related factors (Makari-Judson *et al.*, 2014). There is a 30% increase in the risk of recurrence or death in obese as compared to normal-weight early breast cancer patients (Chan *et al.*, 2014), and increased overall mortality among those with large weight gains after diagnosis (Playdon *et al.*, 2015). It is not clear whether weight loss or prevention of weight gain after diagnosis can reverse these poorer outcomes. Obese patients may have a worse outcome as they have worse prognosis tumours, receive suboptimal treatment or have decreased compliance to therapies. Several ongoing randomised trials are studying whether weight loss (NIHR, 2016) or the insulin-sensitising drug metformin have potential benefits in early-stage breast cancer (Goodwin, 2008).

Unlike other cancer patients, women with advanced breast cancer do not generally develop weight loss and cachexia. These metastatic patients often maintain good energy intakes, which lead to body fat gains but do not prevent declines in lean body mass (Harvie *et al.*, 2005b); heavier women have a worse prognosis. Research is being conducted to see if an energy-restricted diet can delay disease progression among patients with metastatic breast cancer (ISRCTN, 2018).

Evidence-based diet and exercise recommendations after diagnosis

As for prevention, factors such as weight control, energy restriction and exercise have been associated with outcome after diagnosis rather than specific dietary constituents. A 23% reduction in breast cancer relapse has been reported in women losing modest amounts of weight as compared to a control group who gained weight (3% difference between the groups) (Chlebowski *et al.*, 2006). The weight-losing women consumed a low-fat diet (30 g of fat/day; 20% of energy as fat) as compared to control women consuming, on average, 50 g of fat/day (30% of energy as fat). The lack of effect on outcome of a comparable low-fat intervention in another study, in which women did not lose weight (Pierce *et al.*, 2007), suggests that energy restriction and weight loss could be more important than dietary fat restriction. Moderate-fat diets (30–35% energy from fat) are likely to be better than low-fat eating plans (20% energy from fat) for breast cancer patients, as they have proven to be better, in other settings, for limiting energy intake and weight, improving insulin sensitivity and reducing risk of cardiovascular disease (Shai *et al.*, 2008).

There is much interest in the potential anticancer effects of fruit and vegetables, specifically carotenoids and brassicas. However, existing data does not suggest a protective effect (Pierce *et al.*, 2007). Alcohol is consistently linked to risk of developing breast cancer, but not to survival (WCRF, 2014). Physical activity alone does not control weight among breast cancer survivors (Markes *et al.*, 2006). However, physical activity is a vital part of energy-restricted weight control programmes. Exercise has been associated with greater disease-free survival, quality of life, cardiovascular fitness and bone density among breast cancer patients (Battaglini *et al.*, 2014).

Popular dietary practices

Soya and phytoestrogens

Many breast cancer patients increase their intake of soya foods or phytoestrogen supplements, i.e. black cohosh, agnus castus and red clover, in the belief that this will either reduce their risk of breast cancer recurrence or reduce hot flushes. There have been concerns that soya may limit the efficacy of antioestrogen therapies such as tamoxifen (van Duursen *et al.*, 2011). Asian population studies report 10–15 g of soya protein/day to be safe as part of a healthy lifestyle among patients taking tamoxifen (250 mL of soya milk = 7.5 g of soya protein) (Guha *et al.*, 2009; Shu *et al.*, 2009) and aromatase inhibitors (Kang *et al.*, 2010). These studies do not, however, conclusively suggest that soya has benefits for breast cancer patients.

Dairy-free diets

Many breast cancer patients avoid or limit dairy foods after diagnosis. However, this populist approach is not supported by evidence. A recent meta-analyses including 1,566,940 participants and 37,925 breast cancer cases found 10–27% fewer breast cancers among high (>3 servings/day) versus low dairy consumers (<2 serving/day) (Zang *et al.*, 2015). Likewise, a prudent diet that includes low-fat dairy foods has been linked to reduced recurrence and all-cause mortality among breast cancer patients (Kroenke *et al.*, 2005; Kwan *et al.*, 2009).

High-dose vitamin supplements

An estimated 10% of breast cancer patients self-prescribe high-dose antioxidant supplements (beta-carotene, vitamins C and E, and selenium) in the hope that it will provide anti-cancer effects and reduce therapy toxicity. There are concerns that antioxidants may protect tumour cells from the targeted oxidative damage during radiotherapy and certain chemotherapy regimens (i.e. alkylating agents, platinum compounds or anthracycline), and potentially reduce their effectiveness. However, the only report of harm is the reduced efficacy of radiotherapy for smokers with head and lung cancer receiving antioxidant supplements (Harvie, 2014; Yasueda *et al.*, 2016).

Late treatment effects

Lymphoedema (arm swelling) is an undesirable complication following axillary clearance or radiotherapy to the axilla, which can have negative physical and psychological effects. Obesity is a risk factor for the development of lymphoedema, and a small randomised trial suggested that weight loss may reduce arm swelling, and increase overall well-being and quality of life (Shaw *et al.*, 2007).

Bone health

Bone density is an important consideration among patients with chemotherapy-induced menopause or for those prescribed aromatase inhibitors. Lifestyle recommendations to limit reduction in bone density include increasing weight-bearing exercise, reducing alcohol intake, smoking cessation and supplementation with vitamin D (100–1200 IU/day). Calcium supplementation is only advised if dietary intake is <1 g/day (Hadji *et al.*, 2016).

Associated conditions and diseases

Both postmenopausal and premenopausal breast cancer patients have obesity-related comorbidities at the time of diagnosis such as diabetes (10%), heart disease (16%) and hypertension (40%) (Vigen *et al.*, 2016). Recent reports suggest increased rates of diabetes (Lipscombe *et al.*, 2013) and CVD (cardiomyopathy/heart failure, not CHD or stroke) (Armenian *et al.*, 2016) linked to adjuvant treatments. Comorbidities are a major cause of morbidity and mortality among women diagnosed with localised breast cancer. Recent mortality statistics (1973–2012) reported that 30% of mortality was linked to breast cancer, 60% to non-cancer causes, 17% specifically to heart disease and 13% to other primary cancers (Zaorsky *et al.*, 2016). The prevalence of comorbidities and their adverse effect on survival highlights the importance of managing comorbid conditions alongside breast cancer treatments (Barone *et al.*, 2008).

Further reading

WCRF. (2014) *Systematic review on diet, nutrition, physical activity and survival and second cancers in breast cancer survivors*. Available at http://www.wcrf.org/sites/default/files/Breast-Cancer-Survivors-SLR-2014-Report.pdf.

Internet resources

Breast Cancer Care, www.breastcancercare.org.uk
Cancer Research UK, www.cancerresearch.uk.org
Macmillan Cancer Support, https://www.macmillan.org.uk
Memorial Sloan-Kettering Cancer, www.mskcc.org
NICE, www.nice.org.uk
Advanced breast cancer: diagnosis and treatment (CG81)
Breast cancer (early and locally advanced): diagnosis and treatment (CG80)
Familial breast cancer: the classification and care of women at risk of familial breast cancer in primary, secondary and tertiary care (CG164)
Prevent Breast Cancer, https://preventbreastcancer.org.uk
US National Library of Medicine Medline Plus Herbs and Supplements, https://medlineplus.gov/druginfo/herb_All.html

References

Armenian SH, Xu L, Ky B, *et al.* (2016) Cardiovascular disease among survivors of adult-onset cancer: a community-based retrospective cohort study. *J. Clin. Oncol.* 34(10): 1122–1130.
Barone BB, Yeh HC, Snyder CF, *et al.* (2008) Long-term all-cause mortality in cancer patients with pre-existing diabetes mellitus: a systematic review and meta-analysis. *JAMA*. 300(23): 2754–2764.
Battaglini CL, Mills RC, Phillips BL, *et al.* (2014) Twenty-five years of research on the effects of exercise training in breast cancer survivors: a systematic review of the literature. *World J. Clin. Oncol.* 5(2): 177–190.
Brennan SF, Cantwell MM, Cardwell CR, *et al.* (2010) Dietary patterns and breast cancer risk: a systematic review and meta-analysis. *Am. J. Clin. Nutr.* 91(5): 1294–1302.
Burstein HJ, Temin S, Anderson H, *et al.* (2014) Adjuvant endocrine therapy for women with hormone receptor-positive breast cancer: American society of clinical oncology clinical practice guideline focused update. *J. Clin. Oncol.* 32(21): 2255–2269.
Cancer Research UK (CRUK). (2014) *Breast Cancer Rates by Stage at Diagnosis*. https://www.cancerresearchuk.org/health-professional/cancer-statistics/statistics-by-cancer-type/breast-cancer/incidence-invasive#heading-Three. Accessed 19 December 2016.
Cancer Research UK (CRUK). (2016) *Breast Cancer – UK Incidence Statistics*. Available at www.cancerresearch.org.uk. Accessed 19 December 2016.
Chan DS, Vieira AR, Aune D, *et al.* (2014) Body mass index and survival in women with breast cancer – systematic literature review and meta-analysis of 82 follow-up studies. *Ann. Oncol.* 25(10): 1901–1914.
Chaudhary LN, Wen S, Xiao J, *et al.* (2014) Weight change associated with third-generation adjuvant chemotherapy in breast cancer patients. *J. Community Support Oncol.* 12(10): 355–360.
Chlebowski RT, Blackburn GL, Thomson CA, *et al.* (2006) Dietary fat reduction and breast cancer outcome: interim efficacy results from the Women's Intervention Nutrition Study. *J. Natl. Cancer Inst.* 98(24): 1767–1776.
Eliassen AH, Colditz GA, Rosner B, *et al.* (2006) Adult weight change and risk of postmenopausal breast cancer. *JAMA*. 296(2): 193–201.
Goodwin PJ. (2008) Insulin in the adjuvant breast cancer setting: a novel therapeutic target for lifestyle and pharmacologic interventions? *J. Clin. Oncol.* 26(6): 833–834.
Guha N, Kwan ML, Quesenberry CP Jr, *et al.* (2009) Soy isoflavones and risk of cancer recurrence in a cohort of breast cancer survivors: the Life After Cancer Epidemiology study. *Breast Cancer Res. Treat.* 118(2): 395–405.
Hadji P, Coleman RE, Wilson C, *et al.* (2016) Adjuvant bisphosphonates in early breast cancer: consensus guidance for clinical practice from a European Panel. *Ann. Oncol.* 27(3): 379–390.
Harvie M. (2014) Nutritional supplements and cancer: potential benefits and proven harms. *Am. Soc. Clin. Oncol. Educ. Book*. e478–e486.
Harvie M, Howell A, Vierkant RA, *et al.* (2005a) Association of gain and loss of weight before and after menopause with risk of postmenopausal breast cancer in the Iowa women's health study. *Cancer Epidemiol. Biomarkers Prev.* 14(3): 656–661.
Harvie MN, Howell A, Thatcher N, *et al.* (2005b) Energy balance in patients with advanced NSCLC, metastatic melanoma and metastatic breast cancer receiving chemotherapy – a longitudinal study. *Br. J. Cancer* 92(4): 673–680.
Harvie M, Howell A, Evans DG. (2015) Can diet and lifestyle prevent breast cancer: what is the evidence? *Am. Soc. Clin. Oncol. Educ. Book*. 35: e66–e73. doi:00115000e66.
ISRCTN Registry. (2018) *Breast Activity and Healthy Eating After Diagnosis 3*. Available at https://www.isrctn.com/ISRCTN12841416?q=bahead 3 &filters=&sort=&offset=1&totalResults=1&page=1&pageSize=10&searchType=basic-search. Accessed 17 April 2018.
Johansen Taber KA, Morisy LR, Osbahr AJ, *et al.* (2010) Male breast cancer: risk factors, diagnosis, and management (review). *Oncol. Rep.* 24(5): 1115–1120.
Kang X, Zhang Q, Wang S, *et al.* (2010) Effect of soy isoflavones on breast cancer recurrence and death for patients receiving adjuvant endocrine therapy. *CMAJ*. 182(17): 1857–1862.
Kroenke CH, Fung TT, Hu FB, *et al.* (2005) Dietary patterns and survival after breast cancer diagnosis. *J. Clin. Oncol.* 23(36): 9295–9303.
Kwan ML, Weltzien E, Kushi LH, *et al.* (2009) Dietary patterns and breast cancer recurrence and survival among women with early-stage breast cancer. *J. Clin. Oncol.* 27(6): 919–926.
Lipscombe LL, Chan WW, Yun L, *et al.* (2013) Incidence of diabetes among postmenopausal breast cancer survivors. *Diabetologia*. 56(3): 476–483.
Makari-Judson G, Braun B, Jerry DJ, *et al.* (2014) Weight gain following breast cancer diagnosis: Implication and proposed mechanisms. *World J. Clin. Oncol.* 5(3): 272–282.
Markes M, Brockow T, Resch KL. (2006) Exercise for women receiving adjuvant therapy for breast cancer. *Cochrane Database Syst. Rev.* (4): CD005001.
NIHR. (2016) Breast Cancer WEight Loss Study (BWEL Study). *U.S. National Institutes of Health*. Available at https://clinicaltrials.gov/ct2/show/NCT02750826 Accessed 15 November 2018.
Parkin DM, Boyd L, Walker LC. (2011) 16. The fraction of cancer attributable to lifestyle and environmental factors in the UK in 2010. *Br. J. Cancer*. 105(2): S77–S81.
Pierce JP, Natarajan L, Caan B, *et al.* (2007) Influence of a diet very high in vegetables, fruit and fiber and low in fat on prognosis following treatment for breast cancer. *JAMA*. 298(3): 289–298.
Playdon MC, Bracken MB, Sanft TB, *et al.* (2015) Weight gain after breast cancer diagnosis and all-cause mortality: systematic review and meta-analysis. *J. Natl. Cancer. Inst.* 107(12): djv275.
Prevent Breast Cancer. (2016) *Causes of breast cancer (risk factors)*. Available at https://preventbreastcancer.org.uk/about-breast-cancer/causes-of-breast-cancer/. Accessed 15 November 2018.
Renehan AG, Harvie M, Cutress RI, *et al.* (2016) How to manage the obese patient with cancer. *J. Clin. Oncol.* 34(35): 4284–4294.
Scoccianti C, Lauby-Secretan B, Bello PY, *et al.* (2014) Female breast cancer and alcohol consumption: a review of the literature. *Am.*

J. Prev. Med. 46(3 Suppl 1): S16–S25. doi: S0749-3797(13)00646-6 [pii]; 10.1016/j.amepre.2013.10.031 [doi].

Sestak I, Harvie M, Howell A, *et al.* (2012) Weight change associated with anastrozole and tamoxifen treatment in postmenopausal women with or at high risk of developing breast cancer. *Breast Cancer Res. Treat.* 134(2): 727–734.

Shai I, Schwarzfuchs D, Henkin Y, *et al.* (2008) Weight loss with a low-carbohydrate, Mediterranean, or low-fat diet. *N. Engl. J. Med.* 359(3): 229–241.

Shaw C, Mortimer P, Judd PA. (2007) A randomized controlled trial of weight reduction as a treatment for breast cancer-related lymphedema. *Cancer.* 110(8): 1868–1874.

Shu XO, Zheng Y, Cai H, *et al.* (2009) Soy food intake and breast cancer survival. *JAMA.* 302(22): 2437–2443.

Tee MC, Cao Y, Warnock GL, *et al.* (2013) Effect of bariatric surgery on oncologic outcomes: a systematic review and meta-analysis. *Surg. Endosc.* 27(12): 4449–4456.

Torre LA, Bray F, Siegel RL, *et al.* (2015) Global cancer statistics, 2012. *CA Cancer J. Clin.* 65(2): 87–108.

van Duursen MB, Nijmeijer SM, de Morree ES, *et al.* (2011) Genistein induces breast cancer-associated aromatase and stimulates estrogen-dependent tumor cell growth in in vitro breast cancer model. *Toxicology.* 289(2–3): 67–73.

Vigen C, Kwan ML, John EM, *et al.* (2016) Validation of self-reported comorbidity status of breast cancer patients with medical records: the California Breast Cancer Survivorship Consortium (CBCSC). *Cancer Causes Control.* 27(3): 391–401.

Vrieling A, Buck K, Kaaks R, *et al.* (2010) Adult weight gain in relation to breast cancer risk by estrogen and progesterone receptor status: a meta-analysis. *Breast Cancer Res. Treat.* 123(3): 641–649.

WCRF. (2010) *WCRF.* Available at https://www.wcrf.org/sites/default/files/Breast-Cancer-2010-Report.pdf. Accessed 15 November 2018.

WCRF. (2016) *Systematic review on diet, nutrition, physical activity and survival and second cancers in breast cancer survivors.* Available at http://www.wcrf.org/sites/default/files/Breast-Cancer-Survivors-SLR-2014-Report.pdf. Accessed 15 November 2018.

Wu Y, Zhang D, Kang S. (2013) Physical activity and risk of breast cancer: a meta-analysis of prospective studies. *Breast Cancer Res. Treat.* 137(3): 869–882.

Yasueda A, Urushima H, Ito T. (2016) Efficacy and interaction of antioxidant supplements as adjuvant therapy in cancer treatment: a systematic review. *Integr. Cancer Ther.* 15(1): 17–39.

Zang J, Shen M, Du S, *et al.* (2015) The association between dairy intake and breast cancer in Western and Asian populations: A systematic review and meta-analysis. *J. Breast Cancer* 18(4): 313–322.

Zaorsky NG, Churilla TM, Egleston BL, *et al.* (2016) Causes of death among cancer patients. *Ann. Oncol.* 28: 400–407.

7.15.5 Lung cancer

Mhairi Donald

Key points

- People with lung cancer should always be managed as part of a multidisciplinary team.
- Patients experience a wide range of nutritional problems, and require full nutritional assessment at diagnosis and at regular intervals throughout the treatment pathway, to living with and beyond cancer or palliation.
- Dietary adaptations should be implemented to help minimise specific nutritional symptoms and support quality of life.

Lung cancer is the most common type of cancer worldwide. In the UK, it is the most frequent cause of cancer death and the second-most common cancer. Currently, it is more common in men than in women, although the incidence in men is falling as fewer are smoking, while the incidence in women is rising as the number of women smoking has increased. Lung cancer accounts for 13% of all new cancers in the UK (CRUK, 2014). Survival at 1 year has slowly increased in recent years to 38% (National Lung Cancer Audit, 2016), but falls to 10% at 5 years and to 5% at 10 years. Cigarette smoking causes approximately 90% of lung cancers. Other factors thought to contribute are poor diet (lack of fruit and vegetables in particular), and high-dose beta-carotene supplements in smokers have been shown to increase the risk. Industrial carcinogens, air pollutants and arsenic in drinking water, contaminated as result of natural deposits present in the earth or from agricultural and industrial practices, are also risk factors (WCRF, 2014).

Symptoms of lung cancer may include:

- Unexplained cough.
- Persistent or recurrent chest infection.
- Shortness of breath.
- Loss of appetite/weight loss.
- Chest pain.
- Fatigue (NICE, 2015).

There are two main types of primary lung cancer:

- Non–small-cell lung cancer (NSCLC), which accounts for 88% with a median age of 73 years at diagnosis
- Small-cell lung cancer (SCLC), which accounts for 11%, is more aggressive than NSCLC and can spread widely to other organs, including the brain. Median age of 70 years at diagnosis

The early stages of lung cancer do not usually produce symptoms, so the disease is generally at an advanced stage by the time it is diagnosed. It has one of the lowest survival outcomes of any cancer. The association with smoking means patients may also have coexisting, co-morbid problems such as chronic obstructive pulmonary disease (COPD).

Every patient with a diagnosis of lung cancer should have a management plan developed by a lung cancer multidisciplinary team (NICE, 2011). Treatment options are determined by the type and stage of cancer and medical fitness, but may include surgery, chemotherapy, radiotherapy, targeted biological therapies or a combination. There are many side effects associated with these treatments, and nutritional compromises are pronounced.

Nutritional screening

Most patients with lung cancer will have multiple disease-related symptoms, such as breathing difficulties, cough, pain, anorexia, fatigue and weight loss, that are likely to have an effect on nutritional status and overall quality of life. Weight loss is often the first sign of disease in patients with lung cancer, and most patients will experience it as their disease progresses. To combat weight loss and malnutrition, best practice suggests that nutritional screening using a validated tool form part of the initial assessment at the time of diagnosis. In a small study of lung cancer patients at the start of treatment (Khalid *et al.*, 2007), 66% of patients were already reporting symptoms; loss of appetite was the most common, followed by nausea and early satiety. Unintentional weight loss was identified in 28%, with patients who experienced weight loss of 5% or more having significantly more symptoms than patients with no weight loss.

Data on the incidence of weight loss and malnutrition in patients with lung cancer is limited, but there are reported rates of 59% in SCLC and 58% in NSCLC. Weight loss before and during chemotherapy was associated with an increased risk of dose-limiting toxicity, poorer symptom response and survival (Ross *et al.*, 2004). To adequately support a patient's nutritional status, it is important to identify the nutrition impact symptoms and set up individual nutritional management plans.

Treatment options and nutritional implications

Surgery

The type of operation required for lung cancer will depend on the size and position of the tumour. Procedures include a lobectomy (removal of a lobe of the lung), a pneumonectomy (removal of the whole lung) and segmentectomy (removal of a small, wedge-shaped section of cancerous lung and a margin of healthy tissue around the cancer). The outcome of surgery is closely related to the extent of the operation and preoperative lung function. The role of nutrition in predicting the outcome of lung cancer surgery has not been studied extensively. However, one study found that impaired nutritional status was an important predictor of death and the need for postoperative ventilation. Impaired nutritional status was more common in patients with lower body mass index (BMI) and lower fat-free mass (Jagoe *et al.*, 2001). Preoperative nutrition is thought to be beneficial in decreasing complications and chest drain removal time in patients with NSCLC (Kaya *et al.*, 2016), and in improving post-operative recovery (Yuncu & Ozturk, 2014). Emerging evidence suggests that a preoperative pulmonary programme should include nutritional support, and that physical activity may have a beneficial effect on post-operative recovery and morbidity for selected patients (Harada *et al.*, 2013; Misumi *et al.*, 2012; Nakao *et al.*, 2015). A number of thoracic surgery centres have adopted the enhanced recovery programme and have developed guidelines to best support patients undergoing lung resection (White *et al.*, 2013). Any surgical intervention is likely to affect nutritional intake; it may result in reduced appetite, early satiety and fatigue, which in combination contribute to an inadequate nutrient intake. Patients having surgery require ongoing monitoring and nutritional support (see Chapter 6.3, Oral nutritional support).

Radiotherapy

Radiotherapy for lung cancer targets the mediastinal area, which includes the pharynx and the oesophagus, both of which are lined by highly radiosensitive epithelial cells that will be damaged by the treatment. This can lead to a range of radiation-related side effects, including oesophagitis and resulting in dysphagia, epigastric pain, heartburn and taste changes (Cranganu & Camporeale, 2009). At least 30% of lung cancer patients experience weight loss during radiotherapy (Kiss *et al.*, 2014). It is important to relieve the pain and discomfort caused by oesophagitis, to maintain adequate nutrition and hydration. For pain control, adequate analgesics, topical medications (such as sucralfate) and antacids may all need to be considered. Avoiding acidic or spicy ingredients and changing the texture of the diet to soft, semi-solid or nutritious liquids, including oral nutritional supplements, may be recommended. A change in food temperature such as keeping foods cool or at body temperature can also help.

There is paucity of research on the efficacy of dietary support in lung cancer patients receiving radiotherapy; however, in a small pilot study, early and intensive dietary counselling resulted in increased weight, increased fat-free mass, and better physical and functional well-being as compared to those receiving usual care. Patients also reported better satisfaction with nutritional care, suggesting that larger studies are feasible and should be undertaken (Kiss *et al.*, 2016).

Prophylactic cranial radiotherapy may be given to SCLC patients who have limited-stage disease that has not progressed on first-line treatment (NICE, 2011). It is given to the brain to reduce the risk of the lung cancer spreading there. Side effects can include tiredness, headaches, nausea and vomiting.

Chemotherapy

When the tumour is not considered to be resectable, and in advanced SCLC, chemotherapy is considered the mainstay of treatment. Chemotherapy regimens are generally platinum based, with the most common nutrition-related side effects being nausea and vomiting, early satiety, taste changes and dry mouth. A higher risk of developing chemotherapy-related complications and a reduction in treatment response has been associated with patients who are malnourished and have hypoalbuminaemia (Arrieta *et al.*, 2010). Kimura *et al.* (2014) also demonstrated that the presence of cancer cachexia and decreased skeletal muscle mass are associated with poor prognosis in advanced lung NSCLC patients receiving chemotherapy. This highlights the need to identify cachexia management strategies as early as possible.

Targeted biological therapies

Targeted biological therapies are treatments that change the way in which cells signal each other; new blood vessels are manufactured by controlling the growth, by switching off growth, or by stopping the cancer. These are often taken orally and regarded as having less severe side effects. Side effects can include fatigue, diarrhoea, sore mouth, lack of appetite, and skin rashes, which may affect oral intake and nutritional status.

Associated conditions affecting nutrition

Fatigue

Fatigue, pain and dyspnoea (difficult or laboured respiration) have been identified as common symptoms associated with particular distress in lung cancer sufferers. Okuyama *et al.* (2001) found that 59% of patients with advanced lung cancer had experienced clinical fatigue (defined as fatigue that interferes with any daily activities). Clinical fatigue is not generally relieved with rest.

Several factors may contribute to fatigue, including the disease itself. In inoperable NSCLC patients, the presence of a systemic inflammation (identified by elevated C-reactive protein) was associated with increased weight loss, a reduction in performance status, increased fatigue and reduced survival; the greater the inflammatory response, the worse those parameters were affected (Scott *et al.*, 2002). Anaemia and problems in maintaining adequate oral intake may also contribute to fatigue. Supporting adequate oral intake needs to be carefully considered; food and drinks must be nutritious and require minimal preparation effort from the patient. A package of care via social services may be recommended, or support using community meals, ready or prepared meals, and Age UK or the British Red Cross to help with shopping and cooking. Menu planning with an understanding of the patient's social support, and including nutritious snacks, drinks and oral nutritional supplements, should help with physical symptoms and quality of life (see Chapter 6.3, Oral nutritional support). When using oral nutritional supplements, the volume must be considered. In a study of patients with COPD (which has symptoms similar to those of lung cancer), voluntary intake was limited by the volume, frequency and energy density of food portions, as these influenced symptoms such as early satiety and bloating. Weight gain was higher in patients who received 125 mL supplements as against 200 mL cartons, despite their lower total energy contribution (Broekhuizen *et al.*, 2005). Tailored physical activity and energy conservation techniques can also help, and a specialist physiotherapist can plan a programme. An occupational therapist can also advise on the management of fatigue, equipment and alterations at home.

Swallowing difficulties

A dry mouth, as a result of mouth breathing, using oxygen therapy or inhalers, may make chewing and swallowing more difficult. Swallowing difficulties can also be experienced when there is a central tumour or bulky central lymph nodes, where the cancer is squashing on the oesophagus. Recurrent laryngeal nerve palsy has been reported in 2–15% of lung cancer patients, and is more common in left-sided tumours. It is associated with poor expectoration, with coughing and an increased risk of aspiration (Beckles *et al.*, 2003). A modified-consistency diet, to soft, semi-solid or liquid textures, may be recommended to help manage it, or dysphagia may require enteral feeding through the nasogastric route.

Pleural effusion

Cancer cells can spread to the pleura, the membrane that covers the lungs and produces fluid, allowing them to move during breathing. This causes the fluid to build up and press on the lungs, making it difficult for the lungs to expand fully, causing breathlessness. A pleural effusion is usually drained using a chest tube. Persistent effusions may require a permanent indwelling drain to allow ongoing drainage at home. The development of pleural effusions generally signifies incurable disease, so it is important to support symptoms and quality of life. Breathlessness may make it more difficult to eat and swallow; some find it easier to choose foods which are soft and moist, requiring less effort, and eat three small meals and have snacks or nourishing drinks in between.

Supportive and palliative care

Lung cancer is often diagnosed at an advanced stage and can progress rapidly; one in five people with lung cancer will die within 1 month of being diagnosed, and 56% will die within 6 months of diagnosis (Macmillan Cancer Support, 2014). Palliative or best supportive care may need to be implemented from the outset. Patients with NSCLC assigned to early palliative care reported better quality of life and fewer depressive symptoms, and their median survival time post-diagnosis increased by 2.7 months (Temel *et al.*, 2010). The early identification and proactive management of symptoms clearly offered a benefit. Identifying nutrition impact symptoms and offering supportive management strategies are an important focus for dietitians to help support quality of life in this setting (see Chapter 7.16, Palliative and end-of-life care).

Internet resources

British Lung Foundation, www.lunguk.org
Lung Cancer Nutrition, lungcancernutrition.com
National Lung Cancer Forum for Nurses, www.nlcfn.org.uk
The Roy Castle Lung Cancer Foundation, www.roycastle.org

References

Arrieta O, Ortega RMM, Villanueva-Rodriguez G, *et al.* (2010) Association of nutritional status and serum albumin levels with development of toxicity in patients with advanced non-small cell lung cancer treated with paclitaxel-cisplatin chemotherapy: a prospective study. *BMC Cancer.* 10: 50. doi: 10.1186/1471-2407-10-50.

Beckles MA, Spiro SG, Colice GL, Rudd RM. (2003) Initial evaluation of the patient with lung cancer: symptoms, signs, laboratory tests and paraneoplastic syndromes. *Chest* 123(1 Suppl): 97S–104S.

Broekhuizen B, Creutzberg EC, Weling-Scheepers CA, *et al.* (2005) Optimizing oral nutritional drink supplementation in patients with chronic obstructive pulmonary disease. *Br. J. Nutr.* 93: 965–971.

Cancer Research UK (CRUK). (2014) *Cancer Incidence of Lung*. Available at http://www.cancerresearchuk.org/health-professional/cancer-statistics/incidence. Accessed 10 January 2017.

Cranganu A, Camporeale J. (2009) Nutrition aspects of lung cancer. *Nutr. Clin. Pract.* 24(6): 688–700.

Harada H, Yamashita Y, Misumi K, *et al.* (2013) Multidisciplinary team-based approach for comprehensive preoperative pulmonary rehabilitation including intensive nutritional support for lung cancer patients. *PLoS One*. 8(3): e59566. doi: 10.1371/journal.pone.0059566.

Jagoe RT, Goodship TH, Gibson GJ. (2001) The influence of nutritional status on complications after operations for lung cancer. *Ann. Thorac. Surg.* 71(3): 936–943.

Kaya S, Akcam T, Ceylan K, *et al.* (2016) Is preoperative protein-rich nutrition effective on postoperative outcome in non-small cell lung cancer surgery? A prospective randomized study. *J. Cardiothorac. Surg.*11: 14.

Khalid U, Spiro A, Baldwin C, *et al.* (2007) Symptoms and weight loss in patients with gastrointestinal and lung cancer at presentation. *Support. Care Cancer.* 15(1): 39–46.

Kimura M, Naito T, Kenmotsu H, *et al.* (2014) Prognostic impact of cancer in patients with advanced non-small cell lung cancer. *Support. Cancer Care.* Epub 2014. doi: 10.1007/s00520-014-2534-3.

Kiss N, Isenring E, Gough K, *et al.* (2014) The prevalence of weight loss during (chemo)radiotherapy treatment for lung cancer and associated patient- and treatment-related factors. *Clin. Nutr.* 33(6): 1074–1080.

Kiss N, Isenring E, Gough K, *et al.* (2016) Early and intensive dietary counseling in lung cancer patients receiving (chemo) radiotherapy – a pilot randomized controlled trial. *Nutr. Cancer.* 68(6): 958–967.

Macmillan Cancer Support. (2014) *Cancers Unequal Burden. The Reality Behind Improving Cancer Survival Rates*. Available at http://www.macmillan.org.uk/documents/cancersunequalburden_2014.pdf. Accessed 2 June 2017.

Misumi K, Harada H, Yamashita Y, *et al.* (2012) Comprehensive preoperative pulmonary rehabilitation including intensive nutrition support for lung cancer patients. *Chest.* 142: 37A.

Nakao J, Harada H, Handa Y, *et al.* (2015) Clinical benefit of comprehensive preoperative pulmonary rehabilitation including intensive nutritional support for the elderly, low body weight, lung cancer patients. *Respirology.* 20: 64.

National Lung Cancer Audit. (2016) National Lung Cancer Audit Annual Report 2016, January 2017. London: Royal College of Physicians.

NICE (2011) *The diagnosis and treatment of lung cancer. Clinical Guideline 121.* Available at https://www.nice.org.uk/guidance/CG121. Accessed 2 June 2017.

NICE. (2015) *Suspected cancer; recognition and referral*. Available at https://www.nice.org.uk/guidance/NG12. Accessed 2 June 2017.

Okuyama T, Tanaka K, Akechi T, *et al.* (2001) Fatigue in ambulatory patients with advanced lung cancer: prevalence, correlated factors, and screening. *J. Pain Symptom Manage.* 22(1): 554–564.

Ross P, Ashley S, Norton A, *et al.* (2004) Do patients with weight loss have a worse outcome when undergoing chemotherapy for lung cancers? *Br. J. Cancer.* 90(10): 1095–1911.

Scott HR, McMillan DC, Forrest LM, *et al.* (2002) The systemic inflammatory response, weight loss, performance status and survival in patients with inoperable non-small cell lung cancer. *Br. J. Cancer.* 87(3): 264–267.

Temel JS, Greer JA, Muzikansky A, *et al.* (2010) Early palliative care for patients with metastatic non-small cell lung cancer. *N. Engl. J. Med.* 36: 733–742.

WCRF (2014) Lung cancer Available at https://www.wcrf.org/dietandcancer/lung-cancer. Accessed 15 November 2018.

White J, Dixon S, Beattie V. (2013) Guidelines to prepare and support patients undergoing a lung resection. *J. Thorac. Oncol.* 8: S158.

Yuncu G, Ozturk G. (2014) Perioperative enteral nutrition with arginine-omega 3 fatty acids and ribonucleic acid and glutamine supplemented diet could improve postoperative recovery in lung cancer patients. *Clin. Nutr.* 33: S60.

7.15.6 Gynaecological cancers

Mhairi Donald

Key points

- Gynaecological cancers are a diverse group of diseases with differing incidences, treatments and survivorship outcomes.
- Women with gynaecological cancer can experience many nutritional problems and require a full nutritional assessment at diagnosis.
- Ongoing monitoring and responsive dietary management by a dietitian is necessary throughout the treatment pathway, from diagnosis to living with and beyond cancer or palliation.

Gynaecological cancer refers to cancers originating in the female reproductive organs, including the ovaries, cervix, endometrium, vagina and vulva. Gynaecological cancers and their treatments usually have profound and often permanent effects including:

- Bowel, bladder and sexual dysfunction.
- Infertility/onset of early menopause and associated symptoms.
- Changes in body image.

Ovarian cancer

Menstruating women ovulate monthly, and it is thought that ovarian cancer may start when the cells on the surface of the ovary do not repair themselves after ovulation. Ovarian cancer is a leading cause of death in women, and it accounts for 2% of all new cancers in the UK (CRUK, 2013). The incidence rates are higher in postmenopausal women, with the highest rate in the 60–64-year age group. The 5-year survival rate is 46%, and 10-year survival is 35% (CRUK, 2010–2011). There is evidence of an association between overall body fatness (marked by BMI) and ovarian cancer (WCRF/AICR, 2014). Many women present with advanced disease because the symptoms are often attributed to other conditions, e.g. irritable bowel syndrome. Women (especially those aged ≥50 years) should undergo diagnostic tests if they report the following symptoms on a persistent or frequent basis (NICE, 2011):

- Persistent abdominal distension (referred to as bloating).
- Feeling full (early satiety) and or loss of appetite.
- Pelvic or abdominal pain.
- Increased urinary urgency and/or frequency.

Endometrial cancer

Endometrial cancer is an abnormal growth of cells in the lining of the uterus. It accounts for 5% of all new cases of cancer in females (CRUK, 2013), with a 5-year survival rate of 79% and 10-year survival rate of 78% (CRUK, 2010–2011). Risk factors for endometrial cancer include the following:

- Consumption of a high-glycaemic-load diet, overweight or obesity (CRF, 2013).
- Heightened exposure to oestrogen, associated with early menarche and/or late menopause.

Pregnancy lowers the risk of endometrial cancer, and more than one pregnancy will lower the risk further. Risk is also lowered by physical activity (WCRF/AICR, 2013).

Cervical cancer

Cervical cancer can occur in the cells or glands lining the cervix. It accounts for <1% of cancer cases in the UK, with a 5-year survival rate of 67% and a 10-year survival rate of 63% (CRUK, 2014). Risk factors for cervical cancer include:

- Infection with human papilloma virus (HPV), particularly types 16 and 18.
- Unprotected sexual intercourse before the age of 17 years with multiple partners.
- Smoking.
- A weakened immune system, e.g. HIV/AIDS.

Vaccines to protect against the strains of HPV most likely to cause cervical cancer are routinely offered to schoolgirls aged 12–13 years in the UK.

Vulval and vaginal cancers

These are rarer cancers, with a combined incidence rate of 1% of cancer cases in the UK (CRUK, 2014).

Nutrition

Malnutrition in cancer patients is associated with a variety of clinical consequences, including reduced quality of life, decreased response to treatment, increased risk of treatment-induced toxicity and a reduction in overall survival. However, rates of malnutrition are lower with gynaecological cancers than with other cancers. Laky *et al.* (2007) identified malnutrition in 20% of gynaecological cancer patients at diagnosis; the prevalence varied between specific cancer sites, with the highest rate (67%) in ovarian cancer and the lowest rate (6%) in endometrial cancer. In a recent study of hospitalised gynaecological cancer patients, 62% of women were classified using the patient-generated subjective global assessment tool, with moderate or severe malnutrition. The hospital stay was higher and the survival rate lower in the malnourished group, reinforcing the need to consider the nutritional status and care of patients with gynaecological cancer (Rodrigues *et al.*, 2015).

Treatment

The management of gynaecological cancers includes surgery, radiotherapy, brachytherapy, chemotherapy, hormone therapy or a combination of these. The nutritional needs of the patients are likely to vary through the course of treatment. It is important to nutritionally assess and manage the patient at all stages of the cancer journey (AHP Cancer Toolkit–NHS Network, 2012).

Surgery

Surgery is the definitive treatment for endometrial, cervical, ovarian and vulval cancers. The extent of the surgery depends on the stage, size and histology of the tumour, and fitness of the patient. Gynaecological cancer surgery can be a major procedure that may also involve the gastrointestinal or urinary tracts. Sometimes surgery will be done as a laparoscopic keyhole procedure. Surgery is undertaken as part of the enhanced recovery programme (ERP), the underlying principle of which is to minimise the stress responses in the body during surgery, enabling quicker recovery and hospital discharge. The ERP involves preoperative assessment and management to ensure that comorbidities such as anaemia, hypertension or diabetes are managed optimally. It also involves admission on the day of surgery, with minimal periods of preoperative starvation and carbohydrate loading. Postoperative management of women having major abdominal and ovarian surgery with associated bowel resection includes early feeding (fluids or food within 24 hours of surgery). This results in a shorter time to the presence of bowel sounds, allowing women to resume a solid diet without increased complications and shorter hospital stays (Billson *et al.*, 2013; Charoenkwan *et al.*, 2014).

Women with gynaecological cancer will sometimes require the formation of stomas (colostomy, ileostomy and/or urostomy) as a result of surgery for tumour removal, or debulking to deal with the progression or complications of treatment such as obstruction. If the underlying problem cannot be cured, a palliative stoma may be required to make the female patient more comfortable. Individual dietary advice should be offered to patients with stomas to support an adequate fluid intake and a return to a normal mixed diet.

Chemotherapy

Chemotherapy may be used alone, particularly in the management of ovarian cancer, or in combination with radiotherapy for cervical and endometrial cancer. The nutritional symptoms associated with this therapy are oral mucositis, nausea, vomiting, loss of appetite, taste changes and early satiety. Several studies have examined nutritional status and weight changes as prognostic factors for ovarian cancer patients undergoing chemotherapy. Well-nourished patients survived 12.6 months longer than severely malnourished women (Gupta *et al.*, 2008); the risk of death increased by 7% for every 5% loss of body weight (Hess *et al.*, 2007). Improving nutritional status from the start of chemotherapy is also associated with better survival (Gupta *et al.*, 2010). Rutten *et al.* (2016) more recently showed, in a group of advanced ovarian cancer patients who were treated with neoadjuvant chemotherapy prior to debulking surgery, that female patients who maintained or gained skeletal muscle had a better prognosis than those who lost skeletal muscle. More research on the efficacy of nutritional interventions is required, but early implementation of strategies to minimise weight loss and ongoing individualised nutritional input appear to be beneficial.

Radiotherapy

Radiotherapy is predominantly used to treat cervical and endometrial cancer; it can be given externally or internally (brachytherapy), or as a combination of the two. It may be delivered alone or concurrently with chemotherapy, which can increase early toxicity and add to nutritional problems. The radiation treatment can encompass the entire pelvis, which means there may also be damage to the rapidly dividing cells lining the small and large bowel. It can cause side effects, including diarrhoea, irritable bladder, nausea and tiredness. Malnutrition occurs in approximately 33% of radiotherapy recipients, and up to 83% of patients lose weight during treatment (McGough *et al.*, 2004). A recent systematic review to establish the efficacy of low-fat or modified-fat diets, fibre, lactose restriction, and elemental diets showed that there is currently insufficient evidence to recommend nutritional intervention to counteract acute gastrointestinal toxicity during radiotherapy. Evidence for probiotics was more promising, but cannot be introduced into clinical practice without further studies on their safety, particularly in immunocompromised patients (Wedlake *et al.*, 2013). Wedlake *et al.*'s (2017) has subsequently shown that individualised dietetic advice to follow a high-fibre diet during radiotherapy was tolerated by patients and resulted in reduced gastrointestinal toxicity, at the end of radiotherapy and at 1 year post-radiotherapy, as compared to habitual fibre intake. It is important to identify patients at risk of weight loss or specific nutrition-related symptoms to implement individual nutrition support plans and to abandon restrictive non-evidence-based advice to reduce fibre intake.

Associated problems

Bowel obstruction

Bowel obstruction occurs most commonly as a complication of advanced or recurrent ovarian cancer; the bowel may be completely or partially blocked. Blockages can result from the tumour growing into the abdominal area, or mesentery of bowel muscle or nerves, and compromising bowel motility. The optimal management of bowel obstruction remains controversial. Much will depend on the individual clinical picture, nutritional and tumour status, the presence and/or quantity of ascites, and history of chemotherapy or radiotherapy. The goals of treatment for bowel obstruction are to control or relieve symptoms and to optimise quality of life. Treatment may include the following:

- Laparotomy with surgical bypass (Cousins *et al.*, 2016; Pothuri *et al.*, 2003).
- Pharmacological management with drugs such as steroids, prokinetics or the antisecretory agent octreotide with NG drainage (Feuer & Broadley, 2000; Kucukmetin *et al.*, 2010).
- A venting percutaneous endoscopic gastrostomy – offers gastric decompression and drainage, often with the resumption of a modified oral intake (Meyer & Pothuri, 2006).
- Total parenteral nutrition (TPN) – the risks, burdens and benefits of TPN must be discussed when considering its use. It seems to be of most benefit to women who have good performance status (Madhok *et al.*, 2011).
- Low -fibre diet – the efficacy is not well studied, but patients anecdotally report benefits. In theory, less fibre reduces the amount of faeces and wind produced, resulting in a reduction in symptoms such as bloating and stomach cramps (Chan & Power, 2016).

Ascites

The peritoneum is a fine membrane lining the abdomen. It is made up of two layers: one encloses organs such as the small bowel, and the other lines the muscle wall of the abdomen. Ascites is the build-up of excessive fluid in the abdominal cavity between these layers. It is commonly associated with ovarian cancer, as a result of malignant cells shedding into the abdominal cavity and impairing normal drainage. The fluid can also accumulate around the lungs, causing pleural effusion.

The symptoms associated with ascites can significantly reduce quality of life, and they include the following:

- Shortness of breath.
- Anorexia and early satiety
- Nausea, indigestion and heartburn.
- Discomfort and immobility.
- Altered bowel habit.

Percutaneous drainage can offer symptomatic relief and may allow chemotherapy to be instigated. Where ascites builds up rapidly and frequently, a permanent indwelling catheter may help. Women can develop hypoalbuminaemia because of ongoing drainage, and may benefit from support to optimise their intake. The aim of the nutritional management of ascites is to maximise oral intake and quality of life, while minimising any detrimental gastrointestinal effects. This largely involves encouraging frequent, small meals and snacks; fortifying foods with protein and energy; and using low-volume oral nutritional supplements.

Living with and beyond cancer

Although excess body weight does not appear to affect recurrence in endometrial cancer, 72% of endometrial survivors are overweight or obese (von Gruenigen *et al.*, 2008), and their mortality is affected by other comorbidities (e.g. hypertension, cardiac disease and diabetes). A healthy lifestyle after cancer is associated with improved physical and psychological well-being and improved survival. Positive lifestyle changes, including increased exercise and avoiding excess weight, should be encouraged.

Some women will develop late effects of pelvic radiotherapy namely, pelvic radiation disease, which can affect the bladder and/or bowel. In one study, 47% of women reported post-treatment symptoms, which they had tried to manage with dietary changes (Abayomi *et al.*, 2009). Women should be dissuaded from unnecessarily restricting nutritional intake, as this could result in unbalanced diets in the long term. Recent guidance has been developed to aid healthcare professionals looking after patients with pelvic radiation disease. It identified how symptoms are systematically investigated and managed (Andreyev *et al.*, 2014). The guidance recommends that this be done in conjunction with a gastroenterologist, or that women with these effects be referred to a specialist centre.

Internet resources

Jo's Cervical Cancer Trust, www.jostrust.org.uk
Ovacome (The Ovarian Cancer Support Network), www.ovacome.org.uk
Target Ovarian Cancer, www.targetovariancancer.org.uk

References

Abayomi JC, Kirwan J, Hackett AF. (2009) Coping mechanisms used by women in an attempt to avoid symptoms of chronic radiation enteritis. *J. Hum. Nutr. Diet.* 22(4): 310–316.

AHP Cancer Toolkit–NHS Network. (2012) Available at https://www.networks.nhs.uk/nhs-networks/ahp-networks/ahp-qipp-toolkits/AHP_Cancer_Pathway_final%20-3.pdf. Accessed 3 June 2017.

Andreyev J, Muls AC, Norton C, *et al.* (2014) Guidance: the practical management of the gastrointestinal symptoms of pelvic radiation disease. *Front. Gastroenterol.* Epub 2014. doi:10.1136/flgastro-2014-100468.

Billson HA, Holland C, Curwell J, *et al.* (2013) Perioperative nutrition interventions for women with ovarian cancer. *Cochrane Database Syst. Rev.* (9): CD009884. doi: 10.1002/14651858.CD009884.pub2.

Cancer Research UK (CRUK). (2013) *Cancer Incidence of Ovarian, Cervical and Uterine*. Available at http://www.cancerresearchuk.org/health-professional/cancer-statistics/incidence. Accessed 10 January 2017.

Cancer Research UK (CRUK). (2010–2011) Ovarian cancer survival statistics Available at https://www.cancerresearchuk.org/health-professional/cancer-statistics/statistics-by-cancer-type/ovarian-cancer/survival. Accessed 15 November 2018.

Cancer Research UK (CRUK). (2014) Cervical cancer statistics Available at https://www.cancerresearchuk.org/health-professional/cancer-statistics/statistics-by-cancer-type/cervical-cancer. Accessed 15 November 2018.

Chan K, Power J. (2016) Fact Sheet 14 – Blocked Bowel Available at http://www.ovacome.org.uk/wp-content/uploads/2016/02/Fact-sheet-14-BLOCKED-BOWEL.pdf Accessed 3/6/17

Charoenkwan K, Matovinovic E. (2014) Early versus delayed oral fluids and food for reducing complications after major abdominal gynaecological surgery. *Cochrane Database Syst. Rev.* (12): CD004508. doi: 10.1002/14651858.CD004508.pub4

Cousins SE, Tempest E, Feuer DJ. (2016) Surgery for the resolution of symptoms in malignant bowel obstruction in advanced gynaecological and gastrointestinal cancer. *Cochrane Database Syst. Rev.* (1): CD002764. doi: 10.1002/14651858.CD002764.pub2.

CRF. (2015) Ovarian cancer risk. Available at https://www.cancerresearchuk.org/health-professional/cancer-statistics/statistics-by-cancer-type/ovarian-cancer/risk-factors. Accessed 15 November 2018.

Feuer DJ, Broadley KE. (2000) Corticosteroids for the resolution of malignant bowel obstruction in advanced gynaecological and gastrointestinal cancer. *Cochrane Database Syst. Rev.* (2): CD001219. doi: 10.1002/14651858.

Gupta D, Lammersfeld CA, Vashi PG, *et al.* (2008) Can subjective global assessment of nutritional status predict survival in ovarian cancer. *J. Ovarian Res.* 15(1): 5. doi: 10.1186/1757-2215-1-5.

Gupta D, Lis CG, Vashi PG, *et al.* (2010) Impact of improved nutritional status on survival in ovarian cancer. *Support. Care Cancer.* 18(3): 373–381.

Hess LM, Barakat R, Tian C. (2007) Weight change during chemotherapy as a potential prognostic factor for stage III epithelial ovarian carcinoma: a Gynaecological Oncology Group Study. *Gynecol. Oncol.* 107(2): 260–265.

Kucukmetin A, Naik R, Galaal K. (2010) Palliative surgery versus medical management for bowel obstruction in ovarian cancer. *Cochrane Database Syst. Rev.* (7): CD007792. doi: 10.1002/14651858.CD007792.pub2.

Laky B, Janda M, Bauer J, *et al.* (2007) Malnutrition among gynaecological cancer patients. *Eur. J. Clin. Nutr.* 61(5): 642–646.

Madhok BM, Yeluri S, Haigh K, *et al.* (2011) Parenteral nutrition for patients with advanced ovarian malignancy. *J. Hum. Nutr. Diet.* 24(2): 187–191.

McGough C, Baldwin C, Frost G, *et al.* (2004) Role of nutritional intervention in patients treated with radiotherapy for pelvic malignancy. *Br. J. Cancer* 90(12): 2278–2287.

Meyer L, Pothuri B. (2006) Decompressive percutaneous gastrostomy tube use in gynaecologic malignancies. *Curr. Treat. Options Oncol.* 7(2): 111–120.

NICE. (2011) *Ovarian Cancer: The Recognition and Initial Management of Ovarian Cancer. CG 122*. Available at https://www.nice.org.uk/guidance/cg122. Accessed 3 June 2017.

Pothuri B, Vaidya A, Aghajanian C, *et al.* (2003) Palliative surgery for bowel obstruction in recurrent ovarian cancer: an updated series. *Gynecol. Oncol.* 89(2): 306–313.

Rodrigues CS, Lacerda MS, Chaves GV. (2015) Patient generated subjective global assessment as a prognosis tool in women with gynecological cancer. *Nutrition.* 31: 1372–1378.

Rutten I, Dijk D, Kruitwagen R. (2016) Loss of skeletal muscle during neoadjuvant chemotherapy is related to decreased survival in ovarian cancer patients. *J. Cachexia. Sarcopenia Muscle.* 7(4): 458–466. doi: 10.1002/jcsm.12107.

von Gruenigen VE, Courneya KS, Gibbons HE, *et al.* (2008) Feasibility and effectiveness of a lifestyle intervention program in obese endometrial cancer patients: a randomized trial. *Gynecol. Oncol.* 109(1): 19–26.

Wedlake LJ, Shaw C, Whelan K, *et al.* (2013) Systematic review; the efficacy of nutritional interventions to counteract acute gastrointestinal toxicity during therapeutic pelvic radiotherapy. *Aliment. Pharmacol. Ther.* 37(11): 1046–1056.

Wedlake L, Shaw C, McNair H, *et al.* (2017) Randomized controlled trail of dietary fiber for the prevention of radiation-induced gastrointestinal toxicity during pelvic radiotherapy. *Am. J. Clin. Nutr.* 106(3): 849–857.

World Cancer Research Fund/American Institute for Cancer Research (WCRF/AICR). (2013) *Endometrial Cancer. Food, Nutrition, Physical Activity, and the Prevention of Endometrial Cancer.* Available at http://www.wcrf.org/sites/default/files/Endometrial-Cancer-2013-Report.pdf. Accessed 3 June 2017.

World Cancer Research Fund/American Institute for Cancer Research (WCRF/AICR). (2014) *Ovarian Cancer. Food, Nutrition, Physical Activity, and the Prevention of Ovarian Cancer.* Available at http://www.wcrf.org/sites/default/files/Ovarian-Cancer-2014-Report.pdf. Accessed 3 June 2017.

7.15.7 Prostate cancer

Rachel Bracegirdle

Key points

- Prostate cancer is the most common malignancy among men in the UK.
- Diet may play a role in the aetiology of prostate cancer.
- Hormone therapy can cause symptoms of metabolic syndrome and bone thinning; both warrant changes in diet and lifestyle.
- Dietary modifications may be beneficial in managing symptoms of radiation enteritis.

The prostate gland is part of the male reproductive system and makes some of the alkaline fluid that constitutes 20–30% of semen. It is the size of a walnut, located below the bladder and in front of the rectum, with the urethra running through its centre. Prostate cancer is the most common malignancy among men in the UK, with 46,690 new diagnoses made in 2014. This accounted for 26% of all male cancer diagnoses (Cancer Research UK (CRUK), 2014). Survival has tripled over the last 40 years in the UK, with 94% and 85% of men now surviving 1 year and 5 years after diagnosis, respectively (CRUK, 2010–2011). Incidence is greater in developed countries, where approximately 68% of cases occur. The highest incidence is observed in Australia and Northern America, and the lowest in Asia and Africa (Ferlay *et al.*, 2012). Prostate cancer risk increases in migrants to Western countries when compared with those in their native countries. This could be the result of adopting Western dietary practices (Kimura, 2012). Other factors which influence the development of prostate cancer include age, ethnicity and family history. Of newly diagnosed cases, 90% undergo treatment with curative intent (Greene *et al.*, 2005). Treatment may be a combination of surgery, radiotherapy, chemotherapy and hormones. Some adjunct treatments include the use of bisphosphonates and steroids.

Nutrition

Diet plays a role in disease aetiology, supporting nutritional difficulties during treatment and managing the long-term side effects resulting from treatment. The incidence of undernutrition in prostate cancer is relatively low as compared to other cancers, and occurs more commonly in advanced disease (Hébuterne *et al.*, 2014). Weight gain and features of metabolic syndrome are important side effects of hormone treatment; dietetics has a role in survivorship.

Nutrition and aetiology

The World Cancer Research Fund (WCRF) has reviewed evidence on the effect of diet, weight and physical activity on prostate cancer incidence and progression; the findings are summarised in Table 7.15.8 (WCRF/AICR, 2014).

The WCRF expert panel concluded that there is strong evidence to support the judgement of a probable causal relationship between body fatness – as measured by body mass index (BMI), waist circumference and waist–hip ratio – and increased risk of advanced prostate cancer. However, no conclusion could be drawn for the link between body fatness and total or non-advanced prostate cancer. A dose–response meta-analysis showed a statistically significant 8% increased risk of advanced

Table 7.15.8 Influence of dietary components on prostate cancer risk (source: WCRF/AICR Report, 2014. Reproduced with permission from the World Cancer Research Fund International, www.dietandcancerreport.org)

Strength of evidence		Decreases risk	Increases risk
Strong evidence	Convincing	Nil	Nil
	Probable	Nil	Body fatness (advanced prostate cancer). Adult attained height.
Limited evidence	Limited (suggestive)	Nil	Dairy products. Diets high in calcium. Low plasma alpha-tocopherol concentrations. Low plasma selenium concentrations.
	Limited – no conclusion	Cereals (grains) and their products, dietary fibre, potatoes, non-starchy vegetables, fruits, pulses (legumes), processed meat, red meat, poultry, fish, eggs, total fat, saturated fatty acids, monounsaturated fatty acids, polyunsaturated fatty acids, plant oils, sugar (sucrose), sugary foods and drinks, coffee, tea, alcoholic drinks, carbohydrate, protein, vitamin A, retinol, alpha carotene, lycopene, folate, thiamine, riboflavin, niacin, vitamin C, vitamin D, vitamin E supplements, gamma-tocopherol, multivitamins, selenium supplements, iron, phosphorus, calcium supplements, zinc, physical activity, energy expenditure, vegetarian diets, Seventh-day Adventist diets, individual dietary patterns, body fatness (non-advanced prostate cancer), birthweight, energy intake.	
Strong evidence	Substantial effect on risk unlikely	Beta-carotene.	

prostate cancer per 5 kg/m^2 BMI increment. Additionally, a statistically significant 11% increased risk of prostate cancer mortality per 5 kg/m^2 BMI increment was shown in a dose–response meta-analysis (WCRF/AICR, 2014). Several mechanisms have been suggested for the link between body fatness and advanced prostate cancer. Obesity influences hormonal levels and growth factors, which have been proposed to influence cancer risk (De Pergola & Silvestris, 2013). Additionally, obesity could make early detection of prostate cancer difficult (Parekh *et al.*, 2010).

Overall, there is limited evidence to suggest that low plasma selenium concentrations increase the risk of prostate cancer. A meta-analysis showed decreasing prostate cancer incidence with selenium serum or plasma levels over a relatively narrow range, up to 170 ng/mL and selenium toenail concentrations of 0.85–0.94 µg/g (Hurst *et al.*, 2012). However, a selenium status above this range was not found to be protective, and higher concentrations might have adverse effects in terms of increasing risk of other conditions such as diabetes. A protective role for selenium was suggested by the results of the Nutritional Prevention of Cancer (NPC) study. Between 50% and 60% fewer prostate cancer cases were observed in selenium-deficient men taking selenium supplements, as compared to those taking a placebo (Clark *et al.*, 1996; Duffield-Lillico *et al.*, 2003). Conversely, the Selenium and Vitamin E Cancer Prevention Trial (SELECT), a double-blind, randomised controlled trial, found no benefit for selenium supplementation in relation to prostate cancer risk (Klein *et al.*, 2011). At follow-up 3 years after participants stopped supplementation, there was a non-significant increase in prostate cancer in selenium-supplemented groups as compared to placebo. In contrast to the NPC study and the studies in the Hurst *et al.* (2012) meta-analysis, the participants in the SELECT trial were not selenium deficient. A recent Cochrane review concluded that, overall, there is no convincing evidence to suggest that selenium supplements prevent prostate cancer. Further research is required into the effects of selenium in individuals with different nutritional status and genetic backgrounds, as well as the effects of different selenium compounds (Vinceti *et al.*, 2014).

The WCRF/AICR (2014) reported limited evidence to suggest that low plasma alpha-tocopherol concentrations (vitamin E) increase the risk of prostate cancer. Randomised controlled trials investigating vitamin E supplementation have produced inconsistent results. The effect of vitamin E was observed in the Alpha-T, Beta-Carotene (ATBC) Cancer Prevention Study, a randomised, double-blind, placebo-controlled trial where alpha-tocopherol supplementation in smokers showed a reduced prostate cancer incidence (ATBC Study Group, 2003). Conversely, results of the SELECT trial showed a non-statistically significant increase in prostate cancer incidence with vitamin E supplementation (Lippman *et al.*, 2009). The results of additional follow-up 3 years after the participants had stopped supplementation showed that men who had been taking vitamin E supplements had a statistically significant 17% increase in prostate cancer incidence in comparison with men randomised to placebo (Klein *et al.*, 2011). The reasons for the contrasting results for vitamin E in SELECT as compared to the ATBC study are not fully understood. The reduced prostate cancer incidence with vitamin E supplementation in the ATBC study could be due to chance, as it was a secondary finding in a trial not designed to investigate supplementation on prostate cancer. The dose of vitamin E used in SELECT was much higher than in the ATBC study, and could be too high to provide benefit.

There is limited evidence to suggest that dairy products and diets high in calcium increase the risk of prostate cancer. A recent meta-analysis found that high intakes of dairy products and calcium may increase total prostate cancer risk; the risk increased significantly with calcium intakes of >1200 mg/day, but was more pronounced at >2000 mg/day. No increase in risk was found with supplemental or non-dairy calcium (Aune *et al.*, 2015). The limitations of this review include the assessment of observational studies, increasing the potential for confounding variables, and the measurement errors that occurred in dietary assessments. Other studies have found no correlation between calcium and dairy intake, and prostate cancer risk (Huncharek *et al.*, 2008; Koh *et al.*, 2006).

Other foods which have been investigated in relation to prostate cancer risk are shown in Table 7.15.8; however, evidence for these is considered insufficient, weak or variable. Overall, current findings reinforce the importance for the general population of following guidelines for healthy eating as part of prostate cancer prevention.

Treatment

Surgery

A prostatectomy may be undertaken in the curative setting. Preoperative nutritional difficulties are generally uncommon. In the postoperative setting, ileus is an important although infrequent complication, occurring in <5% of all patients, but more commonly following an anastomotic leak with an incidence of 55% (Sukkarie *et al.*, 2007). Where a prolonged ileus occurs, the timely instigation of parenteral nutrition should be considered to support postoperative recovery.

Radiotherapy

Radiotherapy is often used in a curative setting. While treatment is directed at the prostate gland, organs within the pelvis (e.g. the bowel and rectum) sometimes receive radiotherapy. As a consequence of this, gastrointestinal symptoms, including loose stools and a change in bowel habits, may occur due to mucosal damage. This is known as acute radiation enteritis. Temporary changes in bowel motility, lactose intolerance, bile acid malabsorption, bile acid and pancreatic enzyme damage to bowel mucosa, and bacterial overgrowth may also be observed. There is some research showing that dietary modifications may improve the symptoms of acute radiation enteritis, e.g. a low-fat or elemental diet, probiotic supplementation and modifying fibre intake. While the evidence supporting these therapeutic diets is limited and weak due to inadequacies in research methodology, with results confounded by poor compliance in treatment groups, a trial may nonetheless be beneficial in symptomatic patients (McGough *et al.*, 2004; Wedlake *et al.*, 2012a, 2012b). It has been suggested that up to 50% of patients undergoing pelvic radiotherapy experience longer-term gastrointestinal disturbances due to chronic radiation enteritis, causing impaired quality of life. Guidance on managing the acute and chronic gastrointestinal problems arising from cancer treatment is available, including a clearly defined algorithm (Andreyev *et al.*, 2012, 2014). Optimal management of symptoms requires appropriate investigations into symptom causes and the involvement of a multidisciplinary team. Rectal distension can influence the position of the prostate gland and therefore affect radiotherapy treatment. Several methods have been investigated to minimise rectal distension in planning radiotherapy and throughout treatment, including fibre modification and reducing consumption of foods known to cause wind. More research is needed to assess the effectiveness of these interventions, although some centres may already recommend that patients follow advice (McNair *et al.*, 2011; Yahya *et al.*, 2013).

Hormone treatment

Hormone treatment, also referred to as androgen deprivation therapy (ADT), may use antiandrogens, luteinising hormone–releasing hormone agonists, and gonadotrophin-releasing hormone antagonists. Hormones treat prostate cancer by reducing the effects of testosterone in the body to shrink or delay tumour growth and reduce symptoms. Hormone treatment may continue for several years. Nutritional consequences include weight gain and features of metabolic syndrome, e.g. abdominal obesity, increased total body fat mass, dyslipidaemia, increased diabetes risk and hyperinsulinaemia (Morote *et al.*, 2015; Yu *et al.*, 2014). Tailored interventions for weight management and advice on principles of healthy eating can be effective (Demark-Wahnefried *et al.*, 2012; Mohamad *et al.*, 2015) (see Chapter 7.12, Diabetes mellitus and 7.14.3, Dyslipidaemia).

Reduced bone density is another important implication of hormone treatment. Consideration should be given to vitamin D and calcium supplementation. Bisphosphonates may be prescribed to preserve bone density by reducing osteoclast activity and increasing osteoblast activity in bone (see Chapter 7.9.1, Osteoporosis).

Chemotherapy

Chemotherapy is given where cure is no longer possible, and aims to shrink and slow the growth of the cancer, control symptoms such as pain, and improve quality of life. Side effects with potential nutritional implications include stomatitis, taste changes, anorexia, nausea, vomiting, changes in bowel habit, and fatigue. These side effects are temporary and resolve shortly after completing treatment. Short-term dietary changes and oral supplementation may be necessary to help manage eating. Advanced cancer can influence appetite and cause difficulties with eating. Dietary advice and supplementation should be considered with the aim of preserving quality of life. Steroids may sometimes be given with chemotherapy to make treatment more effective, and this can also help improve appetite.

Disease progression and survivorship

Men with prostate cancer can live for many years with the disease. Foods and dietary supplements that have been investigated include processed meats, dairy products, plant-based diets, lycopene and/or tomato, oily fish, vitamin E, beta-carotene, soya/isoflavones, low-fat diets, pomegranate and green tea. Several review articles all provide similar conclusions, in that further research is needed to prove a definitive role for diet in this patient population (Davies *et al.*, 2011; Hackshaw-McGeagh *et al.*, 2015; Ma & Chapman, 2009; Mandair *et al.*, 2014).

Dietary changes can help manage the long-term health implications of hormone treatment and radiotherapy. To reduce the risk of developing comorbidities associated with weight gain and dyslipidaemia, advice on healthy eating and lifestyle measures, including exercise, should be integrated into the patient's care. It is possible that the benefits of this may also extend to a positive impact on disease progression and survival (Davies *et al.*, 2011; Peisch *et al.*, 2016).

There is great consumer interest in the role of diet in disease prevention and management. When a cancer diagnosis is received, diet provides individuals with a readily available method to actively control their own health. While evidence points towards certain correlations between diet and prostate cancer, the lack of high-quality studies and the publication of inconsistent results mean that there is insufficient evidence to translate these into public health or clinical practice recommendations. Individuals may seek advice on diet and prostate cancer, and it is important for dietetic professionals to understand the evidence available. Further research is needed to substantiate current findings. However, the existing knowledge from studies provides a basis for dietitians to give patients and the general public guidance on diet and prostate cancer.

Acknowledgment

The editor acknowledges the prior contribution of Saira Chowdhury.

Internet resources

Prostate Cancer Charity, www.prostatecanceruk.org

References

Andreyev HN, Davidson SE, Gillespie C, *et al.* (2012) Practice guidance on the management of acute and chronic gastrointestinal problems arising as a result of treatment for cancer. *Gut.* 61(2): 179–192.

Andreyev HN, Muls AC, Norton C, *et al.* (2014) Guidance: the practical management of the gastrointestinal symptoms of pelvic radiation disease. *Front. Gastroenterol.* 6(1): 53–72.

ATBC Study Group. (2003) Incidence of cancer and mortality following α-tocopherol and β-carotene supplementation: a post intervention follow-up. *JAMA.* 290(4): 476–485.

Aune D, Navarro Rosenblatt DA, Chan DS, *et al.* (2015) Dairy products, calcium, and prostate cancer risk: a systematic review and meta-analysis of cohort studies. *Am. J. Clin. Nutr.* 101(1): 87–117.

Cancer Research UK (CRUK). (2010–2011) *Prostate Cancer Survival Statistics.* Available at http://www.cancerresearchuk.org/health-professional/cancer-statistics/statistics-by-cancer-type/prostate-cancer#heading-Two. Accessed 16 October 2016.

Cancer Research UK (CRUK). (2014) *Prostate Cancer Incidence Statistics.* Available at http://www.cancerresearchuk.org/health-professional/cancer-statistics/statistics-by-cancer-type/prostate-cancer/incidence#ref. Accessed 4 December 2016.

Clark LC, Combs GF Jr, Turnbull BW, *et al.* (1996) Effects of selenium supplementation for cancer prevention in carcinoma of the skin. A randomized controlled trial: Nutritional Prevention of Cancer Study Group. *JAMA.* 276(24): 1957–1963.

Davies NJ, Batehup L, Thomas R. (2011) The role of diet and physical activity in breast, colorectal, and prostate cancer survivorship: a review of the literature. *Br. J. Cancer.* 105(S1): S52–S73.

De Pergola G, Silvestris F. (2013) Obesity as a major risk factor for cancer. *J. Obes.* 2013: 291546.

Demark-Wahnefried W, Morey MC, Sloane R, *et al.* (2012) Reach out to enhance wellness home-based diet-exercise intervention promotes reproducible and sustainable long-term Improvements in health behaviors, body weight, and physical functioning in older, overweight/obese cancer survivors. *J. Clin. Oncol.* 30(19): 2354–2361.

Duffield-Lillico AJ, Dalkin BL, Reid ME, *et al.* (2003) Selenium supplementation, baseline plasma selenium status and incidence of prostate cancer: an analysis of the complete treatment period of the Nutritional Prevention of Cancer Trial. *BJU Int.* 91: 608–612.

Ferlay J, Soerjomataram I, Ervik M, *et al.* (2012) *Cancer Incidence and Mortality Worldwide: IARC CancerBase (online).* Available at http://globocan.iarc.fr/Pages/fact_sheets_cancer.aspx. Accessed 7 November 2016.

Greene K, Cowan JE, Cooperberg MR. (2005) Who is the average patient presenting with prostate cancer? *Urology.* 6(5): 76–82.

Hébuterne X, Lemarié E, Michallet M, *et al.* (2014) Prevalence of malnutrition and current use of nutrition support in patients with cancer. *JPEN J. Parenter. Enteral. Nutr.* 38(2): 196–204.

Huncharek M, Muscat J, Kupelnick B. (2008) Dairy products, dietary calcium and vitamin D intake as risk factors for prostate cancer: a meta-analysis of 26,769 cases from 45 observational studies. *Nutr. Cancer* 60: 421–441.

Hackshaw-McGeagh LE, Perry RE, Leach VA, *et al.* (2015) A systematic review of dietary, nutritional, and physical activity interventions for the prevention of prostate cancer progression and mortality. *Cancer Causes Control.* 26: 1521–1550.

Hurst R, Hooper L, Norat T, *et al.* (2012) Selenium and prostate cancer: systematic review and meta-analysis. *Am. J. Clin. Nutr.* 96(1): 111–122.

Kimura T. (2012) East meets West: ethnic differences in prostate cancer epidemiology between East Asians and Caucasians. *Chin. J. Cancer.* 31(9): 421–429.

Koh KA, Sesso HD, Paffenbarger RS, *et al.* (2006) Dairy products, calcium and prostate cancer risk. *Br. J. Cancer.* 95(11): 1582–1585.

Klein EA, Thompson IM, Tangen CM, *et al.* (2011) Vitamin E and the risk of prostate cancer. The Selenium and Vitamin E Cancer Prevention Trial (SELECT). *JAMA.* 306(14): 1549–1556.

Lippman SM, Klein EA, Goodman PJ, *et al.* (2009) Effect of selenium and vitamin E on risk of prostate cancer and other cancers. The Selenium and Vitamin E Cancer Prevention Trial (SELECT). *JAMA.* 301(1): 39–51.

Ma RWL, Chapman K. (2009) A systematic review of the effect of diet in prostate cancer prevention and treatment. *J. Hum. Nutr. Diet.* 22(3): 187–199.

Mandair D, Rossi RE, Pericleous M, *et al.* (2014) Prostate cancer and the influence of dietary factors and supplements: a systematic review. *Nutr. Metab.* 11: 30.

McGough C, Baldwin C, Frost G, *et al.* (2004) Role of nutritional intervention in patients treated with radiotherapy for pelvic malignancy. *Br. J. Cancer.* 90(12): 2278–2287.

McNair HA, Wedlake L, McVey GP, *et al.* (2011) Can diet combined with treatment scheduling achieve consistency of rectal filling in patients receiving radiotherapy to the prostate. *Radiother. Oncol.* 101(3): 471–478 (Abstract).

Mohamad H, McNeill G, Haseen F, *et al.* (2015) The effect of dietary and exercise interventions on body weight in prostate cancer patients: a systematic review. *Nutr. Cancer.* 67(1): 43–60.

Morote J, Gómez-Caamaño A, Alvarez-Ossorio JL, *et al.* (2015) The metabolic syndrome and its components in patients with prostate cancer on androgen deprivation therapy. *J. Urol.* 193(6): 1963–1969.

Peisch SF, Van Blarigan EL, Chan JM, *et al.* (2016) Prostate cancer progression and mortality: a review of diet and lifestyle factors. *World J. Urol.* 35(6): 867–874.

Parekh N, Lin Y, Dipaola RS, *et al.* (2010) Obesity and prostate cancer detection: insights from three national surveys. *Am. J. Med.* 123(9): 829–835.

Sukkarie T, Harmon J, Penna F, *et al.* (2007) Incidence and management of anastomotic leakage following laparoscopic prostatectomy with implementation of a new anastomotic technique incorporating posterior bladder neck tailoring. *J. Robot. Surg.* 1: 213–215.

Vinceti M, Dennert G, Crespi CM, *et al.* (2014) Selenium for preventing cancer. *Cochrane Database Syst. Rev.* (3): CD005195.

Wedlake LJ, McGough C, Shaw C, *et al.* (2012a) Clinical trial: efficacy of a low or modified fat diet for the prevention of gastrointestinal toxicity in patients receiving radiotherapy treatment for pelvic malignancies. *J. Hum. Nutr. Diet.* 25: 247–259.

Wedlake LJ, Shaw C, Whelan K, *et al.* (2013) Systematic review: the efficacy of nutritional interventions to counteract acute gastrointestinal toxicity during therapeutic pelvic radiotherapy. *Aliment. Pharmacol. Ther.* 37: 1046–1056.

World Cancer Research Fund International/American Institute for Cancer Research (WCRF/AICR). (2014) *Continuous Update Project Report: Diet, Nutrition, Physical Activity, and Prostate Cancer (Online).* Available at www.wcrf.org/sites/default/files/Prostate-Cancer-2014-Report.pdf. Accessed 27 November 2016.

Yahya S, Zarkar A, Southgate E, *et al.* (2013) Which bowel preparation is best? Comparison of a high-fibre diet leaflet, daily microenema and no preparation in prostate cancer patients treated with radical radiotherapy to assess the effect on planned target volume shifts due to rectal distension. *Br. J. Radiol.* 86(1031): 20130457.

Yu IC, Lin HY, Sparks JD, *et al.* (2014) Androgen receptor roles in insulin resistance and obesity in males: the linkage of androgen-deprivation therapy to metabolic syndrome. *Diabetes.* 63(10): 3180–3188.

7.15.8 Haematological cancers and high-dose therapy

Julie Beckerson

Key points

- High-dose chemotherapy, radiotherapy and haematopoietic stem cell transplants provide potential cure or remission for many blood cancers.
- Treatment-associated side effects such as severe mucositis, nausea and vomiting can lead to rapid deterioration of nutritional status.
- Nutrition support is an important adjunct to high-dose therapy; enteral nutrition support may improve transplant outcomes as compared to parenteral nutrition support.
- Dietary restrictions during neutropenia remain commonplace, although the evidence to support a reduction in infections is lacking.

Haematological cancers involve the blood or lymphatic system and include leukaemia, lymphoma, myeloma, myelodysplastic and myeloproliferative syndromes, and lymphoproliferative disorders. These are rare in children and young adults, but become more common with increasing age, and account for approximately 39,000 or 9% of UK cancer cases per year. Non-Hodgkin's lymphoma, leukaemia and myeloma are the sixth, 12th and 18th most common cancer diagnoses, respectively (Haematological Malignancy Research Network, 2015).

Leukaemia refers to the proliferation and accumulation of abnormal white blood cells in the bone marrow (abnormal blasts). As the disease progresses, abnormal cells spill out of the bone marrow, and infiltrate and damage other tissues. Leukaemia is described as either myeloid or lymphoid, according to the origin of the abnormal cells. Acute and chronic leukaemias are differentiated by the maturity of the cells affected. Acute leukaemia affects immature white blood cells that continue to divide after normal cells have stopped. In chronic leukaemia, mature cells are affected, increasing their lifespan and number in the marrow and circulation.

Lymphoma results from abnormal replication of cells within lymph nodes or other lymphoid tissues, such as the spleen, bone marrow and thymus. It is broadly classified into Hodgkin's or non-Hodgkin's lymphoma, but within these categories there are numerous disease subtypes according to the cell line that multiplies. High-grade lymphomas replicate the quickest, whereas low-grade or indolent lymphomas develop slowly and may be asymptomatic for many years.

Myeloma is a malignant proliferation of monoclonal plasma cells that often secrete large amounts of ineffective antibodies known as paraproteins. In addition to bone marrow involvement, there maybe infiltration of bone, causing osteolytic lesions; kidney damage from elevated plasma paraprotein and/or hypercalcaemia; and isolated lesions known as plasmacytomas.

Diagnosis

The clinical presentation of haematological malignancies frequently reflect the underlying altered haematopoiesis (formation and development of blood cells), where there may be an excess of malignant white blood cells and a suppression of red blood cells and platelets. In leukaemia, ineffective or lack of healthy white blood cells increase susceptibility to infections. Patients may complain of fatigue due to anaemia caused by reduced red blood cells, or increased bruising and bleeding resulting from thrombocytopenia (low platelets). Presenting symptoms such as fever, night sweats and weight loss occur in lymphoma, and may suggest advanced disease. Myeloma patients may also present with bone disease, related to an infiltration of cancer cells, resulting in pathological (non-traumatic) fractures or, in extreme cases, spinal cord compression. Impaired renal function may also be evident due to the excessive numbers of paraproteins produced that must be renally excreted.

Blood tests and bone marrow aspirate are used to determine the type and extent of blood cell abnormalities. Cytogenetic testing of chromosomal changes and immunophenotyping to detect specific molecules on the surface of malignant cells are also used to guide treatment decisions. Other tests include urinary paraprotein, lymph node biopsy, and imaging. Subsequent staging and prognosis of haematological cancers will vary significantly according to the disease subtype.

Treatment

Protocols used in haemato-oncology frequently involve the most intensive and high-dose regimens. In acute leukaemia, disease onset is rapid, and induction chemotherapy must be initiated immediately. However, for some chronic leukaemias, low-grade lymphomas and myeloma, treatment may be delayed until symptoms present. The treatment goals are to control disease and maximise quality of life, while minimising treatment side effects. Bone marrow transplants or, increasingly, stem cell transplants, collectively known as haematopoietic cell transplants (HCTs) may be used. These enable much higher doses of chemotherapy and radiotherapy than those used for the treatment of solid tumours, and have the potential to achieve long-term remission or cure. HCTs are usually performed after several courses of induction chemotherapy to control disease or achieve remission.

There are two main types of HCT, autologous (patients are given back their own cells) and allogeneic (using donor cells). Donor transplants provide the greatest likelihood of long-term remission or cure due to the immunological effects of the donor cells against the host's disease. However, autologous HCT is considered standard care for some conditions, such as myeloma, due to the high morbidity associated with allogeneic transplantation (Shah *et al.*, 2015).

Prior to an infusion of stem cells, a conditioning regimen that may include chemotherapy, radiation and immunosuppressive therapy is given. Cytotoxic agents are given to eradicate tumour cells and destroy host haematopoiesis in preparation for the donor stem cells. Reduced-intensity conditioning (RIC) transplants have been developed for older patients or those less able to withstand high-dose myeloablative chemotherapy. Early toxicities are reduced following these transplants, but there is an increased risk of subsequent relapse for those with poor risk or advanced disease (Wahid, 2013). The choice of HCT depends on the disease, stage, fitness of the recipient, and donor availability.

Consequences of high-dose therapies and stem cell transplant

Neutropenia and infectious complications

Myeloablative therapy causes neutrophil levels to fall, increasing the risk of bacterial sepsis, pneumonia and fungal infections. This is a major cause of morbidity and mortality; therefore, antimicrobial, antifungal and antiviral medications are routinely prescribed. Other preventative measures include contact precautions, hand washing, air filtration and positive pressure isolation rooms. Infection risk is highest in allogeneic HCT, where the period of neutropenia is longer than in autologous HCT. Immunosuppressive therapy and immune reconstitution continue for several months after neutrophil recovery following allogeneic HCT. Viral infections are common during this phase.

Mucositis

All patients undergoing high-dose therapy or HCT are recognised as high risk for developing mucositis. Up to 80% of HCT recipients will experience severe mucositis, frequently requiring intravenous opioid analgesia (Keefe *et al.*, 2007; Rubenstein *et al.*, 2004). Mucositis typically lasts 1–3 weeks, dependent on the conditioning regimen. It can affect any part of the gastrointestinal tract, resulting in mouth or throat pain, ulceration, abdominal pain, nausea, vomiting and diarrhoea. The breakdown of mucosal barriers during mucositis significantly increases infection risk and is associated with worse clinical and economic outcomes (Keefe, 2006; Sonis *et al.*, 2001). Patients at risk of oral mucositis should have regular assessment using a validated tool. There should be an individualised care plan that includes strategies to prevent or reduce the occurrence of mucositis, and treatment plans according to the grade of mucositis and its complications (UK Oral Mucositis in Cancer Group (UKOMiC), 2015).

Organ toxicity

The high-dose chemotherapy and/or radiotherapy used in HCT can cause gastrointestinal, renal, bladder, pulmonary, cardiac, neurological and hepatic complications, resulting in significant morbidity and mortality. Approximately 14% of HCT recipients will develop hepatic veno-occlusive disease (sinusoidal obstructive syndrome), which is characterised by occlusion and injury to hepatic venules and hepatocytes, induced by chemotherapy. It often leads to multi-organ failure and is associated with high mortality rates (Coppell *et al.*, 2010).

Graft versus host disease

Immunosuppression is given to allogeneic HCT patients to avoid the potentially fatal complication of graft-versus-host disease (GvHD). This occurs as a consequence of interactions between mature donor immune cells (T cells) and antigen presenting cells of the recipient. There are two types: acute GvHD, which usually occurs within 100 days of HCT and may affect the skin, gut or liver, manifesting as rash, nausea, vomiting, diarrhoea, ileus and deranged liver function or liver failure; and chronic GvHD, which is a major long-term complication of allogeneic HCT that occurs in 30–70% of transplant recipients. It occurs more than 100 days after transplant and can affect numerous organs and tissues. About 50% of patients will have three or more involved organs (Lee, 2010).

Psychological effects

Extended periods in isolation, separation from family and the experience of transplant have major psychological effects. Reduced attention span and slower cognitive processing can occur as a result of fatigue following high-dose therapy, impacting negatively on mood. Physical side effects from treatment such as severe mucositis or profuse intractable nausea and vomiting can also result in psychological distress that can be both acute and long term (UKOMiC, 2015). Patients may experience significant changes to their appearance. Some changes such as hair and weight loss may be temporary. However, allogeneic HCT recipients who develop GvHD can exhibit severe skin changes and significant muscle wasting that are difficult to reverse.

Survivorship

Continued hospital appointments, fatigue and susceptibility to infection significantly impact rehabilitation after high-dose therapy. Return to normal functioning and improvements in nutritional status can take more than a year after transplantation (Iestra *et al.*, 2002). Patients surviving 5 years after HCT are generally in good health and socially reintegrated. More than 90% of these will have Karnofsky performance scores of 90–100%. However, mortality rates are higher than those expected even 20 years after transplantation, and studies have shown that significant differences in subjective well-being persist for many years when patients are compared with their sibling donors (European Group for Bone Marrow Transplantation 2012).

Nutritional assessment

Nutritional screening is recommended to identify subjects for whom nutritional assessment and care planning is necessary (August *et al.*, 2009). Assessment prior to high-dose treatment is useful to establish pre-existing malnutrition, discuss potential side effects of treatment, develop rapport and improve compliance with recommended interventions (Iestra *et al.*, 2002). High-dose therapies, particularly HCT, have marked effects on metabolic demands and significantly impair nutritional intake. Oral intake declines rapidly in the first 8 days after HCT as a result of gastrointestinal side effects, and many patients consume <60% of their estimated energy requirements (Walrath *et al.*, 2014). As a result, nutritional status declines and does not fully recover when assessed after discharge (Defranchi *et al.*, 2014). Furthermore, reduced physical activity and loss of mobility due to hospitalisation and prolonged isolation result in reduced muscle mass, particularly in a previously active patient.

Anthropometry

Despite prior treatment with induction and consolidation chemotherapy, the majority of patients presenting for HCT are apparently well nourished according to their BMI; there is a negative association with overall survival for those patients with a BMI of $<18.5\,kg/m^2$ (Baumgartner *et al.*, 2017). Conversely, high BMI prior to HCT is linked with acute GvHD, infections and poorer 5-year survival rates (Bulley *et al.*, 2008; Fuji *et al.*, 2009). Studies frequently show reductions in weight or BMI of 5–10% during HCT. However, weights can be inaccurate once treatment has commenced, due to multiple intravenous infusions and changes in organ function. Errors in height can be introduced due to pathological fractures or vertebral collapse in myeloma patients. Other anthropometry or bioelectrical impedance analysis may provide a better indication of nutritional status, although the use of skinfold callipers is limited during thrombocytopenia due to bleeding risk. Functional tests of muscle strength and physical performance can be used to monitor physical activity, which should be promoted for its beneficial effects on treatment outcomes (Arends *et al.*, 2016). There are increasing numbers of studies describing low muscle mass, assessed by CT scanning, in this patient group. The prevalence of sarcopenia prior to allogeneic HCT, using a more robust definition of combined deficits in muscle mass, strength and function, has been estimated at more than 50% (Morishita *et al.*, 2012).

Biochemistry

Regular biochemistry monitoring is essential to detect changes in organ function, mineral and electrolyte imbalances, hyperglycaemia or hyperlipidaemia. Biochemistry alone cannot accurately reflect nutritional status. The underlying disease and complications, such as sepsis and GvHD, will confound the interpretation of albumin. In advanced myeloma, albumin is also lowered at the expense of raised serum paraproteins. Mineral and electrolyte losses are common and often exacerbated by antimicrobial and immunosuppressive drugs, examples of which are shown in Table 7.15.9. Multiple blood transfusions may elevate ferritin levels, indicating iron overload. Repeated hospital stays for treatment can result

Table 7.15.9 Mineral and electrolyte changes with drugs commonly used in stem cell transplantation

Drug	Therapeutic use	Biochemical side effects
Ciclosporin	Immunosuppression	Hyperkalaemia, hypomagnesaemia
Tacrolimus	Immunosuppression	Hyperkalaemia, hypokalaemia
Amphotericin/ AmBisome	Antifungal	Hypokalaemia, hypomagnesaemia
Foscarnet	Antiviral	Hypocalcaemia, other electrolyte disturbances

in suboptimal vitamin D status and low calcium levels, which are of particular relevance for those receiving corticosteroid therapy (Lipkin *et al.*, 2005).

Nutritional requirements

The European Society for Parenteral and Enteral Nutrition (ESPEN) suggests that the energy requirements of cancer patients are comparable to those of healthy individuals, generally ranging 25–30 kcal/day (Arends *et al.*, 2016). This is supported by a small study of 10 acute leukaemia patients undergoing induction chemotherapy (Cereda *et al.*, 2007). Total energy expenditure probably differs between treatments and the presence of complications, although evidence in patients with haematological malignancies is limited. Current UK recommendations for energy suggest disease-specific elevations in basal metabolic rate of 25–34% in leukaemia and 0–25% in lymphoma (Weekes, 2011). However, studies supporting these stress factors include few haematology subjects, and measurements were taken while a proportion of subjects were receiving artificial nutrition (Barak *et al.*, 2002).

Nutritional requirements are raised in acute GvHD, and there may be significant gastrointestinal losses, resulting in a negative balance for many nutrients, including nitrogen. Chronic GvHD patients have an elevated tumour necrosis factor alpha and elevated resting energy expenditure, which may contribute to chronic weight loss (Zauner *et al.*, 2001).

Evidence is lacking to support specific recommendations for nitrogen intake at different stages of treatment. Negative nitrogen balance is likely during high-dose therapy, and the catabolic effects of disease, treatment and complications should be considered when estimating protein requirements. Inactivity as a result of protective isolation and inflammatory consequences of treatment will confer some degree of anabolic resistance to these patients, further supporting a role for higher protein intakes.

Micronutrient requirements may be raised during high-dose therapy due to increased oxidation and tissue damage; however, there is no evidence to support routine antioxidant or trace element supplementation unless there is known deficiency or malnutrition. Fluid losses occur due to gastrointestinal side effects and (to a lesser extent) episodes of pyrexia. However, intravenous input from medications, blood products and electrolyte replacement, together with potential renal or hepatic dysfunction, can predispose patients to fluid overload.

Nutritional intervention in haematopoietic cell transplant

The dietitian and appropriate nutritional support are recognised as vital components of the transplant process (Arends *et al.*, 2016; August *et al.*, 2009). Appropriate nutritional interventions for symptom management during chemotherapy and radiotherapy are discussed in Chapter 7.15.1 (General aspects of cancer). The side effects from HCT that impair nutritional intake are frequently severe and may occur concurrently (Figure 7.15.2); despite aggressive medical management, the HCT patient is often unable to maintain adequate oral nutritional intake.

Artificial nutrition support

Treatment intensity and mucositis are the biggest determinants for artificial nutrition support. Therapy-related nausea, anorexia and mucositis are most severe during myeloablative allogeneic HCT. The use of reduced-intensity transplant-conditioning regimens cause fewer side effects, reducing the need for artificial nutrition. Parenteral nutrition (PN) is recommended in those with severe mucositis, prolonged ileus, intractable vomiting or diarrhoea; in those who are malnourished; or in those for whom it is anticipated that enteral nutrition (EN) will not be tolerated for 7–14 days (Arends *et al.*, 2016; August *et al.*, 2009). It has often been provided during transplantation irrespective of nutritional status. In some units, it remains common practice to commence PN the day after stem cell infusion, and continue for 15–20 days irrespective of nutritional status or intake (Arends *et al.*, 2016). Historically, PN was used extensively due to the high gastrointestinal toxicities of older conditioning regimens and the availability of central access, already established for chemotherapy and stem cell infusion.

Improved pharmacological management of treatment side effects has allowed more safe and effective use of EN during HCT. But there is a lack of randomised data to systematically compare the clinical outcomes of HCT patients receiving EN versus PN (August *et al.*, 2009; Murray & Pindoria, 2008; Thompson & Duffy, 2008). Only two studies have retrospectively analysed the outcomes of HCT patients who were offered tube feeding and where PN was used in instances when this failed. Results suggest an association between EN and less fever, faster engraftment, less infectious mortality and reduced

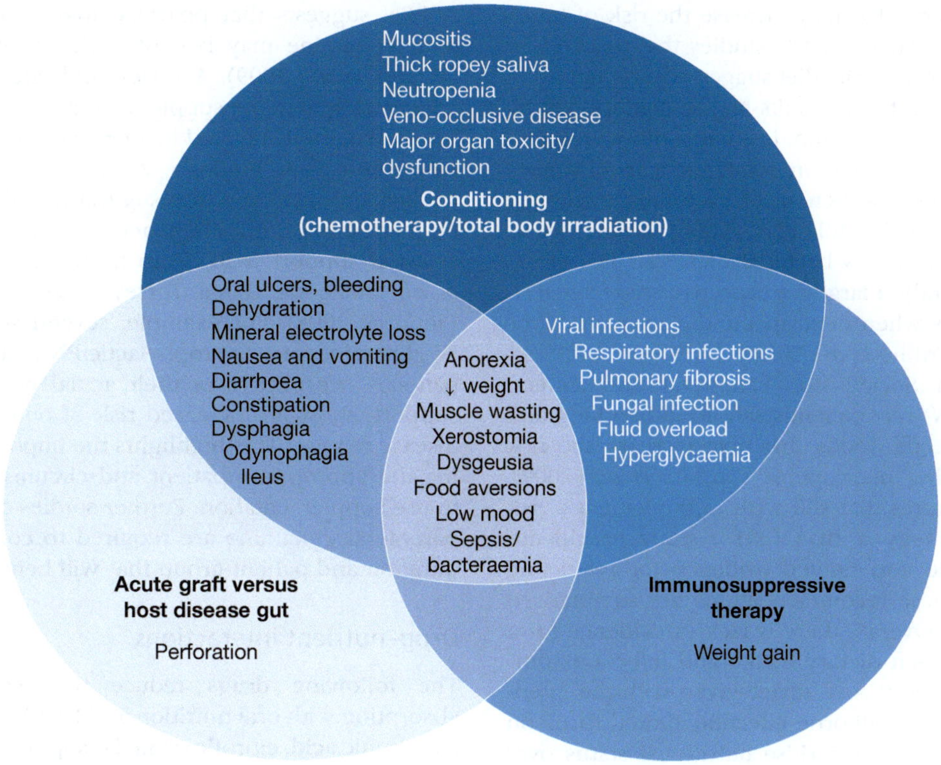

Figure 7.15.2 Side effects of stem cell transplant impacting on nutritional status

risk of GVHD when compared with PN (Guieze *et al.*, 2014; Seguy *et al.*, 2012).

More recently, in a large retrospective cohort study, PN was associated with a significant reduction in mortality at 100 days as compared to those in whom artificial nutrition support could not be established. However, again, the risk was significantly lower in those with adequate oral or enteral tube nutrition. Furthermore, the risk of GvHD was significantly lower in the EN versus PN groups, suggesting that adequate nutrition into the gut may be associated with beneficial effects on HCT outcomes (Beckerson *et al.*, 2018).

The beneficial effects of EN are likely multifactorial. The known infectious risks of PN will be amplified in this immunocompromised group (Black, 2011). During HCT, EN may reduce infectious complications by promoting intestinal recovery, since disruption of the mucosal barrier is thought to contribute to the development of 25–75% of bacteraemias during neutropenia (Stiff, 2001). PN may be considered to be an indirect indication of enteral nutrient deprivation, which itself will compromise multiple elements of the intestinal epithelial barrier. Survival, infections, mucositis and GvHD have been linked to changes in the intestinal microbiome in both mice and human models, but as yet there are no known studies of how the provision of nutritional support may influence the host microbiota during HCT.

Evidence for the optimum enteral feed composition during HCT is lacking; hence, choice should be made according to the usual clinical parameters (Chapter 6.4, Enteral nutrition). Polymeric feeds may be suitable; however, if malabsorption is suspected, then semi-elemental or peptide feeds may be better tolerated (Black, 2011; Lipkin *et al.*, 2005). Enteral feeding tubes must be placed prior to the development of mucositis to avoid pain and further mucosal damage. Thrombocytopenia is common, and tube placement presents a risk of haemorrhage. Local guidelines will vary, but a platelet count of >20 × 109/L may be adequate. Since feeding tubes are sterile, neutropenia *per se* is not a contraindication to their placement. Waiting until the acute emetic effects of conditioning have settled will reduce the risk of tube dislodgement.

Post-pyloric (nasojejunal) feeding may be useful if there is protracted vomiting or gastric stasis: some UK transplant centres have adopted this approach. The prophylactic insertion of gastrostomy or jejunostomy tubes to overcome repeated nasoenteric tube displacements due to vomiting has been tested. However, stoma site infections resulting in peritonitis and associated treatment delays have limited the use of these tubes (Black, 2011).

During gut GvHD, destruction of intestinal crypts, profuse diarrhoea and ulceration can lead to perforation. In severe cases, the most appropriate form of nutrition is PN (Arends *et al.*, 2016). However, EN was shown to be safe and beneficial in a small controlled-cohort study (Imataki *et al.*, 2006), and EN should be considered for low-grade gut GvHD.

SECTION 7

The neutropenic diet

The need for and efficacy of a neutropenic diet is controversial. Damage to the gut mucosal barrier by high-dose therapy, bacterial overgrowth and opioid-related impairment of peristalsis may increase the risk of translocation and bacteraemia. Early studies that placed leukaemia patients on a sterile diet suggested a reduction in infections; however, these results maybe confounded by the use of protective isolation, laminar airflow and antimicrobial gut decontamination. Subsequent small studies have not confirmed the benefit of excluding uncooked fruit and vegetables (DeMille *et al.*, 2006; Gardner *et al.*, 2008) or following a low-bacterial diet (van Tiel *et al.*, 2007). More recently, a large retrospective study suggested less infections when neutropenic dietary restrictions were removed (Trifilio *et al.*, 2012).

The American Society for Parenteral and Enteral Nutrition (ASPEN) recommends safe food handling and avoidance of specific foods that may increase the risk of infection during neutropenia (August *et al.*, 2009). For those UK centres that still wish to implement a risk management strategy, a BDA (2016) study has identified the rationale and limited evidence for restricting certain foods. These recommendations are summarised in Table 7.15.10. Overall, there is lack of evidence for a relationship between dietary intake and infections during high-dose therapy. Any advice given with the intention of minimising foodborne infection should focus on hygienic practices and prioritise nutritional status over theoretical risk.

Glutamine

Radiation- or chemotherapy-induced tissue damage may be attenuated by adequate tissue glutamine, suggesting a potential role in the prevention of tissue toxicity during myeloablative treatments (Wischmeyer, 2003).

Table 7.15.10 Dietary restrictions according to neutrophil count (BDA, 2016)

Neutrophil count	Foods to restrict
$<2.0 \times 10^9$	Mould-ripened or blue-veined cheeses
	Unpasteurised dairy products
	Raw or lightly cooked shellfish
	Raw or undercooked meat, poultry or fish
	Raw or undercooked eggs
	Probiotic products
	Fresh pâté
$<0.5 \times 10^9$	Raw or unpeeled fruit, dried fruit, vegetables and salad
	Unpasteurised fruit or vegetable juices or smoothies
	Water or ice from wells, coolers or bottled water
	Ice cream from ice cream vans
	Fresh nuts
	Uncooked herbs, spices and pepper
	Unpasteurised honey
	Unnecessarily large packets of food items

ASPEN suggests that pharmacological doses of parenteral glutamine may benefit patients undergoing HCT (August *et al.*, 2009). A review indicated the beneficial effects of glutamine-supplemented PN versus standard PN on length of stay and incidence of positive blood cultures (Murray & Pindoria, 2002). However, subsequent studies and meta-analyses suggest that the benefits may be limited to during allogeneic HCT when the need for artificial support is likely to be the greatest (Crowther *et al.*, 2009; da Gama Torres *et al.*, 2008; Murray & Pindoria, 2008). For example, several studies that give IV glutamine and/or prophylactic PN to autologous HCT patients, irrespective of their actual need for nutrition support, show an increased risk of outcomes including disease relapse. This highlights the importance of selecting the appropriate patient and circumstance in which to use supplementation. Further studies of both oral and parenteral glutamine are required to confirm the dose, duration and patient group that will benefit.

Drug–nutrient interactions

The following drugs reduce the bioavailability or absorption with oral nutrition and EN (Wohlt *et al.*, 2009): alendronic acid, ciprofloxacin, lansoprazole, omeprazole, pantoprazole, penicillin v, phenytoin, sucralfate, voriconazole.

Other drugs of note used in this patient group include:

- Ciclosporin – avoid all grapefruit-containing foods.
- Posaconazole – requires concurrent oral nutrition or EN.

Exact recommendations may vary according to formulation and local policy.

References

Arends J, Bachmann P, Baracos V, *et al.* (2016) ESPEN guidelines on nutrition in cancer patients. *Clin. Nutr.* 36(1):11–48.

August DA, Huhmann MB, American Society for Parenteral and Enteral Nutrition (A.S.P.E.N.) Board of Directors. (2009) ASPEN clinical guidelines: nutrition support therapy during adult anticancer treatment and in hematopoietic cell transplantation. *JPEN. J. Parenter. Enteral. Nutr.* 33: 472–500.

Barak N, Wall-Alonso E, Sitrin MD. (2002) Evaluation of stress factors and body weight adjustments currently used to estimate energy expenditure in hospitalized patients. *JPEN. J. Parenter. Enteral. Nutr.* 26: 231–238.

Baumgartner A, Bargetzi A, Zueger N, *et al.* (2017) Revisiting nutritional support for allogeneic hematologic stem cell transplantation-a systematic review. *Bone Marrow Transplant.* 52: 506–513.

BDA. (2016) *Neutropenic Dietary Advice for Haematology Patients.* Available at https://www.bda.uk.com/improvinghealth/healthprofessionals/neutropenic_dietary_advice_for_haematology_patients. Accessed 31 May 2017.

Beckerson J, Szydlo RM, Hickson M, *et al.* (2018) Impact of route and adequacy of nutritional intake on outcomes of allogeneic haematopoietic cell transplantation for haematologic malignancies. *Clin. Nutr.* 10.1016/j.clnu.2018.03.008.

Black G. (2011) Haemato-oncology. In: Shaw C (ed) *Nutrition and Cancer.* Chichester: Wiley Blackwell, pp. 287–310.

Bulley S, Gassas A, Dupuis LL, *et al.* (2008) Inferior outcomes for overweight children undergoing allogeneic stem cell transplantation. *Br. J. Haematol.* 140(2): 214–217.

Cereda E, Turrini M, Ciapanna D, *et al.* (2007) Assessing energy expenditure in cancer patients: a pilot validation of a new wearable device. *JPEN J. Parenter. Enteral Nutr.* 31: 502–507.

Coppell JA, Richardson PG, Soiffer R, *et al.* (2010) Hepatic veno-occlusive disease following stem cell transplantation: incidence, clinical course, and outcome. *Biol. Blood Marrow Transplant.* 16(2): 157–168.

Crowther M, Avenell A, Culligan DJ. (2009) Systematic review and meta-analyses of studies of glutamine supplementation in haematopoietic stem cell transplantation. *Bone Marrow Transplant.* 44: 413–425.

da Gama Torres HO, Vilela EG, da Cunha AS, *et al.* (2008) Efficacy of glutamine-supplemented parenteral nutrition on short-term survival following allo-SCT: a randomized study. *Bone Marrow Transplant.* 41: 1021–1027.

Defranchi RL, Bordalejo A, Canueto I, *et al.* (2014) Evolution of nutritional status in patients with autologous and allogeneic hematopoietic stem cell transplant. *Support Care Cancer* 23: 1341–1347.

DeMille D, Deming P, Lupinacci P, *et al.* (2006) The effect of the neutropenic diet in the outpatient setting: a pilot study. *Oncol. Nurs. Forum.* 33: 337–343.

European Group for Bone Marrow Trans plantation (2012) *Haemopoietic Stem Cell Transplantation*, 6th ed. Paris: European School of Haematology.

Fuji S, Kim SW, Yoshimura K, *et al.* (2009) Possible association between obesity and posttransplantation complications including infectious diseases and acute graft-versus-host disease. *Biol. Blood Marrow Transplant.* 15: 73–82.

Gardner A, Mattiuzzi G, Faderl S, *et al.* (2008) Randomized comparison of cooked and noncooked diets in patients undergoing remission induction therapy for acute myeloid leukemia. *J. Clin. Oncol.* 26: 5684–5688.

Guieze R, Lemal R, Cabrespine A, *et al.* (2014) Enteral versus parenteral nutritional support in allogeneic haematopoietic stem-cell transplantation. *Clin. Nutr.* 33: 533–538.

Haematological Malignancy Research Network. (2015) Incidence. Available at www.hmrn.org/statistics/incidence. Accessed 31 May 2017.

Iestra JA, Fibbe WE, Zwinderman AH, *et al.* (2002) Body weight recovery, eating difficulties and compliance with dietary advice in the first year after stem cell transplantation: a prospective study. *Bone Marrow Transplant.* 29: 417–424.

Imataki O, Nakatani S, Hasegawa T, *et al.* (2006) Nutritional support for patients suffering from intestinal graft-versus-host disease after allogeneic hematopoietic stem cell transplantation. *Am. J. Hematol.* 81: 747–752.

Keefe DM. (2006) Mucositis management in patients with cancer. *Support Cancer Ther.* 3: 154–157.

Keefe DM, Rassias G, O'Neil L, *et al.* (2007) Severe mucositis: how can nutrition help? *Curr. Opin. Clin. Nutri. Metab. Care.* 10: 627–631.

Lee SJ. (2010) Have we made progress in the management of chronic graft-vs-host disease? *Best Pract. Res Clin. Haematol.* 23: 529–535.

Lipkin AC, Lenssen P, Dickson BJ. (2005) Nutrition issues in hematopoietic stem cell transplantation: state of the art. *Nutr. Clin. Pract.* 20(4): 423–439.

Morishita S, Kaida K, Tanaka T, *et al.* (2012) Prevalence of sarcopenia and relevance of body composition, physiological function, fatigue, and health-related quality of life in patients before allogeneic hematopoietic stem cell transplantation. *Support Care Cancer.* 20(12): 3161–3168.

Murray SM, Pindoria S. (2002) Nutrition support for bone marrow transplant patients. *Cochrane Database Syst. Rev.* (2): CD002920.

Murray SM, Pindoria S. (2008) Nutrition support for bone marrow transplant patients. *Cochrane Database Syst. Rev.* (4): CD002920.

Rubenstein EB, Peterson DE, Schubert M, *et al.* (2004) Clinical practice guidelines for the prevention and treatment of cancer therapy-induced oral and gastrointestinal mucositis. *Cancer.* 100(9): 2026–2046.

Seguy D, Duhamel A, Rejeb MB, *et al.* (2012) Better outcome of patients undergoing enteral tube feeding after myeloablative conditioning for allogeneic stem cell transplantation. *Transplantation.* 94(3): 287–294.

Shah N, Callander N, Ganguly S, *et al.* (2015) Hematopoietic stem cell transplantation for multiple myeloma: guidelines from the American Society for blood and marrow transplantation. *Biol. Blood Marrow Transplant.* 21: 1155–1166.

Sonis ST, Oster G, Fuchs H, *et al.* (2001) Oral mucositis and the clinical and economic outcomes of hematopoietic stem-cell transplantation. *J. Clin. Oncol.* 19(8): 2201–2205.

Stiff P. (2001) Mucositis associated with stem cell transplantation: current status and innovative approaches to management. *Bone Marrow Transplant.* 27(S2): S3–S11.

Thompson JL, Duffy J. (2008) Nutrition support challenges in hematopoietic stem cell transplant patients. *Nutr. Clin. Pract.* 23(5): 533–546.

Trifilio S, Helenowski I, Giel M, *et al.* (2012) Questioning the role of a neutropenic diet following hematopoetic stem cell transplantation. *Biol. Blood Marrow Transplant.* 18(9): 1385–1390.

UK Oral Mucositis in Cancer Group (UKOMiC). (2015) *Mouth Care Guidance and Support in Cancer and Palliative Care*, 2nd edn.

van Tiel F, Harbers MM, Terporten PH, *et al.* (2007) Normal hospital and low-bacterial diet in patients with cytopenia after intensive chemotherapy for hematological malignancy: a study of safety. *Ann. Oncol.* 18(6): 1080–1084.

Wahid SF. (2013) Indications and outcomes of reduced-toxicity hematopoietic stem cell transplantation in adult patients with hematological malignancies. *Int. J. Hematol.* 97(5): 581–598.

Walrath M, Bacon C, Foley S, *et al.* (2014) Gastrointestinal side effects and adequacy of enteral intake in hematopoietic stem cell transplant patients. *Nutr. Clin. Pract.* 30: 305–310.

Weekes CE. (2011) Adult macro and micro nutrient requirements. In: Todorovic VE, Micklewright A (eds) *A Pocket Guide to Clinical Nutrition*. Birmingham: BDA, pp. 3.1–3.20.

Wischmeyer PE. (2003) Clinical applications of L-glutamine: past, present, and future. *Nutr. Clin. Pract.* 18(5): 377–385.

Wohlt PD, Zheng L, Gunderson S, *et al.* (2009) Recommendations for the use of medications with continuous enteral nutrition. *Am. J. Health Syst. Pharm.* 66(16): 1458–1467.

Zauner C, Rabitsch W, Schneeweiss B, *et al.* (2001) Energy and substrate metabolism in patients with chronic extensive graft-versus-host disease. *Transplantation.* 71(4): 524–528.

7.15.9 Cancer cachexia

Rhys White and Saira Chowdhury

Key points

- Cachexia is a complex syndrome associated with anorexia and weight loss. It is frequently accompanied by increased muscle catabolism and inflammation.
- There are currently no universally accepted treatments for cancer cachexia. This remains an area of intense research, and it is likely that management will involve a multimodal approach.

The term cachexia is Greek in origin and is a combination of *kakós* (bad) and *hexis* (condition or appearance) (Doehner & Anker, 2002). It is thought to occur in 50–80% of cancer patients, being more common in solid tumours of the lung and GI tract (Argiles *et al.*, 2014a). There is no universally accepted definition for cachexia; however, an international consensus group has established a cancer cachexia framework (Fearon *et al.*, 2011) which is now widely incorporated into cachexia research (see Figure 7.15.3). This group defines cachexia as '*a multifactorial syndrome characterised by an ongoing loss of skeletal muscle mass (with or without loss of fat mass) that cannot be fully reversed by conventional nutritional support and leads to progressive functional impairment*'. The framework group recommends the building of a data-driven approach for a more robust set of diagnostic criteria which will require further validation and application to clinical practice.

The data repository established by the framework group has enabled the development of a validated robust grading system (grades 1–4) for cancer-associated weight loss incorporating the independent prognostic significance of both BMI and percentage weight loss (Martin *et al.*, 2015). Those with the lowest BMI and highest percentage weight loss had the poorest survival. This is a tool that can be easily applied to clinical practice. Further work is now underway to develop additional diagnostic criteria for food intake, inflammation and muscle loss.

Disease process

The pathophysiology is characterised by a negative protein and energy balance driven by a variable combination of anorexia, catabolism and systemic inflammation (Fearon *et al.*, 2011). The inflammatory process drives many of the metabolic alterations that are observed in cachectic patients.

Inflammation

The presence of tumour is detected by the hypothalamus, which results in the expression of proinflammatory cytokines, e.g. tumour necrosis factor-α, interleukin-1 and interleukin-6. These cytokines initiate the inflammatory response, resulting in the hepatic production of acute-phase proteins, most notably C-reactive protein and fibrinogen. Consequently, amino acids are diverted away from skeletal muscle anabolism to the production of acute-phase proteins, while visceral protein mass is preserved (Tisdale, 2002).

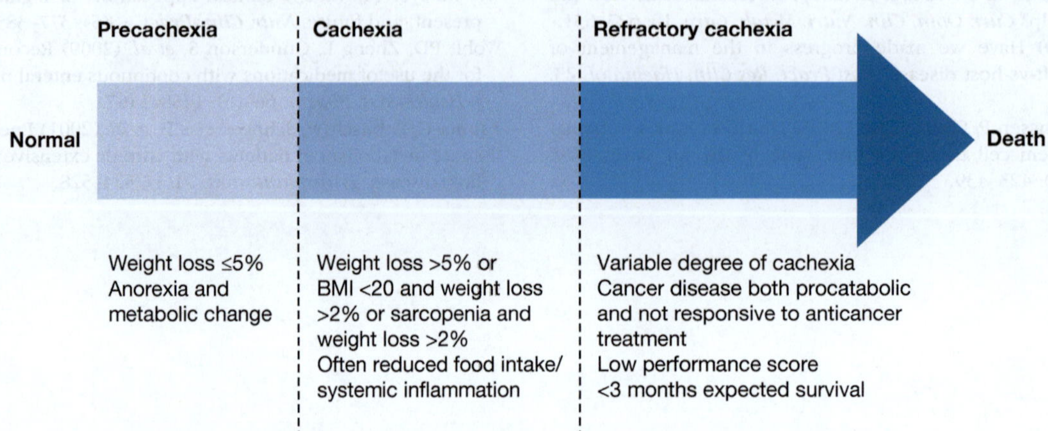

Figure 7.15.3 International consensus cancer cachexia framework classification (Fearon *et al.*, 2011; Reproduced with permission from Elsevier)

Catabolism

Tumour-related factors, e.g. proteolysis-inducing factor and lipid-mobilising factor, are instrumental in mobilising substrates to cause muscle wasting and depletion of fat mass. Proteolysis-inducing factor plays a key role in skeletal atrophy and reduced muscle function by promoting protein degradation, reducing protein synthesis and initiating apoptosis. Skeletal muscle depletion is particularly detrimental as it contributes significantly to functional impairment and reduced quality of life (Dodson *et al.*, 2011). The loss of fat stores, particularly white adipose tissue, occurs due to an escalation in lipolytic activity through the action of lipid-mobilising factor and a decrease in formation of adipose tissue. The cytokines, tumour necrosis factor-α, interleukin-1 and interleukin-6 have also been implicated in adipose tissue depletion. Tumour necrosis factor-α exerts its catabolic effects through an increase in gluconeogenesis and lipolysis; it contributes to insulin resistance, impaired lipogenesis, induction of muscle degradation and inhibition of myogenesis; causes decrease in the synthesis of proteins, lipids and glycogen; and leads to increased interleukin-1 levels (Fearon *et al.*, 2012; Tisdale, 2009).

Increase in resting energy expenditure

In contrast to the starvation state, resting energy expenditure may be increased in the cachectic state, although it is not universally increased across all tumour types. The increase in futile cycle activity occurring in cancer contributes to elevated resting energy expenditure. The anaerobic glycolysis that takes place in cancer cells produces lactate. Lactate is recycled between the tumour and liver through the Cori cycle to generate glucose, which is a highly energy-inefficient process and increases the resting energy expenditure (Argiles *et al.*, 2014b). It is also suggested that white adipose tissue undergoes a browning process to convert to brown adipose tissue, a highly thermogenic tissue, which results in increased lipid mobilisation and energy expenditure (Petruzzelli *et al.*, 2014).

Anorexia

Cytokines, circulating hormones, and the action of neuropeptides and neurotransmitters collectively contribute to the anorexia symptoms of cancer. Raised cytokine levels lead to hyperactivation of the anorexigenic pathways and inhibition of orexigenic pathways, resulting in reduced appetite pathways (Scarlett *et al.*, 2007; Tuca *et al.*, 2013). Fat mass depletion is associated with reduced leptin release, which ordinarily stimulates appetite. However in cachexia, raised levels of tumour necrosis factor-α and interleukin-1 increases plasma leptin levels. This concurrently suppresses the orexigenic pathway and stimulates the anorexigenic pathways, resulting in unopposed anorexia (Sarraf *et al.*, 1997). Some evidence suggests that tumour necrosis factor-α and interleukin-1 mimic leptin signalling, which disrupts the orexigenic response to reduced leptin levels (Bing *et al.*, 2001; Mantovani *et al.*, 2000). Interleukin-1 stimulates hypothalamic serotonin release, which activates orexigenic pathways, causing early satiety and reduced appetite (Heisler *et al.*, 2002; Shintani *et al.*, 1993). The action of serotonin also contributes to thermogenesis in brown tissue, resulting in increased resting energy expenditure (Arruda *et al.*, 2010).

Nutritional assessment

In patients identified as at risk of malnutrition or cachexia, factors such as appetite, dietary intake, muscle mass, strength, physical function, catabolic drivers and psychosocial effects should be assessed to guide nutritional interventions (Arends *et al.*, 2017; Fearon *et al.*, 2011). There is no consensus on the individual methods to assess these domains, although the consensus framework group and the European Society for Clinical Nutrition and Metabolism (ESPEN) provide some examples of possible methods/tools that can be used (Table 7.15.11). Some validated nutritional assessment tools are also available, with Patient Generated Subjective Global Assessment (PG-SGA) being widely used as an assessment of nutritional risk in cancer patients (Bauer *et al.*, 2002).

Management

Cancer cachexia remains largely an untreated condition with limited strong evidence for individual treatments. Treatment should take into account the stage of cachexia and the prognosis of the patient, including whether anti-cancer therapy is planned, in order to ensure that appropriate goals are set. In pre-cachexia, the treatment goals are most likely to relate to reversal/maintenance of weight and muscle loss, whereas, for those in the refractory stage, goals should be focused on alleviating cancer-related symptoms and improving overall well-being (Radbruch *et al.*, 2010). A multidisciplinary approach involving hospital and community professionals, including dietitians, other therapists and palliative care specialists, is essential. Treatment plans should consider both physiological and psychosocial factors and their impact on both, the patients and their carers. Cachexia is particularly distressing and will require sensitive management due to the often conflicting needs and desires of patients and carers.

The main focus of clinical management is to stimulate appetite and/or gut motility, reduction in systemic inflammation and/or hypercatabolism, or to increase muscle mass and/or improve anabolism (Arends *et al.*, 2017). Table 7.15.12 provides examples of drugs currently used in the management of cancer cachexia. Other pharmacological treatments have been researched, including cannabinoids, androgens, non-steroidal anti-inflammatory drugs (NSAIDs) and branched-chain amino acids, but there is currently insufficient consistent clinical data to recommend their use (Arends *et al.*, 2017). Ghrelin, a gastric peptide, has been extensively researched due to its role in regulating growth hormone release, increasing

Table 7.15.11 Possible methods and tools for the assessment of cancer cachexia (source: adapted from Arends *et al.*, 2017; Fearon *et al.*, 2011)

Cachexia domain/parameter	Assessment method/tool(s)
Dietary intake	Simple qualitative assessment
	Food and fluid charts
	Diet history
	Food recall
	Symptoms impacting on dietary intake, e.g. xerostomia, changes in taste and smell, nausea, vomiting, mucositis, diarrhoea, pain, etc.
Body composition	Weight, height and BMI
	Percentage weight loss
	Dual X ray absorptiometry (DXA)
	Anthropometry
	Computed tomography (CT) or magnetic resonance imaging (MRI) scans at lumbar level 3
	Bioelectrical impedance Analysis (BIA)
Physical performance/strength	WHO/ECOG scale or Karnofsky performance status
	Sit to stand / walking tests
	Hand grip dynamometry
	Patient-reported physical functioning (e.g. European Organisation for Research and Treatment of Cancer, or ('EORTC')
Catabolic drivers	C-reactive protein (CRP)
	Albumin
	Glasgow Prognostic Score (GPS)
Psychosocial effects	Routine questions such as 'how much do you feel distressed about your inability to eat' or 'have you experienced feelings of pressure, guilt or relational stress with regard to food intake and weight-loss'

Table 7.15.12 Examples of drugs used in the management of cancer cachexia

Drug	Action	Disadvantages	Further reading
Megestrol acetate and medroxyprogesterone	Increase appetite and body weight, but not fat-free mass.	Increases risk of thromboembolic events, oedema and death.	Ruiz Garcia *et al.* (2013)
		No improvements have been shown in physical function, fatigue or lean body mass.	
		Inconsistent results in relation to impact on quality of life.	
Corticosteroids (glucocorticoids)	Improve appetite/oral intake and quality of life.	Protein breakdown, insulin resistance, water retention, adrenal suppression and infections.	Aoyagi *et al.* (2015)
Prokinetics	Stimulate gastric emptying, so are frequently used to improve early satiety and nausea.	Metoclopramide can cause somnolence, depression, hallucinations and extrapyramidal symptoms, as well as potentially irreversible late dyskinesias.	Arends *et al.* (2017)

appetite and food intake, and inhibiting the production of pro-inflammatory cytokines (Esposito *et al.*, 2015). Anamorelin, an orally active novel ghrelin receptor agonist, has been investigated in a number of double-blind, placebo-controlled trials, and has been shown to improve appetite, body weight and lean body mass as compared to placebo, although overall survival and handgrip strength did not improve (Nishie *et al.*, 2017). It is anticipated that anamorelin will become licenced for clinical use in the future.

Nutritional management

Nutrition support in patients with cachexia may increase body weight where it meets the nutritional deficit. However, it has not been shown to have a demonstrable effect on lean body mass, and therefore does not improve functional status or quality of life where weight loss arises as a result of metabolic disturbances (Dodson *et al.*, 2011; Kotler, 2000). The initiation of artificial nutrition support may reduce carer anxiety and improve a patient's psychological well-being (Bruera & Sweeney, 2000). In the absence of starvation, and where gastrointestinal function and integrity are normal, parenteral nutrition should not be used in catabolic patients (Blum *et al.*, 2010). However, patients with active tumours and significant starvation from bowel obstruction or malabsorptive symptoms do benefit from parenteral nutrition (Hoda *et al.*, 2005). Parenteral nutrition in these conditions may prevent further deterioration in nutritional status, but will not treat cachexia (Bozzetti *et al.*, 1999), and its use should be considered carefully (see Chapter 6.5, Parenteral nutrition). A recent review on supplementing vitamins, minerals, proteins and other nutritional substrates in cancer cachexia concluded that no positive recommendation can currently be made supporting their use, and that further research is needed to ascertain their safety and efficacy (Mochamat *et al.*, 2017). There is emerging evidence to support high protein intakes to facilitate whole-body protein anabolism in cancer patients. While current guidelines recommend protein intakes of at least 1–1.5 g/kg/day (Arends *et al.*, 2017), new evidence suggests that intakes of up to 2 g/kg/day may be required to achieve positive protein balance in the presence of insulin resistance, impaired glucose utilisation and whole-body protein anabolism (Bozzetti & Bozzetti, 2013; Winter *et al.*, 2012). Further research into protein intake at this level is required before it can be translated into a recommendation.

One nutrition intervention in cachectic patients is the prescription of pharmacological doses of eicosapentaenoic acid. Eicosapentaenoic acid is an n-3 polyunsaturated fat, found predominantly in oily fish, and has immune-modulating and anti-inflammatory properties. Trials using eicosapentaenoic acid to treat cancer cachexia demonstrate divergent results. Observed benefits include a reduction in resting energy expenditure and inflammatory mediators. Additional positive outcomes include increases in appetite, energy intake, body weight, lean body mass, quality of life and physical activity; and reduced frequency of reported anorexia, fatigue and neuropathic toxicity in those undergoing chemotherapy (Mocellin *et al.*, 2016; Sanchez-Lara *et al.*, 2014; Trabal *et al.*, 2010). However, these findings are not confirmed by large, randomised clinical trials (Bruera *et al.*, 2003; Fearon *et al.*, 2006). Subsequent systematic reviews have concluded that there is currently insufficient evidence to support the use of eicosapentaenoic acid supplementation in cancer cachexia (Dewey *et al.*, 2007; Mazzotta & Jeney, 2009; Ries *et al.*, 2012). In contrast to these findings, two systematic reviews found that eicosapentaenoic acid supplementation did improve nutritional parameters in weight-losing cancer patients (Colomer *et al.*, 2007) and in patients undergoing chemotherapy and/or radiotherapy (de Aguiar Pastore Silva *et al.*, 2015). International guidelines acknowledge the low-level evidence available to support eicosapentaenoic acid use, but do recommend it as safe for use in patients with advanced cancer undergoing chemotherapy, who are at risk of weight loss or are malnourished. Further research into the role of eicosapentaenoic acid on body composition, quality of life and clinical outcome is recommended (Arends *et al.*, 2017; Bauer *et al.*, 2006).

Exercise and physical activity are also seen as important interventions for cachexia management. Physical activity can reduce muscle catabolism and increase anabolism, and also has the potential to reduce inflammation. However, there are limited studies that have investigated physical activity in cancer cachexia. ESPEN guidelines (Arends *et al.*, 2017) recommend either maintenance of, or an increase in, the physical activity levels of all cancer patients, and that resistance exercise should be incorporated to maintain muscle mass and strength. Given the complex multifactorial nature of cancer cachexia, the most effective management is likely to involve multimodal interventions that include nutrition, exercise and drug therapy. Research is underway investigating these multimodal approaches, and results are eagerly anticipated.

Acknowledgement

The editor acknowledges the prior contribution of Deborah Howland.

Further reading

Shaw C (ed). (2010) *Nutrition and cancer*. Oxford: Wiley Blackwell.

References

Aoyagi T, Terracina KP, Raza A, *et al.* (2015). Cancer cachexia, mechanism and treatment. *World J. Gastrointest. Oncol.* 7(4): 17–29.

Arends J, Bachmann P, Baracos V, *et al.* (2017) ESPEN guidelines on nutrition in cancer patients. *Clin. Nutr.* 36: 11–48.

Argiles J, Busquets S, Stemmler B, *et al.* (2014a) Cancer cachexia; understanding the molecular basis. *Nat. Rev. Cancer.* 14(11): 754–762.

Argiles JM, Fontes-Olivera CC, Toledo M, *et al.* (2014b) Cachexia: a problem of energetic inefficiency. *J. Cachexia. Sarcopenia Muscle.* 5: 279–286.

Arruda AP, Milanski M, Romanatto T, *et al.* (2010) Hypothalamic actions of tumor necrosis factor alpha provide the thermogenic core for the wastage syndrome in cachexia. *Endocrinology.* 151: 683–694.

Bauer J, Capra S, Ferguson M. (2002) Use of the scored Patient-Generated Subjective Global Assessment (PG-SGA) as a nutritional assessment tool in patients with cancer. *Eur. J. Clin. Nutr.* 56: 779–785.

Bauer JD, Ash S, Davidson WL, *et al.* (2006) Evidence based practice guidelines for the nutritional management of cancer cachexia. *Nutr. Diet.* 63: S3–S32.

Bing C, Taylor S, Tisdale MJ, *et al.* (2001) Cachexia in MAC16 adenocarcinoma: suppression of hunger despite normal regulation of leptin, insulin and hypothalamic neuropeptide Y. *J. Neurochem.* 79: 1004–1012.

Blum D, Omlin A, Fearon, K, *et al.* (2010) Evolving classification systems for cachexia: ready for clinical practice? *Support Cancer Care.* 18: 273–279.

Bozzetti F, Bozzetti V. (2013) Is the intravenous administration of amino acid adequate in cancer patients? A critical appraisal of literature. *Clin. Nutr.* 32: 142–146.

Bozzetti F, Gavazzi C, Mariani L, *et al.* (1999) Artificial nutrition in cancer patients: which route, what composition? *World J. Surg.* 23: 577–583.

Bruera E, Sweeney C. (2000) Cachexia and asthenia in cancer patients. *Lancet Oncol.* 1: 138–147.

Bruera E, Strasser F, Palmer JL, *et al.* (2003) Effect of dish oil on appetite and other symptoms in patients with advanced cancer and anorexia/cachexia: a double-blind, placebo-controlled study. *J. Clin. Oncol.* 21: 129–134.

Colomer R, Moreno-Nogueira JM, García-Luna PP, *et al.* (2007) N-3 fatty acids, cancer and cachexia: a systematic review of the literature. *Br. J. Nutr.* 97: 823–831.

de Aguiar Pastore Silva J, Emilia de Souza Fabre M, Waitzberg DL. (2015) Omega-3 supplements for patients in chemotherapy and/or radiotherapy: a systematic review. *Clin. Nutr.* 34: 359–366.

Dewey A, Baughan C, Dean T, *et al.* (2007) Eicosapentaenoic acid (EPA, an omega-3 fatty acid from fish oils) for the treatment of cancer cachexia. *Cochrane Database Syst. Rev.* (4): CD004597.

Dodson S, Baracos VE, Jatoi A, *et al.* (2011) Muscle wasting in cancer cachexia: clinical implications, diagnosis, and emerging treatment strategies. *Ann. Rev. Med.* 62: 265–279.

Doehner W, Anker S. (2002) Cardiac cachexia in early literature: a review of research prior to Medline. *Int. J. Cardiol.* 85: 7–14.

Esposito A, Criscitiello C, Gelao L, *et al.* (2015) Mechanisms of anorexia-cachexia syndrome and rational for treatment with selective ghrelin receptor agonist. *Cancer Treat. Rev.* 41: 793–797.

Fearon KC, Barber MD, Moses AG, *et al.* (2006) Double-blind, placebo-controlled, randomized study of eicosapentaenoic acid diester in patients with cancer cachexia. *J. Clin. Oncol.* 24: 3401–3407.

Fearon K, Strasser F, Anker SD, *et al.* (2011) Definition and classification of cancer cachexia: an international consensus. *Lancet Oncol.* 12(5): 489–495.

Fearon KC, Glass DJ, Guttridge DC. (2012) Cancer cachexia: mediators, signaling, and metabolic pathways. *Cell Metab.* 16(8): 153–166.

Garcia RV *et al.* (2013) Megestrol acetate for treatment of anorexia-cachexia syndrome. *Cochrane Database Syst Rev.* 3: CD004310. doi: 10.1002/14651858.

Heisler LK, Cowley MA, Tecott LH, *et al.* (2002) Activation of central melanocortin pathways by fenfluramine. *Science.* 297: 609–611.

Hoda D, Jatoi A, Burnes J, *et al.* (2005) Should patients with advanced, incurable cancers ever be sent home with total parenteral nutrition? A single institution's 20 year experience. *Cancer.* 103(4): 863–868.

Kotler D. (2000) *Cachexia. Ann. Intern. Med.* 133: 622–634.

Mantovani G, Macciò A, Mura L, *et al.* (2000) Serum levels of leptin and proinflammatory cytokines in patients with advanced-stage cancer at different sites. *J. Mol. Med. (Berl.)* 78: 554–561.

Martin L, Senesse P, Gioulbasanis I, *et al.* (2015) Diagnostic criteria for the classification of cancer-associated weight loss. *J. Clin. Oncol.* 33(1): 90–99.

Mazzotta P, Jeney CM. (2009) Anorexia-cachexia syndrome: a systematic review of the role of dietary polyunsaturated fatty acids in the management of symptoms, survival, and quality of life. *J. Pain Symptom Manage.* 37: 1069–1077.

Mocellin MC, Camargo CQ, Nunes EA, *et al.* (2016) A systematic review and meta-analysis of the N-3 polyunsaturated fatty acids effects on inflammatory markers in colorectal cancer. *Clin. Nutr.* 35: 359–369.

Mochamat, Cuhls H, Marinova M, *et al.* (2017) A systematic review on the role of vitamins, minerals, proteins, and other supplements for the treatment of cachexia in cancer: a European Palliative Care Research Centre cachexia project. *J. Cachexia. Sarcopenia Muscle* 8: 25–39.

Nishie K, Yamamoto S, Nagata C, *et al.* (2017) Anamorelin for advanced non-small-cell lung cancer with cachexia: systematic review and meta-analysis. *Lung Cancer.* 112: 25–34.

Petruzzelli M, Schweiger M, Schreiber R, *et al.* (2014) A switch from white to brown fat increases energy expenditure in cancer associated cachexia. *Cell Metab.* 20: 433–447.

Radbruch L, Elsner F, Trottenberg P, *et al.* (2010) *Clinical practice guidelines on cancer cachexia in advanced cancer patients. Aachen, Department of Palliative Medicine/European Palliative Care Research Collaboration.* Available at http://www.cancercachexia.com/literature-watch/43_clinical-practice-guidelines-on-cancer-cachexia-in-advanced-cancer. Accessed 17 April 2018.

Ries A, Trottenberg P, Elsner F, *et al.* (2012) A systematic review on the role of fish oil for the treatment of cachexia in advanced cancer: an EPCRC cachexia guidelines project. *Palliat. Med.* 26: 294–304.

Sanchez-Lara K, Turcott JG, Juarez-Hernandez E, *et al.* (2014) Effects of an oral nutritional supplement containing eicosapentaenoic acid on nutritional and clinical outcomes in patients with advanced non-small cell lung cancer: randomised trial. *Clin. Nutr.* 33: 1017–1023.

Sarraf P, Frederich RC, Turner EM, *et al.* (1997) Multiple cytokines and acute inflammation raise mouse leptin levels: potential role in inflammatory anorexia. *J. Exp. Med.* 185: 171–175.

Scarlett JM, Jobst EE, Enriori PJ, *et al.* (2007) Regulation of central melanocortin signalling by interleukin-1 beta. *Endocrinology.* 148: 4217–4225.

Shintani F, Kanba S, Nakaki T, *et al.* (1993) Interleukin-1 beta augments release of norepinephrine, dopamine, and serotonin in the rat anterior hypothalamus. *J. Neurosci.* 13: 3574–3581.

Tisdale MJ. (2002) Cachexia in cancer patients. *Nat. Rev. Cancer.* 2: 862–871.

Tisdale MJ. (2009) Mechanisms of cancer cachexia. *Physiol. Rev.* 89: 381–410.

Trabal J, Leyes P, Forga M, *et al.* (2010) Potential usefulness of an EPA-enriched nutritional supplement on chemotherapy tolerability in cancer patients without overt malnutrition. *Nutr. Hosp.* 25: 736–740.

Tuca A, Jimenez-Fonseca P, Gascón P. (2013) Clinical evaluation and optimal management of cancer cachexia. *Crit. Rev. Oncol. Hematol.* 88: 625–636.

Winter A, Macadams J, Chevalier S. (2012) Normal protein anabolic response to hyperaminoacidemia in insulin-resistant patients with lung cancer cachexia. *Clin. Nutr.* 31: 765–773.

7.16 Palliative and end-of-life care

Lucy Eldridge

Key points

- Palliative care is the active holistic care of patients with advanced progressive illness, providing management of pain and other symptoms, as well as psychological, social and spiritual support.
- The primary nutritional objective is to maintain or improve the quality of life.
- Decisions concerning nutrition should always be patient centred, individualised and open to change in line with the patient's condition.
- Artificial nutritional support is a medical intervention, and therefore decision-making should consider benefits, burdens, harms and risks.

Palliative care is the active holistic care of patients with advanced progressive illness. It places equal importance on an individual's physical, emotional, spiritual and social needs (Hospice UK, 2016). The universal definition of palliative care is '*an approach that aims to improve the quality of life of patients and their families facing the problems associated with life-threatening illness, through the prevention and relief of suffering by means of early identification and impeccable assessment and treatment of pain and other problems whether physical, psychosocial or spiritual*' (WHO, 2011). Palliative care is based on several principles (WHO, 2011) that aim to:

- Provide relief from pain and other distressing symptoms.
- Affirm life and regard dying as a normal process.
- Neither hasten nor postpone death.
- Integrate the psychological and spiritual aspects of patient care.
- Offer a support system to help patients live as actively as possible until death.
- Offer a support system to help the family cope during the patient's illness and in their bereavement.
- Use a team approach to address the needs of patients and their families, including bereavement counselling, if indicated.
- Enhance quality of life, and also positively influence the course of illness.

Palliative care is applicable early in the course of illness and in conjunction with other therapies that are intended to prolong life or symptom control, e.g. chemotherapy or radiation therapy. Patients may be in the palliative stage of their disease for months or years. It may be difficult to define what stage a patient has reached, and, although clear that life expectancy is limited, identifying the length of time remaining may be impossible. Patients and carers may associate palliative care specifically with care for dying people, which consequently may have significant implications for acceptability and access (NICE, 2004).

The hospice movement has adapted to the changing needs of the population over the past 50 years and led the way for better end-of-life care throughout the health service (Hospice UK, 2016). The care delivered can be provided at home, in day-care centres, nursing homes and hospitals, as well as within a hospice or palliative care unit. It involves a multi-professional approach that may include healthcare and social professionals, as well as members of charitable, voluntary and independent organisations (NICE, 2004). The aim is to provide care based on individual needs and personal choice. Although palliative care is focused on the patient, providing support to carers is recognised as being an integral part of care.

It is the responsibility of all healthcare and social care professionals who provide day-to-day care to assess and meet the needs of patients and their families within their limits, and know when to seek advice from or refer to a specialist palliative care service (NICE, 2004). Specialist providers of palliative care have the expertise to address patients' complex needs and symptom control management. The role of the dietitian within the palliative care setting is to help identify and address nutritional factors that impair a patient's physical and

Manual of Dietetic Practice, Sixth Edition. Edited by Joan Gandy.

Companion website: www.manualofdieteticpractice.com

psychological well-being, with the primary nutritional objective of maintaining or improving the quality of life for that individual. The dietitian in this setting should:

- Assess the nutritional needs and problems of the patient.
- Establish when nutritional support measures may be appropriate.
- Advise on how the nutritional requirements of the patient may be met.
- Suggest ways in which the nutrition-related problems caused by the physical or psychological effects of the disease or its treatment may be alleviated.
- Provide advice and guidance for carers.
- Liaise with catering services to provide a flexible approach to food provision.
- Identify need for eating aids to assist independent eating.
- Provide training and support for professional colleagues.

Dietitians working in the field of palliative care require good communication skills in order to create an empathic relationship with patients and carers. It is the responsibility of all dietitians involved in the care of those with life-limiting illnesses to facilitate the provision of appropriate nutritional care. They should have access to support and advice within the multidisciplinary team, especially for more complex cases.

Diagnostic criteria and classification

The target population for palliative care is wide and should not be constrained by diagnosis. Although historically associated with cancer, it is now recognised that palliative care equally applies to those with other non-malignant life-limiting conditions, e.g. motor neurone disease, dementia, heart failure, end-stage diabetes and renal disease. In order to provide high-quality palliative care regardless of diagnosis, a whole-system coordinated care pathway 8 approach, involving all providers of palliative care in all locations, has been strongly recommended (DH, 2008). This requires identification of people approaching the end of life; assessing their needs; initiating discussions surrounding preferences and wishes for care; agreeing on a care plan to reflect these; and supporting carers, both during a person's illness and after his or her death (NICE, 2015).

Nutritional aspects

In addition to providing nutrients, nutrition has important psychological, social, spiritual and cultural roles in the palliative stages of illness. Eating can help maintain a sense of normality in a patient's life. As food intake is also associated with health and well-being, it may evoke feelings of fear and despair in those who are struggling to eat. This can have a major effect on an individual's self-esteem and confidence, leading to social isolation and depression. Progressive illness may also affect nutritional status in several ways:

- The psychological effect of being diagnosed with an incurable and progressive illness is profound, especially if the diagnosis is unexpected. The consequent anxiety, depression and, perhaps, sense of hopelessness can markedly impair food intake.
- Worsening symptoms of the disease, particularly those of a fatigue-related, dysphagic or gastrointestinal nature, may make eating physically difficult and lead to associations with discomfort.
- Medication may cause side effects (e.g. nausea, vomiting or diarrhoea) that reduce food intake. Drowsiness induced by sedatives or pain relievers, such as opioids or narcotics, may make patients disinclined to eat.
- Treatments such as chemotherapy or radiotherapy and associated side effects can markedly affect food intake and increase the likelihood of nutritional deficiencies.
- Nutritional requirements may be increased by the physiological effects of the illness (e.g. pyrexia, secondary infection, increasing tumour mass), or by nutrient losses (e.g. malabsorption).
- As the final phase of the illness develops, physiological functions such as gastric emptying, digestion, absorption and peristalsis may decline. Both appetite and the ability to tolerate food will decrease.

Nutritional assessment

It is important that patients are assessed throughout their illness to ensure that nutritional support is proactive instead of reactive, thus ensuring that patients do not enter the terminal phases of their illness in a state of serious nutritional depletion. The assessment of palliative patients will vary according to individual needs, problems and clinical circumstances, but will primarily follow the following stepwise process:

- Defining the clinical condition, prognosis and aim of any medical intervention.
- Assessing eating habits.
- Establishing current nutritional status; it may not always be appropriate to regularly weigh a patient, as this can cause anxiety.
- Identifying nutrition-related problems or barriers to food and fluid intake, and evaluating their physical and psychological impacts.
- Exploring the nutritional concerns of patients and their family and/or carers.
- Discussing with patients and carers dietary goals that are appropriate and achievable.
- Integrating these goals into the care plan in a way that is compatible with medical and nursing objectives.
- Regularly reviewing progress, evaluating the effectiveness of any measures implemented, and modifying them as necessary.

Screening tools and the weighing of patients will vary depending on where the patient is based and local policy and practice; there are no specific palliative care nutrition screening tools. In a palliative care setting, it is important that screening assess both quantitative and qualitative issues, including what food means and how important it is to the individual at any particular stage (Hopkinson *et al.*, 2008). Food issues, especially weight loss, can be more distressing to carers than patients (Hopkinson, 2016). The relevance of biochemistry and weighing patients will depend on the prognosis, the medical intent at that stage of palliative care and the patient's preference.

Nutritional management

The principal objectives are to maximise food enjoyment and minimise food-related discomfort. It is also important to prevent or treat avoidable and unnecessary malnutrition, since this can affect both physical and psychological well-being. However, it is equally important that nutritional support measures not be so invasive or unacceptable to the patient that they impair quality of life. The objectives should always be one or more of the following:

- Retain the ability to derive pleasure from food and the social aspects of eating.
- Retain physical strength long enough to fulfil final wishes and ambitions.
- Have sufficient physical strength to obtain benefit from rehabilitation.
- Retain some control over the disease process through attention to nutrition.
- Die with dignity and not as a result of starvation.

Patients should be encouraged to retain an interest in food, and to regard good nutrition as a positive aid to help maintain strength and improve well-being. Nutritional counselling on both the use of nutrient-dense foods and finding foods the patient enjoys is important, and should consider symptoms, emotional adaptation to illness, and social circumstances (Hopkinson *et al.*, 2011). If nutritional needs are not being met, suggestions to improve intake by increasing the frequency of food consumption and choosing foods of greater nutrient density are useful first steps. Fortification strategies to boost energy intake can be effective, but if these prove inadequate, or food intake is particularly poor, oral supplements may be helpful. However, it is important to be aware that, although nutritional supplements can be useful, they can divert patients from the foods they want to eat. In addition, patients do not always like supplements, and may feel guilty if they are unable to take them (Hill & Hart, 2001). Forcing food on those who have no desire to eat and drink can cause distress (McClement *et al.*, 2003; Strasser *et al.*, 2007).

Patients may have reduced their dietary intake for a variety of reasons; however, simple measures can often make an enormous difference to nutrient intake. Ideally, food should be offered that is attractively presented and of high quality. Menus should be tempting and varied, with snacks that can be provided at any time. The giving and receiving of nourishment is a means of showing love and affection, and food refusal can consequently cause offence and create barriers within the family unit. Involving carers in discussions about the nutritional needs and difficulties of the patient, and establishing realistic expectations, can help defuse problems. Table 7.16.1 gives suggestions that may be particularly helpful for people within palliative care (see Chapter 6.3, Oral nutritional support).

Maintaining good hydration

Good hydration is essential, but it is important that adequate fluid provision not be achieved in a way that impairs appetite and compromises nutrient intake from food. If food intake is generally poor, nutrient-rich sources of fluids should be encouraged. Patients at the end of their lives should have individualised approaches to address their hydration needs (NICE, 2015).

Dysphagia

Dysphagia requires expert assessment and management in order to provide food of an appropriate consistency, while also maintaining nutrient intake (see Chapter 7.3, Dysphagia). It is important to ensure that these are nutrient dense as appropriate. At the end of life, a risk management approach, allowing patients to eat and drink even with an unsafe swallow, is deemed the most appropriate route, and may offer better quality of life (NICE, 2015; Royal College of Physicians (RCP), 2010).

Therapeutic diets

For patients who have pre-existing conditions that require special diets (e.g. diabetes mellitus and hyperlipidaemia), consideration should be given to the appropriateness of the dietary restriction. For individuals in the advanced stages of disease, the restrictions could be relaxed or stopped; however, this needs to be done with reassurance and encouragement. With diabetes, it would be more preferable to adjust medication to manage symptoms than limit diet, especially for those with a poor appetite (Diabetes UK, 2013).

Artificial nutritional support

Artificial nutritional support (ANS) has become part of palliative care and, for selected patients, has the potential to increase both survival and quality of life (Druml *et al.*, 2016). It is often used in individuals who, due to increasing debility, dysphagia or intestinal failure, can only obtain adequate nutrition through enteral or parenteral feeding. However, it is important to remember that, for some, ANS may cause more harm than good. Clinicians need to make a decision based on the perceived benefits, harms, risks and burdens of ANS in individual patient circumstances (Table 7.16.2). Cochrane reviews assessing the effects of ANS (Good *et al.*, 2014a) and hydration (Good *et al.*, 2014b) in palliative patients concluded that there was a lack of randomised controlled studies, and that no recommendations for practices could therefore be made.

There has been an increase in home parenteral nutrition in palliative patients, especially for cancer, and there

Table 7.16.1 Dietary guidance for people with palliative care needs

Symptom	Dietary guidance
Poor appetite	Eat small, frequent, attractively presented foods.
	Eat favourite foods or those found to be most enjoyable.
	Consume fluids after, rather than with, meals to maximise food intake.
	Ensure posture helps rather than hinders eating.
	Eat in surroundings that are as pleasant as possible.
	Eat in the company of others, unless a preference is expressed to eat alone.
	Consider appetite stimulants, e.g. alcohol, megestrol acetate or low-dose steroids.
Sore mouth	Replace salty, spicy or acidic foods with blander, less astringent alternatives.
	Eat soft, moist foods.
	Cold foods are more soothing.
Dry mouth (xerostomia)	Take frequent, small sips of water.
	Suck ice cubes, ice lollies or citrus-flavoured boiled sweets.
	Chew fruit-flavoured sweets.
	Meals should be moist in texture.
	Consider artificial saliva
Taste changes	Problematic foods should be substituted with nutritionally similar alternatives: • Poultry or fish instead of red meat. • Soft drinks or milk instead of tea or coffee. • Boiled sweets or pastilles instead of chocolate. • Experiment with herbs and spices in cooking
Early satiety	Consume small, frequent amounts of nutrient-dense foods.
Belching and/or flatulence	Avoid foods and drinks that exacerbate gas production, e.g.: • Carbonated beverages, beer • Brassicas (broccoli, spinach, cauliflower, Brussels sprouts), peas, beans, sweetcorn, onion and radish.
	Reduce the amount of ingested air by: • Eating slowly. • Keeping the mouth shut when chewing and swallowing. • Avoiding sucking drinks through a straw.
Constipation	Ensure adequate medical intervention.
	Increase fluid intake without compromising nutritional intake.
	Confirm that the patient does not have an intestinal obstruction, or is dehydrated.
	If appropriate, increase fibre-rich foods, but care should be taken with patients whose appetite is decreased.
Diarrhoea	Establish cause.
	Avoid foods that appear to exacerbate symptoms.
	If appropriate, ensure that antidiarrhoeal drugs have been prescribed.
	Encourage a wide variety of foods.
Hypercalcaemia	Do not reduce or restrict dietary sources of calcium.
	Encourage carbonated drinks containing phosphoric acid.

is evidence that it may be beneficial, but only if the following applies:

- Patient cannot be fed orally or enterally.
- If performance status (Karnofsky performance status >50) and quality of life are acceptable, prognosis is >3 months, and therefore it is anticipated that starvation would be the cause of death rather than tumour progression.
- If there is a strong patient and family motivation to undertake the provision of parenteral nutrition at home (Bozzetti *et al.*, 2009).

Ethical and legal considerations

The RCP (2010), the General Medical Council (GMC, 2010) and ESPEN (Druml *et al.*, 2016) provide guidance on end-of-life care, which includes nutritional advice.

Oral nutrition

Oral nutrition and hydration are considered basic care, both ethically and legally, and should always be provided unless actively resisted by the patient. It is important that patients are monitored, and, if a patient refuses food, this issue should be explored with the patient and

Table 7.16.2 Potential benefits, harms, risks and burdens of artificial nutrition support in palliative care (Brotherton & Judd, 2007; Dy, 2006; Raijmakers *et al.*, 2011; Shaw, 2011)

Benefits	Assess for nutrition, fluid and medication.
	May improve quality of life, functional status and a sense of well-being.
	May prevent deterioration and reduce fatigue and chronic nausea.
	Support religious beliefs.
	Decrease the pressure to eat.
Harms	False hope.
	Exacerbation or cause of symptoms, e.g. gastrointestinal, fluid overload or ascites.
	Altered body image.
Risks	Complications of placement, metabolic disturbances, wound infection, abdominal pain, leakage.
	Sepsis.
Burdens	Possibly delays discharge or requires hospital admission.
	Time required for training and/or to arrange home care package.
	Carers have greater responsibility.
	Limitations of activities of daily living and of social life.
	Additional monitoring.

documented (GMC, 2010). Food should not be forced upon a patient where this causes unavoidable choking or aspiration (Lennard-Jones, 1998). For a patient who is at risk of aspiration and who wishes to continue with food or fluid, the risks and benefits should be discussed (NICE, 2015).

Artificial nutritional support

All forms of ANS and hydration are deemed to be medical treatment, and as such can be treated as any other form of medical intervention. It is vital that each patient be considered individually, the goals of care be clear and the resulting decision be a joint one, involving both the care team and the patient. Patients cannot insist on artificial nutrition if their doctor feels it is not in their best interests (GMC, 2010). However, patients' wishes are paramount, and competent patients have the absolute right to decide what nutritional support they will or will not accept, even if it is of clinical benefit and refusal could lead to starvation or exacerbation of their symptoms (Druml *et al.*, 2016). Incompetent patients retain this right through a valid advance refusal (HM Government Mental Capacity Act, 2005; NICE, 2015). In patients for whom death is believed to be inevitable and nutrition intervention is not considered to be of benefit, it can be withheld or withdrawn (GMC, 2010). However, if ANS is withheld or withdrawn, it is important to address the anxieties of patients, relatives and carers. The primary goal of treatment in terminal care is the comfort of the patient; therefore, the decision concerning whether or not to feed must be made on this basis (GMC, 2010; RCP, 2010).

Artificial hydration

In the last few days of life, patients may be too weak to take oral foods and fluids. This may be due in part to declining physical function, but is often attributable to the reduced level of consciousness resulting from the use of sedatives and pain-relieving drugs. The use of intravenous hydration at this stage has been a matter of debate and raises a number of ethical issues (Thorns & Garrard, 2003). The extent to which intravenous fluids offer symptomatic relief is unknown, as it is not possible to conduct comparative studies for ethical reasons. It has been argued that artificial rehydration is necessary to satisfy thirst and other symptoms, such as confusion and headaches (Dalal & Bruera, 2004). Others consider that simpler measures, such as attention to oral hygiene, are sufficient to prevent discomfort. It is also argued that intravenous hydration at this stage is unnecessarily invasive and can cause a physical barrier between patients and their families at an important time (Thorns & Garrard, 2003).

The principal conclusion is that a blanket policy of artificial nutrition and hydration, or no artificial nutrition and hydration, is ethically indefensible. Deciding what is appropriate for each case must be based on an individual basis according to the likely benefits and burdens of such intervention. Good-practice decisions concerning artificial nutrition and hydration should involve a multidisciplinary team, the patient and relatives, and carers.

Acknowledgement

The editor acknowledges the prior contribution of Jane Power.

Further reading

Bruerra E, Higginson I, Von Gunten CF, *et al.* (2016) *Textbook of Palliative Medicine and Supportive Care*, 2nd edn. Cleveland: CRC Press.

Preedy V. (2011) *Diet and Nutrition in Palliative Care*. New York: CRC Press.

Shaw C, Eldridge L. (2015) Nutritional considerations for the palliative care patient. *Int. J. Palliat. Nurs.* 21(1): 7–15.

Watson M, Lucas C, Hoy A, *et al.* (2011) *Palliative Adult Network guidelines*, 3rd edn. Available at www.book.pallcare.info.

Internet resources

BDA Palliative Care Subgroup of the Oncology Group, www.bda.uk.com
Cruse Bereavement Care, www.crusebereavementcare.org.uk
Dying Matters, http://www.dyingmatters.org
European Association for Palliative Care, www.eapcnet.eu
Gold Standards Framework, www.goldstandardsframework.org.uk
Hospice UK, www.hospiceuk.org
Macmillan Cancer Support, www.macmillan.org.uk
Marie Curie Cancer Care, www.mariecurie.org.uk
The National Council for Palliative Care, www.ncpc.org.uk
The Scottish Partnership for Palliative Care, www.palliativecarescotland.org.uk

References

Bozzetti F, Arends J, Lundholm K, *et al.* (2009) ESPEN guidelines on parenteral nutrition: non-surgical oncology. *Clin. Nutr.* 28: 445–454.

Brotherton AM, Judd PA. (2007) Quality of life in adult enteral tube feeding patients. *J. Hum. Nutr. Diet.* 20: 513–522.

Dalal S, Bruera E. (2004) Dehydration in cancer patients: to treat or not to treat. *Support. Oncol.* 2(6): 467–479.

DH. (2008) *End of life care strategy: promoting high quality care for all adults at the end of life.* Available at https://www.gov.uk/government/publications/end-of-life-care-strategy-promoting-high-quality-care-for-adults-at-the-end-of-their-life. Accessed 1/6/17.

Diabetes UK. (2013) *End of life diabetes care. Clinical care recommendations*, 2nd edn. Available at www.diabetes.org.uk/nutrition-guidelines. Accessed January 2017.

Druml C, Ballmer P, Druml W, *et al.* (2016) ESPEN guideline on ethical aspects of artificial nutrition and hydration. *Clin. Nutr.* 35: 545–556.

Dy S. (2006) Enteral and parenteral nutrition in terminally ill cancer patients: a review of the literature. *Am. J. Hosp. Palliat. Med.* 23: 369–377.

General Medical Council (GMC). (2010) *Treatment and care towards the end of life: Good practise in decision making.* Available at www.gmc-uk.org/End_of_life.pdf_32486688.pdf. Accessed 1 June 2017.

Good P, Cavenagh J, Mather M, *et al.* (2014a) Medically assisted nutrition for palliative care in adult patients. *Cochrane Database Syst. Rev.* (4): CD006274.

Good P, Cavenagh J, Mather M, *et al.* (2014b) Medically assisted hydration for palliative care in adult patients. *Cochrane Database Syst. Rev.* (2): CD006273.

HM Government Mental Capacity Act. (2005) Available at https://www.legislation.gov.uk/ukpga/2005/9/contents. Accessed 15 November 2018.

Hill D, Hart K. (2001) A practical approach to nutritional support for patients with advanced cancer. *In. J. Palliat. Nurs.* 7(7): 317–321.

Hopkinson JB. (2016) Food connections: a qualitative exploratory study of weight- and eating-related distress in families affected by advanced cancer. *Eur. J. Oncol. Nurs.* 20: 87–96.

Hopkinson JB, Okamoto I, Addington-Hall JM. (2011) What to eat when off treatment and living with involuntary weight loss and cancer: a systematic search and narrative review. *Support Care Cancer.* 19(1): 1–17.

Hopkinson JB, Wright DNM, Foster C. (2008) Management of weight loss and anorexia. *Ann. Oncol.* 19(S7): 289–293.

Hospice UK. (2016) *Hospice Care in the UK 2016.* Available at https://www.cityhospice.org.uk/Handlers/Download.ashx?IDMF=0a8d2609-f4ba-4e10-ae02-38d2d6d3f4c0. Accessed January 2017.

Lennard-Jones J. (1998) *Ethical and Legal Aspects of Clinical Hydration and Nutrition Support.* Maidenhead: BAPEN.

McClement SE, Degner LF, Harlos MS. (2003) Family beliefs regarding the nutritional care of a terminally ill relative: a qualitative study. *J. Palliat. Med.* 6(5): 737–748.

NICE. (2004) *Guidance on Cancer Services: Improving Supportive and Palliative Care for Adults with Cancer.* London: NICE. Available at www.nice.org.uk. Accessed January 2017.

NICE. (2015) *Care of Dying Adults in the Last Days of Life.* London: NICE. Available at www.nice.org.uk. Accessed January 2017.

Raijmakers N, van Zuylen L, Costantini M, *et al.* (2011) Artificial nutrition and hydration in the last week of life in cancer patients. A systematic literature review of practices and effects. *Ann. Oncol.* 22(7): 1478–1486.

Royal College of Physicians (RCP). (2010) *Oral Feeding Difficulties and Dilemmas. A Guide to Practical Care Particularly Towards the End of Life.* London: RCP.

Shaw C. (2011) Nutrition in palliative care. In: Shaw C (ed) *Nutrition and Cancer.* Oxford: Wiley Blackwell, pp. 173–187.

Strasser F, Binswanger J, Cerny T, *et al.* (2007) Fighting a losing battle: eating-related distress of men with advanced cancer and their female partners. A mixed-methods study. *Palliat. Med.* 21: 129–137.

Thorns A, Garrard E. (2003) Ethical issues in care of the dying. In: Ellershaw J, Wilkinson S (eds) *Care of the Dying. A Pathway to Excellence.* Oxford: Oxford University Press.

WHO. (2011) *WHO Definition of Palliative Care.* Available at www.who.int/cancer/palliative/definition/en/. Accessed January 2017.

7.17 Trauma and critical care

7.17.1 Critical care

Ella Terblanche and Charlotte Proctor

Key points

- Up to 75% of patients survive an intensive care unit (ICU) admission; however, many are left with severe weakness and delayed recovery.
- The critical illness, ICU procedures, equipment and medications all influence nutritional provision and need to be accounted for.
- Enteral feeding is the route of choice, and feeding should commence within 48 hours of admission; the accurate assessment of energy and protein requirements remains controversial.
- An individualised approach to nutrition support is advocated that adjusts to the different phases of critical illness.

Approximately half of all prescribed feed is delivered to patients while in an ICU; however, strategies need to be employed to optimise nutrition delivery. ICUs are modern high-tech units with a vast array of equipment designed to support each of the body systems. The ICU multidisciplinary team (MDT) includes intensivists, medical and nursing staff, pharmacists, dietitians and physiotherapists, as well as access to speech and language therapy, occupational therapy and psychology. There are nationally recognised recommendations for the role of the critical care dietitian and clinical standards for dietetic provision (Masterson & Baudouin, 2015). The critical care dietitian should:

- Lead the development and implementation of nutrition-related protocols and guidelines in association with the MDT.
- Consider nutrition risk, when planning patient-specific nutritional interventions such as parenteral nutrition (PN).
- Lead nutrition-related audit and research to widen the evidence base and to evaluate nutrition-related research.
- Contribute to consultant-led ward rounds and MDT meetings, and have regular consultant communication where nutritional goals and plans are discussed as per the NICE guideline CG83 (NICE, 2009).
- Provide ongoing education and training for clinicians, nurses and allied health professionals (AHPs), and act as a resource for other professionals.
- Contribute to appropriate strategic meetings and clinical governance activities.

Diagnostic criteria and classification

Approximately 249,000 patients a year require admission to English ICUs, and this is increasing annually (NHS, 2015). Patients are classified according to the severity of the illness and the level of support that is needed, rather than their hospital location, e.g. ICU or high-dependency unit (HDU) (Table 7.17.1).

Metabolic response to injury, trauma and sepsis

The changes that occur following stress (injury, trauma or sepsis) are different to those from starvation, as they aim to mobilise tissues for defence and repair in an attempt to survive. Cuthbertson *et al.*'s (2001) pioneering work introduced the terms ebb and flow to describe the metabolic response. The response is complex and involves interactions and physiological responses, including counter-regulatory hormones and cytokines. It is now believed that nutrition support should be individualised to the metabolic demand over the different phases of

SECTION 7

Manual of Dietetic Practice, Sixth Edition. Edited by Joan Gandy.

Companion website: www.manualofdieteticpractice.com

Table 7.17.1 Classification of patients in the acute hospital setting

Classification	Level of support required
Level 0	Patients whose needs can be met through normal ward care in an acute hospital.
Level 1	Patients at risk of their condition deteriorating, or those recently relocated from higher levels of care, whose needs can be met on an acute ward with additional advice and support from the critical care team.
Level 2	Patients requiring more detailed observation or intervention, including support for a single failed organ system or postoperative care, and those stepping down from higher levels of care.
Level 3	Patients requiring advanced respiratory support alone or basic respiratory support, together with support of at least two organ systems.

critical illness, i.e. limiting energy in the early phase and increasing slowly during stabilisation and rehabilitation (McClave *et al.*, 2016; Preiser *et al.*, 2015; Singer *et al.*, 2014).

Ebb phase

This occurs immediately after the injury and lasts approximately 24–48 hours. There is a reduction in metabolic activity and oxygen consumption, and a fall in body temperature. Energy reserves, e.g. glucose from liver glycogen and free fatty acids from adipose tissue, are mobilised, but there is impairment in the ability to use them.

Flow phase

The second phase is called the flow or acute phase, and it is mediated by cytokines, hormones and changes in nutrient metabolism. The length of the flow phase depends on the severity of the injury and the resolution of the traumatic or septic insult. After uncomplicated major surgery, the patient can be expected to enter the anabolic phase within 2–3 weeks, but, with major burns or unresolved sepsis, the breakdown of lean tissue continues for as long as the pathological stimulus is present.

Counter-regulatory hormones

The levels of these hormones (catecholamines, glucagon and cortisol) increase, resulting in increased protein mobilisation and subsequent catabolism. They are responsible for the hyperglycaemia and insulin resistance commonly seen in critically ill patients. Glucagon stimulates gluconeogenesis, cortisol increases net protein catabolism, and the catecholamines lead to glucose intolerance.

Cytokines

Circulating levels of pro-inflammatory and anti-inflammatory cytokines also increase. Interleukin (IL)-1, IL-6 and tumour necrosis factor alpha (TNFα) are the major proinflammatory mediators. They act in conjunction with the various hormones on hepatic and peripheral tissue to increase lean tissue breakdown and loss.

Gluconeogenesis and protein metabolism

Following injury, glucose is an important fuel for the central nervous system, wounds and the immune system, all of which are metabolically active during stress. Glycogen stores are quickly depleted, so the need for available glucose is met from muscle protein breakdown for hepatic gluconeogenesis. Amino acids derived from muscle breakdown are also required for the synthesis of the acute-phase proteins, e.g. C-reactive protein (CRP). During the flow phase, achievement of energy balance, which fails to alleviate catabolism in critically ill patients, is the most that can be hoped for, to attenuate the rate of loss.

Anabolic phase

Eventually, catabolism declines, and the flow phase passes into the anabolic or recovery phase. Metabolic rate decreases, and fluid status and insulin sensitivity return to pre-injury levels, which are usually coupled with an increase in appetite and ambulation. Nutritional therapy should now aim to increase protein synthesis and restore muscle mass.

Disease consequences

Although 75% of patients return home after an ICU stay (NICE, 2009), many are left with delayed recovery, e.g. loss of muscle mass, severe weakness, impaired exercise capacity and fatigue; commonly termed ICU-acquired weakness (ICUAW), which is associated with a longer hospital stay, reduced likelihood to return home after hospital discharge, and reduced long-term survival (Arabi *et al.*, 2017). ICUAW was initially described in patients following acute respiratory distress syndrome (ARDS) (Herridge *et al.*, 2003), but is now considered to affect all patients (Herridge *et al.*, 2016). It is attributed to a combination of the following risk factors (Kress & Hall, 2014):

- Prolonged, controlled mechanical ventilation.
- Persistent systemic inflammation.
- Multi-organ failure.
- Immobilisation.
- Hyperglycaemia.
- Steroids.
- Paralysing agents.

For many ICU survivors, exercise limitations and disability persist at 5 years, and is associated with increased healthcare costs (Herridge *et al.*, 2016); one-third of patients never work again (Herridge *et al.*, 2016). This is not surprising as ICU patients can lose up to 2% of their muscle mass a day (Griffiths & Jones, 1999). Patients can be so weak on discharge to a ward that they are unable to feed themselves. Impaired coughing and swallowing can place them at risk of aspiration, and taste changes can further compromise nutritional status. Poor recovery post-ICU is a major public health issue and the subject of guidelines (NICE, 2009).

Nutritional consequences

Dietitians working in critical care should familiarise themselves with the equipment, procedures, disease process and medications used, to ensure that nutritional assessments and diet therapy are safe and appropriate. Tables 7.17.2 and 7.17.3 give details of the equipment and medications commonly used in the ICU and their nutritional implications. Table 7.17.4 highlights the factors that can increase and decrease energy expenditure.

Nutritional assessment

Anthropometry

Many patients are admitted to the ICU as emergency cases, intubated and sedated, and therefore cannot give their weight or height. Patients are bedbound, and obtaining an accurate weight and height is challenging. Some ICU beds weigh patients, but weights obtained may reflect fluid status and include bed equipment. Oedema and fluid retention can cause weight to increase by 10–20% in a single day (Lowell *et al.*, 1990), thus making anthropometric measures commonly used elsewhere inaccurate. Surrogate measures for height can be used, although these have not been validated for use within the ICU.

Biochemistry

Assessment of biochemistry is carried out frequently, often twice a day, plus blood gas measurements. Many factors during critical illness, e.g. gut losses, diuresis, volume expansion and internal redistribution, and renal replacement therapy alter biochemical values. Low electrolyte levels are not always related to nutritional status or refeeding syndrome. It is common practice to aim for upper limits of potassium, magnesium and phosphate due to their therapeutic properties. Twenty four hours is a long time in the ICU, and blood results from a previous day may be of little help in assessing the current picture. Fluid balance can be radically altered by critical illness owing to the metabolic response to stress, inflammation, malnutrition, drug treatment and organ dysfunction. Assessing fluid needs is complex and difficult to perform. It is best for the ICU medical team to lead the management of fluid requirements, and requires close collaboration within the team, which includes a dietitian (see Chapter 6.6, Parenteral nutrition).

Clinical and nutritional assessment

Identifying which patients are at nutritional risk is a key skill of the critical care dietitian. The process should detect those patients at high risk and most likely to benefit from nutrition support. In a large study where nutritional status was assessed by a dietitian, 55% were shown to be malnourished on admission to the ICU, and this was a significant predictor of 30-day mortality

Table 7.17.2 Commonly used equipment in the intensive care unit (ICU) and their nutritional implications

Equipment	Purpose	Nutritional considerations
Mechanical ventilator	Controls breathing pattern. Different settings to suit patient's needs, e.g. mandatory ventilation (machine doing all the breathing) and spontaneous ventilation (the patient initiates the breaths).	The different settings can either reduce (mandatory ventilation) or increase (spontaneous ventilation) the work of breathing, which influences energy expenditure and energy requirements (Hoher *et al.*, 2008).
Endotracheal tubes (ETT)	Tubes used to provide mechanical ventilation. The ETT is passed through the mouth or nose into the trachea. Used for short-term ventilation.	The tube makes it difficult to coordinate swallowing. Oral intake is usually avoided. Can cause temporary dysphagia when removed.
Tracheostomy	Tracheostomy is inserted into the trachea via the neck. Used for mid- to long-term ventilation.	Swallowing difficulties as listed in the preceding text. In special circumstances, oral trials can be facilitated, usually with the help of an experienced speech and language therapist.
Airflow cooling blanket	Used to decrease body temperature. Aims to achieve body temperature of 35 °C. Used as a treatment following cardiac surgery and after cardiac arrest.	Significantly lowers energy expenditure and energy requirements. Use a predictive equation that takes temperature into consideration (Faisy *et al.*, 2003; Frankenfield *et al.*, 2004).
Continuous renal replacement therapy	Used to treat acute kidney injury in ICU patients. Clears unwanted solutes and large volumes of fluid.	Loss of electrolytes, e.g. phosphate and magnesium. Loss of 5–10 g of protein/day, dependent on modality type. Loss of water-soluble vitamins. Loss of trace elements, e.g. selenium (Cano *et al.*, 2009).

Table 7.17.3 Drug–nutrient interactions

Drug	Nutritional consideration
Opioid analgesia/sedation agents, e.g. fentanyl and morphine	Can cause constipation and decrease gut motility, resulting in reduced gastric emptying.
Propofol	1 kcal/mL – contributes additional energy. Only take into consideration if taken over a prolonged period. Risk of fat overload.
Paralysing agents, e.g. atracurium and pancuronium	Decrease energy expenditure and gut motility.
Phenytoin, rifampicin, ciprofloxacin, raltegravir or penicillin V	If given via the enteral route, require a break from feed to allow drug absorption.
Intravenous fluids, e.g. crystalloids and colloids	Can contribute to sodium overload.
Inotropes and vasopressors, e.g. noradrenaline (norepinephrine), adrenaline (epinephrine), dobutamine and vasopressin	High doses cause a reduction of hepatic, renal and splanchnic blood flow. Can lead to risk of gut ischaemia.
Regional citrate anticoagulation	Infused during continuous renal replacement therapy, can contribute considerable energy intake which should be monitored.
Prokinetics, e.g. metoclopramide and erythromycin	Enhance gut motility and help overcome delayed gastric emptying. Assist in Nasojejunal tube placement.
Sliding-scale insulin therapy	Hypoglycaemia risk with interruptions to feeding.
Stress ulcer prophylaxis, e.g. lansoprazole, esomeprazole, omeprazole and ranitidine	Alters pH and can make nasogastric tube placement confirmation by pH paper unreliable.
Furosemide (loop diuretic)	Increases excretion of potassium, magnesium, sodium, calcium. May need supplementation.
Corticosteroids	Increases glucose levels. Increases sodium and water retention and potassium and calcium excretion.

Table 7.17.4 Factors commonly associated with either an increase or decrease in energy expenditure in hospitalised patients

Factors increasing energy expenditure	Factors reducing energy expenditure
Pyrexia	Sedation, anaesthesia
Disease state – the sicker the patient, the higher the energy expenditure	Age
Surgery	Neuromuscular blocking agents (paralysis), barbiturates, coma
Recovery phase of critical illness	Acute phase of critical illness
Abnormal losses, e.g. wound exudate, diarrhoea and vomiting	Starvation
Infection, chest infection and shivering	Reduced mobility / immobility
Pain	Hypothermia / active cooling
Extraneous movements, e.g. following head injury	
Exercise and rehabilitation	
Dressing changes	

(Mogensen *et al.*, 2015). Several clinical factors will affect the loss of muscle mass, including pre-existing malnutrition, sarcopenia, severity of illness, intensity of the inflammatory response and adequacy of nutrition support provided (Heyland *et al.*, 2011). Due to poor outcomes associated with malnutrition and ICUAW, there is interest in how best to assess nutritional risk. McClave *et al.* (2016) recommend that nutritional risk be assessed for all patients admitted to ICU for whom volitional intake is anticipated to be insufficient. The use of the nutrition risk score (NRS) (Kondrup *et al.*, 2003) or the nutrition risk in critically ill (NUTRIC) score (Heyland *et al.*, 2011) are advocated. The NUTRIC score places emphasis on severity of illness and inflammation in identifying disease-related nutritional risk; it does not include any direct measure of nutritional status. Patients are categorised as high or low risk. A positive association has been shown between nutritional adequacy and 28-day survival in patients with a high score, but this association diminishes with decreasing NUTRIC score (Rahman *et al.*, 2016). The NRS places all ICU patients at high risk due to illness score, and therefore is not very meaningful.

New measures such as ultrasound measurements (Puthucheary *et al.*, 2013) and CT scans (Paris & Mourtzakis, 2016) of muscle mass are described as tools to incorporate into nutritional assessments. There is still more to be done on standardising techniques and ensuring reproducibility and accurate interpretation before they are ready for use in clinical practice (Connolly *et al.*, 2015). At present, it is unknown if muscle mass is influenced by nutritional intake, or if it indicates disease severity (Arabi *et al.*, 2017).

Nutritional management

Timing of initiation of nutrition support

Early nutritional support is commonly defined as commencing 24–48 hours after admission and is routinely recommended in international guidelines (Critical Care Nutrition, 2015; McClave *et al.*, 2016). Early enteral nutrition (EN) can maintain gut integrity, modulate stress and the systemic immune response, attenuate disease severity and reduce mortality and infections (McClave *et al.*, 2016).

Route of nutrient delivery

EN is considered to be the first choice of nutrition support (Critical Care Nutrition, 2015; Kreymann *et al.*, 2006; McClave *et al.*, 2016); however, the delivery is frequently disrupted due to gastrointestinal (GI) intolerance (Wang *et al.*, 2016) or fasting for diagnostic procedures, surgery and airway management, resulting in poor nutrition support delivery (Segaran *et al.*, 2015). Cumulative energy deficits contribute to malnutrition, increased infections, increased ICU and hospital stay and mortality (Elke *et al.*, 2014; Singer *et al.*, 2010). In a recent systematic review, the use of EN was compared with PN, there was no effect on overall mortality, but decreased infectious complications and ICU length of stay (LOS) (Elke *et al.*, 2016). However, differences in the caloric intake between the subgroups may influence the observed effects (Elke *et al.*, 2016).

Historically, there have been important differences between the European and American societies' recommendations for the use of PN in critically ill patients. The European Society for Parenteral and Enteral Nutrition (ESPEN) guidelines (Singer *et al.*, 2009) advocate early use of PN if nutritional needs are not met in 2 days. In contrast, the American perspective is to withhold PN for the first 7 days (McClave *et al.*, 2016). For many decades, PN has been associated with increased infections (Simpson & Doig, 2005); however, the CALORIES trial (Harvey *et al.*, 2014) challenged this perception. In this large study, patients were randomised for receiving EN or PN within 36 hours of ICU admission for the first 5 days. It demonstrated no difference between the patients in terms of 30-day mortality or infectious complications. It should be noted that the targets of 25 kcal/kg/day were not achieved in either the EN or PN group. This study confirms that PN is not harmful in critically ill patients who are fed less than 25 kcal/kg per day. Although the CALORIES trial provides valuable information regarding the optimal route of nutrition support, it does not define the optimal dose or timing of PN.

Two landmark trials have attempted to address the timing of supplemental PN, with conflicting results (Casaer *et al.*, 2011; Heidegger *et al.*, 2013). The EPaN-IC trial compared the impact of early (day 2) PN with late initiation (day 8) to supplement inadequate EN. An increase in infectious episodes and days of mechanical ventilation were reported with early supplemental PN; no differences in 90-day mortality were observed (Casaer *et al.*, 2011). Although this is a large, well-conducted study, the results need to be interpreted with caution, primarily due to the lack of generalisability, as 60% of the patients studied had undergone cardiac surgery. Additionally, they were not malnourished, and less than 50% were still in ICU after day 3. Typically, these are patients who were of low nutritional risk, who would not normally receive nutrition support. Those in the early supplemental PN group received high energy targets. The overfeeding seen in this trial in patients with low nutritional risk may explain the increase in infections and mechanical ventilator days.

Heidegger *et al.* (2013) studied patients receiving EN who did not reach 60% of energy requirements as measured by indirect calorimetry (IC) by day 3. The patients were randomised to receive EN or both EN and supplementary PN from days 4 to 8. A reduction in infections and less days on antibiotics was observed in patients receiving supplementary PN. Doig *et al.* (2013) considered only those patients with relative contraindications to EN and randomised them to receive either standard care or early PN starting on day 1. Early PN resulted in significantly fewer days of mechanical ventilation but no difference in 60-day mortality and infections. In summary, the CALORIES trial (Harvey *et al.*, 2014) identified that PN is not more harmful than EN when excessive energy is avoided. EN remains the first choice; however, if EN fails, either exclusive or supplementary PN should be considered in appropriate patients, i.e. those who are at nutritional risk or malnourished.

What targets should we aim for – hypocaloric feeding or full-energy feeding?

The optimal dose of nutrition support is still unknown. Some advocate full-calorie feeding, and others suggest the use of hypocaloric nutrition, making it confusing to know what to aim for. To add to the confusion, there is no standard definition for terms such as permissive underfeeding, trophic feeding and hypocaloric feeding. All advocate a reduction in energy, but the targets are often different, i.e. 10–20 mL/hour, or 500–1000 kcal/day, or 10 kcal/kg. The arguments for achieving full-energy feeding originate from large observational studies, e.g. Heyland *et al.* (2011) showed that patients who received more than two-thirds of their energy target were much less likely to die as compared to those receiving suboptimal energy. In an earlier study, an increase of 1000 kcal/day was associated with a decrease in mortality and days on ventilation in patients with a BMI of $<25\,kg/m^2$ and $>35\,kg/m^2$, with no benefit in those in the BMI range of $25–35\,kg/m^2$ (Alberda *et al.*, 2009). When the NUTRIC score was used to categorise nutrition risk, those with high scores appeared to benefit most from aggressive nutrition support. However hypocaloric nutrition may not be harmful in those with low nutritional risk (Heyland *et al.*, 2011).

Interest in hypocaloric feeding has increased recently following the EDEN trial (Rice *et al.*, 2012) and the PERMIT trial (Arabi *et al.*, 2015). The EDEN trial was a multicentre randomised controlled trial (RCT) of initial trophic compared with full enteral feeding for up to 6 days in patients with ARDS; it found no significant differences in mortality and days without ventilation. The PERMIT trial randomised patients to permissive underfeeding or standard enteral feeding while maintaining a similar protein intake in both groups. This trial also found no differences in mortality, infections or LOS. A post-hoc analysis identified no differences in outcomes between high and low NUTRIC scores when comparing permissive and standard feeding practices (Arabi *et al.*, 2017), although there are limitations in using the NUTRIC score, as discussed earlier. The meta-analysis from Marik and Hooper (2016) found no differences in the risk of infections, mortality, ICU LOS and mechanical ventilation days, when comparing hypocaloric feeding with standard feeding. Al-Dorzi *et al.* (2016) also undertook a systematic review and meta-analysis of 21 studies, although 15 of these did not set out to measure hypocaloric feeding versus standard feeding. No association was found between the energy dose and hospital mortality. Lower energy intake was associated with lower risk of blood stream infections and renal replacement therapy. This may suggest that hypocaloric feeding is as good as full-energy feeding for some critically ill patients, but is not generalisable for all. Most patients were studied in the early acute phase, and were relatively young and well-nourished. For most of the studies, the energy and protein intake did not reach the recommended amounts for either group, so in fact they are comparing two different forms of underfeeding. The included studies only considered ICU outcomes, and this might be too early to see a benefit from nutrition support or detrimental effects from underfeeding. Long-term follow-up of patients enrolled in the EDEN study shows potential benefits in physical recovery in the full-fed group as compared to the hypocalorically fed group (Needham *et al.*, 2013). The exact amount of energy needed remains unknown. More large-scale RCTs are needed in a range of ICU patients over longer time periods. Optimal might be 70–80% of target requirements; however, due to frequent under-delivery, full-target EN should be the aim (Critical Care Nutrition, 2015; McClave *et al.*, 2016; Zusman *et al.*, 2016).

Overfeeding

Overfeeding macronutrients to critically ill patients can negatively affect organ function, particularly the lungs, liver and kidneys. Any excessive intake, but particularly excessive carbohydrate, can result in hypercapnia (carbon dioxide retention), which potentially prolongs the need for mechanical ventilation (Liposky & Nelson, 1994). Additionally, overfeeding carbohydrate can lead to hyperglycaemia, hypertriglyceridaemia and fat accumulation in the liver. Overfeeding protein can lead to azotaemia, uraemia, hypertonic dehydration and metabolic acidosis if the kidneys are unable to sufficiently adjust urea excretion or acid–base balance. Excessive fat infusions from PN can result in hypertriglyceridaemia and fat overload (Klein *et al.*, 1998). Non-nutrition energy sources can make a significant energy contribution and lead to overfeeding if not taken into consideration. The anaesthetic propofol is administered as a high-lipid infusion (Intralipid), and contributes 1 kcal/mL of additional energy. It can cause hypertriglyceridaemia when used in excessive doses. Additionally, intravenous dextrose and regional citrate anticoagulation, used during continuous renal replacement therapy, can contribute considerable calories and require monitoring to prevent overfeeding from occurring. Intravenous dextrose can contribute considerable energy. The underweight, overweight and elderly are particularly vulnerable to overfeeding, because of the difficulties in assessing their true requirements.

Prediction of energy targets

One of the biggest challenges is the assessment of metabolic rate for critically ill patients. The most accurate method is IC, although few dietitians have access to the equipment. Therefore, standardised equations are used to estimate metabolic rate. Many equations are available, but data are sparse on how they compare against measured energy expenditure (MEE) in a range of patients, e.g. the elderly, malnourished and obese. The energy expenditure (EE) of critically ill patients is variable; it increases and decreases over the different ICU phases, making the prediction of requirements challenging. It is influenced by the impact of critical illness and its many treatments (see Table 7.17.4).

There are a number of critical illness predictive equations such as Swinamer *et al.* (1990), Ireton-Jones *et al.* (1992), Penn State (Frankenfield *et al.*, 2004) and Faisy *et al.* (2003). Except for the Ireton-Jones equation, the others incorporate physiological factors such as temperature and ventilation settings, making them more applicable. The Penn State equation is considered the most accurate when compared to MEE (Frankenfield *et al.*, 2009), and is used by many ICU dietitians. However, there is general agreement that predictive equations are not sufficiently accurate for reliable use in critically ill patients (Fraipont & Preiser, 2013). Significant discrepancies exist between the predicted equations and IC (Tatucu-Babet *et al.*, 2016). For these reasons, international guidance suggests that, in the absence of IC, the targets should be 20–25 kcal/kg in the early phase and 25–30 kcal/kg once stable. For those in the active rehabilitation phase, needs could exceed 30 kcal/kg. Estimated EE should be re-evaluated at least once a week, adjusting to the different stages of critical illness (McClave *et al.*, 2016; Preiser *et al.*, 2015; Singer *et al.*, 2014).

Estimation of protein targets

Optimal protein targets are a challenge to determine during critical illness. The nitrogen balance obtained from 24-hour urine collections does not reflect whole-body protein balance. Protein is synthesised and lost via the liver, gut and immune system, and estimations of these losses are needed. Optimal protein provision matched to the phase of critical illness is thought to influence outcomes of critically ill patients, such as survival, reducing loss of lean body mass (LBM) and maintaining functional outcomes after a prolonged period on intensive care (Wischmeyer, 2013). Losses are greater depending on the severity of illness and increasing number of failing organs (Puthucheary *et al.*, 2013). Loss of LBM can have negative implications on respiratory function and the ability to mobilise, and lead to increased number of days dependent on ventilation, risk of ventilator-acquired pneumonias, increased LOS on the ICU and increased mortality (Sharshar *et al.*, 2009).

Recommendations for target protein requirements range from 1.2 to 2g protein/kg/day (Critical Care Nutrition, 2015; McClave *et al.*, 2016; Singer *et al.*, 2009). The available clinical trials are old and poorly designed. Many studies overfeed or underfeed energy, and often underfeed protein. Hoffer and Bistrian (2012) provide an excellent overview of the existing literature. Currently, the optimal protein requirements are not known; more recent observational studies are therefore guiding current practice in the absence of well-designed, high-quality RCTs. Weijs *et al.* (2014) suggested that a lower mortality is related to a >1.2g/kg early protein intake. An analysis by Nicolo *et al.* (2015) found that ≥80% protein targets (1.2g/kg) was associated with a favourable reduction in 60-day mortality. Importantly, this was independent of energy intake, which could indicate that protein is perhaps more important than energy provision in the early critical care phase. A promising dietetic-led RCT was recently conducted by Ferrie *et al.* (2016) with the aim of comparing standard protein intake with guideline recommendations for parenterally fed patients while crucially controlling for energy. Unfortunately this study did not achieve its aims, but identified an improvement in functionality (using handgrip) at 7 days. It was unfortunately underpowered, but similar studies assessing the impact of protein intake on measurements of functionality will help to define protein requirements in the critically ill.

In ICU patients, 1.2–1.5g protein/kg/day should be aimed for, until further RCTs are published. This should be higher in patients with burns, trauma or increased losses. It is important to assess energy and protein requirements separately depending on the phase of critical illness. Protein modular supplements may need to be used to meet these targets without overfeeding energy. The EFFORT RCT is due to start data collection in 2018, randomising lower or higher protein intake in a large multinational trial which may provide clearer guidance for protein provision in the critically ill.

Nutrition support in obese patients

Assessing the energy and protein requirements of patients with obesity is one of the most problematic and controversial aspects of nutrition support. However, it is agreed that the aim should be a balance between the preservation of muscle mass and avoiding overfeeding and its harmful effects (McClave *et al.*, 2016). The controversy of using predictive equations largely stems from the altered body composition as compared to lean individuals (Kushner & Drover, 2011). Malnutrition can occur in all ICU patients irrespective of BMI, including obesity, as there is a misconception that the adipose stores represent additional nutritional reserves that can be depended upon in times of critical illness. This might not be the case, as the muscle loss observed was similar between those with and without obesity (Segaran *et al.*, 2015). Obesity should never be used as a rationale to withhold nutrition support. Deciding upon which weight to use is challenging as the actual weight does not reflect the amount of metabolically inactive body fat. As a result of the larger fat-free mass (Forbes, 1982, 1987), using ideal body mass (IBW) is likely to underestimate energy needs, and the use of actual body weight (ABW) will overestimate. The use of adjusted body weight (AdjBW) has been proposed (Amato *et al.*, 1995) on the assumption that the obese have a lean body mass that equates to 25% more than that of the non-obese. This approach has not been validated and is not recommended, as the original predictive equations were developed using ABW, and the use of AdjBW for predicting EE in obese patients will result in an underestimation (Frankenfield *et al.*, 2003). As most predictive equations are generated from non-obese patients, and body weight is one of the largest variables in these equations, estimation errors are common when predicting energy expenditure (Kushner & Drover, 2011).

The ASPEN/SCCM guidelines (McClave *et al.*, 2016) recommend that nutrition support not exceed 65–70% of target energy requirements as measured by IC. If IC is not available, they suggest 11–14kcal/kg of ABW for those with a BMI of >30kg/m^2, and 22–25kcal/kg of IBW for patients with a BMI of >50kg/m^2. These are expert consensus recommendations, and are based on the pooled findings of a small number of studies (Dickerson, 2004). Patients experienced shorter ICU lengths of stays and fewer antibiotic days when fed 11–14kcal/kg of ABW as compared to those who received 19–25kcal/kg ABW. This recommendation needs to be interpreted with caution, as only two studies are RCTs, only one was conducted in ICU patients, and all the studies were inadequately powered to evaluate major end points such as morbidity and mortality.

No randomised trials have evaluated a range of protein intakes, so the optimal protein requirements for obese patients remain unknown. The ASPEN/SCCM guidelines (McClave *et al.*, 2016) suggest 2g/kg of IBW for those with a BMI of 30–40kg/m^2, and 2.5g/kg of IBW for those with a BMI of >40kg/m^2. This is based on the same six trials of nutritional support in hospitalised patients

(Dickerson, 2004), as the energy recommendations have the same limitations. They demonstrated that at least 2 g/IBW is required to achieve neutral nitrogen balance. Further studies investigating the target protein intake for obese patients need to be undertaken. Until such time, expert guidelines should be consulted and clinical judgment used.

To conclude, a low-energy, high-protein strategy may not be applicable to all. Not all obese patients will have the same nutritional risk, with some benefiting from restriction while others need more. Individual patient assessment is necessary to assess the nutritional risk and help determine those who are most likely to benefit from nutrition support, as you would with non-obese patients. Predictive equations are inaccurate and can result in significant underfeeding and overfeeding. Indirect calorimetry (IC) remains the best way of ascertaining EE; however, if this is not available, the American guidance (McClave *et al.*, 2016) should be used as a starting place. If the low-energy, high-protein strategy is indicated, it can be challenging to achieve with the current enteral and parenteral formulas.

Feeding protocols

The use of ICU feeding protocols to promote early and safe enteral feeding is encouraged (McClave *et al.*, 2016). Units that follow simple algorithms are able to feed patients earlier and achieve energy goals sooner (Ventura & Waitzberg, 2015). Their use has been shown to increase the number of patients receiving EN; reduce the number receiving PN, or not being fed at all (Heyland *et al.*, 2004); and reduce hospital stay and hospital mortality (Martin *et al.*, 2004). The key to successful implementation is simplicity, as cumbersome protocols are more likely to be ignored or incorrectly applied. Although feeding protocols may vary between institutions, they have the following features in common:

- Aim to promote early, safe EN.
- Provide direction when managing gastric residual volumes (GRVs).
- Advocate use of prokinetics to improve tolerance.
- Recommend alternative routes of feeding if any intolerance persists, e.g. post-pyloric feeding or PN.

Nutrition support should be individualised to the metabolic demand over the different phases of critical illness (Preiser *et al.*, 2015). Therefore, protocols should only be followed for the initial period (e.g. up to 72 hours) before the critical care dietitian performs a nutritional assessment to identify which patients require individualised feeding plans.

Interruptions to feed

The unpredictable nature of critical illness and the medical management frequently lead to disruptions in the delivery of EN. In practice, it is rare for all the prescribed EN to be delivered. Large multicentre studies have found that ICU patients were uniformly underfed, with data from the International Nutrition Survey (2013), showing an average of 64% of energy and 60% of protein prescriptions being received over the first 4 days, increasing to 70% of energy and 60% of protein in those who remained in ICU for 12 days (Nicolo *et al.*, 2015). Frequently cited reasons include fasting for extubation, surgical and airway procedures, loss of access and GI intolerance (Kozeniecki *et al.*, 2016). The introduction of fasting guidelines has been shown to improve the delivery of nutrition (Segaran *et al.*, 2017). All efforts should be made to avoid unnecessarily prolonged fasting.

International guidelines (Critical Care Nutrition, 2015; McClave *et al.*, 2016) also recommend a volume-based feeding (VBF) approach using a daily feed target volume, empowering nursing staff to adjust feeding rates to make up for deficits encountered when interruptions occur. McClave *et al.* (2016) randomised 63 patients to volume-based or rate-based feeding and found that VBF significantly reduced energy deficits without any adverse effects. However, Heyland *et al.* (2016) compared VBF in 126 predominantly medical patients to 982 patients acting as controls. Both cohorts were underfed; the VBF group met 43% of energy requirements vs. 32% in the control group. There was a small improvement in nutritional delivery (8% increase in energy adequacy and 15% protein adequacy), which may not translate into improved clinical outcomes.

The introduction of VBF in UK ICUs is gaining popularity. This change in approach requires support from the ICU MDT. Nursing staff require comprehensive training to have the confidence to implement a new protocol and independently alter the feeding rate, traditionally dictated by a dietitian, protocol or medical team. Close monitoring of blood glucose levels and GI tolerance is required. In practice, inappropriately elevated feeding rates are occasionally calculated, which can lead to overfeeding.

Gastrointestinal dysfunction and enteral feeding intolerance

Critical illness frequently causes GI dysfunction, which contributes to feeding intolerance and poor EN delivery. A working group of the European Society of Intensive Care Medicine (ESICM) has developed useful consensus definitions and guidelines for GI dysfunction (Blaser *et al.*, 2012). Large GRVs have historically been used as a marker of gastric emptying and assumed to reflect EN intolerance. The incidence of feeding intolerance is 38% (5–75%), depending on the definition and threshold used for high GRVs (Blaser *et al.*, 2014; Gungabissoon *et al.*, 2014). The pathophysiology of GI dysfunction is multifactorial, including mechanical ventilation, sepsis, traumatic brain injury sedation, paralysing agents and vasopressors. Feeding intolerance is associated with fewer ventilator-free days, longer ICU stays and increased mortality (Gungabissoon *et al.*, 2014); GRVs are generally higher in more severely ill patients (Hsu *et al.*, 2011).

Significance of gastric residual volume

The reported values for the designated cut-off for withholding feed vary from 200 to 500 mL. The aims of performing regular checks are risk reduction and/or prevention of pulmonary aspiration of gastric contents, which may result in pneumonia. However, GRVs may have little clinical meaning and do not consistently correlate with aspiration risk (McClave *et al.*, 2005), as increasing the GRV cut-off from 200 mL to 400 mL did not increase the risk of aspiration in predominantly surgical patients. Conversely, dropping the GRV cut-off from 400 mL to 200 mL failed to reduce the risk and protect patients from aspiration. The REGANE study (Montejo *et al.*, 2010) compared GRV cut-offs of 200 mL and 500 mL. The mean EN delivery was significantly higher in the intervention group, although the incidence of pneumonia, duration of mechanical ventilation and ICU length of stay were similar in both groups. The patients studied were predominately medical patients who are less likely to experience GI dysfunction.

Non-monitoring versus routine monitoring of gastric residual volumes

The multicentre study by Reignier *et al.* (2013) is the only RCT to evaluate if the risk of ventilator-related pneumonia (VAP) is increased when GRVs are not monitored, as compared to routine GRVs of >250 mL. The trial found no difference in the incidence of VAP between the groups; however, non-monitoring was associated with more vomiting. The nutritional adequacy was greater in the non-monitoring group, but the differences were minimal. Again, the patients were predominately medical rather than surgical, and not in multi-organ failure, so the results are unlikely to be generalisable to all ICU patients.

How frequently should gastric residual volumes be checked?

Williams and Leslie (2010) conducted an RCT comparing GRVs undertaken 4-hourly with variable GRVs of up to 8 hours. Vomiting and regurgitation was significantly increased in the variable checking group. No significant differences were found in the rates of VAP.

Returning or discarding of gastric residual volumes

One study has investigated whether returning GRVs up to 250 mL vs. discarding the GRVs resulted in better outcomes (Juvé-Udina *et al.*, 2009). There was no difference observed in ICU length of stay, diarrhoea, abdominal distention, nausea, vomiting or VAP between the two groups. Fluid balance and serum electrolytes were comparable and not different. There were less episodes of delayed gastric emptying in the return group. Overall, the study concluded that returning GRVs is not associated with more GI complications as compared to discarding them.

Practical application

Based on the evidence available, the rationale for routine GRV monitoring has been questioned; the 2016 ASPEN/SCCM guidelines (McClave *et al.*, 2016) advise that GRVs should not be used as part of routine care. This recommendation may be a little premature and not applicable to all, particularly surgical patients and those with multi-organ failure. The Critical Care Nutrition (2015) have adopted a more cautious approach, suggesting the use of 250–500 mL and a frequency of checking GRVs either 4-hourly or 8-hourly. The evidence for whether to return or discard GRVs is not compelling, and therefore decisions should be made at a unit-level in discussion with the MDT.

Prokinetic agent treatment

The use of prokinetic agents (metoclopramide, erythromycin and domperidone) has been suggested to help overcome feeding intolerance. However, studies have often been small and have methodological weaknesses, such as varying doses of drugs and a range of GRV cut-off values (Booth *et al.*, 2002). The most recent systematic review and meta-analysis (Lewis *et al.*, 2016) examined the efficacy and safety of prokinetic agents in critically ill patients receiving EN. It found that prokinetic agents significantly reduced feeding intolerance and the risk of developing high GRVs, and increased the success of post-pyloric feeding tube placement. However, the impact on other clinical outcomes such as pneumonia, mortality and ICU length of stay is unclear.

There are safety concerns regarding the use of prokinetic agents. Erythromycin, an antibiotic, has the potential to cause serious ventricular arrhythmia and microbial resistance to antibiotics (Booth *et al.*, 2002). Both metoclopramide and erythromycin should be used for the shortest duration required. Metoclopramide use should not exceed 5 days duration, owing to the risk of neurological adverse effects (European Medicine Agency, 2013). International guidance recommends metoclopramide as the first-line prokinetic in ICU due to safety concerns with erythromycin (Critical Care Nutrition, 2015; McClave *et al.*, 2016).

Reducing the risk of aspiration

Preventative measures include (McClave *et al.*, 2016) the following:

- Elevate the head of the bed to ≥45°.
- Consider using prokinetic agents.
- Use continuous enteral feeding.
- Consider the placement of a post-pyloric tube; regularly assess feeding tube placement to ensure that it has remained in the correct position.
- Consider using chlorhexidine mouthwash.

Post-pyloric enteral nutrition

Post-pyloric or small-bowel EN is often considered an effective way of overcoming large GRVs and therefore reducing the risk of aspiration; however, studies to support this assumption are limited. Nasoduodenal or nasojejunal tubes (NJT) are difficult to place and keep in the correct position; endoscopic placement can be time consuming and labour intensive. Self-propelling tubes are available; however, in one study, only 26–38%

of tubes placed in the stomach moved spontaneously into the duodenum, and the majority moved back into the stomach by retroperistalsis (Rees *et al.*, 1988). The use of a fluoroscopic technique to place tubes has been shown to be successful (Welpe *et al.*, 2010); others have achieved success with an electromagnetic tracking system (Taylor *et al.*, 2010).

There is conflicting advice regarding the use of NJTs. The ASPEN/SCCM guidelines (McClave *et al.*, 2016) support their use, while the older European guidelines (Kreymann *et al.*, 2006) concluded that the evidence does not justify general recommendations. Davies *et al.* (2012) found no significant increase in energy delivery with NJTs in patients with mildly elevated GRVs, and minor GI haemorrhage was increased. McClave *et al.* (2016) concluded that there is no difference in mortality or length of stay with small bowel feeding as compared to gastric feeding, despite the reduced risk of pneumonia. The studies described in both guidelines are small and report on differing outcomes. Despite this, more recent international guidelines recommend the use of post-pyloric feeding in those who are intolerant to gastric feeding, providing access can be easily gained.

Glycaemic control

Acute illness or injury may result in hyperglycaemia, insulin resistance and glucose intolerance, collectively termed as stress hyperglycaemia (Marik & Bellomo, 2013). It is thought to be an evolutionarily preserved adaptive response that allows the host to survive during periods of severe stress. Marik and Bellomo (2013) provide an excellent overview and explanations of the pathophysiological responses. Stress hyperglycaemia is not exclusive to patients with pre-existing diabetes, but appears to be related to the extent of critical illness. In most cases, it will resolve as the clinical condition improves.

Currently, there are two quite distinct views on glycaemic control during critical illness, and questions exist on whether tight glycaemic control is warranted. The early trial of van den Berghe *et al.* (2001) showed a significant reduction in the morbidity and mortality of surgical ICU patients with the aggressive use of insulin to maintain normoglycaemia. Favourable outcomes were attributed to the tight control of blood glucose as compared to a control group. It was concluded that this tight glycaemic control resulted in a reduction in mortality of 33% in surgical ICU patients. Since this publication, 14 independent prospective RCTs in various critically ill patient populations as well as a systematic review and meta-analysis (Yamada *et al.*, 2016) have been performed, and all demonstrate no outcome benefit from tight glycaemic control. The Normoglycaemia in Intensive Care Evaluation – Survival Using Glucose Algorithm Regulation (NICE SUGAR) trial (Finfer *et al.*, 2009) has been the largest trial to date, which demonstrated an increase in 90-day mortality in patients randomised to intensive insulin therapy. The type of feeding strategy employed in the trials fundamentally played a role. In the van den Berghe *et al.* (2001) study, participants were given large doses of intravenous glucose in addition to PN within 24 hours of admission, even in those who could tolerate EN. The findings of the NICE-SUGAR trial are more likely to be generalisable to those ICUs that use EN predominately. A moderate range of blood glucose management of 7–10 mmol/L is advised (Critical Care Nutrition, 2015; McClave *et al.*, 2016; Preiser, 2016).

Immune-modulating nutritional support

Enteral formulations

Immune-modulating enteral feeds are characterised by increased quantities of specific nutrients that may have the potential to improve immune function and modulate the inflammatory response. Such nutrients include arginine, n-3 polyunsaturated fatty acids, glutamine, ribonucleic acid (RNA) and antioxidants, including vitamin C and selenium. Currently, the use of immune-modulating EN is not recommended in international guidelines, and their use in UK clinical practice is still controversial. There is not sufficient evidence to support the use of these enteral feeds.

Specific nutrients

Fish oils

The addition of anti-inflammatory fish oils, eicosapentaenoic acid (EPA) and δ-linolenic acid (GLA), and antioxidants to EN has been used to potentially influence clinical outcome. A meta-analysis showed a reduction in mechanical ventilation and ICU days, as well as decreased risk of developing new organ failures and mortality in those who received the EPA/GLA EN (Pontes-Arruda *et al.*, 2008). The studies have several limitations inhibiting their applicability, e.g. lack of power calculations and/or blinding, short trial duration, the sickest patients being excluded, differing levels of EPA and GLA used, and a high-fat, low-carbohydrate control feed being used. More recent studies (Grau-Carmona *et al.*, 2011; Kagan *et al.*, 2015; Rice *et al.*, 2011; Stapleton *et al.*, 2011) have shown a lack of treatment effect. When all trials were aggregated, the use of an EN supplemented with fish oils and antioxidants did not significantly reduce ICU length of stay or the duration of mechanical ventilation or hospital stay as compared to a standard enteral formulation (McClave *et al.*, 2016). As a result, no recommendation for the use of these feeds can be made until further evidence is available.

Arginine

Arginine is one of the most controversial immunomodulatory nutrients. Studies show improvements in clinical outcomes and reduced mortality with arginine supplementation of enteral feeds (Atkinson *et al.*, 1998; Caparros *et al.*, 2001). Galban *et al.* (2000) assessed enteral arginine use in septic patients, finding reduced infections; however, benefits were only seen in patients with moderate critical illness, limiting generalisability to all. Greater mortality and an increase in the inflammatory response have been observed in severely septic patients (Bertolini *et al.*, 2003; Heyland & Samis, 2003). It is proposed that, in severe sepsis, arginine may be converted into nitric oxide, contributing to haemodynamic instability and organ dysfunction. For this reason, recent international guidelines suggest caution or avoidance of arginine in severe sepsis (Critical Care Nutrition, 2015; McClave *et al.*, 2016).

Glutamine

Recent international guidelines (Critical Care Nutrition, 2015; McClave *et al.*, 2016) no longer support the routine supplementation of glutamine via the PN or EN route after considering the results of multicentre trials (REDOXS and Metaplus). The REDOXS trial (Heyland *et al.*, 2013) identified a trend towards increased mortality and no clinical benefit with the use of a high-dose (approximately 50 g per day) enteral and parenteral glutamine. However, glutamine was used in some patients with renal dysfunction, which is cited as a contraindication against the use of IV glutamine. The Metaplus trial (van Zanten *et al.*, 2014) supplemented EN with 30 g glutamine, plus selenium and fish oils, and found no difference in infectious complications or other secondary outcomes, as compared to standard practice and an increase in 6-month mortality.

Previously, benefits such as reductions in mortality, infectious complications, and ICU/hospital length of stay have been demonstrated (Déchelotte *et al.*, 2006; Wischmeyer, 2008). The reduction in infectious complications was seen in resolving multi-organ failure, smaller doses, and patients who were indicated PN and without renal or liver failure. There still remain questions regarding the appropriate dose, timing and route of glutamine; until the international community can be certain that supplemental glutamine does not cause any harm, glutamine should not be routinely used in the critically ill. The RE-ENERGISE trial is currently assessing the clinical outcomes and health-related quality of life regarding use of enteral glutamine on burns patients, with the results due in 2021.

Selenium and antioxidants

The plasma concentration of selenium and other antioxidants are reduced in septic patients, and are associated with a greater number of infectious complications and a higher incidence of mortality (Forceville, 2007). It is not clear if low plasma selenium concentrations are indicative of deficiency or normal metabolism during the acute-phase response. Manzanares *et al.* (2016) conducted a recent meta-analysis with high-dose selenium supplementation (>500 µg/day) and found no differences in mortality, infections, renal function or length of stay. However, a reduction in infectious complications was seen in non-septic patients who did not receive an initial IV bolus. Therefore, international guidelines do not recommend routine parenteral supplementation. More work is needed to determine the optimal dosage, route and frequency (if required at all) for selenium and other anti-oxidants such as zinc, ascorbic acid, vitamin E and beta-carotene before routine supplementation becomes common practice in critically ill patients.

Vitamin and mineral requirements

It is still not well understood if micronutrient requirements are significantly altered during critical illness. If aiming for an intake equal to the reference nutrient intake, the micronutrient needs of most patients can be met if target energy intakes are achieved. However, the target is rarely achieved during ICU stay. Hence, in those who consistently do not receive the target intake, supplementation of vitamins and minerals should be considered (van Zanten, 2015). Patients with major burns, high GI losses, and on continuous renal replacement therapy will have additional vitamin and mineral needs (Berger *et al.*, 2004). McClave *et al.* (2016) make a low-grade recommendation regarding the provision of antioxidant vitamins and trace elements, although they do not provide specific details on route, duration, dose or frequency.

Vitamin D

Interest in vitamin D is increasing as a high prevalence of deficiency (>50%) has been observed in critically ill patients (Amrein *et al.*, 2010). There is a growing body of observational data that describes the association between vitamin D deficiency and increased risk of 28-day mortality as well as sepsis (Moromizato *et al.*, 2014). One RCT has been performed with adequate power (VITdAL-ICU trial), randomising patients to an enteral loading dose followed by monthly or placebo doses (Amrein *et al.*, 2014). Although the trial did not find a difference in the primary outcome of hospital stay, there was a significant decrease in hospital mortality in those with severe deficiency (<30 nmol/L). At present, the data are insufficient to put forward a recommendation for the use of vitamin D supplementation in the critically ill.

Internet resources

American Society for Parenteral & Enteral Nutrition, www.nutritioncare.org

British Dietetic Association Critical Care Specialist Group, www.bda.co.uk

British Society for Parenteral & Enteral Nutrition, www.bapen.org.uk

Critical Care Nutrition, at the Clinical Evaluation Research Unit (CERU), www.criticalcarenutrition.com

European Society for Clinical Nutrition & Metabolism, www.espen.org

Intensive Care Society, www.ics.ac.uk

Scottish Intensive Care Society, www.scottishintensivecare.org.uk

Society of Critical Care Medicine, www.sccm.org

References

Alberda C, Gramlich L, Jones N, *et al.* (2009) The relationship between nutritional intake and clinical outcomes in critically ill patients: results of an international multicenter observational study. *Intensive Care Med.* 35(10): 1728–1737.

Al-Dorzi HM, Albarrak A, Ferwana M, *et al.* (2016) Lower versus higher dose of enteral caloric intake in adult critically ill patients: a systematic review and meta-analysis. *Crit. Care* 20: 358.

Amato P, Keating KP, Quercia RA, *et al.* (1995) Formulaic methods of estimating calorie requirements in mechanically ventilated obese patients: a reappraisal. *Nut. Clin. Pract.* 10(6): 229–232.

Amrein K, Amrein S, Holl A, *et al.* (2010) Vitamin D, parathyroid hormone and serum calcium levels and their association with hospital mortality in critically ill patients. *Crit. Care.* 14: S198.

Amrein K, Schnedl C, Holl A, *et al.* (2014) Effect of high-dose vitamin D_3 on hospital length of stay in critically ill patients with vitamin D deficiency: the VITdAL-ICU randomized clinical trial. *JAMA.* 312(15): 1520–1530.

Arabi YM, Aldawood AS, Haddad SH, *et al.* (2015) Permissive underfeeding or standard enteral feeding in critically ill adults. *N. Eng. J. Med.* 372(25): 2398–2408.

Arabi YM, Casaer MP, Chapman M, *et al.* (2017) The intensive care medicine research agenda in nutrition and metabolism. *Intensive Care Med.* 43: 1239–1256.

Atkinson S, Sieffert E, Bihari D. (1998) A prospective, randomized, double-blind, controlled clinical trial of enteral immunonutrition in the critically ill. Guy's Hospital Intensive Care Group. *Crit. Care Med.* 26(7): 1164–1172.

Berger MM, Shenkin A, Revelly JP, *et al.* (2004) Copper, selenium, zinc, and thiamine balances during continuous venovenous hemodiafiltration in critically ill patients. *Am. J. Clin. Nutr.* 80(2): 410–416.

Bertolini G, Iapichino G, Radrizzani D, *et al.* (2003) Early enteral immunonutrition in patients with severe sepsis: results of an interim analysis of a randomized multicentre clinical trial. *Intensive Care Med.* 29(5): 834–840.

Blaser AR, Malbrain ML, Starkopf J, *et al.* (2012) Gastrointestinal function in intensive care patients: terminology, definitions and management. Recommendations of the ESICM Working Group on Abdominal Problems. *Intensive Care Med.* 38(3): 384–394.

Blaser AR, Starkopf J, Kirsimägi Ü, *et al.* (2014) Definition, prevalence, and outcome of feeding intolerance in intensive care: a systematic review and meta-analysis. *Acta Anaesthesiol. Scand.* 58(8): 914–922.

Booth CM, Heyland DK, Paterson WG. (2002) Gastrointestinal promotility drugs in the critical care setting: a systematic review of the evidence. *Crit. Care Med.* 30(7): 1429–1435.

Cano NJ, Aparicio M, Brunori G, *et al.* (2009) ESPEN guidelines on parenteral nutrition: adult renal failure. *Clin. Nutr.* 28(4): 401–414.

Caparros T, Lopez J, Grau T. (2001) Early enteral nutrition in critically ill patients with a high-protein diet enriched with arginine, fiber, and antioxidants compared with a standard high-protein diet. The effect on nosocomial infections and outcome. *JPEN J. Parenter. Enteral Nutr.* 25(6): 299–308.

Casaer MP, Mesotten D, Hermans G, *et al.* (2011) Early versus late parenteral nutrition in critically ill adults. *N. Engl. J. Med.* 365(6): 506–517.

Connolly B, MacBean V, Crowley C, *et al.* (2015) Ultrasound for the assessment of peripheral skeletal muscle architecture in critical illness: a systematic review. *Crit. Care Med.* 43: 897–905.

Critical Care Nutrition. (2015) *Canadian Critical Care Nutrition Practice Guidelines*. Available at www.criticalcarenutrition.com. Accessed 01 December 2016.

Cuthbertson DP, Valero Zanuy MA, Leon Sanz ML. (2001) Post-shock metabolic response, 1942. *Nutr. Hosp.* 16(5): 176–182.

Davies AR, Morrison SS, Bailey MJ, *et al.* ENTERIC Study Investigators; ANZICS Clinical Trials Group. (2012) A multicenter, randomized controlled trial comparing early nasojejunal with nasogastric nutrition in critical illness. *Crit. Care Med.* 40(8): 2342–2348.

Déchelotte P, Hasselmann M, Cynober L, *et al.* (2006) L-alanyl-L-glutamine dipeptide–supplemented total parenteral nutrition reduces infectious complications and glucose intolerance in critically ill patients: The French controlled, randomized, double-blind, multicenter study. *Crit. Care Med.* 34(3): 598–604.

Dickerson RN. (2004) Specialized nutrition support in the hospitalized obese patient. *Nutr. Clin. Pract.* 19(3): 245–254.

Doig GS, Simpson F, Sweetman EA, *et al.* (2013) Early parenteral nutrition in critically ill patients with short-term relative contraindications to early enteral nutrition: a randomized controlled trial. *JAMA.* 309(20): 2130–2138.

Elke G, Wang M, Weiler N, *et al.* (2014) Close to recommended caloric and protein intake by enteral nutrition is associated with better clinical outcome of critically ill septic patients: secondary analysis of a large international nutrition database. *Crit. Care.* 18(1): 1.

Elke G, van Zanten AR, Lemieux M, *et al.* (2016) Enteral versus parenteral nutrition in critically ill patients: an updated systematic review and meta-analysis of randomized controlled trials. *Crit. Care.* 20(1): 1.

European Medicine Agency. (2013) European medicine agency recommends changes to the use of metoclopramide. Available at https://www.ema.europa.eu/en/medicines/human/referrals/metoclopramide-containing-medicines. Accessed 22 November 2018.

Faisy C, Guerot E, Diehl JL, *et al.* (2003) Assessment of resting energy expenditure in mechanically ventilated patients. *Am. J. Clin. Nutr.* 78(2): 241–249.

Ferrie S, Allman-Farinelli M, Daley M, *et al.* (2016) Protein requirements in the critically ill: a randomized controlled trial using parenteral nutrition. *JPEN. J. Parenter. Enteral Nutr.* 40(6): 795–805.

Finfer S, Chittock DR, Su SY, *et al.* (2009) Intensive versus conventional glucose control in critically ill patients. *N. Engl. J. Med.* 360(13): 1283–1297.

Forbes GB. (1982) Is obesity a genetic disease? *J. Med. Soc. N. J.* 79(1): 47–48.

Forbes GB. (1987) Lean body mass-body fat interrelationships in humans. *Nutr. Rev.* 45(8): 225–231.

Forceville X, Laviolle B, Annane D, *et al.* (2006) Effects of high doses of selenium, as sodium selenite, in septic shock: a placebo-controlled, randomized, double-blind, phase II study. *Critical Care* 2007, 11:R73 (doi: 10.1186/cc5960).

Fraiport V, Preiser JC. (2013) Energy Estimation and Measurement in Critically Ill Patients. *J. Parenter. Enteral Nutr.*37 (6): 705–713.

Frankenfield DC, Coleman A, Alam S, *et al.* (2009) Analysis of estimation methods for resting metabolic rate in critically ill adults. *JPEN J. Parenter. Enteral Nutr.* 33(1): 27–36.

Frankenfield DC, Rowe WA, Smith JS, *et al.* (2003) Validation of several established equations for resting metabolic rate in obese and nonobese people. *J. Am. Die. Assoc.* 103(9): 1152–1159.

Frankenfield D, Smith JS, Cooney RN. (2004) Validation of 2 approaches to predicting resting metabolic rate in critically ill patients. *JPEN. J. Parenter. Enteral Nutr.* 28(4): 259–264.

Galban C, Montejo JC, Mesejo A, *et al.* (2000) An immune-enhancing enteral diet reduces mortality rate and episodes of bacteremia in septic intensive care unit patients. *Crit. Care Med.* 28(3): 643–648.

Grau-Carmona T, Morán-García V, García-de-Lorenzo A, *et al.* (2011) Effect of an enteral diet enriched with eicosapentaenoic acid, gamma-linolenic acid and anti-oxidants on the outcome of mechanically ventilated, critically ill, septic patients. *Clin. Nutr.* 30(5): 578–584.

Griffiths RD, Jones C. (1999) Recovery from intensive care. *BMJ.* 319: 427–429.

Gungabissoon U, Hacquoil K, Bains C, *et al.* (2014) Prevalence, risk factors, clinical consequences, and treatment of enteral feed intolerance during critical illness. *JPEN J. Parenter. Enteral Nutr.* 39(4): 441–448.

Harvey SE, Parrott F, Harrison DA, *et al.*; CALORIES Trial Investigators. (2014) Trial of the route of early nutritional support in critically ill adults. *N. Engl. J. Med.* 371(18): 1673–1684.

Heidegger CP, Berger MM, Graf S, *et al.* (2013) Optimisation of energy provision with supplemental parenteral nutrition in critically ill patients: a randomised controlled clinical trial. *Lancet.* 381(9864): 385–393.

Herridge MS, Cheung AM, Tansey CM, *et al.* (2003) One-year outcomes in survivors of the acute respiratory distress syndrome. *N. Engl. J. Med.* 348(8): 683–693.

Herridge MS, Moss M, Hough CL, *et al.* (2016) Recovery and outcomes after the acute respiratory distress syndrome (ARDS) in

patients and their family caregivers. *Intensive Care Med.* 42(5): 725–738.
Heyland DK, Samis A. (2003) Does immunonutrition in patients with sepsis do more harm than good? *Intensive Care Med.* 29(5): 669–671.
Heyland DK, Dhaliwal R, Day A, *et al.* (2004) Validation of the Canadian clinical practice guidelines for nutrition support in mechanically ventilated, critically ill adult patients: results of a prospective observational study. *Crit. Care Med.* 32(11): 2260–2266.
Heyland DK, Dhaliwal R, Jiang X, *et al.* (2011) Identifying critically ill patients who benefit the most from nutrition therapy: the development and initial validation of a novel risk assessment tool. *Crit. Care* 15(6): 1.
Heyland DK, Lemieux M, Shu L, *et al.* (2016) What is 'best achievable' practice in implementing the enhanced protein-energy provision via the enteral route feeding protocol in intensive care units in the United States? Results of a multicenter, quality improvement collaborative. *JPEN J. Parenter. Enteral Nutr.* 42(2):308–317.
Heyland DK, Muscedere J, Wischmeyer PE, *et al.* (2013) A randomized trial of glutamine and antioxidants in critically ill patients. *N. Engl. J. Med.* 368(16): 1489–1497.
Hoffer LJ, Bistrian BR. (2012) Appropriate protein provision in critical illness: a systematic and narrative review. *Am. J. Clin. Nutr.* 96(3): 591–600.
Hoher JA, Zimermann Teixeira PJ, Hertz F, *et al.* (2008) A comparison between ventilation modes: how does activity level affect energy expenditure estimates? *JPEN J. Parenter. Enteral Nutr.* 32(2): 176–183.
Hsu CW, Sun SF, Lee DL, *et al.* (2011) Impact of disease severity on gastric residual volume in critical patients. *World J. Gastroenterol.* 17(15): 2007–2012.
Ireton-Jones CS, Turner WW Jr, Liepa GU, *et al.* (1992) Equations for the estimation of energy expenditures in patients with burns with special reference to ventilatory status. *J. Burn Care Rehabil.* 13(3): 330–333.
Kagan I, Cohen J, Stein M, *et al.* (2015) Preemptive enteral nutrition enriched with eicosapentaenoic acid, gamma-linolenic acid and antioxidants in severe multiple trauma: a prospective, randomized, double-blind study. *Intensive Care Med.* 41(3): 460–469.
Klein CJ, Stanek GS, Wiles CE III. (1998) Overfeeding macronutrients to critically ill adults: metabolic complications. *J. Am. Diet. Assoc.* 98(7): 795–806.
Kondrup J, Allison SP, Elia M, *et al.* (2003) ESPEN guidelines for nutrition screening (2003). *Clin. Nutr.* 22(4): 415–421.
Kozeniecki M, McAndrew N, Patel JJ. (2016) Process-related barriers to optimizing enteral nutrition in a tertiary medical intensive care unit. *Nutr. Clin. Pract.* 31(1): 80–85.
Kress JP, Hall JB. (2014) ICU-acquired weakness and recovery from critical illness. *N. Engl. J. Med.* 370(17): 1626–1635.
Kreymann KG, Berger MM, Deutz NE, *et al.* (2006) ESPEN guidelines on enteral nutrition: intensive care. *Clin. Nutr.* 25(2): 210–223.
Lewis K, Alqahtani Z, Mcintyre L, *et al.* (2016) The efficacy and safety of prokinetic agents in critically ill patients receiving enteral nutrition: a systematic review and meta-analysis of randomized trials. *Crit. Care* 20(1): 259.
Liposky JM, Nelson LD. (1994) Ventilatory response to high caloric loads in critically ill patients. *Crit. Care Med.* 22(5): 796–802.
Lowell JA, Schifferdecker C, Driscoll DF, *et al.* (1990) Postoperative fluid overload: not a benign problem. *Critical Care Medicine* 18(7): 728–733.
Manzanares W, Lemieux M, Elke G, *et al.* (2016) High-dose intravenous selenium does not improve clinical outcomes in the critically ill: a systematic review and meta-analysis. *Crit. Care* 20(1): 356.
Marik PE, Bellomo R. (2013) Stress hyperglycemia: an essential survival response! *Crit. Care* 17(2): 305.
Marik PE, Hooper MH. (2016) Normocaloric versus hypocaloric feeding on the outcomes of ICU patients: a systematic review and meta-analysis. *Intensive Care Med.* 42(3): 316–323.
Martin CM, Doig GS, Heyland DK, *et al.* (2004) Multicentre, cluster-randomized clinical trial of algorithms for critical-care enteral and parenteral therapy (ACCEPT). *CMAJ.* 170(2): 197–204.
Masterson G, Baudouin S. (2015) General provision of intensive care services 2015. *J. Intensive Care Soc.* 16(1): 9–10.
McClave SA, Taylor BE, Martindale RG, *et al.* (2016) Guidelines for the provision and assessment of nutrition support therapy in the adult critically ill patient: Society of Critical Care Medicine (SCCM) and American Society for Parenteral and Enteral Nutrition (ASPEN). *JPEN J. Parenter. Enteral Nutr.* 40(2): 159–211.
McClave SA, Lukan JK, Stefater JA, *et al.* (2005) Poor validity of residual volumes as a marker for risk of aspiration in critically ill patients. *Crit. Care Med.* 33(2): 324–330.
Mogensen KM, Robinson MK, Casey JD, *et al.* (2015) Nutritional status and mortality in the critically ill. *Crit. Care Med.* 43(12): 2605–2615.
Montejo JC, Minambres E, Bordeje L, *et al.* (2010) Gastric residual volume during enteral nutrition in ICU patients: the REGANE study. *Intensive Care Med.* 36(8): 1386–1393.
Moromizato T, Litonjua AA, Braun AB, *et al.* (2014) Association of low serum 25-hydroxyvitamin D levels and sepsis in the critically ill. *Crit. Care Med.* 42(1): 97–107.
Needham DM, Dinglas VD, Bienvenu OJ, *et al.* (2013) One year outcomes in patients with acute lung injury randomised to initial trophic or full enteral feeding: prospective follow-up of EDEN randomised trial. *BMJ.* 346: f1532.
NHS. (2015) *Hospital Episode Statistics Online. Adult Critical Care England, 2013–2014.* Available at www.hscic.gov.uk/pubs/acc1011. Accessed 28 November 2016.
NICE. (2009) *Rehabilitation after Clinical Illness. CG83.* Available at www.nice.org.uk/cg83. Accessed 3 April 2017.
Nicolo M, Heyland DK, Chittams J, *et al.* (2015) Clinical outcomes related to protein delivery in a critically ill population: a multicenter, multinational observation study. *JPEN J. Parenter. Enteral Nutr.* 40(1): 45–51
Paris M, Mourtzakis M. (2016) Assessment of skeletal muscle mass in critically ill patients: considerations for the utility of computed tomography imaging and ultrasonography. *Curr. Opin. Clin. Nutr. Metab. Care* 19(2): 125–130.
Pontes-Arruda A, Demichele S, Seth A, *et al.* (2008) The use of an inflammation-modulating diet in patients with acute lung injury or acute respiratory distress syndrome: a meta-analysis of outcome data. *JPEN J. Parenter. Enteral Nutr.* 32(6): 596–605.
Preiser JC, van Zanten AR, Berger MM, *et al.* (2015) Metabolic and nutritional support of critically ill patients: consensus and controversies. *Crit. Care.* 19(1): 35.
Preiser JC, Chase JG, Hovorka R et al. (2016) Glucose Control in the ICU: A Continuing Story. *J. Diab. Sci. Tech.* 10(6):1372–1381.
Puthucheary ZA, Rawal J, McPhail M, *et al.* (2013) Acute skeletal muscle wasting in critical illness. *JAMA.* 310: 1591–1600.
Rahman A, Hasan RM, Agarwala R, *et al.* (2016) Identifying critically-ill patients who will benefit most from nutritional therapy: further validation of the 'modified NUTRIC' nutritional risk assessment tool. *Clin. Nutr.* 35(1): 158–162.
Reignier J, Mercier E, Le Gouge A, *et al.* (2013) Effect of not monitoring residual gastric volume on risk of ventilator-associated pneumonia in adults receiving mechanical ventilation and early enteral feeding: a randomized controlled trial. *JAMA.* 309(3): 249–256.
Rice TW, Wheeler AP, Thompson BT, *et al.* (2011) Enteral omega-3 fatty acid, γ-linolenic acid, and antioxidant supplementation in acute lung injury. *JAMA.* 306(14): 1574–1581.
Rice TW, Wheeler AP, Thompson BT, *et al.* (2012) Initial trophic vs full enteral feeding in patients with acute lung injury: the EDEN randomized trial. *JAMA.* 307: 795—803.
Segaran E, Barker I, Hartle A. (2015) Optimising enteral nutrition in critically ill patients by reducing fasting times. *J. Intensive Care Soc.* 7 (1): 38–43.
Segaran E, Wandrag L, Stotz M, *et al.* (2017) Does body mass index impact on muscle wasting and recovery following critical

illness? A pilot feasibility observational study. *J. Hum. Nutr. Diet.* 30(2):227–235

Sharshar T, Bastuji-Garin S, Stevens RD, *et al.* (2009) Presence and severity of intensive care unit-acquired paresis at time of awakening are associated with increased intensive care unit and hospital mortality. *Crit. Care Med.* 37(12): 3047–3053.

Simpson F, Doig GS. (2005) Parenteral vs. enteral nutrition in the critically ill patient: a meta-analysis of trials using the intention to treat principle. *Intensive Care Med.* 31(1): 12–23.

Singer P, Berger MM, van den Berghe G, *et al.* (2009) ESPEN guidelines on parenteral nutrition: intensive care. *Clin. Nutr.* 28(4): 387–400.

Singer P, Pichard C, Heidegger CP, *et al.* (2010) Considering energy deficit in the intensive care unit. *Curr. Opin. Clin. Nutr. Metab. Care.* 13(2): 170–176.

Singer P, Hiesmayr M, Biolo G, *et al.* (2014) Pragmatic approach to nutrition in the ICU: expert opinion regarding which calorie protein target. *Clin. Nutr.* 33(2): 246–251.

Stapleton RD, Martin TR, Weiss NS, *et al.* (2011) A phase II randomized placebo-controlled trial of omega-3 fatty acids for the treatment of acute lung injury. *Crit. Care Med.* 39(7): 1655–1662.

Swinamer DL, Grace MG, Hamilton SM, *et al.* (1990) Predictive equation for assessing energy expenditure in mechanically ventilated critically ill patients. *Crit. Care Med.* 18(6): 657–661.

Tatucu-Babet OA, Ridley EJ, Tierney AC. (2016) Prevalence of underprescription or overprescription of energy needs in critically ill mechanically ventilated adults as determined by indirect calorimetry: a systematic literature review. *JPEN J. Parenter. Enteral Nutr.* 40(2): 212–225.

Taylor SJ, Manara AR, Brown J. (2010) Treating delayed gastric emptying in critical illness: metoclopramide, erythromycin, and bedside (cortrak) nasointestinal tube placement. *JPEN J. Parenter. Enteral Nutr.* 34(3): 289–294.

van den Berghe G, Wouters P, Weekers F, *et al.* (2001) Intensive insulin therapy in the critically ill patients. *N. Engl. J. Med.* 345(19): 1359–1367.

van Zanten AR. (2015) Glutamine and antioxidants: status of their use in critical illness. *Curr. Opin. Clin. Nutr. Metab. Care.* 18(2): 179–186.

van Zanten AR, Sztark F, Kaisers UX, *et al.* (2014) High-protein enteral nutrition enriched with immune-modulating nutrients vs standard high-protein enteral nutrition and nosocomial infections in the ICU: a randomized clinical trial. *JAMA.* 312(5): 514–524.

Ventura AM, Waitzberg DL. (2015) Enteral nutrition protocols for critically ill patients: are they necessary? *Nutr. Clin. Pract.* 30(3): 351–362.

Wang K, McIlroy K, Plank LD, *et al.* (2016) Prevalence, outcomes, and management of enteral tube feeding intolerance: a retrospective cohort study in a tertiary center. *JPEN J. Parenter. Enteral Nutr.* 41(6): 959–967.

Weijs PJ, Stapel SN, de Groot SD, *et al.* (2012) Optimal protein and energy nutrition decreases mortality in mechanically ventilated, critically ill patients a prospective observational cohort study. *JPEN J. Parenter. Enteral Nutr.* 36(1): 60–68.

Welpe P, Frutiger A, Vanek P, *et al.* (2010) Jejunal feeding tubes can be efficiently and independently placed by intensive care unit teams. *JPEN J. Parenter. Enteral Nutr.* 34(2): 121–124.

Williams TA, Leslie GD. (2010) Should gastric aspirate be discarded or retained when gastric residual volume is removed from gastric tubes? *Aust. Crit. Care* 23(4): 215–217.

Wischmeyer PE. (2008) Glutamine: role in critical illness and ongoing clinical trials. *Curr. Opin. Gastroenterol.* 24(2): 190–197.

Wischmeyer PE. (2013) The evolution of nutrition in critical care: how much, how soon? *Crit. Care* 17(1): S7.

Yamada T, Shojima N, Noma H, *et al.* (2016) Glycemic control, mortality, and hypoglycemia in critically ill patients: a systematic review and network meta-analysis of randomized controlled trials. *Intensive Care Med.* 43(1): 1–15.

Zusman O, Theilla M, Cohen J, *et al.* (2016) Resting energy expenditure, calorie and protein consumption in critically ill patients: a retrospective cohort study. *Crit. Care.* 20(1): 367.

7.17.2 Traumatic brain injury

Vicky Davies

Key points

- A number of metabolic and physiological adaptations begin early in the acute phase of traumatic brain injury, but can persist long after rehabilitation.
- Early nutritional support is associated with better outcomes, and full nutritional requirements should be safely met within 5–7 days post-injury.
- Regular monitoring of anthropometry, biochemistry, feed tolerance and nutritional intake is essential to ensure appropriate nutritional management.
- A multidisciplinary approach is key throughout the acute and rehabilitation phases in order to manage the complex features that can influence nutritional status.

Traumatic brain injury (TBI) and head injury are terms that are used to describe an injury to the brain caused by a trauma to the head. Around 1.4 million people visit emergency departments each year in England and Wales following TBI, and, in 2013–2014, there were 162,544 admissions to UK hospitals, equating to 445 cases each day (NICE, 2014). The incidence of TBI is greater in males; men are 1.6 times more likely than women to be admitted to hospital. The primary causes of TBI include falls (22–43%), assaults (30–50%) and road traffic accidents (approximately 25%), with alcohol consumption considered to be involved in up to 65% of adult head injuries

(NICE, 2014). TBI is thought to be the leading cause of disability and mortality in young people, with children under the age of 15 years accounting for 30% of cases (Maas *et al.*, 2008). Prognosis and long-term survival depend on a number of factors, including extent of injury, age, sex and level of functional disability (Brooks *et al.*, 2013).

Definition and classification

Injuries to the brain following trauma can range from mild to severe, where the latter can often have devastating and lifelong effects. Mild cases account for 75–80% of all TBIs (NICE, 2014). The Glasgow Coma Scale (GCS) is used to classify the severity of TBIs (NICE, 2014; Teasdale & Jennett, 1974):

- *Mild TBI* – GCS 13–15. Nausea and dizziness, sometimes preceded by a brief period of unconsciousness. Very unlikely to experience any lasting effects.
- *Moderate TBI* – GCS 9–12. Loss of consciousness for anywhere from 15 minutes to 6 hours, or a short period of post-traumatic amnesia (less than 24 hours) requiring overnight hospital admission for observation. Some residual symptoms may remain.
- *Severe TBI* – GCS <9. An unconscious state lasting longer than 6 hours, or post-traumatic amnesia lasting longer than 24 hours. These patients are likely to be hospitalised for a longer period of time and often require rehabilitation before discharge.

In addition to the level of severity being used to classify TBI, there are also a number of terms relating to the mode and impact of injury that can have clinical and prognostic implications (Table 7.17.5).

Clinical investigation and management

Interventions following the primary insult are aimed at preventing secondary brain injuries through advanced trauma life support and transfer to a major trauma centre that has access to specialist neurosurgical support (NICE, 2014). Initial treatment priorities include resuscitation and pain management with the aim of controlling intracranial pressure (ICP), which may be monitored via a device implanted through the skull (Haddad & Arabi, 2012). Where medical management fails to control ICP effectively, surgical intervention involving the removal of part of the skull (decompressive craniectomy) will be required. Post-operative care and medical management are provided within an intensive care setting (see Chapter 7.17.1, Critical care). A multi-disciplinary team approach is fundamental in the management of patients with TBI.

Metabolic response to injury

TBIs may cause abnormal regulation of nervous, endocrine and inflammatory systems to enable the continuous supply of substrates for cell growth and repair (Agha *et al.*, 2004; Ghirnikar *et al.*, 1998). These changes may be caused by a metabolic response to stress and by direct injury to the brain, the major organ responsible for internal regulation and homeostasis. More recently, it has been hypothesised that metabolic crisis is linked to the occurrence of seizures in patients with TBI as measured through electroencephalography (Vespa *et al.*, 2016). Possible alterations to regulatory systems include:

- Increased production of pro-inflammatory cytokines, tumour necrosis factor alpha (TNFα), interleukin-1β (IL-1β) and interleukin-6 (IL-6) (Charrueau *et al.*, 2009).

Table 7.17.5 Common terms relating to mode and impact of traumatic head injury

Term	Definition
Closed injury	Often referred to as blunt trauma, involving a blow to the head that causes the brain to knock against the skull. Closed injuries are classified as either 'primary' or 'secondary', and are the most common form of TBI.
Primary brain damage	Results from immediate anatomical/physiological insult or mechanical force.
Secondary brain damage	Results from the pathophysiological consequences of primary injury including cerebral oedema, raised intracranial pressure (ICP), hypoxia, haemorrhage, seizures, ischaemia and infection.
Penetrating/open injury	Less common than closed injuries and refers to when an object breaches the skull and coverings of the brain (three membranes collectively known as the meninges), causing direct injury and an open wound.
Cerebral contusion	A region of vascular or neuronal injury (bruising) caused by either direct trauma or rapid rotational movement.
Epidural/extradural haematoma (EDH)	Refers to structural disruption of the skull/dural vessels, leading to bleeding in the space between the dura (outermost membrane of the brain) and the skull.
Subdural haematoma (SDH)	A form of intracranial haemorrhage that occurs beneath the dura, often requiring surgical intervention.
Diffuse axonal injury	Represents diffuse cellular injury to the brain via a shearing force that disrupts the axons (white matter of the brain), following rapid rotational movement or deceleration.
Focal injuries	Specific lesions including contusions, haematomas, infarctions, axonal tears, cranial nerve evulsions and skull fractures.

- Increased circulation of the counter-regulatory hormones – cortisol, glucagon and catecholamines (Vizzini & Aranda-Michel, 2011).
- Production of acute-phase proteins from the liver (Charrueau *et al.*, 2009).
- Increased cardiac output and hypertension, leading to elevated CO_2 production and O_2 consumption (Vizzini & Aranda-Michel, 2011).

Impaired cerebral metabolism

Hyperglycaemia is a common phenomenon in head-injured patients due to a global depression of cerebral metabolic rate and for glucose uptake and utilisation (Jalloh *et al.*, 2015). Hyperglycaemia is further precipitated by circulating counter-regulatory hormones, which are released in response to trauma and cause an increase in gluconeogenesis despite persistent hyperglycaemia (Figure 7.17.1). Blood glucose levels of >11 mmol/L in the first 24 hours post-TBI have been associated with poorer outcomes, including lower GCS 5 days post-injury, increased length of hospital stay and increased mortality (Jeremitsky *et al.*, 2005; Vizzini & Aranda-Michel, 2011). The so-called *energy failure* observed following TBI is associated with a concomitant reduction in oxygen metabolism, increased uptake of lactate and increased release of excitatory neurotransmitters such as glutamate (Jalloh *et al.*, 2015).

A high lactate to pyruvate ratio in the cerebral fluid within the first 72 hours is associated with increased mortality (Timofeev *et al.*, 2011). The accumulation of lactate is thought to be secondary to a combination of mitochondrial dysfunction, hypoxia and impaired energy transfer between cells (Quintard *et al.*, 2016). Evidence is emerging to suggest that lactate can be used by certain cells as an energy substrate for the brain, especially following TBI, where energy demands may exceed supply (Barros, 2013). Infusion of hypertonic sodium lactate in patients following TBI has shown promise in individuals with impaired cerebral oxidative metabolism and may be an evolving therapy (Quintard *et al.*, 2016).

Paroxysmal sympathetic hyperactivity

Paroxysmal sympathetic hyperactivity (PSH), also known as autonomic storming, has been reported to affect up to 33% of patients with severe TBI (Hinson & Sheth, 2012). PSH describes the consequences that TBI can have on the sympathetic and parasympathetic (autonomic) nervous system. It results in a hyper-stress response that can affect a number of processes, including regulation of digestion, perspiration, breathing, temperature and heart rate, and diagnosis can often be delayed due to the varied symptomatology (Meyer, 2014).

Patients with diffuse axonal injury are at highest risk of developing PSH, and symptoms are thought to persist for a prolonged period post-injury, up to as much as 5 years (Baguley *et al.*, 2009). Treatment involves mitigating the clinical signs and symptoms by using pharmacological agents including alpha-agonists, dopaminergic agents and opiates, and early identification and treatment is recommended to avoid the long-term effects of organ dysfunction (Meyer, 2014). Nutritional requirements for patients with PSH may be significantly above their estimated needs despite adjustment for brain injury, and close and frequent monitoring with timely adjustments to nutritional treatment plans is therefore recommended (Caldwell *et al.*, 2014).

Energy expenditure

The frequency of severe hypermetabolism in TBI ranges 31–57% in the first 72 hours (Ott *et al.*, 1994; Raurich & Ibáñez, 1994), and continues for 30 days post-injury (Foley *et al.*, 2008). However, the full extent and duration of hypermetabolism is unknown, owing to the paucity of

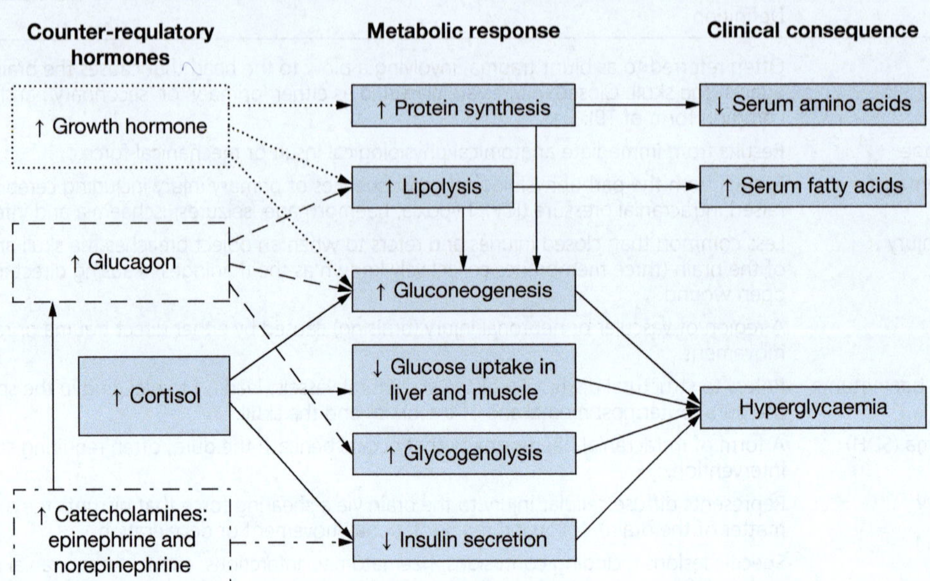

Figure 7.17.1 Metabolic response to traumatic brain injury

evidence for measured energy expenditure beyond the 30-day period. Given the prolonged effects of PDH (Baguley *et al.*, 2009), it is likely that similar patterns would be observed with energy expenditure. Hypermetabolism is defined as the ratio of measured energy expenditure to predicted energy expenditure (PEE), and can be expressed as a percentage of the PEE (Krakau *et al.*, 2007):

- <0.9 (90%) – hypometabolism
- 1.1 (110%) – hypermetabolism
- 1.3 (130%) – severe hypermetabolism

The degree of hypermetabolism is believed to be proportional to the severity of head injury (Fruin *et al.*, 1986). A systematic review found that the mean percentage of PEE ranged from 116% to 200% up to 7 days post-injury in patients without sedation, paralysis or barbiturate-induced coma (Foley *et al.*, 2008). However, in patients receiving these medical interventions, it was 80–123%, suggesting that they may blunt the traditional hypermetabolic response. Coma reduces metabolism, and paralysis reduces motor activity, leading to an overall reduced energy requirement (Bruder *et al.*, 1998; Clifton *et al.*, 1984). Other factors, including the use of morphine, mechanical ventilation and pyrexia, can also affect energy expenditure, and should be considered during nutritional assessment (Bruder *et al.*, 1998; Bursztein *et al.*, 1978; Raurich & Ibáñez, 1994). Energy expenditure is complex and multifactorial, with large variations observed between individuals with similar diagnoses. Consideration of all parameters and appropriate clinical judgement is required when assessing the energy expenditure of individuals following TBI.

Catabolism

Catabolism is observed in the majority of patients with severe TBI during the first 2 weeks post-injury, and is often characterised by an increase in nitrogen excretion (Clifton *et al.*, 1984; Krakau *et al.*, 2007; Young *et al.*, 1988). Negative nitrogen balance ensues, and has generally been observed at between −3 and −16g/day, with excessive losses of up to 30g/day reported (Krakau *et al.*, 2007). This level of protein breakdown can cause a 10% loss of lean body mass within 7 days post-injury, increasing to 10–29% within 2 months (Krakau *et al.*, 2007; Raipal & Johnston, 2009). However, a more recent study concluded that protein catabolism was no greater in TBI patients as compared to other trauma patients (Dickerson *et al.*, 2012). This suggests that critical illness secondary to trauma, regardless of presentation, may be the main determinant of a catabolic state rather than direct injury to the brain.

Gastrointestinal dysfunction

Traumatic injury, and its subsequent treatment, is often associated with abdominal hypoperfusion that can lead to a number of harmful changes to the gastrointestinal tract. Reduced blood flow can result in mucosal ischaemia, villous atrophy and increased gut permeability (Patel *et al.*, 2016). The mechanisms for increased intestinal permeability following TBI are complex, but impairment of vagal motor activity and cortico-pontine regulation, as well as increased TNFα activity, have been implicated (Pruitt *et al.*, 2016). Alterations to the gut microbiome and bacterial translocation have also been cited as causes of gut dysfunction following TBI (Patel *et al.*, 2016).

Gastroparesis is frequently reported in patients with head injury and can occur in up to 80% of patients (Kao *et al.*, 1998). Suppression of vagal nerve activity, alteration of brain–gut peptides and suppression of the enterogastric reflex as a result of increased intracranial pressure are thought to be responsible (Tan *et al.*, 2011). A prospective study of patients with severe TBI in barbiturate-induced comas identified a high risk of significant ileus that was refractory to prokinetic agents and post-pyloric feeding (Bochicchio *et al.*, 2006). The authors concluded that parenteral nutrition should be considered earlier in this patient population if gut dysfunction and subsequent intolerance to enteral nutrition is observed (see Chapter 7.17.1, Critical care).

Nutritional requirements

Estimating nutritional requirements is extremely difficult due to the rapid changes in clinical condition and a wide range of complex symptoms that can dramatically influence energy expenditure. Provision of adequate nutrition can be challenging, and significant energy and protein deficits can occur, particularly during the acute phase (Chapple *et al.*, 2016). An observational study showed that only 58% of energy requirements and 53% of protein requirements were met during the first 12 days of admission (Chapple *et al.*, 2016). For patients with TBI, strategies should be considered that aim to both calculate and deliver optimum nutrition.

Energy

It is recommended that, for patients with TBI, basal energy replacement be achieved within 5–7 days post-injury to reduce mortality (Carney *et al.*, 2017). Indirect calorimetry (IC) is considered the gold standard method of measuring resting energy expenditure (REE) (Cook *et al.*, 2008); however, this may not be realistic in practice. Predictive equations can be used to estimate energy requirements; however, none of these are specific to patients with TBI.

For mechanically ventilated patients in the acute phase of injury, the Penn State equations have been found to be the most accurate, and can better reflect the changes to energy expenditure during the initial treatment period (Frankenfield & Ashcraft, 2012; Savard *et al.*, 2008). However, the use of IC has been shown to have advantages beyond informing energy expenditure. A recent study showed that using the respiratory quotient (RQ) to direct nutritional delivery was associated with clinical improvements in nitrogen balance and substrate utilisation in patients with TBI (Maxwell *et al.*, 2017). Therefore, using IC to target nutritional therapy is likely to be more beneficial than surrogate measures in this population.

While hypocaloric feeding at around 50% of measured energy expenditure may negatively affect nitrogen balance in neurosurgical patients (Berg *et al.*, 2013), overfeeding is associated with poorer outcomes, including prolonged ventilator dependency, hyperglycaemia, metabolic acidosis and impaired liver function (Griffiths, 2007). Excessive energy provision should be avoided in the acute phase of injury when the metabolic dysfunction is likely to be at its peak. Within the critical care setting, energy provision for patients with TBI may reflect that of other trauma patients (see Chapter 7.17.1, Critical care).

For non-ventilated patients, the Scientific advisory Committee on Nutrition recommends the use of the Henry (2005) equations. However, these calculations may often need to be revised to equilibrate energy balance (Caldwell *et al.*, 2014). During the recovery phase, energy provision should be titrated to support increased activity and participation during rehabilitation, and frequent assessment and individualised treatment planning are essential to sufficiently meet fluctuating energy demands. Due to the considerable variability in energy expenditure throughout the course of the injury and the many factors that contribute to its fluctuations, clinical judgement must be used alongside predictive equations to avoid inappropriate dosing of nutrition.

Protein

During the acute phase post-injury, protein provision is aimed at attenuating losses associated with the catabolic response and maintaining a positive nitrogen balance. An early study by Twyman *et al.* (1985) found that providing 2.2 g of protein/kg/day resulted in a positive nitrogen balance (9.9 g of nitrogen retained over 10 days), as compared to 1.5 g of protein/kg/day, which was associated with a negative nitrogen balance (−31.2 g of nitrogen retained over the same period). This finding is supported by other more recent studies which have shown that an increased provision of protein is associated with more favourable outcomes in critically ill patients (Allingstrup *et al.*, 2012; Elke *et al.*, 2014; Weijs *et al.*, 2012). On the contrary, increased nitrogen provision has also been associated with greater nitrogen losses when delivered parenterally (Justo Meirelles & de Aguilar-Nascimento, 2011), and not all patients achieve a positive nitrogen balance in response to high-dose protein infusion (Dickerson *et al.*, 2012).

The precise quantity and timing of protein provision continues to be heavily debated due to conflicting findings; however, the attainment of positive nitrogen balance through high-protein feedings may still be beneficial and should be further evaluated in well-designed randomised trials (Allingstrup *et al.*, 2012; Frankenfield, 2006). Clinicians must also acknowledge the role of sufficient energy provision in maximising nitrogen retention and utilisation (Berg *et al.*, 2013; Maxwell *et al.*, 2016). Provision of high protein levels to meet requirements without adequate energy leads to increased nitrogen loss (Hoffer, 2003). Caution is necessary to avoid excessive energy intake when aiming to meet elevated protein requirements during the acute phase post-injury, as this may lead to the potentially detrimental effects of overfeeding.

In critically ill patients, protein requirements have been recommended at 1.2–2 g/kg/day of actual body weight, with adjustments for ideal body weight used in obese patients (McClave *et al.*, 2016). However, the quality of evidence behind these recommendations is poor, and more research in TBI patients is needed. The role of physical therapy alongside nutritional interventions to maintain optimal muscle mass has recently been considered as an alternative approach to high-dose protein alone, and should be tested in future randomised trials (Heyland *et al.*, 2016).

Micronutrients and immunonutrition

Patients with TBI have increased urinary zinc excretion as well as reduced serum zinc concentration (McClain *et al.*, 1986). Young *et al.* (1996) reported an improved GCS and visceral protein level in a zinc-supplemented group of TBI patients. However, concerns have been raised that accumulation of free zinc may be neurotoxic and has been linked to neuronal death in animal models (Gower-Winter & Levenson, 2012). Portbury and Adlard (2015) have suggested that dysfunction of zinc homeostasis may be linked to the neuronal pathologies observed following TBI, and research trials are needed to determine whether supplementation may offer novel therapeutic advantages.

Dietary reference values (DH, 1991) provide guidance on baseline micronutrient requirements for patients following TBI (see Chapter 17.7.1, Critical care); however, the provision of some nutrients may need to be adjusted according to the phase of injury (Vizzini & Aranda-Michel, 2011). The inability to balance antioxidant production with reactive oxygen species plays a significant role in the pathophysiologic changes that occur following TBI (Abdul-Muneer *et al.*, 2015), and there has been much interest in how antioxidant-rich, immune-enhancing nutrition (IEN) formulas may improve outcomes in these patients.

Enteral formulas supplemented with combinations of nutrients including glutamine, arginine, alanine, n-3 fatty acids and probiotics have been associated with reduced length of ICU stay and mortality in TBI patients (Falcão de Arruda & de Aguilar-Nascimento, 2004; Yang & Xu, 2007). A retrospective study in TBI found that patients receiving IEN formulas had lower rates of bloodborne infections, but length of ICU stay and days on mechanical ventilation were longer (Painter *et al.*, 2015). Guidelines for the management of critically ill patients recommend the use of immune-modulating formulas that include glutamine for patients with trauma (Carney *et al.*, 2017), but the route of administration, timing, dose and severity of injury are likely to influence outcomes in TBI (Scrimgeour & Condlin, 2014).

There are many factors that make interpretation of clinical data in relation to IEN challenging, not least the variation in composition of the formulas tested. Many formulas included in trials have contained n-3 fatty acids in combination with other immune-modulating nutrients, but there have so far been no clinical trials of n-3 as a sole immune-enhancing agent. Both eicosapentaenoic acid (EPA) and docosahexaenoic acid (DHA) are highly augmented within neuronal plasma membranes, and the requirements for these, particularly DHA, may be higher during recovery after TBI to support structural repair (Barrett *et al.*, 2014). Animal models have demonstrated positive effects of DHA supplementation on outcomes following TBI (Wu *et al.*, 2011), and it is hoped that this emerging avenue will be explored further in clinical trials involving humans.

Fluid and electrolytes

During the acute phase of TBI, patients are at high risk of significant disturbances to fluid and electrolyte balance. Antidiuretic hormone (ADH), or arginine vasopressin (AVP), regulates osmotic homeostasis in response to changes in arterial blood volume and serum osmolality (Kalra *et al.*, 2016). In head injury, hypothalamic and/or pituitary damage leads to dysfunction of the hypothalamic–pituitary axis, which may be associated with altered secretion and action of AVP. Some drugs used to treat TBI (e.g. mannitol) can also cause fluid loss through polyuria, and subsequent hypomagnesaemia, hypokalaemia and hypophosphataemia (Polderman *et al.*, 2001). Therapeutic cooling is associated with severe electrolyte depletion as a result of increased urinary excretion during the cooling phase (Soleimanpour *et al.*, 2014). Both the initial insult and subsequent treatments can lead to derangements in fluid and electrolyte balance in patients with TBI.

Hyponatraemia is the most common electrolyte imbalance observed, affecting around 15% of patients, and is associated with increased length of hospital stay and mortality (Hannon & Thompson, 2014). Hyponatraemia is implicated in a number of conditions, and an accurate assessment of blood volume status is required to aid diagnosis (Table 7.17.6). Diabetes insipidus (DI) can occur following TBI as a result of decreased secretion and/or action of AVP (Capatina *et al.*, 2015). DI is characterised by polyuria, a normal or high serum osmolality, hypernatraemia and hypovolaemia, and is associated with increased mortality, especially in those with early onset (Karali *et al.*, 2008). Management involves adequate fluid replacement, with 5% dextrose solution or isotonic saline if there is haemodynamic compromise (Lindner & Funk, 2013). With fluid management being the mainstay of treatment for DI, low-sodium feeds are often unnecessary.

Initiation of feeding

A number of guidelines recommend early initiation of feeding within the first 24–48 hours post-injury, as this has been associated with better outcomes (Bullock & Povlishock, 2007; Kreymann *et al.*, 2006; McClave *et al.*, 2016). Caution is needed during the very acute phase if patients present with haemodynamic instability requiring resuscitation, as feeding may be of detriment (Carney *et al.*, 2017). There is agreement that early feeding (within 24–72 hours), particularly via the enteral route, is beneficial for patients with TBI, and is associated with better outcomes in terms of morbidity and mortality (Bullock & Povlishock, 2007; Cook *et al.*, 2008; Falcão de Arruda & de Aguilar-Nascimento, 2004; McClave *et al.*, 2016).

Route of nutrition

The method of nutritional delivery to patients following TBI will depend on many factors, including severity of

Table 7.17.6 Diagnostic classification and treatment of conditions associated with hyponatraemia (Hannon & Thompson, 2014; Leonard *et al.*, 2015)

Condition	Blood volume status	Diagnostic criteria	Treatment
Syndrome of inappropriate antidiuretic hormone (SIADH) secretion	Euvolaemic	Low serum osmolality. Elevated urinary sodium (>40 mmol/L). Failure to correct hyponatraemia by infusion of 0.9% saline.	Fluid restriction. Exclude hypothyroidism and glucocorticoid deficiency.
Acute adrenocorticotrophic hormone (ACTH) deficiency	Euvolaemic	09:00 h cortisol <300 nmol/L in stressed patient. Hypotension, hypoglycaemia.	Steroid replacement therapy.
Cerebral salt wasting syndrome (CSWS)	Hypovolaemic	Profound diuresis and natriuresis. Low serum osmolality. Hypotension.	Aggressive IV fluids – hypertonic or 0.9% saline. Exclude renal tubular injury.
Inappropriate IV fluids	Hypervolaemic	Positive fluid balance. Oedema, left ventricular failure. Hyperglycaemia.	Diuretics. Stop IV fluids.

injury, GCS, gastrointestinal function, swallow function and any additional injuries or underlying comorbidities. Most patients with severe TBI will require artificial nutritional support during the acute phase of injury before weaning to the oral route as tolerated during recovery. The paucity of research examining the effects of nutritional support following TBI means that decisions for feeding rely heavily on clinical judgement as part of a MDT approach.

Enteral feeding

Enteral feeding is the preferred route in critically ill patients with traumatic injury due to the perceived benefits of maintaining the integrity of intestinal mucosa and reducing bacterial translocation in the gut (Carney *et al.*, 2017; McClave *et al.*, 2016). Up to 92% of patients with acute brain injury will require enteral feeding at some point during their hospitalisation, but intolerance to gastric feedings during the acute phase of injury has been found to be high (Bochicchio *et al.*, 2006; Chapple *et al.*, 2016). Post-pyloric feeding may offer an alternative route for nutrition if gastric feeding is not tolerated; however, this may not always be effective in the presence of significant ileus (Bochicchio *et al.*, 2006).

Parenteral nutrition

Much like other critically ill patients with trauma, parenteral nutrition (PN) is indicated if the patient has a non-functioning gastrointestinal tract and/or is unable to tolerate or achieve adequate nutrition by enteral feeding or oral nutrition support (Bochicchio *et al.*, 2006). A review (Perel *et al.*, 2006) found that PN was associated with better outcomes; however, this may have been as a result of earlier initiation of nutrition, rather than as a result of intravenous delivery. This review also noted a trend towards increased incidence of infection in parenteral feeding when compared with enteral feeding, and also an increased association with hyperglycaemia. Conversely, PN was associated with lower rates of pneumonia. A more detailed discussion on the use of PN in critically ill patients can be found in Chapter 7.17.1 (Critical care).

Oral nutrition support

Observational data from an acute neuro-trauma centre has shown that up to 63% of those admitted to an ICU with moderate to severe brain trauma will commence oral intake before leaving critical care (Chapple *et al.*, 2016). Dysphagia is common, with up to 84% requiring texture modification during acute hospitalisation, and approximately 40% will continue to experience swallowing difficulties on admission to rehabilitation (Brown *et al.*, 2007; Chapple *et al.*, 2016). The complexity of regaining a safe swallow in head-injured patients can be affected by their physical, cognitive, behavioural and communication-related impairments, which can make interventions for oral nutrition support challenging. It has been reported that patients with TBI who are solely ingesting nutrition orally will have significantly greater energy and protein deficits during their entire hospitalisation than those receiving either exclusive or supplementary enteral nutrition (Chapple *et al.*, 2016). Weaning from enteral feeding tubes is likely to be prolonged in these patients due to the complexity of their presentation, and it is recommended that tube feeding only be discontinued when adequate oral intake is achieved.

Disease consequences

Morbidity

Morbidity varies considerably, although long-term effects are extensive and persistent (Tagliaferri *et al.*, 2005). Thornhill *et al.* (2000) found that 29% of patients with severe head injury had a severe disability, and 19% had a moderate disability 1 year post-injury. One study found that 34% of head-injured patients reported difficulties subsequent to their injury, and 11% were medically unfit for employment (McCartan *et al.*, 2008). Consequences can be variable and far reaching, and may include physical disability, neuroendocrine effects, memory impairment and other neuropsychological difficulties.

Post-traumatic amnesia

Post-traumatic amnesia (PTA) generally refers to the subacute phase of recovery immediately after unconsciousness. Features of PTA chiefly concern extensive memory impairment but may also include psychological symptoms (confusion, agitation, anxiety and distress) and behavioural problems, such as uncharacteristic violence, aggression and disinhibition (Marshman *et al.*, 2013). Characteristics of PTA can often be observed alongside dysexecutive syndrome, which relates to impairments of a range of abilities following frontal lobe injury. Due to the heterogeneity of presentations, provision of adequate nutrition and hydration to individuals experiencing PTA can be challenging, and there is little research evidence to suggest the most appropriate strategies. However, liaising with members of the multidisciplinary team who are able to conduct assessments of PTA (e.g. occupational therapists and speech and language therapists) can help to individualise nutritional management plans. Appropriate supervision and support to eat and drink should be provided in view of the overarching memory impairment that these patients often experience.

Hypopituitarism

Due to the unique structure of the hypothalamic–pituitary vasculature and the particular location of anterior pituitary cells, TBI is a leading cause of pituitary dysfunction (Karaca *et al.*, 2016). Around 33–55% of patients with TBI have anterior pituitary hormone deficiencies, which can affect thyroid, adrenal and gonadal axes (Urban *et al.*, 2005). Deficiency in growth hormone is particularly prevalent and is often the first sign of pituitary impairment (Aimaretti *et al.*, 2004a). A recent study found that 9.1% of patients following TBI had growth hormone deficiency, with 21.3% demonstrating abnormalities in at least one of their pituitary axes (Alavi *et al.*, 2016). Hypopituitarism can have an impact on metabolic rate and body weight. To prevent long-term consequences of pituitary dysfunction, early detection and treatment is recommended with regular assessment of pituitary function for up to 12 months following injury (Aimaretti *et al.*, 2004b; Javed *et al.*, 2015).

Chemosensory disturbance

Injury to the brain can result in numerous impairments to the somatosensory system. Olfactory dysfunction has been found to affect over half of patients with more severe presentations of traumatic injury (Gudziol *et al.*, 2014). Taste perception may also be affected, particularly in those patients with direct injury to the tongue or damage to the cranial nerves VII or IX (Reiter *et al.*, 2004). There are a number of challenges in performing routine clinical taste testing, and, as such, the incidence of gustatory dysfunction among patients with TBI is currently unknown (Landis & Lacroix, 2006).

Damage to specific brain regions involved in olfactory and gustatory function may lead to new food aversions. Conversely, case reports have described how pre-morbid aversions may disappear following TBI (Fujii *et al.*, 1998). In both cases, pre-morbid dietary preferences may no longer be relevant; therefore, regular, detailed assessment of potential food aversions due to anosmia (loss of smell) and ageusia (loss of taste) is necessary to minimise the impact on nutritional intake.

Rehabilitation

In rehabilitation, the overarching aim is to help patients regain their functional independence, which may take from many months to several years. Specialist neurological rehabilitation units offer high-intensity rehabilitation as part of a multidisciplinary approach, which can provide earlier physical and cognitive functional gains (Turner-Stokes *et al.*, 2015). Complex specialised rehabilitation units are reserved for patients with highly complex needs, such as those with more severe presentations of TBI who may also have one or more comorbidities, and referrals should be made as early as possible in the acute phase of injury (British Society of Rehabilitation Medicine, 2009) (see Chapter 7.6.6, Neurorehabilitation).

Mortality

Due to significant advances in medical and neurosurgical management over the last 100 years, mortality from TBI has decreased by approximately 50% (Roozenbeek *et al.*, 2013). More recent data from the UK's Trauma Audit and Research Network (TARN) showed that the in-hospital mortality rate for isolated TBI cases was 23.1% in England and Wales (Gabbe *et al.*, 2011). When compared with a dataset from Australia, the UK's mortality rate is 3.5% higher, and this trend is even more pronounced in cases under 65 years of age. The observed differences are considered to be attributable in part to the increased number of cases in Australia that were transferred to a specialist neurosurgical trauma centre, which is now a key recommendation in UK guidelines for the management of TBI (NICE, 2014).

Conclusion

TBIs can have lasting and profound effects on the patient's physical and cognitive functioning. Providing adequate and safe nutritional support early post-injury has been shown to promote better outcomes during recovery. Close monitoring of anthropometry, biochemistry, and the clinical and dietary aspects throughout the acute and rehabilitation stages will help to ensure the patient receives timely and apt adjustments in nutritional care. A multidisciplinary approach is essential for determining appropriate nutritional strategies that can be applied throughout the patient journey.

Acknowledgement

The editor acknowledges the prior contribution of Kirsty-Anna Mclaughlin and Gemma Moore.

Internet resources

Brain Injury Rehabilitation Trust, www.birt.co.uk
Brainwave, www.brainwave.org.uk
Child Brain Injury Trust, www.childbraininjurytrust.org.uk
Headway, www.headway.org.uk
UK Acquired Brain Injury Forum, www.ukabif.org.uk

References

Abdul-Muneer PM, Chandra N, Haorah J. (2015) Interactions of oxidative stress and neurovascular inflammation in the pathogenesis of traumatic brain injury. *Mol. Neurobiol.* 51(3): 966–979.

Agha A, Rogers B, Mylotte D, *et al.* (2004) Neuroendocrine dysfunction in the acute phase of traumatic brain injury. *Clin. Endocrinol. (Oxf).* 60(5): 584–591.

Aimaretti G, Ambrosio MR, Benvenga S, *et al.*; Italian Society of Endocrinology. (2004a) Hypopituitarism and growth hormone deficiency (GHD) after traumatic brain injury (TBI). *Growth Horm. IGF Res.* 14(Suppl A): S114–S117.

Aimaretti G, Ambrosio MR, Di Somma C, *et al.* (2004b) Traumatic brain injury and subarachnoid haemorrhage are conditions at high risk for hypopituitarism: screening study at 3 months after the brain injury. *Clin. Endocrinol. (Oxf).* 61(3): 320–326.

Alavi SA, Tan CL, Menon DK, *et al.* (2016) Incidence of pituitary dysfunction following traumatic brain injury: a prospective study from a regional neurosurgical centre. *Br. J. Neurosurg.* 30(3): 302–306.

Allingstrup MJ, Esmailzadeh N, Wilkens Knudsen A, *et al.* (2012) Provision of protein and energy in relation to measured requirements in intensive care patients. *Clin. Nutr.* 31(4): 462–468.

Baguley IJ, Heriseanu RE, Nott MT, *et al.* (2009) Dysautonomia after severe traumatic brain injury. *Am. J. Phys. Med. Rehabil.* 88(8): 615–622.

Barrett E, McBurney M, Ciappio E. (2014) ω-3 fatty acid supplementation as a potential therapeutic aid for the recovery from mild traumatic brain injury/concussion. *Adv. Nutr.* 5(3): 268–277.

Barros LF. (2013) Metabolic signaling by lactate in the brain. *Trends Neurosci.* 36(7): 396–404.

Berg A, Rooyackers O, Bellander BM, *et al.* (2013) Whole body protein kinetics during hypocaloric and normocaloric feeding in critically ill patients. *Crit. Care* 17(4): R158.

Bochicchio GV, Bochicchio K, Nehman S, *et al.* (2006) Tolerance and efficacy of enteral nutrition in traumatic brain-injured patients induced into barbiturate coma. *JPEN. J. Parenter. Enteral Nutr.* 30(6): 503–506.

British Society of Rehabilitation Medicine. (2009) *BSRM Standards for Rehabilitation Services Mapped on to the National Service Framework for Long-term Conditions*. Available at https://www.bsrm.org.uk/downloads/standardsmapping-final.pdf Accessed 7 March 2019..

Brooks JC, Strauss DJ, Shavelle RM, *et al.* (2013) Long-term disability and survival in traumatic brain injury: results from the National Institute on Disability and Rehabilitation Research Model Systems. *Arch. Phys. Med. Rehabil.* 94(11): 2203–2209.

Brown AW, Malec JF, Diehl NN, *et al.* (2007) Impairment at rehabilitation admission and 1 year after moderate-to-severe traumatic brain injury: a prospective multi-centre analysis. *Brain Inj.* 21(7): 673–680.

Bruder N, Raynal M, Pellissier D, *et al.* (1998) Influence of body temperature, with or without sedation, on energy expenditure in severe head-injured patients. *Crit. Care Med.* 26(3): 568–572.

Bullock MR, Povlishock JT. (2007) Guidelines for the management of severe traumatic brain injury. Editor's Commentary. *J. Neurotrauma*. 24(1): 2 p preceding S1.

Bursztein S, Taitelman U, Myttenaere S, *et al.* (1978) Reduced oxygen consumption in catabolic states with mechanical ventilation. *Critical Care Medicine* 6(3): 162–164.

Caldwell SB, Smith D, Wilson FC. (2014) Impact of paroxysmal sympathetic hyperactivity on nutrition management after brain injury: a case series. *Brain Inj.* 28(3): 370–373.

Capatina C, Paluzzi A, Mitchell R, *et al.* (2015) Diabetes insipidus after traumatic brain injury. *J. Clin. Med.* 4(7): 1448–1462.

Carney N, Totten AM, O'Reilly C, *et al.* (2017) Guidelines for the management of severe traumatic brain injury, fourth edition. *Neurosurgery.* 80(1): 6–15.

Chapple LS, Deane AM, Heyland DK, *et al.* (2016) Energy and protein deficits throughout hospitalization in patients admitted with a traumatic brain injury. *Clin. Nutr.* 35(6): 1315–1322.

Charrueau C, Belabed L, Besson V, *et al.* (2009) Metabolic response and nutritional support in traumatic brain injury: evidence for resistance to renutrition. *J. Neurotrauma.* 26(11): 1911–1920.

Clifton GL, Robertson CS, Grossman RG, *et al.* (1984) The metabolic response to severe head injury. *J. Neurosurg.* 60(4): 687–696.

Cook AM, Peppard A, Magnuson B. (2008) Nutrition considerations in traumatic brain injury. *Nutr. Clin. Pract.* 23(6): 608–620.

DH. (1991) *Dietary Reference Values for Food Energy and Nutrients for the United Kingdom.* (41) London: HSMO.

Dickerson RN, Pitts SL, Maish GO, *et al.* (2012) A reappraisal of nitrogen requirements for patients with critical illness and trauma. *J. Trauma Acute Care Surg.* 73(3): 549–557.

Elke G, Wang M, Weiler N, *et al.* (2014) Close to recommended caloric and protein intake by enteral nutrition is associated with better clinical outcome of critically ill septic patients: secondary analysis of a large international nutrition database. *Crit. Care.* 18(1): R29.

Falcão de Arruda IS, de Aguilar-Nascimento JE. (2004) Benefits of early enteral nutrition with glutamine and probiotics in brain injury patients. *Clin. Sci.* 106(3): 287–292.

Foley N, Marshall S, Pikul J, *et al.* (2008) Hypermetabolism following moderate to severe traumatic acute brain injury: a systematic review. *J. Neurotrauma.* 25(12): 1415–1431.

Frankenfield D. (2006) Energy expenditure and protein requirements after traumatic injury. *Nutr. Clin. Pract.* 21(5): 430–437.

Frankenfield DC, Ashcraft CM. (2012) Description and prediction of resting metabolic rate after stroke and traumatic brain injury. *Nutrition (Burbank, Los Angeles County, Calif.)* 28(9): 906–911.

Fruin AH, Taylon C, Pettis MS. (1986) Caloric requirements in patients with severe head injuries. *Surg. Neurol.* 25(1): 25–28.

Fujii M, Fujita K, Hiramatsu H, *et al.* (1998) Cases of two patients whose food aversions disappeared following severe traumatic brain injury. *Brain Inj.* 12(8): 709–713.

Gabbe BJ, Lyons RA, Lecky FE, *et al.* (2011) Comparison of mortality following hospitalisation for isolated head injury in England and Wales, and Victoria, Australia. *PLoS One*, 6(5): e20545.

Ghirnikar RS, Lee YL, Eng LF. (1998) Inflammation in traumatic brain injury: role of cytokines and chemokines. *Neurochem. Res.* 23(3): 329–340.

Gower-Winter SD, Levenson CW. (2012) Zinc in the central nervous system: From molecules to behavior. *Biofactors.* 38(3): 186–193.

Griffiths RD. (2007) Too much of a good thing: the curse of overfeeding. *Crit. Care* 11(6): 176.

Gudziol V, Hoenck I, Landis B, *et al.* (2014) The impact and prospect of traumatic brain injury on olfactory function: a cross-sectional and prospective study. *Eur. Arch. Otorhinolaryngol.* 271(6): 1533–1540.

Haddad S, Arabi Y. (2012) Critical care management of severe traumatic brain injury in adults. *Scand. J. Trauma Resusc. Emerg. Med.* 20(1): 12.

Hannon MJ, Thompson CJ. (2014) Neurosurgical hyponatremia. *J. Clin. Med.* 3(4): 1084–1104.

Henry CJK. (2005) Basal metabolic rate studies in humans: measurement and development of new equations. *Public Health Nutr.* 8(7A): 1133–1152.

Heyland DK, Stapleton RD, Mourtzakis M, *et al.* (2016) Combining nutrition and exercise to optimize survival and recovery from critical illness: conceptual and methodological issues. *Clin. Nutr.* 35(5): 1196–1206.

Hinson HE, Sheth KN. (2012) Manifestations of the hyperadrenergic state after acute brain injury. *Curr. Opin. Crit. Care* 18(2): 139–145.

Hoffer LJ. (2003) Protein and energy provision in critical illness. *Am. J. Clin. Nutr.* 78(5): 906–911.

Jalloh I, Carpenter KL, Helmy A, *et al.* (2015) Glucose metabolism following human traumatic brain injury: methods of assessment and pathophysiological findings. *Metab. Brain Dis.* 30(3): 615–632.

Javed Z, Qamar U, Sathyapalan T. (2015) Pituitary and/or hypothalamic dysfunction following moderate to severe traumatic brain injury: current perspectives. *Indian J. Endocrinol. Metab.* 19(6): 753–763.

Jeremitsky E, Omert LA, Dunham CM, *et al.* (2005) The impact of hyperglycemia on patients with severe brain injury. *J. Trauma.* 58(1): 47–50.

Justo Meirelles CM, de Aguilar-Nascimento JE. (2011) Enteral or parenteral nutrition in traumatic brain injury: a prospective randomised trial. *Nutr. Hosp.* 26(5): 1120–1124.

Kalra S, Zargar AH, Jain SM, *et al.* (2016) Diabetes insipidus: the other diabetes. *Indian J. Endocrinol. Metab.* 20(1): 9–21.

Kao CH, ChangLai SP, Chieng PU, *et al.* (1998) Gastric emptying in head-injured patients. *Am. J. Gastroenterol.* 93(7): 1108–1112.

Karaca Z, Tanrıverdi F, Ünlühizarcı K, *et al.* (2016) GH and pituitary hormone alterations after traumatic brain injury. *Prog. Mol. Biol. Transl. Sci.* 138: 167–191.

Karali V, Massa E, Vassiliadou G, *et al.* (2008) Evaluation of development of diabetes insipidus in the early phase following traumatic brain injury in critically ill patients. *Crit. Care* 12(2): P130.

Krakau K, Hansson A, Karlsson T, *et al.* (2007) Nutritional treatment of patients with severe traumatic brain injury during the first six months after injury. *Nutrition* 23(4): 308–317.

Kreymann KG, Berger MM, Deutz NE, *et al.* (2006) ESPEN guidelines on enteral Nutrition: intensive care. *Clin. Nutr.* 25(2): 210–223.

Landis BN, Lacroix J-S. (2006) Postoperative/posttraumatic gustatory dysfunction. *Adv. Otorhinolaryngol.* 63: 242–254.

Leonard J, Garrett RE, Salottolo K, *et al.* (2015) Cerebral salt wasting after traumatic brain injury: a review of the literature. *Scand. J. Trauma Resusc. Emerg. Med.* 23(1): 98.

Lindner G, Funk GC. (2013) Hypernatremia in critically ill patients. *J. Crit. Care* 28(2): 216. e11–20.

Maas AI, Stocchetti N, Bullock R. (2008) Moderate and severe traumatic brain injury in adults. *Lancet Neurol.* 7(8): 728–741.

Marshman LAG, Jakabek D, Hennessy M, *et al.* (2013) Post-traumatic amnesia. *J. Clin. Neurosci.* 20(11): 1475–1481.

Maxwell J, Gwardschaladse C, Lombardo G, *et al.* (2017) The impact of measurement of respiratory quotient by indirect calorimetry on the achievement of nitrogen balance in patients with severe traumatic brain injury. *Eur. J. Trauma Emerg. Surg.* 43(6): 775–782 (September).

McCartan DP, Fleming FJ, Motherway C, *et al.* (2008) Management and outcome in patients following head injury admitted to an Irish Regional Hospital. *Brain Inj.* 22(4): 305–312.

McClain CJ, Twyman DL, Ott LG, *et al.* (1986) Serum and urine zinc response in head-injured patients. *J. Neurosurg.* 64(2): 224–230.

McClave SA, Taylor BE, Martindale RG, *et al.* (2016) Guidelines for the provision and assessment of nutrition support therapy in the adult critically ill patient: Society of Critical Care Medicine (SCCM) and American Society for Parenteral and Enteral Nutrition (A.S.P.E.N.). *JPEN. J. Parenter. Enteral Nutr.* 40(2): 159–211.

Meyer K. (2014) Understanding paroxysmal sympathetic hyperactivity after traumatic brain injury. *Surg. Neurol. Int.* 5(14): 490–492.

NICE. (2014) *Head injury: triage, assessment, investigation and early management of head injury in infants, children and adults.* Available at https://www.nice.org.uk/guidance/cg176. Accessed 22 November 2018.

Ott M, Schmidt J, Young B, *et al.* (1994) Nutritional and metabolic variables correlate with amino acid forearm flux in patients with severe head injury. *Crit. Care Med.* 22(3): 393–398.

Painter TJ, Rickerds J, Alban RF. (2015) Immune enhancing nutrition in traumatic brain injury – a preliminary study. *Int. J. Surg.* 21: 70–74.

Patel JJ, Rosenthal MD, Miller KR, *et al.* (2016) The gut in trauma. *Curr. Opin. Crit. Care.* 22(4): 339–346.

Perel P, Yanagawa T, Bunn F, Roberts IG, Wentz R. (2006) Nutritional support for head-injured patients. *Cochrane Database of Systematic Reviews* 4: CD001530.

Polderman KH, Peerdeman SM, Girbes AR. (2001) Hypophosphatemia and hypomagnesemia induced by cooling in patients with severe head injury. *J. Neurosurg.* 94(5): 697–705.

Portbury SD, Adlard PA. (2015) Traumatic brain injury, chronic traumatic encephalopathy, and Alzheimer's disease: common pathologies potentiated by altered zinc homeostasis. *J. Alzheimer's Dis.* 46(2): 297–311.

Pruitt DT, Schmid AN, Kim LJ, *et al.* (2016) Vagus nerve stimulation delivered with motor training enhances recovery of function after traumatic brain injury. *J. Neurotrauma.* 33(9): 871–879.

Quintard H, Patet C, Zerlauth J-B, *et al.* (2016) Improvement of neuroenergetics by hypertonic lactate therapy in patients with traumatic brain injury is dependent on baseline cerebral lactate/pyruvate ratio. *J. Neurotrauma.* 33(7): 681–687.

Rajpal V, Johnston J. (2009) Nutrition management of traumatic brain injury patients. *Support Line* 31(1): 10–19.

Raurich JM, Ibáñez J. (1994) Metabolic rate in severe head trauma. *JPEN. J. Parenter. Enteral Nutr.* 18(6): 521–524.

Reiter ER, DiNardo LJ, Costanzo RM. (2004) Effects of head injury on olfaction and taste. *Otolaryngol. Clin. North Am.* 37(6): 1167–1184.

Roozenbeek B, Maas AIR, Menon DK. (2013) Changing patterns in the epidemiology of traumatic brain injury. *Nat. Rev. Neurol.* 9(4): 231–236.

Savard J-F, Faisy C, Lerolle N, *et al.* (2008) Validation of a predictive method for an accurate assessment of resting energy expenditure in medical mechanically ventilated patients. *Crit. Care Med.* 36(4): 1175–1183.

Scrimgeour AG, Condlin ML. (2014) Nutritional treatment for traumatic brain injury. *J. Neurotrauma.* 31: 989–999.

Soleimanpour H, Rahmani F, Golzari SEJ, *et al.* (2014) Main complications of mild induced hypothermia after cardiac arrest: a review article. *J. Cardiovasc. Thorac. Res.* 6(1): 1–8.

Tagliaferri F, Compagnone C, Korsic M, Servadei F, Kraus J. (2005) A systematic review of brain injury epidemiology in Europe. *Eur. J. Neurosurgery* 148(3): 255–268.

Tan M, Zhu J-C, Yin H-H. (2011) Enteral nutrition in patients with severe traumatic brain injury: reasons for intolerance and medical management. *Br. J. Neurosurg.* 25(1): 2–8.

Teasdale G, Jennett B. (1974) Assessment of coma and impaired consciousness. A practical scale. *Lancet* 2(7872): 81–84.

Thornhill S, Teasdale GM, Murray GD, *et al.* (2000) Disability in young people and adults one year after head injury: prospective cohort study. *BMJ.* 320(7250): 1631–1635.

Timofeev I, Carpenter KL, Nortje J, *et al.* (2011) Cerebral extracellular chemistry and outcome following traumatic brain injury: a microdialysis study of 223 patients. *Brain* 134(2): 484–494.

Turner-Stokes L, Disler PB, Nair A, *et al.* (2015) Multi-disciplinary rehabilitation for acquired brain injury in adults of working age. *Cochrane Database Syst. Rev.* (3): CD004170.

Twyman D, Young AB, Ott L, *et al.* (1985) High protein enteral feedings: a means of achieving positive nitrogen balance in head injured patients. *JPEN. J. Parenter. Enteral Nutr.* 9(6): 679–684.

Urban RJ, Harris P, Masel B. (2005) Anterior hypopituitarism following traumatic brain injury. *Brain Inj.* 19(5): 349–358.

Vespa P, Tubi M, Claassen J, *et al.* (2016) Metabolic crisis occurs with seizures and periodic discharges after brain trauma. *Ann. Neurol.* 79(4): 579–590.

Vizzini A, Aranda-Michel J. (2011) Nutritional support in head injury. *Nutrition.* 27(2): 129–132.

Weijs PJM, Stapel SN, de Groot SD, *et al.* (2012) Optimal protein and energy nutrition decreases mortality in mechanically ventilated, critically ill patients: a prospective observational cohort study. *JPEN. J. Parenter. Enteral Nutr.* 36(1): 60–68.

Wu A, Ying Z, Gomez-Pinilla F. (2011) The salutary effects of DHA dietary supplementation on cognition, neuroplasticity, and membrane homeostasis after brain trauma. *J. Neurotrauma.* 28(10): 2113–2122.

Yang D, Xu J. (2007) Effect of dipeptide of glutamine and alanine on severe traumatic brain injury. *Chin. J. Traumatol.* 10(3): 145–149.

Young AB, Ott LG, Beard D, *et al.* (1988) The acute-phase response of the brain-injured patient. *J. Neurosurg.* 69(3): 375–80.

Young B, Ott L, Kasarskis E, *et al.* (1996) Zinc supplementation is associated with improved neurologic recovery rate and visceral protein levels of patients with severe closed head injury. *J. Neurotrauma.* 13(1): 25–34.

7.17.3 Spinal cord injury

Anthony Twist and Samford Wong

Key points

- Acute post-injury period
  - Energy expenditure is reduced; care needed to avoid overfeeding.
  - Protein requirements may be high.
- Rehabilitation
  - A reduction in energy expenditure increases the risk of excessive weight gain.
  - Neurogenic bowel dysfunction may require dietary fibre intake adjustment.
  - There is a high risk of pressure ulcers; therefore, nutritionally balanced diets are essential.

The UK has 11 spinal cord injury (SCI) centres, which have a total of approximately 460 beds for the rehabilitation of people with a spinal injury; the first UK SCI centre opened in Stoke Mandeville in 1944. The metabolic response to injury is well documented (see Chapter 7.17.1, Critical care), and the prevalence of malnutrition and its effects on the person with SCI have been recognised since the time of Hippocrates (Guttmann, 1973). Prior to the mid-twentieth century, few people with SCI survived more than 2 years. Today, long-term survival closely matches that of the age-matched non-spinal-injury population; the mean age for sustaining SCI appears to be increasing.

As with anyone suffering acute injury necessitating subsequent rehabilitation, dietetic care should be an integral part of their management. Dietetic provision in UK SCI centres is variable, with a whole-time equivalent covering 56–160 beds and variable levels of staffing grades (Wong *et al.*, 2015).

Spinal cord injury definitions

The effects of an SCI depend on which segments of the spinal cord is damaged (see Figure 7.17.2). The American Spinal Injury Association Impairment Scale (ASIA) (see Figure 7.17.3) focuses on 10 sensory points and 10 key muscles to be tested during neurological assessment (ASIA, 2002). The likely consequence of spinal injury may include the following:

- Complete and incomplete lesions:
  - In a complete lesion, all neurological function is lost below the level of the lesion.
  - In an incomplete lesion, there is partial preservation of neurological function, and any combination of motor (muscle), sensory (feeling) or autonomic function may be spared. (Nerves of the autonomic system control those body functions which are not under conscious control.)
  - Brown-Séquard syndrome or central cord syndrome describes the different patterns of incomplete lesions, and the latter usually occurs as a result of neck injuries. These and other syndromes are described in *The ABC of Spinal Cord Injury* (see the 'Further reading' section).
- Paraplegia – function of the lower limbs is lost as a result of damage to the thoracic, lumbar or, to a lesser extent, sacral cord segments.
- Tetraplegia (quadriplegia) – this results from damage to cervical cord segments causing loss of function in all four limbs.
- In both paraplegia and tetraplegia, there is impairment of autonomic function, including bladder and bowel control.
- Muscle wasting – post-injury muscle wasting results in a reduction of lean body mass, and, in the longer term, immobility encourages an increase in total body fat (Rasmann Nuhlicek *et al.*, 1988; Shizgal *et al.*, 1986; Spungen *et al.*, 2003).
- Autonomic dysreflexia (AD) – people with SCI above (thoracic vertebra) the T6 level may experience AD. It is a group of abnormal signs and symptoms triggered by a harmful stimulus below the level of the lesion that causes an increase in autonomic activity (Consortium for Spinal Cord Medicine, 2008). It is characterised by a sudden, severe headache secondary to an uncontrolled elevation of blood pressure, flushing and profuse sweating. If untreated, the hypertension may progress to fatal complications, such as cerebral haemorrhage or acute myocardial infarction. The most common nutrition-related stimuli are an over-distended bladder, bowel impaction, urinary infection and pressure ulcers.

Management

Management within first week of injury

Complex physiological changes occur following spinal cord injury, and these vary with the following:

- Level of the lesion.
- Extent of damage to the spinal cord (as measured by the ASIA scale or Frankel classification).

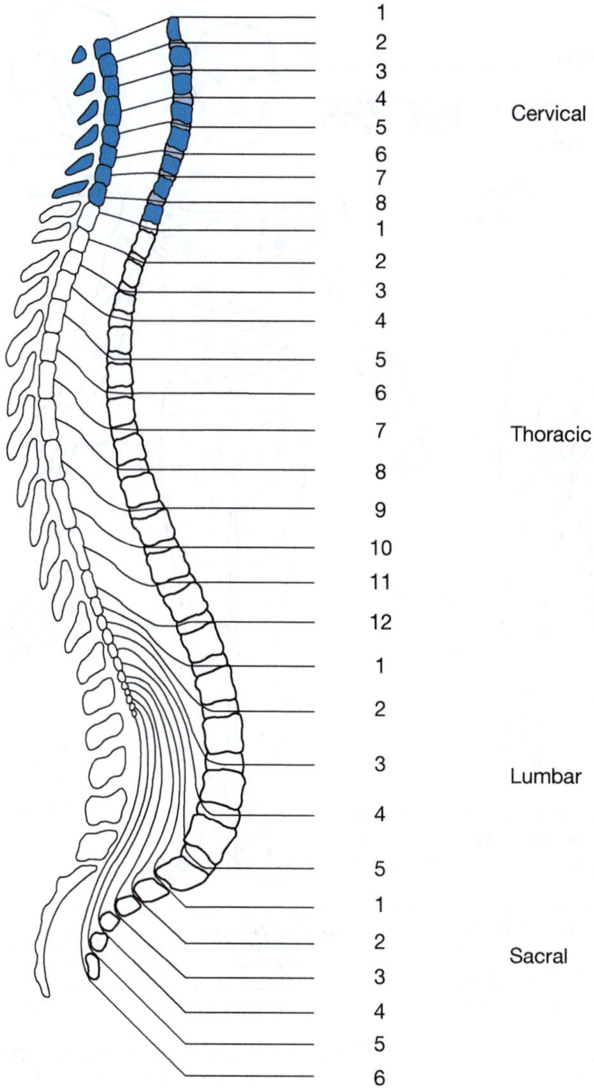

Figure 7.17.2 The spinal cord

- Presence of concomitant injury or illness.
- Time elapsed since injury.

These physiological changes result in a dynamic metabolic state that may adversely affect the nutritional status at any time (Worthington *et al.*, 1993). If left untreated, this catabolic state could lead to loss of lean muscle mass and poorer clinical outcomes, including impaired wound healing, increased risk of infection, increased premature mortality and increased healthcare costs. The association between acute SCI and deterioration in nutritional status can persist for several months post-injury (Marian, 2004).

The presence of delayed gastric emptying and paralytic ileus during this initial post-injury period often preclude or complicate enteral feeding (see Chapter 7.17.1, Critical care). Unfortunately, other priorities in clinical care may result in the neglect of nutritional needs. Additionally, weighing the individual is often difficult, as is the interpretation of anthropometry. However, most people with SCI transferred from general hospital to SCI centres should at least have had a nutritional risk assessment using a validated tool; either the Malnutrition Universal Screening Tool ('MUST'), or a validated, disease-specific screening tool such as the Spinal Nutrition Screening Tool (SNST) (Wong *et al.*, 2012a) (see Appendix A7, Nutrition screening tools). This will help identify the need for further nutritional interventions and should be repeated periodically unless transfer occurs very quickly.

Energy requirements

The energy needs of SCI individuals are unclear (Barco *et al.*, 2002; Cox *et al.*, 1985; Kearns *et al.*, 1992; Nevin *et al.*, 2016a; Peruzzi *et al.*, 1994; Rodriguez *et al.*, 1997). However, in contrast to people with trauma or head injury, it appears that energy expenditure is reduced after SCI (Buchholz & Pencharz, 2004; Sedlock & Laventure, 1990). In fact, measured basal metabolic rate (BMR) has been found to be 14–27% lower than in able-bodied controls (Buchholz & Pencharz, 2004). Two possible mechanisms have been proposed to explain the reduced BMR: a change in body composition, resulting in reduced fat-free mass, and an altered sympathetic nervous system activity. Therefore, predicting energy expenditure with the use of standard equations will tend to overestimate measured requirements by 5–32%, especially in tetraplegia (Cox *et al.*, 1985).

Indirect calorimetry remains the only accurate assessment of resting energy expenditure (REE) for patients after SCI. Nevin *et al.* (2016a) found indirect calorimetry to be an acceptable addition to routine clinical care, despite some patients complaining of claustrophobia (Nevin *et al.*, 2016b). Not all clinical rehabilitation centres will have access to indirect calorimetry (Buchholz & Pencharz, 2004); in its absence, it is recommended to interpret the predicted energy requirements with caution (American Dietetic Association, 2009). Overfeeding should be avoided, since it could have adverse effects on glucose tolerance and lead to respiratory dysfunction due to excessive carbon dioxide production (EAST, 2003). Dietitians must exercise judgement and be alert to emerging research on energy requirements in spinal injury.

Iron

Anaemia is common in acute SCI, even without visible blood losses (Huang *et al.*, 1990). Providing adequate nutritional intake of iron is essential. Adequate vitamin C intake helps improve iron absorption from non-haemoglobin sources.

Vitamins

Laven *et al.* (1989) demonstrated deficiencies in a variety of vitamins, including vitamin C, folate and thiamine, which drop to their lowest level 2 weeks following injury, and remain low for some weeks. They suggested full vitamin screening to ensure that these deficiencies are recognised and rectified. Rice *et al.* (1995) recommended that a daily multivitamin be given to all acute SCI individuals.

Management 2–12 weeks following injury

A SCI individual should be transferred as soon as possible to an SCI centre. The importance of nutritional assessment, early identification of those at nutritional

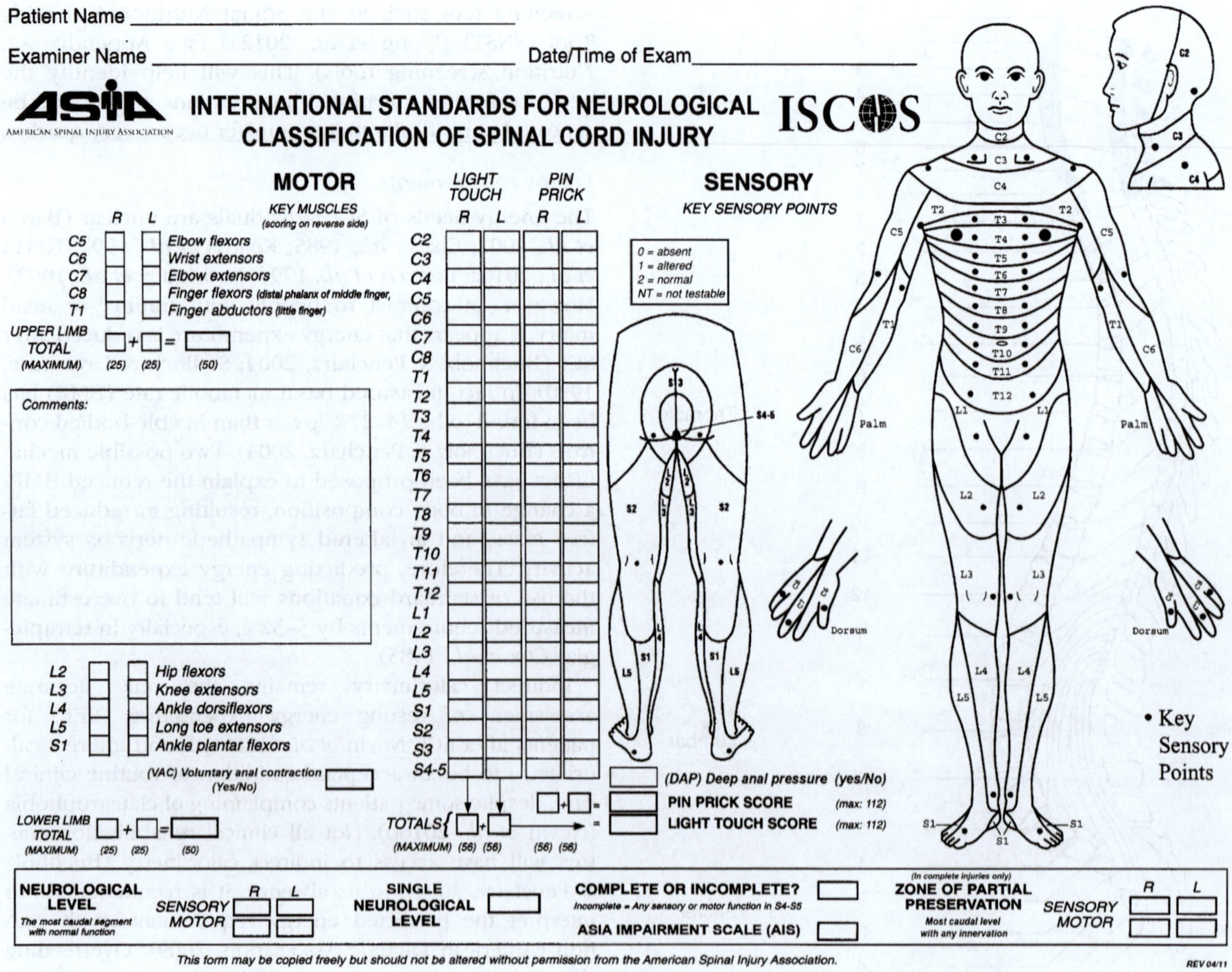

Figure 7.17.3 International standards for neurological classification of spinal cord injury (source: International Standards for Neurological Classification of Spinal Cord Injury, American Spinal Injury Association 2013. Reproduced with permission from the American Spinal Injury Association)

risk, and appropriate nutritional support are being increasingly recognised in these centres (MASCIP, 2010; RCP, 2008). Dietitians who manage people with SCI need to understand the extent of their injuries and acknowledge the profound psychological effects of these injuries. Whenever clinically permissible, SCI individuals should be fed in a semi-recumbent position; this may not be possible if they have not undergone spinal fixation. Caution is needed in feeding SCI individuals in a fully recumbent position. Nutritional status is adversely affected by SCI, particularly during the first 2–4 weeks (Cheshire & Coats, 1966; Laven *et al.*, 1989), and nutritional depletion resulting from the initial metabolic response to trauma may be severe. Negative nitrogen balance after SCI is inevitable, correlating with the level and extent of injury, and may persist for as long as 7 weeks (Hadley, 2002). Acute protein needs are unclear, but 2 g protein/kg/day is suggested (American Dietetic Association, 2009; Kearns *et al.*, 1992; Marian, 2004; Peruzzi *et al.*, 1994).

Gastrointestinal problems arise in both the acute and long-term setting, with paralytic ileus and gastric ulcers commonly occurring during the first 4 weeks post-injury, and lower tract dysfunction thereafter (Frost, 1998). Intestinal paralysis (ileus) is prominent during the acute phase of SCI. Regurgitation and vomiting may occur and result in aspiration pneumonia. The Consortium for Spinal Cord Medicine (2008) recommended considering enteral feeding within 24–48 hours after admission if patients could not meet their nutritional needs orally. The enteral route should be considered before parenteral nutrition due to the increased risk of infectious complications and lower incidence of hyperglycaemia.

Nutritional assessment

The prevalence of malnutrition is common among SCI individuals. A recent study of people admitted to UK SCI centres found that approximately 40% were at risk of undernutrition and 45% were overweight on admission (Wong *et al.*, 2012b). Factors that are likely to reduce dietary intake include associated injuries, e.g. long bone fractures and brain injuries, and pressure ulcers. Other factors are summarised in Table 7.17.7.

Use of disease-specific nutrition screening tool

National and international reports (Council of Europe Committee of Ministers, 2003; NICE, 2006; RCP, 2008) have

SECTION 7

Muscle Function Grading

0 = total paralysis

1 = palpable or visible contraction

2 = active movement, full range of motion (ROM) with gravity eliminated

3 = active movement, full ROM against gravity

4 = active movement, full ROM against gravity and moderate resistance in a muscle specific position.

5 = (normal) active movement, full ROM against gravity and full resistance in a muscle specific position expected from an otherwise unimpaired peson.

5* = (normal) active movement, full ROM against gravity and sufficient resistance to be considered normal if identified inhibiting factors (i.e. pain, disuse) were not present.

NT = not testable (i.e. due to immobilization, severe pain such that the patient cannot be graded, amputation of limb, or contracture of >50% of the range of motion).

ASIA Impairment (AIS) Scale

☐ **A = Complete.** No sensory or motor function is preserved in the sacral segments S4-S5.

☐ **B = Sensory Incomplete.** Sensory but not motor function is preserved below the neurological level and includes the sacral segments S4-S5 (light touch, pin prick at S4-S5: or deep anal pressure (DAP)), AND no motor function is preserved more than three levels below the motor level on either side of the body.

☐ **C = Motor Incomplete.** Motor function is preserved below the neurological level**, and more than half of key muscle functions below the single neurological level of injury (NLI) have a muscle grade less than 3 (Grades 0-2).

☐ **D = Motor Incomplete.** Motor function is preserved below the neurological level**, and at least half (half or more) of key muscle functions below the NLI have a muscle grade ≥ 3.

☐ **E = Normal.** If sensation and motor function as tested with the ISNCSCI are graded as normal in all segments, and the patient had prior deficits, then the AIS grade is E. Someone without an initial SCI does not receive an AIS grade.

**For an individual to receive a grade of C or D, i.e. motor incomplete status, they must have either (1) voluntary anal sphincter contraction or (2) sacral sensory sparing with sparing of motor function more than three levels below the motor level for that side of the body. The Standards at this time allows even non-key muscle function more than 3 levels below the motor level to be used in determining motor incomplete status (AIS B versus C).

NOTE: When assessing the extent of motor sparing below the level for distinguishing between AIS B and C, the ***motor level*** on each side is used; whereas to differentiate between AIS C and D (based on proportion of key muscle functions with strength grade 3 or greater) the ***single neurological level*** is used.

Steps in Classification

The following order is recommended in determining the classification of individuals with SCI.

1. Determine sensory levels for right and left sides.
2. Determine motor levels for right and left sides.
   Note: in regions where there is no myotome to test, the motor level is presumed to be the same as the sensory level, if testable motor function above that level is also normal.
3. Determine the single neurological level.
   This is the lowest segment where motor and sensory function is normal on both sides, and is the most cephalad of the sensory and motor levels determined in steps 1 and 2.
4. Determine whether the injury is Complete or Incomplete.
   (i.e. absence or presence of sacral sparing)
   If voluntary anal contraction = **No** *AND all S4-5 sensory scores =* **0** *AND deep anal pressure =* **No,** *then injury is COMPLETE. Otherwise, injury is incomplete.*
5. Determine ASIA Impairment Scale (AIS) Grade:

Is injury Complete? If **YES,** AIS=A and can record ZPP (lowest dermatome or myotome on each side with some preservation)

NO ↓

Is injury motor Incomplete? If **NO,** AIS=B (Yes=voluntary anal contraction OR motor function more than three levels below the motor level on a given side, if the patient has sensory incomplete classification)

YES ↓

Are at least half of the key muscles below the single neurological level graded 3 or better?

NO ↓ AIS=C

YES ↓ AIS=D

If sensation and motor function is normal in all segments, AIS=E

Note: AIS E is used in follow-up testing when an individual with a documented SCI has recovered normal function. If at initial testing no deficits are found, the individual is neurologically intact; the ASIA Impairment Scale does not apply.

Figure 7.17.3 *(Continued)*

highlighted the importance of nutritional screening as an important step to address malnutrition. The SNST has been developed for use in people with SCI and externally validated (Wong *et al.*, 2012a) (see Appendix A7, Nutrition screening tools). It is based on eight parameters:

- Body mass index (BMI).
- Age.
- Level of SCI.
- Presence of comorbidities.
- Skin conditions.
- Diet.
- Appetite.
- Ability to eat.

Assessing weight loss since injury

The degree of weight loss since SCI is an important indicator of nutritional depletion; most individuals will be able to recall their pre-injury weight. Obtaining current weight can be difficult even if bed-weighing or hoist scales are available, owing to several factors, including unemptied catheter or stoma. Dependence on a ventilator can mean weighing is not feasible. It is recommended that weight be taken on admission, and repeated periodically for those identified to be at nutritional risk (NICE, 2017). In some cases, estimation of weight loss must be done visually; however, it should be borne in mind that muscle wasting may have resulted from denervation following the spinal injury and bed rest rather than nutritional depletion.

Other assessments

Estimates of muscle mass by measurements such as mid-arm muscle circumference are likely to be distorted by the effects of the spinal cord injury and any consequent paraplegia or quadriplegia. Estimates of adiposity by BMI will be dependent on the ability to obtain a meaningful estimate of current body weight. While direct measurement of height is likely to be impossible, a reliable estimate of height can be made by ulnar length measurements (Elia, 2003). A 24-hour urine collection to measure urea nitrogen can be useful in determining protein status (Agarwal *et al.*, 1987). Bioimpedance measurement is potentially useful, although hydration states can fluctuate in the acute period.

Dietary intake

Although it is often possible to obtain estimates of previous and current dietary intake from the SCI individuals, records of food and fluid intake and changes in appetite noted by care staff should also be taken into account. Anecdotally, people with SCI appear to have a reduced dietary intake in SCI centres, but, due to the enforced immobility, they may meet their energy requirement.

Table 7.17.7 Factors that may reduce dietary intake

Category	Factors
Neurological	Extent of SCI
	Pain associated with SCI
	Surgical intervention of spinal cord
Psychological	Depression due to SCI
	Social isolation
	Confusion
Infections	Urinary tract
	Bladder
	Chest
	Catheter-related
	Infected pressure ulcers
	Sepsis
Drugs	Polypharmacy
	Nausea and vomiting
	Diarrhoea
Physical difficulties	Bed rest post-SCI
	Refusal or reluctance to eat and drink
	Mechanical dysphagia due to ventilator
Respiratory	Chest infections
	Ventilating support
	Tracheotomy tube
Gastrointestinal	Neurological or mechanical dysphagia
	Paralytic ileus
	Nausea and vomiting
	Gastrointestinal bleeding
	Diarrhoea or constipation
	Early satiety
	Abdominal injuries
Social	Recreational drug use
	Alcohol abuse
	Stress
	Lack of social support

Table 7.17.8 Guide to weighing individuals with spinal cord injuries

Degree of mobility	Suitable weighing method
Fully mobile SCI individuals	Standing scales
Good balance	Sit down scales
Poor balance	
Wheelchair-dependent	Sit down scales
Able to transfer and can hold legs free from the floor	Wheelchair weighing scales
	Weighbridge
Unable/inconvenient to transfer from wheelchair	Wheelchair weighing scales
	Weighbridge
Able to transfer but cannot hold legs free from chair	
On bed or trolley, can be lifted by hoist	Hoist scale with sling or stretcher attachment
Bed-bound, bed not easily moved	Weighbridge or platform weighing scales
Bed-bound, bed cannot be moved	Bed with weighing device
	Portable bed weighing scales

Manufacturers of this equipment are listed at the end of this chapter.

Management after 12 weeks – continuing rehabilitation phase

The aim of rehabilitation is to enable the individual to develop the maximum potential possible for their disability. For those who have lost weight during the immediate post-injury period, weight regain and restoration of muscle mass is a priority, so that they are able to derive maximum benefit from physiotherapy and occupational therapy sessions. Intake is often improved once a person is able to sit up, but where normal food intake is insufficient, additional nutritious snacks and prescribed oral nutritional supplements may be required. Reduction in energy needs is proportional to the amount of denervated muscle an SCI individual has. The American Dietetic Association (2009) suggested using 22 kcal/kg body weight for those with quadriplegia, and 28 kcal/kg for those with paraplegia, to estimate (with caution) energy needs. If individuals are unable to meet their nutritional needs by oral intake alone, overnight enteral feeding may be a useful method of nutritional support, as this strategy does not interfere with daytime therapy sessions. At this stage of rehabilitation, it is usually easier to measure and monitor SCI individuals than in earlier stages, as shown in Table 7.17.8. However, due to the associated muscle wasting, the ideal range is suggested to be 18.5–22 kg/m^2 (Laughton *et al.*, 2009).

Overweight and obesity

As rehabilitation progresses, becoming overweight is an increasing risk as appetite and food intake return to, or even exceed, pre-injury levels. Body composition changes occur after SCI in response to reduced physical activity, immobilisation and muscle atrophy, resulting in reduced REE. The management of obesity in individuals with SCI is very important due its high prevalence (Groah *et al.*, 2009). There is limited data on the rate of weight gain after SCI in the UK; however, in comparison with the UK national survey data (Henderson *et al.*, 2003), SCI individuals (Groah *et al.*, 2009) seem more likely to become overweight and obese than the able-bodied population (74% and 40%, respectively).

The detrimental health consequences of obesity are well documented (see Chapter 7.13.1, General aspects and prevention of obesity). In long-term SCI individuals, cardiovascular disease (CVD) morbidity and mortality exceeds that caused by renal and pulmonary conditions, with CVD becoming the primary cause of death (Myers *et al.*, 2007). The risk of mortality associated with CVD is twice as high compared with able-bodied individuals (Myers *et al.*, 2007). In addition, overweight SCI individuals are at a higher risk of developing pressure ulcers (Elsner & Gefen, 2008), and have increased difficulties in managing daily life as compared to overweight individuals without SCI (Abresch *et al.*, 2007).

Evidence suggest that a simple dietetic intervention (Chen *et al.*, 2006; Wong *et al.*, 2011) can help individuals with SCI to lose weight without compromising lean body mass. Although the intervention incurs additional cost, it has the potential to significantly decrease long-term healthcare expenditure if health outcome and quality of life are improved. Dietetic intervention, including comprehensive nutrition education and counselling on a cardioprotective diet, should be offered to at-risk individuals. This is particularly important for those who may have previously had little interest or knowledge of nutritional issues. The Multidisciplinary Association of Spinal Cord Injured Professional (MASCIP) has published guidelines for the management of obesity after SCI (2017). As with the general population, the provision of bariatric surgery should be considered if non-surgical interventions have been tried (Wong *et al.*, 2013).

Other nutrition-related problems

Neurogenic bowel dysfunction

Neurogenic bowel dysfunction (NBD) is one of the many impairments that result from SCI and is often quoted as being one of the most distressing problems (Lynch *et al.*, 2000). According to Stiens *et al.* (1997), two patterns of NBD occur post-SCI:

- Upper motor neurone (UMN) or reflexic bowel syndrome, which generally occurs in cervical and thoracic injury. It results in constipation, with faecal retention behind a spastic anal sphincter.
- Lower motor neurone (LMN) or areflexic bowel syndrome, which generally occurs in lumbar or sacral injury where the conus (the conical end of the spinal cord) or nerve roots are damaged. It produces constipation with a high risk of frequent incontinence through a lax external sphincter mechanism.

Each type of NBD requires different bowel management, and adjustments in dietary intake (particularly dietary fibre) may be required to produce an ideal stool consistency. Chemical stimulants are commonly used in UMN when a softer stool is required. A high fibre intake with adequate fluids may be helpful. Manual evacuation is commonly used if a harder or drier stool is required in situations where a reduced fibre intake may be more appropriate. MASCIP have initiated guidelines (2012) that give advice on how to manipulate diet, including insoluble fibre, to alter stool consistency. They acknowledge that good-quality research in this area is lacking, and that an element of trial and error is often required to determine what the individual finds effective.

If enteral feeding is required, it has (anecdotally) been found to be best tolerated by starting with a non-fibre feed and introducing fibre-containing feed gradually to toleration. Finishing on a feed that is a mixture of fibre and non-fibre may be beneficial. Additional fluids may be necessary due to the slower colonic transit time, which results in increased resorption of fluid. In practice, at least 2L or more is usually recommended.

Pressure ulcers

Individuals with SCI are at high risk of pressure ulcers due to the loss of sensation of pressure, skin ischaemia, incontinence, poor nutritional intake and inability or reluctance to change position. Both underweight and overweight increase the likelihood of pressure ulcer development. They can significantly increase nutritional requirements due to the protein-rich exudate, and they also expose tissue to infection. Antibiotic treatment of PU may also reduce food intake as a result of associated side effects. To promote wound healing, a high-protein diet of 1.5–2g/kg/day and higher energy are recommended (Ho *et al.*, 2010) (see Chapter 7.17.6, Wound healing, tissue viability and pressure sores).

Metabolic syndrome

The SCI population is at a higher risk of diabetes mellitus, metabolic syndrome and coronary heart disease due to decreased mobility, increased obesity and, in particular, central obesity. Early lifestyle modification and dietetic intervention targeted towards at-risk individuals to prevent the development of nutrition-related complications should be part of the rehabilitation programme.

Renal calculi

There is a higher risk of renal calculi, primarily as a result of recurrent bladder infections, increased retention of calcium by the bladder and kidneys, and immobility. To help prevent bladder infections, SCI individuals are normally recommended to drink at least 2L water-based fluids per day; restriction of calcium is not indicated (Rice *et al.*, 1995).

Urinary tract infections

Patients take cranberry juice in the belief that it might help in preventing bladder infections; however, there is little research on this topic. A Cochrane review (Jepson *et al.*, 2004) in otherwise healthy adults showed that, while there is some evidence of beneficial effects from regular cranberry consumption in women, the optimum dosage or method of administration (e.g. juice or tablets) remains unknown, and that further better-designed trials are needed. Cranberry juice may enhance the anticoagulant effect of warfarin, and therefore those on warfarin should avoid it. In addition, it may provide significant energy and contribute to weight gain.

Osteoporosis

It has been demonstrated that bone density decreases in the first few weeks after SCI and continues to worsen for 3–8 years (Wilmet *et al.*, 1995). Vitamin D deficiency, disuse or poor circulation could all contribute to the development of this low bone density and increased porosity. A cross-sectional study in men with complete SCI found that bone loss was greatest in the epiphyses, and was reduced by 50% in the femur and 60% in the tibia (Freehafer, 1995). Vitamin D deficiency is common after SCI due to limited sunlight exposure, and vitamin D supplements should be considered. A well-balanced diet incorporating sufficient calcium is recommended (see Chapter 7.9.1, Osteoporosis).

Weighing equipment manufacturers

Arjohuntleigh UK and Ireland, www.arjohuntleigh.com
Avery Weigh-Tronix, www.averyweigh-tronix.com
Marsden Weighing Machine Group Ltd, www.marsden-weighing.co.uk
Seca, www.seca.com

Internet resources

British Association of Spinal Cord Injury Specialist (BASCIS), www.bascis.org.uk
International Spinal Cord Society (ISCOS), www.iscos.org.uk
Multidisciplinary Association of Spinal Cord Injury Professionals (MASCIP), www.mascip.co.uk
Spinal Injuries Association, www.spinal.co.uk
Spinal Injuries Scotland (SIS), www.sisonline.org

Further reading

Campagnolo DI, Kirshbaum S. (2011) *Spinal Cord Medicine*, 2nd edn. Lippincott: Williams and Wilkins.

Grundy D, Swain A. (2002) *The ABC of Spinal Cord Injury*, 4th edn. London: BMJ Publications.

Harrison P. (ed) (2006) *Managing Spinal Cord Injuries: Continuing Care*. Milton Keynes: SIA.

Harrison P. (ed) (2007) *Managing Spinal Cord Injuries: The First 48 Hours*, 2nd edn. Milton Keynes: SIA.

Lin WV. (ed in chief) (2010) *Spinal Cord Medicine Principles and Practice*, 2nd edn. New York. Demos.

Multidisciplinary Association of Spinal Cord Injury Professionals (MASCIP). (2010) *Management of the Older Person with a New Spinal Cord Injury*. Stanmore. MASCIP.

References

Abresch RT, McDonald DA, Widman LM, *et al.* (2007) Impact of spinal cord dysfunction and obesity on the health-related quality of life of children and adolescents. *J. Spinal Cord Med.* 30(S1): S112–S118.

Agarwal N, Lee BY, Del Guercio LRM. (1987) Urinary creatinine excretion in spinal cord injury patients. *Nutrition* 3: 192.

American Dietetic Association. (2009) *Spinal Cord Injury (SCI) Evidence-Based Nutrition Practice Guideline*. Available at www.adaevidencelibrary.com

American Spinal Injury Association (ASIA). (2002) *International Standards for Neurological Classification of Spinal Cord Injury (Revised 2000)*. Chicago: ASIA.

American Spinal Injury Association (ASIA). (2013) International Standards for Neurological Classification of SCI (ISNCSCI) Worksheet. Available at https://asia-spinalinjury.org/wp-content/uploads/2016/02/International_Stds_Diagram_Worksheet.pdf Accessed 7 March 2019.

Barco KT, Smith RA, Peerless JR, *et al.* (2002) Energy expenditure assessment and validation after acute spinal injury. *Nutr. Clin. Pract.* 17: 309–313.

Buchholz AC, Pencharz PB. (2004) Energy expenditure in chronic spinal cord injury. *Curr. Opin. Clin. Nutr. Metab. Care.* 7: 635–639.

Chen Y, Henson S, Jackson AB, *et al.* (2006) Obesity intervention in persons with spinal cord injury. *Spinal Cord.* 44: 82–91.

Cheshire DJE, Coats DA. (1966) Respiratory and metabolic management in acute tetraplegia. *Paraplegia.* 4: 1–23.

Consortium for Spinal Cord Medicine. (2008) *Early Acute Management in Adults with Spinal Cord Injury: A Clinical Practice Guideline for Health-Care Providers*. Washington DC: Paralyzed Veterans of America.

Council of Europe Committee of Ministers. (2003) Resolution RESAP on food and nutritional care in hospitals. Available at https://www.nutritionday.org/cms/upload/pdf/11.resolution/Resolution_of_the_Council_of_Europe.pdf. Accessed 22 November 2018.

Cox SAR, Weiss SM, Posuniak EA, *et al.* (1985) Energy expenditure after spinal cord injury: an evaluation of stable rehabilitating patients. *J. Trauma.* 25: 419–423.

Eastern Association for the Surgery of Trauma (EAST). (2003) Practice Management Guidelines Work Group. Practice management guidelines for nutritional support of the trauma patient. Allentown (PA): EAST.

Elia, M. (2003) The 'MUST' Report. Nutritional Screening of Adults: A Multidisciplinary Responsibility. Development and Use of the 'Malnutrition Universal Screening Tool' ('MUST') for adults. Redditch: BAPEN.

Elsner JJ, Gefen A. (2008) Is obesity a risk factor for deep tissue injury in patients with spinal cord injury? *J. Biomech.* 41: 3322–3331.

Freehafer AA. (1995) Limb fractures in patients with spinal cord injury. *Arch. Phys. Med. Rehabil.* 76: 823–827.

Frost FS. (1998) Spinal cord injury: gastrointestinal implications and management. *Top. Spinal Cord Inj. Rehabil.* 4(2): 56–80.

Groah SL, Nash MS, Ljungberg IH, *et al.* (2009) Nutrient intake and body habits after spinal cord injury: an analysis by sex and level of injury. *J. Spinal Cord Med.* 32: 25–33.

Guttmann L. (1973) *Spinal Cord Injuries: Comprehensive Management and Research*. Oxford: Blackwell Scientific Publications.

Hadley MN. (2002) Nutrition support after spinal cord injury. *Neurosurgery* 50: S81–S84.

Henderson L, Gregory J, Irving K, *et al.* (2003) *The National Diet and Nutritional Survey: Adults aged 19–64 Years. Volume 2: Energy, Protein, Carbohydrates, Fat and Alcohol Intake*. London: HMSO.

Ho CH, Powell HL, Collins JF, *et al.* (2010) Poor nutrition is a relative contraindication to negative pressure wound therapy for pressure ulcers: preliminary observation in patients with spinal cord injury. *Adv. Skin Wound Care.* 23: 508–516.

Huang CT, DeVivo, Stover SL. (1990) Anemia in acute phase of spinal cord injury. *Arch. Phys. Med. Rehabil.* 71(1): 3–7.

Jepson RG, Mihaljevic L, Craig J. (2004) Cranberries for preventing urinary tract infection. *Cochrane Database Syst. Rev.* (2): CD001321.

Kearns PJ, Thompson JD, Werner PC, *et al.* (1992) Nutritional and metabolic response to acute spinal cord injury. *JPEN J. Parenter. Enteral Nutr.* 16(1): 11–15.

Laughton GE, Buchholz AC, Martin Ginis KA, *et al.* (2009) Lowering body mass index cutoffs better identifies obese persons with spinal cord injury. *Spinal Cord.* 47: 757–762.

Laven GT, Huang CT, DeVivo MJ, *et al.* (1989) Nutritional status during the acute stage of spinal cord injury. *Arch. Phys. Med. Rehabil.* 70: 277–282.

Lynch AC, Wong C, Anthony A, *et al.* (2000) Bowel dysfunction following spinal cord injury: a description of bowel function in a spinal cord injured population and comparison with age and gender matched controls. *Spinal Cord.* 38(12): 717–723.

Marian M. (2004) Acute spinal cord injuries: nutrition management. *Support Line.* 26(2): 3–8.

Multidisciplinary Association of Spinal Cord Injury Professionals (MASCIP) – initiated by. (2012) *Guidelines for Management of Neurogenic Bowel Dysfunction in Individuals with Central Neurological Conditions*. Available at https://www.mascip.co.uk/wp-content/uploads/2015/02/CV653N-Neurogenic-Guidelines-Sept-2012.pdf. Accessed 22 November 2018.

Myers J, Lee M, Kiratli J. (2007) Cardiovascular Disease in Spinal Cord Injury: An overview of prevalence, risk, evaluation and management. *Am. J. Phys. Med. Rehabil.* 86: 142–152.

Nevin AN, Steenson J, Vivanti A, *et al.* (2016a) Investigation of measured and predicted resting energy needs in adults after spinal cord injury: a systematic review. *Spinal Cord.* 54: 248–253.

Nevin A, Mayr H, Atresh S, *et al.* (2016b) Feasibility and acceptability of implementing indirect calorimetry into routine clinical care of patients with spinal cord injury. *Top. Spinal Cord Inj. Rehabil.* 22: 269–276.

NICE. (2017) *Nutrition Support in Adults: Oral nutrition Support, Enteral Tube Feeding and Parenteral Nutrition*. Available at https://www.nice.org.uk/Guidance/CG32. Accessed 22 November 2018.

Peruzzi W, Shapiro B, Cane R, *et al.* (1994) Resting energy expenditure in the acute phase of spinal cord injury (oral presentation). *Crit. Care Med.* 22(1): A208.

Rasmann Nuhlicek DN, Spurr GB, Barboriak JJ, *et al.* (1988) Body composition of patients with spinal cord injury. *Eur. J. Clin. Nutr.* 42: 765–773.

Rice HB, Ponichtera-Mulcare JA, Glaser RM. (1995) Nutrition and the spinal cord injured individual. *Clin. Kinesiol.* 49: 21–27.

Rodriguez DJ, Benzel EC, Clevenger FW. (1997) The metabolic response to spinal cord injury. *Spinal Cord.* 35(9): 599–604.

Royal College of Physicians (RCP). (2008) *Chronic Spinal Cord Injury: Management of Patients in Acute Hospital Setting: National Guidelines*. London: Royal College of Physicians.

Sedlock DA, Laventure SJ. (1990) Body composition and resting energy expenditure in long term spinal cord injury. *Paraplegia*. 28: 448–454.

Shizgal HM, Roza A, Leduc B, *et al.* (1986) Body composition in quadriplegic patients. *JPEN J. Parenter. Enteral Nutr.* 10(4): 364–368.

Spinal Injuries Association. (2017) *Understanding SCI*. Available at https://www.spinal.co.uk/living-with-sci/understanding-sci. Accessed 11 January 2017.

Spungen A, Adkins RH, Stewart CA, *et al.* (2003) Factors influencing body composition in persons with spinal cord injury: a cross-sectional study. *J. Appl. Physiol.* 95: 2398–2407.

Stiens SA, Bergman SB, Goetz LL. (1997) Neurogenic bowel dysfunction after spinal cord injury: clinical evaluation and rehabilitative management. *Arch. Phys. Med. Rehabil.* 78(3): S86–101.

Wilmet E, Ismail AA, Heilporn A, *et al.* (1995) Longitudinal study of the bone mineral content and of soft tissue composition after spinal cord section. *Paraplegia*. 33(11): 674–677.

Wong S, Barnes T, Coggrave M, *et al.* (2013) Morbid obesity after spinal cord injury: an ailment not to be treated? *Eur. J. Clin. Nutr.* 67: 998–999.

Wong S, Derry F, Jamous A, *et al.* (2012a) Validation of the spinal nutrition screening tool (SNST) in patients with spinal cord injuries (SCI): result from a multicentre study. *Eur. J. Clin. Nutr.* 66(3): 382–387.

Wong S, Derry F, Jamous A, *et al.* (2012b) The prevalence of malnutrition in spinal cord injuries patients: a UK multicentre study. *Br. J. Nutr.* 108(5): 918–923.

Wong S, Graham A, Grimble G, *et al.* (2011) Spinal Clinic for Obese Out-patient Project (SCOOP) – a 1 year report. *Food Nutr. Sci.* 2: 901–907. doi: 10.4236/fns.2011.28123.

Wong S, Graham A, Hirani SP, *et al.* (2015) Review of dietetic service provision and activity in spinal cord injury centres: a multicentre survey in the UK and Republic of Ireland. *Spinal Cord.* 53: 855–859.

Worthington P, Crowe MA, Armenti V. (1993) Nutritional support for patients with spinal cord injury. *Trauma Qual.* 9(2): 82–92.

7.17.4 Burn injury

Natasha Kershaw and Emily Bridge

Key points

- Severe burn injury elicits one of the most pronounced inflammatory responses likely to be encountered in a clinical setting.
- Severely burned patients benefit from enteral glutamine and antioxidant micronutrient supplementation due to their role in minimising infectious complications and wound healing.
- Modulation of the metabolic response using anabolic pharmacotherapies (e.g. oxandrolone and propranolol) has been found to be safe and beneficial.
- Insulin resistance and related hyperglycaemia are common in major burns; moderate glucose control (6–8 mmol/L) with continuous insulin has been proven safe and beneficial.

In 2014–2015, there were 17,157 reported burn cases across England and Wales, not including patients treated by non-burn specialist services, including emergency units, or those who died from their injuries (Dunn *et al.*, 2016). Depending on the severity of illness and availability of services, burn care may be provided in a range of clinical settings, e.g. general surgical or plastic surgery wards, or intensive care units. Those with severe or complex burn injuries should be managed by a specialist burns service. The length of stay (LOS) for burn critical care patients is typically >3 weeks longer than the general critical care population (Windle, 2006).

Types of burn injuries are diverse and include fat and water scalds; flame, chemical and friction burns; and electrical injuries. Scalds are the most common cause in the very young and elderly (Hettiaratchy & Dziewulski, 2004). This chapter focuses on the management of adults with severe burns; however, the metabolic, physiological consequences and the interventional approaches in paediatric burn populations are similar. Dietetic management of children with severe burns is discussed comprehensively elsewhere (McCarthy & Gurry, 2007) (see Chapter 3.8.26, Burns).

Diagnostic criteria and classification

A major burn injury in adults is defined as one affecting >20% of the total body surface area (TBSA) (Saffle & Graves, 2007). Regular assessment of size, distribution and depth of burn is essential for surgical planning. TBSA is assessed with the aid of pictorial charts (Figure 7.17.4). Wound depth is described as superficial, partial thickness, deep dermal or full thickness. A full-thickness burn may extend into both muscle and bone.

Metabolism and physiology in major burn

Burn shock and hypometabolism

Damaged cells in burnt tissue trigger the release of inflammatory cytokines and other inflammatory mediators. This increases blood flow to the affected areas, so that oxygen, macrophages, and platelets can be delivered. Capillary permeability increases, allowing these key immune molecules and resources to enter the interstitial spaces, and, therefore, gain access to the site of the damaged cells. Large volumes of fluid, as either exudate or bleeding, are then able to leak out of the raw exposed tissue. The fluid that does not escape pools in

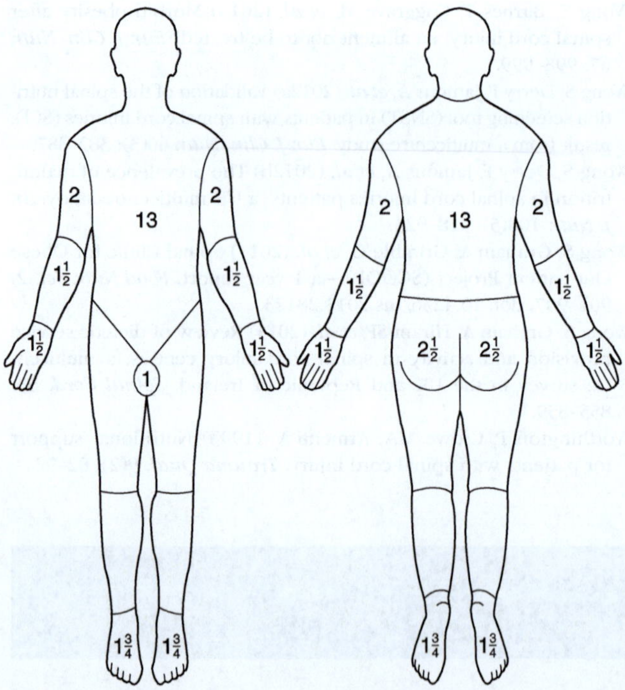

Age	Age (years)					
	0	1	5	10	15	Adult
Head and neck	21	19	15	13	11	9
Thigh	5½	6½	8	9	9	9½
Calf	5	5	5½	6	6½	7

Figure 7.17.4 Percentage of different parts of the body at different ages (source: Kemble & Lamb, 1984. Reproduced with permission from Elsevier)

the interstitial spaces, causing oedema. The combined effect of fluid loss and redistribution results in acute hypovolemia (Rousseau *et al.*, 2013). Hypovolemia causes low cardiac output and poor perfusion to vital organs. Poor perfusion to the kidneys will result in reduced urine output and, potentially, acidosis. Inadequate blood supply to the bowel can result in patches of ischaemic damage. The primary treatment during the burn shock phase is aggressive fluid resuscitation. This further exacerbates both peripheral and bowel oedema. An oedematous bowel is more turgid, which causes it to become more permeable, impairing peristalsis. As a consequence of this, ileus and bacterial translocation are common.

Burn shock usually lasts for 24–48 hours, or until fluid resuscitation is complete. This correlates with the 'ebb' phase of the metabolic response to major burn injury, and, as such, the nutritional requirement will be low (Jeschke *et al.*, 2011).

Hypermetabolism and hypercatabolism

Damaged tissue has a high cellular demand for energy and substrates needed in repair and recycling. Stress hormones promote proteolysis, lipolysis and glycogenolysis in an attempt to satisfy this demand (Jeschke *et al.*, 2011). The amount released from the breakdown of peripheral stores, however, will exceed what the body is able to metabolise at any one time. As a consequence, the body enters into an energy-consuming phase of futile substrate cycling, commonly referred to as the 'flow phase'. Triglyceride–fatty acid cycling will increase by up to 450%, and glycolytic–gluconeogenic cycling by 250% (Jeschke *et al.*, 2008). Over time, the driving forces of this cycling, i.e. the damaged tissue and the resulting inflammatory cytokines, will reduce, as will the levels of catabolism and metabolism. REE is expected to peak at 180% of the basal rate during the acute phase, reduce to 150% once wound closure has been achieved, be 120% at 9 months post-injury, and be 110% at 1 year (Jeschke *et al.*, 2011).

Nutritional assessment and monitoring

Weight and anthropometry

Weight can be difficult to interpret in major burns. During the initial resuscitation phase, dozens of litres of fluid are often given. This usually results in significant oedema that can take several weeks to subside. Many patients require very deep tissue excision, mastectomy or limb amputation, when a limb becomes unsalvageable or fat necrosis has occurred. It is, therefore, important, when possible, to obtain a reported pre-injury weight from a friend, relative or a recent health record. Discussion with the surgeon can also be helpful to estimate tissue loss. When weights are taken, it is better to time them for when the dressings are changed, as they will contribute significantly, especially when soaked with exudate. Trends over time will be easier to interpret than a weight in isolation.

It is important to note that, even with aggressive nutritional support, it is not always possible to limit weight loss to <10%, which is the agreed target set in many UK burns centres (MB ODN, 2016). Around one-third of adults admitted to a UK burn unit were unable to achieve this target, but lost up to 22% of their admission or reported pre-injury weight (Windle, 2004).

Nitrogen balance

Urinary nitrogen output is the result of internal nitrogen processing and so may assist in determining changes in protein economy and metabolism. Urinary urea nitrogen (UUN) is used to assess nitrogen balance (see Chapter 6.1, Nutritional requirements in clinical practice) and the severity of catabolism. In turn, these may help direct nutritional therapy. It is important to note, however, that burn wound exudate is rich in nitrogen. In addition, there is a linear relationship between TBSA and protein-losing enteropathy, as evidenced by the greater protein content in stools (Venkatesh *et al.*, 2004). Patients with a burn injury will, therefore, experience significant additional losses that are not accounted for in the nitrogen balance calculation.

Biochemistry

Serum albumin concentration is a poor marker of nutritional status. Levels are likely to reflect the inflammatory response and physiological insult of the burn injury. Transcapillary escape, wound exudate loss, and reduced albumin synthesis in preference for positive acute-phase protein production will all cause hypoalbuminaemia. Anaemia is common due to blood loss from the burnt tissue and repeated surgery. High levels of inflammatory cytokines will also affect bone marrow suppression (Posluszny & Gamelli, 2011). However, in view of the potential for pre-burn suboptimal nutritional status in some patients, a nutritional cause should be excluded if possible. Serum trace elements are usually low in major burns due to exudate loss and re-distribution. Wound edge biopsy will give a good indication of status, but is not practical or economical in the clinical setting (Berger *et al.*, 2007a).

Clinical management

Treatment begins with the first contact that emergency services make with the patient at the location of the injury. It lasts through a protracted hospital stay and will continue, potentially for years, after the patient has been discharged. The National Burn Care Committee describes these phases of treatment as the '7 Rs': rescue, resuscitation, retrieval, resurfacing of skin, rehabilitation, reconstruction and review (National Burn Care Committee, 2001).

Resurfacing of the skin involves a multitude of techniques, often over several weeks and months. Many injuries will involve wounds that have a mixture of depths. Superficial or partial-thickness wounds will typically heal conservatively, requiring only good wound care and sometimes a temporary skin-substitute dressing. Deep-dermal or full-thickness wounds require surgical intervention, often multiple trips to theatre for serial grafting, lasting several hours each. These procedures have the potential to interrupt feeding, and the practical delivery of feed needs to be considered. Furthermore, the rate of donor site healing, graft take, and remaining wound size will all give an indication of the patient's nutritional needs and the adequacy of provision.

Rehabilitation will begin early in the hospital stay and will take place in the intensive care setting. A substantial part of rehabilitation, however, will occur while the patient is well enough to be off all organ support, awake, and (hopefully) eating and drinking. Promoting adequate oral intake is a team effort. Speech and language therapists may be involved due to the effect of oral, facial or neck scar tissue, or because of complications relating to prolonged intubation and weakness. Occupational therapy and physiotherapy may be required to assist the patient to start self-feeding again (if possible), often with the aid of adapted equipment. Many patients with burns have a pre-existing mental health history. Even those who do not are often greatly affected by burn trauma symptoms and the physical and psychosocial consequences of such an injury. Low mood, anxiety, and paranoia can all affect a patient's ability and willingness to eat and drink; in these circumstances, the psychological services team's contribution is invaluable.

Nutritional management

Routes of feeding and timing of nutritional support

Historically, parenteral nutrition (PN) in burn patients has caused concerns particularly regarding rates of infections, risk of hyperglycaemia, and, ultimately, the overall effect on mortality. However, the CALORIES trial found that PN was no more harmful or beneficial than enteral feeding in critically ill patients (Harvey *et al.*, 2014). While the cohort did not include thermally injured patients, the trial did challenge common concerns associated with PN, such as hyperglycaemia and rate of line infection, and found that it can be a safe method of feeding a critically ill patient (Howells, 2016). Enteral feeding remains the route of choice, and all steps to utilise the gastrointestinal tract should be pursued. Gastroparesis may be managed by prokinetic therapy, or post-pyloric tube placement where this fails (see Chapter 7.4.4, Gastroparesis).

Early initiation of nutritional support in burns patients appears safe, and may confer advantages in terms of avoiding stress ulceration, reducing incidence of wound infections, and, when in combination with early surgical excision of wounds, reduction in skeletal muscle catabolism (Hart *et al.*, 2003; Mosier *et al.*, 2011). In 2013, ESPEN recommended that enteral feeding be commenced within 6–12 hours post-injury, although the feasibility of this being achieved was not discussed. There has been concern regarding the risk of ischaemic injury in initiating enteral nutrition (EN) support in under-perfused patients (Andel *et al.*, 2002). In practice, however, by the time the patient is admitted, fluid resuscitation is usually underway. If a patient has received fluid resuscitation and there is a delay in initiating enteral feeding, there is a risk of paralytic ileus occurring due to widespread oedema affecting the gut (Rousseau *et al.*, 2013).

Bowel management

It is common for burn patients to develop sluggish bowels, often related to high doses of sedation, opioids and oedema in the bowel. A retrospective study has shown that 86.1% of patients had late defecation (>6 days), which was associated with ongoing lower gastrointestinal dysfunction and feeding intolerance, requiring PN (Trexler *et al.*, 2014). Staff should aim for a patient's bowels to be open within 4 days of injury (MB ODN, 2016). Use of a fibre-containing feed (Rousseau *et al.*, 2013) or laxatives should be considered.

Glycaemic management

ESPEN-endorsed recommendations state that optimal glycaemic control should be 5–8 mmol/L (Rousseau *et al.*, 2013). Moderate glycaemic control (6–8 mmol/L) has been shown to be safe, with very few cases of hypoglycaemia and no deleterious clinical consequences (Berger & Pantet, 2016; Stoecklin *et al.*, 2016). Blood glucose values of >10 mmol/L are associated with delayed wound healing, infectious complications, multiple organ failure and higher mortality (Berger & Pantet, 2016).

Nutritional requirements

Energy

Hypermetabolism is a well-documented complication of major burn, and, historically, energy prescriptions of up to 33.4 MJ (8000 kcal)/days were advocated (Wilmore *et al.*, 1971). Since then, more conservative prediction formulae have been developed. These are particularly important in light of more recent knowledge of energy expenditure, complications of overzealous energy provision such as prolonged ventilator dependency, and higher septic mortality rates in critically ill hyperglycaemic patients. Interventions such as early surgery and initiation of nutritional support have contributed to a reduction in the hypermetabolic response (Hart *et al.*, 2003).

Historically, basal metabolic rate (BMR) based equations with added stress factors (based on % TBSA) were used to calculate energy requirements. However, these are inaccurate as they do not account for shifts in metabolic changes that burn patients exhibit (Rousseau *et al.*, 2013). Indirect calorimetry (IC) is the gold standard method of determining energy requirements in adult burn patients (Rousseau *et al.*, 2013). While the use of IC in US burn units has increased over the last 20 years (Graves *et al.*, 2009), IC use is less common in the UK, and ultimately the technique has its own limitations (Simonson & DeFronzo, 1990). In its absence, the Toronto equation is considered a well-validated alternative as it is based on a number of calorimetric studies (Rousseau *et al.*, 2013) (Table 7.17.9).

Protein

Intake of 1.5–2.0 g/kg/day protein has been suggested to ensure adequate provision in adults, following the observations that amino acid oxidation rates can be increased by 50% as compared to healthy individuals (Herndon, 2007; Rousseau *et al.*, 2013). Intakes of 0.24 g nitrogen/kg (1.5 g/kg of protein/day) is likely to improve nitrogen balance in adults with >20% TBSA.

Table 7.17.9 Toronto equation for estimating energy requirements in burns patients (kcal/day) (Allard *et al.*, 1990)

Formula	Comments
REE = −4343 + (10.5 × % TBSA burn) + (0.23 × kcal) + (0.84 × HB) + (114 × t (°C)) − (4.5 × post-burn days). Activity factors: Ventilator-dependent: 1.2. There are no activity factors for non-ventilated patients. Activity factors for the HB and Schofield equations could be used in these patients.	Complex, requires calculation of HB formula, which is an estimate of basal energy expenditure and requires multiplication by a static factor. Takes account of healing over time for spontaneous breathing patients.

REE, resting energy expenditure; kcal, energy intake in the last 24 hours; HB, Harris–Benedict equation; TBSA, total body surface area; t, maximum temperature in 24 hours.

Micronutrient supplementation

Most vitamins, minerals and trace elements play a direct or indirect role in wound healing as they are cofactors for enzyme systems involved in immunity and wound healing, as shown in Table 7.17.10 (see Chapter 7.17.6, Wound healing, tissue viability and pressure sores). In addition, up to 10% of total body zinc and 40% of total body copper may be lost within 7 days of severe burn injury, which increases urinary excretion, contributing significantly to depletion (Gamliel *et al.*, 1996). European adult guidelines (Kreymann *et al.*, 2006) support the use of copper, selenium and zinc supplementation at a dose higher than standard. Administration of 40.4 μmol copper, 2.9 μmol selenium and 406 μmol zinc for 30 days after a burn injury reduces chest infection rates and LOS. Other guidelines suggest reserving specific micronutrient supplementation for correcting deficiency states, and note that regular nutritional therapy often provides well in excess of baseline amounts (Prelack *et al.*, 2007). A recent meta-analysis concluded that the use of parenterally administered combined trace elements (Cu, Se, Zn) reduced overall infectious complications, and found that combined oral and intravenous Zn supplementation may be more beneficial in reducing wound and urinary infections (Kurmis *et al.*, 2016). No adverse outcomes of trace element supplementation have been reported to date (Kurmis *et al.*, 2016). ESPEN-endorsed recommendations regarding doses and length of trace element supplementation (Berger *et al.*, 1994, 1998, 2004, 2007a; Rousseau *et al.*, 2013) are as follows:

- Copper 40–59 μmol.
- Selenium 235–377 μmol.
- Zinc 400–574 μmol.

Suggested prescription duration

- 7–8 days for >20–40% TBSA burns.
- 14 days for >40–60% TBSA burns.
- 30 days for >60% TBSA burns.

In burns patients, 500–1000 mg/day vitamin C is recommended to aid endothelium stabilisation through the promotion of collagen synthesis, to reduce capillary leak, and for fluid resuscitation requirements (Rousseau *et al.*, 2013). Enteral supplementation of up to 1000 mg/day of vitamin C is likely to be safe, and vitamin C toxicity issues are generally minor.

Immune-modulating nutrition

Glutamine

Glutamine acts as a primary fuel source for rapidly dividing cells, including enterocytes, lymphocytes and macrophages (Lin *et al.*, 2013). During acute stress, glutamine

Table 7.17.10 Role of micronutrients in burn wound healing

Micronutrient	Role	Notes
Vitamin A	Epithelialisation and stimulation of fibroblasts. Antioxidant effect prevents damage by free radicals in SIRS.	
B Vitamins	Oxidative pathways. Cofactor for collagen deposition.	
Vitamin C	Cofactor in hydroxylation of proline and lysine. Collagen synthesis. Antioxidant properties protect metalloenzymes from oxidation.	As a free-radical scavenger, may reduce vascular permeability and reduce fluid resuscitation requirements.
Vitamin D	Aids calcium absorption. Optimises wound healing.	10 μg/day usually met through enteral feed or oral nutritional supplements. Consider liver and renal function.
Iron	Promotes collagen synthesis. Optimises tissue perfusion.	Avoid iron supplements in acute illness – possible increased risk of infection and mortality.
Zinc	RNA/DNA replication, lymphocyte function and collagenase enzyme systems.	Up to 10% total body zinc lost via wound exudate.
Copper	Cofactor in the lysyl oxidase enzyme system, essential for collagen synthesis and maturation. Optimises immune function, bone formation and prevention of anaemia as it aids iron absorption.	Up to 40% of total body copper lost via wound exudate.
Selenium	Component of glutathione peroxidase (antioxidant).	Lost through skin following burn injury

SIRS, systemic inflammatory response syndrome; RNA/DNA, ribonucleic acid/deoxy ribonucleic acid.

levels are low (Gore & Jahoor, 2000; Viggiano *et al.*, 2012). Following a major burn, the patient is at particular risk of recurrent sepsis from the various flora and fauna colonised within the cutaneous wounds and bacterial translocation from the gut. Furthermore, ischaemic changes within the bowel due to poor gut perfusion causes it to produce cytokines (Deitch, 2001). Inflammatory mediators then circulate via mesenteric lymph, causing distant organ injury (Deitch, 2001). Glutamine supplementation may help to protect the immunological function of the gut and aid the immune system. Supplementation has been shown to preserve the integrity of the epithelial cells in the gastrointestinal tract, reducing bacterial translocation (Ziegler *et al.*, 2000). Intestinal and extra-intestinal levels of IgA are preserved by reducing incidents of apoptosis within crucial lymphoid tissue, such a Peyer's patches, in the gastrointestinal tract (Fan *et al.*, 2010). IgA assists immune cells to identify and process antigens, thereby responding rapidly to recurrent infectious insults. Glutamine supplementation in animal studies have been shown to attenuate the production of inflammatory cytokines following tissue shock, including post-inhalational injury, septic shock, and ischaemia/reperfusion injury (Li *et al.*, 2013; Singleton & Wischmeyer, 2007; Wischmeyer *et al.*, 2001). Supplementation has been shown to aid tissue recovery and organ function by upregulating the production of heat shock proteins and cellular energy metabolism (Li *et al.*, 2013; Singleton & Wischmeyer, 2007; Wischmeyer *et al.*, 2001; Zhang *et al.*, 2013). Increased rates of wound healing, fewer infectious events, and reduced LOS and mortality have all been observed in this patient population (Lin *et al.*, 2013; Peng *et al.*, 2004, 2005). Treatment practices vary, but typical usage includes 0.3–0.5 g/kg/day of enteral glutamine for 10–21 days (Hall *et al.*, 2012; Rousseau *et al.*, 2013).

However, glutamine use has recently decreased over safety concerns about patients in the critical care setting. The REDOX trial found an increased mortality at 6 months (Heyland *et al.*, 2013). Sub-group analysis showed that increased risk of mortality only occurred in those who had baseline renal dysfunction (Heyland *et al.*, 2015). It is important to note, however, that this trial excluded all patients with burn injuries and consisted of mostly medical patients. Burns patients are commonly found to be depleted of glutamine due to a mismatch between peripheral release and a significantly increased, prolonged central consumption (Gore & Jahoor, 2000). Conversely, the majority of patients studied in the REDOX trial had normal plasma concentrations or even supranormal levels at baseline (Cynobar & De Bandt, 2014). Parenteral delivery of glutamine may also have contributed to even higher plasma levels during the trial period; enteral delivery has a significantly lower systemic uptake (Lin *et al.*, 2013). The findings of the REDOX trial may therefore not be applicable to the burns population.

Following on from this, Heyland and colleagues have now begun a trial investigating enteral glutamine supplementation in burns patients, called the 'Re-energize Trial' (Heyland *et al.*, 2017). This international study will be the largest RCT to take place in the field of burns to date. Once completed, it should give clearer evidence on the safety and efficacy of supplementation in burns. In the meantime, caution is needed if supplementing with glutamine, and it should be avoided in renal insufficiency.

Arginine

Arginine is a conditionally essential amino acid observed to be low in patients with a burn injury (Fan *et al.*, 2010). It is the exclusive substrate for nitric oxide synthesis, and is involved in stimulating the release of anabolic hormones and T-lymphocytes (Fan *et al.*, 2010). Arginine supplementation in animal models showed an increased rate of wound healing in non-burn wounds (Shi *et al.*, 2007). However, human trials have failed to consistently replicate this (Debats *et al.*, 2011). A meta-analysis of studies involving critical care patients who had been given combined immunonutrients and antioxidants found an increase in mortality (Heyland & Samis, 2003). The authors postulated that the likely culprit for the increased mortality was arginine, due to the theoretical potential for harm induced by increased nitric oxide (NO) production and its vasodilatory affects (Heyland & Samis, 2003). It is interesting to note, however, that small-scale studies have failed to observe an increased level of NO with supplementation, and one study showed lower levels during the early resuscitation phase of burn injury (Yan *et al.*, 2007). There is insufficient evidence to justify arginine use in the practice setting (Rousseau *et al.*, 2013).

Omega-3 fatty acids

The use of n-3 fatty acids in critical care is reviewed in Chapter 7.17.1 (Critical care). Research is emerging in burns looking at targeted nutritional therapy using the n-3 fatty acid metabolite resolvin D2. Supplementation with resolvin D2 in animal models has been shown to restore normal neutrophil motility, allowing them to respond appropriately to chemotaxis after major burn (Kurihara *et al.*, 2013). With proper motility, neutrophils migrate to damaged cutaneous tissue to manage microbial insult at the wound site (Kurihara *et al.*, 2013). Activated neutrophils are also discouraged from invading healthy tissue, which would otherwise cause damage to vital organs and extension to the zone of burn wound necrosis (Bohr *et al.*, 2013; Inoue *et al.*, 2016). Resolvin D2 supplementation in animal models has demonstrated reduced pathological changes in kidney and liver samples, reduced incidences of secondary dermal necrosis, and reduced mortality (Bohr *et al.*, 2013; Inoue *et al.*, 2016; Kurihara *et al.*, 2013). The effects in humans have not yet been investigated, and as such use in a clinical practice setting is not yet supported.

Oxandrolone and propranolol

Oxandrolone is an anabolic steroid that is becoming more commonly used to treat patients who have had a major burn. A meta-analysis concluded that oxandrolone was safe for treating severe burns. Significant benefits include lower net weight loss, lean body mass loss, nitrogen loss, donor site healing time, and LOS in the catabolic and rehabilitation phases, without increased mortality, infection, metabolic rate, hyperglycaemia or liver dysfunction rate (Li *et al.*, 2016). Longer-term use was found to lead to a gain in body mass after 6 months, with additional improvements in height, weight, bone mineral content and muscle strength (Li *et al.*, 2016). Recommended doses for adults are 10 mg/12 hours (Rousseau *et al.*, 2013).

Propranolol is a beta-blocker that opposes the action of catecholamines; as such, it reduces cardiac load and the hypermetabolic, catabolic response to a major burn (Atiyeh *et al.*, 2008), thereby reducing lipolysis and increasing muscle metabolism (Finnerty & Herndon, 2013). A lesser incidence of hepatomegaly is seen when patients with a major burn have been treated with propranolol (Finnerty & Herndon, 2013). Dose and delivery will vary, but a suggested starting point would be 10 mg given twice per day to avoid dips in the mean arterial pressure (LeCompte *et al.*, 2017). Dose is then titrated until a 15–20% reduction in heart rate has been achieved (Gauglitz *et al.*, 2011).

Follow-up post-discharge

The majority of patients with burn injuries will not be discharged home until their injuries are sufficiently healed, such that only relatively minor wounds remain and metabolic demands are near to normal. A healthy, well-balanced diet should be advocated. Basal metabolic rate can be raised for up to a year post-injury, and weight should therefore be monitored during outpatient care. Vitamin D synthesis post-injury is reduced as burn patients are advised to stay out of the sun or wear high-factor sun block. Vitamin D levels should be checked at discharge after 3, 6 and 12 months, and deficiencies corrected (MB ODN, 2016).

In some circumstances, patients may be transferred in their healing and rehabilitation phase to a more local hospital and may have sufficient wound remaining to need nutritional support or texture modification. Effective and timely communication between the burn dietitian and the local dietetic service is essential.

Acknowledgement

The editor acknowledges the prior contribution of Mark Windle.

Internet resources

British Burns Association, www.britishburnsassociation.org

References

Allard JP, Pichard C, Hoshino E, *et al.* (1990) Validation of a new formula for calculating the energy requirements of burn patients. *JPEN J. Parenteral Enteral Nutr.* 14: 115–118.

Andel H, Rab M, Andel D, *et al.* (2002) Impact of duodenal feeding on the oxygen balance of the splanchnic region during different phases of severe burn injury. *Burns*. 28: 60–64.

Atiyeh BS, Gunn SWA, Dibo SA. (2008) Nutritional and pharmacological modulation of the metabolic response of severely burned patients. *Ann. Burns Fire Disasters*. 21(2): 63–72.

Berger M, Pantet O. (2016) Nutrition in burn injury: any recent changes? *Curr. Opin. Crit. Care*. 22: 285–291.

Berger M, Baines M, Raffoul W, *et al.* (2007a) Trace element supplements after major burns modulate antioxidant status and clinical course by way of increased tissue trace element concentration. *Am. J. Clin. Nutr.* 85: 1293–1300.

SECTION 7

Berger MM, Binnert C, Chiolero RL, *et al.* (2007b) Trace element supplementation after major burns increases burned skin trace element concentrations and modulates local protein metabolism but not whole-body substrate metabolism. *Am. J. Clin. Nutr.* 85: 1301–1306.

Berger MM, Binnert C, Baines M., *et al.* (2004) Trace element supplements influence protein metabolism and tissue levels after major burns. *Intensive Care Med.* 30(suppl): S61.

Berger M, Cavadini C, Chiolero R, *et al.* (1994) Influence of large intake of trace elements on recovery after major burns. *Nutrition.* 10(4): 327–334.

Berger M, Spertini F, Shenkin A, *et al.* (1998) Trace element supplementation modulates pulmonary infection rates after major burns: a double blind, placebo-controlled trial. *Am. J. Clin. Nutr.* 68: 365–371.

Bohr S, Patel SJ, Sarin D, *et al.* (2013) Resolvin D2 prevents secondary thrombosis and necrosis in a mouse burn wound model. *Wound Repair Regen.* 21(1): 35–43.

Cynobar L, De Bandt JP. (2014) Glutamine in the intensive care unit. *Curr. Opin. Clin. Nutr. Metab. Care* 17(1): 8–104.

Debats IBJG, Koeneman MM, Booi DI, *et al.* (2011) Intravenous arginine and human skin graft donor site healing: a randomized control trial. *Burns.* 37: 420–426.

Deitch EA. (2001) Role of the gut lymphatic system in multiple organ failure. *Curr. Opin. Crit. Care.* 7: 92–98.

Dunn K, Reade C, Dudley-Suthern R. (2016) *International Burn Injury Database. Annual Report (2014/2015).* Available at http://file:///C:/Users?Administrator/Downloads/2014_15%20iBID%20Report.pdf. Accessed 01 December 2016.

Fan J, Meng Q, Gua G, *et al.* (2010) Effect of glutamine added to enteral nutrition on Peyer's patch apoptosis in severely burned mice. *Burns.* 46: 409–417.

Finnerty CC, Herndon DN. (2013) Is propranolol of benefit in pediatric burn patients? *Adv. Surg.* 47:177–197.

Gamliel Z, DeBiasse MA, Demling RH. (1996) Essential microminerals and their response to burn injury. *J. Burn Care Rehabil.* 17: 264–272.

Gauglitz GG, Williams FN, Herndon DN, *et al.* (2011) Burns: where are we standing with Propranolol, Oxandrolone, and the new incretin analogues? *Curr. Opin. Clin. Nutr. Metab. Care.* 14(2): 176–181.

Gore DC, Jahoor F. (2000) Deficiency in peripheral glutamine production in pediatric patients with burns. *J. Burn Care Rehabil.* 21(2): 171.

Graves C, Saffle J, Cochran A. (2009) Actual burn nutrition care practices: an update. *J. Burn Care Res.* 30: 77–82.

Hall KL, Shahrokhi S, Jeschke MG. (2012) Enteral nutrition support in burn care: a review of current recommendations as instituted in the Ross Tilley Burn Centre. *Nutrients.* 4: 1554–1565.

Hart DW, Wolf SE, Chinkes DL, *et al.* (2003) Effects of early excision and aggressive enteral feeding on hypermetabolism, catabolism and sepsis after severe burn. *J. Trauma.* 54: 755–761.

Harvey SE, Parrott F, Harrison DA, *et al.*; CALORIES Trial Investigators. (2014) Trial of the route of early nutritional support in critically ill adults. *N. Eng. J. Med.* 371: 1673–1684.

Herndon DN. (2007) *Total Burn Care*, 3rd edn. Philadelphia: Saunders Elsevier.

Hettiaratchy S, Dziewulski P. (2004) ABC of burns. *Pathophysiology and types of burns. BMJ.* 328: 1427–1429.

Heyland DK, Samis A. (2003) Does immunonutrition in patients with sepsis do more harm than good? *Intensive Care Med.* 29: 669–671.

Heyland DK, Elke G, Cook D, *et al.* (2015) Glutamine and antioxidants in the critically ill patient: a post hoc analysis of a large-scale randomized trial. *JPEN J. Parenter. Enteral Nutr.* 39(4): 401–409.

Heyland D, Muscedere J, Wischmeyer PE, *et al.* (2013) A randomized trial of glutamine and antioxidants in critically ill patients. *N. Engl. J. Med.* 368(16): 1489–1497.

Heyland DK, Wischmeyer P, Jeschke MG, *et al.* (2017) A RandomizeEd trial of ENtERal Glutamine to minimIZE thermal injury (The RE-ENERGIZE Trial): a clinical trial protocol. *Scars Burns Heal.* 3: 1–15.

Howells E. (2016) Feeding the critically ill burn patient. *Complete Nutrition.* 16(4): 18–20.

Inoue Y, Yu YM, Kurihara T, *et al.* (2016) Kidney and liver injuries after major burns in rats are prevented by resolvin D2. *Crit. Care Med.* 6(44): e241–e252.

Jeschke MG, Chinkes DN, Finnerty CC, *et al.* (2008) Pathophysiologic response to severe burn injury. *Ann. Surg.* 248: 387–401.

Jeschke MG, Gauglitz GG, Kulp GA, *et al.* (2011) Long-term persistence of the pathophysiologic response to severe burn injury. *PLoS One.* 6(7): e21245.

Kreymann KG, Berger MM, Deutz C, *et al.* (2006) ESPEN guidelines on enteral nutrition: intensive care. *Clin. Nutr.* 25: 210–223.

Kurihara T, Jones CN, Yu YM, *et al.* (2013) Resolvin D2 restores neutrophil directionality and improves survival after burns. *FASEB J.* 27(6): 2270–2281.

Kurmis R, Greenwood J, Aromataris E. (2016) Trace element supplementation following severe burn injury: a systematic review and meta-analysis. *J. Burn Care Res.* 37(3): 143–159.

LeCompte MT, Rae L, Kahn SA. (2017) A survey of the use of propranolol in burn centers: who, what, when, why. *Burns.* 43: 121–126.

Li H, Guo Y, Yan Z, *et al.* (2016) The efficacy and safety of oxandrolone treatment for patient with severe burns. *Burns.* 42: 717–727.

Li W, Qiu X, Wang J, *et al.* (2013) The therapeutic efficacy of glutamine for rats with smoking inhalation injury. *Int. Immunopharmacol.* 16: 248–253.

Lin JJ, Chung XJ, Yang CY, *et al.* (2013) A meta-analysis of trials using the intention to treat principle for glutamine supplementation in critically ill patients with burn. *Burns.* 39(4): 565–570.

Midland Burn Operational Delivery Network (MB ODN). (2016) *Guidelines for Nutritional Management of Adults and Paediatrics.* Available at http://www.midlandsburnnetwork.nhs.uk. Accessed 4 April 2017.

McCarthy H, Gurry C. (2007) Burns. In: Shaw V, Lawson M. (eds) *Clinical Paediatric Dietetics*, 3rd edn. Oxford: Blackwell Publishing.

Mosier MJ, Pham TN, Klein MB, *et al.* (2011) Early enteral nutrition in burns: compliance with guidelines and associated outcomes in a multicenter study. *J. Burn Care Res.* 32: 104–109.

National Burn Care Committee. (2001) *National Burn Care Review: Standards and Strategy for Burn Care. A Review of Burn Care in the British Isles.* UK: Committee Report.

Peng X, Yan H, You Z, *et al.* (2004) Effects of enteral supplementation with glutamine granules on intestinal mucosal barrier function in severe burned patients. *Burns.* 30: 135–139.

Peng X, Yan H, You Z, *et al.* (2005) Clinical and protein metabolic efficacy of glutamine granules-supplemented enteral nutrition in severely burned patients. *Burns.* 31: 342–346.

Posluszny JA, Gamelli RL. (2011) Anaemia of thermal injury: combined acute blood loss anaemia and anaemia of chronic illness. *J. Burn Care Res.* 31: 229–242.

Prelack K, Dylewski M, Sheridan RL. (2007) Practical guidelines for the nutritional management of burn injury and recovery. *Burns.* 33: 14–24.

Rousseau AF, Losser MR, Ichai C, *et al.* (2013) ESPEN endorsed recommendations: nutritional therapy in major burns. *Clin. Nutr.* 32: 497–502.

Saffle JR, Graves C. (2007) Nutritional support of the burned patient. In: Herndon DN. (ed) *Total Burn Care.* Philadelphia: Saunders Elsevier, pp. 398–419.

Shi HP, Wang SM, Zhang GX, *et al.* (2007) Supplemental L-arginine enhances wound healing following trauma/hemorrhagic shock. *Wound Repair. Regen.* 15: 66–70.

Simonson DC, DeFronzo RA. (1990) Indirect calorimetry: methodological and interpretative problems. *Am. J. Physiol.* 258: E399–E412.

Singleton KD, Wischmeyer PE. (2007) Glutamine's protection against sepsis and lung injury is dependent on heat shock protein 70 expression. *Am. J. Physiol. Regul. Integr. Comp. Physiol.* 292: R1839–R1845.

Stoecklin P, Delodder F, Pantet O, *et al.* (2016) Moderate glycaemic control safe in critically ill adult burn patients: a 15-year cohort study. *Burns.* 42: 63–70.

Trexler ST, Lundy JB, Chung KK, *et al.* (2014) Prevalence and impact of late defecation in the critically ill, thermally injured adult. *J. Burn Care Res.* 35: e224–229.

Venkatesh B, Gough J, Ralston DR, *et al.* (2004) Protein losing enteropathy in critically ill adult patients with burns: a preliminary report. *Intensive Care Med.* 30: 162–166.

Viggiano E, Passavanti MB, Pace MC, *et al.* (2012) Plasma glutamine decreases immediately after surgery and is related to incisiveness. *J. Cell Physiol.* 227(5): 1988–1991.

Wilmore DW, Curreri PW, Spitzer KW, *et al.* (1971) Supranormal dietary intake in thermally injured hypermetabolic patients. *Surg. Gynecol. Obstet.* 132: 881–886.

Windle EM. (2004) Audit of successful weight maintenance in adult and paediatric survivors of thermal injury at a UK regional burn centre. *J. Hum. Nutr. Diet.* 17: 435–441.

Windle EM. (2006) Glutamine supplementation in critical illness: evidence, recommendations and implications for clinical practice in burn care. *J. Burn Care Res.* 27: 764–772.

Wischmeyer PE, Kahana M, Wolfson R, *et al.* (2001) Glutamine reduces cytokine release, organ damage, and mortality in a rat model of endotoxemia. *Shock.* 16(5): 398–402.

Yan H, Peng Z, Huang Y, *et al.* (2007) Effects of early enteral arginine supplementation on resuscitation of severe burn patients. *Burns.* 33: 179–184.

Zhang Y, Yan H, Lv SG, *et al.* (2013) Effects of glycyl-glutamine dipeptide supplementation on myocardial damage and cardiac function in rats after severe burn injury. *Int. J. Clin. Exp. Pathol.* 6(5): 821–830.

Ziegler TR, Bazargan N, Leader LM, *et al.* (2000) Glutamine and the gastrointestinal tract. *Curr. Opin. Clin. Nutr. Metab. Care.* 3(5): 355–362.

7.17.5 Surgery

Rachael Barlow

Key points

- Nutritional support of the surgical patient today is radically different to when a direct causal link between nutrition and surgical outcomes was first demonstrated.
- Surgery initiates physiological stress, the magnitude of which is related to the operative procedure and results in an increase in energy expenditure and protein mobilisation.
- Malnutrition, particularly protein depletion, is associated with a significantly higher risk of postoperative complications.
- Nutritional screening, assessment, preoperative nutritional support, optimal fluid management and early postoperative enteral nutrition are key components of the enhanced recovery after surgery programme – a patient-centred pathway that optimises surgical outcome by improving clinical outcomes and patient experience.

Most of the UK population requires surgery at some point in their lifetime (NCEPOD, 2011). Approximately 3 million surgeries are performed in the UK each year, with an average in-hospital mortality of 0.8–1% (NCEPOD, 2011). Many will be carried out in the elderly and in patients with numerous associated comorbidities and health issues. Moreover, surgical care represents a significant patient safety risk and economic burden for healthcare systems such as the NHS (RCS, 2018). There is such a vast range of surgical procedures now practiced in the UK, along with the diversity of patients undergoing surgery, making it difficult to generalise the metabolic and nutritional responses following surgery. Procedures vary from elective to emergency surgery, and from laparoscopic to prolonged procedures taking many hours. What is clear is that the type and duration of the surgical procedure influences the speed of postoperative recovery.

The role of the dietitian is vital in the management of surgical patients at all stages of the surgical pathway. Postoperative management has been shown to be improved if a dietitian is part of the multidisciplinary team (MDT) (Wood, 2005). However, the health status of the patient and the reason for surgery need to be central to the extent of the involvement of the dietitian. For example, an emergency appendectomy in an otherwise fit, healthy adult has little implication for nutritional intervention, whereas a malnourished, cachectic patient requires nutritional support pre- and post-surgery if compromised nutritional status is not to adversely affect clinical progress. The majority of this chapter focuses on major-surgery patients.

The clinical management of surgical patients has progressed radically over the last 100 years, with the availability of prophylactic antibiotics, intravenous fluids and colloids, increased understanding of anaesthetic agents and analgesics, specialist critical care units (CCU) and an increased understanding of organ function perioperatively. Nutrition is now an integrated component of surgical care, with nutritional support education being a requirement of the training of core surgical trainees (RCS, 2018).

Preoperative malnutrition

Evidence suggests that 25–40% of patients are malnourished on hospital admission (Kruizenga *et al.*, 2005). The implications of malnutrition for the surgical patient centre on the increased risk for both systemic and intestinal immunity (Beattie *et al.*, 2000). Although it is difficult to establish a direct causal relationship, preoperative malnutrition has been associated with a significantly higher risk of postoperative complications (Allison, 2000; Salvino *et al.*, 2004), impaired quality of life (Ferguson *et al.*, 1998) and mortality in older age groups (Rapp-Kesek *et al.*, 2004).

Populations at risk

Many patients presenting for surgery will have chronic diseases, organ dysfunction, cancer, inflammatory bowel disease and associated symptoms such as anorexia, nausea, vomiting, taste changes and change in bowel habit. All causes of nutrient loss and increased metabolic need will influence nutritional status. Typically, high-risk patients include the following:

- Elderly.
- Patients who are undergoing surgery and unlikely to resume oral intake for >5 days.
- Weight loss >10% in 3 months.
- Weight loss >5% in 1 month
  - or BMI <20 kg/m^2.
  - or reduced food intake by 25–50% normal requirements in the preceding week.
- Impaired muscle strength using hand dynamometry.

It must be remembered that malnutrition can occur in obese patients who have low muscle mass. Sarcopenic obesity can be hard to detect, but is important to determine before major surgery. Fat-free mass may be a better predictor of mortality and poor outcomes than BMI (Van Venrooij *et al.*, 2011). However, the use of routine preoperative body composition analysis is not yet routine practice.

Effects of surgery

Any surgical trauma causes physiological stress that is related to the severity of the procedure. Desborough (2000) provides an excellent overview of the complex sequela of events.

Classification of nutritional risk

A variety of tools have been developed to assess the nutritional status of patients awaiting surgery, such as the Mini Nutritional Assessment (MNA), Subjective Global Index (SGI), Nutritional Risk Index (NRI), and Malnutrition Universal Screening Tool ('MUST') (see Chapter 6.2, Malnutrition). It is recommended that all surgical inpatients be screened for nutritional and physical status on admission, and reviewed weekly thereafter (NICE, 2006). The use of body composition analysis and anthropometry should be seen as essential for dietitians assessing preoperative patients to fully understand a patient's body composition risk.

Enhanced recovery after surgery (ERAS) has revolutionised the role of nutritional risk assessment. ERAS stipulates that nutritional risk assessment should occur as early in the patient's treatment pathway as possible, ideally in primary care, or, at the very latest, in the preoperative assessment clinic (1000 Lives Wales, 2017). The logistics of making nutritional risk assessment a core component of the surgical pathway requires excellent engagement with the MDT by the dietitian. A study (Barlow *et al.*, 2017) has developed an optimisation bundle designed to be used by GPs at the time of initial referral for investigation, and includes nutritional risk assessment to enable sign posting for timely nutritional intervention.

Preoperative nutritional support

Optimisation of nutritional status preoperatively reduces postoperative infectious complications (Somanchi *et al.*, 2011; Windsor *et al.*, 2004) and enhances wound healing rates (see Chapter 7.17.6, Wound healing, tissue viability and pressure sores). Pre-operative nutritional interventions in gastrointestinal surgery have been shown to support this (Burden *et al.*, 2012). This review included heterogeneous study participants undergoing immunonutrition, oral supplements and parenteral nutrition (PN). A recent study (Burden *et al.*, 2017) concluded that oral supplementation does positively influence clinical outcomes in colorectal cancer patients with pre-surgery weight loss. As a general role, active nutritional support by the provision of oral nutritional supplements or enteral feeding (EN) should be routinely considered in patients with a BMI of <18.5 kg/m^2, or in those who present with unintentional weight loss of >10% of body weight within the last 3 months. A BMI below 20 kg/m^2 with unintentional weight loss of >5% of body weight within the previous 3–6 months is also predictive of malnutrition (NICE, 2006).

Fasting guidelines

Prolonged preoperative fasting has, until recently, been a time-honoured tradition. However, this is slowly changing, as evidence increases that patients fasted from liquids and solids for an average of 12–14 hours have a compromised fluid and nutritional intake (Crenshaw & Winslow, 2002). It exposes patients to unnecessary starvation, suboptimal stress reduction and intravenous fluid overload preoperatively (Lassen *et al.*, 2005). The rationale for preoperative fasting is to reduce the volume and acidity of gastric contents, thus reducing the risks of intraoperative regurgitation and aspiration of gastric contents into the lungs; yet, evidence supporting this rationale is lacking. Guidelines from the American Society of Anesthesiologists (ASA, 2017) recommend allowing consumption of clear liquids (including fruit juices without pulp) up to 2 hours before elective surgery, a light breakfast (e.g. tea and toast) 6 hours before the procedure, and a heavier meal 8 hours beforehand. These newer practices improve patient comfort and reduce adverse outcomes (Hayhurst & Durieux, 2014; Saqr & Chambers, 2006). Patients considered at high risk of aspiration (obese, diabetic or with gastrointestinal reflux) can follow a similar fasting regimen, but this should be at the anaesthetist's discretion (Jellish *et al.*, 2005; Maltby *et al.*, 2004).

Carbohydrate loading

Carbohydrate loading has gained widespread popularity in the preoperative management of major surgical patients over the past decade. The surge in popularity is due to its integral role in the ERAS Programme (Fearon & Luffman, 2003). The use of carbohydrate-rich drinks prior to surgery has been shown to alter the metabolic state, from a fasted to a fed state. This modulates the postoperative insulin response impacting on insulin sensitivity, leading to improved muscle strength and mass in particularly lean body tissue (Ljungqvist & Søreide, 2003). This has been linked with early mobilisation and rehabilitation (Melis *et al.*, 2006a; Yuill *et al.*, 2005). A detailed review of the physiological action of the mechanism of carbohydrate and insulin resistance is given by Ljungqvist and Søreide (2003).

Practically, carbohydrate solutions should be administered 4–12 hours preoperatively. Caution is required for all diabetic patients, due to possible impaired glycaemic control and impaired gastric emptying; however, the evidence remains conflicting. Protocols should be agreed locally, with detailed discussions taking place between the dietetics department, anaesthetist, diabetologist and the wider clinical team.

Perioperative nutritional support

The routine use of perioperative nutritional support has traditionally been a controversial postoperative therapeutic intervention in surgical patients; however, the advent of the ERAS programme seems to be resolving this. Perioperative nutrition intervention aims to:

- Minimise negative nitrogen balance by avoiding starvation.
- Maintain muscle, immune and cognitive function.
- Optimise postoperative recovery and return to function.

Starting enteral or oral feeding within 24 hours of surgery is associated with optimal clinical outcome (Allison, 2005; Barlow *et al.*, 2011; Kotze, 2011). Immediate postoperative enteral feeding, commenced within 6–12 hours post-procedure, is associated with a significant reduction in postoperative complications, reducing both intensive care unit (ICU) and total hospital length of stay (LOS) (Barlow *et al.*, 2011; Beattie *et al.*, 2000; Gabor *et al.*, 2005; Kreymann *et al.*, 2006; Macfie *et al.*, 2000; Smedley *et al.*, 2004). The recommendation to start early enteral feeding is often tempered by the possibility of postoperative complications. However, Macfie *et al.* (2000) suggest that the introduction of enteral nutrition (EN) does not contribute to complication risk, but allows any pending surgical complications to be detected at an earlier opportunity, allowing remedial surgical or medical intervention to take place. In addition, early enteral feeding post-surgery reduces the risk of anastomotic dehiscence, pneumonia, wound infection and intra-abdominal abscess (Lewis *et al.*, 2001). This has been reiterated in a study (Barlow *et al.*, 2011), which also showed a significant improvement in the time spent in hospital with early enteral feeding.

Several meta-analyses have suggested that normal food intake or EN may be beneficial in reducing infective complications and hospital stay in general surgical patients (Marik & Zaloga, 2001; Møiniche *et al.*, 1995; Schilder *et al.*, 1997). However, the issue of the early introduction of oral food intake in patients with an upper gastrointestinal tract anastomosis is not straightforward. Lassen *et al.* (2005) advocated the use of early oral food after upper gastrointestinal tract resection at will; however, for many patients, this may not be the preferred method. This may not be a viable option for patients with anorexia or in those who lack confidence with eating in the first few days postoperatively. The use of nasojejunal, jejunostomy and other post-pyloric feeding for immediate early EN has been reported to be safe, well tolerated and to have advantages over traditional management with intravenous fluids or PN (Aiko *et al.*, 2001; Sand *et al.*, 1997). For a detailed review of the proposed mechanism of action of early EN, see Kudsk (2002) and Genton and Kudsk (2003). The recommendation for clinical practice should be to use EN (either oral or enteral tube feeding) where the gastrointestinal tract is accessible and functioning.

Immunonutrition

Immune-enhancing supplementation is an expensive alternative to standard formula products. Although the benefit from these has been demonstrated, their cost currently prohibits large-scale implementation into routine practice in the preoperative period for elective surgical patients. Several studies on the use of immunonutrition perioperatively have indicated that immune-enhanced EN is superior to EN in lowering the incidence of infections and complications (Braga *et al.*, 1999, 2002; Daly *et al.*, 1995; Gianotti *et al.*, 2002). The use of preoperative immune-enhancing oral supplementation has been shown to reduce complication rates in colorectal cancer patients (Hegazi *et al.*, 2014; Waitzberg *et al.*, 2006). Burden *et al.* (2011) concluded that there is no advantage in providing routine immunonutritional supplements to all patients, but did suggest that these may be beneficial in patients who lose weight preoperatively (see Chapter 7.11.1, Nutrition and immunity).

Route of feeding

Jejunostomy

Jejunostomy is a surgical procedure by which a tube is situated in the lumen of the proximal jejunum, primarily to administer nutrition, fluid and medication (Sarr,

1988), reducing the need for central venous access for administration of nutrition and drugs (see Chapter 6.4, Enteral nutrition). Clearly, the choice of feeding jejunostomy is crucial, and it may be a major factor in the development of complications, alongside the insertion technique used by the surgeon. The use of aggressive feeding, such as using high rates to initiate the enteral feed, coupled with the rapid increase in rate of the feed and the osmolarity of the feed, are all important (Melis *et al.*, 2006b). Too rapid delivery of EN coupled with the overzealous use of opioids, which slow gastrointestinal peristalsis, could lead to increased intra-abdominal pressure and exacerbate gastrointestinal oedema, reducing splanchnic blood flow and increasing the likelihood of gastrointestinal ischaemia (Melis *et al.*, 2006b). The volume of EN delivered is vital. Watters *et al.* (1997) reported that EN delivered to nutritional requirements within 3 days in major surgical patients leads to respiratory problems secondary to increased abdominal distension. The ESPEN guidelines (2006) state that the '*placement of a needle catheter jejunostomy or naso-jejunal tube is recommended for all candidates for tube feeding undergoing major abdominal surgery*'. Furthermore, recent research (Bowrey *et al.*, 2015) has supported the routine use of jejunostomy inserted at the time of upper gastrointestinal surgery along with benefits for patients following discharge. This study demonstrated that home enteral feeding by jejunostomy was feasible, safe and acceptable to patients and their carers.

Parenteral nutrition

PN is discussed in Chapter 6.5 (Parenteral nutrition).

Postoperative gastrointestinal motility

The three most common reasons for the delay of enteral feed commencement are the absence of bowel sounds (with presumed ileus), risk of gastrointestinal anastomoses dehiscence, and haemodynamic instability, especially in the ICU patient. After surgery, postoperative gastrointestinal dysfunction or ileus is commonly reported to occur. It is thought to occur in 90% of patients undergoing intra-abdominal surgery. Livingston and Passaro (1990) defined ileus as the '*inhibition of propulsive bowel motility, irrespective of pathological mechanisms*'. Ileus is characterised by the development of nausea, vomiting, delayed gastric emptying, bowel distension, decreased bowel sounds, delay in the passage of stools and pain after a surgical procedure (Mythen, 2005). The pathogenesis of ileus is multifactorial. Livingston and Passaro (1990) describe the pathogenesis of ileus; these factors were further elucidated by Mythen (2005).

Traditionally, it has been considered that ileus prevents the safe delivery of EN. Barium studies have demonstrated that small bowel motility continues in the postoperative phase, despite delayed gastric emptying taking 24–48 hours to recover, and colonic motility taking 3–5 days to return (Livingston & Passaro, 1990). Clinicians often use the traditional practice of auscultation of bowel sounds to gain information on intestinal function and motility. However, bowels sounds have not been shown to correlate with motor patterns of function or dysfunction (Madsen *et al.*, 2005). The administration of EN has been shown to promote gastrointestinal motility in several studies (Beier-Holgersen & Boesby, 1996; Stewart *et al.*, 1998). Delivery of EN in clinical practice is not simple. Attention to the feed rate of EN delivery is important, as failure to increase this may not produce a postprandial motility response, and, without this, there will be no normal small bowel contraction and peristalses, resulting in undigested EN passing into the colon. The ERAS programme has changed the perception of nutritional management perioperatively, with nutrition now seen as an integral component of surgical care (Fearon & Luffman, 2004).

Nutrition requirements

It is important to remember that the aim of nutritional support in the surgical patient is to reduce postoperative complications, while optimising recovery and quality of life. Postsurgical energy requirements vary according to the degree of trauma and concurrent clinical factors. After minor surgical procedures, energy expenditure will not be greatly affected, whereas major procedures with resultant sepsis and high output stoma or drain losses potentially increase energy and protein requirements. The quality of nutritional support, rather than quantity, is now considered to be more relevant for postsurgical patients. An intake of 25–35 kcal/kg/day of total energy with 0.8–1.5 g of protein (0.13–0.24 g of nitrogen)/kg/day is a starting point. However, overzealous, aggressive nutritional support is not helpful if it leads to complications.

Fluid requirements

Fluid requirements can be met by 30–35 mL/kg/day, with additional fluid provided to compensate for pyrexia and increased drain, fistulae or stoma losses. Serum biochemistry and anthropometry are usually the only tools available to estimate the nutritional adequacy of a prescribed regimen, but it should be noted that these may not be representative of nutritional status in the postsurgical patient (Bachrach-Lindstrom *et al.*, 2001). It is widely known that postoperative fluid and electrolyte balance has been traditionally suboptimal (Lobo *et al.*, 2001). Suboptimal fluid balance can impair respiratory function and wound healing by affecting tissue oxygenation due to interstitial oedema and gut oedema. Lobo *et al.* (2001) concluded that fluid and sodium restriction in patients undergoing major colonic resection significantly reduced the duration of ileus and improved gut perfusion. Additionally, disturbances in acid–base balance, glucose or electrolytes affect gut function and motility, presumably due to altered cellular mechanics (Wilkes *et al.*, 2001). The British Consensus Guidelines on intravenous fluid therapy for adult surgical patients (GIFTASUP) (Powell-Tuck *et al.*, 2011) provide a useful consensus for the recommendations for perioperative fluid management, and these are now being incorporated into many hospital surgical and critical care units. NICE guidance (2017) for the management of intravenous fluids in the surgical patient offers a basis on which to manage fluid prescription for surgical patients.

Glycaemic control

Postoperative insulin resistance and hyperglycaemia aggravate the inflammatory response, enhancing cytokine production and contributing to the surgical stress that negatively impacts on morbidity and mortality (Ljungqvist *et al.*, 2005). Tight glycaemic control using sliding scale insulin therapy improves outcome (see Chapter 7.17.1, Critical care). This appears to be due to a direct effect of insulin on blood glucose and an indirect effect of insulin in correcting abnormal serum lipid profile, and the downregulation of the catabolic state evoked in the surgically stressed patient (Vanhorebeek *et al.*, 2005). Many ICUs adopting tight glycaemic control protocols require a 24-hour feed schedule to minimise the risk of catastrophic hypoglycaemia.

Nutritional management of surgical complications

Complications in feeding the surgical patient may relate to the presence of the underlying pathology (e.g. Crohn's disease, cachexia, pancreatitis or diabetes), the planned surgical outcome (such as ileostomy formation) or an adverse effect as a result of surgery (wound dehiscence, fistula formation, infection and pyrexia). The use of bariatric surgery as a method of weight management has increased dramatically in recent years, and brings its own nutritional problems (Edwards *et al.*, 2006), including late-developing deficiencies of iron, vitamin B_{12}, calcium and vitamin D, in addition to protein energy malnutrition and fat malabsorption (Malinowski, 2006). The recently published BOMS guidelines should help to alleviate any concerns surrounding vitamin and mineral deficiencies (O'Kane, 2014). The immediate perioperative nutritional input for common complications of surgery is described in the following text. Long-term management of each condition may require a different approach.

Wound healing

The nutritional aspects of wound healing are discussed in Chapter 7.17.6 (Wound healing, tissue viability and pressure sores). Recent studies on the role of nutritional support in wound healing in surgical patients are limited. Schroeder *et al.* (1991) concluded that EN in patients after gastrointestinal resection, as compared to nil by mouth and intravenous fluids, improved collagen synthesis and promoted wound strength. More recently, a meta-analysis (Lewis *et al.*, 2001) demonstrated that anastomotic dehiscence rates were reduced in patients receiving EN. A study by Braga *et al.* (2002) also suggested that EN is not detrimental to anastomotic healing even when early direct passage of nutrients over a fresh intestinal suture has occurred.

Enterocutaneous fistulae

These fistulae are tracts leading from the bowel to the skin surface. Low-residue enteral feeds are well tolerated and do not contribute to losses from distal bowel fistula. Sodium and magnesium replacement may be necessary if the fistula drains small bowel contents. The use of antidiarrhoeal or antisecretory drugs may reduce fistula losses sufficient to allow healing. Enteral feeding with predigested formula may also be successful if a somatostatin analogue (octreotide) is given to reduce gastrointestinal secretions. Nutritional support decreases or modifies the composition of the gastrointestinal secretions and is considered to have a primary therapeutic role in the management of patients with fistula (Dudrick *et al.*, 1999).

Chylothorax

Chylothorax is a rare but serious complication of thoracic surgery or major neck dissection, resulting in damage to the thoracic duct. Drainage of chyle (fat-rich lymph fluid) from the thoracic duct injury into the pleural cavity results in chylothorax, which is relieved by chest drain insertion. Most nutrients, including medium-chain triglycerides (MCTs), are absorbed across the gastrointestinal tract into the portal circulation for transport to the liver. Dietary fats are insoluble in aqueous solutions such as blood, so are packaged into chylomicrons within the intestinal cells, and then travel as chyle in the interstitial fluid within the lymphatic system. Chyle also contains quantities of protein (e.g. albumin, lymphocytes and antibodies), and has an electrolyte composition similar to that of plasma. Chyle flow is reduced by fasting and increased by oral fluids, especially those high in long-chain fatty acids. Intravenous fluids have no effect on chyle flow.

Chylothorax can be managed conservatively by following a very-low-fat diet (ideally <15 g of fat/day) and substituting MCTs for longer-chain fatty acids in enteral or oral diets, or by bypassing the thoracic duct completely and using PN (which can contain long-chain fatty acids). A chest drain relieves the chyle collection. If conservative management fails, ligation of the thoracic duct, traditionally carried out by thoracotomy, is required. The advent of video-assisted thoracoscopic surgery permits a laparoscopic approach to ligation of the thoracic duct (Kumar *et al.*, 2004).

Acute pancreatitis

Early EN modulates the stress response, promotes more rapid resolution of pancreatitis and results in a better outcome as compared to PN (McClave *et al.*, 2006). EN attenuates inflammation, reduces the incidence of septic complications and provides a more cost-effective approach to postsurgical feeding than PN (Louie *et al.*, 2005) (see Chapter 7.4.5, Disorders of the pancreas). The use of antioxidants has been shown to improve outcome (Braganza *et al.*, 2011), but this remains an area of controversy.

Open abdomen

Occasionally, patients undergoing abdominal surgery develop abdominal compartment syndrome, a massive intestinal oedema following abdominal laparotomy that renders the abdomen difficult to close surgically. Closure of the abdomen increases intra-abdominal pressure to such an extent that cardiovascular, respiratory and renal functions are compromised. The abdomen is therefore left open but covered until swelling subsides and surgical closure can be achieved. It is possible to enterally feed a patient with an open abdomen without complication (Cothren *et al.*, 2004).

High-output stomas and intestinal failure

The small intestine is initially maladapted to the uptake of sodium and water, a process usually confined to the large bowel. Net secretion occurs in the upper small intestine to increase the sodium content of luminal fluid and will have the effect of increasing stoma losses. Restricting the intake of salt-poor fluids to <500 mL/day and sipping sodium-rich oral rehydration solution (e.g. WHO rehydration solution, or double-strength Dioralyte or Rehydrat) can reduce small intestine secretions, minimise the fluid load through the small intestine and increase the chance of absorption. Alternatively, patients can take oral salt tablets *pro rata* with salt-poor fluids for a similar effect (see Chapter 7.4.9, Intestinal failure and intestinal resection).

Enhanced recovery after surgery

The ERAS programme was first described by Kehlet and Mogensen (1999). ERAS is an evidence-based multimodal care pathway that has proven earlier recovery for patients undergoing major surgery (Gustafsson *et al.*, 2013; Nygren *et al.*, 2012, 2013; Simpson *et al.*, 2015; Walter *et al.*, 2009; Wind *et al.*, 2006). ERAS is a paradigm shift in surgical care, and it integrates a range of interventions that aims to reduce the loss of and improve the restoration of functional capacity after surgery (Kehlet & Mogensen, 1999). ERAS aims to limit the loss of function, and the program is a package of evidence-based modifications in preoperative, intra-operative and postoperative elements of care to reduce surgical stress and postoperative catabolism (Fearon & Luffman, 2004).

Enhanced recovery is sometimes referred to as fast-track or accelerated surgery, and is supported by a growing base of clinical and research evidence (www.erasuk.org). Optimal nutrition, hydration, pain management and mobilisation, alongside excellent surgical and anaesthetic techniques, represent the core tenets of ERAS (Fearon & Luffman, 2004). Enhanced recovery interventions include the following:

- Optimising the patient's health/medical condition preoperatively, ideally with primary care if surgery is elective.
- Assessing risk and fitness for surgery at preoperative assessment, ideally at least 2–4 weeks prior to surgery.
- Reducing starvation by using carbohydrate-loading drinks up to 2–4 hours before surgery.
- Using minimally invasive surgical techniques where possible.
- Optimal pain relief with the avoidance of opioids where possible.
- Early mobilisation within 6–12 hours of surgery if clinically safe and viable.
- Early enteral or oral nutrition with 4 hours of surgery if clinically safe and viable.

It is well documented that ERAS is clinically effective as well as cost-effective/cost-saving, in that it reduces complications and health services utilisation (e.g. LOS in hospital) without compromising patient safety and health-related quality of life (Adamina *et al.*, 2011; Gouvas *et al.*, 2009; Varadhan *et al.*, 2010). Although ERAS has the potential to make an important contribution to healthcare systems, uptake has been minimal, with fewer than one-third of surgical practices in the UK (Greco *et al.*, 2014). In Wales, recent information concludes that few NHS hospitals are routinely delivering ERAS effectively for patient benefit, and hence are not benefiting from the outcomes listed in the following text.

Since the first consensus ERAS guidelines for colorectal surgery were published in 2005 (http://erassociety.org/about/history/), ERAS guidelines have been published for other major procedures, since the principles of the ERAS pathway apply to many patients undergoing major surgery. In 2010, a non-profit, academic, international, multidisciplinary society was formed: the ERAS Society (http://erassociety.org). The aim was to improve perioperative care through research and education, and to enhance the implementation of best practices worldwide. In several countries, national ERAS groups have been formed and linked to the ERAS Society. Several national ERAS programmes have been launched in the UK (1000Livesplus, DH and Scottish Government). With improved quality of care and reduced harm, hospital stay will become more efficient, and hospitals should benefit from the programme by savings in bed days. The benefits of ERAS implementation include the following:

- Reduction in hospital stay (Varadhan *et al.*, 2010).
- Development of postoperative complications reduced by 40% in patients undergoing colorectal surgery (Varadhan *et al.*, 2010).
- Decreased nursing care and reliance on delayed allied health intervention due to reduction in complication (Nygren *et al.*, 2013).
- Cost-effectiveness – ERAS saved US$2985 (range US$373–5753) per patient, with the probability for ERAS to be cost-effective at close to 100% (Nelson *et al.*, 2016). A study has concluded that every US$1 invested in ERAS would bring US$3.8 in return on that investment (Thanh *et al.*, 2016).
- Reduced the rate of readmission, readmission LOS, emergency department visits and GP visits (Greco *et al.*, 2014). There are wider societal benefits associated with ERAS, such as patients returning to work

sooner and lessened caregiver burden without lowering patients' quality of life (Lv *et al.*, 2012).

- For patients undergoing surgeries as part of multimodal cancer treatment plans, a faster recovery allowed them to initiate adjuvant treatments, improving their oncologic outcomes (Biagi *et al.*, 2011). Work from Cardiff (Chan *et al.*, 2013) has demonstrated an improved survival benefit from using ERAS in patients undergoing upper gastrointestinal cancer surgery.
- Khan *et al.* (2010) performed a systematic review that demonstrated improved health-related quality of life and patient satisfaction.

Nutritional management and ERAS

In summary, the incorporation of nutrition in ERAS is as follows:

- Pretreatment optimisation and prehabilitation, ideally including nutrition within primary care.
- Nutritional screening at preoperative assessment clinic with the introduction of nutritional support/intervention as required.
- Intra-operative and postoperative consideration of nutritional plans with clear document of these plans.
- Early enteral or oral nutrition, ideally within 12 hours of surgery.
- Nutritional advice for discharge and rehabilitation.

Enhanced recovery is dependent on the engagement, commitment and involvement of all members of the MDT at all stages of the patient's care, including general practice, secondary care, surgery and throughout the hospital stay. Nutritional screening, assessment and early EN are key components of the ERAS pathway, and as such the dietitian should play a pivotal role in the development and delivery of ERAS.

Prehabilitation

Prehabilitation is a vital part of the ERAS programme. It is an MDT process that occurs between the time of diagnosis and the beginning of acute treatment. It includes physical and psychological assessments that establish a baseline functional level, identify impairments, and provide interventions that promote physical and psychological health. It is an MDT concept that aims to prepare the patient for pending treatment. It has been proven to:

- Reduce postoperative residual functional disability.
- Reduce morbidity/mortality.
- Improve postoperative quality of life.
- Improve preoperative respiratory function to offer greater surgical options, and therefore improve resection rates.
- Improve nutritional status to prepare patients for treatment phase.
- Manage patient expectations by informing and educating patients.
- Empower patients, giving them ownership of their health and recovery.
- Signpost patients to adjunct services, including smoking cessation and counselling services.

The prehabilitation team should consist of allied health professionals, including physiotherapists, dietitians and occupational therapists.

Internet resources

American Society of Anesthesiologists, www.asahq.org
ERAS Society UK, www.erasuk.org
NHS Improvement, https://www.nhs.uk/conditions/enhanced-recovery/
NHS Scotland,http://www.qihub.scot.nhs.uk/quality-and-efficiency/whole-system-patient-flow/enhanced-recovery.aspx
NHS Wales, www.1000livesplus.wales.nhs.uk
Royal College of Surgeons, https://www.rcseng.ac.uk

References

Adamina M, Kehlet H, Tomlinson GA, *et al.* (2011) Enhanced recovery pathways optimize health outcomes and resource utilization: a meta-analysis of randomized controlled trials in colorectal surgery. *Surgery.* 149: 830–840.

Aiko S, Yoshizumi Y, Sugiura Y, *et al.* (2001) Beneficial effects of immediate enteral nutrition after esophageal cancer surgery. *Surg. Today.* 31(11): 971–978.

Allison SP. (2000) Malnutrition, disease, and outcome. *Nutrition.* 16: 590–593.

Allison SP. (2005) Integrated nutrition. *Proc. Nutr. Soc.* 64(3): 319–323.

American Society of Anesthesiologists (ASA). (2017) Practice Guidelines for Preoperative Fasting and the use of Pharmacologic agents to reduce the risk of pulmonary aspiration. *Anesthesiology.* 3(126): 376–393.

Bachrach-Lindstrom M, Unosson M, Ek AC, *et al.* (2001) Assessment of nutritional status using biochemical and anthropometric variables in a nutritional intervention study of women with hip fracture. *Clin. Nutr.* 20: 217–223.

Barlow R, Price P, Reid TD, *et al.* (2011) Prospective multicentre randomised controlled trial of early enteral nutrition for patients undergoing major upper GI resection. *Clin. Nutr.* 30(5): 560–566.

Barlow R, Perkins C, Mayor SM, *et al.* (2017) *Fit for list? Optimising the health status of patients with suspected cancer in primary care: Is it feasible?* Available at http://www.erasuk.net/uploads/2/6/4/0/26401678/erasukconferencenov16fit_for_list.pdf. Accessed 15 February 2018.

Beattie AH, Prach AT, Baxter JP, *et al.* (2000) A randomised controlled trial evaluating the use of enteral nutritional supplements postoperatively in malnourished surgical patients. *Gut.* 46: 813–818.

Beier-Holgersen R, Boesby S. (1996) Influence of postoperative enteral nutrition on postsurgical infections. *Gut.* 39(96): 833–835.

Biagi JJ, Raphael MJ, Mackillop WJ, *et al.* (2011) Association between time to initiation of adjuvant chemotherapy and survival in colorectal cancer: a systematic review and meta-analysis. *JAMA.* 305(22): 2335–2342. doi: 10.1001/jama.2011.749.

Bowrey DJ, Baker M, Halliday V, *et al.* (2015) A randomised controlled trial of six weeks of home enteral nutrition versus standard care after oesophagectomy or total gastrectomy for cancer: report on a pilot and feasibility study. *Trials.* 16: 531. doi: 10.1186/s13063-015-1053.

Braga M, Gianotti L, Radaelli G, *et al.* (1999) Perioperative immunonutrition in patients undergoing cancer surgery: results of a randomized double-blind phase 3 trial. *Arch. Surg.* 134(4): 428–433.

Braga M, Gianotti L, Nespoli L, *et al.* (2002) Nutritional approach in malnourished surgical patients: a prospective randomized study. *Arch. Surg.* 137(2): 174–180.

Braganza J, Lee SH, McCloy RF, *et al.* (2011) Chronic pancreatitis. *Lancet*. 377: 1184–1197.

Burden ST, Hill J, Shaffer JL, *et al.* (2011) An unblended randomised controlled trial of preoperative oral supplements in colorectal cancer patients. *J. Hum. Nutr. Diet*. 24(5): 441–448.

Burden S, Todd, C, Hill J, *et al.* (2012) Pre-operative nutritional support in patients undergoing gastrointestinal surgery. *Cochrane Database Syst. Rev.* 11: CD008879.

Burden S, Gibson DJ, Lal S, *et al.* (2017) Pre-operative oral nutritional supplementation with dietary advice versus dietary advice alone in weight- losing patients with colorectal cancer: single-blind randomized controlled trial. *J. Cachexia. Sarcopenia Muscle*. 8: 437–446.

Chan DS, Reid TD, White C, *et al.* (2013) Influence of a regional centralised upper gastrointestinal cancer service model on patient safety, quality of care and survival. *Clin. Oncol. (R Coll Radiol)*.

Cothren CC, Moore EE, Ciesla DJ, *et al.* (2004) Postinjury abdominal compartment syndrome does not preclude early enteral feeding after definitive closure. *Am. J. Surg.* 188(6): 653–658.

Crenshaw JT, Winslow EH. (2002) Preoperative fasting: old habits die hard. *Am. J. Nurs.* 102: 36–44.

Daly JM, Weintraub FN, Shou J, *et al.* (1995) Enteral nutrition during multimodality therapy in upper gastrointestinal cancer patients. *Ann. Surg.* 221(4): 327–338.

Desborough JP. (2000) The stress response to trauma and surgery. *Br. J. Anaesth.* 85: 109–117.

Dudrick SJ, Maharaj AR, McKelvey AA. (1999) Artificial nutritional support in patients with gastrointestinal fistulas. *World J. Surg.* 23: 570–576.

Edwards ED, Jacob BP, Gagner M, *et al.* (2006) Presentation and management of common post-weight loss surgery problems in the emergency department. *Ann. Emerg. Med.* 47: 160–166.

Fearon K, Luffman (2003) The nutritional management of surgical patients: enhanced recovery after surgery. *Proc. Nutr. Soc.* 62: 867–881.

Ferguson M, Capra S, Bauer J, *et al.* (1998) Quality of life in patients with malnutrition. *JAMA* 98: A22.

Gabor S, Renner H, Matzi V, *et al.* (2005) Early enteral feeding compared with parenteral nutrition after oesophageal or oesophagogastric resection and reconstruction. *Br. J. Nutr.* 93: 509–513.

Genton L, Kudsk KA. (2003) Interactions between the enteric nervous system and the immune system: role of neuropeptides and nutrition. *Am. J. Surg.* 186(3): 253–258.

Gianotti L, Braga M, Nespoli L, *et al.* (2002) A randomized controlled trial of preoperative oral supplementation with a specialized diet in patients with gastrointestinal cancer. *Gastroenterology*. 122(7): 1763–1770.

Gouvas N, Tan E, Windsor A, *et al.* (2009) Fast-track vs standard care in colorectal surgery: a meta-analysis update. *Int. J. Colorectal Dis.* 24: 1119–1131.

Greco M, Capretti G, Beretta L, *et al.* (2014) Enhanced recovery program in colorectal surgery: a meta-analysis of randomized controlled trials. *World J. Surg.* 38: 1531–1541.

Gustafsson UO, Scott MJ, Schwenk W, *et al.* (2013) Guidelines for perioperative care in elective colonic surgery: Enhanced Recovery After Surgery (ERAS®) Society recommendations. *World J. Surg.* 37: 259–284. doi: 10.1007/s00268-012-1772-0

Hayhurst C, Durieux ME. (2014) Enteral hydration prior to surgery: the benefits are clear. *Anesth. Analg.* 118(6):1163–1164.

Hegazi RA, Hustead DS, Evans DC. (2014) Preoperative standard oral nutrition supplements vs immunonutrition: results of systematic review and meta-analysis. *J. Am. Coll. Surg.* 219(5): 1078–1087.

Jellish WS, Kartha V, Fluder E, *et al.* (2005) Effect of metoclopramide on gastric fluid volumes in diabetic patients who have fasted before elective surgery. *Anesthesiology*. 102(5): 904–909.

Kehlet H, Mogensen T. (1999) Hospital stay of 2 days after open sigmoidectomy with a multimodal rehabilitation programme. *Br. J. Surg.* 86(2): 227–230.

Khan S, Wilson T, Ahmed J, *et al.* (2010) Quality of life and patient satisfaction with enhanced recovery protocols. *Colorectal Dis.* 12(12):1175–1182. doi: 10.1111/j.1463-1318.2009.01997.x.

Kotze V. (2011) Perioperative nutrition: What do we know? *S. Afr. J. Clin. Nutr.* 24(3): S19–S22.

Kreymann KG, Berger MM, Deutz NE, *et al.* (2006) ESPEN guidelines on enteral nutrition: intensive care. *Clin. Nutr.* 25(2): 210–223.

Kruizenga HM, Van Tulder MW, Seidell JC, *et al.* (2005) Effectiveness and cost-effectiveness of early screening and treatment of malnourished patients. *Am. J. Clin. Nutr.* 82: 1082–1089.

Kudsk K. (2002) Current aspects of mucosal immunology and its influence by nutrition. *Am. J. Surg.* 183: 390–398.

Kumar S, Kumar A, Pawar DK. (2004) Thoracoscopic management of thoracic duct injury: is there a place for conservatism? *J. Postgrad. Med.* 50: 57–59.

Lassen K, Hannemann P, Ljungqvist O, *et al.*; Enhanced Recovery After Surgery Group. (2005) Patterns in current perioperative practice: survey of colorectal surgeons in five northern European countries. *BMJ.* 330: 1420–1421.

Lewis SJ, Egger M, Sylvester PA, *et al.* (2001) Early enteral feeding versus 'nil by mouth' after gastrointestinal surgery: systematic review and meta-analysis of controlled trials. *BMJ.* 323: 773–776.

Lives Wales. (2017) Enhanced Recovery After Surgery (ERAS). Available at http://www.1000livesplus.wales.nhs.uk/eras. Accessed 3 August 2017.

Livingston EH, Passaro EP Jr. (1990) Postoperative ileus. *Dig. Dis. Sci.* 35(1): 121–132.

Ljungqvist O, Søreide E. (2003) Preoperative fasting. *Br. J. Surg.* 90: 400–406.

Ljungqvist O, Nygren J, Soop M, *et al.* (2005) Metabolic perioperative management: novel concepts. *Curr. Opin. Crit. Care.* 11: 295–299.

Lobo DN, Dube MG, Neal KR, *et al.* (2001) Problems with solutions: drowning in the brine of an inadequate knowledge base. *Clin. Nutr.* 20(2): 125–130.

Louie BE, Noseworthy T, Hailey D, *et al.* (2005) 2004 MacLean-Mueller prize enteral or parenteral nutrition for severe pancreatitis: a randomized controlled trial and health technology assessment. *Can. J. Surg.* 48: 298–306.

Lv L, Shao YF, Zhou YB. (2012) The enhanced recovery after surgery (ERAS) pathway for patients undergoing colorectal surgery: an update of meta-analysis of randomized controlled trials. *Int. J. Colorectal. Dis.* 27:1549–1554.

Macfie J, Woodcock NP, Palmer MD, *et al.* (2000) Oral dietary supplements in pre- and postoperative surgical patients: a prospective and randomised control trial. *Nutrition.* 16: 723–728.

Madsen D, Sebolt T, Cullen L, *et al.* (2005) Listening to bowel sounds: an evidence-based practice project: nurses find that a traditional practice isn't the best indicator of returning gastrointestinal motility in patients who've undergone abdominal surgery. *Am. J. Nurs.* 105(12): 40–49.

Malinowski SS. (2006) Nutritional and metabolic complications of bariatric surgery. *Am. J. Med. Sci.* 331: 219–225.

Maltby JR, Pytka S, Watson NC, *et al.* (2004) Drinking 300 mL of clear fluid two hours before surgery has no effect on gastric fluid volume and pH in fasting and non-fasting obese patients. *Can. J. Anaesth.* 51: 111–115.

Marik PE, Zaloga GP. (2001) Early enteral nutrition in acutely ill patients: a systematic review. *Crit. Care Med.* 29(12): 2264–2270.

McClave SA, Chang WK, Dhaliwal R, *et al.* (2006) Nutrition support in acute pancreatitis: a systematic review of the literature. *JPEN J. Parenter. Enteral Nutr.* 30(2): 143–156.

Melis GC, van Leeuwen PA, von Blomberg-van der Flier BM, *et al.* (2006a) A carbohydrate-rich beverage prior to surgery prevents surgery-induced immunodepression: a randomized, controlled, clinical trial. *JPEN J. Parenter. Enteral Nutr.* 30: 21–26.

Melis M, Fichera A, Ferguson MK. (2006b) Bowel necrosis associated with early jejunal tube feeding: a complication of postoperative enteral nutrition. *Arch. Surg.* 141(7): 701–704.

Møiniche S, Bülow S, Hesselfeldt P, *et al.* (1995) Convalescence and hospital stay after colonic surgery with balanced analgesia, early oral feeding, and enforced mobilisation. *Eur. J. Surg.* 161(4): 283–288.

Mythen MG. (2005) Postoperative gastrointestinal tract dysfunction. *Anesth. Anal.* 100(1): 196–204.

National Confidential Enquiry into Patient Outcome and Death (NCEPOD). (2011) *Knowing the Risk; A Review of the Peri-Operative Care of Surgical Patients.* Available at www.ncepod.org.uk/2011report2/downloads/POC_fullreport.pdf. Accessed 1 December 2012.

Nelson G, Kiyang LN, Crumley ET, *et al.* (2016) Implementation of Enhanced Recovery After Surgery (ERAS) across a provincial healthcare system: the ERAS Alberta Colorectal Surgery Experience. *World J. Surg.* 40: 1092–1103.

NICE. (2006) *Nutrition Support in Adults. Clinical Guideline 32.* Available at www.nice.org.uk/CG032. Accessed 3 August 2017.

NICE. (2017) *Intravenous Fluid Therapy in Adults in Hospital (CG174).* Available at www.nice.org.uk/Guidance/CG174. Accessed 3 August 2017.

Nygren J, Thacker J, Carli F, *et al.* (2012) Guidelines for perioperative care in elective rectal/pelvic surgery: enhanced recovery after surgery (ERAS®) Society recommendations. *Clin. Nutr.* 31: 801–816.

Nygren J, Thacker J, Carli F, *et al.* (2013) Guidelines for perioperative care in elective rectal/pelvic surgery: Enhanced Recovery After Surgery (ERAS®) Society recommendations. *World J. Surg.* 37: 285–305.

O'Kane M. (2014) *BOMSS guidelines on peri-operative and postoperative biochemical monitoring and micronutrient replacement for patients undergoing bariatric surgery.* Available at http://www.bomss.org.uk/wp-content/uploads/2014/09/BOMSS-guidelines-Final-version1Oct14.pdf. Accessed 17 April 2018.

Powell-Tuck J, Gosling P, Lobo DN, *et al.* (2011) *British Consensus Guidelines on intravenous fluid therapy for adult surgical patients GIFTASUP.* Available at www.bapen.org.uk/pdfs/bapen_pubs/giftasup.pdf. Accessed 2 February 2012.

Rapp-Kesek D, Stahle E, Karlsson TT. (2004) Body mass index and albumin in the preoperative evaluation of cardiac surgery patients. *Clin. Nutr.* 23: 1398–1404.

Royal College of Surgeons (RCS). (2018) Undergraduate curriculum 2015. Available at https://www.rcseng.ac.uk/search/#SearchTerm=curriculum. Accessed 15 February 2018.

Salvino RM, Dechicco RS, Seidner DL. (2004) Perioperative nutrition support: who and how. *Cleve. Clin. J. Med.* 71: 345–351.

Sand J, Luostarinen M, Matikainen M. (1997) Enteral or parenteral feeding after total gastrectomy: prospective randomised pilot study. *Eur. J. Surg.* 163(10): 761–766.

Saqr L, Chambers WA. (2006) Preventing excessive pre-operative fasting: national guideline or local protocol? *Anaesthesia.* 61: 1–3.

Sarr MG. (1988) Needle catheter jejunostomy: an aid to postoperative care of the morbidly obese patient. *Am. Surg.* 54(8): 510–512.

Schilder JM, Hurteau JA, Look KY, *et al.* (1997) A prospective controlled trial of early postoperative oral intake following major abdominal gynecologic surgery. *Gynecol. Oncol.* 67(3): 235–240.

Schroeder D, Gillanders L, Mahr K, *et al.* (1991) Effects of immediate postoperative enteral nutrition on body composition, muscle function, and wound healing. *JPEN J. Parenter. Enteral Nutr.* 15(4): 376–383.

Simpson JC, Moonesinghe SR, Grocott MPW, *et al.* (2015) Enhanced recovery from surgery in the UK: an audit of the enhanced recovery partnership programme 2009–2012. *Br. J. Anaesth.* 115(4): 560–568.

Smedley F, Bowling T, James M, *et al.* (2004) Randomised clinical trial of the effects of preoperative and postoperative oral nutritional supplements on clinical course and cost of care. *Br. J. Surg.* 91: 983–990.

Somanchi M, Tao X, Mullin GE. (2011) The facilitated early enteral and dietary management effectiveness trial in hospitalized patients with malnutrition. *JPEN J. Parenter. Enteral Nutr.* 35(2): 209–216.

Stewart BT, Woods RJ, Collopy BT, *et al.* (1998) Early feeding after elective open colorectal resections: a prospective randomized trial. *Aust. N. Z. J. Surg.* 68(2): 125–128.

Thanh NX, Chuck AW, Wasylak T, *et al.* (2016) An economic evaluation of the Enhanced Recovery After Surgery (ERAS) multisite implementation program for colorectal surgery in Alberta. *Can. J. Surg.* 59(6): 415–421.

van Venrooij LM, van Leeuwen PA, Hopmans W, *et al.* (2011) Accuracy of quick and easy undernutrition screening tools – Short Nutritional Assessment Questionnaire, Malnutrition Universal Screening Tool, and modified Malnutrition Universal Screening Tool – in patients undergoing cardiac surgery. *J. Am. Diet. Assoc.* 111(12):1924–30. doi: 10.1016/j.jada.2011.09.009.

Varadhan KK, Neal KR, Dejong CH, *et al.* (2010) The enhanced recovery after surgery (ERAS) pathway for patients undergoing major elective open colorectal surgery: a meta-analysis of randomized controlled trials. *Clin. Nutr.* 29(4): 434–440.

Waitzberg DL, Saito H, Plank LD, *et al.* (2006) Postsurgical infections are reduced with specialised nutritional support. *World J. Surg.* 30: 1592–1604.

Walter CJ, Collin J, Dumville JC, *et al.* (2009) Enhanced recovery in colorectal resections: a systematic review and meta-analysis. *Int. J. Colorectal Dis.* 11: 344–353.

Watters JM, Kirkpatrick SM, Norris SB, *et al.* (1997) Immediate postoperative enteral feeding results in impaired respiratory mechanics and decreased mobility. *Ann. Surg.* 226(3): 369–377; discussion 377–380.

Weimann A, Braga M, Harsanyi L, *et al.* (2006) ESPEN guidelines on enteral nutrition: Surgery including organ transplantation. *Clin. Nutr.* 25(2): 224–244.

Wilkes NJ, Woolf R, Mutch M, *et al.* (2001) The effects of balanced versus saline-based hetastarch and crystalloid solutions on acid-base and electrolyte status and gastric mucosal perfusion in elderly surgical patients. *Anesth. Anal.* 93(4): 811–816.

Wind J, Polle SW, Jin PHPFK, *et al.* (2006) Systematic review of enhanced recovery programmes in colonic surgery. *Br. J. Surg.* 93: 800–809.

Windsor A, Braga M, Martindale R, *et al.* (2004) Fit for surgery: an expert panel review on optimising patients prior to surgery, with a particular focus on nutrition. *Surgeon.* 2: 315–319.

Wood K. (2005) Audit of nutritional guidelines for head and neck cancer patients undergoing radiotherapy. *J. Hum. Nutr. Diet.* 18: 343–351.

Yuill KA, Richardson RA, Davidson HI, *et al.* (2005) The administration of an oral carbohydrate-containing fluid prior to major elective upper-gastrointestinal surgery preserves skeletal muscle mass postoperatively – a randomised clinical trial. *Clin. Nutr.* 24: 32–37.

7.17.6 Wound healing, tissue viability and pressure sores

Christina Merryfield

Key points

- Malnutrition impairs wound healing.
- Micronutrient status should be checked and deficiencies corrected.
- Micronutrient supplements in the absence of deficiency have no additional benefit.
- It is important to identify other local and systemic factors that may delay or impede healing, e.g. medication, anaemia, smoking and age.

A wound may be described in many ways, by its aetiology, anatomical location and whether it is acute or chronic (Enoch & Price, 2004). A wound is a breakdown in the protective function of the skin, with the loss of continuity of epithelium with or without loss of underlying connective tissue (muscle, bone, nerves) (Leaper & Harding, 1998). Wounds occur following injury to the skin, underlying tissues or organs caused by surgery, trauma, cuts, chemicals, heat or cold, friction, shear force, pressure, or disease, such as leg ulcers or carcinomas (Hutchinson, 1992). A pressure ulcer is defined as a localised injury to the skin and/or underlying tissue, usually over a bony prominence as a result of pressure, or pressure in combination with shear. Several contributing or confounding factors are also associated with pressure ulcers; the significance of these factors has yet to be elucidated (NPUAP, 2014). Wound healing can be defined as the physiology by which the body replaces and restores function to damaged tissues (Shipperley & Martin, 2002).

Diagnostic criteria and classification

Skin wounds commonly result in the exposure of dermal tissues to the environment, haemorrhage, and loss of body fluids (water and plasma), micronutrients and metabolites, thus disturbing intercellular relationships (Lansdown, 2001). Wounds are often divided into acute or chronic, and they heal by primary or secondary intention. Acute wounds result from surgery or trauma and usually have a relatively short, uneventful healing time. Chronic wounds such as leg ulcers, pressure ulcers, diabetic foot ulcers and malignant wounds have prolonged healing times, are prone to episodes of infection and may have increased levels of exudate due to prolonged inflammation (Gray *et al.*, 2006). Common types of chronic wounds are venous, arterial, neuropathic and pressure. Other important causes include malignancy, drug-induced ulcers and vasculitis (Fan Wai-Ping *et al.*, 2010).

Pressure ulcers can be categorised using a validated international NPUAP/EPUAP pressure ulcer classification system. There are four categories/stages, plus two additional stages for suspected deep-tissue injury and unstageable pressure ulcers where the depth is unknown. Stage I and II ulcers are considered the least severe, and stage IV ulcers the most severe. A broad range of skin damage or necrosis may be represented within the stage III classification. The depth of a stage III pressure ulcer depends on the anatomical location, and can be shallow or deep (NPUAP, 2014).

Process of wound healing

The process of wound healing can be divided into three overlapping phases:

- Inflammatory.
- Proliferation.
- Maturation and remodelling.

Some wounds heal with routine wound care; however, those with rough edges and tissue deficit generally take longer to heal. The inflammatory stage occurs during the first few days, and the wound area attempts to restore homeostasis by constricting blood vessels to control bleeding. Platelet aggregation and thromboplastin make a clot, and inflammation occurs. The proliferative stage lasts ≥3 weeks. Granulation occurs and collagen is formed to fill the wound, and new blood vessels are formed. The maturation and remodelling stage may last up to 2 years, during which time new collagen is synthesised, and scar tissue is eventually formed (RCN, 2005).

Healing of wounds involves the activity of an intricate network of blood cells, tissue types, cytokines and growth factors. This results in increased cellular activity, which intensifies the metabolic demand for nutrients (MacKay & Miller, 2003). The aim of wound healing management is to achieve a stable wound that has healthy granulation tissue tone characterised by a well-vascularised wound bed. Good management should remove, or at least minimise, factors that delay healing (Enoch & Harding, 2003).

Disease consequence and public health

In the UK, chronic wounds represent a significant burden to patients and the NHS; approximately 200,000 patients have chronic wounds. Common symptoms of ulceration include pain, exudate and odour; these symptoms are frequently associated with poor sleep, loss of mobility and social isolation. The cost of wound care service in 2014 was estimated at £2165 million, and is predicted to rise to £2377 by 2019 (Dowsett *et al.*, 2014). The prevalence rate of pressure ulcers in 2013 was 4.7%. The daily costs of treating a pressure ulcer without complications in a hospital or long-term care setting are estimated to be £43–374 (NICE, 2014a).

Good nutritional status is essential for wound healing. Ignoring nutritional status may compromise the patient's ability to heal and prolong the stages of wound healing (Russell, 2001). Malnutrition is frequently undetected and untreated, causing a wide range of adverse consequences such as impaired wound healing and, subsequently, increased length of hospital stay. It is estimated that, in England, malnutrition affects 30% of adult admissions to hospital, and about 34% (in winter) of those in hospital wards (BAPEN, 2015). This represents a considerable number of people at risk of poor wound healing (see Chapter 6.2, Malnutrition). A validated nutrition screening tool should be conducted on admission to the healthcare facility or first visit to a community setting to determine individuals at risk or with a pressure sore. Such individuals should be referred to a dietitian for comprehensive nutritional assessment (NPUAP, 2014).

Assessment

Anthropometry

This should include weight, height and calculated body mass index (BMI). Impaired hand grip strength has been shown to be a marker of nutritional status, and is an indicator of increased postoperative complications, increased length of hospitalisation, higher rehospitalisation and decreased physical status (Norman *et al.*, 2011).

Biochemical assessment

It is unlikely that biochemical measurements will provide more information than other indicators such as undesired weight loss, although there may be an association between albumin level and pressure ulcers. Therefore, it is important to consider other factors in nutritional assessment, such as diagnosis, changes in weight status and dietary intake (NPUAP, 2009).

Clinical assessment

The Waterlow pressure ulcer risk assessment tool is frequently used in the UK; it incorporates a scoring system and provides guidance associated with levels of risk status (Waterlow, 2005). The assessment incorporates BMI and a malnutrition screening tool (e.g. 'MUST' (see Chapter 6.2, Malnutrition). Other commonly used tools include the Braden scale, Norton risk assessment scale (NICE, 2014b) and the Pressure Ulcer Scale for Healing (PUSH) produced by the National Pressure Ulcer Advisory Panel, which includes a healing score to monitor the changes in pressure ulcer status.

Dietary assessment

It is fundamental to assess whether the patient has an optimum nutritional status to allow wounds to heal. A diet history and/or food chart at ward level will help to assess the patient's intake.

Clinical investigation and management

Factors that may delay or prevent wound healing can be localised or systemic throughout the body, as shown in Table 7.17.11. All patients are potentially at risk of developing a pressure ulcer. However, pressure ulcers are more likely to occur in the following circumstances (NICE, 2014b):

- Serious illness.
- Neurological conditions.
- Impaired mobility.
- Impaired nutrition, poor posture or a deformity.
- Equipment such as seating or beds which are not specifically designed to provide pressure relief

Pressure ulcer incidence may be higher with increased age, frailty or severity of illness; pressure ulcer history; or significant weight loss and eating difficulties (NPUAP, 2009).

Wound healing assessment is critical for the planning and evaluation of care, and should also include (Gottrup *et al.*, 2007) the following:

- Medical history.
- Cause of tissue damage.
- Medication and allergies.
- Other diseases, e.g. diabetes, vascular disease and immune compromise.
- Lifestyle and environment – obesity, tobacco and/or alcohol use.

Table 7.17.11 Factors that may delay or impede wound healing (Gottrup *et al.*, 2007)

Local factors	Systemic factors
Primary	**Pivotal**
Blood supply (tissue perfusion)	Haemodynamic conditions (perfusion, hypovolaemia, hypoxia, pain, etc.)
Tissue oxygen tension	
Secondary	**Important**
Tissue damage	Age
Mechanical stress of the tissue	Smoking
	Medication
Hypothermia	Diseases
Pain	Nutritional status
Radiation	Anaemia
Infection	Alcoholism
Surgical technique	Radiation
Suture technique and materials	Others (immunological, etc.)
Others (vasculitis, immunological, etc.)	

- Impaired mobility.
- Inadequate social network, carer support.
- Psychological problems.
- Inadequate nutrition and body weight.

An infected pressure ulcer will increase tissue damage, causing further strain, a deeper ulcer and an increase in nutritional demands (Hurd, 2003). The infection requires treatment for the wound to heal.

Nutritional management

Nutritional requirements increase in the presence of a chronic wound, and, if the demand is not met, this can have a significant impact on wound healing. Metabolic demand rises in the presence of a wound due to greatly increased cell activity (Casey, 1998). Optimum nutrition is a key factor in maintaining all phases of wound healing. Protein energy malnutrition (PEM) in the presence of a wound will lead to the loss of lean body mass (LBM) or protein stores, which will impede the healing process (Demling, 2009). A balance of all food groups is required to meet the essential nutrient needs for wound healing. However, if nutritional requirements cannot be achieved by dietary intake, fortified foods and/or high-energy, high-protein oral nutritional supplements should be offered, or alterative feeding if consistent with the individual's goals and wishes (NPUAP, EPUAP & PPPIA, 2014). Nutritional supplements should not be offered specifically to prevent a pressure ulcer in adults whose nutritional intake is adequate (NICE, 2014b). The role of specific nutrients in wound healing is shown in Table 7.17.12.

Macronutrients

Energy demands rise significantly in the presence of a wound. Basal metabolic rate rises by up to 10% following minor surgery, and can rise by ≥100% in severe burns (White & Baxter, 1998). It is estimated that adults

Table 7.17.12 Role of key nutrients in tissue viability and wound healing (Johnston, 2007)

Nutrient	Function	Comments
Fat	Energy. Cell membrane component. Involved in the formation of inflammatory mediators and clotting components.	
Carbohydrate	Energy.	
Protein	Tissue synthesis and repair.	Excess protein can stress the liver and kidney.
Vitamin A	Enhances immune response. Antioxidant. Promotes collagen synthesis and epithelialisation.	Excess toxic.
Vitamin C	Antioxidant. Promotes collagen synthesis and angiogenesis. Enhances iron absorption. Promotes immune function.	Additional vitamin C not beneficial unless deficient.
Selenium	Antioxidant.	Deficiency relatively common.
Copper	Collagen cross-linkage.	Deficiency rare.
Manganese	Component of enzymes needed for tissue regeneration.	Deficiency rare. Magnesium can substitute for manganese when manganese status is poor.
Zinc	Fibroblast proliferation. Component of enzyme systems. Collagen synthesis. Immune function.	Zinc supplement will not accelerate healing if not deficient in patients. Can cause toxicity.
Iron	Promotes collagen synthesis. Improves delivery of oxygen, nutrients and components of healing to tissue. Component of many enzyme systems.	Blood loss can lead to anaemia.
B vitamins	Efficient energy usage. Collagen formation. Component of enzyme systems.	
Vitamin E	Antioxidant. Enhances immune response.	Excess can impair wound healing.
Vitamin K	Blood clotting.	Deficiency very rare.

SECTION 7

with, or at risk of, a pressure ulcer require 30–35 kcal/kg of body weight. Adjustment of energy is also based on weight change or level of obesity (NPUAP, EPUAP & PPPIA, 2014). Activation of the immune system and the action of white blood cells require higher levels of energy. Insufficient energy intake will deplete fat stores and the loss of protective cushioning, thus increasing the likelihood of pressure injuries (Todorovic, 2003). Also, low energy intake is usually associated with a lower intake of micronutrients, and the resultant deficiencies may impair wound healing (Thomas, 2001).

Carbohydrate in the form of glucose is the major fuel for collagen synthesis, and providing sufficient carbohydrate as the primary fuel source is more efficient than glucogenesis from protein and fat (NPUAP, 2009). Fat has a role in cell membrane structure and function. n-3 Fatty acids may have a role in increasing proinflammatory cytokine production at wound sites, and therefore have the potential to affect wound healing during the inflammatory stage (McDaniel *et al.*, 2008). n-3 fatty acids may have a benefit when administered pre- and postoperatively as immune feeds (Moskovitz & Kim, 2002).

Inadequate protein has been shown to delay wound healing by prolonging the inflammatory phase. There is also evidence to suggest that protein intakes above normal may be desirable in order to counteract increased protein losses in highly exuding wounds, and to encourage tissue repair (Cawood *et al.*, 2012). Protein intake should be 1.25–1.5 g protein/kg daily for adults at risk of a pressure ulcer, and adequate protein should be provided for positive nitrogen balance in adults with a pressure ulcer (NPUAP, EPUAP & PPPIA, 2014). Protein malnutrition delays wound healing by impairing collagen synthesis and deposition, and decreasing scar strength (Arnold & Barbul, 2006). Prolonged inadequate protein intake may promote tissue oedema, which delays healing by slowing oxygen diffusion from capillaries to cell membranes. Available nutrients will be drawn to the wound site initially, with lean muscle mass used to provide the amino acids necessary for wound healing. If a patient loses 20% LBM, muscles will compete with wounds for protein; if 30% or more of LBM is lost, the body will prioritise muscle maintenance over wound healing (Acton, 2013). Minor surgery may not significantly increase protein requirement; however, if the patient is already malnourished, wound healing will be adversely affected unless dietary protein intake is increased (MacKay & Miller, 2003). Immunonutrition, in its current formulation, includes supplementation with arginine and/or glutamine, n-3 fatty acids, different vitamins, and trace minerals. Arginine is rapidly depleted during periods of severe stress and is utilised in the synthesis of collagen; maximum safe doses have not been established. Additional research is needed to recommend the use of arginine, alone or combined with other nutrients, for pressure ulcer healing (Chow & Barbul, 2014).

Glutamine's role in pressure ulcer healing may be as a fuel source for fibroblasts and epithelial cells needed for healing; however, supplemental glutamine has not been shown to improve wound healing, and more studies are needed (NPUAP, 2009).

Micronutrients

Micronutrients have a vital role in wound healing; vitamins A, B_1, B_2 and B_6 are vital for energy production and collagen deposition (Woodward *et al.*, 2009). Copper, zinc and selenium have roles in immune function and can be lost in significant amounts from wounds, particularly in the burn exudate and urine of severe burns patients. Patients with total body surface area burns of 30% or greater should be given intravenous supplementation for the first 8 days, and serum levels monitored on a weekly basis (Berger *et al.*, 1998).

Vitamin C is essential for collagen formation and critical for wound healing. An eightfold increase in wound dehiscence has been reported in patients with depleted vitamin C concentrations (Zaloga, 1994). Although data on vitamin C supplementation and chronic wound healing is inconclusive, it is suggested that patients with small wounds or pressure ulcers receive 500–1000 mg daily in divided doses for optimal utilisation (Tanaka & Molnar, 2007). At doses above 1 g/day, absorption falls to less than 50%, and absorbed, unmetabolised ascorbic acid is excreted in the urine (Jacob & Sotoudeh, 2002). However, discretion must be used when recommending vitamin C supplementation, as toxicity may occur in patients who are at risk of oxalate stone formation (Posthauer, 2006). To maximise wound healing but minimise soft tissue damage in renal-failure patients, the suggested maximum recommended intake is 100 mg/day (Clark, 2002; Winkler, 2000). Some studies have shown that vitamin C supplementation at 60–200 mg/day only helps a pressure ulcer to heal if the patient is deficient in vitamin C. Vitamin C supplementation in non-deficient patients has not been shown to accelerate wound healing (Ringsdorf & Cheraskin, 1982).

Adequate concentrations of vitamin A influence the body's therapeutic inflammatory response to wounds (Arnold & Barbul, 2006); it plays a role in cell division, cell differentiation and immune system function. Depletion of vitamin A can result in impaired wound healing and susceptibility to infection (Ross, 2002). It is suggested that vitamin A supplementation for 10–14 days has a unique role in nutritional management in patients with chronic wounds being treated with corticosteroids for inflammatory diseases; however, caution is needed (Stechmiller, 2010).

Zinc has a role in all stages of wound healing (Bradbury, 2006). Deficiency is associated with delayed wound healing by reducing the rate of epithelialisation, and decreasing scar strength and collagen synthesis (Andrews & Gallager-Allred, 1999). Zinc supplementation does not appear to aid the healing of leg ulcers, although it may be beneficial in those with venous legs ulcers and low serum zinc (Wilkinson, 2012). A suggested supplementation for non-healing pressure ulcers is 15 mg/day, and 20–25 mg/day for larger non-healing wounds, but this should be limited to 14 days (Woodward *et al.*, 2009).

Excess zinc supplementation has been shown to interfere with cation absorption, specifically iron and copper (Stechmiller, 2010). There is support for zinc supplementation if zinc deficiency is present, but it should be stopped once the deficiency has been corrected (NPUAP, 2009).

Iron is necessary for the formation of collagen and to support tissue oxygenation at the wound site. Iron also provides oxygen to the site of the wound (Woodward *et al.*, 2009). Low haemoglobin levels need to be corrected before healing can continue effectively (McClemont, 1984).

Fluid

Adequate fluid is required to maintain good skin tone and blood flow, which is critical for the prevention of skin breakdown. A guide of 30–35 mL/kg of body weight/day (minimum of 1500 mL/day) is recommended, but should be adjusted depending on the clinical condition (Todorovic, 2003). Another general formula uses 1 mL/kcal (Clark, 2002). Dehydration is also a major risk factor for the development of pressure sores as the skin becomes inelastic, fragile and more susceptible to breakdown (Horns *et al.*, 2004).

Drug–nutrient interactions

Medications may have a positive or negative effect on wound healing. Corticosteroids inhibit fibroplasia and the formation of granulation tissue. High doses interfere with vascular proliferation and delay epithelialisation. Antiplatelet drugs, including aspirin and other nonsteroidal anti-inflammatory drugs, have a dose-dependent effect since they act as inflammatory mediators. Anticoagulants such as warfarin and heparin inhibit coagulation and adversely affect wounds. Conversely, drugs such as prostacyclin can be used to promote healing in arterial and vasculitic ulcers. Calcium antagonists can help improve blood flow (Sussman, 2007).

Internet resources

Coloplast Wound Care, www.coloplast.co.uk
European Pressure Ulcer Advisory Panel, www.epuap.org
NICE Clinical Guideline (CG179) Pressure Ulcers – Prevention and Treatment, www.nice.org.uk/nicemedia/pdf/CG029publicinfo.pdf
The Waterlow Score, www.judy-waterlow.co.uk
World Wide Wounds, www.worldwidewounds.com

References

Acton C. (2013) The importance of nutrition in wound healing. *Wounds UK*. 9(3): 61–64.

Andrews M, Gallager-Allred C. (1999) The role of zinc in wound healing. *Adv. Wound Care*. 12: 137–138.

Arnold M, Barbul A. (2006) Nutrition and wound healing. *Plast. Reconstr. Surg*. 117: 42S–58S.

Berger MM, Spertini F, Shenkin A, *et al.* (1998) Trace element supplementation modulates infection rates in major burns: a double-blind placebo clinical trial. *Am. J. Clin. Nutr.* 68: 365–371.

Bradbury S. (2006) Wound healing: is oral zinc supplementation beneficial? *Wounds UK*. 2(1): 54–61.

British Association of Parenteral and Enteral Nutrition (BAPEN). (2015) *The cost of malnutrition in England and potential cost savings from nutritional interventions*. Available at www.bapen.org.uk and www.uhs.nhs.uk/nihr-brc. Accessed 9 March 2016.

Casey G. (1998) The importance of nutrition in wound healing. *Nurs. Stand*. 13(3): 51–56.

Cawood AL, Elia M, Stratton RJ. (2012) Systemic review and meta-analysis of the effects of high protein oral nutritional supplements. *Ageing Res. Rev.* 11(2): 278–296.

Chow O, Barbul A. (2014) Immunonutrition: role in wound healing and tissue regeneration. *Adv. Wound Care (New Rochelle)* 3(3): 46–53.

Clark S. (2002) The biochemistry of antioxidants revisited. *Nutr. Clin. Pract*. 17: 5–17.

Demling RH. (2009) Nutrition, anabolism, and the wound healing process: an overview. *Eplasty* 9: 65–94.

Dowsett C, Bielby A, Searle R. (2014) Reconciling increasing wound care demands with available resources. *J. Wound Care*. 23(11):552, 554, 556–558 passim. doi: 10.12968/jowc.2014.23.11.552.

Enoch S, Harding K. (2003) Wound bed preparation: the science behind the removal of barriers to healing. *Wounds Compend. Clin. Res. Pract*. 15(7): 213–229.

Enoch S, Price P. (2004) *Cellular, molecular and biochemical differences in the pathophysiology of healing between acute wounds, chronic wounds and wounds in the aged*. Available at www.worldwidewounds.com.

Fan Wai-Ping L, Rashid M, Enoch S. (2010) Current advances in modern wound healing. *Wounds UK*. 6(3): 22–36.

Gottrup F, Kirsner R, Meaumes S, et al. (2007) *Clinical Wound Assessment – A Pocket Guide*. Minneapolis: Coloplast A/S, p. 6.

Gray D, Cooper P, Timmons J (eds). (2006) *Essential Wound Management. An Introduction for Undergraduates*. London: Wounds UK Limited, p. 6.

Horns D, Bender SA, Ferguson ML, *et al.* (2004) The National Pressure Ulcer Long-term Care Study: Pressure ulcer development in long-term care residents. *J. Am. Geriatr. Soc.* 52: 359–367.

Hurd TA. (2003) Nutrition and wound-care management/prevention. *Wound Care Canada*. 2(2): 20–24.

Hutchinson J. (1992) *The Wound Programme*. Dundee: Centre for Medical Education.

Jacob RA, Sotoudeh G. (2002) Vitamin C function and status in chronic disease. *Nutr. Clin. Care* 5: 66–74

Johnston E. (2007) The role of nutrition in tissue viability. *Wound Essent*. 2: 10–21.

Lansdown ABG. (2001) Nutrition and the healing of skin wounds. Available at https://www.nursinginpractice.com/article/importance-skin-nutrition-wound-healing. Accessed 2 December 2018.

Leaper DJ, Harding KG. (1998) *Wounds: Biology and Management*. Oxford: Oxford University Press, pp. 23–40.

MacKay D, Miller AL. (2003) Nutritional support for wound healing. *Altern. Med. Rev.* 8(4): 359–377.

McClemont E. (1984) Pressure sores. No pressure-no sore. *Nursing (Lond)*. 2(21): suppl 3.

McDaniel JC, Belury M, Ahijevych K, *et al.* (2010) Omega-3 fatty acids effect on wound healing. *Wound Repair Regen*. 16(3):337–345.

Moskovitz AN, Kim YI. (2002) Does perioperative immunonutrition reduce postoperative complications in patients with gastrointestinal cancer undergoing operations? *Nutr. Rev.* 62: 443–447.

National Pressure Ulcer Advisory Panel (NPUAP), European Pressure Ulcer Advisory Panel (EPUAP) and Pan Pacific Pressure Injury Alliance (PPPIA). (2014) *Prevention and Treatment of Pressure Ulcers:* Quick Reference Guide. http://www.npuap.org/wp-content/uploads/2014/08/Quick-Reference-Guide-DIGITAL-NPUAP-EPUAP-PPPIA.pdf. Accessed 2 December 2018.

National Pressure Ulcer Advisory Panel (NPUAP). (2009) The Role of Nutrition in Pressure Ulcer Prevention and Treatment: National Pressure Ulcer Advisory Panel White Paper.

National Pressure Ulcer Advisory Panel (NPUAP). (2014) *PUSH Tool.* Available at http://www.npuap.org/resources/educational-and-clinical-resources/push-tool/. Accessed 14 March 2016.

NICE. (2014a) Costing Statement: Pressure Ulcers Implementing the NICE Guidance on Pressure Ulcers (CG179). https://www.nice.org.uk/guidance/cg179/resources/costing-statement-pdf-248688109. Accessed 2 December 2018.

NICE. (2014b) *Pressure Ulcers: Prevention and Management (CG179).* Available at https://www.nice.org.uk/guidance/cg179/resources/pressure-ulcers-prevention-and-management-35109760631749. Accessed 24 March 2016.

Norman K, Stobäus N, Gonzalez MC, et al. (2011) Hand grip strength: Outcome predictor and marker of nutritional status. *Clin. Nutr.* 30(2): 135–142.

Posthauer ME. (2006) The role of nutrition in wound care. *Adv. Skin Wound Care* 19: 43–52.

Ringsdorf WM Jr, Cheraskin E. (1982) Vitamin C and human wound healing. *Oral Surg. Oral Med. Oral Pathol.* 53: 231–236.

Ross V. (2002) Micronutrient recommendations for wound healing. *Support Line.* 24(4): 3–9.

Royal College of Nursing (RCN). (2005) The Management of Pressure Ulcer's in Primary and Secondary Care. A Clinical Practice Guideline. London: RCN.

Russell L. (2001) The importance of patients' nutritional status in wound healing. *Br. J. Nurs.* 10(6): S42, S44–49.

Shipperley T, Martin C. (2002) The physiology of wound healing: an emergency response. *Nursing Times.net* 98(8): 54.

Stechmiller JK. (2010) Understanding the role of nutrition and wound healing. *Nutr. Clin. Pract.* 25: 61–68.

Sussman G. (2007) The impact of medicines on wound healing. *Pharmacist.* 26(11): 874–878.

Tanaka H, Molnar JA. (2007) Vitamin C and wound healing. In: Molnar JA (ed) *Nutrition and Wound Healing.* Boca Rato, FL: CRC Press, pp. 121–148.

Thomas D. (2001) Issues and dilemmas in the prevention and treatment of pressure ulcers: A review. *J. Gerontol. A Biol. Sci. Med. Sci.* 56(6): M328–M340.

Todorovic V. (2003) Food and wounds: nutritional factors in wound formation and healing. *Clin. Nutr. Update.* 8(2): 6–8.

Waterlow J. (2005) *Pressure Ulcer Prevention Manual.* Available at www.judy-waterlow.co.uk. Accessed 18 July 2012.

White B, Baxter M. (1998) *Hormones and Metabolic Control,* 2nd edn. London: Edward Arnold.

Wilkinson E. (2012) Oral zinc for arterial and venous leg ulcers. *Cochrane Database Syst. Rev.* (8): CD001273.

Winkler MR. (2000) Inquire here: should vitamin C and zinc be administered as supplements for wound healing? *Support Line* 22: 20.

Woodward M, Sussman G, Rice J, et al. (2009) *Nutrition and Wound Healing: Expert Guide for Healthcare Professionals.* Gatwick: Nestle Nutrition Healthcare.

Zaloga GP. (1994) *Nutrition in Critical Care.* St Louis: Mosby.

Appendix A1 Dietary reference values

Energy

Table A1.1 Estimated average requirements (EARs) for energy in children aged 0–18 years (SACN, 2011)

Age	EAR (MJ/day)	
	Boys	Girls
0–3 months	2.6	2.4
4–6 months	2.7	2.5
7–9 months	2.9	2.7
10–12 months	3.2	3.0
1–3 years	4.1	3.8
4–6 years	6.2	5.8
7–10 years	7.6	7.2
11–14 years	9.8	9.1
15–18 years	12.6	10.2

Table A1.2 Estimated average requirements (EARs) according to height and weight at a body mass index (BMI) of 22.5 kg/m^2 and assuming a physical activity level (PAL) of 1.63 (SACN, 2011)

Age (years)	Height (cm)	Weight (kg), BMI = 22.5 kg/m^2	EAR (MJ/day)
Males			
19–24	178	71.5	11.6
25–34	178	71.0	11.5
35–44	176	69.7	11.0
45–54	175	68.8	10.8
55–64	174	68.3	10.8
65–74	173	67.0	9.8
75+	170	65.1	9.6
Females			
19–24	163	29.9	9.1
25–34	163	59.7	9.1
35–44	163	59.9	8.8
45–54	162	59.0	8.8
55–64	161	58.0	8.7
65–74	159	57.2	8.0
75+	155	54.3	7.7

Protein

Table A1.3 Reference nutrient intakes (RNIs) for protein (Department of Health, 1991)

Age	Weight (kg)	RNI (g/day)
0–3 months	5.9	12.5
4–6 months	7.7	12.7
7–9 months	8.8	13.7
10–12 months	9.7	14.9
1–3 years	12.5	14.5
4–6 years	17.8	19.7
7–10 years	28.3	28.3
Males		
11–14 years	43.0	42.1
15–18 years	64.5	55.2
19–50 years	74.0	55.5
50+ years	71.0	53.3
Females		
11–14 years	43.8	41.2
15–18 years	55.5	45.4
19–50 years	60.0	45.0
50+ years	62.0	46.5
Pregnancy		+6.0
Lactation		
0–4 months		+11.0
4+ months		+8.0

Source: Department of Health, (2011). *Dietary Reference Values for Food Energy and Nutrients for the United Kingdom*. Report on Health and Social Subjects 41.

Manual of Dietetic Practice, Sixth Edition. Edited by Joan Gandy.

Companion website: www.manualofdieteticpractice.com

Vitamins

Table A1.4 Reference nutrient intakes (RNIs) for vitamins (Department of Health, 1991; SACN, 2016)

Age	Thiamin (mg/day)	Riboflavin (mg/day)	Niacin[1] (mg/day)	Vitamin B_6[2] (mg/day)	Vitamin B_{12} (µg/day)	Folate (µg/day)	Vitamin C (mg/day)	Vitamin A (µg/day)	Vitamin D[4] (µg/day)
0–3 months	0.2	0.4	3	0.2	0.3	50	25	350	8.5–10[3]
4–6 months	0.2	0.4	3	0.2	0.3	50	25	350	8.5–10[3]
7–9 months	0.2	0.4	4	0.3	0.4	50	25	350	8.5–10[3]
10–12 months	0.3	0.4	5	0.4	0.4	50	25	350	8.5–10[3]
1–3 years	0.5	0.6	8	0.7	0.5	70	30	400	10
4–6 years	0.7	0.8	11	0.9	0.8	100	30	400	10
7–10 years	0.7	1	12	1	1	150	30	400	10
Males									
11–14 years	0.9	1.2	15	1.2	1.2	200	35	600	10
15–18 years	1.1	1.3	18	1.5	1.5	200	40	700	10
19–50 years	1	1.3	17	1.4	1.5	200	40	700	10
50+ years	0.9	1.3	16	1.4	1.5	200	40	700	10
Females									
11–14 years	0.7	1.1	12	1	1.2	200	35	600	10
15–18 years	0.8	1.1	14	1.2	1.5	200	40	600	10
19–50 years	0.8	1.1	13	1.2	1.5	200	40	600	10
50+ years	0.8	1.1	12	1.2	1.5	200	40	600	10
Pregnancy	+0.1[3]	+0.3	[5]	[5]	[5]	+100	+10	+100	10
Lactation									
0–4 months	+0.2	+0.5	+2	[5]	+0.5	+60	+30	+350	10
4+ months	+0.2	+0.5	+2	[5]	+0.5	+60	+30	+350	10

[1] Nicotinic acid equivalent.
[2] Based on protein providing 14.7% of the estimated average requirement (EAR) for energy.
[3] Safe intake.
[4] SACN (2016).
[5] No increment.

Minerals and trace elements

Table A1.5 Reference nutrient intakes (RNIs) for minerals and trace elements (Department of Health, 1991)

Age	Calcium (mg/day)	Phosphorus[1] (mg/day)	Magnesium (mg/day)	Sodium[2] (mg/day)	Potassium[3] (mg/day)	Chloride[4] (mg/day)	Iron[5] (mg/day)	Zinc (mg/day)	Copper (mg/day)	Selenium (μg/day)	Iodine (μg/day)
0–3 months	525	400	55	210	800	320	1.7	4	0.2	10	50
4–6 months	525	400	60	280	850	400	4.3	4	0.3	13	60
7–9 months	525	400	75	320	700	500	7.8	5	0.3	10	60
10–12 months	525	400	80	350	700	500	7.8	5	0.3	10	60
1–3 years	350	270	85	500	800	800	6.9	5	0.4	15	70
4–6 years	450	350	120	700	1100	1100	6.1	6.5	0.6	20	100
7–10 years	550	450	200	1200	2000	1800	8.7	7	0.7	30	110
Males											
11–14 years	1000	775	280	1600	3100	2500	11.3	9	0.8	45	130
15–18 years	1000	775	300	1600	3500	2500	11.3	9.5	1	70	140
19–50 years	700	550	300	1600	3500	2500	8.7	9.5	1.2	75	140
50+ years	700	550	300	1600	3500	2500	8.7	9.5	1.2	75	140
Females											
11–14 years	800	625	280	1600	3100	2500	14.85	9	0.8	45	130
15–18 years	800	625	300	1600	3500	2500	14.85	7	1	60	140
19–50 years	700	550	270	1600	3500	2500	14.85	7	1.2	60	140
50+ years	700	550	270	1600	3500	2500	8.7	7	1.2	60	140
Pregnancy	–[6]	–[6]	–[6]	–[6]	–[6]	–[6]	–[6]	–[6]	–[6]	–[6]	–[6]
Lactation											
0–4 months	+550	+440	+50	–[6]	–[6]	–[6]	–[6]	+6	+0.3	+15	–[6]
4+ months	+550	+440	+50								

[1] Phosphorus (P) RNI is set equal to calcium (Ca) in mmol values; 1 mmol Ca = 40 mg, 1 mmol P = 30.9.
[2] 1 mmol = 23 mg sodium (Na); 1 g salt (NaCl) contains 17.1 mmol, Na.
[3] 1 mmol = 39.1 mg.
[4] Intakes of dietary chloride should equal sodium intakes in molar terms. 1 mmol chloride = 35.5 mg.
[5] Supplements may be required if menstrual losses are high.
[6] No increment.

References

Department of Health. (1991) *Dietary Reference Values for Food and Nutrients for the United Kingdom*. London: HMSO.

SACN. (2011) *Dietary Reference Values for Energy*. London: TSO.

SACN. (2016) *Vitamin D and Health*. London: TSO.

Appendix A2 Dietary data

Conversion factors

Energy

1000 joules = 1 kJ

1000 kJ = 1 MJ

1 kcal = 4.184 kJ [The Royal Society (London) recommended conversion factor]

1 kJ = 0.239 kcal

1 W = 1 joule/second

0.06 W = 1 kJ/ min

86.4 W = 1 kJ/24h

Table A2.1 Nutrient energy yields

Nutrient	kcal/g	kJ/g
Protein	4	17
Fat	9	37
Carbohydrate	3.75	16
Sugar alcohols	2.4	10
Ethyl alcohol	7	29
Glycerol	4.31	18
Medium-chain triglyceride (MCT)	8.4	35

Protein and nitrogen

$$\text{Dietary protein}(g) = \text{dietary nitrogen}(g) \times 6.25$$
$$\text{Dietary nitrogen}(g) = \text{dietary protein}(g) \div 6.25$$

This conversion factor is only appropriate for a mixture of foods. For milk or cereals alone, the factors 6.4 or 5.7 should be used.

Vitamins

Vitamin A

The active vitamin A content of a diet is usually expressed in retinol equivalents.

1 μg of retinol equivalent = 1 μg of retinol or 6 μg of beta – carotene

1 IU of vitamin A = 0.3 μg of retinol or 0.6 μg of beta – carotene

Vitamin D

1 μg of vitamin D = 40 IU

1 IU = 0.025 μg of vitamin D

Nicotinic acid/tryptophan

1 mg of nicotinic acid = 60 mg of tryptophan

Nicotinic acid content mg equivalents = nicotinic acid (mg) + [tryptophan (mg) / 60]

Vitamin E

Vitamin E activity is expressed as D-alpha-tocopherol equivalents. Activity is expressed as international units (IU): 1 IU is equivalent to 0.67 mg D-alpha-tocopherol.

Table A2.2 Mineral content of compounds and solutions

Solution/compound	Mineral content	
1 g of sodium chloride	393 mg of Na	17 mmol of Na
1 g of sodium carbonate	273 mg of Na	12 mmol of Na
1 g of potassium bicarbonate	524 mg of K	13.4 mmol of K
1 g of calcium chloride (hydrated)	273 mg of Ca	7 mmol of Ca
1 g of calcium carbonate	400 mg of Ca	10 mmol of Ca
1 g of calcium gluconate	93 mg of Ca	2.3 mmol of Ca
1 L of normal saline	3450 mg of Na	150 mmol of Na

Manual of Dietetic Practice, Sixth Edition. Edited by Joan Gandy.

Companion website: www.manualofdieteticpractice.com

Food exchange lists

Carbohydrate

Table A2.3 Food portions containing approximately 10 g of carbohydrate (CHO)

Food	Weight (g)	Description
Wholemeal bread	25	1 thin slice/large loaf
White bread	20	1 thin slice/small loaf
Potatoes – boiled	60	1 size of hen's egg
Potatoes – mashed	60	1 scoop
Potatoes – roast	40	1 very small
Sweet potatoes – boiled	50	1 size of hen's egg
Rice – boiled, brown, white	30	¾ tablespoon
Pasta – boiled, e.g. spaghetti, macaroni	50	1 tablespoon
Pulses, e.g. lentils	60	2 tablespoons
Peas – frozen	100	3 tablespoons
Parsnip – boiled	80	1 medium
Sweetcorn – boiled	50	2 tablespoons
Thick soup, e.g. tinned vegetable	100	1 small tin
Thin soup, e.g. minestrone	250	1 standard mug
Sausages	100	2 large sausages
Beef burger, economy	100	1 economy burger
Beef burger, 100% meat = no CHO	–	–
Fish fingers	60	2 fish fingers
Breakfast cereals, e.g. bran flakes	15	2 tablespoons
Breakfast cereals, e.g. wheat bisk type	20	1 bisk
Muesli, no added sugar	15	¾ tablespoon
Porridge – made with water	125	Small average portion
Biscuits – plain digestive	15	1 digestive
Apple, pear	100	1 medium
Orange	120	1 small
Banana	45	½ small banana
Melon – galia, honeydew	200	1 medium slice
Pineapple, fresh	100	1 large slice
Grapes	70	15 large grapes
Orange juice – no added sugar	110	½ average glass
Apple juice – no added sugar	100	½ average glass
Cranberry juice	70	1/3 average glass
Milk – full fat, semi-fat or skimmed	200	1 average glass
Yogurt – low fat, fruit	70	½ small pot
Yogurt – low fat, plain	135	1 small pot
Ice cream – plain dairy, vanilla	50	1 small scoop
Lemonade	170	1 small glass
Lucozade®	60	1/3 average glass
Cola	90	½ average glass
Beer – best bitter	450	¾ pint glass
Lager – premium	400	¾ pint glass
Wine – medium white	330	2½ small wine glasses
Wine – red contains 0.2 g CHO/100 mL	–	–
Crisps	20	¾ small packet
Peanuts – dry roasted	100	1 large packet

Protein

Table A2.4 Approximate protein content of food portions

Food	Portion size	Protein per portion (g)	Approximate energy per portion (kcal)
Milk	180 mL	6	115 (full fat) 85 (semi-skimmed) 60 (skimmed
Cheddar cheese	25 g	6	100
Yoghurt	125 g	6	125
Egg	50 g (one average hen's egg)	6	70
Meat/poultry lean cooked	25 g	6	40
White fish	35 g	6	30
Baked beans	120 g	6	100
Peas	100 g	6	70
Bread (1 large thin slice)	25 g	2	50
Pasta (boiled)	50 g	2	50
Rice (boiled)	100 g	2	140
Most breakfast cereals	25 g	2	90
Digestive biscuits	15 g (one biscuit)	2	70
Potatoes	140 g	2	100
Crisps	30 g	2	160

Potassium

Table A2.5 Food portions containing approximately 4 mmol of potassium

Food	Portion size providing approximately 4 mmol potassium
Milk	100 mL
Yoghurt	60 g
Cheddar cheese	130 g
Egg	100 g (two small eggs)
Meat/fish	50 g
White flour	120 g
Wholemeal flour	45 g
White bread	160 g
Wholemeal bread	70 g
Apple	125 g
Orange with skin	100 g
Grapes/orange without skin	50 g
Potato, boiled	50 g
Orange juice	100 mL
Tomato juice	60 mL

Sodium

Table A2.6 No added salt and 40 mmol of sodium diets

No added salt	40 mmol of sodium diet
This restricts sodium intake to <100 mmol of Na+ per day. A pinch of salt may be used in cooking, but none should be added to food at the table. The following foods must be avoided: • Bacon, ham, sausages, pâté • Tinned fish and meat • Smoked fish and meat • Fish and meat pastes • Tinned and packet soups • Sauce mixes • Tinned vegetables • Bottled sauces and chutneys • Meat and vegetable extracts, stock cubes • Salted nuts and crisps • Soya sauce • Monosodium glutamate • Cheese – up to 100 g/week • Bread – up to 4 slices/day	In addition to the foods listed in the first column, the following restrictions apply: • No salt to be used in cooking or at table • Salt-free butter or margarine must be used • Milk should be restricted to 300 mL/day • Breakfast cereals must be salt free

Table A2.7 Dietary source of calcium grouped according to the 'calcium star' system (BDA, 2014)

	Quantity	Calcium (mg)	Stars (1 star = 60 mg)
Calcium in dairy products			
Milk, all types	200 mL	240	****
Cheese	30 g	220	****
Yoghurt	120 g	200	***
Malted milk drink	25 g serving in 200 mL milk	440–710	*******(+)
Rice pudding	200 g (1/2 large tin)	176	***
Custard	120 mL	120	**
Non-dairy sources of calcium			
Calcium-enriched milk alternatives (rice, soya, oat, nut)	200 mL	240	****
Tofu (only if set with calcium chloride, or calcium sulphate, not nigari)	60 g	200	***
Calcium-fortified bread	1 slice (40 g)	191	* to ***
Sardines (with bones)	1/2 tin (60 g)	258	****
Tinned salmon (with bones)	1/2 tin (52 g)	47	*
Orange	1 medium (120 g)	75	*
Broccoli, boiled	2 spears (85 g)	34	*

Adapted from BDA (2014).). British Dietetic Association. (2014) *Food Fact Sheet: Calcium*. Available at https://www.bda.uk.com/foodfacts/Calcium.pdf. Accessed 6 December 2018.

Appendix 3 Anthropometric and function data

Upper-arm anthropometry

For measurement techniques and discussion, see Chapter 2.2 (Assessment of nutritional status).

Table A3.1 Triceps skinfold thickness (TSF) (data derived from Bishop *et al*., 1981)

	Centiles							
	Mean (mm)	5th	10th	25th	50th	75th	90th	95th
Men								
18–74 years	12.0	4.5	6.0	8.0	11.0	15.0	20.0	23.0
18–24 years	11.2	4.0	5.0	7.0	9.5	14.0	20.0	23.0
25–34 years	12.6	4.5	5.5	8.0	12.0	16.0	21.5	24.0
35–44 years	12.4	5.0	6.0	8.5	12.0	15.5	20.0	23.0
45–54 years	12.4	5.0	6.0	8.0	11.0	15.0	20.0	25.5
55–64 years	11.6	5.0	6.0	8.0	11.0	14.0	18.0	21.5
65–74 years	11.8	4.5	5.5	8.0	11.0	15.0	19.0	22.0
Women								
18–74 years	23.0	11.0	13.0	17.0	22.0	28.0	34.0	37.5
18–24 years	19.4	9.4	11.0	14.0	18.0	24.0	30.0	34.0
25–34 years	21.9	10.5	12.0	16.0	21.0	26.5	33.5	37.0
35–44 years	24.0	12.0	14.0	18.0	23.0	29.5	35.5	39.0
45–54 years	25.4	13.0	15.0	20.0	25.0	30.0	36.0	40.0
55–64 years	24.9	11.0	14.0	19.0	25.0	30.5	35.0	39.0
65–74 years	23.3	11.5	14.0	18.0	23.0	28.0	33.0	36.0

Table A3.2 Mid-upper-arm circumference (MUAC) (data derived from Bishop *et al*., 1981)

	Centiles							
	Mean (mm)	5th	10th	25th	50th	75th	90th	95th
Men								
18–74 years	31.8	26.4	27.6	29.6	31.7	33.9	36.0	37.3
18–24 years	30.9	25.7	27.1	28.7	30.7	32.9	35.5	37.4
25–34 years	30.5	25.3	26.5	28.5	30.7	32.4	34.4	35.5
35–44 years	32.3	27.0	28.2	30.0	32.0	34.4	36.5	37.6
45–54 years	32.7	27.8	28.7	30.7	32.7	34.8	36.3	37.1
55–64 years	32.1	26.7	27.8	30.0	32.0	34.2	36.2	37.6
65–74 years	31.5	25.6	27.3	29.6	31.7	33.4	35.2	36.6

Manual of Dietetic Practice, Sixth Edition. Edited by Joan Gandy.

Companion website: www.manualofdieteticpractice.com

Table A3.2 (*Continued*)

	Centiles							
	Mean (mm)	5th	10th	25th	50th	75th	90th	95th
Women								
18–74 years	29.4	23.2	24.3	26.2	28.7	31.9	35.2	37.8
18–24 years	27.0	22.1	23.0	24.5	26.4	28.8	31.7	34.3
25–34 years	28.6	23.3	24.2	25.7	27.8	30.4	34.1	37.2
35–44 years	30.0	24.1	25.2	26.8	29.2	32.2	36.2	38.5
45–54 years	30.7	24.3	25.7	27.5	30.3	32.9	36.8	39.3
55–64 years	30.7	23.9	25.1	27.7	30.2	33.3	36.3	38.2
65–74 years	30.1	23.8	25.2	27.4	29.9	32.5	35.3	37.2

Table A3.3 Mid-arm-muscle circumference (MAMC) (data derived from Bishop *et al.*, 1981)

$$MAMC(cm) = MAC(cm) - [TSF(mm) \times 0.314]$$

	Centiles							
	Mean (mm)	5th	10th	25th	50th	75th	90th	95th
Men								
18–74 years	28.0	23.8	24.8	26.3	27.9	29.6	31.4	32.5
18–24 years	27.4	23.5	24.4	25.8	27.2	28.9	30.8	32.3
25–34 years	28.3	24.2	25.3	26.5	28.0	30.0	31.7	32.9
35–44 years	28.8	25.0	25.6	27.1	28.7	30.3	32.1	33.0
45–54 years	28.2	24.0	24.9	26.5	28.1	29.8	31.5	32.6
55–64 years	27.8	22.8	24.4	26.2	27.9	29.6	31.0	31.8
65–74 years	26.8	22.5	23.7	25.3	26.9	28.5	29.9	30.7
Women								
18–74 years	22.2	18.4	19.0	20.2	21.8	23.6	25.8	27.4
18–24 years	20.9	17.7	18.5	19.4	20.6	22.1	23.6	24.9
25–34 years	21.7	18.3	18.9	20.0	21.4	22.9	24.9	26.6
35–44 years	22.5	18.5	19.2	20.6	22.0	24.0	26.1	27.4
45–54 years	22.7	18.8	19.5	20.7	22.2	24.3	26.6	27.8
55–64 years	22.8	18.6	19.5	20.8	22.6	24.4	26.3	28.1
65–74 years	22.8	18.6	19.5	20.8	22.5	24.4	26.5	28.1

Estimating height from ulna length (see Figure A3.7)

Table A3.4 Estimates of height from ulna length (Elia, 2003)

Men, height (m)		Ulna length (cm)	Women, height (m)	
<65 years	>65 years		<65 years	>65 years
1.94	1.87	**32.0**	1.84	1.84
1.93	1.86	**31.5**	1.83	1.83
1.91	1.84	**31.0**	1.81	1.81
1.89	1.82	**30.5**	1.80	1.79
1.87	1.81	**30.0**	1.79	1.78
1.85	1.79	**29.5**	1.77	1.76
1.84	1.78	**29.0**	1.76	1.75
1.82	1.76	**28.5**	1.75	1.73
1.80	1.75	**28.0**	1.73	1.71
1.78	1.73	**27.5**	1.72	1.70
1.76	1.71	**27.0**	1.70	1.68
1.75	1.70	**26.5**	1.69	1.66
1.73	1.68	**26.0**	1.68	1.65
1.71	1.67	**25.5**	1.66	1.63
1.69	1.65	**25.0**	1.65	1.61
1.67	1.63	**24.5**	1.63	1.60
1.66	1.62	**24.0**	1.62	1.58
1.64	1.60	**23.5**	1.61	1.56
1.62	1.59	**23.0**	1.59	1.55
1.60	1.57	**22.5**	1.58	1.53
1.58	1.56	**22.0**	1.56	1.52
1.57	1.54	**21.5**	1.55	1.50
1.55	1.52	**21.0**	1.54	1.48
1.53	1.51	**20.5**	1.52	1.47
1.51	1.49	**20.0**	1.51	1.45
1.49	1.48	**19.5**	1.50	1.44
1.48	1.46	**19.0**	1.48	1.42
1.46	1.45	**18.5**	1.47	1.40

Table A3.5 International classification of adult underweight, overweight and obesity according to BMI (WHO, 2016)

Classification	Body mass index (kg/m²)	
	Principal cut-off points	Additional cut-off points
Underweight	<18.50	<18.50
Severe thinness	<16.00	<16.00
Moderate thinness	16.00–16.99	16.00–16.99
Mild thinness	17.00–18.49	17.00–18.49
Normal range	18.50–24.99	18.50–22.99
		23.00–24.99
Overweight	≥25.00	≥25.00
Pre-obese	25.00–29.99	25.00–27.49
		27.50–29.99
Obese	≥30.00	≥30.00
Obese class I	30.00–34.99	30.00–32.49
		32.50–34.99
Obese class II	35.00–39.99	35.00–37.49
		37.50–39.99
Obese class III	≥40.00	≥40.00

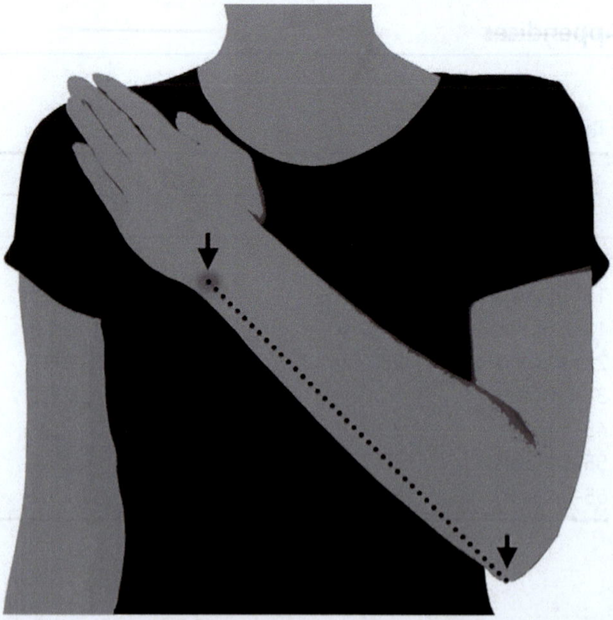

Figure A3.1 How to measure ulna length: Measure between the point of the elbow (olecranon process) and the mid-point of the prominent bone of the wrist (styloid process) (left side, if possible)

Table A3.6 Cut-off points for use in different countries / ethnic groups to identify health risk associated with central obesity. Measurements above these values are associated with increased risk.

Country / ethnic group		
	Waist circumference (cm) (Alberti *et al.*, 2007; NICE, 2013)	
Europids	Men	≥94
	Women	≥80
South Asians	Men	≥90
	Women	≥80
Chinese	Men	≥90
	Women	≥80
Japanese	Men	≥90
	Women	≥80
Ethnic South and Central American	Use South Asian recommendation until more specific data are available.	
Sub-Saharan African	Use European valuess until more specific data are available.	
Eastern Mediterranean and Middle East (Arab) populations	Use European values until more specific data are available.	
	Sagittal abdominal depth (cm)	
Brazil (Duarte Pimentel *et al.*, 2010)	Men	≥23.1
	Women	≥20.1
Sweden (Risérus *et al.*, 2010)	Men	≥22.0
	Women	≥20.0
UK* (Valsamakis *et al.*, 2004)	Men	≥27.6

*Includes White and Indo-Asian participants.

Table A3.7 Normative values for handgrip strength in adults (Dodds *et al.*, 2014)

Age (years)	Handgrip strength centiles (kg)				
	10th	25th	50th	75th	90th
Men					
20	30	35	40	46	52
25	36	41	48	55	61
30	38	44	51	58	64
35	39	45	51	58	64
40	38	44	50	57	63
45	36	42	49	56	61
50	35	41	48	54	60
55	34	40	47	53	59
60	33	39	45	51	56
65	31	37	43	48	53
70	29	34	39	44	49
75	26	31	35	41	45
80	23	27	32	37	42
85	19	24	29	33	38
90	16	20	25	29	33
Women					
20	21	24	28	32	36
25	23	26	30	35	38
30	24	27	31	35	39
35	23	27	31	35	39
40	23	27	31	35	39
45	22	26	30	34	38
50	21	25	29	33	37
55	19	23	28	32	35
60	18	22	27	31	34
65	17	21	25	29	33
70	16	20	24	27	31

Table A3.7 *(Continued)*

Age (years)	Handgrip strength centiles (kg)				
	10th	25th	50th	75th	90th
75	14	18	21	25	28
80	13	16	19	23	26
85	11	14	17	20	23
90	9	11	14	17	20

References

Alberti KGMM, Zimmet P, Shaw J. (2007) International Diabetes Federation: a consensus on type 2 diabetes prevention. *Diabet. Med.* 24: 451–463.

Bishop CW, Bowen PE, Ritchey SJ. (1981) Norms for nutritional assessment of American adults by upper arm anthropometry. *Am. J. Clin. Nutr.* 34: 2530–2539.

Dodds RM, Sydall HE, Cooper R, et al. (2014) Grip strength across the life course: Normative data from twelve British Studies. *PLoS One*. 9: e113637. doi: 10.1371.

Duarte Pimentel G, Portero-McLellan KC, Maesta N, *et al.* (2010) Accuracy of sagittal abdominal diameter as a predictor of abdominal fat among Brazilian adults: a comparison with waist circumference. *Nutr. Hosp.* 25: 656–661.

Elia M. (2003) *Development and Use of the Malnutrition Universal Screening Tool ('MUST') for Adults*. Basingstoke: BAPEN.

NICE. (2013) *BMI: Preventing ill health and premature death in black, Asian and other minority ethnic groups*. Available at https://www.nice.org.uk/guidance/ph46. Accessed 20 February 2017.

Risérus U, de Faire U, Berglund L, *et al.* (2010) Sagittal abdominal diameter as a screening tool in clinical research. *J. Obes.* 2010: 757939. doi: http://doi.org/10.1155/2010/757939.

Valsamakis G, Chetty R, Anwart A, *et al.* (2004) Association of simple anthropometric measures of obesity with visceral fat and the metabolic syndrome in male Caucasian and Indo-Asian subjects. *Diabet. Med.* 21: 1339–1345.

WHO. (2016) *BMI Classification*. comAvailable at http://apps.who.int/bmi/index.jsp?introPage=intro_3.html. Accessed 28 December 2016.

Appendix 4 Predicting energy requirements

For a discussion on stress factors and physical activity levels (PALs) in clinical practice, see Chapter 6.1 (Nutritional requirements in clinical practice) and the specific clinical chapters in Section 7 (Clinical dietetic practice) for detailed discussions as appropriate.

Table A4.1 Basal metabolic rate (BMR) (Henry, 2005; as recommended by SACN, 2011)

	Age (years)	BMR prediction equation (MJ/day)
Males	<3	0.255 (w) – 0.141
	3–10	0.0937 (w) + 2.15
	10–18	0.0769 (w)+ 2.43
	18–30	0.0669 (w) + 2.28
	30–60	0.0592 (w) + 2.48
	>60	0.0563 (w) + 2.15
Females	<3	0.246 (w) – 0.0965
	3–10	0.0842 (w) + 2.12
	10–18	0.0465 (w) + 3.18
	18–30	0.0546 (w) + 2.33
	30–60	0.0407 (w) + 2.90
	>60	0.0424 (w) + 2.38

w, weight in kg.

In 2011, the Scientific Advisory Committee on Nutrition (SACN) published the report *Dietary Reference Values for Energy*. Energy requirements for the UK were last reviewed by the Committee on Medical Aspects of Food Policy (COMA) in their 1991 report *Dietary Reference Values for Food and Energy and Nutrients for the United Kingdom*. Following careful consideration of the evidence, SACN has recommended a revision to the estimated average requirements (EARs) for food energy for infants, children, adolescents and adults. However, these are intended only for use in healthy populations and not individuals or groups who require clinical management. Although exclusive breastfeeding is recommended for about the first 6 months of life, it is recognised that infants are fed in a variety of ways. Therefore, separate recommendations have been made for exclusively breastfed infants, breast milk substitute-fed infants, and those for whom the method of feeding is mixed or unknown. For the full report, refer to SACN (2011), particularly Tables 14 and 15.

References

Henry CJ. (2005) Basal metabolic rate studies in humans: measurement and development of new equations. *Public Health Nutr.* 8: 1133–1152.

SACN. (2011) *Dietary Recommendations for Energy. Working Group Report*. Available at https://www.gov.uk/government/publications/sacn-dietary-reference-values-for-energy. Accessed 6 December 2018.

Manual of Dietetic Practice, Sixth Edition. Edited by Joan Gandy.

Companion website: www.manualofdieteticpractice.com

Appendix 5 Clinical chemistry

mg to mmol	$\frac{\text{mg}}{\text{atomic weight}}$
mmol to mg	mmol × atomic weight

Milliequivalents (mEq)

$$1\text{mEq} = \frac{\text{atomic weight (mg)}}{\text{valency}}\text{M}$$

To convert

mg to mEq	(mg × valency)/atomic weight
mEq to mg	(mEq × atomic weight)/valency

For minerals with a valency of 1, mEq = mmol
For minerals with a valency of 2, mEq = mmol × 2

Laboratory variations

Methods of analysis and standardisations vary considerably from laboratory to laboratory. These differences will influence the quoted reference ranges, and therefore readers are advised to use only those quoted by their local laboratory. Local reference ranges may be at variance with the levels quoted in the following tables.

Correction of serum calcium for low albumin

Corrected serum calcium level (mmol/L)

Table A5.1 Atomic weights and valencies

Mineral	Atomic weight	Valency
Sodium	23.0	1
Potassium	39.0	1
Phosphorus	31.0	2
Calcium	40.0	2
Magnesium	24.3	2
Chlorine	35.4	1
Sulphur	32.0	2
Zinc	65.4	2

Table A5.2 Mineral content of compounds and solutions

Solution/compound	Mineral content	
1 g sodium chloride	393 mg Na	(17.1 mmol Na^+)
1 g sodium bicarbonate	274 mg Na	(12 mmol Na^+)
1 g potassium bicarbonate	390 mg K	(10 mmol K^+)
1 g calcium chloride (dihydrate)	273 mg Ca	(6.8 mmol Ca^{2+})
1 g calcium carbonate	400 mg Ca	(10 mmol Ca^{2+})
1 g calcium gluconate	89 mg Ca	(2.2 mmol Ca^{2+})
1 litre normal saline	3450 mg Na	(150 mmol Na^+)

Table A5.3 Conversion factors for mmol/mg/mEq

Mineral	mg/mmol		mg/mEq		mmol/mEq	
	mg=	mmol=	mg=	mEq=	mmol=	mEq=
Sodium	mmol × 23	mg ÷ 23	mEq × 23	mg ÷ 23	mEq	mmol
Potassium	mmol × 39	mg ÷ 39	mEq × 39	mg ÷ 39	mEq	mmol
Phosphorus	mmol × 31	mg ÷ 31	mEq × 15.5	mg ÷ 15.5	mEq ÷ 2	mmol × 2
Calcium	mmol × 40	mg ÷ 40	mEq × 20	mg ÷ 20	mEq ÷ 2	mmol × 2
Magnesium	mmol × 24.3	mg ÷ 24.3	mEq × 12.15	mg ÷ 12.15	mEq ÷ 2	mmol × 2
Chlorine	mmol × 35.4	mg ÷ 35.4	mEq × 35.4	mg ÷ 35.4	mEq	mmol
Sulphur	mmol × 32	mg ÷ 32	mEq × 16	mg ÷ 16	mEq ÷ 2	mmol × 2
Zinc	mmol × 65.4	mg ÷ 65.4	mEq × 32.7	mg ÷ 32.7	mEq ÷ 2	mmol × 2

Manual of Dietetic Practice, Sixth Edition. Edited by Joan Gandy.

Companion website: www.manualofdieteticpractice.com

$$= \text{measured serum calcium (mmol/L)} + \left(\frac{40 - \text{measured albumin}}{40}\right)$$

An alternative (and possibly more accurate) equation is:
Corrected serum calcium level (mmol/L)

$$= \text{measured serum calcium (mmol/L)} + \left[\left(40 - \text{measured albumin}\right) \times 0.02\right]$$

To be even more accurate, the serum protein level should also be considered:

$$= \text{measured serum calcium (mmol/L)} + \left[\left(72 - \text{measured protein}\right) \times 0.02\right]$$

This corrected calcium value should be added to that obtained from the correction for low albumin, and a mean of the two levels obtained, calculated to two decimal places.

Table A5.4 Adult normal values (adapted from Provan, 2010. *Oxford Handbook of Clinical and Laboratory Investigation*, 3rd edn)

Substance	Value	Substance	Value
Albumin	32–50 g/L	Red cell count	
Bicarbonate	20–29 mmol/L	Males	$4.5–6.5 \times 10^{12}$/L
Bilirubin	<17 μmol/L	Females	$3.8–5.8 \times 10^{12}$/L
Calcium	2.15–2.55 mmol/L	Mean cell haemoglobin (MCH)	27–32 pg
Chloride	97–107 mmol/L	Mean cell volume (MCV)	77–95 fl
Creatinine	60–125 mmol/L	Mean cell haemoglobin concentration	32–36 g/dL
Phosphate	0.7–1.5 mmol/L	White blood count (WBC)	$4.0–11.0 \times 10^{9}$/L
Potassium	3.5–5.0 mmol/L	Neutrophils	$2.0–7.5 \times 10^{9}$/L
Sodium	135–145 mmol/L	Eosinophils	$0.04–0.4 \times 10^{9}$/L
Urate	0.14–0.46 mmol/L	Monocytes	$0.2–0.8 \times 10^{9}$/L
Urea	3.0–6.5 mmol/L	Basophils	$0.0–0.1 \times 10^{9}$/L
		Lymphocytes	$1.5–4.5 \times 10^{9}$/L
		Platelets	$150–400 \times 10^{9}$/L
		Erythrocyte sedimentation rate	2–12 mm/1st hour
		Ferritin (varies with gender and age)	14–200 μg/L
		Ferritin (premenopausal women)	14–148 μg/L
		Serum B_{12}	150–700 ng/L
Haemoglobin		Serum folate	2.0–11.0 μg/L
Males	13.0–18.0 g/dL	Red cell folate	150–700 μg/L
Females	11.5–16.5 g/dL	Prothrombin time (PT)	12–14 s
Haematocrit (PCV)		Activated partial thromboplastin time (APTT)	26.0–33.5 s
Males	0.40–0.52		
Females	0.36–0.47	Thrombin time (TT)	+3 s of control

Table A5.5 Conversion chart for $HbA1_c$ from % to International Federation of Clinical Federation (IFCC) mmol/mol

%	mmol/mol	%	mmol/mol	%	mmol/mol	%	mmol/mol	%	mmol/mol	%	mmol/mol	%	mmol/mol	%	mmol/mol	%	mmol/mol	%	mmol/mol
4.0	20	5.0	31	6.0	42	7.0	53	8.0	64	9.0	75	10.0	86	11.0	97	12.0	108	13.0	119
4.1	21	5.1	32	6.1	43	7.1	54	8.1	65	9.1	76	10.1	87	11.1	98	12.1	109	13.1	120
4.2	22	5.2	33	6.2	44	7.2	55	8.2	66	9.2	77	10.2	88	11.2	99	12.2	110	13.2	121
4.3	23	5.3	34	6.3	45	7.3	56	8.3	67	9.3	78	10.3	89	11.3	100	12.3	111	13.3	122
4.4	25	5.4	36	6.4	46	7.4	57	8.4	68	9.4	79	10.4	90	11.4	101	12.4	112	13.4	123
4.5	26	5.5	37	6.5	48	7.5	58	8.5	69	9.5	80	10.5	91	11.5	102	12.5	113	13.5	124
4.6	27	5.6	38	6.6	49	7.6	60	8.6	70	9.6	81	10.6	92	11.6	103	12.6	114	13.6	125
4.7	28	5.7	39	6.7	50	7.7	61	8.7	72	9.7	83	10.7	93	11.7	104	12.7	115	13.7	126
4.8	29	5.8	40	6.8	51	7.8	62	8.8	73	9.8	84	10.8	95	11.8	105	12.8	116	13.8	127

References

Provan J. (2010) *Oxford Handbook of Clinical and Laboratory Investigation*, 3rd edn. Oxford: Oxford University Press

Appendix 6 Nutritional supplements and enteral feeds

Patients at risk of malnutrition may be prescribed oral nutritional supplements (ONS) or enteral feeds as long as they have a functional gastrointestinal tract. Many of these products are prescribed only in specified clinical circumstances defined by the Advisory Committee on Borderline Substances (ACBS), and are termed ACBS prescribable. Standard ACBS indications are disease-related malnutrition, intractable malabsorption, pre-operative preparation of malnourished patients, dysphagia, proven inflammatory bowel disease, following total gastrectomy, short-bowel syndrome and bowel fistula. The following tables provide a guide to the range of proprietary supplements, feeds and other nutritional support products currently available in the UK.

Product composition within a particular category will differ; some products may be more appropriate than others in particular clinical circumstances. Ongoing product development by the manufacturers inevitably means that, over time, the availability and composition of some products may change, and new products will appear. The information given here is for guidance only, and product details should be checked before clinical usage.

These tables were compiled in October 2017. For current product availability, composition and prescribing indications, consult the British National Formulary (BNF), the Monthly Index of Medical Specialities (MIMS) or the manufacturer's advice. Information on which products are suitable for special diets (e.g. kosher, halal, gluten free, lactose free, vegetarian, vegan) can also be obtained directly from the manufacturers.

A6.1 Adult nutritional supplements and enteral feeds

Note: Many sip feed supplements are available in a variety of flavours to offset taste fatigue. Some, but not all, are nutritionally complete: check compositional details before use. Some products can also be used for tube feeding.

These products can be purchased by patients from supermarkets and chemists, and are useful at times when dietary intake is poor. None are nutritionally complete.

A6.2 Paediatric nutritional supplements and enteral feeds

This appendix is used as a guide, and is not definitive. For further details, see Shaw V. (2015) *Clinical Paediatric Dietetics*, 4th edn. Oxford: Blackwell Publishing. Compiled using data from BNF for Children, 2017.

Manual of Dietetic Practice, Sixth Edition. Edited by Joan Gandy.

Companion website: www.manualofdieteticpractice.com

Table A6.1.1 Prescribable liquid (sip feed) supplements

Product type	Product name (Manufacturer) *Quantity*		Per bottle/can			
			Energy		Protein	Fibre
			kJ	kcal	(g)	(g)
Standard energy	Ensure (Abbott) *250 mL*		1057	251	10.0	0.0
(1 kcal/mL)	Fresubin Original (Fresenius Kabi) *200 mL*		840	200	7.6	0.0
Juice type	Ensure Plus Juce (Abbott) *220 mL*		1403	330	10.6	0.0
(low fat)	Fortijuce (Nutricia Clinical) *200 mL*		1280	300	8.0	0.0
(1.25–1.5 kcal/mL)	Resource Fruit (Nestlé) *200 mL*		1062	250	8.0	0.0
High energy	Ensure Plus Milkshake style (Abbott) *220 mL*		1390	330	13.8	0.0
(1.5–2.4 kcal/mL)	Ensure Plus Savoury (Abbott) *220 mL*		1390	330	14.0	0.0
	Ensure Plus Yoghurt style (Abbott) *220 mL*		1389	330	13.8	0.0
	Ensure Twocal (Abbott) *200 mL*		1675	400	16.8	2.0
	Fortisip Bottle (Nutricia Clinical) *200 mL*		1250	300	11.8	0.0
	Fortisip Compact (Nutricia Clinical) *125 mL*		1261	300	12.0	0.0
	Fortisip Extra (Nutricia Clinical) *200 mL*		1350	320	20.0	0.0
	Fortisip Yogurt Style (Nutricia Clinical) *200 mL*		1260	300	12.0	0.4
	Fresubin 2 kcal Drink (Fresenius Kabi) *200 mL*		1680	400	20.0	0.0
	Fresubin Energy (Fresenius Kabi) *200 mL*		1260	300	11.2	0.0
	Renilon 7.5 (Nutricia Clinical) *125 mL*		1050	250	9.4	0.0
High energy + fibre	Ensure Plus Fibre (Abbott) *200 mL*		1303	310	13.0	5.0
(1.5–2.0 kcal/mL)	Fresubin 2 kcal Fibre Drink (Fresenius Kabi) *200 mL*		1680	400	20	3.2
	Fresubin Energy Fibre (Fresenius Kabi) *200 mL*		1260	300	11.2	4.0
	Fortisip Compact Fibre (Nutricia Clinical) *125 mL*		1256	300	11.8	4.5
	Fortisip Multi Fibre (Nutricia Clinical) *200 mL*		1290	308	12.0	4.4
	Nutrison Energy Multi Fibre (Nutricia Clinical) 20 mL		640	153	6	2.2
	Resource 2.0 Fibre (Nestlé) *200 mL*		1680	400	18.0	5.0
	Fortisip Compact Protein (Nutricia Clinical) 125 mL		1263	300	18	0
	Fresubin Protein Energy Drink (Fresenius Kabi) *200 mL*		1260	300	20.0	0.0
	Resource Protein (Nestlé) *200 mL*		1054	250	18.8	0.0
	Nutricomp Drink Plus (Braun) 200 mL		1264	300	12	<0.2
Thickened	Fresubin Thickened (Fresenius Kabi) *200 mL*		1260	300	20.0	*
(1.5–2.4 kcal/mL)	Syrup (stage 1) and custard (stage 2)					
	Nutilis Complete Stage 1 (Nutricia) *125 mL*		1288	306	12.0	4.0
	Resource Thickened Drink (Nestlé) *114 mL*		435	102	0.0	0.0
	Syrup and custard consistencies					
	SLO Drinks (SLO Drinks)			*	*	*
	Syrup, custard and pudding consistencies					
Powdered	Complan Shake (Complan Foods) *55 g sachet*	*in 200 mL water*	1025	244	8.5	0.0
		in 200 mL whole milk	1621	387	15.6	0.0
	Foodlink Complete (Foodlink)		1612	385*	18.5*	0.0
	Shake per 57 g sachet prepared with 200 mL milk					
	Foodlink Complete with Fibre (Foodlink)		1760	421	19.6	4.5
	Shake per 63 g sachet prepared with 200 mL milk					
	Oral Impact (Nestlé) *74 g in 250 mL water*		*	*	*	
	Vegenat-med Balanced Protein (Vegenat) *110 g sachet*		1924	458	18.0	5.8
	Vegenat-med High Protein (Vegenat) *110 g sachet*		1940	463	23.3	6.0

* Exact composition varies – see manufacturer's data.

Table A6.1.2 Non-prescribable powdered supplements

Product name (Manufacturer) *Quantity*	Per sachet + 200 mL whole milk			
	Energy		Protein	Fibre
	kJ	kcal	(g)	(g)
Complan (Complan Foods) *55 g sachet mixed with water*	1030	244	8.5	0.1

Table A6.1.3 Prescribable solid/semi-solid supplements (dessert style – also useful for dysphagic patients)

Product type	Product name (Manufacturer) *Quantity*	Per bottle/can			
		Energy		Protein	Fibre
		kJ	kcal	(g)	(g)
Solid/semi-solid desserts	Clinutren Dessert (Nestlé) *125 g*	779	187	11	2.9
	Ensure Plus Crème (Abbott) *125 g*	718	171	7.1	0.0
	Forticreme Complete (Nutricia Clinical) *125 g*	844	200	11.9	0.0
	Fortisip Fruit Dessert (Nutricia Clinical) *150 g*	844	200	10.5	3.9
	Fresubin Crème (Fresenius Kabi) *125 g*	945	225	12.5	2.5
	Resource Dessert Energy (Nestlé) *125 g*	839	200	6.0	0.0
	Resource Dessert Fruit (Nestlé) *125 g*	848	200	6.3	1.8

Table A6.1.4 Single nutrient component supplements

Component	Product name (Manufacturer)	Notes, ACBS indications and nutritional values	
Carbohydrate	Caloreen (Nestlé) *powder*	1630 kJ/385 kcal/100 g	Disease-related malnutrition, malabsorption states or other conditions requiring fortification with a high or readily available carbohydrate supplement
	Maxijul Liquid (SHS) *liquid*	850 kJ/200 kcal/100 mL	
	Maxijul Super Soluble (SHS) *powder*	1615 kJ/380 kcal/100 g	
	Polycal (Nutricia Clinical) *powder*	1630 kJ/384 kcal/100 g	
	Polycal Liquid (Nutricia Clinical) *liquid*	1050 kJ/247 kcal/100 mL	
	Resource Optifibre (Nestlé) *powder*	816 kJ/202 kcal and 86 g fibre/100 g	
	S.O.S. 10, 15, 20, 25 (Vitaflo) *powder*	1590 kJ/380 kcal/100 g	
	Vitajoule (Vitaflo) powder	1615 kJ/380 kcal/100 g	
Fat	Calogen (Nutricia Clinical) *liquid* 100% LCT fat emulsion	1850 kJ/450 kcal/100 mL	Disease-related malnutrition, malabsorption states or other conditions requiring fortification with a high-fat supplement
	Calogen Extra Shots (Nutricia Clinical)	1650 kJ/400 kcal/100 mL	
	Fresubin 5 kcal Shot (Fresenius Kabi) *liquid*	2100 kJ/500 kcal/100 mL	
	Liquigen (SHS) *liquid* 97% MCT	1850 kJ/450 kcal/100 mL	Steatorrhoea associated with cystic fibrosis (pancreas), intestinal lymphangiectasia, intestinal surgery, chronic liver disease/cirrhosis and other proven malabsorption syndromes
	Medium-Chain Triglyceride (MCT) Oil (SHS) *liquid* 100% MCT	3515 kJ/855 kcal/100 mL	
Protein	Casilan 90 (Heinz) *powder* 90% protein	1572 kJ/356 kcal/100 g	Disease-related malnutrition, malabsorption states or other conditions requiring fortification with a high-protein supplement
	Protifar (Nutricia Clinical) *powder* 89% protein	1560 kJ/368 kcal/100 g	

Table A6.1.5 Multiple nutrient component supplements

Components	Product name (Manufacturer)	Notes, ACBS indications & nutritional values	
Fat/carbohydrate	MCT Duocal (SHS) *powder*	Conditions requiring extra calories, e.g. fat malabsorption, or where assimilation of LCTs is impaired.	50 g in 150 mL water provides: 1041 kJ/249 kcal, 36 g CHO, 11.6 g fat
	Duocal (SHS) *liquid*	Conditions requiring extra calories	Per 100 mL: 695 kJ/166 kcal, 23.7 g CHO, 7.9 g fat (30% MCT)
Protein/ carbohydrate	ProSource (Nutrinovo) *liquid*	Protein energy malnutrition and patients on a fluid-restricted diet	Per 30 mL: 420 kJ/100 kcal, 10 g protein, 15 g CHO
	Calogen Extra (Nutricia Clinical) *liquid*	High-energy fat emulsion with protein, carbohydrate, vitamins and minerals	Per 100 mL: 1650 kJ/400 kcal, 5 g protein, 4.5 g CHO, 40.3 g fat
Protein/fat/ carbohydrate	Calshake (Fresenius Kabi) *powder*	For increased energy requirements, e.g. patients with cystic fibrosis, cancer or HIV/ AIDS	87 g sachet + 240 mL whole milk provides approx.: 2504 kJ/599 kcal, 11.6 g protein, 68.9 g CHO, 28.3 g fat
	Enshake (Abbott) *powder*	High-energy, high-protein drink, for patients with involuntary weight loss	96.5 g sachet + 240 mL whole milk provides approx.: 2519 kJ/600 kcal, 16 g protein, 78.9 g CHO, 24.7 g fat
	Pro-Cal (Vitaflo) *powder*	Disease-related malnutrition, malabsorption states and other conditions requiring fortification with energy and protein, e.g. burns	15 g sachet provides: 415 kJ/100 kcal, 2 g protein, 4.2 g CHO, 8.3 g fat
	Pro-Cal Shot (Vitaflo) liquid		Per 30 mL: 418 kJ/100 kcal, 2 g protein, 4 g CHO, 8.5 g fat
	Scandishake Mix (Nutricia Clinical) *powder*	High-energy supplement for disease-related malnutrition based on skimmed milk powder, carbohydrate and fat	85 g sachet + 240 mL whole milk provides: 2457 kJ/588 kcal, 11.7 g protein, 66.8 g CHO, 30.4 g fat
	Vitasavoury 300 (Vitaflo) *powder*	Low-volume, high-energy supplements for disease-related malnutrition, malabsorption states or other conditions requiring additional energy and protein	50 g sachet provides: 1281 kJ/309 kcal, 6 g protein, 11.3 g CHO, 26 g fat

CHO, carbohydrate; MCT, medium-chain triglycerides; LCT, long-chain triglycerides.

Table A6.1.6 Food and fluid thickeners (for thickening of food and drinks of patients with dysphagia)

Type of product	Product name (Manufacturer)
Modified maize starch powder*	Multi Thick (Abbott)
	Nutilis (Nutricia Clinical)
	Resource ThickenUp (Nestlé)
	Thick and Easy (Fresenius Kabi)
	Thick and Easy Clear (Fresenius Kabi)
	Thixo-D (Sutherland)
	Vitaquick (Vitaflo)
Maltodextrin and xanthan gum	Resource ThickenUp Clear (Nestlé)

* See individual manufacturer's recommendations for the quantities required to achieve various textures.

Table A6.1.7 Enteral feeds – standard indications

Product type	Product name (Manufacturer)	Per 100 mL			
		Energy		Protein	Fibre
		kJ	kcal	(g)	(g)
Standard energy (1 kcal/mL)	Fresubin Original (Fresenius Kabi)	420	100	3.8	0.0
	Fresubin Original Fibre (Fresenius Kabi)	420	100	3.8	1.5
	Peptamen (Nestlé)	421	100	4.0	0
	Jevity (Abbott)	449	107	4.0	1.8
	Jevity Promote (Abbott)	434	103	5.6	1.7
	Novasource GI Control (Nestlé) 40% MCTs	463	110	4.1	2.1
	Nutrison (Nutricia Clinical)	420	100	4.0	0.0
	Nutrison MCT (Nutricia Clinical) 61% MCTs	420	100	5.0	0.0
	Nutrison Multi Fibre (Nutricia Clinical)	430	103	4.0	1.5
	Osmolite (Abbott)	424	101	4.0	0.0
	Osmolite HP (Abbott)	424	100	6.26	0.0
Nutritionally complete (1.0–1.2 kcal/mL)	Fresubin 1000 Complete (Fresenius Kabi) Complete in 1000 mL	418	100	5.5	2.0
	Fresubin 1200 Complete (Fresenius Kabi) Complete in 1000 mL	500	120	6.0	2.0
	Fresubin 1500 Complete (Fresenius Kabi) Complete in 1500 mL	420	100	3.8	1.5
	Fresubin 1800 Complete (Fresenius Kabi) Complete in 1500 mL	500	120	6.0	2.0
	Fresubin 2250 Complete (Fresenius Kabi) Complete in 1500 mL	630	150	5.6	1.5
	Fresubin Intensive (Fresenius Kabi) Complete in 1000 mL	512	122	10	0.64
	Nutrison 800 Complete Multi Fibre (Nutricia Clinical) Complete in 800 mL	345	83	5.5	1.5
	Nutrison 1000 Complete Multi Fibre (Nutricia Clinical) Complete in 1000 mL	420	100	5.5	2.0
	Nutrison 1200 Complete Multi Fibre (Nutricia Clinical) Complete in 1000 mL	505	120	5.5	2.0
Medium energy (1.2–1.3 kcal/mL)	Jevity Plus (Abbott)	514	122	5.6	2.2
	Jevity Plus HP (Abbott)	551	131	8.1	1.5
	Nutrison Advanced Protison (Nutricia Clinical)	540	128	7.5	1.5
	Nutrison Protein Plus (Nutricia Clinical)	525	125	6.3	0.0
	Nutrison Protein Plus Multi Fibre (Nutricia Clinical)	525	125	6.3	1.5
	Osmolite Plus (Abbott)	508	121	5.6	0.0
	Peptamen HN (Nestle)	559	133	6.6	0.0
High energy (1.5–2.0 kcal/mL)	Twocal (Abbott)	837	200	8.4	1.0
	Fresubin Energy (Fresenius Kabi)	630	150	5.6	0.0
	Fresubin Energy Fibre (Fresenius Kabi)	630	150	5.6	1.5
	Fresubin HP Energy (Fresenius Kabi)	630	150	7.5	0.0
	Jevity 1.5 kcal (Abbott)	649	154	6.4	2.2
	Novasource GI Forte (Nestlé)	649	155	6.0	2.2
	Nutrison Concentrated (Nutricia Clinical)	840	200	7.5	0.0
	Nutrison Energy (Nutricia Clinical)	630	150	6.0	0.0
	Nutrison Energy Multi Fibre (Nutricia Clinical)	640	153	6.0	1.5
	Nutrison Energy Multifibre Vanilla (Nutricia Clinical)	645	154	6.0	2.2
	Osmolite 1.5 kcal (Abbott)	630	150	6.3	0.0
	Peptamen AF (Nestle)	638	152	9.4	0.0

Table A6.1.8 Specialist indication enteral feeds and supplements

Product type	Product name (Manufacturer)	Per 100 mL			
		Energy		Protein	Fibre
		kJ	kcal	(g)	(g)
Amino acid liquid formula	Elemental 028 Extra (SHS) *Sip feed*	360	86	2.5	0.0
Low-sodium liquid formula	*Nutrison Low Sodium (Nutricia Clinical)*	420	100	4.0	0.0
Peptide-based liquid formula	Peptamen (Nestlé)	421	100	4.0	0.0
	Peptamen HN (Nestlé)	559	133	6.6	0.0
	Peptisorb (Nutricia Clinical)	425	100	4.0	0.0
	Perative (Abbott)	552	131	6.7	0.0
	Survimed OPD (Fresenius Kabi)	420	100	4.5	0.0
Soya protein liquid formula	Fresubin Soya Fibre (Fresenius Kabi)	420	100	3.8	2.0
	Nutrison Soya (Nutricia Clinical)	420	100	4.0	0.0
	Nutrison Soya Multi Fibre (Nutricia Clinical)	420	100	4.0	1.5

Table A6.1.9 Specialised formulas for specific clinical conditions

Condition	Notes and ACBS indications	Product (Manufacturer)
Cancer	Pancreatic cancer.	FortiCare (Nutricia Clinical) *liquid*
	Lung cancer undergoing chemotherapy.	Supportan (Fresenius Kabi) *liquid*
	Pancreatic cancer.	ProSure (Abbott) *liquid*
	Contains EPA.	
Crohn's disease	Crohn's disease.	Alicalm (SHS) *powder*
	Active Crohn's disease / nutritional support during Crohn's remission.	Modulen IBD (Nestlé) *powder* (can be flavoured with Flavour Mix (Nestlé) powder)
Epilepsy	Part of ketogenic diet in the management of drug therapy–resistant epilepsy.	KetoCal (SHS) *powder*
Liver disease	Whey protein + BCAA. Chronic liver disease and/or porto-hepatic encephalopathy.	Generaid (SHS) *powder*
Pulmonary	Acute lung injury, ARDS and SIRS.	Oxepa (Abbott) *liquid*
	COPD, cystic fibrosis or respiratory failure.	Pulmocare (Abbott) *liquid*
	Disease-related malnutrition in COPD + BMI <20.	Respifor (Nutricia Clinical) *liquid*
Renal	Chronic renal failure with haemodialysis or continuous ambulatory peritoneal dialysis.	Nepro (Abbott) *liquid*
	Cirrhosis.	
	Chronic renal failure.	Renamil (KoRa) *powder*
	Biochemically proven hypoproteinaemia.	Renapro (KoRa) *powder*
	Patients on dialysis.	
Renal/liver	For use where a high-energy, low-fluid, low-electrolyte diet is required.	Duocal Super Soluble (SHS) *powder*
	Chronic/acute renal failure without dialysis.	Suplena (Abbott) *liquid*
	Chronic/acute liver disease with fluid restriction.	
Short-bowel syndrome	Intractable malabsorption and proven irritable bowel disease.	Elemental 028 Extra (SHS) *powder*
		Glucodrate (Vitaflo) *powder*
Synthetic diets	Mineral and trace element supplement for synthetic diets.	Metabolic Mineral Mixture (SHS) *powder*

ARDS: acute respiratory distress syndrome; BCAA: branched-chain amino acids; COPD: chronic obstructive pulmonary disease; SIRS: Systemic inflammatory response syndrome.

Table A6.1.10 Nutritional supplements for metabolic diseases

Condition	Notes and ACBS indications	Product (Manufacturer)
Glutaric aciduria	Type 1 glutaric aciduria.	XLYS, TRY Glutaridon* (SHS) *powder*
Glycogen storage diseases	Plus other metabolic conditions where a constant glucose supply is essential.	Glycosade (Vitaflo) *powder*
Homocystinuria	Methionine-free protein substitute.	HCU cooler (Vitaflo) *liquid* HCU Express (Vitaflo) *powder*
Hypermethioninaemia	And vitamin B_6 non-responsive homocystinuria.	HCU LV (SHS) *powder*
Hypermethioninaemia or homocystinuria	Essential and nonessential amino acids, except methionine.	XMET Homidon* (SHS) *powder* XMET Maxamum (SHS) *powder*
Isovaleric acidaemia	Essential and nonessential amino acids, except leucine.	XLEU Faladon (SHS) *powder*
Maple syrup urine disease	Use in low-protein diets by mixing with protein substitute, adding to modular feeds, incorporating into other permitted food or drink.	Isoleucine Amino Acid Supplement (Vitaflo) *powder* Valine Amino Acid Supplement (Vitaflo) *powder*
	Essential and nonessential amino acids, except isoleucine, leucine, valine.	MSUD Aid III (SHS) *powder* MSUD cooler (Vitaflo) *liquid* MSUD express (Vitaflo) *powder* MSUD Maxamum (SHS) *powder*
Methylmalonic acidaemia Propionic acidaemia	Essential and nonessential amino acids, except methionine, threonine, valine and low isoleucine.	XMTVI Asadon (SHS) *powder* XMTVI Maxamum (SHS) *powder*
Other errors of protein metabolism	Use in low-protein diets by mixing with protein substitute, adding to modular feeds, incorporating into other permitted food or drink.	Cystine Amino Acid Supplement (Vitaflo) *powder* Leucine Amino Acid Supplement (Vitaflo) *powder* Phenylalanine Amino Acid Supplement (Vitaflo) *powder*
Dietary management of patients with increased risk of infection	For use in post-operative, post-traumatic (e.g. burns) or severely malnourished patients.	Reconvan (Fresenius Kabi) *liquid*
Other inborn errors of metabolism	n-3 supplement containing DHA.	DocOmega (Vitaflo) *powder*
	n-3 and supplement containing AA and DHA.	KeyOmega (Vitaflo) *powder*
Phenylketonuria (PKU)	Phenylalanine-free protein substitute.	Add-Ins (SHS) *powder*
Phenylalanine-free protein substitutes	Ready-to-drink phenylalanine-free liquid product.	Easiphen (SHS) *liquid*
	Phenylalanine-free drink mix.	Lophlex (SHS) *powder*
	For use in maternal PKU where there are low plasma tyrosine concentrations.	L-Tyrosine (SHS) *powder*
	Phenylalanine-free protein supplement.	Milupa PKU 3-advanta (Milupa) *powder*
	Each unit (one sachet, 10 tablets or 20 capsules) provides 10 g amino acids except phenylalanine.	Phlexy-10 Exchange System (SHS) *Capsule/Tablet/Drink*
	Unflavoured blend of essential and nonessential amino acids.	PK Aid-4 (SHS) *powder*
	Ready-to-drink phenylalanine-free protein substitutes, including n-3 LCPs, DHA and EPA.	PKU cooler10 (Vitaflo) *liquid* Provides 10 g of protein equivalent PKU cooler15 (Vitaflo) *liquid* Provides 15 g of protein equivalent PKU cooler20 (Vitaflo) *liquid* Provides 20 g of protein equivalent
	Phenylalanine-free protein substitute.	PKU express (Vitaflo) *powder* 1 x 25 g sachet provides 15 g of protein equivalent
	Phenylalanine-free liquid containing a balanced mixture of essential and nonessential amino acids, carbohydrates, vitamins, trace elements and some minerals.	PKU Lophlex LQ 10 (SHS) *liquid* Provides 10 g of protein equivalent PKU Lophlex LQ 20 (SHS) *liquid* Provides 20 g of protein equivalent
	For use in low-protein diets.	Tyrosine Amino Acid Supplement (Vitaflo) *powder*
	Phenylalanine-free protein substitute drink mix.	XP Maxamum (SHS) *powder*

(Continued)

Table A6.1.10 (*Continued*)

Condition	Notes and ACBS indications	Product (Manufacturer)
Tyrosinaemia	Ready-to-drink, tyrosine- and phenylalanine-free protein substitute.	TYR cooler (Vitaflo) *liquid*
	Unflavoured, powdered tyrosine- and phenylalanine-free protein substitute.	TYR express (Vitaflo) *powder* 25 g sachet provides 15 g of protein equivalent
	Normal plasma methionine concentrations.	XPHEN TYR Tyrosidon (SHS) *powder*
	Above-normal plasma methionine concentrations.	XPTM Tyrosidon (SHS) *powder*
Urea cycle disorders	Except arginase deficiency.	L-Arginine (SHS) *powder*
	Essential amino acid supplement.	Dialamine (SHS) *powder* EAA Supplement (Vitaflo) *powder*
Low-protein milk replacement drinks	Low-protein, low-phenylalanine drink based on cow's milk.	Loprofin PKU Drink (SHS) *liquid*
	Suitable for dietary management of amino acid metabolism disorders.	Milupa lp-drink (Milupa) *powder*
	Liquid blend of carbohydrate and fat.	ProZero (Vitaflo) *liquid*
	Low-protein, low-phenylalanine drink based on milk extracts.	Sno-Pro (SHS) *liquid*
Vitamin and mineral component	For use with restricted diets for PKU and similar amino acid abnormalities.	Phlexy-Vits (SHS) *powder/tablet*
Flavouring preparations	For use with unflavoured protein substitutes.	FlavourPac (Vitaflo) *powder* (blackcurrant, lemon, orange, tropical, raspberry) Modjul Flavour System (SHS) *powder* (blackcurrant, orange, pineapple)

*A source of vitamins, minerals, and trace elements is also required, e.g. Phlexy-Vits.
AA, arachidonic acid; DHA, docosahexaenoic acid; EPA, eicosapentaenoic acid; LCPs, long-chain polyunsaturated fatty acids.

Table A6.1.11 Manufacturers' websites

Abbott, Abbott Laboratories Ltd	www.abbott.co.uk
Complan Foods, Complan Foods Ltd	www.complanfoods.com
Foodlink, Foodlink (UK) Ltd	www.foodlinkltd.co.uk
Fresenius Kabi, Fresenius Kabi Ltd	www.fresenius-kabi.co.uk
Heinz, H. J. Heinz Company Ltd	www.heinz.co.uk
KoRa, KoRa Healthcare Ltd	www.kora-health.com
Milupa, Milupa Aptamil	www.milupa-metabolics.com
Nestlé, Nestlé Nutrition	www.nestlehealthscience.co.uk
Nutricia Clinical, Nutricia Clinical Care	www.nutricia.co.uk
Nutrinovo, Nutrinovo Ltd	www.nutrinovo.com
SLO Drinks, SLO Drinks Ltd	www.slodrinks.com
Sutherland, Sutherland Health Ltd	www.sutherlandhealth.com
Vegenat, Vegenat	http://vegenatnutricion.es/index.php?r=site/index
Vitaflo, Vitaflo International Ltd	www.vitaflo.co.uk

Note: SHS International Ltd is part of Nutricia and no longer has a separate web site.

Table A6.2.1 Paediatric sip feeds

Product type	Product name (Manufacturer)	Per 100 mL ready-to-drink product/ standard dilution				Notes
		Energy		Protein	Fibre	
		kJ	kcal	(g)	(g)	
Low energy <1 kcal/mL	Nutriprem 1 (Cow & Gate) *liquid*	335	80	2.6	0.6	70 mL bottle, formula for low-birth-weight babies <1.8 kg only available in hospital
	Nutriprem 2 (Cow & Gate) *liquid*	310	75	2.0	0.6	Catch-up growth in pre-term infants (less than 35 weeks at birth) and small for gestational-age infants up to 6 months corrected age
	SMA Gold Prem 2 (SMA Nutrition) *powder*	305	73	2.0	0.0	
	SMA High Energy (SMA Nutrition) *liquid*	414	99	2.6	0.0	250 mL carton, disease related malnutrition, malabsorption, growth failure from birth to 18 months
Standard energy (1 kcal/mL)	Clinutren Junior (Nestlé) *powder*	420	100	3.0	0.0	Growth failure*†
	Infatrini (Nutricia Clinical) *liquid*	420	101	2.6	0.6	125 mL bottle failure to thrive, disease-related malnutrition and malabsorption, from birth up to body weight 9 kg
	Paediasure (Abbott) *liquid*	422	101	2.8	0.0	200 mL bottle*†
	Paediasure Fibre (Abbott) *liquid*	424	101	2.8	0.73	
	Paediasure Peptide (Abbott) *liquid*	420	100	3.0	0.0	
	Similac High Energy (Abbott) *liquid*	419	100	2.6	0.4	60 mL and 200 mL bottles increased energy requirements, faltering growth &/or need for fluid restriction, body weight up to 8 kg
High energy (1.5 kcal/mL)	Fortini (Nutricia Clinical) *liquid*	630	150	3.4	0.0	Disease-related malnutrition and growth failure in children of 1–6 years*, body weight 8–20 kg
	Fortini Multifibre (Nutricia Clinical) *liquid*	630	150	3.4	1.5	
	Fortini Smoothie Multifibre (Nutricia Clinical) *liquid*	625	150	3.4	1.4	
	Frebini Energy Drink (Fresenius Kabi) *liquid*	630	150	3.8	0.0	Disease-related malnutrition and growth failure in children of 1–10 years*, body weight 8–30 kg
	Frebini Energy Fibre Drink (Fresenius Kabi) *liquid*	630	150	3.8	1.1	
	Paediasure Plus (Abbott) *liquid*	632	151	4.2	0.0	*†
	Paediasure Plus Fibre (Abbott) *liquid*	635	152	4.2	1.1	*†
	Paediasure Plus Juce (Abbott) *liquid*	638	150	4.2	0.0	Low fat*†
	Resource Junior (Nestlé) *liquid*	630	150	3.0	0.0	For children of 1–10 years*

*Not suitable for use in children aged under 1 year.
†For children aged 1–10 years, body weight 8–30 kg.

Table A6.2.2 Feed thickener

Product name (Manufacturer)	Notes
Carobel Instant (Cow & Gate)	Instant thickening agent, prepared from carob seed flour, suitable from birth. Prescribable for thickening feeds in the treatment of habitual and recurrent vomiting.

Table A6.2.3 Paediatric enteral feeds – standard indications

Product type	Product name (Manufacturer)	Per 100 mL				Notes
		Energy		Protein	Fibre	
		kJ	kcal	(g)	(g)	
Low energy (<1 kcal/mL)	Nutrini Low Energy Multi Fibre (Nutricia Clinical) *liquid*	315	75	2.1	0.8	For ages 1–6 years, except bowel fistula, body weight 8–20 kg
Standard energy (1 kcal/mL)	Clinutren Junior (Nestlé) *powder*	420	100	3.0	0.0	For growth failure*†
	Frebini Original (Fresenius Kabi) *liquid*	420	100	2.5	0.0	
	Frebini Original Fibre (Fresenius Kabi) *liquid*	420	100	2.5	0.8	
	Infatrini (Nutricia Clinical) *liquid*	415	100	2.6	0.8	Failure to thrive, disease-related malnutrition and malabsorption, from birth up to body weight 8 kg
	Nutrini (Nutricia Clinical) *liquid*	420	100	2.8	0.0	For growth failure, for ages 1–6 years, body weight 8–20 kg*
	Nutrini Multi Fibre (Nutricia Clinical) *liquid*	420	100	2.8	0.8	
	Paediasure (Abbott) *liquid*	422	101	2.8	0.0	*†
	Paediasure Fibre (Abbott) *liquid*	424	101	2.8	0.73	
	Similac High Energy (Abbott) *liquid*	419	100	2.6	0.4	Increased energy requirements, faltering growth and/or need for fluid restriction, body weight up to 8 kg
	Tentrini (Nutricia Clinical) *liquid*	420	100	3.3	0.0	For growth failure in children aged 7–12 years, body weight 21–45 kg
	Tentrini Multi Fibre (Nutricia Clinical) *liquid*	420	100	3.3	1.1	
Medium energy (1.2 kcal/mL)	Isosource Junior (Nestlé) *liquid*	513	122	2.7	0.0	For growth failure in children aged 1–6 years, body weight 8–20 kg*
High energy (1.5 kcal/mL)	Frebini Energy (Fresenius Kabi) *liquid*	630	150	3.8	0.0	For growth failure in ages 1–10 years, body weight 8–30 kg*
	Frebini Energy Fibre (Fresenius Kabi) *liquid*	630	150	3.8	1.1	
	Nutrini Energy (Nutricia Clinical) *liquid*	630	150	4.1	0.0	For growth failure in ages 1–6 years, body weight 8–20 kg*
	Nutrini Energy Multi Fibre (Nutricia Clinical) *liquid*	630	150	4.1	0.8	For ages 1–6 years, body weight 8–20 kg* and total gastrectomy, not with bowel fistula
	Paediasure Plus (Abbott) *liquid*	632	151	4.2	0.0	*†
	Paediasure Plus Fibre (Abbott) *liquid*	635	152	4.2	1.1	
	Tentrini Energy (Nutricia Clinical) *liquid*	630	150	4.9	0.0	For growth failure in children aged 7–12 years, body weight 21–45 kg
	Tentrini Energy Multi Fibre (Nutricia Clinical) *liquid*	630	150	4.9	1.1	For children aged 7–12 years, body weight 21–45 kg and proven inflammatory bowel disease

*Not suitable for use in children aged under 1 year.
†For children aged 1–10 years, body weight 8–30 kg.

Table A6.2.4 Specialist paediatric formulas

Formula type	Product name (Manufacturer)	Per 100 mL ready-to-drink product (standard dilution)				Notes
		Energy		Protein	Fibre	
		kJ	kcal	(g)	(g)	
Amino acid based	Emsogen (SHS) *powder*	368	88	2.5	0.0	Short-bowel syndrome, intractable malabsorption, proven inflammatory bowel disease, bowel fistula. Not suitable as sole source of nutrition for children aged 1–5 years*
	Neocate Active (SHS) *powder*	418	100	2.8	0.0	For 1–10 years*
	Neocate Advance (SHS) *powder*	420	100	2.5	0.0	
	Neocate LCP (SHS) *powder*	279	67	1.8	0.0	‡
	Nutramigen Puramino (Mead Johnson) *powder*	290	68	1.9	0.0	
Fructose based	Galactomin 19 (SHS) *powder*	288	69	1.9	0.0	Conditions of glucose plus galactose intolerance
Hydrolysate	Aptamil Pepti 1 (Allergy) (Milupa) *powder*	280	67	1.6	0.6	Established cows' milk protein intolerance, with or without secondary lactose intolerance‡.
	Aptamil Pepti 2 (Allergy) (Milupa) *powder*	285	68	1.6	0.6	Established cows' milk protein allergy or intolerance. Not suitable <6 months; suitable for 6 months–12 years.
	Cow & Gate Pepti-Junior (Cow & Gate) *powder*	275	66	1.8	0.0	Disaccharide and/or whole-protein intolerance, or where amino acids and peptides are indicated in conjunction with medium-chain triglycerides‡.
	Nutramigen Lipil 1 (Mead Johnson) *powder*	280	68	1.9	0.0	Disaccharide and/or whole-protein intolerance where additional medium-chain triglycerides are not included‡.
	Nutramigen Lipil 2 (Mead Johnson) *powder*	285	68	1.7	0.0	Established disaccharide and/or whole-protein intolerance where additional-chain triglycerides are not indicated. Not suitable for <6 months, suitable for 6 months–12 years.
	Nutrini Peptisorb (Nutricia Clinical) *liquid*	420	100	2.8	0.0	For growth failure in ages 1–6 years*, body weight 8–20 kg.
	Pepdite (SHS) *powder*	297	71	2.1	0.0	Disaccharide and/or whole-protein intolerance‡.
	Pepdite 1+ (SHS) *powder*	423	100	3.1	0.0	Disaccharide and/or whole-protein intolerance, or where amino acids or peptides are indicated in conjunction with medium-chain triglycerides. For ages 1–12 years*.
	Peptamen Junior (Nestlé) *liquid*	420	100	3.0	0.0	Short-bowel syndrome, intractable malabsorption, proven inflammatory bowel disease, bowel fistula, in children aged 1–10 years*
	Pregestimil Lipil (Mead Johnson) *powder*	280	68	1.9	0.0	Disaccharide and/or whole-protein intolerance, or where amino acids or peptides are indicated in conjunction with medium-chain triglycerides and hydrolysed casein‡.
Low calcium	Locasol (SHS) *powder*	278	66	1.9	0.0	Conditions of calcium intolerance requiring restriction of calcium and vitamin D intake‡.
MCT-enhanced	Caprilon (SHS) *powder*	277	66	1.5	0.0	Fat 3.6 g (MCT 75%)[d] ‡.
	MCT Pepdite (SHS) *powder*	286	68	2.0	0.0	Fat 2.7 g (MCT 75%)[d] ‡.
	MCT Pepdite +1 (SHS) *powder*	381	91	2.8	0.0	Fat 3.6 g (MCT 75%)[d] for ages 1–12 years*.
	Monogen (SHS) *powder*	310	74	2.2	0.0	LCAD (long-chain acyl-CoA dehydrogenase deficiency), CPTD (carnitine palmitoyltransferase deficiency), primary and secondary lipoprotein lipase deficiency. Fat 2.1 g (MCT 90%)‡.

(Continued)

Table A6.2.4 *(Continued)*

Formula type	Product name (Manufacturer)	Per 100 mL ready-to-drink product (standard dilution)				Notes
		Energy		Protein	Fibre	
		kJ	kcal	(g)	(g)	
Peptide-based	Paediasure Peptide (Abbott) *liquid*	420	100	3.0	0.0	*†
	Peptamen Junior (Nestlé) *liquid*	420	100	3.0	0.0	Short-bowel syndrome, intractable malabsorption, proven inflammatory bowel disease, bowel fistula*†.
Pre-thickened infant feeds	Enfamil AR (Mead Johnson) *powder*	285	68	1.7	0.0	Significant gastro-oesophageal reflux‡.
	SMA Staydown (SMA Nutrition) *powder*	279	67	1.6	0.0	
Residual lactose	Enfamil O-Lac (Mead Johnson) *powder*	280	68	1.4	0.0	Proven lactose intolerance‡.
	Galactomin 17 (SHS) *powder*	295	70	1.7	0.0	Proven lactose intolerance in pre-school children, galactosaemia, and galactokinase deficiency‡.
	SMA LF (SMA Nutrition) *powder*	281	67	1.5	0.0	Proven lactose intolerance‡.
Soya-based	InfaSoy (Cow & Gate) *powder*	275	66	1.6	0.0	Proven lactose and associated sucrose intolerance in pre-school children, galactokinase deficiency, galactosaemia, and proven whole cows' milk sensitivity‡.
	SMA Wysoy (SMA Nutrition) *powder*	280	67	1.8	0.0	

*Not suitable for use in children aged under 1 year;
†For children aged 1–10 years, body weight 8–30 kg;
‡Suitable from birth to 12 years; MCT = medium-chain triglycerides;
d= Disorders in which a high intake of MCT is beneficial. (MCT 75%).

Table A6.2.5 Nutritional supplements for metabolic diseases

Metabolic disease	Product name (Manufacturer)	Age range	Notes
Glutaric aciduria (type 1)	GA1 Anamix Infant (SHS) *powder*	Birth to 3 years	Contains vitamins, minerals, trace elements, essential and nonessential amino acids (except lysine), and low tryptophan.
	GA Gel (Vitaflo) *gel*	6 months–10 years	
	XLYS, Low TRY, Maxamaid (SHS) *powder*	1–8 years	
Glycogen storage disease	Glycosade (Vitaflo) *powder*	>2 years	Also other metabolic conditions where a constant glucose supply is essential.
Homocystinuria	Cystine Amino Acid Supplement (Vitaflo) *powder*		
	HCU cooler (Vitaflo) *liquid*	>3 years	Methionine-free protein substitutes for use as nutritional supplements.
	HCU Express (Vitaflo) *liquid*	>8 years	
	HCU gel (Vitaflo) *powder*	1–10 years	
Hypermethioninaemia or homocystinuria	XMET Homidon (SHS) *powder*		Methionine-free unflavoured powdered drink mixes.
	XMET Maxamaid (SHS) *powder*	1–8 years	
	XMET Maxamum (SHS) *powder*	>8 years	Methionine-free unflavoured powdered drink mix with vitamins, minerals, and trace elements.
	HCU Anamix Infant (SHS) *powder*	Birth to 3 years	Essential and nonessential amino acids except methionine for proven vitamin B_6 non-responsive homocystinuria or hypermethioninaemia.
	HCU LV (SHS) *powder*	>8 years	For hypermethioninaemia or vitamin B_6 non-responsive homocystinuria.
High energy Fat/carbohydrate supplement	Energivit (SHS) *powder*		For children requiring additional energy, vitamins, minerals, and trace elements following a protein-restricted diet.

Table A6.2.5 *(Continued)*

Metabolic disease	Product name (Manufacturer)	Age range	Notes
Hyperlysinaemia	HYPER LYS Anamix Infant (SHS) *powder*	Birth to 3 years	Essential and nonessential amino acids except lysine.
	XLYS Maxamaid (SHS) *powder*	1–8 years	
Isovaleric acidaemia	IVA Anamix Infant (SHS) *powder*	Birth to 3 years	Isovaleric acidaemia and other proven disorders of leucine metabolism.
	XLEU Faladon (SHS) *powder*		XLEU Faladon can be used as part of a modular feed or added as an amino acid supplement to XLEU Analog in the latter stages of weaning.
	XLEU Maxamaid (SHS) *powder*	1–8 years	
Low-protein milk replacement drinks	Loprofin PKU Drink (SHS) *liquid*	>1 year	Low-protein, low-phenylalanine drink based on cow's milk for use in PKU.
	Low-protein drink (Milupa) *powder*	>1 year	For inborn errors of amino acid metabolism.
	Milupa lp-drink (Milupa) *powder*	>1 year	For dietary management of amino acid metabolism disorders.
	ProZero (Vitaflo) *liquid*	>6 months	Liquid blend of carbohydrate and fat.
	Sno-Pro (SHS) *liquid*		Low-protein, low-phenylalanine drink based on milk extracts for PKU, chronic renal failure, and other inborn errors of amino acid metabolism.
Maple syrup urine disease	MSUD Aid III (SHS) *powder*		Also related conditions where intake of branched-chain amino acids must be limited
	MSUD Anamix Infant (SHS) *powder*	Birth to 3 years	
	MSUD Anamix Junior (SHS) *powder*	1–10 years	
	MSUD Anamix Junior LQ (SHS) *liquid*	1–10 years	Liquid format
	MSUD cooler (Vitaflo) *liquid*	>3 years	
	MSUD express (Vitaflo) *powder*	>8 years	
	MSUD Gel (Vitaflo) *powder*	1–10 years	
	MSUD Maxamaid (SHS) *powder*	1–8 years	
	MSUD Maxamum (SHS) *powder*	>8 years	
Methylmalonic acidaemia and propionic acidaemia	MMA/PA Anamix Infant (SHS) *powder*	Birth to 3 years	Essential and nonessential amino acids except methionine, threonine, and valine; low isoleucine content
	XMTVI Asadon (SHS) *powder*	Infants and children	
	XMTVI Maxamaid (SHS) *powder*	1–8 years	
	XMTVI Maxamum (SHS) *powder*	>8 years	
Phenylketonuria PKU	Add-Ins (SHS) *powder*	>4 years	Essential and nonessential amino acids except phenylalanine.
	Easiphen (SHS) *liquid*	>8 years	
	Lophlex (SHS) *powder*	>8 years	
	Milupa PKU 2-prima (Milupa) *powder*	1–8 years	
	Milupa PKU 2-secunda (Milupa) *powder*	9–15 years	
	Milupa PKU 3-advanta (Milupa) *powder*	>15 years	
	Phlexy-10 Exchange System (SHS) *Capsule/Tablet/Drink*	>8 years	Each unit (one sachet, 10 tablets or 20 capsules) provides 10 g amino acids except phenylalanine.
	Phlexy-Vits (SHS) *powder/tablet*	>11 years	Vitamin and mineral component of restricted therapeutic diets in PKU and similar amino acid abnormalities.
	PKU Anamix First Spoon (SHS) *powder*	6 months–5 years	Contains DHA, essential and nonessential amino acids except phenylalanine.
	PKU Anamix Infant (SHS) *powder*	Birth to 3 years	Contains prebiotic oligosaccharides, AA and DHA.
	PKU Anamix Junior (SHS) *powder*	1–10 years	Contains AA, DHA, vitamins and minerals.
	PKU Anamix Junior LQ (SHS) *liquid*	1–10 years	
	PKU cooler 10, 15, 20 (Vitaflo) *liquid*	>3 years	Ready-to-drink phenylalanine-free protein substitutes, contains DHA and EPA, vitamins, minerals, trace elements.
	PKU express (Vitaflo) *powder*	>3 years	Contains essential and nonessential amino acids except phenylalanine, carbohydrate, vitamins, minerals and trace elements.
	PKU gel (Vitaflo) *powder*	1–10 years	

(Continued)

Table A6.2.5 (*Continued*)

Metabolic disease	Product name (Manufacturer)	Age range	Notes
Phenylketonuria	PKU Lophlex LQ 10, 20 (SHS) *liquid*	>4 years	Ready-to-drink, phenylalanine-free, containing essential and nonessential amino acids, carbohydrates, vitamins, trace elements and some minerals.
	PKU Start (Vitaflo) *liquid*	<12 months	Ready-to-feed, phenylalanine-free infant formula, containing essential and non-dispensable amino acids, carbohydrate, fat, vitamins, minerals, trace elements, AA and DHA.
	XP Maxamaid (SHS) *powder* XP Maxamum (SHS) *powder*	1–8 years >8 years	Phenylalanine-free drink mix containing essential and nonessential amino acids, carbohydrate, vitamins, minerals and trace elements.
Tyrosinaemia	Methionine-free TYR Anamix Infant (SHS) *powder*	Birth to 3 years	For proven tyrosinaemia type 1.
	TYR Anamix Infant (SHS) *powder*	Birth to 3 years	Proven tyrosinaemia where plasma-methionine concentrations are normal.
	TYR Anamix Junior (SHS) *powder*	1–10 years	Proven tyrosinaemia.
	TYR Anamix Junior LQ (SHS) *liquid*	>1 year	Tyrosinaemia type 1 (when NTBC is used), type II and III.
	TYR cooler (Vitaflo) *liquid* TYR express (Vitaflo) *powder* TYR Gel (Vitaflo) *Gel*	>3 years >8 years 1–10 years	Contains carbohydrates, minerals, trace elements and vitamins, essential and nonessential amino acids (except tyrosine) and phenylalanine.
	XPHEN TYR Maxamaid (SHS) *powder*	1–8 years	Tyrosinaemia type I (when NTBC is used), type II and III.
Flavouring preparations	FlavourPac (Vitaflo) *powder* Modjul Flavour System (SHS) *powder*	>3 years >6 months	For use with unflavoured protein substitutes.

AA, arachidonic acid; DHA, docosahexaenoic acid; EPA, eicosapentaenoic acid; NTBC, nitisone; PKU, phenylketonuria.

Table A6.2.7 Manufacturers' websites

Abbott, Abbott Laboratories Ltd	www.abbott.co.uk
Cow & Gate, Nutricia Ltd	www.cowandgate.co.uk
Fresenius Kabi, Fresenius Kabi Ltd	www.fresenius-kabi.co.uk
Mead Johnson, Mead Johnson Nutrition	www.meadjohnson.com
Milupa, Milupa Aptamil	www.milupa-metabolics.com
Nestlé, Nestlé Nutrition	www.nestlehealthscience.co.uk
Nutricia Clinical, Nutricia Clinical Care	www.nutricia.co.uk
SMA Nutrition, Pfizer Ltd	www.smanutrition.co.uk
Vitaflo, Vitaflo International Ltd	www.vitaflo.co.uk

Note: SHS International is part of Nutricia and does not have a separate website.

Appendix 7 Nutrition screening tools

This appendix contains screening tools that are discussed in detail in text; many other tools are available that are applicable to dietetic practice. For details on paediatric screening tools, refer to Shaw V (ed.) (2015) *Clinical Paediatric Dietetics*, 4th edn, Wiley Blackwell.

Manual of Dietetic Practice, Sixth Edition. Edited by Joan Gandy.

Companion website: www.manualofdieteticpractice.com

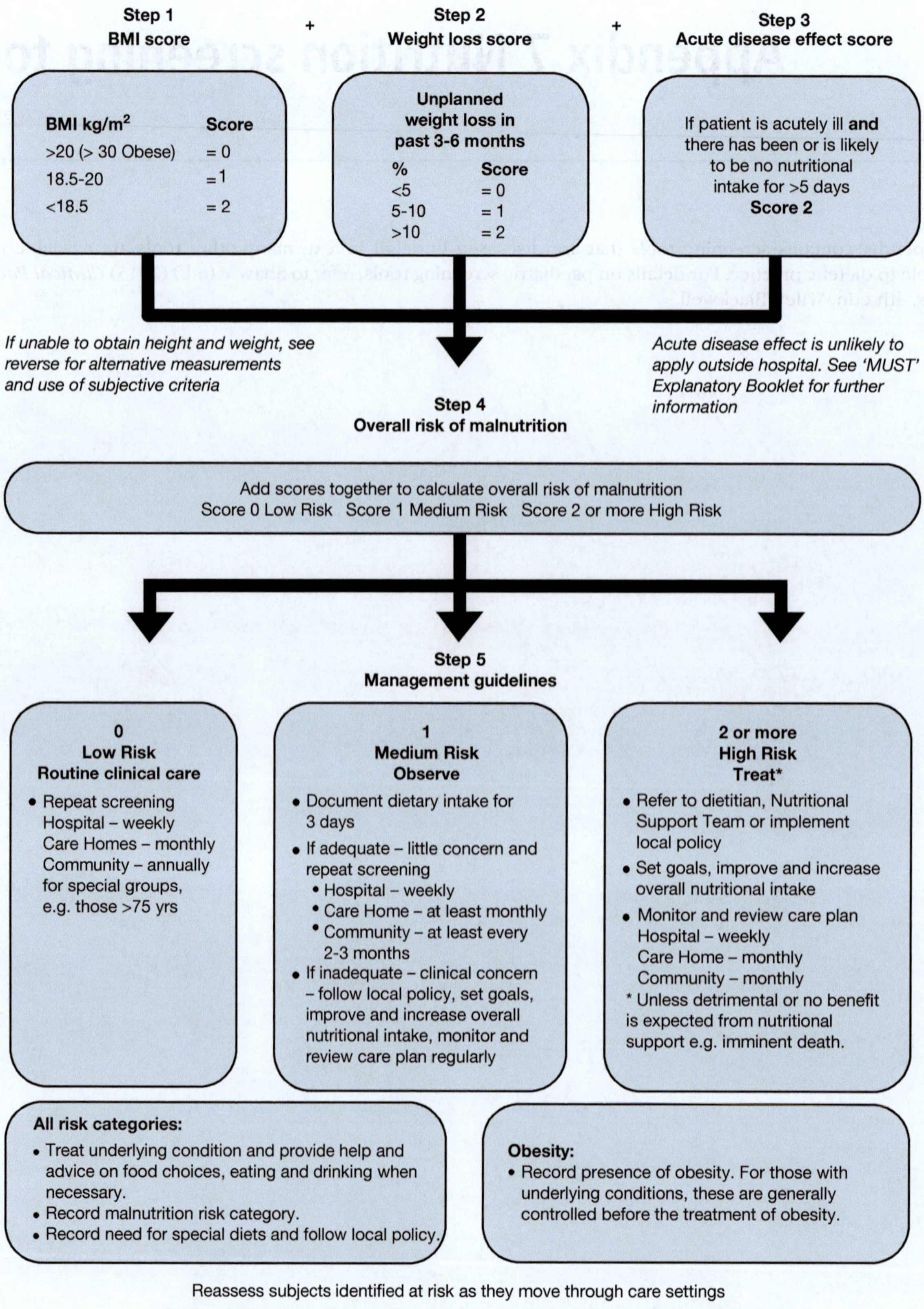

Figure A7.1 Malnutrition Universal Screening Tool 'MUST' (from www.bapen.org.uk/pdfs/must/must_page3.pdf)

Patient's Name
NHS/ID No

Complete all boxes on admission and action as indicated by score

Estimated/reported Weight (kg)	Estimated/reported Height (m)	Body mass index (BMI) (use BMI chart to calculate)

Score each risk factor, using highest score if more than one is relevant.
Total up column scores to obtain final score and record below.

Weight loss in last 3 months and current BMI (choose highest score)	Age (years)	Level of SCI	Other medical conditions	Skin conditions	Diet	Intake	Ability to eat
0 'Minimal' (under 5%) MI ≥22.5 kg/m^2	1 18–30	1 S1–S5	0 None	0 Intact	0 Normal diet and fluids or established NG/PEG feed	0 Eating all meals or tolerating full enteral feed	0 Not applicable as on NG/PEG feed
1 'Some' (5–10%) BMI 18.5–22.5 kg/m^2	2 31–60	2 L1–L5	1 Chronic conditions, e.g. pain/substance abuse	1 Grade 1 ulcer	1 Introductory NG/PEG feed	1 Under half meal or NG/PEG feed tolerated	0 Able to eat independently
3 'Moderate' (11–15%) BMI 16.5–18.4 kg/m^2	3 >60	3 T1–T12	2 Acute trauma, e.g. head injury/ fractures	2 Grade 2 ulcer	2 Modified texture diet	2 Minimal diet or enteral feed	2 Requires some help
4 'Marked' (>15%) BMI <16.4 kg/m^2	4 Under 18	5 C1–C8	3 Within 1 week of surgery/ongoing infection	3 Grade 3 ulcer	3 Nil by mouth for >5 days	3* Vomiting and diarrhoea or not tolerating NG/PEG feed	3 Needs to be fed
			4 Ventilated (non-invasive)	5 Grade 4 ulcer			
			5 Fully ventilated with tracheostomy			Investigate cause and treat	

Date	Column score	Column score	Column score	Column score	Column score	Column score	Column score	Column score	TOTAL SCORE

Figure A7.2 Spinal nutritional screening tool

Transfer total score overleaf and choose appropriate action plan according to identified risk category.

Complete table below to update nutritional risk scores and document weight changes.

Date	Total score	Risk (L/M/H)	Latest weight Actual/estimate	Weight Change (± kg)	Variance and comments	Referred to dietitian	Review date	Nurse's signature

Follow local action plan according to risk score. Document actions in nursing notes.

Score	Risk	Action plan	
10 and under	**Low Rehab**	Encourage healthy food and drink choices Assist with feeding if needed	**Monthly weight if possible** **Repeat score monthly**
	Low Acute	Encourage appropriate menu choices If eating less than half meals complete 3-day food chart and offer two nutritional supplements /sip feeds* a day **If no improvement in eating refer to dietitian**	**Weekly weight if possible** **Repeat score weekly**
11–15	**Moderate Rehab and Acute**	Encourage appropriate menu choices Assist with feeding if needed Complete 3-day food chart. Implement 'Red Tray' Replace missed meals with nutritional supplements /sip feeds* a day **If no improvement in eating refer to dietitian**	**Weekly weight if possible** **Repeat score weekly**
Above 15	**High Rehab and Acute**	Encourage high energy/protein menu choices Assist with feeding if needed Complete 3-day food chart. Implement 'Red Tray' Replace missed meals with nutritional supplements as prescribed by doctor or dietitian **Refer to dietitian**	**Weekly weight if possible** **Repeat score weekly**

Patients N.B.M. for over 5 days or requiring NG/PEG feeding need automatic referral to dietitian. If 'out of hours' feeding regimens for the prevention of refeeding syndrome guidance is available on ....

***Supplement drinks; if the patient has diabetes monitor blood glucose levels and refer to dietitian and diabetes advisor.**
If the patient has renal problems, monitor bloods closely and refer to dietitian and medical team.
If too much weight is being gained or BMI above 30 kg/m²: (1) give patient #Why Weight Matters' diet sheet, (2) Suggest patient attends 'drop-in' weight clinic to monitor weight trend and (3) offer referral to dietitian.

PLEASE RING EXT .... TO FORMALLY REFER PATIENTS TO DIETITIAN FROM NUTRITIONAL SCREENING

Figure A7.2 *(Continued)*

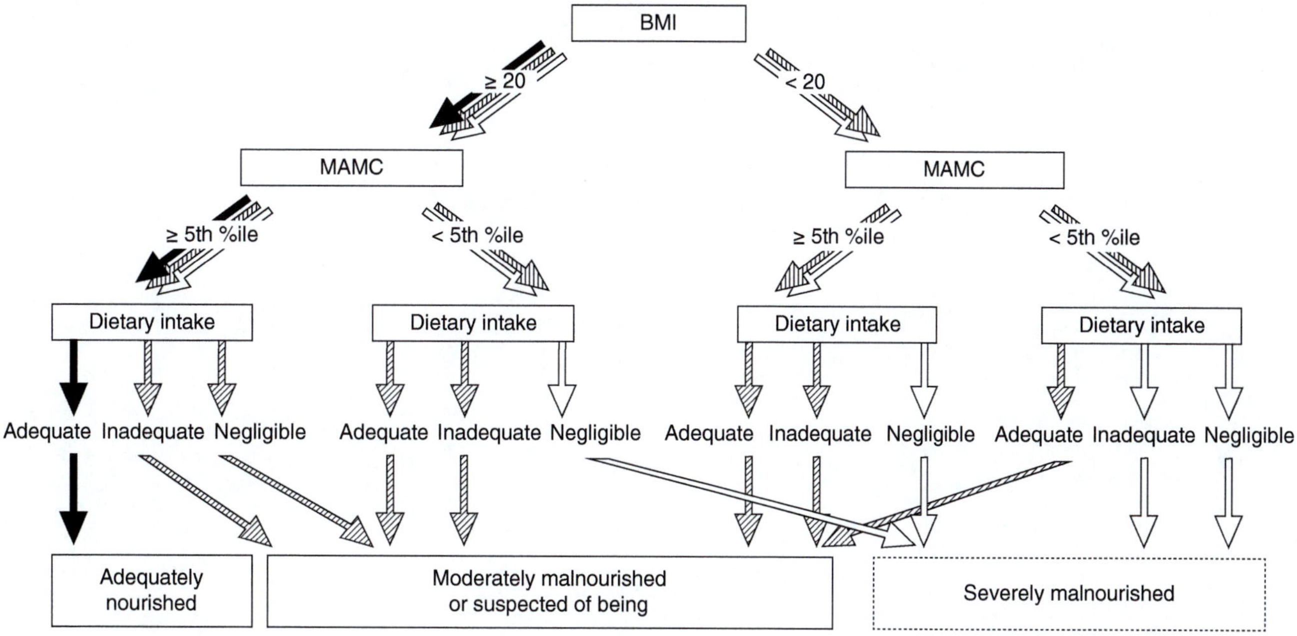

Figure A7.3 Royal Free Hospital Global Assessment (RFH-GA) scheme for determining nutritional status in patients with cirrhosis [from Morgan *et al.* (2006) Derivation and validation of a new global method for assessing nutritional status in patients with cirrhosis. *Hepatology* 44: 823–835].

Note: This figure shows an assessment tool rather than a screening tool but is added for completeness.

Index

Manual of Dietetic Practice, Sixth Edition. Edited by Joan Gandy.

Companion website: www.manualofdieteticpractice.com